Maternal-Fetal and Neonatal Endocrinology

Maternal-Fetal and Neonatal Endocrinology

Physiology, Pathophysiology, and Clinical Management

Edited by

Christopher S. Kovacs
Faculty of Medicine,
Endocrinology, Memorial University of Newfoundland,
St. John's, NL, Canada

Cheri L. Deal
Department of Pediatrics, Université de Montréal;
Pediatric Endocrine and Diabetes Service,
Centre Hospitalier Universitaire Sainte-Justine
Montreal, QC, Canada

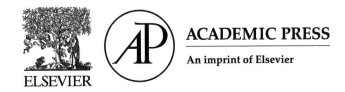

ACADEMIC PRESS

An imprint of Elsevier

Academic Press is an imprint of Elsevier
125 London Wall, London EC2Y 5AS, United Kingdom
525 B Street, Suite 1650, San Diego, CA 92101, United States
50 Hampshire Street, 5th Floor, Cambridge, MA 02139, United States
The Boulevard, Langford Lane, Kidlington, Oxford OX5 1GB, United Kingdom

Notices
Knowledge and best practice in this field are constantly changing. As new research and experience broaden our understanding, changes in research methods, professional practices, or medical treatment may become necessary.

Practitioners and researchers must always rely on their own experience and knowledge in evaluating and using any information, methods, compounds, or experiments described herein. In using such information or methods they should be mindful of their own safety and the safety of others, including parties for whom they have a professional responsibility.

To the fullest extent of the law, neither the Publisher nor the authors, contributors, or editors, assume any liability for any injury and/or damage to persons or property as a matter of products liability, negligence or otherwise, or from any use or operation of any methods, products, instructions, or ideas contained in the material herein.

Library of Congress Cataloging-in-Publication Data
A catalog record for this book is available from the Library of Congress

British Library Cataloguing-in-Publication Data
A catalogue record for this book is available from the British Library

ISBN: 978-0-12-814823-5

For information on all Academic Press publications
visit our website at https://www.elsevier.com/books-and-journals

Cover credit: Front cover painting "Feeling Life" 2018 by Christopher Kovacs based with permission on a reference photo by Vojtech Vlk @ 123RF.com. Back cover painting "Nourishing Life" © 2018 by Christopher Kovacs based with permission on a reference photo by Melisa Chaulk, Happy Valley – Goose Bay, Labrador.

Publisher: Stacy Masucci
Acquisition Editor: Tari K. Broderick
Editorial Project Manager: Carlos Rodriguez
Production Project Manager: Poulouse Joseph
Cover Designer: Mark Rogers

Typeset by SPi Global, India

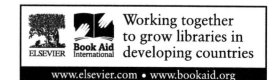

Contents

Section 1
The Mother

Part A
Normal Endocrine Physiology of the Mother During Pregnancy and Lactation

8. Adrenal Cortex and Medulla Physiology During Pregnancy, Labor, and Puerperium

Matthieu St-Jean, Isabelle Bourdeau and André Lacroix

9. Ovarian Function During Pregnancy and Lactation

Jessica A. Ryniec and Elizabeth A. McGee

14. The Onset and Maintenance of Human Lactation and its Endocrine Regulation

Anna Sadovnikova, John J. Wysolmerski and Russell C. Hovey

15. Postpartum Lactational Amenorrhea and Recovery of Reproductive Function and Normal Ovulatory Menstruation

Jerilynn C. Prior

20. Thyroid Cancer During Pregnancy and Lactation

Christopher W. Rowe, Kristien Boelaert and Roger Smith

21. Disorders of Mineral and Bone Metabolism During Pregnancy and Lactation

Christopher S. Kovacs, Marlene Chakhtoura and Ghada El-Hajj Fuleihan

27. Preconception and Pregnancy in Women with Obesity, Postbariatric Surgery, and Polycystic Ovarian Syndrome

Catherine Takacs Witkop

32. Normal Thyroid Development and Function in the Fetus and Neonate

Sarah Lawrence, Julia Elisabeth von Oettingen and Johnny Deladoëy

33. Physiology of Calcium, Phosphorus, and Bone Metabolism During Fetal and Neonatal Development

Christopher S. Kovacs and Leanne M. Ward

34. Developmental Physiology of Carbohydrate Metabolism and the Pancreas

Kathryn Beardsall and Amanda L. Ogilvy-Stuart

35. Developmental Origins and Roles of Intestinal Enteroendocrine Hormones

Venkata S. Jonnakuti, Diana E. Stanescu and Diva D. De Leon

36. Development and Function of the Adrenal Cortex and Medulla in the Fetus and Neonate

Sonir R. Antonini, Monica F. Stecchini and Fernando S. Ramalho

37. Development and Function of the Ovaries and Testes in the Fetus and Neonate

Analía V. Freire, María Gabriela Ropelato and Rodolfo A. Rey

38. Development of Renin-Angiotensin-Aldosterone and Nitric Oxide System in the Fetus and Neonate

Jiaqi Tang, Bailin Liu, Na Li, Mengshu Zhang, Xiang Li, Qinqin Gao, Xiuwen Zhou, Miao Sun, Zhice Xu and Xiyuan Lu

39. Origins of Adipose Tissue and Adipose Regulating Hormones

Declan Wayne, T'ng Chang Kwok, Shalini Ojha, Helen Budge and Michael E. Symonds

39.1.2 White and Brown Adipose Tissue: Physiological Role and Developmental Origins   664
39.1.3 Adipose Tissue Cell Lineage   664
39.2 Brown Adipose Tissue   664
39.2.1 Structure and Physiology   664
39.3 White Adipose Tissue   665
39.3.1 Structure and Physiology   665
39.4 Neonatal and Fetal Adipose Tissue Development   666
39.4.1 The Endocrine System and Adipose Tissue Regulating Hormones   667
39.4.2 Adipose Tissue Regulating Hormones   667
39.5 Cytokines   667
39.5.1 Insulin   667
39.5.2 Ghrelin   667
39.5.3 Glucocorticoids   668
39.5.4 Leptin   669
39.5.5 Others   669
39.5.6 Adiponectin   669
39.5.7 Resistin   670
39.6 Perspectives   670
References   670

40. Fetal and Placental Growth Physiology and Pathophysiology

Victor Han, Bethany Radford and Zain Awamleh

40.1 Normal Physiological Growth of the Fetus and Placenta   673
40.1.1 Normal Growth—Cell-Based   673
40.1.2 Totipotency, Pluripotency, and Differentiation   674
40.1.3 Regulation of Cell Replication and Differentiation   674
40.1.4 Cell Type-Specific Adaptation During Development   675
40.1.5 Regulation of Growth   676
40.2 Developmental Origins of Health and Disease   677
40.3 Placental Growth and Development   677
40.3.1 Evidence from Gene Targeting Studies   678
40.4 Fetal Growth and Development   679
40.4.1 Optimal Fetal Growth   679
40.4.2 Normal Growth—Population-Based   679
40.4.3 Parturition   679
40.4.4 Antenatal Corticosteroid Therapy   681

40.5 Neonatal, Infantile, and Early Childhood Growth and Development   681
40.5.1 Normal Neonatal, Infantile, and Early Childhood Growth   681
40.6 Regulation of Normal Neonatal, Infantile, and Early Childhood Growth   681
40.7 Summary and Clinical Implications   681
References   682

41. Placental Production of Peptide, Steroid, and Lipid Hormones

Jerome F. Strauss, III and Sam A. Mesiano

41.1 Introduction: The Placenta-Maternal Endocrine Interface   685
41.2 Hypothalamic-Pituitary Hormone Analogues   686
41.2.1 Gonadotropin-Releasing Hormone/Gonadotropin   686
41.2.2 Corticotrophin-Releasing Hormone/Pro-Opiomelanocortin Derivatives   688
41.2.3 Somatotropins   689
41.3 Growth Factors   690
41.3.1 Insulin-Like Growth Factors   690
41.3.2 Vascular Endothelial Growth Factor Family   690
41.3.3 Fibroblast Growth Factor Family   690
41.3.4 Transforming Growth Factor β Family   690
41.3.5 Activins and Inhibins   691
41.3.6 Epidermal Growth Factor Family   691
41.4 Adipokines   691
41.5 Steroid Hormones   691
41.5.1 Progesterone   692
41.5.2 Estrogens   694
41.5.3 Glucocorticoid Metabolism   695
41.6 Lipid Mediators   695
41.6.1 Prostanoids   695
41.6.2 Prostanoids and Parturition   697
41.6.3 Prostanoids and Pregnancy-Induced Hypertension/Preeclampsia   698
41.6.4 Other Lipid Mediators   698

Part E
Endocrine Disorders Affecting the Fetus or Neonate

42. Hypothalamic and Pituitary Disorders Affecting the Fetus and Neonate

Manuela Cerbone, Harshini Katugampola and Mehul T. Dattani

43. Fetal and Postnatal Disorders of Thyroid Function

Sarah Elizabeth Lawrence, Julia Elisabeth von Oettingen and Johnny Deladoëy

44. Disorders of Calcium, Phosphorus, and Bone Metabolism During Fetal and Neonatal Development

Christopher S. Kovacs and Leanne M. Ward

45. Pathophysiology and Management of Disorders of Carbohydrate Metabolism and Neonatal Diabetes

Amanda L. Ogilvy-Stuart and Kathryn Beardsall

Part F
New Diagnostic Technologies

52. New Technologies in Pre- and Postnatal Diagnosis

*Anne-Marie Laberge, Aspasia Karalis,
Pranesh Chakraborty and Mark E. Samuels*

Contributors

Numbers in parentheses indicate the pages on which the authors' contributions begin.

Sonir R. Antonini (611), Ribeirao Preto Medical School, University of Sao Paulo, Sao Paulo, Brazil

Zain Awamleh (673), Department of Biochemistry, Schulich School of Medicine & Dentistry, Western University; Children's Health Research Institute, Lawson Health Research Institute and Western University, London, Canada

Sioban Bacon (371), Department of Medicine, Division of Endocrinology and Metabolism, University of Toronto; Division of Endocrinology, Mt. Sinai Hospital, Toronto, ON, Canada

Corin Badiu (15,241), National Institute of Endocrinology "C. I. Parhon"; Department of Endocrinology, "Carol Davila" University of Medicine and Pharmacy, Bucharest, Romania

Kathryn Beardsall (587,783), Department of Paediatrics, University of Cambridge; Neonatal Unit, Rosie Hospital, Cambridge University Hospitals NHS Foundation Trust, Cambridge, United Kingdom

Ingrid J. Block-Kurbisch (53,287), Department of Obstetrics and Gynecology, University of California; Department of Medicine, University of California; Department of Medicine, St. Mary's Medical Center, Dignity Health, San Francisco, CA, United States

Kristien Boelaert (317), Institute of Metabolism and Systems Research, College of Medical and Dental Sciences, University of Birmingham, Birmingham, United Kingdom

Isabelle Bourdeau (101,417), Division of Endocrinology, Department of Medicine and Research Center, Centre hospitalier de l'Université de Montréal (CHUM), Montréal, QC, Canada

Marcello D. Bronstein (39,259), Neuroendocrine Unit, Division of Endocrinology and Metabolism, Hospital das Clínicas, University of São Paulo Medical School; Laboratory of Cellular and Molecular Endocrinology LIM-25, University of São Paulo Medical School, São Paulo, Brazil

Helen Budge (663), Division of Child Health, Obstetrics and Gynaecology, University of Nottingham, Nottingham, United Kingdom

Manuela Cerbone (527,709), Great Ormond Street Hospital for Children NHS Foundation Trust; University College London Great Ormond Street Institute of Child Health, London, United Kingdom

Marlene Chakhtoura (329), Calcium Metabolism and Osteoporosis Program, WHO Collaborating Center for Metabolic Bone Disorders, Faculty of Medicine, American University of Beirut—Medical Center, Beirut, Lebanon

Pranesh Chakraborty (941), Department of Pediatrics, Department of Biochemistry, Microbiology and Immunology, Newborn Screening Ontario, Children's Hospital of Eastern Ontario, University of Ottawa, Ottawa, ON, Canada,

Diana Maria Chitimus (15,241), Division of Physiology and Neuroscience, Department of Functional Sciences, "Carol Davila" University of Medicine and Pharmacy, Bucharest, Romania

Gertrude Costin (813), Department of Pediatrics, Icahn School of Medicine at Mount Sinai, New York, NY, United States

Mehul T. Dattani (527,709), Great Ormond Street Hospital for Children NHS Foundation Trust; University College London Great Ormond Street Institute of Child Health, London, United Kingdom

Diva D. De Leon (599,805), The Children's Hospital of Philadelphia, Perelman School of Medicine at the University of Pennsylvania, Philadelphia, PA, United States

Cheri L. Deal (913), Department of Pediatrics, Université de Montréal; Pediatric Endocrine and Diabetes Service, Centre Hospitalier Universitaire Sainte Justine, Montreal, QC, Canada

Johnny Deladoëy (563,735), CHU Sainte-Justine, Université de Montréal, Montréal, QC, Canada

Lois E. Donovan (389), Division of Endocrinology and Metabolism, Department of Medicine; Department of

Obstetrics and Gynaecology, Cumming School of Medicine, University of Calgary, Calgary, AB, Canada

Ghada El-Hajj Fuleihan (329), Calcium Metabolism and Osteoporosis Program, WHO Collaborating Center for Metabolic Bone Disorders, Faculty of Medicine, American University of Beirut—Medical Center, Beirut, Lebanon

Denice S. Feig (371), Department of Medicine, Division of Endocrinology and Metabolism, University of Toronto; Division of Endocrinology, Mt. Sinai Hospital, Toronto, ON, Canada

Analía V. Freire (625), Centro de Investigaciones Endocrinológicas "Dr. César Bergadá" (CEDIE), CONICET-FEI-División de Endocrinología, Hospital de Niños Ricardo Gutiérrez, Buenos Aires, Argentina

Qinqin Gao (643,869), Institute for Fetology, First Hospital of Soochow University, Suzhou, China

Audrey Garneau (521), Department of Obstetrics and Gynecology, University of Kentucky College of Medicine, Lexington, KY, United States

Andrea Glezer (39,259), Neuroendocrine Unit, Division of Endocrinology and Metabolism, Hospital das Clínicas, University of São Paulo Medical School; Laboratory of Cellular and Molecular Endocrinology LIM-25, University of São Paulo Medical School, São Paulo, Brazil

Veronica Gomez-Lobo (505), Department of Obstetrics and Gynecology, MedStar Washington Hospital Center; Children's National Health System and Medstar Washington Hospital Center, Washington, DC, United States

Romina P. Grinspon (841), Centro de Investigaciones Endocrinológicas "Dr. César Bergadá" (CEDIE), CONICET-FEI-División de Endocrinología, Hospital de Niños Ricardo Gutiérrez, Buenos Aires, Argentina

Victor Han (673), Division of Neonatal-Perinatal Medicine, Department of Paediatrics, Schulich School of Medicine & Dentistry, Western University; Department of Biochemistry, Schulich School of Medicine & Dentistry, Western University; Children's Health Research Institute, Lawson Health Research Institute and Western University, London, Canada

Russell C. Hovey (189), Department of Animal Science, University of California, Davis, CA, United States

Raquel Soares Jallad (39,259), Neuroendocrine Unit, Division of Endocrinology and Metabolism, Hospital das Clínicas, University of São Paulo Medical School; Laboratory of Cellular and Molecular Endocrinology LIM-25, University of São Paulo Medical School, São Paulo, Brazil

Venkata S. Jonnakuti (599,805), The Children's Hospital of Philadelphia, Perelman School of Medicine at the University of Pennsylvania, Philadelphia, PA, United States

Aspasia Karalis (941), Medical Genetics, Department of Pediatrics, CHU Sainte-Justine and Université de Montréal, Montreal, QC, Canada

Harshini Katugampola (527,709), Great Ormond Street Hospital for Children NHS Foundation Trust; University College London Great Ormond Street Institute of Child Health, London, United Kingdom

Asma Khalil (455), Department of Fetal Medicine; Molecular & Clinical Sciences Research Institute, St. George's University of London, London, United Kingdom

Md. Wasim Khan (75), Division of Endocrinology, Diabetes and Metabolism, Department of Medicine, University of Illinois at Chicago, Chicago, IL, United States

Ahmed Khattab (813), Division of Pediatric Endocrinology, Rutgers-Robert Wood Johnson Medical School, Child Health Institute of New Jersey, New Brunswick, NJ, United States

Christopher S. Kovacs (61,329,573,755), Faculty of Medicine, Endocrinology, Memorial University of Newfoundland, St. John's, NL, Canada

T'ng Chang Kwok (663,891), Division of Child Health, Obstetrics and Gynaecology, University of Nottingham, Nottingham, United Kingdom

Anne-Marie Laberge (941), Medical Genetics, Department of Pediatrics, CHU Sainte-Justine and Université de Montréal, Montreal, QC, Canada

André Lacroix (101,417), Division of Endocrinology, Department of Medicine and Research Center, Centre hospitalier de l'Université de Montréal (CHUM), Montréal, QC, Canada

David C.W. Lau (147), Departments of Medicine, Biochemistry and Molecular Biology, University of Calgary Cumming School of Medicine, Calgary, AB, Canada

Sarah Elizabeth Lawrence (563,735), Children's Hospital of Eastern Ontario, Ottawa, ON, Canada

Brian T. Layden (75), Division of Endocrinology, Diabetes and Metabolism, Department of Medicine, University of Illinois at Chicago; Jesse Brown Veterans Affairs Medical Center, Chicago, IL, United States

Diana Le Duc (547), Institute of Human Genetics, University of Leipzig Hospitals and Clinics, Leipzig, Germany Department of Evolutionary Genetics, Max Planck Institute for Evolutionary Anthropology, Leipzig, Germany

Na Li (643,869), Institute for Fetology, First Hospital of Soochow University, Suzhou, China

Xiang Li (643,869), Institute for Fetology, First Hospital of Soochow University, Suzhou, China

Alexis Light (505), Department of Obstetrics and Gynecology, MedStar Washington Hospital Center, Washington, DC, United States

Bailin Liu (643,869), Institute for Fetology, First Hospital of Soochow University, Suzhou, China

Xiyuan Lu (643,869), Institute for Fetology, First Hospital of Soochow University, Suzhou, China

Eugenie R. Lumbers (129), School of Biomedical Sciences and Pharmacy, Hunter Medical Research Institute, University of Newcastle, New Lambton, NSW, Australia

Anne Macdonald (813), Department of Pediatrics, Icahn School of Medicine at Mount Sinai, New York, NY, United States

Marcio Carlos Machado (39,259), Neuroendocrine Unit, Division of Endocrinology and Metabolism, Hospital das Clínicas, University of São Paulo Medical School; Laboratory of Cellular and Molecular Endocrinology LIM-25, University of São Paulo Medical School; Endocrinology Service, AC Camargo Cancer Center, São Paulo, Brazil

Elizabeth A. McGee (117), Director of Reproductive Endocinology and Infertility, Obstetrics, Gynecology and Reproductive Sciences, University of Vermont, Larner College of Medicine, Burlington, VT, United States

Sam A. Mesiano (685), Department of Reproductive Biology, Case Western Reserve University; Department of Obstetrics and Gynecology, University Hospitals Cleveland Medical Center, Cleveland, OH, United States

Geetha Mukerji (371), Department of Medicine, Division of Endocrinology and Metabolism, University of Toronto; Division of Endocrinology, Women's College Hospital, Toronto, ON, Canada

Cathy M. Murray (159), Division of Endocrinology and Metabolism, Faculty of Medicine, Memorial University of Newfoundland, St. John's, NL, Canada

Mithra L. Narasimhan (813), Department of Pediatrics, Icahn School of Medicine at Mount Sinai, New York, NY, United States

Maria New (813), Department of Pediatrics, Icahn School of Medicine at Mount Sinai, New York, NY, United States

Amanda L. Ogilvy-Stuart (587,783), Neonatal Unit, Rosie Hospital, Cambridge University Hospitals NHS Foundation Trust, Cambridge, United Kingdom Neonatal

Unit, Cambridge University Hospitals NHS Foundation Trust, Cambridge, United Kingdom

Shalini Ojha (663,891), Division of Medical Sciences and Graduate Entry Medicine School of Medicine, University of Nottingham Neonatal Intensive Care Unit, Derby Teaching Hospitals NHS Foundation Trust, Derby, United Kingdom

Christine J. Orr (159), Division of Endocrinology and Metabolism, Faculty of Medicine, Memorial University of Newfoundland, St. John's, NL, Canada

Anca Maria Panaitescu (15,241), Department of Obstetrics and Gynecology, "Carol Davila" University of Medicine and Pharmacy, Filantropia Clinical Hospital, Bucharest, Romania

Georgios E. Papadakis (7,217), Service of Endocrinology, Diabetes and Metabolism, CHUV, Lausanne University Hospital, Lausanne, Switzerland

Francesca Gabriela Paslaru (241), Department of Neurosurgery, "Bagdasar-Arseni" Clinical Emergency Hospital, Bucharest, Romania

Jonathan Paul (169), Medicine and Public Health, University of Newcastle, Newcastle, NSW, Australia

Gheorghe Peltecu (15,241), Department of Obstetrics and Gynecology, "Carol Davila" University of Medicine and Pharmacy, Filantropia Clinical Hospital, Bucharest, Romania

Jason Phung (169), Obstetrics & Gynaecology, John Hunter Hospital, Newcastle, NSW, Australia

Nelly Pitteloud (7,217), Service of Endocrinology, Diabetes and Metabolism, CHUV, Lausanne University Hospital, Lausanne, Switzerland

Jerilynn C. Prior (207), Centre for Menstrual Cycle and Ovulation Research, Division of Endocrinology, Department of Medicine, University of British Columbia; School of Population and Public Health, University of British Columbia; BC Women's Health Research Institute, Vancouver, BC, Canada

Zoe E. Quandt (287), Department of Medicine, Division of Endocrinology and Metabolism, University of California, San Francisco, CA, United States

Bethany Radford (673), Department of Biochemistry, Schulich School of Medicine & Dentistry, Western University; Children's Health Research Institute, Lawson Health Research Institute and Western University, London, Canada

Fernando S. Ramalho (611), Ribeirao Preto Medical School, University of Sao Paulo, Sao Paulo, Brazil

Rodolfo A. Rey (625,841), Centro de Investigaciones Endocrinológicas "Dr. César Bergadá" (CEDIE), CONICET-FEI-División de Endocrinología, Hospital de Niños Ricardo Gutiérrez; Departamento de Histología, Biología Celular, Embriología y Genética, Facultad de Medicina, Universidad de Buenos Aires, Buenos Aires, Argentina

María Gabriela Ropelato (625), Centro de Investigaciones Endocrinológicas "Dr. César Bergadá" (CEDIE), CONICET-FEI-División de Endocrinología, Hospital de Niños Ricardo Gutiérrez, Buenos Aires, Argentina

Adrian Eugen Rosca (547), Division of Physiology and Neuroscience, Department of Functional Sciences, "Carol Davila" University of Medicine and Pharmacy, Bucharest, Romania

Christopher W. Rowe (317), Department of Endocrinology, John Hunter Hospital; School of Medicine and Public Health, University of Newcastle, Newcastle, NSW, Australia

Jessica A. Ryniec (117), Reproductive Endocrinology and Infertility, University of Vermont, Burlington, VT, United States

Anna Sadovnikova (189), Department of Animal Science, University of California, Davis, CA, United States

Kirsten E. Salmeen (53,287), Department of Obstetrics and Gynecology, Kaiser Permanente; Department of Obstetrics and Gynecology, University of California, San Francisco, CA, United States

Mark E. Samuels (941), Department of Medicine, Centre de Recherche du CHU Ste-Justine, Université de Montréal, Montreal, QC, Canada

Sahar Sherf (411), Division of Endocrinology, UCLA David Geffen School of Medicine, Los Angeles, CA, United States

Jien Shim (91), Division of Endocrinology, UCLA David Geffen School of Medicine, Los Angeles, CA, United States

Roger Smith (169,317), Endocrinology, University of Newcastle; Department of Endocrinology, John Hunter Hospital, Newcastle, NSW, Australia School of Medicine and Public Health, University of Newcastle, Newcastle, NSW, Australia

Diana E. Stanescu (599,805), The Children's Hospital of Philadelphia, Perelman School of Medicine at the University of Pennsylvania, Philadelphia, PA, United States

Brett Stark (505), Department of OBGYN and Reproductive Science, University of California San Francisco, San Francisco, CA, United States

Monica F. Stecchini (611), Ribeirao Preto Medical School, University of Sao Paulo, Sao Paulo, Brazil

Matthieu St-Jean (101,417), Division of Endocrinology, Department of Medicine and Research Center, Centre hospitalier de l'Université de Montréal (CHUM), Montréal, QC, Canada

Jerome F. Strauss, III (685), Department of Obstetrics and Gynecology, Division of Reproductive Biology and Research, Virginia Commonwealth University, Richmond, VA, United States

Miao Sun (643,869), Institute for Fetology, First Hospital of Soochow University, Suzhou, China

Michael E. Symonds (663,891), Division of Child Health, Obstetrics and Gynaecology; Nottingham Digestive Disease Centre and Biomedical Research Centre, The School of Medicine, University of Nottingham, Nottingham, United Kingdom

Jiaqi Tang (643,869), Institute for Fetology, First Hospital of Soochow University, Suzhou, China

Rosemary Townsend (455), Department of Fetal Medicine; Molecular & Clinical Sciences Research Institute, St. George's University of London, London, United Kingdom

Suzana Elena Voiculescu (241,547), Division of Physiology and Neuroscience, Department of Functional Sciences, "Carol Davila" University of Medicine and Pharmacy, Bucharest, Romania

Julia Elisabeth von Oettingen (563,735), McGill University Health Centre, Montreal, QC, Canada

Leanne M. Ward (573,755), Department of Pediatrics, Faculty of Medicine, University of Ottawa; Division of Endocrinology, Children's Hospital of Eastern Ontario, Ottawa, ON, Canada

Declan Wayne (663), Division of Child Health, Obstetrics and Gynaecology, University of Nottingham, Nottingham, United Kingdom

Catherine Takacs Witkop (485), Uniformed Services University of the Health Sciences, Bethesda, MD, United States

John J. Wysolmerski (189), Section of Endocrinology and Metabolism, Department of Internal Medicine, Yale School of Medicine, New Haven, CT, United States

Cheng Xu (7,217), Service of Endocrinology, Diabetes and Metabolism, CHUV, Lausanne University Hospital, Lausanne, Switzerland

Zhice Xu (643,869), Institute for Fetology, First Hospital of Soochow University, Suzhou, China; Center for Perinatal Biology, Loma Linda University, Loma Linda, CA, United States

Jennifer M. Yamamoto (389), Division of Endocrinology and Metabolism, Department of Medicine; Department of Obstetrics and Gynaecology, Cumming School of Medicine, University of Calgary, Calgary, AB, Canada

Jessica S. Yang (805), The Children's Hospital of Philadelphia, Perelman School of Medicine at the University of Pennsylvania, Philadelphia, PA, United States

Steven L. Young (521), Division of Reproductive Endocrinology and Infertility, Department of Obstetrics and Gynecology and Department of Cell Biology and Physiology, University of North Carolina School of Medicine, Chapel Hill, NC, United States

Run Yu (91,411), Division of Endocrinology, UCLA David Geffen School of Medicine, Los Angeles, CA, United States

Ana-Maria Zagrean (15,241,547), Division of Physiology and Neuroscience, Department of Functional Sciences, "Carol Davila" University of Medicine and Pharmacy, Bucharest, Romania

Leon Zagrean (15), Division of Physiology and Neuroscience, Department of Functional Sciences, "Carol Davila" University of Medicine and Pharmacy, Bucharest, Romania

Mengshu Zhang (643,869), Institute for Fetology, First Hospital of Soochow University, Suzhou, China

Xiuwen Zhou (643,869), Institute for Fetology, First Hospital of Soochow University, Suzhou, China

Preface

Why compile a textbook that focuses on maternal-fetal and neonatal endocrinology? If the answer isn't self-evident, we can explain why from our own clinical experiences. And judging by comments we've received from colleagues and patients around the world, we're not alone in this.

Endocrinologists and internists are called upon by obstetricians to diagnose and manage women who have endocrine disorders that either predate pregnancy or present for the first time during pregnancy. The presentation and management of endocrine diseases can differ substantially during pregnancy, and even during lactation. Medications may cross the placenta and affect the fetus or enter breastmilk and affect the neonate. Altered endocrine physiology in the mother can affect the developing fetus or neonate, with interventions needed prior to birth (e.g., fetal Graves' disease) or after (maternal hypercalcemia during pregnancy, leading to neonatal hypocalcemia and hypoparathyroidism). Endocrine disorders can also primarily develop in the fetus and present in the neonate, and these presentations may differ from the classical ones that occur in adults. Sometimes there is not a disorder at all, but rather normal physiological changes of pregnancy [e.g., low total serum calcium and suppressed parathyroid hormone (PTH)] or lactation [enlarged pituitary gland on magnetic resonance imaging (MRI)] are misinterpreted to indicate disease states.

Clinicians generally have a good understanding of the management of diabetes and thyroid disorders during pregnancy and know where to turn when they need help. However, other endocrine disorders are seen less often during pregnancy or postpartum and may be overlooked, and the nuances of their management during these times periods are far less well appreciated.

With advances in prenatal diagnosis and treatment, physicians must also be prepared to expertly address the implications of a diagnosis because this may influence subsequent decision-making and guidance given. When a prenatal diagnosis of Turner syndrome or Klinefelter syndrome is made on amniocentesis, pediatric endocrinologists and other physicians must be aware that the postnatal karyotype will often show mosaicism. Consequently, the newborn and child may have very few or less severe stigmata of either condition. It is also critical to appreciate that when fetal genitalia seen on ultrasound do not correlate with the karyotype, this is usually perceived as an emergency by the parents, families, and healthcare team. Additional genetic studies may be needed prenatally or in the newborn.

Does primary adrenal insufficiency require any alteration in the dosing of glucocorticoids or mineralocorticoids during pregnancy or labor? How do changes in maternal physiology affect the management of hypoparathyroidism during pregnancy, and then in a different way during lactation? If a mother has X-linked hypophosphatemic rickets, how will this affect her pregnancy or her breastmilk, and if her baby inherits the condition, when should it begin to show evidence of it? Diagnostic tools may no longer be valid in pregnancy, such as the renin:aldosterone ratio to distinguish primary from secondary aldosteronism, or the calcium:creatinine clearance ratio that distinguishes familial hypocalciuric hypercalcemia from primary hyperparathyroidism. Imaging studies involving contrast or radiation exposure generally cannot be done. Medical and surgical treatments may be contraindicated or limited. For every endocrine disorder, reproduction may affect the presenting signs and symptoms, diagnosis, and management.

When should prenatal treatment be considered if you are entertaining a diagnosis of severe dyshormonogenesis in a fetus with a large goiter? What are the norms for clitoral and penile length in premature newborns, and what clinical signs should orient us when assessing ambiguous genitalia in a newborn? If severe, refractory hypoglycemia occurs in a newborn, what treatment options do we have while awaiting a diagnosis? What signs should make us suspect central adrenal failure in a newborn, and what are its genetic and syndromic causes? Why does growth hormone deficiency usually not affect linear growth until after the first year of life, and in what syndromes may you encounter it?

Finding answers to all these questions is not always easy. In most textbooks of endocrinology, the impact of pregnancy, postpartum, and lactation are given a line or two at the end of a chapter, or overlooked. Similarly, prenatal diagnoses and treatment of the various fetal endocrine diseases are usually covered in chapters on making a postnatal diagnosis, and normative data for fetal organ growth and function are provided only in specialized texts or journal articles. Therefore, there is a clear need for a formalized source of maternal-fetal and neonatal endocrinology. The only prior textbook was Tulchinsky and Little's *Maternal-Fetal Endocrinology*, last published in 1994 and far less comprehensive in scope.

The essay by Krista Rideout that opens this book illustrates and humanizes the problems that some of these women and their partners have faced in getting expert advice or input. Their endocrine disorders would otherwise be well understood and managed, except during pregnancy and lactation, which seems to create a black box for many clinicians.

Finally, as examiners for the certification examination in endocrinology and metabolism offered by the Royal College of Physicians and Surgeons of Canada, both of the editors of this book have made a point each year of including questions that address the impact of pregnancy on an endocrine disorder, or discuss differential diagnoses and treatment of fetal syndromes with an endocrine component or endocrinopathies presenting in the neonate. Candidates who scored poorly have argued that the questions were unfair: Why should they be expected to know about any other endocrine disorders during pregnancy? Why, indeed? If the consultant endocrinologist does not know how to manage a pheochromocytoma or hypoparathyroidism during pregnancy, or counsel a family on the impact of uncontrolled maternal Graves' disease on fetal outcomes including neurological development, who will do this? And how will that happen?

All of the preceding discussion contributes to why we have recognized for some time that there is a need for a single source that contains everything you'd ever wanted to know—and shouldn't be afraid to ask—about endocrine physiology or pathophysiology during pregnancy, lactation, and fetal/neonatal development. Because most endocrine disorders are seen much less often during pregnancy—especially if the disorder reduces the likelihood of conceiving—this creates an experience and knowledge gap and the need for a formalized reference source.

This textbook should appeal to adult and pediatric endocrinologists, internists, obstetricians and gynecologists, maternal-fetal medicine specialists, pediatricians, neonatologists, residents, fellows, nurses, and allied health professionals in all these overlapping specialties.

This book is divided into two halves, "Mother" and "Child." In turn, each half is subdivided into two sections, with the first covering normal changes in endocrine physiology and the second half covers the pathophysiology and treatment of endocrine disorders. The physiology chapters begin with a bulleted list of key clinical changes, while the pathophysiology sections begin with a summary list of common clinical problems. If you want to know how adrenal physiology and hormones levels are altered during normal pregnancy or fetal development, you will find this information in the respective physiology sections. If you want to know how to manage hyperthyroidism during pregnancy or in the fetus or neonate, you will find those topics covered in the respective pathophysiology sections. Novel chapters complete our content, such as "Fertility, Pregnancy, and Chest Feeding in Transgendered Individuals" and "New Technologies in Prenatal and Postnatal Diagnosis," which includes a discussion of the ethical dilemmas that these technologies may create.

We're delighted that that we gathered expertise from around the globe, across different specialties, spanning basic through translational to clinical research, and from MDs and PhDs, to cover all the relevant topics we could think of.

Your feedback is invited for a next edition, especially if there are topics we overlooked, despite the comprehensiveness of this book.

Editors
Christopher S. Kovacs
Cheri L. Deal

Acknowledgments and Dedication

A book like this cannot come about without an enormous debt of gratitude and thanks to be offered to many people:

- Tari Broderick at Elsevier first asked if I had any ideas for a textbook. When I surprised her by saying yes, she wouldn't let go. Tari even kick-started things by initiating the written proposal.
- Cheri Deal stepped up to coedit with me when I realized that the scope required expert input from a pediatric endocrinologist. I'm ever grateful to Cheri for taking on this enormous task.
- I would also like to thank all the authors who contributed to this book, and a network of colleagues, too numerous to mention, who suggested names of candidate authors.
- Thank you to all the staff at Elsevier who were involved in the production of this book.
- Among the many graduate students and postdocs who have contributed to the success of my lab, I would like to particularly acknowledge Janine Woodrow, Charlene (Noseworthy) Simmonds, Sandra Cooke-Hubley, Yue Ma, Brittany Gillies, K. Berit Sellars, and Brittany A. Ryan.

As is true for many academic physicians, I am a clinician, researcher, and teacher. But my work as a professional artist predates my medical career, and I'm delighted to bring the two careers together by creating the two paintings that grace the interior and cover of this book. More recently, I have written and edited literary works, including a biography and essays of literary analysis and criticism. I could not have developed these various talents and skills, or got to where I am today, without the help, guidance, support, and love from many people.

Of course, this includes my parents (Marylin and Simon Kovacs), my wife (Susan MacDonald), and my children (Caileigh and Jamieson).

But there are many other people who have had a significant impact on my career and development, whether it be within medicine, research, creative writing, or visual arts; by serving as teachers, supervisors, mentors, and colleagues; or providing encouragement, friendship, love, and support. Some have done all these things. These are the people for whom this book is dedicated. Most are living, but regrettably some are now deceased. I've listed them in the order that I recall meeting them, starting with the artist who taught me:

William Wegman, Michael Campbell, Peter Lee, Don Beaudois, Edmund R. Yendt, Margot and Wilson MacDonald, Connie L. Chik, Anthony R. Ho, Henry M. Kronenberg, Beate Lanske, Ernestina Schipani, John Wysolmerski, John D. Harnett, A. Brenda Galway, Carol J. Joyce, Anthony C. Karaplis, David Goltzman, T. John Martin, Robert Gagel, Clifford J. Rosen, Neva J. Fudge, Alan Goodridge, Beth J. Kirby, Natalie A. Sims, Dave Grubbs, Ann Crimmins, Lisa D. Dawe, René St-Arnaud, and Krista L. Rideout.

Among these people, I must give a particular shout-out, dedication, and deep bow of thanks to the two mentors who have supported and guided my career: Henry M. (Hank) Kronenberg at Harvard Medical School/Massachusetts General Hospital, and T. John (Jack) Martin at the University of Melbourne/St. Vincent's Institute. This book could not exist without the two of you helping me gain the inspiration, knowledge, critical insight, confidence, and hubris to take on such a monumental task. I salute you both.

I've gained, matured, benefited, and learned from my interactions with all of these people and more. Any mistakes made along the way remain my own responsibility.

Thank you all.

Christopher S. Kovacs

Acknowledgments and Dedication by Cheri L. Deal

It has been an honor to be included in the editing of this book, the brainchild of Chris Kovacs. I have to start by thanking the people at Elsevier, for their professionalism and their patience! You have been the drivers. Behind me is also my very patient and supportive husband of 41 years, Thierry Neubert, and our now adult kids (Kimberly and Jacqueline), who have steadfastly stood by me during the many years of training, research, and clinical practice needed to develop the expertise for this task.

I would like to acknowledge my enormous debt of gratitude to my most important mentors, including George Rothblat, Hugh Tyson, Marie-Anne Fieldes (deceased), Harvey Guyda, Cindy Goodyer, Charlotte Branchaud (deceased), Constantin Polychronakos, Ron Rosenfeld, Claude Roy (deceased), Elizabeth Rousseau, Michel Weber (deceased), and André Lacroix. Not all of these names belong to physicians and/or scientists in the field of endocrinology, but all of them nurtured my intellect, instilled and reinforced a love of the scientific method, supported my career, and encouraged the pursuit of excellence in academic medicine.

To all of my students over the years (and getting older means that there are now too many to mention individually), know that you have also inspired me, nourished my brain, and helped me learn how to teach effectively. I only hope that I have also managed to show you the joy in problem-solving and in going that extra mile to improve the lives of our patients.

Thanks also goes to my terrific pediatric endocrine, diabetes, and bone metabolism team (including Guy Van Vliet, who hired me all those years ago, Celine Huot, Nathalie Alos, Rachel Scott, Johnny Deladoey, Patricia Olivier, Melanie Henderson, Lyne Chiniara, Louis Geoffroy, and Monique Gonthier). I so appreciate our daily stimulating discussions, weekly presentations, and constant help with the enormous clinical load at our center—all of this has helped feed my research and teaching over the years. There are also other unsung heroes in our hospital that deserve mention: our colleagues who participate in the multidisciplinary teams at the Mother-Child Sainte-Justine University Teaching Hospital and who are critical to the diagnosis and treatment of the many complex endocrine, metabolic and developmental conditions seen by pediatric endocrinologists. *All* of you are why I have *stayed* at the Sainte-Justine and the University of Montreal for my career in pediatric endocrinology and diabetes.

Lastly, I would like to honor all my patients and their families who have continued to teach me throughout my career. To you, a very big and humble thank-you.

Cheri L. Deal

When Endocrine Disorders Disrupt Pregnancy: Perspectives of Affected Mothers

Krista L. Rideout

Manager, Clinical Research, Department of Research and Innovation, Eastern Regional Health Authority, St. John's, NL, Canada

I'm pregnant!

You're pregnant!

These simple statements have so much significance for women, especially for a first-time mother who is new to pregnancy and motherhood. Whether the pregnancy is planned or unplanned, it is a major life event, full of many emotions: happiness, excitement, fear, surprise, anticipation, and uncertainty, to name a few. During pregnancy, we experience a shift in our identity. We start to become more maternal, and our bodies go through some of the biggest physical and psychological changes we will ever experience. We ask ourselves many questions related to these changes: *Will we lose ourselves in motherhood? Will the changes to our bodies ever reverse? Will we age before our time?*

As expectant moms, we always worry—*What if something goes wrong?*

We have so many concerns circling through our thoughts. Fear of miscarriage, fetal abnormalities, and pregnancy complications. *Will I have a vaginal birth or a caesarian section? Will I breastfeed or bottle-feed? Will I need an epidural, or can I do it naturally? Will my baby be all right?* We find ourselves daydreaming about the baby's sex, possible names for a boy or girl, and when we will tell family and friends. We may hold back these thoughts early in pregnancy as a way of protecting ourselves in case something goes wrong. Many women worry about planning for the new family member too early, as it may be tempting fate.

Often, many of our worries about miscarriage and fetal abnormalities pass when we reach the second trimester, or after the first ultrasound is completed.

But what if your fears are realized?

Something is wrong—you have a medical condition that could put you and your baby at risk. In the context of this book, that might be an endocrine condition that could have major implications for your health and that of your baby.

Diabetes during pregnancy is common enough that most physicians should be able to effectively manage it or refer to an endocrinologist or diabetologist for expert advice. But having said that, hypothyroidism is also very common in pregnancy, affecting 5%–10% of women, and yet most physicians seem unaware that women need higher doses of thyroid hormone during pregnancy. If a mother has marked hypothyroidism, that can have effects on fetal brain development, lead to a lower IQ, and cause other problems for her baby. And so, even common endocrine problems can be mismanaged or overlooked in pregnancy.

What if a woman has a rarer endocrine disorder that the family physician or obstetrician has never managed? What if her doctors cannot recognize the signs and symptoms? How will these women be able to get medical help and advice?

I will now share with you stories of women who experienced living with endocrine disorders during pregnancy, postpartum, or while breastfeeding. These stories highlight the importance of proper diagnosis and management, recognizing the real and perceived risks, collaboration of multiple disciplines, and finding the best advice or person to optimize the outcomes for mom and baby. These stories also highlight how things can go wrong when the health-care team doesn't recognize an endocrine disorder is present, or its implications.

Meet Maggie,[1] who has had Von Hippel-Lindau disease since the age of three. She inherited it from her mother, who died suddenly and tragically shortly after delivery, from an intracranial hemorrhage. A diagnosis was never officially made.

---

[1] All names have been changed.

However, when Maggie's maternal aunt also suddenly passed away, her autopsy revealed Von Hippel-Lindau disease. Maggie and her maternal grandfather were then diagnosed.

Von Hippel-Lindau disease is an autosomal dominant condition that includes hemangioblastomas in the central nervous system, pheochromocytomas, and renal cell carcinomas. It can cause sudden death from bleeding into the brain, which is made more likely through hypertensive crises caused by pheochromocytomas. This is what is suspected to have happened with Maggie's mom.

A *pheochromocytoma* is a catecholamine-producing tumor of the adrenal glands that releases adrenaline or noradrenaline, causing severe hypertension and paroxysms. This is an extremely rare condition that can be life-threatening to the mother and her fetus. The resulting high blood pressure and fast heart rhythms can cause sudden death in a seemingly healthy young woman, especially in association with labor and delivery, or anesthesia for a caesarian section.

Maggie has multiple health problems secondary to Von Hippel-Lindau disease. By the time she was 10 years old, she had her first surgery, a partial adrenalectomy to remove a right-sided pheochromocytoma. During her teenage years, Maggie vividly remembers having uncontrollable mood swings. She felt as though she had little control over her emotions. She had headaches and clammy hands constantly. All of these things can be due to catecholamine excess. When she was 16, another right-sided pheochromocytoma and a left-sided pheochromocytoma were removed. After the surgeries, the majority of her symptoms resolved. Her adrenals were gone, so she required lifelong adrenal hormone replacement.

With her early diagnosis and interventions, it looked like Maggie would avoid the fatal problem that her mom experienced.

In her early 20s, Maggie found out that she was pregnant. Given her history, her pregnancy involved multiple disciplines, including an endocrinologist, neurologist, anesthetist, and a high-risk obstetrician. Despite having her adrenals removed, toward the end of her pregnancy, Maggie developed a pheochromocytoma outside the adrenals (a paraganglioma), enlargement of intracranial lesions, and hydrocephalus. The nightmare situation that her mom experienced was still possible!

She was started on special medications to ensure proper blood pressure control throughout the pregnancy. Amniocentesis was conducted at 35 weeks to determine fetal lung maturity, and she was scheduled for a caesarian section. A vaginal birth was not an option because the pushing could cause an increase in intracranial pressure. After delivery, she was transferred to the intensive care unit (ICU) for monitoring, given her continued risk of hypertension. She was monitored for 24 h before being transferred to the obstetrical floor.

Maggie gave birth to a healthy baby girl. Her pregnancy and delivery went better than expected, considering her medical history and the potential risks she was facing. She went through an extremely stressful time that was emotionally straining, given the circumstances of her mother's death. Despite this, she felt that she received the best possible care during her pregnancy and delivery. She also worried about her baby, who had a 50% chance of inheriting the condition (prenatal diagnosis wasn't possible then). Before her daughter's third birthday, Maggie received the upsetting news that her child was affected too.

Early recognition is key for identifying and managing pheochromocytoma during pregnancy. However, this can be very difficult because half of patients diagnosed with pheochromocytoma have no symptoms. Further, even when symptoms are present, they often mimic normal pregnancy symptoms, such as headaches, irritability, sweating, fast heart rate, nausea, and vomiting. Maggie's story illustrates how collaboration, extensive planning, and monitoring have a great influence on maternal and fetal outcomes. Her mom experienced the worst possible outcome of a pheochromocytoma in pregnancy—sudden death from a brain hemorrhage that could have been avoided. If it had not been for her mother and aunt, whose deaths made her diagnosis possible, Maggie might have suffered the same fate during labor and delivery.

Now I'd like to tell you about Tracie, who had three different endocrine diseases associated with pregnancy.

Eight months after her first baby was born, she started experiencing symptoms of dizziness and forgetfulness. She felt cold all the time and had trouble breastfeeding. Her family physician told her that she was depressed. However, Tracie disagreed, and she was eventually found to be markedly hypothyroid. Her first issue was the onset of postpartum hypothyroidism that was delayed in diagnosis because her physician attributed everything to postpartum depression.

Despite adequate treatment with Synthroid, Tracie developed neck pain that she described as "being choked." She found a lump in her neck, and her daughter's pediatrician confirmed that it was in her thyroid. When the family physician palpated her neck and dismissed the issue, Tracie persisted and requested an ultrasound.

In this way, Tracie was diagnosed with thyroid cancer, her second endocrine condition. She was in total shock and went through an extremely hard time, especially because she had to discontinue breastfeeding. She had a total thyroidectomy, and unfortunately all her parathyroid glands were damaged. Then she had postsurgical hypoparathyroidism, her third endocrine disorder. She was eventually discharged home on calcitriol and calcium.

Tracie now had hypothyroidism, hypoparathyroidism, and thyroid cancer. She and her husband wanted a second child. Of course, they had major concerns considering all the issues she had after her first pregnancy. *Would everything go OK with another pregnancy? Would the pregnancy cause regrowth of my cancer? Would the calcium affect the baby's bone development? Is pregnancy safe after radioactive iodine treatment?* Given all these concerns, Tracie consulted a maternal fetal specialist.

Hypoparathyroidism during pregnancy can result in maternal and fetal complications. Complications for the mother can include miscarriage, preterm labor, and hypocalcemia leading to seizures. One of the major challenges of managing this condition is trying to maintain normal calcium levels because inadequate supplementation in the mother can cause hyperparathyroidism in the fetus. This results in a weakened skeleton that can fracture in the womb.

Tracie became pregnant with her second child. She wanted to ensure that she could breastfeed this baby because she had to wean early with her first child. Her specialist, however, told her that she couldn't breastfeed because calcitriol was contraindicated, and she must never stop it.

Tracie decided to do her own research online and found Dr. Christopher Kovacs, in connection with review articles that he'd written on this subject. She emailed him requesting his advice on her situation. He responded that she likely would not need calcitriol while she breastfed because her breasts would make parathyroid hormone-related protein after delivery. This hormone tends to normalize calcium metabolism in breastfeeding women with hypoparathyroidism. She was extremely grateful that she found Dr. Kovacs, but was left feeling confused because she had two specialists giving her conflicting information.

Her second pregnancy and delivery went well. She delivered a baby girl, who had mild jaundice but otherwise was healthy. She wanted so badly to breastfeed, but her baby would not latch. Instead, she resorted to pumping and bottle-feeding the breastmilk. Her calcitriol dose had not been changed, as Dr. Kovacs had recommended. Two days after delivery, her calcium started to rise, followed by severe cramping in her feet and trouble walking. Her blood work revealed that her blood calcium was exceptionally high. Her calcium, calcitriol, and magnesium supplements were stopped. She was followed closely by an endocrinologist, and her calcium levels normalized for the remainder of lactation. It was expected that her blood calcium would drop with weaning, but her levels remained normal.

Tracie has been 7 years without requiring calcitriol, likely because her breasts have continued to make parathyroid hormone-related protein. She does not miss the side effects of aching bones, mood swings, and oral paresthesia. She still has occasional symptoms, such as leg cramping and numbness and tingling in her limbs. These symptoms are usually associated with a gastrointestinal illness, and she says she can easily live with them. Tracie's advice for other women is to know yourself, listen to your body, be your own advocate, and when in doubt, get a second opinion. Tracie felt that she received some misinformation throughout her pregnancies, and she is happy that she took her own health seriously enough to seek additional advice.

Tracie was not alone in being looked after by specialists who did not know that breastfeeding causes the release of parathyroid hormone-related protein from the breasts, which in turn causes the skeleton to partly break down and release calcium.

Debbie was diagnosed with Hodgkin's disease shortly after her first menstrual period at age 13. The chemotherapy caused ovarian failure, and she never experienced another period. Her hematologist told her that she could never become pregnant. Unfortunately, she was not treated with hormone replacement either, and she developed osteoporosis. In her early 30s, she unexpectedly became pregnant, and it took a while for her to realize the truth of the matter because she had been told it was impossible. The joy of delivering a healthy baby was marred during the first couple of days by the lactation consultant, nurses, and physicians on the obstetrical ward, who berated her that if she didn't breastfeed, she wasn't a good mother. Debbie told them that she couldn't breastfeed. She said that her bones wouldn't be able to tolerate it because calcium comes out of the skeleton to make milk. She told them to ask her endocrinologist. Instead, the obstetrical resident went off to do some research and discovered that Debbie was actually correct. She was happily permitted to bottle-feed her baby and was no longer worried about her bones being harmed.

Unlike Tracie, who had hypoparathyroidism causing hypercalcemia, I'd like to tell you about Mary, who had the opposite problem: hypercalcemia due to hyperparathyroidism. She also had a delayed diagnosis and cure of her condition.

Mary had her first baby in 2014. Shortly after her daughter's birth, and while breastfeeding, she started having symptoms of tiredness and muscle and bone pain. Her family members, friends, and physician told her that the symptoms she was experiencing were a normal part of having a baby. She didn't believe this and persisted with her doctors. She requested to have her vitamin D blood level checked, and while doing so, her serum calcium was also measured. She turned out to have high blood calcium and parathyroid hormone levels, consistent with primary hyperparathyroidism.

She saw several endocrinologists, who apparently suggested taking vitamin D, which seems paradoxical because it could worsen her problem. Her symptoms did not improve. She had parathyroid surgery in 2015, but they couldn't find the troublesome gland. She remained hypercalcemic.

Mary did some research and found several articles from Dr. Kovacs. She emailed him to get his opinion. He explained that there wasn't enough information to know for certain whether her hypercalcemia was due entirely to primary hyperparathyroidism, or how much it was aggravated by breastfeeding and the production of parathyroid hormone-related protein. The doctors wouldn't measure her blood levels. She decided to wait up to a year after she finished breastfeeding to see if the hypercalcemia would resolve. But it persisted, which suggested that primary hyperparathyroidism and not breastfeeding was the cause. She brought this information back to her endocrinologist. She was eventually referred to another surgeon, who removed the parathyroid adenoma that was the culprit. Since then, her calcium levels have been fine.

Mary's case shows the recurring issue of how the symptoms of pregnancy or postpartum overlap with symptoms of endocrine conditions, and thus they can be ignored by clinicians. She had to persist on her own to get advice from someone who could puzzle out what must be going on. In her case, the breastfeeding would have contributed to the rise in blood calcium and probably provoked her initial symptoms. It was necessary for her to stop breastfeeding to be certain whether the hypercalcemia was due to the parathyroids and not the production of breastmilk. In her case, it was a parathyroid that was the source of the problem all along, but there were difficulties localizing it.

The final story to be told here is about Kristie, who had hyperthyroidism that onset after her first child was born. The pregnancy and delivery were normal. Postpartum, she started having several health issues. She was constantly sweating, shaking, anxious, and struggling with breastfeeding. She expressed her concerns to her family doctor, the public health nurse, and a nurse at the breastfeeding clinic, but they reassured her that this was very normal and common in new moms. Seven or eight months passed, and she continued to experience worsening symptoms. On several occasions, she had to pull over while driving because she was so shaky and dizzy. Her family physician finally ordered blood work that revealed hyperthyroidism. She was started on methimazole and a beta blocker, and then referred to endocrinology.

Hyperthyroidism is the overproduction of thyroid hormone. Graves' disease (which Kristie has) is an autoimmune disorder and one of the most common causes of hyperthyroidism in women. Uncontrolled hyperthyroidism in pregnancy can lead to miscarriage, low birth weight, preeclampsia, and even thyroid storm if not treated. Thyroid hormone from the mother is also a critical component of fetal brain development in early pregnancy. An additional concern about Graves' disease is that it is caused by an antibody that can cross the placenta and lead to fetal hyperthyroidism.

Kristie's major concern was having another baby. She had many fears now: *Would she miscarry? Would her baby have Graves' disease? Would the baby be affected by the medication she was taking?* Her endocrinologist discussed the medications she could use during pregnancy for her hyperthyroidism, potential effects on the baby, and that it is possible for her condition to improve or get worse during pregnancy. She switched to propylthiouracil due to the risk of methimazole causing congenital malformations.

When Kristie became pregnant, she was followed closely by endocrinology and high-risk obstetrics specialists, with more frequent ultrasound monitoring of her baby. She was very lucky; before the third trimester, her Graves' disease was in remission, the stimulating antibody was undetectable, and the propylthiouracil was stopped. Her baby was born healthy, and she breastfed without concern. But around 4 months postpartum, her levels started to rise again, and she had to restart the methimazole. She had minimal symptoms this time because it was caught early; however, she did have to stop breastfeeding because her breastmilk dried up. Breastfeeding with hyperthyroidism can be a challenge, as it can cause issues with the milk supply and letdown, as well as with the medication getting into the breastmilk.

A diagnosis of hyperthyroidism in pregnancy and the postpartum period can be difficult, as some of the symptoms are common in normal pregnancies, such as tachycardia, sweating, fatigue, and anxiety. Symptoms can also mimic postpartum depression or the baby blues. In Kristie's case, her symptoms and concerns were dismissed as being a normal part of the postpartum period. Kristie's advice for other women is that they should listen to their bodies and to be persistent with their medical providers if necessary.

A woman's body undergoes rapid endocrine and metabolic changes during pregnancy to support the growth of the fetus. These changes are crucial for its development. However, these changes can lead to problems during pregnancy and postpartum if they become unbalanced. Endocrine disorders in pregnancy provide a unique challenge to all health-care providers, as disease signs and symptoms may be difficult to distinguish from the normal changes that occur during pregnancy. This is exactly what happened to many of the women whose stories I've shared with you. Their stories underscore the importance of a textbook like this. The issues span mother and baby and require multidisciplinary involvement. This includes physicians, nurses, and allied health professionals from endocrinology, pediatrics, neonatology, obstetrics, and genetics, who may use this book as a reference when diagnosing and treating women during the preconception, pregnancy, and postpartum periods.

Consistent take-home messages from these women, who experienced endocrine illnesses during pregnancy and postpartum, is to be your own advocate. Prioritizing your health is nonnegotiable. Recognize that symptoms of disease can be mistakenly dismissed as being just the result of normal pregnancy, postpartum, and breastfeeding. For example, how can you distinguish fatigue that is due to being up all night with a newborn from fatigue that might be a clue to an endocrine disorder or other illness? If you are not satisfied with your current diagnosis and treatment, get a second opinion. Listen to your own body. If you feel things are not right, be persistent. You are the only one who truly knows how you feel. Bear in mind that many of the health-care providers you encounter may have no experience with the manifestations or management of endocrine diseases during pregnancy and breastfeeding. For these reasons, don't be afraid to do your own research of reputable medical journals.

Remember the initial declaration, "I'm pregnant! You're pregnant!" Despite any endocrine disorders that may precede or develop during pregnancy, in the end, we want every woman to be able to proudly announce:

"I have a beautiful, healthy baby!"

When you are Told That Your Fetus or Newborn has an Endocrine Condition: Perspectives of the Parents

Cheri L. Deal* and Catalina Maftei[†]

*Department of Pediatrics, Université de Montréal; Pediatric Endocrine and Diabetes Service, Centre Hospitalier Universitaire Sainte Justine, Montréal, QC, Canada, [†]Department of Pediatrics, Université de Montréal and Genetics Service, Centre Hospitalier Universitaire Sainte Justine, Montréal, QC, Canada

when you are in the dark, it is easy to feel overwhelmed…(but) know that this child can be a gift
…it was the not knowing the diagnosis that was the hardest…
…the endocrinology service feels like family to us…

This chapter tells the story of three sets of parents, who graciously agreed to be interviewed in order to remind us of what, for them, has been the most significant aspects of the diagnostic and treatment odyssey of their children, now on the brink of adulthood. What comes out loudly and clearly are their fears and confusion as they tried to understand all the explanations given. "*Endocrinology is not simple*," in the words of one of them, and yet having a firm diagnosis helps relieve the anxiety. What else goes into being able to move forward when confronted with a lifelong condition with endocrine and other health consequences?

Meet our first family—who, following an amniocentesis performed at the beginning of the second trimester for advanced maternal age, were reassured *that all was normal*. This was their second pregnancy, and their healthy 5-year-old girl was as happy as her parents to learn that she would have a sibling. They had chosen not to learn the sex of the baby, so they were a bit surprised when the physicians attending the delivery seemed mystified by the arrival of a perfect little girl. Thinking back on the moment that they were told why—that this baby was expected to be a little boy based on the karyotype—"*It was a very solemn parade that entered the room: our treating obstetrician, a geneticist, a pediatrician, 2 residents and 2 nurses. I (Father) was told to sit down. Our baby was not in the room at the moment because she was undergoing a blood test. We were really worried – was something terribly wrong? Would we lose her before knowing her?*" The family learned that there appeared to be a "sex reversal," and that more tests were necessary to understand why. "*The explanation was given by the physician who delivered the baby and was no doubt correct, but we were unprepared for this type of news.*"

Although complete androgen insensitivity was suspected from the onset, the initial sequencing results missed a splice site mutation in the androgen receptor, which led to a gene-by-gene approach until, with the persistence of our Endocrine Service, whole exome sequencing finally did pick it up. During this time, for the family who understood that their daughter had "*seemingly normal, functional intra-abdominal testes and no uterus*," it took them "*a lot of reading and assimilation before we understood what this diagnosis meant. This was definitely helped by our referral to Dr. Deal by the geneticist, when our daughter was 8 weeks old. Endocrinology informed us the most, and kept us up to date with test results, confirmation of the diagnosis and changing attitudes and treatment approaches.*"

However, this family's journey did not stop there. Shortly after this daughter was born, it was discovered that their 5-year-old daughter had also been born after an amniocentesis, done privately, that was interpreted as normal. The results, it seemed, had not been transferred to the hospital where this little girl was delivered. More important, this child underwent bilateral hernia repair at age 2 months. "*The geneticist went back and discovered that the amniocentesis of our first born was also 46,XY, and therefore she, too, was affected by the same genetic condition. Imagine our shock now. But Dr. Deal immediately put us in contact with a psychologist for the family, who was extremely helpful in seeing us through this period and who followed us over several years.*"

This very proactive family used documents given to them by our team, as well as rapidly consulting the Internet, particularly for their older child, to be reassured as to the experiences of others. However, when asked the question as to when their stress, graded as 4.5/5 during the first few weeks/months following the diagnosis and perturbing their sleep, began to be manageable, they agreed that *"our stress slowly diminished as we gradually accepted this new reality. Since our daughters were in good health both physically and mentally, our apprehension slowly disappeared."*

What "pearls" have these parents left with us?

- *"What has been the best and the worst experiences? The best have been with Dr. Deal. The appointments are always conducted with the greatest respect, the information given was always pertinent and permitted our daughters to slowly come to understand androgen insensitivity. They have had a lasting relationship with their doctor. The worst was to be told a diagnosis in the hospital by our obstetrician, 3 days after a caesarian delivery. We also did not like being seen by physicians that we did not know on a few visits. We think that it is important for our girls to build a relationship with one physician."*
- *"Although many pieces of information we have learned over the year were important, by far the most is learning about the health problems associated with the syndrome, and facing ANY risk of cancer no matter how small, if the gonads are left in. We needed to know that their life expectancy would be the same as a child without androgen insensitivity, and we needed to talk about gender identity and sexuality."*
- *"Did we discuss recurrence risk? Not a problem since our family was complete, and since our two daughters are infertile. But as the endocrinologist has often said, there are many ways to have a family!"*

Our second family also wrestled with a genetic diagnosis, which brings with it a diagnosis of infertility (namely, Turner syndrome). How did they learn about this?

We were out of the country when the story started with my wife losing blood, around the 12th week of her pregnancy with our second child. We had an ultrasound done immediately and they told us that the fetal heartbeat was still strong, but that we should have an ultrasound when we got back home. We were scared for the baby.

The bleeding stopped after a couple of days, and the pregnancy seemed to proceed normally. Hoping to have good news as soon as possible, the parents sought out a private radiology clinic to have a repeat ultrasound at 16 weeks of pregnancy. *"This was when we were told that something was wrong with the baby – that there was extra skin on the neck and that we needed to have an amniocentesis."* After this, they repeated the ultrasound in the University Center and were told that the nuchal translucency was increased. An amniocentesis was performed at 21 weeks.

(Mother) You have to understand that I still had a bit of a language barrier (being of European origin), so I needed careful explanations. When we were told by the obstetrician that the baby's chromosomes were 45,X meaning that there was one chromosome missing, I did understand the basics. He was very scientific, very matter of fact, and he said that our daughter had Turner Syndrome and that we needed another ultrasound with a fetal heart specialist. He offered us the choice of a therapeutic abortion although we were trying to get our head around the name of the condition. Was it a disease? I just wanted to know if her brain was okay, that she would not be a vegetable.

"We did see a geneticist at 22 weeks and other consultations were organised but it was at 23 weeks when we saw the pediatric cardiologist who did the fetal cardiac ultrasound and who reassured us that all would be well with her intelligence although she would eventually need surgery for her heart since she had a coarctation of the aorta. We were also told to go see a pediatric endocrinologist." Their stress level dropped since they were, as they put it, optimistic by nature, but they were determined to find out as much as possible, and they remember feeling as if it was *"us against the world"* and noting that *"when you are in the dark, it is easy to feel overwhelmed."*

They sought information from as many sources as possible, including their family doctor, who *"showed us really terrible pictures in a textbook,"* and by chance, while waiting to see the pediatric endocrinologist, they learned about a support group meeting of the Turner Syndrome Association in another city. "(Father) *This was a turning point for us, and we were able to see children and young girls living very successfully with this condition, as well as speak to their parents. We also met with Dr. Deal, who was speaking at the conference and who answered our questions, confirming our gut feeling that we and our little girl would do just fine."*

Early after birth, their attention was focused on immediate health issues, including a severe aortic arch atresia that needed surgery on day 2 of life. More doctors were seen—orthopedics, a confirmation of the karyotype by genetics, close cardiology, and cardiac surgery follow-up. Later, it was the ear infections, some hearing loss, and the ear surgery for tubes.

"We took it one day at a time and dealt mostly with the medical issues. Then when she was in first grade, we met with the psychologist from the Endocrine Clinic for her first evaluation. We knew our daughter was smart but she was having difficulty in French and in Math and was impulsive." The psychologist helped the school to tailor her pedagogical support, but more important, *"offered lots of family counselling. She was great, and she validated us as parents. She saw us with, and without our daughter, she saw just our daughter, she saw our two daughters together, and she saw the entire family. Everybody had a chance to speak."*

For us, our daughter's infertility was less of an issue than some of her medical problems, and we spoke openly with her all along the way as did the Endocrinology team. We wanted to have anticipatory guidance, and be kept aware of the treatment options. In fact, we turned down growth hormone therapy since her height prognosis was very good, given that we are tall parents.

What else do they want to share with others?

- *"There is often a sentiment of guilt when you start talking about genetics, which, quite frankly, I still don't understand. It is so important to let this guilt go, particularly for Turner Syndrome which is not anyone's fault."*
- *"We only felt that we had all the right tools to make the right decisions for our child after meeting with the endocrinologist. Most importantly, we learned it's a syndrome not a disease."*
- *"Things have so changed over the years, that now you can get lots of good information on the internet. Chat groups can be a great support for kids and parents. You need to reach out to the right people, not panic, know that this child can be a gift."*
- *"And please doctors, make sure that the family has ALL the relevant information before being given the option of have a therapeutic abortion."*

What happens when you learn that your severely dehydrated baby has congenital adrenal hyperplasia (CAH), which could have been clinically detected much earlier, even without neonatal screening? How do you feel when your 1-in-64 chance of having three affected babies with CAH actually comes true? How does it change your vision of the disease? How do you integrate research evidence with your choice of prenatal therapy? What would you ask health teams to do differently?

Meet family number three, who spent many painful weeks trying to understand why their first baby was not gaining weight rapidly enough. The pregnancy went well, and they were the proud parents of a 4.21-kg baby boy. They were seen by the local clinic nurse often in the first few weeks because she came frequently to take weight measurements; despite breast-feeding every 1–2 h during the day, with a good mild letdown, this perfect newborn took 18 days to regain his birth weight. He continued to have a relatively poor but consistent weight gain, interspersed with frequent crying episodes, even with breastmilk supplementation and frequent nursing. The community nurse offered encouragement and reassured them because he looked otherwise well and was not vomiting or sleeping excessively; he was just not gaining weight rapidly, going from the 95th down to the 50th percentile over 8 weeks. *"We kept being told he was going to be tall and lean since we were athletic and not overweight!"*

(Mother) Our baby was seen twice by a family physician as well, but it was only at the age of 10 weeks that the clinic agreed that he was failing to thrive, and he would require hospitalisation in a pediatric unit. We were very worried, and the diagnosis was not yet clear even though many tests were performed. I was doing everything I could to keep him fed round the clock. On arrival to a community hospital, our son was very thin but not hyperpigmented as all the doctors noted; he did nothing but cry and try to nurse and, by this time, was vomiting periodically.

This was not a consanguineous family, but the pediatrician had wisely thought about a putative diagnosis of CAH with a sodium of 130 mmol/L and normal potassium; therefore, at 11 weeks of age, bloods for determination of serum 17-OH progesterone and electrolytes were drawn. Contact was made with our hospital center before the baby was transferred to us with a sodium of 128 mmol/L and with a potassium of 5.5 mmol/L, which shortly climbed to 7.0 mmol/L. *"They put in a pick line, gave him IV hydrocortisone, and within 12 hours we had a different baby entirely."*

(Mother) I remember the day after our arrival in Montreal, the pediatric endocrinologist came into our baby's hospital room, a Saturday morning, and sat on the bed nearby where I was trying to sleep. I was very stressed, fearful of the future, and exhausted. He told me that salt-wasting congenital adrenal hyperplasia was, indeed, confirmed and spent over an hour with me, drawing pictures, explaining what causes this condition, what it will mean for my son and for our family. As soon as we had a diagnosis I was reassured; I had time to ask my questions and process the information. It was the not knowing the diagnosis that was the hardest.

Gradually, the family met the other members of the Endocrine team, and talk of having a future pregnancy came up. At the time, the turnaround time for 21-hydroxylase gene sequencing (a mutation being the most likely cause of CAH) was very long, and few centers did it, so the parents accepted to complete another test. This indirect test (HLA typing) could potentially determine if the fetus and the older son are sharing the same genetic information in the region of the 21-hydroxylase gene, in the hope that the parents could make informed decisions about an experimental treatment with prenatal dexamethasone. This test predicted that the next fetus would also have CAH. After very long discussions with the high-risk pregnancy obstetrician, adult endocrinologist, the pediatric endocrinology team, and a geneticist, *"we decided to move forward with prenatal dexamethasone treatment. We understood it was experimental but we learned about the published results to date and spoke about the theoretical risks."*

For their second pregnancy, dexamethasone treatment was started at week 3, and an early amniocentesis at 14 weeks confirmed that it was a girl. *"I was lucky, because apart from the stretch marks, I had very little side effects of the treatment, even continuing it up until the delivery and after, when I was tapered. No diabetes, no hypertension, no mood issues."* Then, 27 months after receiving their firstborn into their arms, the parents welcomed a beautiful little girl.

As the pediatric endocrinologist on duty at the time (Dr. Deal), I remember thinking that she was so perfect, I had to make sure that she was actually affected since, linkage disequilibrium aside, seeing hormonal and genetic results was believing! Here, 17-hydroxyprogesterone and androstenedione levels were diagnostic by day 2, and thanks to connections with researchers in Lyon who were interested in this condition, we eventually confirmed that she was also a compound heterozygote for two deleterious mutations. Good genotype-phenotype correlations were already available predicting salt-losing CAH, with significant virilisation in females.

By pregnancy number 3, this family was at ease with CAH.

(Mother) *"Given the success of our second pregnancy and continued health of both our kids, I of course wanted dexamethasone treatment for our next baby."* Early amniocentesis confirmed that the fetus was a boy, so this time, treatment was stopped at week 14 of pregnancy. However, genotype again confirmed they were expecting a third child with CAH, and as before, 17-hydroxyprogesterone and androstenedione levels confirmed that the diagnosis and treatment was started on day 4. When asked how they felt about now having three affected kids, here was their response: *"they are all the same, so there is no room for jealousy or for not taking their medication."*

This family's story started before the widespread use of neonatal screening for CAH, and before the heated discussions and consensus guidelines about prenatal steroid exposure. The parents now know that medicine evolves, and that as their children become adults, we are happy to note that their health is excellent. Their developmental trajectories and school achievements have been normal as expected by their family, as we and their parents have confirmed. They have expressed that their biggest concern was that the health professionals initially did not think it abnormal that the weight gain was so slow. *"I just wanted to be referred to an expert, and in this case it should have led to an earlier consultation with a pediatric endocrinologist. The endocrinology service feels like family to us; you have been there to see our children grow up and you have made sure that they understand their condition. You always answer our phone calls and you guided us during the childhood illnesses, and this has keep all of them out of the hospital once they were diagnosed."*

And their last words of wisdom to doctors and health professionals:

*(Mother) knowing what it feels like **not** knowing a diagnosis, and how having the **certainty** of a genetic diagnosis allows you to accept and move on so that you can focus on the best treatment, I would hope that early diagnosis would make life easier for families today. I also had a very good colleague whose husband had congenital adrenal hyperplasia and she was a critical support person for me in those very early days after the diagnosis of our first child. I would encourage physicians to approach their patients' families who are at ease and more experienced with their children's' diagnoses to ask them to be that support for others. Firsthand experience from non-medical people, even if every family is different, allows for human contact —which is everything.*

It is our hope, and no doubt that of all the authors who have contributed to this book, that the lessons offered through these cases will be of use to physicians and health professionals dealing with endocrine diagnoses in a fetus or newborn. Enjoy!

Section 1

The Mother

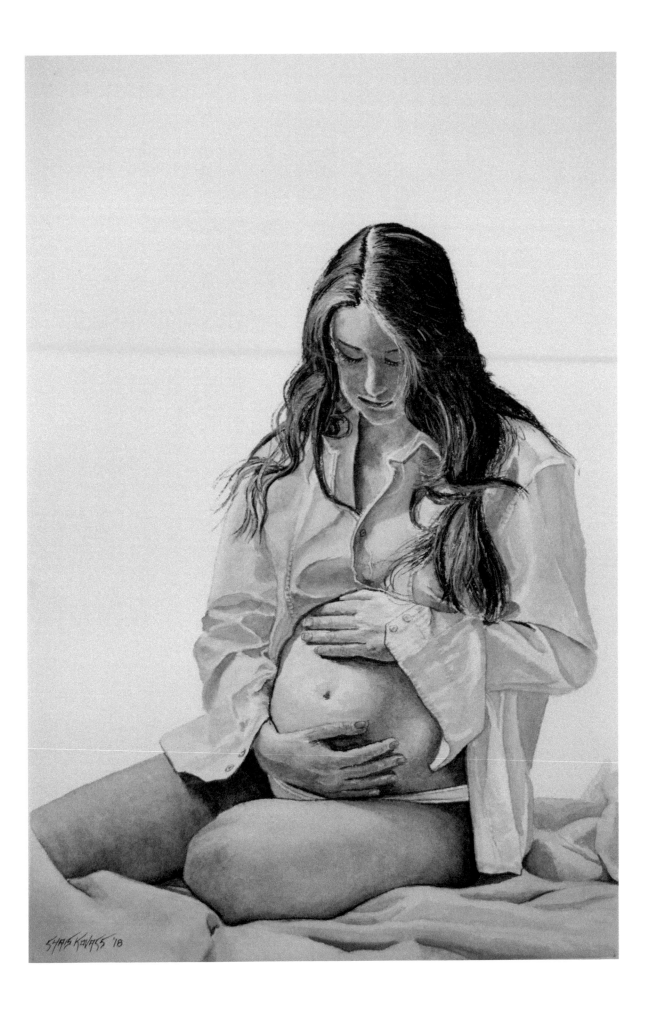

Normal Endocrine Physiology of the Mother During Pregnancy and Lactation

Chapter 1

Normal Endocrine Physiology of Hypothalamic Hormones During Ovulation, Pregnancy, and Lactation

Cheng Xu, Georgios E. Papadakis and Nelly Pitteloud

Service of Endocrinology, Diabetes and Metabolism, CHUV, Lausanne University Hospital, Lausanne, Switzerland

> **Key Clinical Changes**
> - Hypothalamic pulsatile GnRH secretion induces different patterns of follicle stimulating hormone (FSH) and luteinizing hormone (LH) release from the pituitary, which is critical to induce follicular maturation, ovulation, and maintenance of the corpus luteum during menstrual cycles.
> - Kisspeptin neurons are the gatekeeper of gonadotropin-releasing hormone (GnRH) neurons, and they mediate negative and positive feedback of sex steroids to the hypothalamus.
> - Placental secretion of kisspeptin and GnRH acts in a paracrine manner to ensure implantation and evolution of a pregnancy.
> - Peripherally produced oxytocin is important for the contractility of myometrium during parturition.
> - Maternal hypothalamic secretion of oxytocin is involved in the maintenance of lactation.
> - Oligo- or amenorrhea during breastfeeding is induced by inhibition of the maternal hypothalamic kisspeptin-GnRH neuron system.

Pregnancy is a complex physiologic condition involving the interaction of the neuroendocrine system of the maternal brain and the fetal-placental unit. Maternal changes in the hypothalamic-pituitary axes are well established and are considered critical for the maternal homeostasis necessary to induce ovulation, as well as maintaining an ongoing pregnancy and subsequent lactation. In this chapter, we will discuss the pivotal role of hypothalamic hormones in ovulation, pregnancy, and lactation.

1.1 HYPOTHALAMIC FUNCTION DURING OVULATION

1.1.1 GnRH

1.1.1.1 Pulsatility of GnRH

GnRH is the pivotal hormone of the hypothalamic-pituitary-gonadal (HPG) axis. GnRH is a decapeptide secreted by a subgroup of neurons (termed *GnRH neurons*), located in the arcuate nucleus (ARC) and preoptic area (POA) in the hypothalamus. Pulsatile secretion of GnRH from the hypothalamus induces the secretion of gonadotropins (FSH and LH) in the pituitary. Gonadotropins in turn stimulate gametogenesis and the production of sex steroids in the gonads.

The periodicity and amplitude of GnRH pulses determine the secretion pattern of LH and FSH, as demonstrated by experimental studies of monkeys in which the hypothalamus was lesioned and GnRH was replaced by exogenous administration.[1] Continuous infusion of GnRH decreases both LH and FSH levels, indicating that the pulsatility of GnRH secretion is critical to the regulation of pituitary responsiveness. Rapid GnRH pulses (i.e., 1 pulse of GnRH per hour) increase LH secretion, while slower pulses (i.e., 1 pulse every 3 h) favor the secretion of FSH. The concentration of GnRH is high in the central portal system but is not measurable in the circulation due to the low concentration and short half-life. The correlation of GnRH and LH pulses has been shown to be in a 1:1 ratio under physiological conditions by animal

Maternal-Fetal and Neonatal Endocrinology. https://doi.org/10.1016/B978-0-12-814823-5.00001-5

experiments in which blood samples were collected simultaneously from the portal and peripheral blood.[2] Thus, the LH pulsatile pattern, which can be determined by sampling every 10 min, can be used to reflect GnRH pulsatility in humans.[3]

1.1.1.2 GnRH Pulsatile Pattern Throughout the Ovulatory Cycle

Human studies using frequent sampling of LH in healthy female volunteers have revealed different GnRH pulsatile patterns throughout the menstrual cycle.[4, 5] Briefly, the average GnRH pulse frequency is around 1 pulse every 90 min in the early follicular phase, which increases the secretion of FSH. The frequency gradually increases to 1 pulse every 60 min by the late follicular phase to promote LH secretion. GnRH pulse frequency decreases markedly during the luteal phase to approximately 1 pulse every 4 h, leading to a lower level of gonadotropins. Although the dynamics of GnRH pulses are extrapolated from indirect data on LH measurement in female volunteers, exogenous pulsatile GnRH treatment using this regimen in patients with functional or congenital GnRH deficiency can successfully restore ovulation, thus validating the hypothesis.[6] Such a GnRH pulsatility pattern is important to induce the dynamic changes of gonadotropin levels, which are critical to achieve follicular development, ovulation, and preparation for possible pregnancy.

1.1.2 Kisspeptin

Although the fundamental role of GnRH in the initiation and maintenance of HPG axis activity has long been recognized, our knowledge of its upstream regulation system has been expanded only recently. GnRH neurons receive a variety of inputs from upstream afferent neurons, such as stimulatory (e.g., glutamate and norepinephrine) and inhibitory drives [e.g., gamma-aminobutyric acid (GABA) and endogenous opioid peptides].[7] These afferent systems can integrate the information from steroid hormones and metabolic cues to stimulate or suppress GnRH neuron activity.[8] The kisspeptin pathway plays a critical role in transmitting these signals, serving as the "gatekeeper" for the reawakening of GnRH neuron network at puberty, as well as the regulator of GnRH neurons and gonadotropin secretion.[9]

Kisspeptin is composed of 145 amino acids encoded by the *KISS1* gene. It can be broken into fragments: kisspeptin-54, kisspeptin-14, kisspeptin-13, and kisspeptin-10. Functional active kisspeptin fragments contain the 10 amino acids of the carboxy-terminal (amino acids 112–121), which are important for receptor binding and function.[10] Kisspeptin is the natural ligand of *KISS1R*, originally known as G protein-coupled receptor 54 (GPR54). Mutations in *KISS1R* genes were identified in patients with congenital GnRH deficiency in 2003,[11, 12] and subsequently, a large number of biological and animal studies have been performed to elucidate the role of the kisspeptin pathway in the control of the GnRH neuronal network.[9]

Intracerebroventricular injection and peripheral administration of kisspeptins have been shown to increase gonadotropin secretion in animal models (mouse, rat, sheep, monkey, etc.) with sexual dimorphism.[9] Such sexual dimorphism also exists in humans, as revealed by physiological studies performed in healthy volunteers. In males, either bolus or continuous infusion of kisspeptin can elicit LH secretion,[13, 14] while the effect in females depends on the stages of the menstrual cycle.[13] Kisspeptin can stimulate gonadotropin secretion only during the follicular and preovulatory phases, and it exhibits its greatest effect on LH at the preovulatory phase.[15] Furthermore, the role of kisspeptin has been confirmed in patients with functional GnRH deficiency. In patients with hypothalamic amenorrhea, whose GnRH neuron network is functionally inhibited by exogenous factors, administration of kisspeptin can acutely stimulate the secretion of gonadotropins.[16, 17] However, tachyphylaxis has been observed during chronic treatment. Finally, kisspeptin injection is now used to trigger ovulation in a stimulation regimen, confirming its key role in the generation of LH surge[18, 19] (this point will be discussed further in Chapter 16).

The mechanism of kisspeptin in the regulation of the menstrual cycle and ovulation has been explored in animal models. Kisspeptin-expressing neurons are mainly found in two hypothalamic nuclei: the ARC and the anteroventral periventricular nucleus (AVPV), but they exhibit different physiological roles in those locations. Using optogenetic approaches in genetic modified mouse models, it recently was shown that Kiss1-expressing neurons in ARC are key components of the GnRH pulse generator, essential for GnRH secretion, and they mediate negative feedback of estrogens.[20] In contrast, the positive feedback of estrogens, which induces the ovulatory LH surge, is mediated by Kiss1 neurons located in the AVPV.[21]

1.2 ADAPTIVE RESPONSES OF HYPOTHALAMIC HORMONES DURING PREGNANCY

Gestational adaptations during pregnancy aim at maintaining early pregnancy, ensuring adequate nutritional support to the developing fetus, and preparing for parturition. Maternal endocrine adaptations involve the hypothalamus, pituitary, parathyroid, thyroid, adrenal glands, and ovary, and are linked to the interactions of the fetal-placental-maternal unit.

The hypothalamus regulates much of the endocrine system by coordinating input from multiple signals from peripheral hormones, and output via the hypothalamic-pituitary axis through the secretion of hypothalamic hormones. The activity of various hypothalamic-pituitary axes directly affect the functions of the thyroid, adrenals, and gonads, and influence growth, lactation, and water balance.

Hypothalamic hormones include stimulatory hormones, such as GnRH, corticotropin-releasing hormone (CRH), growth hormone-releasing hormone (GHRH), thyrotropin-releasing hormone (TRH), and inhibitory hormones such as somatostatin (SST) and prolactin-inhibiting factors (mainly dopamine). In contrast to the nonpregnant state, when the hypothalamic hormones are highly concentrated in the portal system and undetectable in the peripheral circulation, the circulating concentrations of many of these hormones rise during pregnancy. However, such changes in concentration are mainly due to secretions from the placenta.[22]

Importantly, the placenta produces a plethora of hormones, which are similar or analogous to maternal hypothalamic-pituitary hormones. These hormones are primarily released into the maternal circulation and can bind to cognate receptors on maternal cells. Therefore, the placenta acts as a secondary neuroendocrine control center to adjust maternal physiology, usually in favor of supporting the needs of the fetus.[23]

In this section, we will focus on the physiological changes on the maternal hypothalamic-pituitary-gonadal and hypothalamic-pituitary-GH axes, as well as the hypothalamic hormones that are secreted by the posterior pituitary: anti-diuretic hormone (ADH) and oxytocin. Placental secretion of these hormones and their role on maternal changes during pregnancy also will be discussed. Changes in the hypothalamic-pituitary-thyroid axis and hypothalamic-pituitary-adrenal (HPA) axis will be discussed in Chapters 4 and 8, respectively.

1.2.1 GnRH and Kisspeptin

1.2.1.1 Maternal GnRH and Kisspeptin

From early pregnancy, gonadotropin levels are very low, reflecting decreased functioning of maternal GnRH and Kisspeptin neurons. Maternal LH and FSH levels are inhibited by the high levels of progesterone secreted first by the corpus luteum, and then by the placenta.[24]

1.2.1.2 Placental GnRH

GnRH produced by human placenta is identical to hypothalamic GnRH.[25] Using radioimmunoassays, circulating GnRH is detectable in pregnant women, which is higher in early gestation than in late gestation.[26] This pattern of placental GnRH secretion correlates closely with human chorionic gonadotropin (hCG) levels observed during pregnancy. GnRH has been shown to stimulate hCG secretion in superfused placenta explants[27] and perifused placental cells,[28] although the precise mechanism is unclear. These data suggest that GnRH plays a role in regulating hCG production and that placental GnRH is essential for the establishment and maintenance of early pregnancy.[29] In addition, the association between low GnRH levels in maternal circulation and prematurity was observed in the few cases that have been studied, suggesting that GnRH levels may be indicative of placental dysfunction.[26]

1.2.1.3 Placental Kisspeptin

Kisspeptin and its receptor, *KISS1R*, were first studied in the placenta due to the high level of expression there.[30] The circulating kisspeptin increases throughout gestation and decreases dramatically postpartum, further confirming the placental origin of secretion.[31] Several studies in rodent models and humans have demonstrated the vital role of kisspeptin during pregnancy. Using *Kiss1* knockout mice (mice in which *Kiss1* has been inactivated), it has been shown that the kisspeptin pathway is important for implantation and decidualization by regulating the uterine endothelium.[32, 33] In humans, the *KISS1* gene is highly expressed in placental tissues obtained during the first trimester and at full term.[34] Lower kisspeptin levels correlate with subsequent small gestational age at delivery,[35] the development of preeclampsia and intrauterine growth restriction,[36] incidence of type 1 diabetes, gestational hypertension, and gestational diabetes.[37] In addition, kisspeptin levels can be used to predict the risk of miscarriage.[38] Thus, normal secretion of placental kisspeptin appears important to ensure a successful and safe pregnancy.

1.2.2 GHRH and Somatostatin

The hypothalamic-pituitary-GH axis is regulated by two hypothalamic hormones: the stimulating hormone GHRH and the inhibitory hormone SST. As for the other hormones discussed previously, it is important to distinguish the origin of increased GH levels during pregnancy, whether it is from the maternal pituitary gland or from the placenta. During early pregnancy, GH measured in maternal blood is secreted in a pulsatile pattern from the pituitary. However, in late pregnancy, the majority of circulating GH is derived from the placenta and remains constant over time.[39] Placental GH is secreted constitutively and does not respond to GHRH.[40] However, it appears to be regulated by maternal glucose levels such that reduced GH levels have been observed in diabetic pregnant women with hyperglycemia.[41] Conversely, maternal hypoglycemia is a primary stimulator of placental GH secretion, which would subsequently increase maternal blood glucose and thus protect the fetus from nutrient deficiency.[39] Thus, regulation of the hypothalamic-pituitary-GH axis, especially of the placental GH, is critical in pregnancy.

1.2.3 Antidiuretic Hormone

There are only a very few studies that focused on the role of ADH (or vasopressin) during normal pregnancy. It has been shown that ADH plasma concentration in pregnant women do not differ from nonpregnant women, despite a decrease of approximately 10 mOsmol/kg.[42]

1.2.4 Oxytocin

Parturition is controlled by multiple hormones that affect the contractility of the myometrium and the integrity of the uterine cervix. While the withdrawal of progesterone and the activation of estrogen play a pivotal role in the initiation of parturition, oxytocin (OT) is the most potent stimulator of uterine contraction to promote labor and postpartum hemostasis.

OT is a 9-amino-acid peptide that is synthesized in the paraventricular (PVN) and supraoptic (SON) nuclei of the hypothalamus and released by the posterior pituitary. OT is also produced in a number of peripheral tissues, including the ovaries. The oxytocin receptor gene (*OXTR*) is expressed in various tissues, including brain, uterus, kidney, ovary, testis, thymus, heart, vascular endothelium in both mice[43] and humans (GTEx portal database, https://gtexportal.org/home/gene/OXTR). Despite the widespread clinical use of OT during labor, the site of OT secretion and its mechanism of action during parturition were uncertain for a long time.

1.2.4.1 Maternal OT

Increased OT pulses frequency and duration have been detected after spontaneous labor by sampling at 1-min intervals in parturient women.[44] Vaginal distention is a principal stimulus for the release of pituitary OT in human labor via a neurologic feedback mechanism known as the *Ferguson reflex*. After birth, pituitary OT contributes to uterine involution, and especially the tonic contraction of the myometrium needed for postpartum hemostasis. OT also affects the preparation of the breast for lactation (see Section 1.3, later in this chapter).

1.2.4.2 Peripheral OT

During pregnancy, synthesis of OT by human intrauterine tissues of both fetal and maternal origin (amnion, chorion, and decidua) has been detected.[45] In addition, the content and expression of the OT receptor (*OXTR*) in human myometrium and decidua increases gradually toward the end of pregnancy and then rises significantly in association with the onset of labor.[46] Putting these data together, intrauterine production of OT with the upregulation of *OXTR* expression may play a significant paracrine role in regulating uterine contraction at parturition, especially in the absence of significant changes of maternal circulating OT levels.[47]

1.2.4.3 Insights from OT Deficiency Models

Genetically modified mouse models with oxytocin deficiency provided more insights into the roles of OT in reproduction. Homozygous female mice with oxytocin knockout ($Oxt^{-/-}$) or oxytocin receptor knockout ($Oxtr^{-/-}$) exhibit no defects in either fertility or delivery of their litters,[48–51] suggesting that oxytocin is not indispensable during parturition.

In human, no loss-of-function mutation has been reported in the genes encoding oxytocin or oxytocin receptors. OT deficiency in other hypothalamic-pituitary pathologies is difficult to determine because the measurement of OT is not used in routine clinical settings. A moderate but significant decrease in OT levels was reported in a small number of patients with craniopharyngioma or hypopituitarism.[52, 53] However, there was no measurement of OT levels during parturition in these patients. Several reports described spontaneous labor onset and uneventful vaginal delivery without pharmacological intervention in patients with either panhypophysectomy or panhypopituitarism.[54, 55] Although biochemical confirmation of OT deficiency in these patients is lacking, they are very likely to exhibit impaired central OT secretion. These data further support the observation from the animal studies that maternal OT is not critical for parturition, and its deficiency can probably be compensated for by other mechanisms.

1.3   ADAPTIVE RESPONSES OF HYPOTHALAMIC HORMONES TO LACTATION

1.3.1   Lactation and Breastfeeding

During pregnancy, mammary glands grow, preparing the alveoli for lactation under the stimulation of high levels of lactogenic hormones such as prolactin, human placental lactogen, and placental growth hormone. The high concentration of progesterone during pregnancy blocks lactogenesis. Following delivery, the circulating estradiol and progesterone levels decrease, while the high prolactin concentration persists, which results in the production of all of the components of milk.[56] Milk production also requires the synergistic action of GH, insulin, thyroxine, and cortisol, which will be discussed predominantly in Chapter 14. Among the maternal hypothalamic hormones, oxytocin release and suppression of dopamine play an important role in the maintenance of lactation.

Episodic oxytocin secretion from the posterior pituitary during suckling causes the contraction of the myoepithelial cells of the mammary acini and ducts, inducing the flow of milk. The suckle-induced stimuli send sensory signals originating in the nipple through thoracic nerves 4, 5, and 6 to the central nervous system. Intranuclear release of oxytocin in PVN and SON is critical for generating the pulsatile pattern of systemic oxytocin secretion.[57, 58] Activation of noradrenergic, histaminergic, and excitary amino acids is necessary for suckling-induced release of central oxytocin during lactation.[59] In addition, oxytocin can be released by visual and auditory stimuli.

Female $Oxt^{-/-}$ and $Oxtr^{-/-}$ mice exhibit defects in milk ejection in response to their pups sucking, leading to the postnatal death of pups within 24 h without milk spot in their stomachs.[48–51] The histological study of mammary glands in homozygous female mice showed normal mammary development during gestation and normal postpartum milk production. The intraperitoneal injection of OT in female $Oxt^{-/-}$ mice can restore the milk ejection and rescue the pups.[48, 49] Similarly, all the offspring of $Oxtr^{-/-}$ mice were successfully fostered to the wild-type female mice.[51] These studies elegantly confirmed the indispensable role of OT in normal lactation (milk ejection). Interestingly, all the reported patients with theoretically OT deficiency (either panhypophysectomy or panhypopituitarism) failed lactation after their delivery.[54, 55] This can be due to double defects in both PRL and OT.

The suckling-induced signals also induce the release of prolactin, in part by suppressing dopamine secretion in the hypothalamus. In lactating women, the basal prolactin levels are elevated during the first 6 weeks postpartum, with peaks at each session of breastfeeding.[60, 61] From 7 to 28 weeks postpartum, basal prolactin levels are in the normal range; however, the spike in prolactin levels persists during suckling.[60, 61]

Homozygous female Prl knockout ($Prl^{-/-}$) mice exhibit irregular estrus cycles and are totally infertile.[62] They exhibit abnormal mammary gland development and morphology. However, lactation is not possible to evaluate due to infertility. In humans, isolated PRL deficiency (OMIM 264110) is a rare condition, reported in only six patients.[63–65] The genetic cause is not yet identified. A recent report demonstrated an autoimmune etiology in one patient with isolated PRL deficiency.[65] In contrast to the Prl-deficient mice, the fertility in these patients was either unaffected or could be induced by clomiphene treatment.[63–65] Indeed, all these patients exhibit puerperal alactogenesis. Lactation was successfully induced by subcutaneous injection recombinant PRL in one patient.[65] In addition, lactation failure is reported in patients with combined pituitary hormone deficiency harboring mutations in $PROP1$, the gene that affects the development of all lineage precursors of the anterior pituitary.[66]

Lactation can be induced in transgendered men and women who wish to breastfeed or chestfeed by using combined hormonal treatment, including a dopamine antagonist (which induces PRL) or recombinant PRL, together with estradiol and progesterone. This will be discussed in more detail in Chapter 28.

1.3.2   Breastfeeding and Amenorrhea

During exclusive breastfeeding, approximately 40% of women will remain amenorrheic up to 6 months postpartum,[67] and the risk of becoming pregnant during the first 6 months following birth is less than 3%.[68] Lactation suppresses both kisspeptin activity and GnRH secretion that lead to oligoovulation or anovulation through different mechanisms. Physiological studies in animal models provided molecular insights into this process. In rats, lactation reduces the expression of kisspeptin in ARC and the projection of $Kiss1$ fibers to the median eminence, which may contribute to decreased GnRH release and reproductive dysfunction.[69, 70] Further, direct neural signals from the breast to the AVPV and ARC of hypothalamus also reduce kisspeptin activity.[71] In mice, chronic prolactin administration reduces $Kiss1$

expression in both rostral periventricular regions of the third ventricle (RP3V) and ARC via phosphorylation of STAT5. During lactation, the suppression of *Kiss1* messenger ribonucleic acid (mRNA) in the RP3V can be partially reversed by bromocriptine treatment, which lowers the prolactin levels. These data suggest that prolactin contributes to the GnRH deficit during lactational amenorrhea by suppressing kisspeptin activity.[72]

It is important to note that the degree of GnRH deficiency during lactation is modulated by the intensity of the breast-feeding, the nutritional status, and the body mass index (BMI) of the mother.[73–75] As lactation represents a metabolic energy burden, this correlation highlights the tight crosstalk between metabolism and central reproductive control.

REFERENCES

1. Wildt L, Hausler A, Marshall G, Hutchison JS, Plant TM, Belchetz PE, et al. Frequency and amplitude of gonadotropin-releasing hormone stimulation and gonadotropin secretion in the rhesus monkey. *Endocrinology* 1981;**109**(2):376–85.
2. Clarke IJ, Cummins JT. The temporal relationship between gonadotropin releasing hormone (GnRH) and luteinizing hormone (LH) secretion in ovariectomized ewes. *Endocrinology* 1982;**111**(5):1737–9.
3. Seminara SB, Hayes FJ, Crowley Jr WF. Gonadotropin-releasing hormone deficiency in the human (idiopathic hypogonadotropic hypogonadism and Kallmann's syndrome): pathophysiological and genetic considerations. *Endocr Rev* 1998;**19**(5):521–39.
4. Adams JM, Taylor AE, Schoenfeld DA, Crowley Jr WF, Hall JE. The midcycle gonadotropin surge in normal women occurs in the face of an unchanging gonadotropin-releasing hormone pulse frequency. *J Clin Endocrinol Metab* 1994;**79**(3):858–64.
5. Reame N, Sauder SE, Kelch RP, Marshall JC. Pulsatile gonadotropin secretion during the human menstrual cycle: evidence for altered frequency of gonadotropin-releasing hormone secretion. *J Clin Endocrinol Metab* 1984;**59**(2):328–37.
6. Martin K, Santoro N, Hall J, Filicori M, Wierman M, Crowley Jr WF. Clinical review 15: management of ovulatory disorders with pulsatile gonadotropin-releasing hormone. *J Clin Endocrinol Metab* 1990;**71**(5):1081a–g.
7. Sisk CL, Foster DL. The neural basis of puberty and adolescence. *Nat Neurosci* 2004;**7**(10):1040–7.
8. Gordon CM. Clinical practice. Functional hypothalamic amenorrhea. *N Engl J Med* 2010;**363**(4):365–71.
9. Pinilla L, Aguilar E, Dieguez C, Millar RP, Tena-Sempere M. Kisspeptins and reproduction: physiological roles and regulatory mechanisms. *Physiol Rev* 2012;**92**(3):1235–316.
10. Clarke SA, Dhillo WS. Kisspeptin across the human lifespan: evidence from animal studies and beyond. *J Endocrinol* 2016;**229**(3):R83–98.
11. Seminara SB, Messager S, Chatzidaki EE, Thresher RR, Acierno Jr JS, Shagoury JK, et al. The GPR54 gene as a regulator of puberty. *N Engl J Med* 2003;**349**(17):1614–27.
12. de Roux N, Genin E, Carel JC, Matsuda F, Chaussain JL, Milgrom E. Hypogonadotropic hypogonadism due to loss of function of the KiSS1-derived peptide receptor GPR54. *Proc Natl Acad Sci U S A* 2003;**100**(19):10972–6.
13. Jayasena CN, Nijher GM, Comninos AN, Abbara A, Januszewski A, Vaal ML, et al. The effects of kisspeptin-10 on reproductive hormone release show sexual dimorphism in humans. *J Clin Endocrinol Metab* 2011;**96**(12):E1963–72.
14. Dhillo WS, Chaudhri OB, Patterson M, Thompson EL, Murphy KG, Badman MK, et al. Kisspeptin-54 stimulates the hypothalamic-pituitary gonadal axis in human males. *J Clin Endocrinol Metab* 2005;**90**(12):6609–15.
15. Dhillo WS, Chaudhri OB, Thompson EL, Murphy KG, Patterson M, Ramachandran R, et al. Kisspeptin-54 stimulates gonadotropin release most potently during the preovulatory phase of the menstrual cycle in women. *J Clin Endocrinol Metab* 2007;**92**(10):3958–66.
16. Jayasena CN, Nijher GM, Chaudhri OB, Murphy KG, Ranger A, Lim A, et al. Subcutaneous injection of kisspeptin-54 acutely stimulates gonadotropin secretion in women with hypothalamic amenorrhea, but chronic administration causes tachyphylaxis. *J Clin Endocrinol Metab* 2009;**94**(11):4315–23.
17. Jayasena CN, Nijher GM, Abbara A, Murphy KG, Lim A, Patel D, et al. Twice-weekly administration of kisspeptin-54 for 8 weeks stimulates release of reproductive hormones in women with hypothalamic amenorrhea. *Clin Pharmacol Ther* 2010;**88**(6):840–7.
18. Abbara A, Clarke S, Islam R, Prague JK, Comninos AN, Narayanaswamy S, et al. A second dose of kisspeptin-54 improves oocyte maturation in women at high risk of ovarian hyperstimulation syndrome: a phase 2 randomized controlled trial. *Hum Reprod* 2017;**32**(9):1915–24.
19. Abbara A, Jayasena CN, Christopoulos G, Narayanaswamy S, Izzi-Engbeaya C, Nijher GM, et al. Efficacy of Kisspeptin-54 to trigger oocyte maturation in women at high risk of ovarian hyperstimulation syndrome (OHSS) during in vitro fertilization (IVF) therapy. *J Clin Endocrinol Metab* 2015;**100**(9):3322–31.
20. Clarkson J, Han SY, Piet R, McLennan T, Kane GM, Ng J, et al. Definition of the hypothalamic GnRH pulse generator in mice. *Proc Natl Acad Sci U S A* 2017;**114**(47):E10216–23.
21. Garcia-Galiano D, Pinilla L, Tena-Sempere M. Sex steroids and the control of the Kiss1 system: developmental roles and major regulatory actions. *J Neuroendocrinol* 2012;**24**(1):22–33.
22. Newbern D, Freemark M. Placental hormones and the control of maternal metabolism and fetal growth. *Curr Opin Endocrinol Diabetes Obes* 2011;**18**(6):409–16.
23. Costa MA. The endocrine function of human placenta: an overview. *Reprod BioMed Online* 2016;**32**(1):14–43.
24. Petraglia F, Florio P, Nappi C, Genazzani AR. Peptide signaling in human placenta and membranes: autocrine, paracrine, and endocrine mechanisms. *Endocr Rev* 1996;**17**(2):156–86.
25. Khodr GS, Siler-Khodr TM. Placental luteinizing hormone-releasing factor and its synthesis. *Science* 1980;**207**(4428):315–7.
26. Siler-Khodr TM, Khodr GS, Valenzuela G. Immunoreactive gonadotropin-releasing hormone level in maternal circulation throughout pregnancy. *Am J Obstet Gynecol* 1984;**150**(4):376–9.

27. Barnea ER, Kaplan M, Naor Z. Comparative stimulatory effect of gonadotrophin releasing hormone (GnRH) and GnRH agonist upon pulsatile human chorionic gonadotrophin secretion in superfused placental explants: reversible inhibition by a GnRH antagonist. *Hum Reprod* 1991;**6**(8):1063–9.
28. Currie WD, Steele GL, Yuen BH, Kordon C, Gautron JP, Leung PC. Luteinizing hormone-releasing hormone (LHRH)- and (hydroxyproline9)LHRH-stimulated human chorionic gonadotropin secretion from perifused first trimester placental cells. *Endocrinology* 1992;**130**(5):2871–6.
29. Sasaki K, Norwitz ER. Gonadotropin-releasing hormone/gonadotropin-releasing hormone receptor signaling in the placenta. *Curr Opin Endocrinol Diabetes Obes* 2011;**18**(6):401–8.
30. Kotani M, Detheux M, Vandenbogaerde A, Communi D, Vanderwinden JM, Le Poul E, et al. The metastasis suppressor gene KiSS-1 encodes kisspeptins, the natural ligands of the orphan G protein-coupled receptor GPR54. *J Biol Chem* 2001;**276**(37):34631–6.
31. Horikoshi Y, Matsumoto H, Takatsu Y, Ohtaki T, Kitada C, Usuki S, et al. Dramatic elevation of plasma metastin concentrations in human pregnancy: metastin as a novel placenta-derived hormone in humans. *J Clin Endocrinol Metab* 2003;**88**(2):914–9.
32. Calder M, Chan YM, Raj R, Pampillo M, Elbert A, Noonan M, et al. Implantation failure in female Kiss1 −/− mice is independent of their hypogonadic state and can be partially rescued by leukemia inhibitory factor. *Endocrinology* 2014;**155**(8):3065–78.
33. Zhang P, Tang M, Zhong T, Lin Y, Zong T, Zhong C, et al. Expression and function of kisspeptin during mouse decidualization. *PLoS ONE* 2014;**9**(5).
34. Bilban M, Ghaffari-Tabrizi N, Hintermann E, Bauer S, Molzer S, Zoratti C, et al. Kisspeptin-10, a KiSS-1/metastin-derived decapeptide, is a physiological invasion inhibitor of primary human trophoblasts. *J Cell Sci* 2004;**117**(Pt 8):1319–28.
35. Smets EM, Deurloo KL, Go AT, van Vugt JM, Blankenstein MA, Oudejans CB. Decreased plasma levels of metastin in early pregnancy are associated with small for gestational age neonates. *Prenat Diagn* 2008;**28**(4):299–303.
36. Armstrong RA, Reynolds RM, Leask R, Shearing CH, Calder AA, Riley SC. Decreased serum levels of kisspeptin in early pregnancy are associated with intra-uterine growth restriction and pre-eclampsia. *Prenat Diagn* 2009;**29**(10):982–5.
37. Cetkovic A, Miljic D, Ljubic A, Patterson M, Ghatei M, Stamenkovic J, et al. Plasma kisspeptin levels in pregnancies with diabetes and hypertensive disease as a potential marker of placental dysfunction and adverse perinatal outcome. *Endocr Res* 2012;**37**(2):78–88.
38. Jayasena CN, Abbara A, Izzi-Engbeaya C, Comninos AN, Harvey RA, Gonzalez Maffe J, et al. Reduced levels of plasma kisspeptin during the antenatal booking visit are associated with increased risk of miscarriage. *J Clin Endocrinol Metab* 2014;**99**(12):E2652–60.
39. Alsat E, Guibourdenche J, Couturier A, Evain-Brion D. Physiological role of human placental growth hormone. *Mol Cell Endocrinol* 1998;**140**(1–2):121–7.
40. de Zegher F, Vanderschueren-Lodeweyckx M, Spitz B, Faijerson Y, Blomberg F, Beckers A, et al. Perinatal growth hormone (GH) physiology: effect of GH-releasing factor on maternal and fetal secretion of pituitary and placental GH. *J Clin Endocrinol Metab* 1990;**71**(2):520–2.
41. McIntyre HD, Serek R, Crane DI, Veveris-Lowe T, Parry A, Johnson S, et al. Placental growth hormone (GH), GH-binding protein, and insulin-like growth factor axis in normal, growth-retarded, and diabetic pregnancies: correlations with fetal growth. *J Clin Endocrinol Metab* 2000;**85**(3):1143–50.
42. Lindheimer MD, Davison JM. Osmoregulation, the secretion of arginine vasopressin and its metabolism during pregnancy. *Eur J Endocrinol* 1995;**132**(2):133–43.
43. Gimpl G, Fahrenholz F. The oxytocin receptor system: structure, function, and regulation. *Physiol Rev* 2001;**81**(2):629–83.
44. Fuchs AR, Romero R, Keefe D, Parra M, Oyarzun E, Behnke E. Oxytocin secretion and human parturition: pulse frequency and duration increase during spontaneous labor in women. *Am J Obstet Gynecol* 1991;**165**(5 Pt 1):1515–23.
45. Chibbar R, Miller FD, Mitchell BF. Synthesis of oxytocin in amnion, chorion, and decidua may influence the timing of human parturition. *J Clin Invest* 1993;**91**(1):185–92.
46. Fuchs AR, Fuchs F, Husslein P, Soloff MS. Oxytocin receptors in the human uterus during pregnancy and parturition. *Am J Obstet Gynecol* 1984;**150**(6):734–41.
47. Casey ML, MacDonald PC. Biomolecular processes in the initiation of parturition: decidual activation. *Clin Obstet Gynecol* 1988;**31**(3):533–52.
48. Nishimori K, Young LJ, Guo Q, Wang Z, Insel TR, Matzuk MM. Oxytocin is required for nursing but is not essential for parturition or reproductive behavior. *Proc Natl Acad Sci U S A* 1996;**93**(21):11699–704.
49. Young 3rd WS, Shepard E, Amico J, Hennighausen L, Wagner KU, LaMarca ME, et al. Deficiency in mouse oxytocin prevents milk ejection, but not fertility or parturition. *J Neuroendocrinol* 1996;**8**(11):847–53.
50. Takayanagi Y, Yoshida M, Bielsky IF, Ross HE, Kawamata M, Onaka T, et al. Pervasive social deficits, but normal parturition, in oxytocin receptor-deficient mice. *Proc Natl Acad Sci U S A* 2005;**102**(44):16096–101.
51. Brunton PJ, Russell JA, Douglas AJ. Adaptive responses of the maternal hypothalamic-pituitary-adrenal axis during pregnancy and lactation. *J Neuroendocrinol* 2008;**20**(6):764–76.
52. Gebert D, Auer MK, Stieg MR, Freitag MT, Lahne M, Fuss J, et al. De-masking oxytocin-deficiency in craniopharyngioma and assessing its link with affective function. *Psychoneuroendocrinology* 2018;**88**:61–9.
53. Daughters K, Manstead ASR, Rees DA. Hypopituitarism is associated with lower oxytocin concentrations and reduced empathic ability. *Endocrine* 2017;**57**(1):166–74.
54. Shinar S, Many A, Maslovitz S. Questioning the role of pituitary oxytocin in parturition: spontaneous onset of labor in women with panhypopituitarism—a case series. *Eur J Obstet Gynecol Reprod Biol* 2016;**197**:83–5.
55. Volz J, Heinrich U, Volz-Koster S. Conception and spontaneous delivery after total hypophysectomy. *Fertil Steril* 2002;**77**(3):624–5.
56. Neville MC, Casey C, Hay Jr WW. Endocrine regulation of nutrient flux in the lactating woman. Do the mechanisms differ from pregnancy? *Adv Exp Med Biol* 1994;**352**:85–98.
57. Bergquist F, Ludwig M. Dendritic transmitter release: a comparison of two model systems. *J Neuroendocrinol* 2008;**20**(6):677–86.
58. Lipschitz DL, Crowley WR, Armstrong WE, Bealer SL. Neurochemical bases of plasticity in the magnocellular oxytocin system during gestation. *Exp Neurol* 2005;**196**(2):210–23.

59. Bealer SL, Armstrong WE, Crowley WR. Oxytocin release in magnocellular nuclei: neurochemical mediators and functional significance during gestation. *Am J Phys Regul Integr Comp Phys* 2010;**299**(2):R452–8.

60. Tyson JE, Friesen HG. Factors influencing the secretion of human prolactin and growth hormone in menstrual and gestational women. *Am J Obstet Gynecol* 1973;**116**(3):377–87.

61. Noel GL, Suh HK, Frantz AG. Prolactin release during nursing and breast stimulation in postpartum and nonpostpartum subjects. *J Clin Endocrinol Metab* 1974;**38**(3):413–23.

62. Horseman ND, Zhao W, Montecino-Rodriguez E, Tanaka M, Nakashima K, Engle SJ, et al. Defective mammopoiesis, but normal hematopoiesis, in mice with a targeted disruption of the prolactin gene. *EMBO J* 1997;**16**(23):6926–35.

63. Falk RJ. Isolated prolactin deficiency: a case report. *Fertil Steril* 1992;**58**(5):1060–2.

64. Kauppila A, Chatelain P, Kirkinen P, Kivinen S, Ruokonen A. Isolated prolactin deficiency in a woman with puerperal alactogenesis. *J Clin Endocrinol Metab* 1987;**64**(2):309–12.

65. Iwama S, Welt CK, Romero CJ, Radovick S, Caturegli P. Isolated prolactin deficiency associated with serum autoantibodies against prolactin-secreting cells. *J Clin Endocrinol Metab* 2013;**98**(10):3920–5.

66. Voutetakis A, Sertedaki A, Livadas S, Maniati-Christidi M, Mademtzis I, Bossis I, et al. Ovulation induction and successful pregnancy outcome in two patients with Prop1 gene mutations. *Fertil Steril* 2004;**82**(2):454–7.

67. Campbell OM, Gray RH. Characteristics and determinants of postpartum ovarian function in women in the United States. *Am J Obstet Gynecol* 1993;**169**(1):55–60.

68. Kennedy KI, Visness CM. Contraceptive efficacy of lactational amenorrhoea. *Lancet* 1992;**339**(8787):227–30.

69. True C, Kirigiti M, Ciofi P, Grove KL, Smith MS. Characterisation of arcuate nucleus kisspeptin/neurokinin B neuronal projections and regulation during lactation in the rat. *J Neuroendocrinol* 2011;**23**(1):52–64.

70. Yamada S, Uenoyama Y, Deura C, Minabe S, Naniwa Y, Iwata K, et al. Oestrogen-dependent suppression of pulsatile luteinising hormone secretion and kiss1 mRNA expression in the arcuate nucleus during late lactation in rats. *J Neuroendocrinol* 2012;**24**(9):1234–42.

71. Higo S, Aikawa S, Iijima N, Ozawa H. Rapid modulation of hypothalamic Kiss1 levels by the suckling stimulus in the lactating rat. *J Endocrinol* 2015;**227**(2):105–15.

72. Brown RS, Herbison AE, Grattan DR. Prolactin regulation of kisspeptin neurones in the mouse brain and its role in the lactation-induced suppression of kisspeptin expression. *J Neuroendocrinol* 2014;**26**(12):898–908.

73. The World Health Organization Multinational Study of Breast-feeding and Lactational Amenorrhea. I. Description of infant feeding patterns and of the return of menses. World Health Organization Task Force on Methods for the Natural Regulation of Fertility. *Fertil Steril* 1998;**70**(3):448–60.

74. Rahman M, Mascie-Taylor CG, Rosetta L. The duration of lactational amenorrhoea in urban Bangladeshi women. *J Biosoc Sci* 2002;**34**(1):75–89.

75. Wasalathanthri S, Tennekoon KH. Lactational amenorrhea/anovulation and some of their determinants: a comparison of well-nourished and under-nourished women. *Fertil Steril* 2001;**76**(2):317–25.

Chapter 2

The Pineal Gland and its Function in Pregnancy and Lactation

Ana-Maria Zagrean*, Diana Maria Chitimus*, Corin Badiu[†,‡], Anca Maria Panaitescu[§], Gheorghe Peltecu[§] and Leon Zagrean*

*Division of Physiology and Neuroscience, Department of Functional Sciences, "Carol Davila" University of Medicine and Pharmacy, Bucharest, Romania, [†]National Institute of Endocrinology "C. I. Parhon", Bucharest, Romania, [‡]Department of Endocrinology, "Carol Davila" University of Medicine and Pharmacy, Bucharest, Romania, [§]Department of Obstetrics and Gynecology, "Carol Davila" University of Medicine and Pharmacy, Filantropia Clinical Hospital, Bucharest, Romania

---

Key Clinical Changes

- The circadian rhythm in serum melatonin concentrations is maintained in pregnancy and lactation.
- The nocturnal serum concentration of melatonin increases gradually during pregnancy and returns to pregestational values postpartum.
- Melatonin crosses the placenta unaltered or is excreted in the breast milk, thus signaling photoperiodicity in the fetus or the breastfed infant, respectively.
- The pineal gland undergoes morphological, structural, and biochemical changes in pregnancy.
- Placenta is an important source for extrapineal melatonin.
- Melatonin's free-radical scavenging and antioxidant/antinitridergic capacities play an important role in the female reproductive function (Table 2.1).

2.1 INTRODUCTION

The pineal gland or pineal body, also referred to as the *epiphysis cerebri*, is a neuroendocrine gland mainly known for its nocturnal melatonin production and release and for its roles as a circadian oscillator and important regulator of physiological functions.

First described in humans by Galen of Pergamon (A.D.), its central position in the brain inspired René Descartes to consider it the "seat of the soul" about 1500 years later.

Melatonin (*N*-acetyl-5-methoxytryptamine) is the molecule connecting two phenomena: terrestrial life and sunlight. The evolution of melatonin synthesis and function from unicellular organisms to the appearance of the pineal gland, as well as its connection to the nervous system, are driven by the need to develop a hormonal connection between each organism and environmental lighting.[7]

Although melatonin was generated near the beginning of life, scientists noticed its physiological implications barely a century ago[8] and identified it only in the mid-20th century.[9] After isolation from bovine pineal extract, Lerner proposed the term *melatonin* for the active pineal factor that prevents darkening of frog skin by a melanocyte-stimulating hormone.[9] Following this finding, many studies have demonstrated the presence of melatonin in organisms living in different environments and with different levels of organization, from unicellular[10] to plants,[11] insects,[12] and mammals, particularly humans.

Pineal melatonin, also named a "timekeeper endocrine messenger,"[13] is a hormone carrying a photoperiodic signal triggered by the endogenous clock, the suprachiasmatic nucleus (SCN). Melatonin is intimately involved in physiology, modulating circadian rhythms and regulating sleep/wake cycles and seasonal rhythmicity in mammalian species. It plays important roles in regulating and timing neuroendocrine, reproductive, cardiovascular, immune and nervous system

Maternal-Fetal and Neonatal Endocrinology. https://doi.org/10.1016/B978-0-12-814823-5.00002-7

15

TABLE 2.1 Table of normal ranges for melatonin and its metabolites in humans

Parameter	Period	Age (years)	Serum (pg/mL)	CSF (pg/mL)	FF (pg/mL)
N-Acetylserotonin[a]	Morning	18–70	6.8	n.a.	n.a.
Melatonin	Nighttime[b]	3–10	100–216	28.6±7.0[c]	n.a
		10–20	54.3–86.1		
		20–50[d]	52.3–149.5		
		>50	15.3–27.8		
	Daytime	n.a.	2–20[e] (10.0±1.4)[f]	8.69±2.75[g]	36.5±4.8[f]

Parameter	Period	Age (years)	Urine (ng/h)
6-Sulfatoxymelatonin[h]	Nighttime	20–35	1017–6074
		35–50	598–3612
		51–65	861–2421
	Daytime	20–35	182–1130
		35–50	202–1140
		51–65	139–725

[a]Blood concentration measured in healthy subjects by liquid chromatography-mass spectrometry (LC-MS/MS).[1]
[b]Blood concentration measured in healthy subjects by radioimmunoassay (RIA).[2]
[c]Nighttime samples collected from the lumbar cistern; free and bound melatonin assayed by high-performance liquid chromatography (HPLC).[3]
[d]Consistent data with more recent studies where peak endogenous melatonin levels did not exceed 200pg/mL over 20years of age. No significant correlation between age and peak endogenous melatonin levels within either age group was reported.[4]
[e]See Ref. 5.
[f]Comparative measurements in blood versus follicular fluid (FF) in healthy women, by RIA.[5]
[g]Daytime samples collected from the cerebrospinal fluid (CSF) from the third cerebral ventricle; free melatonin measured by RIA.[3]
[h]Urine concentration measured in healthy subjects by enzyme-linked immunosorbent assay (ELISA).[6]
(Data collected from multiple studies.)

functions. Moreover, melatonin is a free-radical scavenger with potent antioxidant activity, intervening to balance the oxidative challenge that accompanies physiological and pathological circumstances.

Much of the data regarding the pineal gland have arisen from animal studies, and so some caution is warranted in correlating these data with normal human physiology. Also, melatonin has been shown to be produced in small amounts in extrapineal sites such as the skin, gastrointestinal tract, retina, bone marrow cells, placenta, and ovaries[14–18] and also in virtually every nucleated cell from various tissues and organs, wherein it functions in paracrine or autocrine ways to influence homeostatic balance.[19]

Considering that melatonin is involved in the regulation of whole-body physiology and affects reproductive function, appetite, body weight, and behavior, the function of the pineal gland during gestation and lactation should be of high interest and relevant to both maternal and fetal physiology. This is supported by an association between low plasma levels of melatonin and the incidence of preeclampsia and fetal growth restriction, as well as by evidence of an increased success rate of in vitro fertilization when melatonin has also been used.[20]

2.2 ANATOMY OF THE PINEAL GLAND

The pineal gland is an unpaired neuroendocrine organ located in the midline of the brain, in a groove flanked by the thalamic bodies. It is connected to the roof of the third ventricle by a small pineal stalk consisting of two lamina, rostral and caudal. In humans, the pineal is part of the epithalamus, a component of the diencephalon, together with the medial and the lateral habenulas (Figs. 2.1 and 2.2). The pineal is covered by a pial capsule and hangs in the cerebrospinal fluid (CSF) of the pineal recess, having direct contact with the third ventricle. Superiorly, it relates to the internal cerebral veins and the great cerebral vein of Galen, being located right above the superior colliculi of the midbrain.[7] In rodents, the pineal gland is located superficially, between the cerebral cortex and the cerebellum, connected by the pineal stalk to its more profound component situated in the epithalamic region. The pineal gland in the human adult weighs between 0.1 and 0.2 g and

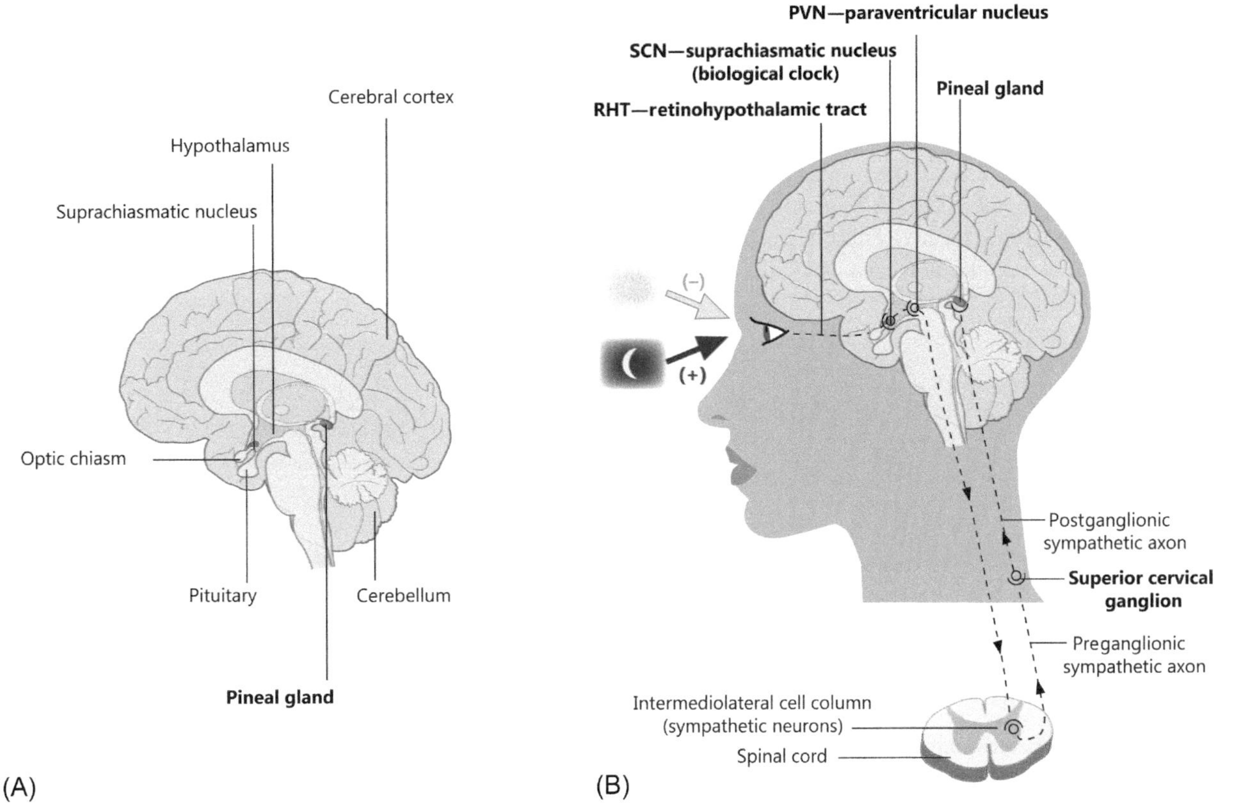

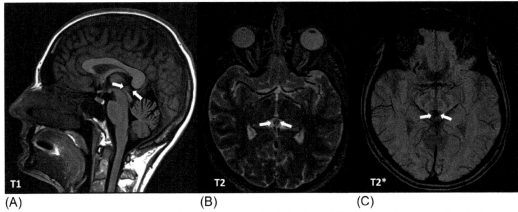

FIG. 2.1 Pineal gland: anatomical relationships and functional connections. (A) The anatomical relationships; (B) the neural pathways that interconnect: the retina, the retinohypothalamic tract (RHT), the central biological clock in the suprachiasmatic nucleus (SCN), the paraventricular nucleus (PVN), the superior cervical ganglion (SCG), and the pineal gland.

FIG. 2.2 3T MRI sequences at the level of the pineal gland *(arrows)* in sagittal T1 (A), axial T2 (B), and axial T2* (C), showing hypointense T2* signal consistent with calcification of the pineal gland in an asymptomatic 40-year-old woman. *(From the personal collection of Dr. A.M. Zagrean.)*

measures about 5–12 mm × 2–4 mm × 3–5 mm in size, sometimes displaying a round-shaped or pine-cone appearance, which gave the name *pineal* to this gland.

Aging is frequently related to the accumulation of calcareous deposits (*acervuli*) within the pineal, giving it an authentic radiographic feature; they usually appear as layered concretions of salts in the intracellular and intercellular compartments.[21] Thus, the pineal gland becomes visible on a simple skull X-ray, computed tomography (CT) or magnetic resonance imaging (MRI) scan (Fig. 2.2), providing an imaging marker for the midsagittal plane. Early pineal gland calcification occurs in 40% of patients between 17 and 29 years of age.[22]

The impact, if any, of these calcifications on pineal function is not well understood, but they do not significantly interfere with melatonin synthesis. Brain tumors or swelling can shift the pineal off the midline, serving as a diagnostic marker in radiologic imaging.

The pineal develops from the second month of gestation, as an ependymal envagination from the posterior part of the roof of the third cerebral ventricle, superior to the tegmental plate, as discussed in detail in Chapter 31.

Together with the subcommisural organ, the area postrema, the subfornical organ, the vascular organ of lamina terminalis, the median eminence, and the pituitary gland, the pineal gland belongs to the circumventricular organs, which are devoid of the blood-brain barrier. This characteristic allows these tissues to easily sense signals from the periphery and respond to feedback regulation mechanisms by releasing bioactive molecules toward the periphery, thereby contributing to homeostasis.

2.2.1 Vascularization

The pineal vasculature is very rich, with numerous capillaries distributed in the pineal parenchyma, which supply the necessary blood for the demanding metabolic activity of hormonal synthesis. This feature is illustrated by a nocturnal increase in pineal blood flow, when melatonin is secreted and released.[23]

The pineal blood supply is provided by branches deriving from the posteromedial choroidal artery from the posterior cerebral artery. The three identified pineal arteries vascularize different regions of the gland and are reported in the research literature as lateral, rostral, and middle pineal arteries.[24] The venous blood is drained into the internal cerebral veins and Rosenthal basal veins, ultimately reaching the great cerebral vein of Galen.

2.2.2 Innervation

The pineal gland receives mainly sympathetic innervation via the conarian nerves, which contain norepinephrine (NE)-secreting fibers originating in the superior cervical ganglions (SCGs) and carrying inputs from the circadian pacemaker in the hypothalamus, the suprachiasmatic nuclei (SCN). SCNs receive inputs via the retinohypothalamic tract (RHT) from ganglion cells in the retina, responding to the environmental lighting. The pineal also receives parasympathetic fibers from the otic and pterygopalatine ganglia.

In spite of its intimate rapport with the midbrain, the pineal receives through the pineal stalk a central innervation consisting of a few afferent fibers from other brain areas, such as the hypothalamus, visual structures, or limbic forebrain.[25, 26] In mammals, these fibers distribute unevenly in the pineal gland and, depending on their central origin, contain a variety of neuropeptides, such as vasopressin, oxytocin, substance P, somatostatin, vasoactive intestinal peptide (VIP), histidine isoleucine peptide,[26, 27] neuropeptide Y (NPY),[28] and neurotransmitters, such as gamma-aminobutyric acid (GABA) or glutamate. In humans, nerve fibers containing enkephalins originate in neuronal-like cells that exist throughout the pineal.[28]

Most of the nerve fibers reaching the pineal terminate in the perivascular spaces, near pinealocytes, and rarely make synapticlike contacts with the pineal cells. The pineal receptors include α1- and β-adrenergic receptors, but also GABA-ergic, glutamatergic, 2-dopaminergic, cholinergic, and possibly serotoninergic receptors, as well as receptors for peptides and steroids. β-Adrenergic receptors are crucial to determining the circadian regulation of melatonin synthesis. Their expression, transcription, and translation exhibit a circadian rhythm.[29]

2.2.3 Cellular Composition

The predominant cell type is the pinealocyte (95% of the pineal cells), a raspberrylike cell, which is a modified neuron with neuroendocrine properties that is responsible for secreting melatonin. Melatonin secretion occurs at a 24-h rhythm driven by the endogenous clock located in the SCN, and is accompanied by increased circulating levels of melatonin during night. Compared with the pinealocytes in submammals, which have photoreceptor properties analogous with those in retinal photoreceptors and thus act as endogenous biological clocks,[30] pinealocytes in mammals do not display direct photosensitivity. Instead, their response to light is through a neural pathway connecting the retina, as described later in this chapter.

The pinealocytes are mainly concentrated in the pineal core and relatively dispersed throughout the pineal cortex. Histologically, the pinealocyte is identified by staining enzymes involved in melatonin production, but also by staining other molecules, like S-antigen, which is highly expressed both in the retina and the pineal gland.[31]

Regarding its ultrastructure, the pinealocyte has numerous cytoplasmic processes, a rich Golgi apparatus with associated secretory vesicles, and a granular endoplasmic reticulum with vacuoles of flocculated material. It is assumed that the clear vesicles are the expression of neurosecretions, while the vacuoles containing flocculated material form directly from the endoplasmic reticulum and correspond to an ependymal type of secretion. Indolamines and various neuropeptides, such as arginine-vasotocin and angiotensin II, were identified by immunocytochemistry in pinealocytes.

Glial cells are also present with the pineal, among which are glial fibrillary acidic protein (GFAP)-positive interstitial cells, perivascular phagocytes, and microglia with possible antigen-presenting activity.[26]

Phylogenetically, pinealocytes are related to photoreceptor cells, which explains why the pineal was initially called "the third eye." However, in humans, these photoreceptor functions have been lost. The remnant photoperiod control is through the connection from the SCN via the RHT.

The main control of melatonin synthesis is through the sympathetic innervation discussed previously, and is mediated by the two mentioned neurotransmitters NE and NPY. Melatonin synthesis is controlled on a genetic basis according to a circadian rhythm entrained by a light/dark cycle clock,[32] as described next.

2.3 ROLE OF THE PINEAL GLAND IN HUMAN PHYSIOLOGY

The pineal gland in mammals and humans acts mainly as a neuroendocrine modulator of circadian-related functions, including the sleep-wake cycle, body temperature variations, and feeding behavior. The rhythmical daily transcriptional-translational feedback mechanism driven by environmental light is signaled through retinal input and conveyed to the biological clock (SCN) as described previously. In humans, this pattern entrains a cyclical variation of other physiological parameters, such as plasma cortisol, heart rate, and erythropoiesis.

The pineal gland secretes mainly melatonin, an indolic hormone. In smaller amounts, it also secretes peptide hormones such as arginine-vasotocin, angiotensin, and renin. The isolation and characterization of these hormones have revealed a new understanding of the pineal gland's endocrine physiology and pathophysiology.[27, 33]

In mammals with seasonal reproduction, the pineal gland plays an important role in the adaptation of the reproductive function to environmental conditions. In humans, the pineal melatonin influences reproduction by regulating seasonal changes in gonadal activity, shown by circadian variation in ovulation, commonly in the morning during summer, and in the evening during winter. The circadian biorhythms and environmental conditions also modulate cerebral excitability, with an impact on human behavior through changes in pineal melatonin, an effect demonstrated by the reversal of menopause-related depression after melatonin administration.[34]

Melatonin and pineal peptides generate systemic effects on cardiovascular, immunological, and bone physiology.[21, 35] However, as mentioned earlier, most data regarding pineal function come from animal studies, and it is not clear yet which of these pieces of information can be generalized to humans.

Melatonin plays roles in learning and memory and exerts protective effects on the fetal hippocampus. In experimental conditions, with lead and ethanol coexposure in pregnant rats, melatonin significantly reversed the learning and memory deficit in rat pups.[36] Melatonin similarly protected against adverse effects of diclofenac on the newborn rat brain, specifically in the dentate gyrus of the hippocampus.

Cardiovascular function in humans displays circadian variations that might reflect actions of melatonin. During nighttime, there are increased melatonin levels accompanied by a significantly lower heart rate, blood pressure, and cardiac output, as well as increased peripheral vascular resistance.[37] Myocardial infraction and stroke have an increased incidence early in the morning, when melatonin levels are low.[21, 38] Interestingly, in coronary heart disease patients, nocturnal melatonin levels were lower and NE levels were higher, as compared to healthy controls.[21] A potential mechanism for these associations is that melatonin is a free-radical scavenger and promotes cellular antioxidant activity and may exert a protective effect in cardiovascular patients. It may also have a protective effect in pregnant women exposed to hemodynamic changes, especially during the third trimester.

Melatonin's role in the immune system is well documented, and it has been especially studied in immunodeficiency conditions. Melatonin has a direct effect on immune cells (e.g., increasing leukocyte production and regulating T- and B-cell apoptosis), thus contributing to the initiation of the immune response. Melatonin also lowers the transcription of proinflammatory cytokines, reduces prostaglandin synthesis (e.g., PGE-2), and diminishes leukocyte adhesion on the endothelial vascular layer and their migration, thus inhibiting acute inflammatory reactions.[39]

Melatonin is also involved in bone homeostasis by stimulating osteoblast proliferation, differentiation, and bone formation, while inhibiting bone resorption.[35] It has been shown in vitro to stimulate the synthesis of type I collagen, the main organic component of extracellular bone matrix, as well as the expression of sialoprotein, osteocalcin, and alkaline phosphatase.[40] Melatonin was found in the bone marrow, where it also could function as an autacoid. Moreover, melatonin's bone-protecting effect is exerted by its free-radical scavenger and antioxidant properties, which may alter osteoclast activity and bone resorption. Studies in mice and humans have shown that melatonin could act as a regulator of bone mass through melatonin type 2 (MT2) receptors.[41, 42]

Melatonin exerts effects on female reproductive function by acting on the pituitary, hypothalamus, ovaries, and placenta. The effect of melatonin on ovarian function is supported by the finding of high levels of melatonin in follicular fluid (FF) by the expression of melatonin receptors in granulosa cells, as well as by demonstrated modulation of ovarian steroidogenesis, especially progesterone.[43] The contribution of melatonin to normal follicular function and oocyte development is also suggested through its free radical scavenger and antioxidant features.[44]

The extensive functions of pineal melatonin are summarized in Fig. 2.3.

FIG. 2.3 The spectrum of melatonin roles in human physiology.

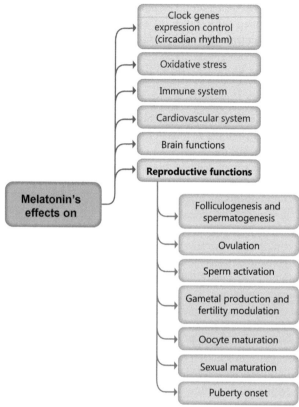

2.3.1 Melatonin

2.3.1.1 Melatonin Biosynthesis and Regulation

Pineal hormones were first known as pineal factors, and it was not until 1958 that one of them was isolated as the indoleamine melatonin (*N*-acetyl-5-methoxytryptamine) (Fig. 2.4).[9] Out of all the pineal products, melatonin has received the most attention, deriving its name from its ability to alter the color of frog skin and on its chemical relation to serotonin (5-HT, 5-hydroxytryptamine).[21] The elucidation of the chemical structure of melatonin allowed its synthesis, and subsequent studies clarified its physiological role and metabolism.

Despite many fanciful theories regarding the role of the pineal gland, it is now understood that its main function is to integrate information about the current state of the light/dark cycle from the environment, and to modulate release of melatonin into the blood in response.

2.3.1.1.1 Biosynthesis

The first major step in pineal indole biosynthesis is the conversion of tryptophan, which is taken up by pinealocytes from the circulation. There are four enzymatic steps in the process:

1. Conversion of the amino acid tryptophan to 5-hydroxytryptophan (5-HTP)
   Enzyme: tryptophan hydroxylase 1 (TPOH).
   Particularities: TPHO is the rate-limiting enzyme of serotonin production and exhibits increased activity during the night.

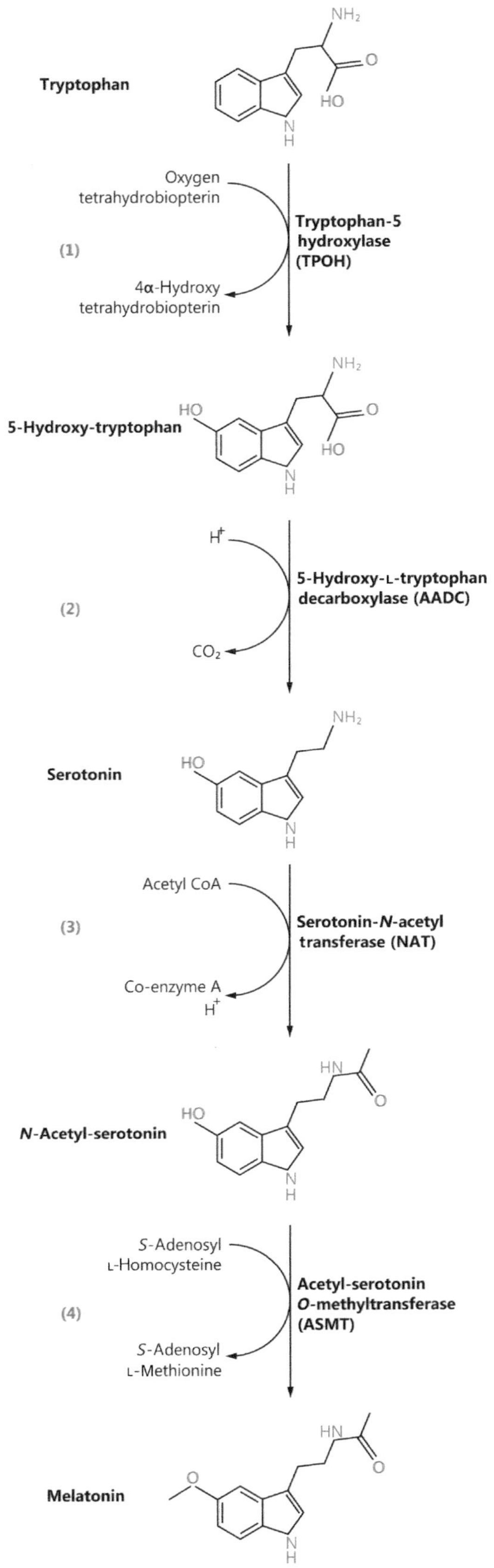

FIG. 2.4 Melatonin molecular structure and biosynthesis pathway.

Tryptophan

Oxygen
tetrahydrobiopterin

(1)

**Tryptophan-5
hydroxylase
(TPOH)**

4α-Hydroxy
tetrahydrobiopterin

5-Hydroxy-tryptophan

H^+

(2)

**5-Hydroxy-L-tryptophan
decarboxylase (AADC)**

CO_2

Serotonin

Acetyl CoA

(3)

**Serotonin-N-acetyl
transferase (NAT)**

Co-enzyme A
H^+

N-Acetyl-serotonin

S-Adenosyl
L-Homocysteine

(4)

**Acetyl-serotonin
O-methyltransferase
(ASMT)**

S-Adenosyl
L-Methionine

Melatonin

2. Synthesis of 5-hydroxytryptamine (5-HT or serotonin)

   Enzyme: aromatic amino acid decarboxylase 5-hydroxytryptamine (AADC).

   Particularities: AADC is a cytoplasmic enzyme with low substrate specificity, sensitive only to prolonged darkness.

3. Formation of *N*-acetylserotonin (NAS) following the transfer of an acetyl group from acetyl CoA

   Enzyme: arylalkylamine *N*-acetyltransferase (AANAT, or for short, NAT).

   Particularities: NAT is the rate-limiting enzyme in the formation of melatonin and is subjected to a complex mechanism of regulation, integrated by the SCN.

4. Melatonin is formed after the methylation of a hydroxyl group at carbon 5 from *S*-adenosyl methionine

   Enzyme: hydroxyindole-*O*-methyltransferase (HIOMT) (also termed *N-acetylserotonin methyltransferase,* or *ASMT*).[45]

   Particularities: HIOMT catalyzes the *O*-methylation of other hydroxyindole compounds (i.e., 5-hydroxytryptophan, 5-hydroxytryptamine, 6-hydroxy-tryptophol, and 5-hydroxyindole acetic acid). Some of the resulting compounds, 5-methoxy-tryptophan and 5-methoxitryptamine, have been identified in the blood, and *O*-acetyl-5-methoxy-tryptophan appears to be the primary compound released into circulation.

All four enzymatic derivatives of tryptophan follow a circadian pattern of release in the rat pineal gland, with higher levels at night. Unlike NAS and melatonin, which are barely detectable during the daytime,[46] both 5-HTP and serotonin display high levels during the day.[47]

2.3.1.1.2   The Release and Metabolism of Melatonin

Melatonin is not stored in the pineal gland in appreciable amounts. Shortly after synthesis, it is released from pinealocytes mainly into the peripheral circulation, but also into the CSF. Measurable amounts of melatonin in the blood and CSF reflect the production of pineal melatonin at night. It is a highly lipophilic molecule; about 70% of it is bound to albumin, while the rest remains in a free state that freely crosses cellular membranes. After intravenous administration, melatonin's half-life is about 30 min, but a biphasic elimination pattern with half-lives of about 3 and 45 min has also been observed for oral intake.[48, 49]

Melatonin is metabolized primarily in the liver, but also in the kidney, undergoing hydroxylation and then conjugation into sulfate and glucuronide. Liver and kidney pathologies (e.g., cirrhosis and chronic renal failure) are known to alter clearance rates.[21] In humans, the main metabolite is 6-sulfatoxymelatonin (aMT6s); its urinary concentration accounts for up to 90% of administered melatonin.[6, 49] Approximately 1% of melatonin is excreted in the native state.[50]

Some melatonin is metabolized to NAS, which can point to a feedback system in controlling melatonin production. NAS, recently measured in serum, is a potentially active indole derivative, suggesting that the conversion process may have physiological significance.[1]

2.3.1.1.3   Patterns and Regulation of Melatonin Secretion

The synthesis and secretion of pineal hormones reveal evidence of both central and local control,[47] as discussed next.

Central control   The pineal gland is connected to the biological clock in the SCN, the main circadian oscillator, via a multisynaptic pathway. The general signaling circuit involves input from the SCN to the paraventricular nuclei (PVN), intermediolateral (IML) columns of the spinal cord, SCG, and finally the pineal gland (Fig. 2.5).[47]

Light information received by the retina enables the synchronization of the SCN clock via the RHT. SCN fibers pass to the PVN in the hypothalamus, and reticular formation conveys the signal to the intermediolateral cell columns of the spinal cord, which contain preganglionic sympathetic neurons.

Depending on the existence of the light stimulus, the two possible pathways either promote or inhibit NAT activity, as follows:

a. Provided there is a light stimulus, the SCN neuron releases GABA, leading to an inhibitory postsynaptic potential (IPSP) in the PVN in the hypothalamus. The signal to the pineal is interrupted, and no melatonin is produced.

b. In the absence of a light signal, the SCN neuron generates an excitatory postsynaptic potential (EPSP) by releasing glutamate, thus activating the PVN. Both SCGs conduct the nervous impulse through postganglionic fibers, which terminate in NE synapses. NE stimulates the pinealocytes via β-adrenergic and α-adrenergic receptors, regulating cyclic adenosine monophosphate (cAMP) synthesis. cAMP promotes NAT activity during melatonin biosynthesis.

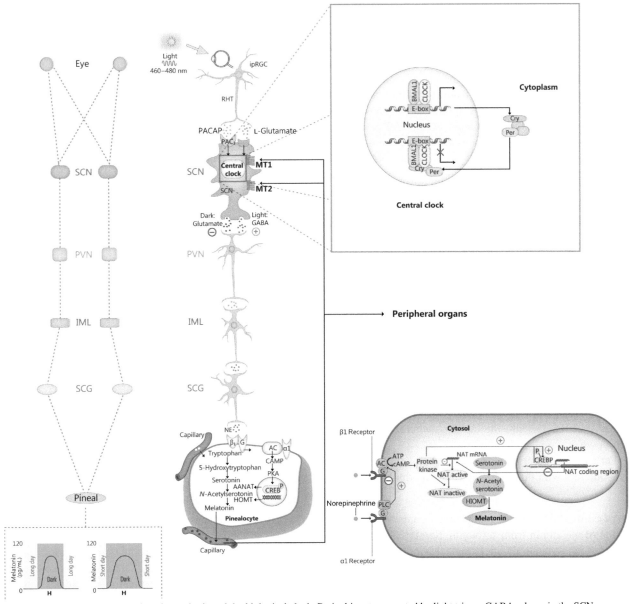

FIG. 2.5 Central control on melatonin synthesis and the biological clock. Retinal inputs generated by light trigger GABA release in the SCN neurons, leading to an inhibitory response in the hypothalamic PVN, thereby blocking melatonin production. In the absence of light, the SCN neurons generate an excitatory response by releasing glutamate, thus activating the PVN. Both SCGs conduct the nervous impulse through postganglionic fibers, which terminate in norepinephrinergic synapses. Norepinephrine (NE) stimulates the pinealocytes via β-adrenergic and α-adrenergic receptors, regulating cAMP synthesis. cAMP promotes N-acetyltransferase (AANAT/NAT) activity during melatonin biosynthesis. *AC*, Adenyl Cyclase; *BMAL1*, brain and muscle Arnt-like protein-1; *cAMP*, cyclic AMP; *CLOCK*, circadian locomotor output cycles kaput; *CREBP*, cAMP response element binding protein; *Cry*, cryptochrome; *E-Box*, enhancer box; *HIOMT*, hydroxyindole-O-methyltransferase; *IML*, intermediolateral cell column; *IpRGC*, intrinsically photosensitive retinal ganglion cell; *MT1*, melatonin receptor 1; *MT2*, melatonin receptor 2; *PACAP*, pituitary adenyl cyclase activating protein; *Per*, Period; *PKA*, protein kinase A; *PLC*, phospholipase C; *RHT*, retinal-hypothalamic tract.

The α-adrenergic receptors play a role in the potentiation of the β-adrenergic activity through a sharp increase in Ca^{2+} activity and the activation of protein kinase C (PKC) and prostaglandins.[51] Phosphorylation of specific serine residues of the NAT molecule by protein kinase A (PKA) boosts its activity. Ultimately, synergistic β- and α-adrenergic stimulation result in an elevation of intracellular cAMP.

Activation of inducible cAMP early repressor gene (ICER) might represent a control mechanism for limiting nocturnal melatonin production (in the rat at least). There are also suggestions of a parasympathetic regulatory mechanism based on the observation that rat pinealocytes express all the elements of a glutamatergic system, and that administration of glutamate inhibits NAT activity.[52]

The response of the mammalian pineal to light during nighttime depends on the intensity, wavelength, and duration of the light, reaching maximum inhibition for a wavelength interval of 460–480 nm.[53] Blue light exposure, used more often at night due to the proliferation of energy-efficient lighting (LEDs) and electronic devices, seems to be more chronodisruptive, desynchronizing the circadian rhythms and inducing the strongest inhibition of melatonin synthesis.[53] Other factors, such as temperature, precipitations, magnetic fields, and food can be involved in the regulation of melatonin synthesis, thereby influencing fertility.[54] Also, NAT activity is suppressed by some exogenous stimuli (stress factors), immobilization, swimming in cold or warm water, exposure to heat, noise, hunger, and other inputs. Although catecholamine secretion increases as a result of stress factors, NAT activity is inhibited as catecholamine presynaptic reuptake mechanisms intervene.

The role of the clock genes located in the SCN has been carefully researched in past decades. Two transcription factors, BMAL1 (brain and muscle Arnt-like protein-1) and CLOCK (circadian locomotor output cycles kaput), form a heterodimer that activates the transcription of the genes for two proteins, Per (Period) and Cry (Cryptochrome). Cry and Per, along with other proteins, form a repressor complex that translocates back into the nucleus, allowing the Per-Cry complex to shut off the transcription of these genes in a negative feedback loop, creating the oscillator.

The SCN generates circadian rhythms through a set of positive and negative feedback loops of transcription and translation.[55, 56] Bilateral SCN lesions obliterate the circadian rhythms of melatonin synthesis and secretion, demonstrating that the SCN is the melatonin rhythm generator.[57] On the other hand, with constant exposure to darkness, the approximate 24-h cycle of the SCN will keep melatonin and serotonin synthesis on this schedule, but serum levels of the hormones will not continue to convey information about light and darkness. Liu and Borjigin suggested that the circadian pacemaker may be an elastic structure that can decompress and compress under varying photic conditions.[58]

BMAL1 and CLOCK bind to the E-box (Enhancer box) in the promoter region of the genes for Per and Cry, among other proteins. In the presence of these two positive transcription factors, Per and Cry, messenger ribonucleic acid (mRNA) translation is enhanced. The cytoplasmic levels of the proteins increase and form a complex that is further translocated into the nucleus, where Cry-Per represses transcription so that further synthesis of the genes is shut down.

Per and Cry undergo protein degradation, no longer promoting the repression, and the cycle restarts. Other regulatory loops interact with this one, stabilizing its rhythmicity.

Local control The pineal gland receives adrenergic innervation, as previously discussed, which leads to the nightly formation of melatonin from serotonin. Serotonin is present at high levels in the pineal gland during the day and increases further at night due to the increased activity of TPOH, the rate-limiting enzyme of serotonin production. The posttranslational control by phosphorylation of TPOH is also stimulated through the adrenergic mechanism.[59] The synchronization of the two rate-limiting enzymes for humans has not yet been explained. In the presence of active melatonin synthesis, which consumes its precursors, the concentrations of 5-HTP and serotonin in the rat pineal gland drop below their daytime levels.[60]

Classically, NAT has been considered the rate-limiting enzyme of melatonin production. During daytime, it limits melatonin synthesis due to its low activity. However, for most of the night, NAT does not limit melatonin production. In humans, mutations in HIOMT that determine deficiencies in the last step of melatonin synthesis and lower melatonin levels, were found in patients with Alzheimer's disease[61, 62] and autism spectrum disorders.[63]

2.3.1.2 Melatonin Receptors

Melatonin exerts systemic effects either through specific receptors or independently. The two melatonin receptors, MT1 and MT2, are seven typical membrane-spanning G protein-coupled receptors that share about 60% amino acid homology. A third protein, 45% identical to the melatonin receptors, has been isolated in the human pituitary; however, its ligand remains unknown.[21] The two receptors are distinguished based on their binding affinity for melatonin, with the MT1 receptor's affinity being approximately fivefold greater than that of MT2 (Fig. 2.6). Throughout the human body, melatonin receptors are widely distributed; some of the relevant organs are listed in Fig. 2.6. Recent studies have correlated modified MT2 expression in human osteoblasts with the development of scoliosis.[42]

Location		Receptor type
Ovary		MT1
Uterus (myometrium)		MT1
Adrenal cortex		MT1
Liver		MT1
Pancreas		MT1
Spleen		MT1
Brain	Cerebellum, Hippocampus, Ventral tegmental area, Substantia Nigra	MT1
	SCN and hypothalamus	MT1, MT2
Placenta		MT1, MT2
Testis		MT1, MT2
Breast		MT1, MT2
Cardiovascular system (heart and blood vessels)		MT1, MT2
Immune system		MT1, MT2
Retina		MT1, MT2
Kidney		MT1, MT2
Pituitary		MT2
Gastrointestinal system		MT2
Adipose tissue		MT2

FIG. 2.6 Melatonin receptors MT1 and MT2 distribution in humans. *(Modified after Norman AW, Henry HL. The pineal gland.* Hormones *2015;351–61.)*

MT1 and MT2 are both G-protein-coupled receptors and, depending on the cell type, they launch one of two intracellular pathways (Fig. 2.7):

a. G_i inhibits adenyl cyclase, which further decreases cAMP, leading to a diminished PKA activity;

b. G_q promotes phospholipase C (PLC) activity, leading to the cleavage of phosphatidyl inositol diphosphate (PIP2) into inositol triphosphate (IP3) and diacylglycerol (DAG). These second messengers stimulate increased intracellular Ca^{2+} and PKC, respectively.

Through either decreased cAMP or increased intracellular Ca^{2+}, melatonin exerts most of its functions on gene expression, transcription, and translation.

2.3.1.2.1 Melatonin Effects on Reproductive Function through MT1 and MT2 Melatonin Receptors

Melatonin signaling via MT1 and MT2 receptors modulates reproductive function in both females and males. Its correlation with gonadotropins and steroid hormones provides good insight into the role that melatonin may play in folliculogenesis, sexual maturation, puberty onset, pregnancy, and menopause. Melatonin indirectly influences gonadal function through gonadotropin-releasing hormone (GnRH) and gonadotropin secretion; however, a direct effect is not excluded because melatonin might be synthesized in gonads.[34]

In mammals, the distribution of melatonin receptors throughout the hypothalamic-pituitary-gonadal (HPG) axis hints at the possible role that it may play in the reproductive function, particularly regarding GnRH release. The cAMP-mediated signaling supposedly decreases the Ca^{2+} influx though voltage-mediated channels and its release from intracellular stores, which further suppresses GnRH-induced gonadotropin secretion.[64, 65]

Melatonin levels differ substantially before and after puberty, and this finding suggested that melatonin may regulate the onset of puberty through its effects on the hypothalamus. These effects are supported by the presence of melatonin receptors on gonadotropin-inhibitory-hormone (GnIH)-producing cells, which increase their secretion during short days,[66] thus providing melatonin with a role to suppress GnRH release. Before puberty, concentrations of melatonin are high and may

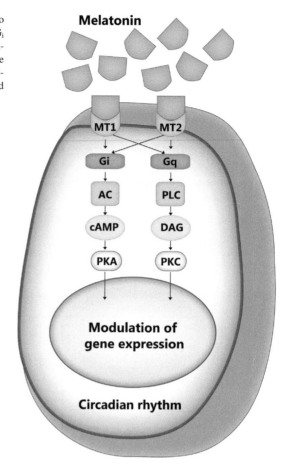

FIG. 2.7   Coupled G-protein MT1 and MT2 signaling pathways. Melatonin binding to MT1 and MT2 receptors launch the corresponding intracellular pathways: (i) the G_i pathway inhibits adenyl cyclase (AC), which further decreases cAMP, leading to diminished PKA activity; (ii) the G_q pathway promotes PLC activity, leading to the cleavage of phosphatidyl inositol diphosphate (PIP2) into inositol triphosphate (IP3) and diacylglycerol (DAG). These second messengers stimulate increased intracellular Ca^{2+} and PKC, respectively.

prevent hypothalamic activation. However, by the onset of puberty, there is a decline in serum levels of melatonin, which may trigger the pivotal release of GnRH. Maximal melatonin concentrations have been found during adolescence, followed by a steady decline with aging.[2]

Melatonin receptors are present in the ovarian granulosa and theca cells, which are known to promote steroid hormone production, as well as being found in mature follicles and the corpus luteum. Melatonin via its free-radical scavenger and antioxidant properties may be directly involved in the normal maturation and protection of oocytes. Melatonin concentrations are higher in human ovarian follicular fluid than in plasma, likely due not only to transport of melatonin from the bloodstream, but to local synthesis, predominantly by granulosa cells.[67]

In the ovary, it appears that the main signaling pathway that influences steroidogenesis is via cAMP and through the expression of the steroidogenic acute regulatory protein (StAR).

The follicle produces different sex steroids depending on its stage in development. In humans, melatonin has been shown to modulate the follicular response to gonadotropins (particularly LH) by elevating expression of its receptor in the granulosa cells. Another stimulation pathway of melatonin for follicular development is via IGF-1.[34] Melatonin upregulates IGF-1 expression, which in turn contributes (along with gonadotropins) to follicular growth.[67]

The MT1 receptor has been identified in myometrial cell membranes and displays significant upregulation during labor. Melatonin is believed to synergize with oxytocin to promote and coordinate muscle contractions[68] (Fig. 2.8).

Melatonin receptors play a different role in the villous trophoblast syncytialization in the human placenta. Both MT1 and MT2 are expressed during all trimesters of pregnancy.[69] MT1 mRNA and protein are significantly more expressed in the first trimester of pregnancy compared to the second and third trimesters. Increased expression of MT1 during syncytiotrophoblast formation is associated with cellular apoptosis, contrasting with the role of MT2 in promoting villous cytotrophoblast development and differentiation.[69]

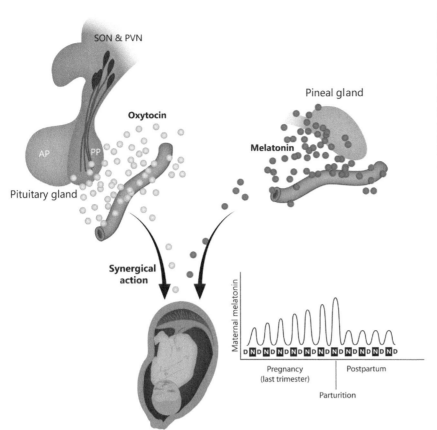

FIG. 2.8 Nocturnal melatonin blood levels gradually increase during gestation and return to pregestational levels after parturition. Melatonin and oxytocin act synergistically on the uterus for a more powerful myometrial contraction during initiation of parturition, which frequently occurs during the night, when melatonin secretion is increased. *AP*, anterior pituitary; *PP*, posterior pituitary; *PVN*, paraventricular nucleus; *SON*, supraoptic nucleus. *(Modified after Reiter RJ, Tan DX, Galano A. Melatonin: exceeding expectations.* Physiology *2014;29(5):325–33.)*

With respect to male reproduction function, melatonin receptors have been identified in several testicular cells. Its actions on Leydig cells modulate testicular maturation, while in vitro experiments on Sertoli cells have shown favorable effects on spermatogenesis by lowering lactate production and increasing glucose consumption.[70, 71]

Given that MT1 and MT2 receptors have been identified in almost all tissues, it is not possible to clearly separate the effects of pineal melatonin from those of extrapineal melatonin. However, only pineal melatonin has been shown to be synthesized and released in response to the circadian rhythm.

2.3.1.3 Melatonin and Biorhythms

Melatonin production varies in different species; however, its nocturnal acrophase, synchronized with increased NAT activity, characterizes most mammals, including humans. Hourly serum melatonin levels[2] and urinary 6-sulfatocymelatonin[6] fluctuations have been measured. During the evening, melatonin levels increase until the maximum is reached, usually between 1 a.m. and 4 a.m., followed by a decrease to minimal levels during the daytime.

The secretion of melatonin is not pulsatile, as occurs with other hormones such as GnRH. A seasonal biorhythm has been demonstrated in various mammalian species. In humans, however, the seasonal changes in melatonin concentration are still debatable: some authors suggest that during the luteal phase, the serum concentration is higher than during the follicular phase.[34] Moreover, it has been suggested that low melatonin levels contribute to the ovulatory rise in body temperature.[34] During the year, increased melatonin values were reported during dark periods in winter[72] associated with the lengthening of the nocturnal melatonin peak.[73]

The physiological concentration of melatonin may vary in different body fluids and cellular compartments, as it is locally produced (e.g., ovary, placenta, liver).[74]

Mean serum levels of melatonin vary considerably during the lifetime, displaying great variations in the amplitude of the nocturnal peaks among individuals. The highest values have been reported so far in children aged 1–3 years (329.5 ± 42 pg/mL), while the mean values for each age category progressively decline, following the illustrating pattern in Fig. 2.9.[2] Other epidemiological studies have found maximal nocturnal values are reached between the fourth and seventh year of age.[4]

FIG. 2.9   Melatonin nocturnal variations in different age groups. Pineal melatonin signals the photoperiodicity and is secreted during the night, reaching maximum blood levels in the middle of darkness. Peak melatonin levels are attained during childhood. The graph illustrates the aging-related decline of mean nocturnal melatonin levels in humans.

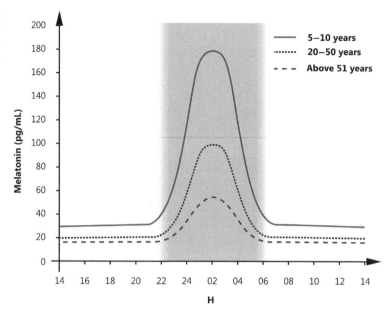

2.3.1.3.1   Circadian Rhythm

The endogenous component in the control of melatonin production displays the relative independence of melatonin production from ambient light exposure. In other words, serotonin-*N*-acetyltransferase (NAT), the major enzyme regulating melatonin biosynthesis, which determines both the onset and termination of hormone synthesis, has a biorhythm independent of but synchronized with environmental light exposure. This endogenous rhythm of NAT and melatonin is neurogenic, but not proprietary to pinealocytes. The initiation of melatonin secretion, synchronized with the occurrence of night (twilight) and suppressed by the appearance of light (dawn), presents two distinct moments of this process, which is mediated by the SCN. A biphasic control mechanism has been postulated with at least two separate oscillators, which differentiate sensitively in the evening and in the morning, thereby determining the initiation and suppression of melatonin production by the NAT enzyme.

The two endogenous oscillators (initiation and determination) interact with each other through phase relationships and are externally synchronized to the day/night astronomical rhythm. The location of the two endogenous oscillators has not been specified, but the SCN appears to be involved. The SCN functions as a synchronized endogenous clock, especially with the day/night cycle, regulating the rhythm of melatonin synthesis to circadian light signals (photoperiod), thus allowing the measurement of the photoperiod time (daytime) through the circadian biorhythm of melatonin.

The control of pineal functions exerted by both external environmental factors (e.g., light and temperature) and the endogenous clock is transmitted through pineal innervation. The pineal acts, therefore, as a neuroendocrine transducer that converts a photoneural signal into a hormonal signal (melatonin), and the pinealocyte is a photoneuroendocrine cell.

Melatonin administration is associated with a decrease in core body temperature, while the distal temperature elevates, suggesting an increase in heat loss. Endogenous melatonin contributes to a nocturnal decrease in body temperature, leading to the hypothesis that pineal resection might be related to insomnia.[21]

2.3.1.3.2   Melatonin and Sleep During Pregnancy and Lactation

The sleep patterns during pregnancy and postpartum are commonly altered, resulting in poor sleep. They are accompanied by hormonal changes, fluctuations in mood and anxiety, along with the transition from pregnancy into the first few postpartum months, and the need to face the newborn's unpredictable sleep patterns. Altered sleep cycles during pregnancy cause insomnia in 62% of pregnant women,[75] especially during the third trimester, and contribute to excessive daytime sleepiness, fatigue, and possibly postpartum depression.

Cortisol and melatonin concentrations vary during pregnancy, with evidence of interdependent patterns. A decreased cortisol-to-melatonin ratio has been found in poor sleepers, which might be useful for differentiating depression from sleep disturbances in pregnancy.[76] During the first trimester, rising progesterone levels and specific behavior disturbances such as a frequent need to urinate are related to increased tiredness. In pregnant and nonpregnant women, the peak of melatonin occurs around the midpoint of sleeping time, calculated by using the mean of bedtime and wake-up time. The midpoint of sleep time and melatonin peak values should be interpreted clinically, considering the influence of coexistent factors such as night-shift work, weekdays versus weekends, and even supplemental vitamin intake. The midpoint of sleep was significantly higher in the first trimester of pregnant women compared to the control group.[77]

2.3.1.3.3 Rhythmicity in the Female Reproductive Function

In mammals and seasonal breeders, melatonin has been shown to modulate reproductive activity by conveying the seasonal and circadian fluctuations of the shortness of the day. The female menstrual cycle is dictated by a very strict pattern in GnRH and gonadotropin secretion. Either by acting on the GnIH-secreting cells or directly blocking the GnRH effect on gonadotropin discharge, melatonin is associated with a general suppressive action.

Whether the pineal is either antigonadotropic or progonadotropic is debatable. The overall changing of the duration of the nocturnal melatonin message entrains the hypothalamic-pituitary-gonadal axis differently depending on the time of the year.[34]

Melatonin's potential beneficial actions during menopause have been investigated with the purpose of alleviating hot flushes, mood disturbances, vulvovaginal atrophy, muscle weakness, bone mass loss, and sexual dysfunction.[78] Exogenous melatonin administration proved to reverse hormonal and menopause-related neurovegetative disturbances, as well as menopause-related depression.[78]

2.3.2 Other Pineal Hormones

In addition to the indolamine hormone melatonin, the pineal contains peptide hormones. Pineal peptide hormones, for which chemical formulas have been proposed and whose physiological role has been studied, are arginine-vasotocin and angiotensin. The identification of angiotensin is preceded by the discovery of pineal renin.[79, 80] Consequently, angiotensins were identified by immunohistochemistry in the pineal gland.[81] In humans, arginine-vasopressin, arginine-vasotocin, and oxytocin have been identified by radioimmunoassay (RIA) in the pineal gland.[82]

Vasotocin is the only pineal peptide hormone whose amino acid sequence has been established by mass spectrometry and whose presence in mammals and humans has a phylogenetic explanation. It is a nonapeptide with the cyclic nucleus of oxytocin and the side chain of vasopressin.

Vasopressin itself is present in the pineal gland, from where it has been isolated and purified, and its local synthesis has been confirmed by in situ hybridization. Vasopressin appears to be located only in pineal nerve fibers, but it is present in relatively large amounts compared to vasotocin. This leads to crossreactivity in relevant identification tests. For this reason, after vasopressin was detected in the pineal gland, many authors were skeptical about the presence of vasotocin in mammals. In mammals, vasotocin was replaced by vasopressin, but it appears to persist transiently in the fetus (in sheep and humans) within the neurohypophysis, and in adult mammals within the cerebral epiphysis.[27]

The renin-angiotensin system was highlighted in the pineal gland by biological and radioimmunological methods. Initially, Haulica et al. demonstrated biologically the presence of a high concentration of renin in animals and humans.[80] Demonstration of the de novo synthesis of renin and angiotensin in pineal cell cultures, as well as an increase in its production from newborn to adult (rat), with inverse evolution to vasotocin activities, allowed the development of the hypothesis that angiotensin is a pineal hormone, probably involved in thirst, central blood pressure regulation, and the synthesis of serotonin and melatonin.

Some biologically active peptides isolated from the mammalian pineal gland originate in the SCG, hypothalamus, and other areas of the central nervous system; these either occur in neurons of cerebral origin, or are captured from the general circulation: oxytocin, VIP, NPY and substance P, endorphins, enkephalins, delta-sleep-inducing peptide and somatostatin, and histidine-isoleucine peptide. The physiological role of these peptides in the pineal organ is not elucidated; it is assumed that these peptides influence the pineal synthetic activity and transmit neuromodulatory information from the brain or target organs.[83]

2.4 SPECIFIC FUNCTIONS OF THE PINEAL GLAND DURING PREGNANCY AND LACTATION

The pineal gland undergoes structural and functional changes during pregnancy and lactation. In rats, there is a documented increase in cytoplasmic organelles (e.g., the number of Golgi bodies and dense-core vesicles) in the second half of the pregnancy.[84] In humans, a rise in the pineal activity during pregnancy is illustrated by an increase in plasma melatonin[14] and by elevated excretion of melatonin metabolites in urine in the near term.[85]

Serum melatonin levels are higher in the third trimester of pregnancy than in the first and the second trimesters, and also higher than in nonpregnant women.[86, 87] A clear diurnal rhythm in serum melatonin concentrations is maintained for both early and late pregnancy.[87] During pregnancy, from the earliest stages of embryo development, melatonin acts as an early maternal-fetal endocrine signal that is transferred unaltered from the maternal to the fetal circulation, resulting in fetal plasma values of melatonin equivalent to those of the mother[88] (Fig. 2.10).

The presence of melatonin in amniotic fluid is the subject of various hypotheses: increased pineal activity during the third trimester, the potential local production by the amniotic membrane cells, or even leakage from placenta or fetal tissues.[89] The fetus is exclusively dependent upon the maternal pineal production of melatonin b the fetal pineal gland only matures at only around 9–12 weeks postpartum.[90, 91] Even though the human placenta is an additional source of melatonin,[92] it has been demonstrated that it acts mostly locally as an autocoid or paracoid, without being involved in the regulation of the fetal circadian rhythm.[74]

Melatonin treatment during gestation resulted in an increased endothelial relaxation of umbilical arteries in a mouse model of fetal growth restriction.[93] Also, melatonin is involved in gestation maintenance by stimulating synthesis of progesterone and sustaining the uterine quiescence, thus preventing preterm delivery in a murine model of preterm birth.[94] The implications of melatonin in human pregnancy and lactation will be discussed next.

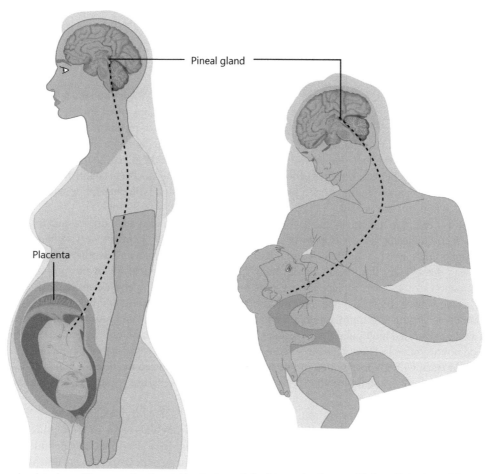

Pineal gland

Placenta

FIG. 2.10 Maternal melatonin readily crosses the placental barrier to reach the fetus, or is taken up with the milk by the suckling newborn, in order to signal the ambient lighting conditions.

2.4.1   Role of the Pineal Gland in Fertility and Reproduction

Circadian rhythms and fertility are interconnected, with melatonin being involved in the hormonal synchronization mechanism. Circadian clocks are documented not only in the brain, but also in peripheral tissues, with important roles for ovulation, nidation, and the progress of gestation. A genetic basis for the circadian clock (Per1, Per3, Cry1, Clock, and Bmal1) has been demonstrated not only in the SCN, but also in other central nervous system or peripheral tissues, including the pituitary and ovaries.[32]

Melatonin regulates reproductive seasonal variations in many animal species, while in primates, seasonal reproduction does not apply.[95] Changes in day length are detected by pineal and are reflected in melatonin secretion, with downregulation of the gonadal axis during winter.

In humans, these variations are less important, but still, in northern populations with long winter nights, reproductive vitality is season-related.[72] Interestingly, human births occur more frequently at night, when the levels of melatonin are higher,[68] which illustrates a possible role of melatonin and circadian signals in that process.

Melatonin has been shown to affect the female reproductive tract, depending on the menstrual phase,[95] by acting on the GnIH-secreting cells or directly blocking the GnRH effect on gonadotropin discharge. A correlation between melatonin and gonadotropins and/or sexual steroids was described, which reflects on puberty onset, sexual maturation, ovulation, and menopause as discussed previously.[23, 95]

Administration of melatonin and synthetic progesterone leads to decreased LH secretion, thereby blocking ovulation and the luteal phase increase in progesterone, without affecting FSH or inhibiting estradiol.[96] Daily administration of melatonin (300 mg) during 4 months caused a decrease in LH mean values compared to the control, its effect being consistent with that of the double administration of melatonin and synthetic progesterone.[97] This may represent an evolutionary remnant of ovulation inhibition during the winter months, designed to prevent delivery of offspring in an unfavorable environment when resources are less available.

2.4.1.1   Antioxidant Properties of Melatonin and Reproductive Function

Melatonin has important free-radical scavenging and antioxidant properties[34] and it has been the subject of investigation of reproductive medical conditions where oxidative stress is known to be involved, including infertility and preeclampsia/eclampsia. Melatonin has a good safety profile in both animals and human studies, with no demonstrable teratogenic effects, and it can be administered throughout pregnancy.[98] Furthermore, melatonin does not have sedative effects, nor does it have hepatic or kidney toxicity; on the contrary, it may have a cytoprotective action.[99] Melatonin, however, is limited to use in patients with autoimmune conditions, given its immune stimulation proprieties.

Melatonin's antioxidant effects through direct and indirect mechanisms, well documented up to date,[100] make this molecule a cellular protector against highly toxic oxygen- and nitrogen-derived free radicals (e.g., peroxynitrite anion, hydroxyl radical, hypochlorous acid) and other chemical substances.[101] Melatonin's small amphipathic (i.e., lipophilic and hydrophilic) molecule can readily gain access to subcellular sites where free radicals (including mitochondria) are generated, and directly scavenge the reactive oxygen and nitrogen species, a process that implies single electron transfer, hydrogen transfer, and radical adduct formation.[5, 100] Also, melatonin acts by inducing the expression and increasing the activity of antioxidant enzymes (glutathione peroxidase, glutathione reductase, superoxide dismutase, catalase), reducing the activity of prooxidant enzymes while also improving mitochondrial function.[100] Through these actions, melatonin proved to be an efficient anticarcinogenic agent.[100]

Melatonin's role in protecting the ovary, placenta, and fetus has been well researched.[102, 103] The main damage caused by reactive oxygen species (ROS) is the lipid peroxidation of cell membranes.

During ovulation, reactive oxygen and nitrogen species are highly generated. The amount of ROS influences the maturation of the oocytes by controlling the expression of relevant genes. On the other hand, a significant increase in ROS may result in damage to oocyte and granulosa cell membrane and structure. Thus, this strict control of the oxidative environment is mandatory. In addition, melatonin can have a regulatory function in fertilization and embryo development.[104]

In pregnant women, the placenta is a significant source of peroxidized lipids, increasing the mean blood levels of such lipids. The antioxidant role of melatonin exerts a protective effect by preserving the integrity of both placenta and fetus against ROS.[105]

2.4.2   Role of Pineal in Pregnancy and Maternal-Fetal Communication

During pregnancy and postpartum, maternal circadian rhythms are responsible for the programming of fetal and newborn circadian rhythms (Fig. 2.11). Maternal melatonin may play a major role in influencing the development of the fetus

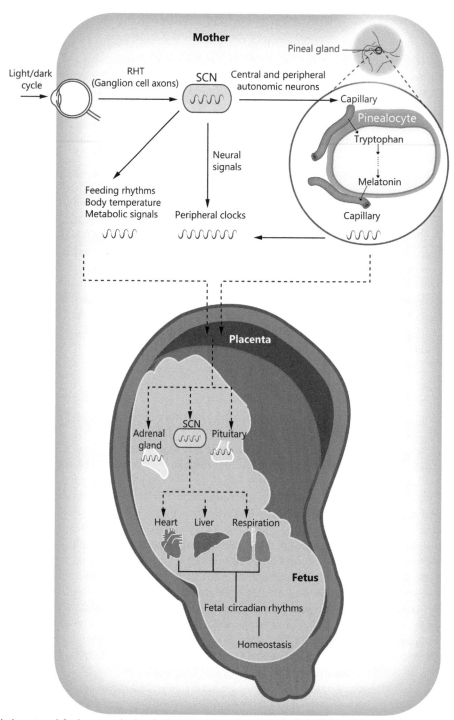

FIG. 2.11 Melatonin in maternal-fetal communication. In the maternal compartment, the light/dark cycle controls SCN activity, and thus melatonin secretion in the pinealocyte. Feeding rhythms, body temperature, and general metabolism of the mother are also influenced by the SCN, eventually influencing fetal homeostasis. Local production of melatonin occurs in the placenta but has no documented effect on the programming of fetal circadian rhythm. In the fetal compartment, maternal melatonin and its impact on maternal homeostasis influences the maturation of the fetal SCN and the adrenal corticosteroid rhythm. *(Modified after Reiter RJ, Tan DX, Galano A. Melatonin: exceeding expectations. Physiology 2014;29(5):325–33.)*

because it readily crosses the placenta. Studies have documented that the cycle of melatonin in the maternal blood is mimicked in the fetal circulation.[88] Current data suggest that the circadian-generating architecture in the fetus, particularly in the SCN, is entrained by the maternal melatonin cycle.[5] Maternal melatonin elicits an entraining effect on the fetal hypothalamus by acting on melatonin receptors in the fetal suprachiasmatic nuclei. The nonhuman fetal clock genes are essentially imprinted by melatonin, meaning that the expression of fetal clock genes changes when the melatonin-releasing pattern is altered by exposure of the mother to continuous light. Interestingly, these changes are reversed by daily parenteral melatonin administration to the mother.[106] Also, human fetuses display 24-h rhythms in temperature and oxygen consumption by 32–33 weeks of gestation.[107]

Disturbances of the fetal circadian system may have long-term consequences in the offspring. Women who engage in shift work during pregnancy have altered melatonin cycles and have an increased incidence of spontaneous abortions, premature deliveries, and low-birth-weight infants.[108] Also, a disturbed light/dark cycle in late pregnancy or during the perinatal period may have major effects on subsequent behavioral and metabolic functions,[89] possibly being involved in the development of conditions such as metabolic syndrome, obesity, attention deficit-hyperactivity disorder, or autism spectrum disorders.[109, 110]

2.4.3 Role of Pineal During Labor

Labor occurs primarily in the night or early morning hours.[34] Human myometrium is a target for melatonin. Melatonin has been demonstrated to act synergistically with oxytocin to enhance the contractility of human myometrial smooth muscle cells by acting on the same intracellular signaling pathway (Fig. 2.8). In vitro, melatonin increases myometrial oxytocin sensitivity and myometrial contractility through MT2 receptors via the PLC/PKC/myosin light-chain kinase (MLCK) signaling pathway, and further boosts the expression of the gap junction protein Cx43 through a PKC-dependent pathway, promoting intercellular connectivity.[68] Therefore, some studies point to a significant role for circulating melatonin in the timing and degree of uterine contractions in late-term pregnancy and delivery.[111, 112] Considering the excessive urban exposure to light during the night, including in hospital environments, there is a tendency toward melatonin deficiency and chronodisruption, with deleterious impacts during pregnancy and labor. These circumstances urge measures for pregnant women to keep a regular light/dark cycle and sleep/wake cycle, particularly during the last trimester.[112]

2.4.4 Role of Pineal in Lactation

Melatonin is a normal component of nighttime human milk and possibly plays a role in communicating the time of the day to the newborn. Melatonin in the milk exhibits a pronounced daily rhythm, with high levels during the night and undetectable levels during the day,[113] reflecting serum fluctuations. Even though it only reaches up to one-third of the serum level,[114] melatonin levels in breast milk are stable after 3–4 days postpartum despite the disturbed circadian sleep-wake cycle of the breastfeeding mother.

Melatonin concentrations are low in newborns and increase after 3 months, when a diurnal rhythm is detectable. The maximum secretion level is reached at 2–3 years of life and then declines to adult levels. By the 12th week of postnatal life, the pineal gland of the newborn begins melatonin production. However, the first 3 months of a baby's life coincide with a disturbed sleep rhythm, usually accompanied by infant colic.

Melatonin's highest levels in nocturnal breast milk may have a hypnotic effect on the infant and signal photoperiodicity. Also, it acts as a relaxing factor on the smooth muscle of the gastrointestinal tract. Thus, nighttime breast milk may improve infants' sleep and reduce colic, compared to artificial formulas that lack melatonin.[114] To better improve infants' sleep quality, it is recommended for nocturnal breastfeeding to occur in the dark in order to maintain a high melatonin content in breast milk.

Melatonin was found in bovine milk in low concentrations of 5–25 pg/mL, showing a diurnal pattern parallel with its serum levels, with maximum values at midnight and lower at noon. These findings reinforce the recommendation that nighttime milk as a valuable source of melatonin.[115]

Moreover, breast milk contains tryptophan, the melatonin precursor, which is important for melatonin synthesis in infants, especially after 3 months of life. The tryptophan level in milk follows a circadian rhythm with a peak around 3 a.m., followed by a peak in the urinary melatonin metabolite, 6-sulfatoxymelatonin, around 6 a.m. in infants that were exclusively breast-fed.[116]

The pineal may play a supplementary role in stimulating prolactin release, and thus lactation. There is a correlation between the concentrations of melatonin and prolactin in pregnant or lactating women. Both intravenous and oral administration of melatonin stimulate prolactin release.[117]

2.5 CONCLUSIONS

The pineal is a neuroendocrine gland and a circadian oscillator that produces melatonin during night, consecutive to sympathetic stimulation received from the biological clock (SCN) via GCNs. Melatonin exerts systemic effects either through specific melatonin receptors or independently. It influences female reproductive function and maintains a circadian rhythm during pregnancy and lactation, temporarily increasing in concentration during gestation and labor. Melatonin might synergize with oxytocin during labor, promoting uterine contractility.

Maternal melatonin signals photoperiodicity by crossing the placenta to the fetus, and by passage in the breast milk to the neonate. Melatonin is a free-radical scavenger and may exert protective antioxidant effects, countering the oxidative challenge that accompanies the high metabolic demands during pregnancy, labor and lactation.

REFERENCES

1. Dunand M, Grund B, Eugster PJ, Ivanyuk A, Fogarasi-Szabo N, Bardinet C, et al. Serotonin, melatonin and their metabolites measured in plasma by a new LC-MS/MS assay in healthy volunteers. *Clin Ther* 2017;**39**(8):e40–1.
2. Waldhauser F, Weiszenbacher G, Tatzer E, Gisinger B, Waldhauser M, Schemper M, et al. Alternations in nocturnal serum melatonin levels in humans with growth and aging. *J Clin Endocrinol Metab* 1988;**66**(3):648–52.
3. Tan DX, Manchester LC, Sanchez-Barcelo E, Mediavilla MD, Reiter RJ. Significance of high levels of endogenous melatonin in mammalian cerebrospinal fluid and in the central nervous system. *Curr Neuropharmacol* 2010;**8**:162–7.
4. Zhdanova IV, Cantor ML, Leclair OU, Kartashov AI, Wurtman RJ. Behavioral effects of melatonin treatment in non-human primates. *Sleep Res Online* 1998;**1**(3):114–8.
5. Reiter RJ, Tan DX, Galano A. Melatonin: exceeding expectations. *Physiology* 2014;**29**(5):325–33.
6. Mahlberg R, Tilmann A, Salewski L, Kunz D. Normative data on the daily profile of urinary 6-sulfatoxymelatonin in healthy subjects between the ages of 20 and 84. *Psychoneuroendocrinology* 2006;**31**(5):634–41.
7. Klein DC. The pineal gland and melatonin. In: *Endocrinology: adult and pediatric*. W.B. Saunders; 2016. p. 312–322.e5.
8. McCord CP, Allen FP. Evidences associating pineal gland function with alterations in pigmentation. *J Exp Zool* 1917;**23**(1):207–24.
9. Lerner AB, Case JD, Takahashi Y, Lee TH, Mori W. Isolation of melatonin, the pineal gland factor that lightens melanocytes 1. *J Am Chem Soc* 1958;**80**(10):2587.
10. Poggeler B, Balzer I, Hardeland R, Lerchl A. Pineal hormone melatonin oscillates also in the dinoflagellate Gonyaulax polyedra. *Naturwissenschaften* 1991;**78**(6):268–9.
11. Dubbels R, Reiter RJ, Klenke E, Goebel A, Schnakenberg E, Ehlers C, et al. Melatonin in edible plants identified by radioimmunoassay and by high performance liquid chromatography-mass spectrometry. *J Pineal Res* 1995;**18**(1):28–31.
12. Vivien-Roels B, Pevet P, Beck O, Fevre-Montange M. Identification of melatonin in the compound eyes of an insect, the locust (Locusta migratoria), by radioimmunoassay and gas chromatography-mass spectrometry. *Neurosci Lett* 1984;**49**(1–2):153–7.
13. Simonneaux V, Ribelayga C. Generation of the melatonin endocrine message in mammals: a review of the complex regulation of melatonin synthesis by norepinephrine, peptides, and other pineal transmitters. *Pharmacol Rev* 2003;**55**(2):325–95.
14. Pang SF, Tang PL, Tang GWK, Yam AWC, Ng KW. Plasma levels of immunoreactive melatonin, estradiol, progesterone, follicle stimulating hormone, and β-human chorionic gonadotropin during pregnancy and shortly after parturition in humans. *J Pineal Res* 1987;**4**(1):21–31.
15. Slominski A, Wortsman J, Tobin DJ. The cutaneous serotoninergic/melatoninergic system: securing a place under the sun. *FASEB J* 2005;**19**(2):176–94.
16. Bubenik GA. Gastrointestinal melatonin: localization, function, and clinical relevance. *Dig Dis Sci* 2002;**47**(10):2336–48.
17. Conti A, Conconi S, Hertens E, Skwarlo-Sonta K, Markowska M, Maestroni JM. Evidence for melatonin synthesis in mouse and human bone marrow cells. *J Pineal Res* 2000;**28**(4):193–202.
18. Carrillo-Vico A, Calvo JR, Abreu P, Lardone PJ, García-Mauriño S, Reiter RJ, et al. Evidence of melatonin synthesis by human lymphocytes and its physiological significance: possible role as intracrine, autocrine, and/or paracrine substance. *FASEB J* 2004;**18**(3):537–9.
19. Tan D-X, Manchester LC, Hardeland R, Lopez-Burillo S, Mayo JC, Sainz RM, et al. Melatonin: a hormone, a tissue factor, an autocoid, a paracoid, and an antioxidant vitamin. *J Pineal Res* 2003;**34**(1):75–8.
20. Rizzo P, Raffone E, Benedetto V. Effect of the treatment with myo-inositol plus folic acid plus melatonin in comparison with a treatment with myo-inositol plus folic acid on oocyte quality and pregnancy outcome in IVF cycles. A prospective, clinical trial. *Eur Rev Med Pharmacol Sci* 2010;**14**(6):555–61.
21. Macchi MM, Bruce JN. Human pineal physiology and functional significance of melatonin. *Front Neuroendocrinol* 2004;**25**(3–4):177–95.
22. Smith AB, Rushing EJ, Smirniotopoulos JG. From the archives of the AFIP: lesions of the pineal region: radiologic-pathologic correlation. *RadioGraphics* 2010;**30**(7):2001–20.
23. Oliveira PF, Sousa M, Monteiro MP, Silva B, Alves MG. Pineal gland and melatonin biosynthesis. In: *Encyclopedia of reproduction*. Elsevier; 2018. p. 465–71.
24. Kahilogullari G, Ugur HC, Comert A, Brohi RA, Ozgural O, Ozdemir M, et al. Arterial vascularization of the pineal gland. *Childs Nerv Syst* 2013;**29**(10):1835–41.
25. Møller M. Presence of a pineal nerve (nervus pinealis) in the human fetus: a light and electron microscopical study of the innervation of the pineal gland. *Brain Res* 1978;**154**(1):1–12.

26. Møller M, Baeres FM. The anatomy and innervation of the mammalian pineal gland. *Cell Tissue Res* 2002;**309**(1):139–50.
27. Møller M, Badiu C, Coculescu M. Arginine vasotocin mRNA revealed by in situ hybridization in bovine pineal gland cells. *Cell Tissue Res* 1999;**295**(2):225–9.
28. Møller M, Phansuwan-Pujito P, Badiu C. Neuropeptide Y in the adult and fetal human pineal gland. *Biomed Res Int* 2014;**2014**:1–7.
29. Møller M. Peptidergic cells in the mammalian pineal gland. Morphological indications for a paracrine regulation of the pinealocyte. *Biol Cell* 1997;**89**(9):561–7.
30. Falcón J, Guerlotté JF, Voisin P, Collin J-PH. Rhythmic melatonin biosynthesis in a photoreceptive pineal organ: a study in the pike. *Neuroendocrinology* 1987;**45**(6):479–86.
31. Perentes E, Rubinstein LJ, Herman MM, Donoso LA. *S*-Antigen immunoreactivity in human pineal glands and pineal parenchymal tumors. A monoclonal antibody study. *Acta Neuropathol* 1986;**71**(3–4):224–7.
32. Badiu C. Genetic clock of biologic rhythms. *J Cell Mol Med* 2003;**7**(4):408–16.
33. Badiu C, Badiu L, Coculescu M, Vilhardt H, Møller M. Presence of oxytocinergic neuronal-like cells in the bovine pineal gland: an immunocytochemical and in situ hybridization study. *J Pineal Res* 2001;**31**(3):273–80.
34. Oliveira PF, Sousa M, Monteiro MP, Silva B, Alves MG. Pineal gland and regulatory function. In: *Encyclopedia of reproduction*. 2nd ed. vol. 1. Elsevier; 2018. p. 472–7.
35. Cardinali D, Ladizesky MG, Boggio V, Cutrera RA, Mautalen C. Melatonin effects on bone: experimental facts and clinical perspectives. *J Pineal Res* 2003;**34**(2):81–7.
36. Cardinali D, Vigo D, Olivar N, Vidal M, Brusco L. Melatonin therapy in patients with Alzheimer's disease. *Antioxidants (Basel)* 2014;**3**(2):245–77.
37. Veerman DP, Imholz BP, Wieling W, Wesseling KH, van Montfrans GA. Circadian profile of systemic hemodynamics. *Hypertension* 1995;**26**(1):55–9.
38. Behar S, Halabi M, Reicher-Reiss H, Zion M, Kaplinsky E, Mandelzweig L, et al. Circadian variation and possible external triggers of onset of myocardial infarction. SPRINT Study Group. *Am J Med* 1993;**94**(4):395–400.
39. Zbella EA. The pineal gland. In: *Principles in medical therapy in pregnancy. Series in cognitive and neural systems,* New York, NY: Sprinder U. Springer; 1985. p. 269–71.
40. Nakade O, Koyama H, Ariji H, Yajima A, Kaku T. Melatonin stimulates proliferation and type I collagen synthesis in human bone cells in vitro. *J Pineal Res* 1999;**27**(2):106–10.
41. Sharan K, Lewis K, Furukawa T, Yadav VK. Regulation of bone mass through pineal-derived melatonin-MT2 receptor pathway. *J Pineal Res* 2017;**63**(2):1–12.
42. Yim APY, Yeung HY, Sun G, Lee KM, Ng TB, Lam TP, et al. Abnormal skeletal growth in adolescent idiopathic scoliosis is associated with abnormal quantitative expression of melatonin receptor, MT2. *Int J Mol Sci* 2013;**14**(3):6345–58.
43. Reiter RJ, Tan D-X, Manchester LC, Paredes SD, Mayo JC, Sainz RM. Melatonin and reproduction revisited. *Biol Reprod* 2009;**81**(3):445–56.
44. Tamura H, Takasaki A, Taketani T, Tanabe M, Lee L, Tamura I, et al. Melatonin and female reproduction. *J Obstet Gynaecol Res* 2014;**40**(1):1–11.
45. Borjigin J, Li X, Snyder SH. The pineal gland and melatonin: molecular and pharmacologic regulation. *Annu Rev Pharmacol Toxicol* 1999;**39**(1):53–65.
46. Benloucif S, Burgess HJ, Klerman EB, Lewy AJ, Middleton B, Murphy PJ, et al. Measuring melatonin in humans. *J Clin Sleep Med* 2008;**4**(1):66–9.
47. Borjigin J, Samantha Zhang L, Calinescu AA. Circadian regulation of pineal gland rhythmicity. *Mol Cell Endocrinol* 2012;**349**(1):13–9.
48. Arendt J. Melatonin and the pineal gland: influence on mammalian seasonal and circadian physiology. *Rev Reprod* 1998;**3**(1):13–22.
49. Arendt J, Deacon S, English J, Hampton S, Morgan L. Melatonin and adjustment to phase shift. *J Sleep Res* 1995;**4**:74–9.
50. Kovács J, Brodner W, Kirchlechner V, Arif T, Waldhauser F. Measurement of urinary melatonin: a useful tool for monitoring serum melatonin after its oral administration. *J Clin Endocrinol Metab* 2000;**85**(2):666–70.
51. Chik CL, Ho AK, Brown GM. Effect of food restriction on 24-h serum and pineal melatonin content in male rats. *Acta Endocrinol* 1987;**115**(4):507–13.
52. Moriyama Y, Hayashi M, Yamada H, Yatsushiro S, Ishio S, Yamamoto A. Synaptic-like microvesicles, synaptic vesicle counterparts in endocrine cells, are involved in a novel regulatory mechanism for the synthesis and secretion of hormones. *J Exp Biol* 2000;**203**(Pt 1):117–25.
53. Bonmati-Carrion MA, Arguelles-Prieto R, Martinez-Madrid MJ, Reiter R, Hardeland R, Rol MA, et al. Protecting the melatonin rhythm through circadian healthy light exposure. *Int J Mol Sci* 2014;**15**(12):23448–500.
54. Lee BM. Light exposure, melatonin secretion, and menstrual cycle parameters: an integrative review. *Biol Res Nurs* 2007;**9**(1):49–69.
55. Mendoza J, Challet E. Brain clocks: from the suprachiasmatic nuclei to a cerebral network. *Neuroscience* 2009;**15**(5):477–88.
56. Welsh DK, Takahashi JS, Kay SA. Suprachiasmatic nucleus: cell autonomy and network properties. *Annu Rev Physiol* 2010;**72**:551–77.
57. Kalsbeek A, Fliers E, Franke AN, Wortel J, Buijs RM. Functional connections between the suprachiasmatic nucleus and the thyroid gland as revealed by lesioning and viral tracing techniques in the rat. *Endocrinology* 2000;**141**(10):3832–41.
58. Liu T, Borjigin J. Reentrainment of the circadian pacemaker through three distinct stages. *J Biol Rhythm* 2005;**20**(5):441–50.
59. Huang Z, Liu T, Chattoraj A, Ahmed S, Wang MM, Deng J, et al. Posttranslational regulation of TPH1 is responsible for the nightly surge of 5-HT output in the rat pineal gland. *J Pineal Res* 2008;**45**(4):506–14.
60. Sun X, Deng J, Liu T, Borjigin J. Circadian 5-HT production regulated by adrenergic signaling. *Proc Natl Acad Sci* 2002;**99**(7):4686–91.
61. Liu R-Y, Zhou J-N, van Heerikhuize J, Hofman MA, Swaab DF. Decreased melatonin levels in postmortem cerebrospinal fluid in relation to aging, Alzheimer's disease, and apolipoprotein E-ε4/4 genotype [1]. *J Clin Endocrinol Metab* 1999;**84**(1):323–7.
62. Mishima K, Tozawa T, Satoh K, Matsumoto Y, Hishikawa Y, Okawa M. Melatonin secretion rhythm disorders in patients with senile dementia of Alzheimer's type with disturbed sleep-waking. *Biol Psychiatry* 1999;**45**(4):417–21.
63. Melke J, Goubran Botros H, Chaste P, Betancur C, Nygren G, Anckarsäter H, et al. Abnormal melatonin synthesis in autism spectrum disorders. *Mol Psychiatry* 2008;**13**(1):90–8.

64. Ishii H, Tanaka N, Kobayashi M, Kato M, Sakuma Y. Gene structures, biochemical characterization and distribution of rat melatonin receptors. *J Physiol Sci* 2009;**59**(1):37–47.

65. Zemkova H, Vanecek J. Dual effect of melatonin on gonadotropin-releasing-hormone-induced Ca signaling in neonatal rat gonadotropes. *Neuroendocrinology* 2001;**74**(4):262–9.

66. Ubuka T, Bentley GE. Identification, localization, and regulation of passerine GnRH-I messenger RNA. *J Endocrinol* 2009;**201**(1):81–7.

67. Tamura H, Nakamura Y, Terron MP, Flores LJ, Manchester LC, Tan DX, et al. Melatonin and pregnancy in the human. *Reprod Toxicol* 2008;**25**(3):291–303.

68. Sharkey JT, Puttaramu R, Word RA, Olcese J. Melatonin synergizes with oxytocin to enhance contractility of human myometrial smooth muscle cells. *J Clin Endocrinol Metab* 2009;**94**(2):421–7.

69. Soliman A, Lacasse AA, Lanoix D, Sagrillo-Fagundes L, Boulard V, Vaillancourt C. Placental melatonin system is present throughout pregnancy and regulates villous trophoblast differentiation. *J Pineal Res* 2015;**59**(1):38–46.

70. Rocha CS, Martins AD, Rato L, Silva BM, Oliveira PF, Alves MG. Melatonin alters the glycolytic profile of Sertoli cells: implications for male fertility. *Mol Hum Reprod* 2014;**20**(11):1067–76.

71. Rocha CS, Rato L, Martins AD, Alves MG, Oliveira PF. Melatonin and male reproductive health: relevance of darkness and antioxidant properties. *Curr Mol Med* 2015;**15**(4):299–311.

72. Kauppila A, Kivelä A, Pakarinen A, Vakkuri O. Inverse seasonal relationship between melatonin and ovarian activity in humans in a region with a strong seasonal contrast in luminosity. *J Clin Endocrinol Metab* 1987;**65**(5):823–8.

73. Lacoste V, Wetterberg L. Individual variations of rhythms in morning and evening types with special emphasis on seasonal differences. In: *Light and biological rhythms in man*. Pergamon; 1993. p. 287–304.

74. Reiter RJ, Tan DX. What constitutes a physiological concentration of melatonin? *J Pineal Res* 2003;**34**(1):79–80.

75. Abbott SM, Attarian H, Zee PC. Sleep disorders in perinatal women. *Best Pract Res Clin Obstet Gynaecol* 2014;**28**(1):159–68.

76. Suzuki S, Dennerstein L, Greenwood KM, Armstrong SM, Sano T, Satohisa E. Melatonin and hormonal changes in disturbed sleep during late pregnancy. *J Pineal Res* 1993;**15**(4):191–8.

77. Yan Z. *A study on factors affecting sleep during pregnancy in clinical trials*. 2017. p. 1167 (Arts & Sciences Electronic Theses and Dissertations). https://openscholarship.wustl.edu/art_sci_etds/1167https://doi.org/10.7936/K7ZS2VWM.

78. Bellipanni G, DI Marzo F, Blasi F, Di Marzo A. Effects of melatonin in Perimenopausal and menopausal women: our personal experience. *Ann N Y Acad Sci* 2005;**1057**(1):393–402.

79. Hăulică I, Brănişteanu D, Roşca V, Stratone A, Berbeleu V, Bălan G, et al. A renin-like activity in pineal gland and hypophysis. *Physiologie* 1975;**12**(1):21–4.

80. Hăulică I, Ianovici I, Roşca V, Ionescu G. Presence of isorenin in human pineal gland. *Endocrinologie* 1979;**17**(4):277–9.

81. Badiu C. Morphological evidence for a intrinsic angiotensin system in the bovine pineal gland. *Acta Endocrinol* 2006;**2**(4):389–401.

82. Geelen G, Allevard-Burguburu AM, Gauquelin G, Xiao YZ, Frutoso J, Gharib CL, et al. Radioimmunoassay of arginine vasopressin, oxytocin and arginine vasotocin-like material in the human pineal gland. *Peptides* 1981;**2**(4):459–66.

83. Møller M, Ravault JP, Cozzi B. The chemical neuroanatomy of the mammalian pineal gland: neuropeptides. *Neurochem Int* 1996;**28**(1):23–33.

84. Lew GM. Morphological and biochemical changes in the pineal gland in pregnancy. *Life Sci* 1987;**41**(24):2589–96.

85. Grishchenko VI, Demidenko DI, Koliada LD. Dynamics of melatonin excretion in women at the end of pregnancy, during normal labor and during the postpartum period. *Akush Ginekol (Mosk)* 1976;**5**:27–9.

86. Nakamura Y, Tamura H, Kashida S, Takayama H, Yamagata Y, Karube A, et al. Changes of serum melatonin level and its relationship to feto-placental unit during pregnancy. *J Pineal Res* 2001;**30**(1):29–33.

87. Kivelä A. Serum melatonin during human pregnancy. *Acta Endocrinol* 1991;**124**(3):233–7.

88. Okatani Y, Okamoto K, Hayashi K, Wakatsuki A, Tamura S, Sagara Y. Maternal-fetal transfer of melatonin in pregnant women near term. *J Pineal Res* 1998;**25**(3):129–34.

89. Reiter RJ, Rosales-Corral SA, Manchester LC, Tan D-X. Peripheral reproductive organ health and melatonin: ready for prime time. *Int J Mol Sci* 2013;**14**(4):7231–72.

90. Voiculescu SE, Zygouropoulos N, Zahiu CD, Zagrean AM. Role of melatonin in embryo fetal development. *J Med Life* 2014;**7**(4):488–92.

91. Voiculescu SE, Le Duc D, Roşca AE, Zeca V, Chiţimuş DM, Arsene AL, et al. Behavioral and molecular effects of prenatal continuous light exposure in the adult rat. *Brain Res* 2016;**1650**:51–9.

92. Lanoix D, Beghdadi H, Lafond J, Vaillancourt C. Human placental trophoblasts synthesize melatonin and express its receptors. *J Pineal Res* 2008;**45**(1):50–60.

93. Renshall L, Wareing M, Cowley E, Cottrell E, Sibley C, Greenwood S, et al. Melatonin supplementation during pregnancy increases fetal abdominal circumference and umbilical artery relaxation in a mouse model of fetal growth restriction. *Placenta* 2016;**45**:102–3.

94. Schander J, Bariani MV, Rubio APD, Correa F, Jensen F, Franchi AM. New strategies to prevent preterm birth. *Placenta* 2017;**51**:106–7.

95. Fernando S, Rombauts L. Melatonin: shedding light on infertility?—a review of the recent literature. *J Ovarian Res* 2014;**7**(1):1–14.

96. Cohen M, Small RA, Brzezinski A. Hypotheses: melatonin/steroid combination contraceptives will prevent breast cancer. *Breast Cancer Res Treat* 1995;**33**(3):257–64.

97. Voordouw BC, Euser R, Verdonk RE, Alberda BT, de Jong FH, Drogendijk AC, et al. Melatonin and melatonin-progestin combinations alter pituitary-ovarian function in women and can inhibit ovulation. *J Clin Endocrinol Metab* 1992;**74**(1):108–17.

98. Miller SL, Yawno T, Alers NO, Castillo-Melendez M, Supramaniam VG, VanZyl N, et al. Antenatal antioxidant treatment with melatonin to decrease newborn neurodevelopmental deficits and brain injury caused by fetal growth restriction. *J Pineal Res* 2014;**56**(3):283–94.

99. Tavakoli M. Kidney protective effects of melatonin. *J Nephropharmacol* 2014;**3**(1):7–8.

100. Zhang H-M, Zhang Y. Melatonin: a well-documented antioxidant with conditional pro-oxidant actions. *J Pineal Res* 2014;**57**(2):131–46.

101. Gilad E, Cuzzocrea S, Zingarelli B, Salzman AL, Szabó C. Melatonin is a scavenger of peroxynitrite. *Life Sci* 1997;**60**(10):PL169–74.

102. Tamura H, Takasaki A, Taketani T, Tanabe M, Kizuka F, Lee L, et al. Melatonin as a free radical scavenger in the ovarian follicle. *Endocr J* 2013;**60**(1):1–13.

103. Maldonado MD, Murillo-Cabezas F, Terron MP, Flores LJ, Tan DX, Manchester LC, et al. The potential of melatonin in reducing morbidity-mortality after craniocerebral trauma. *J Pineal Res* 2007;**42**(1):1–11.

104. Ishizuka B, Kuribayashi Y, Murai K, Amemiya A, Itoh MT. The effect of melatonin on in vitro fertilization and embryo development in mice. *J Pineal Res* 2000;**28**(1):48–51.

105. Dikic SD, Jovanovic AM, Dikic S, Jovanovic T, Jurisic A, Dobrosavljevic A. Melatonin: a "Higgs boson" in human reproduction. *Gynecol Endocrinol* 2015;**31**(2):92–101.

106. Torres-Farfan C, Rocco V, Monsó C, Valenzuela FJ, Campino C, Germain A, et al. Maternal melatonin effects on clock gene expression in a non-human primate fetus. *Endocrinology* 2006;**147**(10):4618–26.

107. Bauer M, Mazza E, Jabareen M, Sultan L, Bajka M, Lang U, et al. Assessment of the in vivo biomechanical properties of the human uterine cervix in pregnancy using the aspiration test. *Eur J Obstet Gynecol Reprod Biol* 2009;**144**:S77–81.

108. Mahoney MM. Shift work, jet lag, and female reproduction. *Int J Endocrinol* 2010;**2010**.

109. Ma N, Hardy DB. The fetal origins of the metabolic syndrome: can we intervene? *J Pregnancy* 2012;**2012**:1–11.

110. Hardeland R, Madrid JA, Tan D-X, Reiter RJ. Melatonin, the circadian multioscillator system and health: the need for detailed analyses of peripheral melatonin signaling. *J Pineal Res* 2012;**52**(2):139–66.

111. Olcese J. Circadian clocks and pregnancy. *Front Endocrinol (Lausanne)* 2014;**5**:123.

112. Reiter RJ, Tan DX, Korkmaz A, Rosales-Corral SA. Melatonin and stable circadian rhythms optimize maternal, placental and fetal physiology. *Hum Reprod Update* 2014;**20**(2):293–307.

113. Illnerová H, Buresová M, Presl J. Melatonin rhythm in human milk. *J Clin Endocrinol Metab* 1993;**77**(3):838–41.

114. Cohen Engler A, Hadash A, Shehadeh N, Pillar G. Breastfeeding may improve nocturnal sleep and reduce infantile colic: potential role of breast milk melatonin. *Eur J Pediatr* 2012;**171**(4):729–32.

115. Jouan PN, Pouliot Y, Gauthier SF, Laforest JP. Hormones in bovine milk and milk products: a survey. *Int Dairy J* 2006;**16**(11):1408–14.

116. Cubero J, Valero V, Sánchez J, Rivero M, Parvez H, Rodríguez AB, Barriga C. The circadian rhythm of tryptophan in breast milk affects the rhythms of 6-sulfatoxymelatonin and sleep in newborn. *Neuro Endocrinol Lett* 2005;**26**(6):657–61.

117. Wright J, Aldhous M, Franey C, English J, Arendt J. The effects of exogenous melatonin on endocrine function in man. *Clin Endocrinol* 1986;**24**(4):375–82.

Chapter 3

Pituitary Physiology During Pregnancy and Lactation

Raquel Soares Jallad*,†, Andrea Glezer*,†, Marcio Carlos Machado*,†,‡ and Marcello D. Bronstein*,†

*Neuroendocrine Unit, Division of Endocrinology and Metabolism, Hospital das Clínicas, University of São Paulo Medical School, São Paulo, Brazil, †Laboratory of Cellular and Molecular Endocrinology LIM-25, University of São Paulo Medical School, São Paulo, Brazil, ‡Endocrinology Service, AC Camargo Cancer Center, São Paulo, Brazil

Key Clinical Changes

- During pregnancy, the maternal pituitary gland, especially the adenohypophysis, undergoes a physiologic increase in size secondary to lactotroph hyperplasia.
- The enlargement of the anterior pituitary and reduced stores of arginine vasopressin (AVP) contribute to the bright spot of the posterior pituitary on T1-weighted magnetic resonance imaging (MRI) disappearing during pregnancy.
- Circulating maternal growth hormone (GH) levels increase, due mainly to tonic secretion of GH by the placenta, which becomes the predominant GH form in maternal blood after midpregnancy.
- Normal pregnancy is considered a state of hypercortisolism due to physiological activation of the hypothalamic-pituitary-adrenal (HPA) axis.
- Corticosteroid-binding globulin (CBG) production rises due to high levels of estradiol; in turn, serum total cortisol is increased and urinary-free cortisol increases up to threefold.
- There is a modest and transitory decrease of maternal thyrotropin (TSH) around 9–13 weeks of pregnancy, which coincides with the peak placental production of human chorionic gonadotropin (hCG).
- Pregnancy is characterized by increased total body water, expanded plasma volume, a 10-mOsm/kg decrease in serum osmolality, and a reset of the osmostat so that AVP secretion and thirst occur at a lower serum osmolality.

3.1 ANTERIOR PITUITARY GLAND

3.1.1 Introduction

During pregnancy, there is an integration of three complex and physiological neuroendocrine compartments: maternal, placental, and fetal. Each plays a critical role in maintaining the health of the embryo/fetus, placenta, and mother up to delivery. Some hormones are found circulating in nonpregnant women and others are hormones produced and released only during pregnancy. The maternal hormonal milieu is important for the establishment of a receptive endometrium, implantation, and maintenance of early pregnancy.

The pituitary gland is composed of three parts: the anterior lobe (adenohypophysis); intermediate lobe (present in many species, but involutes in humans after the first trimester of gestation, and so is absent in the adult pituitary); and posterior lobe (neurohypophysis).[1] The adenohypophysis constitutes the majority of the pituitary gland and is composed primarily of five hormone-producing cell types (thyrotropes, lactotropes, corticotropes, somatotropes, and gonadotropes), secreting thyrotropin (TSH), prolactin (PRL), adrenocorticotropin (ACTH), growth hormone (GH) and the gonadotropins (luteinizing hormone [LH] and follicle-stimulating hormone [FSH]), respectively.[1] The posterior lobe stores an antidiuretic hormone (ADH-vasopressin) and oxytocin secreted by the hypothalamic supraoptic paraventricular nucleus[1] (Fig. 3.1).

The hypothalamic-PRL axis and HPA axis are central to reproductive function, including conception, pregnancy maintenance, parturition, and breastfeeding. The PRL and ACTH levels in the maternal circulation increase throughout

Maternal-Fetal and Neonatal Endocrinology. https://doi.org/10.1016/B978-0-12-814823-5.00003-9

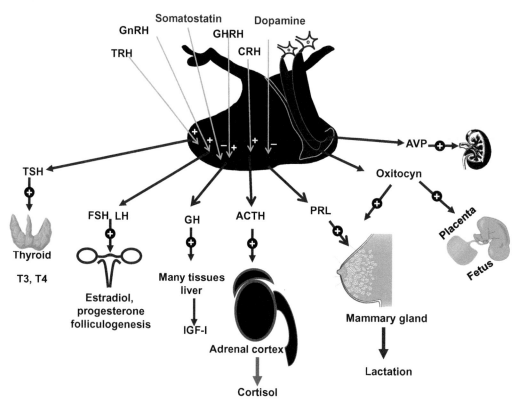

FIG. 3.1 Schematic representation of hypothalamic-pituitary hormones and their target glands and systemic actions. The hypothalamic-PRL and HPA axes are central to reproductive function, from conception to breastfeeding. The PRL and ACTH levels in the maternal circulation increase throughout pregnancy until term. Both hormones in the maternal circulation originate primarily from the maternal pituitary, with small contributions from the maternal decidua. The other maternal pituitary hormones make only minor contributions during pregnancy.

pregnancy until term. Both hormones in the maternal circulation originate primarily from the maternal pituitary, with small contributions from the maternal decidua. As for the other maternal pituitary hormones, they make only a minor contribution during pregnancy.[1] Most maternal circulant levels of GH are derived from the placenta (GH-V), with a marked reduction in maternal pituitary GH (GH-N).[2] There is a modest decline in circulating TSH levels in the first trimester, followed by normalization.[3,4] Maternal serum LH and FSH levels decreased during pregnancy and remain until term.[5] This chapter is designed to review in detail the physiological adaptations (anatomical and functional) that occur in the maternal pituitary gland in response to the demands of pregnancy.

3.1.2 Anatomical Changes in Pituitary Gland

During pregnancy, the maternal pituitary gland, especially the adenohypophysis, undergoes a physiologic increase in size that can be assessed radiologically[6–8] and histologically.[9,10]

In the nonpregnant state, the pituitary gland weighs between 0.5 and 1.0 g.[1] During pregnancy, it increases in size from the first month and continues to increase until the third semester[6–8] (Fig. 3.2). Serial cranial MRI shows an overall increase in its three dimensions, and its shape changes.[6–8] The height of the pituitary gland is correlated to gestational age.[8] The pituitary gland develops a convex, dome-shaped superior surface, which may impinge on the optic chiasm.[6–8] Usually, in normal pregnancy, the physiological pituitary enlargement does not extend above the sella to the optic chiasm. However, in some cases, pituitary enlargement can lead to bitemporal hemianopia in healthy pregnant women.[11] Comparing to the nonpregnant state, the T1 signal intensity of the adenohypophysis increases at the end of the third trimester.[6,7]

Immunohistochemical studies have shown that the cellular composition of the adenohypophysis changes during pregnancy.[9] Hyperplasia and hypertrophy of lactotrophs begin early in pregnancy and are responsible for the increase in the pituitary's size.[12,13] In nonpregnant women, lactotrophs account for 20% of the pituitary, whereas by term, they account for about 40%–60% of these cells.[9,12] Gestational hyperestrogenemia have been associated with the majority of these changes.[12] With respect to the other pituitary cells, the number of somatotrophic and gonadotrophic cells decline,

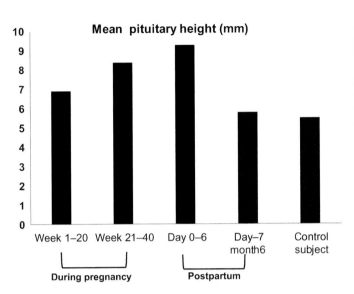

FIG. 3.2 Pituitary volumetric changes throughout pregnancy. The progressive pituitary increase is mainly due to estrogen-induced lactotroph hyperplasia. There is an increase in size and shape of the pituitary gland during pregnancy. However, in the late postpartum period, no statistically significant differences in gland size or shape could be detected compared to nonpregnant control subjects. *(Based on Elster AD, Sanders TG, Vines FS, Chen MY. Size and shape of the pituitary gland during pregnancy and post partum: measurement with MR imaging. Radiology 1991;181(2):531–5.)*

while corticotrophic and thyrotrophic cells remain stable.[9,12–14] Several weeks to months after the end of pregnancy (delivery or abortion), the number of lactotropes gradually decreases, accompanied by involution of the pituitary's size.[6,7]

3.1.3   Functional Changes of Pituitary Gland

3.1.3.1   Hypothalamic-PRL Axis

PRL is a polypeptide with a classical function to promote mammary gland differentiation during pregnancy and ensure milk production after delivery.[13–15] Lactotrophs, which are specialized cells of the anterior pituitary gland, synthesize and secrete PRL.[15] Although PRL has autocrine and paracrine actions and >300 functions,[16] its role in humans is not very well understood.

PRL, GH, and placental lactogen (PL) belong to the same protein family and share genetic, structural, binding, and functional properties.[15] The *PRL* gene, localized on chromosome 6, is composed of five exons and four introns.

PRL can be classified according to its molecular weight in three isoforms: monomeric (mPRL), dimeric or big-prolactin (bPRL), and macroprolactin or big-big prolactin (bbPRL).[17] Monomeric PRL has 199 amino acids, weighs 23 KDa, and usually accounts for 80%–95% of total serum PRL. Here, bPRL is composed of two mPRLs connected by a disulfide bond and representing about 10% of total serum PRL. Further, bbPRL usually is composed by immunoglobulin G (IgG) bound specifically to mPRL, weighs >150 KDa, and represents <5% of total serum PRL.[17,18] Macroprolactinemia occurs when bbPRL is the major circulating PRL isoform. Although gel filtration chromatography is the gold standard for macroprolactinemia diagnosis, polyethyleneglycol-(PEG) precipitation is the method of choice for screening due to lower cost and easier performance. Using PEG precipitation, about 25% of hyperprolactinemic individuals presents with macroprolactinemia.[19] Macroprolactin has low biological activity in vivo and in vitro,[16] in species-specific bioassays unless it is associated with high levels of mPRL.[20,21] It is a benign situation with no need of sellar imaging evaluation and treatment.[22,23] The pathophysiology of macroprolactinemia is not known. Some authors showed that PRL posttranslational modifications, as phosphorylation, could be involved in the generation of IgG against mPRL.[24] Autoimmunity was not associated with macroprolactinemia.[24]

Unlike all other pituitary hormones, PRL secretion is predominantly under the inhibitory control of dopamine produced by the tuberoinfundibular dopamine (TIDA) neurons, located in the arcuate nucleus of the hypothalamus.[15] Pituitary stalk integrity is crucial to maintaining the tonic dopamine inhibition over lactotrophs. There are five dopamine receptors, but only subtypes 2 (DR2) and 4 (DR4) are found in the pituitary gland.[19] Dopamine reduces PRL gene expression[25,26] reduces PRL secretion,[27] and suppresses lactotroph proliferation induced by estradiol.[26] PRL can control its own secretion in a short-loop feedback by stimulating the TIDA neurons.[15]

After systemic administration, PRL can be found in the hypothalamus, despite the fact that its high molecular weight impairs the passage through the blood brain barrier.[28] Some authors advocate that PRL reaches the brain through a saturable carrier-transport system, independent of the PRL receptor.[29]

Serum PRL increases throughout pregnancy, and hyperprolactinemia is maintained until lactation by three major changes in the regulatory pathways controlling PRL secretion. First, placental lactogen secreted by the placenta[30] activates PRL receptors, and its secretion is not under negative feedback control. Second, during late pregnancy[31] and lactation,[32] the TIDA neurons are less sensitive to PRL in the short-loop negative feedback. Third, during lactation, suckling of the nipple by the neonate increases PRL secretion due to a decrease of TIDA neuronal activity,[33] possibly associated with the release of one or more PRL releasing factors.[34] Suckling stimulates somatosensory afferent information from the nipples through the spinal cord to the hypothalamus,[35] possibly stimulating dynorphin neurons that suppress the activity of TIDA neurons via parathyroid hormone receptor 2.[36] These changes are essential for the maintenance of lactation competency.[29,37]

Moreover, PRL transport into the brain is increased during lactation, pointing to the enhancement of PRL action on the central nervous system in this period.[29,37] Animals lacking a functional PRL receptor exhibit profound deficits in expression of maternal care,[38] although animals with a disrupted PRL gene exhibit some maternal behaviors,[39] possibly through activation of PRL receptors by placental lactogen.

Hyperprolactinemia also decreases the acute stress response.[40,41] Although the site of action through which PRL mediates this action is not known, it is likely to involve the paraventricular nucleus and the HPA axis. In both males and nonpregnant female rats, PRL has dose-dependent anxiolytic actions.[41]

In several types of animals, a link between reduced maternal care and depressivelike state or alterations of emotional behavior in the offspring were reported. As the activation of oxytocin and PRL systems during lactation attenuate HPA axis activation by stress, alterations in those systems could contribute to affective disorders in the postpartum period.[42] Low levels of PRL were described in women with postpartum depressive disorder.[43] Bromocriptine administration in the early stages of pregnancy in rats reduced PRL levels and was associated with depressive-like state and impairment of maternal behavior.[44] The role of PRL in controlling maternal behavior and responses must be clarified in humans.

Estrogens play an important role in physiological hyperprolactinemia during pregnancy because they stimulate the PRL gene expression,[45] stimulate the secretion of stored PRL, cause hyperplasia in lactotrophs,[46] and inhibit the tone of TIDA neurons.[47] Moreover, many neurons express both PRL receptors and estrogen receptor alpha,[48] reinforcing estradiol's role in regulating PRL receptor expression in neurons. [49]

Pituitary enlargement in pregnancy is primarily due to estrogenic stimulation of lactotrophs; accordingly, circulating PRL levels in pregnancy have been found to correlate with estriol,[50] estradiol, and progesterone levels.[51] Lactotroph cells normally occupy about one-fifth of the pituitary but account for half of pituitary cells by the end of pregnancy. In a healthy pregnant woman, the pituitary increases in size and volume by 45% in the first trimester alone, and by the end of pregnancy, there is an overall increase of 136%[7] (Fig. 3.2). At 3 days after delivery, the maximum size of the pituitary is reached, returning to prepregnancy size by 6 months postpartum.[7] Similarly, PRL levels may increase to over 100–400 ng/mL by the end of a normal pregnancy. [52]

Hu et al. evaluated serum PRL levels by electrochemiluminescence immunoassay in 378 healthy pregnant women among the first (1–13 weeks), second (14–27 weeks), and third (≥28 weeks) trimesters.[53] PRL increased with gestational age with median levels of 78, 144, and 305 ng/mL in each trimester, reaching the highest values in the third trimester as compared to both women in other periods of pregnancy and nonpregnant women [53] (Fig. 3.3A).

During lactation, fertility is impaired, depending on the frequency and intensity of suckling episodes. In lactating rats, there is increased expression of PRL receptors in the hypothalamus, where GnRH neurons are localized.[54] It is possible that PRL is involved in the suckling-induced suppression of fertility during lactation, as hyperprolactinemia inhibits gonadotrophin secretion. On the other hand, it is possible that some threshold level of PRL may be necessary for normal reproduction. Although women with PRL levels suppressed to 5 ng/mL had no change in their pulsatile LH/FSH secretion, they had lower luteal phase progesterone and higher end of follicular phase estrogen. [55] However, there are four documented cases of patients with isolated PRL deficiency and no fertility impairments were reported, suggesting that PRL deficiency likely has no major impact on fertility.[56]

Another possible role of PRL during pregnancy and lactation is appetite stimulation. The upregulation of PRL receptor expression in lactating rats in the various hypothalamic nuclei associated with appetite regulation may enable a lactating female to be significantly more sensitive than a nonpregnant female to the orexigenic effects of PRL. Hyperprolactinemia may play an important role in the hyperphagia of pregnancy and lactation.[57]

Hyperprolactinemia stimulates appetite and feeding[58] via the paraventricular nucleus.[58] Freemark et al. demonstrated that PRL receptor-deficient mice have lower body weight and reduced fat mass compared with wild-type controls, pointing to PRL's role in the regulation of body weight[59] in the long term, whereas initial analyses did not report this finding.[60] PRL administration increased food intake in nonpregnant condition in various animal species.[29,61] Additionally, hyperprolactinemia might stimulate food intake[62] in healthy pregnancy in humans. The proposed mechanism is leptin resistance induced by PRL.[29] However, data supporting the notion that hyperprolactinemia induces increased food intake in nonpregnant women have not been reported.

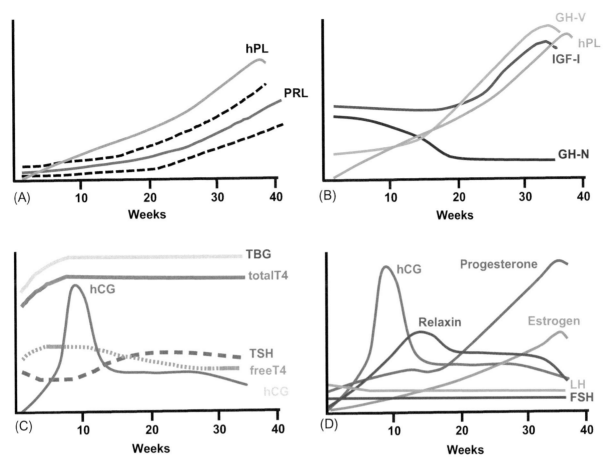

FIG. 3.3 Hormonal changes during normal pregnancy. (A) Maternal PRL axis: PRL gradually increases, mainly due to estrogen stimulation of lacto-trophs. (B) Maternal GHRH-GH-IGF-I axis: In the first trimester of healthy pregnancy, GH-N (maternal pituitary) is the predominant form in blood, decreasing progressively after week 15. During the same period, GH-V (placental) becomes detectable in maternal plasma and increases throughout the second and third trimesters, reaching maximum levels between weeks 35 and 37. In the second half of gestation, GH-N declines and by 30 weeks, its secretion is suppressed to very low values or even below the limit of detection. Thus, GH-V becomes the predominant GH, stimulating hepatic synthesis of IGF-I after midpregnancy. (C) Maternal HPT (hypothalamic-pituitary-thyroid) axis: During healthy pregnancy, there is a modest and transient decrease of maternal TSH, around 9–13 weeks of pregnancy, which coincides with the peak placental production of hCG. Thyroid function is adapted by TBG increase. Therefore, the pregnant woman remains euthyroid because although the concentration of total thyroid hormone increased, it was bound to TBG, so that its free fraction remained normal. (D) Maternal HPG (hypothalamic-pituitary-gonadal) axis: FSH and LH levels are suppressed by feedback inhibition from elevated levels of estrogen and progesterone (initially from the corpus luteum and decidua and later from the placenta), PRL (from the maternal pituitary), inhibin (from the corpus luteum and placenta), and hCG.

PRL plays a role in adipogenesis and adipocyte differentiation, modulating lipid metabolism and stimulating leptin production.[63,64] In the pancreas, PRL promotes growth of islets during fetal development and increases insulin secretion.[65,66] PRL promotes lipid mobilization from fat stores to provide fatty acids to the mammary gland,[67] thereby enhancing milk production during lactation. PRL also plays a role in carbohydrate metabolism adaptation during pregnancy by inducing the proliferation of beta cells, stimulating insulin synthesis, and lowering the glycemic threshold that stimulates insulin secretion.[62] Recently, some authors found that higher PRL levels were associated with reduced glucose tolerance in the third trimester of pregnancy in 69 healthy pregnant women, suggesting the possible independent role of PRL in the pathogenesis of gestational diabetes.[68]

3.1.3.2 GHRH-Insulin-Like Growth Factor-I Axis

The human *GH* gene family is a cluster of five highly related genes, localized in a s66-kb segment of chromosome 17 (17q22-24).[2,69–72] This locus includes five closely related genes: two genes coding for GH: *GH1* (human pituitary GH gene, pituitary GH gene, or *GH-N* gene) and *GH2* (human placental growth hormone variant, placental *GH* gene or *GH-V* gene)[2,69,70] and three genes encoding human chorionic somatomammotropins (hCS): *hCS-A* (or *CSH1*), *hCS-B* (or *CSH2*), and *hCSL* (or *CSHL1*).[71] With the exception of the *GH1* gene, the other four are expressed exclusively in the placenta. All of these genes share 91%–99% of their DNA sequences.[2,69,70]

The *GH1* gene encodes pituitary GH. There are two isoforms of different molecular weights. GH-N *22K* is the main form produced by the pituitary gland in men and nonpregnant women, and in acromegaly; it is also in a recombinant form used for GH replacement therapy. GH-N *20K* represents <10% circulating GH in normal individuals and shows a slight increase in acromegaly. GH-N isoforms are detectable only in maternal blood.[2,69,70] The *GH2* gene produces placental GH.[73,74] It is a protein containing 191 amino acids with a molecular weight of 22.3 kDa. GH-V differs in 13 amino acids from GH-N.[73] There are at least three isoforms, with weights of 22, 24, and 26 kDa.[73] GH-V binds with high affinity to GH receptors, but with low affinity to PRL receptors.[74] GH-V does not cross the placental barrier, so it is only detectable in maternal blood.[74] GH-V plays a key role in maternal adaptation to pregnancy. Maternal GH-V concentrations are closely related to fetal growth in humans.[75] GH-V has also been proposed as a potential candidate to mediate the insulin resistance observed later in pregnancy.[62,76,77]

The *hCS-A* and *hCS-B* genes are identical and encode human placental lactogen (hPL).[71,78,79] The *hCSL* gene has a high degree of homology with *hCS-A* and *hCS-B*; however, it is considered a pseudogene.[80] Further, hCS binds with high affinity to PRL receptors but with low affinity to GH receptors, suggesting that it functions largely as a lactogen rather than as a somatogen in pregnancy.[71,78] Also, hPL is a single-chain polypeptide of 191 amino acids with two disulfide bridges and has a 96% homology with hGH.[71,78]

In the first trimester of normal pregnancy, GH-N is secreted in a pulsatile fashion from the maternal anterior pituitary, as it is the predominant form in maternal blood.[2] GH-N does not cross the placenta. Thereafter, pituitary GH production decreases progressively from about week 15.[2] During the same period, nonpulsatile secretion of GH-V from the placenta becomes detectable in maternal plasma.[71,81] After 5 weeks of pregnancy, GH-V increases progressively throughout the second and third trimesters of pregnancy, reaching maximum levels between weeks 35 to 37.[71,81] In the second half of gestation, maternal GH-N declines, and by 30 weeks, its secretion is suppressed to very low values or even below the limit of detection.[82] Therefore, by the third trimester, release of GH-N in response to either insulin-induced hypoglycemia or arginine stimulation is markedly attenuated, suggesting that GH-V secretion cannot be rescued by this stimulus.[82,83] This phenomenon occurs concomitantly with increased GH-V levels. It is postulated that GH-V stimulates the secretion of hepatic IGF-I, which through the negative feedback contributes to the suppression of GH-N, such that GH-N is replaced completely by GH-V at approximately 20 weeks.[84,85] Thus, GH-V expressed by the placenta becomes the predominant GH in the mother to stimulate hepatic synthesis of IGF-I after midpregnancy[85,86] (Fig. 3.3B).

In summary, circulating maternal GH levels begin to increase at around 10 weeks' gestation, plateau at approximately 28 weeks, and can remain elevated for several months postpartum. The majority of circulating GH-like activity is derived from placental GH-V (85%), followed by placental hPL 12%) and pituitary GH-N (3%).[87]

The regulation of GH and hCS synthesis is not fully understood. It is clear that GH-V is not regulated by the same mechanisms that modulate GH-N pituitary secretion. Unlike the pulsatile secretion of GH-N, secretion of GH-V is tonic and not regulated by GH-releasing hormone (GHRH).[83] It is dependent on placental mass and thus gestational age as well.[88] GH-V also does not appear to be regulated by ghrelin.[89]

GH-N and GH-V share similar somatotrophic, lactogenic, and lipolytic properties.[77,87,89] Their binding affinities for GH-binding protein (GHBP) are similarly high.[74,90] GHBP is secreted by the liver and adipose tissue and declines gradually during the course of human pregnancy, reaching approximately 40% of prepregnant values between the first or the beginning of the second quarter and term.[74,90,91] The binding of GH to its hepatic receptor stimulates the secretion of IGF-I, the main mediator of the effects of GH.[92–94] However, GH-V binds the PRL receptor poorly, and its lactogenic affects are greatly reduced compared with GH-N.[95]

In normal pregnancy, IGF-I levels show modest reduction during the first trimester, likely due to the decrease in GH-N and to reduced hepatic sensitivity to GH caused by hyperestrogenemia of pregnancy.[95–97] During the second half of normal pregnancy (24–25 weeks), GH-N, GH-V, and IGF-I secretion changes: GH-N progressively declines, reaching undetectable levels in the third trimester, whereas GH-V secretion and IGF-I levels progressively increase up to delivery.[97] The twofold-to-threefold increase in IGF-I levels is due to GH-V stimulation, which replaces GH-N as the primary stimulus for IGF-I production during pregnancy.[77,87,89] High circulating levels of GH-V and IGF-I maintain pregnancy in a mildly acromegalic state. Normal pregnant women may exhibit some clinical features similar to those observed in patients with acromegaly, such as facial changes due to edema, paresthesias in the hands (carpal tunnel symptoms), and increased sensation in hands and feet.

3.1.3.3 HPA Axis and Pregnancy

Normal pregnancy is considered a state of hypercortisolism due to physiological activation of the HPA axis. Nevertheless, there are no specific clinical manifestations of Cushing's syndrome, such as large purple striae, proximal muscle weakness, and easy bruising.

Classically, corticotropin-releasing hormone (CRH) is synthetized in the hypothalamus. However, CRH has also been identified in thecal and stromal cells, as well as in cells of the ovarian corpora luteum.[98] The epithelial cells of the endometrium have shown CRH receptors that mediate its effects on the maturation of the fetal adrenal, fetal-placental unit, and placenta itself. The placental CRH has a molecular structure that is indistinguishable from the hypothalamic form.[99]

CRH and ACTH levels rise in the first trimester due to placental CRH and ACTH secretion. However, CRH-binding protein levels also increase during this period.[100] Because of ACTH stimulation, the maternal adrenal glands become hypertrophic. The result of these hormonal changes is a small increase of cortisol levels (serum, salivary, and urinary), which becomes more relevant as pregnancy progresses. Nevertheless, cortisol secretion maintains a pulsatile and circadian secretion.

Corticosteroid-binding globulin (CBG) production rises due to high levels of estradiol, reaching the highest levels at term. This causes an overestimation of serum total cortisol measured at plasma. However, serum-free cortisol also increases near 1.6-fold by the 11th week of normal pregnancy due to pregnancy-induced HPA activation.[101] Consequently, urinary-free cortisol increases up to threefold the nonpregnant. Value.[102] On the other hand, the placenta expresses the enzyme 11ß hydroxysteroid dehydrogenase type 2, which inactivates cortisol by converting it to cortisone, thereby protecting the fetus from high maternal cortisol levels.[103]

ACTH and cortisol responses after dynamic tests change during pregnancy. Administration of human CRH (1 µg/kg) during normal pregnancy does not cause a significant rise in ACTH and cortisol levels, as would be expected; the response to CRH improves a few weeks after delivery.[104] However, higher doses of human CRH (2 µg/kg) can produce a rise in ACTH and cortisol beginning from the third trimester.[105,106] Another alteration during pregnancy is an attenuation of the suppression of cortisol during the low-dose dexamethasone suppression test.[103]

About the fourth day postpartum, maternal CRH, ACTH, and cortisol gradually return to prepregnancy levels. The adrenal glands are suppressed, similar to early recovery of successfully operated patients with Cushing's disease, and gradually return to the prepregnancy state by 12 weeks after delivery.[107] This transient period of adrenal insufficiency might be related to mood disorders and autoimmune diseases frequently observed in postpartum women.

3.1.3.4   Hypothalamic-Pituitary-Thyroid (HPT) Axis

The hypothalamic-pituitary-thyroid axis (HPT) is responsible for controlling the synthesis and secretion of two thyroid hormones: triiodothyronine (T3) and tetraiodothyronine or thyroxine (T4).[17] Thyrotropin-releasing hormone (TRH), produced in the hypothalamus, acts on thyrotrophs of the adenohypophysis to stimulate the synthesis and release of thyroid-stimulating hormone (TSH), which stimulates the thyroid gland to secrete T4 and T3.[17] The axis is controlled by negative feedback on the hypothalamus and pituitary, which is exerted by thyroid hormones. Thyroid hormones are transported in the blood and noncovalently attached to three proteins: thyroxine-binding globulin (TBG), albumin, and transthyretin or thyroxine-binding prealbumin. TBG is the most abundant carrier protein, carrying two-thirds of T4 serum.[17] The free or metabolically active fraction represents about 0.04% of T4 and 0.5% of T3.[17]

During gestation, important changes in the physiology of the pituitary-thyroid axis occur, mainly due to the increase in chorionic gonadotrophin (hCG) and thyroxin-binding globulin (TBG) levels.[4,108–111] The most striking change in the first trimester is suppression of TSH, which coincides with increased levels of hCG. This hormone increases in early pregnancy, peaks between the 9th and 13th week of gestation, and then normalizes at up to 20 weeks gestation.[4,108–112] It is secreted by the placenta and presents homology with TSH, in its alpha subunit. In this way, hCG acts as a stimulating hormone of the thyroid gland.[113] This thyrotrophic action of hCG was recognized in a case report of hyperplacentosis.[114] In this instance, the normal pregnant woman with increased placental volume, high values of hCG, and hyperthyroidism, saw a resolution of the postpartum hyperthyroidism only, with a hysterectomy.[114] In general, the thyrotrophic action of hCG is transient and there is no need for treatment. This is because after the first trimester, there is a reduction in hCG levels and an increase in TSH levels. Normal values of TSH are observed at the beginning of the second trimester and remain within normal range until term[4,108–111] (Fig. 3.3C).

The increase in TBG also favors TSH normalization. In the first trimester, elevated estrogen levels increase serum concentrations of TBG. This increase occurs both by the direct stimulation of its production and by the production of the sialized isoform protein, which degrades less rapidly in the liver.[108] As a consequence, there is an increase in total T4 and T3 concentrations. The rapid and marked increase in TBG (two times the normal level) is accompanied by a tendency to reduce T4 and free T3 and stimulation of the HPT axis.[108,110] Changes in free T3 and T4 levels are mild and transient and are not usually detected in routine exams[108,110] (Fig. 3.3C).

In summary, in gestation, the normal TSH response to TRH is generally preserved.[108,110] During the first trimester, hCG stimulates maternal thyroid function, resulting in an increased production of thyroid hormones which, through negative feedback, decrease TSH. Even during the first trimester, elevated levels of TBG lead to a decrease in the levels of free T3 and free T4, and consequently an increase in TSH. At the end of the first trimester, there is a reduction in hCG levels. Therefore, the decrease in TSH is mild and transient once the increase of TBG and the reduction of hCG favor the return of the TSH values to normal levels, which remain stable until the moment of delivery. Thyroid function adapts to the increase in TBG. Therefore, the normal pregnant woman remains euthyroid because although the concentration of total thyroid hormone has increased, most of it is bound to TBG; however, the free fraction remains normal[108,110] (Fig. 3.3C).

3.1.3.5 Hypothalamic-Pituitary-Gonadal (HPG) Axis

At the beginning of each cycle, when menstruation occurs, there is pituitary release of small amounts of FSH and LH (small pulses), which together cause the growth and maturation of the ovarian follicles.[17] The growth of these follicles induces the increase of estrogen production. This is secreted at an increasing rate, stimulating endometrial proliferation, and reaches its peak approximately in the middle of the cycle.[17] High estrogen concentration initially reduces the pulse of LH and FSH and then causes a sudden increase (a preovulatory outbreak) of these two hormones, stimulating ovulation (follicle rupture and egg release).[17] After ovulation, the residual elements of the ruptured follicle form the development of the corpus luteum-secreting estrogen and high amounts of progesterone in order to maintain gestation until the placenta can assume this function.[17]

When the fertilization occurs during the menstrual cycle, the embryo reaches the uterus and the placenta secretes a hormone called human chorionic gonadotropin (hCG), which prevents degeneration of the corpus luteum.[17] This has the function of maintaining the production of progesterone and estrogen, hormones critical to the maintenance of pregnancy. The placenta quickly begins to synthesize estrogen and progesterone, which gradually replace the hormones secreted by the corpus luteum. This serves to prevent ovulation.[17]

The ovarian production of these hormones inhibited the pituitary production of LH and FSH, preventing the stimulation of new ovarian follicles and, consequently, ovulation throughout the gestation period. There is, therefore, a blockage of the menstrual cycle. At the end of pregnancy, the corpus luteum disintegrates and decreases the amount of progesterone, causing the contraction of the uterus that facilitates the expulsion of the fetus during childbirth. After delivery, a new menstrual cycle begins, as can be seen in Fig. 3.3D.

Immunohistochemical studies show a reduction of gonadotrophic cells during pregnancy, which normalizes at 1 year after delivery.[17] Decreased pituitary responsiveness to GnRH is observed in parallel with a decrease in basal gonadotropin levels, starting from 6 to 7 weeks and remaining undetectable into the puerperium.[115,116] All these changes are due to feedback inhibition from elevated circulating levels of estrogen and progesterone (initially from the corpus luteum and decidua and later from the placenta), PRL (from the maternal pituitary), inhibin (from the corpus luteum and placenta), and hCG [may also have a direct suppressive effect on LH (but not FSH) secretion][115,116] (Fig. 3.3D).

Immunohistochemical studies show a reduction of gonadotrophic cells during pregnancy, which normalizes at 1 year after delivery.[9]

After delivery, the serum concentrations of these suppressive substances fall, and consequently, maternal gonadotropin secretion resumes, along with responsiveness to GnRH.[115,116] The LH and FSH responses to GnRH stimulation are actually exaggerated in the second postpartum month before returning to normal.[115,116]

3.1.3.6 Posterior Pituitary Gland

Antidiuretic hormone (ADH-arginine-vasopressin) and oxytocin are produced in the hypothalamus and stored in the neurohypophysis. The human placenta does not allow the passage of oxytocin and ADH.

Water balance is controlled by thirst and the secretion of AVP, which in turn is primarily regulated by serum osmolality. In pregnancy, water metabolism is altered, with increased total body water and an expanded plasma volume (>1.5 times normal), while serum osmolality physiologically decreases by 10 mOsm/kg compared to nonpregnant women. Thus, the osmolar threshold for AVP secretion deviates to a lower level, which may be due to chorionic gonadotrophin resetting the fixed point of the osmostat. Moreover, the thirst threshold decreases in pregnancy. Hence, AVP secretion and thirst occur at a lower serum osmolality.[117–119]

Physiologically, there is a real increase of AVP levels during pregnancy, aiming to maintain sufficient antidiuretic activity and fluid balance. However, the plasma levels of AVP during pregnancy are similar to nonpregnant levels due to threefold-to-fourfold increased metabolic clearance. This increased clearance is caused by a placental enzyme called vasopressinase, which degrades both AVP and oxytocin. The level of this enzyme increases 1000-fold during pregnancy, and its physiological role is unknown. Additionally, a marked increase in the production of renal prostaglandin E2 and glomerular filtration rate may contribute to increase in urinary output.[119]

During pregnancy, oxytocin is also produced by the amnion, chorion, and decidua.[120,121] Serum oxytocin concentrations increase gradually during gestation and reach peak values after labor begins, remaining elevated until the fetus is expelled.[122,120] Its half-life is 1–3 min, with plasma removal performed primarily by the kidneys and liver and by the breast tissue.[122,120] During pregnancy, there is a plasma inactivation of oxytocin by the placental enzyme oxytocinase, which increases exponentially, reaching its peak value at the end of pregnancy.[122,120] Therefore, oxytocinase acts as a physiological regulator of plasma oxytocin levels in pregnant women.[122,120] Oxytocin acts through oxytocin receptors.[123,124] When pregnancy begins, there are no receptors in the uterus for oxytocin.[123,124] These receptors appear gradually during pregnancy. When oxytocin binds to them, it causes contraction of the uterine smooth muscle, as well as stimulation of prostaglandin production by the uterus, which will activate the uterine smooth muscle.[123,124]

Labor depends on both the secretion of oxytocin and the production of prostaglandins because without them, there will not be adequate dilatation of the cervix and consequently, labor will not progress normally.[123–125] The triggering factors of labor are not well known, but it is established that when the fetal hypothalamus reaches a certain degree of maturation, it stimulates the fetal pituitary to release ACTH. This hormone acts on the adrenal fetus, increasing the secretion of cortisol and other hormones, which stimulate the placenta to secrete prostaglandins.[125] There are possible inhibitory factors of labor, such as the estrogen/progesterone ratio and the level of relaxin, a hormone produced by the corpus luteum of the ovary and the placenta.[125,126]

Progesterone maintains its high levels throughout pregnancy, being one of the factors responsible for maintaining the state of uterine quiescence throughout pregnancy. Among the various effects of progesterone, we can highlight the following: decreased estrogen receptors, inhibition of oxytocin synthesis, decreased gap junction formation, increased beta receptor synthesis, decreased intracellular calcium, and increased calcium in the sarcoplasmic vessels. Estrogen, in turn, unlike progesterone, increases intracellular actin and myosin synthesis, gap junction formation in the myometrium, and synthesis of oxytocin and prostaglandin (prostaglandin F2-alpha) receptors. Additionally, estrogens act directly on myometrial cells, increasing sensitivity to oxytocin. In the last stage of pregnancy, estrogen tends to increase more than progesterone, increasing the estrogen/progesterone ratio and, consequently, the expression of oxytocin receptors by myometrial cells, as well as their sensitivity to oxytocin.[126]

The level of relaxin increases to the maximum before giving birth and then falls rapidly. It increases the number of receptors for oxytocin. Thus, at the end of gestation, the gravid uterus is susceptible to the contractile action of oxytocin. The primary stimulus for the release of oxytocin is the mechanical distension of the cervix caused by the passage of the fetus. There is stimulation of the sensory nerve endings of the birth canal wall and reflex release of oxytocin, which significantly potentiates the uterine contractions, making them faster, more coordinated, and more intense until the labor is completed. Therefore, the greater participation of oxytocin would not be manifest in the physiological induction of labor, but in the expulsion of the fetus and the placenta.[126]

For the milk ejection, a second endocrine mechanism is also involved, originating from the suction of the newborn and leading to pulsatile oxytocin secretion from the neurophypophysis.[40] This stimulates the contraction of the myoepithelial cell network in the alveoli and in the small mammary ducts, promoting milk outflow.[40]

Milk ejection is performed by the stimulation of oxytocin in the myoepithelial cells that surround the breast alveoli and contract, causing milk excretion.[40] Oxytocin also acts in the smooth muscle cells in the breast, promoting compression of the breast and erection of the papilla—events that contribute to the mechanism of milk ejection.[40]

REFERENCES

1. Melmed S. *Williams textbook of endocrinology.* 13th ed. Philadelphia, PA: Elsevier; 2016.
2. Frankenne F, Closset J, Gomez F, Scippo ML, Smal J, Hennen G. The physiology of growth hormones (GHs) in pregnant women and partial characterization of the placental GH variant. *J Clin Endocrinol Metab* 1988;**66**(6):1171–80.
3. Ballabio M, Poshychinda M, Ekins RP. Pregnancy-induced changes in thyroid function: role of human chorionic gonadotropin as putative regulator of maternal thyroid. *J Clin Endocrinol Metab* 1991;**73**(4):824–31.
4. Grün JP, Meuris S, De Nayer P, Glinoer D. The thyrotrophic role of human chorionic gonadotrophin (hCG) in the early stages of twin (versus single) pregnancies. *Clin Endocrinol (Oxf)* 1997;**46**(6):719–25.
5. Fowler PA, Evans LW, Groome NP, Templeton A, Knight PG. A longitudinal study of maternal serum inhibin-A, inhibin-B, activin-A, activin-AB, pro-alphaC and follistatin during pregnancy. *Hum Reprod* 1998;**13**(12):3530–6.
6. Gonzalez JG, Elizondo G, Saldivar D, Nanez H, Todd LE, Villarreal JZ. Pituitary gland growth during normal pregnancy: an in vivo study using magnetic resonance imaging. *Am J Med* 1988;**85**(2):217–20.
7. Dinç H, Esen F, Demirci A, Sari A, Resit Gümele H. Pituitary dimensions and volume measurements in pregnancy and post partum. *MR assessment Acta Radiol* 1998;**39**(1):64–9.
8. Elster AD, Sanders TG, Vines FS, Chen MY. Size and shape of the pituitary gland during pregnancy and post partum: measurement with MR imaging. *Radiology* 1991;**181**(2):531–5.
9. Scheithauer BW, Sano T, Kovacs KT, Young WF, Ryan N, Randall RV. The pituitary gland in pregnancy: a clinicopathologic and immunohistochemical study of 69 cases. *Mayo Clin Proc* 1990;**65**(4):461–74.

10. Hinshaw DB, Hasso AN, Thompson JR, Davidson BJ. High resolution computed tomography of the post partum pituitary gland. *Neuroradiology* 1984;**26**(4):299–301.

11. Park AJ, Haque T, Danesh-Meyer HV. Visual loss in pregnancy. *Surv Ophthalmol* 2000;**45**(3):223–30.

12. Goluboff LG, Ezrin C. Effect of pregnancy on the somatotroph and the prolactin cell of the human adenohypophysis. *J Clin Endocrinol Metab* 1969;**29**(12):1533–8.

13. Asa SL, Penz G, Kovacs K, Ezrin C. Prolactin cells in the human pituitary. A quantitative immunocytochemical analysis. *Arch Pathol Lab Med* 1982;**106**(7):360–3.

14. Hennighausen L, Robinson GW. Information networks in the mammary gland. *Nat Rev Mol Cell Biol* 2005;**6**(9):715–25.

15. Freeman ME, Kanyicska B, Lerant A, Nagy G. Prolactin: structure, function, and regulation of secretion. *Physiol Rev* 2000;**80**(4):1523–631.

16. Goffin V, Binart N, Touraine P, Kelly PA. Prolactin: the new biology of an old hormone. *Annu Rev Physiol* 2002;**64**:47–67.

17. Melmed S, Polonsky KS, Larsen PR, Kronenberg H. *Williams textbook of endocrinology.* 13th ed. Philadelphia, PA: Elsevier; 2016.

18. Suh HK, Frantz AG. Size heterogeneity of human prolactin in plasma and pituitary extracts. *J Clin Endocrinol Metab* 1974;**39**(5):928–35.

19. Hattori N, Ishihara T, Saiki Y, Shimatsu A. Macroprolactinaemia in patients with hyperprolactinaemia: composition of macroprolactin and stability during long-term follow-up. *Clin Endocrinol (Oxf)* 2010;**73**(6):792–7.

20. Bronstein MD. Editorial: is macroprolactinemia just a diagnostic pitfall? *Endocrine* 2012;**41**(2):169–70.

21. Glezer A, Soares CR, Vieira JG, Giannella-Neto D, Ribela MT, Goffin V, et al. Human macroprolactin displays low biological activity via its homologous receptor in a new sensitive bioassay. *J Clin Endocrinol Metab* 2006;**91**(3):1048–55.

22. Gibney J, Smith TP, McKenna TJ. The impact on clinical practice of routine screening for macroprolactin. *J Clin Endocrinol Metab* 2005;**90** (7):3927–32.

23. Hauache OM, Rocha AJ, Maia AC, Maciel RM, Vieira JG. Screening for macroprolactinaemia and pituitary imaging studies. *Clin Endocrinol (Oxf)* 2002;**57**(3):327–31.

24. Shimatsu A, Hattori N. Macroprolactinemia: diagnostic, clinical, and pathogenic significance. *Clin Dev Immunol* 2012;**2012**:167132.

25. Valerio A, Belloni M, Gorno ML, Tinti C, Memo M, Spano P. Dopamine D2, D3, and D4 receptor mRNA levels in rat brain and pituitary during aging. *Neurobiol Aging* 1994;**15**(6):713–9.

26. Ishida M, Mitsui T, Yamakawa K, Sugiyama N, Takahashi W, Shimura H, et al. Involvement of cAMP response element-binding protein in the regulation of cell proliferation and the prolactin promoter of lactotrophs in primary culture. *Am J Physiol Endocrinol Metab* 2007;**293**(6):E1529–37.

27. Lledo PM, Legendre P, Zhang J, Israel JM, Vincent JD. Effects of dopamine on voltage-dependent potassium currents in identified rat lactotroph cells. *Neuroendocrinology* 1990;**52**(6):545–55.

28. Brown RS, Kokay IC, Herbison AE, Grattan DR. Distribution of prolactin-responsive neurons in the mouse forebrain. *J Comp Neurol* 2010;**518** (1):92–102.

29. Grattan DR. 60 YEARS OF NEUROENDOCRINOLOGY: the hypothalamo-prolactin axis. *J Endocrinol* 2015;**226**(2):T101–22.

30. Soares MJ, Müller H, Orwig KE, Peters TJ, Dai G. The uteroplacental prolactin family and pregnancy. *Biol Reprod* 1998;**58**(2):273–84.

31. Grattan DR, Averill RL. Absence of short-loop autoregulation of prolactin during late pregnancy in the rat. *Brain Res Bull* 1995;**36**(4):413–6.

32. Arbogast LA, Voogt JL. The responsiveness of tuberoinfundibular dopaminergic neurons to prolactin feedback is diminished between early lactation and midlactation in the rat. *Endocrinology* 1996;**137**(1):47–54.

33. Selmanoff M, Gregerson KA. Suckling decreases dopamine turnover in both medial and lateral aspects of the median eminence in the rat. *Neurosci Lett* 1985;**57**(1):25–30.

34. Nagy G, Mulchahey JJ, Smyth DG, Neill JD. The glycopeptide moiety of vasopressin-neurophysin precursor is neurohypophysial prolactin releasing factor. *Biochem Biophys Res Commun* 1988;**151**(1):524–9.

35. Berghorn KA, Le WW, Sherman TG, Hoffman GE. Suckling stimulus suppresses messenger RNA for tyrosine hydroxylase in arcuate neurons during lactation. *J Comp Neurol* 2001;**438**(4):423–32.

36. Dobolyi A, Dimitrov E, Palkovits M, Usdin TB. The neuroendocrine functions of the parathyroid hormone 2 receptor. *Front Endocrinol (Lausanne)* 2012;**3**:121.

37. Grattan DR. Behavioural significance of prolactin signalling in the central nervous system during pregnancy and lactation. *Reproduction* 2002;**123** (4):497–506.

38. Lucas BK, Ormandy CJ, Binart N, Bridges RS, Kelly PA. Null mutation of the prolactin receptor gene produces a defect in maternal behavior. *Endocrinology* 1998;**139**(10):4102–7.

39. Horseman ND, Zhao W, Montecino-Rodriguez E, Tanaka M, Nakashima K, Engle SJ, et al. Defective mammopoiesis, but normal hematopoiesis, in mice with a targeted disruption of the prolactin gene. *EMBO J* 1997;**16**(23):6926–35.

40. Carter DA, Lightman SL. Oxytocin responses to stress in lactating and hyperprolactinaemic rats. *Neuroendocrinology* 1987;**46**(6):532–7.

41. Torner L, Toschi N, Pohlinger A, Landgraf R, Neumann ID. Anxiolytic and anti-stress effects of brain prolactin: improved efficacy of antisense targeting of the prolactin receptor by molecular modeling. *J Neurosci* 2001;**21**(9):3207–14.

42. Torner L. Actions of prolactin in the brain: from physiological adaptations to stress and neurogenesis to psychopathology. *Front Endocrinol (Lausanne)* 2016;**7**:25.

43. Abou-Saleh MT, Ghubash R, Karim L, Krymski M, Bhai I. Hormonal aspects of postpartum depression. *Psychoneuroendocrinology* 1998;**23** (5):465–75.

44. Larsen CM, Grattan DR. Prolactin, neurogenesis, and maternal behaviors. *Brain Behav Immun* 2012;**26**(2):201–9.

45. Lieberman ME, Maurer RA, Claude P, Wiklund J, Wertz N, Gorski J. Regulation of pituitary growth and prolactin gene expression by estrogen. *Adv Exp Med Biol* 1981;**138**:151–63.

46. Nolan LA, Levy A. The trophic effects of oestrogen on male rat anterior pituitary lactotrophs. *J Neuroendocrinol* 2009;**21**(5):457–64.

47. Morel GR, Carón RW, Cónsole GM, Soaje M, Sosa YE, Rodríguez SS, et al. Estrogen inhibits tuberoinfundibular dopaminergic neurons but does not cause irreversible damage. *Brain Res Bull* 2009;**80**(6):347–52.
48. Furigo IC, Kim KW, Nagaishi VS, Ramos-Lobo AM, de Alencar A, Pedroso JA, et al. Prolactin-sensitive neurons express estrogen receptor-α and depend on sex hormones for normal responsiveness to prolactin. *Brain Res* 2014;**1566**:47–59.
49. Lerant A, Freeman ME. Ovarian steroids differentially regulate the expression of PRL-R in neuroendocrine dopaminergic neuron populations: a double label confocal microscopic study. *Brain Res* 1998;**802**(1–2):141–54.
50. Ferriani RA, Silva-de-Sá MF, de-Lima-Filho EC. A comparative study of longitudinal and cross-sectional changes in plasma levels of prolactin and estriol during normal pregnancy. *Braz J Med Biol Res* 1986;**19**(2):183–8.
51. Ylikorkala O, Kivinen S, Reinilä M. Serial prolactin and thyrotropin responses to thyrotropin-releasing hormone throughout normal human pregnancy. *J Clin Endocrinol Metab* 1979;**48**(2):288–92.
52. Bajwa SK, Bajwa SJ, Mohan P, Singh A. Management of prolactinoma with cabergoline treatment in a pregnant woman during her entire pregnancy. *Indian J Endocrinol Metab* 2011;**15**(Suppl 3):S267–70.
53. Hu Y, Ding Y, Yang M, Xiang Z. Serum prolactin levels across pregnancy and the establishment of reference intervals. *Clin Chem Lab Med* 2018;**56**(5):803–7.
54. Pi X, Grattan DR. Expression of prolactin receptor mRNA is increased in the preoptic area of lactating rats. *Endocrine* 1999;**11**(1):91–8.
55. Molitch ME. Endocrinology in pregnancy: management of the pregnant patient with a prolactinoma. *Eur J Endocrinol* 2015;**172**(5):R205–13.
56. Cocks Eschler D, Javanmard P, Cox K, Geer EB. Prolactinoma through the female life cycle. *Endocrine* 2018;**59**(1):16–29.
57. Moore BJ, Brasel JA. One cycle of reproduction consisting of pregnancy, lactation or no lactation, and recovery: effects on fat pad cellularity in ad libitum-fed and food-restricted rats. *J Nutr* 1984;**114**(9):1560–5.
58. Sauvé D, Woodside B. Neuroanatomical specificity of prolactin-induced hyperphagia in virgin female rats. *Brain Res* 2000;**868**(2):306–14.
59. Freemark M, Fleenor D, Driscoll P, Binart N, Kelly P. Body weight and fat deposition in prolactin receptor-deficient mice. *Endocrinology* 2001;**142**(2):532–7.
60. Bole-Feysot C, Goffin V, Edery M, Binart N, Kelly PA. Prolactin (PRL) and its receptor: actions, signal transduction pathways and phenotypes observed in PRL receptor knockout mice. *Endocr Rev* 1998;**19**(3):225–68.
61. Perez Millan MI, Luque GM, Ramirez MC, Noain D, Ornstein AM, Rubinstein M, et al. Selective disruption of dopamine D2 receptors in pituitary lactotropes increases body weight and adiposity in female mice. *Endocrinology* 2014;**155**(3):829–39.
62. Newbern D, Freemark M. Placental hormones and the control of maternal metabolism and fetal growth. *Curr Opin Endocrinol Diabetes Obes* 2011;**18**(6):409–16.
63. Ben-Jonathan N, Hugo ER, Brandebourg TD, LaPensee CR. Focus on prolactin as a metabolic hormone. *Trends Endocrinol Metab* 2006;**17**(3):110–6.
64. Carré N, Binart N. Prolactin and adipose tissue. *Biochimie* 2014;**97**:16–21.
65. Freemark M, Avril I, Fleenor D, Driscoll P, Petro A, Opara E, et al. Targeted deletion of the PRL receptor: effects on islet development, insulin production, and glucose tolerance. *Endocrinology* 2002;**143**(4):1378–85.
66. Brelje TC, Stout LE, Bhagroo NV, Sorenson RL. Distinctive roles for prolactin and growth hormone in the activation of signal transducer and activator of transcription 5 in pancreatic islets of langerhans. *Endocrinology* 2004;**145**(9):4162–75.
67. Barber MC, Clegg RA, Finley E, Vernon RG, Flint DJ. The role of growth hormone, prolactin and insulin-like growth factors in the regulation of rat mammary gland and adipose tissue metabolism during lactation. *J Endocrinol* 1992;**135**(2):195–202.
68. Ekinci EI, Torkamani N, Ramchand SK, Churilov L, Sikaris KA, Lu ZX, et al. Higher maternal serum prolactin levels are associated with reduced glucose tolerance during pregnancy. *J Diabetes Investig* 2017;**8**(5):697–700.
69. Barsh GS, Seeburg PH, Gelinas RE. The human growth hormone gene family: structure and evolution of the chromosomal locus. *Nucleic Acids Res* 1983;**11**(12):3939–58.
70. Hirt H, Kimelman J, Birnbaum MJ, Chen EY, Seeburg PH, Eberhardt NL, et al. The human growth hormone gene locus: structure, evolution, and allelic variations. *DNA* 1987;**6**(1):59–70.
71. Jacquemin P, Oury C, Peers B, Morin A, Belayew A, Martial JA. Characterization of a single strong tissue-specific enhancer downstream from the three human genes encoding placental lactogen. *Mol Cell Biol* 1994;**14**(1):93–103.
72. Igout A, Van Beeumen J, Frankenne F, Scippo ML, Devreese B, Hennen G. Purification and biochemical characterization of recombinant human placental growth hormone produced in Escherichia coli. *Biochem J* 1993;**295**(Pt. 3):719–24.
73. Scippo ML, Frankenne F, Hooghe-Peters EL, Igout A, Velkeniers B, Hennen G. Syncytiotrophoblastic localization of the human growth hormone variant mRNA in the placenta. *Mol Cell Endocrinol* 1993;**92**(2):R7–13.
74. Baumann G, Dávila N, Shaw MA, Ray J, Liebhaber SA, Cooke NE. Binding of human growth hormone (GH)-variant (placental GH) to GH-binding proteins in human plasma. *J Clin Endocrinol Metab* 1991;**73**(6):1175–9.
75. Daughaday WH, Trivedi B, Winn HN, Yan H. Hypersomatotropism in pregnant women, as measured by a human liver radioreceptor assay. *J Clin Endocrinol Metab* 1990;**70**(1):215–21.
76. MacLeod JN, Worsley I, Ray J, Friesen HG, Liebhaber SA, Cooke NE. Human growth hormone-variant is a biologically active somatogen and lactogen. *Endocrinology* 1991;**128**(3):1298–302.
77. Liao S, Vickers MH, Stanley JL, Ponnampalam AP, Baker PN, Perry JK. The placental variant of human growth hormone reduces maternal insulin sensitivity in a dose-dependent manner in C57BL/6J mice. *Endocrinology* 2016;**157**(3):1175–86.
78. Handwerger S, Freemark M. The roles of placental growth hormone and placental lactogen in the regulation of human fetal growth and development. *J Pediatr Endocrinol Metab* 2000;**13**(4):343–56.

79. Parks JS, Nielsen PV, Sexton LA, Jorgensen EH. An effect of gene dosage on production of human chorionic somatomammotropin. *J Clin Endocrinol Metab* 1985;**60**(5):994–7.

80. Misra-Press A, Cooke NE, Liebhaber SA. Complex alternative splicing partially inactivates the human chorionic somatomammotropin-like (hCS-L) gene. *J Biol Chem* 1994;**269**(37):23220–9.

81. Eriksson L, Frankenne F, Edèn S, Hennen G, Von Schoultz B. Growth hormone 24-h serum profiles during pregnancy—lack of pulsatility for the secretion of the placental variant. *Br J Obstet Gynaecol* 1989;**96**(8):949–53.

82. Lønberg U, Damm P, Andersson AM, Main KM, Chellakooty M, Lauenborg J, et al. Increase in maternal placental growth hormone during pregnancy and disappearance during parturition in normal and growth hormone-deficient pregnancies. *Am J Obstet Gynecol* 2003;**188**(1):247–51.

83. de Zegher F, Vanderschueren-Lodeweyckx M, Spitz B, Faijerson Y, Blomberg F, Beckers A, et al. Perinatal growth hormone (GH) physiology: effect of GH-releasing factor on maternal and fetal secretion of pituitary and placental GH. *J Clin Endocrinol Metab* 1990;**71**(2):520–2.

84. Eriksson L, Frankenne F, Edèn S, Hennen G, von Schoultz B. Growth hormone secretion during termination of pregnancy. Further evidence of a placental variant. *Acta Obstet Gynecol Scand* 1988;**67**(6):549–52.

85. Caufriez A, Frankenne F, Englert Y, Golstein J, Cantraine F, Hennen G, et al. Placental growth hormone as a potential regulator of maternal IGF-I during human pregnancy. *Am J Physiol* 1990;**258**(6 Pt. 1):E1014–9.

86. Igout A, Frankenne F, L'Hermite-Balériaux M, Martin A, Hennen G. Somatogenic and lactogenic activity of the recombinant 22 kDa isoform of human placental growth hormone. *Growth Regul* 1995;**5**(1):60–5.

87. Chen EY, Liao YC, Smith DH, Barrera-Saldaña HA, Gelinas RE, Seeburg PH. The human growth hormone locus: nucleotide sequence, biology, and evolution. *Genomics* 1989;**4**(4):479–97.

88. Freemark M. Placental hormones and the control of fetal growth. *J Clin Endocrinol Metab* 2010;**95**(5):2054–7.

89. Fuglsang J, Skjaerbaek C, Espelund U, Frystyk J, Fisker S, Flyvbjerg A, et al. Ghrelin and its relationship to growth hormones during normal pregnancy. *Clin Endocrinol (Oxf)* 2005;**62**(5):554–9.

90. Massa G. Growth hormone-binding proteins during human pregnancy: maternal, fetal and neonatal data. *Proc Soc Exp Biol Med* 1994;**206**(3):316–9.

91. McIntyre HD, Serek R, Crane DI, Veveris-Lowe T, Parry A, Johnson S, et al. Placental growth hormone (GH), GH-binding protein, and insulin-like growth factor axis in normal, growth-retarded, and diabetic pregnancies: correlations with fetal growth. *J Clin Endocrinol Metab* 2000;**85**(3):1143–50.

92. Chellakooty M, Vangsgaard K, Larsen T, Scheike T, Falck-Larsen J, Legarth J, et al. A longitudinal study of intrauterine growth and the placental growth hormone (GH)-insulin-like growth factor I axis in maternal circulation: association between placental GH and fetal growth. *J Clin Endocrinol Metab* 2004;**89**(1):384–91.

93. Corbacho AM, Martínez De La Escalera G, Clapp C. Roles of prolactin and related members of the prolactin/growth hormone/placental lactogen family in angiogenesis. *J Endocrinol* 2002;**173**(2):219–38.

94. Ryan EA, Enns L. Role of gestational hormones in the induction of insulin resistance. *J Clin Endocrinol Metab* 1988;**67**(2):341–7.

95. Verhaeghe J. Does the physiological acromegaly of pregnancy benefit the fetus? *Gynecol Obstet Invest* 2008;**66**(4):217–26.

96. Hills FA, English J, Chard T. Circulating levels of IGF-I and IGF-binding protein-1 throughout pregnancy: relation to birthweight and maternal weight. *J Endocrinol* 1996;**148**(2):303–9.

97. Persechini ML, Gennero I, Grunenwald S, Vezzosi D, Bennet A, Caron P. Decreased IGF-1 concentration during the first trimester of pregnancy in women with normal somatotroph function. *Pituitary* 2015;**18**(4):461–4.

98. Lindsay JR, Jonklaas J, Oldfield EH, Nieman LK. Cushing's syndrome during pregnancy: personal experience and review of the literature. *J Clin Endocrinol Metab* 2005;**90**(5):3077–83.

99. Carr BR, Parker CR, Madden JD, MacDonald PC, Porter JC. Maternal plasma adrenocorticotropin and cortisol relationships throughout human pregnancy. *Am J Obstet Gynecol* 1981;**139**(4):416–22.

100. Behan DP, Linton EA, Lowry PJ. Isolation of the human plasma corticotrophin-releasing factor-binding protein. *J Endocrinol* 1989;**122**(1):23–31.

101. Demey-Ponsart E, Foidart JM, Sulon J, Sodoyez JC. Serum CBG, free and total cortisol and circadian patterns of adrenal function in normal pregnancy. *J Steroid Biochem* 1982;**16**(2):165–9.

102. Jung C, Ho JT, Torpy DJ, Rogers A, Doogue M, Lewis JG, et al. A longitudinal study of plasma and urinary cortisol in pregnancy and postpartum. *J Clin Endocrinol Metab* 2011;**96**(5):1533–40.

103. Odagiri E, Ishiwatari N, Abe Y, Jibiki K, Adachi T, Demura R, et al. Hypercortisolism and the resistance to dexamethasone suppression during gestation. *Endocrinol Jpn* 1988;**35**(5):685–90.

104. Schulte HM, Weisner D, Allolio B. The corticotrophin releasing hormone test in late pregnancy: lack of adrenocorticotrophin and cortisol response. *Clin Endocrinol (Oxf)* 1990;**33**(1):99–106.

105. Linton EA, Perkins AV, Hagan P, Poole S, Bristow AF, Tilders F, et al. Corticotrophin-releasing hormone (CRH)-binding protein interference with CRH antibody binding: implications for direct CRH immunoassay. *J Endocrinol* 1995;**146**(1):45–53.

106. Suda T, Iwashita M, Ushiyama T, Tozawa F, Sumitomo T, Nakagami Y, et al. Responses to corticotropin-releasing hormone and its bound and free forms in pregnant and nonpregnant women. *J Clin Endocrinol Metab* 1989;**69**(1):38–42.

107. Pivonello R, De Martino MC, Auriemma RS, Alviggi C, Grasso LF, Cozzolino A, et al. Pituitary tumors and pregnancy: the interplay between a pathologic condition and a physiologic status. *J Endocrinol Invest* 2014;**37**(2):99–112.

108. Glinoer D. The regulation of thyroid function in pregnancy: pathways of endocrine adaptation from physiology to pathology. *Endocr Rev* 1997;**18**(3):404–33.

109. Glinoer D. Increased TBG during pregnancy and increased hormonal requirements. *Thyroid* 2004;**14**(6):479–80. [author reply 80-1].

110. Glinoer D. Personal considerations on the 2011 American thyroid association and the 2007 endocrine society pregnancy and thyroid disease guidelines. *Thyroid* 2011;**21**(10):1049–51.

111. Ye X, Shi L, Huang H. Longitudinal study about the function of pituitary-thyroid axis in pregnancy. *Zhonghua Fu Chan Ke Za Zhi* 2001;**36**(9):527–30.

112. Nisula BC, Ketelslegers JM. Thyroid-stimulating activity and chorionic gonadotropin. *J Clin Invest* 1974;**54**(2):494–9.

113. Yoshimura M, Nishikawa M, Yoshikawa N, Horimoto M, Toyoda N, Sawaragi I, et al. Mechanism of thyroid stimulation by human chorionic gonadotropin in sera of normal pregnant women. *Acta Endocrinol* 1991;**124**(2):173–8.

114. Ginsberg J, Lewanczuk RZ, Honore LH. Hyperplacentosis: a novel cause of hyperthyroidism. *Thyroid* 2001;**11**(4):393–6.

115. Szymańska K, Kałafut J, Rivero-Müller A. The gonadotropin system, lessons from animal models and clinical cases. *Minerva Ginecol* 2018;**70**(5):561–87.

116. Ntali G, Capatina C, Grossman A, Karavitaki N. Clinical review: functioning gonadotroph adenomas. *J Clin Endocrinol Metab* 2014;**99**(12):4423–33.

117. Wallia A, Bizhanova A, Huang W, Goldsmith SL, Gossett DR, Kopp P. Acute diabetes insipidus mediated by vasopressinase after placental abruption. *J Clin Endocrinol Metab* 2013;**98**(3):881–6.

118. Marques P, Gunawardana K, Grossman A. Transient diabetes insipidus in pregnancy. *Endocrinol Diabetes Metab Case Rep* 2015;**2015**.

119. Kalelioglu I, Kubat Uzum A, Yildirim A, Ozkan T, Gungor F, Has R. Transient gestational diabetes insipidus diagnosed in successive pregnancies: review of pathophysiology, diagnosis, treatment, and management of delivery. *Pituitary* 2007;**10**(1):87–93.

120. Prevost M, Zelkowitz P, Tulandi T, Hayton B, Feeley N, Carter CS, et al. Oxytocin in pregnancy and the postpartum: relations to labor and its management. *Front Public Health* 2014;**2**:1.

121. Chibbar R, Miller FD, Mitchell BF. Synthesis of oxytocin in amnion, chorion, and decidua may influence the timing of human parturition. *J Clin Invest* 1993;**91**(1):185–92.

122. Fuchs AR, Romero R, Keefe D, Parra M, Oyarzun E, Behnke E. Oxytocin secretion and human parturition: pulse frequency and duration increase during spontaneous labor in women. *Am J Obstet Gynecol* 1991;**165**(5 Pt. 1):1515–23.

123. Blanks AM, Shmygol A, Thornton S. Regulation of oxytocin receptors and oxytocin receptor signaling. *Semin Reprod Med* 2007;**25**(1):52–9.

124. Romero R, Sibai BM, Sanchez-Ramos L, Valenzuela GJ, Veille JC, Tabor B, et al. An oxytocin receptor antagonist (atosiban) in the treatment of preterm labor: a randomized, double-blind, placebo-controlled trial with tocolytic rescue. *Am J Obstet Gynecol* 2000;**182**(5):1173–83.

125. Findlay AL. The control of parturition. *Res Reprod* 1972;**4**(5). Chart.

126. Vannuccini S, Bocchi C, Severi FM, Challis JR, Petraglia F. Endocrinology of human parturition. *Ann Endocrinol (Paris)* 2016;**77**(2):105–13.

Chapter 4

Thyroid Physiology During Pregnancy, Postpartum, and Lactation

Kirsten E. Salmeen* and Ingrid J. Block-Kurbisch[†,‡,§]

*Department of Obstetrics and Gynecology, Kaiser Permanente, San Francisco, CA, United States, [†]Department of Medicine, University of California, San Francisco, CA, United States, [‡]Department of Obstetrics and Gynecology, University of California, San Francisco, CA, United States, [§]Department of Medicine, St. Mary's Medical Center, Dignity Health, San Francisco, CA, United States

> **Key Clinical Changes in Pregnancy**
> - Increased estradiol level
> - Transient human chorionic gonadotropin (hCG)-mediated stimulation of thyroid gland
> - Increased thyroid-binding globulin (TBG)
> - Suppressed and subsequently rising thyroid-stimulating hormone (TSH)
> - Increased saturation of TBG with thyroid hormone
> - Decreased free thyroid hormone
> - Increased iodine clearance and need

4.1 INTRODUCTION

The maternal thyroid gland must adapt rapidly after conception to accommodate the sudden increase in maternal metabolic needs and to deliver thyroid hormone to the developing fetus. An adequate maternal thyroid response soon after conception is among the more critical maternal physiologic adaptations to pregnancy, and changes in maternal thyroid function are observed in very early pregnancy (within the first month). Among other functions, thyroid hormone is necessary to produce changes in maternal cardiac output and blood volume, fat stores, cholesterol metabolism, and synthesis of pituitary hormones—all of which undergo dramatic changes during pregnancy. Moreover, for the first 10–12 weeks of pregnancy until its own thyroid gland begins to function, the embryo/fetus is dependent upon the maternal thyroid hormone to drive metabolic activity (most critically, axonal growth, myelination, and cell differentiation within the brain and central nervous system).

The primary expected, normal, and physiologic changes in thyroid function that occur after conception include a substantial increase in TGB; substantial increases in total T3 and T4, which require adequate iodine concentrations to produce; and a first-trimester reduction in TSH, or thyrotropin.[1] These changes are driven by increased estrogen levels and by the presence of hCG, which closely resembles TSH in structure and thus has weak TSH-like activity.[2]

For healthcare providers who care for women during pregnancy, knowledge about the normal, physiological changes in thyroid function is necessary to avoid overdiagnosing hyperthyroidism or underdiagnosing subclinical hypothyroidism, both common errors made by practitioners who are unfamiliar with normal thyroid function during pregnancy. Such errors can result in substantial anxiety for patients and their families, and they are easily avoided by understanding the normal response of the thyroid gland during pregnancy.

4.2 PREGNANCY

4.2.1 Early Adaptation of Thyroid Function

The changes that occur within the HPT axis to adapt to pregnancy are geared toward increasing the available supply of thyroid hormones—thyroxine (T4) and triiodothyronine (T3)—to accommodate increased maternal and fetal demands.

As is the case outside of pregnancy as well, under healthy conditions, there is a tightly regulated balance of thyroid hormone concentrations, which is mediated by negative inhibition by the thyroid hormones, thyroid hormone-binding globulins and activity of deiodinases.[3]

The thyroid hormones have receptors in most organ systems of the body and mediate essentially all metabolic functions. Under usual circumstances, the production and release of thyroid hormones from the thyroid gland are stimulated by thyroid-stimulating hormone (TSH or thyrotropin), which is released from the anterior pituitary gland. TSH release is regulated by thyrotropin-releasing hormone (TRH), which is emitted from the hypothalamus. The thyroid hormones give negative feedback at the level of both the hypothalamus and pituitary, inhibiting secretion of TRH and TSH, respectively. TSH regulates essentially all steps in the production and release of thyroid hormones, including signaling the uptake of iodine needed to produce hormones, hormone synthesis, and hormone release.[3]

Thyroid hormones are synthesized in the thyroid gland by iodination of tyrosine residues on thyroglobulin, a process known as *organification*. The iodine required for the synthesis of thyroid hormones is obtained from the diet. Iodide is consumed and oxidized to iodine by the enzyme thyroid peroxidase (TPO). Iodination of specific tyrosine molecules yields monoiodinated tyrosine (MIT) and diiodinated tyrosine (DIT). Coupling of MIT to DIT or vice versa by the enzyme thyroid peroxidase (TPO) makes triiodothyronine (T3) and tetraiodothyronine (T4, which is synonymous with thyroxine). T3, and T4 are released directly into circulation from the thyroid gland. Although T3 exhibit considerably greater activity due to an approximately 100-fold higher affinity for thyroid receptors as compared to T4, the thyroid releases primarily T4. The majority of available T3 in circulation is generated by conversion of T4 to T3 by type 2 deiodinase (D2). >99% of thyroid hormone in circulation is bound to thyroid hormone-binding globulins, including thyroxine-binding globulin (TBG), trans-thyretin, and albumin. Only 0.03% of T4 and 0.3% of T3 circulate in free form. Upregulation and downregulation of these binding hormones, especially TBG, play an important role in the early thyroidal response to pregnancy.

Conception is associated with two primary hormonal changes that drive the thyroidal response to pregnancy: increased estrogen concentrations and synthesis of hCG from the placenta.[4] The effects of these hormonal changes on thyroid function are described later in this chapter. Other changes include increased maternal plasma volume and renal blood flow with increased glomerular filtration, which leads to increased renal clearance of iodine. Additionally, there is transplacental loss of iodine. Peripheral thyroid hormone metabolism is enhanced as a result of increased transfer to the feto-placental unit and by placental deiodination (Table 4.1).

In women who have adequate iodine stores and normal thyroid function, the thyroid is readily able to adapt to pregnancy with minimal increase in the size of the gland (10%–20%).[5,6]

The recognition of thyroid enlargement as an early indication of pregnancy dates to ancient Egypt and has been well described by many authors since then. Placing a ribbon around a woman's neck each morning and waiting until it broke or no longer fit completely was used as a pregnancy test.[7,8]

Measurement of thyroid hormones in healthy pregnancies is typically notable for a transient first-trimester decline in TSH, followed by a slight increase in basal TSH values and a marginal decrease (10%–15%) in free T3 and T4 levels[9] (Fig. 4.1). Although variation from a woman's nonpregnant thyroid function is expected during pregnancy, and the range of normal values change, most healthy pregnant women maintain TSH and free T3/T4 levels within the expected non-pregnant ranges. The most profound thyroid response to pregnancy can be detected in measurements of total T3 and T4, which increase by 30%–100%.[10]

TABLE 4.1 Factors contributing to adaptation of thyroid function in pregnancy

Maternal physiologic changes	Effect
Increased estradiol level	Increased TBG level with decreased clearance Increased Total T4/T3 levels Decreased Free T4/T3 levels
hCG stimulation of thyroid gland	Thyroid volume increase Increased TH production Decreased TSH in early pregnancy
Increased plasma volume and GFR Transplacental transfer of Iodine	Increased renal clearance of iodine Fetal thyroid hormone production
Transplacental transfer of T4 Placental diodination of T4	Increased peripheral metabolism of T4 Rise in TSH in the second half of gestation

Maternal thyroid hormones

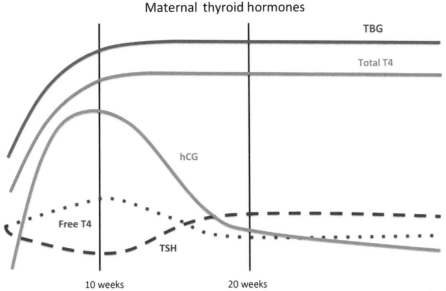

FIG. 4.1 Adaptation of maternal thyroid function in pregnancy. *(Modified from Burrow GN, Fisher DA, Larsen PR. Maternal and fetal thyroid function. N Engl J Med 1994;331(16):1072–8.)*

4.2.2 Role of Iodine, Beta-HCG, and TBG

4.2.2.1 *Iodine*

In healthy, nonpregnant adults, total iodine content is approximately 15–20 mg, with >70% contained within the thyroid gland.[11] Within the gastrointestinal tract, dietary iodine is converted to the iodide ion, which is absorbed very efficiently (>90%). When the dietary iodine supply is adequate, <20% of absorbed iodine is taken up by the thyroid gland, and >90% is eventually excreted in urine, making urinary iodine concentration (UIC) the best measure of recent iodine intake.[12,13] The iodine content of foods is determined by the iodine content of soil, which varies across the world.[11] Common sources of nonsupplemented dietary iodine include seaweed, certain types of fish, and eggs. However, the bulk of dietary iodine comes from supplemented foods, including iodized salt, cereals, and pastas. Many multivitamin dietary supplements (including many prenatal vitamins) also contain iodine.

Although the salivary glands are also able to concentrate iodine in saliva,[14] the main physiologically identified role of iodine is the synthesis of thyroid hormones, and thus, dietary requirements for iodine are determined by T4 needs. If iodine content is inadequate, the thyroid cannot generate adequate thyroid hormones. In adults, iodine deficiency can result in goiter, hypothyroidism, and impaired mental function. For fetuses and young children, the implications of iodine deficiency can include increased mortality and permanent cognitive disability. In fact, iodine deficiency is the leading cause of potentially preventable cognitive disability worldwide.[1] Severe iodine deficiency during pregnancy (defined as a population median UIC < 50 μg/L)[15] can result in fetal demise or cretinism (severe restriction of growth and cognitive development). Mild and moderate deficiency (defined by a population median UIC of 50–150 μg/L)[15] can result in fetal growth restriction and increased rates of speech and hearing deficits and cognitive disability.[13] Fortunately, in response to initiatives to increase the availability of iodized salt by the World Health Organization (WHO) over the past 30 years, there has been a substantial reduction in rates of congenital cretinism and associated low cognitive function.[13] The simple intervention of iodizing salt has been associated with an estimated 75% reduction in low intelligence.[16]

For nonpregnant adults, both the U.S. Institute of Medicine (IOM) and the WHO recommend an average iodine intake of 150 μg/day.[17] In pregnancy, however, iodine requirements increase >50% owing to the increased need for thyroid hormones to meet both maternal and fetal demands, iodine transfer to the fetus, and increased renal clearance due to increased glomerular filtration.[18] Although most women living in iodine-replete countries and following a typical diet have adequate dietary iodine intake, iodine supplementation is recommended for all pregnant women to ensure appropriate iodine concentrations to allow for adequate thyroid hormone production. The U.S. Department of Health and Human Services recommends a daily iodine intake of 220 μg. The WHO and the American Thyroid Association recommend a slightly higher amount (250 μg/day).[17,19]

Importantly, excessive iodine intake also can have deleterious effects on fetuses during pregnancy. Most adults tolerate excessive iodine intake due to a homeostatic mechanism called the *Wolff-Chaikoff effect*, which inhibits organification and the release of thyroid hormones following ingestion of a large iodine load.[20] In normal adults, escape from the Wolff-Chaikoff effect occurs after several days, and normal thyroid hormone production resumes.[21] However, fetuses have an immature Wolff-Chaikoff effect and thus can become hypothyroid if maternal iodine intake is chronically excessive. This may occur among women who have been advised that iodine is an important supplement during pregnancy and who inadvertently oversupplement. Cases of fetal goiter and hypothyroidism caused by excessive maternal iodine intake have been reported.[22] The American Thyroid Association recommends avoiding sustained dietary iodine supplementation exceeding 500 µg/day.[15]

In summary, appropriate iodine intake during pregnancy is critical for the formation of normal concentrations of thyroid hormones. All pregnant women should consume between 220 and 500 µg/day of dietary iodine.

4.2.2.2 Human Chorionic Gonadotropin

Pregnancy is heralded by the placental formation of hCG, known as "the pregnancy hormone." HCG is detectable in maternal plasma approximately 7 days after ovulation, corresponding with blastocyst implantation and doubles approximately every 48 h until it peaks at approximately 100,000 mIU/mL. Also, hCG levels begin to decline after approximately 10 weeks and reach a nadir of approximately 10,000 mIU/mL at approximately 15 weeks.

There is significant structural overlap between hCG and the anterior pituitary hormones, including luteinizing hormone, follicle-stimulating hormone, and TSH. These glycoprotein hormones share the same alpha subunit and have unique beta subunits (both urine and serum pregnancy tests rely on detection of the beta-subunit of hCG to identify when a pregnancy has been conceived).

The structural overlap between hCG and TSH, as well as similarities in hCG and TSH receptors, result in the ability of hCG to act like TSH and weakly stimulate TSH receptors, with a potency of approximately 1/1000 that of TSH.[23] During the first trimester, hCG activity is associated with partial inhibition of the pituitary-thyroid axis, with a transient lowering of serum TSH. Changes in serum TSH are linearly and inversely related to concentrations of hCG.[5] Inhibition of the pituitary-thyroid axis by hCG acts to increase thyroid hormone production, which has been quantified in studies of pregnant women with varying levels of hCG. A 10,000 IU/L increase in hCG has been associated with a 0.6-pmol/L increase in T4 and a 0.1-mU/mL reduction in TSH.[7] Typically, this hCG-mediated increase in thyroid hormone production is fairly mild and is not clinically detectable with an abnormal TSH or elevated free T3/T4. However, in approximately 20% of normal pregnant women, TSH may be transiently suppressed to below the lower limit of normal.[24] Assuming that the patient is asymptomatic and free T4 levels are normal, it is important that these women not be diagnosed with hyperthyroidism as this normal, physiologic response to pregnancy will spontaneously resolve as hCG levels decline and the parental anxiety associated with a diagnosis is unnecessary. Follow-up TSH levels can be obtained later in pregnancy to reassure patients and providers that there is no clinically important thyroid disorder.

Rarely, gestational thyrotoxicosis (defined by suppressed TSH and increased free T4) can occur in women with exceptionally high hCG levels (as may occur in women with molar pregnancies or multiples).[25]

4.2.2.3 Thyroxine-Binding Globulin

There is a rapid and marked increase in serum TBG, driven by estradiol, which occurs soon after conception and is maintained until the end of pregnancy. During menstrual cycles, when a woman does not conceive, estrogen levels fall rapidly after ovulation. However, when conception occurs, estrogen levels remain elevated. Increased estrogen levels drive increased production of TBG by the liver. Elevated estrogen levels also result in increased sialylation (the process whereby sialic acid groups are added to a molecule), which in turn reduces hepatic clearance and prolongs the half-life of TBG.[26] These factors result in at least a twofold increase in TBG concentrations, from approximately 15 mg/L to approximately 30 mg/L. This increase occurs very soon after conception and plateaus by 12–14 weeks, after which time a new pregnant-state thyroid hormone homeostasis has been established.[2] Increased serum TBG results in a slight reduction of free T3 and T4, which reduces inhibition at the level of the hypothalamus and pituitary, resulting in increased release of TSH and driving increased production of thyroid hormones.[9]

4.2.3 Uteroplacental Transport

Maternal physiologic changes in thyroid function have been well established since the 1980s. Mechanisms of uteroplacental transport of thyroid hormones, on the other hand, remain less well understood. In a sentinel paper published in

1989, Vulsma and colleagues concluded that there is placental transfer of maternal thyroid hormones by demonstrating serum T4 levels at 20%–50% of maternal levels in infants born with thyroid agenesis.[27] Furthermore, thyroid hormone has been identified in amniotic fluid before fetal thyroid production commences at around 18 weeks.[28]

Three deiodinases catalyze deiodination of the thyroid hormones in human tissue—namely, type 1 (D1), type 2 (D2), and type 3 (D3). D2 converts T4 to T3 and D3 inactivates T3 by converting it to T2 or T4 by converting it to reverse T3 (which is inactive). Both D2 and D3 are expressed within the human placenta and act to control the concentration of maternal thyroid hormone that is transported.[2] To date, six thyroid hormone transport proteins have been identified in placental tissue. In addition to the synthesis of deiodinases and transport proteins, the placenta synthesizes thyroid hormone distributor proteins, including transthyretin, albumin, alpha-1 antitrypsin, and alpha-1-acid glycoprotein.[29] These proteins likely also play a key role in maintaining appropriate levels of thyroid hormone in the fetus.[30]

Fetal thyroid hormone production starts at approximately 18 weeks; thus, maternal to fetal transport of iodine is necessary. Although the precise mechanisms of iodine transport have not been completely elucidated, there is evidence that the placenta is able to store iodine in a concentration-dependent manner.[31] Additionally, sodium-iodide symporters (which simultaneously transport sodium and iodide ions from extracellular fluid into cells via active transport) and pendrin (an ion exchanger expressed in many types of cells) have been identified in human placental trophoblasts.[32–35] Sodium-iodide symporters have also been identified in mammary gland tissue, resulting in the secretion of iodine in breast milk, which is critical for neonatal hormone synthesis.[36]

Although there is more to be learned about the specific details of uteroplacental transport of iodine and maternal thyroid hormones, it is clear that there are a number of redundant mechanisms that operate with a high degree of precision to maintain appropriate levels of both iodine and thyroid hormone in the developing fetus.

4.2.4 Implications for Fetal Neurodevelopment

In 1888, the Clinical Society of London reported the association of hypothyroidism with intellectual abnormalities and stressed the importance of the thyroid gland in assuring normal brain development.[37] As described previously, iodine deficiency (or, rarely, iodine excess) resulting in hypothyroidism is a leading cause of congenital disability worldwide. Clinically significant hypothyroidism from any cause during pregnancy has been associated with cognitive disability in offspring. These effects are likely because thyroid receptors are widely distributed throughout the fetal brain and nervous system. Thyroid hormone appears to regulate processes associated with terminal brain differentiation, such as dendritic and axonal growth, synaptogenesis, neuronal migration, and myelination.[38] Induced hypothyroidism in rats leads to diminished synthesis of messenger ribonucleic acid (mRNA) for several myelin-associated proteins.[39]

The specific clinical effects of hypothyroidism during pregnancy are described in Chapter 19.

4.2.5 Trimester-Specific TFTs and Interpretation

Generally, for most healthy women, thyroid function tests (TFTs) remain close to or within the normal ranges during pregnancy.[9] With the exception of a transiently reduced TSH in the first trimester, any substantial departure from normal thyroid function values warrants further follow-up to ensure that there is no clinically significant thyroid disease.

As described previously, a minor downward shift in TSH is expected with an anticipated 0.1–0.2 mU/L reduction in the lower limit of normal and a 0.5–1.0 mU/L reduction in the upper limit of normal.[15] This reduction is most notable during the first trimester, when the HPT axis is suppressed by hCG. Up to 20% of healthy women with normal pregnancies may have a TSH that is undetectable. Importantly, free T3 and free T4 should remain within the normal range for these women. While most studied populations demonstrate a reduction in TSH, there is variability by race/ethnicity.[40–43]

Importantly, assays used to measure free T4 may be less accurate during pregnancy due to changes in binding proteins. Increases in TBG and decreases in albumin concentrations may cause immunoassays used in commercial labs to be unreliable.[44]

As a consequence of these factors, the American Thyroid Association recommends that when possible, population-based, trimester-specific, and laboratory-specific reference ranges for TFT should be used.[15] When these values are not available, an upper value of 2.5–3.0 for TSH is recommended (Table 4.2). Additionally, measuring total T4 (using a trimester-specific reference range) can be more reliable than measuring free T4 when highly accurate measurement of T4 is needed (as may be the case for isolated hypothyroxinemia or other conditions described in Chapter 19).

TABLE 4.2 Normal thyroid function values during pregnancy in iodine-sufficient populations[15,53,54]

	First trimester	Second trimester	Third trimester
TSH (mU/mL)	0.1–2.5	0.2–3.0	0.3–3.0
Free T4 (ng/dL)	0.8–1.2	0.6–1.0	0.5–0.8
Total T4 (mcg/dL)	6.5–10.1	7.5–10.3	6.3–9.7
Free T3 (pg/mL)	4.1–4.4	4.0–4.2	Not reported
Total T3 (ng/dL)	97–149	123–162	Not reported
TBG (mg/dL)	1.8–3.2	2.8–4.0	2.6–4.2

4.3 POSTPARTUM PERIOD AND LACTATION

The rate of normalization of thyroid hormone function to prepregnancy levels is not well described. However, the hormonal milieu that drives changes in the HPT axis normalizes quickly postpartum (e.g., estrogen levels rapidly return to prepregnancy levels). Further, thyroid hormone requirements for the mother return to prepregnancy requirements. However, the prevalence of thyroid disease (particularly postpartum thyroiditis and Graves' disease) are increased postpartum. Additionally, although it is not found in most women with postpartum depression, some studies have suggested an association between postpartum depression and hypothyroidism and inferred from the evidence that treatment may improve depressive symptoms.[45–48]

Normal values for thyroid hormones during lactation are also not well described, although one small study demonstrated an increase in TSH from pregnancy values and a reduction in total and free T4 from pregnancy values in lactating women. A wide range of values were compatible with successful breastfeeding, although thyroid disorders have been associated with low milk supply and abnormal letdown, and circulating T3 and T4 are correlated with milk production.[49,50] Additionally, animal studies have demonstrated that induced hypothyroidism decreases milk supply.[51,52] The American Thyroid Association recommends that women experiencing poor lactation without another identified cause should have their TSH measured, and also suggests treating both subclinical and overt hypothyroidism, given the potential impact on milk supply and letdown.[15]

Adequate iodine intake during breastfeeding is also critical in order to transmit appropriate amounts of iodine to the baby for thyroid hormone production. Inadequate iodine intake among breastfeeding mothers can result in neonatal hypothyroidism and developmental abnormalities in neonates. The recommended daily allowance of iodine for breastfeeding women is 290 μg.[15]

REFERENCES

1. Organization WH. Indicators for assessing iodine deficiency disorders and their control programmes. In: *Report of a Joint WHO/UNICEF/ICCIDD consultation.* Geneva: WHO; 1993.
2. Burrow GN, Fisher DA, Larsen PR. Maternal and fetal thyroid function. *N Engl J Med* 1994;**331**(16):1072–8.
3. Molina P. *Endocrine physiology.* 5th ed. McGraw-Hill Education; 2018.
4. Glinoer D. The regulation of thyroid function in pregnancy: pathways of endocrine adaptation from physiology to pathology. *Endocr Rev* 1997;**18**(3):404–33.
5. Glinoer D, de Nayer P, Bourdoux P, Lemone M, Robyn C, van Steirteghem A, et al. Regulation of maternal thyroid during pregnancy. *J Clin Endocrinol Metab* 1990;**71**(2):276–87.
6. Berghout A, Wiersinga W. Thyroid size and thyroid function during pregnancy: an analysis. *Eur J Endocrinol* 1998;**138**(5):536–42.
7. Belchetz PE. Thyroid disease in pregnancy. *Br Med J* 1987;**294**(6567):264–5.
8. Forbes TR. Early pregnancy and fertility tests. *Yale J Biol Med* 1957;**30**(1):16–29.
9. Glinoer D. What happens to the normal thyroid during pregnancy? *Thyroid* 1999;**9**(7):631–5.
10. Guillaume J, Schussler GC, Goldman J. Components of the total serum thyroid hormone concentrations during pregnancy: high free thyroxine and blunted thyrotropin (TSH) response to TSH-releasing hormone in the first trimester. *J Clin Endocrinol Metab* 1985;**60**(4):678–84.
11. Zimmermann MB. The effects of iodine deficiency in pregnancy and infancy. *Paediatr Perinat Epidemiol* 2012;**26**(Suppl. 1):108–17.
12. Zimmermann MB, Jooste PL, Pandav CS. Iodine-deficiency disorders. *Lancet* 2008;**372**(9645):1251–62.
13. World Health Organization. Dept. of Nutrition for Health and Development ICfCoIDD, UNICEF. *Assessment of iodine deficiency disorders and monitoring their elimination: a guide for programme managers.* 2nd ed. Geneva: World Health Organization; 2012.

14. Venturi S, Venturi M. Iodine in evolution of salivary glands and in oral health. *Nutr Health* 2009;**20**(2):119–34.
15. Alexander EK, Pearce EN, Brent GA, Brown RS, Chen H, Dosiou C, et al. Guidelines of the american thyroid association for the diagnosis and management of thyroid disease during pregnancy and the postpartum. *Thyroid* 2017;**27**(3):315–89.
16. N A MA, V C TW. *Effect and safety of salt iodization to prevent iodine deficiency disorders: a systematic review with meta-analyses*. Geneva: WHO eLibrary of Evidence for Nutrition Actions (eLENA); 2014.
17. Micronutrients IoMPo. *Dietary reference intakes for vitamin A, vitamin K, arsenic, boron, chromium, copper, iodine, iron, manganese, molybdenum, nickel, silicon, vanadium, and zinc.* Washington, DC: National Academies Press (US) Copyright 2001 by the National Academy of Sciences; 2001. All rights reserved.
18. Glinoer D. Pregnancy and iodine. *Thyroid* 2001;**11**(5):471–81.
19. Andersson M, de Benoist B, Delange F, Zupan J. Prevention and control of iodine deficiency in pregnant and lactating women and in children less than 2-years-old: conclusions and recommendations of the technical consultation. *Public Health Nutr* 2007;**10**(12a):1606–11.
20. Wolff J, Chaikoff IL. Plasma inorganic iodide as a homeostatic regulator of thyroid function. *J Biol Chem* 1948;**174**(2):555–64.
21. Eng PH, Cardona GR, Fang SL, Previti M, Alex S, Carrasco N, et al. Escape from the acute Wolff-Chaikoff effect is associated with a decrease in thyroid sodium/iodide symporter messenger ribonucleic acid and protein. *Endocrinology* 1999;**140**(8):3404–10.
22. Thomas JV, Collett-Solberg PF. Perinatal goiter with increased iodine uptake and hypothyroidism due to excess maternal iodine ingestion. *Horm Res* 2009;**72**(6):344–7.
23. Yamazaki K, Sato K, Shizume K, Kanaji Y, Ito Y, Obara T, et al. Potent thyrotropic activity of human chorionic gonadotropin variants in terms of 125I incorporation and de novo synthesized thyroid hormone release in human thyroid follicles. *J Clin Endocrinol Metab* 1995;**80**(2):473–9.
24. Glinoer D, De Nayer P, Robyn C, Lejeune B, Kinthaert J, Meuris S. Serum levels of intact human chorionic gonadotropin (HCG) and its free alpha and beta subunits, in relation to maternal thyroid stimulation during normal pregnancy. *J Endocrinol Invest* 1993;**16**(11):881–8.
25. Grun JP, Meuris S, De Nayer P, Glinoer D. The thyrotropic role of human chorionic gonadotropin in the early stages of twin (versus single) pregnancies. *Clin Endocrinol Oxf Jun* 1997;**46**(6 SRC—BaiduScholar):719–25.
26. Ain KB, Mori Y, Refetoff S. Reduced clearance rate of thyroxine-binding globulin (TBG) with increased sialylation: a mechanism for estrogen-induced elevation of serum TBG concentration. *J Clin Endocrinol Metab* 1987;**65**(4):689–96.
27. Vulsma T, Gons MH, de Vijlder JJ. Maternal-fetal transfer of thyroxine in congenital hypothyroidism due to a total organification defect or thyroid agenesis. *N Engl J Med* 1989;**321**(1):13–6.
28. Calvo RM, Jauniaux E, Gulbis B, Asunción M, Gervy C, Contempré B, et al. Fetal tissues are exposed to biologically relevant free thyroxine concentrations during early phases of development. *J Clin Endocrinol Metab* 2002;**87**(4):1768–77.
29. McKinnon B, Li H, Richard K, Mortimer R. Synthesis of thyroid hormone binding proteins transthyretin and albumin by human trophoblast. *J Clin Endocrinol Metab* 2005;**90**(12):6714–20.
30. Landers K, Richard K. Traversing barriers—how thyroid hormones pass placental, blood-brain and blood-cerebrospinal fluid barriers. *Mol Cell Endocrinol* 2017;**458**:22–8.
31. Burns R, Azizi F, Hedayati M, Mirmiran P, O'Herlihy C, Smyth PPA. Is placental iodine content related to dietary iodine intake? *Clin Endocrinol (Oxf)* 2011;**75**(2):261–4.
32. Dohan O, De la Vieja A, Paroder V, Riedel C, Artani M, Reed M. The sodium/iodide symporter (NIS): characterization, regulation and medical significance. *Endocr Rev Feb* 2003;**24**(1 SRC—BaiduScholar):48–77.
33. Burns R, O'Herlihy C, Smyth PPA. Regulation of iodide uptake in placental primary cultures. *Eur Thyroid J* 2013;**2**(4):243–51.
34. Bidart JM, Lacroix L, Evain-Brion D, Caillou B, Lazar V, Frydman R, et al. Expression of Na+/I- symporter and Pendred syndrome genes in trophoblast cells. *J Clin Endocrinol Metab* 2000;**85**(11):4367–72.
35. Mitchell AM, Manley SW, Morris JC, Powell KA, Bergert ER, Mortimer RH. Sodium iodide symporter (NIS) gene expression in human placenta. *Placenta* 2001;**22**(2–3):256–8.
36. Tazebay UH, Wapnir IL, Levy O, Dohan O, Zuckier LS, Zhao QH, et al. The mammary gland iodide transporter is expressed during lactation and in breast cancer. *Nat Med* 2000;**6**(8):871–8.
37. Ord WM. Report of a committee of the clinical society of London nominated December, to investigate the subject of myxedema. *Transactions of the Clinical Society of London* 1888;**14 SRC-BaiduScholar**:1–215.
38. Oppenheimer JH, Schwartz HL. Molecular basis of thyroid hormone-dependent brain development. *Endocr Rev* 1997;**18**(4):462–75.
39. Rodriguez-Pena A, Ibarrola N, Iniguez MA, Munoz A, Bernal J. Neonatal hypothyroidism affects the timely expression of myelin-associated glycoprotein in the rat brain. *J Clin Invest* 1993;**91**(3 SRC—BaiduScholar):812–8.
40. Yan Y-Q, Dong Z-L, Dong L, Wang F-R, Yang X-M, Jin X-Y, et al. Trimester- and method-specific reference intervals for thyroid tests in pregnant Chinese women: methodology, euthyroid definition and iodine status can influence the setting of reference intervals. *Clin Endocrinol (Oxf)* 2011;**74**(2):262–9.
41. Li C, Shan Z, Mao J, Wang W, Xie X, Zhou W, et al. Assessment of thyroid function during first-trimester pregnancy: what is the rational upper limit of serum TSH during the first trimester in Chinese pregnant women? *J Clin Endocrinol Metab* 2014;**99**(1):73–9.
42. Marwaha RK, Chopra S, Gopalakrishnan S, Sharma B, Kanwar RS, Sastry A, et al. Establishment of reference range for thyroid hormones in normal pregnant Indian women. *BJOG* 2008;**115**(5):602–6.
43. Moon H-W, Chung H-J, Park C-M, Hur M, Yun Y-M. Establishment of trimester-specific reference intervals for thyroid hormones in Korean pregnant women. *Ann Lab Med* 2015;**35**(2):198–204.
44. Lee RH, Spencer CA, Mestman JH, Miller EA, Petrovic I, Braverman LE, et al. Free T4 immunoassays are flawed during pregnancy. *Am J Obstet Gynecol* 2009;**200**(3):260.e1–6.

45. Hendrick V, Altshuler LL, Suri R. Hormonal changes in the postpartum and implications for postpartum depression. *Psychosomatics* 1998;**39**(2):93–101.

46. Harris B, Othman S, Davies JA, Weppner GJ, Richards CJ, Newcombe RG, et al. Association between postpartum thyroid dysfunction and thyroid antibodies and depression. *BMJ* 1992;**305**(6846):152–6.

47. Harris B, Oretti R, Lazarus J, Parkes A, John R, Richards C, et al. Randomised trial of thyroxine to prevent postnatal depression in thyroid-antibody-positive women. *Br J Psychiatry* 2002;**180**(Apr.):327–30.

48. Pop VJ, de Rooy HA, Vader HL, van der Heide D, van Son M, Komproe IH, et al. Postpartum thyroid dysfunction and depression in an unselected population. *N Engl J Med* 1991;**324**(25):1815–6.

49. Motil KJ, Thotathuchery M, Montandon CM, Hachey DL, Boutton TW, Klein PD, et al. Insulin, cortisol and thyroid hormones modulate maternal protein status and milk production and composition in humans. *J Nutr* 1994;**124**(8):1248–57.

50. Stuebe AM, Meltzer-Brody S, Pearson B, Pedersen C, Grewen K. Maternal neuroendocrine serum levels in exclusively breastfeeding mothers. *Breastfeed Med* 2015;**10**(4):197–202.

51. Hapon MB, Varas SM, Giménez MS, Jahn GA. Reduction of mammary and liver lipogenesis and alteration of milk composition during lactation in rats by hypothyroidism. *Thyroids* 2007;**17**(1):11–8.

52. Thrift TA, Bernal A, Lewis AW, Neuendorff DA, Willard CC, Randel RD. Effects of induced hypothyroidism on weight gains, lactation, and reproductive performance of primiparous Brahman cows. *J Anim Sci* 1999;**77**(7):1844–50.

53. Medici M, Korevaar TIM, Visser WE, Visser TJ, Peeters RP. Thyroid function in pregnancy: what is normal? *Clin Chem* 2015;**61**(5):704–13.

54. Lockitch G. *Handbook of diagnostic biochemistry and Hematology in normal pregnancy.* Boca Raton: CRC Press; 1993.

Chapter 5

Physiology of Calcium, Phosphorus, and Bone Metabolism During Pregnancy, Lactation, and Postweaning

Christopher S. Kovacs

Faculty of Medicine, Endocrinology, Memorial University of Newfoundland, St. John's, NL, Canada

Key Clinical Changes

- Albumin-corrected serum calcium and ionized calcium remain normal during pregnancy, whereas the fall in the uncorrected serum calcium should not be mistaken for hypocalcemia.
- Pregnancy is characterized by low parathyroid hormone (PTH) and high concentrations of calcitriol, PTH-related protein (PTHrP), and estradiol.
- Intestinal calcium absorption doubles during pregnancy to meet the fetal demand for this vital mineral.
- Lactation is characterized by low PTH and estradiol, normal calcitriol, and high levels of PTHrP.
- The skeleton is resorbed during lactation to provide much of the calcium content of milk, but it is restored after weaning to its prior bone density and apparent strength.

5.1 INTRODUCTION

Female physiology adapts during pregnancy and lactation to meet the added nutritional demands of the fetus and neonate. The average full-term fetus has about 30 g of calcium, 20 g of phosphorus, and 0.80 g of magnesium.[1] About 80% of this mineral is accreted during the third trimester after active transport across the placenta. The rate of accretion increases from 60 mg/day of calcium at week 24 to between 300 and 350 mg/day during the last 6 weeks.[1] In each hour of those final weeks, the placenta draws 5%–10% of the calcium and phosphorus present in the mother's plasma. This could provoke hypocalcemia, were it not for maternal physiology adapting to defend against the fetal demand by increasing the influx of minerals to the maternal circulation.

The average breastfed baby consumes 780 mL/day of milk during the first 6 months.[1] Combined with an average calcium content of 260 mg/L, this means a total calcium intake of about 200 mg/day. About 60%–70% of calcium is absorbed from human milk, thereby making about 120–140 mg of calcium available each day.[1] From this intake, the neonatal skeleton accretes approximately 100 mg/day of calcium. There is considerable individual variability in neonatal demand for breast milk and, therefore, breast-milk output. Furthermore, women who nurse twins and triplets have double and triple the milk and calcium output of women nursing singletons, respectively.[1]

From 6 to 12 months of age, the breastfed infant consumes less milk and more solid foods. The average milk consumption is 600 mL/day, which has a modestly lower calcium content of 200 mg/L.[1] This means women can be expected to lose about 120 mg/day of calcium from ongoing milk production.

These estimates of average calcium output—from 300 to 350 mg/day during the third trimester, 200 mg/day during the first 6 months of lactation, and 120 mg/day during late lactation—may seem modest and easily obtained through normal intake and intestinal absorption. However, fractional calcium absorption is typically about 25% of intake in healthy adults who consume 1000–1200 mg/day of calcium.[2] But if normal efficiency of intestinal calcium absorption were relied upon, an extra 1200 mg of calcium would need to be consumed to provide 300 mg/day during the third trimester, whereas breastfeeding women would need to consume an extra 800 mg/day during the first 6 months of lactation. And yet data from the U.S. National Health and Nutrition Examination Survey (NHANES) and Statistics Canada show that between ages 18 and

50, the 50th percentile for calcium intake ranges from 800 to 1000 mg/day in both populations,[3] for an expected fractional absorption of only 200–250 mg/day. Consequently, if the nonpregnant rate of intestinal calcium absorption were in force, most women do not consume adequate calcium to meet the additional needs of their babies.

This is where specific adaptations are invoked during pregnancy and lactation to meet the increased calcium and mineral requirements, but without requiring women to consume more mineral than normal. During pregnancy, intestinal absorption doubles, whereas during lactation, skeletal resorption increases to provide calcium to milk.

Due to space limitations on the reference list, a comprehensive review containing citations to over 1000 papers will be preferentially cited.[1]

5.2 SKELETAL AND MINERAL PHYSIOLOGY DURING PREGNANCY

Theoretically, maternal physiology could adapt to the demands of pregnancy by increasing intestinal calcium absorption, decreasing renal calcium excretion, and increasing skeletal resorption of calcium. However, the principal adaptation is a twofold increase in intestinal calcium absorption. This is accompanied by renal calcium wasting and some resorption of calcium from the skeleton.

5.2.1 Changes in Mineral Ions and Calciotropic and Phosphotropic Hormones

Fig. 5.1 depicts the progressive changes in serum calcium, phosphorus, and calciotropic hormone levels during normal human pregnancy. Most laboratories do not provide pregnancy-specific reference ranges, and thus relative changes are schematically depicted.

5.2.1.1 *Calcium and Phosphorus*

Serum calcium declines 5%–10% during pregnancy, such that the mean value in many cohorts falls below normal, thereby suggesting hypocalcemia.[1] However, this is an artifact caused by the decline in serum albumin, which itself is a consequence of normal expansion of the intravascular volume. The fall in serum calcium is physiologically unimportant. It should not be mistaken for hypocalcemia.

The albumin-corrected serum calcium and ionized calcium do not change during pregnancy, as shown by many longitudinal and cross-sectional studies.[1] Similarly, both values remain normal in women bearing twins. These findings underscore why either of these two parameters must be used during pregnancy, while the unadjusted serum calcium should be ignored.

Serum phosphorus and magnesium also remain unchanged during pregnancy.[1]

5.2.1.2 *Parathyroid Hormone*

The older literature is fraught with claims that pregnancy is a physiological state of secondary hyperparathyroidism. This erroneous notion came about when the fall in unadjusted serum calcium was misinterpreted as true hypocalcemia, and increased PTH was found with early assays.[1] But the decline is serum calcium is an artifact, and those early PTH assays measured biologically inactive fragments of PTH that accumulate during pregnancy.

Modern two-site immunoradiometric assays capture mainly active forms of PTH. In longitudinal and cross-sectional studies of North American and European women who consumed a diet adequate in calcium, PTH is typically suppressed to the lower end of the normal range or below it during the first trimester.[1] It may remain suppressed or increase to midnormal by term. This is true for twin pregnancies.

Conversely, the data are more variable for pregnant women from Asia and Africa. Some studies found suppression of PTH during pregnancy, while others reported that PTH did not decline, and in still others, it was above normal.[1] When PTH does not suppress during pregnancy, it is likely an indicator that the traditional diet in these regions is low in vitamin D or calcium, or high in phytate (which blocks calcium absorption). Low calcium intake or reduced calcium absorption will provoke secondary hyperparathyroidism.

5.2.1.3 *PTH-Related Protein*

PTH-related protein (PTHrP) progressively increases across the three trimesters, as shown in several longitudinal studies.[1] This increase has been detected as early as 3–13 weeks, and reaches triple that value or more by term. A few case reports have not detected PTHrP at all, but this is likely due to improper sample collection and processing that permits PTHrP's rapid degradation in serum, as discussed elsewhere.[1]

PTHrP probably comes predominantly from the breasts and placenta, as suggested by cases of PTHrP-mediated hypercalcemia (pseudohyperparathyroidism) during pregnancy (see Chapter 21). But PTHrP is also produced by many other

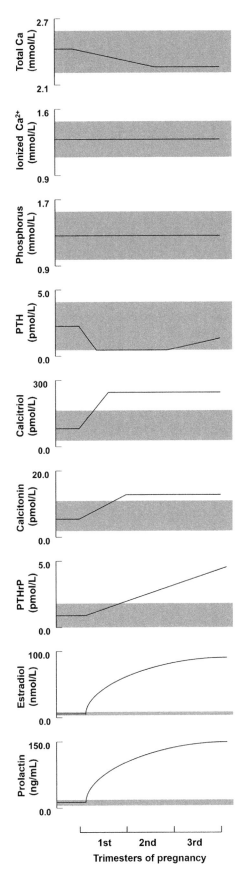

FIG. 5.1 Schematic depiction of longitudinal changes in calcium, phosphorus, and calciotropic hormone levels during human pregnancy. *Shaded regions* depict the approximate normal ranges. PTH does not decline in women with low calcium or high phytate intake, and it may even rise above normal. Calcidiol values are not depicted; most longitudinal studies indicate that the levels are unchanged by pregnancy but may vary due to seasonal variation in sunlight exposure and changes in vitamin D intake. FGF23 values cannot be plotted due to lack of data. *(Reproduced with permission from Kovacs CS. Maternal mineral and bone metabolism during pregnancy, lactation, and post-weaning recovery. Physiol Rev 2016;96(2):449–547.)*

tissues, including the parathyroids, amnion, decidua, myometrium, and umbilical cord.[1] The rise in circulating PTHrP appears physiologically important and contributes to why maternal calcium and bone metabolism improve during pregnancy in women with hypoparathyroidism (see Chapter 21).

PTHrP's gradual rise parallels a similar increase in calcitriol (as discussed next). This may imply that PTHrP is partly responsible for stimulating renal 1α-hydroxylase (Cyp27b1) to produce calcitriol.[1]

5.2.1.4 Calcitriol and Calcidiol

Longitudinal and cross-sectional studies have found that serum calcitriol increases at least twofold to threefold, reaching its highest levels in the third trimester.[1] Most studies did not measure free calcitriol, but because vitamin D-binding protein increases only 20%–40% during pregnancy as albumin falls significantly, free calcitriol is increased during all three trimesters.[1] When singleton and twin pregnancies are compared, the increases in calcitriol and vitamin D binding protein have been indistinguishable.

PTH is the dominant stimulator of Cyp27b1; hypoparathyroidism results in very low calcitriol levels. But PTH is usually suppressed to low values during pregnancy as calcitriol is increased, which indicates that other factors must stimulate Cyp27b1. These potentially include PTHrP, estradiol, prolactin, and placental lactogen, for which there are animal and limited human data confirming their ability to stimulate calcitriol production.[1] It has often been assumed that the placental production of calcitriol accounts for the doubling or tripling of serum calcitriol. This is incorrect, as shown by animal studies, and by the observation that anephric women on dialysis have very low endogenous calcitriol levels, even while pregnant.[4] Serum calcidiol or 25-hydroxyvitamin D (25OHD), the substrate from which calcitriol is made, does not change appreciably during pregnancy unless due to changes in diet or seasonal exposure to sunlight.[1]

The doubling or tripling of calcitriol during pregnancy is not an indication of maternal vitamin D deficiency or insufficient calcium intake. Supplementation with up to 5000 IU/day of vitamin D during pregnancy did not alter maternal serum calcium, albumin-corrected calcium, phosphorus, PTH, or the rise in calcitriol.[5–8] Instead, the increase in free and bound calcitriol appears to be a programmed response to pregnancy. In one study, mean calcitriol levels reached a plateau at a 25OHD level of 100 nmol/L, regardless of vitamin D intake.[6] This may reflect the maximal capacity of renal Cyp27b1 to convert 25OHD into calcitriol, balanced against increasing catabolism of 25OHD and calcitriol by Cyp24a1.

5.2.1.5 Calcitonin

Serum levels of calcitonin typically increase during pregnancy and may exceed the normal range.[1] This may result in part from stimulation by increased concentrations of estradiol, estrone, and estriol, and from extrathyroidal production in the breasts and placenta. Totally thyroidectomized women have similar calcitonin levels during pregnancy as intact women.[9]

5.2.1.6 Fibroblast Growth Factor-23 (FGF23)

Intact fibroblast growth factor-23 (FGF23) levels during human pregnancy have not been reported. Within 24h after delivery, mean values were similar to nonpregnant controls.[10]

5.2.1.7 Sex Steroids and Other Hormones

Estradiol increases up to 100-fold, estriol and estrone increase to a lesser extent, and progesterone increases up to 10-fold.[1] There is also a 10-fold or greater increase in prolactin, 10- to 100-fold increase in placental lactogen, 25-fold increase in placental growth hormone, and suppression of pituitary growth hormone.[1] IGF-I decreases to 50% of basal values during the second trimester and then rises to twofold to threefold above nonpregnant values by term.[1] Oxytocin increases modestly to peak levels near term.[1]

5.2.2 Upregulation of Intestinal Absorption of Calcium and Phosphorus

Stable calcium isotopes (^{48}Ca, ^{44}Ca, ^{42}Ca) and mineral balance studies have been carried out in pregnant women.[1] These have consistently demonstrated that fractional absorption of calcium doubles as early as 12 weeks of gestation, and this increase is maintained to term. Animal models have shown a similar doubling of calcium, phosphorus, and magnesium absorption.[1]

The doubling to tripling of serum calcitriol during normal pregnancy has been assumed to explain the doubling in efficiency of intestinal calcium absorption. Compelling animal data indicate that increased intestinal calcium absorption cannot be fully due to calcitriol, and that the increase still will develop in the absence of calcitriol or its receptor.[1]

This implies that other factors (possibly prolactin, placental lactogen, and growth hormone, among others) may stimulate calcium absorption by enterocytes. However, no clinical studies have examined either intestinal calcium absorption in women with vitamin D deficiency or genetic disorders of vitamin D physiology in which calcitriol is not synthesized or the vitamin D receptor is absent.

The doubling in fractional absorption of calcium is the major maternal adaptation to meet the fetal requirement for calcium; in fact, it provides more mineral than needed. Moreover, animal and human data indicate that most of the calcium in the fetal skeleton at term is absorbed from the maternal diet during pregnancy.[1]

5.2.3   Altered Renal Mineral Handling

There is a physiological increase in creatinine clearance and glomerular filtration rate during normal pregnancy. From at least week 12 onward, 24-h urine calcium excretion increases significantly. Mean values are typically at the upper limit of normal or in the hypercalciuric range.[1] Fasting urine calcium is usually normal or low, confirming that the 24-h increase in urine calcium is due to absorptive hypercalciuria,[1] which means that the doubling of intestinal calcium absorption increases the renal filtered load, and thereby excretion of calcium. Note that random spot urines have been used in some studies, but these are neither sensitive enough nor timed appropriately (especially when done fasting or before meals) to detect absorptive hypercalciuria.

Absorptive hypercalciuria is an obligatory, physiological consequence of pregnancy, in which the kidneys dump excess calcium that is not required. Unfortunately, this contributes to an increased risk of kidney stones during pregnancy.

Hypocalciuria during pregnancy has been associated with preeclampsia, pregnancy-induced hypertension, and low (equal to nonpregnant values) serum calcitriol.[11–14] The combination of low calcitriol, hypocalciuria, and reduced creatinine clearance is likely secondary to disturbed renal function rather than being a cause of the hypertension. Consistent with this, a longitudinal study found that calcitriol levels were appropriately increased early in pregnancy and became low after hypertension and proteinuria developed.[15] On the other hand, calcium supplementation is effective at reducing the risk of preeclampsia or pregnancy-induced hypertension, but only in women with the lowest intakes of calcium.[16] High-dose vitamin D supplementation is ineffective.[6,7,17–19]

5.2.4   Altered Skeletal Turnover and Mineral Metabolism

The doubling of intestinal calcium absorption during the first trimester occurs months prior to the fetal demand for mineral during the third trimester. This results in a positive calcium balance for women by midpregnancy,[20] which in turn should mean that skeletal mineral content is increased by that point in time. However, there are no studies of bone mineral content (BMC) or density (BMD) at this time, due to concerns about fetal radiation exposure. By term, the calcium balance is generally neutral.

Biochemical markers of bone formation and resorption can be used to infer relative changes in bone turnover, but there are confounding problems with their use during pregnancy, as discussed elsewhere.[1] In general, bone resorption markers are low in the first trimester but increase to as much as twice the normal level by term. Bone formation markers are also typically low during the first trimester and either have remained low or risen to the normal range or above by term. Total alkaline phosphatase rises markedly due to placental production and is not an indicator of relative bone formation rates during pregnancy.

Dual X-ray absorptiometry (DXA) measurements of BMD and BMC of the hip and spine have been done, but typically 1–8 months before planned pregnancy and 1–6 weeks after delivery.[1] These generally small studies have shown either no change or as much as a 5% decrease in lumbar spine bone density when prepregnancy and postpregnancy values are compared. The long interval between baseline measurements and pregnancy leaves residual uncertainty as to whether any perceived changes in BMD occurred during pregnancy. The largest study of 92 women found that BMD decreased by 1.8% at the lumbar spine, 3.2% at the total hip, and 2.4% at the whole body.[21] Whether all of these small changes in BMD are fully attributable to pregnancy is also unclear because all women went on to breastfeed before the day 15 ± 7 postpartum measurement, which causes bone loss (see Section 5.3).

Overall, it is conceivable that BMC increases by midpregnancy, which is consistent with the positive calcium balance, and bone resorption follows during the third trimester, leaving a net result of either no change or a small decrease in BMC or BMD. Dozens of studies have examined whether pregnancy has any associations over the long term with low bone mass for age or fragility fractures. Most studies have found that parity is associated with either a neutral or a protective effect against low BMD or fractures.[1]

5.3 SKELETAL AND MINERAL PHYSIOLOGY DURING LACTATION AND POSTWEANING RECOVERY

In contrast to pregnancy, intestinal calcium absorption is normal during lactation. The principal adaptations to meet the calcium requirements of milk production are increased resorption of the maternal skeleton and renal calcium conservation.

5.3.1 Changes in Mineral Ions and Calciotropic Hormones

Fig. 5.2 depicts the progressive changes in serum calcium, phosphorus, and calciotropic hormone levels during normal human lactation. Only relative changes are shown due to the fact that most laboratories do not report lactation-specific values.

5.3.1.1 Calcium and Phosphorus

Serum calcium (adjusted for albumin or not) and ionized calcium remain normal during lactation.[1] Longitudinal studies have shown that albumin-corrected and ionized calcium levels increase slightly but remain within the normal range, and may be increased further in women nursing twins. Hypercalcemia can occur as a consequence of normal lactation (see the section on pseudohyperparathyroidism in Chapter 21).

Serum phosphorus also increases during lactation, and in numerous studies, the mean values rose above normal.[1] Women nursing twins may have even higher serum phosphorus. Magnesium has been normal or modestly increased.

The increases in circulating calcium and phosphorus are due to upregulated skeletal resorption (as discussed next), which brings calcium and phosphorus into the circulation. Renal calcium and phosphorus conservation also contributes to these increases.

During postweaning, serum calcium, phosphorus, and magnesium are normal.

5.3.1.2 Parathyroid Hormone

As with pregnancy, lactation was originally thought to be a state of physiological secondary hyperparathyroidism. However, modern intact PTH assays have consistently found suppressed or even undetectable concentrations of PTH in North American and European women who are breastfeeding exclusively or near-exclusively.[1] On the other hand, C-terminal assays show increased levels due to accumulation of these nonfunctioning metabolites.[1]

Whether PTH becomes suppressed during lactation is also dependent upon calcium intake and ethnicity. Increased circulating PTH has been seen during lactation in some studies of women from regions of Africa and Asia where low calcium, high phytate, and low vitamin D intakes are more prevalent.[1] This has also been seen in a single study in which African American and Caucasian women from North America were compared to each other, which suggests ethnic differences in the PTH response to lactation.[22]

During the postweaning interval, when the skeleton is reclaiming mineral content, PTH is normal or may increase modestly.[1]

5.3.1.3 Parathyroid Hormone-Related Protein

PTHrP is best known as the cause of humoral hypercalcemia of malignancy, but similarly high plasma concentrations develop in healthy breastfeeding women, while 1000–10,000 times higher values are found in milk.[1] Most studies have found the circulating concentrations of PTHrP to be significantly increased in lactating women compared to nonpregnant women or bottle-feeding controls.[1] It is secreted by the breasts, in which it plays a physiological role in regulating skeletal resorption and renal calcium handling (see Sections 5.3.4–5.3.6, later in this chapter). Plasma PTHrP increases after suckling and correlates positively with the ionized calcium and negatively with PTH, while higher concentrations predict greater bone loss.[1] PTHrP's systemic effects consistently cause hypoparathyroid women to become normocalcemic while breastfeeding, while higher PTHrP concentrations have caused lactational hypercalcemia (pseudohyperparathyroidism) in otherwise healthy women (see Chapter 21).[1]

During postweaning, PTHrP becomes undetectable in the circulation. How quickly this develops is quite variable and not well documented. Its disappearance provokes hypocalcemia in hypoparathyroid women and signals the need to restart supplemental calcium and calcitriol.[1] However, this may occur before weaning or around the time of weaning, while in other scenarios, sustained production of PTHrP by the breasts results in normocalcemia persisting for months to years afterward.

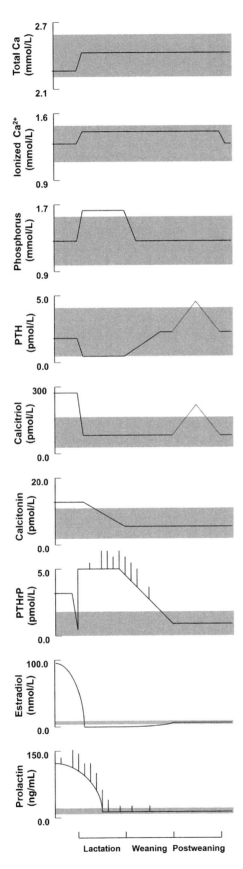

FIG. 5.2 Schematic depiction of longitudinal changes in calcium, phosphorus, and calciotropic hormone levels during lactation and postweaning skeletal recovery in women. Normal adult values are indicated by the shaded areas. PTH does not decline in women with low calcium or high phytate intake, and may even rise above normal. Calcidiol values are not depicted; most longitudinal studies indicate that the levels are unchanged by lactation but may vary due to seasonal variation in sunlight exposure and changes in vitamin D intake. PTHrP and prolactin surge with each suckling episode, and this is represented by upward spikes. FGF23 values cannot be plotted due to lack of data. Very limited data suggest that calcitriol and PTH may increase during postweaning, and the lines are *dashed* to reflect this uncertainty. *(Reproduced with permission from Kovacs CS. Maternal mineral and bone metabolism during pregnancy, lactation, and post-weaning recovery. Physiol Rev 2016;96(2):449–547.)*

5.3.1.4 Calcitriol and Calcidiol

Free and total calcitriol fall rapidly from the high values during pregnancy to nonpregnant values during the puerperium, and remain there throughout lactation.[1] Very limited data suggest that calcitriol may be higher in women nursing twins, and that calcitriol might increase above normal during postweaning.[1]

Numerous studies have shown that 25OHD levels are unchanged during up to 12 months of breastfeeding.[1] Milk normally contains very low amounts of vitamin D and 25OHD, so it does not represent a drain on maternal vitamin D stores.

The fall in calcitriol from the high levels of pregnancy may result from the loss of such factors as the high concentrations of estradiol and placental lactogen.[1] Conversely, PTHrP reaches its highest levels during lactation, and yet calcitriol is not increased, which suggests that PTHrP is not responsible for the rise in calcitriol during pregnancy or that it requires the high concentrations of estradiol that occur during pregnancy to have its effects.

5.3.1.5 Calcitonin

Calcitonin has been inconsistently increased or normal among studies of lactating women, with no clear explanation for the discrepancies.[1] Women nursing twins had higher serum calcitonin than women nursing singletons.[23] The lactating breast produces calcitonin and secretes it into breast milk at 45 times its concentration in blood. Consequently, thyroidectomized and thyroid-intact women have the same mean calcitonin concentration while breastfeeding.[9]

5.3.1.6 Fibroblast Growth Factor-23

No measurements of FGF23 during lactation have been reported. Because women have high serum phosphorus and low PTH while breastfeeding, this might provoke higher FGF23 to compensate. Conversely, it also could imply that low FGF23 concentrations are present, contributing to the increased serum phosphorus.

5.3.1.7 Sex Steroids and Other Hormones

Breastfeeding women typically have high levels of prolactin and very low estradiol and progesterone.[1] Loss of the placenta causes an initial fall in progesterone and estradiol, which is a signal to turn on lactogenesis. Suckling and increased prolactin suppress ovarian function by flattening and inhibiting the release of gonadotropin-releasing hormone (GnRH) by the hypothalamus.

Estradiol reaches low values equivalent to menopause during early lactation, after which it may remain low or gradually increase toward normal levels. Menstrual cycles can resume in women who continue to breastfeed nearly exclusively. Basal prolactin declines to normal as the postpartum days pass, but each suckling episode causes a spike in prolactin. These prolactin surges contribute to ongoing ovarian suppression and milk production.

Oxytocin spikes in the maternal circulation within a few minutes of the baby being put to the breast. Because the oxytocin receptor is expressed by osteoblasts and osteoclasts,[1] it conceivably plays a role in bone metabolism.

5.3.2 Calcium Pumping and Secretion in Mammary Tissue

The hormonal regulation of milk production has mainly been elucidated through animal studies; this topic is discussed in more detail in Chapter 14. In brief, PTHrP is expressed by mammary epithelial cells and plays a key role in maintaining the supply of calcium for milk production, largely by stimulating systemic bone resorption and renal tubular conservation of calcium.[1] The calcium-sensing receptor is expressed in breast tissue and appears to directly control the calcium content of milk by inhibiting local production of PTHrP and stimulating the expression and activity of a calcium pump—specifically, plasma membrane bound type 2 calcium-ATPase (PMCA2).[1] In turn, PMCA2 may also be locally regulated by PTHrP, serotonin, and calcitriol.[1] The calcium-sensing receptor's inhibition of PTHrP may serve to prevent milk production from provoking maternal hypocalcemia, but this effect must be modest because lactation-induced hypocalcemia occurs in rodents and cows.

Among studies done in breastfeeding women, the PTHrP concentration of milk, as well as of maternal blood, correlates with the calcium content of milk.[1] Calcium supplementation does not affect the PTHrP content of milk.[24] Similarly, extremes of high or low calcium intake and high or low vitamin D intake have no effect on milk calcium content.[1]

Little vitamin D, 25OHD, or calcitriol is present in milk.[1] Consequently, breastfeeding is a risk factor for vitamin D deficiency and rickets in babies who receive little or no sunlight exposure. Why is the vitamin D-related content of milk so low? Humans naturally synthesize vitamin D in skin but cannot develop vitamin D toxicity by that route because limited precursor is produced each day. However, it is possible to become vitamin D toxic from oral ingestion. Therefore, neonatal physiology is likely also designed to obtain vitamin D primarily from sunlight exposure. The low vitamin D content of milk avoids excess intake by the baby and depletion of maternal vitamin D stores.

FGF23 may play a role in regulating the phosphorus content of milk, which was reduced to about half the normal level in two women who had high levels of FGF23 due to X-linked hypophosphatemic rickets (XLH).[25,26] However, the low serum phosphorus in XLH may the cause of the reduced phosphorus in milk, as opposed to the implication that FGF23 directly regulates phosphorus transport into mammary epithelial cells.

5.3.3 Intestinal Mineral Absorption

Calcium balance studies, including those that administered stable isotopes of calcium, have shown that intestinal calcium absorption is maintained at the normal (nonpregnant) rate during lactation, or about half the value found during pregnancy.[1] This coincides with the fall in calcitriol to normal values and supports the idea that high levels of calcitriol contribute to the increased efficiency of calcium absorption during pregnancy.

Women typically consume extra calcium while breastfeeding. Randomized trials and cohort studies have shown that this does not alter milk calcium content or the magnitude of bone resorbed during lactation; however, it does increase urine calcium excretion.[1] Consequently, consuming extra calcium does not appear to confer any benefit during lactation.

Furthermore, high-dose vitamin D supplementation (4000–6400 IU/day) results in very high 25OHD at 160 nmoL/L (64 ng/mL), but it does not affect breast milk calcium content.[27–29] This confirms that vitamin D and calcitriol play no role in determining the calcium content of milk. Also, two studies showed that intestinal calcium absorption increased modestly during postweaning,[30, 31] which should contribute to restoring skeletal mineral content.

5.3.4 Reduced Renal Excretion of Calcium

In contrast to pregnancy, glomerular filtration rate drops during lactation, the tubular maximum for calcium increases, and the fractional excretion of calcium falls to hypocalciuric values in 24-h urine collections.[1] This effect is consistent with the actions of PTHrP.

Urine phosphorus excretion is normal or increased in 24-h urine collections, which is also likely due to the phosphaturic actions of PTHrP.[1] A significant increase in the tubular maximum for phosphate has been found in many studies, which indicates that the kidneys conserve phosphorus in spite of PTHrP's phosphaturic effect.[1]

The renal responses to lactation serve to conserve calcium for milk production, while excreting excess phosphorus from skeletal resorption and intestinal absorption. Hypocalciuria and renal calcium conservation persist during postweaning, whereas renal phosphorus handling returns to normal.[1]

5.3.5 Increased Skeletal Resorption and Osteocytic Osteolysis During Lactation

Studies in lactating rodents have shown that substantial bone resorption occurs during lactation in order to provide needed calcium for milk.[1] Rats and mice typically lose 20%–30% of skeletal mineral content during 3 weeks of lactation. This results from increased osteoclast-mediated bone resorption in addition to osteocytic osteolysis, a process through which osteocytes resorb mineral from their lacunae. Lactation substantially reduces bone strength.

Available data from breastfeeding women are consistent with the animal data, in that hormonally programmed resorption of the maternal skeleton occurs.[1] Bone resorption and formation markers increase markedly, with resorption markers displaying the most marked increases.[1] Longitudinal studies have shown that BMD and BMC decline 5%–10% after 3–6 months of lactation, with the greatest (5%–10%) losses in the trabecular-rich spine, modest (0%–5%) losses at the hip, femur, and distal radius, and the smallest (0%–2%) changes at purely cortical sites such as the entire body.[1] The median loss of BMD in these studies is about 6%–8% of BMD from the lumbar spine, with half or less of that lost from the appendicular skeleton.

These quoted ranges reflect mean changes from each study, but individual women can vary from a small gain to a 20% decline in the lumbar spine BMD.[1] Lactation can cause normal women to reach an osteoporotic level of BMD. In women who do not breastfeed, small gains in BMD occur, which may indicate recovery from losses incurred during pregnancy.[1]

In theory, women who breastfeed for extended periods may experience even greater bone loss. However, less milk is produced as the postpartum months pass, and skeletal recovery (at least in terms of BMD regain) begins despite ongoing lactation in some women.[1]

High-resolution peripheral quantitated tomography (HR-pQCT) can resolve the microarchitecture of bone. It cannot examine the spine, which is where the most marked skeletal resorption occurs. However, HR-pQCT has demonstrated that in women who lactate for extended intervals, trabecular thickness, cortical thickness, and cortical volume all decline, while trabecular number increases.[32,33]

Several blinded, randomized interventional studies and cohort studies have shown that increased dietary or supplemental intake of calcium does not alter the magnitude of bone resorbed during lactation.[1] Conversely, very low calcium intake (<300 mg/day) did not influence maternal bone loss, changes in bone resorption markers, or calcium content of breast milk.[1] Skeletal resorption appears to be programmed by hormonal signals during lactation and independent extremes of calcium intake. Instead, skeletal losses are increased by greater breast milk output and more intense or exclusive lactation.[1]

5.3.6 Breast-Brain-Bone Circuit-Controlling Bone Metabolism During Lactation

During lactation, there is an important physiological interaction and cross-talk among breast, brain, and bone, with breast tissue being the central controller. The summary model is shown and described in Fig. 5.3.

Animal studies have shown that the relative deficiency of estradiol, as well as high levels of PTHrP originating in mammary tissue, are two dominant factors that explain the increased bone resorption that occurs during lactation.[1] The available human data are consistent with these findings.

Lactational bone loss is more rapid than can be accounted for by estradiol deficiency alone.[1] Bone loss has also continued in women who breastfeed after their menses resumed,[34,35] which implies that estradiol deficiency is no longer present.

Studies on the effects of GnRH analog-induced estradiol deficiency support the notion that estradiol deficiency alone cannot explain lactational bone loss. Further, 6 months of marked estradiol deficiency in reproductive-age women causes only 2%–4% reductions in BMD of the spine, with no losses at cortical sites, in contrast to greater loss of BMD during lactation at both trabecular and cortical sites. It is the combination of increased PTHrP and low estradiol (and possibly other factors as well) that stimulate more rapid bone loss during lactation.

5.3.7 Bone Formation and Skeletal Recovery Postweaning

Animal studies have consistently shown that following lactation, an anabolic phase occurs during which skeletal mineral content and microarchitecture improve in the long bones and are restored to normal in the vertebrae.[1] Bone strength returns to prepregnancy values at all skeletal sites. This anabolism is accomplished by upregulation of osteoblast numbers and activity, while osteocytes restore mineral content in their lacunae.

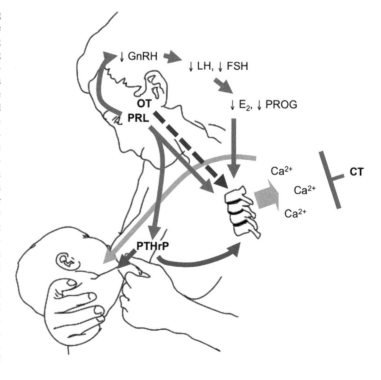

FIG. 5.3 Breast-brain-bone circuit controls lactation. Suckling and prolactin (PRL) both inhibit the hypothalamic GnRH pulse center, which in turn suppresses the gonadotropins [luteinizing hormone (LH) and follicle-stimulating hormone (FSH)], leading to low levels of the ovarian sex steroids [estradiol (E_2) and progesterone (PROG)]. Prolactin may also have direct effects on its receptor in bone cells. PTHrP production and release from the breast are stimulated by suckling, prolactin, low estradiol, and the calcium receptor. PTHrP enters the bloodstream and combines with systemically low estradiol levels to markedly upregulate bone resorption and (at least in rodents) osteocytic osteolysis. Increased bone resorption releases calcium and phosphate into the bloodstream, which then reaches the breast ducts and is actively pumped into the breast milk. PTHrP also passes into milk at high concentrations, but the question of whether swallowed PTHrP plays a role in regulating calcium physiology of the neonate is uncertain. In addition to stimulating milk ejection, oxytocin (OT) may directly affect osteoblast and osteoclast function *(dashed line)*. Calcitonin (CT) may inhibit skeletal responsiveness to PTHrP and low estradiol, given that mice lacking calcitonin lose twice the amount of bone during lactation as normal mice. Not depicted is that calcitonin may also act on the pituitary to suppress prolactin release, and within breast tissue to reduce PTHrP expression and lower the milk calcium content. *(Modified with kind permission ©2005 Springer Science and Business Media B.V. Kovacs CS. Calcium and bone metabolism during pregnancy and lactation. J Mammary Gland Biol Neoplasia 2005;10(2):105–18.)*

In women, bone mass and mineralization increase after weaning, leading to partial or full recovery of the losses invoked by lactation. Longitudinal studies using DXA have shown that bone density returns to normal by 12 months postweaning.[1]

HR-pQCT studies of the radius and ultradistal femur have shown improvements in trabecular microarchitecture and cortical parameters after weaning, but with some persistent deficits.[32,33] The cross-sectional diameter of the femur has increased after lactation or postweaning recovery, accompanied by recovery of cortical bone area, in a few studies.[36,37] An increase in cross-sectional diameter or volume will improve bone strength and compensate for any permanent loss of trabecular microarchitecture.

Lactation does not cause long-term impairment of skeletal mass, density, or strength. Dozens of epidemiologic studies have found neutral or protective associations of lactation with peak bone mass, BMD, and fracture risk.[1] Fractures do occur rarely during lactation (see Chapter 21); consequently, lactational bone loss is not always benign. However, in most women, fracturing is of no consequence because the skeleton is later restored to its prior mineralization and strength.

The factors that regulate skeletal recovery after weaning remain unknown. Animal studies have shown that recovery occurs despite absence of the main calciotropic hormones, including PTH, calcitriol, or its receptor, PTHrP, and calcitonin.[1,38–42] Restoration of ovarian function should slow or halt bone resorption, but by itself, it cannot explain the speed or magnitude of skeletal recovery.[1] Estradiol acts on osteoclasts to suppress bone resorption, and in turn, formation is suppressed.[1] Moreover, in the aforementioned studies of reproductive-age women who lost bone mass during GnRH analog therapy, most do not restore it afterward despite recovering ovarian function.[43–53]

Earlier resumption of menses correlated with an earlier return to baseline BMD in a few studies, but this does not imply that recovery of estradiol or ovarian function explains skeletal recovery.[1] Instead, earlier resumption of menses identifies women who likely breastfed less intensively and for a shorter duration, lost less bone, and will recover to baseline sooner. Calcium supplementation during postweaning may improve bone mass accrual,[54] unlike the lack of effect that it has during lactation. In addition, increased weight-bearing exercise is conceivably beneficial to improve bone mass during the postweaning interval.[1]

5.4   CONCLUSIONS

Pregnancy and lactation differ in the adaptations invoked to meet the challenges for increased delivery of minerals (Fig. 5.4). A doubling of intestinal calcium and phosphorus absorption during pregnancy meets the fetal mineral demand.

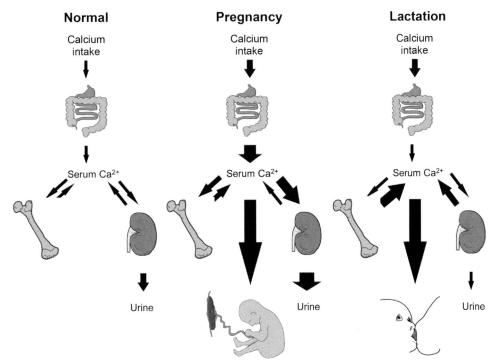

FIG. 5.4   Comparison of the adaptive processes of calcium and bone homeostasis during human pregnancy and lactation compared to normal (nonpregnant, nonlactating). The thickness of *arrows* indicates a relative increase or decrease with respect to normal. *(Modified with permission ©1997 The Endocrine Society. Kovacs CS, Kronenberg HM. Maternal-fetal calcium and bone metabolism during pregnancy, puerperium, and lactation. Endocr Rev 1997;18(6):832–72.)*

During lactation, an uncoupling of bone turnover favors marked skeletal resorption to provide much of the calcium for milk, regardless of oral calcium intake. After weaning, bone turnover uncouples in the reverse direction to favor net bone formation and return the skeleton to apparently normal strength.

These adaptations affect how disorders of bone and mineral metabolism may present, and they must be managed, as discussed in Chapter 21.

REFERENCES

1. Kovacs CS. Maternal mineral and bone metabolism during pregnancy, lactation, and post-weaning recovery. *Physiol Rev* 2016;**96**(2):449–547.
2. Hunt CD, Johnson LK. Calcium requirements: new estimations for men and women by cross-sectional statistical analyses of calcium balance data from metabolic studies. *Am J Clin Nutr* 2007;**86**(4):1054–63.
3. Institute of Medicine. *Dietary reference intakes for calcium and vitamin D*. Washington, DC: The National Academies Press; 2011.
4. Turner M, Barre PE, Benjamin A, Goltzman D, Gascon-Barre M. Does the maternal kidney contribute to the increased circulating 1,25-dihydroxyvitamin D concentrations during pregnancy? *Miner Electrolyte Metab* 1988;**14**:246–52.
5. Delvin EE, Salle BL, Glorieux FH, Adeleine P, David LS. Vitamin D supplementation during pregnancy: effect on neonatal calcium homeostasis. *J Pediatr* 1986;**109**:328–34.
6. Hollis BW, Johnson D, Hulsey TC, Ebeling M, Wagner CL. Vitamin D supplementation during pregnancy: double-blind, randomized clinical trial of safety and effectiveness. *J Bone Miner Res* 2011;**26**(10):2341–57.
7. Wagner CL, McNeil R, Hamilton SA, Winkler J, Rodriguez Cook C, Warner G, et al. A randomized trial of vitamin D supplementation in 2 community health center networks in South Carolina. *Am J Obstet Gynecol* 2013;**208**(2). 137.e1–13.
8. Roth DE, Al Mahmud A, Raqib R, Akhtar E, Perumal N, Pezzack B, et al. Randomized placebo-controlled trial of high-dose prenatal third-trimester vitamin D3 supplementation in Bangladesh: the AViDD trial. *Nutr J* 2013;**12**(1):47.
9. Bucht E, Telenius-Berg M, Lundell G, Sjoberg HE. Immunoextracted calcitonin in milk and plasma from totally thyroidectomized women. Evidence of monomeric calcitonin in plasma during pregnancy and lactation. *Acta Endocrinol* 1986;**113**:529–35.
10. Ohata Y, Arahori H, Namba N, Kitaoka T, Hirai H, Wada K, et al. Circulating levels of soluble alpha-Klotho are markedly elevated in human umbilical cord blood. *J Clin Endocrinol Metab* 2011;**96**(6):E943–7.
11. Pedersen EB, Johannesen P, Kristensen S, Rasmussen AB, Emmertsen K, Moller J, et al. Calcium, parathyroid hormone and calcitonin in normal pregnancy and preeclampsia. *Gynecol Obstet Invest* 1984;**18**:156–64.
12. Frenkel Y, Barkai G, Mashiach S, Dolev E, Zimlichman R, Weiss M. Hypocalciuria of preeclampsia is independent of parathyroid hormone level. *Obstet Gynecol* 1991;**77**:689–91.
13. Seely EW, Wood RJ, Brown EM, Graves SW. Lower serum ionized calcium and abnormal calciotropic hormone levels in preeclampsia. *J Clin Endocrinol Metab* 1992;(74):1436–40.
14. Lalau JD, Jans I, el Esper N, Bouillon R, Fournier A. Calcium metabolism, plasma parathyroid hormone, and calcitriol in transient hypertension of pregnancy. *Am J Hypertens* 1993;**6**:522–7.
15. Halhali A, Villa AR, Madrazo E, Soria MC, Mercado E, Diaz L, et al. Longitudinal changes in maternal serum 1,25-dihydroxyvitamin D and insulin like growth factor I levels in pregnant women who developed preeclampsia: comparison with normotensive pregnant women. *J Steroid Biochem Mol Biol* 2004;**89–90**(1–5):553–6.
16. Hofmeyr GJ, Lawrie TA, Atallah AN, Duley L, Torloni MR. Calcium supplementation during pregnancy for preventing hypertensive disorders and related problems. *Cochrane Database Syst Rev* 2014;**6**:CD001059.
17. Christian P, Khatry SK, Katz J, Pradhan EK, LeClerq SC, Shrestha SR, et al. Effects of alternative maternal micronutrient supplements on low birth weight in rural Nepal: double blind randomised community trial. *BMJ* 2003;**326**(7389):571.
18. Christian P, West KP, Khatry SK, Leclerq SC, Pradhan EK, Katz J, et al. Effects of maternal micronutrient supplementation on fetal loss and infant mortality: a cluster-randomized trial in Nepal. *Am J Clin Nutr* 2003;**78**(6):1194–202.
19. Perez-Lopez FR, Pasupuleti V, Mezones-Holguin E, Benites-Zapata VA, Thota P, Deshpande A, et al. Effect of vitamin D supplementation during pregnancy on maternal and neonatal outcomes: a systematic review and meta-analysis of randomized controlled trials. *Fertil Steril* 2015;**103** (5):1278–88 [e4].
20. Heaney RP, Skillman TG. Calcium metabolism in normal human pregnancy. *J Clin Endocrinol Metab* 1971;**33**(4):661–70.
21. Moller UK, Við Streym S, Mosekilde L, Rejnmark L. Changes in bone mineral density and body composition during pregnancy and postpartum. A controlled cohort study. *Osteoporos Int* 2012;**23**(4):1213–23.
22. Carneiro RM, Prebehalla L, Tedesco MB, Sereika SM, Gundberg CM, Stewart AF, et al. Evaluation of markers of bone turnover during lactation in African-Americans: a comparison with Caucasian lactation. *J Clin Endocrinol Metab* 2013;**98**(2):523–32.
23. Greer FR, Lane J, Ho M. Elevated serum parathyroid hormone, calcitonin, and 1,25-dihydroxyvitamin D in lactating women nursing twins. *Am J Clin Nutr* 1984;**40**:562–8.
24. Cross NA, Hillman LS, Forte LR. The effects of calcium supplementation, duration of lactation, and time of day on concentrations of parathyroid hormone-related protein in human milk: a pilot study. *J Hum Lact* 1998;**14**(2):111–7.
25. Jonas AJ, Dominguez B. Low breast milk phosphorus concentration in familial hypophosphatemia. *J Pediatr Gastroenterol Nutr* 1989;**8**(4):541–3.
26. Reade TM, Scriver CR. Hypophosphatemic rickets and breast milk. *N Engl J Med* 1979;**300**(24):1397.

27. Hollis BW, Wagner CL. Vitamin D requirements during lactation: high-dose maternal supplementation as therapy to prevent hypovitaminosis D for both the mother and the nursing infant. *Am J Clin Nutr* 2004;**80**(6 Suppl):1752S–1758S.

28. Basile LA, Taylor SN, Wagner CL, Horst RL, Hollis BW. The effect of high-dose vitamin D supplementation on serum vitamin D levels and milk calcium concentration in lactating women and their infants. *Breastfeed Med* 2006;**1**(1):27–35.

29. Wagner CL, Hulsey TC, Fanning D, Ebeling M, Hollis BW. High-dose vitamin D3 supplementation in a cohort of breastfeeding mothers and their infants: a 6-month follow-up pilot study. *Breastfeed Med* 2006;**1**(2):59–70.

30. Kalkwarf HJ, Specker BL, Heubi JE, Vieira NE, Yergey AL. Intestinal calcium absorption of women during lactation and after weaning. *Am J Clin Nutr* 1996;**63**(4):526–31.

31. Ritchie LD, Fung EB, Halloran BP, Turnlund JR, Van Loan MD, Cann CE, et al. A longitudinal study of calcium homeostasis during human pregnancy and lactation and after resumption of menses. *Am J Clin Nutr* 1998;**67**(4):693–701.

32. Brembeck P, Lorentzon M, Ohlsson C, Winkvist A, Augustin H. Changes in cortical volumetric bone mineral density and thickness, and trabecular thickness in lactating women postpartum. *J Clin Endocrinol Metab* 2015;**100**(2):535–43.

33. Bjornerem A, Ghasem-Zadeh A, Wang X, Bui M, Walker SP, Zebaze R, et al. Irreversible deterioration of cortical and trabecular microstructure associated with breastfeeding. *J Bone Miner Res* 2017;**32**(4):681–7.

34. Sowers M, Corton G, Shapiro B, Jannausch ML, Crutchfield M, Smith ML, et al. Changes in bone density with lactation. *JAMA* 1993;**269**(24):3130–5.

35. Funk JL, Shoback DM, Genant HK. Transient osteoporosis of the hip in pregnancy: natural history of changes in bone mineral density. *Clin Endocrinol (Oxf)* 1995;**43**(3):373–82.

36. Specker B, Binkley T. High parity is associated with increased bone size and strength. *Osteoporos Int* 2005;**16**(12):1969–74.

37. Wiklund PK, Xu L, Wang Q, Mikkola T, Lyytikainen A, Volgyi E, et al. Lactation is associated with greater maternal bone size and bone strength later in life. *Osteoporos Int* 2012;**23**(7):1939–45.

38. Kirby BJ, Ma Y, Martin HM, Buckle Favaro KL, Karaplis AC, Kovacs CS. Upregulation of calcitriol during pregnancy and skeletal recovery after lactation do not require parathyroid hormone. *J Bone Miner Res* 2013;**28**(9):1987–2000.

39. Gillies BR, Ryan BA, Tonkin BA, Poulton IJ, Ma Y, Kirby BJ, et al. Absence of calcitriol causes increased lactational bone loss and lower milk calcium but does not impair post-lactation bone recovery in Cyp27b1 null mice. *J Bone Miner Res* 2017;**33**(1):16–26.

40. Fudge NJ, Kovacs CS. Pregnancy up-regulates intestinal calcium absorption and skeletal mineralization independently of the vitamin D receptor. *Endocrinology* 2010;**151**(3):886–95.

41. Kirby BJ, Ardeshirpour L, Woodrow JP, Wysolmerski JJ, Sims NA, Karaplis AC, et al. Skeletal recovery after weaning does not require PTHrP. *J Bone Miner Res* 2011;**26**(6):1242–51.

42. Woodrow JP, Sharpe CJ, Fudge NJ, Hoff AO, Gagel RF, Kovacs CS. Calcitonin plays a critical role in regulating skeletal mineral metabolism during lactation. *Endocrinology* 2006;**147**(9):4010–21.

43. Revilla R, Revilla M, Hernandez ER, Villa LF, Varela L, Rico H. Evidence that the loss of bone mass induced by GnRH agonists is not totally recovered. *Maturitas* 1995;**22**:145–50.

44. Roux C, Pelissier C, Listrat V, Kolta S, Simonetta C, Guignard M, et al. Bone loss during gonadotropin releasing hormone agonist treatment and use of nasal calcitonin. *Osteoporos Int* 1995;**5**:185–90.

45. Fogelman I, Fentiman I, Hamed H, Studd JW, Leather AT. Goserelin (Zoladex) and the skeleton. *Br J Obstet Gynaecol* 1994;**101**(Suppl 10):19–23.

46. Mukherjee T, Barad D, Turk R, Freeman R. A randomized, placebo-controlled study on the effect of cyclic intermittent etidronate therapy on the bone mineral density changes associated with six months of gonadotropin-releasing hormone agonist treatment. *Am J Obstet Gynecol* 1996;**175**:105–9.

47. Taga M, Minaguchi H. Reduction of bone mineral density by gonadotropin-releasing hormone agonist, nafarelin, is not completely reversible at 6 months after the cessation of administration. *Acta Obstet Gynecol Scand* 1996;**75**:162–5.

48. Newhall-Perry K, Holloway L, Osburn L, Monroe SE, Heinrichs L, Henzl M, et al. Effects of a gonadotropin-releasing hormone agonist on the calcium-parathyroid axis and bone turnover in women with endometriosis. *Am J Obstet Gynecol* 1995;**173**:824–9.

49. Orwoll ES, Yuzpe AA, Burry KA, Heinrichs L, Buttram Jr. VC, Hornstein MD. Nafarelin therapy in endometriosis: long-term effects on bone mineral density. *Am J Obstet Gynecol* 1994;**171**:1221–5.

50. Rico H, Arnanz F, Revilla M, Perera S, Iritia M, Villa LF, et al. Total and regional bone mineral content in women treated with GnRH agonists. *Calcif Tissue Int* 1993;**52**:354–7.

51. Paoletti AM, Serra GG, Cagnacci A, Vacca AM, Guerriero S, Solla E, et al. Spontaneous reversibility of bone loss induced by gonadotropin-releasing hormone analog treatment. *Fertil Steril* 1996;**65**:707–10.

52. Howell R, Edmonds DK, Dowsett M, Crook D, Lees B, Stevenson JC. Gonadotropin-releasing hormone analogue (goserelin) plus hormone replacement therapy for the treatment of endometriosis: a randomized controlled trial. *Fertil Steril* 1995;**64**:474–81.

53. Uemura T, Mohri J, Osada H, Suzuki N, Katagiri N, Minaguchi H. Effect of gonadotropin-releasing hormone agonist on the bone mineral density of patients with endometriosis. *Fertil Steril* 1994;**62**:246–50.

54. Kalkwarf HJ, Specker BL, Bianchi DC, Ranz J, Ho M. The effect of calcium supplementation on bone density during lactation and after weaning. *N Engl J Med* 1997;**337**(8):523–8.

Chapter 6

Gestational Glucose Metabolism: Focus on the Role and Mechanisms of Insulin Resistance

Md. Wasim Khan* and Brian T. Layden*,†

*Division of Endocrinology, Diabetes and Metabolism, Department of Medicine, University of Illinois at Chicago, Chicago, IL, United States, †Jesse Brown Veterans Affairs Medical Center, Chicago, IL, United States

---

Key Clinical Changes

- Pregnancy requires redirecting maternal metabolism to adapt to shunting glucose to the fetus.
- Early pregnancy is characterized by enhanced insulin sensitivity, followed by progressive insulin resistance (IR) in the second and third trimesters.
- Insulin resistance is the result of increased secretion of pregnancy hormones such as human placental lactogen, growth hormone, progesterone, and prolactin.
- Fasting glucose levels decrease during pregnancy in spite of enhanced gluconeogenesis.
- β-cell hyperplasia results in progressive increase in insulin production in both the fasting and postprandial states.
- Maternal insulin resistance (IR) and lower fasting glucose levels result in lipolysis and hypertriglyceridemia, allowing preferential fat use for fuel.

6.1 INTRODUCTION

The fact that metabolism reprograms and fashions itself to successfully combat the stress of pregnancy in the living organism is a miraculous event. The metabolic reprogramming of pregnancy is a dynamic process. Other similar reprogramming occurs in physiological states (i.e., growth), and nonphysiological conditions such as cancer. Not so long ago, pregnancy was thought of as a phenomenon in which the growing fetus was considered a parasite to the health of the mother. However, recent research has shown us how the complex processes of pregnancy and lactation lead to reprogramming of the nutritional balance between the mother and fetus, a process that is tightly regulated by the interplay of hormones to allocate nutrients precisely between the two. As pregnancy progresses, the metabolic rewiring becomes more complex, as it deals with the traffic of nutrients to and from the mother and fetus. In short, this rewiring of maternal metabolism during the entire period of pregnancy has the following purposes:

- To provide the growing fetus with the necessary micronutrients and macronutrients required for development and to prepare it for birth
- To adequately meet the increased nutrient demands of the mother
- To build up maternal energy and metabolite stores that are sufficient to meet the demands of labor and lactation

During early gestation and midgestation, there is increased maternal food intake that is directed toward storage and development of the maternal structures responsible for gestation.[1,2] Concurrent with increased food intake, there is a significant increase in insulin production that boosts the overall anabolism (particularly lipogenesis), while inhibiting lipid oxidation.[1,2] Insulin sensitivity, however, changes as pregnancy proceeds, with high sensitivity in the early stages and a progressive reduced sensitivity (insulin resistance) toward the end of gestation. In the late stages of gestation, food intake continues to increase, but there is a shift from anabolism to catabolism as a means to mobilize energy to support the growth

Maternal-Fetal and Neonatal Endocrinology. https://doi.org/10.1016/B978-0-12-814823-5.00006-4

and development of the fetus and maternal tissues such as breast and liver.[1] This shift in metabolism from anabolic to catabolic is brought about, in part, by striking changes in insulin sensitivity.

Understanding the shifts in nutrient balance and metabolism during pregnancy has direct implications to how pregnancy is clinically managed. Moreover, the incidence of gestational diabetes mellitus (GDM), which is diabetes that develops during pregnancy, has doubled over the last 6–8 years in parallel with the obesity epidemic. GDM carries long-term implications for the subsequent development of type 2 diabetes in the mother, as well as increased risk for obesity and glucose intolerance in the offspring. Due to the increasing threat of GDM, understanding the complex regulation of insulin action and carbohydrate metabolism during pregnancy in physiological and pathophysiological conditions is a very relevant topic to explore. In this chapter, we focus on gestational glucose metabolism, the cellular mechanisms governing IR, and insulin secretion during normal pregnancy.

6.2 GESTATIONAL GLUCOSE METABOLISM AND THE ROLE OF INSULIN

6.2.1 An Overview

Glucose is the principal energy substrate and macromolecular building block for the placenta and fetus, making it essential for growth and development. It is the major substrate that is placentally transferred from mother to fetus, and it has been shown (in studies on rats) that it cannot be synthesized de novo from placentally transferred substrates in the fetus.[1,2] During pregnancy, the changes in glucose homeostasis are governed by heightened insulin production, accompanied by increased IR.[3] Therefore, it is a complex set of mechanisms that work together to keep glucose metabolism relatively constant. Broadly, there are three major points of regulation of glucose metabolism: (1) maintenance of maternal glucose levels by increasing rates of glucose production and development of relative maternal glucose intolerance and IR; (2) transfer of maternal glucose to the fetus by the placenta, which is buffered by placental glucose utilization; and (3) production of insulin by the developing fetal pancreas, which enhances glucose utilization and thus increases glucose demand by the fetus during late gestation. The majority of physiological and pathophysiological research on glucose metabolism during pregnancy has focused on its modulation, regulation, and flux.

6.2.2 Glucose Homeostasis During the Stages of Pregnancy

Both basal and postprandial glucose levels undergo gradual changes over the entire course of pregnancy to meet the nutritional and anabolic demands of the mother and fetus. Studies have shown that throughout each trimester, there are significant progressive alterations in women who have normal glucose tolerance.[5,6] Basal glucose, insulin, and gluconeogenesis levels show no significant differences in early pregnancy. However, by the third trimester, maternal blood glucose is lower and insulin levels double compared to nongravid women. There is a significant elevation in postprandial glucose concentration, with about a 16%–30% increase in hepatic glucose production to maintain maternal glucose levels at 15%–20% higher levels than in the fetus. The flux of glucose to the fetus is counteracted by hyperphagia in the mother, as well as maternal metabolism reprograming to reduce consumption of glucose by her own tissues.[4] Fasting plasma glucose levels significantly decline despite increased hepatic glucose production over the course of pregnancy, through complex mechanisms that are still poorly understood.[5] The most probable causative factors for this are (1) increased plasma volume in early pregnancy, (2) increased glucose utilization by mother and fetus, (3) inadequate hepatic gluconeogenesis, and (4) a lower glucose set point.

6.2.3 Insulin Sensitivity During the Stages of Pregnancy

Peripheral insulin sensitivity is one of the major drivers of overall glucose homeostasis, and it is under dynamic regulation throughout pregnancy.[7] Insulin levels are regulated by the balance of insulin production by the pancreas and its subsequent clearance and insulin sensitivity within maternal muscle, liver, and fat tissues.[3] Overall, insulin lowers plasma glucose by increasing cellular uptake and inhibiting hepatic glucose production after meals, while reduced insulin action leads to lipolysis, fatty acid oxidation, and gluconeogenesis. During pregnancy, there is increased fasting hepatic gluconeogenesis, despite lower fasting glucose, and increased insulin production, which supports a decline in maternal insulin sensitivity as pregnancy progresses.[8] It is noteworthy that hepatic glucose production is due to gluconeogenesis and glycogenolysis, so whether gluconeogenesis (which also depends on availability of substrates such as alanine) remains unaltered during pregnancy is not entirely clear.[2]

There is enhanced insulin sensitivity, accompanied by lipid accumulation in fat depots during the first weeks after embryonic implantation, due to decreased growth hormone levels resulting from modifications in the placental region.[1,9,10] After this period of increased sensitivity to insulin, circulating levels of human placental lactogens, placentally derived human growth hormone (pGH), progesterone, cortisol, prolactin, and other hormones increase and contribute to reducing insulin sensitivity in peripheral tissues, such as adipocytes and skeletal muscle. This occurs during the second and third trimesters of pregnancy, but the highest levels of IR occur in the third trimester. In late stages of normal pregnancy, there is a reduction of insulin-regulated glucose disposal of up to 50% due to heightened IR, which the body tries to counterbalance through an approximate 200%–250% increase in insulin production.[11] This period is characterized by reduced utilization of glucose by the mother and enhanced maternal hepatic glucose production.[6,12]

6.3 CELLULAR MECHANISMS FOR IR IN PREGNANCY

Pregnancy is characterized by radical changes in insulin sensitivity during the course of pregnancy and these changes do not reflect a pathological condition. Rather, they represent a necessary and indispensable adaptation to meet the energy demands of the fetus and to prepare the mother for delivery and lactation. In fact, IR developing in pregnancy is likely to be a physiological event that favors glucose supply to the fetus. The reduced insulin-mediated utilization of glucose switches maternal energy metabolism from metabolizing carbohydrates to lipid substrates—specifically, free fatty acids (FFAs)—thereby redirecting carbohydrates toward the fetal tissues. In late gestation, maternal adipose stores decline, while postprandial levels of FFAs build up in circulation, and insulin action is reduced by up to 60% compared to nonpregnant women.[13] The molecular basis of dynamic changes in IR during pregnancy is incompletely understood. Thus far, studies have brought forward many causative factors of IR during pregnancy, ranging from defects in insulin signaling to the interplay of hormones and adipocytokines (Fig. 6.1). Here, we will discuss what is known about IR during pregnancy, focusing on the most recognized causative factors to date.

6.3.1 Placental Hormones and Adipocytokines in IR During Pregnancy

During the later stages of pregnancy, one of the chief tissues contributing to whole-body glucose homeostasis is skeletal muscle, and it becomes insulin resistant along with adipose tissue.[14] Pregnancy hormones derived from the placenta, as well as various other maternal adipocytokines secreted during pregnancy, are believed to play important roles in this reprogramming (Table 6.1). However, studies indicate that with the exception of tumor necrosis factor (TNF)-α, changes in placental hormones do not solely mediate maternal IR.[14] Instead, a combination of factors lead to changes in insulin sensitivity during pregnancy. We will discuss the most important of these and how they are thought to play a role in developing IR during pregnancy.

A pregnancy-specific hormone, human placental lactogen (hPL), has been reported to increase up to 30-fold throughout the course of pregnancy, and it has been shown to induce pancreatic insulin production.[15] There are studies that show the positive association of hPL with peripheral IR; however, the results of these studies are variable.[16] Another important pregnancy hormone implicated in IR is placental growth hormone (GH-V), which differs from pituitary growth hormone by only 13 amino acids. GH-V levels also go up by 6-fold to 8-fold during pregnancy, and it replaces pituitary growth hormone in the maternal circulation by 20 weeks of gestation.[17] Similar to the well-documented role of pituitary growth hormone on insulin sensitivity, when pGH was overexpressed in transgenic mice to reach levels comparable to the third trimester of pregnancy, significant peripheral IR was observed.[18] Recent studies indicate that one particularly important effect of pGH in the context of IR is to enhance the expression of the p85α subunit of phosphatidylinositol (PI) 3-kinase in skeletal muscles in pregnant and nonpregnant women.[19] The p85α subunit of PI 3-kinase acts as a dominant-negative competitor to the formation of PI 3-kinase heterodimer with the p110 subunit, thereby inhibiting PI 3-kinase activity and subsequently preventing further insulin signaling, which leads to increased IR.[20] More work is needed to clarify how these specific hormones work together during pregnancy.

There has also been a focus on the role of maternal secreted factors such as leptin, adiponectin, TNF-α, interleukin-6, and resistin (collectively known as *adipocytokines*) in mediating IR during pregnancy. TNF-α is a cytokine produced from monocytes, macrophages, T-cells, neutrophils, fibroblasts, and adipocytes.[14] A positive correlation has been reported between TNF-α and hyperinsulinemia in obese animals and humans.[21,22] In in vitro culture studies, TNF-α causes an increase in IR in rat and human skeletal muscle cells.[38] There is also evidence that local TNF-α found in skeletal muscle may act in a paracrine fashion to increase IR.[23] The most probable mechanism by which TNF-α impairs insulin signaling is by increasing serine phosphorylation of insulin receptor substrate (IRS)-1[21] and diminishing insulin receptor tyrosine kinase activity.[24] Some studies have reported a correlation in changes in insulin sensitivity with plasma TNF-α from early

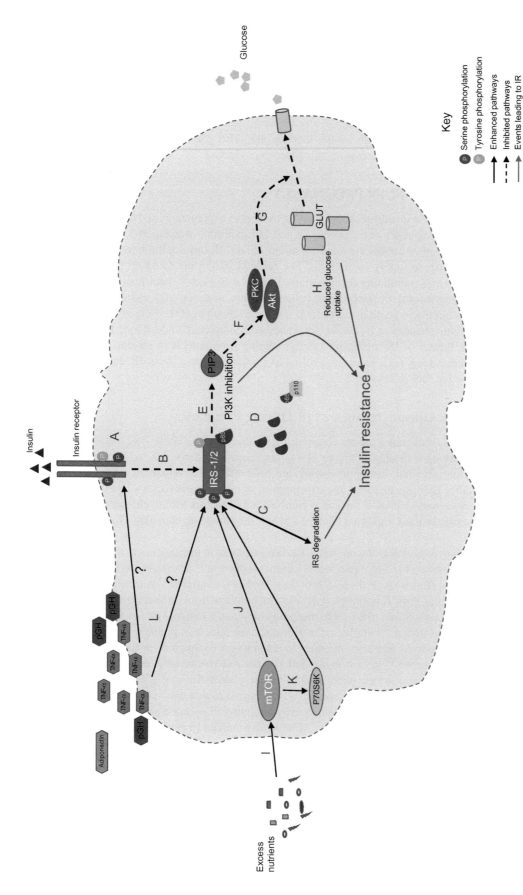

FIG. 6.1 Summary of potential mechanisms that cause IR during pregnancy. Despite increased insulin production, there is increased phosphorylation at serine residues of insulin receptors (A), which leads to decreased IRS-1 activation. (B) Increased serine phosphorylation of IRS-1 (C) leads to the degradation of IRS-1. Additionally, IRS-1 can be bound by increased levels of p85, which competes with the p85–p110 heterodimers (D), which leads to decreased phosphorylation and decreased activation of the PI3kinase (E). Decreased PI3K activity dampens Akt and PKC activity, leading to reduced glucose uptake (F–H). Excess nutrients that are a hallmark of pregnancy activate the cellular nutrient sensor mTOR, which phosphorylates IRS at tyrosine residues (I–J). Active mTOR further phosphorylates its downstream effector, S6 kinase (K), which phosphorylates and inhibits IRS-1 in a feedback loop. Finally, the increased levels of TNF-α and pGH with decreased adiponectin levels inhibit the insulin receptor and IRS (L) via mechanisms that are not completely understood.

TABLE 6.1 Hormonal effects on maternal metabolism

Hormone/ adipocytokine	Levels through gestation	Effects	
		Early gestation to midgestation	Late gestation
Estradiol	Progressively increased	Increased triglyceride levels	Increased triglyceride levels
Progesterone	Progressively increased	Enhanced food intake, lipogenesis, and IR	Enhances food intake, lipogenesis, and IR
Prolactin	Progressively increased	Enhanced food intake, lipogenesis	Enhanced food intake and insulin production
pGH	Increased after midgestation	–	Enhanced insulin/IGF-1 production and IR
TNF-α	Progressively increased	–	Enhanced IR
Leptin	Progressively increased	Controversial; thought to increase nutrient transfer to fetus	Controversial; thought to increase nutrient transfer to fetus and mobilize fat depots
Adiponectin	Decreased in late gestation	Enhanced IR	Enhanced IR
Resistin	Progressively increased	Enhanced IR	Enhanced IR
Visfatin	Progressively increased or remains unaltered	Controversial (maternal-fetal glucose transfer); possibly enhances insulin sensitivity	Controversial (maternal-fetal glucose transfer); possibly enhances insulin sensitivity

to late gestation.[14] These studies point out that circulating TNF-α may be produced by the placenta and skeletal muscle to induce or exacerbate IR through mechanisms that remain to be determined.[14]

As adiposity increases during pregnancy, there is enhanced secretion of pro-inflammatory cytokines from adipose tissue,[25,26] suggesting that their release may play an important role in the development of IR. Adiponectin is the most abundant adipokine, secreted exclusively by adipose tissue. Low plasma levels of adiponectin correlate with IR in obesity, type 2 diabetes, and GDM.[27,28] Recent studies have shown that expression of adiponectin messenger ribonucleic acid (mRNA) in white adipose tissue and secretion of adiponectin both decline with advancing gestation, even in lean women,[29] which suggests that pregnancy-associated factors reduce adiponectin levels. Skeletal muscle and liver have adiponectin receptors.[30] Adiponectin signals via cyclic adenosine monophosphate (cAMP) activated protein kinase to stimulate glucose uptake in skeletal muscle and reduce hepatic glucose production. Therefore, diminished adiponectin concentrations likely lead to reduced glucose uptake in skeletal muscle and increased hepatic glucose production. Additionally, the buildup of TNF-α and other proinflammatory mediators in the adipose tissue due to IR appears to suppress the transcription of adiponectin,[31,32] which may contribute to the lower levels of adiponectin observed in serum.

6.3.2 Role of Reduced Glucose Transport

The primary action and effect of insulin is to increase glucose uptake into insulin-responsive tissues (muscle, liver, and adipose). Upon insulin action at its receptor, glucose is transported across the cell membrane by glucose transporters (GLUTs) by the facilitated transport process.[14] There are 14 known glucose transporter isoforms, each of which plays a specific role in glucose metabolism, which is further determined by its pattern of tissue expression, substrate specificity, transport kinetics, and regulated expression in various physiological conditions. Researchers have studied the effect of pregnancy and gestational diabetes on glucose transport specifically in muscle, which is the major insulin responsive tissue responsible for glucose uptake. In one study involving nonpregnant women, pregnant women without GDM, and pregnant women with GDM that were matched for body mass index (BMI), age, and ethnicity (90% Caucasian), freshly isolated muscle fibers obtained during an elective cesarean delivery was used to calculate the ability of insulin to stimulate glucose transport.[33]

This study demonstrated that the skeletal muscle fibers of pregnant women experienced a 40% reduction in insulin-stimulated glucose transport compared to nonpregnant women, and this impairment in insulin-mediated glucose uptake was reduced 65% in GDM subjects.[33] This impairment in insulin-mediated glucose uptake was not due to any change in total GLUT4 expression in skeletal muscle between pregnant women with and without GDM.[34] Similar to this study, others have shown that glucose transport in isolated adipocytes was also markedly reduced in normal pregnant women and further reduced in obese women with GDM.[35] Taken together, these studies have shown that IR contributes to reduced glucose uptake into insulin-sensitive tissues during pregnancy.

6.3.3 Changes in the Insulin-Signaling Pathway

When insulin binds to the insulin receptor, it stimulates the phosphorylation of at least six tyrosine residues in the ß-subunit of the receptor.[36] This is the initial step in insulin signaling. Maximal tyrosine phosphorylation is required to achieve full activation of the pathway, but this is repressed in GDM subjects, which is possibly the result of an endogenous inhibitory pathway for receptor signaling.[33] The autophosphorylation of these tyrosine residues activates the receptor for dock intracellular protein, IRS-1, which is the major docking protein in human skeletal muscle. Once IRS-1 is phosphorylated on its tyrosine residues, it activates the recruitment process of the PI 3-kinase, which is a crucial moment in insulin signaling.[38] Physiologically, these phosphorylation events are balanced by the activity of cellular and membrane-bound protein tyrosine phosphatases, which carry out the dephosphorylation reactions, serve as a negative regulator of insulin signaling, and potentially alter or reduce insulin sensitivity in human and animal models.[39,40] However, research indicates that the levels of the major protein phosphatase (the PTP1B protein) is not altered in pregnancy.[41]

In contrast to tyrosine phosphorylation at the insulin receptor, which stimulates insulin signaling, phosphorylation of the serine/threonine residues act as a dampening signaling mechanism.[14] Exploring this in pregnancy, investigators measured the activity of the partially purified insulin receptors isolated from skeletal muscles of women in late gestation after insulin treatment, and they found a significant reduction in activity of the insulin receptors.[37] Subsequently, these authors pretreated these insulin receptors with alkaline phosphatase (to remove phosphorylation), and found that the ability of insulin to activate phosphorylation of tyrosine residues on the insulin receptor was restored to normal in muscles from pregnant women, but only partially restored in muscles from GDM subjects.[37] These data suggest that during pregnancy, there may be some posttranslational modification of the insulin receptor, induced by a serine kinase, which may be dampening insulin signaling. Additionally, the cytokine TNF-α (whose levels increase during pregnancy) has been documented to act directly as a serine/threonine kinase to inhibit both the insulin receptor and IRS-1 tyrosine phosphorylation,[41] thereby leading to increased IR. Another factor is elevated serine phosphorylation (Serine 307/312 for mice/humans) of IRS-1 dampens insulin action on both the insulin receptor and IRS-1, and leads to impaired glucose uptake.[42] The serine kinases that are responsible for this phosphorylation event remain unknown; however, there are a number of potential candidates ranging from JNK1, protein kinase C, mammalian target of rapamycin (mTOR), and p70S6K1.[43–45] As an example, JNK1 is known to be activated by cytokines such as TNF-α (which increase in late gestation), and other kinases such as mTOR and p70S6K1, which are downstream of the insulin-signaling pathway. These factors may provide a feedback inhibition loop in insulin-resistant conditions such as pregnancy, when nutrients are in excess.[46,47]

For IRS-1 to activate the PI 3 kinase, IRS-1 must dock the p-85α and p110 heterodimers of the PI 3 kinase.[48] This association of IRS-1 and PI 3-kinase brings the latter into close proximity to its phospholipid substrates, resulting in the formation of phosphoinositol-3,4,5-phosphate, which is critical for downstream signaling to Akt, and protein kinase C, which regulates glucose uptake.[48] Studies have found that the protein levels of p85α were higher (1.5–2 fold) in skeletal muscle and adipose tissue of pregnant non-GDM and GDM subjects compared with obese nonpregnant women.[33,49] These levels returned to normal in these subject groups a month after delivery.[20] It is possible that excess p85α subunits compete with p85α–p110 heterodimers binding to IRS-1, thereby dampening insulin signaling.

6.3.4 Role of Adipose Tissue

As stated previously, there is no change in the levels of GLUT4 protein in skeletal muscle; however, researchers have found that both GLUT4 levels and insulin-induced translocation of GLUT4 to plasma membranes are significantly downregulated in the adipose tissue of pregnant women, and the decrease is more significant in pregnant GDM subjects.[50,51] One of the most significant molecular changes in adipose tissue during pregnancy includes a reduction in the peroxisome proliferator-activated receptor (PPAR)-γ,[14] a transcription factor that is highly expressed in adipose tissue. PPAR-γ is considered a central regulator of the adipogenic program because it plays essential roles in fat cell differentiation, insulin sensitivity, and lipid storage.[52,53] Linda et al., reported a 40%–50% decrease in PPARγ mRNA and protein levels in abdominal white adipose tissue from both obese pregnant control subjects and obese GDM subjects at term, compared with obese non-pregnant subjects.[49] One hypothesis is that during gestation, the increased levels of the inflammatory cytokine TNF-α downregulates PPARγ expression in 3T3-L1 cells and can inhibit adipocyte differentiation.[54,55] These observations have led to the hypothesis that placental growth hormone plays an important role during pregnancy in accelerating the transition from lipid storage to lipolysis, along with IR. Together, these studies indicate that adipose tissue IR could lead to important metabolic profile changes such as FFA release and cytokine expression, which may play a major role in the mechanisms underlying IR by increasing nutrient availability and transfer to the fetus.

6.4 ROLE OF β-CELL ADAPTATIONS IN PREGNANCY

As mentioned previously, glucose provides the majority of fetal energy and building block needed.[56,57] However, there is a challenge because glucose transport across the placenta is a passive process. It is achieved by the use of facilitative glucose transporters and depends on the concentration gradient across the maternal and fetal circulations.[56–58] In early gestation, the β-cells from the developing fetus lower their glucose concentration gradient by maintaining high basal levels of insulin secretion and lowering sensitivity to glucose.[59] The main challenge arrives during late gestation, when fetal growth is at its peak and more maternal glucose is needed for the fetus. In response to the increased demand for glucose, the placenta secretes hormones that enhance maternal IR and hepatic gluconeogenesis, thereby raising maternal glucose levels to maintain an optimal gradient.[60] This enhanced IR leads to adaptations that result in growth of the pool of maternal β-cells and their insulin-secreting capactiy.[92–101] Together, increased maternal IR and β-cell adaptations ensure a steady supply of nutrients to the fetus until the end of gestation, after which the β-cells return to their prepregnancy size and number.[61–65]

6.4.1 β-Cell Response to Placental Lactogens

Researchers have shown that β-cell adaptation is not a result of heightened IR in the mother, but this compensation takes place before the development of IR.[61,62] Increased β-cell proliferation in pregnancy parallels the increased production of lactogens of both pituitary and placental origin.[61] This has been shown to be true in rodents, where prolactin treatment significantly drives β-cell proliferation, and enhances glucose-stimulated secretion of insulin both in vitro and in vivo.[61,62,66]

To strengthen these early observations, studies also have shown that an intact prolactin receptor (PRLR), whose expression increases in β-cells during pregnancy, is essential for adaptations during pregnancy.[67–71] Among the genes activated by the PRLR-signaling cascade that are of particular importance in pregnancy are tryptophan hydroxylase 1 and 2 (TPH 1 and 2), which control the rate-limiting step in the synthesis of serotonin.[71–75] During pregnancy, Tph1 RNA is reported to increase up to 3-fold in the islets of mice.[71–75] Thus, during pregnancy, β-cells appear to produce higher amounts of serotonin during pregnancy.[71,73,75] This study also shows that when tryptophan is removed from the diet, or with pharmacologic inhibition of TPH, the diminished serotonin signaling reduces β-cell expansion, which in turn results in further impairment of glucose tolerance in pregnant mice.[71] Serotonin also has been shown to increase insulin secretion in response to glucose during pregnancy.[76] However, the exact function of serotonin secreted from the maternal islets during pregnancy is uncertain. Contradictory evidence has arisen in part because of the various experimental models and conditions used in these studies.[77] Furthermore, mammals have many serotonin receptors, and many of them are expressed in different types of islet cells, with dynamically regulated expression throughout pregnancy.[71] However, there is convincing evidence that, at least in mouse models, serotonin secreted during pregnancy drives β-cell expansion and proliferation.[71]

Serotonin binds to ionotropic Htr3a receptors, which function as serotonin-gated cationic channels and allow a leak of extracellular Na$^+$ ions along the concentration gradient into the β-cell. This, thereby, induces mild depolarization of the membrane and lowers the threshold for insulin secretion upon a glucose stimulus.[76] It also has been shown that in pregnant mice, blocking Htr3a signaling reduces insulin secretion by the β-cell and induces glucose intolerance. This does not occur in nonpregnant mice, thereby indicating that Htr3a has a pregnancy-specific role.[76] A hypothetical role of β-cell serotonin is somewhat similar to that of glucokinase. As glucokinase senses glucose levels in the β-cells, TPH can act as a sensor of protein levels because tryptophan is an essential amino acid, with the lowest levels in most types of diets. Additionally, TPH has a Km for tryptophan that is similar to its physiological concentration in tissues, and it controls the rate-limiting step in serotonin synthesis. Therefore, levels of serotonin produced by β-cells during pregnancy may closely reflect dietary protein intake.[78] Taken together, placental lactogens drive β-cell-specific serotonin synthesis in pregnancy, which in turn drives β-cell expansion and proliferation and insulin secretion. This may be one of the mechanisms to fine-tune the β-cell nutrient response during pregnancy.

6.4.2 Other Pathways Mediating β-Cell Expansion in Pregnancy

The fact that a complete loss of islet serotonin signaling does not produce a complete halt in β-cell proliferation in pregnant mice[71] indicates that complementary pathways must exist for β-cell adaptations. These pathways are likely providing refinement, critical constraint, and redundancy to provide a well-balanced reprogramming of β-cell physiology in pregnancy. The changes in glucose levels and the demand for insulin as IR begins to develop could provide cues for the serotonin-driven β-cell proliferation.[79-81] Other fine-tuning mechanisms include increased levels of glucokinase (the β-cell glucose sensor), cAMP, and junction coupling, which may play important roles in the final release of insulin from the β-cells, all of which have been suggested to be coordinated by PRLR signaling.[82-84]

PRLR signaling has also been shown to activate other signaling cascades such as the Ras/Rap/MAPK, PI3K/AKT/mTOR, and Raf/MEK/ERK, although their exact mechanism in β-cell adaptations remains unclear.[67,85-88] In pregnant rats, islet endothelial cells, which secrete abundant hepatocyte growth factor, proliferate before β-cell expansion takes place.[89] Additionally, several transcription factors such as Foxd3 have been implicated in β-cell expansion during pregnancy. Targeted deletion of pancreatic Foxd3 reduced β-cell expansion during pregnancy; however, it also has been shown that Foxd3 expression normally decreases in pregnancy.[90] In contrast, expression of FoxM1, which is a cell cycle-associated transcription factor, increases in β-cells of the mouse during pregnancy,[91] whereas pancreatic deletion of FoxM1 reduces β-cell expansion during pregnancy.[91,92] Taken together, all these changes, together with β-cell adaptations, counterbalance IR during late pregnancy and ensure adequate insulin secretion.

6.5 PLACENTAL HORMONES AND ADIPOCYTOKINES IN THE CONTROL OF MATERNAL METABOLISM

Maternal hormones produced by the placenta and pituitary are the prime factors that orchestrate metabolic reprogramming of maternal metabolism. As discussed previously, hormones and cytokines play major roles in modulating insulin sensitivity and β-cell adaptations throughout pregnancy. In this section, we will take a closer look at how the levels of these hormones change during pregnancy and orchestrate changes in maternal metabolism (Table 6.1).

6.5.1 Early Gestation to Midgestation

There are three main changes in hormone production from the placenta and maternal pituitary gland that control metabolic reprogramming during early gestation to midgestation. First, in humans placental estradiol and progesterone production increases exponentially after 6 weeks of gestation. Studies in mice have shown that estradiol is important for placental angiogenesis, an essential process for feto-placental nutrient transport.[93,94] Progesterone has been shown to stimulate maternal food intake,[95] and in combination with free cortisol and TNF-α (which increase in late gestation), it attenuates insulin action in adipose tissue and skeletal muscle, thereby giving rise to IR.[96-98] Second, there is a progressive increase in the amounts of prolactin and hPL secreted by the pituitary and decidua.[99] Third, GH-N (pituitary growth hormone) levels decline throughout early pregnancy and are undetectable at 24 weeks of gestation; conversely, the level of GH-V (placental growth hormone) rises sharply after midgestation until delivery.[100-102] The fall in GH-N levels may enhance maternal insulin sensitivity and, together with progesterone and prolactin, promote maternal lipid accumulation.[99] The rise in progesterone, prolactin, and hPL increase maternal food intake in early gestation, after which levels of leptin (produced by maternal adipose tissues and placenta) contribute to maternal hyperphagia.[99,103-105] These changes drives maternal white adipose tissue accumulation, which is an essential source of energy and serves as a reservoir for energy during lactation.[99] The lactogens may also promote fat deposition by inducing the expression of PPAR-γ and adipogenesis in preadipocyte precursors.[99,104,106]

6.5.2 Late Gestation

GH-V levels rise sharply after midgestation. Together with increased TNF-α, cortisol, progesterone, and decreased levels of adiponectin, these contribute to increased IR, thereby further increasing insulin production. Despite these changes, lipolysis increases and adipose stores are mobilized during fasting.[18,107-109] The size of the placenta and maternal glucose levels regulate GH-V secretion, with fasting and hypoglycemia weakly stimulating its production and glucose administration in vivo and in vitro inhibiting its secretion.[110] Therefore, it is thought that GH-V acts as an insulin antagonist that impairs the utilization of glucose by the mother, thereby enhancing glucose delivery to the developing fetus.[99] GH-V has also been shown to control maternal IGF-1 production, which promotes maternal tissue growth and placental blood flow.[4,30-32] In late gestation, the effects of leptin are blunted by lactogenic hormones, giving rise to central leptin resistance. This in turn enables the mother to maintain high calorie intake despite the tremendous increase in lipid levels in the body.[99] Together, these somatogenic and lactogenic hormones work together to regulate the metabolic adaptations that occur during pregnancy.

6.5.3   Role of Adipocytokines

Pregnancy-induced IR has mainly been attributed to the interplay of placental and maternal hormones, although the underlying mechanisms are not completely understood.[111,112] Recent investigations have shifted the focus to several new potential mediators of IR, including adipose tissue-derived hormones (*adipocytokines*) that include leptin, adiponectin, TNF-α, interleukin 6 (IL-6), resistin, and visfatin.[113–115] Given the importance of adipose tissue and its hormones in terms of adequate metabolic control and energy homeostasis, this section will summarize the findings concerning the role of adipocytokines in pregnancy.

Leptin is an important metabolic hormone, mainly synthesized in white adipose tissue. It is known to influence insulin secretion, glucose utilization, glycogen synthesis, and fatty acid metabolism.[113,116] It is released into the circulation in proportion to the amount of lipid stores, and it acts at hypothalamic receptors, thereby decreasing nutrient intake and simultaneously increasing energy expenditure, mainly in the form of fat catabolism.[113,116] As already described, leptin levels rise in the maternal circulation during the third trimester of pregnancy and decrease to prepregnancy concentrations around parturition.[113,116] Although the origin and potential role of the increase in leptin concentration remain to be established, there is evidence to suggest that the placenta, rather than maternal adipose tissue, makes a substantial contribution to the increase of maternal leptin concentrations in pregnancy.[117] One possible function of the increased maternal leptin levels may be to enhance the mobilization of maternal fat stores, thereby increasing availability and transplacental transfer of lipid substrates to the fetus.[113,116] Leptin is also known to regulate placental growth, nutrient transfer, angiogenesis, and trophoblast invasion.[118]

Adiponectin is the most abundant adipose-tissue-specific protein, which has been reported to have anti-inflammatory, antiatherogenic, and insulin-sensitizing properties.[29] It is secreted by adipocytes as multimeric complexes with a high-molecular-weight (HMW) oligomer and a low-molecular-weight (LMW) hexamer.[119–122] LMW hexamers account for the majority of systemic circulating adiponectins.[119–122] In contrast to other adipocytokines, studies have found that circulating adiponectin concentrations decline progressively throughout pregnancy, consistent with decreased insulin sensitivity.[28–32] Studies have shown that adiponectin, and in particular HMW oligomer levels, are positively correlated with insulin sensitivity in humans and rodents.[119–122] Adiponectin is now considered an important adipose tissue-generated signal that modulates insulin sensitivity, and it may play an important role in gestational metabolism.

Resistin is a novel hormone, abundantly expressed in monocytes and macrophages and to a lesser extent by adipocytes, which is thought to contribute to impaired glucose tolerance.[122–123] It is expressed by the placenta (induced by insulin) and its levels increase substantially in the third trimester, during which it is thought to play a role in the regulation of maternal energy metabolism.[124–125] It may contribute to the decline in insulin sensitivity in mid-to-late pregnancy and the development of postprandial hyperglycemia, which may be beneficial for fetal growth.[125]

Visfatin is a recently described adipocytokine; consequently, its role in pathophysiology is not well established. It is highly expressed in visceral as compared to subcutaneous adipose tissue, and it promotes adipogenesis by exerting effects that mimic insulin action.[125] Visfatin mRNA and protein are expressed in human fetal membranes and placenta; therefore, it is thought that visfatin could play a role in the transfer of glucose from the maternal to fetal circulations.[125–127] It has been shown that visfatin levels go up in the omental fat of pregnant women, but not in serum, suggesting that visfatin may act locally as a paracrine/autocrine agent rather than as a hormone.[125–127] Moreover, there is evidence that, together with leptin, visfatin can counteract IR. Therefore, it is possible that the pregnancy-induced increase in visfatin acts to counteract it.[125]

As discussed in Section 6.2.1, studies have suggested the role of a chronic inflammatory process in adipose tissue that may also contribute to pregnancy-induced IR.[96] Inflammatory cytokines, such as TNF-α and IL-6 (produced by adipose tissue monocytes and macrophages), may be important mediators of IR.[96] Several studies have reported a rise in TNF-α and IL-6 during pregnancy (mainly due to placental production), which may contribute to pregnancy-associated IR.[120,121]

6.6   LACTATION: A POSTPREGNANCY CHALLENGE

Lactation, along with pregnancy, imposes a metabolically challenging event. As discussed with the onset of pregnancy, a combination of increased insulin secretion, increased circulating lipids, and consequently increased visceral adiposity leads to maternal IR. When lactation starts, a shift in metabolism occurs, which alters resource allocation (particularly triglycerides) from storage to milk synthesis. Lactation results in improved glucose handling and improved insulin sensitivity, with a concomitant drop in β-cell proliferation. Lipid metabolism is decreased in metabolically active tissues, and lipid stores are mobilized to facilitate lipid transport to the mammary gland for milk synthesis.[128,129] Therefore, it has been proposed that lactation aids in reducing postpartum adiposity and potentially reduces the risk of obesity.[128,129] Stuebe and Rich-Edwards put forward this interesting hypothesis, known as the *reset hypothesis,* which states that lactation resets the metabolic reprogramming that occurs during pregnancy and thereby reduces the prevalence of metabolic disease.[128,129]

A breastfed infant receives approximately 800 mL/day of milk from the mother, which provides 560 kcal (40% from lactose).[130,131] Therefore, the mother must consume these excess calories to maintain physiological energy balance and maintain her body stores of fat and protein during lactation. Existing research from animals and humans show that the primary source of milk lactose is glucose from maternal plasma.[130,131] In the fed state, this surplus of glucose supply is met by (1) increasing the dietary intake of carbohydrates, (2) enhancing endogenous glucose production by glycogenolysis rather than gluconeogenesis, (3) reducing splanchnic extraction of dietary glucose, and (4) reducing glucose oxidation, storage, or both by the mother. While in the fasting or prolonged starvation states, the lactating mother produces more glucose, reduces their own use of glucose by increasing use of FFA and ketone bodies, develops hypoglycemia, and/or decreases lactose synthesis and, thus, milk production.[130]

Pregnancy induces IR, leading to glucose intolerance as explained previously, whereas data from animal and human studies suggest that lactation plays a role in the resetting of glucose homeostasis back to normal postpregnancy levels. Lactation has been shown to decrease both glucose levels and IR during the postpartum period in animals, while repeated pregnancies without lactation appear to disrupt glucose homeostasis.[131–133] In studies involving a nondiabetic human population, it was found that there were significant differences in metabolic parameters between lactating and nonlactating women. Insulin levels were lower and carbohydrate utilization and total energy expenditure were higher in lactating mothers.[131–133] Several other studies have investigated whether breastfeeding has beneficial effects on maternal glucose homeostasis in human GDM subjects. Studies have found that glucose metabolism were significantly improved in the lactating group in terms of better glucose disposal and insulin sensitivity.[134–136] Numerous studies suggest that lactation reduces the risk of progression to T2DM in GDM subjects;[134–142] however, the exact mechanism is still elusive. There are a good number of hypotheses that discuss probable pathways underlying these protective effects, such as the following:

1. Studies in rats show that lactation decreases blood glucose and plasma insulin concentrations in the postpartum period by 20% and 35%, compared with nonlactating rats. The mammary gland expresses insulin receptors and is extremely sensitive to insulin during lactation. Therefore, it has been suggested that the lower plasma insulin concentrations during lactation are primarily due to increased insulin sensitivity as a result of increased glucose disposal by the mammary gland.[143–144]

2. In a human study, results indicated glucose in the circulation could be preferentially diverted to the mammary glands via a noninsulin-independent pathway to meet the demands of milk production, which may reduce the glucose load on the pancreas and thereby preserve long-term insulin production.[145]

3. Hormones such as prolactin are thought to play a role in the regulation of insulin secretion and glucose homeostasis by downregulating menin, which is a protein that inhibits islet cell proliferation by histone-methylation, leading to impaired glucose tolerance during pregnancy. However, how this may occur during lactation is currently unclear.[146]

4. Insulin action drives intracellular lipids from insulin-responsive tissues (e.g., liver and muscle) to insulin-sensitive adipocytes, thereby building up adiposity, which is further aggravated in GDM. Lactation may improve this situation by mobilizing lipids derived from the liver and muscle (nonadipose tissues) into milk production rather than making more adipocytes.[147]

6.7 FUTURE PERSPECTIVES

The advent of new technologies has vastly improved our understanding of maternal glucose metabolism during pregnancy; there have been genomewide association studies that have brought forward new candidates such as the novel hexokinase HKDC1, which is associated with gestational glucose metabolism.[148–151] These studies have also identified genes that are important in peripheral IR and ß-cell function during pregnancy.[152] Similarly, recent advances in metabolomics has enabled the scientific community to bring forward high-throughput identification of metabolites that are associated with glycemic traits during pregnancy.[153,154] And finally, there is the exciting new avenue of the gut microbiome as a novel environmental factor that potentially affects the metabolism of the host.[154–157] Research has revealed how these commensal microorganisms not only harvest energy from undigested food, but also either act as nutrient sensors themselves or regulate them.[154–157] Taken together, these advancements have put forward valuable new data, provoked new questions, and challenged existing dogmas. Exploring these fresh avenues, we can shed new light on how glucose metabolism is dynamically regulated during pregnancy, which will help us uncover mechanisms that drive GDM.

REFERENCES

1. Newbern D, Freemark M. Placental hormones and the control of maternal metabolism and fetal growth. *Curr Opin Endocrinol Diabetes Obes* 2011;**18**:409–16.
2. Herrera E, Lasuncion MA, Palacin M, Zorzano A, Bonet B. Intermediary metabolism in pregnancy first theme of the Freinkel era. *Diabetes* 1991;**40** (Suppl. 2):83–8.
3. Hadden DR, McLaughlin C. Normal and abnormal maternal metabolism during pregnancy. *Semin Fetal Neonatal Med* 2009;**14**:6–71.
4. Leturque A, Ferre P, Burnol A-F, Kande J, Maulard P, Girard J. Glucose utilization rates and insulin sensitivity in vivo in tissues of virgin and pregnant rats. *Diabetes* 1986;**35**:172–7.
5. Catalano PM, Tyzbir ED, Roman NM, Amini SB, Sims EA. Longitudinal changes in insulin release an insulin resistance in nonobese pregnant women. *Am J Obstet Gynecol* 1991;**165**:1667–72.
6. Catalano PM, Tyzbir ED, Wolfe RR, Roman NM, Amini SB, Sims EA. Longitudinal changes in basal hepatic glucose production and suppression during insulin infusion in normal pregnant women. *Am J Obstet Gynecol* 1992;**167**:913–9.
7. Angueira AR, Ludvik AE, Reddy TE, Wicksteed B, Lowe Jr. WE, Layden BT. New insights into gestational glucose metabolism: lessons learned from 21st century approaches. *Diabetes* 2015;**64**:327–34.
8. Sivan E, Chen X, Homko CJ, Reece EA, Boden G. Longitudinal study of carbohydrate metabolism in healthy obese pregnant women. *Diabetes Care* 1997;**20**:1470–5.
9. Di Cianni G, Miccoli R, Volpe L, Lencioni C, Del Prato S. Intermediate metabolism in normal pregnancy and in gestational diabetes. *Diabetes Metab Res Rev* 2003;**19**:259–70.
10. Ramos MP, Crespo-Solans MD, del Campo S, Cacho J, Herrera E. Fat accumulation in the rat during early pregnancy is modulated by enhanced insulin responsiveness. *Am J Physiol Endocrinol Metab* 2003;**285**:E318–28.
11. Catalano PM, Huston L, Amini SB, Kalhan SC. Longitudinal changes in glucose metabolism during pregnancy in obese women with normal glucose tolerance and gestational diabetes mellitus. *Am J Obstet Gynecol* 1999;**180**:903–16.
12. Connolly CC, Papa T, Smith MS, Lacy DB, Williams PE, Moore MC. Hepatic and muscle insulin action during late pregnancy in the dog. *Am J Phys Regul Integr Comp Phys* 2007;**292**:447–52.
13. Catalano PM, Huston L, Amini SB, Kalhan SC. Longitudinal changes in glucose metabolism during pregnancy in obese women with normal glucose tolerance and gestational diabetes mellitus. *Am J Obstet Gynecol* 1999;**180**:903–16.
14. Barbour LA, McCurdy CE, Hernandez TL, Kirwan JP, Catalano PM, Friedman JE. Cellular mechanisms for insulin resistance in normal pregnancy and gestational diabetes. *Diabetes Care* 2007;**30**(Suppl 2):S112–9.
15. Brelje TC, Scharp DW, Lacy PE, Ogren L, Talamantes F, Robertson M, Friesen HG, Sorenson RL. Effect of homologous placental lactogens, prolactins, and growth hormones on islet B-cell division and insulin secretion in rat, mouse, and human islets: implication for placental lactogen regulation of islet function during pregnancy. *Endocrinology* 1993;**132**:879–87.
16. Ryan EA, Enns L. Role of gestational hormones in the induction of insulin resistance. *J Clin Endocrinol Metab* 1988;**67**:341–7.
17. Handwerger S, Freemark M. The roles of placental growth hormone and placental lactogen in the regulation of human fetal growth and development. *J Pediatr Endocrinol Metab* 2000;**13**:343–56.
18. Barbour LA, Shao J, Qiao L, Pulawa LK, Jensen DR, Bartke A, Garrity M, Draznin B, Friedman JE. Human placental growth hormone causes severe insulin resistance in transgenic mice. *Am J Obstet Gynecol* 2002;**186**:512–7.
19. Bandyopadhyay GK, Yu JG, Ofrecio J, Olefsky JM. Increased p85/55/50 expression and decreased phosphatidylinositol 3-kinase activity in insulin-resistant human skeletal muscle. *Diabetes* 2005;**54**:2351–9.
20. Barbour LA, Mizanoor Rahman S, Gurevich I, Leitner JW, Fischer SJ, Roper MD, Knotts TA, Vo Y, McCurdy CE, Yakar S, Leroith D, Kahn CR, Cantley LC, Friedman JE, Draznin B. Increased P85alpha is a potent negative regulator of skeletal muscle insulin signaling and induces in vivo insulin resistance associated with growth hormone excess. *J Biol Chem* 2005;**280**:37489–94.
21. Peraldi P, Hotamisligil GS, Buurman WA, White MF, Spiegelman BM. Tumor necrosis factor (TNF)-alpha inhibits insulin signaling through stimulation of the p55 TNF receptor and activation of sphingomyelinase. *J Biol Chem* 1996;**271**:13018–22.
22. Hotamisligil GS, Peraldi P, Budavari A, Ellis R, White MF, Spiegelman BM. IRS-1- mediated inhibition of insulin receptor tyrosine kinase activity in TNF-alpha- and obesity-induced insulin resistance. *Science* 1996;**271**:665–8.
23. Ofei F, Hurel S, Newkirk J, Sopwith M, Taylor R. Effects of an engineered human anti-TNF-alpha antibody (CDP571) on insulin sensitivity and glycemic control in patients with NIDDM. *Diabetes* 1996;**45**:881–5.
24. Peraldi P, Spiegelman B. TNF-alpha and insulin resistance: summary and future prospects. *Mol Cell Biochem* 1998;**182**:169–75.
25. Coppack SW. Pro-inflammatory cytokines and adipose tissue. *Proc Nutr Soc* 2001;**60**:349–56.
26. Lyon CJ, Law RE, Hsueh WA. Minireview: adiposity, inflammation, and atherogenesis. *Endocrinology* 2003;**144**:2195–200.
27. Worda C, Leipold H, Gruber C, Kautzky-Willer A, Knofler M, Bancher-Todesca D. Decreased plasma adiponectin concentrations in women with gestational diabetes mellitus. *Am J Obstet Gynecol* 2004;**191**:2120–4.
28. Cseh K, Baranyi E, Melczer Z, Kaszas E, Palik E, Winkler G. Plasma adiponectin and pregnancy-induced insulin resistance. *Diabetes Care* 2004;**27**:274–5.

29. Catalano PM, Hoegh M, Minium J, Huston- Presley L, Bernard S, Kalhan S, Hauguel- De Mouzon S. Adiponectin in human pregnancy: implications for regulation of glucose and lipid metabolism. *Diabetologia* 2006;**49**:1677–85.

30. Hara K, Yamauchi T, Kadowaki T. Adiponectin: an adipokine linking adipocytes and type 2 diabetes in humans. *Curr Diab Rep* 2005;**5**:136–40.

31. Bruun JM, Lihn AS, Verdich C, Pedersen SB, Toubro S, Astrup A, Richelsen B. Regulation of adiponectin by adipose tissue derived cytokines: in vivo and in vitro investigations in humans. *Am J Physiol Endocrinol Metab* 2003;**285**:E527–33.

32. Fasshauer M, Kralisch S, Klier M, Lossner U, Bluher M, Klein J, Paschke R. Adiponectin gene expression and secretion is inhibited by interleukin-6 in 3T3–L1 adipocytes. *Biochem Biophys Res Commun* 2003;**301**:1045–50.

33. Friedman JE, Ishizuka T, Shao J, Huston L, Highman T, Catalano P. Impaired glucose transport and insulin receptor tyrosine phosphorylation in skeletal muscle from obese women with gestational diabetes. *Diabetes* 1999;**48**:1807–14.

34. Garvey WT, Maianu L, Hancock JA, Golichowski AM, Baron A. Gene expression of GLUT4 in skeletal muscle from insulin resistant patients with obesity, IGT, GDM, and NIDDM. *Diabetes* 1992;**41**:465–75.

35. Garvey WT, Birnbaum MJ. Cellular insulin action and insulin resistance. *Bailliere Clin Endocrinol Metab* 1993;**7**:785–873.

36. White MF, Shoelson SE, Keutmann H, Kahn CR. A cascade of tyrosine autophosphorylation in the beta-subunit activates the phosphotransferase of the insulin receptor. *J Biol Chem* 1988;**263**:2969–80.

37. Shao J, Catalano PM, Yamashita H, Ishizuka T, Friedman JE. Vanadate enhances but does not normalize glucose transport and insulin receptor phosphorylation in skeletal muscle from obese women with gestational diabetes mellitus. *Am J Obstet Gynecol* 2000;**183**:1263–70.

38. Backer JM, Myers Jr. MG, Shoelson SE, Chin DJ, Sun XJ, Miralpeix M, Hu P, et al. Phosphatidylinositol 3-kinase is activated by association with IRS-1 during insulin stimulation. *EMBO J* 1992;**11**:3469–79.

39. Goldstein BJ, Li PM, Ding W, Ahmad F, Zhang WR. Regulation of insulin action by protein tyrosine phosphatases. *Vitam Horm* 1998;**54**:67–96.

40. Elchebly M, Payette P, Michaliszyn E, Cromlish W, Collins S, Loy AL, et al. Increased insulin sensitivity and obesity resistance in mice lacking the protein tyrosine phosphatase-1B gene. *Science* 1999;**283**:1544–8.

41. Shao J, Catalano PM, Yamashita H, Ruyter I, Smith S, Youngren J, et al. Decreased insulin receptor tyrosine kinase activity and plasma cell membrane glycoprotein- 1 overexpression in skeletal muscle from obese women with gestational diabetes mellitus (GDM): evidence for increased serine/threonine phosphorylation in pregnancy and GDM. *Diabetes* 2000;**49**:603–10.

42. Moeschel K, Beck A, Weigert C, Lammers R, Kalbacher H, Voelter W, et al. Protein kinase C-zeta-induced phosphorylation of Ser318 in insulin receptor substrate-1 (IRS-1) attenuates the interaction with the insulin receptor and the tyrosine phosphorylation of IRS-1. *J Biol Chem* 2004;**279**:25157–63.

43. Li Y, Soos TJ, Li X, Wu J, Degennaro M, Sun X, et al. Protein kinase C theta inhibits insulin signaling by phosphorylating IRS1 at Ser(1101). *J Biol Chem* 2004;**279**:45304–7.

44. Tzatsos A, Kandror KV. Nutrients suppress phosphatidylinositol 3-kinase/Akt signaling via raptor-dependent mTOR mediated insulin receptor substrate 1 phosphorylation. *Mol Cell Biol* 2006;**26**:63–76.

45. Um SH, Frigerio F, Watanabe M, Picard F, Joaquin M, Sticker M, et al. Absence of S6K1 protects against age- and diet-induced obesity while enhancing insulin sensitivity. *Nature* 2004;**431**:200–5.

46. Barbour LA, McCurdy CE, Hernandez TL, De la Houssaye BE, Draznin B, Friedman JE. Reduced IRS-1 and increased serine IRS-1 phosphorylation in skeletal muscle of women with GDM (Abstract). *Diabetes* 2006;**55**(Suppl. 1):A39.

47. Shah OJ, Hunter T. Turnover of the active fraction of IRS1 involves raptor-mTOR and S6K1-dependent serine phosphorylation in cell culture models of tuberous sclerosis. *Mol Cell Biol* 2006;**26**:6425–34.

48. Biddinger SB, Kahn CR. From mice men: insights into the insulin resistance syndromes. *Annu Rev Physiol* 2006;**68**:123–58.

49. Catalano PM, Nizielski SE, Shao J, Preston L, Qiao L, Friedman JE. Downregulated IRS-1 and PPAR gamma in obese women with gestational diabetes: relationship to FFA during pregnancy. *Am J Physiol Endocrinol Metab* 2002;**282**:E522–33.

50. Okuno S, Akazawa S, Yasuhi I, Kawasaki E, Matsumoto K, Yamasaki H, et al. Decreased expression of the GLUT4 glucose transporter protein in adipose tissue during pregnancy. *Horm Metab Res* 1995;**27**:231–4.

51. Garvey WT, Maianu L, Zhu JH, Brechtel-Hook G, Wallace P, Baron AD. Evidence for defects in the trafficking and translocation of GLUT4 glucose transporters in skeletal muscle as a cause of human insulin resistance. *J Clin Invest* 1998;**101**:2377–86.

52. Brun RP, Spiegelman BM. PPAR gamma and the molecular control of adipogenesis. *J Endocrinol* 1997;**155**:217–8.

53. Schoonjans K, Staels B, Auwerx J. The peroxisome proliferator activated receptors (PPARs) and their effects on lipid metabolism and adipocyte differentiation. *Biochim Biophys Acta* 1996;**1302**:93–109.

54. Masternak MM, Al-Regaiey KA, Del Rosario Lim MM, Jimenez-Ortega V, Panici JA, Bonkowski MS, et al. Effects of caloric restriction and growth hormone resistance on the expression level of peroxisome proliferator-activated receptors superfamily in liver of normal and long-lived growth hormone receptor/ binding protein knockout mice. *J Gerontol A Biol Sci Med Sci* 2005;**60**:1394–8.

55. Nilsson L, Binart N, Bohlooly YM, Bramnert M, Egecioglu E, Kindblom J, et al. Prolactin and growth hormone regulate adiponectin secretion and receptor expression in adipose tissue. *Biochem Biophys Res Commun* 2005;**331**:1120–6.

56. Hay Jr. WW. Energy and substrate requirements of the placenta and fetus. *Proc Nutr Soc* 1991;**50**:321–36.

57. Battaglia FC. Principal substrates of fetal metabolism: fuel and growth requirements of the ovine fetus. *CIBA Found Symp* 1978;**63**:57–74.

58. Baumann MU, Deborde S, Illsley NP. Placental glucose transfer and fetal growth. *Endocrine* 2002;**19**:13–22.

59. Espinosa de los M, Driscoll SG, Steinke J. Insulin release from isolated human fetal pancreatic islets. *Science* 1970;**168**:1111–2.

60. Nolan CJ, Proietto J. The feto-placental glucose steal phenomenon is a major cause of maternal metabolic adaptation during late pregnancy in the rat. *Diabetologia* 1994;**37**:976–84.

61. Parsons JA, Brelje TC, Sorenson RL. Adaptation of islets of Langerhans to pregnancy: increased islet cell proliferation and insulin secretion correlates with the onset of placental lactogen secretion. *Endocrinology* 1992;**130**:1459–66.

62. Sorenson RL, Brelje TC. Adaptation of islets of Langerhans to pregnancy: beta-cell growth, enhanced insulin secretion and the role of lactogenic hormones. *Horm Metab Res* 1997;**29**:301–7.

63. Karnik SK, Chen H, McLean GW, Heit JJ, Gu X, Zhang AY, et al. Menin controls growth of pancreatic beta-cells in pregnant mice and promotes gestational diabetes mellitus. *Science* 2007;**318**:806–9.

64. Butler AE, Cao-Minh L, Galasso R, Rizza RA, Corradin A, Cobelli C, et al. Adaptive changes in pancreatic beta cell fractional area and beta cell turnover in human pregnancy. *Diabetologia* 2010;**53**:2167–76.

65. Rieck S, Kaestner KH. Expansion of beta-cell mass in response to pregnancy. *Trends Endocrinol Metab* 2010;**21**:151–8.

66. Brelje TC, Scharp DW, Lacy PE, Ogren L, Talamantes F, Robertson M, et al. Effect of homologous placental lactogens, prolactins, and growth hormones on islet B-cell division and insulin secretion in rat, mouse, and human islets: implication for placental lactogen regulation of islet function during pregnancy. *Endocrinology* 1993;**132**:879–87.

67. Amaral ME, Cunha DA, Anhe GF, Ueno M, Carneiro EM, Velloso LA, et al. Participation of prolactin receptors and phosphatidylinositol 3-kinase and MAP kinase pathways in the increase in pancreatic islet mass and sensitivity to glucose during pregnancy. *J Endocrinol* 2004;**183**:469–76.

68. Huang C, Snider F, Cross JC. Prolactin receptor is required for normal glucose homeostasis and modulation of beta-cell mass during pregnancy. *Endocrinology* 2009;**150**:1618–26.

69. Rawn SM, Huang C, Hughes M, Shaykhutdinov R, Vogel HJ, Cross JC. Pregnancy hyperglycemia in prolactin receptor mutant, but not prolactin mutant, mice and feeding-responsive regulation of placental lactogen genes implies placental control of maternal glucose homeostasis. *Biol Reprod* 2015;**93**:75.

70. Goyvaerts L, Lemaire K, Arijs I, Auffret J, Granvik M, Van Lommel L, et al. Prolactin receptors and placental lactogen drive male mouse pancreatic islets to pregnancy-related mRNA changes. *PLoS One* 2015;**10**:.

71. Kim H, Toyofuku Y, Lynn FC, Chak E, Uchida T, Mizukami H, et al. Serotonin regulates pancreatic beta cell mass during pregnancy. *Nat Med* 2010;**16**:804–8.

72. Rieck S, White P, Schug J, Fox AJ, Smirnova O, Gao N, et al. The transcriptional response of the islet to pregnancy in mice. *Mol Endocrinol* 2009;**23**:1702–12.

73. Schraenen A, Lemaire K, de Faudeur G, Hendrickx N, Granvik M, Van Lommel L, et al. Placental lactogens induce serotonin biosynthesis in a subset of mouse beta cells during pregnancy. *Diabetologia* 2010;**53**:2589–99.

74. Layden BT, Durai V, Newman MV, Marinelarena AM, Ahn CW, Feng G, et al. Regulation of pancreatic islet gene expression in mouse islets by pregnancy. *J Endocrinol* 2010;**207**:265–79.

75. Goyvaerts L, Schraenen A, Schuit F. Serotonin competence of mouse beta cells during pregnancy. *Diabetologia* 2016;**59**:1356–63.

76. Ohara-Imaizumi M, Kim H, Yoshida M, Fujiwara T, Aoyagi K, Toyofuku Y, et al. Serotonin regulates glucose- stimulated insulin secretion from pancreatic beta cells during pregnancy. *Proc Natl Acad Sci U S A* 2013;**110**:19420–5.

77. Zawalich WS, Tesz GJ, Zawalich KC. Are 5-hydroxytryptamine-preloaded beta-cells an appropriate physiologic model system for establishing that insulin stimulates insulin secretion? *J Biol Chem* 2001;**276**:37120–3.

78. Baeyens L, Hindi S, Sorenson RL, German MS. β-cell adaptation in pregnancy. *Diabetes Obes Metab* 2016;**18**(1):63–70.

79. Dadon D, Tornovsky-Babaey S, Furth-Lavi J, Ben-Zvi D, Ziv O, Schyr-Ben-Haroush R, et al. Glucose metabolism: key endogenous regulator of beta-cell replication and survival. *Diabetes Obes Metab* 2012;**14**(3):101–8.

80. Berger M, Scheel DW, Macias H, Miyatsuka T, Kim H, Hoang P, et al. Gαi/o-coupled receptor signaling restricts pancreatic beta-cell expansion. *Proc Natl Acad Sci U S A* 2015;**112**:2888–93.

81. Guettier JM, Gautam D, Scarselli M, Ruiz de Azua I, Li JH, Rosemond E, et al. A chemical-genetic approach to study G protein regulation of beta cell function in vivo. *Proc Natl Acad Sci U S A* 2009;**106**:19197–202.

82. Weinhaus AJ, Stout LE, Sorenson RL. Glucokinase, hexokinase, glucose transporter 2, and glucose metabolism in islets during pregnancy and prolactin-treated islets in vitro: mechanisms for long term up-regulation of islets. *Endocrinology* 1996;**137**:1640–9.

83. Weinhaus AJ, Bhagroo NV, Brelje TC, Sorenson RL. Role of cAMP in upregulation of insulin secretion during the adaptation of islets of Langerhans to pregnancy. *Diabetes* 1998;**47**:1426–35.

84. Cunha DA, Amaral ME, Carvalho CP, Collares-Buzato CB, Carneiro EM, Boschero AC. Increased expression of SNARE proteins and synaptotagmin IV in islets from pregnant rats and in vitro prolactin treated neonatal islets. *Biol Res* 2006;**39**:555–66.

85. Amaral ME, Ueno M, Carvalheira JB, Carneiro EM, Velloso LA, Saad MJ, et al. Prolactin-signal transduction in neonatal rat pancreatic islets and interaction with the insulin signaling pathway. *Horm Metab Res* 2003;**35**:282–9.

86. Zahr E, Molano RD, Pileggi A, Ichii H, Jose SS, Bocca N, et al. Rapamycin impairs in vivo proliferation of islet beta-cells. *Transplantation* 2007;**84**:1576–83.

87. Hughes E, Huang C. Participation of Akt, menin, and p21 in pregnancy- induced beta-cell proliferation. *Endocrinology* 2011;**152**:847–55.

88. Chamberlain CE, Scheel DW, McGlynn K, Kim H, Miyatsuka T, Wang J, et al. Menin determines KRAS proliferative outputs in endocrine cells. *J Clin Invest* 2014;**124**:4093–101.

89. Johansson M, Mattsson G, Andersson A, Jansson L, Carlsson PO. Islet endothelial cells and pancreatic beta-cell proliferation: studies in vitro and during pregnancy in adult rats. *Endocrinology* 2006;**147**:2315–24.

90. Plank JL, Frist AY, LeGrone AW, Magnuson MA, Labosky PA. Loss of Foxd3 results in decreased beta-cell proliferation and glucose intolerance during pregnancy. *Endocrinology* 2011;**152**:4589–600.

91. Zhang H, Zhang J, Pope CF, Crawford LA, Vasavada RC, Jagasia SM, et al. Gestational diabetes mellitus resulting from impaired beta-cell compensation in the absence of FoxM1, a novel downstream effector of placental lactogen. *Diabetes* 2010;**59**:143–52.

92. Zhang H, Ackermann AM, Gusarova GA, Crawford LA, Vasavada RC, Jagasia SM, et al. The FoxM1 transcription factor is required to maintain pancreatic beta-cell mass. *Mol Endocrinol* 2006;**20**:1853–66.

93. Das A, Mantena SR, Kannan A, Evans DB, Bagchi MK, Bagchi IC. De novo synthesis of estrogen in pregnant uterus is critical for stromal decidualization and angiogenesis. *Proc Natl Acad Sci U S A* 2009;**106**:12542–7.

94. Reynolds LP, Borowicz PP, Caton JS, Vonnahme KA, Luther JS, Buchanan DS, et al. Uteroplacental vascular development and placental function: an update. *Int J Dev Biol* 2010;**54**:355–66.

95. Augustine RA, Grattan DR. Induction of central leptin resistance in hyperphagic pseudopregnant rats by chronic prolactin infusion. *Endocrinology* 2008;**149**:1049–55.

96. Kirwan JP, Hauguel-De Mouzon S, Lepercq J, Challier JC, Huston-Presley L, Friedman JE, et al. TNF-a is a predictor of insulin resistance in human pregnancy. *Diabetes* 2002;**51**:2207–13.

97. Mastorakos G, Ilias I. Maternal and fetal hypothalamic-pituitary–adrenal axes during pregnancy and postpartum. *Ann N Y Acad Sci* 2003;**997**:136–49.

98. Ryan EA, Enns L. Role of gestational hormones in the induction of insulin resistance. *J Clin Endocrinol Metab* 1988;**67**:341–7.

99. Freemark M. Regulation of maternal metabolism by pituitary and placental hormones: roles in fetal development and metabolic programming. *Horm Res* 2006;**65**(3):41–9.

100. Barbour LA, Shao J, Qiao L, Leitner W, Anderson M, Friedman JE, et al. Human placental growth hormone increases expression of the p85 regulatory unit of phosphatidylinositol 3-kinase and triggers severe insulin resistance in skeletal muscle. *Endocrinology* 2004;**145**:1144–50.

101. Caufriez A, Frankenne F, Hennen G, Copinschi G. Regulation of maternal IGF-I by placental GH in normal and abnormal human pregnancies. *Am J Phys* 1993;**265**:E572–7.

102. Mastorakos G, Ilias I. Maternal and fetal hypothalamic-pituitary-adrenal axes during pregnancy and postpartum. *Ann N Y Acad Sci* 2003;**997**:136–49.

103. Grueso E, Rocha M, Puerta M. Plasma and cerebrospinal fluid leptin levels are maintained despite enhanced food intake in progesterone treated rats. *Eur J Endocrinol* 2001;**144**:659–65.

104. Freemark M, Fleenor D, Driscoll P, Binart N, Kelly P. Body weight and fat deposition in prolactin receptor-deficient mice. *Endocrinology* 2001;**142**:532–7.

105. Flint DJ, Binart N, Kopchick J, Kelly P. Effects of growth hormone and prolactin on adipose tissue development and function. *Pituitary* 2003;**6**:97–102.

106. Fleenor D, Oden J, Kelly PA, Mohan S, Alliouachene S, Pende M, et al. Roles of the lactogens and somatogens in perinatal and postnatal metabolism and growth: studies of a novel mouse model combining lactogen resistance and growth hormone deficiency. *Endocrinology* 2005;**146**:103–12.

107. Butte NF, Wong WW, Treuth MS, Ellis KJ, O'Brian Smith E. Energy requirements during pregnancy based on total energy expenditure and energy deposition. *Am J Clin Nutr* 2004;**79**:1078–87.

108. Wlodek ME, Westcott KT, O'Dowd R, Serruto A, Wassef L, Moritz KM, et al. Uteroplacental restriction in the rat impairs fetal growth in association with alterations in placental growth factors including PTHrP. *Am J Phys Regul Integr Comp Phys* 2005;**288**:R1620–7.

109. Lacroix MC, Guibourdenche J, Frendo JL, Muller F, Evain-Brion D. Human placental growth hormone—a review. *Placenta* 2002;**23**(**A**):S87–94.

110. Freemark M, Avril I, Fleenor D, Driscoll P, Petro A, Opara E, et al. Targeted deletion of the PRL receptor: effects on islet development, insulin production, and glucose tolerance. *Endocrinology* 2002;**143**:1378–85.

111. Ryan EA, Enns L. Role of gestational hormones in the induction of insulin resistance. *J Clin Endocrinol Metab* 1988;**67**(2):341–7.

112. Catalano PM, Roman-Drago NM, Amini SB, Sims EA. Longitudinal changes in body composition and energy balance in lean women with normal and abnormal glucose tolerance in pregnancy. *Am J Obstet Gynecol* 1998;**179**(1):156–65.

113. Masuzaki H, Ogawa Y, Sagawa N, et al. Nonadipose tissue production of leptin: leptin as a novel placenta-derived hormone in humans. *Nat Med* 1997;**3**(9):1029–33.

114. Chen J, Tan B, Karteris E, Hosoda K, Matsumoto T, Mise H, et al. Secretion of adiponectin by human placenta: differential modulation of adiponectin and its receptors by cytokines. *Diabetologia* 2006;**49**(6):1292–302.

115. Yura S, Sagawa N, Itoh H, Kakui K, Nuamah MA, Korita D, et al. Resistin is expressed in the human placenta. *J Clin Endocrinol Metab* 2003;**88**(3):1394–7.

116. Wauters M, Considine RV, Van Gaal LF. Human leptin: from an adipocyte hormone to an endocrine mediator. *Eur J Endocrinol* 2000;**143**(3):293–311.

117. Henson M, Swan K, O'Neil JS. Expression of placental leptin and leptin receptor transcripts in early pregnancy and at term. *Obstet Gynecol* 1998;**92**(6):1020–8.

118. Sagawa N, Yura S, Itoh H, Kakui K, Takemura M, Nuamah MA, et al. Possible role of placental leptin in pregnancy: a review. *Endocrine* 2002;**19**(1):65–71.

119. Pajvani UB, Du X, Combs TP, Berg AH, Rajala MW, Schulthess T, et al. (2003) Structure – function studies of the adipocyte-secreted hormone Acrp30/adiponectin. Implications for metabolic regulation and bioactivity. *J Biol Chem* 2003;**278**:9073–85.

120. Tschritter O, Fritsche A, Thamer C, Haap M, Shirkavand F, Rahe S, et al. Plasma adiponectin concentrations predict insulin sensitivity of both glucose and lipid metabolism. *Diabetes* 2003;**52**:239–43.

121. Lara-Castro C, Luo N, Wallace P, Klein RL, Garvey WT. Adiponectin multimeric complexes and the metabolic syndrome trait cluster. *Diabetes* 2006;**55**:249–59.

122. Steppan CM, Bailey ST, Bhat S, Brown EJ, Banerjee RR, Wright CM, et al. The hormone resistin links obesity to diabetes. *Nature* 2001;**409**(6818):307–12.
123. Steppan CM, Lazar MA. Resistin and obesity-associated insulin resistance. *Trends Endocrinol Metab* 2002;**13**(1):18–23.
124. Lappas M, Yee K, Permezel M, Rice GE. Release and regulation of leptin, resistin and adiponectin from human placenta, fetal membranes, and maternal adipose tissue and skeletal muscle from normal and gestational diabetes mellitus-complicated pregnancies. *J Endocrinol* 2005;**186**(3):457–65.
125. Nien JK, Mazaki-Tovi S, Romero R, Kusanovic JP, Erez O, Gotsch F, et al. Resistin: a hormone which induces insulin resistance is increased in normal pregnancy. *J Perinat Med* 2007;**35**(6):513–21.
126. Morgan SA, Bringolf JB, Seidel ER. Visfatin expression is elevated in normal human pregnancy. *Peptides* 2008;**29**(8):1382–9.
127. Telejko B, Kuzmicki M, Zonenberg A, Szamatowicz J, Wawrusiewicz-Kurylonek N, Nikolajuk A, et al. Visfatin in gestational diabetes: serum level and mRNA expression in fat and placental tissue. *Diabetes Res Clin Pract* 2009;**84**(1):68–75.
128. Hyatt HW, Zhang Y, Hood WR, Kavazis AN. Lactation has persistent effects on a mother's metabolism and mitochondrial function. *Sci Rep* 2017;**7**:.
129. Stuebe AM, Rich-Edwards JW. The reset hypothesis: lactation and maternal metabolism. *Am J Perinatol* 2009;**26**:81.
130. Sunehag AL, Louie K, Bier JL, Tigas S, Haymond MW. Hexoneogenesis in the human breast during lactation. *J Clin Endocrinol Metab* 2001;**87**:297–301.
131. Butte NF, Hopkinson JM, Mehta N, Moon JK, Smith EO. Adjustments in energy expenditure and substrate utilization during late pregnancy and lactation. *Am J Clin Nutr* 1999;**69**:299–307.
132. Jones RG, Ilic V, Williamson DH. Physiological significance of altered insulin metabolism in the conscious rat during lactation. *Biochem J* 1984;**220**:455–60.
133. Burnol AF, Leturque A, Ferre P, Kande J, Girard J. Increased insulin sensitivity and responsiveness during lactation in rats. *Am J Phys* 1986;**251**(5 Pt 1):E537–41.
134. O'Reilly M, Avalos G, Dennedy MC, O'Sullivan EP, Dunne FP. Breast-feeding is associated with reduced postpartum maternal glucose intolerance after gestational diabetes. *Ir Med J* 2012;**105**:31–6.
135. Gunderson EP, Hedderson MM, Chiang V, Crites Y, Walton D, Azevedo RA, et al. Lactation intensity and postpartum maternal glucose tolerance and insulin resistance in women with recent GDM: the SWIFT cohort. *Diabetes Care* 2012;**35**:50–6.
136. O'Reilly MW, Avalos G, Dennedy MC, O'Sullivan EP, Dunne F. Atlantic DIP: high prevalence of abnormal glucose tolerance post partum is reduced by breast-feeding in women with prior gestational diabetes mellitus. *Eur J Endocrinol* 2011;**165**:953–9.
137. Much D, Beyerlein A, Roßbauer M, Hummel S, Ziegler AG. Beneficial effects of breastfeeding in women with gestational diabetes mellitus. *Mol Metab* 2014;**13**(3):284–92.
138. Much D, Beyerlein A, Kindt A, Krumsiek J, Stückler F, Rossbauer M, et al. Lactation is associated with altered metabolomic signatures in women with gestational diabetes. *Diabetologia* 2016;**59**(10):2193–202.
139. Gunderson EP. The role of lactation in GDM women. *Clin Obstet Gynecol* 2013;**56**(4):844–52.
140. Gunderson EP, Hurston SR, Ning X, Lo JC, Crites Y, Walton D, et al. Lactation and progression to type 2 diabetes mellitus after gestational diabetes mellitus: a prospective cohort study. *Ann Intern Med* 2015;**163**(12):889–98.
141. S C-C, Weisnagel SJ, Tchernof A, Robitaille J. Relationship between lactation duration and insulin and glucose response among women with prior gestational diabetes. *Eur J Endocrinol* 2013;**168**(4):515–23.
142. Tanase-Nakao K, Arata N, Kawasaki M, Yasuhi I, Sone H, Mori R, et al. Potential protective effect of lactation against incidence of type 2 diabetes mellitus in women with previous gestational diabetes mellitus: a systematic review and meta-analysis. *Diabetes Metab Res Rev* 2017;**33**(4).
143. Burnol AF, Leturque A, Ferre P, Kande J, Girard J. Increased insulin sensitivity and responsiveness during lactation in rats. *Am J Phys* 1986;**251**:E537–41.
144. Jones RG, Ilic V, Williamson DH. Physiological significance of altered insulin metabolism in the conscious rat during lactation. *Biochem J* 1984;**220**:455–60.
145. Butte NF, Hopkinson JM, Mehta N, Moon JK, Smith EO. Adjustments in energy expenditure and substrate utilization during late pregnancy and lactation. *Am J Clin Nutr* 1999;**69**:299–307.
146. Karnik SK, Chen H, McLean GW, Heit JJ, Gu X, Zhang AY, et al. Menin controls growth of pancreatic beta-cells in pregnant mice and promotes gestational diabetes mellitus. *Science (New York, NY)* 2007;**318**:806–9.
147. Ramos-Roman MA. Prolactin and lactation as modifiers of diabetes risk in gestational diabetes. *Horm Metab Res* 2011;**43**:593–600.
148. Tigas S, Sunehag A, Haymond MW. Metabolic adaptation to feeding and fasting during lactation in humans. *J Clin Endocrinol Metab* 2002;**87**(1):302–7.
149. Cho YM, Kim TH, Lim S, Choi SH, Shin HD, Lee HK, et al. Type 2 diabetes-associated genetic variants discovered in the recent genome-wide association studies are related to gestational diabetes mellitus in the Korean population. *Diabetologia* 2009;**52**:253–61.
150. Robitaille J, Grant AM. The genetics of gestational diabetes mellitus: evidence for relationship with type 2 diabetes mellitus. *Genet Med* 2008;**10**:240–50.
151. Freathy RM, Hayes MG, Urbanek M, Lowe LP, Lee H, Ackerman C, et al. HAPO Study Cooperative Research Group. Hyperglycemia and adverse pregnancy outcome (HAPO) study: common genetic variants in GCK and TCF7L2 are associated with fasting and postchallenge glucose levels in pregnancy and with the new consensus definition of gestational diabetes mellitus from the International Association of Diabetes and Pregnancy Study Groups. *Diabetes* 2010;**59**:2682–9.

152. Zhang C, Bao W, Rong Y, Yang H, Bowers K, Yeung E, et al. Genetic variants and the risk of gestational diabetes mellitus: a systematic review. *Hum Reprod Update* 2013;**19**:376–90.

153. Kwak SH, Kim SH, Cho YM, Go MJ, Cho YS, Choi SH, et al. A genome-wide association study of gestational diabetes mellitus in Korean women. *Diabetes* 2012;**61**:531–41.

154. Scholtens DM, Muehlbauer MJ, Daya NR, Stevens RD, Dyer AR, Lowe LP, et al. HAPO Study Cooperative Research Group. Metabolomics reveals broad-scale metabolic perturbations in hyperglycemic mothers during pregnancy. *Diabetes Care* 2014;**37**:158–66.

155. Menni C, Fauman E, Erte I, Perry JR, Kastenmüller G, Shin SY, et al. Biomarkers for type 2 diabetes and impaired fasting glucose using a nontargeted metabolomics approach. *Diabetes* 2013;**62**:4270–6.

156. Bäckhed F, Ding H, Wang T, Hooper LV, Koh GY, Nagy A, et al. The gut microbiota as an environmental factor that regulates fat storage. *Proc Natl Acad Sci U S A* 2004;**101**:15718–23.

157. Karlsson F, Tremaroli V, Nielsen J, Bäckhed F. Assessing the human gut microbiota inp metabolic diseases. *Diabetes* 2013;**62**:3341–9.

Chapter 7

Gut Hormones in Pregnancy and Lactation

Jien Shim and Run Yu

Division of Endocrinology, UCLA David Geffen School of Medicine, Los Angeles, CA, United States

Key Clinical Changes
- Gut hormones regulate gastrointestinal motility, gastric acidity, digestive enzyme secretion, and nutrient absorption.
- The roles of gut hormones in body weight regulation and metabolism are being recognized.
- The circulating concentrations of some gut hormones are altered during pregnancy or lactation, but this has not been studied for all such hormones.
- The specific functions of gut hormones in pregnancy and lactation are largely unclear, but gut hormones probably contribute to meeting the increased nutrient requirements during pregnancy and lactation.

7.1 INTRODUCTION TO GUT HORMONES

The first hormones ever discovered were two gastrointestinal hormones: secretin and gastrin.[1] In 1902, two British physiologists, Ernest Henry Starling and William Maddock Bayliss, discovered that pancreatic bicarbonate secretion significantly increased when a substance from the duodenal mucosa (secretin) was injected into the blood, regardless of whether the pancreas was innervated. In 1905, John Sydney Edkins, another British physiologist, discovered a chemical extracted from the gastric mucosa that stimulated gastric acid secretion, and called it *gastrin*.[2] That year, Starling coined the term *hormone*, derived from the Greek word *ormao*, which translates to "arise to activity."[3] The discovery of these two gastrointestinal hormones marked the beginning of the field of endocrinology.

Although the first two hormones ever discovered were gastrointestinal, subsequent discoveries of corticosteroids, insulin, pituitary hormones, and sex steroids steered interest away from gastrointestinal hormones. However, in recent years, with the rising epidemic of obesity and metabolic syndrome, interest in gastrointestinal hormones has been growing, as these hormones have been shown to play significant roles in food intake and energy balance.[4] To date, more than 30 gut hormones have been discovered, and the number continues to grow.[5] In this chapter, we illustrate the normal physiology of gastrointestinal hormones and their roles in pregnancy and lactation. We will use the terms *gastrointestinal hormones* and *gut hormones* interchangeably.

7.2 INDIVIDUAL GUT HORMONES DURING PREGNANCY AND LACTATION

7.2.1 Gastrin

Gastrin is a 34-amino-acid peptide, whose major function is to stimulate gastric acid secretion by acting on the cholecystokinin 2 (CCK2) receptor of gastric parietal cells and enterochromaffin-like (ECL) cells.[6] The ECL cells secrete histamine in response to gastrin stimulation, and histamine acts on the H2 receptor of parietal cells, which provide a stronger stimulus for parietal cell acid secretion than direct gastrin action. Gastrin is produced by the G cells of the gastric antrum and secreted in response to a meal. A precursor peptide, preprogastrin, is processed intracellularly to form progastrin, which is further cleaved to form gastrin. High stomach pH (low acidity) stimulates gastrin secretion, while low stomach pH (high acidity) and fasting inhibit its secretion. In clinical settings, proton pump inhibitor use is commonly associated with hypergastrinemia. Diarrhea, abdominal pain, and peptic ulcers characterize Zollinger-Ellison syndrome, which is caused by gastrinoma (Table 7.1).

Gastrin levels are unchanged during normal pregnancy.[7] When compared with nonpregnant women who were undergoing elective gynecologic surgery, pregnant women undergoing cesarian section have greater and more acidic gastric

TABLE 7.1 Common gastrointestinal hormones and their roles in pregnancy and lactation

Hormones	Known main functions	Roles in pregnancy and lactation (in humans unless stated otherwise)
Gastrin	• Stimulates gastric acid secretion	• Unchanged levels during pregnancy • Elevated levels during lactation (in rats)
Ghrelin	• Stimulates growth hormone release • Induces appetite • Increases gastric motility	• Possible role in embryonic implantation and myometrium relaxation • Elevated levels in hyperemesis gravidarum, gestational diabetes mellitus, and pregnancy-induced hypertension • Stimulates prolactin secretion
Leptin	• Regulates food intake • Controls energy balance	• Elevated levels during pregnancy • Elevated levels in gestational diabetes mellitus and preeclampsia • Direct correlation with maternal body mass index
Somatostatin	• Inhibits growth hormone secretion • Inhibits gastrointestinal hormone secretions • Inhibits pancreatic exocrine secretion • Inhibits gastrointestinal motility • Inhibits splanchnic blood flow	• Elevated levels during pregnancy • Decreased levels during suckling • Higher levels in breast milk than in maternal serum
Secretin	• Promotes pancreatic and bicarbonate secretion • Inhibits gastrin and gastric acid secretion • Inhibits gastric motility at low levels • Stimulates gastric motility at high levels • Increases bile flow • Increases lower esophageal sphincter tone • Increases insulin secretion in response to glucose	• Elevated levels during pregnancy
Cholecystokinin	• Promotes gallbladder contraction • Increases pancreatic enzyme secretion	• Elevated levels in pregnancy • Elevated levels in lactating cows
Motilin	• Stimulates gastrointestinal smooth muscle contractions to induce peristalsis	• Elevated levels in pregnancy and lactation
Gastric inhibitory peptide (GIP)	• Promotes glucose-dependent insulin secretion	• Elevated levels during pregnancy and lactation in rodents
Glucagon-like peptide-1 (GLP-1)	• Promotes glucose-dependent insulin secretion • Slows gastric emptying • Decreases appetite	• Decreased levels in gestational diabetes mellitus • Present in breast milk
Glucagon-like peptide-2 (GLP-2)	• Inhibits gastric motility • Inhibits gastric acid secretion • Promotes intestinal crypt cell proliferation • Promotes intestinal blood flow	• Unknown
Oxyntomodulin	• Inhibits gastric acid secretion • Promotes weight loss	• Unknown
Fibroblast growth factor 19 (FGF19)	• Promotes glucose uptake in adipocytes • Promotes hepatic glycogen synthesis • Inhibits gluconeogenesis	• Decreased levels in women with gestational diabetes mellitus and PCOS

content without any difference in serum gastrin levels.[8] Although pregnancy is associated with gastrointestinal symptoms, such as dyspepsia and constipation, levels of gastrin and cholecystokinin (CCK) do not differ in pregnant women in the first and third trimesters and 4–6 months postpartum.[9]

Gastrin has not been studied in human lactation, but it has been studied in lactating rats.[10] Unlike in humans, serum gastrin concentration was suppressed during pregnancy in rats, greatly increased during lactation, and returned to normal levels at the time of weaning. The ECL cells are activated during lactation, which correlated with increased gastrin levels. Hypergastrinemia during lactation may be due to increased food intake; however, further studies are necessary to better elucidate the mechanism of elevated gastrin secretion during lactation.

7.2.2 Ghrelin

Ghrelin is a 28-amino-acid peptide with many physiological actions, but it is known mainly for its growth hormone (GH)-releasing and appetite-inducting activities.[11] Other actions of ghrelin include increasing gastric mobility, gastric emptying, and gastric acid secretion, decreasing insulin secretion, increasing IGF-1 secretion, increasing lipogenesis at adipose tissue, and increasing cardiac contractility.[12] It is secreted mostly by the P/D1 cells of the stomach and the duodenum, but also by the pancreas, pituitary, kidney, and placenta. Ghrelin binds to growth hormone secretagogue receptor (GHS-R), a G-protein-coupled receptor, which is expressed in both the central nervous system and peripheral tissues.[13,14] Ghrelin's action on GHS-R of the pituitary stimulates GH release. This GH axis is different from the better-known hypothalamic-pituitary axis involving the growth hormone-releasing hormone (GHRH) and GHRH receptor in the pituitary, which when activated, leads to high levels of GH. The appetite-stimulating activities of ghrelin is demonstrated by reductions in its levels following gastrectomy and its weight-gain effects in cachectic patients.[15,16]

Ghrelin's role in growth hormone-releasing activity has been implicated in studies involving human subjects. Healthy infants born small for gestational age have a higher concentration of ghrelin compared with normal infants or those large for gestational age, suggesting that ghrelin plays a role in neonatal or fetal growth.[17] In rodents, maternal ghrelin has a significant role in fetal development. Ghrelin treatment increases fetal birth weight even when maternal food intake is restricted.[18] Oral GHS, which binds to GHS-R, mimicking endogenous ghrelin activity, increases GH levels in adults.[19] Although GHS-R mutations have been found in individuals with isolated growth hormone deficiency and short stature, individuals with normal height have also been shown to have variants of GHS-R, suggesting that ghrelin is not solely responsible for short stature syndrome.[13]

Ghrelin's role in pregnancy and lactation has been implicated in many human and animal studies. First, ghrelin has been detected in both mouse and human placenta, suggesting a role in embryonic implantation.[20] Ghrelin and its receptor GHS-R expression in the human myometrium suggest its role in relaxation of the myometrium during pregnancy by upregulation of its expression, and contraction of the myometrium during labor by downregulation of its expression. High levels of ghrelin are observed in pregnant women with hyperemesis gravidarum, along with estradiol, suggesting a role in energy metabolism in pregnancy.[21] Also, elevated levels of ghrelin are found in the second trimester of pregnant women with gestational diabetes mellitus (GDM) compared with those without GDM and nonpregnant healthy women, which may be associated with increased weight gain during the second trimester.[22] In contrast, another study reported no association of ghrelin levels in pregnancy with insulin resistance.[23] During oral glucose tolerance tests, pregnant women with GDM have higher ghrelin messenger ribonucleic acid (mRNA) expression in the placenta compared with those without GDM.[24] However, there are no differences in the levels of ghrelin before or after the glucose load.

Ghrelin may have a role in cardiovascular physiology during pregnancy, as women with pregnancy-induced hypertension have higher levels of ghrelin than normal pregnant women.[25] Interestingly, in one study looking at patients with severe preeclampsia, there is a negative correlation between serum ghrelin levels and blood pressure, suggesting that high levels of ghrelin may be a compensatory mechanism to lower blood pressure in patients with preeclampsia.[26]

Ghrelin stimulates prolactin secretion, and it is present in breast milk, even in the colostrum.[27,28] Ghrelin-induced prolactin secretion can be blocked by bromocriptine, a dopamine receptor agonist.[29] Interestingly, maternal serum levels of ghrelin do not differ between lactating and nonlactating women, but in GDM mothers, ghrelin levels are lower than in non-GDM mothers.[27] The detailed mechanism of ghrelin-prolactin interaction has yet to be determined.

7.2.3 Leptin

Leptin is an anorexigenic peptide hormone, mainly produced by adipocytes; thus, it is also known as an *adipokine*.[30] It maintains energy balance and controls fat metabolism by acting on the leptin receptor (OB-R) in the central nervous system, predominantly in the hypothalamus. Leptin is encoded by the *ob* gene, located on chromosome 7q31.3, and inactivating mutations lead to leptin deficiency, and thereby a rare form of severe obesity.[31] In contrast, most human obesity is not associated with leptin deficiency at all. Instead, increased circulating levels of free leptin are found in individuals with higher body mass index (BMI), suggesting leptin resistance.[32]

In addition to its role in the regulation of food intake and energy balance, leptin is known for its role in reproduction and fetal development. Increased leptin levels are observed in pregnant women. Leptin levels increase in late pregnancy but fall soon after parturition, suggesting that leptin is also a placental hormone.[33] Its role in reproduction and fertility has been studied in mice and humans. Leptin knockout (KO) mice are infertile, but they are able to reproduce after the injection of recombinant leptin.[34] In contrast, women with history of recurrent pregnancy loss have similar leptin levels during the implantation window (day 22 of menstrual cycle) as healthy, fertile women, arguing against leptin's role in the first trimester of pregnancy.[35]

Leptin levels have been measured in different types of pathologic states related to reproduction. Obese pregnant women have higher levels of leptin than normal pregnant women.[36] In addition, polycystic ovarian syndrome (PCOS), endometriosis, and GDM have also been associated with hyperleptinemia.[37] Elevated leptin levels are also seen in women with preeclampsia, and the levels correlate with the severity of the disease.[38]

Obesity in the mother has been linked to obesity in the offspring, and therefore, leptin content in human breast milk has been studied in obese and nonobese mothers.[39] Maternal BMI is directly correlated with breast milk leptin levels. Breast milk leptin levels decrease by one-third between 1 month and 6 months postpartum, which is likely attributed to maternal weight loss. In addition, there is an inverse relationship between breast milk leptin levels and infant length, percent fat, total fat mass, and trunk fat mass at 6 months of age. Further studies are necessary to better understand the relationship among maternal obesity, leptin levels in breast milk, and infant health.

7.2.4 Somatostatin

Somatostatin is an inhibitory hormone that has many effects in the central nervous system and the gastrointestinal system.[40] In the gastrointestinal system, it is secreted by various cells, including neural, endocrine, and enteroendocrine cells. In the central nervous system, it is mainly known to inhibit growth hormone release. In addition, somatostatin receptor ligands, which have longer half-lives than the endogenous somatostatin, are used for the treatment of acromegaly and other neuroendocrine tumors.[41] In the gastrointestinal system, somatostatin inhibits most gastrointestinal hormone secretions, pancreatic exocrine secretions, gastrointestinal motility, and splanchnic blood flow. Therefore, in clinical practice, it is commonly used for the treatment of secretory diarrhea associated with human immunodeficiency virus (HIV), vasoactive intestinal polypeptide-secreting tumor (VIPoma), and carcinoid syndrome, as well as for treatment of gastrointestinal bleeding by reducing splanchnic blood flow.[42,43]

Most of the recent somatostatin research in pregnancy has revolved around the treatment of neuroendocrine tumors with somatostatin analogs. There has not been a lot of investigation of somatostatin and its physiology during pregnancy and lactation. Somatostatin levels increase and peak in late pregnancy, as well as during the first few weeks of the postpartum period, which may be a response to increased gastric acid during pregnancy and postpartum.[44]

During lactation, suckling is associated with a decrease in maternal somatostatin levels, but they return to normal after suckling concludes.[45] A negative correlation is found between somatostatin and prolactin levels during suckling, suggesting somatostatin's possible role in prolactin secretion and lactation. Four times higher levels of somatostatin have been found in breast milk compared with maternal plasma levels, which suggests that an active transport mechanism may be involved in somatostatin transfer in the mammary gland rather than passive diffusion.[46] However, the exact role of somatostatin in breast milk is unknown.

7.2.5 Secretin

Secretin is a 27-amino-acid peptide that is produced and secreted by the S cells of the small intestine and colon.[47] Its primary action is to promote pancreatic fluid and bicarbonate secretion. It also inhibits gastrin and gastric acid secretion, gastric motility, and gastrin release. At higher levels, it increases bile flow, gastrointestinal motility, lower esophageal sphincter tone, and insulin secretion in response to glucose.

Secretin has not been well studied in pregnancy and lactation. One study showed that secretin levels increase during pregnancy and peak around 36 weeks. Given its already-known function in gastrointestinal physiology, increased levels of secretin in pregnancy may suggest its role in gastrointestinal motility and acid secretion in pregnancy. Secretin levels return to normal, nonpregnant levels just a few days postpartum.[48] In mice, secretin expression is noted during embryonic days 5–8 at the implantation site, suggesting a role in mouse decidualization.[49]

7.2.6 Cholecystokinin

CCK is well known for its function in gallbladder contraction and pancreatic enzyme secretion.[50] Its other roles include stimulating insulin secretion, delaying gastric emptying, and regulating food intake. CCK is secreted by the enteroendocrine I cells of the small intestine in response to intake of nutrients, especially proteins and fats, and its receptors are distributed throughout the gastrointestinal tract, as well as in the central and peripheral nervous systems. It is commonly known for its use in hepatobiliary iminodiacetic acid (HIDA) scanning to evaluate the gallbladder radiographically.[51]

CCK has been studied for its relationship to weight loss. CCK levels decrease after diet-induced weight loss.[52] Its levels are also low in patients with bulimia nervosa, celiac disease, and delayed gastric emptying.[53] Therefore, CCK has been studied as a weight-loss drug, but 24-week treatment with the CCK-A receptor agonist GI181771X had no significant effects on weight loss or waist circumference in a randomized, double-blind, placebo-control trial.[54]

Common gastrointestinal symptoms in pregnancy, including heartburn, indigestion, and constipation, may be associated with gastrointestinal and biliary motility, but only a few studies have examined CCK's role in pregnancy. High levels of CCK are observed in pregnant women, suggesting its possible involvement in causing gastrointestinal symptoms.[7] There is a higher incidence of cholesterol gallstones and impaired gallbladder motility during pregnancy, but in one study, CCK levels had no association with gallbladder volume in pregnant women.[55]

CCK has been studied in lactating dairy cows, and its levels are elevated in the beginning of lactation, followed by a gradual decrease.[56] CCK, however, has not been studied in human lactation. Further studies are necessary to investigate its function in lactation.

7.2.7 Motilin

Motilin is a 22-amino-acid hormone, released by the enteroendocrine M cells of the duodenum and proximal jejunum.[57] It is secreted in a cyclical pattern during the interdigestive periods between meals. It stimulates gastrointestinal smooth muscle contractions in the esophagus, stomach, small intestine, and colon. Motilin induces phase III contraction of the migrating motor complex of the intestine that promotes peristaltic waves. Therefore, motilin agonists have been implicated in clinical use to enhance gastric emptying.[58] For example, erythromycin, which is a macrolide antibiotic commonly used for gastroparesis treatment, is a motilin receptor agonist. Recently, a new motilin agonist, camicinal, has been shown to accelerate gastric emptying and increase glucose absorption in feed-intolerant, critically ill patients in a randomized, double-blind, placebo-controlled trial.[59]

Motilin has been studied in pregnant women. In one observational study, motilin levels increase during pregnancy and peak in the third trimester and postpartum.[44] Motilin levels are not altered in women with hyperemesis gravidarum compared with nonpregnant women.[21]. These studies suggest that motilin may not play a major role in gastrointestinal physiology in pregnancy, and the significance of rising motilin levels in later stages of pregnancy is unclear. In lactating women, circulating levels of motilin are higher than in nonlactating women.[60] Motilin is also present in human breast milk. Further studies are necessary to characterize motilin's role in lactation and neonatal development.

7.2.8 Gastric Inhibitory Peptide

Gastric inhibitory peptide (GIP), also known as *glucose-dependent insulinotropic polypeptide,* is an incretin hormone, along with glucagonlike peptide-1 (GLP-1), discussed next.[61] Incretin hormones potentiate insulin secretion after meal ingestion in a glucose-dependent manner.

GIP is primarily secreted from enteroendocrine K cells in the duodenum and proximal jejunum. There is also a small amount of production in the central nervous system. Obesity and insulin resistance are associated with increased GIP secretion.[62]

In pregnant rodents, plasma GIP levels are unchanged but intestinal GIP stores are increased.[63] Moreover, GIP levels are elevated during lactation. Thus, it may play a role in pregnancy and lactation. In humans, incretin hormones have been studied in adult offspring of pregnant women with GDM and type 1 diabetes mellitus, but there is no difference in GIP levels at baseline or during an oral glucose tolerance test, suggesting its limited role in the offspring's development of glucose intolerance.[64]

7.2.9 Glucagonlike Peptide-1

GLP-1 is an insulinotropic peptide produced by the enteroendocrine L cells.[65] An incretin hormone, GLP-1, like GIP, is secreted shortly in response to a carbohydrate meal and promotes insulin secretion, thus also promoting the release of glucose-dependent insulin. It also slows gastric emptying and decreases appetite. It acts on the central nervous system by binding to receptors in the arcuate nucleus of the hypothalamus, promoting satiety. GLP-1 receptor agonists, which have longer half-lives than endogenous GLP-1, are now drugs commonly used to treat diabetes mellitus and obesity.

GLP-1 secretion is lower in pregnant women with GDM than in normal pregnant women.[66] In addition, maternal GLP-1 levels negatively correlate with fetal abdominal circumference.[67] Individuals born to mothers with GDM or type 1 diabetes mellitus have lower levels of fasting GLP-1 in adulthood compared with those without intrauterine exposure to hyperglycemia.[64] This suggests that in utero exposure to hyperglycemia may cause glucose intolerance in the offspring by mechanisms involving GLP-1.

GLP-1 is present in human breast milk. In 4–5-week postpartum mothers, GLP-1 and fat concentrations are higher in hindmilk than in foremilk, unlike two other anorexigenic hormones, leptin and peptide YY.[68] GLP-1 concentration in hindmilk is negatively correlated with infant weight gain from birth to 6 months. However, further studies are necessary to determine whether breast-milk hormones remain biologically active and play a significant role in the infant.

7.2.10   Glucagonlike Peptide-2

Glucagonlike peptide-1 (GLP-2) is a 33-amino-acid peptide, produced by the enteroendocrine L cells of the ileum and large intestine, as well as the brainstem.[69] It is secreted in response to luminal nutrients. It inhibits gastric motility and acid secretion, and stimulates intestinal crypt cell proliferation and intestinal blood flow. Clinically, it has been implicated in the treatment of short bowel syndrome.[70] Teduglutide is a synthetic GLP-2 analog that causes significant reduction in the parenteral nutrition support volume requirement in patients with short bowel syndrome with intestinal failure.[71]

GLP-2 has not been studied in pregnancy or lactation.

7.2.11   Oxyntomodulin

Oxyntomodulin (OXM) is a type of enteroglucagon, a group of chemicals produced in the gut that have glucagonlike immunoreactivity.[72] OXM contains the full glucagon sequence, plus an additional short sequence of amino acids. It is secreted by the L cells of the intestine in response to luminal nutrients, including proteins, carbohydrates, and lipids. At the pancreas, it binds to glucagon and GLP-1 receptors, but at a significantly lower affinity (by 50–100 times) than glucagon in pigs and rodents.[73,74] In the stomach, OXM has been shown to inhibit gastric acid secretion, but the exact mechanism is unknown, as it also can have the opposite effect of stimulating acid secretion in isolated parietal cells in vitro.[75] Finally, like GLP-1, OXM has been studied for its weight-loss effects. When injected for 4 weeks, it causes a 2.3-kg weight loss in humans and increases energy expenditure.[76]

Due to its weak effect on glucagon and GLP-1 receptors, it seems to have limited biological significance. Its coagonist effect on the two receptors is of interest, however, because the downstream effects of activation of the glucagon and GLP-1 receptors are somewhat opposite. The hypoglycemic effects on the glucagon receptor can be opposed by the effect on GLP-1 receptor, while augmenting weight-loss potential by both receptors.[72]

OXM has not been studied in pregnancy or lactation.

7.2.12   Fibroblast Growth Factor 19

Fibroblast growth factor 19 (FGF19) is a gut hormone with pleiotropic effects.[77] It is secreted by the small intestine in response to feeding. FGF19 has insulinlike actions, such as promoting glucose uptake in adipocytes, synthesizing hepatic glycogen, and inhibiting gluconeogenesis. It also has a role in bile acid homeostasis and hepatic protein metabolism. Lower FGF19 levels are observed in patients with type 2 diabetes mellitus and obese patients, suggesting that FGF19 plays a role in weight loss.[78] High levels of FGF19 after bariatric surgery are associated with good postoperative outcomes, including remission of type 2 diabetes mellitus.[79]

With regard to FGF19's role in pregnancy, one study assessed FGF19 levels in pregnant women with GDM.[80] High levels of insulin are associated with lower levels of FGF19. In GDM, a highly insulin-resistant state with hyperinsulinism, low levels of FGF19 are seen, compared with those in healthy pregnant women matched for maternal and gestational age. Interestingly, a history of PCOS, another insulin-resistant state, is independently associated with lower FGF19 levels, regardless of the presence of GDM. The exact mechanisms behind the association of an insulin-resistant state and low FGF19 levels are not known.

FGF19's role in lactation has not been well studied.

7.3 CONCLUSION

There are many gut hormones, each with distinct roles that are not limited to gastrointestinal and neuroendocrine systems. Recent studies stress the importance of their roles in growth, metabolism, and appetite regulation. There have been attempts to elucidate their roles in pregnancy and lactation, but most have only suggested associations by the measurement of hormone levels during pregnancy and lactation. More research is needed to better understand gut hormone physiology in pregnancy and lactation.

REFERENCES

1. Bayliss WM, Starling EH. The mechanism of pancreatic secretion. *J Physiol* 1902;**28**:325–53.
2. Edkins JS. The chemical mechanism of gastric secretion. *J Physiol* 1905;**34**:133–44.
3. Starling EH. The Croonian lecture on the chemical correlation of the function of the body. *Lancet* 1905;**II**:339–41.
4. Wabitsch M. Gastrointestinal hormones induced the birth of endocrinology. *Endocr Dev* 2017;**32**:1–7.
5. Rehfeld JF. The changing concept of gut endocrinology. *Endocr Dev* 2017;**32**:8–19.
6. Dockray GJ, Varro A, Dimaline R, Wang T. The gastrins: their production and biological activities. *Annu Rev Physiol* 2001;**63**:119–39.
7. Frick G, Bremme K, Sjogren C, et al. Plasma levels of cholecystokinin and gastrin during the menstrual cycle and pregnancy. *Acta Obstet Gynecol Scand* 1990;**69**:317–20.
8. Hong JY, Park JW, Oh JI. Comparison of preoperative gastric contents and serum gastrin concentrations in pregnant and nonpregnant women. *J Clin Anesth* 2005;**17**:451–5.
9. Chiloiro M, Darconza G, Piccioli E, et al. Gastric emptying and orocecal transit time in pregnancy. *J Gastroenterol* 2001;**36**:538–43.
10. Vigen RA, Chen D, Syversen U, et al. Serum gastrin and gastric enterochromaffin-like cells during estrous cycle, pregnancy and lactation, and in response to estrogen-like agents in rats. *J Physiol Pharmacol* 2011;**62**:335–40.
11. Kojima M, Kangawa K. Ghrelin: structure and function. *Physiol Rev* 2005;**85**:495–522.
12. Perchard R, Clayton PE. Ghrelin and growth. *Endocr Dev* 2017;**32**:74–86.
13. Korbonits M, Goldsteone AP, Gueorquiev M, et al. Ghrelin—a hormone with multiple functions. *Front Neuroendocrinol* 2004;**25**:27–68.
14. Kojima M, Hosoda H, Date Y, et al. Ghrelin is a growth hormone-releasing acylated peptide from stomach. *Nature* 1999;**402**:656–60.
15. Ariyasu H, Takaya K, Tagami T, et al. Stomach is a major source of circulating ghrelin, and feeding state determines plasma ghrelin-like immuno-reactivity levels in humans. *J Clin Endocrinol Metab* 2001;**86**:4753–8.
16. Mansson JV, Alves FD, Biolo A, et al. Use of ghrelin in cachexia syndrome: a systematic review of clinical trials. *Nutr Rev* 2016;**74**:659–69.
17. Fidanci K, Meral C, Suleymanoglu S, et al. Ghrelin levels and postnatal growth in healthy infants 0–3 months of age. *J Clin Res Pediatr Endocrinol* 2010;**2**:34–8.
18. Nakahara K, Nakagawa M, Baba Y, et al. Maternal ghrelin plays an important role in rat fetal development during pregnancy. *Endocrinology* 2006;**147**:1333–42.
19. Chapman IM, Pescovitz OH, Murphy G, et al. Oral administration of growth hormone releasing peptide-mimetic MK-677 stimulates the GH/insulin-like growth factor-I axis in selected GH-deficient adults. *J Clin Endocrinol Metab* 1997;**82**:3455–63.
20. Angelidis G, Dafopoulos K, Messini CI, et al. Ghrelin: new insights into female reproductive system-associated disorders and pregnancy. *Reprod Sci* 2012;**19**:903–10.
21. Oruc AS, Mert I, Akturk M, et al. Ghrelin and motilin levels in hyperemesis gravidarum. *Arch Gynecol Obstet* 2013;**288**:710–9.
22. Palik E, Baranyi E, Melczer Z, et al. Elevated serum acylated ghrelin and resistin levels associate with pregnancy-induced weight gain and insulin resistance. *Diabetes Res Clin Pract* 2007;**76**:351–7.
23. Riedl M, Maier C, Handisura A, et al. Insulin resistance has no impact on ghrelin suppression in pregnancy. *J Intern Med* 2007;**262**:458–65.
24. Telejko B, Kuzmicki M, Zonenberg A, et al. Ghrelin in gestational diabetes: serum level and mRNA expression in fat and placental tissue. *Exp Clin Endocrinol Diabetes* 2010;**118**:87–92.
25. Makino Y, Hosoda H, Shibata K, et al. Alteration of plasma ghrelin levels associated with the blood pressure in pregnancy. *Hypertension* 2002;**39**:781–4.
26. Aydin S, Guzel SP, Kumru S, et al. Serum leptin and ghrelin concentrations of maternal serum, arterial, and venous cord blood in healthy and pre-eclamptic pregnant women. *J Physiol Biochem* 2008;**64**:51–9.
27. Aydin S, Ozkan Y, Erman F, et al. Presence of obestatin in breast milk: relationship among obestatin, ghrelin, and leptin in lactatin women. *Nutrition* 2008;**24**:689–93.
28. Wren AM, Small CJ, Fribbens CV, et al. The hypothalamic mechanisms of the hypophysiotropic action of ghrelin. *Neuroendocrinology* 2002;**76**:316–24.
29. Messini CI, Dafopoulos K, Chalvatzas N, et al. Blockage of ghrelin-induced prolactin secretion in women by bromocriptine. *Fertil Steril* 2010;**94**:1478–81.
30. Park H, Ahima RS. Physiology of leptin: energy homeostasis, neuroendocrine function and metabolism. *Metabolism* 2015;**64**:24–34.
31. Wasim M, Awan FR, Najam SS, et al. Role of leptin deficiency, inefficiency, and leptin receptors in obesity. *Biochem Genet* 2016;**54**:565–72.
32. Hamed EA, Zakary MM, Ahmed NS, et al. Circulating leptin and insulin in obese patients with and without type 2 diabetes mellitus: relation to ghrelin and oxidative stress. *Diabetes Res Clin Pract* 2011;**94**:434–41.

33. Gonzalez RR, Simon C, Caballero-Campo P, et al. Leptin and reproduction. *Hum Reprod Update* 2000;**6**:290–300.
34. Chehab FF, Lim ME, Lu R. Correction of the sterility defect in homozygous obese female mice by treatment with the human recombinant leptin. *Nat Genet* 1996;**12**:318–20.
35. Serazin V, Duval F, Wainer R, et al. Are leptin and adiponectin involved in recurrent pregnancy loss? *J Obstet Gynaecol Res* 2018;**44**:1015–22. https://doi.org/10.1111/jog.13623.
36. Misra VK, Trudeau S. The influence of overweight and obesity on longitudinal trends in maternal serum leptin levels during pregnancy. *Obesity* 2011;**19**:416–21.
37. Toulis KA, Goulis DF, Farmakiotis D, et al. Adiponectin levels in women with polycystic ovary syndrome: a systematic review and a meta-analysis. *Hum Reprod Update* 2009;**15**:297–307.
38. Hogg K, Blair JD, von Dadelszen P, et al. Hypomethylation of the LEP gene in placenta and elevated maternal leptin concentration in early onset pre-eclampsia. *Mol Cell Endocrinol* 2013;**367**:64–73.
39. Fields DA, George B, Williams M, et al. Associations between human breast milk hormones and adipocytokines and infant growth and body composition in the first 6 months of life. *Pediatr Obes* 2016;**12**:78–85.
40. Low MJ. Clinical endocrinology and metabolism. The somatostatin neuroendocrine system: physiology and clinical relevance in gastrointestinal and pancreatic disorders. *Best Pract Res Clin Endocrinol Metab* 2004;**18**:607–22.
41. Melmed S. New therapeutic agents for acromegaly. *Nat Rev Endocrinol* 2016;**12**:90–8.
42. Harris AG, O'Dorisio TM, Woltering EA, et al. Consensus statement: octreotide dose titration in secretory diarrhea. Diarrhea Management Consensus Development Panel. *Dig Dis Sci* 1995;**40**:1464.
43. Valenzuela JE, Schubert T, Fogel MR, et al. A multicenter, randomized, double-blind trial of somatostatin in the management of acute hemorrhage from esophageal varices. *Hepatology* 1989;**10**:958.
44. Holst N, Jenssen TG, Burhol PG. Plasma concentrations of motilin and somatostatin are increased in late pregnancy and postpartum. *Br J Obstet Gynaecol* 1992;**99**:338–41.
45. Goldstein A, Armony-Sivan R, Rozin A, et al. Somatostatin levels during infancy, pregnancy, and lactation: a review. *Peptides* 1995;**16**:1321–6.
46. Werner H, Amarant T, Millar RP, et al. Immunoreactive and biologically active somatostatin in human and sheep milk. *Eur J Biochem* 1985;**148**:353–7.
47. Afroze S, Meng F, Jensen K, et al. The physiological roles of secretin and its receptor. *Ann Transl Med* 2013;**1**:29.
48. Holst N, Jenssen TG, Burhol PG, et al. Plasma secretin concentrations during normal human pregnancy, delivery and postpartum. *Br J Obstet Gynaecol* 1989;**96**:424–7.
49. Huang Z, Wang T, Qi Q, et al. Progesterone regulates secretin expression in mouse uterus during early pregnancy. *Reprod Sci* 2014;**21**:724–32.
50. Owyang C, Logsdon CD. New insights into neurohormonal regulation of pancreatic secretion. *Gastroenterology* 2004;**127**:957.
51. Ziessman HA. Cholecystokinin cholescintigraphy: clinical indications and proper methodology. *Radiol Clin North Am* 2001;**39**:997.
52. Sumithran P, Prendergast LA, Delbridge E, et al. Long-term persistence of hormonal adaptations to weight loss. *N Engl J Med* 2011;**365**:1597–604.
53. Geracioti Jr TD, Liddle RA. Impaired cholecystokinin secretion in bulimia nervosa. *N Engl J Med* 1988;**319**:683.
54. Jordan J, Greenway FL, Leiter LA, et al. Stimulation of cholecystokinin-A receptors with GI181771X does not cause weight loss in overweight or obese patients. *Clin Pharmacol Ther* 2008;**83**:281–7.
55. Radberg G, Asztely M, Cantor P, et al. Gastric and gallbladder emptying in relation to the secretion of cholecystokinin after a meal in late pregnancy. *Digestion* 1989;**42**:174–80.
56. Svennersten-Sjaunja K, Olsson K. Endocrinology of milk production. *Domest Anim Endocrinol* 2005;**29**:241–58.
57. Itoh Z. Motilin and clinical application. *Peptides* 1997;**18**:593–608.
58. Sanger GJ, Furness JB. Ghrelin and motilin receptors as drug targets for gastrointestinal disorders. *Nat Rev Gastroenterol Hepatol* 2016;**13**:38–48.
59. Chapman MJ, Deane AM, O'Connor SL, et al. The effect of camicinal (GSK962040), a motilin agonist, on gastric emptying and glucose absorption in feed-intolerant critically ill patients: a randomized, blinded, placebo-controlled clinical trial. *Crit Care* 2016;**20**:232.
60. Liu J, Qiao X, Qian W, et al. Motilin in human milk and its elevated plasma concentration in lactating women. *J Gastroenterol Hepatol* 2014;**19**:1187–91.
61. Salera M, Giacomoni P, Pironi L, et al. Gastric inhibitory polypeptide release after oral glucose: relationship to glucose intolerance, diabetes mellitus, and obesity. *J Clin Endocrinol Metab* 1982;**55**:329–36.
62. Muscelli E, Mari A, Casolaro A, et al. Separate impact of obesity and glucose tolerance on the incretin effect in normal subjects and type 2 diabetic patients. *Diabetes* 2008;**57**:1340–8.
63. Moffett RC, Irwin N, Francis JM, et al. Alterations in glucose-dependent insulinotropic polypeptide and expression of genes involved in mammary gland and adipose tissue lipid metabolism during pregnancy and lactation. *PLoS One* 2013;**13**.
64. Kelstrup L, Clausen TD, Mathiesen ER, et al. Incretin and glucagon levels in adult offspring exposed to maternal diabetes in pregnancy. *J Clin Endocrinol Metab* 2015;**100**:1967–75.
65. Holst JJ. The physiology of glucagon-like peptide 1. *Physiol Rev* 2007;**87**:1409–39.
66. Lencioni C, Resi V, Romero F, et al. Glucagon-like peptide-1 secretion in women with gestational diabetes mellitus during and after pregnancy. *J Endocrinol Invest* 2011;**34**:287–90.
67. Valsamakis G, Margeli A, Vitoratos N, et al. The role of maternal gut hormones in normal pregnancy: fasting plasma active glucagon-like peptide 1 level is a negative predictor of fetal abdomen circumference and maternal weight change. *Eur J Endocrinol* 2010;**162**:897–903.
68. Schueler J, Alexander B, Hart AM, et al. Presence and dynamics of leptin, GLP-1, and PYY in human breast milk at early postpartum. *Obesity* 2013;**21**:1451–8.

69. Yusta B, Huang L, Munroe D, et al. Enteroendocrine localization of GLP-2 receptor expression in humans and rodents. *Gastroenterology* 2000;**119**:744–55.

70. Kim ES, Keam SJ. Teduglutide: a review in short bowel syndrome. *Drugs* 2017;**77**:345–52.

71. Jeppesen PB, Pertkiewicz M, Messing B, et al. Teduglutide reduces need for parenteral support among patients with short bowel syndrome with intestinal failure. *Gastroenterology* 2012;**143**:1472–81.

72. Pocai A. Action and therapeutic potential of oxyntomodulin. *Mol Metab* 2013;**3**:241–51.

73. Baldissera FG, Holst JJ, Knuhtsen S, et al. Oxyntomodulin (glicetin-(33-69)): pharmacokinetics, binding to liver cell membranes, effects on isolated perfused pig pancreas, and secretion from isolated perfused lower small intestine of pigs. *Regul Pept* 1988;**21**:151–66.

74. Baggio LL, Huang Q, Brown TJ, et al. Oxyntomodulin and glucagon-like-peptide-1 differentially regulate murine food intake and energy expenditure. *Gastroenterology* 2004;**127**:546–58.

75. Holst JJ, Wewer Albrechtsen NJ, Nordskov Gabe MB, et al. Oxyntomodulin: actions and role in diabetes. *Peptides* 2018;**100**:48–53.

76. Wynne K, Park AJ, Small CJ, et al. Subcutaneous oxyntomodulin reduces body weight in overweight and obese subjects: a double-blind, randomized, controlled trial. *Diabetes* 2005;**54**:2390–5.

77. Wu AL, Coulter S, Liddle C, et al. FGF19 regulates cell proliferation, glucose and bile acid metabolism via FGFR4-dependent and independent pathways. *PLoS One* 2011;**18**.

78. Mraz M, Lacinova Z, Kavalkova P, et al. Serum concentrations of fibroblast growth factor 19 in patients with obesity and type 2 diabetes mellitus: the influence of acute hyperinsulinemia, very-low calorie diet and PPAR-alpha agonist treatment. *Physiol Res* 2011;**60**:627–36.

79. Martinez de la Escalera L, Kyrou I, Vrbikova J, et al. Impact of gut hormone FGF-19 on type-2 diabetes and mitochondrial recovery in a prospective study of obese diabetic women undergoing bariatric surgery. *BMC Med* 2017;**15**:34.

80. Wang D, Zhu W, Li J, et al. Serum concentrations of fibroblast growth factors 19 and 21 in women with gestational diabetes mellitus: association with insulin resistance, adiponectin, and polycystic ovary syndrome history. *PLoS One* 2013;**8**.

Chapter 8

Adrenal Cortex and Medulla Physiology During Pregnancy, Labor, and Puerperium

Matthieu St-Jean, Isabelle Bourdeau and André Lacroix

Division of Endocrinology, Department of Medicine and Research Center, Centre hospitalier de l'Université de Montréal (CHUM), Montréal, QC, Canada

---

Key Clinical Changes

- Hypothalamo-pituitary-adrenal (HPA) axis is upregulated in pregnancy, with elevation in total and free cortisol, increased sensitivity of the adrenals to ACTH, and refractoriness to negative feedback by glucocorticoids.
- The placenta plays a major role in the regulation of the HPA axis by its production of CRH and ACTH throughout pregnancy, and by acting as a protective barrier for the fetus against the hypercortisolism of pregnancy.
- The HPA axis maintains its circadian variation during pregnancy, but the diurnal variation may be partially blunted.
- Pregnancy is associated with an upregulation of almost all the components of the Renin-Angiotensin-Aldosterone System (RAAS) to counteract the mineralocorticoid antagonists and kaliuretic effects of progesterone and to preserve the hemodynamic stability in pregnancy.
- Total testosterone, free testosterone, and SHBG increase during pregnancy, but DHEAS, a substrate for placental estrogen synthesis, decreases by 50%.
- Catecholamine levels are unchanged throughout pregnancy, and the placenta possesses MAO and COMT, which inactivate catecholamines and protect the fetus against excess catecholamine.

The adrenal glands are composed of two embryologically distinct parts: the outer adrenal cortex and the inner adrenal medulla. The adrenal cortex is composed of three zones of cells that synthesize, through multiple enzymatic steps, the different steroid hormones from cholesterol.[1] Each layer expresses specific steroidogenic enzymes that differentiate their function. The outer zona glomerulosa (ZG) specifically contains CYP11B2, or aldosterone synthase, which is responsible for aldosterone synthesis.[1] ZG is devoid of 17-α-hydroxylase, which is necessary for cortisol and androgen synthesis. Aldosterone synthesis is regulated by three principal secretagogues: angiotensin II, potassium, and to a lesser extent adrenocorticotropic hormone (ACTH).[1] The zona fasciculata (ZF) is the most prominent part of the adrenal cortex, producing mainly cortisol, but also androgens (mostly dehydroepiandrosterone sulfate (DHEAS) and androstenedione).[1] The inner zona reticularis (ZR) produces mostly androgens (i.e., DHEAS and androstenedione) due to its higher 17.20 lyase activity, but it makes cortisol as well. The synthesis of cortisol and androgens is regulated by ACTH, which is produced by the corticotroph cells of the anterior pituitary gland under the pulsatile control of hypothalamic corticotropin-releasing hormone (CRH) and of vasopressin.[1] The adrenal medulla produces and releases catecholamines (mostly norepinephrine and epinephrine). During pregnancy, maternal adrenal glands undergo minimal changes in weight and size, but the ZF enlarges.[2,3]

This chapter will review the physiological changes occurring in the adrenal glands during pregnancy. We will mostly focus on the changes in glucocorticoid and mineralocorticoid physiology. We also present a brief overview of the alterations occurring in the adrenal androgens and catecholamines during pregnancy.

8.1 GLUCOCORTICOID PHYSIOLOGY IN PREGNANCY, LABOR, AND PUERPERIUM

8.1.1 Plasma CRH and CRH-bp: Origin and Roles During Pregnancy

CRH is a 41-amino-acid peptide synthesized and released by the paraventricular nucleus neurons of the hypothalamus. Its principal functions is to regulate the anterior pituitary corticotrope synthesis of POMC and release of ACTH and β-endorphin into the bloodstream.[4] Maternal plasma CRH levels increase exponentially from the eighth week of pregnancy and onward to levels which are up to 1000 times those found in nonpregnant women.[5–8] After 35 weeks of gestation, there is a sharp increase in the plasma levels of CRH with a mean peak, ranging from 1462 to 4346 pg/mL between 38 and 40 weeks of pregnancy.[9–11] Most of plasma CRH is not of hypothalamic origin as it is rapidly degraded by enzymes in the pituitary gland.[12] CRH was isolated from the placenta in 1988.[13] Placental CRH was shown to be identical to the hypothalamic CRH in structure, immunoreactivity, and bioactivity.[4,6] CRH messenger ribonucleic acid (mRNA) was demonstrated in human placental extracts between 7 and 40 weeks of gestation.[14,15] A 20-fold increase of CRH mRNA is found in placental extracts 5 weeks prior to parturition, which parallels the marked elevation of plasma CRH.[15] CRH synthesis was demonstrated in vitro by superfusion studies of human placenta fragments.[16] Thus, the placenta is the major source of circulating CRH during pregnancy.[4]

Compared to the massive rise in CRH, ACTH, and cortisol levels increase modestly during pregnancy,[4] despite a demonstration that placental CRH is a secretagogue for pituitary and placental ACTH.[17,18] Two explanations for this discrepancy were proposed. The human CRH-binding protein (CRH-bp), a 322-amino-acid glycoprotein, attenuates the bioactivity of CRH by binding free CRH.[4,6,12,19] CRH-bp binds human CRH (hCRH), but not ovine CRH (oCRH).[20] CRH-bp levels are similar to nonpregnant women during the first two trimesters, but they fall by 50% between weeks 38 and 40 of pregnancy.[21] As CRH-bp does not increase in early pregnancy, its biosynthesis is not upregulated by estrogen.[6,21] In vitro, CRH-bp inhibits the ACTH-releasing-activity of the placenta but not of pituitary corticotropes of rat, supporting its inhibitory role on the bioactivity of the placental CRH, but it allows maternal stress response in late pregnancy.[22] Second, there is a possible partial desensitization of maternal corticotrophs after chronic stimulation by placental CRH,[4] as shown in vivo in rats[23] and in vitro in ovine pituitary cells.[24]

The regulation of placental CRH production is incompletely understood. Opposite to their effects on corticotropes, glucocorticoids stimulate the expression of the *CRH* gene and CRH production in the placenta.[12,25,26] This increase in CRH can stimulate pituitary ACTH release and result in increased cortisol secretion, which in turn can stimulate placental CRH release, resulting in a feed-forward mechanism.[26] Estrogens, progesterone, and nitric oxide have an inhibitory action on CRH release by the placenta.[26] In human placental culture cells, norepinephrine, acetylcholine, angiotensin II, Interleukine-1, oxytocin, and arginine vasopressin (AVP) stimulate the production of CRH[27]; the contribution of these factors on placental CRH production in vivo is unknown.

During pregnancy, in addition to playing an important regulator role of the hypothalamic-pituitary axis (HPA), CRH may play other functions.[4,5] CRH stimulates estrogen biosynthesis in cultured human placental cells.[12] CRH produced by the embryo and endometrium facilitates decidualization and implantation by modulating the antirejection process and regulating endometrial invasion.[5] CRH acts as a clock that determines pregnancy duration, and it is usually higher in women with spontaneous labor compared with those requiring induction.[4,28] In women with impending premature delivery, higher levels of CRH indicate that labor will begin within a day.[4] CRH is probably involved in the transition of the upper myometrium from a initial relaxed state to one sensitive to contractile signals from oxytocin and prostaglandins at term.[4] CRH stimulates prostaglandin E2 production, which favors cervical ripening and myometrial contractions.[4] CRH also regulates the expression of glucose transporters (GLUT), which facilitates placental glucose transport.[4] Of the 14 GLUT family proteins,[29] GLUT1 and GLUT3 are essential for glucose transport from the maternal circulation to the fetus through the placenta.[4] Placental GLUT1 expression is increased by locally produced CRH acting via CRH-R1,[29] while binding CRH-R2 downregulates GLUT1 in the placenta.[4,29] Higher CRH levels in later stages of pregnancy may bind mainly to CRH-R1 in order to increase GLUT1 expression and glucose transport to the growing fetus, but this remains to be demonstrated.[4]

8.1.2 CRH Receptors

There are two isoforms of the CRH receptor (CRH-R): CRH-R1 and CRH-R2.[4–6,12] Both belong to the seven transmembrane, G-protein-coupled superfamily and are positively coupled to adenylate cyclase.[12] Both isoforms of CRH-R share 70% sequence homology, but they have different pharmacologic profiles.[6,12,14] CRH-receptors (CRH-Rs) are expressed in numerous peripheral tissues, including the placenta, endometrium, central nervous system, heart, muscle, skin, and lymphatic organs.[6,14] CRH has 10 times higher affinity for CRH-R1 than CRH-R2.[12] CRH binds to CRH-R1 of the corticotroph cells,[5,12] where the ACTH response is modulated by the number of CRH-Rs. Factors such as immobilization, stress, adrenalectomy, administration of CRH, AVP, and glucocorticoids reduce the number of CRH-Rs in corticotrophs.[5,12] CRH and AVP have an additive effect on the levels of CRH-Rs on corticotrophs.[5] During pregnancy and labor, CRH-R1 and CRH-R2 expression in the myometrium enables CRH and CRH-like peptides to modulate myometrial contractility.[30] The CRH-R1 subtype mediates the inhibition of CRH on myometrial contractility, causing relaxation of myometrial cells.[4] In contrast, CRH-R2 promotes smooth muscle contraction.[12]

8.1.3 Urocortin in Pregnancy: Their Origin and Possible Role

The urocortins (UCN) UCN1 and UCN2 are 40-amino-acid peptides of members of the CRH peptide family, and they share 34%–45% sequence homology with CRH.[6,31,32] UCN3 has also been described, but its role during pregnancy is unknown. UCN levels during pregnancy are constant until onset of labor, when they increase.[6,33] UCN circulates in plasma bound to CRH-bp.[31] Free UCN exerts its action through its binding with CRH-R1 and CRH-R2. UCN binds with six times greater affinity to CRH-R1 and 40 times greater affinity to CRH-R2 than CRH.[31] UCN1 can bind to both CRH-R1 and CRH-R2, but UCN2 can only bind to CRH-R2.[34] UCN1 is expressed in anterior pituitary, cerebellum, heart, gastrointestinal tract, fetal membranes, placenta, decidua, chorion, and amnion.[34,35] UCN1 was demonstrated in vitro to increase uterine contractility induced by endometrial prostaglandins.[6,31] UCN1 also increases the secretion of prostaglandin E2 by the trophoblasts, and it decreases the expression of 15-hydroxyprostaglandin dehydrogenase (PGDH), an enzyme that usually metabolizes the prostaglandins.[31,36] All these effects are inhibited by astressin, a CRH-R2 inhibitor. Therefore, the prostaglandins increase induced by UCN1 is explained by a CRH-R2-mediated effect.[36] Also, UCN1 can increase ACTH and cortisol secretion in healthy humans[35] and ACTH release by human placental cells in culture.[37]

UCN2 is expressed in multiple organs, including the brain, colon, small intestine, stomach, thyroid, adrenal, heart, skeletal muscles, and vascular endothelial cells.[32] During pregnancy, UCN2 is also found in the maternal decidua, trophoblast, fetal membranes, and myometrium.[32,37] UCN2 was demonstrated to stimulate estradiol release by trophoblast cell cultures in the presence of DHEAS, androstenedione, or testosterone.[32] At term, the expression of UCN2 gene is significantly higher in human laboring gestational tissues compared to nonlaboring gestational tissues (placenta, fetal membranes, and myometrium).[32] Like UCN1, UCN2 also decreases PDGH expression, which probably contributes to increased concentrations of prostaglandins.[36] UCN2 also accelerates the procontractile effect of prostaglandin F2α (PGF$_{2\alpha}$), likely by upregulating the expression of the PGF$_{2\alpha}$ receptor and the myometrial expression of proinflammatory cytokines.[32] The upregulation of proinflammatory cytokines within the laboring myometrium stimulates uterine contractions and potentiates the prostaglandin-induced uterine contractions.[32] However, UCN2 does not have a direct effect on line contraction in myometrial cells. Therefore, UCN2 plays an indirect role on the enhancement of myometrial cell contraction through the production of proinflammatory cytokines and the accentuation of the contractile response to prostaglandins.[32] UCN2 is also proposed to be a regulator of the placental vascular tone, given that it is expressed in endothelial cells in the placental villi.[37] Unlike UCN1, UCN2 does not induce ACTH secretion in either rat pituitary cells.[38] or cultured human placental cells.[37] Because UCN2 binds to CRH-R2 only and UCN1 and CRH bind to CRH-R1 and CRH-R1, the ACTH release action was attributed to activation of CRH-R1.[37]

8.1.4 Plasma ACTH: Origin and Roles During Pregnancy

ACTH is a 39-amino-acid peptide that is secreted by the pituitary corticotropes following posttranslational proteolytic cleavage of its precursor peptide proopiomelanocortin (POMC).[6,39] The cleavage of POMC can give rise to related peptides, including β-endorphin, β-lipotropin, and α-MSH.[6,39] In men and nonpregnant women, β-endorphin, β-lipotropin, and ACTH follow a similar diurnal rhythm, and their phasic secretion is under a common central control.[40] The principal action of ACTH is through its binding with melanocortin 2 receptor (MC2R) to stimulate the synthesis and release of glucocorticoids from the adrenal ZF.[41] ACTH is unable to cross the placenta, so its effects are limited to the mother.[6]

ACTH levels increase twofold by the end of the second half of pregnancy compared to the first trimester.[8,33,39,42–45] Some studies reported that the basal levels of ACTH during pregnancy were higher[39,46] compared to nongravid women, and others reported that they were lower.[45,47]

In the second half of pregnancy, the ACTH rises in spite of the elevated level of free cortisol, suggesting that there is another source of ACTH besides the pituitary that is not subject to negative feedback by cortisol.[6,45] Term placenta extracts contain ACTH and immunoreactive β-endorphin and β-lipoprotein.[43,48,49] These peptides arise from POMC in the placenta.[6,48,49] CRH stimulates the secretion of peptides containing the ACTH sequence in primary culture of human placental cells, and this effect is reversed by a CRH antagonist.[18] Glucocorticoids that usually suppress the secretion of pituitary ACTH have no influence on the release of ACTH by the placenta.[18] In vitro, human placental ACTH is bioactive to the same extent in early and late gestation.[50]

8.1.5 Cortisol-Binding Globulin: Changes in Levels and Isoforms During Pregnancy and its Possible Role in Pregnancy

Cortisol-binding globulin (CBG), or transcortin, is a 50–60-kDA transport glycoprotein that binds cortisol and progesterone with high affinity.[51] CBG synthesis occurs mainly in the liver,[52,53] but also in the endometrium, corpus luteum, and placenta, where CBG mRNA is expressed.[54–57] Approximatively 90% of circulating cortisol is bound to CBG, 5% to albumin and 5% is free.[51,58] During pregnancy, CBG levels increases progressively two- to threefold following stimulation by the circulating estrogen,[59] similarly to women taking oral contraceptives.[60–62] CBG levels during the second half of pregnancy are threefold higher than in nonpregnant patients.[60,63] The primary role of CBG is to protect steroid hormones from catabolism and to deliver them to target cells.[64] CBG contains six sites for N-glycosylation, and there is an average of five sites occupied by biantennary or triantennary oligosaccharides with variable additional terminal sialic acid residues, leading to different glycoforms.[65] A pregnancy-associated glycoform of CBG is produced by an altered posttranslational modulation of CBG protein[66] under the influence of estradiol[51]; this glycoform has only triantennary oligosaccharides and represents 10% of total CBG during pregnancy.[65,66] This specific type of CBG is usually present at 6 months of pregnancy and has a 60-fold increased binding affinity for syncytiotrophoblast cell membranes compared to normal CBG.[66] It might facilitate the specific delivery of steroids to the developing fetus because 25% of the fetal cortisol in late pregnancy is of maternal origin,[67] and it may also possibly play a role in the regulation of glucocorticoid-induced placental CRH release.[51,64–66] In the postpartum period, there are inconsistent data for the kinetics of CBG. Some studies demonstrate normalization of CBG levels at 3–6 weeks postpartum,[61,63,68] whereas other reported elevated levels until 3–6 months postpartum.[60,69] This persistence of CBG in the postpartum period might be explained by an increase in its half-life[51,66] or a continued secretion of the pregnancy-associated variant by the maternal organism.[66]

8.1.6 Total and Free Cortisol Levels During Pregnancy

Pregnancy is a state characterized by an elevation of plasma total cortisol, plasma free cortisol, urine free cortisol, and salivary cortisol.[6] Plasma total cortisol, which comprises the level of bound cortisol (to CBG and albumin) and unbound cortisol (also termed *free cortisol*), increases progressively during pregnancy[6,45,60,61,63,70–75] in parallel to the CBG increase.[63] This increase was shown to start as early as the 11th to 12th week of gestation and is maintained throughout pregnancy.[63,71] During the third trimester of pregnancy, total cortisol levels are increased two- to threefold compared to nonpregnant women (Tables 8.1–8.6).[60,71,73,78–80]

TABLE 8.1 Variation of the different components of the hypothalamo-pituitary adrenal axis and feto-placental unit during pregnancy and pregnancy

Parameters	Change during pregnancy (T3 vs T1)	Changes in pregnancy compared to normal nonpregnant women	Time for normalization in postpartum
Placental CRH	Progressive increase with a sharp increase after 35 weeks	Increase by 1000-fold	≤24h
CRH-bp	Unchanged until 38 weeks of pregnancy, where it falls to 50% of those levels	Same than nongravid women until 38 weeks of gestation where it falls to 50% of those levels	NA
ACTH (pituitary +placental)	Increased by 2-fold	Inconsistent (up or down depending on the study)	≤24h
Plasma total cortisol	Increases progressively by 1.5- to 2-fold	Increased by 2- to 3-fold	<1 week to ≤3 months
Plasma free cortisol	Increased progressively by 1.3-to 3-fold	Increased by 1.5- to 3-fold	<1 week
24-h urinary free cortisol excretion	Increased progressively by 1.5- to 2-fold	Increased by 2- to 3-fold	≤2–3 months
Late-night free salivary cortisol	Increased	Equivocal results (mostly increased)	NA
CBG	Increased by 2- to 3-fold during pregnancy	Increased by 3-fold in late pregnancy	Variable (3–6 weeks until 3–6 months depending on the study)

NA, not assessed.

TABLE 8.2 Normal values for mean morning total cortisol observed during pregnancy and postpartum

References	Assays	Trimesters	Values (nmol/L)	Nonpregnant values (nmol/L)
Ambroziak et al.[73] Mean (2.5%– 97.5%)	Elecsys 2010 (Hitachi, Japan)	T1	586.2 (281.7–954.8)	484.9 (274.8–721.4)
		T2	833.1 (456.8–1305.4)[a]	
		T3	973.5 (406.6–1464.5)[a]	
		PP	487.4 (293.8–706.2)	
Jung et al.[60] Mean ± SD	LC-MSMS	T1	577 ± 30[a]	364 ± 28
		T2	878 ± 28[a]	
		T3	1043 ± 41[a]	
		PP (2–3 months)	486 ± 38[a]	
Suri et al.[75] Mean ± SD	Chemiluminescence enzyme immunoassay	T1	257 ± 61[b]	NA
		T2	400 ± 119[b,c]	
		T3	458 ± 116[b,c]	
		PP (11–14 weeks)	251 ± 132[b]	
Abou-Samra et al.[71] (not the same patient assessed at each trimester) Mean ± SD	Radiocompetition after chromatographic separation	T1	452 ± 88[a]	303 ± 55
		T2	675 ± 160[a]	
		T3	924 ± 201[a]	

[a]Different than the nonpregnant values.
[b]The values of the study in µg/dL were converted to nmol/L by using the conversion factor: 1 µg/dL = 27.59 nmol/L.
[c]Different than the postpartum and T1.
NA, not assessed.

TABLE 8.3 Normal values for mean morning free serum cortisol observed during pregnancy and postpartum

References	Assays	Trimesters	Values (nmol/L)	Nonpregnant values (nmol/L)
Jung et al.[60] Mean ± SD	Equilibrium dialysis	T1	14.5 ± 1.2	12.2 ± 1.6
		T2	17.2 ± 1.4[a]	
		T3	19.6 ± 1.5[a]	
		PP (2–3 months)	12.3 ± 2.0	
Abou-Samra et al.[71] Mean ± SD	Equilibrium dialysis	T1	11.9 ± 3.3	11.0 ± 2.8
		T2	18.5 ± 6.1[a]	
		T3	34.2 ± 7.5[a]	

[a]Different than the nonpregnant values.

TABLE 8.4 Normal values for mean morning salivary cortisol observed during pregnancy and postpartum[a]

References	Assays	Trimesters	Values (nmol/L)	Nonpregnant values (nmol/L)
Ambroziak et al.[73] Mean (2.5%–97.5%)	Elecsys 2010 (Hitachi, Japan)	T1	18.4 (7.2–34.2)	18.5 (5.27–37.8)
		T2	19.6 (6.9–36.4)	
		T3	21.9 (8.9–39.7)	
		PP (3 months)	13.8 (4.08–26.01)	
Suri et al.[75] Mean ± SD	Enzyme-linked immunoassay (Salimetrics, State College, PA)	T1	5.79 ± 2.76[a]	NA
		T2	9.93 ± 4.69[a,b]	
		T3	12.97 ± 4.97[a,b]	
		PP	6.06 ± 4.69[a]	

[a]The values of the study in μg/dL were converted to nmol/L by using the conversion factor: 1 μg/dL = 27,59 nmol/L.
[b]Different than the first trimester and postpartum.
NA, not assessed.

TABLE 8.5 Normal values for mean late-night/midnight salivary cortisol observed during pregnancy and postpartum

References	Assays	Trimesters	Values (nmol/L)	Nonpregnant values (nmol/L)
Manetti et al.[76] Mean ± SD	RIA (Immunotech, Marseille, France)	T2 and T3	6.64 ± 3.67[a,b]	3.78 ± 1.57
Lopes et al.[77] Median (min–max)	ELISA—Cortisol (expanded range)	T1	2.20 (0.55–6.90)[c]	1.93 (0.83–4.14)
		T2	2.76 (0.55–7.73)[c]	
		T3	4.13 (1.93–9.38)[a,c]	
Ambroziak et al.[73] Mean (2.5%–97.5%)	Elecsys 2010 (Hitachi, Japan)	T1	4.4 (1.8–9.1)	4.6 (1.1–9.0)
		T2	4.6 (1.7–9.8)	
		T3	5.6 (1.3–13.5)	
		PP (3 months)	3.0 (1.0–5.3)	

[a]Different than the nonpregnant values.
[b]The values of the study in ng/mL were converted to nmol/L by using the conversion factor: 1 ng/mL = 2759 nmol/L.
[c]The values of the study in μg/dL were converted to nmol/L by using the conversion factor: 1 μg/dL = 27.59 nmol/L.
NA, not assessed.

TABLE 8.6 Normal values for mean 24-h urinary free cortisol excretion observed during pregnancy and postpartum

Parameters	Assays	Trimester	Values (nmol/day)	Nonpregnant values (nmol/day)
Jung et al.[60] Mean ± SD	LC-MSMS	T1	135 ± 10[a]	78 ± 12
		T2	187 ± 13[a]	
		T3	242 ± 15[a]	
		PP (2–3 months)	75 ± 9	
Chico et al.[60a] Mean ± SD	RIA	T1	262 ± 118	NA
		T2	463 ± 256[b]	
		T3	424 ± 210[b]	

[a]Different than the nonpregnant values.
[b]Different than the first trimester.
NA, not assessed.

Free cortisol increases progressively during pregnancy in parallel to total cortisol. Plasma free cortisol was shown to be increased in pregnancy, especially during the second and third trimesters.[60,63,71,81] Plasma free cortisol levels, measured by equilibrium dialysis during the third trimester, increase 1.5- to 3-fold compared to nonpregnant controls.[60,71] Progressive elevation in urinary free cortisol (UFC) were also noted during pregnancy, which also parallel the increase in total cortisol.[79] During the third trimester, the 24h UFC values are two to three times higher than in nonpregnant patients.[60,79,82] Even if the glomerular filtration rate is increased during pregnancy, it does not seem to explain the elevated UFC excretion.[83] Free salivary cortisol showed a strong correlation with total or free plasma cortisol.[72,75,84] However, studies on the measure of salivary cortisol levels during pregnancy are inconsistent, showing both increased[61,74–77,85] or normal levels.[72,73] Manetti et al.[76] and Lopes et al.[77] showed that late-night salivary cortisol (LNSC) was higher in patients in the third trimester of pregnancy than in nonpregnant patients. However, Ambroziak et al.,[73] recently showed that morning salivary cortisol and LNSC were not different in pregnant patients compared to nonpregnant controls, no matter the trimester. However, in this study, LNSC is 20% higher in the third trimester of pregnancy than in the controls, and it is also higher than in the postpartum period, but it was not statistically significant.[73] In the study of Lopes et al.[77] the LNSC sampling during the third trimester were done at 40 weeks of pregnancy compared to 31 weeks as found by Ambroziak et al.[73] Given the fact that free cortisol is higher at the end of the third trimester, it seems appropriate to say that LNSC is probably higher for patients in the third trimester of pregnancy than for nonpregnant patients, but the extent of this increase might depend on the timing of the samples during the third trimester.

8.1.7 Diurnal Variation of the HPA Axis and the Feto-Placental Unit During Pregnancy

The secretion of placental CRH does not exhibit a circadian rhythm.[5,6,69] There is no relation between the diurnal variation of CRH and the diurnal variation of ACTH or cortisol.[69,85] The circadian rhythm of ACTH is maintained during pregnancy,[39,47,69,85] and it parallels the diurnal variation of β-endorphin.[39] The highest values of ACTH are in the morning, around 8 a.m., and the lowest are at midnight.[39,69] There is a close correlation between the levels of ACTH and cortisol during the third trimester, and ACTH precedes cortisol secretion by 30 min.[69] Total and free cortisol also preserved a day-night variation during pregnancy, but it may be partly blunted.[45,61,63,69,82,85–88] Also, in the morning, the peak in cortisol was demonstrated to be an hour later in pregnant patients (8 a.m. instead of 7 a.m.) than nongravid women.[74]

Some explanations were suggested to explain the lack of correlation between the diurnal variation of CRH and ACTH or cortisol. It was suggested that a nonpulsatile CRH stimulation could still produce a pulsatile pattern of ACTH and cortisol secretion.[69] This hypothesis is supported by the fact that during a continuous infusion of ovine CRH in normal humans, the secretion of ACTH and cortisol remained pulsatile.[69] Another explanation is that vasopressin, which is secreted in pulsatile fashion with a circadian rhythm, might regulate the circadian and pulsatile ACTH release by the pituitary during pregnancy and be potentiated by the chronically high level of circulating CRH.[69,89] Goland et al.[89] have demonstrated that in pregnant baboons, the secretion of ACTH and cortisol in response to vasopressin is higher in late pregnancy, when the level of CRH is higher, than in early pregnancy. Therefore, even if the secretion of CRH is nonpulsatile, it appears to be a major regulator of ACTH and cortisol during pregnancy.[6,69]

8.1.8 Physiologic Hypercortisolism of Pregnancy: Particular Regulation of the HPA Axis During Pregnancy

The higher level of free cortisol during pregnancy results in a greater exposure of maternal tissues to glucocorticoids.[60,82,85,86,88] This progressive elevation in free and total cortisol and its metabolite levels that is seen in pregnancy can result from an upregulation of the HPA axis in addition to the estrogen-stimulated CBG elevation.[6,60] The upregulation of the HPA axis maybe secondary to a resistance of the HPA axis to cortisol.[6,88] It was found that during pregnancy, the HPA axis is resistant to suppression by dexamethasone.[43,79,88] Progesterone, which increases progressively by threefold between the first and third trimester of pregnancy,[71] might be implicated in that process, given that progesterone levels in late pregnancy correlate with salivary cortisol.[85] Progesterone competes with cortisol for the binding with CBG.[63,85] However, the effect of progesterone on the glucocorticoid receptor in vitro is unclear, with some studies reporting an agonist action[90,91] and other and antagonist action.[71,92,93] Therefore, high levels of progesterone can contribute to the increase in free cortisol by its reduction of the cortisol-CBG binding.[71,85]

Other mechanisms have been proposed to explain the rise in free cortisol during pregnancy.[60] As described previously, during the second half of pregnancy, there is an increase in plasma CRH and ACTH,[44,45] which are autonomous[6,45,60] and possibly of placental origin.[13,18] This increase in CRH and ACTH might also upregulate the HPA axis. Also, the adrenal glands have increased responsiveness to ACTH during pregnancy, as demonstrated by the higher cortisol response to synthetic ACTH compared to nonpregnant women.[6,88,94,95] Brown et al.[95] found that the mean maximum cortisol response to continued ACTH infusion in a normal three-trimester pregnancy was 963 nmol/L compared to 507 nmol/L in the nonpregnant controls. One study was done to evaluate the response of the adrenal in pregnancy to an intravenous bolus of 1 μg of cortrosyn[96]; 6 pregnant women who were at a mean of 31.4 ± 2.3 weeks of pregnancy reached a peak cortisol value of 1215 nmol/L (99% IC 917–1535 nmol/L) at a mean of 27.4 ± 1.6 min.[96] However, no nonpregnant control groups have been studied. Suri et al.[75] examined the response of serum cortisol and salivary cortisol to a 250-μg cortrosyn intravenous bolus in pregnant women through pregnancy and at 3 months postpartum. They demonstrated that the response of salivary cortisol to the intravenous bolus of cortrosyn increases progressively during pregnancy when compared to the postpartum period. However, the response of the total serum cortisol was only higher in the second trimester compared to the postpartum state.[75] All these data confirmed that pregnancy represents a state where the adrenal glands have a higher sensitivity to ACTH compared to nonpregnant women and the postpartum period.

8.1.9 Specific Role of Glucocorticoids During Pregnancy and the Impact of Excessive Fetal Glucocorticoid Exposure

Glucocorticoids are important during the various phases of pregnancy. In early pregnancy, glucocorticoids have been shown to promote the establishment of gestation.[97] They inhibit immune rejection responses during the peri-implantation windows, and they also play a beneficial role in the induction of decidualization in early pregnancy.[97] Also, glucocorticoids play an important role in late fetal development, such as lung maturation.[6] However, prolonged exposure to excessive levels of glucocorticoids is detrimental to placental and fetal development.[98] Fetal exposure to excessive amounts of glucocorticoids during pregnancy leads to intrauterine growth retardation and may lead to the development of chronic disease, such as hypertension and diabetes, later in life.[99]

8.1.10 Fetus Protection Against the High Maternal Glucocorticoids Levels During Pregnancy

The fetus is protected during gestation from the effects of maternal hypercortisolism by the 11-βhydroxysteroid dehydrogenase 2 (11-βHSD 2) enzyme located in the syncytial trophoblastic cells.[6] Here, 11-βHSD 2 catalyzes the conversion of cortisol to its inactive metabolite cortisone.[100] Also, 11-βHSD 2 expression is already observable in the placenta at 3 weeks postconception, but its activity at that time was not assessed.[101] Its expression increases exponentially to more than 56-fold between weeks 4–6 and weeks 35–40 of gestation.[102] Cortisol and CRH upregulates the expression of 11-βHSD 2 in villous trophoblastic cells, which may represent a mechanism of self-defense to counteract maternal hypercortisolism.[97,103] The capacity of 11-βHSD 2 is high enough to ensure that the fetal cortisol levels are much lower than maternal levels during gestation.[6] However, despite the efficacy of 11-βHSD 2, 25% of the fetal cortisol is of maternal origin at term.[104] Mutations or epigenetic modifications of the gene encoding 11-βHSD 2, which diminish the function of the enzyme, is associated with a significant reduction in birth weight.[99] Dexamethasone and betamethasone, which are synthetic glucocorticoids, are poor substrates for 11-βHSD 2, and they can cross the placental barrier without being inactivated following maternal administration.[99]

8.1.11 Change in the HPA Axis and Cortisol Levels During Parturition and in the Postpartum

Peak CRH levels occurs within 48 h prior to delivery, and it decreases during labor.[28] In contrast to the decreasing level of CRH during labor, ACTH increases markedly by 10- to 15-fold during labor and delivery, demonstrating that the HPA axis is not completely suppressed.[6,28,39,45] The increase in ACTH levels is higher in women who had oxytocin-induced labor than those who underwent spontaneous labor or elective caesarean, which suggests that oxytocin can possibly potentiate the CRH-stimulated ACTH release from corticotropes.[28,105] Also, ACTH levels immediately after vaginal delivery are higher than those found in elective caesarean delivery.[39] The level of ACTH in the elective caesarean reached their peak 30 min after delivery, reflecting the stress associated with the surgery.[39] During labor, levels of total and free cortisol sharply increase to values that are almost double those that are seen in the third trimester.[45,80,106,107] The increase in cortisol is higher in vaginal delivery when compared to elective caesarean delivery, which reflects the stress induced by the onset of labor.[106]

In the postpartum period, CRH and ACTH fall rapidly toward the nonpregnant range within 24 h.[10,44] After delivery, total and free cortisol levels slowly decrease to the nonpregnant range over a period of several days in some studies.[61,85] However, a recent study showed a delay in the normalization of total cortisol of up to 3 months.[60] The time for normalization of UFC in the postpartum period is not well defined. However, it is known that at 2–3 months after delivery, UFC is normalized.[60] The possible explanations for the normalization delay of total cortisol might be the longer half-life or the continued biosynthesis of pregnancy-associated CBG in the postpartum period, given that the free cortisol was normalized at that time.[60,73] The circadian rhythm of ACTH and cortisol is also maintained in the early postpartum period.[39,85] In the postpartum period, the abnormal cortisol suppression after 1 mg of dexamethasone may persist for up to 2–3 weeks.[108] This finding is consistent with the fact that total cortisol probably requires 2 weeks to months to normalize in the postpartum period, but the time for normalization varies between individuals, given that some women have normal dexamethasone test 5 days after delivery.[109]

8.2 MINERALOCORTICOID PHYSIOLOGY IN PREGNANCY, LABOR, AND PUERPERIUM

Normal pregnancy is characterized by a decrease in blood pressure despite a 45% expansion of the intravascular volume and an increase in cardiac output of 25%–50%, explained by a decrease in peripheral vascular resistance.[6,110] Mineralocorticoids and the renin-angiotensin system (RAS) play an important role in these adaptations.[110] Here, we will describe briefly changes in the RAS and aldosterone physiology during pregnancy (see Chapter 10 for more detail).

The RAS is a hormone-signaling cascade implicated in the regulation of blood pressure and systemic electrolyte balance.[111] In the context of diminished circulating blood volume, the juxtaglomerular apparatus, in the afferent arteriole of the kidney, senses the diminished renal perfusion and increases renin secretion. Renin, an enzyme, cleaves the angiotensinogen, a protein synthesized by the liver, to produce angiotensin I (ANG-I). ANG-I, a biologically inactive peptide, is then cleaved by the angiotensin-converting enzyme (ACE), expressed by endothelium particularly in the lungs, to the biologically active angiotensin II (ANG-II).[111] ANG-II exerts its action through binding with two major angiotensin receptors, AT1R and AT2R, which are seven-transmembrane, G-protein-coupled receptors that have 34% sequence homology and similar affinity for ANG-II. The AT1R is the predominant ANG-II receptor in adults and is responsible for the majority of the ANG-II effects.[111] AT1R is localized in several tissues, such as blood vessels, kidneys, adrenals, heart, and the central and peripheral autonomic nervous systems.[112] ANG-II, by its binding with AT1R, induced vasoconstriction, increased sympathetic activity, aldosterone production, and release by the ZG.[6,111]

Progesterone and estradiol concentrations increase progressively in the maternal blood during pregnancy, mostly as a result of placental production.[6,113] Progesterone acts as a mineralocorticoid receptor antagonist. It reduces sodium reabsorption in the distal tubule, and it also causes smooth muscle relaxation, which contribute to reduce systemic vascular resistance.[6,114] Progesterone is also associated with an antikaliuretic effect.[115]

8.2.1 RAS Modifications During Pregnancy

Pregnancy is associated with an upregulation of all components of the RAS, partly to counteract the effects of progesterone.[111,116] Plasma renin activity (PRA) increases early in the first trimester until the 20th week of pregnancy and reaches values threefold to sevenfold greater than the normal range, after which it remains stable until delivery.[6,113,117] Approximatively 50% of the increase in plasma renin activity during pregnancy is explained by the increase in synthesis of the renin substrate, angiotensinogen, and the other 50% represents the real increase in renin concentration.[113] The concentration of plasma renin is higher in pregnant women at 28–38 weeks of pregnancy compared to nonpregnant women.[118] Extrarenal production of renin by the ovaries and the maternal decidua probably contributes to the early increase in renin.[119] Other factors that might explain the increase in renin are the hemodynamic changes of the pregnancy, which include the prostaglandin-induced peripheral vasodilatation and the arteriovenous shunt effect of the uteroplacental unit. These changes lead to decreased blood pressure, and the RAS could be activated to maintain organ perfusion and blood pressure.[113]

Progesterone elevation might also contribute to the renin elevation by its previously described effects.[6,120] The ovary also secretes prorenin during pregnancy.[6,121] Prorenin is the precursor of renin in renin-producing cells.[119] The maternal plasma levels of prorenin reach their maximum at 8–12 weeks of gestation, which reaches 10 times the nonpregnant levels.[121] To become active, prorenin requires being in an open conformation.[122] Some authors suggested that binding of prorenin to the prorenin soluble receptor is activated and participates in the generation of ANG-I from angiotensinogen.[121] However, a recent study reported that in physiological conditions (pH of 7.4 and temperature of 37°C), only a small percentage ($\approx 1\%$) of prorenin is in the open conformation.[122] Thus, prorenin contribution to the increased activity of the RAS in pregnancy remains to be determined.

Angiotensinogen in pregnancy paralleled the renin increase; there is an increase in the first trimester until the 20th week, where it reaches a plateau until delivery.[6,113,123] Angiotensinogen synthesis by the liver is stimulated by estradiol during pregnancy, which is supported by the demonstration of estradiol-induced, hepatic angiotensinogen synthesis in animal models, and a polymorphism in the estradiol response element of the angiotensinogen gene is negatively associated with angiotensinogen levels during pregnancy.[111,113,116,124,125] The placenta might also contribute, as angiotensinogen mRNA and protein are found in human placental tissues.[6,119] There is a high-molecular-weight angiotensinogen that circulates specifically in the plasma of pregnant women. The levels of this high-molecular-weight angiotensinogen increases throughout pregnancy and constitutes about 16% of the total angiotensinogen.[121] However, the role of this specific form of angiotensinogen remains unknown.[6]

ACE activity remains constant during pregnancy, but the levels are lower than in nonpregnant women.[121] This is the only component of the RAS that is decreased during pregnancy.[111] ANG-II plasma levels correlate with the plasma levels of ANG-I, which is consistent with the fact that angiotensin-converting enzymes have no limiting role in the synthesis of ANG-II.[117] ANG-II levels increase throughout pregnancy, reaching maximal values in the third trimester.[117] ANG-II concentrations in the third trimester are 50% above the nonpregnant values.[121] Several studies have revealed immunoreactivity for ANG-II in the placenta.[119] As demonstrated by the higher levels of ANG-II in the second half of pregnancy, activation of renin-angiotensin-aldosterone system (RAAS) is higher in the second and third trimesters of pregnancy, despite the early increase in PRA and its substrate angiotensinogen.[117] However, blood pressure in pregnancy remains normal despite this increase in ANG-II levels because ANG-II efficacy is reduced through changes in AT1R sensitivity, elevated progesterone levels, and elevated prostacyclin levels, which cause vasodilatation.[126]

The placental RAS plays key roles in the implantation, placentation, and development of the uteroplacental and umbilicoplacental circulation, as well as regulation of uteroplacental vascular resistance, but they also contribute to the activity of the circulating maternal RAS.[119,121]

8.2.2 Aldosterone Levels During Pregnancy

In normal pregnancy, plasma and urinary aldosterone increase progressively, in parallel with progesterone, with levels being five- to sevenfold more during the first trimester and 10- to 20-fold more at the end of the third trimester.[6,80,113,117,123] Plasma aldosterone circulates mostly unbound to plasma protein.[6] Plasma aldosterone correlates with the levels of urinary aldosterone, but the proportional increase in urinary aldosterone during the second and third trimesters is twice the increase in plasma aldosterone.[113] The relationship between PRA and plasma aldosterone is dissociated during the second and third trimesters of pregnancy.[127] This particular findings suggest that either the adrenals are more sensitive to ANG-II or that other factors known to regulate aldosterone secretion in normal patients, such as norepinephrine, ACTH, and digitalis-like factor, contribute to the elevation in aldosterone.[127] ACTH which increases during pregnancy may contribute to the increased aldosterone secretion.[127] In twin pregnancies, the plasma aldosterone and PRA were reported in one study to be higher in the second trimester, but they decrease during the third trimester to lower levels than normal singleton pregnancy.[128] However, there are no explanations for these findings. Potassium levels remain normal in pregnancy despite the elevation in aldosterone levels, probably because of the mineralocorticoids' antagonist action of progesterone.[114] Urinary excretion of sodium and potassium remains constant throughout pregnancy.[123] The plasmatic aldosterone concentration (PAC) and PRA ratio increase in the third trimester of pregnancy, as aldosterone increases more than PRA during the second half of pregnancy.[128]

Aldosterone is an important factor for fetus development, as demonstrated with a blockade of the mineralocorticoid receptor in animal models that resulted in inhibition of organogenesis.[129]

8.2.3 Regulation of RAAS During Pregnancy

The physiological regulation of RAAS is intact during pregnancy, as the response of plasma renin to posture or intravenous or oral saline loading is similar to that of nonpregnant women.[118,127,130] Aldosterone also maintains a normal response to diuretics, volume depletion, and administration of mineralocorticoids.[6]

8.2.4 Other Mineralocorticoids

During pregnancy, the levels of corticosterone, deoxycortisol, and cortisone increase by two- to threefold, in parallel with cortisol.[80] The plasma levels of 11-deoxycorticosterone (DOC), a potent mineralocorticoid, increases progressively during pregnancy to reach a peak (60–100 ng/100 mL) in the third trimester.[6,114] DOC elevation might contribute to the sodium retention of pregnancy.[114] During pregnancy, it appears that most of DOC is produced from the 21-hydroxylation of progesterone in an extraadrenal source.[123] The fetoplacental unit probably contributes to the circulating maternal DOC levels because concentrations of DOC have been shown to be elevated in mixed cord blood.[131]

8.2.5 RAAS in the Postpartum Period

In the postpartum period, the levels of all the component of the RAAS decrease rapidly within 3 days[128] and return to nonpregnant values 6 weeks later.[117]

8.2.6 RAAS in Pregnancy-Associated Hypertension

RAAS modifications are observed during pregnancy-associated hypertension or preeclampsia. The level of plasma renin, ANG-I, ANG-II, and aldosterone are reduced compared to healthy pregnant patients.[117,126,128] The reduced ANG-II levels are not explained by diminished activity of ACE in preeclampsia compared to normal pregnancy.[111] Reduced RAAS might explain the reduced circulating volume that is found in preeclampsia.[128] However, in gestational hypertension, the sensitivity to ANG-II on the adrenal glands or vessels is increased through AT1R heterodimers.[111,126] Based on animal studies, the implication of autoantibodies directed against the AT1R is also suggested in the pathophysiology of preeclampsia.[126] Preeclampsia is a state of dysregulated RAAS, but the triggering factors that lead to these modifications remain to be defined.[111]

8.3 ADRENAL SEX STEROIDS DURING PREGNANCY

Total testosterone levels increase progressively from the first trimester to term.[132–134] In the normal state, testosterone mostly circulates in plasma bound to proteins; 38% is bound to albumin and 60% is bound to sex hormone-binding globulin (SHBG).[135] During the third trimester of pregnancy, testosterone is bound 95.4% with SHBG, 0.82% with CBG, and 3.55% with albumin.[136] Only free testosterone, a small fraction of the total testosterone, can cross the placenta membrane and interact with the androgen receptor.[133] The increase in total testosterone can be partially explained by an early increase in estrogen-induced SHBG synthesis by the liver.[133] SHBG increases through all pregnancy, reaching its peak, which is almost six times the nonpregnant value, in the third trimester.[132,133,135,136] Also, the binding capacity of SHBG increases in pregnancy.[135] Free testosterone and bioavailable testosterone also increase significantly throughout pregnancy, but levels of bioavailable testosterone stay in the normal nonpregnant range in most (but not all) pregnant women.[133,136] Androstenedione levels are more variable between studies.[132] Some reported a significant increase during the end of the third trimester compared to nonpregnant women,[133] while others reported an early significant increase in the first trimester without further changes during pregnancy,[137] and some have reported a nonsignificant increase in the third trimester.[135,136] Androstenedione concentrations during pregnancy display a high interindividual variation,[134,135] which may explain the differences between the studies. DHEAS decreases by 50% compared to nonpregnant levels during the first half of pregnancy and remains stable thereafter.[133,135,137] DHEAS metabolic clearance rate increases by fivefold starting at midpregnancy, probably because it is a substrate for the increasing placental estradiol synthesis throughout pregnancy.[133] However, even if the maternal level of DHEAS are lower in the second half of pregnancy than nonpregnant patients, it was demonstrated that the production rate of DHEAS by the maternal adrenal glands almost doubled during pregnancy.[3,133] Therefore, higher metabolic clearance rather than decreased production explains the decreased level of DHEAS during pregnancy. Androgens are probably implicated in parturition.[133] In vivo and in vitro studies have demonstrated that androgens promote cervical remodeling, and they also have an inhibitory action on myometrial contraction.[133]

It is suggested that the ovaries are the major contributors to the circulating level of testosterone and androstenedione in pregnancy, given that the level of these androgens during pregnancy are lower in women with premature ovarian failure and assisted-reproduction pregnancy compared to normal pregnant women.[133] In contrast, DHEAS is produced only by the maternal adrenal glands, similar to nonpregnant women.[133] In animal models, fetectomy, which removes the fetal precursor (DHEAS) of the placental estradiol synthesis without modifying the metabolic clearance rate of DHEAS, have resulted in an increase in maternal DHEAS plasma levels, and the administration of estradiol in these animals decreases the maternal DHEAS levels. This suggests that the placental production of estradiol probably downregulates the adrenal production of androgens by the mother.[133] The placenta also has the capacity to produce androgens de novo; syncitiotrophoblasts express the enzyme CYP17, which converts C21 steroids to C19 steroids such as testosterone. The activity of this latter enzyme was confirmed in vitro.[133]

The fetus is protected against the virilizing effects of maternal androgens in pregnancy by the physiological increase in SHBG, which binds and inactivates androgens; the elevation of the progesterone levels, which compete for the androgen receptor binding and inhibits the 5α-reductase conversion of testosterone to its more potent dihydrotestosterone; and by the presence of aromatase complex in the placenta, which converts testosterone and androstenedione to estradiol or estrone.[133]

The importance of the placenta aromatase in these protective mechanisms against maternal androgen has been confirmed by the finding that aromatase deficiency in the placenta results in virilized fetuses.[133]

In the postpartum period, the total testosterone decreases, but the time for normalization is unknown.[132,136] Bioavailable testosterone levels were normalized 4 days postpartum.[136] SHBG decreases progressively in the postpartum period to levels that are 25% lower by the fourth day postpartum compared to level at the end of the third trimester.[136] Androstenedione also decreases in the postpartum period compared to values in the third trimester.[136,138] DHEAS increases to values similar to nonpregnant women 1 month postpartum.[139]

8.4 CATECHOLAMINE PHYSIOLOGY DURING PREGNANCY

Secretion of catecholamines is not increased during pregnancy, as demonstrated by plasma and urinary catecholamine levels, which are not increased at all, or only slightly, during pregnancy.[140] Even in the context of hypertension or pre-eclampsia, plasma catecholamines are only slightly elevated [140] or not at all,[141] and urinary catecholamines are normal.[142] Maternal catecholamines do not cross the placental barrier easily. Even in the context of high circulating concentrations of catecholamines in the maternal plasma such as a pheochromocytoma, the umbilical cord blood contains <10% of the maternal concentration.[143] The placental cells have noradrenaline transporters that enable intracellular uptake of catecholamines, and they also contain catecholamine-metabolizing enzymes such as monoamine oxidase (MAO) and catechol-*O*-methyltransferase (COMT), which inactivate catecholamines.[144] However, excess catecholamines during pregnancy, as in patients with pheochromocytoma, might induce vasoconstriction in the placental vascular bed and may be responsible for placental abruption and intrauterine hypoxia.[140]

REFERENCES

1. Arlt W, Stewart PM. Adrenal corticosteroid biosynthesis, metabolism, and action. *Endocrinol Metab Clin N Am* 2005;**34**(2):293–313.
2. Lekarev O, New MI. Adrenal disease in pregnancy. *Best Pract Res Clin Endocrinol Metab* 2011;**25**(6):959–73.
3. Monticone S, Auchus RJ, Rainey WE. Adrenal disorders in pregnancy. *Nat Rev Endocrinol* 2012;**8**(11):668–78.
4. Thomson M. The physiological roles of placental corticotropin releasing hormone in pregnancy and childbirth. *J Physiol Biochem* 2013;**69**(3):559–73.
5. Mastorakos G, Ilias I. Maternal and fetal hypothalamic-pituitary-adrenal axes during pregnancy and postpartum. *Ann N Y Acad Sci* 2003;**997**:136–49.
6. Lindsay JR, Nieman LK. The hypothalamic-pituitary-adrenal axis in pregnancy: challenges in disease detection and treatment. *Endocr Rev* 2005;**26**(6):775–99.
7. Goland RS, Wardlaw SL, Stark RI, Brown Jr LS, Frantz AG. High levels of corticotropin releasing hormone immunoreactivity in maternal and fetal plasma during pregnancy. *J Clin Endocrinol Metab* 1986;**63**:1199–203.
8. Laatikainen T, Virtanen T, Räisänen I, Salminen K. Immunoreactive corticotropin-releasing factor and corticotropin during pregnancy, labor and puerperium. *Neuropeptides* 1987;**10**:343–53.
9. Goland RS, Wardlaw SL, Blum M, Tropper PJ, Stark RI. Biologically active corticotropin-releasing hormone in maternal and fetal plasma during pregnancy. *Am J Obstet Gynecol* 1988;**159**(4):884–90.
10. Campbell EA, Linton EA, Wolfe CD, Scraggs PR, Jones MT, Lowry PJ. Plasma corticotropin-releasing hormone concentrations during pregnancy and parturition. *J Clin Endocrinol Metab* 1987;**64**:1054–9.
11. Goland RS, Jozak S, Conwell I. Placental corticotropin-releasing hormone and the hypercortisolism of pregnancy. *Am J Obstet Gynecol* 1994;**171**(5):1287–91.
12. Nezi M, Mastorakos G, and Mouslech Z. n.d. Corticotropin releasing hormone and the immune/inflammatory response. [Endotext [Internet]], 2018.
13. Sasaki A, Tempst P, Liotta AS, Margioris AN, Hood LE, Kent SB, et al. Isolation and characterization of a corticotropin-releasing hormone-like peptide from human placenta. *J Clin Endocrinol Metab* 1988;**67**(4):768–73.
14. Sehringer B, Zahradnik HP, Simon M, Ziegler R, Noethling C, Schaefer WR. mRNA expression profiles for corticotrophin-releasing hormone, urocortin, CRH-binding protein and CRH receptors in human term gestational tissues determined by real-time quantitative RT-PCR. *J Mol Endocrinol* 2004;**32**(2):339–48.
15. Frim DM, Robinson BG, Smas CM, Division E, Hospital W. Characterization and gestational regulation of corticotropin-releasing hormone messenger RNA in human placenta. *J Clin Invest* 1988;**82**(July):287–92.
16. Thomson M, Chan EC, Falconer J, Madsen G, Smith R. Secretion of corticotropin-releasing hormone by superfused human placental fragments. *Gynecol Endocrinol* 1988;**2**:87–100.
17. Schulte HM, Healy DL. Corticotropin releasing hormone- and adreno-corticotropin-like immunoreactivity in human placenta, peripheral and uterine vein plasma. *Horm Metab Res Suppl* 1987;**16**:44–6.
18. Petraglia F, Sawchenko PE, Rivier J, Vale W. Evidence for local stimulation of ACTH secretion by corticotropin-releasing factor in human placenta. *Nature* 1987;**328**:717–9.
19. Linton EA, Wolfe CD, Behan DP, Lowry PJ. A specific carrier substance for human corticotrophin releasing factor in late gestational maternal plasma which could mask the ACTH-releasing activity. *Clin Endocrinol* 1988;**28**:315–24.

20. Orth DN, Mount CD. Specific high-affinity binding protein for human corticotropin-releasing hormone in normal human plasma. *Biochem Biophys Res Commun* 1987;**143**(2):411–7.

21. Linton EA, Perkins AV, Woods RJ, Eben F, Wolfe CD, Behan DP, et al. Corticotropin releasing hormone-binding protein (CRH-BP): plasma levels decrease during the third trimester of normal human pregnancy. *J Clin Endocrinol Metab* 1993;**76**(1):260–2.

22. Linton EA, Behan DP, Saphier PW, Lowry PJ. Corticotropin-releasing hormone (CRH)-binding protein: reduction in the adrenocorticotropin-releasing activity of placental but not hypothalamic CRH. *J Clin Endocrinol Metab* 1990;**70**(6):1574–80.

23. Tizabi Y, Aguilera G. Desensitization of the hypothalamic-pituitary-adrenal axis following prolonged administration of corticotropin-releasing hormone or vasopressin. *Neuroendocrinology* 1992;**56**(5):611–8.

24. Thomson M, Chan EC, Falconer J, Madsen G, Geraghty S, Curryer N, et al. Desensitization of superfused isolated ovine anterior pituitary cells to human corticotropin-releasing factor. *J Neuroendocrinol* 1990;**2**:181–7.

25. Karalis K, Goodwin G, Majzoub JA. Cortisol blockade of progesterone: a possible molecular mechanism involved in the initiation of human labour. *Nat Med* 1996;**2**:556–60.

26. Smith R. Parturition. *N Engl J Med* 2007;**356**(3):271–83.

27. Petraglia F, Sutton S, Vale W. Neurotransmitters and peptides modulate the release of immunoreactive corticotropin-releasing factor from cultured human placental cells. *Am J Obstet Gynecol* 1989;**160**(1):247–51.

28. Ochędalski T, Zylinńska K, Laudański T, Lachowicz A. Corticotrophin-releasing hormone and ACTH levels in maternal and fetal blood during spontaneous and oxytocin-induced labour. *Eur J Endocrinol* 2001;**144**(2):117–21.

29. Gao L, Lv C, Xu C, Li Y, Cui X, Gu H, Ni X. Differential regulation of glucose transporters mediated by CRH receptor type 1 and type 2 in human placental trophoblasts. *Endocrinology* 2012;**153**(3):1464–71.

30. Karteris E, Markovic D, Chen J, Hillhouse EW, Grammatopoulos DK. Identification of a novel corticotropin-releasing hormone type 1β-like receptor variant lacking exon 13 in human pregnant myometrium regulated by estradiol-17β and progesterone. *Endocrinology* 2010;**151**(10):4959–68.

31. Vitale SG, Laganà AS, Rapisarda AMC, Scarale MG, Corrado F, Cignini P, et al. Role of urocortin in pregnancy: an update and future perspectives. *World J Clin Cases* 2016;**4**(7):165.

32. Voltolini C, Battersby S, Novembri R, Torricelli M, Severi FM, Petraglia F, et al. Urocortin 2 role in placental and myometrial inflammatory mechanisms at parturition. *Endocrinology* 2015;**156**(2):670–9.

33. Glynn LM, Schetter CD, Chicz-DeMet A, Hobel CJ, Sandman CA. Ethnic differences in adrenocorticotropic hormone, cortisol and corticotropin-releasing hormone during pregnancy. *Peptides* 2007;**28**(6):1155–61.

34. De Bonis M, Torricelli M, Severi FM, Luisi S, De Leo V, Petraglia F. Neuroendocrine aspects of placenta and pregnancy. *Gynecol Endocrinol* 2012;**28**(Suppl 1):22–6.

35. Davis ME, Pemberton CJ, Yandle TG, Lainchbury JG, Rademaker MT, Nicholls MG, et al. Urocortin-1 infusion in normal humans. *J Clin Endocrinol Metab* 2004;**89**(3):1402–9.

36. Gao L, Lu C, Xu C, Tao Y, Cong B, Ni X. Differential regulation of prostaglandin production mediated by corticotropin-releasing hormone receptor type 1 and type 2 in cultured human placental trophoblasts. *Endocrinology* 2008;**149**(6):2866–76.

37. Imperatore A, Florio P, Torres PB, Torricelli M, Galleri L, Toti P, et al. Urocortin 2 and urocortin 3 are expressed by the human placenta, deciduas, and fetal membranes. *Am J Obstet Gynecol* 2006;**195**(1):288–95.

38. Nemoto T, Iwasaki-Sekino A, Yamauchi N, Shibasaki T. Regulation of the expression and secretion of urocortin 2 in rat pituitary. *J Endocrinol* 2007;**192**(2):443–52.

39. Räisänen I. Plasma levels and diurnal variation of beta-endorphin, beta-lipotropin and corticotropin during pregnancy and early puerperium. *Eur J Obstet Gynecol Reprod Biol* 1988;**27**(1):13–20.

40. Petraglia F, Facchinetti F, Parrini D, Micieli G, De Luca S, Genazzani AR. Simultaneous circadian variations of plasma ACTH, beta-lipotropin, beta-endorphin and cortisol. *Horm Res* 1983;**17**(3):147–52.

41. Clark BJ. ACTH action on StAR biology. *Front Neurosci* 2016;**10**(December):1–7.

42. Klimek M. Comparative analysis of ACTH and oxytocinase plasma concentration during pregnancy. *Neuro Endocrinol Lett* 2005;**26**(4):337–41.

43. Rees LH, Burke CW, Chard T, Evans W, Letchworth A. Possible placental origin of ACTH in normal human pregnancy. *Nature* 1975;**254**(5501):620–2.

44. Okamoto E, Takagi T, Makino T, Sata H, Iwata I, Nishino E, et al. Immunoreactive corticotropin-releasing hormone, adrenocorticotropin and cortisol in human plasma during pregnancy and delivery and postpartum. *Horm Metab Res* 1989;**21**:566–72.

45. Carr BR, Parker Jr. CR, Madden JD, MacDonald PC, Porter JC. Maternal plasma adrenocorticotropin and cortisol relationships throughout human pregnancy. *Am J Obstet Gynecol* 1981;**139**:416–22.

46. Genazzani AR, Petraglia F, Parrini D, Nasi A, Angioni G, Facchinetti F, et al. Lack of correlation between amniotic fluid and maternal plasma contents of B-endorphin, B-lipotropin, and adrenocorticotropic hormone in normal and pathologic pregnancies. *Am J Obstet Gynecol* 1984;**148**:198–203.

47. Mukherjee K, Swyer GI. Plasma cortisol and adrenocorticotrophic hormone in normal men and non-pregnant women, normal pregnant women and women with pre-eclampsia. *J Obstet Gynaecol Br Commonw* 1972;**79**(6):504–12.

48. Odagiri EMI, Sherrell BJ, Mount CD, Nicholson WE, Orth DN. Human placental immunoreactive corticotropin, lipotropin, and B-endorphin: evidence for a common precursor. *Proc Natl Acad Sci USA* 1979;**76**(4):2027–31.

49. Ng ML, Healy DL, Rajna A, Fullerton M, O'Grady C, Funder JW. Presence of pro-opiomelanocortin peptides and corticotropin-releasing factor in human placenta. *Malays J Pathol* 1996;**18**(1):59–63.

50. Waddell BJ, Burton P. Release of bioactive ACTH by perifused human placenta at early and late gestation. *J Endocrinol* 1993;**136**(2):345–53.

51. Mihrshahi R, Lewis JG, Ali SO. Hormonal effects on the secretion and glycoform profile of corticosteroid-binding globulin. *J Steroid Biochem Mol Biol* 2006;**101**(4–5):275–85.

52. Khan MS, Adent D, Rosner W. Humancorticosteroid binding globulin is secreted by a hepatoma-derived cell line. *J Steroid Biochem* 1984; **20**(2):677–8.

53. Hammond G, Smith C, Goping I, Underhill D, Harley M, Reventos J, et al. Primary structure of human corticosteroid binding globulin, deduced from hepatic and pulmonary cDNAs, exhibits homology with serine protease inhibitors. *Proc Natl Acad Sci U S A* 1987;**84**(15):5153–7.

54. Misao R, Iwagaki S, Sun WS, Fujimoto J, Saio M, Takami T, et al. Evidence for the synthesis of corticosteroid-binding globulin in human placenta. *Horm Res* 1999;**51**(4):162–7.

55. Miska W, Peña P, Villegas J, Sanchez R. Detection of a CBG-like protein in human Fallopian tube tissue. *Andrologia* 2004;**36**(1):41–6.

56. Misao R, Hori M, Ichigo S, Fujimoto J, Tamaya T. Corticosteroid-binding globulin mRNA levels in human uterine endometrium. *Steroids* 1994; **59**(10):603–7.

57. Misao R, Nakanishi Y, Fujimoto J, Iwagaki S, Tamaya T. Levels of sex hormone-binding globulin and corticosteroid-binding globulin mRNAs in corpus luteum of human subjects: correlation with serum steroid hormone levels. *Gynecol Endocrinol* 1999;**13**(2):82–8.

58. Nenke MA, Zeng A, Meyer EJ, Lewis JG, Rankin W, Johnston J, et al. Differential effects of estrogen on corticosteroid-binding globulin forms suggests reduced cleavage in pregnancy. *J Endocr Soc* 2017;**1**:202–10 (March 2017).

59. Rosenthal HE, Slaunwhite Jr WR, Sandberg AA. Transcortin: a corticosteroid-binding protein of plasma. X. Cortisol and progesterone interplay and unbound levels of these steroids in pregnancy. *J Clin Endocrinol Metab* 1969;**29**:352–67.

60. Jung C, Ho JT, Torpy DJ, Rogers A, Doogue M, Lewis JG, et al. A longitudinal study of plasma and urinary cortisol in pregnancy and postpartum. *J Clin Endocrinol Metab* 2011;**96**(5):1533–40.

60a. Chico A, Manzanares JM, Halperin I, Martinez de Osaba MJ, Adelantado J, Webb SM. Cushing's disease and pregnancy: Report of six cases. *Eur J Obstet Gynecol Reprod Biol* 1996;**64**:143–6.

61. Scott EM, McGarrigle HH, Lachelin G. The increase in plasma and saliva cortisol levels in pregnancy is not due to the increase in corticosteroid-binding globulin levels. *J Clin Endocrinol Metab* 1990;**71**:639–44.

62. Potter JM, Mueller UW, Hickman PE. Corticosteroid binding globulin in normotensive and hypertensive human pregnancy. *Clin Sci* 1987;**72**:725–35.

63. Demey-Ponsart E, Foidart JM, Sulon J, Sodoyez JC. Serum CBG, free and total cortisol and circadian patterns of adrenal function in normal pregnancy. *J Steroid Biochem* 1982;**16**:165–9.

64. Benassayag C, Souski I, Mignot T-M, Robert B, Hassid J, Duc-Goiran P, et al. Corticosteroid-binding globulin status at the fetomaternal interface during human term pregnancy1. *Biol Reprod* 2001;**64**(3):812–21.

65. Mitchell E, Torpy DJ, Bagley CJ. Pregnancy-associated corticosteroid-binding globulin: high resolution separation of glycan isoforms. *Horm Metab Res* 2004;**36**(6):357–9.

66. Strel'chyonok OA, Avvakumov GV. Specific steroid-binding glycoproteins of human blood plasma: novel data on their structure and function. *J steroid Biochem* 1990;**35**(5):519–34.

67. Murphy BEP. Human fetal serum cortisol levels related to gestational age: evidence of a midgestational fall and a steep late gestational rise independent of sex or mode of delivery. *Am J Obstet Gynecol* 1982;**144**:276–82.

68. Sandberg AA, Slaunwhite R, Carter AC. Transcortin: a corticosteroid-binding protein of plasma. III. The effects of various steroids. *J Clin Invest* 1960;**39**:1914–26.

69. Magiakou MA, Mastorakos G, Rabin D, Margioris AN, Dubbert B, Calogero AE, et al. The maternal hypothalamic-pituitary-adrenal axis in the third trimester of human pregnancy. *Clin Endocrinol* 1996;**44**(4):419–28.

70. Phocas I, Sarandakou A, Rizos D. Maternal serum total cortisol levels in normal and pathologic pregnancies. *Int J Gynaecol Obstet* 1990;**31**(1):3–8.

71. Abou-Samra AB, Pugeat M, Dechaud H, Nachury L, Bouchareb B, Fevre-Montange M, et al. Increased plasma concentration of N-terminal beta-lipotrophin and unbound cortisol during pregnancy. *Clin Endocrinol* 1984;**20**(2):221–8.

72. Abrao ALP, Leal SC, Falcao DP. Salivary and serum cortisol levels, salivary alpha-amylase and unstimulated whole saliva flow rate in pregnant and non-pregnant. *Rev Bras Ginecol Obstet* 2014;**36**(2):72–8.

73. Ambroziak U, Kondracka A, Bartoszewicz Z, Krasnodębska-Kiljańska M, Bednarczuk T. The morning and late-night salivary cortisol ranges for healthy women may be used in pregnancy. *Clin Endocrinol* 2015;**83**(6):774–8.

74. Meulenberg P, Hofman J. The effect of oral contraceptive use and pregnancy on the daily rhythm of cortisol and cortisone. *Clin Chim Acta* 1990; **190**(3):211–21.

75. Suri D, Moran J, Hibbard JU, Kasza K, Weiss RE. Assessment of adrenal reserve in pregnancy: defining the normal response to the adrenocorticotropin stimulation test. *J Clin Endocrinol Metab* 2006;**91**(10):3866–72.

76. Manetti L, Rossi G, Grasso L, Raffaelli V, Scattina I, Del Sarto S, et al. Usefulness of salivary cortisol in the diagnosis of hypercortisolism: comparison with serum and urinary cortisol. *Eur J Endocrinol* 2013;**168**(3):315–21.

77. Lopes LML, Francisco RPV, Galletta MAK, Bronstein MD. Determination of nighttime salivary cortisol during pregnancy: comparison with values in non-pregnancy and Cushing's disease. *Pituitary* 2016;**19**(1):30–8.

78. Mizutani S, Sakura H, Akiyama H, Kobayashi H. Simultaneous determinations of total cortisol and progesterone during late pregnancy by radioimmunoassay. *Radioisotopes* 1982;**31**:185–9.

79. Odagiri E, Ishiwatari N, Abe Y, Jibiki K, Adachi T, Demura R, et al. Hypercortisolism and the resistance to dexamethasone suppression during gestation. *Endocrinol Jpn* 1988;**35**(5):685–90.

80. Dorr HG, Heller A, Versmold HT, Sippell WG, Hermann M, Bidlingmaier F, et al. Longitudinal study of progestins, mineralocorticoids, and glucocorticoids throughout human pregnancy. *J Clin Endocrinol Metab* 1989;**68**:863–8.

81. Ho JT, Lewis JG, O'Loughlin P, Bagley CJ, Romero R, Dekker GA, et al. Reduced maternal corticosteroid-binding globulin and cortisol levels in pre-eclampsia and gamete recipient pregnancies. *Clin Endocrinol* 2007;**66**(6):869–77.

82. Cousins L, Rigg L, Hollingsworth D, Meis P, Halberg F, Brink G, et al. Qualitative and quantitative assessment of the circadian rhythm of cortisol in pregnancy. *Am J Obstet Gynecol* 1983;**145**:411–6.

83. Mikkelsen AL, Felding C, Hasselbalch H. Urinary free cortisol during pregnancy. *Acta Obstet Gynecol Scand* 1984;**63**:253–6.

84. Meulenberg PM, Hofman J. Differences between concentrations of salivary cortisol and cortisone and of free cortisol and cortisone in plasma during pregnancy and postpartum. *Clin Chem* 1990;**36136**(1):70–5.

85. Allolio B, Hoffman J, Winkelmann W, Kusche M, Schulte HM. Diurnal salivary cortisol patterns during pregnancy and after delivery. *Clin Endocrinol* 1990;**33**:279–89.

86. Burke CW, Roulet F. Increased exposure of tissues to cortisol in late pregnancy. *Br Med J* 1970;**1**(5697):657–9.

87. Nolten WE, Lindheimer MD, Rueckert PA, Oparil S, Ehrlich EN. Diurnal patterns and regulation of cortisol secretion in pregnancy. *J Clin Endocrinol Metab* 1980;**51**:466–72.

88. Nolten WE, Rueckert P. Elevated free cortisol index in pregnancy: possible regulatory mechanisms. *Am J Obstet Gynecol* 1981;**139**:492–8.

89. Goland RS, Wardlaw SL, MacCarter G, Warren WB, Stark RI. Adrenocorticotropin and cortisol responses to vasopressin during pregnancy. *J Clin Endocrinol Metab* 1991;**73**:257–61.

90. Pijnenburg-Kleizen KJ, Engels M, Mooij CF, Griffin A, Krone N, Span PN, et al. Adrenal steroid metabolites accumulating in congenital adrenal hyperplasia lead to transactivation of the glucocorticoid receptor. *Endocrinology* 2015;**156**(10):3504–10.

91. Moore NL, Hickey TE, Butler LM, Tilley WD. Multiple nuclear receptor signaling pathways mediate the actions of synthetic progestins in target cells. *Mol Cell Endocrinol* 2012;**357**(1–2):60–70 [Internet].

92. Rousseau GG, Baxter JD, Tomkins GM. Glucocorticoid receptors: relations between steroid binding and biological effects. *J Mol Biol* 1972;**67**(1):99–115.

93. Rupprecht R, Reul JM, van Steensel B, Spengler D, Söder M, Berning B, et al. Pharmacological and functional characterization of human miner-alocorticoid and glucocorticoid receptor ligands. *Eur J Pharmacol* 1993;**247**(2):145–54 [Internet].

94. Johnstone FD, Campbell S. Adrenal response in pregnancy to long-acting tetracosactrin. *J Obs Gynaecol Br Commonw* 1974;**81**(5):363–7.

95. Brown MA, Thou STP, Whitworth JA. Stimulation of aldosterone by ACTH in normal and hypertensive pregnancy. *Am J Hypertens* 1995;**8**:260–7.

96. McKenna DS, Wittber GM, Nagaraja HN, Samuels P. The effects of repeat doses of antenatal corticosteroids on maternal adrenal function. *Am J Obstet Gynecol* 2000;**183**(3):669–73.

97. Yang Q, Wang W, Liu C, Wang Y, Sun K. Compartmentalized localization of 11β-HSD 1 and 2 at the feto-maternal interface in the first trimester of human pregnancy. *Placenta* 2016;**46**:63–71.

98. Gennari-Moser C, Khankin EV, Schüller S, Escher G, Frey BM, Portmann CB, et al. Regulation of placental growth by aldosterone and cortisol. *Endocrinology* 2011;**152**(1):263–71.

99. Drake AJ, Tang JI, Nyirenda MJ. Mechanisms underlying the role of glucocorticoids in the early life programming of adult disease. *Clin Sci* 2007;**113**(5):219–32.

100. Benediktsson R, Calder AA, Edwards CRW, Seckl JR. Placental 11β-hydroxysteroid dehydrogenase: a key regulator of fetal glucocorticoid exposure. *Clin Endocrinol* 1997;**46**(2):161–6.

101. Salvante KG, Milano K, Kliman HJ, Nepomnaschy PA. Placental 11 β-hydroxysteroid dehydrogenase type 2 (11β-HSD2) expression very early during human pregnancy. *J Dev Orig Health Dis* 2017;**8**(2):149–54.

102. McTernan CL, Draper N, Nicholson H, Chalder SM, Driver P, Hewison M, et al. Reduced placental 11β-hydroxysteroid dehydrogenase type 2 mRNA levels in human pregnancies complicated by intrauterine growth restriction: an analysis of possible mechanisms. *J Clin Endocrinol Metab* 2001;**86**(10):4979–83.

103. Fahlbusch FB, Ruebner M, Volkert G, Offergeld R, Hartner A, Menendez-Castro C, et al. Corticotropin-releasing hormone stimulates expression of leptin, 11beta-HSD2 and syncytin-1 in primary human trophoblasts. *Reprod Biol Endocrinol* 2012;**10**:1–9.

104. Beitins IZ, Bayard F, Ances IG, Kowarski A, Migeon CJ. The metabolic clearance rate, blood production, interconversion and transplacental passage of cortisol and cortisone in pregnancy near term. *Pediatr Res* 1973;**7**(5):509–19.

105. Ochedalski T, Lachowicz A. Maternal and fetal hypothalamo-pituitary-adrenal axis: different response depends upon the mode of parturition. *Neuro Endocrinol Lett* 2004;**25**(4):278–82.

106. Willcox DL, Yovich JL, McColm SC, Phillips J. Progesterone, cortisol and oestradiol-17β in the initiation of human parturition: sartitioning between free and bound hormone in plasma. *Br J Obstet Gynaecol* 1985;**92**(1):65–71.

107. Talbert LM, Pearlman WH, Potter H. Maternal and fetal serum levels of total cortisol and cortisone, unbound cortisol, and corticosteroid-binding globulin in vaginal delivery and cesarean section. *Am J Obstet Gynecol* 1977;**129**(7):781–7.

108. Smith R, Owens PC, Brinsmead MW, Singh B, Hall C. The nonsuppressibility of plasma cortisol persists after pregnancy. *Horm Metab Res* 1987;**19**(1):41–2.

109. Owens PC, Smith R, Brinsmead MW, Hall C, Rowley M, Hurt D, et al. Postnatal disappearance of the pregnancy-associated reduced sensitivity of plasma cortisol to feedback inhibition. *Life Sci* 1987;**41**:1745–50.

110. West CA, Sasser JM, Baylis C. The enigma of continual plasma volume expansion in pregnancy: critical role of the renin-angiotensin-aldosterone system. *Am J Physiol Ren Physiol* 2016;**311**(6):F1125–34.

111. Irani RA, Xia Y. Renin angiotensin signaling in normal pregnancy and preeclampsia. *Semin Nephrol* 2011;**31**(1):47–58.

112. Zhuo J, Moeller I, Jenkins T, Chai SY, Allen AM, Ohishi M, et al. Mapping tissue angiotensin-converting enzyme and angiotensin AT1, AT2 and AT4 receptors. *J Hypertens* 1998;**16**(12 SUPPL):2027–37.

113. Wilson M, Morganti AA, Laragh JH. Blood pressure, the renin-aldosterone system and sex steroids throughout normal pregnancy. *Am J Med* 1980;**68**(January):97–104.

114. Kamoun M, Mnif MF, Charfi N, Kacem FH, Naceur BB, Mnif F, et al. Adrenal diseases during pregnancy: pathophysiology, diagnosis and management strategies. *Am J Med Sci* 2014;**347**(1):64–73.

115. Ehrlich EN, Lindheimer MD. Effect of administered mineralocorticoids or ACTH in pregnant women. Attenuation of kaliuretic influence of mineralocorticoids during pregnancy. *J Clin Invest* 1972;**51**(6):1301–9.

116. Landau E, Amar L. Primary aldosteronism and pregnancy. *Ann Endocrinol (Paris)* 2016;**77**(2):148–60.

117. Langer B, Grima M, Coquard C, Bader AM, Schlaeder G, Imbs JL. Plasma active renin, angiotensin I, and angiotensin II during pregnancy and in preeclampsia. *Obstet Gynecol* 1998;**91**(2):196–202.

118. Nielsen LH, Ovesen P, Hansen MR, Brantlov S, Jespersen B, Bie P, et al. Changes in the renin-angiotensin-aldosterone system in response to dietary salt intake in normal and hypertensive pregnancy. A randomized trial. *J Am Soc Hypertens* 2016;**10**(11):881–890.e4.

119. Nielsen AH, Schauser KH, Poulsen K. The uteroplacental renin—angiotensin system. *Placenta* 2000;**21**(21):468–77.

120. Oparil S, Ehrlich EN, Lindheimer MD. Effect of progesterone on renal sodium handling in man: relation to aldosterone excretion and plasma renin activity. *Clin Sci Mol Med* 1975;**49**(2):139–47.

121. Lumbers ER, Pringle KG. Roles of the circulating renin-angiotensin-aldosterone system in human pregnancy. *AJP Regul Integr Comp Physiol* 2014;**306**(2):R91–101.

122. Martini AG, Krop M, Saleh L, Garrelds IM, Jan Danser AH. Do prorenin-synthesizing cells release active, open prorenin? *J Hypertens* 2017;**35**(2):330–7.

123. Eschler DC, Kogekar N, Pessah-Pollack R. Management of adrenal tumors in pregnancy. *Endocrinol Metab Clin N Am* 2015;**44**(2):381–97.

124. Klett C, Ganten D, Hellmann W, Kaling M, Ryffel GU, Weimar-Ehl T, et al. Regulation of hepatic angiotensinogen synthesis and secretion by steroid hormones. *Endocrinology* 1992;**130**(6):3660–8.

125. Morgan L, Crawshaw S, Baker PN, Broughton Pipkin F, Kalsheker N. Polymorphism in oestrogen response element associated with variation in plasma angiotensinogen concentrations in healthy pregnant women. *J Hypertens* 2000;**18**(5):553–7.

126. Riester A, Reincke M. Mineralocorticoid receptor antagonists and management of primary aldosteronism in pregnancy. *Eur J Endocrinol* 2015;**172**(1):R23–30.

127. Bentley-Lewis R, Graves SW, Seely E. The renin-aldosterone response to stimulation and suppression during normal pregnancy. *Hypertens Pregnancy* 2005;**24**(1):1–18.

128. Koyama T, Yamada T, Furuta I, Morikawa M, Yamada T, Minakami H. Plasma aldosterone concentration and plasma renin activity decrease during the third trimester in women with twin pregnancies. *Hypertens Pregnancy* 2012;**31**(4):419–26.

129. Mirshahi M, Ayani E, Nicolas C, Golestaneh N, Ferrari P, Valamanesh F, et al. The blockade of mineralocorticoid hormone signaling provokes dramatic teratogenesis in cultured rat embryos. *Int J Toxicol* 2002;**21**:191–9.

130. Weinberger MH, Kramer NJ, Grim CE, Petersen L. The effect of posture and saline loading on plasma renin activity and aldosterone concentration in pregnant, non-pregnant and estrogen-treated women. *J Clin Endocrinol Metab* 1977;**44**(1):69–77.

131. Brown RD, Strott CA, Liddle GW. Plasma deoxycorticosterone in normal and abnormal pregnancy. *J Clin Endocrinol Metab* 1972;**35**(5):736–42.

132. Kuijper EAM, Ket JCF, Caanen MR, Lambalk CB. Reproductive hormone concentrations in pregnancy and neonates: a systematic review. *Reprod BioMed Online* 2013;**27**(1):33–63.

133. Makieva S, Saunders PTK, Norman JE. Androgens in pregnancy: roles in parturition. *Hum Reprod Update* 2014;**20**(4):542–59.

134. Villarroel C, Salinas A, López P, Kohen P, Rencoret G, Devoto L, et al. Pregestational type 2 diabetes and gestational diabetes exhibit different sexual steroid profiles during pregnancy. *Gynecol Endocrinol* 2017;**33**(3):212–7.

135. Leary PO, Boyne P, Flett P, Beilby J, James I. Longitudinal assessment of changes in reproductive hormones during normal pregnancy. *Clin Chem* 1991;**37**(5):667–72.

136. Kerlan V, Nahoul K, Le Martelot MT, Bercovici JP. Longitudinal study of maternal plasma bioavailable testosterone and androstanediol glucuronide levels during pregnancy. *Clin Endocrinol* 1994;**40**(2):263–7.

137. Soldin OP, Guo T, Weiderpass E, Tractenberg RE, Hilakivi-Clarke L, Soldin SJ. Steroid hormone levels in pregnancy and 1 year postpartum using isotope dilution tandem mass spectrometry. *Fertil Steril* 2005;**84**(3):701–10.

138. Serin IS, Kula M, Basbug M, Ünllühizarci K, Güçer S, Tayyar M. Androgen levels of preeclamptic patients in the third trimester of pregnancy and six weeks after delivery. *Acta Obstet Gynecol Scand* 2001;**80**(11):1009–13.

139. Tagawa N, Hidaka Y, Takano T, Shimaoka Y, Kobayashi Y, Amino N. Serum concentrations of dehydroepiandrosterone and dehydroepiandrosterone sulfate and their relation to cytokine production during and after normal pregnancy. *Clin Chim Acta* 2004;**340**(1–2):187–93.

140. Lenders J. Pheochromocytoma and pregnancy: a deceptive connection. *Eur J Endocrinol* 2012;**166**(2):143–50.

141. Pedersen EB, Christensen NJ, Christensen P, Johannesen P, Kornerup HJ, Kristensen S, et al. Preeclampsia – a state of prostaglandin deficiency? Urinary prostaglandin excretion, the renin-aldosterone system, and circulating catecholamines in preeclampsia. *Hypertension* 1983;**5**(1):105–11.

142. Pedersen EB, Christensen NJ, Christensen P, Johannesen P, Kornerup HJ, Kristensen S, et al. Prostaglandins, renin, aldosterone, and catecholamines in preeclampsia. *Acta Medica Scand Suppl* 1983;**677**:40–3.

143. Dahia PL, Hayashida CY, Strunz C, Abelin N, Toledo SP. Low cord blood levels of catecholamine from a newborn of a pheochromocytoma patient. *Eur J Endocrinol* 1994;**130**(3):217–9.

144. Saarikoski S. Effect of oestrogens and progesterone on the metabolic inactivation of noradrenaline in the human placenta. *Placenta* 1988;**9**(5):507–12.

Chapter 9

Ovarian Function During Pregnancy and Lactation

Jessica A. Ryniec* and Elizabeth A. McGee†

*Reproductive Endocrinology and Infertility, University of Vermont, Burlington, VT, United States, †Director of Reproductive Endocinology and Infertility, Obstetrics, Gynecology and Reproductive Sciences, University of Vermont, Larner College of Medicine, Burlington, VT, United States

Key Clinical Changes

- The ovary produces the corpus luteum, which produces estradiol and progesterone to support the endometrium, zygote, and embryo in the early phases of pregnancy.
- In a nonfertile cycle, the pituitary no longer supports the corpus luteum after 14 days postovulation, and this leads to its regression and falling sex steroid levels.
- In a fertile cycle, ongoing production of hCG by the conceptus leads to the corpus luteum, maintaining its viability and production of sex steroids until the placenta subsequently takes over.
- The role or function of the ovary in the second or third trimester has not been well studied, and therefore it remains uncertain.
- Return of ovarian function and ovulation occurs weeks to months after parturition, with the longest intervals in women who breastfeed intensely for prolonged intervals.

9.1 INTRODUCTION

The main function of the ovary during pregnancy in humans is endocrine support during implantation and the first trimester, at which point this role is taken over by the placenta. This early pregnancy support is carried out mainly by the corpus luteum of the ovary. Thus, essential to a discussion of the important role of the ovary in pregnancy are the events that occur in the ovary, leading up to ovulation and maternal detection of pregnancy. This chapter will begin by discussing those events and will continue with the expected changes in ovarian function and hormones that occur during pregnancy, postpartum, and lactation in humans. We have also included data and references to other mammals where it is useful in understanding ovarian function and physiology, or where there is insufficient information in humans.

9.2 OVARIAN HORMONE CHANGES DURING OVULATION, LUTEINIZATION, IMPLANTATION, EARLY PREGNANCY, AND LUTEOLYSIS

9.2.1 Ovulation

In each ovarian cycle, a cohort of follicles progresses through selection, and a species-specific number of dominant ovulatory follicles ultimately arises. The ovulatory quotient is determined through an intricate selection process that culminates in dominance and ovulation.[1] Follicles are responsive to follicle-stimulating hormone (FSH) early in their development, but they do not become gonadotropin dependent for survival until sometime in the antral stage, often just prior to the cycle in which they join the selected cohort.[2] As estradiol levels rise with development of the dominant follicle and its increased aromatase activity,[3] negative feedback inhibits FSH secretion and fewer mature follicles in the cohort cease to develop. The dominant follicle develops luteinizing hormone (LH) receptors on its granulosa cells and is therefore less susceptible to the reduction in FSH levels.[1] Not only do these follicles express LH receptors, allowing them to respond to the LH surge, but they also enhance cyclic adenosine monophosphate (cAMP) response to LH, leading to the events of ovulation and luteinization (which is the transformation of the dominant follicle into a corpus luteum).[4] The dominant follicle also has increased blood flow relative to the less dominate follicles in the cohort.[1] Numerous growth factors and cytokines are also involved in the continued survival of the dominant follicle.[2]

The LH surge drives ovulation, which is accompanied by the further upregulation of LH receptors in granulosa cells in preovulatory follicles.[5,6] Luteogenesis requires a response in multiple cell types, including the theca, granulosa, and cumulus cells, as well as the ovarian stromal cells, and is focused on the preovulatory follicles because they are most responsive to LH.[7]

Progesterone also likely plays a key role in the process, as evidenced in rodent studies. In rats, ovulation is dependent on the LH-timed increase in progesterone, and furthermore, the progesterone receptor is upregulated in granulosa cells by LH.[8] Progesterone receptor knockout mice do not ovulate and are infertile.[9] For ovulation, progesterone regulates the expression of a number of essential proovulatory genes, including metalloproteinases.[10]

As ovulation is a process by which the oocyte is released not only from the follicle, but also from the ovary, the breakdown of multiple extracellular matrices must occur. To be released from the ovary and into the pelvis, as occurs in humans, the oocyte must traverse the mural granulosa layer, the basement membrane, the theca layer, and the stroma between the follicle, finally reaching the germinal epithelium. A coordinated dance of regulatory molecules allows focal degeneration of these layers in the formation of the stigma of the ovary.[10,11] Metalloproteinases play a major role in this degradative process, and therefore they are crucial for ovulation.[11] The matrix metalloproteinase family includes collagenases, gelatinases, stromelysins, and membrane-type enzymes. The initial increase in these enzymes (mainly collagenase and gelatinase) occurs in response to LH stimulation.

There is also a body of literature supporting the role of inflammation and prostaglandin in the ovulatory process in many species.[12] Specifically, the 72-kDa form of prostaglandin synthase (Cox-2), the rate-limiting step in prostaglandin synthesis, is increased in granulosa cells of ovulatory follicles in rats by an LH surge,[13] and suppression of prostaglandins can block ovulation in rodents. Deletion of Cox-2 results in failure of the release of the oocyte from the follicle in mice.[14] However, the exact role of prostaglandins in humans has yet to be fully elucidated.

9.2.2   Formation of the Corpus Luteum

Following ovulation, the corpus luteum is formed from the mural granulosa cells, extracellular matrix, and theca cells in a process termed *luteogenesis*. During this process, there is a rapid ingrowth of blood vessels into the previously avascular granulosa layer of the follicle, as well as reorganization of the cell-to-cell relationships between granulosa and theca cells, with differentiation of both cell types into luteal cells with a high capacity for steroid production.

An important step in the formation of the corpus luteum includes its own vascularization, driven by vascular endothelial growth factor (VEGF) and fibroblast growth factor (FGF) from the granulosa cells.[15] This vascularization allows important molecules, such as low-density lipoprotein (LDL) for progesterone production, access to the corpus luteum, as well as for secretion of granulosa and theca products into the circulation[16] (each steroidogenic cell abuts a microvascular bundle; see Fig. 9.1). The exact mechanisms governing this process are not yet completely defined. As stated previously, VEGF is

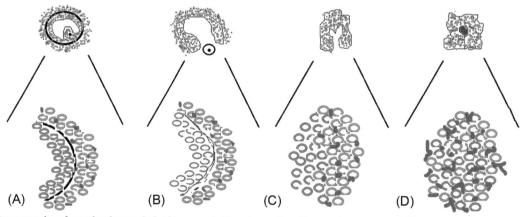

FIG. 9.1   Representation of vascular changes during luteogenesis. Granulosa cells and theca cells are represented by *orange* and *green* respectively, blood vessels are represented in *red*. (A) Day 0—prior to ovulation, vasculature is confined to the thecal layer. (B) Day 1—ovulation, vasculature still restricted to the thecal layer, basement membrane degrading. (C) Day 2–3—following ovulation, the thecal layer collapses into the granulosa layer with the blood supply following. (D) Day 5–6— following ovulation there is intensive angiogenesis with blood vessels branching and spreading throughout the corpus luteum.

present, is highly expressed in the corpus luteum during luteinization, and is intimately involved in the process.[15,17] Expression of VEGF is activated by the LH surge and is likely modulated by insulinlike growth factors.[18] While its mechanism of action is not clearly defined in luteal cells, it is well established through antagonist studies performed in rhesus monkeys that VEGF acts locally, directly affecting the corpus luteum, and is essential for normal development and function.[19]

Certain estradiol metabolites are also involved in the angiogenic process during corpus luteum formation. These include 4-hydroxyestrone and 16-ketoestradiol.[20] These metabolites are higher in the early and midluteal phases and increase with the administration of hCG. Each was shown to increase VEGF secretion supporting their proangiogenic role.[20]

The corpus luteum is composed of both granulosa lutein and theca lutein cells. Much of the evidence of the structural changes that occur during luteinization comes from the study of granulosa cells, but it is likely that changes within the theca cells are similar, as they also become more steroidogenic during this process.[21]

Following ovulation, granulosa cell hypertrophy, and the gap junctions that serve as intracellular connections regress prior to tissue remodeling, as evidenced in cows.[21,22] The internal structures of the cells change to become highly active steroidogenic centers. The mitochondria of the luteal cells are varied in size and shape, are larger in pregnancy and located more centrally in the cell. The cristae of the mitochondria tend to take on the tubular form, increasing the ratio of matrix to intracristal space, increasing the area of inner membrane that is exposed to the matrix. The enzymes responsible for conversion of cholesterol to pregnenolone are located in these mitochondria.[21] The smooth endoplasmic reticulum also further develops within luteal cells, a feature consistent among steroid-producing cells. The increased amount of smooth endoplasmic reticulum is often found peripherally in luteal cells, and similar to the mitochondria take on a branched tubular form. They often become centered on a mitochondrion, excluding other organelles from this steroid-producing region, and it is hypothesized that this allows ease of transfer of molecules between these two structures involved in various steps of steroid synthesis.[21] The smooth endoplasmic reticulum in luteal cells also appears more closely adjacent to the Golgi cisternae, although the role of the Golgi is poorly defined in steroid-producing cells. Finally, the nuclei of luteal cells have well-developed nucleoli and dispersed chromatin, consistent with a cell undergoing extensive deoxyribonucleic acid (DNA) translation and ribonucleoprotein synthesis.[21]

Not only do the internal structures of the luteal cells change, but there also are changes to the surface as well.[21] Projections develop on the surface of these cells, increasing the total cell surface, and in the space between adjacent luteal cells, basal lamina is lacking. Tight junctional complexes develop between cells for intracellular connections. These changes may serve to improve cell-to-cell communication in the corpus luteum.

Terminal differentiation of the luteinized granulosa cells leads to an increased ability to make progesterone, which is important for support of early pregnancy through increased storage of cholesterol and amplification of the conversion of cholesterol to progesterone in the steroidogenic pathway.[23] In humans, the granulosa cells also maintain their ability to make estradiol from androgen precursors, as they continue to express aromatase. Although macaque studies have revealed that progestogenic enzymes such as CYP11A1 and HSD3B2 are upregulated, whereas those involved in androgen and estradiol synthesis (CyP17A1 and CYP19A1, respectively), are relatively reduced.[24,25] The overall increase in steroidogenesis is supported by an increase in steroidogenic acute regulatory protein (StAR), the rate-limiting step in steroidogenesis, the expression of which increases markedly immediately following follicular rupture.[24,25]

Much less is known about the specific structural and functional changes within theca lutein cells, but studies suggest an important role in estradiol synthesis in the corpus luteum. One such study revealed that estradiol synthesis decreases concurrently with a transient decrease in theca lutein cells during corpus luteum development, whereas estradiol synthesis increases in the mature and regressing corpus luteum when theca lutein cells are more abundant. Production of estradiol was also higher in areas of the corpus luteum where there were both granulosa and theca lutein cells present, suggesting the two types of luteal cells continue to interact for this to occur.[26]

Galectin-1 binds to sugar chains on cells, including human luteal cells, and is thought to function as a luteotrophic agent promoted by both hCG and prostaglandin E2. This binding leads to an increase in 3-beta-hydroxysteroid dehydrogenase expression in granulosa lutein cells.[27] Galectin-1 is localized to healthy granulosa lutein cells, but the related galectin-3 is found more in macrophages and regressing granulosa lutein cells, leading to the proposal that this galectin switch has a role in luteal survival and regression in humans.[27] Numerous other local and circulating cytokines and growth factors may also augment the expression of 3-beta-hydroxysteroid dehydrogenase and promote progesterone production in the new corpus luteum. These include adiponectin and platelet-derived growth factor.[28,29]

Other peptides that are synthesized by the corpus luteum include oxytocin, relaxin, inhibin, and activin. Oxytocin is felt to have a paracrine luteotropic effect and is produced following the LH surge, supporting this theory.[30] The corpus is also the sole source of relaxin during pregnancy, and it is secreted in a stage-dependent manner.[31] Inhibin A is secreted in early gestation in women, although its role is unclear.[32]

9.2.3 Corpus luteum Regression

The corpus luteum is a temporally limited structure and eventually regresses and resolves in a process termed *luteolysis* or *regression*. There is both functional (disrupted progesterone production) and structural (degeneration of cells) luteolysis, which occur following a nonfertile ovarian cycle, or at the point in gestation when its survival is no longer supported. Functional luteal regression happens more quickly than structural.

In a nonfertile luteal cycle, corpus luteum regression begins with the reduction of gonadotropin secretion from the pituitary. This occurs approximately 14 days following ovulation in humans. Vascularization decreases, StAR protein expression decreases and there is a corresponding decrease in progesterone synthesis, leading to functional regression. *Functional luteal regression* is the reduction in the ability of the corpus luteum to secrete progesterone and other hormones at the levels needed to sustain early pregnancy. The corpus luteum structurally involutes through both autophagy and apoptosis.[33] Factors involved in luteal function and regression are summarized in Table 9.1 and discussed next.

While prostaglandins are involved in ovulation, one specific prostaglandin, PGF2-alpha, is also critical for luteolysis. In sheep models, increased pituitary oxytocin causes low levels of PGF2-alpha to be released by the uterus, which in turn leads to increased release of corpus luteal oxytocin. With luteal release of oxytocin, large amounts of PGF2-alpha are released, leading to luteal regression.[44] In pigs, there are PGF2-alpha receptors present starting in the early luteal phase, but they are

TABLE 9.1 Functional and structural luteotropic and luteolytic factors[15,17–20,27–30,34–43]

	Luteotropic	Luteolytic
Functional	LH – Increased StAR – Increased P450c22 – Increased 2B-HSD – Increased P450arom FSH Prolactin IGF-1 Progesterone Oxytocin hCG	Decreased gonadotropin Decreased StAR 2-Methoxyestradiol
Structural	VEGF FGF Eosinophils T lymphocytes TIMP-1	Macrophages T lymphocytes PGF2-α Oxytocin Apoptosis – TNF-α – FAS-ligand – Caspases – BCL-2 – SLIT – p53 – AP1 – Interferon-gamma Autophagy – Beclin 1 – LC3-II – Lamp 1 MMPs 2-Methoxyestradiol

not sensitive until days 12–13.[34] In humans, it has been hypothesized that luteal oxytocin may stimulate ovarian production of ovarian PGF2-alpha, and the combination of both substances reduces blood flow and promotes apoptosis.

There also could be a role for estradiol or its metabolites in luteolysis.[45] Specifically, 2-methoxyestradiol has been shown to be antiangiogenic and is found in higher levels in the late luteal phase. It has been shown to downregulate transcription of VEGF, decreasing angiogenesis, which leads to hypoxia and luteal regression.[20] In fertile cycles, 2-methoxyestradiol is decreased with rising hCG, further supporting its role in luteolysis.[20]

Bone morphogenic proteins (BMPs) also may play a role in promoting functional luteal regression.[35] Expression of BMP2, BMP4, and BMP6 are suppressed by hCG in human luteal cells and are low in intact, healthy corpus luteum (CL). However, reduction in hCG allows upregulation of expression of the BMPs, which can reduce the expression and function of 3βHSD, as well as other steroidogenic enzymes. The remodeling that occurs with luteolysis is partly an immune-mediated process. In animal studies, as soon as ovulation occurs, there is a recruitment of eosinophils and T lymphocytes into the corpus luteum, and these subsequently attract and activate macrophages.[46,47] In cows, there is a higher proportion of CD8 T cells in the corpus luteum, specifically gamma-delta CD8 cells, and these can secrete either proinflammatory or anti-inflammatory cytokines. There is a variation in the specific subset of T cells that are expressed at different points of the luteal phase. This suggests a role in immunoregulation, which may be initially luteotropic and then luteolytic.[36] First, T regulatory cells that suppress lymphocyte function dominate and promote the survival of the corpus luteum. Subsequently, during luteolysis, luteal cells activate T lymphocyte proliferation, leading to the release of proinflammatory cytokines that inhibit steroidogenesis and initiate apoptosis. In fertile cycles, this change does not occur, and the gamma-delta CD8 cells remain in higher numbers, preventing luteal regression. Macrophages promote cell death through apoptosis and activate and secrete matrix metalloproteinases (MMPs) involved in structural degradation of the corpus luteum. They also inhibit steroidogenesis through the release of reactive oxygen species and the tumor necrosis factor alpha (TNF-α). They are found in higher numbers in the regressing corpus luteum and are reduced in fertile cycles with luteal rescue, which further supports their luteolytic effect.[35]

The role of apoptosis in luteal regression is central across multiple species, including rodents, domestic animals, and primates. Factors that may be particularly important include TNF-α and Fas ligand.[37,38] These initiate the extrinsic apoptotic pathway, which leads to caspase activation, subsequent DNA fragmentation, and cell death.[34] The intrinsic pathway involves the BCL-2 family, also leading to caspases that lead to further cell destruction. Other factors that peak during luteal regression include certain Slit proteins, p53, activating protein-1, and interferon-gamma.[34]

In addition to apoptosis, autophagy plays a role in human, primate, rodent, and domestic animal luteolysis in both fertile and nonfertile cycles.[39] The specific role of autophagy, however, is not well defined, and further research is required. Research into the role of autophagy in the process of luteal regression in the pig may be informative regarding the factors involved.[39] This study demonstrated the presence of autophagosomes and autophagic proteins throughout the luteal phase, with an increase in autolysosomes and autophagy-related proteins late in the luteal phase. It appears that important proteins include Beclin 1, LC3-II, and Lamp 1, which is consistent with previous studies on autophagy in other cells.

Just as MMPs play a major role in ovulation, they also participate in the degradation of the extracellular matrix in luteolysis.[35] The main MMPs involved in luteolysis include interstitial collagenase, gelatinase A, and gelatinase B. These can be inhibited by tissue inhibitors of metalloproteinases (TIMPs) in response to the regulatory factors that rescue the corpus luteum as discussed next.[35]

9.2.4 Rescue of the Corpus Luteum

In humans, if pregnancy occurs, the corpus luteum persists as the main source of progesterone for the first 6–8 weeks of gestation until the placenta takes over this role. Further, hCG is responsible for this rescue and maintenance of the corpus luteum. It protects the corpus luteum by decreasing apoptotic factors and increasing survival factors.[33] One such survival factor is TIMP-1, which is known to inhibit the metalloproteinases that cause structural breakdown of the corpus luteum. Its role in rescue of the corpus luteum, however, may be more complicated, as the presence of TIMP-1 does not vary greatly through the cycle and MMPs may be present even when TIMP-1 is highly expressed.[35] This is likely because of cellular localization, as TIMP-1 is highly expressed in the granulosa lutein cells, whereas MMPs are expressed in the stromal cells.

LH is also responsible for maintenance of the corpus luteum in pregnancy, and pulsatile release of LH leads to a pulsatile release of progesterone.[40] The role of LH is further supported as the LH receptor remains active and binding is maintained in early pregnancy.[41] It has a number of important roles, including regulation of LDL entry into the cell, facilitating steroidogenesis.[42] LH action may also enhance steroidogenesis by upregulating components of other signaling systems that augment or work synergistically with LH signaling.[28]

Pituitary prolactin is another hormone that is supportive of the corpus luteum, and this occurs in multiple ways. The first is by increasing expression of the LH receptor on the corpus luteum, thus propagating LH effects, and the second is by repressing 20-alpha-hydroxysteroid dehydrogenase, which is a key enzyme in the downstream metabolic pathway of progesterone.[43]

9.2.5 Function of the Corpus Luteum

The corpus luteum acts as an endocrine organ that supports early pregnancy and is the source of estradiol and progesterone during the luteal phase of the cycle. The LH surge that leads to ovulation upregulates the genes encoding StAR, P450c22, 3β-HSD, and P450arom (as well as many other factors); this in turn leads to production of progesterone and estradiol by the corpus luteum.[48,49] The granulosa lutein cells have demonstrated production of progesterone and estradiol, whereas the theca lutein cells produce androgen precursors and 17-alpha-hydroxyprogesterone.

In humans, the progesterone produced by the corpus luteum is responsible for the maintenance of pregnancy for the first 7 embryonic weeks, after which progesterone production is mainly controlled by the placenta. The corpus luteum produces 25–30 mg/day of progesterone, which can act in endocrine, paracrine, and autocrine fashion, as discussed later in this chapter.

The corpus luteum also manufactures estradiol and androgens that are required for pregnancy; however, the placenta becomes the major source of these hormones and the ovary contributes only minimally. Locally produced estradiol does play a role in luteolysis, as discussed later in this chapter. It is also responsible for synthesis of endometrial progesterone receptors, allowing progesterone-mediated changes to the endometrium.

Relaxin is a peptide hormone produced by the ovary, with unclear function in early pregnancy. It is mainly produced by the large luteal cells of the corpus luteum. Of the three relaxin proteins, RLN2 is produced by the corpus luteum. The highest levels are noted in the late luteal phase and into the first trimester of pregnancy, but its function is not fully understood.[50] It is possible that it contributes to the process of decidualization of the endometrium and assists in the suppression of uterine contractions.

9.2.6 Progesterone for Development of Lining, Promoting Quiescence, Delaying Transit, and Facilitating Implantation

Prior to pregnancy, progesterone causes the endometrium to convert to a secretory pattern that is highly vascularized and produces secretions that encourage a favorable intrauterine environment. This is a process of predecidualization. With pregnancy, the lining of the endometrium becomes decidualized, closing the window for implantation. This change in the lining is caused by a progesterone-mediated change in gene expression as well.[51]

Once fertilization occurs, the embryo must travel through a proximal fallopian tube into the uterine cavity for implantation. There are estradiol and progesterone receptors along the fallopian tubes, and estradiol and progesterone are thought to alter tubal motility, facilitating the embryo's movement into the uterus.[52] While some of these hormones may be produced by the cumulus cells surrounding the embryo itself, the ovary may also continue to produce hormones in a paracrine fashion.[52]

Another role for progesterone includes decreasing uterine contractions, facilitating implantation. Previous work with embryo transfers indicated that higher levels of progesterone lead to both lower uterine contraction rates and a change in the pattern of contractions. This relative quenching of the uterine contractions may enhance the ability of the embryo to interact with the endometrium and enhance implantation events.[53]

9.2.7 Shift from Ovary to Uterus/Placenta

Placental *competence,* or the time in which the placenta becomes the primary source of steroid hormones over the ovary, has been found to occur between 6 and 10 weeks of gestation in the human.[54] Estradiol levels increased starting at 6–8 weeks, despite a constant level of supplementation in agonadal patients. Additionally, pregnanediol excretion increased between weeks 5–14, and this was more pronounced in agonadal patients upon supplementation than those with spontaneous pregnancies.[54] Finally, 17-alpha-hydroxyprogesterone levels are an indicator of the function of the corpus luteum, since 17-alpha-hydroxylase enzyme is not expressed in the placenta. Levels of this hormone start to decline after the fifth week of gestation, while progesterone levels continue to rise.[55] The timeline of the luteal-placental shift is further supported by reports of luteectomy that results in miscarriage prior to 7 weeks of gestation.[56]

9.3 OVARIAN HORMONES IN PREGNANCY

Very little is known about ovarian function after the luteal-placental shift. This is a very difficult developmental time for research, due both to its complexity and ethical limitations in study design. Some older studies of surgically removed corpora lutea have shown that the 3-βHSD enzyme activity needed for progesterone production exists at high levels up to 12 weeks' gestation, drops to about half from 14 to 20 weeks' gestation, and is minimally detectable from the late third trimester up to 72h postpartum. However, other dehydrogenases remain active in the corpus luteum, which reflects its continued physical (if not functional) viability throughout pregnancy.[57]

9.4 OVARIAN STRUCTURAL CHANGES WITH PREGNANCY

9.4.1 Anatomic Changes to the Ovary During Pregnancy

During pregnancy, ovulation is suppressed and new dominant follicles do not develop, although smaller follicles continue to grow and regress. The development and structure of the corpus luteum have been discussed previously; however, many other structural changes occur within the ovary during pregnancy.

The vasculature supplying and draining the ovaries during pregnancy is dramatically different during pregnancy, similar in nature to the changes in uterine blood flow.[58] It has been observed that the average diameter of the ovarian vascular pedicle can increase from 9.03 to 25.85mm (a 2.86-fold increase, although technical difficulties may limit the accuracy of these results).[58] The same study revealed decreased oxygen saturation in ovarian vein blood in pregnant women compared with nonpregnant women (66.38% vs 92.1%). In addition, the anatomy of the ovarian vessels was altered, with increased caliber of the vessels, smooth muscle hypertrophy, and a loosening of the vessel wall stroma. The capacity of the ovarian veins was increased by 60 times by term.[58]

9.4.2 Ovarian Cysts of Pregnancy

Ovarian cysts are common in the first trimester, but the majority of these are physiological and resolve without intervention (71.9%).[59] The reported prevalence of adnexal masses in pregnancy is 1%–25%.[60] Even for those that persist, expectant management is felt to be safe, and in a longitudinal study by Condous, it was demonstrated that only 0.13% required acute intervention during pregnancy. There were no malignancies in the Condous study, but some studies found ovarian neoplasms during pregnancy.[61,62] These studies have detected malignancy in between 1% and 3% of adnexal masses removed during pregnancy. This may be higher than the true risk, however, because the fact that the patients had a surgical indication during pregnancy put them at higher risk of malignancy due to there likely being more concerning features present in the ovarian mass. Leiserowitz calculated an incidence of ovarian cancer in 1/56,000 deliveries, with a clinically significant ovarian tumor in 1/23,800 deliveries when also considering borderline tumors. While rare, ovarian cancer in pregnancy is also associated with better clinical outcomes and less aggressive tumors.[62]

There are a number of cystic lesions in pregnancy that may be hormonally active and have systemic effects. The two most common of these are pregnancy luteoma and hyperreacto luteinalis, both of which are characterized by ovarian secretion of androgens, which can lead to varying degrees of maternal hyperandrogenism with hirsutism, acne, and alopecia. In extreme cases, virilization with clitoromegaly and deepening of the voice can occur.[63]

Pregnancy luteoma is most commonly found in multiparous, reproductive-age women and are usually found incidentally during routine ultrasound, presenting as a solid ovarian mass. They arise as a proliferation of stroma cells. They can be bilateral in up to 50% of cases. A total of 60% of women experience hyperandrogenism, with one-third of these mothers exhibiting the clinical features of androgen excess. Two-thirds of women who experience virilization may demonstrate fetal virilization as well. Because they occur under the influence of hCG, they resolve postpartum, but recurrence is common.[63]

Hyperreactio luteinalis is also most commonly detected incidentally in multiparous, reproductive-age women, with a "spoke wheel" or cystic appearance detected via ultrasound. They arise from the theca interna layer due to hypertrophy and luteinization. This is more common in women with high hCG levels, such as with a multiple pregnancy or molar gestation. As opposed to pregnancy luteoma, more than 90% are bilateral. Only 20% lead to maternal virilization, and no cases have been reported of fetal virilization. These also resolve either during pregnancy or postpartum.[63]

9.5 LACTATION EFFECTS ON THE OVARY

During pregnancy, estradiol, progesterone, and other factors prepare the breast for lactation; however, as discussed previously, estradiol and progesterone come mainly from the placenta, not from the ovaries. Progesterone at this point actually blocks lactogenesis, but following delivery, the high levels of estradiol and progesterone from the placenta drop, and pituitary prolactin is elevated, stimulating milk production. During breastfeeding, ovarian estradiol and progesterone are suppressed.

9.5.1 Suppression

Gonadotropin-releasing hormone (GnRH) is inhibited by multiple systems, notably those involved with kisspeptin/neurokinin B, which are activated by suckling.[64] This occurs via the activation of multiple systems, including the dopamine, serotonin, gamma-aminobutyric acid, and corticotropin-releasing factor systems. Prolactin itself also directly suppresses kisspeptin and stimulates dopamine, which ultimately inhibits GnRH in mice.[65]

In women, the inhibition of GnRH prevents release of FSH/LH and thus prevents ovulation and leads to low ovarian hormone production, resulting in oligo-ovulation or anovulation. With a certain level of nursing frequency, serum prolactin is high enough to suppress LH surges, and thus ovarian function. In fact, compared to normally cycling women who had a preovulatory estradiol level of 250–300 pg/mL, exclusively breastfeeding women who are amenorrheic have estradiol levels as low as 20–40 pg/mL. This is evolutionarily advantageous because lactation can be an energy burden, and returning to fertility would not benefit a mother who cannot support both her own energy needs and the needs of an infant. The degree of suppression of GnRH depends on maternal nutrition, intensity of lactation, and body mass/composition.[66,67] In a situation where the needs of lactation and daily living exceed the level of energy available, amenorrhea or oligomenorrhea can occur and persist for an extended period.

9.5.2 Return of Ovulation

In women who have not breastfed, the average return of ovulation occurred between 45 and 94 days postpartum, as detected by urinary pregnanediol levels,[68] although some women with suppressed lactation can ovulate as soon as 14 days postpartum. Return to ovulation in a fully breastfeeding woman can occur much later in the postpartum period, with an average of 112 days to first ovulation in this group, but lactational amenorrhea can last up to 1 year with exclusive breastfeeding,[69] although this fact may be more related to the intensity of breastfeeding (number of feeds per day and volume of milk output) rather than exclusivity alone.

Lactational amenorrhea has been investigated as a contraceptive method, and in women who are exclusively breastfeeding and remain amenorrheic, the risk of pregnancy is less than 3% in the first 6 months.[70] After 6 months, pregnancy rates increase even among exclusively breastfeeding women; therefore, an alternative method of contraception is recommended by that time. A highly reliable modern contraceptive method that is compatible with lactation is recommended for most women, such as an intrauterine device (IUD) or progesterone-only methods.

9.5.3 Other Effects of Lactation on the Ovary

Lactation and breastfeeding have other benefits in terms of the ovaries. Given the low circulating estradiol level in amenorrheic, breastfeeding women, it may decrease the severity or the risk of endometriosis. In a study that evaluated laparoscopically detected endometriosis compared with reproductive history, including lactation, there was an 80% decrease in endometriosis risk with greater than 23 months of lactation (total lifetime duration).[71]

The effects of lactation and breastfeeding on breast cancer risk have been extensively studied, with a well-established protective effect that increases with the length of breastfeeding.[72] Less well studied is the effect of breastfeeding on ovarian cancer, but a protective effect also may exist. A large meta-analysis revealed a 9% reduction in ovarian cancer for every 5 months of breastfeeding.[73] This is postulated to be related to decreased ovulation (some ovarian cancer theories relate risk to the number of ovulations) and suppression of gonadotropins.

9.6 CONCLUSION

The ovary is a critical organ for fertility, not just as a source of female gametes but also as a driving force to prepare the endometrium for implantation and to support early gestation. The role of the ovary in mid- and late gestation is largely unknown, although it is still capable of steroidogenesis. The return of cyclic ovarian function postpartum is highly variable, depending on a number of factors. This timing is of great interest in promoting global health issues of optimizing lactation and supporting an interpregnancy interval that optimizes the health of both mother and siblings.

REFERENCES

1. Zeleznik. The physiology of follicle selection. *Reprod Biol Endocrinol* 2004;**2**:31.
2. McGee EA, Hsueh AJ. Initial and cyclic recruitment of ovarian follicles. *Endocr Rev* 2000;**21**(2):200–14.
3. Lephart ED, Doody KJ, Mcphaul MJ, Simpson ER. Inverse relationship between ovarian aromatase cytochrome P450 and 5α-reductase enzyme activities and mRNA levels during the estrous cycle in the rat. *J Steroid Biochem Mol Biol* 1992;**42**(5):439–47.
4. Jonassen JA, Bose K, Richards JS. Enhancement and desensitization of hormone-responsive adenylate cyclase in granulosa cells of preantral and antral ovarian follicles: effects of estradiol and follicle-stimulating hormone. *Endocrinology* 1982;**111**:74–9.
5. Knobil E. The neuroendocrine control of the menstrual cycle. *Recent Prog Horm Res* 1980;**36**:53–88.
6. Richards JS. Maturation of ovarian follicles: actions and interactions of pituitary and ovarian hormones on follicular cell differentiation. *Physiol Rev* 1980;**60**:51–89.
7. Richards JS, Pangas SA. The ovary: basic biology and clinical implications. *J Clin Invest* 2010;**120**:963–72.
8. Brannstrom M, Janson PO. Progesterone is a mediator in the ovulatory process of the in vitro-perfused rat ovary. *Biol Reprod* 1989;**40**:1170–8.
9. Lydon JP, DeMayo F, Funk CR. Mice lacking progesterone receptor exhibit reproductive abnormalities. *Genes Dev* 1995;**9**:2266–78.
10. Liu K, Wahlberg P, Hagglund AC, Ny T. Expression pattern and functional studies of matrix degrading proteases and their inhibitors in the mouse corpus luteum. *Mol Cell Endocrinol* 2003;**205**(1–2):131–40.
11. Curry Jr TE, Osteen KG. The matrix metalloproteinase system: changes, regulation, and impact throughout the ovarian and uterine reproductive cycle. *Endocr Rev* 2003;**24**(4):428–65.
12. Espey LL. Ovulation as an inflammatory reaction—a hypothesis. *Biol Reprod* 1980;**22**:73–106.
13. Sirois J, Simmons DL, Richards JS. Hormonal regulation of messenger ribonucleic acid encoding a novel isoform of prostaglandin endoperoxide H synthase in rat preovulatory follicles. *J Biol Chem* 1992;**267**(16):11586–92.
14. Tilley SL, Audoly LP, Hicks EH. Reproductive failure and reduced blood pressure in mice lacking the EP2 prostaglandin E2 receptor. *J Clin Invest* 1999;**103**(11):1539–45.
15. Robinson RS, Woad KJ, Hammond AJ, Laird M, Hunter MG, Mann GE. Angiogenesis and vascular function in the ovary. *Reproduction* 2009;**138**:869–81.
16. Christenson LK, Stouffer RL. Proliferation of microvascular endothelial cells in the primate corpus luteum during the menstrual cycle and simulated early pregnancy. *Endocrinology* 1996;**137**:367–74.
17. Fraser HM, Lunn SF. Regulation and manipulation of angiogenesis in the primate corpus luteum. *Reproduction* 2001;**121**:355–62.
18. Martinez-Chequer JC, Stouffer RL, Hazzard TM, Patton PE, Molskness TA. Insulin-like growth factors-1 and -2, but not hypoxia, synergize with gonadotropin hormone to promote vascular endothelial growth factor-A secretion by monkey granulosa cells from preovulatory follicles. *Biol Reprod* 2003;**68**:1112–8.
19. Hazzard TM, XU F, Stouffer RL. Injection of soluble vascular endothelial growth factor receptor 1 into the preovulatory follicle disrupts ovulation and subsequent luteal function in the rhesus monkey. *Endocrinology* 2002;**67**:1305–12.
20. Henriquez S, Kohen P, Xu X, Veenstra TD, Munoz A, Palomino WA, Strauss JF, Devoto L. Estrogen metabolites in human corpus luteum physiology: differential effects on angiogenic activity. *Fertil Steril* 2016;**106**(1):230–7.
21. Enders AC. Cytology of the corpus luteum. *Biol Reprod* 1973;**8**:158–82.
22. Berisha B, Bridger P, Toth A, Kliem H, Meyer HH, Schams D, Pfarrer C. Expression and localization of gap junctional connexins 26 and 43 in bovine periovulatory follicles and in corpus luteum during different functional stages of oestrous cycle and pregnancy. *Reprod Domest Anim* 2009;**44**:295–302.
23. Christenson LK, Devoto L. Cholesterol transport and steroidogenesis by the corpus luteum. *Reprod Biol Endocrinol* 2003;**1**:90.
24. Bogan RL, Murphy MJ, Stouffer RL, Hennebold JD. Systematic determination of differential gene expression in the primate corpus luteum during the luteal phase of the menstrual cycle. *Mol Endocrinol* 2008;**123**:333–9.
25. Xu F, Stouffer RL, Muller J, et al. Dynamics of the transcriptome in the primate ovulatory follicle. *Mol Hum Reprod* 2011;**17**:152–65.
26. Mori T, Nihnobu K, Takeuchi S, Onho Y, Tojo S. Interrelation between luteal cell types in steroidogenesis in vitro of human corpus luteum. *J Steroid Biochem* 1983;**19**(1):811–5.
27. Nio-Kobayashi J, Boswell L, Amano M, Iwanaga T, Duncan WC. The loss of luteal progesterone production in women is associated with a galactin switch via α2,6-sialylation of glycoconjugates. *J Clin Endocrinol Metabol* 2014;**99**(12):4616–24.
28. Wickham E, Tao T, Nestler J, McGee E. Activation of the LH receptor up regulates the type 2 adiponectin receptor in human granulosa cells. *J Assist Reprod Genet* 2013;**30**(7):963–8.
29. Sleer LS, Taylor CC. Platelet derived growth factors and receptors in the rat corpus luteum: localization and identification of an effect on luteogenesis. *Biol Reprod* 2007;**76**(3):391–400.
30. Eispanier A, Jurdzinski A, Hodges JK. A local oxytocin system is part of the luteinization process in the preovulatory follicle of the marmoset monkey (Callithrix jacchus). *Biol Reprod* 1997;**57**:16–26.
31. Sherwood OD. Relaxin's physiological roles and other diverse actions. *Endocr Rev* 2004;**25**:205–34.

32. Knight PG, Satchell L, Glister C. Intra-ovarian roles of activins and inhibins. *Mol Cell Endocrinol* 2012;**359**:53–65.

33. Del Canto F, Sierralta W, Kohen P, Munoz A, Strauss III JF, Devoto L. Features of natural and gonadotropin-releasing hormone antagonist-induced corpus luteum regression and effects of in vivo human chorionic gonadotropin. *J Clin Endocrinol Metab* 2007;**92**:4436–43.

34. Przygrodzka E, Witek KJ, Kaczmarek MM, Andronowska A, Ziecik AJ. Expression of factors associated with apoptosis in the porcine corpus luteum throughout the luteal phase of the estrous cycle and early pregnancy: their possible involvement in acquisition of luteolytic sensitivity. *Theriogenology* 2015;**83**(4):535–45.

35. Duncan WC. The human corpus luteum: remodeling during luteolysis and maternal recognition of pregnancy. *Rev Reprod* 2000;**5**:12–7.

36. Poole DH, Pate JL. Luteal microenvironment directs resident T lymphocyte function in cows. *Biol Reprod* 2012;**86**(2):29. 1–10.

37. Peluffo MC, Young KA, Hennebold JF, Stouffer RL. Expression and regulation of tumor necrosis factor (TNF) and TNF-receptor family members in the macaque corpus luteum during the menstrual cycle. *Mol Reprod Dev* 2009;**76**:367–78.

38. Quirk SM, Cowan RG, Joshi SG, Henrikson KP. Fas antigen-mediated apoptosis in human granulosa/luteal cells. *Biol Reprod* 1995;**52**:279087.

39. Grzesiak M, Michalik A, Rak A, Knapczyk-Stwora K, Pieczonka A. The expression of autophagy-related proteins within the corpus luteum lifespan in pigs. *Domest Anim Endocrinol* 2018;**64**:9–16.

40. Filicori M, Butler JP, Crowley Jr WF. Neuroendocrine regulation of the corpus luteum in the human. Evidence for pulsatile progesterone secretion. *J Clin Investig* 1984;**73**(6):1638–47.

41. Duncan WC, McNeilly AS, Fraser HM, Illingworth PJ. Luteinizing hormone receptor in the human corpus luteum: lack of down-regulation during maternal recognition of pregnancy. *Hum Reprod* 1996;**11**(10):2291–7.

42. Brannian JD, Shiigi SM, Stouffer RL. Gonadotropin surge increases fluorescent-tagged low-density lipoprotein uptake by Macaque granulosa cells from preovulatory follicles. *Biol Reprod* 1992;**47**(3):355–60.

43. Gibori G, Richards JS. Dissociation of two distinct luteotropic effects of prolactin: regulation of luteinizing hormone-receptor content and progesterone secretion during pregnancy. *Endocrinology* 1978;**102**:767–74.

44. McCracken JA, Custer EE, Lamsa JC. Luteolysis: a neuroendocrine-mediated event. *Physiol Rev* 1999;**79**:263.

45. Gore BZ, Caldwell BV, Speroff L. Estrogen-induced human luteolysis. *J Clin Endocrinol Metab* 1973;**36**(3):615–7.

46. Murdoch WJ. Treatment of sheep with prostaglandin F2 alpha enhances production of a luteal chemoattractant for eosinophils. *Am J Reprod Immunol* 1987;**15**:52–6.

47. Kirsch TM, Friedman AC, Vogel RL. Macrophages in corpora lutea of mice: characterization and effects on steroid secretion. *Biol Reprod* 1981;**25**:629–38.

48. Vande Wiele RL, Bogumil J, Dyrenfurth I, Ferin M, Jewelewicz R, Warren M, Rizkallah T, Mikhail G. Mechanisms regulating the menstrual cycle in women. *Recent Prog Horm Res* 1970;**26**:63–103.

49. McRae RS, Johnston HM, Mihm M, O'Shaughnessey PJ. Changes in mouse granulosa cell gene expression during early luteinization. *Endocrinology* 2005;**146**(1):309–17.

50. Quagliarello J, Steinetz BG, Weiss G. Relaxin secretion in early pregnancy. *Obstet Gynecol* 1979;**53**(1):62–3.

51. Young SL. Oestrogen and progesterone action on endometrium: a translational approach to understanding endometrial receptivity. *Reprod Biomed Online* 2013;**27**(5):497–505.

52. Punnonen R, Lukola A. Binding of estrogen and progestin in the human fallopian tube. *Fertil Steril* 1981;**36**(5):610–4.

53. Fanchin R, Righini C, de Ziegler D, Olivennes F, Ledee N, Frydman R. Effects of vaginal progesterone administration on uterine contractility at the time of embryo transfer. *Fertil Steril* 2001;**75**(6):1136–40.

54. Schneider MA, Davies MC, Honour JW. The timing of placental competence in pregnancy after oocyte donation. *Fertil Steril* 1993;**59**:1059.

55. Tulchinsky D, Hobel CJ. Plasma human chorionic gonadotropin, estrone, estradiol, progesterone, and 17 alpha-hydroxyprogesterone in human pregnancy. 3. Early normal pregnancy. *Am J Obstet Gynecol* 1973;**117**(7):884–93.

56. Caspo AI, Pulkkinen MO, Wiest WG. Effects of luteectomy and progesterone replacement therapy in early pregnant patients. *Am J Obstet Gynecol* 1973;**115**:759–65.

57. Strauss III JF, Mastroianni Jr L, Stambaugh R. Human ovarian enzymes during pregnancy. *J Clin Endocrinol Metab* 1973;**36**(1):192–5.

58. Hodgkinson CP. Physiology of the ovarian veins during pregnancy. *Obstet Gynecol* 1953;**1**(1):26–37.

59. Condous G, Khalid A, Okaro A, Bourne T. Should we be examining the ovaries in pregnancy? Prevalence and natural history of adnexal pathology detected at first-trimester sonography. *Ultrasound Obstet Gynecol* 2004;**24**(1):62–6.

60. Schwartz N, Timor-Tritsch IE, Wang E. Adnexal masses in pregnancy. *Clin Obstet Gynecol* 2009;**52**(4):570–85.

61. Leiserowitz GS, Xing G, Cress R, Brahmbhatt B, Dalyrymple JL, Smith LH. Adnexal masses in pregnancy: how often are they malignant? *Gynecol Oncol* 2006;**101**(2):315–21.

62. Whitecar MP, Turner S, Higby MK. Adnexal masses in pregnancy: a review of 130 cases undergoing surgical management. *Am J Obstet Gynecol* 1999;**181**(1):19–24.

63. Phelan N, Conway GS. Management of ovarian disease in pregnancy. *Best Pract Res Clin Endocrinol Metab* 2011;**25**(6):985–92.

64. True C, Kirigiti M, Ciofi P, Grove KL, Smith MS. Characterisation of arcuate nucleus kisspeptin/neurokinin B neuronal projections and regulation during lactation in the rat. *J Neuroendocrinol* 2011;**23**(1):52–64.

65. Brown RS, Herbison AE, Grattan DR. Effect of prolactin and lactation on A15 dopamine neurons in the rostral preoptic area of female mice. *J Neuroendocrinol* 2015;**27**(9):708–17.

66. The World Health Organization. The World Health Organization multinational study of breast-feeding and lactational amenorrhea. II. Factors associated with the length of amenorrhea. World health organization task force on methods for the natural regulation of fertility. *Fertil Steril* 1998;**70**(3):461–71.

67. Wasalathanthri S, Tennekoon KH. Lactational amenorrhea/anovulation and some of their determinants: a comparison of well-nourished and under-nourished women. *Fertil Steril* 2001;**76**(2):317–25.

68. Jackson MD, Glasier A. Return of ovulation and menses in postpartum nonlactating women: a systematic review. *Obstet Gynecol* 2011;**117**(3):657–62.

69. Perez A, Vela P, Masnick GS, Potter RG. First ovulation after childbirth: the effect of breast-feeding. *Am J Obstet Gynecol* 1972;**114**(8):1041–7.

70. Kennedy KI, Visness CM. Contraceptive efficacy of lactational amenorrhea method. *Lancet* 1992;**339**:227–30.

71. Missmer SA, Hankinson SE, Spiegelman D, Barbieri RL, Malspeis S, Willett WC, Hunger DJ. Reproductive history and endometriosis among pre-menopausal women. *Obstet Gynecol* 2004;**104**:965–74.

72. Collaborative Group on Hormonal Factors in Breast Cancer. Breast cancer and breastfeeding: collaborative reanalysis of individual data from 47 epidemiological studies in 30 countries, including 50302 women with breast cancer and 96973 women without the disease. *Lancet* 2002;**360**(9328):187–95.

73. Luan NN, Wu QJ, Gong TT, Vogtmann E, Wang YL, Lin B. Breastfeeding and ovarian cancer risk: a meta-analysis of epidemiologic studies. *Am J Clin Nutr* 2013;**98**(4):1020–31.

Chapter 10

The Physiological Roles of the Renin-Angiotensin Aldosterone System and Vasopressin in Human Pregnancy

Eugenie R. Lumbers

School of Biomedical Sciences and Pharmacy, Hunter Medical Research Institute, University of Newcastle, New Lambton, NSW, Australia

Key Clinical Changes

- Pregnancy is characterized by marked upregulation of maternal circulating and intrarenal maternal renin-angiotensin systems in order to offset the actions of relaxin, oestrogens, and progesterone on the cardiovascular system and kidneys.
- Rising levels of oestrogens stimulate the production of angiotensinogen by the liver. High levels of angiotensinogen are responsible for the increase in angiotensin II levels in early gestation. Later, plasma renin levels increase above those measured in the luteal phase of the menstrual cycle, and angiotensin II levels increase further.
- The vasoconstrictor actions of angiotensin II, mediated by its interaction with the angiotensin II-AT_1 receptor, are attenuated in pregnancy because of downregulation of the receptor by angiotensin, and possibly because angiotensin II, acting via the AT_2 receptor, and angiotensin-(1–7) produced from angiotensin II are vasodilators.
- The ovarian renin-angiotensin system is involved in folliculogenesis and ovulation. The ovary contributes to the high levels of prorenin found in maternal blood in early pregnancy.
- Placental and decidual renin-angiotensin systems may promote implantation and uteroplacental blood flow. Deficiencies in their production could contribute to impaired placental development, preeclampsia, and preterm birth.

10.1 INTRODUCTION

Both a tissue system and a circulating renin-angiotensin system (RAS) are essential for a normal pregnancy outcome. While the intense activation of the circulating renin-angiotensin-aldosterone in human pregnancy is well described, significant roles for the ovarian, placental, and other intrauterine RASs have been overlooked, as has a potential role of a renal RAS located within the renal tubules. This chapter describes the physiology of these RASs in normal pregnancy. Mention is also made to pregnancy-specific hypertension (preeclampsia) because this form of hypertension is associated with marked changes in the circulating renin-angiotensin-aldosterone system(cRAAS).

The kidneys and reproductive tract share a common embryological origin, so it is not surprising that cells from the kidneys and gonads share similar molecular functional properties. Renin-angiotensin systems are present in all organs involved in internal fertilization (i.e., the genital tract, ovary, and placenta).[1]

The chapter is divided into the following sections:

- The renin-angiotensin components and pathways for the generation of angiotensin peptides
- Regulation and actions of the cRAAS and the intrarenal RAS in pregnancy
- Reproductive tract renin-angiotensin systems

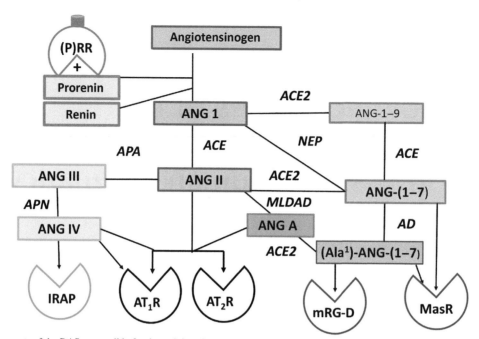

FIG. 10.1 Components of the RAS responsible for the activity of circulating and tissue RASs in pregnancy. (P)RR is the prorenin receptor. Renin, or prorenin binding to the (P)RR, can cleave ANG1 from AGT. ANG I is converted to ANG II by a dipeptidyl carboxypeptidase, ACE. ANG II can act on either an ANG II AT1R or AT2R. The interaction of ANG II with its AT2R opposes actions of ANG II mediated via its AT1R. ANG II can be converted by aminopeptidase A (APA) to Ang III, which is converted to ANG IV. ANG IV acts on IRAP. ANG II is converted by the monopeptidyl carboxypeptidase ACE2 to ANG-(1–7), which acts on its own G protein-coupled receptor (MasR) and has actions similar to those of ANG II mediated via AT2R. ANG II can be converted by mononuclear leucocyte-derived aspartate decarboxylase (MLDAD) to ANG A, which can then be converted by ACE2 to (Ala1)-ANG-(1–7). ANG-(1–7) can also be converted by aspartic decarboxylase (AD) to (Ala1)-ANG-(1–7), also known as almandine, which can act on the MasR and on the Mas receptor-related, G-protein-coupled receptor member D (mRG-D). ANG peptides can often interact with different ANG receptors (see also [2]).

10.2 RENIN-ANGIOTENSIN COMPONENTS AND PATHWAYS FOR GENERATION OF ANGIOTENSIN PEPTIDES

Fig. 10.1 presents an overview of the pathways within the RAS that generate angiotensin (ANG) peptides. ANG peptides affect a number of systems in a variety of tissues. In pregnancy, they are involved in fertility, in the regulation of cardio-vascular and renal function, and in reproductive tissue growth and development.

The complexity of the RAS pathways and difficulties in the quantitation of the proteins and peptides that constitute them[2] can result in inconsistencies in the values quoted for the circulating peptides. These inconsistencies are possibly related to the antibodies used to measure the peptides,[3] the variable efficiency with which angiotensins are protected from endogenous proteases, or both.

10.2.1 Renin and Prorenin

While the activity of the cRAAS is controlled by the concentrations of active renin released by the kidney and angiotensinogen (AGT) released from the liver, this is not the case for other RASs except the maternal intrarenal renin-angiotensin system (IRAS) because only the kidney secretes active renin. In all other tissues, prorenin is secreted. The renin gene expresses a protein (now known as *prorenin*, but originally described as *inactive renin*[4]) that has no catalytic activity on its own because its prosegment is folded over the AGT binding site. For prorenin to become active, this prosegment of the 42-kDa prorenin molecule must either be cleaved catalytically by endopeptidases, such as trypsin, plasmin, cathepsin D, or kallikrein,[5,6] or unfolded out of the active site by low temperatures or low pH and irreversibly activated by proteases. These processes are known as *cryoactivation*[7] and *acid activation*.[4] Unfolding of the prosegment also occurs when prorenin binds to its prorenin receptor ((P)RR). The physiological roles of the (P)RR, intracellular acidification, and tissue proteases in activating tissue prorenin are still largely unknown, even though they can be readily demonstrated in vitro. There is only a small rate of spontaneous conversion of prorenin to active renin.[8]

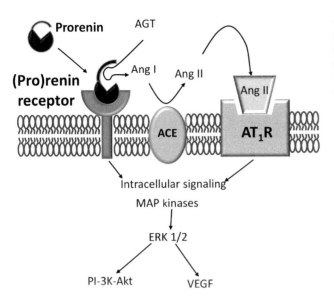

FIG. 10.2 Interactions between prorenin and the (P)RR. Not only does binding of prorenin to the (P)RR activate prorenin so that it can catalyze the formation of ANG I from AGT, but it also activates the (P)RR, leading to the stimulation of intracellular-signaling pathways (e.g., MAPK kinases and Wnt–B-catenin), independent of ANG II. Also, (P)RR is an integral component of a membrane-bound H^+-vacuolar-ATPase.

10.2.2   (Pro)renin Receptor

In 2002, a novel (P)RR was discovered.[9] Prorenin is activated catalytically by binding to a (P)RR, which also can bind active renin. It not only activates the catalytic potential of prorenin, but also has biological actions that are similar to ANG II and independent of its formation (e.g., stimulation of ERK 1/2-signaling pathways) (Fig. 10.2). (P)RR is an essential component of a vacuolar-H^+ATPase (ATP6AP2), and it has a number of other actions, such as activation of Wnt-signaling.[10] Some of these actions of (P)RR are enhanced by prorenin binding to it.[9]

Activation of tissue RAS pathways (other than the intrarenal RAS) must involve the activation of constitutively secreted prorenin. This could be spontaneous, as a very small proportion (about 1.5%) of plasma prorenin exhibits spontaneous catalytic activity.[8] Prorenin also could be activated by endogenous proteases. In plasma, these proteases that activate prorenin in vitro are inhibited.[11] This may not be the case in tissues, but the physiological role of proteolytic activation of prorenin in tissue ANG peptide production is unknown.

At this time, the only known potential pathway for biological regulation of tissue RASs by activation of prorenin would appear to result from binding of prorenin to (P)RR and exposing its catalytic site. It has been argued that the Kd of the interaction between (P)RRs and prorenin is in the nanomolar range, while plasma prorenin levels are only in the picomolar range.[8] Therefore, it is unlikely that plasma prorenin bound to (P)RR can catalyze the production of significant levels of ANG II from plasma AGT. This may not be the case for tissue renin-angiotensin systems, as levels of prorenin in some tissues can be very high.[12,13]

10.2.3   Soluble (P)RR

(P)RR is a membrane-bound receptor. The extracellular domain of the (P)RR can be cleaved from (P)RR by furin,[14] and other proteases and circulates in blood as soluble (P)RR (s(P)RR). Further, s(P)RR can be cleaved from (P)RR which is located on trophoblast (placental cells), by furin, so it is possible that levels in maternal pregnant plasma are influenced by its release from the placenta (unpublished obs). Circulating levels of s(P)RR are increased in preeclampsia.[15]

Plasma s(P)RR may play a physiological role in pregnancy, and in particular in preeclampsia, because it affects the rate at which renin catalyzes oxidized AGT, as discussed next.[16]

10.2.4   Angiotensinogen

Native AGT is a 62-kDa protein, although there are high-molecular-weight (HMW) forms (polymers, as discussed later in this chapter). Therefore, the molecular weight of circulating AGT can vary. Monomeric AGT is a protein of 61.5 kDa or 65.5 kDa (depending on glycosylation) produced by the liver.[17] Polymeric forms of AGT alter the rate of the renin-AGT reaction.

The cleavage site for renin (Leu[10]-Val[11]; Fig. 10.3) in human AGT (hAGT) is held in an inaccessible position, which is probably why the human renin-hAGT interaction is species specific; AGT, however, can be cleaved by other endogenous

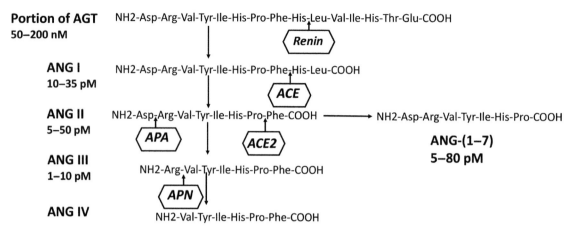

FIG. 10.3 Pathways for the formation of ANG peptides, showing sites of cleavage by proteases and accredited values for ANG peptides in nonpregnant plasma.[2] ACE and ACE2 are ACEs 1 and 2, respectively. APA and APN are aminopeptidases A and N. Cleavage of the C-terminal and N-terminal ends produces ANG peptides with biological activity (see also Figs. 10.1 and 10.4). Note the low levels of active peptides relative to high concentrations of AGT (angiotensinogen).

proteases (such as cathepsin D and trypsin). AGT can exist in blood in both oxidized and reduced forms.[16] ANG I is released more readily from oxidized AGT (Km = 0.86 ± 0.05 μM) than from reduced AGT (Km = 2.9 ± 0.3 μM).[16] When (P)RR is present in solution, the reaction between renin and oxidized AGT is further accelerated because Km is reduced to 0.22 ± 0.09 μM. The reaction rate of renin and reduced AGT is unchanged.[16] In preeclampsia, the levels of both oxidized AGT and s(P)RR are increased.[15,16] Conformational changes in the AGT molecule, such as the Met235T SNP, also increase the accessibility of renin to the AGT's site of cleavage[16]; this SNP is associated with an increased risk of preeclampsia.

Only 10 amino acids from AGT form ANG I; the rest of the molecule remains intact (des-(ANG1)–angiotensinogen[18]). This raises the question as to whether AGT and its HMW product that results from renin catalysis could perform other actions that may be significant in pregnancy.

AGT is a member of the family of serine protease inhibitors known as *serpins*.[19] It is an acute phase-reactant protein and could play a role in suppression of inflammation, as does α1-antitrypsin, which inhibits neutrophil elastase.[20] Like other hepatic proteins that are released in response to IL-6, hepatic AGT expression is stimulated by IL-6.[21] Maintenance of a pregnancy depends on suppression of the maternal immune response to the presence of foreign material (i.e., the fetus and placenta). Rising levels of AGT throughout gestation may ensure a healthy pregnancy outcome, not only because they drive the production of ANG II (and so play a major role in maternal fluid and electrolyte homeostasis), but also because AGT or HMW forms of AGT (i.e., HMW-AGT polymers) limit inflammation. AGT and des-(ANG I)-AGT are also antiangiogenic.[22] These actions of AGT and its breakdown product could counterbalance the proliferative and proangiogenic actions of ANG II.[23]

HMW forms of AGT (140 and 100kDa) account for about 3%–5% of total AGT in plasma in nonpregnant women.[24] There are, however, HMW-AGTs in plasma that are polymers of the proform of eosinophil major basic protein (proMBP) and Cd3g complement that are specific to pregnancy.[25] Levels of HMW-AGT rise throughout gestation and account for about 16% of total AGT; they are higher in women with pregnancy-induced hypertension.[26] The reaction of HMW-AGT with renin is slow.[27] HMW-AGTs were first described by Gordon and Sachin[28] and quantified by Tewksbury and Dart.[26] Five distinct forms exist in the extrafetal tissues (i.e., amnion, chorion, and placenta), while only three exist in maternal plasma.[29] The proform of eosinophil major basic protein (proMBP) with which AGT complexes is highly expressed in the extravillous trophoblast of the placenta.[30] Low levels of proMBP predict Down syndrome and a poor pregnancy outcome.[27]

10.2.5 Angiotensin Converting Enzyme

Angiotensin-converting enzyme (ACE) is a zinc-dependent membrane bound dipeptidase that removes His-Leu from ANG I to form ANG II (Fig. 10.3). There are two forms of ACE: somatic and testicular. Somatic ACE is found in the vascular endothelium, lungs, and other tissues; 90% is membrane bound. It has two catalytic sites on its COOH and NH2-terminal arms.[31] Polymorphisms of the ACE gene exist that affect levels of expression of ACE proteins. The most well described is an insertion/deletion polymorphism. The polymorphism is a 287-bp *alu*-repeat. Levels of ACE are higher in subjects with the D allele and its presence has been associated with cardiovascular disease and preeclampsia.[32]

10.2.6 ACE2

ACE2, like ACE, is a carboxypeptidase with which it has a 42% homology.[33] Its gene is located on the X chromosome, while ACE1 is located on Chr 17. It is a receptor for the SARS virus.[34] ACE2 can cleave an amino acid from the COOH terminal end of ANG I to form ANG 1–9, which is then cleaved by ACE to form ANG-(1–7). Alternatively, ACE2 can remove an amino acid from ANG II, forming ANG-(1–7) (Fig. 10.3). This is the major catalytic pathway for formation of ANG-(1–7).[35] Like ACE, ACE2 is a membrane-bound ectoenzyme, so it is shed into the circulation, but its location is restricted to the kidney, heart, and testis.[33] In pregnancy, ACE2 is expressed in the villous syncytiotrophoblast of the placenta.[36–38]

10.2.7 ANG Peptides and their Receptors

The pathways via which ANG peptides are formed was displayed in Fig. 10.1. Fig. 10.3 shows their amino acid sequences and sites of proteolysis. It also describes the most accurately quantitated levels on ANG peptides in nonpregnant plasma. In pregnancy levels of ANG peptides change dramatically (Fig. 10.7). ANG I has no known biological activity.

The angiotensins act via G protein-coupled receptors (GPCRs; Fig. 10.4).[39] ANG IV is also a ligand for insulin-regulated aminopeptidase (IRAP), which is identical to oxytocinase.[40] GPCRs are part of the cell membrane and have seven transmembrane domains. Binding of an extracellular ligand to an active GPCR initiates conformational changes in the receptor and activation of intracellular signaling via a number of pathways.[41]

For many years, ANG II and its type I receptor subtype (AT$_1$R) held preeminence in mediating the actions of the RAS (e.g., stimulation of aldosterone synthesis and secretion, actions within the central nervous system and adrenal medulla that affect cardiac output and blood pressure, and direct actions on the heart and peripheral blood vessels) (Fig. 10.4; see also Fig. 10.8). Therefore, blocking formation of ANG II or its AT$_1$R have become major therapeutic strategies for treating hypertension and cardiac failure.

Over time, the discovery of the angiotensin type II receptor subtype (AT$_2$R), the peptide ANG-(1–7) and its specific G protein-coupled Mas receptor, and the biological effects of ANG III and ANG IV have made inroads into the preeminence of the Ang II/AT$_1$R interaction and its downstream effects (Fig. 10.1).

The complexity of RAS pathways has been further enhanced by the recognition that ANG can be modified in vivo at its N-terminal by decarboxylation of aspartic acid and converted to Ala^1-ANG II or ANG A.[42] ANG A can bind to AT$_1$R and has a similar affinity to ANG II, although in vivo effects mediated by this interaction have yet to be demonstrated.[42] ANG A also can be converted to alamandine or Ala^1-ANG-(1–7) via ACE2. Alamandine can act on both MasR and Mas receptor-related G-protein-coupled receptor member D (mRGD).[43] The significance of these N-terminal decarboxylated ANG peptides in pregnancy is unknown.

There is increasing evidence that ANG II/AT$_2$R- and ANG-(1–7)/MasR-mediated pathways counteract effects mediated by the ANG II/AT$_1$R interaction, and that they are involved in maintaining maternal and fetal health.

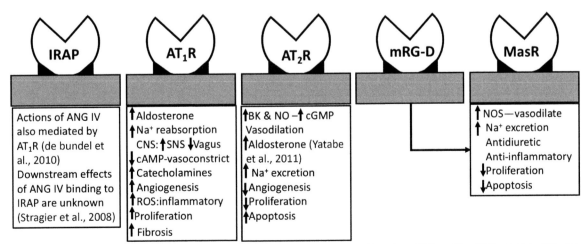

FIG. 10.4 Physiological actions produced by activation of the four types of ANG receptors with various ANG peptides. *BK*, bradykinin; *NO*, nitric oxide; *NOS*, nitric oxide synthase; *ROS*, reactive oxygen species; *CNS*, central nervous system; *SNS*, sympathetic nervous system.

The hypertensinogenic/proliferative AT_1R pathway is linked to the vasodilator/antifibrotic AT_2R-MasR pathway, not only through the actions of ANG II and ANG A on the AT_2R-MasR pathway, but also by their conversion to peptides that act on the Mas pathway (see Figs. 10.1 and 10.4). Therefore, the greatly increased activity of the RAS in pregnancy must involve activation of both these pathways, which suggests that a balance between the opposing actions of the two pathways is required for a normal pregnancy outcome. The placenta may be a major source of circulating ANG-(1–7) in pregnancy. ACE2 is abundantly expressed in the human placenta.[36,37] Knocking out the *ACE2* gene in mice causes a loss of placental ACE2 activity and a fall in plasma ANG-(1–7) levels.[44]

10.2.8 Actions of ANG Peptides

Fig. 10.4 shows the actions of ANG peptides mediated by their interactions with known ANG receptors. Fig. 10.8 summarizes the physiological actions in pregnancy of ANG II.

There is considerable overlap in the ability of ANG peptides to interact with various ANG receptors (see Fig. 10.1). Therefore, they can have actions similar to those mediated by ANG II or ANG-(1–7). The physiological roles of most ANG peptides, apart from ANG II and ANG-(1–7), are unknown, particularly their role in pregnancy. Any effects of a peptide depend on its levels, its affinity, and its intrinsic activity for a given receptor. ANG peptides interacting with AT_1R might act as competitive agonists or partial antagonists of ANG II. Not only do a range of ANG peptides interact with the various G protein-coupled receptors to produce the effects described in Fig. 10.4, but they also modulate the activity of the RAS pathway itself. For example, ANG II inhibits renin release and expression of its own AT_1R, but it stimulates AGT production by the liver and renal proximal tubule.[45,46]

10.3 REGULATION AND ACTIONS OF THE cRAAS AND IRAS IN PREGNANCY

10.3.1 Changes in cRAAS in Human Pregnancy

10.3.1.1 Prorenin and Renin

Levels of both active renin and prorenin are elevated in the second half of the menstrual cycle following ovulation. Active renin is released from the kidney, but the rise in plasma prorenin could result from either renal or ovarian release.[47,48] The striking rise in plasma prorenin in early pregnancy to a maximum that is about 10 times nonpregnant levels (Fig. 10.5) at 8–12 weeks' gestation[49,50] occurs because prorenin is released from the ovary.

Bearing in mind that active renin is only produced by the kidney and the reaction between renin and AGT is of the first order, it is probable that the estrogen-induced increase in AGT in early gestation results in the production of sufficient ANG II to maintain blood volume and blood pressure. After 20 weeks' gestation, however, this AGT-dependent increase in ANG II is insufficient to meet maternal homeostatic demand. As a result, active renin is secreted by the kidney and plasma renin levels rise progressively until term (Fig. 10.5). Interestingly, plasma renin activity is elevated early in gestation and does not increase in parallel with either plasma renin or AGT, but ANG II levels are maximal in late gestation.[50,51]

FIG. 10.5 Plasma prorenin (●) and plasma active renin levels (o) throughout pregnancy. Prorenin and renin are expressed as u*Units*/mL of the MRC renin standard.[49] Prorenin was measured after activation by trypsin.[49] Mean values are shown. (*Redrawn from Derkx FH, Alberda AT, de Jong FH, Zeilmaker FH, Makovitz JW, Schalekamp MA. Source of plasma prorenin in early and late pregnancy: observations in a patient with primary ovarian failure. J Clin Endocrinol Metab 1987;65(2):349-54.*)

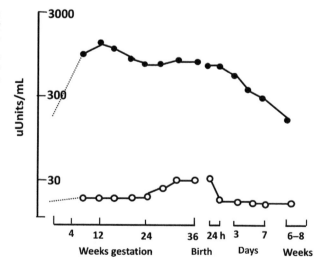

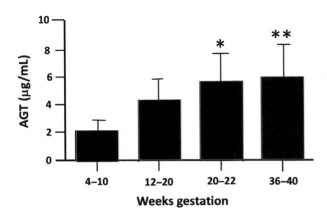

FIG. 10.6   AGT levels (µg/mL) in maternal plasma throughout pregnancy. AGT levels were lower in early gestation compared with levels measured after 20 weeks. *$P < 0.035$ and **$P < 0.001$. *(Redrawn from data used by Skinner SL, Lumbers ER, Symonds EM. Analysis of changes in the renin-angiotensin system during pregnancy.* Clin Sci *1972;42(4):479–88.)*

10.3.1.2   Prorenin Receptor and s(P)RR

(P)RR is localized to the villous syncytiotrophoblast of the placenta.[15,36] Soluble prorenin receptor levels in plasma are 32 ± 10.6 ng/mL,[15] and are higher than those measured in nonpregnant plasma (median 23.5; interquartile range 20.9–26.5 ng/mL[52]). Placental (P)RR expression does not correlate with plasma s(P)RR levels, but s(P)RR levels do correlate with blood pressure and are higher in preeclampsia.[15]

10.3.1.3   Angiotensinogen

Both AGT (Fig. 10.6) and ANG II levels rise progressively throughout pregnancy.[51] The significance of the increase in AGT in human pregnancy[50] has been underestimated. Skinner in 1993[53] emphasized that "at all stages of pregnancy, angiotensinogen is the most important factor determining plasma renin activity and presumably ANG II production."

Estrogens stimulate the production of AGT by the liver. The correlation coefficient between circulating AGT and estradiol-17ß is 0.60, and for AGT and estriol, it is 0.68.[54]

10.3.1.4   ACE and ACE2

Plasma ACE levels are lower in second- and third-trimester indigenous pregnant women compared with nonindigenous nonpregnant women.[55] Others also have reported lower levels of ACE activity in pregnancy that either do not change across gestation[56,57] or rise toward term.[58] This may not be the case in preeclampsia.[56]

The placenta expresses ACE2, which may contribute to the high levels of Ang-(1–7) measured in pregnancy.[37] Human plasma ACE2 activity is difficult to measure because of a low-molecular weight inhibitor.[59]

10.3.1.5   ANG II and ANG-(1–7)

ANG II is the major immunoreactive ANG peptide in pregnancy. Levels measured by radioimmunoassay (RIA) increase from $29.2 + 12.6$ pg/mL(sd) to $41.3 + 11.3$ pg/mL.[3] When individual ANG peptides were separated prior to assay, levels of ANG II were lower in both nonpregnant and pregnant women (9.0 ± 5.9 pmol/L and 20.4 ± 14.9 (sd) pmol/L).[3]

Fig. 10.7 shows that by the third trimester, both ANG II and ANG-(1–7) are greatly increased compared with both nonpregnant and preeclamptic women. Interestingly, the ratio of both ANG II and ANG-(1–7) relative to their precursor ANG I in the third trimester was lower than the ratio measured in nonpregnant women. Because ACE levels are lower and the conversion of ANG II to ACE2 is the major pathway for formation of ANG-(1–7), a lower level of ACE in pregnant plasma could account for the reduction in these ratios.[56] Surprisingly, the ratio of ANG-(1–7) to ANG II was less in third-trimester pregnant women than in nonpregnant women, despite the presence of placental ACE2 and high urinary ANG-(1–7) levels.[56,60] At 15 weeks' gestation, Sykes et al. found that there was sexual dimorphism in the ANG-(1–7)/ANG II ratio; it was lower in women carrying female fetuses.[61]

10.3.2   Regulation and Actions of the cRAAS in Pregnancy

While pregnancy does not begin with ovulation, ovarian function from the time of ovulation orchestrates preparation of the uterus for implantation and modification of maternal cardiovascular and renal function to optimize fetal growth and development.

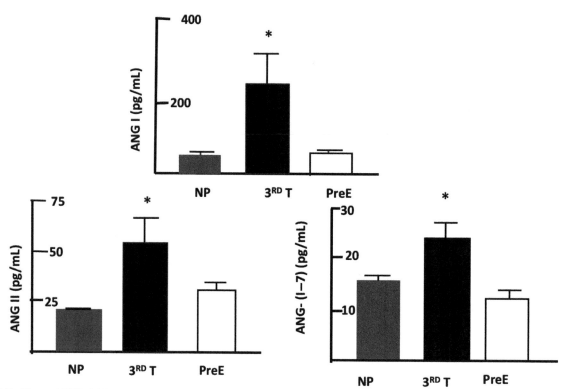

FIG. 10.7   Plasma ANG I, ANG II, and ANG-(1–7) levels (pg/mL) in nonpregnant women (NP) in normotensive women in the third trimester of pregnancy (3RD T) and in women who developed preeclamspia (PreE, *n* = 15). In the third trimester of pregnancy, the levels of all three ANG peptides are higher than those found in NP women and in women with preeclampsia *P < 0.05. *(Redrawn from Merrill DC, Karoly M, Chen K, Ferrario CM, Brosnihan KB. Angiotensin-(1–7) in normal and preeclamptic pregnancy. Endocrine 2002;18(3):239–45.)*

The mature ovarian follicle contains renin (99% as prorenin), and circulating levels of prorenin correlate with the number of ovarian follicles in women in whom hCG, FSH, and LH have been used to induce ovulation.[62] Derkx et al.[49] showed that in a woman with primary ovarian failure in whom pregnancy was induced by embryo transfer, circulating prorenin levels were only about 17% of those found in normal pregnant women, but levels of active renin were the same.

Fig. 10.8 shows how the ovary influences the activity of the cRAAS.

10.3.2.1   Ovarian Prorenin

The role of prorenin released from the ovary is unknown, as plasma levels even in pregnancy are too low to generate ANG I from AGT.[8] Progesterone acts on mineralocorticoid receptors, and so it is an aldosterone antagonist and potentially increases salt excretion, activating release of renin from the kidney. Other actions of progesterone and its metabolites may attenuate this natriuretic action.[63]

10.3.2.2   Relaxin

The ovarian hormone (relaxin) plays a major role in the relaxation of the maternal cardiovascular system in early pregnancy.[64,65] Relaxin is responsible for a pregnancy-induced increase in renal blood flow (RBF) and glomerular filtration rate (GFR).[66] One of its vasodilator actions may be mediated by the activation of two matrix metalloproteinases (MMPs), MMP-2 and MMP-9, located in endothelial caveolae. MMP-2 may cleave endothelin 1–32 from big endothelin. Endothelin 1–32 binds to a receptor (ET$_B$), raises intracellular calcium, and stimulates production of nitric oxide and prostacyclin. Therefore, relaxin, which reaches a peak at the end of the first trimester, is thought to cause a marked fall in systemic vascular resistance (SVR). At the same time, MMP-2 and MMP-9 are gelatinases and, through vascular remodeling, increase global arterial compliance, which reaches a peak at the same time as SVR reaches its nadir. MMP-9 seems to reduce myogenic tone in small vessels.

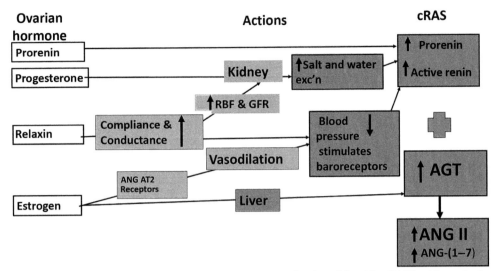

FIG. 10.8   Ovarian hormones, which in the late menstrual cycle and in pregnancy regulate the activity of the cRAAS and the production of ANG peptides. Some actions are direct (e.g., the effect of estrogens on hepatic synthesis and release of AGT). Others are indirect (e.g., effects of relaxin on the kidney and vasculature, altering blood pressure and renal sodium excretion).

The effect of relaxin is to cause underfilling of the maternal cardiovascular system and a marked rise in cardiac output so that the fall in arterial pressure is minimized. These cardiovascular events in early gestation are anticipatory, in that they occur before there is increased demand.

10.3.2.3   Estrogens

In early pregnancy, activation of the RAAS is linked to the effects of relaxin by estrogen- induced production of AGT and ANG II, providing a fail-safe mechanism that expands blood volume and offsets the natriuretic effects of the high glomerular filtration rate (GFR) and of progesterone.[63,66,67]

Increased ANG II levels resulting from the increase in AGT feed back and suppress active renin release, such that in early pregnancy levels are similar to those seen in the midluteal phase of the menstrual cycle. After 20 weeks' gestation, with increasing growth of the conceptus and increased metabolism, mechanisms that normally balance renin activity to homeostatic demand (i.e., renal sympathetic nerve activity, renal perfusion pressure, and tubular sodium flow) now come into play and active renin levels rise.

Later in gestation, increased activity of the ANG-(1–7)-MasR and ANG II/AT_2R, the kallikrein-kinin system and prostacyclin may contribute to the low vascular resistance characteristic of pregnancy.[68]

No other physiological state is characterized by as significant an increase in circulating levels of renin, AGT, ANG II, and aldosterone as that which occurs in pregnancy. The increased activity of this system is essential to counteract the effects of pregnancy induced by the ovarian hormones on maternal cardiovascular and renal function, as displayed in Fig. 10.8.

10.3.3   Actions of ANG Peptides in Pregnancy (Fig. 10.9)

The cardiovascular and renal actions of ANG II, acting via its AT_1R, maintain blood volume and uteroplacental perfusion (Fig. 10.9). To optimize these effects, the vasoconstrictor action of ANG II via the vascular AT_1R is downregulated in pregnancy. Thus, ANG II's ability to constrict blood vessels and increase blood pressure are reduced.[69,70] Also, upregulation of the ANG II/AT_2R in uterine vessels.[71,72] and increased levels of ANG-(1–7) suggest that in pregnancy, there are other changes within the RAS pathways that offset ANG II-induced vasoconstriction.

A study carried out in indigenous South American women who were pregnant compared the impact on the cRAAS of the innate changes associated with pregnancy with the effects of dietary salt intake. At the time of the study, Yanamamo women were on a very-low-sodium diet (urinary sodium; 0.7 ± 0.4 mmol/L). Pregnant Yanamamo women had plasma renin activities of 25.6 ± 6.4 ng/mL/h and urinary aldosterone-to-creatinine ratios of 459.4 ± 38.8. These levels were 5.1 times and 10.7 times those measured in lactating Yanamamo women (5.0 ± 2.6 ng/mL/h and 43.1 ± 36.7, respectively) on the same diet and reflect the nondietary-dependent demands of pregnancy on RAAS (Fig. 10.8). Pregnant Yanamamo women also had urinary aldosterone-to-creatinine ratios that were 3.6 times greater than in Guyami women, who had a higher salt intake

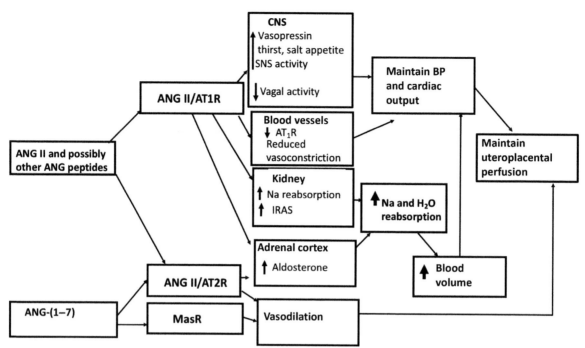

FIG. 10.9 Actions of ANG II that maintain maternal fluid and electrolyte balance and uteroplacental blood flow.

(urinary sodium 77.8 ± 30 mmol/L) and lower urinary aldosterone/creatinine (128.2 ± 97.2). This shows that pregnancy-induced changes in cardiovascular and renal function place a greater demand on the RAAS than does a low dietary salt intake.[73]

10.3.3.1 Vasopressin

Retention of both sodium and water is required to fill the maternal cardiovascular system. This can be achieved by increasing salt and water intake and by reducing salt excretion. ANG II increases both salt appetite and water intake—the latter through its ability to stimulate vasopressin.[74] Increased sodium reabsorption in the proximal parts of the nephron is accompanied by parallel increases in water reabsorption. In the distal nephron, vasopressin controls the permeability of the renal tubule. Vasopressin is secreted from neurohypophysis and is regulated by both osmoreceptors and low-pressure baroreceptors, as well as by ANG II[74,75] (Fig. 10.9). Vasopressin increases the number of water channels (aquaporins) in the renal-collecting duct and regulates the amount of water flowing into the medulla from which it is reabsorbed.

Plasma osmolality is lower in the luteal phase of the menstrual cycle; it declines further (by about 10 mosm/kg) until 10 weeks' gestation and remains low thereafter. Relaxin causes this early reduction in plasma osmolality by resetting osmoreceptors so that plasma arginine vasopressin (AVP) levels are no different from those measured in nonpregnant women, despite the lower plasma osmolality.[76,77] From the first trimester of pregnancy onward, there is also increased thirst perception and increased water intake.[78] Interestingly, in preeclampsia, there are increased levels of vasopressin (assessed by the measurement of copeptin, a protein by-product of its synthesis and release).[79] Because vasopressin is a very powerful vasoconstrictor, which also inhibits cardiac output through its effects on cardiac vagal activity,[80] it is not surprising that copeptin is a postulated biomarker for the diagnosis of preeclampsia. High levels of vasopressin could affect uteroplacental perfusion, mimicking animal models of preeclampsia caused by restricting uterine perfusion in the pregnant animal.[81]

10.3.3.2 The Intrarenal RAS

The kidney, which is the source of active circulating renin, also has within its renal tubules all the components of the RAAS to form ANG II.[82] Furthermore, the collecting duct contains renin, prorenin, and (P)RR.[83] ANG II and IL-6 stimulate intrarenal production of AGT,[46] and the ANG II formed interacts with AT_1Rs in the proximal tubule, increasing sodium reabsorption.

In the distal nephron, active renin and prorenin are located in the principal cells. ANG II stimulates renin synthesis in the principal cells of the collecting duct (CD). The (P)RR is an essential component of the vacuolar-H^+ ATPase, and it is located in the intercalated cells. Prorenin may interact with the (P)RR and play a role in the acidification of urine in the distal nephron; ANG II has been shown to stimulate acidification of urine.[84] Also, s(P)RR promotes the reabsorption of water via stimulation of aquaporin 2.[85] No studies have been carried out to see if these distal components of the IRAS are more active in pregnancy, but the high levels of ANG II (i.e., increased 12-fold) in pregnant urine might suggest that they are involved in regulating renal function in pregnancy,[68] while the 20-fold increase in ANG-(1–7)[68] suggests that it contributes to renal vasodilation.

Furthermore, the urinary AGT-to-creatinine ratio may be a biomarker for increased intrarenal production of ANG II.[86] In normal pregnant women, urinary AGT-to-creatinine ratios were higher than in nonpregnant women and increased with increasing gestation.[55] This ratio was decreased in nonindigenous pregnant women with pregnancy complications.[55] This study provides indirect evidence that increased activity of the maternal IRAS contributes to a healthy pregnancy outcome.

10.4   REPRODUCTIVE TRACT RASs (Fig. 10.10)

10.4.1   The Ovarian Renin-Angiotensin System

Pregnancy would not occur without an ovarian renin-angiotensin system (OVRAS), which, like follicle growth and ovulation, is controlled by the pituitary gonadotrophins. Blockade of the OVRAS inhibits ovulation overactivity, which may be involved in the pathogenesis of polycystic ovarian syndrome (PCOS) and ovarian hyperstimulation syndrome.

Growth of the ovarian follicle begins at the end of the luteal phase of the previous menstrual cycle, and a number of follicles develop until about days 5–7 of the next cycle. After this time, one of the follicles becomes dominant, maturing into the mature Graafian follicle containing the oocyte and its surrounding cloud of cumulus cells. Rupture of the follicular wall releases the oocyte and the accompanying cumulus; the follicle collapses and forms the corpus luteum, which secretes both estrogen and progesterone. Finally, the corpus luteum degenerates and becomes the corpus albicans.

Levels of reninlike activity and ANG II immunoreactivity in follicular fluid increase during the follicular phase of the menstrual cycle, culminating in a peak that immediately follows the midcycle peaks of the LH and FSH.[87] This is reflected

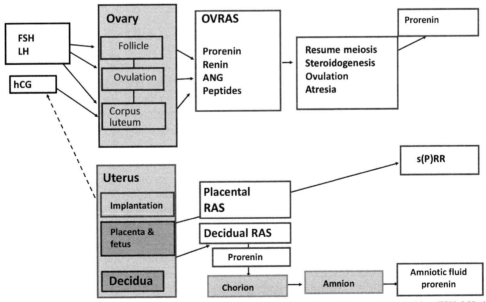

FIG. 10.10   Interrelationships between ovarian and intrauterine renin-angiotensin systems. The pituitary gonadotrophins (FSH, LH) drive maturation of the ovarian follicle, ovulation, and formation of the corpus luteum. Follicular growth and development is accompanied by production of increasing amounts of prorenin, which is either activated by plasmin and/or interacts with its (P)RR to affect ovulation, steroidogenesis, and follicular atresia. Ovarian prorenin escapes into the maternal circulation. Following implantation, the developing trophoblast drives ovarian prorenin production through chorionic gonadotrophin (hCG). The placental RAS is probably associated with the growth and development of the placenta in early gestation. The placenta may shed s(P)RR into the maternal circulation, which can affect the rate of formation of ANG II by renin acting on oxidized AGT. The decidual RAS secretes prorenin, which may affect cellular function in the chorion and amnion, and is the source of the high levels of prorenin found in amniotic fluid throughout gestation.

in a periovulatory rise in plasma prorenin levels, but not active renin, which increases later in the luteal phase of the cycle.[88] Tissue proteases that are essential for ovulation also influence follicular ANG production. The activity of plasmin (a serine protease) is controlled by the ratio of the plasminogen activator (PA) to plasminogen activator inhibitor (PAI). The PA is produced by the granulosa cells; it is essential for breakdown of the follicle and hence for ovulation. IGF-1 also stimulates PA. PAI, which inhibits proteolysis, is produced by thecal cells. PAI is inhibited by FSH.[1] Follicular prorenin may be activated by plasmin[89] and may cleave ANG I from intrafollicular AGT (the synthesis of which is possibly stimulated by estrogen). Plasmin may directly catalyze ANG 1 formation from AGT. Increasing levels of PA are associated with increased levels of active renin and ANG II.[1]

A number of actions of ANG peptides appear to be important in the life of the ovarian follicle. ANG II, along with estradiol, vascular endothelial growth factor (VEGF), and fibroblast growth factor (FGF), are important in the neovascularization associated with development of the corpus luteum.[90,91] ANG peptides play a role in regulating steroidogenesis.[91,92] ANG II has been shown to stimulate progesterone production[91] and inhibit the aromatization of androgens, increasing the androgen-to-estrogen ratio in the follicular fluid and as such promoting follicular atresia.[93] The density of AT_1 and AT_2 receptors in luteal cells and in the microvascular endothelium falls in the midluteal phase of the cycle and then rises in the late luteal phase; it also is high in atretic follicles. ANG II, acting via the AT_2R, induces apoptosis,[94] which is blocked by an AT_2R-specific antagonist.[95] Also, ANG II, acting via the AT_2R, induces self-expression of the receptor.[95]

As stated previously, a role of the OVRAS in ovulation is well described. In vitro studies using animal ovaries show that saralasin, which inhibits ANG II, blocks ovulation[96,97]; ANG II appears to induce ovulation through effects on prostaglandin production.[98]

With ovulation, the oocyte resumes meiosis, which has been arrested by cyclic adenosine monophosphate (cAMP) produced by the follicular cell wall, which is transported across the cumulus to the oocyte. Oocyte arrest in meiosis depends on contact with the follicular cell wall. LH causes closure of gap junctions in cumulus cells, a reduction in cyclic guanosine monophosphate (cGMP), activation of phosphodiesterase, and a reduction in cAMP. The oocyte normally resumes meiosis when it and its surrounding cumulus detach from the follicle cell wall.

Both ANG II and follicular prorenin that interacts with its prorenin receptor and independent of ANG II formation[99] stimulate meiosis. Both stimulate ERK1/2 cell signaling (Fig. 10.2). They do not have additive effects, but the fact that these parallel pathways exist suggests that OVRAS plays a significant role in stimulating of the resumption of meiosis. Prorenin is confined to cumulus cells, with (P)RR found on both cumulus cells and in the oocyte.

10.4.2 Intrauterine RASs

Human pregnancy would not be maintained without the intrauterine RASs. In the nonpregnant state, all the components of the RAS necessary for the formation of ANG peptides are present in the endometrium, both in stroma and in the epithelium.[100,101] Their expression shows cyclical changes, indicating control either by maternal steroid hormones or by gonadotrophins. In the late stage of the menstrual cycle, there is decidualization of endometrial stromal cells. Associated with decidualization, there is increased expression of stromal cell RAS.[102]

Once ovulation has occurred, the oocyte and its cloud of cumulus cells are shed into the abdominal cavity, picked up by the fimbriated ends of the fallopian tube and transported toward the uterine cavity. After fertilization and resumption of mitosis, a blastocyst is formed, which completely embeds within the decidual lining of the uterine wall. The blastocyst cavity has the highest levels of extrarenal renin ever reported.[12] Implantation and placentation involve proliferation, migration, and invasion by the extravillous trophoblast into the decidua, with the innermost portion forming the placenta. Early development of the placenta occurs in a hypoxic milieu. Its morphogenesis also depends on proliferation and invasion by the trophoblast and angiogenesis. In these early stages of placental development, components of the placental RAS are very highly expressed.[38] ANG II stimulates the proliferative activity of trophoblast,[103] as well as influencing the expression of angiogenic factors such as VEGF.[104,105] Shallow or inadequate placentation is associated with abnormal pregnancy outcomes such as intrauterine growth retardation, preterm birth, and preeclampsia.

While we can attribute a functional role to the trophoblastic prorenin receptor/prorenin-angiotensin system in placentation, the contribution of the decidual renin-angiotensin system to fetal health and well-being is unknown. The decidua is the source of the very high prorenin levels found in the chorion, amnion, and amniotic fluid found in late gestation.[13,106] Angiotensin stimulates neovascularization. This effect is readily demonstrated in the chick chorioallantoic membrane.[107,108] It is tempting to suggest that decidual prorenin influences the vascularity of the chorionic villi, which has been shown to be altered in human placentas collected from pathological pregnancies.[109]

At term, there is sexual dimorphism in the expression of decidual RAS.[110] Expression of prorenin is much higher than in decidua collected from women who have had a female fetus than from those carrying a male fetus. After labor, levels of prorenin expression are the same.[110] Decidual explants from women carrying female fetuses produce more renin protein and express the anti-inflammatory ACE2-MasR pathway to a greater extent than decidua from women carrying male fetuses.[110] The ANG II/AT$_1$R pathway stimulates NF-kB pathways, and thus stimulates production of proinflammatory cytokines.[111] The ACE2-Ang-(1–7)-MasR pathway is associated with an anti-inflammatory cytokine profile. The prevalence of proinflammatory mediators is associated with parturition.[112] Spontaneous preterm birth and premature rupture of the membranes leading to preterm birth are much more common if the infant is male. The higher level of expression of the anti-inflammatory ACE2-Ang-(1–7)-MasR pathway may protect the female fetus from preterm birth.

Overexpression of the prorenin receptor can cause fibrosis.[113] High levels of decidual prorenin flooding the amnion and binding to its prorenin receptor may well help maintain the integrity of the amnion. In female fetal membranes, there is a higher level of expression of (P)RR.[114] Thus, the greater level of expression of the decidual prorenin-ANG II-ANG-(1–7) system also may protect female infants from preterm parturition and premature rupture of the fetal membranes.

In conclusion, increased activity of maternal circulating and tissue RASs is essential for normal pregnancy. Exactly how these systems are involved in maternal reproductive health is yet to be fully defined, except for the role of the cRAAS in maternal fluid and electrolyte homeostasis, and therefore in maintaining uteroplacental perfusion.

ACKNOWLEDGMENTS

I would like to acknowledge the help of Dr. Amanda Boyce and Dr. Kirsty Pringle in reading and editing this manuscript, and Dr. Pringle for help with the diagrams.

REFERENCES

1. Palumbo A, Avila J, Naftolin F. The ovarian renin-angiotensin system (OVRAS): a major factor in ovarian function and disease. *Reprod Sci* 2016;**23**(12):1644–55.
2. Chappell MC. Biochemical evaluation of the renin-angiotensin system: the good, bad, and absolute? *Am J Physiol Heart Circ Physiol* 2016;**310**(2):H137–52.
3. Hanssens M, Keirse MJ, Spitz B, Van Assche FA. Measurement of individual plasma angiotensins in normal pregnancy and pregnancy-induced hypertension. *J Clin Endocrinol Metab* 1991;**73**(3):489–94.
4. Lumbers ER. Activation of renin in human amniotic fluid by low pH. *Enzymologia* 1971;**40**(6):329–36.
5. Morris BJ, Lumbers ER. The activation of renin in human amniotic fluid by proteolytic enzymes. *Biochim Biophys Acta* 1972;**289**(2):385–91.
6. Inagami T, Okamoto H, Ohtsuki K, Shimamoto K, Chao J, Margolius HS. Human plasma inactive renin: purification and activation by proteases. *J Clin Endocrinol Metab* 1982;**55**(4):619–27.
7. Sealey JE, Moon C, Laragh JH, Alderman M. Plasma prorenin: cryoactivation and relationship to renin substrate in normal subjects. *Am J Med* 1976;**61**(5):731–8.
8. Batenburg WW, Krop M, Garrelds IM, de Vries R, de Bruin RJ, Burckle CA, et al. Prorenin is the endogenous agonist of the (pro)renin receptor. Binding kinetics of renin and prorenin in rat vascular smooth muscle cells overexpressing the human (pro)renin receptor. *J Hypertens* 2007;**25**(12):2441–53.
9. Nguyen G, Delarue F, Burckle C, Bouzhir L, Giller T, Sraer JD. Pivotal role of the renin/prorenin receptor in angiotensin II production and cellular responses to renin. *J Clin Invest* 2002;**109**(11):1417–27.
10. Nguyen G. Renin, (pro)renin and receptor: an update. *Clin Sci (Lond)* 2011;**120**(5):169–78.
11. Travis J, Salvesen GS. Human plasma proteinase inhibitors. *Annu Rev Biochem* 1983;**52**:655–709.
12. Itskovitz J, Rubattu S, Levron J, Sealey JE. Highest concentrations of prorenin and human chorionic gonadotropin in gestational sacs during early human pregnancy. *J Clin Endocrinol Metab* 1992;**75**(3):906–10.
13. Skinner SL, Lumbers ER, Symonds EM. Renin concentration in human fetal and maternal tissues. *Am J Obstet Gynecol* 1968;**101**(4):529–33.
14. Cousin C, Bracquart D, Contrepas A, Corvol P, Muller L, Nguyen G. Soluble form of the (pro)renin receptor generated by intracellular cleavage by furin is secreted in plasma. *Hypertension* 2009;**53**(6):1077–82.
15. Narita T, Ichihara A, Matsuoka K, Takai Y, Bokuda K, Morimoto S, et al. Placental (pro)renin receptor expression and plasma soluble (pro)renin receptor levels in preeclampsia. *Placenta* 2016;**37**:72–8.
16. Zhou A, Carrell RW, Murphy MP, Wei Z, Yan Y, Stanley PL, et al. A redox switch in angiotensinogen modulates angiotensin release. *Nature* 2010;**468**(7320):108–11.
17. Tewksbury DA, Kaiser SJ, Burrill RE. A study of the temporal relationship between plasma high molecular weight angiotensinogen and the development of pregnancy-induced hypertension. *Am J Hypertens* 2001;**14**(8 Pt 1):794–7.
18. Bouhnik J, Clauser E, Strosberg D, Frenoy JP, Menard J, Corvol P. Rat angiotensinogen and des(angiotensin I)angiotensinogen: purification, characterization, and partial sequencing. *Biochemistry* 1981;**20**(24):7010–5.

19. Hilgenfeldt U, Kellermann W, Kienapfel G, Jochum M. Relationship between angiotensinogen, alpha 1-protease inhibitor elastase complex, antithrombin III and C-reactive protein in septic ARDS. *Eur J Clin Pharmacol* 1990;**38**(2):125–31.

20. Zuo L, Pannell BK, Zhou T, Chuang CC. Historical role of alpha-1-antitrypsin deficiency in respiratory and hepatic complications. *Gene* 2016;**589** (2):118–22.

21. Lai HS, Lin WH, Lai SL, Lin HY, Hsu WM, Chou CH, et al. Interleukin-6 mediates angiotensinogen gene expression during liver regeneration. *PLoS One* 2013;**8**(7).

22. Brand M, Lamande N, Larger E, Corvol P, Gasc JM. Angiotensinogen impairs angiogenesis in the chick chorioallantoic membrane. *J Mol Med (Berl)* 2007;**85**(5):451–60.

23. Hunyady L, Catt KJ. Pleiotropic AT1 receptor signaling pathways mediating physiological and pathogenic actions of angiotensin II. *Mol Endocrinol* 2006;**20**(5):953–70.

24. Tewksbury DA. Angiotensinogen. *Fed Proc* 1983;**42**(10):2724–8.

25. Oxvig C, Haaning J, Kristensen L, Wagner JM, Rubin I, Stigbrand T, et al. Identification of angiotensinogen and complement C3dg as novel proteins binding the proform of eosinophil major basic protein in human pregnancy serum and plasma. *J Biol Chem* 1995;**270**(23):13645–51.

26. Tewksbury DA, Dart RA. High molecular weight angiotensinogen levels in hypertensive pregnant women. *Hypertension* 1982;**4**(5):729–34.

27. Weyer K, Glerup S. Placental regulation of peptide hormone and growth factor activity by proMBP. *Biol Reprod* 2011;**84**(6):1077–86.

28. Gordon DB, Sachin IN, Dodd VN. Heterogeneity of renin substrate in human plasma: effect of pregnancy and oral contraceptives. *Proc Soc Exp Biol Med* 1976;**153**(2):314–8.

29. Tewksbury DA. Quantitation of five forms of high molecular weight angiotensinogen from human placenta. *Am J Hypertens* 1996;**9**(10 Pt 1):1029–34.

30. Overgaard MT, Oxvig C, Christiansen M, Lawrence JB, Conover CA, Gleich GJ, et al. Messenger ribonucleic acid levels of pregnancy-associated plasma protein-A and the proform of eosinophil major basic protein: expression in human reproductive and nonreproductive tissues. *Biol Reprod* 1999;**61**(4):1083–9.

31. Dzau VJ, Bernstein K, Celermajer D, Cohen J, Dahlof B, Deanfield J, et al. Pathophysiologic and therapeutic importance of tissue ACE: a consensus report. *Cardiovasc Drugs Ther* 2002;**16**(2):149–60.

32. Gonzalez-Garrido JA, Garcia-Sanchez JR, Tovar-Rodriguez JM, Olivares-Corichi IM. Preeclampsia is associated with ACE I/D polymorphism, obesity and oxidative damage in Mexican women. *Pregnancy Hypertens* 2017;**10**:22–7.

33. Donoghue M, Hsieh F, Baronas E, Godbout K, Gosselin M, Stagliano N, et al. A novel angiotensin-converting enzyme-related carboxypeptidase (ACE2) converts angiotensin I to angiotensin 1-9. *Circ Res* 2000;**87**(5):E1–9.

34. Kuba K, Imai Y, Rao S, Gao H, Guo F, Guan B, et al. A crucial role of angiotensin converting enzyme 2 (ACE2) in SARS coronavirus-induced lung injury. *Nat Med* 2005;**11**(8):875–9.

35. Vickers C, Hales P, Kaushik V, Dick L, Gavin J, Tang J, et al. Hydrolysis of biological peptides by human angiotensin-converting enzyme-related carboxypeptidase. *J Biol Chem* 2002;**277**(17):14838–43.

36. Marques FZ, Pringle KG, Conquest A, Hirst JJ, Markus MA, Sarris M, et al. Molecular characterization of renin-angiotensin system components in human intrauterine tissues and fetal membranes from vaginal delivery and cesarean section. *Placenta* 2011;**32**(3):214–21.

37. Valdes G, Neves LA, Anton L, Corthorn J, Chacon C, Germain AM, et al. Distribution of angiotensin-(1–7) and ACE2 in human placentas of normal and pathological pregnancies. *Placenta* 2006;**27**(2–3):200–7.

38. Pringle KG, Tadros MA, Callister RJ, Lumbers ER. The expression and localization of the human placental prorenin/renin-angiotensin system throughout pregnancy: roles in trophoblast invasion and angiogenesis? *Placenta* 2011;**32**(12):956–62.

39. Mehta PK, Griendling KK. Angiotensin II cell signaling: physiological and pathological effects in the cardiovascular system. *Am J Physiol Cell Physiol* 2007;**292**(1):C82–97.

40. Albiston AL, Mustafa T, McDowall SG, Mendelsohn FA, Lee J, Chai SY. AT4 receptor is insulin-regulated membrane aminopeptidase: potential mechanisms of memory enhancement. *Trends Endocrinol Metab* 2003;**14**(2):72–7.

41. Erlandson SC, McMahon C, Kruse AC. Structural basis for G protein-coupled receptor signaling. *Annu Rev Biophys* 2018;**47**:1–18.

42. Jankowski V, Vanholder R, van der Giet M, Tolle M, Karadogan S, Gobom J, et al. Mass-spectrometric identification of a novel angiotensin peptide in human plasma. *Arterioscler Thromb Vasc Biol* 2007;**27**(2):297–302.

43. Hrenak J, Paulis L, Simko F. Angiotensin A/alamandine/MrgD axis: another clue to understanding cardiovascular pathophysiology. *Int J Mol Sci* 2016;**17**(7):1098.

44. Bharadwaj MS, Strawn WB, Groban L, Yamaleyeva LM, Chappell MC, Horta C, et al. Angiotensin-converting enzyme 2 deficiency is associated with impaired gestational weight gain and fetal growth restriction. *Hypertension* 2011;**58**(5):852–8.

45. Herrmann HC, Dzau VJ. The feedback regulation of angiotensinogen production by components of the renin-angiotensin system. *Circ Res* 1983;**52** (3):328–34.

46. Kobori H, Harrison-Bernard LM, Navar LG. Expression of angiotensinogen mRNA and protein in angiotensin II-dependent hypertension. *J Am Soc Nephrol* 2001;**12**(3):431–9.

47. Skinner SL, Lumbers ER, Symonds EM. Alteration by oral contraceptives of normal menstrual changes in plasma renin activity, concentration and substrate. *Clin Sci* 1969;**36**(1):67–76.

48. Sealey JE, Cholst I, Glorioso N, Troffa C, Weintraub ID, James G, et al. Sequential changes in plasma luteinizing hormone and plasma prorenin during the menstrual cycle. *J Clin Endocrinol Metab* 1987;**65**(1):1–5.

49. Derkx FH, Alberda AT, de Jong FH, Zeilmaker FH, Makovitz JW, Schalekamp MA. Source of plasma prorenin in early and late pregnancy: observations in a patient with primary ovarian failure. *J Clin Endocrinol Metab* 1987;**65**(2):349–54.
50. Skinner SL, Lumbers ER, Symonds EM. Analysis of changes in the renin-angiotensin system during pregnancy. *Clin Sci* 1972;**42**(4):479–88.
51. Baker PN, Broughton Pipkin F, Symonds EM. Platelet angiotensin II binding and plasma renin concentration, plasma renin substrate and plasma angiotensin II in human pregnancy. *Clin Sci (Lond)* 1990;**79**(4):403–8.
52. Nguyen G, Blanchard A, Curis E, Bergerot D, Chambon Y, Hirose T, et al. Plasma soluble (pro)renin receptor is independent of plasma renin, prorenin, and aldosterone concentrations but is affected by ethnicity. *Hypertension* 2014;**63**(2):297–302.
53. Skinner SL. The renin-angiotensin system in fertility and normal human pregnancy. In: Robertson JIS, Nicholls GM, editors. The renin-angiotensin system. vol. 50. UK: Gower Medical Publishing; 1993. p. 50.1–50.16.
54. Immonen I, Siimes A, Stenman UH, Karkkainen J, Fyhrquist F. Plasma renin substrate and oestrogens in normal pregnancy. *Scand J Clin Lab Invest* 1983;**43**(1):61–5.
55. Pringle KG, de Meaultsart CC, Sykes SD, Weatherall LJ, Keogh L, Clausen DC, et al. Urinary angiotensinogen excretion in Australian indigenous and non-indigenous pregnant women. *Pregnancy Hypertens* 2018;**12**:110–7.
56. Merrill DC, Karoly M, Chen K, Ferrario CM, Brosnihan KB. Angiotensin-(1–7) in normal and preeclamptic pregnancy. *Endocrine* 2002;**18**(3):239–45.
57. Goldkrand JW, Fuentes AM. The relation of angiotensin-converting enzyme to the pregnancy-induced hypertension-preeclampsia syndrome. *Am J Obstet Gynecol* 1986;**154**(4):792–800.
58. Oats JN, Broughton Pipkin F, Symonds EM, Craven DJ. A prospective study of plasma angiotensin-converting enzyme in normotensive primigravidae and their infants. *Br J Obstet Gynaecol* 1981;**88**(12):1204–10.
59. Lew RA, Warner FJ, Hanchapola I, Yarski MA, Ramchand J, Burrell LM, et al. Angiotensin-converting enzyme 2 catalytic activity in human plasma is masked by an endogenous inhibitor. *Exp Physiol* 2008;**93**(5):685–93.
60. Valdes G, Germain AM, Corthorn J, Berrios C, Foradori AC, Ferrario CM, et al. Urinary vasodilator and vasoconstrictor angiotensins during menstrual cycle, pregnancy, and lactation. *Endocrine* 2001;**16**(2):117–22.
61. Sykes SD, Pringle KG, Zhou A, Dekker GA, Roberts CT, Lumbers ER, et al. The balance between human maternal plasma angiotensin II and angiotensin 1–7 levels in early gestation pregnancy is influenced by fetal sex. *J Renin Angiotensin Aldosterone Syst* 2014;**15**(4):523–31.
62. Itskovitz J, Sealey JE, Glorioso N, Rosenwaks Z. Plasma prorenin response to human chorionic gonadotropin in ovarian-hyperstimulated women: correlation with the number of ovarian follicles and steroid hormone concentrations. *Proc Natl Acad Sci U S A* 1987;**84**(20):7285–9.
63. Quinkler M, Meyer B, Oelkers W, Diederich S. Renal inactivation, mineralocorticoid generation, and 11beta-hydroxysteroid dehydrogenase inhibition ameliorate the antimineralocorticoid effect of progesterone in vivo. *J Clin Endocrinol Metab* 2003;**88**(8):3767–72.
64. Conrad KP. Maternal vasodilation in pregnancy: the emerging role of relaxin. *Am J Physiol Regul Integr Comp Physiol* 2011;**301**(2):R267–75.
65. Conrad KP, Davison JM. The renal circulation in normal pregnancy and preeclampsia: is there a place for relaxin? *Am J Physiol Renal Physiol* 2014;**306**(10):F1121–35.
66. Abduljalil K, Furness P, Johnson TN, Rostami-Hodjegan A, Soltani H. Anatomical, physiological and metabolic changes with gestational age during normal pregnancy: a database for parameters required in physiologically based pharmacokinetic modelling. *Clin Pharmacokinet* 2012;**51**(6):365–96.
67. Quinkler M, Meyer B, Bumke-Vogt C, Grossmann C, Gruber U, Oelkers W, et al. Agonistic and antagonistic properties of progesterone metabolites at the human mineralocorticoid receptor. *Eur J Endocrinol* 2002;**146**(6):789–99.
68. Valdes G, Kaufmann P, Corthorn J, Erices R, Brosnihan KB, Joyner-Grantham J. Vasodilator factors in the systemic and local adaptations to pregnancy. *Reprod Biol Endocrinol* 2009;**7**:79.
69. Lumbers ER. Peripheral vascular reactivity to angiotensin and noradrenaline in pregnant and non-pregnant women. *Aust J Exp Biol Med Sci* 1970;**48**(5):493–500.
70. Magness RR, Cox K, Rosenfeld CR, Gant NF. Angiotensin II metabolic clearance rate and pressor responses in nonpregnant and pregnant women. *Am J Obstet Gynecol* 1994;**171**(3):668–79.
71. McMullen JR, Gibson KJ, Lumbers ER, Burrell JH, Wu J. Interactions between AT1 and AT2 receptors in uterine arteries from pregnant ewes. *Eur J Pharmacol* 1999;**378**(2):195–202.
72. McMullen JR, Gibson KJ, Lumbers ER, Burrell JH. Selective down-regulation of AT2 receptors in uterine arteries from pregnant ewes given 24-h intravenous infusions of angiotensin II. *Regul Pept* 2001;**99**(2–3):119–29.
73. Oliver WJ, Neel JV, Grekin RJ, Cohen EL. Hormonal adaptation to the stresses imposed upon sodium balance by pregnancy and lactation in the Yanomama Indians, a culture without salt. *Circulation* 1981;**63**(1):110–6.
74. Johnson AK, Thunhorst RL. The neuroendocrinology of thirst and salt appetite: visceral sensory signals and mechanisms of central integration. *Front Neuroendocrinol* 1997;**18**(3):292–353.
75. Sandgren JA, Linggonegoro DW, Zhang SY, Sapouckey SA, Claflin KE, Pearson NA, et al. Angiotensin AT1A receptors expressed in vasopressin-producing cells of the supraoptic nucleus contribute to the osmotic control of vasopressin. *Am J Physiol Regul Integr Comp Physiol* 2018;**314**:R770–80.
76. Weisinger RS, Burns P, Eddie LW, Wintour EM. Relaxin alters the plasma osmolality-arginine vasopressin relationship in the rat. *J Endocrinol* 1993;**137**(3):505–10.
77. Lindheimer MD, Davison JM. Osmoregulation, the secretion of arginine vasopressin and its metabolism during pregnancy. *Eur J Endocrinol* 1995;**132**(2):133–43.
78. L AFaO. Thirst perception and fluid intake in pregnant female humans in the three trimesters of pregnancy. wwweajournalsorg, 2017;**5**:33–48.

79. Sandgren JA, Scroggins SM, Santillan DA, Devor EJ, Gibson-Corley KN, Pierce GL, et al. Vasopressin: the missing link for preeclampsia? *Am J Physiol Regul Integr Comp Physiol* 2015;**309**(9):R1062–4.

80. Caine AC, Lumbers ER, Reid IA. The effects and interactions of angiotensin and vasopressin on the heart of unanaesthetized sheep. *J Physiol* 1985;**367**:1–11.

81. Fushima T, Sekimoto A, Minato T, Ito T, Oe Y, Kisu K, et al. Reduced uterine perfusion pressure (RUPP) model of preeclampsia in mice. *PLoS One* 2016;**11**(5).

82. Kobori H, Nangaku M, Navar LG, Nishiyama A. The intrarenal renin-angiotensin system: from physiology to the pathobiology of hypertension and kidney disease. *Pharmacol Rev* 2007;**59**(3):251–87.

83. Gonzalez AA, Prieto MC. Roles of collecting duct renin and (pro)renin receptor in hypertension: mini review. *Ther Adv Cardiovasc Dis* 2015;**9**(4):191–200.

84. Advani A, Kelly DJ, Cox AJ, White KE, Advani SL, Thai K. The (pro)renin receptor: site-specific and functional linkage to the vacuolar H+-ATPase in the kidney. *Hypertension* 2009;**54**(2):261–9.

85. Lu X, Wang F, Xu C, Soodvilai S, Peng K, Su J, et al. Soluble (pro)renin receptor via beta-catenin enhances urine concentration capability as a target of liver X receptor. *Proc Natl Acad Sci U S A* 2016;**113**(13):E1898–906.

86. Nishiyama A, Kobori H. Independent regulation of renin-angiotensin-aldosterone system in the kidney. *Clin Exp Nephrol* 2018;**22**:1231–9.

87. Lightman A, Tarlatzis BC, Rzasa PJ, Culler MD, Caride VJ, Negro-Vilar AF, et al. The ovarian renin-angiotensin system: renin-like activity and angiotensin II/III immunoreactivity in gonadotropin-stimulated and unstimulated human follicular fluid. *Am J Obstet Gynecol* 1987;**156**(4):808–16.

88. Sealey JE, Atlas SA, Glorioso N, Manapat H, Laragh JH. Cyclical secretion of prorenin during the menstrual cycle: synchronization with luteinizing hormone and progesterone. *Proc Natl Acad Sci U S A* 1985;**82**(24):8705–9.

89. Lumbers ER, editor. *The ovary*. New York: C.V. Mosby; 1993.

90. Hayashi K, Miyamoto A, Berisha B, Kosmann MR, Okuda K, Schams D. Regulation of angiotensin II production and angiotensin receptors in microvascular endothelial cells from bovine corpus luteum. *Biol Reprod* 2000;**62**(1):162–7.

91. Kobayashi S, Berisha B, Amselgruber WM, Schams D, Miyamoto A. Production and localisation of angiotensin II in the bovine early corpus luteum: a possible interaction with luteal angiogenic factors and prostaglandin F2 alpha. *J Endocrinol* 2001;**170**(2):369–80.

92. Morris RS, Francis MM, Do YS, Hsueh WA, Lobo RA, Paulson RJ. Angiotensin II (AII) modulation of steroidogenesis by luteinized granulosa cells in vitro. *J Assist Reprod Genet* 1994;**11**(3):117–22.

93. Feral C, Le Gall S, Leymarie P. Angiotensin II modulates steroidogenesis in granulosa and theca in the rabbit ovary: its possible involvement in atresia. *Eur J Endocrinol* 1995;**133**(6):747–53.

94. Acosta E, Pena O, Naftolin F, Avila J, Palumbo A. Angiotensin II induces apoptosis in human mural granulosa-lutein cells, but not in cumulus cells. *Fertil Steril* 2009;**91**(Suppl 5):1984–9.

95. Tanaka M, Ohnishi J, Ozawa Y, Sugimoto M, Usuki S, Naruse M, et al. Characterization of angiotensin II receptor type 2 during differentiation and apoptosis of rat ovarian cultured granulosa cells. *Biochem Biophys Res Commun* 1995;**207**(2):593–8.

96. Kuo TC, Endo K, Dharmarajan AM, Miyazaki T, Atlas SJ, Wallach EE. Direct effect of angiotensin II on in-vitro perfused rabbit ovary. *J Reprod Fertil* 1991;**92**(2):469–74.

97. Sahin Y, Kontas O, Muderris II, Cankurtaran M. Effects of angiotensin converting enzyme inhibitor cilazapril and angiotensin II antagonist saralasin in ovarian hyperstimulation syndrome in the rabbit. *Gynecol Endocrinol* 1997;**11**(4):231–6.

98. Yoshimura Y, Karube M, Oda T, Koyama N, Shiokawa S, Akiba M, et al. Locally produced angiotensin II induces ovulation by stimulating prostaglandin production in in vitro perfused rabbit ovaries. *Endocrinology* 1993;**133**(4):1609–16.

99. Dau AM, da Silva EP, da Rosa PR, Bastiani FT, Gutierrez K, Ilha GF, et al. Bovine ovarian cells have (pro)renin receptors and prorenin induces resumption of meiosis in vitro. *Peptides* 2016;**81**:1–8.

100. Li XF, Ahmed A. Dual role of angiotensin II in the human endometrium. *Hum Reprod* 1996;**11**(Suppl 2):95–108.

101. Li XF, Ahmed A. Compartmentalization and cyclic variation of immunoreactivity of renin and angiotensin converting enzyme in human endometrium throughout the menstrual cycle. *Hum Reprod* 1997;**12**(12):2804–9.

102. Lumbers ER, Wang Y, Delforce SJ, Corbisier de Meaultsart C, Logan PC, Mitchell MD, et al. Decidualisation of human endometrial stromal cells is associated with increased expression and secretion of prorenin. *Reprod Biol Endocrinol* 2015;**13**:129.

103. Araki-Taguchi M, Nomura S, Ino K, Sumigama S, Yamamoto E, Kotani-Ito T, et al. Angiotensin II mimics the hypoxic effect on regulating trophoblast proliferation and differentiation in human placental explant cultures. *Life Sci* 2008;**82**(1–2):59–67.

104. Sanchez-Lopez E, Lopez AF, Esteban V, Yague S, Egido J, Ruiz-Ortega M, et al. Angiotensin II regulates vascular endothelial growth factor via hypoxia-inducible factor-1alpha induction and redox mechanisms in the kidney. *Antioxid Redox Signal* 2005;**7**(9–10):1275–84.

105. Delforce SJ, Wang Y, Van-Aalst ME, Corbisier de Meaultsart C, Morris BJ, Broughton-Pipkin F, et al. Effect of oxygen on the expression of renin-angiotensin system components in a human trophoblast cell line. *Placenta* 2016;**37**:1–6.

106. Shaw KJ, Do YS, Kjos S, Anderson PW, Shinagawa T, Dubeau L, et al. Human decidua is a major source of renin. *J Clin Invest* 1989;**83**(6):2085–92.

107. Le Noble FA, Hekking JW, Van Straaten HW, Slaaf DW, Struyker Boudier HA. Angiotensin II stimulates angiogenesis in the chorio-allantoic membrane of the chick embryo. *Eur J Pharmacol* 1991;**195**(2):305–6.

108. Le Noble FA, Schreurs NH, van Straaten HW, Slaaf DW, Smits JF, Rogg H, et al. Evidence for a novel angiotensin II receptor involved in angiogenesis in chick embryo chorioallantoic membrane. *Am J Physiol* 1993;**264**(2 Pt. 2):R460–5.

109. Mayhew TM, Charnock-Jones DS, Kaufmann P. Aspects of human fetoplacental vasculogenesis and angiogenesis. III. Changes in complicated pregnancies. *Placenta* 2004;**25**(2–3):127–39.

110. Wang Y, Pringle KG, Sykes SD, Marques FZ, Morris BJ, Zakar T, et al. Fetal sex affects expression of renin-angiotensin system components in term human decidua. *Endocrinology* 2012;**153**(1):462–8.

111. Ruiz-Ortega M, Bustos C, Hernandez-Presa MA, Lorenzo O, Plaza JJ, Egido J. Angiotensin II participates in mononuclear cell recruitment in experimental immune complex nephritis through nuclear factor-kappa B activation and monocyte chemoattractant protein-1 synthesis. *J Immunol* 1998;**161**(1):430–9.

112. Haddad R, Tromp G, Kuivaniemi H, Chaiworapongsa T, Kim YM, Mazor M, et al. Human spontaneous labor without histologic chorioamnionitis is characterized by an acute inflammation gene expression signature. *Am J Obstet Gynecol* 2006;**195**(2):394. e1–24.

113. Nguyen G, Danser AH. Prorenin and (pro)renin receptor: a review of available data from in vitro studies and experimental models in rodents. *Exp Physiol* 2008;**93**(5):557–63.

114. Pringle KG, Conquest A, Mitchell C, Zakar T, Lumbers ER. Effects of fetal sex on expression of the (pro)renin receptor and genes influenced by its interaction with prorenin in human amnion. *Reprod Sci* 2015;**22**(6):750–7.

Chapter 11

Central Role of Adipose Tissue in Pregnancy and Lactation

David C.W. Lau

Departments of Medicine, Biochemistry and Molecular Biology, University of Calgary Cumming School of Medicine, Calgary, AB, Canada

> **Key Clinical Changes**
> - Insulin sensitivity decreases by 40%–50% of prepregnancy levels as pregnancy advances to facilitate nutrient flow for optimal fetal growth and development.
> - Maternal fat accretion is accompanied by increased release of adipokines that play a role in modulating intermediary metabolism and insulin resistance.
> - Glucose homeostasis is maintained throughout a normal pregnancy by increased insulin secretion through β-cell hypertrophy and hyperplasia.
> - Changes in maternal metabolism and insulin resistance return to prepregnancy states in postpartum.
> - Lactation may be associated with short- and long-term cardiovascular benefits in the mother.
> - Excessive adiposity preconception and gestational weight gain during pregnancy are associated with adverse pregnancy outcomes and fetal anomalies.

11.1 INTRODUCTION

Pregnancy is characterized by complex metabolic and hormonal adaptations of the mother to meet the increasing physiological and energy demands needed to provide adequate nutrient flow for growth and development of the fetus, as well as during labor, delivery, and lactation.[1] While maternal body weight and body fat increase in a normal pregnancy, increased maternal weight at conception and excessive gestational weight gain are associated with increased risk of pregnancy complications, such as gestational diabetes, preeclampsia, abnormal fetal growth, and anomalies. Hence, an understanding of the mechanisms of body fat regulation and the changes in intermediary metabolism during pregnancy and lactation will not only provide insights into the physiology of a normal pregnancy, but also lead to optimal management of pregnancy and successful outcomes.

This chapter focuses on the changes in carbohydrate, protein, and lipid metabolism during pregnancy and lactation, as well as the central role of adipose tissue and its adipocytokines in altering maternal intermediary metabolism and insulin sensitivity in normal and complicated pregnancies.

11.2 OVERVIEW OF MATERNAL METABOLISM DURING PREGNANCY

Complex metabolic and hormonal adaptations occur in the mother during pregnancy to make glucose the principal fuel substrate readily available to the fetus to facilitate optimum fetal development. During early gestation in the first trimester of pregnancy, maternal changes in intermediary metabolism lead to the development of an anabolic state with increased fat stores. Insulin sensitivity decreases by 40%–50% in the second and third trimesters, but it returns to the prepregnancy state within days following delivery or during lactation.[1]

Maternal-Fetal and Neonatal Endocrinology. https://doi.org/10.1016/B978-0-12-814823-5.00011-8

11.2.1 Glucose Metabolism

Maternal glucose metabolism gradually changes over the course of pregnancy to favor a steady supply of glucose to the growing fetus. In the early phase of pregnancy, fasting glucose is unchanged and maintained at about 5 mmol/L (90 mg/dL), with rates of hepatic glucose production matched by rates of glucose uptake in the brain, red blood cells, and splanchnic tissues.[2] A median decrease in fasting glucose of 0.11 mmol/L (2 mg/dL) was observed between 6 and 10 weeks of gestation, suggesting increased insulin sensitivity in early maternal adaptation before any significant embryonic or fetal growth, resulting in a lower glucoregulatory set point in the liver. As pregnancy progresses from the first to the second trimester, a modest decline in fasting glucose continues in women with normal weight, despite an increase in hepatic glucose production. These changes are accompanied by increased fasting insulin levels, indicating an insulin resistance state. By using the euglycemic-hyperinsulinemic clamp study, it has been estimated that insulin sensitivity is reduced by 10% in early gestation, and by about 55%–60% in the third trimester of pregnancy.[3] The reduced insulin-mediated glucose utilization switches the maternal energy metabolism from glucose to free fatty acids, thereby channeling glucose to the fetus.

The progressive insulin-resistant state that develops during a normal pregnancy is similar to that observed in type 2 diabetes, with impaired insulin action occurring mainly at the postreceptor-signaling pathways. The degree of insulin resistance is influenced by maternal adiposity and genetic factors, which is higher in women with obesity, and even greater in women with obesity and gestational diabetes (GDM).[3]

Despite the progressive increase in insulin resistance throughout pregnancy, glucose homeostasis is maintained by a concomitant increase in insulin secretion by about twofold in the third trimester. Both first- and second-phase insulin response to intravenous glucose challenge are increased with advancing gestion in healthy pregnant women.[3] Following delivery, insulin secretion returns to normal prepregnancy levels. Interestingly, insulin secretion has been noted to increase early in the second trimester before significant insulin resistance develops, suggesting the possibility of β-cell hypertrophy or hyperplasia. Indeed, maternal β-cell hypertrophy and hyperplasia are observed in normal pregnancy in response to high levels of circulating human placental lactogen (also known as *human chorionic somatomammotropin*), prolactin, progesterone, cortisol, and growth hormone to adapt to the increasing demands for enhanced insulin secretion.[4]

11.2.2 Lipid Metabolism

While changes in glucose metabolism are considered the primary metabolic adaptation during pregnancy, significant alterations in lipid metabolism also occur to promote fat accretion in early pregnancy and midpregnancy, as well as enhanced fat mobilization in late pregnancy. Lipid metabolism appears to differ between lean and obese women with normal glucose metabolism. In lean women lipogenesis occurs in the first trimester as a result of increased levels of estrogen, progesterone and insulin, whereas lipolysis is seen late in the third trimester (34–36 weeks). Human placental lactogen, also known as *chorionic somatomammotropin*, appears to be the principal hormone inducing lipolysis and fat mobilization. Pregnant women with obesity demonstrate lipolysis in both early and late gestation, and this difference is attributable to a greater degree of insulin resistance in obese compared with nonobese women.[3] Plasma lipid levels initially fall in the first 8 weeks of gestation but tend to increase progressively beginning in the first trimester. Plasma triglyceride are two to four times higher than the prepregnancy levels, whereas total cholesterol levels increase by 25%–50% in the third trimester. Free fatty acid levels are higher during pregnancy and increase further in late pregnancy, partly due to insulin's inability to suppress lipolysis. Free fatty acids in turn can impair β-cell insulin secretion and further augment the insulin-resistant state in the third trimester.[3] Following parturition, the plasma free fatty acids fall to nonpregnancy levels within a few days and triglycerides in 2 weeks.

11.2.3 Protein Metabolism

During pregnancy, circulating amino acid levels, notably the gluconeogenic amino acids (alanine, serine, and threonine), tend to decrease in both the fasting and postprandial state, mainly due to increased hepatic uptake and de novo gluconeogenesis. Pregnancy is associated with a decrease in total α-amino nitrogen, a lower rate of urea synthesis, and a lower rate of branched-chain amino acid transamination. These adaptive changes lead to overall conservation of nitrogen and increased protein synthesis.[5] Positive nitrogen balance is observed throughout pregnancy. Increased amino acid utilization by maternal and fetal tissues indicates increased protein anabolism, which account for about 60% increase in the body weight that occurs in pregnancy.[5,6]

11.2.4 Changes in the Postpartum Period

Following childbirth, both glucose and insulin levels return to nonpregnancy values within a few days. Plasma free fatty acids also fall to nonpregnancy levels within a few days and triglycerides in about 2 weeks. Within 1 h after delivery of the placenta, the placental growth hormone level disappears from the maternal circulation.[7] Following a normal pregnancy, the changes in maternal metabolism return to the nonpregnant state fairly quickly, but that in part depends on whether lactation occurs.

11.3 ROLE OF ADIPOSITY IN PREGNANCY

Maternal body fat, or adiposity, increases substantively in a normal pregnancy and accounts for about 30% of gestational weight gain. The increase in maternal body fat is known to alter maternal metabolism and physiology in both normal and complicated pregnancies, but its relationship remains to be fully elucidated. In early gestation, insulin sensitivity is increased to promote maternal fat storage and total body fat. The increased body fat accretion provides an energy source for both the fetus and the mother, particularly during late pregnancy and lactation. It has been estimated that nonobese women gain about 3.5 kg of fat in the first 15 weeks of a normal pregnancy.[3] Lean women gain more adipose tissue during pregnancy than those women with obesity before conception, and this fact is largely due to increased insulin resistance in obese women.[8] Body fat remains stable during the first 6 weeks of gestation and thereafter is followed by increased adiposity, mainly in subcutaneous adipose tissue.[9] Body fat distribution also differs in lean compared with obese women who are pregnant, with more subcutaneous fat accretion in the former and a greater proportion of intra-abdominal fat in obese women. Intra-abdominal fat, more commonly referred to as *visceral fat*, is metabolically more active than subcutaneous fat, and it preferentially releases a larger number of adipocytokines, many of which can adversely affect glucose, protein, and lipid metabolism, leading to the development of insulin resistance, type 2 diabetes, atherogenic dyslipidemia, hypertension, inflammation, and other clinical features associated with increased cardiometabolic risk.[10] It is not surprising that nonobese women with the top quartile of visceral adipose tissue, depth quantified by ultrasonography in the first trimester, were noted to be significantly associated with the development of glucose intolerance in later pregnancy.[11] There was no association between subcutaneous fat depth and glucose intolerance, in keeping with the tenet that visceral fat is implicated in insulin resistance during pregnancy.

A more recent study also used ultrasonography to estimate changes in adipose tissue distribution during five different gestational periods (12, 16, 20, 32, and 37 weeks) in 400 women with normal pregnancies. There was a gradual shift in fat redistribution from early to late gestation, with decreased subcutaneous fat accretion and increased visceral fat accumulation.[12] The increase in visceral fat accretion during pregnancy is also confirmed in a prospective multicenter study, which examined adiposity and fat distribution during pregnancy in 14 women. Childbearing was associated with a threefold increase in visceral fat accumulation from preconception to postpartum when compared to 108 women not bearing children.[13] This effect was not due to overall excess total body fat deposition, but rather a greater accumulation of visceral fat relative to abdominal subcutaneous fat. The authors concluded that childbearing may be an important contributor to enlargement of the visceral fat depot, independent of an overall increase in adiposity.[13] The search for underlying mechanisms for visceral fat expansion during pregnancy has led to a study of the gene expression of the KEGG cytokine-signaling pathway, which describes signaling cascades arising from adipocyte-derived cytokines implicated in insulin resistance and sensitivity. Omental and subcutaneous fat tissue samples were obtained from 14 healthy nonobese pregnant women at time of elective cesarean section delivery. The authors found that adiponectin and insulin receptor substrate-1 (IRS-1), both key genes mediating insulin sensitivity, were among six genes involved in the KEGG adipocytokine-signaling pathway that were significantly downregulated in the omental relative to subcutaneous fat depot.[14] It appears that differential gene expression in adipose tissue is a mechanism whereby adipose tissue influences gestational insulin resistance in a normal pregnancy to ensure optimal fetal growth and development. As will be discussed in the ensuing section on adipocytokines, adiponectin is an adipocyte-derived, insulin-sensitizing protein, the expression and secretion of which decreases significantly in late gestation.

Adipose tissue morphology and function also influence gestational insulin resistance.[15] Svensson et al. investigated the size, number, and lipolytic activity of adipocytes, and adipokine release in fat biopsies obtained from 22 normal-weight and 11 obese women in the first and third trimesters of pregnancy.[15] Fat mass was found to positively correlate with insulin resistance, assessed by the homeostasis model of insulin resistance (HOMA-IR). HOMA-IR increased in both groups of women between the first and third trimesters, and they remained normoglycemic. Adipocyte size, but not number, increased in the normal-weight women, whereas the group of obese women had more of the large adipocytes between the first and third trimesters.[15] Lipolytic activity and circulating adipocyte fatty acid-binding protein (AFABP) levels increased in both groups of women. Adiponectin release was reduced in the normal-weight group. The authors concluded that fat mass and the proportion of large adipocytes were strongly correlated with HOMA-IR in the third trimester, and this significantly contributed to the increased gestational insulin resistance in obese women compared with normal-weight women.

11.4 ADIPOCYTOKINES IN PREGNANCY

Adipose tissue is now widely accepted as an active metabolic organ that secretes over 600 peptide mediators that are collectively known as *adipocytokines*, or *adipokines* for short.[16] Adipokines are dysregulated in obesity and exert paracrine and endocrine effects, leading to a variety of metabolic and vascular complications, such as insulin resistance, type 2 diabetes, dyslipidemia, hypertension, inflammation, and atherothrombotic diseases.[10] In addition to adipose tissue, the placenta is a rich source of adipokines. Working together, adipokines from maternal adipose tissue and the placenta may play an important role in the modulation of maternal and fetal metabolism, which ultimately influences fetal development and growth. The relevant adipokines that have been associated with normal and complicated pregnancies will be discussed later in this chapter (see Table 11.1).

TABLE 11.1 Changes in metabolic parameters, hormones, and adipokine levels in pregnancy

	Early pregnancy		Late pregnancy	
	Lean	Obese	Lean	Obese
Lean body mass[1]	↔	↔	↑	↑
Fat mass[1]	↔	↔	↑	↑
Insulin sensitivity[3]	↑/↔	↔/↑	↓	↓↓
Fasting glucose[2]	↑	↓	↓	↑
Hepatic glucose production[3]	↔	↑	↑	↑
Fasting insulin[3]	↔	↑	↑	↑
Insulin sensitivity[3]	↑	↔/↑	↓	↓↓
Free fatty acids[1,3]	↑	↓	↓	↑
Lipogenesis[1,3]	↑	↔	↔	↔
Lipolysis[1,3]	↓	↑	↑	↑↑
Adipokines				
Leptin[17]	↔	↑	↑	↑↑
Adiponectin[17]	↔	↓	↓	↓↓
Resistin[17]	↔	↔	↑	↑
TNF-α[18]	↔	↔	↑	↑/↑↑
AFABP[19]	↔	↑	↔	↑
Vaspin[20]	↓	↓	↓	↓
Visfatin[21]	↔	↔	↔/↓	↔
ANGPTL8[22]	↔	↑	↑	↑↑

Pregnancy is associated with complex metabolic and hormonal adaptations of the mother in order to meet the physiological and energy demands to provide adequate nutrient flow for optimal fetal growth and development. Changes in key metabolic parameters, glucose, and lipid metabolism occur in the first trimester (early pregnancy) and second and third trimesters (late pregnancy), and they vary depending on whether the mother is normal weight (Lean) or has prepregnant obesity (Obese). Adipose tissue is an active metabolic organ that secretes a large number of peptide mediators that are collectively known as *adipocytokines*, or *adipokines*. Adipokines from maternal adipose tissue and the placenta may play an important role in modulating fetal development and growth. Changes in the serum levels of the relevant adipokines that have been associated with normal and complicated pregnancies are listed. References are cited in parentheses.
TNF-α, tumor necrosis factor-α; *AFABP*, adipocyte fatty acid-binding protein; *ANGPTL8*, angiopoietin-like protein 8.

11.4.1 Leptin

Leptin is the first and best-known 16.2-kDa adipokine and hormone that is involved in body weight regulation by suppressing appetite centrally in the arcuate nucleus of the hypothalamus.[16] Leptin or leptin receptor deficiency causes hyperphagia and severe obesity. Serum leptin levels correlate with body fat mass and are higher in women than men. Leptin also exerts other metabolic and endocrine effects that influence glucose and lipid metabolism. It suppresses insulin secretion from pancreatic β-cells and plays a role in insulin resistance.

Circulating leptin levels in pregnancy are correlated with adiposity and are twofold higher in women with class 3 obesity (with body mass index (BMI) > 40 kg/m^2) compared with women with normal BMI.[17] Leptin levels continue to rise by twofold to threefold throughout the three trimesters in a normal pregnancy. Leptin and leptin receptors are expressed in the placenta and placental leptin secretion is increased by 1.5–2-fold in the second and third trimesters. Placental leptin is a significant source of maternal circulating levels, which peak at 22–27 weeks at about 30 μg/L and later decline to about 25 μg/L at 34–39 weeks of gestation.[23] Increased leptin levels have been reported in women with GDM, preeclampsia, and severe pregnancy-induced hypertension.[17] A meta-analysis of eight prospective studies indicated that leptin levels were 7.25 μg/L higher among women who later developed GDM than women who did not.[24] Leptin secretion from the placenta is also increased in GDM and is thought to contribute to the regulation of fetal growth, independent of maternal glucose levels.[25,26] Because insulin stimulates leptin secretion in adipocytes, it is feasible that hyperinsulinemia in GDM might further augment leptin levels.[25]

11.4.2 Adiponectin

Adiponectin is a 30-kDa hormone abundantly produced by adipocytes. It exerts pleiotropic effects on a broad array of physiological processes, including energy homeostasis, vascular function, systemic inflammation, and cell growth. The plasma level of adiponectin ranges from 5 to 30 μg/mL and is higher in women than men.[23] One of its most important functions appears to be an insulin-sensitizing agent that stimulates insulin gene expression and secretion. Adiponectin levels are inversely correlated in obesity and insulin-resistant states and reflect whole-body insulin sensitivity. Circulating adiponectin levels are lower in people with obesity, polycystic ovarian syndrome (PCOS), impaired glucose tolerance, or type 2 diabetes. Decreased adiponectin level, or hypoadiponectinemia, is associated with an increased risk for developing type 2 diabetes in otherwise healthy people. During normal pregnancy, circulating adiponectin levels decline in late gestation by about 40%, in keeping with a 25% increase in maternal fat mass and progressive insulin resistance.[17,27] A study examined first-trimester adipokine levels in 59 nulliparous women. Of the 30 women who developed GDM in later pregnancy, their adiponectin levels were 40% lower than the 29 healthy controls.[28] Women with first-trimester adiponectin levels at less than 25th-percentile of normal were 10 times more likely to develop GDM. The plasma levels of the other two adipokines, resistin and interleukin-6, were not different between the GDM and control groups.[28] A meta-analysis of nine prospective studies demonstrated that adiponectin levels in the first or early second trimester of pregnancy were 2.25 μg/mL lower among women who later developed GDM than women who did not.[24] Finally, a systematic review and meta-analysis analyzed the accuracy of circulating adiponectin for predicting GDM when levels were measured prior to the diagnosis. Circulating adiponectin in the first trimester had a diagnostic odds ratio of 6.6, with 60% sensitivity and 81% specificity.[29]

Adiponectin is also expressed and secreted by the syncytiotrophoblast cells in the placenta in late pregnancy, and its secretion is differentially regulated by such circulating cytokines as leptin, interleukin-6, and tumor necrosis factor-α (TNF-α).[25,26]

A causal role of adiponectin in the development of GDM has recently been studied in a pregnant mouse model with and without adiponectin deficiency. Adiponectin gene knockout dams developed glucose intolerance and hyperlipidemia in late pregnancy, as well as increased fetal weight, similar to what is observed in GDM.[30] The metabolic defects were restored with adiponectin reconstitution, supporting a potential role of adiponectin in modulating maternal β-cell adaptation in pregnant mice. It remains to be determined whether similar physiological adaptation also occurs in human pregnancy.

11.4.3 Resistin

Resistin is a proinflammatory 12.5-kDa adipokine whose name is derived from its ability to resist insulin action. It is upregulated in obesity and induces insulin resistance and thrombotic states. Studies on resistin levels during early and late gestation failed to demonstrate significant differences between women with normal pregnancies and those who developed GDM or preeclampsia.[17,19,26,28,31]

Resistin is expressed in the placenta, but resistin levels do not appear to differ in normal and abnormal pregnancies, raising doubt if it plays any role in maternal adaptation and fetal growth during pregnancy.[19]

11.4.4 Tumor Necrosis Factor-α

TNF-α is a proinflammatory adipokine that impairs insulin signaling and inhibits insulin secretion by β-cells. It is expressed and secreted mainly by monocytes and macrophages, and its expression is also found in low levels in adipose tissue. TNF-α induces insulin resistance in skeletal muscle and adipose tissue by reducing insulin receptor tyrosine kinase activity and increasing serine phosphorylation of insulin receptor substrate-1 in the insulin-signaling pathway. Plasma TNF-α levels correlate with body fat mass and insulin resistance.[32] TNF-α levels tend to rise in the third trimester in a normal pregnancy, but high levels from early gestation are associated with subsequent GDM and pregnancy with preeclampsia.[18] TNF-α is also expressed and produced in the placenta, and most of it is released into the maternal circulation.[26]

11.4.5 Adipocyte Fatty Acid-Binding Protein

AFABP is a member of the fatty acid-binding protein superfamily expressed in adipocytes and the placenta. AFABP induces insulin resistance by upregulating hepatic glucose production, and high circulating levels of AFABP independently predict the risk of cardiometabolic risk and type 2 diabetes.[26] AFABP levels were found in three studies to be elevated in women with GDM compared with women with normal pregnancies.[15,26] However, a prospective study in 123 nondiabetic women, 52 of whom developed GDM, failed to show any change in AFABP levels in the second or third trimesters, and there was no difference in levels between women who developed GDM and those who did not.[19]

11.4.6 Vaspin

Vaspin (visceral adipose tissue-derived serpin) is a 45.2-kDa protein that belongs to a superfamily of serine protease inhibitors. It is expressed and secreted predominantly by visceral adipose tissue but is also present in the placenta. It increases insulin sensitivity and has anti-inflammatory and antiatherogenic properties. Circulating vaspin levels are low compared with other adipokines. The levels are higher in women than in men and increase in obesity. Two case-controlled studies have reported that serum vaspin levels were significantly higher in women with GDM than in women with normal pregnancy, which were positively associated with insulin resistance, as assessed by the HOMA-IR method.[20,33] Vaspin messenger ribonucleic acid (mRNA) and protein expression levels in subcutaneous and visceral fat, but not smooth muscle tissue, were both significantly higher in women with GDM.[20] How vaspin contributes to the insulin resistance and pathophysiology of GDM remains unclear.

11.4.7 Visfatin

Visfatin, a 52-kDa adipokine also known as *pre-B-cell colony enhancing factor,* is expressed at high levels in visceral and omental fat, and low levels in subcutaneous and epicardial fat, and is also secreted in low levels by the placenta. It increases insulin sensitivity and has anti-inflammatory and antiatherogenic properties. Circulating visfatin levels correlate with body fat mass and are increased in obese people and people with type 2 diabetes.[26] Circulating visfatin levels in a normal pregnancy increase from the first to the second trimester, and they decrease between 27 and 34 weeks.[21] Maternal visfatin levels are higher in women with GDM compared with normal women.[34] Women with a normal pregnancy but who delivered large-for-gestational-age (LGA) neonates also have higher median visfatin levels.[34] In a nested case-controlled study, a first-trimester visfatin level was found to predict GDM independent of BMI, ethnicity, and parity.[35]

11.4.8 Angiopoietin-Like Protein 8

Angiopoietin-like protein 8 (ANGPTL8) is a novel adipokine implicated in lipid and glucose homeostasis by promoting islet β-cell proliferation. ANGPTL8 levels decreased progressively during pregnancy, although they remained higher than levels in the postpartum period.[22]

ANGPTL8 levels in early pregnancy were considerably higher in women who developed GDM than those who maintained normal glucose tolerance.[36,37] Importantly, women in the highest quartile of ANGPTL8 concentration had an 8.75-fold higher risk of developing GDM than women in the lowest quartile.[37]

In a cross-sectional observational study of women with or without GDM and their offspring, ANGPTL8 levels were higher in venous cord blood than in maternal blood and were significantly lower in women with GDM than in healthy women. Small-for-gestational-age (SMA) infants with low fat mass had the highest ANGPTL8 cord blood levels. Studies in vitro revealed that ANGPTL8 was secreted by brown adipocytes, and its expression was increased in experimental models of conversion of white to brown fat. In addition, ANGPTL8 induced the expression of markers of brown adipocytes. The high levels of ANGPTL8 found in fetal life, together with its relationship with newborn adiposity and brown adipose tissue, point to ANGPTL8 as a potential new player in the modulation of the thermogenic machinery during the fetal-neonatal transition.[22]

11.4.9   Other Adipokines

A number of other adipokines that are associated with obesity and insulin resistance have been studied in pregnancies. They include retinol-binding protein-4 (RBP4), chemerin, FGF21, apelin, progranulin, lipocalcin 2, and omentin. None of these proteins appear to be dysregulated during pregnancy, and none of them are associated with or predict GDM.[19,26]

11.5   MECHANISMS OF ADAPTIVE INSULIN RESISTANCE IN PREGNANCY

Insulin sensitivity in early pregnancy increases to allow for maternal fat accretion and fetal growth.[1] Insulin sensitivity starts to decline by 12–14 weeks and continues into the second and third trimesters to about 40%–50% of prepregnancy values. In late gestation, maternal fat depots contract, while postprandial free fatty acid levels increase because of the reduced ability of insulin to suppress whole-body lipolysis. The development of maternal insulin resistance in the second and third trimesters in a normal pregnancy is essential to provide adequate flow of nutrients (notably glucose) for growth and development of the fetus.

The adaptive insulin resistance in a normal pregnancy is complex and multifactorial. Higher circulating levels of maternal hormones (mainly progesterone, prolactin, and cortisol) contribute to insulin resistance starting from about week 6 of gestation (see Table 11.2). Maternal progesterone causes insulin resistance by decreasing insulin binding and glucose transport, as well as impairing insulin suppression of hepatic glucose production. Plasma cortisol levels increase by about twofold during pregnancy, and cortisol induces insulin resistance at the postreceptor defects by impairing insulin receptor phosphorylation and IRS-1, leading to increased hepatic glucose production. On the other hand, adiposity and many adipokines, including but not limited to leptin, TNF-α, AFABP, resistin, and adiponectin, can further modulate insulin resistance.

The placenta becomes a major source of insulin resistance during the second trimester due to a significant rise in placental growth hormone and human placental lactogen.[7] Placental growth hormone increases by six to eight times, and human placental lactogen increases by about 30-fold during pregnancy. Placental growth hormone (PGH) is secreted from the human placental syncytiotrophoblast exclusively into the maternal circulation, where it promotes maternal fat mobilization and spares glucose for the fetus. PGH impairs glucose utilization and induces maternal insulin resistance by stimulating lipolysis and hepatic gluconeogenesis. The increase in PGH levels, in concert with cortisol, progesterone, TNF-α, and decreased adiponectin levels, greatly augments maternal insulin resistance. PGH levels in pregnant women correlate with the birth weight of their offspring. The in vitro PGH secretion in a human trophoblast model was found to be inhibited by cortisol, leptin, and ghrelin but increased by visfatin, highlighting the complex interplay between adipokines and maternal hormones on fetoplacental growth.[38] Human placental lactogen also plays a role in adaptive insulin resistance by increasing β-cell hypertrophy and hyperplasia to augment insulin secretion as a compensatory response to maintain glucose homeostasis.[7]

At the cellular level, insulin mediates its action through binding to the α-subunit of the heterotetrameric cell surface insulin receptors and activates the intracellular tyrosine kinase domain of the β subunit, which then undergoes tyrosine autophosphorylation[39] (Table 11.2). Autophosphorylation results in activation of the tyrosine kinase activity of the receptor. The activated IR kinase phosphorylates substrate proteins on the tyrosine residues, which serve as docking sites for downstream effectors. Insulin receptor substrate-1 is the most abundant protein in muscle and fat that mediates the metabolic and growth-promoting functions of insulin via the downstream-signaling pathway involving phosphatidylinositol 3-kinase (PI3-K). Defects in insulin postreceptor signaling are largely responsible for the decreased insulin sensitivity in muscle, liver, and adipose tissue. Decreased insulin receptor phosphorylation, downregulation of IRS-1 expression by increased serine phosphorylation, and increased level of p85α subunit of phosphatidyl inositide 3-kinase, can lead to impaired insulin action in the target tissues.[39] For example, TNF-α interferes with insulin receptor autophosphorylation by increasing serine phosphorylation of IRS-1, and thereby downregulating insulin sensitivity. Many of the

TABLE 11.2 Factors affecting insulin resistance in pregnancy

	Mechanism of action	Effect on IR
Cellular insulin action in muscle, liver, and fat		↑
	↓ Insulin receptor binding	
	↓ Glucose transport (GLUT4)	
	↓ Receptor autophosphorylation	
	↓ Tyrosine kinase activity	
	↓ Insulin receptor substrate-1	
	↑ Serine phosphorylation	
	↑ p85α subunit of PI 3-kinase	
Adipokines		↑
Leptin	↑ Insulin sensitivity, ↓ insulin secretion	↑
Resistin	↓ Glucose uptake, insulin action	↑
TNF-α	↓ Receptor autophosphorylation, ↓ IRS-1	↑
AFABP	↑ Hepatic gluconeogenesis	↑
Adiponectin	↑ Insulin sensitivity, ↓ glucose production	↓
Vaspin	↑ Insulin sensitivity	↓
Visfatin	↑ Insulin sensitivity	↓
Maternal hormones		
Prolactin	↑ β-cell hypertrophy and hyperplasia	↓
Progesterone	↓ Insulin receptor binding, ↓ GLUT4, ↑ hepatic gluconeogenesis	↑
Cortisol	↓ Receptor autophosphorylation, ↓ IRS-1, ↑ hepatic gluconeogenesis	↑
Placental hormones		
Human placental lactogen	↑ β-cell hypertrophy and hyperplasia	↓
Placental growth hormone	↑ Hepatic gluconeogenesis	↑

Insulin sensitivity in early pregnancy increases to allow maternal fat accretion and fetal growth. Insulin sensitivity starts to decline by 12–14 weeks and continues into the second and third trimesters to about 40%–50% of prepregnancy values. The development of maternal insulin resistance in the second and third trimesters in a normal pregnancy is essential to provide adequate flow of nutrients for fetal growth and development. The cellular changes in insulin action in muscle, liver, and adipose tissue that lead to insulin resistance are listed. The effects of key adipokines and maternal and placental hormones on insulin resistance are also listed.

IR, insulin resistance; GLUT4, glucose transporter-4; PI 3-kinase, phosphatidylinositol 3-kinase; TNF-α, tumor necrosis factor-α; IRS-1, insulin receptor substrate-1; AFABP, adipocyte fatty acid-binding protein.

abovementioned cellular defects in insulin-stimulated glucose transport, as well as the downstream insulin postreceptor-signaling cascade pathways, were found to be exaggerated in women with GDM.[3,40] In addition, changes in maternal and placental-derived adipokines further augment insulin resistance in GDM. To counter rising insulin resistance, maternal β-cells increases its capacity to secrete insulin by about two to two-and-a-half times through hypertrophy and hyperplasia.[4] Inadequate β-cell adaptation to the increasing demand for insulin secretion, together with severe insulin resistance, can lead to the development of glucose intolerance in later gestation and the subsequent GDM, as well as increased future risk for type 2 diabetes in susceptible women.

11.6 ADIPOKINES AND FETAL GROWTH

The placenta is a complex fetal organ that supports and nurtures optimal fetal growth and development through diverse mechanisms. The discovery that the placenta is a rich source of (as well as a target for) a large number of adipokines that regulate insulin action and insulin resistance suggests potential interplay between the placenta and adipose tissue in modulating maternal metabolism in normal and complicated pregnancies associated with GDM and preeclampsia.[41]

Leptin, adiponectin, resistin, TNF-α, and other adipokines are secreted by the placenta and may influence maternal insulin resistance, and to some extent regulate fetal growth. The presence of leptin and adiponectin receptors in the placenta suggests that these adipokines may exert paracrine and autocrine pathways involved in placenta and fetal growth.[18,26] Umbilical leptin concentrations in newborns at term positively correlated with placental weight and fetal growth. On the other hand, neonates deficient in leptin have normal morphology and birth weight, suggesting that leptin plays a limited role as a placental and/or fetal growth factor but may influence other metabolic processes in the fetoplacental unit.[42]

Cord serum of term neonates contain high concentrations of adiponectin, which positively correlate with birth weight. It has been speculated that adiponectin might influence fetal growth through its augmented effect on insulin sensitivity.[42] Further, placental adiponectin secretion has been shown to be differentially regulated, possibly via paracrine pathways, by other adipokines like leptin and TNF-α.[26]

Finally, fetal adipose tissue development, which is regulated by hormones, nutrients, and adipokines during fetal growth, can alter developmental programming and have long-lasting influence on offspring.[42]

11.7   CHANGES IN MATERNAL ADIPOSITY DURING LACTATION

For maternal metabolism, pregnancy does not end with delivery but instead follows lactation. During pregnancy, adaptive insulin resistance occurs with resultant changes in intermediary metabolism, leading to increased adiposity, especially visceral fat accumulation, and increased plasma lipid and triglyceride levels. These changes gradually return to normal in the postpartum state, but are more quickly reset upon lactation.

At some time during the third trimester, the changing hormonal profile gradually shifts maternal metabolism from an anabolic to a more catabolic state to support fetal growth. The lactogenic hormones (prolactin, human placental lactogen, and growth hormone) promote fat mobilization from adipose tissue, while simultaneously stimulating mammary gland growth and development in preparation for lactation. Increased prolactin and oxytocin secretion suppresses the hypothalamic pituitary-gonadal (HPG) axis, leading to decreased production of progesterone and a lower progesterone-to-estrogen ratio, both of which are known to inhibit the lactogenic effects of prolactin.[43] Prolactin also suppresses lipogenesis in the liver and adipose tissue and increases delivery of lactate and fatty acids to the mammary gland for milk production.

Lactation requires an increased supply of nutrients to ensure the preferential use of nutrients by the mammary gland. Lactation mobilizes adipose tissue by promoting lipolysis through depot-specific regulation of fat cell metabolism to produce milk. Basal lipolysis is increased during lactation and is associated with decreased lipoprotein lipase (LPL) activity, mainly in the femoral (but not the abdominal adipose) depots.[44] On the other hand, LPL activity is increased in the mammary gland, leading to milk production. In lactating animals, adipocytes are smaller and have lower LPL activity than those of nonlactating animals, and the regional differences in LPL activity appear to correlate with changes in body fat distribution.[45] In addition, increased hormone sensitive lipase activity, as well as augmented responsiveness to β-2 adrenergic stimulation, allow coordinated mobilization of fat from adipose tissue to channel fatty acids to the mammary gland.

Because lactation is partly attributed to fat mobilization, women who breastfeed would be expected to lose some weight. Among 45 lactating women monitored for 4 months postpartum, a daily average of 156 kcal was estimated to be derived from fat stores, resulting in body-weight loss of 5.3 kg.[46] Another study estimated that 480 kcal/day is required for lactation.[45] However, how much weight women lose with lactation are dependent on the dietary intake and energy expenditure. Mean weight loss in lactating women from affluent countries is about 0.8 kg/month in the first 6 months, which is much greater than women from underprivileged populations (0.1 kg).[47] These data suggest that rather than mobilizing fat stores, women in developed countries compensate for increasing demands of lactation by increasing dietary intake and decreasing physical activity. On the other hand, women who breastfed for longer than 3 months reported greater weight loss than women who breastfed for 3 months or less, raising the possibility that the hormonal changes on appetite due to lactation might lead to increased fat mobilization.

Several studies have examined the effect of lactation on body fat distribution and composition. Longitudinal studies of skinfold thickness show fat accumulation in the supra-iliac and thigh regions during pregnancy and mobilization from these fat depots postpartum.[45] With respect to longer-term association of lactation and changes in adiposity, the studies have been inconclusive, with some demonstrating favorable but small differences in body weight and BMI with lactation. Findings from randomized clinical trials yielded evidence that lactation from 4 to 6 months postpartum was associated with greater weight loss among mothers in Honduras.[45] Whether these observations can be extended to developed countries remain to be determined.

Taken together, data from animal and human studies infer that lactation is associated with favorable changes in adiposity, glucose, and lipid homeostasis that persist long after lactation. Epidemiological and observational studies have reported that women who have breastfed have lower risks of visceral adiposity, type 2 diabetes, hypertension, dyslipidemia, and cardiovascular morbidity and mortality.[48] A recent systematic review of 21 clinical trials suggested that breastfeeding confers short- and long-term cardiovascular benefits for mothers.[49] The authors cautioned that the results were based on a small number of observational studies and need to be confirmed by prospective randomized clinical trials. While awaiting further research, the U.S. Obesity Society issued a position statement on breastfeeding and obesity. The Obesity Society encouraged women to breastfeed for the first 6 months of an infant's life, with continued breastfeeding through the first year and beyond, as desired by mother and child.[50]

11.8 MATERNAL OBESITY AND PREGNANCY OUTCOMES

Women with obesity or a previous history of GDM have a greater risk of delivering LGA offspring. This is most likely the consequence of excessive shunting of nutrients to facilitate fetal growth and fat accretion when the progression of maternal insulin resistance is not balanced by appropriate maternal β-cell adaptation in order to secrete more insulin.

Excess adiposity in women at preconception, as well as gestational weight gain that develops during pregnancy, not only affects fetal growth but also the subsequent health of offspring through epigenetic mechanisms.[40] Increased adiposity before pregnancy and/or increased weight gain during pregnancy have been associated in pregnancy with increased incidence of GDM, preeclampsia, high blood pressure, low birth weight, macrosomia, preterm births, higher rates of cesarean sections and fetal deaths for any reason, LGA infants, and SGA infants. Importantly, excessive adiposity during pregnancy can adversely influence the insulin-resistant state, which has been linked to abnormal fetal growth such as macrosomia or low birth weight.

11.9 ADIPOSE TISSUE TRANSCRIPTOME AND METABOLOMICS IN PREGNANCY

With the availability of new high-throughput technologies, genomics and metabolomics are being applied to profile the mechanisms underlying the changes in maternal metabolism during pregnancy.[51] This area of research is in its infancy, but it holds great promise to provide new insights that lead to innovative approaches to manage normal and complicated pregnancies, such as those of women with GDM and preeclampsia.

11.10 SUMMARY AND CONCLUSION

Pregnancy involves complex and profound metabolic and hormonal adaptations of the mother to meet the increasing physiological and energy demands to provide adequate nutrient flow for growth and development of the fetus, as well as during labor, delivery, and lactation. Adaptive insulin resistance begins in the latter part of the first trimester and progresses until the delivery of the newborn, after which it returns to normal within a few days postpartum. Maternal and fetal hormones, nutrients, and adipokines contribute to the development of insulin resistance, while glucose homeostasis is maintained by augmented insulin secretion via β-cell hypertrophy and hyperplasia. The increase in adipose tissue mass during pregnancy parallels the increase in adaptive insulin resistance, suggesting a causal link between adiposity and decreased insulin sensitivity.

Adiposity and adipokines are now recognized to play an important role in modulating the metabolic and hormonal changes in normal and complicated pregnancies. Excess adiposity in women at preconception, as well as gestational weight gain that develops during pregnancy, affects not only fetal growth, but also the subsequent health of offspring through epigenetic mechanisms. Lactation appears to confer short- and long-term benefits for mothers, and breastfeeding for the first 6 months of an infant's life should be encouraged and supported. Effort is now focused on the optimal management of pregnancy to avoid excessive weight gain and the adverse outcomes associated with excess maternal adiposity.

REFERENCES

1. Hadden DR, McLaughlin C. Normal and abnormal maternal metabolism during pregnancy. *Semin Fetal Neonatal Med* 2009;**14**(2):66–71.
2. Mills JL, Jovanovic L, Knopp R, et al. Physiological reduction in fasting plasma glucose concentration in the first trimester of normal pregnancy: the diabetes in early pregnancy study. *Metab Clin Exp* 1998;**47**(9):1140–4.
3. Lain KY, Catalano PM. Metabolic changes in pregnancy. *Clin Obstet Gynecol* 2007;**50**(4):938–48.
4. Baeyens L, Hindi S, Sorenson RL, German MS. β-Cell adaptation in pregnancy. *Diabetes Obes Metab* 2016;**18**(Suppl 1):63–70.

5. Kalhan SC. Protein metabolism in pregnancy. *Am J Clin Nutr* 2000;**71**(5 Suppl):1249S–55S.

6. Di Cianni G, Miccoli R, Volpe L, Lencioni C, Del Prato S. Intermediate metabolism in normal pregnancy and in gestational diabetes. *Diabetes Metab Res Rev* 2003;**19**(4):259–70.

7. Newbern D, Freemark M. Placental hormones and the control of maternal metabolism and fetal growth. *Curr Opin Endocrinol Diabetes Obes* 2011;**18**(6):409–16.

8. Ehrenberg HM, Huston-Presley L, Catalano PM. The influence of obesity and gestational diabetes mellitus on accretion and the distribution of adipose tissue in pregnancy. *Am J Obstet Gynecol* 2003;**189**(4):944–8.

9. Sidebottom AC, Brown JE, Jacobs DRJ. Pregnancy-related changes in body fat. *Eur J Obstet Gynecol Reprod Biol* 2001;**94**:216–23.

10. Lau DCW, Dhillon B, Yan H, et al. Adipokines: molecular links between obesity and atheroslcerosis. *Am J Physiol Heart Circ Physiol* 2005;**288**(5):H2031–41.

11. Martin AM, Berger H, Nisenbaum R, et al. Abdominal visceral adiposity in the first trimester predicts glucose intolerance in later pregnancy. *Diabetes Care* 2009;**32**(7):1308–12.

12. Selovic A, Serac J, Missoni S. Changes in adipose tissue distribution during pregnancy estimated by ultrasonography. *J Matern Fetal Neonatal Med* 2016;**29**(13):2131–7.

13. Gunderson EP, Sternfeld B, Wellons MF, et al. Childbearing may increase visceral adipose tissue independent of overall increase in body fat. *Obesity (Silver Spring)* 2008;**16**:1078–84.

14. Ogunyemi D, Xu J, Mahesan A, et al. Differentially expressed genes in adipocytokine signaling pathway of adipose tissue in pregnancy. *J Diabetes Mellitus* 2013;**3**(2):86–95.

15. Svensson H, Wetterling L, Bosaeus M, et al. Body fat mass and the proportion of very large adipocytes in pregnant women are associated with gestational insulin resistance. *Int J Obes (Lond)* 2015;**40**:646–53.

16. Fasshauer M, Blüher M. Adipokines in health and disease. *Trends Pharmacol Sci* 2015;**36**(7):461–70.

17. Hendler I, Balckwell SC, Mehta SH, Whitty JE, Russell E, Sorokin Y, et al. The levels of leptin, adiponectin, and resistin in normal weight, overweight, and obese pregnant women with and without preeclampsia. *Am J Obstet Gynecol* 2005;**193**:979–83.

18. Valsamakis G, Kumar S, Creatsas G, Mastorakos G. The effects of adipose tissue and adipocytokines in human pregnancy. *Ann NY Acad Sci* 2010;**1205**:76–81.

19. Guelfi KJ, Ong MJ, Li S, et al. Maternal circulating adipokine profile and insulin resistance in women at high risk of developing gestational diabetes mellitus. *Metab Clin Exp* 2017;**75**:54–60.

20. Tang Y, Qiao P, Qu X, et al. Comparison of serum vaspin levels and vaspin expression in adipose tissue and smooth muscle tissue in pregnant women with and without gestational diabetes. *Clin Endocrinol (Oxf)* 2017;**87**(4):344–9.

21. Mazaki-Tovi S, Romero R, Kusanovic JP, et al. Maternal visfatin concentration in normal pregnancy. *J Perinat Med* 2009;**37**:206–17.

22. Martinez-Perez B, Ejarque M, Gutierrez C, et al. Angiopoietin-like protein 8 (ANGPTL8) in pregnancy: a brown adipose tissue-derived endocrine factor with a potential role in fetal growth. *Transl Res* 2016;**178**:1–12.

23. Zavalza-Gomez AB, Anaya-Prado R, Rincon-Sanchez AR, et al. Adipokines and insulin resistance during pregnancy. *Diabetes Res Clin Pract* 2008;**80**(1):8–15.

24. Bao W, Baecker A, Song Y, et al. Adipokine levels during the first or early second trimester of pregnancy and subsequent risk of gestational diabetes mellitus: a systematic review. *Metab Clin Exp* 2015;**64**(6):756–64.

25. Al-Badri MR, Zantout MS, Azar ST. The role of adipokines in gestational diabetes mellitus. *Ther Adv Endocrinol Metab* 2015;**6**(3):103–8.

26. Fasshauer M, Blüher M, Stumvoll M. Adipokines in gestational diabetes. *Lancet Diabetes Endocrinol* 2014;**2**:488–99.

27. Catalano PM, Hoegh M, Minium J, et al. Adiponectin in human pregnancy: implications for regulation of glucose and lipid metabolism. *Diabetologia* 2006;**49**(7):1677–85.

28. Lain KY, Daftary AR, Ness RB, Roberts JM. First trimester adipocytokine concentrations and risk of developing gestational diabetes later in pregnancy. *Clin Endocrinol (Oxf)* 2008;**69**(3):407–11.

29. Iliodromiti S, Sassarini J, Kelsey TW, et al. Accuracy of circulating adiponectin for predicting gestational diabetes: a systematic review and meta-analysis. *Diabetologia* 2016;**59**:692–9.

30. Qiao L, Wattez JS, Lee S, et al. Adiponectin deficiency impairs maternal metabolic adaptation to pregnancy in mice. *Diabetes* 2017;**66**(5):1126–35.

31. Lobo TF, Torloni MR, Gueuvoghlanian-Silva BY, et al. Resistin concentration and gestational diabetes: a systematic review of the literature. *J Reprod Immunol* 2013;**97**(1):120–7.

32. Barbour LA, McCurdy CE, Hernandez TL, et al. Cellular mechanisms for insulin resistance in normal pregnancy and gestational diabetes. *Diabetes Care* 2007;**30**(Suppl 2):S112.

33. Jia X, Wang S, Ma N, et al. Comparative analysis of vaspin in pregnant women with and without gestational diabetes mellitus and healthy non-pregnant women. *Endocrine* 2015;**48**(2):533–40.

34. Mazaki-Tovi S, Romero R, Kusanovic JP, et al. Visfatin in human pregnancy: maternal gestational diabetes vis-à-vis neonatal birthweight. *J Perinat Med* 2009;**37**(3):218.

35. Ferreira AFA, Rezende JC, Vaikousi E, et al. Maternal serum visfatin at 11-13 weeks of gestation in gestational diabetes mellitus. *Clin Chem* 2011;**57**:609–13.

36. Ebert T, Kralisch S, Wurst U, et al. Betatrophin levels are increased in women with gestational diabetes mellitus compared to healthy pregnant controls. *Eur J Endocrinol* 2015;**173**(1):1–7.

37. Huang Y, Chen X, Chen X, et al. Angiopoietin-like protein 8 in early pregnancy improves the prediction of gestational diabetes. *Diabetologia* 2018;**61**(3):574–80.

38. Zeck W, Widberg C, Maylin E, et al. Regulation of placental growth hormone secretion in a human trophoblast model—the effects of hormones and adipokines. *Pediatr Res* 2008;**63**:353.

39. Pessin JE, Saltiel AR. Signaling pathways in insulin action: molecular targets of insulin resistance. *J Clin Invest* 2000;**106**(2):165–9.

40. Friedman JE. Obesity and gestational diabetes mellitus pathways for programming in mouse, monkey, and man—where do we go next? The 2014 Norbert Freinkel award lecture. *Diabetes Care* 2015;**38**(8):1402–11.

41. Desoye G, Hauguel-de Mouzon S. The human placenta in gestational diabetes mellitus.The insulin and cytokine network. *Diabetes Care* 2007;**30** (Suppl 2):S120–6.

42. Briana DD, Malamitsi-Puchner A. The role of adipocytokines in fetal growth. *Ann NY Acad Sci* 2010;**1205**(1):82–7.

43. McNamara JP, Huber K. Metabolic and endocrine role of adipose tissue during lactation. *Ann Rev Anim Biosci* 2018;**6**(1):177–95.

44. Rebuffé-Scrive M, Enk L, Crona N, et al. Fat cell metabolism in different regions in women. Effect of menstrual cycle, pregnancy, and lactation. *J Clin Invest* 1985;**75**(6):1973–6.

45. Stuebe AM, Rich-Edwards JW. The reset hypothesis: lactation and maternal metabolism. *Am J Perinatol* 2009;**26**(1):81–8.

46. Butte NF, Garza C, Stuff JE, et al. Effect of maternal diet and body composition on lactational performance. *Am J Clin Nutr* 1984;**39**(2):296–306.

47. Butte NF, Hopkinson JM. Body composition changes during lactation are highly variable among women. *J Nutr* 1998;**128**(2):381S–5S.

48. Schwarz EB. Invited commentary: breastfeeding and maternal cardiovascular health-weighing the evidence. *Am J Epidemiol* 2015;**181**(12):940–3.

49. Nguyen B, Jin K, Ding D. Breastfeeding and maternal cardiovascular risk factors and outcomes: a systematic review. *PLOS One* 2017;**12**(11).

50. Oken E, Fields DA, Lovelady CA, Redman LM. TOS scientific position statement: breastfeeding and obesity. *Obesity* 2017;**25**(11):1864–6.

51. Lowe Jr WL, Karban J. Genetics, genomics and metabolomics: new insights into maternal metabolism during pregnancy. *Diabet Med* 2014;**31** (3):254–62.

Chapter 12

Hormonal Regulation of the Menstrual Cycle and Ovulation

Cathy M. Murray and Christine J. Orr

Division of Endocrinology and Metabolism, Faculty of Medicine, Memorial University of Newfoundland, St. John's, NL, Canada

Key Clinical Changes

- Pulsatile secretion of GnRH with a specific frequency and amplitude is required for normal secretion of the pituitary gonadotropins.
- Estradiol, progesterone, and inhibin from the ovary, and activin and follistatin from the pituitary, modulate the secretion of LH and FSH.
- Estradiol is low early in the follicular phase, begins to rise slowly about 1 week before ovulation, and surges at midcycle, with ovulation and peak levels of LH and FSH.
- The ovary produces a fertilizable ovum; the follicle from which it is released (the corpus luteum) becomes the dominant source of sex steroids during the second half of the cycle.
- If fertilization does not take place, the corpus luteum regresses, estradiol and progesterone levels fall, and the functional endometrial tissue is sloughed off.
- If conception does occur, the endometrium is maintained by progesterone, allowing successful implantation of the embryo and pregnancy.

12.1 INTRODUCTION

The coordinated functions of the hypothalamus, pituitary, ovaries, and endometrium regulate ovulation and the menstrual cycle. The cyclic changes in pituitary gonadotropins and steroid hormones stimulate changes in the ovary to coordinate follicle maturation, ovulation, and development of the corpus luteum.[1] Similar cyclic changes in the endometrium prepare it for implantation of the developing embryo or shredding of the menstrual endometrium if pregnancy does not occur.

12.2 FUNCTION OF THE HYPOTHALAMUS

The hypothalamus is responsible for the pulsatile secretion of gonadotrophin-releasing hormone (GnRH) under the negative feedback of other factors, including ovarian hormones.[2] Serotonin, dopamine, norepinephrine, and opioids produced in the brain may affect the regulation of GnRH secretion.

GnRH is synthesized in the neuronal bodies of the arcuate nucleus of the medial basal hypothalamus.[3] The axons from these neurons project to the medial eminence and end in the capillaries that empty into the portal veins. This low-flow transport system along the pituitary stalk connects the hypothalamus to the anterior pituitary, forming the hypophyseal portal circulation.[2] GnRH travels to the anterior pituitary, where it binds to target cell receptors on the pituitary gonadotrophs, stimulating the release of the two gonadotrophins, luteinizing hormone (LH) and follicle-stimulating hormone (FSH).

The pulsatile secretion of GnRH within a specific frequency and amplitude is required for normal gonadotropin secretion.[4] The pulsatile rhythm of GnRH and, in turn, gonadotrophin secretion is critical to controlling gonadal activity and the reproductive axis. GnRH's ability to upregulate its receptors on pituitary gonadotrophs requires a physiologic periodicity of 60–90 minutes, whereas slower or faster frequencies result in anovulation.[5,6] The pulsatility of GnRH is also responsible for the activation of gene expression of the gonadotropin subunits, dimerization of subunits, and glycosylation in the gonadotrophs.[7]

The pulse frequency in GnRH is responsible for changes in FSH and LH levels and ratios, as well as ovarian function during the two phases of the menstrual cycle (Fig. 12.1A). More rapid pulse frequency of GnRH promotes LH secretion, while slower pulse frequencies promote FSH secretion. The variations in GnRH-pulse frequency are regulated partly by ovarian steroid hormone feedback. The GnRH-pulse frequency is increased by estradiol and decreased by progesterone. Estradiol feeds back on GnRH to suppress both FSH and LH, but also to coordinate a preovulatory surge in LH (Fig. 12.1B). Estradiol regulates the GnRH neurons directly, through estrogen receptor-β to suppress gene expression, and indirectly through estradiol-sensitive afferent neurons to transiently overcome this suppression. These mechanisms allow estradiol to variously inhibit or stimulate GnRH secretion and to regulate follicular maturation and the preovulatory surge in LH.[8]

Locally released neurotransmitters also regulate GnRH pulsatility. GnRH release is stimulated by norepinephrine and inhibited by dopamine.[9] Opioids such as β-endorphin inhibit GnRH release.[10] The negative feedback of ovarian steroids on gonadotropins seems to be partially mediated by endogenous opioids; and ovarian steroids alter endogenous opioid activity.[11] Kisspeptins and their receptor, GPR54, also affect the regulation of GnRH secretion and are important for sexual development and function.[12]

Any central nervous system disorder that interferes with local neurotransmitter regulation of GnRH pulsatility can cause anouvlatory cycles.[4] This includes isolated gonadatrophin deficiency, infection, suprasellar tumors, and head trauma. Functional hypothalamic anovulation is the most common cause of hypothalamic anovulation. It is associated with excessive exercise, abrupt weight loss from caloric restriction, malnutrition, and emotional distress, which affect brain function and slow the GnRH pulse generator, leading to low FSH, LH, and estradiol. Medications that alter norepinephrine, dopamine, and serotonin, such as sedatives, antidepressants, stimulants, and antipsychotics, affect the menstrual cycle by altering GnRH release.[2] Opioids also reduce GnRH pulsatile secretion. Elevated prolactin from pituitary tumors or medications, or associated with hypothyroidism, also interferes with GnRH pulsatility, causing anovulation.

12.3   FUNCTION OF THE PITUITARY

The gonadotropin-releasing cells, or *gonadotrophs*, compose 7%–15% of anterior pituitary cells and synthesize LH and FSH in response to GnRH from the hypothalamus.[13] Gonadotrophs express cell surface GnRH receptors that are G protein coupled.[14] The GnRH receptor predominantly signals via Gq/11.[15] However, signal transduction can occur via other G proteins, and a number of downstream cascades are activated by GnRH, including protein kinase C, calcium, and tyrosine kinase-dependent pathways.[16]

LH and FSH are both comprised of two noncovalently bonded protein subunits, called α and β. Each has a distinct β and a shared α subunit, which is also common with thyroid-stimulating hormone (TSH) and human chorionic gonadotropin (hCG).[2] The unique β-subunit confers the specific activity that is characteristic of each αβ heterodimer, whether it is LH, FSH, TSH, or hCG. Upon binding of GnRH to the GnRH receptor, the subunit genes are transcribed and translated to subunit messenger ribonucleic acid (mRNA). Posttranslational modifications of precursor subunits occur with subunit folding and combination, followed by hormone packaging and secretion. Further, α and β subunit production is partially regulated by negative feedback from estradiol produced by the ovary, which helps to regulate the pulsatile release of GnRH.[17] Estradiol, estrone, and estriol are all C18 steroids, which are commonly referred to as *estrogen*.[2] Estrone and estriol are weak estrogens and must be converted to estradiol for total estrogen activity.

From the viewpoint of the hypothalamus and pituitary, the menstrual cycle is divided into follicular and luteal phases.[1] Menses signals the start of the follicular phase, which ends with the preovulatory surge of LH and ovulation; the luteal phase follows, ending on the first day of menses (Fig. 12.1). The ovaries release estradiol, progesterone, and inhibin, while the pituitary releases activin and follistatin, all of which modulate the secretion of LH and FSH during the menstrual cycle.[2] The regression of the corpus luteum (the site of ovum release) from the preceding cycle results in a drop in estradiol and progesterone, which via loss of negative feedback leads to increased FSH.[1] The slight rise in FSH triggers new follicular growth for the next cycle. The lower levels of estradiol at the beginning of the cycle exert a negative feedback effect on release of LH. Estradiol levels rise later in the follicular phase a positive feedback loop causes a surge in LH and ovulation. During the subsequent luteal phase, LH and FSH are suppressed by negative feedback from estradiol and progesterone, which are largely secreted by the corpus luteum. This inhibition continues until near the end of the luteal phase, when the corpus luteum regresses and estradiol levels fall if pregnancy does not occur.

Inhibin, activin, and follistatin have selective effects on FSH.[18] All are produced in the ovary, with activin and follistatin also being produced in extragonadal tissues. They can exert autocrine-paracrine effects on FSH. Inhibin B is secreted by the ovarian granulosa cells under the control of FSH during the follicular phase. Inhibin A is under the control of LH and secreted by the corpus luteum in the luteal phase. Inhibins act with estradiol to inhibit FSH secretion. Activin stimulates FSH production and release. Follistatin negatively regulates these effects by binding to activin and preventing it from binding with the activin receptor at the cell membrane of gonadotrophs.

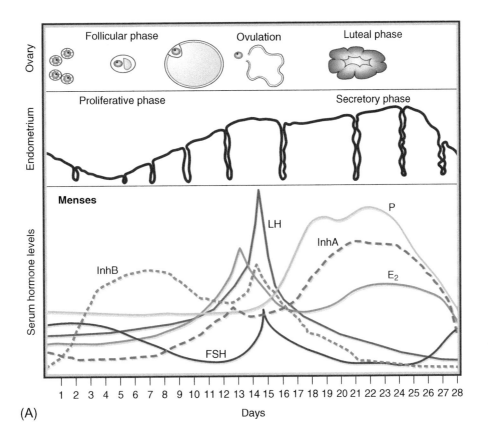

(A)

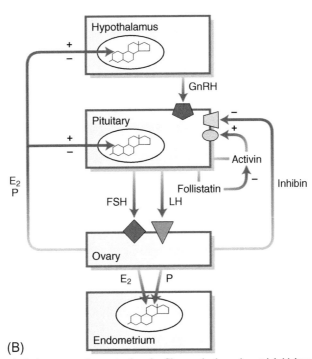

(B)

FIG. 12.1   (A) Hormone activities and levels during a normal menstrual cycle. Changes in the endometrial thickness and serum hormone levels in the ovarian follicle during a 28-day menstrual cycle. (B) Endocrine interactions in the female reproductive axis. Some of the well-characterized endocrine interactions among the hypothalamus, pituitary, ovary, and endometrium for regulation of the menstrual cycle are depicted. *E₂*, estradiol; *FSH*, follicle-stimulating hormone; *GnRH*, gonadotropin-releasing hormone; *Inh*, inhibin; *LH*, luteinizing hormone; *P*, progesterone. *(Courtesy of* Williams textbook of endocrinology, *11th Edition, 2008.)*

LH and FSH are released into the general circulation to act as true endocrine hormones. The pulse frequency of LH is approximately every 90 minutes in the early follicular phase, every 60–70 minutes in the late follicular phase, every 100 minutes in the early luteal phase, and every 200 minutes in the late luteal phase.[19] The serum levels of FSH and LH are proportional to their rate of secretion and serum half-lives, which in turn are regulated by content of carbohydrate residues.[20] The higher the content of carbohydrate residue, especially sialic acid, the lower the rate of metabolism and the longer the serum half-life of the gonadotropin. The higher sialic acid content of FSH is responsible for its slower clearance from the circulation compared to LH. FSH has a serum half-life of 3–4 h, as opposed to LH at 20 minutes; the half-life of hCG is 24 hours.

12.4 OVARIES

The ovaries are responsible for the production and periodic release of oocytes and the production of estradiol and progesterone, which prepare the endometrium for implantation[2] (Fig. 12.1). The ovarian follicle comprises an ovum surrounded by granulosa and theca cells. LH stimulates the theca cells of the ovary to produce androstenedione. Androstenedione diffuses to the granulosa cells, where it is a substrate for aromatase P450 for conversion to estrone and then estradiol. It is a precursor to both estrone and testosterone, which can be converted to estradiol by aromatase P450. FSH receptors on the granulosa cells of the ovary allow FSH to control estradiol production from androgens, inhibin B production, and follicular growth and development.

The ovary consists of an outer cortex, which contains the surface germinal epithelium and follicles, a central medulla containing the stroma, and a hilum, which is the area of attachment to the mesovarium. The hilum contains nerves, blood vessels, and hilus cells, which have the potential to become active in steroidogenesis. The tunica albuginea, the outermost portion of the cortex, is covered in germinal epithelium, which is a single layer of cuboidal cells. The follicles in the inner part of the cortex are imbedded in the stroma, and these follicles contain oocytes (Fig. 12.2). During each cycle, one dominant follicle is recruited for ovulation. After ovulation, the follicle transforms into the corpus luteum, which becomes the dominant site of sex steroid production during the luteal phase. If pregnancy does not occur, the corpus luteum regresses to a corpus albicans, and sex steroid production plummets. The interstitial cells within stromal tissue have the ability to respond to LH or hCG to produce androstenedione. In polycystic ovarian syndrome (PCOS), low constant levels of FSH continuously stimulate follicular growth, but not full maturation and ovulation, thereby extending the follicular life span. Under the influence of increased LH, this leads to cysts, thickened stroma, and increased androstendione production.

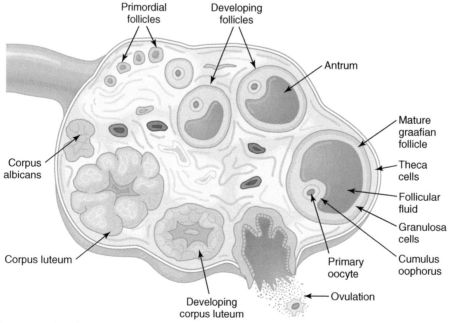

FIG. 12.2   Schematic representation of the sequence of events occurring in the ovary during a complete follicular cycle. *(Adapted from Yen SC, Jaffe R, editors.* Reproductive endocrinology, *Philadelphia: Saunders; 1978. Courtesy of Hacker and Moore's* Essentials of Obstetrics and Gynecology, *6th Edition, 2016.)*

The follicular development within each menstrual cycle originates during fetal development. Oogenesis does not occur in adults; instead, all the oocytes have formed between 8 and 13 weeks of fetal development and are arrested at the prophase of the first meiotic division until the time of ovulation, decades later. As discussed in more detail in Chapter 37, the internal structure of the ovary is also determined during fetal development. Primary follicles form between 20 and 24 weeks of fetal development and consist of cuboidal follicular cells surrounded by stromal cells. In the menstrual cycles prior to ovulation, primary follicles are recruited to develop. A zona pellucida forms around the ovum as granulosa cells proliferate, transforming it into a secondary follicle. The proliferation of cells outside the basal lamina forms the theca.[2]

The formation of a tertiary follicle occurs, with continued hypertrophy of the theca and appearance of a fluid-filled antrum among the granulosa cells. Tertiary follicles develop during the menstrual cycles before ovulation, and this will occur despite the absence of the pituitary because it is controlled by ovarian mechanisms. The ovulatory follicle is recruited at the time of the transition of the luteal phase of the previous cycle to the early follicular phase of the current cycle. The time to achieve the preovulatory phase is about 85 days. Multiple follicles reach the tertiary stage, but only one normally realizes the potential of releasing its ovum. Unless the follicle is recruited by FSH, it undergoes atresia with its cohort of follicles. The follicle recruited by FSH develops into a mature or Graaffian follicle by rapidly increasing in size, due to increased antral fluid volume and the accumulation of granulosa cells forming the cumulus oophorus. The Graaffian follicle is ready for ovulation.

As noted earlier, the follicular phase is characterized by low levels of estradiol that rise slowly about 1 week before ovulation.[1] Estradiol reaches a maximum about 1 day before the midcycle LH surge, followed by a precipitous drop.[1] The marked LH and lesser FSH surges usually trigger one dominant follicle to ovulate during the menstrual cycle.[2] LH or its surrogate hCG is required for rupture of the follicle; increased local prostaglandin biosynthesis within the follicle may mediate the ovulatory effect of LH.[21] The follicle enlarges rapidly, protrudes to the surface of the ovarian cortex, and then ruptures, with extrusion of the egg-cumulus complex into the peritoneal cavity. Ovulation occurs 36–44 hours after the midcycle LH surge.

The dominant follicle reorganizes after ovulation to form the corpus luteum. Capillaries and fibroblasts of the surrounding stroma proliferate to penetrate the basal lamina. Angiogenic growth factors in the follicular fluid, such as vascular endothelial growth factor and basic fibroblast growth factor, guide this rapid revascularization.[22] The granulosa and theca cells undergo luteinization, with the granulosa cells transforming into granulosa-lutein cells (large cells) and the theca cells becoming theca-lutein cells (small cells).[23]

The corpus luteum is the major source of sex steroids secreted by the ovary in the postovulatory phase of the cycle, with as much as 40 mg/day of progesterone secreted in the midluteal phase.[24] During the luteal phase, the serum concentrations of estradiol and progesterone increase to reach their maximum at 5–7 days after ovulation, and then they return to baseline before menses.[1] The basement membrane of the corpus luteum is penetrated by blood vessels that supply the granulosa-lutein cells with low-density lipoprotein (LDL) to serve as a substrate for progesterone production.[25] LH regulates steroidogenesis in the corpus luteum throughout its functional life span, which may last until the end of the current cycle or for the entire duration of a pregnancy.[26] The entry of cholesterol into mitochondria, which is regulated by steroidogenic acute regulatory protein (StAR), is the rate-limiting step in progesterone production.[27]

The corpus luteum generally has a life span of 14 ± 2 days, and then regresses to a corpus albicans, which is an avascular scar. But if pregnancy occurs, the LH surrogate hCG is secreted by the gestational trophoblasts and preserves the ability of the corpus luteum to produce progesterone in early gestation until the placenta is able to produce sufficient hormones to support the pregnancy.[28] The corpus luteum increases to twice its prepregnancy size during the first 6 weeks of gestation due to the proliferation of blood vessels and connective tissue, as well as hypertrophy of the luteinized granulosa and theca cells. This is later followed by regression, such that the corpus luteum at term is only half the size that it was during the menstrual cycle.

12.5   ENDOMETRIUM

The endometrium is the mucosal layer of the uterus, and it is an extraordinary tissue, given its capability for monthly cyclical changes, capacity for growth, response to ovarian hormones, high number of receptors, and unique biochemical characteristics. It is a multilayered tissue that functions to enable implantation and support pregnancy. The endometrium is controlled by ovarian hormones, which prepare the intrauterine environment for implantation of an embryo and direct the endometrial shedding and hemorrhage in the small spiral arteries, resulting in menstruation.[29]

Endometrial tissue is divided morphologically into the functionalis layer, made of the upper two-thirds of tissue, and the basalis layer, the lower third of endometrial tissue.[30] Each layer is composed of stromal cells, with deep invaginations covered by a thin layer of epithelial cells. The entire endometrium contains spiral arteries and capillaries (Fig. 12.3).

The endometrium has high concentrations of estrogen and progesterone receptors, with estradiol inducing growth of the endometrium and progesterone enhancing cellular differentiation.[30] Low levels of these hormones lead to sloughing of the functionalis endometrial tissue and menses. After the functionalis layer is shed, the basalis layer allows growth of a new functionalis layer for the next cycle. While the functionalis layer undergoes cyclical growth and shedding, the basalis remains unchanged during each cycle of menstruation.

Each cycle of endometrial change is divided into phases describing the tissue changes that occur in response to hormonal impulses. These are the proliferative (or *estrogenic*) phase, characterized by proliferation induced by estrogenic stimulation. The secretory (or *progestational*) phase is characterized by progesterone-responsive changes in the endometrium, including stimulation of glandular cells containing glycogen and mucus. Finally, the menstrual phase is characterized by the shedding of endometrial functionalis tissue in response to declining hormone levels.[31]

New endometrial growth occurs at the onset of each ovarian cycle, with early growth corresponding to the ovarian follicular phase (Fig. 12.1A). This preovulatory early proliferative phase is dominated by high levels of estradiol secreted by ovarian granulosa cells. At this stage, the endometrium contains undeveloped glandular epithelium and endometrial tissue (Fig. 12.4). Estrogen receptor-alpha (ER-α) is the primary mediator of estradiol's activity on the endometrium, resulting in the proliferation and thickening of endometrial epithelial cells and the growth of tissue. Estradiol-ER-α complexes bind to DNA sites and allow gene transcription, causing cellular growth and growth of new ERs and progesterone receptors (PRs), types A and B. In this phase, estradiol acts to make new tissue that is responsive to both estradiol and progesterone.[30] There is intensive mitosis in both the epithelium and stroma.

In the next advanced proliferative phase, both progesterone receptors A and B are present in endometrial tissue. Progesterone receptor B is believed to be more biologically important. Progesterone acts to diminish the activity of estradiol by decreasing the number of estrogen receptors, decreasing the tissue levels of estradiol by enhancing its conversion to estrone, and by enhancing estrogen inactivation through increasing sulfation.[30] Progesterone action causes differentiation of endometrial tissue, with peak PR levels during the advanced proliferative phase. Progesterone receptor levels decline before onset of the luteal phase, which is characterized in part by high levels of circulating progesterone. The proliferative phase results in cellular proliferation of the epithelial lining, endometrial glands, and stromal tissue. There is growth of the spiral arteries, which have elongated and grown lightly into the stroma. At this stage, the endometrial glands are straight, with narrow lumens, and do not have a secretory function.[31]

The early secretory phase begins following ovulation. The secretory phase is characterized by the maturation and development of endometrial tissue, the stroma becomes edematous, and the glands become rich with glycogen in anticipation of providing nutrition to a growing embryo. The midsecretory phase is characterized histologically by the development of mucus in the glands and edema in the stromal tissue (Fig. 12.5). Importantly, in the cycle of conception, it is the midsecretory phase in which implantation occurs.[32] In the late secretory phase, marked constriction of spiral arterioles results in

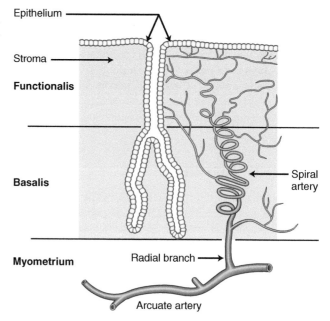

FIG. 12.3 Functional anatomy of the endometrium. The endometrium is a multilayered mucosa specially designed for the implantation and support of pregnancy. A single, continuous layer of epithelial cells line the surface of the stroma and penetrate the stroma, with deep invaginations almost all the way down to the myometrium-endometrium junction. The entire thickness of the endometrium is penetrated by spiral arteries and their capillaries. Spiral arteries originate from the radial branches of the arcuate arteries, which arise from uterine arteries. The superficial layer (functionalis) is shed during menstruation, whereas the permanent bottom layer (basalis) gives rise to the regeneration of endometrium after each menstruation. The striking changes in the spiral arteries (i.e., coiling, stasis, and vasodilation, followed by intense vasoconstriction) are consistently observed before the onset of every menstruation episode. *(Courtesy of* Williams Textbook of Endocrinology, *12th Edition, 2011.)*

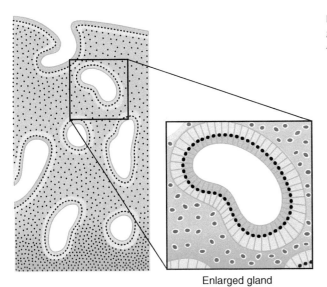

FIG. 12.4 Early proliferative phase endometrium. Note the regular, tubular glands lined by psuedostratified columnar cells. *(Courtesy of Hacker and Moore's Essentials of Obstetrics and Gynecology, 6th Edition, 2016.)*

Enlarged gland

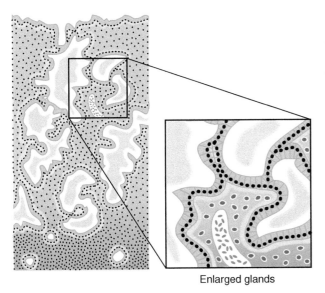

FIG. 12.5 Late secretory phase endometrium. Note the tortuous, saw-toothed appearance of the endometrial glands with secretions in the lumens. The stroma is edematous and necrotic during this stage, leading to sloughing of the endometrium at the time of menstruation. *(Courtesy of Hacker and Moore's Essentials of Obstetrics and Gynecology, 6th Edition, 2016.)*

Enlarged glands

tissue ischemia, followed by leukocyte infiltration and eventual extravasation of red blood cells, with subsequent progression to menstruation.[31]

The menstrual phase represents the termination of this physiologic cycle. Menstruation results from a decline in ovarian steroids and from blockade of progesterone action. The decline in ovarian steroids, demise of the corpus luteum, and resistance to remaining progesterone result in the onset of menstruation and sloughing of the functionalis layer.[32]

When conception occurs, the endometrium does not undergo ischemic change. Instead, decidualization results, with growth of decidua tissue beginning after implantation. This process is influenced by the ongoing presence of progesterone. Endometrial cells become round decidual cells, achieving a depth of 5–10 mm during pregnancy. The basal layer of decidual cells, the decidua basalis, ultimately become the formation plate of the placenta. The presence of progesterone is essential for healthy endometrial tissue that is receptive to implantation.

12.6   FERTILIZATION/IMPLANTATION

During each cycle, several ovarian follicles mature, but only one will become dominant and result in ovulation. The dominant follicle has adequate FSH receptors to grow despite falling gonadotropin levels in the midproliferative phase.[32] Following ovulation, the ovum adheres to the surface of the ovary. The fimbriated end of the fallopian tube sweeps over the ovary to pick up the ovum.[33] Movement into the fallopian tube relies on both muscular contractions and cilia on the fimbrial surface. These cilia have adhesive sites that interact with follicular cells surrounding the ovum to allow ovum transport into the fallopian tube.[33] The ovum passes through the fallopian tubes to reach the uterus about 48–72 h after ovulation. An ovum remains fertilizable for 12–24 h, so fertilization must occur within the oviduct.[34] In fact, fertilization usually occurs in the ampullary region of the oviduct.[33]

High estradiol levels at the time of ovulation result in favorable changes to cervical mucus, allowing easy passage of introduced sperm. The average ejaculate contains 2–5 mL of semen and 200–300 million sperm. The high number of sperm compensates for various sources of loss: only 50%–90% are morphologically normal, a large volume are lost through the introitus following coitus, they may fail to pass through the cervix or uterus, and others may enter the incorrect fallopian tube. Despite the high number of sperm in each ejaculate, only a few hundred get close to the ovum.[31]

Sperm cells must undergo a process called *capacitation* to successfully fertilize the ovum. Capacitation is the functional maturation of spermatozoa, and it includes an acrosome reaction, in which the membrane surrounding the spermatozoa is altered for penetration of the ovum. There is variation in the timing of capacitation of sperm within a single ejaculate, leading to a heterogeneous group of spermatozoa, which in turn increases the likelihood that a spermatozoon capable of fertilization will reach the ovum at the appropriate time.[35]

Fertilization occurs after a single sperm cell successfully penetrates the outer layer of the ovum (or *corona radiata*) and the inner layer (or *zona pellucida*) surrounding the ovum cell membrane.[34] When membranes of the spermatozoon and ovum fuse, this triggers a response in the zona pellucida that normally prevents more sperm from reaching the ovum. Fusion of the haploid cells, each of which contain 22 autosomes and 1 sex chromosome, creates a new cell with 46 chromosomes called a *zygote*.[36] Cell division and replication proceeds in the following 24 h to begin the embryonic period. By 3–4 days following fertilization, the embryo is called a *morula*, usually defined as a spherical, 16-cell mass.[36] The embryo typically leaves the oviduct and enters the uterus about 3 days after fertilization.[30]

The endometrium produces glycogen-rich vacuoles at the base of the glands during the secretory phase, just after ovulation. As progesterone levels increase, glycogen-containing vacuoles ascend toward the gland lumina. The contents of the glands are released into the endometrial cavity to provide energy to the free-floating embryo.[29] By days 4–5 after fertilization, the embryo has developed into a *blastocyst*. An inner cavity within the blastocyst contains the *trophoblasts*, which will be responsible for placental development, and an inner-cell mass, which will become the fetus.

During this blastocyst stage, the cell layer surrounding the embryo will break down, allowing implantation of the embryo into the endometrial lining.[32] Although the embryo reaches the cavity approximately 3 days after fertilization occurs, it does not implant until approximately 1 week after fertilization.[37] There is a narrow window of opportunity for this implantation to occur, with endometrial tissue receptive to embryo implantation only at days 20–24 of a 28-day menstrual cycle.[30] Animal studies suggest the endometrium is most receptive to blastocyst implantation where the usual negative surface charge has been reduced. This reduction in negative charge improves blastocyst attachment by reducing the repulsive charge between blastocyst and endometrial lining.[30]

The hormonal regulation of implantation is discussed in more detail in Chapter 29. The stages of early implantation are apposition, attachment, and invasion.[32] Surface epithelial cells lining the uterine cavity are the initial site of interaction between the endometrium and embryo.[29] There must be synchronous and normal development of both the endometrium and embryo in order for successful implantation to occur. Integrins, a class of proteins involved in cell-to-cell adherence, peak within endometrium at the time of implantation.[31] At the outset of implantation, the blastocyst sheds the zona pellucida and exposes a number of adhesion molecules. These complement adhesion molecules on the endometrial tissue, thereby facilitating early blastocyst attachment.[32] Thus, both electrical charge and surface adhesion contribute to blastocyst adherence.

As the embryo comes into contact with uterine epithelium, junctional complexes are formed between the uterine epithelium and embryo, preventing the embryo from being dislodged.[33] Once adhered to endometrial tissue, the embryonic cells continue to multiply and differentiate further into both trophoblast and inner-cell mass. The inner-cell mass differentiates into a dorsal ectoderm plate and an underlying ventral endoderm. A space forms between the trophoblast and inner-cell mass, which will become the amniotic cavity. The decidua basalis develops at the site of implantation, while a decidua capsularis forms a cellular layer over the developing embryo, separating it from the rest of the uterine cavity. The decidua vera is the remaining lining of the uterine cavity. The decidua vera and capsularis fuse by the 16th week of gestation. The decidua basalis is invaded by trophoblastic giant cells, which appear at the time of implantation and give rise to maternal serum hCG, signaling the beginning of pregnancy.

REFERENCES

1. Gambone JC. Female reproductive physiology. In: Hacker NK, Gambone JC, Hobel CJ, editors. *Hacker and Moore's essentials of obstetrics and gynecology.* Philadelphia, PA: Elsevier; 2016. p. 37–49.
2. Bulun SE, Adashi EY. The physiology and pathology of the female reproductive axis. In: Kronenburg HM, Melmed S, Polonsky KS, Larsen PR, editors. *Williams textbook of endocrinology.* Philadelphia, PA: Saunders Elsevier; 2008. p. 541–614.
3. Seeburg PH, Adelman JP. Characterization of cDNA for precursor of human luteinizing hormone releasing hormone. *Nature* 1984;**311**:666–8.
4. Knobil E. The neuroendocrine control of the menstrual cycle. *Recent Prog Horm Res* 1980;**36**:53–88.
5. Gross KM, Matsumoto AM, Southworth MB, Bremner WJ. Evidence for decreased luteinizing hormone-releasing hormone pulse frequency in men with selective elevation of follicle-stimulating hormone. *J Clin Endocrinol Metab* 1985;**60**:197–202.
6. Van Vugt DA, Diefenbach WD, Alston E, Ferin M. Gonadotropin-releasing hormone pulses in third ventricular cerebrospinal fluid of ovariectomized rhesus monkeys: correlation with luteinizing hormone pulses. *Endocrinology* 1985;**117**:1550–8.
7. Haisenleder DJ, Dalkin AC, Ortolano Gam Marchall JC, Shupnik MA. A pulsatile gonadotropin-releasing hormone stimulus is required to increase transcription of the gonadotropin subunit genes: evidence for differential regulation of transcription by pulse frequency in vivo. *Endocrinology* 1991;**128**:509–17.
8. Petersen SL, Ottem EN, Carpenter CD. Direct and indirect regulation of gonadotropin-releasing hormone neurons by estradiol. *Biol Reprod* 2003;**69**:1771–8.
9. Herbison AE. Noradrenergic regulation of cyclic GnRH secretion. *Rev Reprod* 1997;**2**:1–6.
10. Gindoff PR, Ferin M. Endogenous opioid peptides modulate the effect of corticotropin-releasing factor on gonadotropin release in the primate. *Endocrinology* 1987;**121**:837–42.
11. Shoupe D, Montz FJ, Lobo RA. The effects of estrogen and progestin on endogenous opioid activity in oophorectomized women. *J Clin Endocrinol Metab* 1985;**60**:178–83.
12. Gottsch ML, Clifton DK, Steiner RA. Kisspeptin-GPR54 gene signaling in the neuroendocrine reproductive axis. *Mol Cell Endocrinol* 2006;**254–255**:91–6.
13. Childs GV, Hyde C, Naor Z, Catt K. Heterogeneous luteinizing hormone and follicle-stimulating hormone storage patterns in subtypes of gonadotropes separated by centrifugal elutriation. *Endocrinology* 1983;**113**:2120–8.
14. Childs GV. Functional ultrastructure of gonadotropes: a review. *Curr Top Neuroendocrinol* 1986;**7**:49–97.
15. Milar RP, Lu ZL, Pawson AJ, Flanagan CA, Morgan K, Maudsley SR. Gonadotropin-releasing hormone receptors. *Endocr Rev* 2004;**25**:235–75.
16. Cheng CK, Leung PC. Molecular biology of gonadotropin-releasing hormone (GnRH)-I, GnRH-II, and their receptors. *Endocr Rev* 2005;**26**:283–306.
17. Shupnik MA. Gonadotropin gene modulation by steroids and gonadotropin releasing hormone. *Biol Reprod* 1996;**54**:279–86.
18. Gregory SJ, Kaiser UB. Regulation of gonadotropins by inhibin and activin. *Semin Reprod Med* 2004;**22**:253–67.
19. Filicori M, Santoro N, Merriam GR, Crowley Jr WF. Characterization of the physiological pattern of episodic gonadotropin secretion throughout the human menstrual cycle. *J Clin Endocrinol Metab* 1986;**62**:1136–44.
20. de Leeuw R, Mulders J, Voortman G, Rombout F, Damm J, Kloosterboer L. Structure-function relationship of recombinant follicle stimulating hormone (Puregon). *Mol Hum Reprod* 1996;**2**:361–9.
21. Bauminger A, Lindner HR. Periovulatory changes in ovarian prostaglandin formation and their hormonal control in the rat. *Prostaglandins* 1975;**9**:737–51.
22. Kamat BP, Brown LF, Manseau EJ, Senger DR, Dvorak HF. Expression of vascular permeability factor/vascular endothelial growth factor by human granulosa and theca lutein cells. Role in corpus luteum development. *Am J Pathol* 1995;**146**:157–65.
23. Ohara A, Mori T, Taii S, Ban C, Narimoto K. Functional differentiation in steroidogenesis of two types of luteal cells isolated from mature human corpora luteal of menstrual cycle. *J Clin Endocrinol Metab* 1987;**65**:1192–200.
24. Carr BR, MacDonald PC, Simpson ER. The role of lipoproteins in the regulation of progesterone secretion by the human corpus luteum. *Fertil Steril* 1982;**38**:303–11.
25. Beers WH, Strickland S, Reich E. Ovarian plasminogen activator: relationship to ovulation and hormonal regulation. *Cell* 1975;**6**:387–94.
26. Duncan WC, McNeilly AS, Fraser HM, Illingworth PJ. Luteinizing hormone receptor in the human corpus luteum: lack of down-regulation during maternal recognition of pregnancy. *Hum Reprod* 1996;**11**:2291–7.
27. Strauss 3rd JF, Christenson LK, Devoro L, Martinez F. Providing progesterone for pregnancy: control of cholesterol flux to the side-chain cleavage system. *J Reprod Fertil Suppl* 2000;**55**:3–12.
28. Casper RF, Yen SS. Induction of luteolysis in the human with a long-acting analog of luteinizing hormone-releasing factor. *Science* 1979;**205**:408–10.
29. Yen SSC, Jaffe RB. *Reproductive endocrinology; physiology, pathophysiology and clinical management.* 3rd ed. W.B. Saunders Company; 1991.
30. Melmed S, Polonsky K, Larsen PR, Kronenberg HM. *Williams textbook of endocrinology.* 12th ed. Saunders Elsevier; 2011.
31. Hacker N, Moore JG, Gambone JC. *Essentials of obsetetrics and gynecology.* 6th ed. Elsevier Saunders; 2016.
32. Franasiak JM, Scott Jr RT. *Recurrent implantation failure; etiologies and clinical management.* Springer International Publishing; 2018.
33. Creasy R, Resnik R. *Maternal fetal medicine principles and practice.* 2nd ed. W.B. Saunders Company; 1989.
34. Watson-Whitmyre M. *Conception.* Salem Press Encyclopedia of Science; 2013.
35. Schoni-Affolter F, Dubuis-Grieder C, Strauch E. *Human embryology: the path of the sperm cells to the oocyte—capacitation.* The Swiss Virtual Campus Online, Universities of Fribourg, Lausanne, and Bern; 2007. Available from: *http://www.embryology.ch/indexen.html*.
36. Reece EA, Hobbins JC, Mahoney MJ, Petrie RH. *Medicine of the fetus and mother.* J.B. Lippincott Company; 1992.
37. Herbst AL, Mishell DR, Stenchever MA, Droegemueller W. *Comprehensive gynecology.* 2nd ed. Mosby Year Book; 1992.

Chapter 13

Maintenance of Pregnancy and Parturition

Jason Phung*, Jonathan Paul† and Roger Smith‡

*Obstetrics & Gynaecology, John Hunter Hospital, Newcastle, NSW, Australia, †Medicine and Public Health, University of Newcastle, Newcastle, NSW, Australia, ‡Endocrinology, University of Newcastle, Newcastle, NSW, Australia

---

Key Clinical Changes

- Human pregnancy exhibits functional progesterone withdrawal and estrogen activation.
- The gene expression of contraction-associated proteins is favored at the time of human labor.
- Inflammation in pregnancy is associated with infection from microorganisms and sterile inflammation related to cellular senescence and damage.
- Novel initiators of labor, including cell-free fetal DNA and exosomes released from the placenta and fetal membranes, may provide new insight into the mechanisms of labor and be useful biomarkers for preterm labor.

13.1 ESTABLISHMENT OF PREGNANCY

Successful establishment of pregnancy begins with implantation of a viable blastocyst into a progesterone- and human chorionic gonadotropin (hCG)-primed endometrium. This process requires a two-way interaction between the maternal uterus and the semiallograft blastocyst. Implantation occurs only during a narrow window of time when the endometrium is most receptive to a blastocyst. In humans, this is during the midsecretory phase (6–10 days following ovulation on day 14), corresponding to days 20–24 of a 28-day menstrual cycle. Understanding the mechanics of embryo implantation has clinical implications, as implantation failure can lead to recurrent pregnancy loss and infertility. The natural success rate of implantation and establishment of pregnancy in humans is 25%–30% per cycle. Furthermore, only half of human embryos transferred during in vitro fertilization (IVF) will successfully implant.[1]

A typical menstrual cycle lasts 28 days and begins with menses (day 0). The proliferative phase (follicular phase) following menses is characterized by the pulsatile release of gonadotropin releasing hormone (GnRH) from the hypothalamus, acting on the anterior pituitary gland to release follicle-stimulating hormone (FSH) and luteinizing hormone (LH). FSH causes folliculogenesis in the ovaries, with subsequent selection of a dominant follicle. FSH also acts on ovarian granulosa cells to convert androgens (released from thecal cells in response to LH) into estrogen (estradiol). There is a surge of FSH and LH on day 14, leading to ovulation from the dominant follicle. The secretory phase (luteal phase) is characterized by endometrial thickening and formation of the corpus luteum from the ruptured dominant follicle after ovulation has occurred. The corpus luteum supplies progesterone and estrogen, which steadily increases into the midluteal phase, where the window of receptivity opens. In the absence of blastocyst implantation during this window, luteolysis occurs along with subsequent hormone withdrawal, and menstruation ensues. It is thought that hCG released by the blastocyst aids in making the endometrium receptive to implantation. In baboon studies, hCG administration directly modulates the function of endometrial stromal and epithelial cells.[2] Successful implantation of a blastocyst during this time allows the embedded blastocyst to continue to produce hCG, which maintains the corpus luteum. This ensures an ongoing supply of progesterone and estrogen to support the establishment of pregnancy until the placenta develops. Furthermore, hCG also prevents uterine contractions through stimulating the production of cyclic adenosine monophosphate (cAMP) within the myocytes, which prevents displacement of the conceptus in early gestation.[3] In turn, cAMP also stimulates hCG production within the trophoblasts of the blastocyst.[4]

Estrogen and progesterone mediate changes to the endometrium and cause the activation of the blastocyst required for implantation. Most of the data on hormonal regulation of endometrial receptivity and pregnancy establishment has been obtained from animal studies. Studies in mice show that progesterone receptor A (encoded by the *PGR* gene) and a preimplantation estrogen rise through estrogen receptor (ER) binding (encoded by the *ESR1* gene) is vital for blastocyst activation and successful implantation.[5] Progesterone and cAMP decidualize the endometrium, allowing trophoblast invasion

Maternal-Fetal and Neonatal Endocrinology. https://doi.org/10.1016/B978-0-12-814823-5.00013-1

and development of the placenta. Estrogen appears to be the dominant mediator of stromal changes to the endometrium that are required for implantation.[6] Even animals that seemingly only require progesterone for successful implantation have evidence of aromatase production from blastocysts, suggesting that endogenous production of estrogen from androgens circumvents the need for maternal estrogen supply.[7,8] Following successful implantation, progesterone and cAMP maintain myometrial quiescence, while estrogen stimulates growth of the uterus by myometrial cell proliferation and hypertrophy to accommodate the growing fetus.

13.2   THE CERVIX AND ITS CHANGES IN PREGNANCY

The cervix is the opening of the uterus, composed of fibrous connective tissue (80%–85%)[9] and contractile smooth muscle (10%).[10] Its tensile strength is related to the organization of collagen within the extracellular matrix (ECM), which allows it to resist pressure from the growing fetus and remain closed throughout pregnancy. Other important components of ECM include proteoglycans, hyaluronan, and elastin. The cervix also protects the pregnancy against microbial invasion by secreting thick mucus from endocervical cells, which make up 50% of the tissue mass during pregnancy. These endocervical cells also secrete defensins and are able to activate inflammation and local immune responses to bacteria and their toxins.[11] Due to the difficulties in obtaining cervical biopsy during human pregnancy, our understanding of cervical remodeling in pregnancy is based on studies in rats.[11]

Structural remodeling of the ECM begins in early pregnancy and is key to allowing the cervix to withstand the increasing load from pregnancy. This initial process of remodeling is called *cervical softening* (see Fig. 13.1); this is a misleading term, as *softening* refers to the ECM rather than the softening of the cervix itself (which, in fact, remains firm throughout most of pregnancy). There is a decrease in collagen concentration, leading to increased tissue compliance while still maintaining tissue integrity.[11] Cervical competency, which is key to a successful pregnancy, relies on the slow occurrence of the process of cervical softening. Studies in rodents have demonstrated that relaxin, an insulinlike factor, promotes cervical softening[12]; however, the role of relaxin in cervical remodeling in human pregnancy is not fully characterized.[13]

In rat pregnancy, cervical softening ultimately leads to *cervical ripening* (see Fig. 13.1), which refers to a range of dynamic changes to the cervix itself rather than the ECM (although changes within the ECM also occur). The cervical changes include *effacement* (shortening), softening, and dilation. These changes are present in human cervix in the days (and sometimes weeks) leading up to human parturition.[11,14] The ECM remodeling that occurs in rat cervical ripening includes increases in glycosaminoglycans (e.g., hyaluronan) and aquaporin channels, resulting in increased tissue hydration that causes collagen dispersion in the cervix.[11,15] Hyaluronan, a glycosaminoglycan, also weakens the binding of collagen to scaffolding glycoproteins in the ECM (e.g., fibronectin).[16] Dispersed collagen fibers are subsequently more susceptible to degradation by proteases such as matrix metalloproteinases (MMPs).

MMPs are a group of proteases that have various target substrates: MMP-1 and MMP-8 are collagenases, MMP-2 and MMP-9 are gelatinases, and MMP-3 is a stromelysin.[17] The transcripts of these MMPs are increased in cervical tissue from

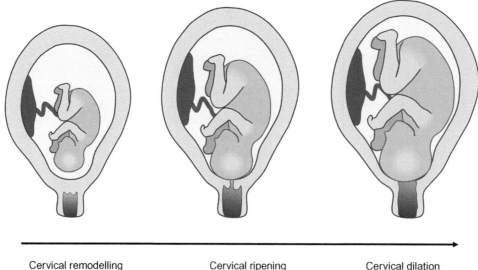

Cervical remodelling   Cervical ripening   Cervical dilation

FIG. 13.1   Cervical remodeling, ripening, and dilation.

pregnant women at term, implicating that they play a role in the remodeling of the cervix prior to the onset of labor.[18,19] These MMPs appear to be regulated by leukocytes and inflammatory cytokines, such as IL-8, IL-1β, IL-6, and tumor necrosis factor-alpha (TNF-α),[20] which are also upregulated at the time of labor.[21] The role of inflammation in labor is discussed later in this chapter.

What is known about the regulation of cervical remodelling in human pregnancy is largely based on animal studies. A body of evidence from mice experiments suggests that hormonal regulation (particularly progesterone withdrawal) is key to initiating cervical ripening and dilation.[22] In pregnant mice, local metabolism of progesterone is important for labor, as the majority of mice deficient in 5a reductase type I do not labor secondary to failure of cervical ripening.[23] There is evidence of local hormone metabolism in the human cervix.[24] Further, 17β-hydroxysteroid dehydrogenase (17βHSD) type 2 is found in the pregnant human cervix and converts 20α-hydroxyprogesterone to bioactive progesterone, and estradiol to the less biologically active estrone. 17βHSD levels drop during labor and is thought to play a role in localized progesterone withdrawal that facilitates cervical remodeling in humans.[24] Following labor, the cervix undergoes a reparative process that restores the cervix to its prepregnancy state.

13.3 MAINTAINING QUIESCENCE IN THE PREGNANT UTERUS

13.3.1 Human Chorionic Gonadotropin

As the fetus grows with gestation, so does the uterus. Key hormones in the establishment of pregnancy continue to increase with advancing gestation, including estrogen (both estradiol and estriol), progesterone, and hCG.[25,26] A successful pregnancy relies on quiescence in the myometrium, so that uterine contraction is delayed until the fetus has completed growth and maturation at term.

A number of factors are important in maintaining uterine quiescence. First, circulating hCG levels continue to gradually rise in the second and third trimesters of pregnancy,[25] where it acts on hCG receptors in the myometrium to maintain myometrium relaxation by inhibiting the production of gap junctions required for labor.[27] Evidence implicating its direct role in myometrial relaxation comes from in vitro studies demonstrating hCG administration to human myometrium tissue strips in pregnancy led to reduced oxytocin-induced contractility.[28] hCG also indirectly maintains quiescence by stimulating cAMP, whose role in maintenance of pregnancy is discussed later in this chapter.[3] Furthermore, there is a decrease in hCG levels 2 weeks prior to the onset of labor,[25] as well as a reduced number of myometrial hCG receptors in labor compared to nonlabor states.[29] This temporal relationship suggests that hCG contributes to pregnancy quiescence, and its declining activity may play a role in parturition in humans.

13.3.2 Progesterone

Progesterone is a steroid hormone important to establishing and maintaining pregnancy. During the menstrual cycle, progesterone inhibits contractions and thickens the lining of the endometrium, allowing blastocyst implantation. Progesterone is initially supped by the corpus luteum in early pregnancy and subsequently by the developing placenta from approximately 7 weeks gestation. Following the establishment of pregnancy, progesterone acts to prolong gestation and maintain uterine quiescence in many species, including humans.

George Corner, and later Arpad Csapo, first described the concept of a "progesterone block" in the 1940s and 1950s, when they observed that progesterone prevented stimulation of contractions with oxytocin in animal models. That is, the presence of progesterone created a block against drivers of uterine contractions and labor. This progesterone-dependent delay in uterine contraction allows fetal growth and development. Metaphorically, progesterone acts as a biological brake to the onset of labor, which, once lifted, enables the uterus to undergo transformation from a noncontractile phenotype into a contractile phenotype.

Progesterone prolongs pregnancy predominantly through anti-inflammatory effects.[30] In vitro studies have demonstrated that progesterone blocks various inflammatory pathways and works to supress inflammation-induced *PTGS2* expression (and hence inhibits prostaglandin production).[31,32] Progesterone also reduces the activation of activator protein 1 (AP-1), a transcription factor expressed in response to human myometrial stretch and thought to be important in labor initiation.[33,34] Progesterone also increases the expression of *ZEB1* and *ZEB2*, which have shown repressive activity over both the *OXTR* and *GJA1* genes, which encode the oxytocin receptor (OTR) and connexin-43 proteins, respectively.[35]

A great body of evidence from animal models shows that decreased progesterone production from the ovary or placenta leads to a reduction in circulating progesterone levels, and hence a reduction in its blocking effects on myometrial contractility. Removing the progesterone block lifts the brake on parturition toward the end of gestation. In rats, mice, rabbits, goats, and pigs, progesterone supply is primarily dependent on the corpus luteum; and luteolysis due to the action of $PGF_{2\alpha}$ results in a measurable drop in systemic progesterone, which coincides with labor. In sheep, active conversion of progesterone to estrogen via 17α-hydroxylase within the placenta appears to be the main driver of labor. There is no measurable drop in progesterone levels that precedes labor in human pregnancy. In fact, serum progesterone levels increase with gestation and during labor. Despite this observation, mifepristone, a prostaglandin analog with antiprogestin effects administered at any point throughout human gestation, initiates cervical ripening and subsequent uterine contractions, leading to expulsion of the conceptus. As such, a functional progesterone withdrawal has been hypothesized as an alternative means to remove the progesterone block in human pregnancy. How this is achieved and the mechanisms that regulate this process in normal and pathological labor remain unknown. A number of hypotheses have been put forward: a loss of progesterone receptors (PRs), increase in progesterone metabolism, local production of antiprogestogens, sequestration of progesterone into cellular lipoproteins, unidirectional binding to proteins, and localization to the fetal membranes.[36,37] The most widely reported hypothesis on functional progesterone withdrawal in human pregnancy revolves around the interplay among the various PR isoforms.[38]

Classically, the PR functions as a transcription factor when it is liganded by progesterone. Once liganded, the PR translocates into the nucleus, where it binds to progesterone-specific promoter sequences on target genes to activate or inhibit their transcription, which appears to occur in a tissue-dependent manner. However, recent studies suggest that unliganded PR is also able to function as a transcription factor.[39] In humans, PR transcripts exist as two major isoforms that are encoded by the same gene but driven by different promotors.[40] The PR-B protein is a strong activator of progesterone-dependent genes and appears to drive the transcription of genes that aid in uterine quiescence. The PR-A protein is a truncated form of PR-B, lacking the first 164 amino acids at the N-terminal where the activator element 3 (AF3) is located.[41] Progesterone receptor A (PR-A) has a predominantly inhibitory function to gene transcription, and when coexpressed with progesterone receptor B (PR-B), it represses PR-B activity.[36] Progesterone receptor C (PR-C) is a third isoform, which is a truncated form of PR-B that lacks a DNA-binding domain and is found only in the cytosolic fraction.[42] Due to its missing DNA-binding site, it lacks transactivation ability but is able to bind to PR-B transcripts, rendering it biologically inactive. In vitro studies using an immortalized pregnant human cell line showed that overexpression of *PR-C* represses activity of PR-B.[42] PR-C was also upregulated in myometrium from women in labor.[42]

As repression of PR-B action appears to be the predominant mechanism by which progesterone withdrawal occurs in human and primate parturition,[38,43] understanding the regulation of PR-A throughout gestation is important. Prostaglandins (PGE_2 more so than $PG_{2\alpha}$), released in response to inflammation, increase both PR-A and PR-B messenger ribonucleic acid (mRNA) abundance in myometrium.[44] There appears to be higher PR-A expression relative to PR-B, leading to an increased PR-A-to-PR-B ratio, and thus an overall progesterone-reducing effect.[44] An important observation during human labor is that despite the fact that there is increased circulating progesterone, there is a decrease in progesterone levels in the nucleus and the majority of PR is unliganded during labor.[39] There is a corresponding increase in the progesterone-metabolizing enzyme, 20a hydroxysteroid dehydrogenase (20aHSD), which leads to localized progesterone withdrawal that encourages uncoupling of PR to its ligand.[39] In studies using immortalized human myometrial cells in pregnancy, liganded PR-B localizes to the nucleus and liganded PR-A is found in the cytoplasm. In their unliganded state, PR-A is found predominantly in the nucleus and PR-B was found only in the cytoplasm.[39] Taken together, liganded PR-B predominates within the nucleus and encourages myometrial quiescence throughout pregnancy. However, at the time of labor when PR are unliganded, PR-A is the predominant isoform found within the nucleus, where it favors the transformation of the myometrium into a contractile phenotype (see Fig. 13.2). For instance, unliganded PR-A functions as a transcription factor to activate GJA1, a known contraction-associated protein (discussed later in this chapter).[39]

A number of epigenetic changes, including histone modification at PR-A promotor regions and cytokine-mediated stabilization of PR-A stability, also work to increase the transrepressive activity of PR-A.[45–48]

13.3.3 Cyclic Adenosine Monophosphate

cAMP is a diffusible second messenger generated by the conversion of adenosine triphosphate (ATP) by adenylate cyclase (AC) enzymes. AC activation occurs in response to ligand binding to nuclear G-protein-coupled receptors (GPCRs). cAMP signaling is involved in a number of cellular pathways and is tightly regulated by AC activation, but also through phosphodiesterase (PDE) enzymes, which degrade free cAMP. Classically, cAMP binds to protein kinase A (PKA), which releases a catalytic subunit that is free to phosphorylate various targets, including the transcription factor cAMP response element-binding protein (CREB).

In the myometrium, cAMP is thought to induce relaxation through the inhibition of calcium signaling by PKA-led phosphorylation of PLC and the inactivation of myosin light chain kinase (MLCK), which prevent the phosphorylation of

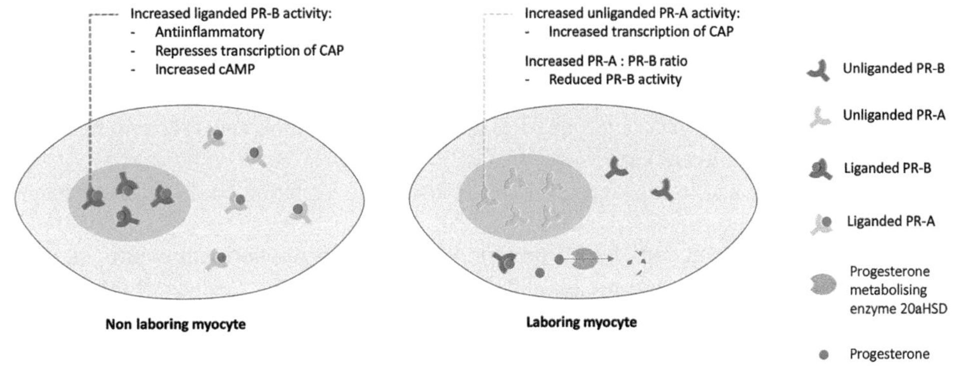

Increased liganded PR-B activity:
- Antiinflammatory
- Represses transcription of CAP
- Increased cAMP

Increased unliganded PR-A activity:
- Increased transcription of CAP

Increased PR-A : PR-B ratio
- Reduced PR-B activity

Unliganded PR-B

Unliganded PR-A

Liganded PR-B

Liganded PR-A

Progesterone metabolising enzyme 20aHSD

Progesterone

Non laboring myocyte

Laboring myocyte

FIG. 13.2 Localization and unliganding of PR-A and PR-B during labor. PR-A increased relative to PR-B during labor.

myosin, which is required for smooth muscle contraction.[49] PKA-activated transcription factors also has been shown to repress inflammatory pathways,[50] and reduce the expression of *OXTR*.[51] Furthermore, cAMP enhances the binding of PR-B to the progesterone response element (PRE) of progesterone-dependent genes, increasing their expression, and subsequently the progesterone block effect as well.[52]

13.4 REQUIREMENTS FOR LABOR CONTRACTIONS IN THE UTERUS

13.4.1 Corticotropin-Releasing Hormone

The term *placental clock* refers to placenta-derived corticotropin-releasing hormone (CRH) and its role in determining the length of human pregnancy.[53] In the nonpregnant state, CRH is a stress peptide hormone released from the hypothalamus as part of the hypothalamic-pituitary-adrenal (HPA) axis. CRH acts on the anterior pituitary to release adrenocorticotropic hormone (ACTH), which in turn acts on the adrenal glands to stimulate the release of cortisol, a glucocorticoid stress hormone (see Fig. 13.3).

Placental CRH is secreted by trophoblasts during human pregnancy and is first detectable by radioimmunoassay (RIA) early in the second trimester.[53] CRH levels rise with gestation in an exponential manner, peaking at the onset of labor.[26,53,54] This sudden increase in CRH level coincides with a reduction in CRH-binding hormone (CRH-BP), an endogenous inhibitor that renders CRH biologically inactive.[55–58] Reductions in CRH-BP levels occur approximately 30 days

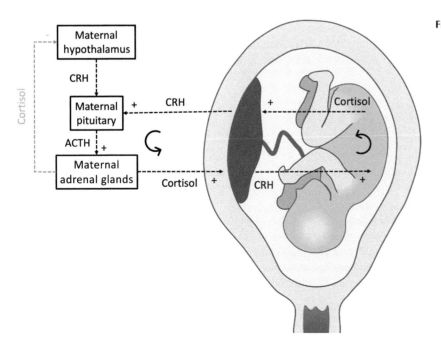

FIG. 13.3 A CRH feed-forward loop.

prior to the onset of labor, which contributes to increases in overall bioactive CRH.[53,55] Multiple studies have demonstrated that an increase in maternal serum CRH levels in the early third trimester is associated with preterm birth.[59,60] Furthermore, serial measurements of maternal CRH levels with advancing gestation have found the following:

- Women who delivered preterm had higher levels of CRH at any given gestation and a faster rate of increase with gestation compared to women who delivered at term.[53]
- Women who delivered postterm had lower levels of CRH at any given gestation compared to women that labored at term.[53]
- CRH levels do not increase in women who deliver preterm in the context of chorioamnionitis, suggesting the pathogenesis of PTB in these women differs to those that labor spontaneously in the absence of infection.[61]

While these results would suggest early processes in the placenta could play a role in determining the length of human pregnancy, heterogeneity between women that deliver preterm limits the use of CRH as a predictive test. Some have investigated the usefulness of a single CRH level in the third trimester,[60] while others have assessed the predictor of serial measurements[62]; however, overall CRH has moderate sensitivity (63%) and modest specificity (52%) when applied as a screening tool.[63]

While cortisol downregulates CRH production in the hypothalamus in a negative feedback loop within the HPA axis, it upregulates CRH production in the placenta in a feed-forward system during pregnancy. Placental CRH is also released into the fetal circulation,[64] where it stimulates the fetal adrenal glands to produce cortisol, from the outer definitive zone,[65] and dehydroepiandrosterone sulfate (DHEAS), from the inner fetal zone.[66] Fetal contributions of cortisol add to the feed-forward loop stimulating further CRH production, eventually resulting in the aforementioned CRH surge. DHEAS, on the other hand, is the precursor for the placental production of estradiol and the substrate for liver 16-hydroxylase. Here, 16-hydroxylated DHEAS is the precursor for placental production of estriol. Furthermore, increasing cortisol production by the fetal adrenal glands is necessary for fetal lung development and maturation. In mice, maturation of the fetal lungs also produces proinflammatory phospholipids and surfactant protein A, which have been found to permeate the amniotic fluid, where they are able to attract immune cells that initiate inflammatory pathways seen at the time of labor.[67]

While there is no doubt that CRH is important in regulating human gestational length, its exact role in the uterus is not fully characterized. Its production is primarily driven by binding of CREB to the CRH gene, which is stimulated by mediators of uterine quiescence (cAMP and PR-B), as discussed previously, but also by mediators of uterine contractions (PR-A and estrogen).[68,69] Studies of human myometrial tissue strips showed that at lower physiological concentrations, CRH caused reduced contractions in human myometrium strips from preterm and term women.[70] This relaxation effect was enhanced 3.5-fold by progesterone supplementation.[70] This tocolytic effect appears to be related to cAMP production, which increases upon activation of the CRH receptor in myometrium through increased adenylyl cyclase (AC) (see Section 13.3.3). At higher concentrations of CRH, its receptor becomes desensitized, leading to reduced CRH receptors coupling to $G\alpha_s$ protein, subsequently reduced AC activation, and thus impaired cAMP production.[71] Furthermore, CRH may have synergistic roles with oxytocin[72] and prostaglandin $F_{2\alpha}$[73] in myometrial contractility; however, high doses of CRH were not able to induce or enhance contractions.[70,74] CRH, therefore, plays a paradoxical role in maintaining uterine quiescence throughout gestation, but it also may aid the transition of myometrium into a contractile phenotype during labor.[75]

13.4.2 Estrogen

Three types of estrogen are produced in humans—estrone (E1), estradiol (E2), and estriol (E3)—which have varying degrees of potency in their interaction with ERs. Estradiol and estriol are the predominant estrogens produced during pregnancy, with estradiol considered to have higher estrogenic activity than estriol. In early pregnancy, the corpus luteum and the maternal ovaries supply estradiol and from the eighth week of gestation, production is taken over by the placenta. However, the placenta is an incomplete steroid-generating organ, in that it lacks the ability to produce DHEAS due to an absence of the enzyme 17α-hydroxylase (P450c17). Because DHEAS and its hydroxylated form, 16-hydroxy-DHEAS, are important precursors required for estrogen synthesis, the placenta relies on maternal and fetal contributions of these substrates. DHEAS produced predominantly by the maternal adrenal is converted to estradiol in the placenta.[76] On the other hand, DHEAS produced by the fetal adrenals undergoes hydroxylation in the fetal liver by 16α-hydroxylase to form 16-OH-DHEAS, which is converted to estriol in the placenta. Production of DHEAS increases with gestation and is regulated by CRH, which is discussed elsewhere in this chapter.

Throughout gestation, estradiol and estriol both steadily increase in equimolar concentrations.[26] At equimolar concentrations, estradiol and estriol block one another's actions through the formation of heterodimers. However, when the ratio of estriol to estradiol exceeds 10:1, there is an increase of estrogenic activity, as estriol is able to form homodimers.[77] In a longitudinal study measuring hormones in pregnancy, there is a rise in the ratio of estriol to estradiol at the time of parturition (driven by rising placenta CRH production, which acts directly on the fetal adrenal to stimulate DHEAS synthesis), demonstrating a functional activation of estrogen toward labor.[26] Interestingly, in the case of fetal death, levels of estriol fall as estradiol levels remain elevated, resulting in a change in ratio that favors estradiol, which also results in the activation of labor.[4,26] This redundant mechanism may be an evolutionary mechanism to preserve maternal life even with fetal death. Switching to an estrogenic environment upregulates a number of contraction-associated proteins, including gap junction alpha-1 protein (encoded by the *GJA1* gene and also known as *connexin 43*),[78,79] OTR (encoded by the *OXTR* gene)[80] and prostaglandin-synthesizing enzymes (see Section 13.4.4).[38] These changes occur upon ligand binding to ESR1 receptors, which displays upregulation at the time of labor.[38]

In vitro studies have also examined estrogen action through the seven-transmembrane receptor GPR30, encoded by *GPER1*. *GPER1* transcripts are found in pregnant human myometrium, and the GPR30 protein is localized to the cell membrane of myometrium.[81] Treatment of pregnant human myometrial strips with the GPR30 agonist, G-1, and estradiol enhanced the phosphorylation of heat shock protein 27 (HSP27) and oxytocin-induced contractility.[81,82] These changes facilitate myometrial contractility by stabilizing actin filaments and increasing calcium signaling, respectively.

Estradiol is also responsible for the rapid expansion and growth of the uterus throughout gestation,[83] which allows accommodation of the growing fetus. The effect of the growing fetus on the uterine wall during human pregnancy is not well understood. Studies in pregnant mice provide insights into myometrial growth patterns in pregnancy, changing from hyperplasia to hypertrophy at midgestation.[84] This is about the same time that the fetus is most spherical and thought to be exerting the greatest tension on the uterine wall.[84,85] As the uterus slows its growth, there is an increase in intrauterine tension. This leads to a combination of stretch, hypoxia, and reduced blood flow that activates caspase enzymes, particularly caspase 3.[85] Caspase 3 (encoded by the *CASP3* gene) contributes to uterine quiescence in mouse pregnancy by cleaving smooth muscle actin in a progesterone-dependent manner.[86] *CASP3* transcripts reduce at the end of mouse gestation, which coincide with reduced progesterone levels and restoration of full-length actin.[84]

Myometrial stretch is also an important initiator of human labor, as women with multiple gestations[87] or polyhydramnios (where there is uterine overdistention) are at higher risk of PTB.[87,88] Evidence suggests that myometrial stretch activates mitogen-activated protein kinases (MAPKs), which are a group of enzymes that phosphorylate serine and threonine amino acids in order to modulate extracellular signals that direct gene expression of contraction-associated genes that favor a contractile phenotype in the uterus.[33] While there is increasing stretch-activated expression of prolabor genes with advancing gestation, most pregnancies do not deliver until term. Furthermore, estrogen levels throughout early gestation to midgestation in human pregnancy are already significantly higher than humans in nonpregnant states. Despite this, the uterus does not switch to a contractile phenotype until the end of pregnancy. This is likely due to progesterone blocking. Upon withdrawal of progesterone's effects, the uterus is able to respond to a multitude of stimuli (including estrogen and myometrial stretch) that enable it to transform from a quiescent to a contractile state. Premature withdrawal of progesterone, therefore, may contribute to premature labor. Evidence of this is observed in studies in which abrupt progesterone withdrawal by ovariectomy in mice leads to PTB, which is associated with an increase in oxytocin and labor.[89]

13.4.3 Oxytocin and the OTR

Sir Henry Dale first discovered oxytocin when one of his studies elicited uterine contractions following the administration of posterior pituitary extracts in pregnant cats.[90] The modern-day use of synthetic oxytocin to cause uterine contractions to induce labor comes from a body of research that is still predominantly from animal studies. There is an increase in oxytocin levels at the time of labor in animal studies (involving rodents, rhesus monkeys, and sheep) that is not consistently reproducible in human labor.[91–96] In women, oxytocin is released from the posterior pituitary in a pulsatile manner and has a relatively short half-life and high clearance rate[97] by placental oxytocinase.[98] Oxytocin binds to the OTR, a protein that increases in expression in the myometrium with advancing gestation.[99,100] While it would seem logical that OTR expression would increase at the time of labor, there is no consensus in the published literature, with some studies showing decreased myometrial expression,[101,102] and others showing increased expression with the onset of labor.[103–105] Interestingly, the action of oxytocin and OTR is not a requirement for labor onset in mice,[106] nor in humans, as reports exist of women with panhypopituitarism who labored spontaneously.[107] The mechanisms of how oxytocin affects smooth muscle contractility is covered in the following discussion.

Besides the myometrium, oxytocin and OTR are found in chorion-amnion and decidua,[108] where it stimulates the production of prostaglandins. In vitro studies demonstrate oxytocin treatment of human amnion cells stimulated the synthesis of prostaglandin E_2 (PGE_2),[109] while the treatment of human decidua cells resulted in increased prostaglandin $F_{2\alpha}$ ($PGF_{2\alpha}$)

production.[110] These prostaglandins are lipid molecules that play vital roles in parturition by encouraging smooth muscle contractions. The mechanism by which oxytocin increases prostaglandin production appears to be the activation of cytoplasmic phospholipase A$_2$ that causes release of a 20-carbon unsaturated fatty acid called *arachidonic acid (AA)*.[111] Prostaglandin G/H synthase (PTGS), or cyclooxygenase, is the group of enzymes that then convert AA into prostaglandin G$_2$ (PGG$_2$), which is then immediately converted to prostaglandin H$_2$ (PGH$_2$), the substrate for production of various prostaglandins, including PGE$_2$, PGF$_{2\alpha}$, and PGD$_2$, as well as prostacyclin (PGI$_2$) and thromboxane (TxA2).[110–113] There is increased AA metabolism at the time of labor,[114] leading to increased prostaglandin action that promotes myometrial contractility.

13.4.4 Prostaglandins and Prostaglandin Receptors

In human pregnancy, the majority of prostaglandin is produced in amnion cells by *PTGS2* (and not its other isoforms).[115,116] Evidence indicating the role of PTGS2 in these processes include increased concentrations of prostaglandin in amniotic fluid of pregnant women[117,118] and increased transcripts of *PTGS2* in human myometrium,[119] chorion-amnion,[114,116,120] and decidua at the time of labor.[121] Furthermore, myometrial stretch and proinflammatory mediators, such as lipopolysaccharide (LPS), IL-1β, and TNF-α, stimulate increased PTGS2 production in vitro and in animal studies, suggesting that inflammation at the onset of labor coincides with an increase in prostaglandin activity.

Prostaglandins are also used clinically to ripen the cervix for induction of labor, and its analog, misoprostol, is commonly used for termination of pregnancy or induction of labor following midgestation fetal demise. PTGS2 inhibitors like celecoxib delay labor in animal models[122]; however, in human pregnancy, the use of a PTGS inhibitor called *indomethacin* causes premature closure of the ductus arteriosus in the fetal heart, reducing its use as a treatment for preterm labor.[123]

A prostaglandin inactivator, prostaglandin dehydrogenase (PGDH), is present in human chorion and trophoblastic cells. It causes irreversible conversion of PGE$_2$ and PGF$_{2\alpha}$ into their biologically inactive forms. Prostaglandins are primarily produced by the amnion, so the fact that PGDH are produced in high quantities in adjacent tissue suggests that it plays a role in the regulation of prostaglandins during pregnancy. Studies have demonstrated that PGDH may be stimulated by progesterone, while CRH, estrogen, and other inflammatory mediators stimulate *PTGS2*. The balance of the opposing actions of PGDH and PTGS2 (and their respective regulators), therefore, may determine whether a contractile or quiescent state is achieved in the uterus. The balance favors contractility at the time of labor.

An understanding of prostaglandin effect, therefore, is important in uncovering the pathway to parturition. Prostaglandins exhibit various effects upon binding to specific GPCRs in target tissue. There are four PGE$_2$ receptors: EP1, EP2, EP3, and EP4, and two receptors for PGF2α, FP (types a and β). EP1 and FP promote contraction by increasing intracellular Ca^{2+} levels, whereas EP4 has a relaxing effect through stimulation of cAMP. EP2 and EP3 have dual actions that promote contraction and relaxation—in particular, EP2 receptor working via G$_{\alpha s}$ to promote cAMP signaling maintains myometrial quiescence, while EP2 working via G$_{\alpha q/11}$ promotes Ca^{2+} signaling and myometrial contractility. Differences in expression of the four PGE$_2$ receptors are observed in the myometrium during labor,[124] and thus regulation of these receptors is likely to determine the balance between uterine quiescence and contractility.

13.4.5 Calcium Signaling and Myometrial (Smooth Muscle) Contractility

Despite its uncertain role in the initiation of parturition, oxytocin is a powerful uterotonic that is used in clinical practice to induce and augment labor, as well as in the prophylaxis and treatment of postpartum hemorrhage. OXTR is a rhodopsin-type GPCR. Activation of the G$_{q/11}$ protein activates phospholipase C-β, which hydrolyzes phosphatidylinositol bisphosphate (PIP$_2$) to form inositol triphosphate (IP$_3$) and diacylglycerol (DAG). IP$_3$ binds to receptors on the sarcoplasmic reticulum, causing release of Ca^{2+} into the cytosol. The increase in intracellular Ca^{2+} results in four Ca^{2+} ions binding to calmodulin, forming a Ca^{2+}-calmodulin complex that activates the enzyme MLCK, which phosphorylates serine-19 of the regulatory myosin light chain (MLC). Phosphorylated MLC is then able to interact with actin filaments in an ATP-dependent manner known as *cross-bridge cycling*, generating force and contraction. This process is reversed by MLC phosphatase (MLCP). DAG activates protein kinase C (PKC), which phosphorylates MLCP into its inactive form. DAG also stimulates an inhibitor of MLCP called *C-kinase-activated protein phosphatase-1 inhibitor 17 kDa (CPI-17)*. Together, PKC increases the phosphorylation of MLC by reducing the action of MLCP. On the other hand, activation of the G$_{12/13}$ protein triggers activation of Rho kinase (ROCK). ROCK is able to phosphorylate myosin-binding subunit 1 (MYPT1) of MLCP, which inactivates its ability to dephosphorylate MLC. This pathway is independent of Ca^{2+} and is activated upon oxytocin binding.[125]

Transient increases in intracellular Ca^{2+}, therefore, are required for cross-bridge cycling and smooth muscle contraction. Excessive cytosolic Ca^{2+} leads to cellular damage and apoptosis. Therefore, Ca^{2+} signaling is tightly regulated through numerous transporters and ion pumps. The resting membrane potential in uterine smooth muscle lies between -35 and $-80\,mV$ and is a reflection of ionic concentrations across the cell membrane, particularly Ca^{2+}, Na^+, K^+, and Cl^-.[126] This resting membrane potential is maintained via an ATPase-dependent Na^+-K^+ channel that pumps three Na^+ ions across the cell membrane into the extracellular space in exchange for two K^+ ions. These K^+ ions then passively diffuse out of the cell via K^+ channels (which are opened by β-sympathomimetics), creating a negatively charged intracellular environment that is refractory to depolarization. Therefore, $K+$ channels maintain uterine quiescence and their diminished activity at parturition encourages uterine contractility.[127] Binding of oxytocin and prostaglandins to their respective receptors causes the opening of ligand-operated Ca^{2+} channels, promoting intracellular increases in Ca^{2+}. The increase in intracellular Ca^{2+} levels lowers the electronegativity of the cell, which activates voltage-gated Ca^{2+} channels, further increasing the influx of Ca^{2+} into the cell. This leads to depolarization of the cell and activation of contraction mechanisms. Other nonselective cation channels may also be involved in the regulation of uterine contractility, including transient receptor potential vanilloid 4 (TRPV4) channels. When activated by agonists in pregnant rats, these channels allow increase cytosolic calcium levels in myometrium and increase uterine contractility.[128] These channels are increased in the myometrium in pregnant women compared to nonpregnant women, but their role in parturition has yet to be defined.

13.4.6   Gap Junctions

The phenomenon discussed previously occurs in each individual myocyte cell—but how does a collective group of myocytes depolarize in unison? Unlike the smooth muscles of the gastrointestinal (which possess interstitial cells of Cajal, which are able to generate rhythmic action potentials) or the myocytes of the heart (which are controlled by the sinoatrial node), there is no equivalent pacemaker in the uterus to orchestrate myometrial contractions. However, labor is characterized by strong, regular, and rhythmic contractions, which is possible due to myometrial electrical coupling through gap junctions. At the time of parturition, myocytes become increasingly connected via the gap junction protein, connexin-43 (see Fig. 13.4). Regulation of connexin-43 in early pregnancy occurs through a progesterone-induced transcription factor called *zinc finger E-box-binding homeobox 1 (ZEB1)*, which works to inhibit the formation of gap junctions.[35] However, as term approaches, the formation of gap junctions increases dramatically. Leading up to labor,

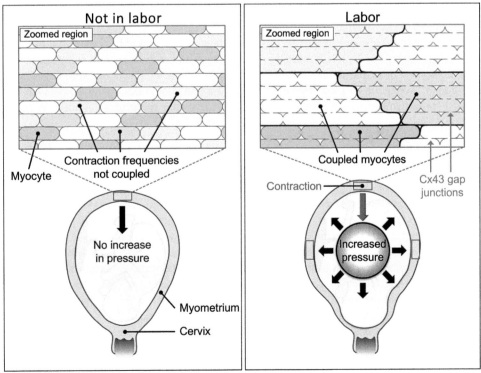

FIG. 13.4   Increased gap-junction connections between myocytes at the time of labor.

decreasing progesterone activity reduces ZEB1 activity, and increasing estrogen activity activates micro-RNA (miRNA) that also works to inhibit ZEB1.[129] When a threshold of myocyte connectivity is reached that allows a sufficiently large area of myometrium to depolarize in unison, there is a rise in intrauterine pressure that stretches the uterine walls as a whole; the stretch causes depolarization of the rest of the uterus leading to synchronous contractions.[130] Prior to reaching this threshold, nonpainful contractions experienced by women in the third trimester, called *Braxton-Hicks contractions*, may represent patches of uterine activity in the presence of insufficient gap-junction connectivity. These contractions increase in frequency toward term and are often referred to as *practice contractions*.

13.4.7 Micro-RNA

A family of miRNAs, miR-200, has also been shown to regulate parturition processes.[35] Here, miRNA is noncoding, single-stranded RNA that is 19–25 nucleotides in length[50] and regulates at least a third of the human genome. It binds to the 3′ untranslated region of mRNA to regulate gene repression, predominantly at the posttranscriptional level. Further, miR-200 downregulates ZEB1 and ZEB2 transcription factors, which repress the expression of contraction-associated proteins such as *GJA1* and *OTXR*.[35] Furthermore, miR-200a (a member of the miR-200 family) also increases during labor, where it inhibits STAT5B,[131] a transcriptional factor that represses 20aHSD and its progesterone-metabolizing activity.[132] Deletion of the *STAT5B* gene in mice leads to sustained high levels of circulating progesterone and causes a delay in labor.[132]

Also, miRNA expression profiles are altered through exogenous oxytocin administration in pregnant women,[133] and various miRNA changes at midgestation have been associated with spontaneous preterm birth.[134] Taken together, it appears that miRNAs are important in both normal and preterm labor.

13.5 INFLAMMATION IN PREGNANCY

13.5.1 Sterile and Nonsterile (Microbial) Inflammation and the Innate Immune System

Inflammation is a result of activation of the innate immune system—the first line of defense against harm.[135] It leads to leucocyte infiltration and production of cytokines and chemokines that alter gene expression to affect protective mechanisms of the host in response to perceived harm. This protective response is mediated by antigen-presenting immune cells that contain pattern-recognition receptors (PRRs), such as toll-like-receptors (TLRs).[136] These PRRs recognize potential pathogenic components, such as bacterial nucleic acids, lipoproteins, glycoproteins, and components of bacterial membranes, including peptidoglycans, lipoteichoic acid, lipopolysaccharide, and glycosylphatidylinositol. These components are collectively known as *pathogen-associated molecular patterns (PAMPs)*. The innate immune system can also be activated by cellular damage in the absence of microorganisms, which can be caused by trauma and ischemia. These components are called *damage-associated molecular patterns (DAMPs)*[137] and include protein components derived from the nucleus, cytoplasm, exosomes, or extracellular matrix, or within plasma, as well as nonprotein DAMPs, such as nucleic acids, ATP, and uric acid. Activation of PRRs by either PAMPs or DAMPs initiates cellular pathways and alters gene expression to produce proinflammatory chemokines, cytokines, and other molecules required to mount an immune response.

13.5.2 Inflammation in Parturition

The fetus is a semiallograft and relies on tight regulation of maternal cytokines at the maternal-fetal interface as a means of allowing pregnancy to continue without fetal cells being attacked by the maternal immune system. Progesterone appears to exert anti-inflammatory effects that allow maternal tolerance of the fetus, which begins in early gestation through the action of the leukemia inhibitory factor (LIF),[138] while throughout gestation, the production of the anti-inflammatory cytokine, IL-10, at the maternal-fetal interface suppresses proinflammatory cytokines.[139,140] This tolerance, however, appears to be lost or withdrawn at the time of labor, which coincides with an excess production of inflammatory markers. This has been demonstrated by studies showing an increase in neutrophils and macrophages in the cervix and myometrium during labor,[141] as well as an increase in the proinflammatory chemokines that promote the migration of these leucocytes into the chorion-amnion, decidua, amniotic fluid, placenta, cervix, and myometrium.[142,143]

Inflammation can also be a response to infection.[144] Microorganisms gain access to the otherwise-sterile amniotic cavity via ascending the genitourinary tract[145] or via hematogenous spread, as in the case of periodontal infection.[146,147] In fact, microbial-associated intra-amniotic inflammation has been causally linked to PTB, as a number of bacterial components are recognized to initiate inflammation at the onset of labor.[148] Inflammation stimulates the release of numerous proinflammation cytokines and chemokines that contribute to various aspects of parturition, reflected in their contributions to (1) remodeling of the cervix to allow dilation, (2) weakening of fetal membranes leading to membrane rupture, and (3) initiating rhythmic contractions.

In the cervix, infiltration of leucocytes leads to the production of IL-8, IL-1β, IL-6, and TNF-α.[149,150] MMP-1, MMP-2, MMP-3, MMP-8, and MMP-9 transcripts are increased in cervical biopsies from pregnant women at term.[18,19] IL-1β and TNF-α are able to increase the production of MMPs (in particular, MMP-1, MMP-3, and MMP-9) and proteases (cathepsin), which work to break down the extracellular matrix of collagen and elastin within the cervix.[20] IL-1β also represses the production of an inhibitor of MMP-2, called the *tissue inhibitor of metalloproteinase 2 (TIMP-2)*.[20] IL-8 is a chemotactic to neutrophils and also acts to increase the production of MMP-8.[151] Together, these processes lead to softening, shortening, and dilation of the cervix.

In the fetal membranes, similar degradation of the extracellular matrix leads to reduced membrane integrity, increasing the likelihood of spontaneous rupture. This is facilitated by IL-1β- and TNF-α-induced increases in MMP-9 and reduction in TIMP-2.[152,153] Furthermore, in vitro treatment of amnion and chorion cells with IL-1β and TNF-α leads to increased PGE$_2$ in a PTGS2-dependent manner.[154,155] PGE$_2$ produced by the amnion further increases MMP-9 levels to perpetuate the effects described previously.[156] IL-1β and TNF-α also reduce the production of PGDH, the inactivator of PGS, within the chorion.[157]

Perhaps unsurprisingly, transcripts of IL-1β and TNF-α are also increased in the myometrium at the time of labor.[149] In the myometrium, these cytokines cause phospholipid metabolism and the production of arachidonic acid,[158] which are the substrates required for PTGS to produce prostaglandins.[159] IL-1β also appears to stimulate expression of *PTGS2* through inflammatory pathways.[160] Increased IL-6 levels in the myometrium work to increase expression of *OXTR*,[161] and alongside IL-1β, they also increase the secretion of oxytocin from myometrial cells in vitro.[162] IL-8, which is consistently increased in the myometrium at the time of both term and preterm labor, appears to attract more leucocytes to propagate the effects of IL-1β.[151]

With advancing gestation, the likelihood of infection-associated PTB decreases. Work by Romero and colleagues found that prior to 25 weeks, microbial-associated intra-amniotic inflammation was more common, while sterile intra-amniotic inflammation was more common from 25 to 33 weeks of gestation.[144] DAMPs, such as high-mobility group box 1 (HMGB1), are elevated in patients with sterile intra-amniotic inflammation with intact membranes,[163] but mechanisms behind sterile intra-amniotic inflammation are not well defined. Certainly, a number of other mechanisms have been postulated to contribute to sterile inflammation, including oxidative stress (leading to cellular necrosis, apoptosis, or senescence), cell-free DNA, mechanical stretch, bleeding (e.g., antepartum hemorrhage or placental abruption), and release of fetal surfactant protein A into amniotic fluid.

13.6 OTHER MECHANISMS INVOLVED IN THE ACTIVATION OF PARTURITION

13.6.1 Oxidative Stress, Aging, and Senescence

Aging is the increasing probability of frailty, malfunction, and death that occurs because of accumulation of damage to molecules, cells, and tissues over a lifetime. Cells that undergo a terminal state of arrest but are still viable and functioning are in a state of senescence, which is distinct from cellular apoptosis. Cellular senescence is triggered by numerous stimuli, including oxidative stress, telomere shortening, and mitochondrial dysfunction—factors that often coexist. Senescence of fetal membrane cells as a result of cumulative oxidative stress has been postulated to release inflammatory mediators that may contribute to labor.[164] Menon et al. have demonstrated numerous markers of oxidative stress and cellular senescence in fetal membranes at term, including structural changes to mitochondria, endoplasmic reticulum, and the nucleus associated with senescence; increased expression of p38 mitogen-activated protein kinase stress-responsive kinases; and increased proportion of cells that are positive for senescence-associated beta-galactosidase.[165]

Cellular senescence is also associated with the release of inflammatory markers called *senescence-associated secretory proteins (SASPs)*,[166,167] which include cytokines, chemokines, growth factors, enzymes that degrade the matrix, and cell adhesion molecules and inhibitors.[166] Due to the degree of overlap between SASPs and inflammatory mediators seen during parturition (including IL-1β, IL-6, IL-8, TNF-α, and MMPs),[166,168,169] there is biological plausibility that SASPs released in response to cellular senescence may be a contributing factor to the inflammatory response seen at the onset of labor. Furthermore, SASPs such as MMPs could contribute to the weakening and spontaneous rupture of membranes that are seen in women at term. Interestingly, the concept of premature senescence of fetal membranes may be involved in the pathophysiology of premature rupture of membranes (PPROM) and subsequent preterm birth.[170]

While the evidence of fetal membrane senescence contributing to human parturition may seem plausible, local inflammation confined to the fetal membrane is unlikely to be sufficient to initiate contractions in the myometrium. SASP and DAMP signals released from fetal membranes are thought to be able to effect changes in adjacent tissue, such as the myometrium, decidua, or cervix, by either direct chemical diffusion or by encapsulation and transportation in exosomes.[171] As some SASPs and DAMPs are readily inactivated by acetylation and oxidation,[172] diffusion is unlikely to enable safe trafficking of these molecules to other tissues. On the other hand, exosome transportation enables protected transportation across the fetal-maternal interface. Exosomes are cell-derived vesicles that are created in the process of exocytosis. Placental-derived exosomes increase in maternal blood with gestation and are able to carry a number of molecules, including SASP and DAMP, in a highly stable manner. Whether they are transported from one compartment to another through blood circulation or directly through tissue layers is still under investigation.[171] Tracking of exosomes in human pregnancy has not been well studied, but the hypothesis that SASP/DAMP created from fetal membranes can be delivered to myometrium and cervix tissue where they activate inflammatory pathways is being investigated as an initiator of parturition.

13.6.2 Cell-Free Fetal Dna

Cell-free fetal DNA (cffDNA) is extracellular DNA of fetal origin that is found in the maternal circulation in a fraction ranging between 3.4% and 6.2% of total cell-free DNA that increases with gestation.[173] Its use has predominantly been in noninvasive prenatal screening for aneuploidy, but cffDNA fractions were noted to be higher in women who delivered preterm.[174,175] Higher cffDNA measured in the second trimester also increased the odds of delivery before 34 weeks (OR 22.0 95% CI 5.02–96.9).[176] The link between cffDNA and inflammation was hypothesized to be through activation of TLR-9, a PRR that recognized hypomethylated DNA, usually from bacterial DNA.[177] Also, cffDNA is hypomethylated and released from senescent placental and fetal membranes. Hence, recognition by TLR-9 provided a framework to suggest increasing cffDNA with gestation-activated sterile inflammation seen at the time of labor. This hypothesis was underpinned by animal data demonstrating that cffDNA injected into pregnant mice led to labor—effects that were mitigated in TLR9-deficient mice.[178] It has since been demonstrated that women in labor actually have a higher proportion of methylated cffDNA compared to nonlaboring women.[179] This seemingly refutes the hypothesis of TLR-9 activation; however, hypomethylation increases from 28 to 36 weeks, and the total amount of cffDNA in laboring women is higher than in nonlaboring women. Hence, it remains possible that there is a relative increase in TLR-9 activation at the time of labor.[179]

13.7 A SUMMARY OF HUMAN PARTURITION

In early pregnancy, progesterone, estrogen, and hCG are key hormones that enable endometrium priming, blastocyst activation, implantation, and placental decidualization. The action of progesterone is a brake on the uterus, which halts contractions until the fetus has completed development and maturation. It functions to inhibit the expression of contraction-associated proteins (OXTR, GJA1, and PTGS2), which are required in order for the myometrium of the uterus to contract during labor.

Mechanistically, progesterone inhibits inflammatory pathways, decreases stretch-activated transcription factors, and increases ZEB1/ZEB2, which work to repress contraction-associated proteins. Secondary messenger cAMP works to inactivate MLCK, a key kinase that phosphorylates myosin to enable interaction with actin. It also inhibits PLC, a key molecule in calcium signaling required for smooth muscle contraction. Further, cAMP enhances the progesterone block effect by increasing the binding of liganded PR-B to PRE-promotors on progesterone-dependent genes. In addition, cAMP is stimulated by hCG and CRH, both of which increase with gestational age and decline just prior to the onset of labor.

As increasing levels of CRH contributes to myometrial quiescence by increasing levels of cAMP, it also stimulates the production of fetal DHEAS, which is hydroxylated in the fetal liver before being converted to estriol by the placenta. Similarly, the placenta also produces estradiol from maternally derived DHEAS in equimolar concentrations to estriol, which causes the formation of biologically inactive heterodimers. Prior to the onset of labor, biologically active estriol homodimers are formed as production of estriol outstrips that of estradiol, leading to a functional activation of estrogen. There is also an upregulation of ER-a receptors in the myometrium.

Through the ER-α receptor, estrogen increases the expression of contraction-associated proteins. Oxytocin and prostaglandins increase intracellular Ca^{2+}, which combines with calmodulin to activate MLCK, which in turn is able to phosphorylate myosin. Phosphorylated myosin is able to interact with actin filaments in an ATP-dependent manner to cause smooth muscle contraction. The increase in myocyte connectivity via gap-junction proteins (e.g., connexin 43) allows a cluster of myocytes to depolarize in unison and function as coupled oscillators. As myocytes are increasingly connected toward labor, patches of myometrium are able to contract in unison to generate sufficient force to cause increases in intra-uterine pressure, which provides a global stimulus for all myocytes within the uterus to contract in unison.

The expression of contraction-associated proteins is further increased by inflammatory markers that are released in response to a number of stimuli, including microbial infection, uterine stretch, haemorrhage, and trauma in the setting of placental abruption, cellular senescence in fetal membranes, or inflammatory mediators such as surfactant proteins from the developing fetal lungs. Importantly, all of these stimuli are more likely to occur toward term, when the majority of women go into labor. Their presence attracts leukocytes and other immune cells, which release further inflammatory mediators, making parturition a highly inflammatory process. Inflammation also increases the production of MMPs and decreases their inhibitors in order to accelerate the cervical-ripening process, leading to cervical ripening and eventually dilation to allow passage of the fetus at birth.

At the same time as the observed inflammatory process, human parturition is characterized by a functional withdrawal of progesterone in the setting of increasing circulating progesterone levels. PR-A is able to inhibit the activity of PR-B (which is the predominant isoform that maintains pregnancy quiescence), and its expression is increased relative to PR-B at the time of labor. There is also increased hydroxysteroid dehydrogenase (HSD) enzyme activity, causing cellular metabolism of progesterone and leading to PR to become unliganded from progesterone during labor. Unliganded PR-A is able to act as a transcription factor in order to increase the expression of contraction-associated proteins in the myometrium.

The exact pathway leading to progesterone withdrawal is unclear; however, attractive hypotheses include functional estrogen activation and inflammation-led activation. It is also unclear whether hormonal processes (such as functional progesterone withdrawal and estrogen activation) initiate the process of labor, and therefore, inflammation is a consequence of labor; or whether inflammation is the initiating process that drives the hormonal changes that lead to labor.

REFERENCES

1. Dekel N, Gnainsky Y, Granot I, Racicot K, Mor G. The role of inflammation for a successful implantation. *Am J Reprod Immunol* 2014;**72**(2):141–7.
2. Fazleabas AT, Donnelly KM, Srinivasan S, Fortman JD, Miller JB. Modulation of the baboon (*Papio anubis*) uterine endometrium by chorionic gonadotrophin during the period of uterine receptivity. *Proc Natl Acad Sci U S A* 1999;**96**(5):2543–8.
3. Fanchin R, Ayoubi J-M, Righini C, Olivennes F, Schönauer LM, Frydman R. Uterine contractility decreases at the time of blastocyst transfers. *Hum Reprod* 2001;**16**(6):1115–9.
4. Smith R, Paul J, Maiti K, Tolosa J, Madsen G. Recent advances in understanding the endocrinology of human birth. *Trends Endocrinol Metab* 2012;**23**(10):516–23.
5. Paria BC, Huet-Hudson YM, Dey SK. Blastocyst's state of activity determines the "window" of implantation in the receptive mouse uterus. *Proc Natl Acad Sci U S A* 1993;**90**(21):10159–62.
6. Winuthayanon W, Hewitt SC, Orvis GD, Behringer RR, Korach KS. Uterine epithelial estrogen receptor alpha is dispensable for proliferation but essential for complete biological and biochemical responses. *Proc Natl Acad Sci U S A* 2010;**107**(45):19272–7.
7. Hoversland RC, Dey SK, Johnson DC. Aromatase activity in the rabbit blastocyst. *J Reprod Fertil* 1982;**66**(1):259–63.
8. Reese J, Wang H, Ding T, Paria BC. The hamster as a model for embryo implantation: insights into a multifaceted process. *Semin Cell Dev Biol* 2008;**19**(2):194–203.
9. Danforth DN. The distribution and functional activity of the cervical musculature. *Am J Obstet Gynecol* 1954;**68**(5):1261–71.
10. Buckingham JC, Buethe Jr. RA, Danforth DN. Collagen-muscle ratio in clinically normal and clinically incompetent cervices. *Am J Obstet Gynecol* 1965;**91**:232–7.
11. Word RA, Li XH, Hnat M, Carrick K. Dynamics of cervical remodeling during pregnancy and parturition: mechanisms and current concepts. *Semin Reprod Med* 2007;**25**(1):69–79.
12. Sherwood OD. Relaxin's physiological roles and other diverse actions. *Endocr Rev* 2004;**25**(2):205–34.
13. Goldsmith LT, Weiss G. Relaxin in human pregnancy. *Ann N Y Acad Sci* 2009;**1160**:130–5.
14. Bishop EH. Pelvic scoring for elective induction. *Obstet Gynecol* 1964;**24**:266–8.
15. Winkler M, Rath W. Changes in the cervical extracellular matrix during pregnancy and parturition. *J Perinat Med* 1999;**27**(1):45–60.
16. Straach KJ, Shelton JM, Richardson JA, Hascall VC, Mahendroo MS. Regulation of hyaluronan expression during cervical ripening. *Glycobiology* 2005;**15**(1):55–65.
17. Nagase H, Visse R, Murphy G. Structure and function of matrix metalloproteinases and TIMPs. *Cardiovasc Res* 2006;**69**(3):562–73.
18. Sennström MB, Brauner A, Byström B, Malmström A, Ekman G. Matrix metalloproteinase-8 correlates with the cervical ripening process in humans. *Acta Obstet Gynecol Scand* 2003;**82**(10):904–11.
19. Stygar D, Wang H, Vladic YS, Ekman G, Eriksson H, Sahlin L. Increased level of matrix metalloproteinases 2 and 9 in the ripening process of the human cervix. *Biol Reprod* 2002;**67**(3):889–94.
20. Watari M, Watari H, DiSanto ME, Chacko S, Shi GP, Strauss 3rd. JF. Pro-inflammatory cytokines induce expression of matrix-metabolizing enzymes in human cervical smooth muscle cells. *Am J Pathol* 1999;**154**(6):1755–62.
21. Osmers RGW, Blaser J, Kuhn W, Tschesche H. Interleukin-8 synthesis and the onset of labor. *Obstet Gynecol* 1995;**86**(2):223–9.

22. Timmons B, Akins M, Mahendroo M. Cervical remodeling during pregnancy and parturition. *Trends Endocrinol Metab* 2010;**21**(6):353–61.

23. Mahendroo MS, Porter A, Russell DW, Word RA. The parturition defect in steroid 5alpha-reductase type 1 knockout mice is due to impaired cervical ripening. *Mol Endocrinol* 1999;**13**(6):981–92.

24. Andersson S, Minjarez D, Yost NP, Word RA. Estrogen and progesterone metabolism in the cervix during pregnancy and parturition. *J Clin Endocrinol Metab* 2008;**93**(6):2366–74.

25. Edelstam G, Karlsson C, Westgren M, Lowbeer C, Swahn ML. Human chorionic gonadatropin (hCG) during third trimester pregnancy. *Scand J Clin Lab Invest* 2007;**67**(5):519–25.

26. Smith R, Smith JI, Shen X, Engel PJ, Bowman ME, McGrath SA, et al. Patterns of plasma corticotropin-releasing hormone, progesterone, estradiol, and estriol change and the onset of human labor. *J Clin Endocrinol Metab* 2009;**94**(6):2066–74.

27. Ambrus G, Rao CV. Novel regulation of pregnant human myometrial smooth muscle cell gap junctions by human chorionic gonadotropin. *Endocrinology* 1994;**135**(6):2772–9.

28. Slattery MM, Brennan C, O'Leary MJ, Morrison JJ. Human chorionic gonadotrophin inhibition of pregnant human myometrial contractility. *BJOG Int J Obstet Gynaecol* 2001;**108**(7):704–8.

29. Zuo J, Lei ZM, Rao CV. Human myometrial chorionic gonadotropin/luteinizing hormone receptors in preterm and term deliveries. *J Clin Endocrinol Metab* 1994;**79**(3):907–11.

30. Tan H, Yi L, Rote NS, Hurd WW, Mesiano S. Progesterone receptor-A and -B have opposite effects on proinflammatory gene expression in human myometrial cells: implications for progesterone actions in human pregnancy and parturition. *J Clin Endocrinol Metab* 2012;**97**(5):719–30.

31. Lei K, Chen L, Georgiou EX, Sooranna SR, Khanjani S, Brosens JJ, et al. Progesterone acts via the nuclear glucocorticoid receptor to suppress IL-1β-induced COX-2 expression in human term myometrial cells. *PLoS One* 2012;**7**(11):e50167.

32. Hardy DB, Janowski BA, Corey DR, Mendelson CR. Progesterone receptor plays a major antiinflammatory role in human myometrial cells by antagonism of nuclear factor-kappaB activation of cyclooxygenase 2 expression. *Mol Endocrinol* 2006;**20**(11):2724–33.

33. Sooranna SR, Lee Y, Kim LU, Mohan AR, Bennett PR, Johnson MR. Mechanical stretch activates type 2 cyclooxygenase via activator protein-1 transcription factor in human myometrial cells. *Mol Hum Reprod* 2004;**10**(2):109–13.

34. MacIntyre DA, Lee YS, Migale R, Herbert BR, Waddington SN, Peebles D, et al. Activator protein 1 is a key terminal mediator of inflammation-induced preterm labor in mice. *FASEB J* 2014;**28**(5):2358–68.

35. Renthal NE, Chen C-C, Williams KC, Gerard RD, Prange-Kiel J, Mendelson CR. miR-200 family and targets, ZEB1 and ZEB2, modulate uterine quiescence and contractility during pregnancy and labor. *Proc Natl Acad Sci U S A* 2010;**107**(48):20828–33.

36. Pieber D, Allport VC, Hills F, Johnson M, Bennett PR. Interactions between progesterone receptor isoforms in myometrial cells in human labor. *Mol Hum Reprod* 2001;**7**(9):875–9.

37. Westphal U, Stroupe SD, Cheng SL. Progesterone binding to serum proteins. *Ann N Y Acad Sci* 1977;**286**:10–28.

38. Mesiano S, Chan EC, Fitter JT, Kwek K, Yeo G, Smith R. Progesterone withdrawal and estrogen activation in human parturition are coordinated by progesterone receptor A expression in the myometrium. *J Clin Endocrinol Metab* 2002;**87**(6):2924–30.

39. Nadeem L, Shynlova O, Matysiak-Zablocki E, Mesiano S, Dong X, Lye S. Molecular evidence of functional progesterone withdrawal in human myometrium. *Nat Commun* 2016;**7**:11565.

40. Giangrande PH, McDonnell DP. The A and B isoforms of the human progesterone receptor: two functionally different transcription factors encoded by a single gene. *Recent Prog Horm Res* 1999;**54**:291–313 discussion -4.

41. Sartorius CA, Melville MY, Hovland AR, Tung L, Takimoto GS, Horwitz KB. A third transactivation function (AF3) of human progesterone receptors located in the unique N-terminal segment of the B-isoform. *Mol Endocrinol* 1994;**8**(10):1347–60.

42. Condon JC, Hardy DB, Kovaric K, Mendelson CR. Up-regulation of the progesterone receptor (PR)-C isoform in laboring myometrium by activation of nuclear factor-kappaB may contribute to the onset of labor through inhibition of PR function. *Mol Endocrinol* 2006;**20**(4):764–75.

43. Haluska GJ, Wells TR, Hirst JJ, Brenner RM, Sadowsky DW, Novy MJ. Progesterone receptor localization and isoforms in myometrium, decidua, and fetal membranes from rhesus macaques: evidence for functional progesterone withdrawal at parturition. *J Soc Gynecol Investig* 2002;**9**(3):125–36.

44. Madsen G, Zakar T, Ku CY, Sanborn BM, Smith R, Mesiano S. Prostaglandins differentially modulate progesterone receptor-A and -B expression in human myometrial cells: evidence for prostaglandin-induced functional progesterone withdrawal. *J Clin Endocrinol Metab* 2004;**89**(2):1010–3.

45. Chai SY, Smith R, Zakar T, Mitchell C, Madsen G. Term myometrium is characterized by increased activating epigenetic modifications at the progesterone receptor-A promoter. *Mol Hum Reprod* 2012;**18**(8):401–9.

46. Ke W, Chen C, Luo H, Tang J, Zhang Y, Gao W, et al. Histone deacetylase 1 regulates the expression of progesterone receptor A during human parturition by occupying the progesterone receptor A promoter. *Reprod Sci* 2016;**23**(7):955–64.

47. Amini P, Michniuk D, Kuo K, Yi L, Skomorovska-Prokvolit Y, Peters GA, et al. Human parturition involves phosphorylation of progesterone receptor-A at serine-345 in myometrial cells. *Endocrinology* 2016;**157**(11):4434–45.

48. Peters GA, Yi L, Skomorovska-Prokvolit Y, Patel B, Amini P, Tan H, et al. Inflammatory stimuli increase progesterone receptor-A stability and transrepressive activity in myometrial cells. *Endocrinology* 2017;**158**(1):158–69.

49. Yuan W, López Bernal A. Cyclic AMP signalling pathways in the regulation of uterine relaxation. *BMC Pregnancy Childbirth* 2007;**7**(Suppl 1):S10.

50. Chen L, Lei K, Malawana J, Yulia A, Sooranna SR, Bennett PR, et al. Cyclic AMP enhances progesterone action in human myometrial cells. *Mol Cell Endocrinol* 2014;**382**(1):334–43.

51. Yulia A, Singh N, Lei K, Sooranna SR, Johnson MR. Cyclic AMP effectors regulate myometrial oxytocin receptor expression. *Endocrinology* 2016;**157**(11):4411–22.

52. Price SA, Bernal AL. Uterine quiescence: the role of cyclic AMP. *Exp Physiol* 2001;**86**(2):265–72.

53. McLean M, Bisits A, Davies J, Woods R, Lowry P, Smith R. A placental clock controlling the length of human pregnancy. *Nat Med* 1995;**1**(5):460–3.

54. Campbell EA, Linton EA, Wolfe CD, Scraggs PR, Jones MT, Lowry PJ. Plasma corticotropin-releasing hormone concentrations during pregnancy and parturition. *J Clin Endocrinol Metab* 1987;**64**(5):1054–9.

55. Linton EA, Perkins AV, Woods RJ, Eben F, Wolfe CD, Behan DP, et al. Corticotropin releasing hormone-binding protein (CRH-BP): plasma levels decrease during the third trimester of normal human pregnancy. *J Clin Endocrinol Metab* 1993;**76**(1):260–2.

56. Potter E, Behan DP, Fischer WH, Linton EA, Lowry PJ, Vale WW. Cloning and characterization of the cDNAs for human and rat corticotropin releasing factor-binding proteins. *Nature* 1991;**349**(6308):423–6.

57. Behan DP, Linton EA, Lowry PJ. Isolation of the human plasma corticotrophin-releasing factor-binding protein. *J Endocrinol* 1989;**122**(1):23–31.

58. Orth DN, Mount CD. Specific high-affinity binding protein for human corticotropin-releasing hormone in normal human plasma. *Biochem Biophys Res Commun* 1987;**143**(2):411–7.

59. Korebrits C, Ramirez NM, Watson L, Al E. Maternal CRH is increased with impending preterm birth. *J Clin Endocrinol Metab* 1998;**83**(5):1585–91.

60. Wadhwa PD, Garite TJ, Porto M, Glynn L, Chicz-Demet A, Dunkel-Schetter C, et al. Placental corticotropin-releasing hormone (CRH), spontaneous preterm birth, and fetal growth restriction: a prospective investigation. *Am J Obstet Gynecol* 2004;**191**(4):1063–9.

61. Warren WB, Patrick SL, Goland RS. Elevated maternal plasma corticotropin-releasing hormone levels in pregnancies complicated by preterm labor. *Am J Obstet Gynecol* 1992;**166**(4):1198–204 [discussion 204–7].

62. McGrath S, McLean M, Smith D, Bisits A, Giles W, Smith R. Maternal plasma corticotropin-releasing hormone trajectories vary depending on the cause of preterm delivery. *Am J Obstet Gynecol* 2002;**186**(2):257–60.

63. Ruiz RJ, Gennaro S, O'Connor C, Dwivedi A, Gibeau A, Keshinover T, et al. CRH as a predictor of preterm birth in minority women. *Biol Res Nurs* 2016;**18**(3):316–21.

64. Goland RS, Jozak S, Warren WB, Conwell IM, Stark RI, Tropper PJ. Elevated levels of umbilical cord plasma corticotropin-releasing hormone in growth-retarded fetuses. *J Clin Endocrinol Metab* 1993;**77**(5):1174–9.

65. Yoon BH, Romero R, Jun JK, Maymon E, Gomez R, Mazor M, et al. An increase in fetal plasma cortisol but not dehydroepiandrosterone sulfate is followed by the onset of preterm labor in patients with preterm premature rupture of the membranes. *Am J Obstet Gynecol* 1998;**179**(5):1107–14.

66. Smith R, Mesiano S, Chan EC, Brown S, Jaffe RB. Corticotropin-releasing hormone directly and preferentially stimulates dehydroepiandrosterone sulfate secretion by human fetal adrenal cortical cells. *J Clin Endocrinol Metab* 1998;**83**(8):2916–20.

67. Condon JC, Jeyasuria P, Faust JM, Mendelson CR. Surfactant protein secreted by the maturing mouse fetal lung acts as a hormone that signals the initiation of parturition. *Proc Natl Acad Sci U S A* 2004;**101**(14):4978–83.

68. Ni X, Hou Y, Yang R, Tang X, Smith R, Nicholson RC. Progesterone receptors A and B differentially modulate corticotropin-releasing hormone gene expression through a cAMP regulatory element. *Cell Mol Life Sci* 2004;**61**(9):1114–22.

69. Ni X, Nicholson RC, King BR, Chan EC, Read MA, Smith R. Estrogen represses whereas the estrogen-antagonist ICI 182780 stimulates placental CRH gene expression. *J Clin Endocrinol Metab* 2002;**87**(8):3774–8.

70. Tyson EK, Smith R, Read M. Evidence that corticotropin-releasing hormone modulates myometrial contractility during human pregnancy. *Endocrinology* 2009;**150**(12):5617–25.

71. Grammatopoulos DK. Insights into mechanisms of corticotropin-releasing hormone receptor signal transduction. *Br J Pharmacol* 2012;**166**(1):85–97.

72. Petraglia F, Benedetto C, Florio P, D'Ambrogio G, Genazzani AD, Marozio L, et al. Effect of corticotropin-releasing factor-binding protein on prostaglandin release from cultured maternal decidua and on contractile activity of human myometrium in vitro. *J Clin Endocrinol Metab* 1995;**80**(10):3073–6.

73. Benedetto C, Petraglia F, Marozio L, Chiarolini L, Florio P, Genazzani AR, et al. Corticotropin-releasing hormone increases prostaglandin F2 alpha activity on human myometrium in vitro. *Am J Obstet Gynecol* 1994;**171**(1):126–31.

74. Simpkin JC, Kermani F, Palmer AM, Campa JS, Tribe RM, Linton EA, et al. Effects of corticotrophin releasing hormone on contractile activity of myometrium from pregnant women. *Br J Obstet Gynaecol* 1999;**106**(5):439–45.

75. Grammatopoulos D, Stirrat GM, Williams SA, Hillhouse EW. The biological activity of the corticotropin-releasing hormone receptor-adenylate cyclase complex in human myometrium is reduced at the end of pregnancy. *J Clin Endocrinol Metab* 1996;**81**(2):745–51.

76. Kaludjerovic J, Ward WE. The interplay between estrogen and fetal adrenal cortex. *J Nutr Metab* 2012;**2012**:837901.

77. Melamed M, Castano E, Notides AC, Sasson S. Molecular and kinetic basis for the mixed agonist/antagonist activity of estriol. *Mol Endocrinol* 1997;**11**(12):1868–78.

78. Petrocelli T, Lye SJ. Regulation of transcripts encoding the myometrial gap junction protein, connexin-43, by estrogen and progesterone. *Endocrinology* 1993;**133**(1):284–90.

79. Lye SJ, Nicholson BJ, Mascarenhas M, MacKenzie L, Petrocelli T. Increased expression of connexin-43 in the rat myometrium during labor is associated with an increase in the plasma estrogen:progesterone ratio. *Endocrinology* 1993;**132**(6):2380–6.

80. Chibbar R, Wong S, Miller FD, Mitchell BF. Estrogen stimulates oxytocin gene expression in human chorio-decidua. *J Clin Endocrinol Metab* 1995;**80**(2):567–72.

81. Maiti K, Paul JW, Read M, Chan EC, Riley SC, Nahar P, et al. G-1-activated membrane estrogen receptors mediate increased contractility of the human myometrium. *Endocrinology* 2011;**152**(6):2448–55.

82. MacIntyre DA, Tyson EK, Read M, Smith R, Yeo G, Kwek K, et al. Contraction in human myometrium is associated with changes in small heat shock proteins. *Endocrinology* 2008;**149**(1):245–52.

83. Anderson JN, Peck Jr. EJ, Clark JH. Estrogen-induced uterine responses and growth: relationship to receptor estrogen binding by uterine nuclei. *Endocrinology* 1975;**96**(1):160–7.

84. Shynlova O, Oldenhof A, Dorogin A, Xu Q, Mu J, Nashman N, et al. Myometrial apoptosis: activation of the caspase cascade in the pregnant rat myometrium at midgestation. *Biol Reprod* 2006;**74**(5):839–49.

85. Shynlova O, Dorogin A, Lye SJ. Stretch-induced uterine myocyte differentiation during rat pregnancy: involvement of caspase activation. *Biol Reprod* 2010;**82**(6):1248–55.

86. Jeyasuria P, Wetzel J, Bradley M, Subedi K, Condon JC. Progesterone-regulated caspase 3 action in the mouse may play a role in uterine quiescence during pregnancy through fragmentation of uterine myocyte contractile proteins. *Biol Reprod* 2009;**80**(5):928–34.

87. Chauhan SP, Scardo JA, Hayes E, Abuhamad AZ, Berghella V. Twins: prevalence, problems, and preterm births. *Am J Obstet Gynecol* 2010;**203** (4):305–15.

88. Petrozella LN, Dashe JS, McIntire DD, Leveno KJ. Clinical significance of borderline amniotic fluid index and oligohydramnios in preterm pregnancy. *Obstet Gynecol* 2011;**117**(2 Pt 1):338–42.

89. Ou CW, Chen ZQ, Qi S, Lye SJ. Increased expression of the rat myometrial oxytocin receptor messenger ribonucleic acid during labor requires both mechanical and hormonal signals. *Biol Reprod* 1998;**59**(5):1055–61.

90. Dale HH. On some physiological actions of ergot. *J Physiol* 1906;**34**(3):163–206.

91. Thornton S, Davison JM, Baylis PH. Plasma oxytocin during the first and second stages of spontaneous human labor. *Acta Endocrinol* 1992;**126** (5):425–9.

92. Leake RD, Weitzman RE, Glatz TH, Fisher DA. Plasma oxytocin concentrations in men, nonpregnant women, and pregnant women before and during spontaneous labor. *J Clin Endocrinol Metab* 1981;**53**(4):730–3.

93. Dawood MY, Ylikorkala O, Trivedi D, Fuchs F. Oxytocin in maternal circulation and amniotic fluid during pregnancy. *J Clin Endocrinol Metab* 1979;**49**(3):429–34.

94. de Geest K, Thiery M, Piron-Possuyt G, Vanden DR. Plasma oxytocin in human pregnancy and parturition. *J Perinat Med* 1985;**13**(1):3–13.

95. Fuchs AR, Romero R, Keefe D, Parra M, Oyarzun E, Behnke E. Oxytocin secretion and human parturition: pulse frequency and duration increase during spontaneous labor in women. *Am J Obstet Gynecol* 1991;**165**(5 Pt 1):1515–23.

96. Chard T, Gibbens GL. Spurt release of oxytocin during surgical induction of labor in women. *Am J Obstet Gynecol* 1983;**147**(6):678–80.

97. Thornton S, Davison JM, Baylis PH. Effect of human pregnancy on metabolic clearance rate of oxytocin. *Am J Phys* 1990;**259**(1 Pt. 2):R21–4.

98. Burd JM, Davison J, Weightman DR, Baylis PH. Evaluation of enzyme inhibitors of pregnancy associated oxytocinase: application to the measurement of plasma immunoreactive oxytocin during human labor. *Acta Endocrinol* 1987;**114**(3):458–64.

99. Kimura T, Takemura M, Nomura S, Nobunaga T, Kubota Y, Inoue T, et al. Expression of oxytocin receptor in human pregnant myometrium. *Endocrinology* 1996;**137**(2):780–5.

100. Fuchs AR, Fuchs F, Husslein P, Soloff MS. Oxytocin receptors in the human uterus during pregnancy and parturition. *Am J Obstet Gynecol* 1984;**150** (6):734–41.

101. Helmer H, Hackl T, Schneeberger C, Knofler M, Behrens O, Kaider A, et al. Oxytocin and vasopressin 1a receptor gene expression in the cycling or pregnant human uterus. *Am J Obstet Gynecol* 1998;**179**(6 Pt. 1):1572–8.

102. Liedman R, Hansson SR, Igidbashian S, Akerlund M. Myometrial oxytocin receptor mRNA concentrations at preterm and term delivery—the influence of external oxytocin. *Gynecol Endocrinol* 2009;**25**(3):188–93.

103. Blanks AM, Vatish M, Allen MJ, Ladds G, de Wit NC, Slater DM, et al. Paracrine oxytocin and estradiol demonstrate a spatial increase in human intrauterine tissues with labor. *J Clin Endocrinol Metab* 2003;**88**(7):3392–400.

104. Wathes DC, Borwick SC, Timmons PM, Leung ST, Thornton S. Oxytocin receptor expression in human term and preterm gestational tissues prior to and following the onset of labor. *J Endocrinol* 1999;**161**(1):143–51.

105. Chan EC, Fraser S, Yin S, Yeo G, Kwek K, Fairclough RJ, et al. Human myometrial genes are differentially expressed in labor: a suppression subtractive hybridization study. *J Clin Endocrinol Metab* 2002;**87**(6):2435–41.

106. Nishimori K, Young LJ, Guo Q, Wang Z, Insel TR, Matzuk MM. Oxytocin is required for nursing but is not essential for parturition or reproductive behavior. *Proc Natl Acad Sci U S A* 1996;**93**(21):11699–704.

107. Shinar S, Many A, Maslovitz S. Questioning the role of pituitary oxytocin in parturition: spontaneous onset of labor in women with panhypopituitarism—a case series. *Eur J Obstet Gynecol Reprod Biol* 2016;**197**:83–5.

108. Chibbar R, Miller FD, Mitchell BF. Synthesis of oxytocin in amnion, chorion, and decidua may influence the timing of human parturition. *J Clin Invest* 1993;**91**(1):185–92.

109. Terzidou V, Blanks AM, Kim SH, Thornton S, Bennett PR. Labor and inflammation increase the expression of oxytocin receptor in human amnion. *Biol Reprod* 2011;**84**(3):546–52.

110. Wilson T, Liggins GC, Whittaker DJ. Oxytocin stimulates the release of arachidonic acid and prostaglandin F2 alpha from human decidual cells. *Prostaglandins* 1988;**35**(5):771–80.

111. Funk CD. Prostaglandins and leukotrienes: advances in eicosanoid biology. *Science* 2001;**294**(5548):1871–5.

112. Husslein P, Fuchs AR, Fuchs F. Oxytocin and the initiation of human parturition. I. Prostaglandin release during induction of labor by oxytocin. *Am J Obstet Gynecol* 1981;**141**(6):688–93.

113. Pasetto N, Zicari A, Piccione E, Lenti L, Pontieri G, Ticconi C. Influence of labor and oxytocin on in vitro leukotriene release by human fetal membranes and uterine decidua at term gestation. *Am J Obstet Gynecol* 1992;**166**(5):1500–6.

114. Bennett PR, Slater D, Sullivan M, Elder MG, Moore GE. Changes in amniotic arachidonic acid metabolism associated with increased cyclo-oxygenase gene expression. *Br J Obstet Gynaecol* 1993;**100**(11):1037–42.

115. Slater D, Allport V, Bennett P. Changes in the expression of the type-2 but not the type-1 cyclo-oxygenase enzyme in chorion-decidua with the onset of labor. *BJOG Int J Obstet Gynaecol* 2005;**105**(7):745–8.

116. Zakar T, Olson DM, Teixeira FJ, Hirst JJ. Regulation of prostaglandin endoperoxide H2 synthase in term human gestational tissues. *Acta Physiol Hung* 1996;**84**(2):109–18.

117. Satoh K, Yasumizu T, Fukuoka H, Kinoshita K, Kaneko Y, Tsuchiya M, et al. Prostaglandin F2 alpha metabolite levels in plasma, amniotic fluid, and urine during pregnancy and labor. *Am J Obstet Gynecol* 1979;**133**(8):886–90.

118. Romero R, Munoz H, Gomez R, Parra M, Polanco M, Valverde V, et al. Increase in prostaglandin bioavailability precedes the onset of human parturition. *Prostaglandins Leukot Essent Fat Acids* 1996;**54**(3):187–91.

119. Slater DM, Dennes WJ, Campa JS, Poston L, Bennett PR. Expression of cyclo-oxygenase types-1 and -2 in human myometrium throughout pregnancy. *Mol Hum Reprod* 1999;**5**.

120. Hirst JJ, Teixeira FJ, Zakar T, Olson DM. Prostaglandin endoperoxide-H synthase-1 and -2 messenger ribonucleic acid levels in human amnion with spontaneous labor onset. *J Clin Endocrinol Metab* 1995;**80**(2):517–23.

121. Mitchell MD, Edwin S, Romero RJ. Prostaglandin biosynthesis by human decidual cells: effects of inflammatory mediators. *Prostaglandins Leukot Essent Fat Acids* 1990;**41**(1):35–8.

122. Sakai M, Tanebe K, Sasaki Y, Momma K, Yoneda S, Saito S. Evaluation of the tocolytic effect of a selective cyclooxygenase-2 inhibitor in a mouse model of lipopolysaccharide-induced preterm delivery. *Mol Hum Reprod* 2001;**7**(6):595–602.

123. Moise Jr. KJ, Huhta JC, Sharif DS, Ou CN, Kirshon B, Wasserstrum N, et al. Indomethacin in the treatment of premature labor. Effects on the fetal ductus arteriosus. *N Engl J Med* 1988;**319**(6):327–31.

124. Astle S, Thornton S, Slater DM. Identification and localization of prostaglandin E2 receptors in upper and lower segment human myometrium during pregnancy. *Mol Hum Reprod* 2005;**11**(4):279–87.

125. Cario-Toumaniantz C, Reillaudoux G, Sauzeau V, Heutte F, Vaillant N, Finet M, et al. Modulation of RhoA—Rho kinase-mediated Ca(2+) sensitization of rabbit myometrium during pregnancy—role of Rnd3. *J Physiol* 2003;**552**(Pt 2):403–13.

126. Wray S, Arrowsmith S. Uterine smooth muscle A2—Hill, Joseph A. In: Olson EN, editor. *Muscle*. Boston/Waltham: Academic Press; 2012. p. 1207–16 Chapter 90.

127. Parkington HC, Stevenson J, Tonta MA, Paul J, Butler T, Maiti K, et al. Diminished hERG K+ channel activity facilitates strong human labor contractions but is dysregulated in obese women. *Nat Commun* 2014;**5**:4108.

128. Ying L, Becard M, Lyell D, Han X, Shortliffe L, Husted CI, et al. The transient receptor potential vanilloid 4 channel modulates uterine tone during pregnancy. *Sci Transl Med* 2015;**7**(319).

129. Renthal NE, Williams KC, Mendelson CR. MicroRNAs—mediators of myometrial contractility during pregnancy and labor. *Nat Rev Endocrinol* 2013;**9**(7):391–401.

130. Smith R, Imtiaz M, Banney D, Paul JW, Young RC. Why the heart is like an orchestra and the uterus is like a soccer crowd. *Am J Obstet Gynecol* 2015;**213**(2):181–5.

131. Williams KC, Renthal NE, Condon JC, Gerard RD, Mendelson CR. MicroRNA-200a serves a key role in the decline of progesterone receptor function leading to term and preterm labor. *Proc Natl Acad Sci U S A* 2012;**109**(19):7529–34.

132. Piekorz RP, Gingras S, Hoffmeyer A, Ihle JN, Weinstein Y. Regulation of progesterone levels during pregnancy and parturition by signal transducer and activator of transcription 5 and 20alpha-hydroxysteroid dehydrogenase. *Mol Endocrinol* 2005;**19**(2):431–40.

133. Cook JR, MacIntyre DA, Samara E, Kim SH, Singh N, Johnson MR, et al. Exogenous oxytocin modulates human myometrial microRNAs. *Am J Obstet Gynecol* 2015;**213**(1):65.e1–9.

134. Gray C, McCowan LM, Patel R, Taylor RS, Vickers MH. Maternal plasma miRNAs as biomarkers during mid-pregnancy to predict later spontaneous preterm birth: a pilot study. *Sci Rep* 2017;**7**(1):815.

135. Janeway C. Immunogenicity signals 1,2,3 … and 0. *Immunol Today* 1989;**10**(9):283–6.

136. Arthur JS, Ley SC. Mitogen-activated protein kinases in innate immunity. *Nat Rev Immunol* 2013;**13**(9):679–92.

137. Matzinger P. The danger model: a renewed sense of self. *Science* 2002;**296**:301–5.

138. Aisemberg J, Vercelli CA, Bariani MV, Billi SC, Wolfson ML, Franchi AM. Progesterone is essential for protecting against LPS-induced pregnancy loss. LIF as a potential mediator of the anti-inflammatory effect of progesterone. *PLoS One* 2013;**8**(2):e56161.

139. Bennett WA, Lagoo-Deenadayalan S, Whitworth NS, Stopple JA, Barber WH, Hale E, et al. First-trimester human chorionic villi express both immunoregulatory and inflammatory cytokines: a role for interleukin-10 in regulating the cytokine network of pregnancy. *Am J Reprod Immunol* 1999;**41**:70–8.

140. Bennett WA, Lagoo-Deenadayalan S, Whitworth NS, Brackin MN, Hale E, Cowan BD. Expression and production of interleukin-10 by human trophoblast: relationship to pregnancy immunotolerance. *Early Pregnancy* 1997;**3**:190–8.

141. Thomson AJ, Telfer JF, Young A, Campbell S, Stewart CJ, Cameron IT, et al. Leukocytes infiltrate the myometrium during human parturition: further evidence that labor is an inflammatory process. *Hum Reprod* 1999;**14**(1):229–36.

142. Kayisli UA, Mahutte NG, Arici A. Uterine chemokines in reproductive physiology and pathology. *Am J Reprod Immunol* 2002;**47**(4):213–21.

143. Tang M-X, Hu X-H, Liu Z-Z, Kwak-Kim J, Liao A-H. What are the roles of macrophages and monocytes in human pregnancy? *J Reprod Immunol* 2015;**112**:73–80.

144. Romero R, Miranda J, Chaemsaithong P, Chaiworapongsa T, Kusanovic JP, Dong Z, et al. Sterile and microbial-associated intra-amniotic inflammation in preterm prelabor rupture of membranes. *J Matern Fetal Neonatal Med* 2015;**28**(12):1394–409.

145. Kim MJ, Romero R, Gervasi MT, Kim JS, Yoo W, Lee DC, et al. Widespread microbial invasion of the chorioamniotic membranes is a consequence and not a cause of intra-amniotic infection. *Lab Invest* 2009;**89**(8):924–36.

146. Leon R, Silva N, Ovalle A, Chaparro A, Ahumada A, Gajardo M, et al. Detection of *Porphyromonas gingivalis* in the amniotic fluid in pregnant women with a diagnosis of threatened premature labor. *J Periodontol* 2007;**78**(7):1249–55.

147. Fardini Y, Chung P, Dumm R, Joshi N, Han YW. Transmission of diverse oral bacteria to murine placenta: evidence for the oral microbiome as a potential source of intrauterine infection. *Infect Immun* 2010;**78**(4):1789–96.

148. Romero R, Grivel J-C, Tarca AL, Chaemsaithong P, Xu Z, Fitzgerald W, et al. Evidence of perturbations of the cytokine network in preterm labor. *Am J Obstet Gynecol* 2015;**213**(6) 836.e1–836.e18.

149. Osmann I, Young A, Ledingham MA, Thomson AJ, Jordan F, Greer IA, et al. Leukocyte density and pro-inflammatory cytokine expression in human fetal membranes, decidua, cervix, and myometrium before and during labor at term. *Mol Hum Reprod* 2003;**9**:41–5.

150. Young A, Thomson AJ, Ledingham MA, Jordan F, Greer IA, Norman JE. Immunolocalization of proinflammatory cytokines in myometrium, cervix, and fetal membranes during human parturition at term. *Biol Reprod* 2002;**66**:445–9.

151. Peltier MR. Immunology of term and preterm labor. *Reprod Biol Endocrinol* 2003;**1**(1):122.

152. Xu P, Alfaidy N, Challis JR. Expression of matrix metalloproteinase (MMP)-2 and MMP-9 in human placenta and fetal membranes in relation to preterm and term labor. *J Clin Endocrinol Metab* 2002;**87**:1353–61.

153. Riley SC, Leask R, Denison FC, Wisely K, Calder AA, Howe DC. Secretion of tissue inhibitors of matrix metalloproteinases by human fetal membranes, decidua and placenta at parturition. *J Endocrinol* 1999;**162**:351–9.

154. Pollard JK, Thai D, Mitchell MD. Evidence for a common mechanism of action of interleukin-1β, tumor necrosis factor-α, and epidermal growth factor on prostaglandin production in human chorion cells. *Am J Reprod Immunol* 1993;**30**:146–53.

155. Romero R, Durum SK, Dinarello CA, Oyarzun E, Hobbins JC, Mitchell MD. Interleukin-1 stimulates prostaglandin biosynthesis by human amnion. *Prostaglandins* 1989;**37**:13–22.

156. McLaren J, Taylor DJ, Bell SC. Prostaglandin E2-dependent production of latent matrix metalloproteinase-9 in cultures of human fetal membranes. *Mol Hum Reprod* 2000;**6**:1033–40.

157. Patel FA, Clifton VL, Chwalisz K, Challis JR. Steroid regulation of prostaglandin dehydrogenase activity and expression in human term placenta and chorio-decidua in relation to labor. *J Clin Endocrinol Metab* 1999;**84**:291–9.

158. Molnar M, Romero R, Hertelendy F. Interleukin-1 and tumor necrosis factor stimulate arachidonic acid release and phospholipid metabolism in human myometrial cells. *Am J Obstet Gynecol* 1993;**169**:825–9.

159. Pollard JK, Mitchell MD. Intrauterine infection and the effects of inflammatory mediators on prostaglandin production by myometrial cells from pregnant women. *Am J Obstet Gynecol* 1996;**174**:682–6.

160. Belt AR, Baldassare JJ, Molnar M, Romero R, Hertelendy F. The nuclear transcription factor NF-κB mediates interleukin-1β-induced expression of cyclooxygenase-2 in human myometrial cells. *Am J Obstet Gynecol* 1999;**181**:359–66.

161. Rauk PN, Friebe-Hoffmann U, Winebrenner LD, Chiao JP. Interleukin-6 up-regulates the oxytocin receptor in cultured uterine smooth muscle cells. *Am J Reprod Immunol* 2001;**45**:148–53.

162. Friebe-Hoffmann U, Chiao JP, Rauk PN. Effect of IL-1β and IL-6 on oxytocin secretion in human uterine smooth muscle cells. *Am J Reprod Immunol* 2001;**46**:226–31.

163. Romero R, Miranda J, Chaiworapongsa T, Korzeniewski SJ, Chaemsaithong P, Gotsch F, et al. Prevalence and clinical significance of sterile intra-amniotic inflammation in patients with preterm labor and intact membranes. *Am J Reprod Immunol* 2014;**72**(5):458–74.

164. Menon R. Human fetal membranes at term: dead tissue or signalers of parturition? *Placenta* 2016;**44**:1–5.

165. Menon R, Bonney EA, Condon J, Mesiano S, Taylor RN. Novel concepts on pregnancy clocks and alarms: redundancy and synergy in human parturition. *Hum Reprod Update* 2016;**22**(5):535–60.

166. Behnia F, Taylor BD, Woodson M, Kacerovsky M, Hawkins H, Fortunato SJ, et al. Chorioamniotic membrane senescence: a signal for parturition? *Am J Obstet Gynecol* 2015;**213**(3) 359.e1-.e16.

167. Polettini J, Behnia F, Taylor BD, Saade GR, Taylor RN, Menon R. Telomere fragment induced amnion cell senescence: a contributor to parturition? *PLoS One* 2015;**10**(9).

168. Coppe JP, Desprez PY, Krtolica A, Campisi J. The senescence-associated secretory phenotype: the dark side of tumor suppression. *Annu Rev Pathol* 2010;**5**:99–118.

169. Keelan JA, Blumenstein M, Helliwell RJ, Sato TA, Marvin KW, Mitchell MD. Cytokines, prostaglandins and parturition—a review. *Placenta* 2003;**24**(Suppl A):S33–46.

170. Menon R, Boldogh I, Hawkins HK, Woodson M, Polettini J, Syed TA, et al. Histological evidence of oxidative stress and premature senescence in preterm premature rupture of the human fetal membranes recapitulated in vitro. *Am J Pathol* 2014;**184**(6):1740–51.

171. Menon R, Mesiano S, Taylor RN. Programmed fetal membrane senescence and exosome-mediated signaling: a mechanism associated with timing of human parturition. *Front Endocrinol* 2017;**8**:196.

172. Zandarashvili L, Sahu D, Lee K, Lee YS, Singh P, Rajarathnam K, et al. Real-time kinetics of high-mobility group box 1 (HMGB1) oxidation in extracellular fluids studied by in situ protein NMR spectroscopy. *J Biol Chem* 2013;**288**(17):11621–7.

173. Lo YM, Tein MS, Lau TK, Haines CJ, Leung TN, Poon PM, et al. Quantitative analysis of fetal DNA in maternal plasma and serum: implications for noninvasive prenatal diagnosis. *Am J Hum Genet* 1998;**62**(4):768–75.

174. Leung TN, Zhang J, Lau TK, Hjelm NM, Lo YM. Maternal plasma fetal DNA as a marker for preterm labor. *Lancet* 1998;**352**(9144):1904–5.

175. Farina A, LeShane ES, Romero R, Gomez R, Chaiworapongsa T, Rizzo N, et al. High levels of fetal cell-free DNA in maternal serum: a risk factor for spontaneous preterm delivery. *Am J Obstet Gynecol* 2005;**193**(2):421–5.

176. Dugoff L, Barberio A, Whittaker PG, Schwartz N, Sehdev H, Bastek JA. Cell-free DNA fetal fraction and preterm birth. *Am J Obstet Gynecol* 2016;**215**(2) 231.e1-7.

177. Phillippe M. Cell-free fetal DNA, telomeres, and the spontaneous onset of parturition. *Reprod Sci* 2015;**22**(10):1186–201.

178. Scharfe-Nugent A, Corr SC, Carpenter SB, Keogh L, Doyle B, Martin C, et al. TLR9 provokes inflammation in response to fetal DNA: mechanism for fetal loss in preterm birth and preeclampsia. *J Immunol* 2012;**188**(11):5706–12.

179. Herrera CA, Stoerker J, Carlquist J, Stoddard GJ, Jackson M, Esplin S, et al. Cell-free DNA, inflammation, and the initiation of spontaneous term labor. *Am J Obstet Gynecol* 2017;**217**(5) 583.e1-e8.

Chapter 14

The Onset and Maintenance of Human Lactation and its Endocrine Regulation

Anna Sadovnikova*, John J. Wysolmerski[†] and Russell C. Hovey*

*Department of Animal Science, University of California, Davis, CA, United States, [†]Section of Endocrinology and Metabolism, Department of Internal Medicine, Yale School of Medicine, New Haven, CT, United States

---

Key Clinical Changes

- Breast development begins during embryogenesis and is coordinately regulated with sexual maturation.
- During pregnancy, the breast epithelium begins to differentiate in response to rising levels of ovarian and pituitary hormones, enabling the synthesis and accumulation of certain milk constituents, including immunoglobulins.
- The rapid drop in circulating progesterone levels directs the onset of secretion and the sustained, copious synthesis of various milk components by the luminal epithelium after parturition. Oxytocin induces milk ejection by its actions on the surrounding myoepithelium.
- Sustained lactation requires a host of maternal adaptations, including changes in glucose, lipid, and mineral metabolism that partition nutrients to the mammary gland for milk production.

14.1 BREAST DEVELOPMENT AND LACTOGENESIS

A future mother begins the path toward successful breastfeeding at the first signs of her own breast development in utero. As she develops sexually, so too does the cellular and morphological makeup of her breasts, in anticipation of the significant endocrine cues that accompany a pregnancy. After birth, acute endocrine switching directs the breast epithelium to assume full and sustained lactation that is capable of supporting and nourishing the newborn by providing the wondrously complex mixture of nutrients present in milk (Fig. 14.1A).

14.1.1 Embryogenesis

Breast development in the human fetus is first evident around 5 weeks of gestation, when the symmetrical milk lines first become visible.[1] By 15–18 weeks, the primary epithelial bud invaginates at the future site of the breast,[1] and by week 20, the future galactophores that drain to the nipple are present as 15–25 independent ductal cords.[2] At birth, the mammary ducts vary in their structure, ranging from relatively simple and elongated tubes to more branched ducts bearing terminal lobules and nascent alveoli.[3] Maternal hormones in the fetal circulation can induce differentiation of the mammary epithelium in the fetus so that 80%–90% of newborns secrete a colostrum-like "witch's milk".[1,4] These secretions generally resolve as the circulating levels of maternal hormones in the newborn decline.[5]

14.1.2 Puberty

The mammary epithelium remains relatively dormant during Tanner Stage 1 until the onset of puberty. The first sign of breast development arises during Tanner Stage 2 as a palpable subareolar bud composed of proliferating epithelial and

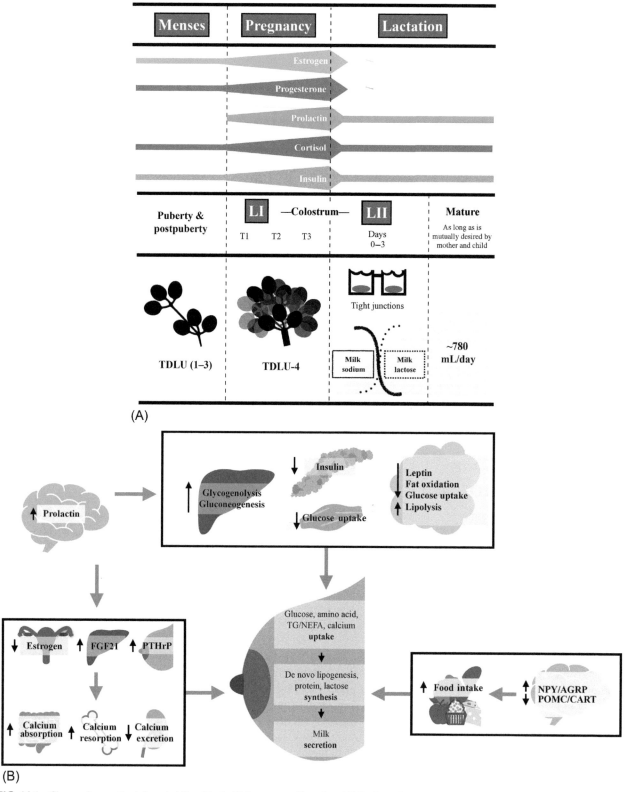

FIG. 14.1 Changes in a mother's breasts (A) and body (B) in support of lactation. (A) During puberty and pregnancy, epithelial cells within the breasts undergo growth and morphological development in response to ovarian secretions. As pregnancy continues, additional stimulation by insulin, corticoids, and lactogenic hormones promotes cellular differentiation that leads to the accumulation of secretion (LI) that becomes the immunoglobulin-rich colostrum available at birth. LII ensues only once the placenta is expelled and the circulating levels of progesterone drop sufficiently to induce tight junction closure and a marked increase in lactose synthesis. Sustained lactation then requires the ongoing contributions of hormones, including insulin,

(Continued)

stromal cells, which lies adjacent to mammary adipocytes that enlarge due to their accumulation of fat. These breast changes occur between 8 and 13 years, roughly 2 years before menarche.[6,7]

With the onset of puberty, epithelial structures develop simultaneously through elongation of the ducts as the result of increased proliferation in terminal end buds, as well as from the development of terminal ductal lobular units (TDLUs) that are arranged as ductules clustered around the ends of ducts.[1,6] Lobules first begin to form at the periphery of the breast around 1–2 years after the first menses,[8] where the complexity of TDLU structures increases with age due to hormone-induced ductal branching during each menstrual cycle.[6]

Epithelial ducts and TDLU structures are surrounded by a fibrous, intralobular stroma, which in turn is surrounded by adipose tissue within each lobule. These lobules are separated by collagenous interlobular connective tissue that provides physical support, as well as connection to the pectoralis fascia via Cooper's ligaments. While breast tissue in males does not normally develop due to low levels of estrogen, some adolescent males experience transient breast development with physiologic gynecomastia due to alterations along the hypothalamic-pituitary-gonadal (HPG) axis, the dopaminergic-prolactin (PRL) pathway, chronic diseases, or various medications.[9]

14.1.3 Pregnancy

During the first trimester, the breast epithelium continues to proliferate,[10,11] giving rise to larger and further-lobulated TDLU-4.[6] These lobules contain an abundance of alveoli, each comprised of a single layer of secretory luminal cells surrounded by a meshwork of contractile myoepithelial cells that aid in milk ejection. The extent of development between the 15–25 independent lobules within the breast can vary significantly. Breast development also varies among women, although the change in total breast volume during pregnancy does not predict milk output during lactation.[12] However, several case reports have described women with inadequate milk production due to breast hypoplasia, also referred to as insufficient glandular tissue (IGT).[13] The pathophysiology or prevalence of IGT is unknown, although its diagnosis includes widely spaced, tubular breasts with the majority of glandular tissue localized in the subareolar region.[13] Likewise, the amount of epithelial tissue in obese mothers may be reduced as a negative consequence of increased fat deposition within the breasts, as occurs in rodents.[14] This reduction in secretory tissue may factor into the higher incidence of lactation failure seen in obese women.

14.1.4 Lactogenesis I/Secretory Differentiation

By the second trimester, the breast epithelium enters a phase of secretory differentiation often referred to as lactogenesis I (LI). At the cytological level, epithelial cells begin to assume a differentiated phenotype characterized by apical-basal polarization, increased abundance of organelles required for milk synthesis and secretion, and the formation of cytoplasmic lipid droplets. These cellular changes are also associated with the onset of transcriptional activation for certain genes involved in the signaling pathways, enzymes, and protein constituents required for milk synthesis.[15] In rodents, these changes include the onset of measurable casein transcription, although the ontogeny of casein expression within the human breast has not been mapped in detail. The secretion that accumulates within the alveolar lumenae during LI is destined to become the colostrum available to the infant at birth, which includes an abundance of secretory IgA synthesized by plasma cells that reside within the interstitium of the breast and that are derived from B-lymphocytes that migrate from peripheral sites such as the lung and intestine.[16] Clinically, the initiation of LI is marked by the presence of lactose and α-lactalbumin in urine, which leak from the alveolar lumenae into the maternal circulation via the paracellular pathway, which does not close until parturition. The appearance of lactose in the urine varies among subjects, ranging from about 12 weeks to 21–22 weeks of pregnancy.[12,17,18] Around the same time, blood flow to the breast increases,[19] which corresponds to an increase in breast temperature recorded in some women between 15 and 32 weeks of pregnancy.[12]

FIG. 14.1, cont'd   corticoids, PRL and the supporting provision of nutrients detailed in (B). The onset of lactation also initiates a complex interplay of maternal adaptations that modulate nutrient uptake and partitioning, as well as reproduction. Increased dietary intake and uptake provide a major source of glucose, lipids, amino acids, and micronutrients for milk synthesis. Peripheral changes in the skeleton, kidney, and small intestine ensure sufficient bioavailability of calcium. Changes in mobilization of lipid from peripheral adipose tissue follows a period of lipogenesis during pregnancy. These changes are coordinated by a complex interplay of endocrine signaling from the hypothalamus and peripheral tissues. At the same time, lactational amenorrhea ensues as the result of suppressed gonadotropic signaling to the ovaries. *LI*, lactogenesis I; *LII*, lactogenesis II; *T1*, first trimester; *T2*, second trimester; *T3*, third trimester; *TDLU*, terminal ductal lobular unit; *MLs*, milliliters; *FGF21*, fibroblast growth factor 21; *TG/NEFA*, triglycerides/non-esterified fatty acids; *NPY/AGRP*, neuropeptide Y/Agouti-related peptide; *POMC/CART*, pro-opiomelanocortin/cocaine-and amphetamine-related transcript.

14.2 ENDOCRINE REGULATION OF BREAST DEVELOPMENT, LI, AND COLOSTROGENESIS

14.2.1 Estrogens and Progestogens

Estrogens are the key driver of epithelial proliferation during the menstrual cycle and gestation, as evidenced by the fact that exogenous estrogen stimulates full development of breast tissue in women[20] and men.[21] Estrogens also prime the epithelial response to the mitogenic effects of progesterone.[22,23] The maximal proliferative response in the breast during late pregnancy and the luteal phase of the menstrual cycle matches the combined elevated levels of estrogen and progesterone during these states.[24] Interestingly, the proliferating cells within the breast during puberty and pregnancy are not usually those that express estrogen or progesterone receptors (ER and PR, respectively), leading to the proposal that estrogen and progesterone act through paracrine mechanisms to stimulate division in adjacent cells.[24] The response to these sex steroids is modulated by their nuclear receptors in epithelial cells, where the level of ER-α increases during early pregnancy and then declines thereafter.[11] The ER-β form of the receptor does not appear to play a role in mammary development.[25] By contrast, the expression of PR-B is relatively static in both nonpregnant and pregnant women,[22] whereas the expression of PR-A declines throughout pregnancy.[11]

14.2.2 Prolactin

Pituitary-derived PRL is essential for breast development and differentiation during pregnancy. PRL binds to the extracellular domain of its dimerizing receptor (PRLR), leading to activation of Jak2, which then phosphorylates downstream targets, including signal transducers and activators of transcription (STAT)-5. In turn, STAT-5 activates gene transcription in concert with other transcription factors, especially Elf5 and NF1B, all of which interact as "pioneering" transcription regulators involved in chromatin remodeling necessary for the coordinated activation of the multigene transcriptional programs required for secretory differentiation.[26,27] While the levels of the PRLR in the human breast epithelium have not been assessed during gestation, its gene expression level in nonhuman primates is elevated throughout pregnancy and lactation.[28]

PRL clearly plays a role during LI, given that urinary lactose output most closely mimics changes in circulating PRL. Hyperprolactinemia induces galactorrhea in men and women following estrogen-primed development,[20,21] whereas a pharmacologic block of PRL using dopamine agonists impairs the onset of lactation.[29] PRL is also likely a key driver of IgA synthesis, given its accumulation in the secretion of patients with galactorrhea induced by dopamine receptor antagonists.[4] By contrast, urinary lactose output is unrelated to the level of a PRL-like molecule, placental lactogen.[12]

14.2.3 Other Endocrine Requirements for LI

Glucocorticoids facilitate epithelial growth and differentiation during pregnancy and LI.[30] After binding their ligands, cytoplasmic glucocorticoid receptors (GRs) enter the nucleus to bind target response elements in the promoters of various milk protein genes to increase their transcription in concert with the actions of PRL.[30] Similar responses have been described during the differentiation of human breast epithelium in vitro.[31] In vitro studies also emphasize that insulin, in combination with GC and PRL, is essential for the synthesis of specific milk proteins during LI.[32] Recent experiments in mice support the notion that insulin, acting directly on epithelial cells through its receptor A and B isoforms, stimulates the mammary epithelium to proliferate and to enter LI.[33] However, the role of insulin, as well as the insulinlike growth factors, in modulating human breast growth and differentiation during pregnancy remains an important yet unresolved question.

14.3 THE COLOSTRAL PHASE

During the first 24h postpartum, the newborn consumes small volumes of colostrum (1–5 mL per feed) over 8–12 feedings.[34–36] The lactose content of colostrum (around 5.1%) is lower than in mature milk, whereas its sodium content is higher. The fat content varies from 1.5% to 3% and includes fatty acids synthesized by the epithelium de novo. The protein content of colostrum is around 2%, including an abundance of IgA.[31,37] Despite the small volumes involved, these early, small feedings are also rich in a range of bioactive and immunomodulatory proteins, including a diversity of oligosaccharides required for maturation of the infant gut and immune system.[38] While there are no rapid changes in the concentrations of lactose or sodium in the maternal blood, urine, or milk in the first 24h postpartum, there are increases in the transcriptional activity of the mammary epithelium.[39–41] By 24h postpartum, the transcription of genes responsible for fatty acid and lipid transport and the de novo synthesis, packaging, and secretion of milk fat, as well as galactose synthesis and transport to the Golgi, is increased.[39]

14.4 LACTOGENESIS II

The onset of copious milk production is referred to as lactogenesis II (LII) or secretory activation. During LII, the synthetic capacity of the mammary epithelium increases dramatically, with milk volume increasing from <100 mL during the first 24 h postpartum to approximately 500 mL by day 5.[17,31,36,42,43] The onset of LII also coincides with pronounced changes in the synthesis and secretion of various milk components, creating a transitory period of differential milk composition, often referred to as the phase of transitional milk. Women often report breast "fullness" or "milk coming in" around 60 h postpartum, followed by uncomfortable breast engorgement.[17,31,42,44,45] However, this experience is not universal, and many women cannot pinpoint the exact timing of increased milk production.[17,42] Moreover, the nuanced shift from breast fullness to discomfort to engorgement has not been defined.[45] Within the epidemiological literature, the onset of LII is subjectively defined as having occurred by 72 h,[46,47] which likely fails to address individual variation among mothers. Importantly, LII occurs independent of whether the breast is stimulated via suckling, pumping, or hand expression.[31,48] At the molecular level, the expression of genes responsible for lipid and carbohydrate synthesis peaks between 72 and 96 h postpartum.[39–41]

14.4.1 Lactose Biosynthesis

Lactose is the principal osmole that draws water into breast milk, and therefore, lactose production is the main determinant of milk volume. Lactose synthesis increases acutely between 24 and 72 h postpartum, and during this time, its concentration in milk increases from about 10 mM to 90–150 mM. This dramatic rise in lactose content also leads to increased levels of lactose in plasma and urine; blood lactose concentrations increase from 10 μM at birth to 30 μM by 72 h postpartum, while the rate of urinary lactose excretion increases several times, from 1.5 mmol/day at 36 weeks of gestation to 2–10 mmol/day by 3 days postpartum.[12,17] At the same time, the sudden increase in milk volume can increase alveolar lumen pressure within and cause backflow of lactose into the interstitium, especially when the mammary glands are engorged or infrequently emptied.[49]

14.4.2 Tight Junction Closure

Tight junctions (TJs) that reside along the lateral borders between epithelial cells become aligned and sealed in response to a declining level of progesterone in the presence of cortisol and either placental lactogen or PRL.[50] Once sealed, TJs prevent the paracellular movement of ions between the alveolar lumen and the interstitial space, while also polarizing the epithelium to induce unidirectional, basal-to-apical secretion and increasing the efficiency of milk synthesis and secretion.[50,51] Thus, the onset of LII can be defined in part by the loss of TJ permeability. As the concentration of lactose in breast milk increases between days 1 and 3 postpartum, the milk sodium (Na) concentration concurrently declines from ~58 to ~20 mM.[17,31,39,42,52] Even though the Na levels in breast milk fall precipitously, the increasing concentrations of lactose and potassium (K) (from ~10 to 20 mM) in milk maintain their osmolarity.[31]

14.4.3 Clinical/Diagnostic Determinants of LII

The most common biochemical markers used to track the onset of LII include milk components such as Na, K, or the Na:K ratio, lactose, citrate, glucose, or total protein content. Alternatively, or in addition, measures of blood or urine lactose, α-lactalbumin, and progesterone can be informative.[12,17,31,42,53,54] There are no standardized guidelines for defining the onset of LII, although Hartmann and colleagues recently sought to specify the ideal combination of these measures.[55] A formal definition of LII would be of immense clinical value, given that its delayed onset is associated with compromised breastfeeding initiation and poor breastfeeding outcomes.[47,56]

One approach to define the onset of LII has been to set cutoffs for the concentration of lactose, citrate, and glucose in milk at 110 mM, 1 mM, and 0.5 mM, respectively. These threshold values were derived by estimating the time at which the specified metabolite reached a predetermined concentration of at least two standard deviations above the initial mean concentration on day 1 of lactation, and two standard deviations below the final plateau concentration on day 3.[42] Using these metrics, healthy women reached the milk lactose cutoff by 31 h postpartum on average. The Na:K ratio in milk is another sensitive measure of TJ closure during LII. Lemay et al. classified the milk Na:K ratio into tertiles (>2.0, 0.6–2.0, and <0.6) to define colostrum, transitional milk, and mature milk, respectively.[41] Using this approach, the authors demonstrated that using a fixed postpartum time point (e.g., 72h) to define the onset of LII may be misleading, as the Na:K ratios did not correspond with self-reported feelings of breast fullness.[41] Considering the prevalence of obesity, diabetes, and intrapartum IV fluid use that can confound breast changes and sensations, it is unclear whether self-reporting of breast fullness can accurately predict the onset of LII.[47,57–59] The question of whether breast fullness and engorgement around LII are unique phenomena remains unclear, as does the nature of their relationship to the physiology of LII.[35,45]

14.5 ENDOCRINOLOGY OF LII

14.5.1 Progesterone

The initiation of LII occurs in response to the rapid decline in circulating progesterone levels after delivery of the placenta, as emphasized by the fact that women fail to initiate lactation until after any retained placental fragments are removed.[54,60,61] Progesterone has a plasma half-life of 5–7min and is rapidly metabolized by the maternal liver.[62] The concentration of progesterone in milk decreases by 65% within the first 24h after a normal delivery and becomes undetectable by 72h postpartum.[39,54]

Prior to LII, progesterone binds PR-B in the lactating mammary gland,[44] which blocks heterodimerization of STAT5 and the GR, while also competitively inhibiting GR binding to its response element and interfering with deoxyribonucleic acid (DNA) loop formation between the enhancer and promoter.[26,63–65] Once progesterone levels decline and its inhibitory effect is removed, PRL, cortisol, insulin, and their downstream effectors are able to coordinately and rapidly activate the transcription of the full complement of milk protein genes, including α-lactalbumin, leading to the onset of lactose synthesis and the subsequent movement of water across the epithelium.

14.5.2 Glucocorticoids

Glucocorticoids participate in the initiation of LII and have been shown to influence the sealing of TJ,[50,66] the upregulation of protein synthesis, and the regulation of genes for key metabolic enzymes and proteins.[30] While GCs are clearly essential for LII, their effect during established lactation may also be dose-dependent, given that high doses of exogenous GC suppress milk production in humans and cows.[67–69] In two recent case reports, GC administered to lactating women for musculoskeletal pain suppressed milk production.[68,69] Antenatal GC administered to women at risk for preterm delivery may lead to precocious LII and reduced milk production.[70,71] Given that many women suffer from posttraumatic stress disorder, postpartum depression, anxiety, or gestational diabetes mellitus (GDM), which are all associated with cortisol dysregulation, perturbations in endogenous cortisol levels have the potential to negatively affect lactation success.

14.5.3 Insulin and Glucose Metabolism

While there is no specific demonstrated role for insulin during LII, mice lacking epithelial insulin receptors have a limited capacity to lactate.[33] Epidemiological evidence suggests that dysregulated maternal glucose metabolism or the combination of poor glucose control and systemic inflammation, as occurs in overweight or obese mothers with either type 1 or GDM, is a major reason for failed onset of LII.[72] Women with type 1 (insulin-dependent) diabetes mellitus took an additional 27h to reach a comparable level of milk lactose relative to healthy women.[42] However, the degree to which insulin homeostasis independently influences the onset of LII in obese or diabetic mothers is unclear.[72] In the SWIFT cohort study, only a third of the women with GDM experienced delayed LII, indicating that insulin dysregulation sometimes (but not always) delays LII.[73] It is important to recognize that this population is also at an increased likelihood of emergency cesarean-section delivery, neonatal hypoglycemia, and blunted PRL secretion during breastfeeding, all of which interfere with the success of early breastfeeding initiation.[74,75] Given that GDM mothers are likely to face a delay in the onset of LII, they are now advised to practice antenatal expression of colostrum to ensure that the newborn has access to adequate milk.[76]

14.5.4 Oxytocin

Oxytocin is the principal hormone involved in the milk ejection reflex. Physical stimulation of the nipple activates somatosensory afferent neurons that initiate the release of oxytocin from the posterior pituitary.[77] In turn, oxytocin binds to receptors on myoepithelial cells that are positioned as a basketlike network around alveolar structures and longitudinally along the ducts.[78] Once bound, oxytocin induces contraction of myoepithelial cells and subsequent flow of milk from the alveolar lumen toward the nipple. Synthetic oxytocin is frequently used in labor induction and acceleration, but its effect on

LII or breastfeeding initiation has not been systematically studied.[79,80] Oxytocin nasal spray is used by some mothers to increase milk production; however, it has not been shown to increase breast milk synthesis.[81,82]

14.5.5 PRL and Growth Hormone

PRL helps sustain lactation, as highlighted by the extensive use of antidopaminergic galactogogues such as domperidone to promote or improve milk supply.[82] Conversely, suppression of serum PRL by dopamine agonists such as cabergoline works to suppress excess milk production.[29] A role for estrogen in the sustenance of PRL release can be inferred from the finding that the antiestrogen tamoxifen inhibited lactation and the breast pumping-induced release of PRL.[83] PRL levels also rise after breastfeeding—more so during early lactation, and to different extents among women.[84] Similar to other mammals, growth hormone (GH) has a galactopoietic effect on mothers with insufficient milk production, with milk yield increases by upward of 30%.[85] It is important to note that human growth hormone activates the human PRLR, so any effect of GH may in fact mimic the effect of PRL.

14.5.6 Induction of Lactation

While the ability to induce lactation has been widely demonstrated in a range of mammals, there is no standard protocol for women. As more women choose surrogacy, adoption, relactation, or supporting a pregnant same-sex partner, there is greater need for a standardized, evidence-based protocol. Reports for induction successes are sporadic, including a transgender woman who was able to induce lactation and exclusively support the nutritional needs of her infant for 6 weeks.[86] (For more information, see also Chapter 28.) Multiple case reports describe first priming the breast tissue with estrogen/progesterone from an oral contraceptive and then slowly increasing the dose of domperidone to increase serum PRL. At least a few months before the baby is due, steroidal supplementation is replaced with a frequent pumping regimen. Domperidone is then continued throughout the breastfeeding period and is frequently combined with herbal galactogogues such as fenugreek and milk thistle.[87,88] Hormonal priming may not be required, given the production of normal milk by women who hyperstimulated their breasts.[31]

14.6 ESTABLISHED LACTATION

14.6.1 Breast Size and Milk Production

The daily synthetic capacity of the breast is dictated by factors including the amount of glandular tissue, individual genetic and epigenetic variations, and the requirements of the newborn. While the output of breast milk varies substantially among women, the average breast milk production from 1 to 6 months postpartum is between 600 and 800 mL/day.[89] From 1 to 6 months postpartum, the median and maximum breast milk intake by the newborn per feeding increases as the frequency of feeding decreases, so that the daily output of breast milk remains stable.[90,91] Milk output is the same between breasts, but differs among women.[92] Importantly, breast milk production or composition cannot be estimated from a single collection.[91,92]

14.6.2 Milk Synthesis and Composition

Following the successful transition through LII, epithelial cells have the capacity for sustained lactation, or galactopoiesis, which is realized through the continued synthesis of various milk components via specific, defined pathways. For a more detailed analysis of breast milk synthesis and its minor components, the reader is directed to several excellent reviews.[38,93–95]

(1) *Carbohydrate*: Breast milk contains a relatively constant concentration of lactose throughout lactation (about 6.2%),[37] which is synthesized from circulating maternal glucose transported into epithelial cells by GLUT1 and other glucose transporters. The ability of epithelial cells to synthesize lactose stems from their expression of the tissue-specific modifier protein, α-lactalbumin, which modifies the activity of galactosyl-transferase so as to complex glucose to the newly formed galactose. Human milk also contains various oligosaccharides (0.1%–0.2%) formed from lactose as the result of a series of glycosyltransferase activities[94] that help establish a healthy infant gut microbiome.[96] The packaging of lactose and other carbohydrates into Golgi-derived secretory vesicles creates an osmotic gradient that ultimately draws water into breast milk to modulate its volume.

(2) *Proteins*: Whereas colostrum and transitional milk have higher protein content than mature milk due to their immunoglobulin content, the protein content of mature breast milk is lower and declines somewhat during lactation (from 1.8% during the first week to approximately 0.9%–1.0% by 3–4 months).[37] Most proteins in mature breast milk are synthesized by epithelial cells and can be separated into protein classes—the precipitable caseins (β-, κ-, and αS1-casein), the soluble whey proteins, and proteins associated with the milk-fat globule membrane. The caseins and epithelial-derived whey proteins are packaged into secretory vesicles prior to their secretion from the apical surface via exocytosis. Depending on the stage of lactation, the whey:casein ratio can vary from about 80:20 in early lactation to 50:50 in late lactation.[38] Other abundant proteins in human milk include lactoferrin, lysozyme, haptocorrin, and lactoperoxidase, which likely play important roles in neonatal health and the prevention of intrammamary infection.[38] Breast milk also contains an array of bioactive proteins that have been implicated in the local regulation of breast function, infant neonatal programming, or maternally optimized infant health.[38]

(3) *Lipids*: The fat in breast milk exists primarily in the form of triglycerides synthesized by epithelial cells after the uptake of fatty acids from the the diet and maternal stores, and from short- and medium-chain fatty acids synthesized de novo from glucose.[97] Triglyceride is secreted in the form of milk-fat globules enveloped in apical membrane, which have an average diameter of 4 μm.[98] The average size of the milk fat globule also changes appreciably during the onset of lactation, from an average diameter of 8.9 μm in colostrum to an average diameter of 2.8 μm by 96 h postpartum.[98]

The fat content of human milk, which averages around 3.7%, varies appreciably between women.[92] The breast storage volume and time after feeding also dictate fat content,[92] as does the lactation stage. The total fat content of breast milk declines between 1 and 4 months, and then increases by 12 months.[92] The concentration of fat in breast milk is also greater in residual milk within the breast (ranging from 5.9% to 10.9%) than that collected at the start of breastfeeding (2.2%–4.0%), consistent with the recent finding that oxytocin-stimulated milk letdown facilitates the expulsion of large milk-fat globules from the apical surface of epithelial cells.[99]

14.6.3 Local Regulation of Milk Synthesis

The mammary epithelium changes its rate of synthesis as milk accumulates between feedings, potentially due to a variety of local mechanisms. Although Geddes et al. did not detect a direct relationship between blood flow and milk production, the study did find that blood flow to the breasts was less in those producing limited milk.[100] Others suggested that the intraluminal accumulation of a certain milk component, a so-called feedback inhibitor of lactation, or FIL, could progressively signal to suppress milk secretion,[101] but such a molecule has never been purified or identified. Alternatively, epithelium-derived serotonin, which was first identified from the ability of PRL to regulate tryptophan hydroxylase activity, may fulfill some of these same actions,[102] where in one study, women taking a selective serotonin reuptake inhibitor were more likely to experience a delay in the onset of LII.[47]

14.6.4 Oral Contraceptives

The effect of ovarian hormones on milk production has been a topic of continued interest, given that women may choose to take oral contraceptives during lactation. Various estrogens administered to women at high doses have been consistently shown to suppress milk yield,[103] while progestin-only methods have no effect unless administered immediately postpartum.[104,105] In line with our understanding of the effects of steroids on lactogenesis, a recent Cochrane review concluded that "the evidence is inadequate to make evidence-based recommendations regarding hormonal contraceptive use for lactating women."[106]

14.7 ADAPTATIONS OF MATERNAL METABOLISM

The demands of milk production, on top of a mother's own requirements, place considerable stress on all aspects of maternal metabolism, a challenge that requires the reorganization of maternal neuroendocrine signaling, as well as peripheral hormone action. Although there are species-specific differences in the exact mix of adaptations, the metabolic needs of lactation are generally met through maternal alterations in food intake, energy expenditure, and catabolism of accumulated metabolic stores (Fig. 14.1B).

14.7.1 Food Intake

With the exception of some marine mammals, most lactating mothers increase food intake to offset some of the energy exported during milk production.[107] Lactating rodents uniformly increase their food intake threefold to fourfold,[107–109] a hyperphagic response that is proportional to suckling intensity. Food intake then rapidly decreases within 48 h of abrupt weaning. Hyperphagia appears to be the result of neuroendocrine changes triggered by the suckling reflex, and it is reinforced by hormonal changes resulting from suckling, negative energy balance, or both.

Appetite is regulated in the hypothalamus by the opposing actions of orexigenic (appetite-stimulating) neurons that express neuropeptide Y (NPY) and agouti-related peptide (AGRP), and anorexogenic (appetite-inhibiting) neurons that express pro-opiomelanocortin (POMC) and cocaine- and amphetamine-related transcript (CART).[107,110] In lactating rats, suckling activates NPY/AGRP expression in the arcuate and dorsomedial nuclei of the hypothalamus, while simultaneously suppressing the expression of POMC/CART in the arcuate nucleus.[107,109–112] These coordinate changes in the expression and secretion of appetite-regulating peptides mediate the increased food consumption caused by suckling. Lactation also suppresses circulating insulin and leptin levels in rodents, both of which can also regulate the production of NPY/AGRP.[108,109,113] Finally, PRL, which is produced in response to the inhibition of hypothalamic dopamine production and elevation of NPY by suckling, has also been shown to stimulate appetite in rodents, and thus elevated PRL levels may also reinforce the hyperphagia noted in lactating rats.[107,110,114]

Nursing women also experience an increase in appetite, albeit to a lesser extent than rodents.[115–117] There are no detailed studies of the regulation of hypothalamic feeding centers in nursing women. While leptin and insulin levels decline in women during lactation relative to pregnancy, there is also no documentation of the clear suppression of these hormones as has been noted in lactating rats.[108,109,118,119] One carefully performed, longitudinal study that compared lactating and nonlactating mothers matched for body mass index (BMI) did not find any change in circulating cortisol, insulin, ghrelin, or adiponectin in nursing women 3 or 6 months postpartum, but it did find elevated circulating levels of peptide YY (PYY) and PRL.[119] Therefore, while mild to modest hyperphagia accompanies nursing, the neural and endocrine regulation of appetite in nursing women is not well understood. However, because hyperprolactinemia in other settings does stimulate appetite and weight gain, elevated PRL may contribute to hyperphagia in nursing women.[120–122]

14.7.2 Reproductive Function

Lactation is associated with central hypogonadotropic hypogonadism and the cessation of cyclic ovarian function, which is mediated through extensive crosstalk between the hypothalamic circuits that regulate appetite and gonadotropin-releasing hormone (GnRH) secretion.[107,110,111] Suckling inhibits GnRH gene expression, as well as the pulsatile secretion of GnRH and luteinizing hormone (LH),[110,112] thereby inhibiting estrogen production and preventing ovulation. Like hyperphagia, the suppression of estrogen and gonadotrophin levels correlates with suckling intensity.[110–112]

A key regulator of GnRH secretion is kisspeptin (Kiss1), which is produced by neurons in the arcuate and anteroventral periventricular nuclei in the hypothalamus.[110,123] Kiss1 signaling interacts in complicated ways with peripheral estrogen levels to regulate both basal GnRH pulsatility and the estrogen-induced ovulatory surge of GnRH/LH.[110,124] In rodents, Kiss1 messenger ribonucleic acid (mRNA) levels and Kiss1 release are suppressed during lactation,[109–111,125] although it is not clear whether this relates to brainstem activation in response to suckling or to changes in peripheral metabolism. Given that suckling intensity and timing are important factors in regulating ovulation during lactation, and because Kiss1 signaling is a central modulator of GnRH secretion, it is likely that suckling directly suppresses Kiss1 signaling in some fashion. The hypothalamic systems that regulate appetite and energy balance also modulate GnRH secretion.[107,110,111] Hypothalamic orexigenic peptides and peripheral metabolic signals, such as decreased insulin and leptin levels, likely interact to inhibit GnRH expression and pulsatile secretion.[110] Finally, increased PRL levels also reinforce hypogonadism by inhibiting GnRH pulsatility, perhaps by inhibiting Kiss1 expression.[126–128]

Like rodents, lactating women also have suppressed LH pulses, which appears to be related to suckling intensity, pattern, and timing.[116,129,130] Several studies have confirmed that the return of menses and ovulation is delayed by nursing and that nursing intensity is important to maintaining amenorrhea. The frequency and duration of nursing episodes, as well as the introduction of supplemental feeding, correlate with the return of menses and fertility, consistent with the idea that suckling frequency and intensity inhibit ovarian function.[116,129,130] Lactation also enhances the negative feedback of estrogen on LH and follicle-stimulating hormone (FSH) secretion in women and blocks the ability of estrogen to induce an LH surge, perhaps by suppressing Kiss1 signaling as outlined previosuly. Suppressed ovulation also correlates with sustained high levels of PRL during lactation.[128] Unlike studies in rodents, leptin levels do not appear to correlate with LH levels or the return of ovarian function in lactating women.[116,128–130]

14.7.3 Glucose Metabolism

Milk production is associated with a large increase in glucose uptake by the mammary gland. In ruminants, mammary glucose uptake consumes 60%–85% of the total amount of glucose that enters the maternal circulation.[131] This dramatic increase in glucose uptake requires adaptations to provide enough glucose for milk synthesis and avoiding maternal hypoglycemia. These adaptations vary with the species, but they generally include some combination of increased gluconeogenesis, decreased maternal glucose utilization, and increased food intake.[115,131,132] In ruminants, the glucose demands of lactation are met by a sharp increase in the rate of gluconeogenesis, and gluconeogenic precursors are supplied both from the diet and from maternal stores.[131] In addition, glucose uptake by myocytes and adipocytes is suppressed during lactation, as is adipocyte lipogenesis.[131] Maternal glucose metabolism in rodents has been studied less, although they also likely experience increased rates of gluconeogenesis, glycogenolysis, or both.[108,109,133] Nursing women have lower blood glucose and insulin levels, despite having an increase in glucose production compared to postpartum women who are not lactating.[115,116]

Insulin sensitivity is also increased in lactating women, especially compared to the relative insulin resistance noted during pregnancy.[115,116] Glucose tolerance testing suggests that stimulated insulin responses, as well as basal insulin secretion, are decreased in lactating women.[115,134–137] Lactating women subjected to a short fast met the demands for milk production, primarily by increasing the rate of glycogenolysis by 50%.[137] However, after a more prolonged fast, their rate of gluconeogenesis increased alongside that of lipolysis and ketogenesis.[138] Glucose levels declined more rapidly with fasting in lactating women, leading to hypoglycemia after 30 h. While insulin levels were similarly suppressed in lactating and nonlactating women after fasting, glucagon levels were significantly higher in the lactating subjects.[138]

The endocrine control of adaptations in glucose metabolism during lactation is not fully understood. It is likely that lower levels of insulin and increased insulin sensitivity are prime drivers for the increased rates of glucose production, whether by stimulating increased glycogenolysis, gluconeogenesis, or both in target tissues.[109,115,116,135–137] Both GH and PRL also modulate glucose metabolism, likely by increasing insulin resistance in peripheral tissues[114,139–141] to direct glucose toward the mammary gland in support of milk production.[115,131] Interestingly, oxytocin has been described to increase insulin sensitivity as well as insulin release, which seems at odds with the reported decreased insulin levels and responses in lactating women and rodents.[142] An abundance of research literature highlights the correlations between maternal body mass and nutrition, the levels of milk adiponectin and other adipokines, and neonatal metabolic programming,[115,131,143–145] although less emphasis has been placed on the potential role of these factors on maternal metabolism during lactation. Maternal adiponectin levels in cows and women are decreased in early lactation which, at least in ruminants, may help to retain insulin insensitivity.[131,146,147] Furthermore, hepatic production of fibroblast growth factor-21 (FGF21) is increased during lactation,[133,148,149] which theoretically might increase fatty acid oxidation and augment insulin sensitivity, thereby reducing gluconeogenesis.[148] However, neither increased fat oxidation nor suppressed gluconeogenesis is typical of the maternal adaptations to lactation, and it has also been shown that hepatic FGF21 is transported into milk and affects neonatal gut function.[150] Thus, a more dominant function of FGF21 during lactation may be to coordinate maternal and neonatal metabolism. Finally, concentrations of both GLP1 and GIP are elevated during lactation in ruminants and rodents, although the contribution of these gut peptides to insulin secretion is not clear, given that insulin levels are decreased in these species during lactation.[131,151–153]

14.7.4 Lipid Metabolism

In most lactating mothers, milk triglycerides are derived from some combination of dietary fat, the mobilization of maternal fat stores and the de novo synthesis of triglycerides by mammary epithelial cells.[93,132,154] Elephant seals, some whales, and some hibernating mammals undergo prolonged fasting during lactation and rely almost exclusively on increased lipolysis so as to mobilize maternal fat stores for milk lipids.[132,154,155] Lactating mice and women mobilize some fat, especially early in lactation, but they also utilize dietary fatty acids and the synthesis of lipids from glucose and amino acid precursors derived from the diet to generate milk triglycerides.[115–117,132,154,155] In the fasting state, lipolysis likely dominates, while in the fed state, the mammary gland extracts fatty acids from circulating chylomicrons and very-low-density lipoproteins through the actions of lipoprotein lipase (LPL), which is upregulated in the mammary gland during lactation.[154,156,157] Lactating women have been estimated to lose about 2 kg of fat over the first 6 months postpartum, primarily from the trunk and thighs, as well as from suprailiac and subscapular fat depots.[158–161] Nursing is also associated with a more rapid decline in circulating triglycerides and an increase in total high-density lipoprotein (HDL) levels, as well as the ratio of HDL to total cholesterol (see also Chapter 11).[115]

As noted previously for glucose metabolism, PRL can cause insulin resistance in adipose tissue and the liver, while augmenting the effect of insulin on glucose uptake and the synthesis and secretion of triglyceride by mammary epithelial cells.[22,40,114,121,132,139,141,157,162–165] Altering insulin action in this tissue-selective manner would direct the precursors of lipid synthesis to the mammary gland. In addition, adipocytes express PRLR, and PRL inhibits adipocyte LPL, acetyl-CoA carboxylase, and fatty acid synthase activity, all of which are involved in adipose tissue lipogenesis.[114,163,166,167] However, the effects of PRL on adipocytes are complex, and this may stimulate adipocyte differentiation and lipogenesis during other states.[114,139,163] This raises the intriguing possibility that PRL may increase fat storage during pregnancy and help to mobilize that same stored fat during lactation. In addition to insulin and PRL, thyroid hormone levels are at least permissive for the altered lipid metabolism during lactation. Hypothyroid, lactating rats had lower milk triglyceride levels due to decreased hepatic export of trigylcerides, decreased mammary LPL activity, and triglyceride uptake by mammary epithelial cells, as well as a decrease in de novo milk fat synthesis.[168] Finally, increased circulating FGF21 levels in both cows and mice during lactation[133,150] may affect systemic lipid metabolism, although the potential contribution of this hormone to the metabolic adaptations during lactation have not been fully explored.[148]

14.7.5   Calcium and Bone Metabolism

Neonatal growth represents the most rapid rate of skeletal elongation during postnatal life, and milk must provide all the calcium required for bone mineralization until offspring are weaned.[169,170] As a result, the production of milk includes a massive requirement for calcium supply to the mammary gland that stresses maternal bone and mineral metabolism. This supply comes from several, likely redundant sources. First, as noted previously, food intake is increased during lactation and dietary calcium is an important source of calcium for milk production.[171] Calcium absorption is clearly upregulated during pregnancy, although studies differ as to whether it remains elevated during lactation. Calcium balance studies in lactating women suggest that, after parturition, the rates of calcium absorption return to a prepregnancy value, whereas some rodent studies suggest that intestinal calcium absorption remains elevated after parturition.[172–178] Calcium reabsorption by the kidneys is elevated during lactation so that a higher proportion of the filtered load is reclaimed, leading to reduced urinary calcium levels.[172,175,176,179,180] Therefore, even if fractional calcium absorption by the intestine is not elevated during lactation, the combination of increased calcium intake and increased renal reabsorption will raise the bioavailable calcium derived from dietary sources.

Another source of calcium for milk production is the maternal skeleton. Overall rates of bone turnover are elevated during lactation, but bone resorption outstrips bone formation so that bone mass declines rapidly and calcium is liberated into the systemic circulation.[169,170] Nursing women lose between 5% and 10% of their bone mass over 6 months, while rodents lose up to one-third of their skeletal mass over a 21-day lactation period. Bone loss in both species is influenced by suckling intensity.[169,170] Dietary calcium, skeletal calcium stores, and increased urinary retention of calcium all provide redundancy to maintain milk calcium content and to prevent maternal hypocalcemia. The relative importance of these sources is likely context dependent, although several lines of evidence underscore that redundancy is important.

First, in otherwise well-nourished women, augmentation of dietary calcium has little effect on bone loss and the liberation of skeletal calcium, suggesting that bone resorption occurs constitutively despite the availability of sufficient dietary calcium.[169,181,182] Second, while inhibition of bone resorption is well tolerated in lactating mice, simultaneous restriction of dietary calcium, together with an inhibition of bone resorption, leads to severe maternal hypocalcemia and death.[171] Finally, genetic inhibition of calcitriol production (and presumably dietary calcium absorption) leads to reduced maternal calcium levels, milk calcium content and increased bone loss in lactating mice.[179] Together, these data suggest that the constitutive mobilization of skeletal calcium contributes to milk calcium and that bone resorption becomes quantitatively more important during times when dietary calcium availability is reduced.

The regulation of calcium and bone metabolism during lactation is complex (see also Chapter 5). Although calcitriol levels are reduced during lactation as compared to pregnancy, studies of Cyp27b1-null mice suggest that calcium absorption during lactation may remain partly dependent on vitamin D.[179] Several studies have shown that PRL also upregulates intestinal calcium absorption during pregnancy and lactation, and it appears that PRL and vitamin D interact to upregulate expression of TRPV6 and calbindin-D(9k), which are both involved in transepithelial transport of calcium across enterocytes.[169,178,179,183–185]

The stimulation of bone resorption during lactation appears to involve the actions of PRL, serotonin, parathyroid hormone-related protein (PTHrP), estrogen, and FGF21.[133,183–190] Estrogen deficiency is well known to be an important driver of accelerated bone loss in postmenopausal women, and interested readers are referred to recent reviews on the involved mechanisms.[191,192] It is worth pointing out in the context of this discussion that lactation is the principal period of prolonged hypoestrogenemia that occurs during a woman's reproductive life. Thus, the skeletal consequences of suckling-induced suppression of GnRH secretion and low estrogen levels are likely a preserved evolutionary adaptation so that postmenopausal osteoporosis essentially results from the reactivation of lactation physiology by estrogen deficiency. PTHrP, a relative of parathyroid hormone that acts on the same receptor,[170] is produced by mammary epithelial cells during lactation in response to systemic PRL and local mammary serotonin production and is secreted into the systemic circulation.[170,187,189,190] PTHrP interacts with its receptors on cells in the osteoblast lineage to activate RANKL signaling and synergizes with low estrogen levels to stimulate osteoclastic bone resorption in both mice and women.[170,171,189,190] Furthermore, the production of PTHrP is coordinated with the delivery of calcium to mammary epithelial cells by calcium-sensing receptors, which inhibits PTHrP production when activated, defining a negative feedback loop between calcium delivery and PTHrP production.[180,193,194] Interestingly, PTHrP production and the suppression of estrogen levels are both regulated, at least in part, by suckling intensity, which may be a principal way that skeletal calcium mobilization is coordinated with milk production.[170] Finally, the work of Bornstein and colleagues has demonstrated that lactation-related bone loss requires the hepatic production of FGF21, given that bone mass is preserved in FGF21-null mice.[133] It is not clear how FGF21 signaling might interact with estrogen or PTHrP levels during lactation, but FGF21 has been shown to regulate bone cell activity in other settings, although recent studies have questioned the degree to which it affects bone cell activity in nonlactating but obese mice.[39,195]

REFERENCES

1. Howard BA, Gusterson BA. Human breast development. *J Mammary Gland Biol Neoplasia* 2000;**5**:119–37.
2. Dabelow A. Die Milchdruse. In: Mollendorff W, Bargmann W, editors. *Handbuch der Mikroskopischen Anatomie Des Menschen*. Berlin: Springer-Verlag; 1957. p. 277–485.
3. Anbazhagan R, Bartek J, Monaghan P, Gusterson BA. Growth and development of the human infant breast. *Am J Anat* 1991;**192**:407–17.
4. Yap PL, Mirtle CL, Harvie A, McClelland DB. Milk protein concentrations in neonatal milk (witch's milk). *Clin Exp Immunol* 1980;**39**:695–7.
5. Madlon-Kay DJ. 'Witch's milk'. Galactorrhea in the newborn. *Am J Dis Child* 1986;**140**:252–3.
6. Russo J, Russo I. Development of the human mammary gland. In: Neville MC, Daniel CW, editors. *The mammary gland: development, regulation and function*. New York: Plenum; 1987. p. 67–93.
7. Emmanuel M, Bokor BR. Tanner stages. In: *StatPearls*. Treasure Island, FL: StatPearls Publishing; 2018.
8. Monaghan P, Perusinghe NP, Cowen P, Gusterson BA. Peripubertal human breast development. *Anat Rec* 1990;**226**:501–8.
9. Ladizinski B, Lee KC, Nutan FNU, Higgins HW, Federman DG. Gynecomastia: etiologies, clinical presentations, diagnosis, and management. *South Med J* 2014;**107**:44–9.
10. Suzuki R, Atherton AJ, O'Hare MJ, Entwistle A, Lakhani SR, Clarke C. Proliferation and differentiation in the human breast during pregnancy. *Differentiation* 2000;**66**:106–15.
11. Taylor D, Pearce CL, Hovanessian-Larsen L, et al. Progesterone and estrogen receptors in pregnant and premenopausal non-pregnant normal human breast. *Breast Cancer Res Treat* 2009;**118**:161–8.
12. Cox DB, Kent JC, Casey TM, Owens RA, Hartmann PE. Breast growth and the urinary excretion of lactose during human pregnancy and early lactation: endocrine relationships. *Exp Physiol* 1999;**84**:421–34.
13. Arbour MW, Kessler JL. Mammary hypoplasia: not every breast can produce sufficient milk. *J Midwifery Womens Health* 2013;**58**:457–61.
14. Flint DJ, Travers MT, Barber MC, Binart N, Kelly PA. Diet-induced obesity impairs mammary development and lactogenesis in murine mammary gland. *Am J Physiol Endocrinol Metab* 2005;**288**:E1179–87.
15. Neville MC, McFadden TB, Forsyth I. Hormonal regulation of mammary differentiation and milk secretion. *J Mammary Gland Biol Neoplasia* 2002;**7**:49–66.
16. Butler JE. Immunoglobulins of the mammary secretions. In: Larson BL, Smith VR, editors. *Lactation: a comprehensive treatise*. New York: Academic Press; 1974. p. 217–55.
17. Arthur PG, Kent JC, Potter JM, Hartmann PE. Lactose in blood in nonpregnant, pregnant, and lactating women. *J Pediatr Gastroenterol Nutr* 1991;**13**:254–9.
18. Flynn FV, Harper C, De Mayo P. Lactosuria and glycosuria in pregnancy and the puerperium. *Lancet* 1953;**265**:698–704.
19. Thoresen M, Wesche J. Doppler measurements of changes in human mammary and uterine blood flow during pregnancy and lactation. *Acta Obstet Gynecol Scand* 1988;**67**:741–5.
20. Tyson JE, Khojandi M, Huth J, Andreassen B. The influence of prolactin secretion on human lactation. *J Clin Endocrinol Metab* 1975;**40**:764–73.
21. Huggins C, Dao TL. Lactation induced by luteotrophin in women with mammary cancer; growth of the breast of the human male following estrogenic treatment. *Cancer Res* 1954;**14**:303–6.
22. Chen CC, Stairs DB, Boxer RB, et al. Autocrine prolactin induced by the Pten-Akt pathway is required for lactation initiation and provides a direct link between the Akt and Stat5 pathways. *Genes Dev* 2012;**26**:2154–68.
23. Atashgaran V, Wrin J, Barry SC, Dasari P, Ingman WV. Dissecting the biology of menstrual cycle-associated breast Cancer risk. *Front Oncol* 2016;**6**:267.
24. Hilton HN, Graham JD, Clarke CL. Minireview: progesterone regulation of proliferation in the normal human breast and in breast cancer: a tale of two scenarios? *Mol Endocrinol* 2015;**29**:1230–42.

25. Warner M, Huang B, Gustafsson JA. Estrogen receptor beta as a pharmaceutical target. *Trends Pharmacol Sci* 2017;**38**:92–9.

26. Stöcklin E, Wissler M, Gouilleux F, Groner B. Functional interactions between Stat5 and the glucocorticoid receptor. *Nature* 1996;**383**:726–8.

27. Shin HY, Willi M, HyunYoo K, et al. Hierarchy within the mammary STAT5-driven Wap super-enhancer. *Nat Genet* 2016;**48**:904–11.

28. Stute P, Sielker S, Wood CE, et al. Life stage differences in mammary gland gene expression profile in non-human primates. *Breast Cancer Res Treat* 2012;**133**:617–34.

29. Rolland R, de Goeij W, Nappi C, et al. Single dose cabergoline versus bromocriptine in inhibition of puerperal lactation: randomised, double blind, multicentre study. *BMJ* 1991;**302**:1367–71.

30. Casey TM, Plaut K. The role of glucocorticoids in secretory activation and milk secretion, a historical perspective. *J Mammary Gland Biol Neoplasia* 2007;**12**:293–304.

31. Kulski JK, Hartmann PE. Changes in human milk composition during the initiation of lactation. *Aust J Exp Biol Med Sci* 1981;**59**:101–14.

32. Bolander Jr. FF, Nicholas KR, Van Wyk JJ, Topper YJ. Insulin is essential for accumulation of casein mRNA in mouse mammary epithelial cells. *Proc Natl Acad Sci U S A* 1981;**78**:5682–4.

33. Neville MC, Webb P, Ramanathan P, et al. The insulin receptor plays an important role in secretory differentiation in the mammary gland. *Am J Physiol Endocrinol Metab* 2013;**305**:E1103–14.

34. Santoro W, Martinez FE, Ricco RG, Jorge SM. Colostrum ingested during the first day of life by exclusively breastfed healthy newborn infants. *J Pediatr* 2010;**156**:29–32.

35. Saint L, Smith M, Hartmann PE. The yield and nutrient content of colostrum and milk of women from giving birth to 1 month post-partum. *Br J Nutr* 1984;**52**:87–95.

36. Neville MC, Keller R, Seacat J, et al. Studies in human lactation: milk volumes in lactating women during the onset of lactation and full lactation. *Am J Clin Nutr* 1988;**48**:1375–86.

37. Gidrewicz DA, Fenton TR. A systematic review and meta-analysis of the nutrient content of preterm and term breast milk. *BMC Pediatr* 2014;**14**:216.

38. Lonnerdal B. Bioactive proteins in human milk-potential benefits for preterm infants. *Clin Perinatol* 2017;**44**:179–91.

39. Wei W, Dutchak PA, Wang X, et al. Fibroblast growth factor 21 promotes bone loss by potentiating the effects of peroxisome proliferator-activated receptor gamma. *Proc Natl Acad Sci U S A* 2012;**109**:3143–8.

40. Mohammad MA, Haymond MW. Regulation of lipid synthesis genes and milk fat production in human mammary epithelial cells during secretory activation. *Am J Physiol Endocrinol Metab* 2013;**305**:E700–16.

41. Lemay DG, Ballard OA, Hughes MA, Morrow AL, Horseman ND, Nommsen-Rivers LA. RNA sequencing of the human milk fat layer transcriptome reveals distinct gene expression profiles at three stages of lactation. *PLoS One* 2013;**8**.

42. Arthur PG, Smith M, Hartmann PE. Milk lactose, citrate, and glucose as markers of lactogenesis in normal and diabetic women. *J Pediatr Gastroenterol Nutr* 1989;**9**:488–96.

43. Kent JC, Mitoulas LR, Cregan MD, Ramsay DT, Doherty DA, Hartmann PE. Volume and frequency of breastfeedings and fat content of breast milk throughout the day. *Pediatrics* 2006;**117**:e387–95.

44. Dewey KG, Nommsen-Rivers LA, Heinig MJ, Cohen RJ. Risk factors for suboptimal infant breastfeeding behavior, delayed onset of lactation, and excess neonatal weight loss. *Pediatrics* 2003;**112**:607–19.

45. Berens P, Brodribb W. ABM clinical protocol #20: engorgement, revised 2016. *Breastfeed Med* 2016;**11**:159–63.

46. Chapman DJ, Pérez-Escamilla R. Maternal perception of the onset of lactation is a valid, public health indicator of lactogenesis stage II. *J Nutr* 2000;**130**:2972–80.

47. Marshall AM, Nommsen-Rivers LA, Hernandez LL, et al. Serotonin transport and metabolism in the mammary gland modulates secretory activation and involution. *J Clin Endocrinol Metab* 2010;**95**:837–46.

48. Kulski JK, Hartmann PE, Martin JD, Smith M. Effects of bromocriptine mesylate on the composition of the mammary secretion in non-breast-feeding women. *Obstet Gynecol* 1978;**52**:38–42.

49. Stelwagen K, Farr VC, McFadden HA, Prosser CG, Davis SR. Time course of milk accumulation-induced opening of mammary tight junctions, and blood clearance of milk components. *Am J Physiol* 1997;**273**:R379–86.

50. Nguyen DA, Parlow AF, Neville MC. Hormonal regulation of tight junction closure in the mouse mammary epithelium during the transition from pregnancy to lactation. *J Endocrinol* 2001;**170**:347–56.

51. Itoh M, Bissell MJ. The organization of tight junctions in epithelia: implications for mammary gland biology and breast tumorigenesis. *J Mammary Gland Biol Neoplasia* 2003;**8**:449–62.

52. Cregan MD, De Mello TR, Kershaw D, McDougall K, Hartmann PE. Initiation of lactation in women after preterm delivery. *Acta Obstet Gynecol Scand* 2002;**81**:870–7.

53. Peaker M, Linzell JL. Citrate in milk: a harbinger of lactogenesis. *Nature* 1975;**253**:464.

54. Kulski JK, Smith M, Hartmann PE. Perinatal concentrations of progesterone, lactose and alpha-lactalbumin in the mammary secretion of women. *J Endocrinol* 1977;**74**:509–10.

55. Boss M, Gardner H, Hartmann PE. Normal human lactation: Closing the gap. *F1000Res* 2018;**7**:801.

56. Brownell E, Howard CR, Lawrence RA, Dozier AM. Delayed onset lactogenesis II predicts the cessation of any or exclusive breastfeeding. *J Pediatr* 2012;**161**:608–14.

57. DeSisto CL. Prevalence estimates of gestational diabetes mellitus in the United States, Pregnancy Risk Assessment Monitoring System (PRAMS), 2007–2010. *Prev Chronic Dis* 2014;**11**.

58. Deputy NP. Prevalence and trends in prepregnancy normal weight—48 States, New York City, and District of Columbia, 2011–2015. *MMWR Morb Mortal Wkly Rep* 2018;**66**:1402–7.

59. Kujawa-Myles S, Noel-Weiss J, Dunn S, Peterson WE, Cotterman KJ. Maternal intravenous fluids and postpartum breast changes: a pilot observational study. *Int Breastfeed J* 2015;**10**:18.

60. Neifert MR, McDonough SL, Neville MC. Failure of lactogenesis associated with placental retention. *Am J Obstet Gynecol* 1981;**140**:477–8.

61. Anderson AM. Disruption of lactogenesis by retained placental fragments. *J Hum Lact* 2001;**17**:142–4.

62. Short RV, Eton B. Progesterone in blood. *J Endocrinol* 1959;**18**:418–25.

63. Kabotyanski EB, Rijnkels M, Freeman-Zadrowski C, Buser AC, Edwards DP, Rosen JM. Lactogenic hormonal induction of long distance interactions between beta-casein gene regulatory elements. *J Biol Chem* 2009;**284**:22815–24.

64. Buser AC, Gass-Handel EK, Wyszomierski SL, et al. Progesterone receptor repression of prolactin/signal transducer and activator of transcription 5-mediated transcription of the beta-casein gene in mammary epithelial cells. *Mol Endocrinol* 2007;**21**:106–25.

65. Wyszomierski SL, Rosen JM. Cooperative effects of STAT5 (signal transducer and activator of transcription 5) and C/EBPbeta (CCAAT/enhancer-binding protein-beta) on beta-casein gene transcription are mediated by the glucocorticoid receptor. *Mol Endocrinol* 2001;**15**:228–40.

66. Zettl KS, Sjaastad MD, Riskin PM, Parry G, Machen TE, Firestone GL. Glucocorticoid-induced formation of tight junctions in mouse mammary epithelial cells in vitro. *Proc Natl Acad Sci U S A* 1992;**89**:9069–73.

67. Hartmann PE, Kronfeld DS. Mammary blood flow and glucose uptake in lactating cows given dexamethasone. *J Dairy Sci* 1973;**56**:896–902.

68. McGuire E. Sudden loss of milk supply following high-dosetriamcinolone (Kenacort) injection. *Breastfeed Rev* 2012;**20**:32.

69. Babwah TJ, Nunes P, Maharaj RG. An unexpected temporary suppression of lactation after a local corticosteroid injection for tenosynovitis. *Eur J Gen Pract* 2013;**19**:248–50.

70. Wiener Y, Tomashev R, Berlin M, Melcer Y, Maymon R. Breast engorgement induced by antenatal betamethasone therapy in a woman after mammoplasty. *Breastfeed Med* 2017;**12**:659–60.

71. Henderson JJ, Hartmann PE, Moss TJM, Doherty DA, Newnham JP. Disrupted secretory activation of the mammary gland after antenatal glucocorticoid treatment in sheep. *Reproduction* 2008;**136**:649–55.

72. De Bortoli J, Amir LH. Is onset of lactation delayed in women with diabetes in pregnancy? A systematic review. *Diabet Med* 2016;**33**:17–24.

73. Matias SL, Dewey KG, Quesenberry Jr. CP, Gunderson EP. Maternal prepregnancy obesity and insulin treatment during pregnancy are independently associated with delayed lactogenesis in women with recent gestational diabetes mellitus. *Am J Clin Nutr* 2014;**99**:115–21.

74. Chu SY, Kim SY, Schmid CH, et al. Maternal obesity and risk of cesarean delivery: a meta-analysis. *Obes Rev* 2007;**8**:385–94.

75. Rasmussen KM, Kjolhede CL. Prepregnant overweight and obesity diminish the prolactin response to suckling in the first week postpartum. *Pediatrics* 2004;**113**:e465–71.

76. Forster DA, Moorhead AM, Jacobs SE, et al. Advising women with diabetes in pregnancy to express breastmilk in late pregnancy (diabetes and antenatal milk expressing [DAME]): a multicentre, unblinded, randomised controlled trial. *Lancet* 2017;**389**:2204–13.

77. Uvnas-Moberg K, Eriksson M. Breastfeeding: physiological, endocrine and behavioural adaptations caused by oxytocin and local neurogenic activity in the nipple and mammary gland. *Acta Paediatr* 1996;**85**:525–30.

78. Gudjonsson T, Adriance MC, Sternlicht MD, Petersen OW, Bissell MJ. Myoepithelial cells: their origin and function in breast morphogenesis and neoplasia. *J Mammary Gland Biol Neoplasia* 2005;**10**:261–72.

79. Erickson EN, Emeis CL. Breastfeeding outcomes after oxytocin use during childbirth: an integrative review. *J Midwifery Womens Health* 2017;**62**:397–417.

80. Budden A, Chen LJ, Henry A. High-dose versus low-dose oxytocin infusion regimens for induction of labour at term. *Cochrane Database Syst Rev* 2014; CD009701.

81. Fewtrell MS, Loh KL, Blake A, Ridout DA, Hawdon J. Randomised, double blind trial of oxytocin nasal spray in mothers expressing breast milk for preterm infants. *Arch Dis Child Fetal Neonatal Ed* 2006;**91**:F169–74.

82. Forinash AB, Yancey AM, Barnes KN, Myles TD. The use of galactogogues in the breastfeeding mother. *Ann Pharmacother* 2012;**46**:1392–404.

83. Masala A, Delitala G, Lo Dico G, Stoppelli I, Alagna S, Devilla L. Inhibition of lactation and inhibition of prolactin release after mechanical breast stimulation in puerperal women given tamoxifen or placebo. *Br J Obstet Gynaecol* 1978;**85**:134–7.

84. Stuebe AM, Meltzer-Brody S, Pearson B, Pedersen C, Grewen K. Maternal neuroendocrine serum levels in exclusively breastfeeding mothers. *Breastfeed Med* 2015;**10**:197–202.

85. Milsom SR, Rabone DL, Gunn AJ, Gluckman PD. Potential role for growth hormone in human lactation insufficiency. *Horm Res* 1998;**50**:147–50.

86. Reisman T, Goldstein Z. Case report: induced lactation in a transgender woman. *Transgend Health* 2018;**3**:24–6.

87. Wilson E, Perrin MT, Fogleman A, Chetwynd E. The intricacies of induced lactation for same-sex mothers of an adopted child. *J Hum Lact* 2015;**31**:64–7.

88. Szucs KA, Axline SE, Rosenman MB. Induced lactation and exclusive breast milk feeding of adopted premature twins. *J Hum Lact* 2010;**26**:309–13.

89. Dewey KG, Lonnerdal B. Milk and nutrient intake of breast-fed infants from 1 to 6 months: relation to growth and fatness. *J Pediatr Gastroenterol Nutr* 1983;**2**:497–506.

90. Kent JC, Hepworth AR, Sherriff JL, Cox DB, Mitoulas LR, Hartmann PE. Longitudinal changes in breastfeeding patterns from 1 to 6 months of lactation. *Breastfeed Med* 2013;**8**:401–7.

91. Khan S, Hepworth AR, Prime DK, Lai CT, Trengove NJ, Hartmann PE. Variation in fat, lactose, and protein composition in breast milk over 24 hours: associations with infant feeding patterns. *J Hum Lact* 2013;**29**:81–9.

92. Mitoulas LR, Kent JC, Cox DB, Owens RA, Sherriff JL, Hartmann PE. Variation in fat, lactose and protein in human milk over 24 h and throughout the first year of lactation. *Br J Nutr* 2002;**88**:29–37.

93. McManaman JL. Lipid transport in the lactating mammary gland. *J Mammary Gland Biol Neoplasia* 2014;**19**:35–42.

94. Newburg DS. Glycobiology of human milk. *Biochemistry (Mosc)* 2013;**78**:771–85.

95. Allen LH, Donohue JA, Dror DK. Limitations of the evidence base used to set recommended nutrient intakes for infants and lactating women. *Adv Nutr* 2018;**9**:295S–312S.

96. Bode L. The functional biology of human milk oligosaccharides. *Early Hum Dev* 2015;**91**:619–22.

97. Mohammad MA, Sunehag AL, Haymond MW. De novo synthesis of milk triglycerides in humans. *Am J Physiol Endocrinol Metab* 2014;**306**: E838–47.

98. Michalski MC, Briard V, Michel F, Tasson F, Poulain P. Size distribution of fat globules in human colostrum, breast milk, and infant formula. *J Dairy Sci* 2005;**88**:1927–40.

99. Masedunskas A, Chen Y, Stussman R, Weigert R, Mather IH. Kinetics of milk lipid droplet transport, growth, and secretion revealed by intravital imaging: lipid droplet release is intermittently stimulated by oxytocin. *Mol Biol Cell* 2017;**28**:935–46.

100. Geddes DT, Aljazaf KM, Kent JC, et al. Blood flow characteristics of the human lactating breast. *J Hum Lact* 2012;**28**:145–52.

101. Peaker M, Wilde CJ. Feedback control of milk secretion from milk. *J Mammary Gland Biol Neoplasia* 1996;**1**:307–15.

102. Marshall AM, Hernandez LL, Horseman ND. Serotonin and serotonin transport in the regulation of lactation. *J Mammary Gland Biol Neoplasia* 2014;**19**:139–46.

103. Pomerance J. Steroid contraception and its effects on lactation are a public health dilemma. *Health Serv Rep* 1972;**87**:611–6.

104. Kapp N, Curtis K, Nanda K. Progestogen-only contraceptive use among breastfeeding women: a systematic review. *Contraception* 2010;**82**:17–37.

105. Tepper NK, Phillips SJ, Kapp N, Gaffield ME, Curtis KM. Combined hormonal contraceptive use among breastfeeding women: an updated systematic review. *Contraception* 2016;**94**:262–74.

106. Wijden CV, Manion C. Lactational amenorrhoea method for family planning. *Cochrane Database Syst Rev* 2015;**10**:https://doi.org/10.1002/14651858.CD001329.pub2.

107. Smith MS, Grove KL. Integration of the regulation of reproductive function and energy balance: lactation as a model. *Front Neuroendocrinol* 2002;**23**:225–56.

108. Crowley WR, Ramoz G, Torto R, Kalra SP. Role of leptin in orexigenic neuropeptide expression during lactation in rats. *J Neuroendocrinol* 2004;**16**:637–44.

109. Xu J, Kirigiti MA, Grove KL, Smith MS. Regulation of food intake and gonadotropin-releasing hormone/luteinizing hormone during lactation: role of insulin and leptin. *Endocrinology* 2009;**150**:4231–40.

110. Smith MS, True C, Grove KL. The neuroendocrine basis of lactation-induced suppression of GnRH: role of kisspeptin and leptin. *Brain Res* 2010;**1364**:139–52.

111. Muroi Y, Ishii T. A novel neuropeptide Y neuronal pathway linking energy state and reproductive behavior. *Neuropeptides* 2016;**59**:1–8.

112. Xu J, Kirigiti MA, Cowley MA, Grove KL, Smith MS. Suppression of basal spontaneous gonadotropin-releasing hormone neuronal activity during lactation: role of inhibitory effects of neuropeptide Y. *Endocrinology* 2009;**150**:333–40.

113. Crowley WR, Ramoz G, Torto R, Keefe KA, Wang JJ, Kalra SP. Neuroendocrine actions and regulation of hypothalamic neuropeptide Y during lactation. *Peptides* 2007;**28**:447–52.

114. Ben-Jonathan N, Hugo ER, Brandebourg TD, LaPensee CR. Focus on prolactin as a metabolic hormone. *Trends Endocrinol Metab* 2006;**17**:110–6.

115. Gunderson EP. Impact of breastfeeding on maternal metabolism: implications for women with gestational diabetes. *Curr Diab Rep* 2014;**14**:460.

116. Heinig MJ, Dewey KG. Health effects of breast feeding for mothers: a critical review. *Nutr Res Rev* 1997;**10**:35–56.

117. Stuebe AM, Rich-Edwards JW. The reset hypothesis: lactation and maternal metabolism. *Am J Perinatol* 2009;**26**:81–8.

118. Butte NF, Hopkinson JM, Nicolson MA. Leptin in human reproduction: serum leptin levels in pregnant and lactating women. *J Clin Endocrinol Metab* 1997;**82**:585–9.

119. Vila G, Hopfgartner J, Grimm G, et al. Lactation and appetite-regulating hormones: increased maternal plasma peptide YY concentrations 3–6 months postpartum. *Br J Nutr* 2015;**114**:1203–8.

120. Baptista T, Lacruz A, de Mendoza S, et al. Body weight gain after administration of antipsychotic drugs: correlation with leptin, insulin and reproductive hormones. *Pharmacopsychiatry* 2000;**33**:81–8.

121. Doknic M, Pekic S, Zarkovic M, et al. Dopaminergic tone and obesity: an insight from prolactinomas treated with bromocriptine. *Eur J Endocrinol* 2002;**147**:77–84.

122. Greenman Y, Tordjman K, Stern N. Increased body weight associated with prolactin secreting pituitary adenomas: weight loss with normalization of prolactin levels. *Clin Endocrinol (Oxf)* 1998;**48**:547–53.

123. Oakley AE, Clifton DK, Steiner RA. Kisspeptin signaling in the brain. *Endocr Rev* 2009;**30**:713–43.

124. Harter CJL, Kavanagh GS, Smith JT. The role of kisspeptin neurons in reproduction and metabolism. *J Endocrinol* 2018;**238**:R173–83.

125. Yamada S, Uenoyama Y, Kinoshita M, et al. Inhibition of metastin (kisspeptin-54)-GPR54 signaling in the arcuate nucleus-median eminence region during lactation in rats. *Endocrinology* 2007;**148**:2226–32.

126. Bachelot A, Binart N. Reproductive role of prolactin. *Reproduction* 2007;**133**:361–9.

127. Sangeeta Devi Y, Halperin J. Reproductive actions of prolactin mediated through short and long receptor isoforms. *Mol Cell Endocrinol* 2014;**382**:400–10.

128. Sonigo C, Bouilly J, Carre N, et al. Hyperprolactinemia-induced ovarian acyclicity is reversed by kisspeptin administration. *J Clin Invest* 2012;**122**:3791–5.

129. Labbok MH. Postpartum sexuality and the lactational amenorrhea method for contraception. *Clin Obstet Gynecol* 2015;**58**:915–27.

130. McNeilly AS. Lactational endocrinology: the biology of LAM. *Adv Exp Med Biol* 2002;**503**:199–205.

131. Bell AW, Bauman DE. Adaptations of glucose metabolism during pregnancy and lactation. *J Mammary Gland Biol Neoplasia* 1997;**2**:265–78.

132. Anderson SM, Rudolph MC, McManaman JL, Neville MC. Key stages in mammary gland development. Secretory activation in the mammary gland: it's not just about milk protein synthesis!. *Breast Cancer Res* 2007;**9**:204.

133. Bornstein S, Brown SA, Le PT, et al. FGF-21 and skeletal remodeling during and after lactation in C57BL/6J mice. *Endocrinology* 2014;**155**:3516–26.

134. Hubinont CJ, Balasse H, Dufrane SP, et al. Changes in pancreatic B cell function during late pregnancy, early lactation and postlactation. *Gynecol Obstet Invest* 1988;**25**:89–95.

135. Lenz S, Kuhl C, Hornnes PJ, Hagen C. Influence of lactation on oral glucose tolerance in the puerperium. *Acta Endocrinol (Copenh)* 1981;**98**:428–31.

136. Motil KJ, Thotathuchery M, Montandon CM, et al. Insulin, cortisol and thyroid hormones modulate maternal protein status and milk production and composition in humans. *J Nutr* 1994;**124**:1248–57.

137. Tigas S, Sunehag A, Haymond MW. Metabolic adaptation to feeding and fasting during lactation in humans. *J Clin Endocrinol Metab* 2002;**87**:302–7.

138. Mohammad MA, Sunehag AL, Chacko SK, Pontius AS, Maningat PD, Haymond MW. Mechanisms to conserve glucose in lactating women during a 42-h fast. *Am J Physiol Endocrinol Metab* 2009;**297**:E879–88.

139. Ben-Jonathan N, Hugo E. Prolactin (PRL) in adipose tissue: regulation and functions. *Adv Exp Med Biol* 2015;**846**:1–35.

140. Kim SH, Park MJ. Effects of growth hormone on glucose metabolism and insulin resistance in human. *Ann Pediatr Endocrinol Metab* 2017;**22**:145–52.

141. Shibli-Rahhal A, Schlechte J. The effects of hyperprolactinemia on bone and fat. *Pituitary* 2009;**12**:96–104.

142. Elabd S, Sabry I. Two birds with one stone: possible dual-role of oxytocin in the treatment of diabetes and osteoporosis. *Front Endocrinol (Lausanne)* 2015;**6**:121.

143. Badillo-Suarez PA, Rodriguez-Cruz M, Nieves-Morales X. Impact of metabolic hormones secreted in human breast milk on nutritional programming in childhood obesity. *J Mammary Gland Biol Neoplasia* 2017;**22**:171–91.

144. Catli G, Olgac Dundar N, Dundar BN. Adipokines in breast milk: an update. *J Clin Res Pediatr Endocrinol* 2014;**6**:192–201.

145. Newburg DS, Woo JG, Morrow AL. Characteristics and potential functions of human milk adiponectin. *J Pediatr* 2010;**156**:S41–6.

146. Asai-Sato M, Okamoto M, Endo M, et al. Hypoadiponectinemia in lean lactating women: prolactin inhibits adiponectin secretion from human adipocytes. *Endocr J* 2006;**53**:555–62.

147. Giesy SL, Yoon B, Currie WB, Kim JW, Boisclair YR. Adiponectin deficit during the precarious glucose economy of early lactation in dairy cows. *Endocrinology* 2012;**153**:5834–44.

148. BonDurant LD, Potthoff MJ. Fibroblast growth factor 21: a versatile regulator of metabolic homeostasis. *Annu Rev Nutr* 2018;**38**:173–96.

149. Schoenberg KM, Giesy SL, Harvatine KJ, et al. Plasma FGF21 is elevated by the intense lipid mobilization of lactation. *Endocrinology* 2011;**152**:4652–61.

150. Gavalda-Navarro A, Hondares E, Giralt M, Mampel T, Iglesias R, Villarroya F. Fibroblast growth factor 21 in breast milk controls neonatal intestine function. *Sci Rep* 2015;**5**:13717.

151. Faulkner A, Martin PA. The concentrations of some gut polypeptides are elevated during lactation in ruminants. *Comp Biochem Physiol B Biochem Mol Biol* 1997;**118**:563–8.

152. Faulkner A, Martin PA. Changes in the concentrations of glucagon-like peptide-1(7-36)amide and gastric inhibitory polypeptide during the lactation cycle in goats. *J Dairy Res* 1998;**65**:433–41.

153. Moffett RC, Irwin N, Francis JM, Flatt PR. Alterations of glucose-dependent insulinotropic polypeptide and expression of genes involved in mammary gland and adipose tissue lipid metabolism during pregnancy and lactation. *PLoS One* 2013;**8**.

154. Rudolph MC, Neville MC, Anderson SM. Lipid synthesis in lactation: diet and the fatty acid switch. *J Mammary Gland Biol Neoplasia* 2007;**12**:269–81.

155. Crocker DE, Champagne CD, Fowler MA, Houser DS. Adiposity and fat metabolism in lactating and fasting northern elephant seals. *Adv Nutr* 2014;**5**:57–64.

156. Farhadian M, Rafat SA, Hasanpur K, Ebrahimi M, Ebrahimie E. Cross-species meta-analysis of transcriptomic data in combination with supervised machine learning models identifies the common gene signature of lactation process. *Front Genet* 2018;**9**:235.

157. Jensen DR, Gavigan S, Sawicki V, Witsell DL, Eckel RH, Neville MC. Regulation of lipoprotein lipase activity and mRNA in the mammary gland of the lactating mouse. *Biochem J* 1994;**298**(Pt 2):321–7.

158. Brewer MM, Bates MR, Vannoy LP. Postpartum changes in maternal weight and body fat depots in lactating vs nonlactating women. *Am J Clin Nutr* 1989;**49**:259–65.

159. Butte NF, Hopkinson JM. Body composition changes during lactation are highly variable among women. *J Nutr* 1998;**128**:381S–581S.

160. McClure CK, Catov J, Ness R, Schwarz EB. Maternal visceral adiposity by consistency of lactation. *Matern Child Health J* 2012;**16**:316–21.

161. Wosje KS, Kalkwarf HJ. Lactation, weaning, and calcium supplementation: effects on body composition in postpartum women. *Am J Clin Nutr* 2004;**80**:423–9.

162. Boxer RB, Stairs DB, Dugan KD, et al. Isoform-specific requirement for Akt1 in the developmental regulation of cellular metabolism during lactation. *Cell Metab* 2006;**4**:475–90.

163. Carre N, Binart N. Prolactin and adipose tissue. *Biochimie* 2014;**97**:16–21.

164. Rudolph MC, Russell TD, Webb P, Neville MC, Anderson SM. Prolactin-mediated regulation of lipid biosynthesis genes in vivo in the lactating mammary epithelial cell. *Am J Physiol Endocrinol Metab* 2011;**300**:E1059–68.

165. Shao Y, Wall EH, McFadden TB, et al. Lactogenic hormones stimulate expression of lipogenic genes but not glucose transporters in bovine mammary gland. *Domest Anim Endocrinol* 2013;**44**:57–69.

166. Barber MC, Clegg RA, Finley E, Vernon RG, Flint DJ. The role of growth hormone, prolactin and insulin-like growth factors in the regulation of rat mammary gland and adipose tissue metabolism during lactation. *J Endocrinol* 1992;**135**:195–202.

167. Ling C, Svensson L, Oden B, et al. Identification of functional prolactin (PRL) receptor gene expression: PRL inhibits lipoprotein lipase activity in human white adipose tissue. *J Clin Endocrinol Metab* 2003;**88**:1804–8.

168. Hapon MB, Varas SM, Gimenez MS, Jahn GA. Reduction of mammary and liver lipogenesis and alteration of milk composition during lactation in rats by hypothyroidism. *Thyroid* 2007;**17**:11–8.

169. Kovacs CS. Maternal mineral and bone metabolism during pregnancy, lactation, and post-weaning recovery. *Physiol Rev* 2016;**96**:449–547.

170. Wysolmerski JJ. Interactions between breast, bone, and brain regulate mineral and skeletal metabolism during lactation. *Ann N Y Acad Sci* 2010;**1192**:161–9.

171. Ardeshirpour L, Dumitru C, Dann P, et al. OPG treatment prevents bone loss during lactation but does not affect milk production or maternal calcium metabolism. *Endocrinology* 2015;**156**:2762–73.

172. Beggs MR, Appel I, Svenningsen P, Skjodt K, Alexander RT, Dimke H. Expression of transcellular and paracellular calcium and magnesium transport proteins in renal and intestinal epithelia during lactation. *Am J Physiol Renal Physiol* 2017;**313**:F629–40.

173. Boass A, Lovdal JA, Toverud SU. Pregnancy- and lactation-induced changes in active intestinal calcium transport in rats. *Am J Physiol* 1992;**263**:G127–34.

174. DeSantiago S, Alonso L, Halhali A, Larrea F, Isoard F, Bourges H. Negative calcium balance during lactation in rural Mexican women. *Am J Clin Nutr* 2002;**76**:845–51.

175. Moser-Veillon PB, Mangels AR, Vieira NE, et al. Calcium fractional absorption and metabolism assessed using stable isotopes differ between post-partum and never pregnant women. *J Nutr* 2001;**131**:2295–9.

176. Specker BL, Vieira NE, O'Brien KO, et al. Calcium kinetics in lactating women with low and high calcium intakes. *Am J Clin Nutr* 1994;**59**:593–9.

177. Toraason M. Calcium flux in vivo in the rat duodenum and ileum during pregnancy and lactation. *Am J Physiol* 1983;**245**:G624–7.

178. Van Cromphaut SJ, Rummens K, Stockmans I, et al. Intestinal calcium transporter genes are upregulated by estrogens and the reproductive cycle through vitamin D receptor-independent mechanisms. *J Bone Miner Res* 2003;**18**:1725–36.

179. Gillies BR, Ryan BA, Tonkin BA, et al. Absence of calcitriol causes increased lactational bone loss and lower milk calcium but does not impair post-lactation bone recovery in Cyp27b1 null mice. *J Bone Miner Res* 2018;**33**:16–26.

180. Mamillapalli R, VanHouten J, Dann P, et al. Mammary-specific ablation of the calcium-sensing receptor during lactation alters maternal calcium metabolism, milk calcium transport, and neonatal calcium accrual. *Endocrinology* 2013;**154**:3031–42.

181. Kalkwarf HJ, Specker BL, Bianchi DC, Ranz J, Ho M. The effect of calcium supplementation on bone density during lactation and after weaning. *N Engl J Med* 1997;**337**:523–8.

182. Kalkwarf HJ, Specker BL, Ho M. Effects of calcium supplementation on calcium homeostasis and bone turnover in lactating women. *J Clin Endocrinol Metab* 1999;**84**:464–70.

183. Ajibade DV, Dhawan P, Fechner AJ, Meyer MB, Pike JW, Christakos S. Evidence for a role of prolactin in calcium homeostasis: regulation of intestinal transient receptor potential vanilloid type 6, intestinal calcium absorption, and the 25-hydroxyvitamin D(3) 1alpha hydroxylase gene by prolactin. *Endocrinology* 2010;**151**:2974–84.

184. Charoenphandhu N, Wongdee K, Krishnamra N. Is prolactin the cardinal calciotropic maternal hormone? *Trends Endocrinol Metab* 2010;**21**:395–401.

185. Suntornsaratoon P, Wongdee K, Goswami S, Krishnamra N, Charoenphandhu N. Bone modeling in bromocriptine-treated pregnant and lactating rats: possible osteoregulatory role of prolactin in lactation. *Am J Physiol Endocrinol Metab* 2010;**299**:E426–36.

186. Ardeshirpour L, Brian S, Dann P, VanHouten J, Wysolmerski J. Increased PTHrP and decreased estrogens alter bone turnover but do not reproduce the full effects of lactation on the skeleton. *Endocrinology* 2010;**151**:5591–601.

187. Hernandez LL, Gregerson KA, Horseman ND. Mammary gland serotonin regulates parathyroid hormone-related protein and other bone-related signals. *Am J Physiol Endocrinol Metab* 2012;**302**:E1009–15.

188. Laporta J, Keil KP, Weaver SR, et al. Serotonin regulates calcium homeostasis in lactation by epigenetic activation of hedgehog signaling. *Mol Endocrinol* 2014;**28**:1866–74.

189. VanHouten JN, Dann P, Stewart AF, et al. Mammary-specific deletion of parathyroid hormone-related protein preserves bone mass during lactation. *J Clin Invest* 2003;**112**:1429–36.

190. VanHouten JN, Wysolmerski JJ. Low estrogen and high parathyroid hormone-related peptide levels contribute to accelerated bone resorption and bone loss in lactating mice. *Endocrinology* 2003;**144**:5521–9.

191. Almeida M, Laurent MR, Dubois V, et al. Estrogens and androgens in skeletal physiology and pathophysiology. *Physiol Rev* 2017;**97**:135–87.

192. Khosla S, Monroe DG. Regulation of bone metabolism by sex steroids. *Cold Spring Harb Perspect Med* 2018;**8**.

193. Kim W, Wysolmerski JJ. Calcium-sensing receptor in breast physiology and Cancer. *Front Physiol* 2016;**7**:440.

194. VanHouten J, Dann P, McGeoch G, et al. The calcium-sensing receptor regulates mammary gland parathyroid hormone-related protein production and calcium transport. *J Clin Invest* 2004;**113**:598–608.

195. Li X, Stanislaus S, Asuncion F, et al. FGF21 is not a major mediator for bone homeostasis or metabolic actions of PPARalpha and PPARgamma agonists. *J Bone Miner Res* 2017;**32**:834–45.

Chapter 15

Postpartum Lactational Amenorrhea and Recovery of Reproductive Function and Normal Ovulatory Menstruation

Jerilynn C. Prior

Centre for Menstrual Cycle and Ovulation Research, Division of Endocrinology, Department of Medicine, University of British Columbia, Vancouver, BC, Canada

School of Population and Public Health, University of British Columbia, Vancouver, BC, Canada

BC Women's Health Research Institute, Vancouver, BC, Canada

Key Clinical Changes

- Postpartum lactational amenorrhea is highly variable in different populations and cultures but serves several purposes: providing infant nutrition, ensuring decreased fecundability, and preserving maternal energy balance.
- Recovery from lactational amenorrhea is related to many factors: frequency and duration of lactation, lactation as the exclusive source of infant nutrition, prolactin levels, maternal age or parity, and others yet to be well described.
- Ovulation occurs before first menstruation 8%–33% of the time, but the adequacy and fecundability of that ovulation is not well documented.
- Women are well documented to be protected from osteoporosis during lactational amenorrhea despite weight loss and the increased demands of caring for a totally dependent infant. The reasons are still obscure but may relate to short progesterone pulses rising to luteal phase equivalent levels or luteal phase progesterone levels that may be higher than in controls. More comprehensive clinical and epidemiological research is needed.
- The pattern of recovery of normal-length menstrual cycles and normal length, sufficient progesterone-level luteal phases after lactational amenorrhea may or may not be similar to the recovery after other causes of hypothalamic amenorrhea, but further detailed prospective research is still necessary.

15.1 DESCRIPTION OF POSTPARTUM OR LACTATIONAL AMENORRHEA AND RELATIVE INFERTILITY

Women have been conceiving, delivering, and breastfeeding their newborn infants throughout human history. It has also been known for centuries, and by peoples with no written language, that it is usual for the lactating new mother not to menstruate for a period of time following delivery (lactational amenorrhea), and also to have a period of time during which, despite heterosexual sexual activity, she is unable or less likely to become pregnant (lactational decreased fecundability). The hunter-gatherer !Kung women of the Kalahari Desert lactated on demand, and multiple times day and night, for 5 years on average, by which time the youngest child was eating other foods and the mother was pregnant again[1, 2] (Fig. 15.1). These peoples used no contraception and had no prepared milk formula, so the life of the infant depended upon breast milk. On average, a woman would bear about three children, spaced about 5 years apart, as a result of breastfeeding on demand.[1] Konner and Worthman, in their study of the !Kung women's breastfeeding patterns, concluded that it was the short interbreastfeeding interval, rather than the total number of lactational minutes per day, that determined the return of ovulation/menstruation.[3] They postulated that when the half-life of serum prolactin allowed it to dip into the nonlactating/normal menstrual-cycle range between breastfeeding bouts, then reproductive function would be activated.[3]

In the !Kung hunter-gatherers' life, women needed to walk >20 km/day to forage for the herbs, grubs, and insects that provided the bulk of the calories needed for her family (because hunting seemed to be a rare activity).[1] The role played by this energy expenditure, the contribution of suckling on demand, the seasonal relative decreased food availability for these African peoples of the desert, and their contributions to the length of amenorrhea and lactational infertility are difficult to

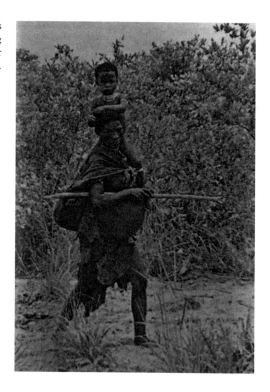

FIG. 15.1 A !Kung woman of the Kalahari Desert carrying her youngest child, who is nearly 5 years old, and her digging stick, plus a bag of gathered foodstuffs while walking about 20 km/day. She is approximately 7 months pregnant and still nursing her youngest child. *(From Lee RB. The !Kung San: men, women and work in a foraging society. London: Cambridge University Press; 1979. Reprinted with permission.)*

sort out. But all of these variables likely are important. By contrast, the well-fed 20th-century Scottish woman who chooses to bottle feed, who has no requirement to walk long distances daily, and likely has a higher body mass index (BMI) than a !Kung woman (Fig. 15.1), will begin menstruating within 2 months postpartum, and ovulate and likely become fertile during her second postpartum cycle.[4]

The World Health Organization (WHO) has recommended that women exclusively breastfeed, with no supplemental calories from any source, for the first 6 months of the neonate's life.[5] The purpose of this chapter is to review what is known about the overall recovery, timing, and pattern of restoration of regular-length menstrual cycles, normal luteal phase lengths, and thus presumed fertility in women who are postpartum and lactating. In particular, this chapter will focus on answering a current puzzle: Why is it that the universal months of menstrual cycle and ovulatory disturbances related to lactational amenorrhea/subclinical ovulatory disturbances do not cause clinically important bone loss or increased fracture risk?[6, 7] By contrast, although the phenomenon of amenorrhea is in common, hypothalamic reproductive disturbances related to immaturity of the reproductive axis in adolescence,[8, 9] such as delayed menarche, are negatively related to total hip areal bone mineral density (BMD).[10] Hypothalamic amenorrhea/oligomenorrhea/ovulatory disturbances associated with energy imbalance related to sports or eating disorders, emotional/social stress, or illness are also proved to cause increased risks for osteoporosis,[11] and increased rates of bone loss are documented even in normal-weight women with abnormal cycles and/or ovulation despite sufficient calcium.[12]

Lactational menstrual cycle and fertility disturbances serve the important physiological purposes of ensuring adequate nutrition for the infant, protecting the nuclear family (mother-father-infant/other children) from the demands of an early-arriving new baby, and protecting the entire population more broadly in cases when a mother's work (food gathering) is essential for the nutrition of the entire community, as with the hunter-gatherer !Kung people.[1, 2] In addition, it is likely that the pattern of recovery from reproductive suppression during lactation may provide information about the reversibility of menstrual cycle and ovulatory disturbances in other circumstances for women.[13, 14] Thus, a dynamic understanding of lactational amenorrhea/infertility and its recovery is an important topic related to women's health.

15.1.1 Anthropology and Epidemiology

Different populations of women—in various climates and regions of the world, at varying altitudes and latitudes, and with various options for nonlactational ways of feeding infants (such as bottle-fed, milk-like formula, or mother-chewed human food[15]), varying energetic demands, various ages at childbirth, and the availability of effective contraception—will have different experiences with postpartum or lactational amenorrhea. There has not yet been a systematic, comprehensive evaluation of all the potentially relevant variables (e.g., maternal weight, energetic demands, and social stress) that may interact with recovery from postpartum or lactational amenorrhea and its relative infertility. An example of the multitude of potentially interacting variables that relate to women's reproduction is evident in a thorough review from 2009.[16] Furthermore, most studies of lactational amenorrhea and its recovery are in very highly selected populations and report small numbers of women. One of the larger studies was from rural and urban women in Pakistan ($n - 1098$),[17] but the majority of studies with actual prospective data (rather than recall) are quite small and usually report results for fewer than 40 women. Although asking women to recall for how long they breastfed may seem suspect, recent epidemiological data show that women's 20–22-year-old memories about the duration of lactation are quite accurate and precise to within 2 weeks.[18]

There are numerous subtle (but likely important) differences in these populations. For example, in Muslim women from Pakistan, postpartum amenorrhea lasted a mean of 3.2 months longer than in those who did not lactate,[17] but it was recorded to be as short as 2–3 weeks in bottle-feeding Inuit women in the Alaskan arctic.[15] The role of culture in lactation practices is a topic that is not often researched, but Niehoff and Meister,[19] in an international survey, reported that Muslim women were expected to breastfeed for 2 years. In other societies (also reported by Niehoff and Meister), abstinence from sexual activity was expected for varying durations of time postpartum.[19] Finally, in yet other cultural groups, if a woman became pregnant while still lactating, it was assumed that she was an adulterer and was severely punished![19]

15.1.2   Endocrinology of Lactational Amenorrhea and Recovery

Although estradiol and progesterone levels drop dramatically after childbirth, and that is an adequate explanation for initial postpartum amenorrhea, the endocrinology of continued lactation is interesting and complex and can be covered here only briefly. Gonadotrophin levels differ in their responses during prospective observations postpartum; follicle-stimulating hormone (FSH) levels rise to normal menstrual cycle levels by about 4 weeks.[20] However, luteinizing hormone (LH) levels were not restored to normal with evidence of follicular activity (based on higher estrogen urinary excretions in weekly urine tests), nor with the first menstruation,[20] but increased to usual menstrual cycle levels only during normal, ovulatory cycles. In later sections, we will focus specifically on measures that prospectively document the reestablishment of ovulation and a normal luteal phase length postpartum in lactating and nonlactating women.

After prolactin, the anterior pituitary hormone that stimulates breast tissue to produce milk, was discovered and assays were developed to measure this hormone, we quickly learned that serum prolactin levels were high during both lactational amenorrhea and its associated decreased fecundability or infertility.[21] We also know that women with prolactin-producing pituitary adenomas commonly experience abnormal menstrual cycles and ovulatory disturbances that improve once the prolactin level is normalized.[22] In addition, it is clear that estradiol directly stimulates pituitary lactotroph production of prolactin,[23] and this explains the increased pituitary size during pregnancy. Finally, we have learned that there are direct effects of an infant's mechanical activity of breast suckling on prolactin production mediated through neuroendocrine pathways.[24]

Much more is now known about the menstrual cycle and reproductive effects of prolactin,[21] including that there may be a prolactin spike at orgasm in both men and women. We also now know that prolactin is made in other reproductive tissues, including the normal human myometrium[25] and uterine myofibromas,[26] as well as likely in luteal granulosa cells.[21] It also appears that co-peaking of LH and prolactin is needed before estradiol and progesterone production from the corpus luteum will be stimulated to peak simultaneously.[27] It is unclear however, what determines this co-pulsing of LH and prolactin. Thus, there are still many practical unanswered questions related to the roles of prolactin in initial formation of the corpus luteum[28] (by inhibiting apoptosis), and in the recovery of menstruation and normal ovulation[27] during or following postpartum lactation. It is likely, however, that prolactin levels must drop into normal menstrual-cycle ranges at least part of the time, potentially as a consequence of longer intervals between bouts of breastfeeding,[3] before menstrual cycles or ovulation can develop. Soules also made the important finding that in normally menstruating women, there was no relationship between serum progesterone and prolactin levels.[29]

Estrogen and progesterone measured in various ways have prospectively been studied during many months postpartum, in many studies. The Edinburgh group measured 24-h or first morning urine samples (sometimes adjusted for creatinine and sometimes not) for pregnanediol glucuronide (PdG) and total estrogens (E1C).[4, 20, 30] They ascertained levels in six healthy women with normal cycling and ovulating (but their criteria for normality were not defined) and used absolute levels of each urinary steroid to indicate ovulation (PdG) and follicular activity (E1C), respectively. However, urinary steroids inevitably undergo metabolism (Cytochrome P450 by Cyp 3A4), and the activity of this enzyme differs on a genetic basis for most women. It has been shown, for example, that this enzyme's activity is systematically higher (and consequently urinary steroid levels are lower) in East Asian women.[31, 32] Furthermore, in a study of >600 women collecting twice-weekly first morning urines for PdG over a single cycle, we found that the follicular phase levels of some were higher than the luteal phase levels of others.[33] Therefore, although these urinary steroid data likely indicate *something*, their importance is not entirely clear, and it is unlikely that they are diagnostic of normal ovulation. The appropriate use of urinary PdG for the diagnosis and timing of ovulation is based on a threefold rise within women from the follicular to the luteal phase[34] or the phenomenon of dropping levels of E1C and rising levels of PdG.[35]

The best study of ovarian progesterone levels during postpartum and lactational amenorrhea and its recovery is by researchers in Galway, Ireland, who collected daily salivary values[36] measured by enzyme immunoassay (EIA) in 30 postpartum women, of whom 10 were not lactating. Using data from normally ovulatory cycles as documented to be normal by serial midcycle vaginal ultrasounds in 41 normal controls, they set the salivary progesterone threshold at 251 pmol/L.[36] Although this Irish postpartum cohort did not breastfeed very long (an average of 4 months), and almost half started the infant on solid feeds by 3 months, 35% of the women ovulated before their first flow, and 55% of their first menstrual cycles were anovulatory. It is interesting that the ovulation-before-flow phenomenon occurred in none of the bottle-feeding women.[36] This study also documented that a higher percentage of first cycles were ovulatory in bottle-feeding (70%) than in lactating (45%) women, and that lactating and nonlactating women showed a decreasing percentage in the first three cycles over time of luteal phases that were short or insufficient.[36]

15.1.3 Key Variables Related to Duration of Lactational Amenorrhea and of Ovulatory Disturbances

The various prospective studies of the duration of amenorrhea in breastfeeding women postpartum have described some of these variables, but no one study has indicated all of them (based on other studies of women's reproduction[16]) that are likely important. As a way of summarizing and comparing several studies in varying environments, with women from a range of ethnicities and at various times in the past, Table 15.1 presents the key variables in four studies of Inuit, Caucasian Irish and Scottish, and Pakistani women who are a mixture of rural and urban residents. As the table shows, not all studies even include the mean age and parity of the women, and none have their BMIs or energy expenditures. Few have the sex of the baby, and only the Bolaji study[36] included the baby's birthweight. They do all have in common that they studied healthy women, on no hormonal contraception, and who have delivered a singleton baby at a known date. Unfortunately, the "ovulation" data in the Edinburgh study are using PdG interpretation methods that are not robust.

TABLE 15.1 Descriptive and comparative demographic, lactational, and reproductive variables in prospective or retrospective studies of lactational amenorrhea in different ethnic groups, environments, and life circumstances

	Galway[36]	Edinburgh[4]	Pakistan[17]	Barrow[15]
Total number of women	30	37	1098	299
Lactating women-number	20	27	941	242
Mean lactation (mo.)	4.1	10	12.2–19	7
Amenorrhea (mo.)	4	8.1	9.5–14.1	9.5
Supplement start-mo.	3 (in 45%)	ND[a]	ND[a]	6
Demand nursing (Y/N)	N	ND[a]	Y?	Y
Mean age	31	27–40	15–44	29
Parity number	2.8	ND[a]	1–7	6
Sex of baby (M/F)	1.3:1	ND[a]	ND[a]	ND[a]
% Ovul before flow	23	35	7.3% preg	ND[a]
BMI (kg/m²)	ND[a]	ND[a]	ND[a]	ND[a]
% First flow ovulatory	45	45	ND[a]	ND[a]
Rural/urban	Urban	Urban	40:60	Rural

[a]ND means not documented or not described.

It is well documented that following childbirth, bottle-feeding women have earlier recovery of menstrual cycles than do breastfeeding women. One of the few studies that has prospectively documented the postpartum day of first menstruation in a large population of lactating or nonlactating women (the latter who are not treated with drugs to prevent breast engorgement) is a study by Berman in the Alaskan arctic.[15] These data have been plotted as a frequency distribution in Fig. 15.2. Note that the mode or most frequent number of women starting menstruation on a certain day postpartum differs significantly between breastfeeding and bottle-feeding women,[15] although both populations demonstrate a typical bimodal distribution. These data illustrate that there must be complex nutritional, energetic, hormonal, and other differences between lactating and nonlactating women.

It is likely that all the variables that are known to be related to hypothalamic amenorrhea, such as BMI, weight loss (but sometimes weight gain to reach obesity), social/psychological stress,[37] meeting the energy needs for physical activity as well as for nursing, and reproductive maturation (maternal age and parity), are important in the duration of lactational amenorrhea.[38] Yet no study on postpartum breastfeeding and amenorrhea has documented all of these variables as well as the commonly reported ones related to suckling duration, intervals, min/day, supplemental feeding, and prolactin levels.

The idea that nutritional balance (so that energy intake covers energy expenditure needs) is important in the onset of menstruation following lactational amenorrhea is suggested by the data of Harvard anthropologist, Peter Ellison, showing a gradual increase from low C-peptide levels (a molecule that is made in the same quantity as insulin) to levels of about 130% of eventual mean menstrual-cycle levels.[39] This overshoot occurs about 2 months before the first return of flow. Ellison also showed that the absolute C-peptide levels systematically and positively varied with the baseline BMI of the postpartum mother.[39]

Current data from multiple studies suggest that some characteristics of a baby's suckling and feeding habits are related to the maintenance or the completion of lactational amenorrhea. The tightest correlations seem to be with the total time of breast feeding/day, with nighttime breastfeeding, or with the presence or lack of calories from non-breastmilk sources. From the available data,[4, 36] it appears that women need to continue to nurse for >60 min/day, ideally at frequent intervals, and not to feed their babies any solid foods in order for lactational amenorrhea to continue. So, again, the relationship appears to be to caloric balance. It has also been postulated that longer duration between suckling episodes might allow prolactin levels to decrease into the normal range, and thus allow reproductive activation.[3]

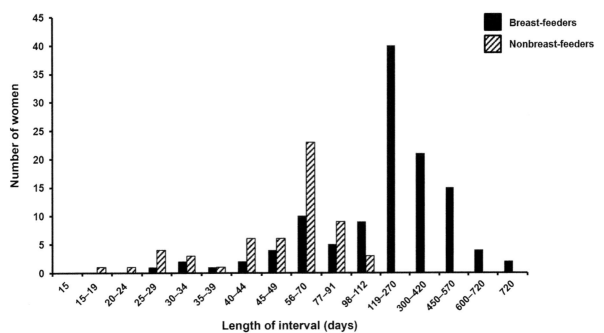

FIG. 15.2   This frequency distribution graph is derived from the data of Berman[15] and shows the duration of postpartum amenorrhea in Inuit women from the Alaskan arctic who are breastfeeding on demand ($n = 242$) versus bottle-feeding women ($n = 57$).

15.2 PARALLELS WITH RESEARCH ON MENSTRUAL CYCLE RECOVERY FROM AMENORRHEA OF OTHER CAUSES

A number of studies have shown that hypothalamic amenorrhea will recover to normal menstrual cycles when the higher cortisol levels have decreased into the normal range,[40] along with the caloric intake matching the energy expenditure.[41] The pattern of menstrual cycle recovery from amenorrhea is typically one of long or irregular cycles without ovulation, followed by normal-cycle intervals with short luteal or luteal insufficient phases, followed by ovulatory menstruation.[14] This pattern appears different than recovery from lactational amenorrhea because such a high percentage of women with lactational amenorrhea appear to experience ovulation prior to the onset of the first flow. This can be seen in 7%–35% of all lactating women with amenorrhea. Two studies suggest that this predominantly occurs in women over age 30 and in those who have previously borne more children,[17, 30] indicating some maturational influence. Once flow begins, the progesterone levels gradually increase in subsequent cycles,[36] and the pattern of ovulatory disturbances gradually resolves to normal luteal phase lengths and progesterone levels with subsequent cycling.[30]

15.3 NEED FOR FURTHER RESEARCH

The first need in prospective observational studies of maternal reproductive recovery from postpartum lactational amenorrhea is to integrate the hormonal variables (prolactin, LH, progesterone, estradiol, and cortisol) with energy balance variables such as body weight and its changes, energy expenditures (both from physical activity and with the calories provided through breast milk), and C-peptide or fasting insulin. In addition, these energetic and hormonal variables need to be

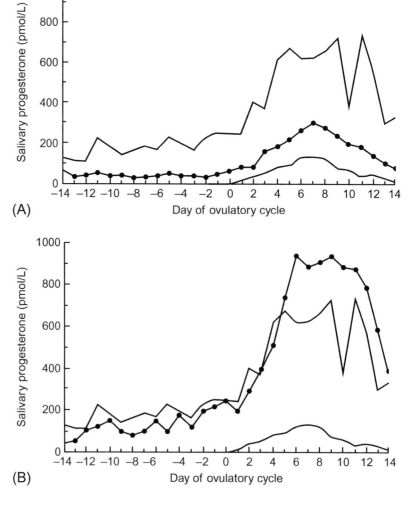

FIG. 15.3 These two graphs of salivary progesterone levels across the normal menstrual cycle show the data (A) from healthy control women ($n = 41$) with the mean as a *dotted line* and *solid lines* for the upper and lower 95% CI limits. By contrast are the data (B) from one woman in an early cycle during recovery from postpartum amenorrhea, whose mean luteal phase salivary progesterone levels exceed the upper 95% CI by >5%. *(From Bolaji II, Tallon DF, Meehan FP, O'Dwyer EM, Fottrell PF. The return of postpartum fertility monitored by enzyme-immunoassay for salivary progesterone. Gynecol Endocrinol 1992;6(1):37–48. Reprinted with permission.)*

integrated with women's daily perceptions of social stress, feelings of self-worth and energy, as well as environmental variables (physical/psychological abuse, and health-related quality of life).

For the purposes of knowing when lactational amenorrhea will no longer be sufficient for contraception, it is important that some simple measure (perhaps salivary progesterone[36]) is available in order to predict that ovulation will occur before flow. There may also be subtle signs that women could perceive that we have not yet thought of—perhaps the development of axillary breast tenderness in the absence of nipple or front-of-breast sensitivity, for example.[33]

We started this discussion with a question about why lactational amenorrhea and ovulatory disturbances during recovery are not associated with bone loss or increased fracture risk.[7] What is interesting in the Bolaji data,[36] as shown in Fig. 15.3, is that 1 of the 20 lactating women had an overshoot of luteal phase progesterone production to more than the upper 95% confidence interval (CI) of controls. In addition, in the same study, a graphed daily profile of salivary progesterone levels over three anovulatory menstrual cycles in a single woman showed at least 3 days on which sporadic values for salivary progesterone were higher than the ovulatory threshold values before the first flow; this occurred in all three nonovulatory cycles, with several 1-day spikes of progesterone into the ovulatory range[36] preceding flow. Based on evidence that progesterone directly stimulates osteoblastic bone formation in women,[42] and that cyclic progesterone effectively increases BMD in normal-weight women with hypothalamic amenorrhea[12] and ovulatory disturbances within regular cycles, it is likely that these bursts of ovulatory progesterone values and an overshoot in 5% of the studied cycles may be relevant to preserved bone integrity, despite lactational amenorrhea. Further investigation of this hypothesis is needed.

REFERENCES

1. Lee RB. *The !Kung San: men, women and work in a foraging society.* London: Cambridge University Press; 1979.
2. Shostak M. *Nisa: the life and words of a !Kung woman.* New York: Vintage Books; 1981.
3. Konner M, Worthman C. Nursing frequency, gonadal function, and birth spacing among !Kung hunter-gatherers. *Science* 1980;**207**:788–91.
4. Howie PW, McNeilly AS, Houston MJ, Cook A, Boyle H. Fertility after childbirth: post-partum ovulation and menstruation in bottle and breast feeding mothers. *Clin Endocrinol* 1982;**17**(4):323–32.
5. World Health Organization. *Global strategy for infant and young child feeding. The optimal duration of exclusive breastfeeding.* Geneva: World Health Organization; 2001. Report No.: A54/INF.DOC./4.
6. Kovacs CS. The skeleton is a storehouse of mineral that is plundered during lactation and (fully?) replenished afterwards. *J Bone Miner Res* 2017;**32**(4):676–80.
7. Kovacs CS. Maternal mineral and bone metabolism during pregnancy, lactation, and post-weaning recovery. *Physiol Rev* 2016;**96**(2):449–547.
8. Vollman RF. The menstrual cycle. In: Friedman EA, editor. *Major Problems in Obstetrics and Gynecology.* 1st ed. vol. 7. Toronto: W.B. Saunders Company; 1977. p. 11–193.
9. Metcalf MG, Skidmore DS, Lowry GF, MacKenzie JA. Incidence of ovulation in the years after the menarche. *J Endocrinol* 1983;**97**(2):213–9.
10. Goshtasebi A, Berger C, Barr SI, Kovacs CS, Towheed T, Davison KS, et al. Adult premenopausal bone health related to reproductive characteristics – population-based data from the Canadian Multicentre Osteoporosis Study (CaMos). *Int J Environ Res Public Health* 2018;**15**(5).
11. Gordon CM, Ackerman KE, Berga SL, Kaplan JR, Mastorakos G, Misra M, et al. Functional hypothalamic amenorrhea: an Endocrine Society Clinical Practice Guideline. *J Clin Endocrinol Metab* 2017;**102**(5):1413–39.
12. Prior JC, Vigna YM, Barr SI, Rexworthy C, Lentle BC. Cyclic medroxyprogesterone treatment increases bone density: a controlled trial in active women with menstrual cycle disturbances. *Am J Med* 1994;**96**:521–30.
13. Prior JC, Ho Yeun B, Clement P, Bowie L, Thomas J. Reversible luteal phase changes and infertility associated with marathon training. *Lancet* 1982;**1**:269–70.
14. Prior JC. Luteal phase defects and anovulation: adaptive alterations occurring with conditioning exercise. *Semin Reprod Endocrinol* 1985;**3**:27–33.
15. Berman ML, Hanson K, Hellman IL. Effect of breast-feeding on postpartum menstruation, ovulation, and pregnancy in Alaskan Eskimos. *Am J Obstet Gynecol* 1972;**114**(4):524–34.
16. Vitzthum VJ. The ecology and evolutionary endocrinology of reproduction in the human female. *Am J Phys Anthropol* 2009;**140**(Suppl 49):95–136.
17. Khan T, Siraj M. Duration of lactation, lactational amenorrhea and incidence of pregnancy in Pakistani women. *J Pak Med Assoc* 1998;**36**:63–5.
18. Natland ST, Andersen LF, Nilsen TI, Forsmo S, Jacobsen GW. Maternal recall of breastfeeding duration twenty years after delivery. *BMC Med Res Methodol* 2012;**12**:179.
19. Niehoff A, Meister N. The cultural characteristics of breast-feeding: a survey. *J Trop Pediatr* 1972;**18**:16–20.
20. Glasier A, McNeilly AS, Howie PW. Fertility after childbirth: changes in serum gonadotrophin levels in bottle and breast feeding women. *Clin Endocrinol* 1983;**19**(4):493–501.
21. Egli M, Leeners B, Kruger TH. Prolactin secretion patterns: basic mechanisms and clinical implications for reproduction. *Reproduction* 2010;**140**(5):643–54.
22. Melmed S, Casanueva FF, Hoffman AR, Kleinberg DL, Montori VM, Schlechte JA, et al. Diagnosis and treatment of hyperprolactinemia: an Endocrine Society clinical practice guideline. *J Clin Endocrinol Metab* 2011;**96**(2):273–88.

23. Prior JC, Cox TA, Fairholm D, Kostashuk E, Nugent R. Testosterone-related exacerbation of prolactin-producing macroadenoma: possible role for estrogen. *J Clin Endocrinol Metab* 1987;**64**:391–4.

24. Gordon K, Hodgen GD, Richardson DW. Postpartum lactational anovulation in a nonhuman primate (Macaca fascicularis): endogenous opiate mediation of suckling-induced hyperprolactinemia. *J Clin Endocrinol Metab* 1992;**75**(1):59–67.

25. Walters CA, Daly DC, Chapitis J, Kuslis ST, Prior JC, Kusmik WF, et al. Human myometrium: a potential source of prolactin. *Am J Obstet Gynecol* 1983;**147**:639–44.

26. Chapitis J, Riddick DH, Betz LM, Brumsted JR, Gibson M, Prior JC, et al. Physicochemical characterization and functional activity of fibroid prolactin produced in cell culture. *Am J Obstet Gynecol* 1988;**158**:846–53.

27. Hinney B, Henze C, Wuttke W. Regulation of luteal function by luteinizing hormone and prolactin at different times of the luteal phase. *Eur J Endocrinol* 1995;**133**(6):701–17.

28. Perks CM, Newcomb PV, Grohmann M, Wright RJ, Mason HD, Holly JM. Prolactin acts as a potent survival factor against C2-ceramide-induced apoptosis in human granulosa cells. *Hum Reprod* 2003;**18**(12):2672–7.

29. Soules MR, Bremner WJ, Steiner RA, Clifton DK. Prolactin secretion and corpus luteum function in women with luteal phase deficiency. *J Clin Endocrinol Metab* 1991;**72**:986–92.

30. McNeilly AS, Howie PW, Houston MJ, Cook A, Boyle H. Fertility after childbirth: adequacy of post-partum luteal phases. *Clin Endocrinol* 1982;**17**(6):609–15.

31. Lin Y, Anderson GD, Kantor E, Ojemann LM, Wilensky AJ. Differences in the urinary excretion of 6-beta-hydroxycortisol/cortisol between Asian and Caucasian women. *J Clin Pharmacol* 1999;**39**(6):578–82.

32. Bedford JL, Prior JC, Barr SI. A prospective exploration of cognitive dietary restraint, subclinical ovulatory disturbances, cortisol and change in bone density over two years in healthy young women. *J Clin Endocrinol Metab* 2010;**95**(7):3291–9.

33. Prior JC, Konishi C, Hitchcock CL, Kingwell E, Janssen P, Cheung AP, et al. Does molimina indicate ovulation? Prospective data in a hormonally documented single-cycle in spontaneously menstruating women. *Int J Environ Res Public Health* 2018;**15**(5).

34. O'Connor KA, Brindle E, Miller RC, Shofer JB, Ferrell RJ, Klein NA, et al. Ovulation detection methods for urinary hormones: precision, daily and intermittent sampling and a combined hierarchical method. *Hum Reprod* 2006;**21**(6):1442–52.

35. Baird DD, McDonnaughey R, Weinberg CR, Musey PI, Collins DC, Kesner JS, et al. Application of a method for estimating day of ovulation using urinary estrogen and progesterone metabolites. *Epidemiology* 1995;**6**:547–50.

36. Bolaji II, Tallon DF, Meehan FP, O'Dwyer EM, Fottrell PF. The return of postpartum fertility monitored by enzyme-immunoassay for salivary progesterone. *Gynecol Endocrinol* 1992;**6**(1):37–48.

37. Nepomnaschy PA, Sheiner E, Mastorakos G, Arck PC. Stress, immune function, and women's reproduction. *Ann N Y Acad Sci* 2007;**1113**:350–64.

38. Prior JC. Physical exercise and the neuroendocrine control of reproduction. *Baillieres Clin Endocrinol Metab* 1987;**1**:299–317.

39. Ellison PT, Valeggia CR. C-peptide levels and the duration of lactational amenorrhea. *Fertil Steril* 2003;**80**(5):1279–80.

40. Berga SL, Loucks TL. Use of cognitive behavior therapy for functional hypothalamic amenorrhea. *Ann N Y Acad Sci* 2006;**1092**:114–29.

41. Mountjoy M, Sundgot-Borgen J, Burke L, Carter S, Constantini N, Lebrun C, et al. The IOC consensus statement: beyond the Female Athlete Triad—Relative Energy Deficiency in Sport (RED-S). *Br J Sports Med* 2014;**48**(7):491–7.

42. Prior JC. Progesterone for the prevention and treatment of osteoporosis in women. *Climacteric* 2018;**21**:366–74.

Part B

Maternal Endocrine Disorders During Pregnancy and Lactation

Chapter 16

Hypothalamic Disorders During Ovulation, Pregnancy, and Lactation

Georgios E. Papadakis, Cheng Xu and Nelly Pitteloud

Service of Endocrinology, Diabetes and Metabolism, CHUV, Lausanne University Hospital, Lausanne, Switzerland

Common Clinical Problems

- Functional hypothalamic amenorrhea is a common cause of anovulatory infertility, which can be reversed with moderation of precipitating factors. Cognitive behavioral therapy should be offered to affected women.
- GnRH pulsatile therapy is the first-line treatment for fertility induction in women with functional hypothalamic amenorrhea and congenital hypogonadotropic hypogonadism, due to its efficacy and safety.
- Craniopharyngioma, as well as its subsequent surgical treatment, can lead to morbid hypothalamic obesity, for which adequate treatments are not yet well established.
- In contrast to pituitary adenomas, and particularly prolactinomas, enlargement of craniopharyngioma during pregnancy is rare, but not impossible.
- Women with hypothalamic disorders, particularly infiltrative diseases, should be monitored during pregnancy for inaugural or worsening of preexisting diabetes insipidus.
- Lactation may be impaired in women with extensive hypothalamic and pituitary damage, as well as in patients with history of cranial irradiation.

16.1 FUNCTIONAL HYPOTHALAMIC AMENORRHEA

Functional hypothalamic amenorrhea (FHA) is an acquired form of gonadotropin-releasing hormone (GnRH) deficiency, leading to hypogonadotropic hypogonadism (HH) for which no organic causes are identified.[1,2] It is typically induced by external stressors, such as caloric deficits, psychological distress, and/or excessive physical activity. The term *functional* refers to the potential of reversibility after correction or moderation of the triggering factor. In adult women, FHA, along with polycystic ovarian syndrome (PCOS), are the most common causes of anovulation, accounting each for roughly one-third of cases of secondary amenorrhea.[3] In addition, its frequency is increasing in adolescents.[4]

16.1.1 Physiopathology and Precipitating Factors

The mainstay of pathophysiology in FHA is suppressed activity of hypothalamic GnRH neurons, leading to decreased GnRH secretion and GnRH-induced luteinizing hormone (LH) pulsatility.[4] In particular, the frequency of LH pulses is markedly reduced, while their amplitude seems conserved. Insufficient levels of LH and follicle-stimulating hormone (FSH) are unable to sufficiently stimulate estradiol production and follicle growth in the ovaries.

Homeostasis of GnRH neurons is modulated by multiple stimulatory and inhibitory signals, either directly or via mediation by the kisspeptin/neurokinin B/dynorphin neurons. In FHA, the deficit of GnRH drive is the result of several neuroendocrine alterations, secondary to the external stressors. Among them, overactivity of the hypothalamic-pituitary-adrenal (HPA) axis is a constant finding in all forms of FHA[5–8] and leads to increased secretion of corticotropin-releasing hormone (CRH), high cortisol levels (but without disruption of its diurnal rhythm), and elevated endogenous opioids. CRH has been shown to decrease GnRH release and LH levels in both in vitro and animal models.[9,10] HPA axis overactivity has been documented in nutritional deprivation,[11] intense physical activity (typically in female athletes), and psychosocial stressors,[12] and it is responsible for reductions in GnRH drive.

Maternal-Fetal and Neonatal Endocrinology. https://doi.org/10.1016/B978-0-12-814823-5.00016-7

Low leptin is a primary feature, particularly in weight-loss and exercise-induced FHA forms,[13] and administration of recombinant leptin has been shown to restore ovulation.[14] There is increasing evidence that other metabolic cues, such as ghrelin and neuropeptide Y (NPY), are elevated in states of energy deficit and negatively influence GnRH secretion, thus contributing to AHF.[15]

In addition to the well-established link with the aforementioned environmental triggers, women who develop FHA may have a genetic predisposition.[16] Sequencing of genes causing congenital GnRH deficiency in an FHA cohort of 55 women revealed loss-of-function heterozygous mutations of four genes (*FGFR1*, *PROKR2*, *GNRHR*, and *KAL1*). These mutations were detected in seven FHA patients, while no variant was detected in a cohort of 422 controls with normal menstrual cycles, including a subset of women that were exercising for a significant amount of time (>5 h per week). Interestingly, four of the FHA patients harboring mutations of the congenital hypogonadotropic hypogonadism (CHH) genes had delayed puberty (age at onset of menarche ≥15 years).

16.1.2 Clinical Manifestations

Menstrual dysfunction is the classical manifestation in women with FHA and reflects the underlying suppression of the hypothalamic-pituitary-gondal (HPG) axis. Typically, women present with secondary amenorrhea or oligomenorrhea. Depending on the age of diagnosis, FHA may also present with primary amenorrhea and delayed puberty in adolescents with eating disorders or excessive exercise.[17] Recently published guidelines by the Endocrine Society suggest diagnostic assessment for FHA in adolescents and women with oligomenorrhea, defined as between-menses intervals repeatedly exceeding 45 days or absence of menses for more than 3 months.[2] The cutoff of 45 days can distinguish FHA from physiologic postmenarchal menstrual variation due to delayed maturation of the HPG axis in adolescents.[18,19] It is important to stress that a subset of women with FHA have milder menstrual dysfunction and can present with infertility due to anovulatory eumenorrhea or isolated luteal phase defects (of insufficient or otherwise shortened duration).[20] Although they are expected to be frequent due to marked hypoestrogenism, vasomotor symptoms such as hot flashes seem to be rare in FHA, according to a study in oligoamenorrheic athletes.[21] Accompanying neuroendocrine changes in FHA women, such as increased activity of the hypothalamic beta-endorphins, may be protective against such symptoms. On the other hand, sexual dysfunction often ensues in FHA patients[22] and is considered of mixed origin due to hormonal deficits (i.e., hypoestrogenemia and hypoandrogenemia) and increased incidence of anxiety disorders and depression.

Symptoms related to the underlying precipitating factor may also be observed. When FHA is caused by energy deficits, a large spectrum of associated manifestations may be seen, varying from a mild or moderately restrictive diet to severe eating disorders, including tendencies to binge and/or purge.[23] Similarly, in the stress-induced form of FHA, anxiety or mood disorders can be a primary complaint and also can be accompanied by cognitive dysfunction and certain problematic personality traits.[24]

Fractures can occur in cases of long-standing FHA, which compromises bone density and strength. The most common finding is stress fractures, mostly seen in female athletes.[25,26] Low-energy fractures at classical osteoporotic sites, as well as spine deformities such as kyphosis and scoliosis due to multiple vertebral fractures, have also been reported.

Finally, some data indicate that women with FHA have increased cardiovascular risk due to endothelial dysfunction, secondary to both hypoestrogenism and other neuroendocrine alterations.[17] Further research, with prospective studies and sufficiently long follow-up, is needed to elucidate the link between FHA and cardiovascular health.

16.1.3 Diagnostic Evaluation and Differential Diagnosis

The diagnosis of FHA is based on the demonstration of HH in the setting of a precipitating factor with temporal association to the onset of an oligoamenorrheic state. The presence of previously intact menstrual cycles further strengthens the probability of FHA. It has been traditionally considered as an exclusion diagnosis, though recent guidelines recommend less extensive diagnostic workup in cases with a clear precipitating factor, such as weight loss, excessive exercise, or increased stress.[2]

The differential diagnosis of FHA is large and depends on the age and type of menstrual dysfunction (primary versus secondary amenorrhea). In adult women with secondary amenorrhea, after formally ruling out a pregnancy, it is reasonable and relatively simple to exclude common causes such as hyperprolactinemia, thyroid dysfunction, and primary ovarian insufficiency. In women who are malnourished or who report associated gastrointestinal symptoms, organic disorders such as celiac disease, inflammatory bowel disease (Crohn's disease, ulcerative colitis), and other chronic inflammatory and infectious states should be ruled out before rendering a diagnosis of FHA. PCOS is an equally frequent cause of secondary amenorrhea, and interestingly, its coexistence with FHA is underestimated.[27,28] The hyperandrogenic symptoms of PCOS are typically absent in patients with concomitant FHA but can be unmasked after weight gain or pulsatile GnRH therapy.[29] A precise diagnosis is crucial and may have both therapeutic (increased risk of ovarian hyperstimulation syndrome (OHSS) when treated with exogenous gonadotropins)[30] and prognostic implications (less resumption of regular menses despite recovery from FHA).[31] Additional workup to exclude other causes of secondary amenorrhea should be limited to cases with clinical suspicion, absence of clear triggering factors, and/or absence of menses recovery despite adequate moderation of the precipitating factor.

16.1.3.1 Medical History and Physical Exam

Obtaining a targeted medical history focused on highlighting the precipitating factors leading to FHA is crucial and should include weight changes (both recent and across the life span), history of binging and purging, quantitative and qualitative assessment of exercise, and presence of stressors. Mood disorders, as well as high-risk attitudes such as perfectionism and a competitive and ambitious professional lifestyle, should be identified. It is important that clinicians assess whether women with FHA have completed puberty by inquiring the age of first menses and assessing breast development. Of importance, FHA in adolescents can manifest with delayed and incomplete puberty, thus mimicking congenital GnRH deficiency. The presence of anosmia or hyposmia points toward a congenital cause of amenorrhea such as Kallmann syndrome (KS).[32] A full family history for reproductive issues such as delayed puberty, primary or secondary amenorrhea, and infertility can also be informative.

In search of other potential diagnoses, clinicians should question patients about the presence of galactorrhea, which could indicate concomitant hyperprolactinemia. Severe and unusual headaches, unexplained nausea and vomiting, and changes in vision can be manifestations of an intracranial tumor, causing hypopituitarism. Evocative symptoms of thyroid dysfunction should be queried, along with complaints consistent with androgen excess such as acne, hirsutism, and male-type alopecia. Other potentially relevant information includes a history of head trauma or cranial irradiation, cyclic abdominal pain in women with primary amenorrhea, history of low-grade fever, nocturnal sweating, and unexplained weight loss, which could imply an infiltrative disorder such as tuberculosis or sarcoidosis. Finally, a detailed history of all medications is needed, with a special focus on opioids (particularly methadone), which directly inhibit GnRH secretion,[33] and antipsychotics (particularly risperidone), which inhibit the HPG axis via dopamine antagonism and subsequent hyperprolactinemia.[34]

A physical exam should be targeted to exclude alternative diagnoses[3] by searching for galactorrhea and signs of other pituitary hypersecretion, such as acromegaly and Cushing's disease. Clinically, thyroid hyperfunction or hypofunction may be apparent by changes in Achilles tendon reflexes and other signs. Signs of androgen excess and insulin resistance (acanthosis nigricans) are common in women with PCOS and congenital adrenal hyperplasia (CAH). External gynecologic examination can reveal clitoromegaly, which is characteristic of virilizing adrenal or ovarian tumors. A detailed gynecologic checkup is more crucial in women with suspected FHA and primary amenorrhea to evaluate for imperforate hymen or other anatomic defects.

16.1.3.2 Laboratory Assessment

Following exclusion of pregnancy by measuring β-human chorionic gonadotropin (β-hCG), a comprehensive workup of an adult or adolescent woman with suspected FHA should include a blood count and a complete chemistry panel, including fasting glucose, lipid profile, and liver function tests. Sedimentation rate and C-reactive protein (CRP) levels should be measured only in patients with symptoms and signs implying a systemic illness, as described previously. Initial hormonal assessment includes measurement of serum thyroid-stimulating hormone (TSH) and free T4, prolactin, estradiol (E2), and gonadotropins (LH, FSH).

The classic biochemical constellation of FHA consists of low (or even undetectable) E2 associated with low-normal or low LH and FSH. Very low or undetectable values of LH and FSH point toward an organic or congenital cause of amenorrhea. It has been traditionally suggested that low-frequency GnRH pulses in women with FHA favor FSH over LH secretion, as suggested by a LH/FSH ratio <1. However, this is not a consistent finding, and LH/FSH ratios >1 can be seen, especially in women with concomitant PCOS-like features. Total testosterone and androgen profiling, including dehydroepiandrosterone sulfate (DHEAS) and androstenedione, should be performed in all women with hyperandrogenic symptoms. If clinical or biochemical hyperandrogenism is present, clinicians should measure morning 17-hydroxyprogesterone to screen for late-onset CAH, which can be clinically indistinguishable from PCOS. Antimüllerian hormone (AMH) levels are an indirect index of the primary follicle number and will be elevated or high-normal when FHA coexists with PCOS.[35] The added value of GnRH stimulation testing is still a matter of debate. The majority of women with FHA will exhibit a normal gonadotropin response (defined as a twofold-to-threefold increase in LH and FSH), consistent with partial GnRH deficiency. Blunted responses may be seen in severe and long-standing cases, such as anorexia nervosa; however, flat responses are rare, in contrast with pituitary causes or severe congenital GnRH deficiency without prior priming.

In our clinical practice, we frequently perform a biochemical screening for hypopituitarism, which, in the case of pathologic findings, will justify adding brain magnetic resonance imaging (MRI). However, testing for pituitary hypersecretion syndromes other than prolactinoma (acromegaly, Cushing) should be limited to patients with clinical symptoms and signs of growth-hormone or cortisol excess. Serum leptin levels, if commercially available, can be informative of fat tissue deficiency, particularly in athletic women with normal body mass index (BMI) but expansion of the muscular compartment. Correlation with body composition has been shown in FHA women with eating disorders,[36] as well as in those with excessive exercise, although no clear cutoff can differentiate between eumenorrheic and amenorrheic athletes.[37]

16.1.3.3 Imaging Studies

There is a consensus that a brain MRI is not routinely necessary in patients with suspected FHA.[2] The latter should be performed where there are red flag symptoms indicating a brain mass (i.e., severe headaches, problems with vision, symptoms of increased intracranial pressure), if there is history of brain trauma preceding the development of symptoms, or when no precipitating factor can be elicited despite a detailed clinical history and physical examination. An MRI should also be performed when there is clinical and/or biochemical evidence of hyperprolactinemia, acromegaly, and/or hypercortisolism, or changes in thirst and urination suggestive of diabetes insipidus. Signs of hypopituitarism in the hormonal workup can prompt a pituitary MRI, although clinicians should remember that FHA could be accompanied by functional disturbances of the hypothalamic-pituitary-thyroid (HPT) axis, which mimic central hypothyroidism.[38] Finally, brain imaging could be considered in cases with persistent HH despite adequate treatment or moderation of the external trigger, although the actual likelihood of a significant finding on MRI in this context has never been studied.

A bone mineral density (BMD) scan by dual X-ray absorptiometry (DXA) is indicated for women with 6 or more months of amenorrhea or a long-standing history of irregular menses, especially in the presence of an eating disorder, low BMI, or both. It is important to stress that bone impairment in these patients is not solely the reflection of increased bone resorption due to hypoestrogenism, but includes also a reduction of bone formation in both weight-loss and exercise-induced FHA.[39,40] This is probably due to the associated relative hypercortisolism and other endocrine alterations that contribute to the chronic hypercatabolic state. More important, a higher risk of fracture has been shown in FHA women with both eating disorders[41] and excessive exercise,[25,42] thus justifying early screening by DXA.

As expected, there is a preferential loss of BMD at the lumbar spine (a trabecular-rich site), as in other forms of hypogonadal osteoporosis. Although the available evidence points toward a deterioration of bone quality (microarchitecture) in addition to bone quantity (BMD),[43,44] the use of tools assessing bone structure, such as high-resolution peripheral quantitative computed tomography (CT), is not widespread in clinical practice. Specific data on bone morbidity of women with stress-induced FHA are lacking, but screening these women with DXA seems reasonable given the known deleterious effects of hypoestrogenism. Clinicians should be aware that the same DXA scan can provide data about body composition, including lean and adipose tissue mass. This can be informative, especially in exercise-induced FHA.

16.1.4 Management

Treatment of patients with FHA requires a multidisciplinary approach. The main objectives are (1) to reverse the causal precipitating factors by promoting weight gain, exercise reduction, and/or alleviation of psychosocial stress; (2) to prevent and treat complications of hypoestrogenism, such as delayed puberty and suboptimal bone mass accrual in adolescents, and osteoporosis in adults; and (3) to restore fertility either by spontaneous recovery of ovulation after removal of precipitating factors, or by medically inducing ovulation. These approaches do not cover severe anorexia nervosa, which is at the extreme end of FHA and which may require inpatient treatment according to well-established recommendations.[45]

Clinicians should take into account that although FHA has different etiologies and management must be individualized, a combination of etiologic factors may be present and contributing to different degrees, thus rendering a holistic approach more effective. For instance, in weight-loss and exercise-induced FHA, there are very often underlying behavioral troubles even in the absence of overt psychological distress, and these patients can benefit from psychological support.

The pathophysiology of the disease should be discussed with the affected women. Correction of the energy imbalance by increasing caloric intake, decreasing exercise intensity, or both should be recommended. Women should be warned that these changes will lead to some weight gain. Referring the patient to a dietitian will allow individualized counseling to increase caloric intake, which might be better accepted in the long run than standardized diet regimens. Increased energy availability through diet, exercise moderation, or both has been shown to improve menstrual dysfunction and restore ovulation in women with anorexia nervosa,[46] as well as in dancers and athletes with FHA.[47,48] It is important to inform patients that amenorrhea may persist several months after the reversal of the precipitating factor and that at least 6–12 months of weight stabilization are needed in some cases.

Ongoing psychological support by an experienced psychiatrist or psychologist is crucial to treating underlying stress and promoting behavioral change to accept the modification of other factors such as caloric intake and physical activity.[2] Of note, in some cases menses may never resume despite adequate weight gain, exercise reduction, and weight stabilization, thereby highlighting the potential role of stress, which may be both clinically evident and subclinical. Among the various psychological approaches, efficacy data favor the use of cognitive behavioral therapy (CBT) on the basis of a small randomized controlled trial (RCT) of 16 women with FHA who received CBT versus standard observation for 20 weeks.[49] The investigators excluded women with depression, eating disorders, or any psychiatric disorders other than personality disorders, as well as underweight women and those engaging in excessive exercise (>10 h/week). FHA in these women was attributed to problematic psychological attitudes such as higher levels of perfectionism, higher need for social approval, and altered attitudes toward eating. A total of six of eight women in the CBT-treated group recovered ovulation, in comparison with only one out of eight in the observation group. Consistent with these findings, the same group demonstrated in a secondary analysis 10 years later that CBT was accompanied by decreased cortisol and increased leptin levels,[50] thus indicating that CBT has a favorable impact on the neuroendocrine alterations of FHA, and not only on the HPG axis.

In adolescents and women who did not experience resumption of ovulatory cycles after 6–12 months of multidisciplinary management, including weight normalization, exercise reduction if relevant, counseling with a dietician, and CBT, then estrogen replacement should be considered. Potential advantages of this treatment are the induction of menses, which can reduce associated stress in some women, as well as benefiting bone health. Oral contraceptive pills (OCPs) are not a suitable choice for this population, as these have not been shown to increase BMD,[51,52] and they have an inhibitory effect on endogenous ovarian function, even in women with previously regular menses.[53] On the contrary, ovarian hormone therapy with use of transdermal E2 has shown more potent effects on both mature and prepubertal bone.[54] The latter has been attributed to the fact that transdermal E2, in contrast to oral estrogens, do not go through a first hepatic pass, and thus they do not downregulate IGF-1 secretion by the liver.[55] Despite these data, there is no study demonstrating the antifracture efficacy of transdermal hormone replacement therapy (HRT). In addition, bone health may not be sufficiently protected if the underlying energy deficit continues. Therefore, clinicians should ensure that patients are not falsely reassured by the restoration of withdrawal bleeding with ovarian hormone therapy and hence neglect the causal factors that led to FHA.

Another medical option to increase BMD is bisphosphonate treatment; however, its use in premenopausal women is not recommended due to concerns for teratogenic effects in future pregnancies. Some encouraging data exist for recombinant parathyroid hormone (PTH), teriparatide, an osteoanabolic agent that significantly increased spine BMD in an RCT in women with anorexia nervosa,[56] and which also has been shown to improve fracture healing in selected cases of FHA patients.[57]

A treatment that showed promising results in the past but has not found a role in current clinical practice is the use of human recombinant leptin or synthetic analogs such as metreleptin. In a small study of 8 women with FHA and prior weight stabilization, recombinant leptin dosed for 2–3 months increased LH pulsatility and E2 levels, and improved multiple aspects of ovarian function, including inducing recovery of ovulatory cycles in 3 women.[14] Although this study confirmed the importance of leptin for the adequate function of the HPG axis, it did not lead to widespread use because of significant loss of weight and body fat in the treatment group, caused by a subjective decrease in appetite. The latter was considered an undesirable complication for these patients. Similar results were also seen in subsequent studies with metreleptin.[58]

Ovulation induction treatment for FHA patients will be discussed later in this chapter, in Section 16.1.4.

16.1.5 FHA: Pregnancy and Lactation

Most research literature regarding FHA and pregnancy focuses on increased risks in women with eating disorders. It is crucial that reproductive endocrinologists and gynecologists ensure that BMI is greater than $18.5–19$ kg/m^2 before initiating treatment to induce ovulation. Adequate control of the eating disorder, as well as close psychological follow-up, are also highly recommended. These measures will increase the chance of successful ovulation induction and reduce risks during the subsequent pregnancy. Low BMI before conception (<20 kg/m^2) is indeed associated with a fourfold-higher probability of preterm labor.[59] Women with eating disorders, and in particular anorexia nervosa, are at risk for miscarriage, fetal loss, small-for-gestational-age babies, and delivery by cesarean section for extremely low weight.[60–62] In a prospective follow-up of a cohort of 246 women with eating disorders (anorexia nervosa or bulimia nervosa), 49 live births were reported, with the majority of women having healthy babies but having an increased incidence of postpartum depression (34.7%).[63] Little is known about the risk of adverse events during pregnancy in other subgroups, such as exercise-related or stress-induced FHA. Finally, there are no systematic published reports on outcomes of FHA women during lactation. As prolactin levels are not affected in FHA, it is theoretically possible that women with well-controlled FHA can breastfeed properly, but specific data are needed.

16.2 CONGENITAL HYPOGONADOTROPIC HYPOGONADISM

CHH, also termed *idiopathic hypogonadotropic hypogonadism* or *isolated GnRH deficiency,* is a rare genetic disorder with HH of hypothalamic origin. It is characterized by defective GnRH secretion or action, leading to absent or incomplete puberty, anovulation, and infertility.[32] CHH can be accompanied by other anomalies, the more frequent being anosmia in approximately 50% of patients. It has been traditionally thought to exhibit a male predominance (male/female ratio of 4:1 or 5:1),[64,65] with a prevalence between 1 in 10,000 to 1 in 48,000 according to different studies.[66,67] Nevertheless, recent work suggests that the sex ratio is closer to 2:1.[68,69] One possible explanation of this difference is underdiagnosis of female patients due to treatment with OCPs without prior adequate investigation. Alternatively, some cases of partial CHH may be falsely considered as FHA or PCOS, due to mild clinical presentations.[70] In this chapter, we will only discuss the different aspects of CHH in females, focusing on its impact on ovulation, pregnancy, and lactation.

16.2.1 Genetics

Since its first description by Dr. Franz Kallmann in 1944,[71] our understanding of the genetics underlying CHH has largely evolved. It is now evident that CHH is a complex and heterogeneous genetic disease, with evidence implicating more than 30 genes identified to date[72,73] that account, however, for roughly 50% of cases. These genes can be classified into groups depending on their impact on GnRH neurons, such as genes causing (1) defects in GnRH neuron fate specification or migration, (2) abnormal neuroendocrine secretion and homeostasis, and (3) gonadotrope defects (i.e., *GNRHR* encoding the receptor of GnRH).[32,72,74] In addition to the absence of identifiable genetic causes in approximately half of cases, genetic counseling is complicated in CHH patients due to (1) potential modes of inheritance (X-linked, autosomal dominant, and autosomal recessive); (2) the frequent presence of incomplete penetrance and variable expressivity, even among members of the same family; and (3) potential oligogenicity, first documented in 2007, with proven loss-of-function mutations in two CHH genes acting in synergy.[75] With the exception of the prototype gene of CHH, *KAL1* (or *ANOS1*), whose transmission mode is X-linked (females harboring heterozygous mutations are asymptomatic carriers), almost all other genes can be found in female CHH probands.

16.2.2 Clinical Manifestations and Associated Phenotypes

16.2.2.1 Hallmarks of CHH in Infancy

CHH being a congenital disease, it is present since birth, and symptoms vary across the life span. Interestingly, the HPG axis is physiologically active (pulsatile GnRH secretion) during late fetal life and for approximately 6 months postnatally before switching to relative quiescence during childhood due to mechanisms yet to be discovered.[76,77] This period of transient activation of HPG axis is called *mini-puberty*. In girls, elevated GnRH-induced gonadotropin levels result in an increase in E2 levels after 1 week of age, with associated increased folliculogenesis.[77,78] The high circulating E2 levels in girls may lead to palpable breast tissue during mini-puberty.[79] In contrast with boys, in which defective mini-puberty due to CHH may manifest with cryptorchidism and/or micropenis, there are no clinical signs of GnRH deficiency in female infants. This limits the diagnosis of CHH at this phase to female infants of an affected parent, revealed as part of neonatal screening.

16.2.2.2 Hallmarks of CHH in Childhood and Adolescence

Childhood is a physiologically hypogonadal period, rendering biochemical confirmation of CHH impossible during this phase. The diagnosis can be suspected in some girls who report lack of smell, although the latter often passes unnoticed. In adolescence, primary amenorrhea is the main complaint in nearly 90% of CHH women.[68,69,80] In the remaining women, CHH can manifest as (1) very few, isolated episodes of vaginal bleeding during adolescence before chronic "secondary" amenorrhea sets in (primary-secondary amenorrhea)[68,80,81]; or (2) less frequently, as chronic oligomenorrhea or anovulatory oligomenorrhea.[82,83] The majority of studies have shown that absent breast development at diagnosis is observed only in a minority of CHH women.[68,80,84] Pubarche also shows great variability, ranging from absent to almost normal pubic hair.[68,80] The reports of absent public hair in CHH women are surprising, given that adrenarche, which is the onset of production of adrenal androgens (i.e., DHEA, androstenedione), is conserved in these patients and thus should allow some degree of pubarche.[85] The few available pieces of data on growth of CHH women indicate that their final height is similar to that of the reference population.[86,87]

16.2.2.3 Hallmarks of CHH in Adulthood

Although the diagnosis of CHH is typically made during adolescence in males, it can be more easily missed in females, especially if a gynecologist or pediatrician does not perform a detailed etiologic workup and they receive estrogen pills for contraception, which will complete breast development and induce regular vaginal bleeding. These types of patients will likely be investigated later in adulthood, when infertility, absence of menses, or both become evident after withdrawal of OCP. Other less common complaints may include bone loss and osteoporotic fractures, especially if the affected patient did not receive regular ovarian hormone treatment. There are no published reports of female CHH patients being first diagnosed after the age of menopause. Specific data on the natural history of CHH in older women are lacking.

An underestimated clinical symptom of female CHH patients is increased psychological distress, associated with the diagnosis of this congenital disorder. A recent online survey suggested that CHH women have a negative perception of their health status, with increased prevalence of depression.[88] The same study showed that patients often feel that their care providers have a tendency to undervalue the psychological consequences of their defective pubertal development.

16.2.2.4 CHH Reversal

It has been well established that a subset of CHH patients can exhibit a spontaneous recovery of the function of the HPG axis. This revolutionary discovery, indicative of the plasticity of the HPG axis, was initially demonstrated in CHH males (about 10%–20% in males)[89] and was subsequently described in several female CHH patients.[90] Patients with reversal exhibit different degrees of GnRH deficiency (from mild to severe), and many harbor mutations in known CHH genes. To date, there are no clear clinical factors for predicting reversible CHH. Prior treatment with sex steroids was the only common denominator in the various studies. External sex steroids may have epigenetic effects, triggering the maturation of the GnRH neuronal network in a subgroup of patients, as the expression of critical genes for GnRH ontogeny is sex-steroid responsive.[91] Importantly, endocrinologists should take into account that some patients will eventually relapse into a state of GnRH deficiency[90,92]; therefore, long-term monitoring of reproductive function is needed.

16.2.2.5 CHH-Associated Phenotypes

As discussed previously, anosmia (i.e., lack of sense of smell) is the most frequent nonreproductive phenotype in CHH patients, observed in approximately 50% of cases.[64] The cooccurrence of these phenotypes (CHH and anosmia) is termed *Kallmann syndrome (KS)*. Other phenotypes, associated with CHH at a lower prevalence, include mirror movements (synkinesia), unilateral renal agenesis, eye movement disorders, sensori-neural hearing loss, midline brain defects (including absent corpus callosum), cleft lip/palate, dental agenesis, skeletal defects, and cardiovascular defects.[32] Three large, but retrospective studies have evaluated the prevalence of these associated phenotypes in CHH, although no systematic screening for these phenotypes was performed.[64,65,93]

16.2.3 Diagnostic Evaluation and Differential Diagnosis

16.2.3.1 Clinical Assessment

As discussed previously, mini-puberty, the transient activation of the HPG axis during infancy, provides a window of opportunity to diagnose CHH by performing hormonal testing at 4–12 weeks of life.[82,94–100] However, this screening is rarely performed in female infants due to lack of typical clinical signs suggesting a CHH diagnosis.[32,87,98] The diagnosis of CHH is very challenging during childhood, which is a physiologically hypogonadal period. The diagnosis is typically made in adolescence due to primary amenorrhea or absent pubertal development associated with a biochemical constellation of low or undetectable E2 levels and low/normal serum levels of gonadotropins. Exclusion of other organic causes of HH is necessary before rendering a CHH diagnosis in a female patient (as discussed later in this chapter).

The diagnostic workup of a patient with presumed CHH should include targeting evaluation for CHH-associated phenotypes, which, if present, will strengthen the probability of a CHH diagnosis and have an impact on genetic counseling. In particular, a standardized olfactory test should be performed to search for anosmia or decreased sense of smell.[65] Formal smell testing is critical, as 50% of CHH patients with a self-reported normal sense of smell are in fact found to be hyposmic or anosmic by standardized testing.[101] Also, an audiogram should be systematically performed to search for sensori-neural hearing impairment, which in some cases can be only mild or unilateral, and thus clinically unnoticed. A physical exam should be performed by an experienced endocrinologist and should focus on the presence of signs such as bimanual syn-kinesia (mirror movements), dental agenesis, history of midline defects (particularly cleft lip and/or palate), skeletal anom-alies (such as scoliosis, polydactyly, and clinodactyly) and pigmentation defects. Unilateral renal agenesis or malformation of the urinary tract should be assessed by renal ultrasound, especially in women with KS. Syndromic forms of CHH can encompass other malformations (e.g., coloboma in CHARGE syndrome), as previously reviewed.[32]

16.2.3.2 Biochemical and Hormonal Testing

Most CHH women have very low circulating gonadotropin levels,[84,102,103] and exhibit apulsatile patterns of LH secretion.[102] Circulating estradiol levels are usually low or in the lower end of the normal range during the follicular phase. It is crucial to implement sensitive assays with a low detection threshold.[84,104] The use of insensitive estradiol assays may result in confusion with other causes of anovulation.[104] Low circulating androgen levels (androstenedione and testosterone) are reported in women with CHH, despite normal circulating DHEAS concentrations.[84] Pituitary response to the GnRH stimulation has been evaluated in only a few case reports of CHH women, who exhibited blunted peak LH responses in comparison with normal women.[83,87] Inhibin B and AMH are two other biomarkers that can be informative in this setting. Inhibin B is secreted by the granulosa cells and correlates with the number of antral follicles.[105] Low Inhibin B concentrations, in the range of prepubertal girls, have been reported in CHH women.[106-108] Mean serum AMH concen-trations are also significantly lower in women with CHH than in healthy women,[84] although two-thirds of patients exhibit serum AMH levels within the normal range. Both pulsatile GnRH and gonadotropin administration can lead to fertility and will be accompanied by an increase in serum AMH levels, even in CHH women with very low baseline values. Thus, in contrast with other causes of infertility, low AMH should not be considered a poor fertility prognostic factor in CHH women. Finally, the biochemical workup of CHH women should rule out hyperprolactinemia, which is a common cause of HH, as well as other pituitary defects, indicative of combined pituitary hormone deficiency.[109,110] Thus, we recommend a baseline measurement of prolactin, free T4, TSH, morning cortisol, and IGF1 in all women with suspected CHH, as well as analysis of growth curve in adolescents. In cases of suspected pituitary insufficiency, dynamic challenge tests may be necessary.[109]

16.2.3.3 Radiological Examination

Pelvic ultrasound is not mandatory at diagnosis of CHH, but it should be performed before initiating a fertility treatment or as indicated by the classic gynecological follow-up. Studies in CHH women demonstrated a significant reduction in mean ovarian volume (OV) compared to healthy adult women of a similar age.[68,80,84,111] Notably, the decrease in OV is greater in KS than in normosmic CHH, suggesting a more severe GnRH deficiency.[80] The only study that has quantified the number of ovarian antral follicles (AFs) showed a significant decrease in the average number of AFs compared to normal, age-matched women, consistent with the low level of AMH.[84] However, both OV and AFs respond favorably to gonadotropin stimulation in female CHH.

Brain MRI should be performed at baseline to exclude hypothalamic-pituitary lesions and to assess for defects in the olfactory bulbs, corpus callosum, semilunar canals, cerebellum, and midline.[112] KS patients typically exhibit unilateral or bilateral olfactory bulb agenesis, olfactory tract agenesis, and/or gyrus malformation.[113] However, a few KS patients have normal olfactory structures despite clinically confirmed anosmia.

CHH women should have BMD measured via DXA.[32] Bone quality can be evaluated by processing a trabecular bone score (TBS) or by performing high-resolution peripheral quantitative computed tomography (HR-pQCT), although neither technique has been validated in this population. Bone workup should be done at baseline and repeated at least 2 years after ovarian hormone treatment to assess the beneficial effect of sex steroids on bone mass and to guide subsequent monitoring. It is potentially interesting that during the same DXA scan, body composition parameters can be obtained to assess total and regional adiposity.

16.2.3.4 Differential Diagnosis

CHH is a diagnosis of exclusion, and extensive workup is needed to rule out structural causes; FHA; organic causes of malnutrition, such as celiac disease; and opioid-induced HH. Every expansive process affecting the hypothalamic-pituitary axis may lead to acquired HH. Classic examples are tumors (i.e., pituitary adenomas, CPs), irradiation, surgery, apoplexy, or infiltrative diseases such as sarcoidosis and histiocytosis. Less commonly, head trauma or subarachnoid hemorrhage can also lead to HH.[114-116] Nevertheless, most patients with these structural causes will have multiple pituitary hormone deficiencies.[115] In order to rule out a structural cause, we typically perform a brain MRI in all women with suspected CHH. The latter is particularly mandatory in cases of other pituitary insufficiencies (including diabetes insipidus), hyperprolactinemia, or symptoms of mass effect (headache, visual impairment, or visual field defect). It is worth mentioning that hereditary hemochromatosis, a potential cause of isolated HH in men, is rarely accompanied by such reproductive phenotype (amenorrhea) in women.[117]

FHA is a reversible form of GnRH deficiency that is often induced by stressors such as caloric deficits, psychological distress, and/or excessive exercise (see Section 16.1.1). In adolescents, the frequency of FHH is rising (3%–5% of young women),[17] and can manifest as primary amenorrhea,[4] complicating its distinction from CHH. In addition, a shared genetic basis of CHH and FHA in women has been described,[16] thus sheds doubt on the ability of genetic testing to differentiate between both entities. Clinicians should actively search for the aforementioned characteristic triggers and monitor the recovery of reproductive function after adequate moderation of the stressors. Another important element is the eventual presence of CHH-associated phenotypes such as congenital anosmia, which would strongly point toward the diagnosis of KS.

Organic causes of malnutrition such as celiac disease, inflammatory bowel disease (e.g., Crohn's disease, and ulcerative colitis), and other chronic inflammatory and infectious states can mimic CHH and FHA. Consequently, adequate testing to rule out the aforementioned conditions should be undertaken in case of suspicious symptoms such as low fever, unexplained weight loss and/or gastrointestinal complaints.

Opioid use is another major cause of reversible HH in both males and females.[33,118] In the central nervous system (CNS), endogenous opioids inhibit pulsatile GnRH release,[119] resulting in low LH levels, which in turn reduce sex steroid production.[33,120–122] Opioid misuse and addiction is a rapidly increasing public health problem, and it will probably become a growing diagnostic issue, particularly among adolescents and young adults.[123]

16.2.4 Management

With appropriate ovarian hormone treatment, CHH women can develop secondary sexual characteristics, maintain normal estrogen levels, and have a satisfactory sex life. There are several regimens that can be orally or transdermally administered. The choice of treatment depends on the therapeutic goal, the timing, and the personal preference of each patient. It is important to know that RCTs of hormonal treatment in CHH are lacking and data from observational studies are scarce.

16.2.4.1 Neonatal CHH in Females

Following a presumed CHH diagnosis in a female infant (due to positive family history leading to a biochemical screening), there are not enough data to propose treatment with ovarian hormones or gonadotropins in such patients, as the consequences of severe GnRH deficiency during late fetal period and mini-puberty in females is unclear.

16.2.4.2 Induction of Female Secondary Sexual Characteristics

The therapeutic objectives in this setting are (1) to achieve breast development, (2) to ensure external and internal genital organ maturity and other aspects of female appearance, and (3) to promote psychosexual development with respect to emotional life and sexuality.[88] In addition, puberty induction increases uterine size, which is important for future pregnancies. Finally, adequate ovarian hormone treatment will optimize growth in order to achieve a final height close to the predicted parental mean target and will promote normal BMD accrual.[124,125] Most therapeutic regimens inducing feminization in CHH arise from expert opinions,[32,125–128] partly due to the paucity of CHH patients.[124,128–131] Further, regimens have often mirrored ovarian hormone treatment implemented in other hypogonadal states, such as Turner syndrome.[132]

In practice, it is reasonable to prioritize transdermal estrogen for pubertal induction based on the favorable risk-benefit profile of this formulation in adults, as well as some data indicating lower risk of cardiovascular events.[124] In addition, a recent RCT in a small number of hypogonadal girls showed that transdermal estradiol resulted in higher E2 levels and more effective feminization than oral conjugated equine estrogen.[131] Transdermal E2 is often started at low doses (e.g., 0.05–0.07 µg/kg nocturnally, from age 11 years), with the goal of mimicking the estrogen rise that occurs during early puberty. In older CHH girls, higher starting doses (0.08–0.12 µg/kg) have been suggested.[124,125,133] The estradiol dosage should then be increased gradually over 12–24 months. After maximizing breast development and/or after the breakthrough bleeding, cyclic progestin is added. In the majority of CHH females, combined estrogen-progestin (E-P) therapy is effective to induce harmonious development of the breasts and genitals. These favorable changes likely contribute to a more satisfactory emotional and sexual life.[88] Finally, estrogen therapy is successful in inducing a growth spurt and increases BMD in the majority of CHH female adolescents.[134]

16.2.4.3   Treatment of Hypogonadism in Adult Women

E-P replacement is required in adult CHH females for maintaining bone health, improving emotional and sexual life, avoiding symptoms of hypoestrogenism (such as hot flashes), and promoting general well-being. Estradiol can be given either orally (at a dose of 1–2 mg) or transdermally (50 μg daily by patch or two pumps of gel daily), with a cyclic progestin (e.g.,. micronized progesterone 200 mg or dydrogesterone 10 mg daily during the last 14 days of the cycle) administered to avoid endometrial hyperplasia. The treatment should be maintained at least until the natural age of menopause. E-P treatment induces monthly withdrawal bleeding but does not restore ovulation. We recommend HRT regimens over OCP for several reasons. CHH females do not need contraception due to the associated infertility, though some caution is needed given the documented cases of reversal in female CHH patients (Section 16.2.3.1). Moreover, the bone effect of ethinylestradiol, the estrogen component of the vast majority of OCPs, is less established than the effect of 17β-estradiol (the estrogen component of ovarian hormone regimens). In line with this recommendation, a 2-year RCT comparing ovarian hormone treatment to OCPs in women with primary ovarian insufficiency revealed significantly higher BMD of the lumbar spine in the former group.[135]

16.2.4.4   Induction of Fertility in CHH Women

Fertility can be achieved with medical induction of ovulation by pulsatile GnRH or gonadotropines, in a similar way as in women with FHA. The modalities of these treatments are detailed in Section 16.1.4, later in this chapter.

16.2.4.5   CHH: Pregnancy and Lactation

Available evidence on pregnancy outcomes in women with CHH are very scarce, with a paucity of data regarding CHH and lactation. In a recent study characterizing the clinical presentation and treatment outcomes of 138 Chinese CHH women, some evidence was reported on pregnancy outcomes of 16 patients who were seeking fertility and for which sufficient follow-up was available.[68] Successful achievement of pregnancy (whether using gonadotropins or IVF) was observed in 81.3% of patients, with a live birth rate of 68.8%, which seems close to what would be expected in the general population. In practically the only published report of obstetric outcomes in female CHH probands harboring homozygous or compound heterozygous mutations in the gene encoding Kisspeptin receptors (*KISS1R*), Pallais et al. described several uncomplicated pregnancies, including some with vaginal delivery and documented lactation.[136] Finally, a recent retrospective study on obstetric outcomes of CHH women undergoing IVF with intracytoplasmic sperm injection (ICSI) revealed high live birth rates per cycle compared with age-matched controls with tubal infertility (31.6% and 24.6% respectively),[137] consistent with the fact that CHH diagnosis does not seem to confer high risk on a subsequent pregnancy.

16.3   ORGANIC LESIONS OF THE HYPOTHALAMUS

16.3.1   Tumors and Other Expansive Entities

Hypothalamic dysfunction results in different combinations of endocrine, metabolic, and neurologic symptoms and may be caused by a large spectrum of pathological disorders.[138] Among them, hypothalamic tumors are a relatively frequent cause. CPs are more common in children and young adults, while primary CNS tumors, such as gliomas and epidermoid and dermoid tumors, are more prevalent in older adults.[139] Ovulation can be disturbed in women harboring these tumors due to either secondary hypogonadism or hyperprolactinemia.

16.3.1.1   CP and Ovulation Disorders

CP is a rare, histologically benign, but locally aggressive neoplasm that is thought to originate from epithelial remnants of Rathke's pouch along a line from the nasopharynx to the diencephalon, although the majority arise from the suprasellar region.[140] A recent study estimated an incidence rate of 1.7 per 1 million persons-years in the United States between 2004 and 2008.[141] Typically, a bimodal age distribution is seen with a first peak in children and young adults <20 years old and a second peak in older adults aged 40–70 years.[141,142] Two main histologic types have been described, with distinct molecular genetic patterns: adamantinomatous and papillary CP (with the former more common in the younger group and the latter more common in the older group), which are associated with mutations in the *CTNNB1* (encoding beta-catenin) and *BRAF* genes, respectively.[143]

The initial manifestations of a CP can vary widely, and symptoms may be present for more than a year before the proper diagnosis is established.[144] In childhood, typical complaints are headaches, visual impairment, polyuria/polydipsia, growth retardation, and/or significant weight gain.[145] Gonadotropin deficiency is seen in 40% of patients and can manifest as absent or stalled puberty in adolescents.[146] The impairment of the HPG axis can be of hypothalamic, pituitary, or mixed origin, depending on the localization of the tumor and the compression of surrounding structures. In adults, the diagnosis is usually made due to headaches or vision loss; however, undiagnosed endocrine insufficiencies often precede these manifestations and are identified only retrospectively. Hypogonadism manifesting as loss of libido in men and amenorrhea in women is frequent.

The diagnosis of CP is suggested by the imaging and confirmed after histologic assessment of the resected tumor. A partially cystic and calcified suprasellar or parasellar lesion is consistent with CP upon MRI.[144] Calcifications in the suprasellar region are seen in 60%–80% of patients and may be easier to visualize via CT than MRI. One or more cysts are present in approximately 75% of cases. The differential diagnosis includes other tumors in the parasellar area, such as pituitary adenoma, meningioma, optic glioma, germinoma, lymphoma, metastasis, and nonneoplastic cysts (Rathke's, pars intermedia, and arachnoid) as well as infiltrative disorders, such as sarcoidosis and histiocytosis.[139]

The optimal management method is still under debate and depends on the surgical expertise of each center. A radical surgical approach aiming for total resection of the tumor has been the traditionally recommended management, with overall good survival rates but to the detriment of reduced quality of life in approximately 50% of long-term survivors.[147] This is due to sequelae, notably morbid hypothalamic obesity and neurobehavioral impairment with affective dysfunction. More recently, a conservative initial approach aiming mainly to decompress mass effects and consisting in planned partial resection (hypothalamus-sparing surgery), followed by adjuvant stereotactic radiosurgery, has been gaining in popularity. The latter has been shown to offer similar long-term disease control with less postoperative hypothalamic obesity,[148,149] and in some non-RCTs, it is associated with even better survival outcomes.[141]

An issue of rising interest in patients with CP is the presence of oxytocin (OT) deficiency and the relevance of an eventual replacement. OT levels were found to be selectively reduced in survivors of childhood-onset CP, with surgical lesions of the anterior hypothalamus.[150] A recent study of 26 adult CP patients revealed similar OT levels compared with age-matched controls, despite the presence of both anterior and posterior pituitary deficiency in 60% of affected patients.[151] Expression of OT in peripheral organs such as the heart, thymus, testes, uterus, and ovaries was considered a potential explanation. Lower baseline OT levels were detected in the subset of patients with MRI-confirmed hypothalamic damage. On the other hand, exercise-induced stimulated OT levels were globally reduced in CP patients. Therapeutic implications of these findings are under investigation. A pilot study with 10 CP patients indicated the positive effects of nasal OT administration on emotion perception in the subset of patients with postsurgery damage of the anterior hypothalamus.[152] Increased desire for socialization and improvement in affection following OT administration has also been reported.[153] A recently published case report described a promising therapeutic response to intranasal OT in a 13-year-old boy with hypothalamic obesity and hyperphagia post-CP resection.[154] Whether this finding will be reproduced in female patients remains to be confirmed.

16.3.1.2 CP: Pregnancy and Lactation

In contrast with the well-established physiologic increase in the size of the pituitary gland and the respective risk for enlargement of preexisting prolactinomas,[155] CP patients are traditionally not considered at risk for progression during pregnancy. Some cases of rapid recurrence, tumor enlargement, or both have been reported.[156,157] There is evidence suggesting the expression of estrogen and progesterone receptors in these tumors,[158,159] which, if confirmed, could offer a possible pathophysiologic explanation for the aforementioned cases. Despite presumed OT deficiency in CP patients with total hypophysectomy[160] or extensive panhypopituitarism following surgery and irradiation,[161] spontaneous labor without OT administration was possible. Interestingly, lactation was unsuccessful in both cases, in line with the animal data postulating the primordial role of OT for milk ejection. However, prolactin deficiency was reported in one case,[161] which could account for the inability to lactate. Prolonged galactorrhea and amenorrhea may be seen postpartum in cases of hyperprolactinemia due to compression of the pituitary stalk or extensive hypothalamic damage by the tumor, with sparing of the pituitary gland.

16.3.1.3 Other Hypothalamic Tumors and Links with Ovulation, Pregnancy, and Lactation

Other hypothalamic tumors, as well as primary CNS tumors involving the hypothalamus (including primary CNS lymphoma), have variable presentations depending on the age of the patient and their size and exact localization. Various degrees of hypopituitarism, with hypogonadism and amenorrhea in some cases, can be present. In children, precocious puberty can be the sole endocrine manifestation of certain tumors, such as hypothalamic hamartomas.[162] Interestingly, endocrine dysfunction, though frequently missed or underappreciated, seems to precede the development of neuro-ophthalmic symptoms in children with CNS tumors.[163]

16.3.2 Infiltrative and Inflammatory Disorders

Among the systematic diseases that affect the hypothalamo-pituitary unit, hypothalamic involvement is a frequent finding in sarcoidosis and Langerhans' cell histiocytosis (LCH), whereas hemochromatosis is typically associated with direct pituitary impairment.

16.3.2.1 Hypothalamic Sarcoidosis and its Effect on Ovulation, Pregnancy, and Lactation

Sarcoidosis is a chronic, multiorgan disease characterized by the formation of immune, noninfectious granulomas that more frequently involve the lungs, skin, and lymph nodes.[164] Hypothalamo-pituitary sarcoidosis, though rare, is the most common intracranial involvement[165] and can be the first presentation of neurosarcoidosis.[166] Traditionally, diabetes insipidus was thought to be the classic endocrine dysfunction in patients with sarcoidosis. Nevertheless, in a multicenter series of 24 patients with hypothalamo-pituitary sarcoidosis, including 10 females, anterior pituitary dysfunction was more common (>90%) than diabetes insipidus (50%).[167] Regarding potential causes of anovulation, gonadotropin insufficiency was present in all but three participants, with hyperprolactinemia in half of the studied patients. Similar findings were reported in an older observation of nine patients with sarcoidosis-associated hypothalamo-pituitary involvement.[168] Clinicians should remember that sarcoidosis can also directly affect the female reproductive tract, with involvement of the uterus, ovaries, and/or fallopian tubes, which can manifest in some cases as amenorrhea.[165]

The hypothalamic defects in patients with neurosarcoidosis is strongly supported by reports demonstrating intact pituitary responsiveness to synthetic hypothalamic-releasing factors, including thyrotropin-releasing hormone (TRH) and GnRH.[169] Despite regression of radiologic lesions with corticosteroid or other immunosuppressive agents, recuperation of endocrine abnormalities in these patients is rare.[167] Other reported symptoms linked to the hypothalamic dysregulation include development of morbid obesity, dysregulation of body temperature, insomnia, personality changes, and an impaired counterregulatory hormonal response to hypoglycemia.[165] Note that polydipsia and polyuria in patients with neurosarcoidosis are not solely attributable to diabetes insipidus, but can also be the consequence of disturbed thirst mechanisms from hypothalamic involvement.[170]

As with most autoimmune disorders, sarcoidosis mostly improves or remains stable during pregnancy.[171] Isolated cases of maternal death have been observed and were attributed to either cardiac arrest[172,173] or neurosarcoidosis.[174] Moreover, several reports suggest an increased risk of obstetric and neonatal complications.[175,176] However, all available studies are retrospective, include small numbers of pregnant women, and do not differentiate between the impacts of the disease and the adverse effects of the therapeutic agents used. The most recent and large to-date study assessed 678 pregnancies in women with presumed diagnosis of sarcoidosis, comparing them with more than 7 million births in controls. This study detected increased risk of preeclampsia, eclampsia, and premature delivery, as well as higher incidence of cesarian delivery and postpartum bleeding.[176] Increased risk of thromboembolic complications was also observed, supporting the prescription of prophylactic anticoagulation in these women. In contrast to these data, a smaller French study did not detect any negative outcomes except for increased risk of low birth weight.[177] Interestingly, in this study, all cases of sarcoidosis adequately treated before pregnancy did not exhibit signs of reactivation during pregnancy, but an increased risk of relapse was noted during lactation.

16.3.2.2 LCH and its Effect on Ovulation, Pregnancy, and Lactation

LCH is another rare systemic disease, characterized by proliferation and infiltration of multiple well-differentiated dendritic cells, called *Langerhans' cells,* which belong to the monocyte-macrophage system.[178] It is more frequent in young boys (peak age 1–4 years),[179] but it can also occur in adults.[180] The hypothalamic-pituitary unit is involved in approximately half of the cases, with the primary neuroendocrine disturbance being diabetes insipidus.[181] Anterior pituitary disturbances have also been described, including gonadotropin deficiency and hyperprolactinemia,[182,183] which could lead to oligoanovulation. Interestingly, resolution gonadotropin deficiency following treatment of LCH with corticosteroids has been reported.[184] Suggestive symptoms of hypothalamic dysfunction, such as hyperphagic obesity, temperature dysregulation, and behavioral changes, can also develop.[183,185]

Reported cases of coexistence of LCH with pregnancy are rare and almost exclusively concern cases of pulmonary LCH. Pregnancy does not appear to influence the progression of the lung disease. However, diabetes insipidus may appear during pregnancy or worsen, thus requiring increased surveillance, with adjustment of desmopressin doses as needed.[186,187] There are no data suggesting worse obstetric or neonatal outcomes.[188] Similar to patients with CP, spontaneous onset of labor is generally observed despite presumed OT deficiency.[161,189] Successful lactation has been reported in most cases,[188,189] unless complete panhypopituitarism with prolactin deficiency are present.[161] In some isolated cases, women exhibited relapse of the disease during the postpartum period, although this finding has not been consistent.[186]

16.3.3   Iatrogenic Lesions

16.3.3.1   Radiotherapy

Hypothalamic hormone deficiency is common after radiation therapy for brain tumors or nasopharyngeal carcinomas in children or adults.[190,191] Endocrine deficiencies can also ensue in patients receiving prophylactic cranial radiotherapy for leukemia, total-body irradiation in the setting of hematopoietic stem cell transplantation for hematologic malignancies, and whole-brain irradiation for lung cancer metastasis.[192] Radiation-induced damage can be due to injury at the level of the hypothalamus, resulting in secondary deficiencies, or due to direct decreases in the secretion of anterior pituitary hormones.[193,194] There is a clear dose-dependent effect regarding the expected endocrine deficits. Children treated with radiation doses $\geq 18\,Gy$ to the hypothalamic-pituitary axis are at risk for GH deficiency and central precocious puberty. Those having received doses $>30–40\,Gy$ are mostly at risk for multiple anterior pituitary hormone deficiencies such as LH, FSH, TSH, and adrenocorticotropic hormone (ACTH). The risk of hypothalamic-pituitary dysfunction after cranial radiation is also time dependent and may not become apparent until many years after treatment. Indeed, the risk seem to persist or even increase up to 10 years after irradiation.[192] In a retrospective study of 748 adult survivors of childhood cancer who were treated with cranial radiation and followed for a mean of 27 years, the prevalence of anterior pituitary hormone deficiencies was 46.5%, 10.8%, 7.5%, and 4% for GH, LH/FSH, TSH, and ACTH, respectively.[195] In a metanalysis of 18 studies on 813 adult patients treated by radiation for nonpituitary tumors (mainly for nasopharyngeal cancer), hypopituitarism was also prevalent, with mean frequencies of 45%, 30%, 25%, and 22% for GH, LH/FSH, TSH, and ACTH deficiencies, respectively, as well as a 34% prevalence for hyperprolactinemia.[196] Consequently, high clinical suspicion for relevant symptoms and systematic screening of the pituitary axis is needed for at-risk survivors of childhood cancer,[197] and a similar attitude is reasonable for patients who received radiotherapy during adulthood. Endocrine deficiencies after radiotherapy are generally irreversible. Hypothalamic injury can also be accompanied by increased risk of obesity, abnormalities in thirst mechanism, and changes in personality, particularly with increasing doses of radiotherapy in children.[138] History of cranial irradiation increases the risk of secondary neoplasms in these patients, which should be considered when addressing treatment of hypopituitarism, given that some data imply increased risk of secondary malignancies in GH-treated childhood cancer survivors.[198]

16.3.3.2   Cranial Irradiation and its Impact on Pregnancy and Lactation

The impact of radiotherapy on future fertility is mostly mediated by the disrupted function of the hypothalamic-pituitary axis, leading to HH, hyperprolactinemia, and anovulation. These deficits are generally treatable, and most women will be able to conceive by ovulation induction via gonadotropin administration. Potential adverse events during a future pregnancy mostly depend on whether the patient also received pelvic radiotherapy (e.g., as part of total body irradiation), which can cause uterine damage, premature ovarian failure, or both.[199] These women have elevated risk for pregnancy-related complications, including spontaneous miscarriages, preterm labor and delivery, low birthweight, and placental abnormalities. Thus, female cancer patients previously treated with pelvic or abdominal irradiation should be closely monitored during pregnancy.

Concerning the effect of isolated cranial irradiation on obstetric and neonatal outcomes, specific data are available from the review of the Childhood Cancer Survivor Study (CCSS). Among the 1915 women reporting 4029 pregnancies in this study, a small subgroup (499 pregnancies) were observed in women having received only cranial irradiation. A slightly but significantly increased risk for miscarriage was seen in comparison with women with no history of radiation therapy: risk ratio (RR) (95% confidence interval (CI)) of 1.40 (1.02–1.94).[200] The latter was further increased when spinal irradiation was added.

No clinically significant impact on breastfeeding capacity of women is expected unless there is radiation-induced hypopituitarism with extensive destruction of lactotroph cells and subsequence prolactin deficiency. Surprisingly, a retrospective analysis of an Australian cohort of women having received cranial radiotherapy of 24 Gy for CNS prophylaxis during treatment of acute lymphoblastic leukemia in childhood reported lactation failure in 10 out of 12 women who produced offspring.[201] These women previously had had regular menses and conceived spontaneously. Subsequent pregnancies went to term and were followed by spontaneous labor. Among the 10 women who did not achieve lactation, all reported absent breast development during the pregnancy, and only three women produced colostrum postpartum. No hormonal profiling was available during or after these pregnancies. In another case series including one female patient with postradiation anterior and posterior pituitary insufficiency, spontaneous onset of labor was also noted, which argues against a major role of presumed OT deficiency for parturition.[161] The patient was unable to initiate breastfeeding, as milk was not produced, consistent with very low postpartum levels of prolactin. Further research is needed to confirm whether disturbed lactation is a frequent occurrence in women with history of cranial irradiation.

16.3.3.3 Postsurgery and Posttraumatic

All patients who undergo surgery affecting the hypothalamic-pituitary area are at increased risk for hormonal abnormalities and altered reproductive function. Hormonal abnormalities often occur concomitantly. All anterior pituitary hormones can be affected, with GH deficiency being the most common. In contrast to the defects postirradiation or postchemotherapy, surgical trauma to the hypothalamus can cause central diabetes insipidus relatively often, due to deficiency of ADH.[202] Similar neuroendocrine alterations are observed after traumatic brain injury.[203] When focusing specifically on hypothalamic complications of cranial surgery, the latter have been mostly studied in patients with CP. In these patients, multiple postoperative complications have been reported, such as hyperphagic obesity, hypersomnolence, and behavioral and social impairment.[204–206] There are no specific considerations regarding the morbidity of pregnancy and lactation in women with postsurgical hypothalamic dysfunction, other than the usual management of hypopituitarism during pregnancy.

16.3.3.4 Drug-Related

Most drugs leading to central oligoanovulation either act solely on the pituitary gland, such as several novel anticancer medications (immune checkpoint inhibitors), or inhibit the HPG axis by antagonizing the dopaminergic system and causing hyperprolactinemia (typically antipsychotics).[207] Two exceptions that exert at least part of their effects via the hypothalamus are opioids and corticosteroids.

Opioid use (including methadone) for pharmacologic reasons or due to underlying addiction is a major cause of reversible HH, and its incidence is likely to increase in the following years.[33,123] In the CNS, endogenous opioids inhibit pulsatile GnRH release,[119,121] in line with well-established close anatomical links between beta-endorphin and GnRH neuronal systems.[208] As expected, exogenous opioids suppress LH secretion and cause clinically evident hypogonadism, though with higher incidence in males than females.[120] Further, opioids can affect the HPG axis by inducing hyperprolactinemia.[121] No effect on maternal OT levels was found by the administration of exogenous morphine or naloxone, an opiate antagonist, in late pregnancy.[209] The safety of opioid use during pregnancy is unclear; there are concerns regarding increased risk of CNS defects, as well as other congenital malformations in the offspring.[210] Moreover, neonatal withdrawal syndrome in the early postpartum is a major concern when the mother has used opioids long term and during the week prior to delivery.[211]

Corticosteroids are another drug class that exerts its action at least partly on the hypothalamus. Exogenous hydrocortisone administration significantly reduced LH pulse frequency in 11 eumenorrheic women, suggesting altered hypothalamic GnRH secretion.[212] The direct action of glucocorticoids at the hypothalamic level was further supported by animal studies showing reversal of glucocorticoid-induced gonadotropin deficiency by intermittent administration of GnRH.[213]

Regarding safety during pregnancy, both prednisone and dexamethasone cross the placenta, but the latter reaches higher concentrations in the fetus because of less efficient metabolism by the placenta. Glucocorticoid therapy during pregnancy may increase the risk of premature rupture of membranes and intrauterine growth restriction,[214] as well as the incidence of pregnancy-induced hypertension and gestational diabetes.[215] The lowest possible dose of glucocorticoid should be used during pregnancy. Women who received more than 20 mg of prednisone per day for more than 3 weeks in the 6 months prior to delivery should be assumed to have suppression of HPA function and receive stress doses of glucocorticoids during labor and delivery. Glucocorticoids are excreted into breast milk, but they are considered compatible with breastfeeding unless high doses (e.g., >20 mg of prednisone per day) are used.[216]

16.4 OVULATION INDUCTION IN PATIENTS WITH HH OF HYPOTHALAMIC ORIGIN

HH of hypothalamic origin accounts for 35% of patients with anovulatory infertility and is among the few treatable causes of infertility. Although the underlying mechanisms of FHA and CHH are different, both conditions are caused by GnRH deficiency. Therefore, GnRH replacement or gonadotropins can successfully restore ovulation and fertility. The therapeutic choice will depend on the expertise of each center and the availability of medical resources.

In contrast to male CHH patients, who need 18–24 months to induce testicular maturation and spermatogenesis under GnRH/gonadotropin treatment, the ovulation in female CHH patients can be induced from the first cycle of treatment. It is important to note that low levels of AMH in patients with FHA or CHH reflect a lack of HPG axis activation rather than a sign of poor ovarian reserve. Thus, such patients should be offered ovulation induction treatment when fertility is desired.

In this section, we will discuss in detail the treatment regimens of GnRH and gonadotropin therapy in FHA and CHH, as well as the advances in kisspeptin as the potential novel molecular treatment for fertility.

16.4.1 Pulsatile GnRH Treatment

Pulsatile GnRH therapy via a pump was first proposed in the 1980s.[217–219] Pulsatile GnRH restores the physiological secretion of pituitary gonadotropins, which in turn induces ovulation. Compared to gonadotropin treatment, this type of therapy is a more physiological way to induce ovulation in women with GnRH deficiency, and it has been shown to be associated with reduced risk of multiple pregnancy and OHSS.[220–222] Therefore, pulsatile GnRH treatment is recommended as the first-line therapy for fertility in both FHA and CHH patients.[2,32]

As discussed in Section 1.1.1.1 of Chapter 1, various GnRH pulse frequencies can distinctly stimulate the secretion of FSH and LH observed in experimental conditions.[223] The GnRH pulse frequency in humans during normal menstrual cycles were determined by frequent LH sampling in a large series of healthy female volunteers.[224] LH pulses, and thus presumed GnRH pulses, were observed at a frequency of 1 pulse every 90 min at the early follicular phase, which promotes the secretion of FSH. This frequency is accelerated to every 60 min at the late follicular phase to stimulate the preovulatory surge. After ovulation, LH pulses are slowed to every 90 min at the early luteal phase, and then every 4 h progressively at the late luteal phase. This change will favor FSH secretion over LH. This observation forms the basis of exogenous pulsatile GnRH therapy.

The classical treatment is to use an intravenous pulsatile GnRH pump with dynamic change of frequency across the cycle, mimicking the physiological observation. This treatment will successfully induce ovulation in both FHA and CHH patients.[225] The continuation of GnRH pulses after ovulation is able to ensure progesterone release by the corpus luteum.[222,226] An optimized progesterone level is mandatory for embryo implantation. Once pregnancy occurs, the endogenous secretion of hCG from the placenta begins, and GnRH pulse treatment can be discontinued. No adverse effects in early pregnancy have been reported.[227]

Subsequently, variations of this protocol were developed, such as using constant GnRH pulse frequency of 90 min throughout the follicular phase, subcutaneous administration of GnRH, and replacement of GnRH with hCG injections (subcutaneous injections of 1500 IU every 3 days for three times) for the support of corpus luteum during the luteal phase.[228] These alternative protocols aimed to offer more flexibility and convenience for patients in their daily lives, simplify clinical care and follow-up, and reduce the cost of the treatment. They were subsequently shown to effectively induce follicular maturation, LH surge, ovulation, and progesterone secretion.[228,229]

The success rate of intravenous GnRH pulsatile therapy was shown to be 90% of the ovulation rate per cycle, and 27.6% of the conception rate per ovulatory cycle.[225] It is slightly lower at 70% of ovulation rate per cycle when administered subcutaneously.[230] However, subcutaneous administration has the advantage of avoiding the risk of phlebitis, which is reported in 1.5% of patients treated intravenously.[222] The number of cycles needed to obtain a pregnancy is quite variable, ranging from one to six cycles.[222,228] The cumulative incidence of pregnancy after six cycles after GnRH treatment is 96%, which is higher than with gonadotropins (72%).[225]

The rate of multiple pregnancy with GnRH pulsatile therapy is approximately 5%–8%, which is slightly higher than the general population (1%–2%), but much lower than with gonadotropin treatment (15%–30%).[225,231] OHSS is rarely reported with GnRH pulsatile treatment.[225] Only when hCG is administered to trigger ovulation is mild OHSS observed (in 1.9% of cases). Therefore, midcycle hCG injection in women treated with pulsatile GnRH therapy should be avoided. The incidence of OHSS is reported to be 2%–3% in gonadotropin therapy, and as high as 20%–30% in IVF treatment.[232]

In CHH patients with severe GnRH deficiency, the gonadotropin response to GnRH pulsatile treatment can be delayed, as their pituitary has not received priming of GnRH previously.[32] Despite this fact, 60% of CHH women can achieve ovulation during their first cycle of intravenous GnRH pulsatile treatment (75 ng/kg/pulse) within 20 days of treatment.[233] In 30% of CHH females, pituitary resistance is present at the first cycle, requiring increased GnRH doses and longer stimulation.[233] Notably, pulsatile GnRH pump can be effective even in the presence of GnRH resistance, such as in women with CHH who harbor partial loss-of-function mutations in *GNRHR*.[233,234]

The GnRH agonist used in the pulsatile GnRH treatment is gonadorelin acetate (Lutrelef, manufactured by Ferring©, Saint-Prex, Switzerland), which is a synthetically produced GnRH with a very short half-life (about 4 min when injected intravenously). The pump system to deliver pulsatile GnRH depends on the availability in different countries. In many European centers, the Crono FE pump (CANÈ SpA Medical Technology©, Rivoli, Italy) is often used. Crono FE is an ambulatory drug delivery pump designed to deliver subcutaneous or intravenous pulsatile infusion. Otherwise, Ferring©

has developed a LutrePulse system, consisting with injection device (pod) and remote control (LutrePulse Manager) for subcutaneous administration.

16.4.2 Gonadotropin Treatment

Although GnRH pulsatile therapy is recommended as the first-line treatment for ovulation induction in FHA or CHH patients, its use has been overlooked, partly due to its unavailability in many countries, including the United States.[2,229] In this context, ovulation can also be achieved with gonadotropin treatment (FSH treatment followed by hCG or recombinant LH to trigger ovulation). However, in both FHA and CHH, women usually require a small dose of LH in addition to FSH during the follicular phase.[32,225,235] In these women, LH will stimulate the theca cells to produce androgens, which form the substrate used by granulosa cells for the production and secretion of estradiol.[84, 236–238] In practice, subcutaneous hMG (human menopausal gonadotropins, containing both FSH and hCG) is often used at doses of 75–150 IU/day to induce follicular maturation. The follicular growth is monitored by ultrasound every other day, along with the measurement of serum estradiol. The starting dose of hMG is often increased or decreased depending on the ovarian response. This follow-up schema minimizes the risk of multiple follicle stimulation and OHSS. Once a dominant follicle (>18 mm) is seen via ultrasound, a high dose of hCG (5000 IU or 6500 IU) is administered to trigger ovulation. After ovulation, progesterone production can be stimulated by either repeated hCG injections or direct administration of progesterone during the postovulatory phase until the end of the luteal phase.

The different rates of efficacy and complications of gonadotropin therapy in comparison with GnRH pulsatile treatment have been discussed previously, in Section 16.4.1. It is important to note that a few CHH patients exhibit pituitary resistance, which cannot be overcome by increasing doses of GnRH stimulation. In such cases, gonadotropin therapy can be successful in bypassing the pituitary resistance and inducing ovulation.[238,239]

16.4.3 The Role of Kisspeptin in the Ovulation Induction Treatment

As discussed in Section 16.1, the kisspeptin pathway is a critical upstream stimulator of GnRH neurons. Experiments in malnourished prepubertal female rats with central administration of kisspeptin showed gonadotropin responses, which led to induction of puberty.[240] In human studies, a single subcutaneous injection of kisspeptin can trigger ovulation in a standard IVF protocol using an FSH recombinant/GnRH antagonist, and this treatment has been shown to reduce the risk of OHSS.[241]

Several studies have explored the use of kisspeptin for ovulation restoration in FHA women. Subcutaneous administration of kisspeptin (Kp-54) has been shown to increase serum LH levels. However, despite gonadotropin responsiveness, follicular growth or change in the endometrium thickness was not observed. In addition, administration over 2 weeks can possibly lead to a chronic desensitization.[242,243] In contrast, intravenous administration seems to induce LH pulsatility without desensitization. In summary, the effectiveness of kisspeptin treatment for ovulation induction in FHA patients has not been proven, so this treatment is not yet recommended for induction of fertility.[2]

In CHH females, the use of kisspeptin was only reported in three cases for the purpose of a physiological study in the research setting. A 12-h continuous intravenous infusion of kisspeptin was shown to be successful in inducing LH pulsatile secretion in a female patient with homozygous loss-of-function mutation in TACR3.[244] In another study including two female CHH patients, the bolus of kisspeptin injection failed to induce LH secretion.[245] Indeed, these patients harbored loss-of-function mutations in known CHH genes: one was compound heterozygous for mutations in GNRHR, and the other harbored a heterozygous mutation in FGFR1. These genetic defects interrupt the integrity of the HPG axis and may explain the unresponsiveness of LH to kisspeptin stimulation. In summary, the use of kisspeptin in CHH females remains obscure.

16.4.4 The Place of IVF in the Fertility Treatment of HH Patients

IVF is not recommended as the first-line therapy in patients with FHA or CHH, as ovulation induction by pulsatile GnRH or gonadotropins usually restores fertility. However, if conception fails after repeated successful induced ovulations in FHA/CHH females, IVF may be considered as an alternative treatment for fertility.[246,247]

16.4.5 Summary

The prognosis of fertility in FHA and CHH women is excellent, despite low baseline AMH levels. GnRH pulsatile treatment should be considered as the first-line treatment due to its higher efficacy for ovulation and pregnancy rate, as well as its lower risk of multiple pregnancy and OHSS compared to gonadotropin treatment. When a GnRH pump is not available, gonadotropin treatment can be an efficient alternative. In addition, gonadotropin treatment can bypass the pituitary resistance to restore ovulation, which may occur in a small number of CHH patients. Despite the success of kisspeptin in IVF, its use for ovulation induction in patients with FHA and CHH is not yet recommended.

REFERENCES

1. Gordon CM. Clinical practice. Functional hypothalamic amenorrhea. *N Engl J Med* 2010;**363**(4):365–71.
2. Gordon CM, Ackerman KE, Berga SL, Kaplan JR, Mastorakos G, Misra M, et al. Functional hypothalamic amenorrhea: an endocrine society clinical practice guideline. *J Clin Endocrinol Metab* 2017;**102**(5):1413–39.
3. Practice Committee of the American Society for Reproductive M. Current evaluation of amenorrhea. *Fertil Steril* 2006;**86**(5 Suppl 1):S148–55.
4. Liu JH, Bill AH. Stress-associated or functional hypothalamic amenorrhea in the adolescent. *Ann N Y Acad Sci* 2008;**1135**:179–84.
5. Villanueva AL, Schlosser C, Hopper B, Liu JH, Hoffman DI, Rebar RW. Increased cortisol production in women runners. *J Clin Endocrinol Metab* 1986;**63**(1):133–6.
6. Biller BM, Federoff HJ, Koenig JI, Klibanski A. Abnormal cortisol secretion and responses to corticotropin-releasing hormone in women with hypothalamic amenorrhea. *J Clin Endocrinol Metab* 1990;**70**(2):311–7.
7. Berga SL, Daniels TL, Giles DE. Women with functional hypothalamic amenorrhea but not other forms of anovulation display amplified cortisol concentrations. *Fertil Steril* 1997;**67**(6):1024–30.
8. Laughlin GA, Dominguez CE, Yen SS. Nutritional and endocrine-metabolic aberrations in women with functional hypothalamic amenorrhea. *J Clin Endocrinol Metab* 1998;**83**(1):25–32.
9. Gambacciani M, Yen SS, Rasmussen DD. GnRH release from the mediobasal hypothalamus: in vitro inhibition by corticotropin-releasing factor. *Neuroendocrinology* 1986;**43**(4):533–6.
10. Petraglia F, Sutton S, Vale W, Plotsky P. Corticotropin-releasing factor decreases plasma luteinizing hormone levels in female rats by inhibiting gonadotropin-releasing hormone release into hypophysial-portal circulation. *Endocrinology* 1987;**120**(3):1083–8.
11. Loucks AB, Thuma JR. Luteinizing hormone pulsatility is disrupted at a threshold of energy availability in regularly menstruating women. *J Clin Endocrinol Metab* 2003;**88**(1):297–311.
12. Marcus MD, Loucks TL, Berga SL. Psychological correlates of functional hypothalamic amenorrhea. *Fertil Steril* 2001;**76**(2):310–6.
13. Warren MP, Voussoughian F, Geer EB, Hyle EP, Adberg CL, Ramos RH. Functional hypothalamic amenorrhea: hypoleptinemia and disordered eating. *J Clin Endocrinol Metab* 1999;**84**(3):873–7.
14. Welt CK, Chan JL, Bullen J, Murphy R, Smith P, DePaoli AM, et al. Recombinant human leptin in women with hypothalamic amenorrhea. *N Engl J Med* 2004;**351**(10):987–97.
15. Navarro VM, Kaiser UB. Metabolic influences on neuroendocrine regulation of reproduction. *Curr Opin Endocrinol Diabetes Obes* 2013;**20**(4):335–41.
16. Caronia LM, Martin C, Welt CK, Sykiotis GP, Quinton R, Thambundit A, et al. A genetic basis for functional hypothalamic amenorrhea. *N Engl J Med* 2011;**364**(3):215–25.
17. Meczekalski B, Katulski K, Czyzyk A, Podfigurna-Stopa A, Maciejewska-Jeske M. Functional hypothalamic amenorrhea and its influence on women's health. *J Endocrinol Investig* 2014;**37**(11):1049–56.
18. Flug D, Largo RH, Prader A. Menstrual patterns in adolescent Swiss girls: a longitudinal study. *Ann Hum Biol* 1984;**11**(6):495–508.
19. Legro RS, Lin HM, Demers LM, Lloyd T. Rapid maturation of the reproductive axis during perimenarche independent of body composition. *J Clin Endocrinol Metab* 2000;**85**(3):1021–5.
20. De Souza MJ, Miller BE, Loucks AB, Luciano AA, Pescatello LS, Campbell CG, et al. High frequency of luteal phase deficiency and anovulation in recreational women runners: blunted elevation in follicle-stimulating hormone observed during luteal-follicular transition. *J Clin Endocrinol Metab* 1998;**83**(12):4220–32.
21. Hammar ML, Hammar-Henriksson MB, Frisk J, Rickenlund A, Wyon YA. Few oligo-amenorrheic athletes have vasomotor symptoms. *Maturitas* 2000;**34**(3):219–25.
22. Dundon CM, Rellini AH, Tonani S, Santamaria V, Nappi R. Mood disorders and sexual functioning in women with functional hypothalamic amenorrhea. *Fertil Steril* 2010;**94**(6):2239–43.
23. Fries H, Nillius SJ, Pettersson F. Epidemiology of secondary amenorrhea. II. A retrospective evaluation of etiology with special regard to psychogenic factors and weight loss. *Am J Obstet Gynecol* 1974;**118**(4):473–9.
24. Giles DE, Berga SL. Cognitive and psychiatric correlates of functional hypothalamic amenorrhea: a controlled comparison. *Fertil Steril* 1993;**60**(3):486–92.
25. Warren MP, Brooks-Gunn J, Hamilton LH, Warren LF, Hamilton WG. Scoliosis and fractures in young ballet dancers. Relation to delayed menarche and secondary amenorrhea. *N Engl J Med* 1986;**314**(21):1348–53.
26. Barrack MT, Gibbs JC, De Souza MJ, Williams NI, Nichols JF, Rauh MJ, et al. Higher incidence of bone stress injuries with increasing female athlete triad-related risk factors: a prospective multisite study of exercising girls and women. *Am J Sports Med* 2014;**42**(4):949–58.
27. Robin G, Gallo C, Catteau-Jonard S, Lefebvre-Maunoury C, Pigny P, Duhamel A, et al. Polycystic ovary-like abnormalities (PCO-L) in women with functional hypothalamic amenorrhea. *J Clin Endocrinol Metab* 2012;**97**(11):4236–43.
28. Sum M, Warren MP. Hypothalamic amenorrhea in young women with underlying polycystic ovary syndrome. *Fertil Steril* 2009;**92**(6):2106–8.

29. Mattle V, Bilgyicildirim A, Hadziomerovic D, Ott HW, Zervomanolakis I, Leyendecker G, et al. Polycystic ovarian disease unmasked by pulsatile GnRH therapy in a subgroup of women with hypothalamic amenorrhea. *Fertil Steril* 2008;**89**(2):404–9.

30. Shoham Z, Conway GS, Patel A, Jacobs HS. Polycystic ovaries in patients with hypogonadotropic hypogonadism: similarity of ovarian response to gonadotropin stimulation in patients with polycystic ovarian syndrome. *Fertil Steril* 1992;**58**(1):37–45.

31. Wang JG, Lobo RA. The complex relationship between hypothalamic amenorrhea and polycystic ovary syndrome. *J Clin Endocrinol Metab* 2008;**93** (4):1394–7.

32. Boehm U, Bouloux PM, Dattani MT, de Roux N, Dode C, Dunkel L, et al. Expert consensus document: European Consensus Statement on congenital hypogonadotropic hypogonadism-pathogenesis, diagnosis and treatment. *Nat Rev Endocrinol* 2015;**11**(9):547–64.

33. Reddy RG, Aung T, Karavitaki N, Wass JA. Opioid induced hypogonadism. *BMJ* 2010;**341**:c4462.

34. Bushe C, Yeomans D, Floyd T, Smith SM. Categorical prevalence and severity of hyperprolactinaemia in two UK cohorts of patients with severe mental illness during treatment with antipsychotics. *J Psychopharmacol* 2008;**22**(2 Suppl):56–62.

35. Christiansen SC, Eilertsen TB, Vanky E, Carlsen SM. Does AMH reflect follicle number similarly in women with and without PCOS? *PLoS One* 2016;**11**(1).

36. Bruni V, Dei M, Morelli C, Schettino MT, Balzi D, Nuvolone D. Body composition variables and leptin levels in functional hypothalamic amenorrhea and amenorrhea related to eating disorders. *J Pediatr Adolesc Gynecol* 2011;**24**(6):347–52.

37. Corr M, De Souza MJ, Toombs RJ, Williams NI. Circulating leptin concentrations do not distinguish menstrual status in exercising women. *Hum Reprod* 2011;**26**(3):685–94.

38. Berga SL, Mortola JF, Girton L, Suh B, Laughlin G, Pham P, et al. Neuroendocrine aberrations in women with functional hypothalamic amenorrhea. *J Clin Endocrinol Metab* 1989;**68**(2):301–8.

39. Misra M, Soyka LA, Miller KK, Herzog DB, Grinspoon S, De Chen D, et al. Serum osteoprotegerin in adolescent girls with anorexia nervosa. *J Clin Endocrinol Metab* 2003;**88**(8):3816–22.

40. Ihle R, Loucks AB. Dose-response relationships between energy availability and bone turnover in young exercising women. *J Bone Miner Res* 2004;**19**(8):1231–40.

41. Rigotti NA, Neer RM, Skates SJ, Herzog DB, Nussbaum SR. The clinical course of osteoporosis in anorexia nervosa. A longitudinal study of cortical bone mass. *JAMA* 1991;**265**(9):1133–8.

42. Ackerman KE, Cano Sokoloff N, DE Nardo Maffazioli G, Clarke HM, Lee H, Misra M. Fractures in relation to menstrual status and bone parameters in young athletes. *Med Sci Sports Exerc* 2015;**47**(8):1577–86.

43. Ackerman KE, Nazem T, Chapko D, Russell M, Mendes N, Taylor AP, et al. Bone microarchitecture is impaired in adolescent amenorrheic athletes compared with eumenorrheic athletes and nonathletic controls. *J Clin Endocrinol Metab* 2011;**96**(10):3123–33.

44. Lawson EA, Miller KK, Bredella MA, Phan C, Misra M, Meenaghan E, et al. Hormone predictors of abnormal bone microarchitecture in women with anorexia nervosa. *Bone* 2010;**46**(2):458–63.

45. Golden NH, Katzman DK, Sawyer SM, Ornstein RM, Rome ES, Garber AK, et al. Update on the medical management of eating disorders in adolescents. *J Adolesc Health* 2015;**56**(4):370–5.

46. Dempfle A, Herpertz-Dahlmann B, Timmesfeld N, Schwarte R, Egberts KM, Pfeiffer E, et al. Predictors of the resumption of menses in adolescent anorexia nervosa. *BMC Psychiatry* 2013;**13**:308.

47. Dueck CA, Matt KS, Manore MM, Skinner JS. Treatment of athletic amenorrhea with a diet and training intervention program. *Int J Sport Nutr* 1996;**6**(1):24–40.

48. Lagowska K, Kapczuk K, Jeszka J. Nine-month nutritional intervention improves restoration of menses in young female athletes and ballet dancers. *J Int Soc Sports Nutr* 2014;**11**(1):52.

49. Berga SL, Marcus MD, Loucks TL, Hlastala S, Ringham R, Krohn MA. Recovery of ovarian activity in women with functional hypothalamic amenorrhea who were treated with cognitive behavior therapy. *Fertil Steril* 2003;**80**(4):976–81.

50. Michopoulos V, Mancini F, Loucks TL, Berga SL. Neuroendocrine recovery initiated by cognitive behavioral therapy in women with functional hypothalamic amenorrhea: a randomized, controlled trial. *Fertil Steril* 2013;**99**(7):2084–91. e1.

51. Warren MP, Brooks-Gunn J, Fox RP, Holderness CC, Hyle EP, Hamilton WG, et al. Persistent osteopenia in ballet dancers with amenorrhea and delayed menarche despite hormone therapy: a longitudinal study. *Fertil Steril* 2003;**80**(2):398–404.

52. Cobb KL, Bachrach LK, Sowers M, Nieves J, Greendale GA, Kent KK, et al. The effect of oral contraceptives on bone mass and stress fractures in female runners. *Med Sci Sports Exerc* 2007;**39**(9):1464–73.

53. Westhoff CL, Torgal AH, Mayeda ER, Stanczyk FZ, Lerner JP, Benn EK, et al. Ovarian suppression in normal-weight and obese women during oral contraceptive use: a randomized controlled trial. *Obstet Gynecol* 2010;**116**(2 Pt 1):275–83.

54. Misra M, Katzman D, Miller KK, Mendes N, Snelgrove D, Russell M, et al. Physiologic estrogen replacement increases bone density in adolescent girls with anorexia nervosa. *J Bone Miner Res* 2011;**26**(10):2430–8.

55. Weissberger AJ, Ho KK, Lazarus L. Contrasting effects of oral and transdermal routes of estrogen replacement therapy on 24-hour growth hormone (GH) secretion, insulin-like growth factor I, and GH-binding protein in postmenopausal women. *J Clin Endocrinol Metab* 1991;**72** (2):374–81.

56. Fazeli PK, Wang IS, Miller KK, Herzog DB, Misra M, Lee H, et al. Teriparatide increases bone formation and bone mineral density in adult women with anorexia nervosa. *J Clin Endocrinol Metab* 2014;**99**(4):1322–9.

57. Zhang D, Potty A, Vyas P, Lane J. The role of recombinant PTH in human fracture healing: a systematic review. *J Orthop Trauma* 2014;**28**(1):57–62.

58. Sienkiewicz E, Magkos F, Aronis KN, Brinkoetter M, Chamberland JP, Chou S, et al. Long-term metreleptin treatment increases bone mineral density and content at the lumbar spine of lean hypoleptinemic women. *Metabolism* 2011;**60**(9):1211–21.

59. Moutquin JM. Socio-economic and psychosocial factors in the management and prevention of preterm labour. *BJOG* 2003;**110**(Suppl 20):56–60.
60. Bulik CM, Sullivan PF, Fear JL, Pickering A, Dawn A, McCullin M. Fertility and reproduction in women with anorexia nervosa: a controlled study. *J Clin Psychiatry* 1999;**60**(2):130–5. quiz 5-7.
61. Group ECW. Nutrition and reproduction in women. *Hum Reprod Update* 2006;**12**(3):193–207.
62. Mazer-Poline C, Fornari V. Anorexia nervosa and pregnancy: having a baby when you are dying to be thin–case report and proposed treatment guidelines. *Int J Eat Disord* 2009;**42**(4):382–4.
63. Franko DL, Blais MA, Becker AE, Delinsky SS, Greenwood DN, Flores AT, et al. Pregnancy complications and neonatal outcomes in women with eating disorders. *Am J Psychiatry* 2001;**158**(9):1461–6.
64. Waldstreicher J, Seminara SB, Jameson JL, Geyer A, Nachtigall LB, Boepple PA, et al. The genetic and clinical heterogeneity of gonadotropin-releasing hormone deficiency in the human. *J Clin Endocrinol Metab* 1996;**81**(12):4388–95.
65. Quinton R, Duke VM, Robertson A, Kirk JM, Matfin G, de Zoysa PA, et al. Idiopathic gonadotrophin deficiency: genetic questions addressed through phenotypic characterization. *Clin Endocrinol* 2001;**55**(2):163–74.
66. Fromantin M, Gineste J, Didier A, Rouvier J. Impuberism and hypogonadism at induction into military service. Statistical study. *Probl Actuels Endocrinol Nutr* 1973;**16**:179–99.
67. Laitinen EM, Vaaralahti K, Tommiska J, Eklund E, Tervaniemi M, Valanne L, et al. Incidence, phenotypic features and molecular genetics of Kallmann syndrome in Finland. *Orphanet J Rare Dis* 2011;**6**:41.
68. Tang RY, Chen R, Ma M, Lin SQ, Zhang YW, Wang YP. Clinical characteristics of 138 Chinese female patients with idiopathic hypogonadotropic hypogonadism. *Endocr Connect* 2017;**6**(8):800–10.
69. Bonomi M, Vezzoli V, Krausz C, Guizzardi F, Vezzani S, Simoni M, et al. Characteristics of a nationwide cohort of patients presenting with isolated hypogonadotropic hypogonadism (IHH). *Eur J Endocrinol* 2018;**178**(1):23–32.
70. Hietamaki J, Hero M, Holopainen E, Kansakoski J, Vaaralahti K, Iivonen AP, et al. GnRH receptor gene mutations in adolescents and young adults presenting with signs of partial gonadotropin deficiency. *PLoS One* 2017;**12**(11).
71. Kallmann FJ, Schoenfeld WA, Barrera SE. The genetic aspects of primary eunuchoidism. *Am J Ment Defic* 1944;**XLVIII**:203–36.
72. Maione L, Dwyer AA, Francou B, Guiochon-Mantel A, Binart N, Bouligand J, et al. Genetics in endocrinology: genetic counseling for congenital hypogonadotropic hypogonadism and Kallmann syndrome: new challenges in the era of oligogenism and next-generation sequencing. *Eur J Endocrinol* 2018;**178**(3):R55–80.
73. Stamou MI, Cox KH, Crowley Jr WF. Discovering genes essential to the hypothalamic regulation of human teproduction using a human disease model: adjusting to life in the "-omics" era. *Endocr Rev* 2016;**2016**(1):4–22.
74. Seminara SB, Hayes FJ, Crowley Jr WF. Gonadotropin-releasing hormone deficiency in the human (idiopathic hypogonadotropic hypogonadism and Kallmann's syndrome): pathophysiological and genetic considerations. *Endocr Rev* 1998;**19**(5):521–39.
75. Pitteloud N, Quinton R, Pearce S, Raivio T, Acierno J, Dwyer A, et al. Digenic mutations account for variable phenotypes in idiopathic hypogonadotropic hypogonadism. *J Clin Invest* 2007;**117**(2):457–63.
76. Waldhauser F, Weissenbacher G, Frisch H, Pollak A. Pulsatile secretion of gonadotropins in early infancy. *Eur J Pediatr* 1981;**137**(1):71–4.
77. Kuiri-Hanninen T, Haanpaa M, Turpeinen U, Hamalainen E, Seuri R, Tyrvainen E, et al. Postnatal ovarian activation has effects in estrogen target tissues in infant girls. *J Clin Endocrinol Metab* 2013;**98**(12):4709–16.
78. Kuiri-Hanninen T, Kallio S, Seuri R, Tyrvainen E, Liakka A, Tapanainen J, et al. Postnatal developmental changes in the pituitary-ovarian axis in preterm and term infant girls. *J Clin Endocrinol Metab* 2011;**96**(11):3432–9.
79. Schmidt IM, Chellakooty M, Haavisto AM, Boisen KA, Damgaard IN, Steendahl U, et al. Gender difference in breast tissue size in infancy: correlation with serum estradiol. *Pediatr Res* 2002;**52**(5):682–6.
80. Shaw ND, Seminara SB, Welt CK, Au MG, Plummer L, Hughes VA, et al. Expanding the phenotype and genotype of female GnRH deficiency. *J Clin Endocrinol Metab* 2011;**96**(3):E566–76.
81. de Roux N, Young J, Misrahi M, Genet R, Chanson P, Schaison G, et al. A family with hypogonadotropic hypogonadism and mutations in the gonadotropin-releasing hormone receptor. *N Engl J Med* 1997;**337**(22):1597–602.
82. Sarfati J, Bouvattier C, Bry-Gauillard H, Cartes A, Bouligand J, Young J. Kallmann syndrome with FGFR1 and KAL1 mutations detected during fetal life. *Orphanet J Rare Dis* 2015;**10**:71.
83. Brioude F, Bouligand J, Trabado S, Francou B, Salenave S, Kamenicky P, et al. Non-syndromic congenital hypogonadotropic hypogonadism: clinical presentation and genotype-phenotype relationships. *Eur J Endocrinol* 2010;**162**(5):835–51.
84. Bry-Gauillard H, Larrat-Ledoux F, Levaillant JM, Massin N, Maione L, Beau I, et al. Anti-Mullerian hormone and ovarian morphology in women with isolated hypogonadotropic hypogonadism/Kallmann syndrome: effects of recombinant human FSH. *J Clin Endocrinol Metab* 2017;**102**(4):1102–11.
85. Giton F, Trabado S, Maione L, Sarfati J, Le Bouc Y, Brailly-Tabard S, et al. Sex steroids, precursors, and metabolite deficiencies in men with isolated hypogonadotropic hypogonadism and panhypopituitarism: a GCMS-based comparative study. *J Clin Endocrinol Metab* 2015;**100**(2):E292–6.
86. Dickerman Z, Cohen A, Laron Z. Growth in patients with isolated gonadotrophin deficiency. *Arch Dis Child* 1992;**67**(4):513–6.
87. Hero M, Laitinen EM, Varimo T, Vaaralahti K, Tommiska J, Raivio T. Childhood growth of females with Kallmann syndrome and FGFR1 mutations. *Clin Endocrinol* 2015;**82**(1):122–6.
88. Dzemaili S, Tiemensma J, Quinton R, Pitteloud N, Morin D, Dwyer AA. Beyond hormone replacement: quality of life in women with congenital hypogonadotropic hypogonadism. *Endocr Connect* 2017;**6**(6):404–12.
89. Raivio T, Falardeau J, Dwyer A, Quinton R, Hayes FJ, Hughes VA, et al. Reversal of idiopathic hypogonadotropic hypogonadism. *N Engl J Med* 2007;**357**(9):863–73.

90. Sidhoum VF, Chan YM, Lippincott MF, Balasubramanian R, Quinton R, Plummer L, et al. Reversal and relapse of hypogonadotropic hypogonadism: resilience and fragility of the reproductive neuroendocrine system. *J Clin Endocrinol Metab* 2014;**99**(3):861–70.

91. Kim J, Semaan SJ, Clifton DK, Steiner RA, Dhamija S, Kauffman AS. Regulation of Kiss1 expression by sex steroids in the amygdala of the rat and mouse. *Endocrinology* 2011;**152**(5):2020–30.

92. Santhakumar A, Miller M, Quinton R. Pubertal induction in adult males with isolated hypogonadotropic hypogonadism using long-acting intramuscular testosterone undecanoate 1-g depot (Nebido). *Clin Endocrinol* 2014;**80**(1):155–7.

93. Costa-Barbosa FA, Balasubramanian R, Keefe KW, Shaw ND, Al-Tassan N, Plummer L, et al. Prioritizing genetic testing in patients with Kallmann syndrome using clinical phenotypes. *J Clin Endocrinol Metab* 2013;**98**(5):E943–53.

94. Main KM, Schmidt IM, Skakkebaek NE. A possible role for reproductive hormones in newborn boys: progressive hypogonadism without the postnatal testosterone peak. *J Clin Endocrinol Metab* 2000;**85**(12):4905–7.

95. Grumbach MM. A window of opportunity: the diagnosis of gonadotropin deficiency in the male infant. *J Clin Endocrinol Metab* 2005;**90**(5):3122–7.

96. Main KM, Schmidt IM, Toppari J, Skakkebaek NE. Early postnatal treatment of hypogonadotropic hypogonadism with recombinant human FSH and LH. *Eur J Endocrinol* 2002;**146**(1):75–9.

97. Bougneres P, Francois M, Pantalone L, Rodrigue D, Bouvattier C, Demesteere E, et al. Effects of an early postnatal treatment of hypogonadotropic hypogonadism with a continuous subcutaneous infusion of recombinant follicle-stimulating hormone and luteinizing hormone. *J Clin Endocrinol Metab* 2008;**93**(6):2202–5.

98. Xu C, Lang-Muritano M, Phan-Hug F, Dwyer AA, Sykiotis GP, Cassatella D, et al. Genetic testing facilitates prepubertal diagnosis of congenital hypogonadotropic hypogonadism. *Clin Genet* 2017;**92**(2):213–6.

99. Lambert AS, Bougneres P. Growth and descent of the testes in infants with hypogonadotropic hypogonadism receiving subcutaneous gonadotropin infusion. *Int J Pediatr Endocrinol* 2016;**2016**:13.

100. Villanueva C, Jacobson-Dickman E, Xu C, Manouvrier S, Dwyer AA, Sykiotis GP, et al. Congenital hypogonadotropic hypogonadism with split hand/foot malformation: a clinical entity with a high frequency of FGFR1 mutations. *Genet Med* 2015;**17**(8):651–9.

101. Lewkowitz-Shpuntoff HM, Hughes VA, Plummer L, Au MG, Doty RL, Seminara SB, et al. Olfactory phenotypic spectrum in idiopathic hypogonadotropic hypogonadism: pathophysiological and genetic implications. *J Clin Endocrinol Metab* 2012;**97**(1):E136–44.

102. Pitteloud N, Hayes FJ, Boepple PA, DeCruz S, Seminara SB, Mac Laughlin DT, et al. The role of prior pubertal development, biochemical markers of testicular maturation, and genetics in elucidating the phenotypic heterogeneity of idiopathic hypogonadotropic hypogonadism. *J Clin Endocrinol Metab* 2002;**87**(1):152–60.

103. Young J. Approach to the male patient with congenital hypogonadotropic hypogonadism. *J Clin Endocrinol Metab* 2012;**97**(3):707–18.

104. Rosner W, Hankinson SE, Sluss PM, Vesper HW, Wierman ME. Challenges to the measurement of estradiol: an endocrine society position statement. *J Clin Endocrinol Metab* 2013;**98**(4):1376–87.

105. Andersen CY, Schmidt KT, Kristensen SG, Rosendahl M, Byskov AG, Ernst E. Concentrations of AMH and inhibin-B in relation to follicular diameter in normal human small antral follicles. *Hum Reprod* 2010;**25**(5):1282–7.

106. Kottler ML, Chou YY, Chabre O, Richard N, Polge C, Brailly-Tabard S, et al. A new FSHbeta mutation in a 29-year-old woman with primary amenorrhea and isolated FSH deficiency: functional characterization and ovarian response to human recombinant FSH. *Eur J Endocrinol* 2010;**162**(3):633–41.

107. Tommiska J, Toppari J, Vaaralahti K, Kansakoski J, Laitinen EM, Noisa P, et al. PROKR2 mutations in autosomal recessive Kallmann syndrome. *Fertil Steril* 2013;**99**(3):815–8.

108. Sehested A, Juul AA, Andersson AM, Petersen JH, Jensen TK, Muller J, et al. Serum inhibin A and inhibin B in healthy prepubertal, pubertal, and adolescent girls and adult women: relation to age, stage of puberty, menstrual cycle, follicle-stimulating hormone, luteinizing hormone, and estradiol levels. *J Clin Endocrinol Metab* 2000;**85**(4):1634–40.

109. Higham CE, Johannsson G, Shalet SM. Hypopituitarism. *Lancet* 2016;**388**(10058):2403–15.

110. Kelberman D, Rizzoti K, Lovell-Badge R, Robinson IC, Dattani MT. Genetic regulation of pituitary gland development in human and mouse. *Endocr Rev* 2009;**30**(7):790–829.

111. Tsilchorozidou T, Conway GS. Uterus size and ovarian morphology in women with isolated growth hormone deficiency, hypogonadotrophic hypogonadism and hypopituitarism. *Clin Endocrinol* 2004;**61**(5):567–72.

112. Sarfati J, Saveanu A, Young J. Pituitary stalk interruption and olfactory bulbs aplasia/hypoplasia in a man with Kallmann syndrome and reversible gonadotrope and somatotrope deficiencies. *Endocrine* 2014;**49**(3):865–6.

113. Hacquart T, Ltaief-Boudrigua A, Jeannerod C, Hannoun S, Raverot G, Pugeat M, et al. Reconsidering olfactory bulb magnetic resonance patterns in Kallmann syndrome. *Ann Endocrinol (Paris)* 2017;**78**(5):455–61.

114. Basaria S. Male hypogonadism. *Lancet* 2014;**383**(9924):1250–63.

115. Silveira LF, Latronico AC. Approach to the patient with hypogonadotropic hypogonadism. *J Clin Endocrinol Metab* 2013;**98**(5):1781–8.

116. Schneider HJ, Kreitschmann-Andermahr I, Ghigo E, Stalla GK, Agha A. Hypothalamopituitary dysfunction following traumatic brain injury and aneurysmal subarachnoid hemorrhage: a systematic review. *JAMA* 2007;**298**(12):1429–38.

117. Kelly TM, Edwards CQ, Meikle AW, Kushner JP. Hypogonadism in hemochromatosis: reversal with iron depletion. *Ann Intern Med* 1984;**101**(5):629–32.

118. Abs R, Verhelst J, Maeyaert J, Van Buyten JP, Opsomer F, Adriaensen H, et al. Endocrine consequences of long-term intrathecal administration of opioids. *J Clin Endocrinol Metab* 2000;**85**(6):2215–22.

119. Bottcher B, Seeber B, Leyendecker G, Wildt L. Impact of the opioid system on the reproductive axis. *Fertil Steril* 2017;**108**(2):207–13.

120. Fraser LA, Morrison D, Morley-Forster P, Paul TL, Tokmakejian S, Larry Nicholson R, et al. Oral opioids for chronic non-cancer pain: higher prevalence of hypogonadism in men than in women. *Exp Clin Endocrinol Diabetes* 2009;**117**(1):38–43.

121. Vuong C, Van Uum SH, O'Dell LE, Lutfy K, Friedman TC. The effects of opioids and opioid analogs on animal and human endocrine systems. *Endocr Rev* 2010;**31**(1):98–132.

122. O'Rourke Jr. TK, Wosnitzer MS. Opioid-induced androgen deficiency (OPIAD): diagnosis, management, and literature review. *Curr Urol Rep* 2016;**17**(10):76.

123. Collins FS, Koroshetz WJ, Volkow ND. Helping to end addiction over the long-term: the research plan for the NIH HEAL initiative. *JAMA* 2018;**320** (2):129–30.

124. Kenigsberg L, Balachandar S, Prasad K, Shah B. Exogenous pubertal induction by oral versus transdermal estrogen therapy. *J Pediatr Adolesc Gynecol* 2013;**26**(2):71–9.

125. Dunkel L, Quinton R. Transition in endocrinology: induction of puberty. *Eur J Endocrinol* 2014;**170**(6):R229–39.

126. de Muinck Keizer-Schrama SM. Introduction and management of puberty in girls. *Horm Res* 2007;**68**(Suppl 5):80–3.

127. Divasta AD, Gordon CM. Hormone replacement therapy and the adolescent. *Curr Opin Obstet Gynecol* 2010;**22**(5):363–8.

128. Hindmarsh PC. How do you initiate oestrogen therapy in a girl who has not undergone puberty? *Clin Endocrinol* 2009;**71**(1):7–10.

129. Kiess W, Conway G, Ritzen M, Rosenfield R, Bernasconi S, Juul A, et al. Induction of puberty in the hypogonadal girl–practices and attitudes of pediatric endocrinologists in Europe. *Horm Res* 2002;**57**(1–2):66–71.

130. Drobac S, Rubin K, Rogol AD, Rosenfield RL. A workshop on pubertal hormone replacement options in the United States. *J Pediatr Endocrinol Metab* 2006;**19**(1):55–64.

131. Shah S, Forghani N, Durham E, Neely EK. A randomized trial of transdermal and oral estrogen therapy in adolescent girls with hypogonadism. *Int J Pediatr Endocrinol* 2014;**2014**(1):12.

132. Klein KO, Rosenfield R, Santen RJ, Gawlik A, Backeljauw P, Gravholt CH, et al. Estrogen replacement in Turner syndrome: literature review and practical considerations. *J Clin Endocrinol Metab* 2018;**103**(5):1790–803.

133. Norjavaara E, Ankarberg-Lindgren C, Kristrom B. Sex steroid replacement therapy in female hypogonadism from childhood to young adulthood. *Endocr Dev* 2016;**29**:198–213.

134. MacGillivray MH. Induction of puberty in hypogonadal children. *J Pediatr Endocrinol Metab* 2004;**17**(Suppl 4):1277–87.

135. Cartwright B, Robinson J, Seed PT, Fogelman I, Rymer J. Hormone replacement therapy versus the combined oral contraceptive pill in premature ovarian failure: a randomized controlled trial of the effects on bone mineral density. *J Clin Endocrinol Metab* 2016;**101**(9):3497–505.

136. Pallais JC, Bo-Abbas Y, Pitteloud N, Crowley Jr WF, Seminara SB. Neuroendocrine, gonadal, placental, and obstetric phenotypes in patients with IHH and mutations in the G-protein coupled receptor, GPR54. *Mol Cell Endocrinol* 2006;**254–255**:70–7.

137. Mumusoglu S, Ata B, Turan V, Demir B, Kahyaoglu I, Aslan K, et al. Does pituitary suppression affect live birth rate in women with congenital hypogonadotrophic hypogonadism undergoing intra-cytoplasmic sperm injection? A multicenter cohort study. *Gynecol Endocrinol* 2017;**33** (9):728–32.

138. Jameson JL, De Groot LJ. *Endocrinology: adult and pediatric*. 7th ed. W.B. Saunders; 2016.

139. Gardner DG, Greenspan FS, Shoback DM. In: David G, editor. *Greenspan's basic & clinical endocrinology*. Gardner and Dolores Shoback; 2018.

140. Petito CK, DeGirolami U, Earle KM. Craniopharyngiomas: a clinical and pathological review. *Cancer* 1976;**37**(4):1944–52.

141. Zacharia BE, Bruce SS, Goldstein H, Malone HR, Neugut AI, Bruce JN. Incidence, treatment and survival of patients with craniopharyngioma in the surveillance, epidemiology and end results program. *Neuro-Oncology* 2012;**14**(8):1070–8.

142. Bunin GR, Surawicz TS, Witman PA, Preston-Martin S, Davis F, Bruner JM. The descriptive epidemiology of craniopharyngioma. *J Neurosurg* 1998;**89**(4):547–51.

143. Brastianos PK, Taylor-Weiner A, Manley PE, Jones RT, Dias-Santagata D, Thorner AR, et al. Exome sequencing identifies BRAF mutations in papillary craniopharyngiomas. *Nat Genet* 2014;**46**(2):161–5.

144. Garnett MR, Puget S, Grill J, Sainte-Rose C. Craniopharyngioma. *Orphanet J Rare Dis* 2007;**2**:18.

145. Muller HL. Childhood craniopharyngioma—current concepts in diagnosis, therapy and follow-up. *Nat Rev Endocrinol* 2010;**6**(11):609–18.

146. Muller HL. Childhood craniopharyngioma. *Pituitary* 2013;**16**(1):56–67.

147. Sughrue ME, Yang I, Kane AJ, Fang S, Clark AJ, Aranda D, et al. Endocrinologic, neurologic, and visual morbidity after treatment for craniopharyngioma. *J Neuro-Oncol* 2011;**101**(3):463–76.

148. Yang I, Sughrue ME, Rutkowski MJ, Kaur R, Ivan ME, Aranda D, et al. Craniopharyngioma: a comparison of tumor control with various treatment strategies. *Neurosurg Focus* 2010;**28**(4).

149. Elowe-Gruau E, Beltrand J, Brauner R, Pinto G, Samara-Boustani D, Thalassinos C, et al. Childhood craniopharyngioma: hypothalamus-sparing surgery decreases the risk of obesity. *J Clin Endocrinol Metab* 2013;**98**(6):2376–82.

150. Daubenbuchel AM, Hoffmann A, Eveslage M, Ozyurt J, Lohle K, Reichel J, et al. Oxytocin in survivors of childhood-onset craniopharyngioma. *Endocrine* 2016;**54**(2):524–31.

151. Gebert D, Auer MK, Stieg MR, Freitag MT, Lahne M, Fuss J, et al. De-masking oxytocin-deficiency in craniopharyngioma and assessing its link with affective function. *Psychoneuroendocrinology* 2018;**88**:61–9.

152. Hoffmann A, Ozyurt J, Lohle K, Reichel J, Thiel CM, Muller HL. First experiences with neuropsychological effects of oxytocin administration in childhood-onset craniopharyngioma. *Endocrine* 2017;**56**(1):175–85.

153. Cook N, Miller J, Hart J. Parent observed neuro-behavioral and pro-social improvements with oxytocin following surgical resection of craniopharyngioma. *J Pediatr Endocrinol Metab* 2016;**29**(8):995–1000.

154. Hsu EA, Miller JL, Perez FA, Roth CL. Oxytocin and naltrexone successfully treat hypothalamic obesity in a boy post-craniopharyngioma resection. *J Clin Endocrinol Metab* 2018;**103**(2):370–5.

155. Molitch ME. Prolactinoma in pregnancy. *Best Pract Res Clin Endocrinol Metab* 2011;**25**(6):885–96.

156. Maniker AH, Krieger AJ. Rapid recurrence of craniopharyngioma during pregnancy with recovery of vision: a case report. *Surg Neurol* 1996;**45**(4):324–7.

157. Aydin Y, Can SM, Gulkilik A, Turkmenoglu O, Alatli C, Ziyal I. Rapid enlargement and recurrence of a preexisting intrasellar craniopharyngioma during the course of two pregnancies. Case report. *J Neurosurg* 1999;**91**(2):322–4.

158. Thapar K, Stefaneanu L, Kovacs K, Scheithauer BW, Lloyd RV, Muller PJ, et al. Estrogen receptor gene expression in craniopharyngiomas: an in situ hybridization study. *Neurosurgery* 1994;**35**(6):1012–7.

159. Honegger J, Renner C, Fahlbusch R, Adams EF. Progesterone receptor gene expression in craniopharyngiomas and evidence for biological activity. *Neurosurgery* 1997;**41**(6):1359–63. discussion 63–4.

160. Volz J, Heinrich U, Volz-Koster S. Conception and spontaneous delivery after total hypophysectomy. *Fertil Steril* 2002;**77**(3):624–5.

161. Shinar S, Many A, Maslovitz S. Questioning the role of pituitary oxytocin in parturition: spontaneous onset of labor in women with panhypopituitarism—a case series. *Eur J Obstet Gynecol Reprod Biol* 2016;**197**:83–5.

162. Jaruratanasirikul S, Thaiwong M. Outcome of gonadotropin-releasing analog treatment for children with central precocious puberty: 15-year experience in southern Thailand. *J Pediatr Endocrinol Metab* 2011;**24**(7–8):519–23.

163. Taylor M, Couto-Silva AC, Adan L, Trivin C, Sainte-Rose C, Zerah M, et al. Hypothalamic-pituitary lesions in pediatric patients: endocrine symptoms often precede neuro-ophthalmic presenting symptoms. *J Pediatr* 2012;**161**(5):855–63.

164. Iannuzzi MC, Rybicki BA, Teirstein AS. Sarcoidosis. *N Engl J Med* 2007;**357**(21):2153–65.

165. Porter N, Beynon HL, Randeva HS. Endocrine and reproductive manifestations of sarcoidosis. *QJM* 2003;**96**(8):553–61.

166. Bullmann C, Faust M, Hoffmann A, Heppner C, Jockenhovel F, Muller-Wieland D, et al. Five cases with central diabetes insipidus and hypogonadism as first presentation of neurosarcoidosis. *Eur J Endocrinol* 2000;**142**(4):365–72.

167. Langrand C, Bihan H, Raverot G, Varron L, Androdias G, Borson-Chazot F, et al. Hypothalamo-pituitary sarcoidosis: a multicenter study of 24 patients. *QJM* 2012;**105**(10):981–95.

168. Bihan H, Christozova V, Dumas JL, Jomaa R, Valeyre D, Tazi A, et al. Sarcoidosis: clinical, hormonal, and magnetic resonance imaging (MRI) manifestations of hypothalamic-pituitary disease in 9 patients and review of the literature. *Medicine (Baltimore)* 2007;**86**(5):259–68.

169. Stuart CA, Neelon FA, Lebovitz HE. Hypothalamic insufficiency: the cause of hypopituitarism in sarcoidosis. *Ann Intern Med* 1978;**88**(5):589–94.

170. Stuart CA, Neelon FA, Lebovitz HE. Disordered control of thirst in hypothalamic-pituitary sarcoidosis. *N Engl J Med* 1980;**303**(19):1078–82.

171. Selroos O. Sarcoidosis and pregnancy: a review with results of a retrospective survey. *J Intern Med* 1990;**227**(4):221–4.

172. Reuhl J, Schneider M, Sievert H, Lutz FU, Zieger G. Myocardial sarcoidosis as a rare cause of sudden cardiac death. *Forensic Sci Int* 1997;**89**(3):145–53.

173. Wallmuller C, Domanovits H, Mayr FB, Laggner AN. Cardiac arrest in a 35-year-old pregnant woman with sarcoidosis. *Resuscitation* 2012;**83**(6):e151–2.

174. Maisel JA, Lynam T. Unexpected sudden death in a young pregnant woman: unusual presentation of neurosarcoidosis. *Ann Emerg Med* 1996;**28**(1):94–7.

175. Haynes de Regt R. Sarcoidosis and pregnancy. *Obstet Gynecol* 1987;**70**(3 Pt 1):369–72.

176. Hadid V, Patenaude V, Oddy L, Abenhaim HA. Sarcoidosis and pregnancy: obstetrical and neonatal outcomes in a population-based cohort of 7 million births. *J Perinat Med* 2015;**43**(2):201–7.

177. Chapelon Abric C, Ginsburg C, Biousse V, Wechsler B, de Gennes C, Darbois Y, et al. Sarcoidosis and pregnancy. A retrospective study of 11 cases. *Rev Med Interne* 1998;**19**(5):305–12.

178. Carpinteri R, Patelli I, Casanueva FF, Giustina A. Pituitary tumours: inflammatory and granulomatous expansive lesions of the pituitary. *Best Pract Res Clin Endocrinol Metab* 2009;**23**(5):639–50.

179. Maria Postini A, del Prever AB, Pagano M, Rivetti E, Berger M, Asaftei SD, et al. Langerhans cell histiocytosis: 40 years' experience. *J Pediatr Hematol Oncol* 2012;**34**(5):353–8.

180. Girschikofsky M, Arico M, Castillo D, Chu A, Doberauer C, Fichter J, et al. Management of adult patients with Langerhans cell histiocytosis: recommendations from an expert panel on behalf of Euro-Histio-Net. *Orphanet J Rare Dis* 2013;**8**:72.

181. Shioda Y, Adachi S, Imashuku S, Kudo K, Imamura T, Morimoto A. Analysis of 43 cases of Langerhans cell histiocytosis (LCH)-induced central diabetes insipidus registered in the JLSG-96 and JLSG-02 studies in Japan. *Int J Hematol* 2011;**94**(6):545–51.

182. Kaltsas GA, Powles TB, Evanson J, Plowman PN, Drinkwater JE, Jenkins PJ, et al. Hypothalamo-pituitary abnormalities in adult patients with langerhans cell histiocytosis: clinical, endocrinological, and radiological features and response to treatment. *J Clin Endocrinol Metab* 2000;**85**(4):1370–6.

183. Makras P, Alexandraki KI, Chrousos GP, Grossman AB, Kaltsas GA. Endocrine manifestations in Langerhans cell histiocytosis. *Trends Endocrinol Metab* 2007;**18**(6):252–7.

184. Makras P, Papadogias D, Kontogeorgos G, Piaditis G, Kaltsas GA. Spontaneous gonadotrophin deficiency recovery in an adult patient with Langerhans cell histiocytosis (LCH). *Pituitary* 2005;**8**(2):169–74.

185. Amato MC, Elias LL, Elias J, Santos AC, Bellucci AD, Moreira AC, et al. Endocrine disorders in pediatric—onset Langerhans cell histiocytosis. *Horm Metab Res* 2006;**38**(11):746–51.

186. DiMaggio LA, Lippes HA, Lee RV. Histiocytosis X and pregnancy. *Obstet Gynecol* 1995;**85**(5 Pt 2):806–9.

187. Fuks L, Kramer MR, Shitrit D, Raviv Y. Pulmonary Langerhans cell histiocytosis and diabetes insipidus in pregnant women: our experience. *Lung* 2014;**192**(2):285–7.

188. Ogburn Jr PL, Cefalo RC, Nagel T, Okagaki T. Histiocytosis X and pregnancy. *Obstet Gynecol* 1981;**58**(4):513–5.

189. Clark A, Houlden RL. Oxytocin deficiency and spontaneous onset of labor and lactation in langerhans cell histiocytosis. *AACE Clinical Case Reports* 2018;**4**(5):e394–7 [September/October 2018].

190. Constine LS, Woolf PD, Cann D, Mick G, McCormick K, Raubertas RF, et al. Hypothalamic-pituitary dysfunction after radiation for brain tumors. *N Engl J Med* 1993;**328**(2):87–94.

191. Lam KS, Wang C, Yeung RT, Ma JT, Ho JH, Tse VK, et al. Hypothalamic hypopituitarism following cranial irradiation for nasopharyngeal carcinoma. *Clin Endocrinol* 1986;**24**(6):643–51.

192. Sathyapalan T, Dixit S. Radiotherapy-induced hypopituitarism: a review. *Expert Rev Anticancer Ther* 2012;**12**(5):669–83.

193. Samaan NA, Bakdash MM, Caderao JB, Cangir A, Jesse Jr RH, Ballantyne AJ. Hypopituitarism after external irradiation. Evidence for both hypothalamic and pituitary origin. *Ann Intern Med* 1975;**83**(6):771–7.

194. Darzy KH. Radiation-induced hypopituitarism. *Curr Opin Endocrinol Diabetes Obes* 2013;**20**(4):342–53.

195. Chemaitilly W, Li Z, Huang S, Ness KK, Clark KL, Green DM, et al. Anterior hypopituitarism in adult survivors of childhood cancers treated with cranial radiotherapy: a report from the St Jude Lifetime Cohort study. *J Clin Oncol* 2015;**33**(5):492–500.

196. Appelman-Dijkstra NM, Kokshoorn NE, Dekkers OM, Neelis KJ, Biermasz NR, Romijn JA, et al. Pituitary dysfunction in adult patients after cranial radiotherapy: systematic review and meta-analysis. *J Clin Endocrinol Metab* 2011;**96**(8):2330–40.

197. Sklar CA, Antal Z, Chemaitilly W, Cohen LE, Follin C, Meacham LR, et al. Hypothalamic-pituitary and growth disorders in survivors of childhood cancer: an endocrine society clinical practice guideline. *J Clin Endocrinol Metab* 2018;**103**(8):2761–84.

198. Krzyzanowska-Mittermayer K, Mattsson AF, Maiter D, Feldt-Rasmussen U, Camacho-Hubner C, Luger A, et al. New neoplasm during GH replacement in adults with pituitary deficiency following malignancy: a KIMS analysis. *J Clin Endocrinol Metab* 2018;**103**(2):523–31.

199. Wo JY, Viswanathan AN. Impact of radiotherapy on fertility, pregnancy, and neonatal outcomes in female cancer patients. *Int J Radiat Oncol Biol Phys* 2009;**73**(5):1304–12.

200. Green DM, Whitton JA, Stovall M, Mertens AC, Donaldson SS, Ruymann FB, et al. Pregnancy outcome of female survivors of childhood cancer: a report from the childhood cancer survivor study. *Am J Obstet Gynecol* 2002;**187**(4):1070–80.

201. Johnston K, Vowels M, Carroll S, Neville K, Cohn R. Failure to lactate: a possible late effect of cranial radiation. *Pediatr Blood Cancer* 2008;**50**(3):721–2.

202. Schreckinger M, Walker B, Knepper J, Hornyak M, Hong D, Kim JM, et al. Post-operative diabetes insipidus after endoscopic transsphenoidal surgery. *Pituitary* 2013;**16**(4):445–51.

203. Capatina C, Paluzzi A, Mitchell R, Karavitaki N. Diabetes insipidus after traumatic brain injury. *J Clin Med* 2015;**4**(7):1448–62.

204. Snow A, Gozal E, Malhotra A, Tiosano D, Perlman R, Vega C, et al. Severe hypersomnolence after pituitary/hypothalamic surgery in adolescents: clinical characteristics and potential mechanisms. *Pediatrics* 2002;**110**(6).

205. Muller HL. Paediatrics: surgical strategy and quality of life in craniopharyngioma. *Nat Rev Endocrinol* 2013;**9**(8):447–9.

206. Zada G, Kintz N, Pulido M, Amezcua L. Prevalence of neurobehavioral, social, and emotional dysfunction in patients treated for childhood craniopharyngioma: a systematic literature review. *PLoS One* 2013;**8**(11).

207. Molitch ME. Drugs and prolactin. *Pituitary* 2008;**11**(2):209–18.

208. Dudas B, Merchenthaler I. Close anatomical associations between beta-endorphin and luteinizing hormone-releasing hormone neuronal systems in the human diencephalon. *Neuroscience* 2004;**124**(1):221–9.

209. Lindow SW, van der Spuy ZM, Hendricks MS, Nugent FA, Dunne TT. The effect of morphine and naloxone administration on maternal oxytocin concentration in late pregnancy. *Clin Endocrinol* 1993;**39**(6):671–5.

210. Broussard CS, Rasmussen SA, Reefhuis J, Friedman JM, Jann MW, Riehle-Colarusso T, et al. Maternal treatment with opioid analgesics and risk for birth defects. *Am J Obstet Gynecol* 2011;**204**(4) 314 e1-11.

211. Devlin LA, Davis JM. A practical approach to neonatal opiate withdrawal syndrome. *Am J Perinatol* 2018;**35**(4):324–30.

212. Saketos M, Sharma N, Santoro NF. Suppression of the hypothalamic-pituitary-ovarian axis in normal women by glucocorticoids. *Biol Reprod* 1993;**49**(6):1270–6.

213. Dubey AK, Plant TM. A suppression of gonadotropin secretion by cortisol in castrated male rhesus monkeys (Macaca mulatta) mediated by the interruption of hypothalamic gonadotropin-releasing hormone release. *Biol Reprod* 1985;**33**(2):423–31.

214. Guller S, Kong L, Wozniak R, Lockwood CJ. Reduction of extracellular matrix protein expression in human amnion epithelial cells by glucocorticoids: a potential role in preterm rupture of the fetal membranes. *J Clin Endocrinol Metab* 1995;**80**(7):2244–50.

215. Ostensen M, Khamashta M, Lockshin M, Parke A, Brucato A, Carp H, et al. Anti-inflammatory and immunosuppressive drugs and reproduction. *Arthritis Res Ther* 2006;**8**(3):209.

216. Ost L, Wettrell G, Bjorkhem I, Rane A. Prednisolone excretion in human milk. *J Pediatr* 1985;**106**(6):1008–11.

217. Leyendecker G, Struve T, Plotz EJ. Induction of ovulation with chronic intermittent (pulsatile) administration of LH-RH in women with hypothalamic and hyperprolactinemic amenorrhea. *Arch Gynecol* 1980;**229**(3):177–90.

218. Leyendecker G, Wildt L. From physiology to clinics—20 years of experience with pulsatile GnRH. *Eur J Obstet Gynecol Reprod Biol* 1996;**65**(Suppl):S3–12.

219. Leyendecker G, Wildt L, Hansmann M. Pregnancies following chronic intermittent (pulsatile) administration of Gn-RH by means of a portable pump ("Zyklomat")—a new approach to the treatment of infertility in hypothalamic amenorrhea. *J Clin Endocrinol Metab* 1980;**51**(5):1214–6.

220. Martin KA, Hall JE, Adams JM, Crowley Jr WF. Comparison of exogenous gonadotropins and pulsatile gonadotropin-releasing hormone for induction of ovulation in hypogonadotropic amenorrhea. *J Clin Endocrinol Metab* 1993;**77**(1):125–9.

221. Mason P, Adams J, Morris DV, Tucker M, Price J, Voulgaris Z, et al. Induction of ovulation with pulsatile luteinising hormone releasing hormone. *Br Med J (Clin Res Ed)* 1984;**288**(6412):181–5.

222. Christou F, Pitteloud N, Gomez F. The induction of ovulation by pulsatile administration of GnRH: an appropriate method in hypothalamic amenorrhea. *Gynecol Endocrinol* 2017;**33**(8):598–601.

223. Wildt L, Hausler A, Marshall G, Hutchison JS, Plant TM, Belchetz PE, et al. Frequency and amplitude of gonadotropin-releasing hormone stimulation and gonadotropin secretion in the rhesus monkey. *Endocrinology* 1981;**109**(2):376–85.

224. Filicori M, Santoro N, Merriam GR, Crowley Jr WF. Characterization of the physiological pattern of episodic gonadotropin secretion throughout the human menstrual cycle. *J Clin Endocrinol Metab* 1986;**62**(6):1136–44.

225. Martin K, Santoro N, Hall J, Filicori M, Wierman M, Crowley Jr. WF. Clinical review 15: management of ovulatory disorders with pulsatile gonadotropin-releasing hormone. *J Clin Endocrinol Metab* 1990;**71**(5). 1081a–g.

226. Letterie GS, Coddington CC, Collins RL, Merriam GR. Ovulation induction using s. c. pulsatile gonadotrophin-releasing hormone: effectiveness of different pulse frequencies. *Hum Reprod* 1996;**11**(1):19–22.

227. Messinis IE. Ovulation induction: a mini review. *Hum Reprod* 2005;**20**(10):2688–97.

228. Christin-Maitre S, de Crecy M. Pregnancy outcomes following pulsatile GnRH treatment: results of a large multicenter retrospective study. *J Gynecol Obstet Biol Reprod (Paris)* 2007;**36**(1):8–12.

229. Tranoulis A, Laios A, Pampanos A, Yannoukakos D, Loutradis D, Michala L. Efficacy and safety of pulsatile gonadotropin-releasing hormone therapy among patients with idiopathic and functional hypothalamic amenorrhea: a systematic review of the literature and a meta-analysis. *Fertil Steril* 2018;**109**(4):708–19. e8.

230. Homburg R, Eshel A, Armar NA, Tucker M, Mason PW, Adams J, et al. One hundred pregnancies after treatment with pulsatile luteinising hormone releasing hormone to induce ovulation. *BMJ* 1989;**298**(6676):809–12.

231. Fauser BC, Devroey P, Macklon NS. Multiple birth resulting from ovarian stimulation for subfertility treatment. *Lancet* 2005;**365**(9473):1807–16.

232. Papanikolaou EG, Pozzobon C, Kolibianakis EM, Camus M, Tournaye H, Fatemi HM, et al. Incidence and prediction of ovarian hyperstimulation syndrome in women undergoing gonadotropin-releasing hormone antagonist in vitro fertilization cycles. *Fertil Steril* 2006;**85**(1):112–20.

233. Abel BS, Shaw ND, Brown JM, Adams JM, Alati T, Martin KA, et al. Responsiveness to a physiological regimen of GnRH therapy and relation to genotype in women with isolated hypogonadotropic hypogonadism. *J Clin Endocrinol Metab* 2013;**98**(2):E206–16.

234. Seminara SB, Beranova M, Oliveira LM, Martin KA, Crowley Jr WF, Hall JE. Successful use of pulsatile gonadotropin-releasing hormone (GnRH) for ovulation induction and pregnancy in a patient with GnRH receptor mutations. *J Clin Endocrinol Metab* 2000;**85**(2):556–62.

235. Schoot DC, Harlin J, Shoham Z, Mannaerts BM, Lahlou N, Bouchard P, et al. Recombinant human follicle-stimulating hormone and ovarian response in gonadotrophin-deficient women. *Hum Reprod* 1994;**9**(7):1237–42.

236. Couzinet B, Lestrat N, Brailly S, Forest M, Schaison G. Stimulation of ovarian follicular maturation with pure follicle-stimulating hormone in women with gonadotropin deficiency. *J Clin Endocrinol Metab* 1988;**66**(3):552–6.

237. Schoot DC, Coelingh Bennink HJ, Mannaerts BM, Lamberts SW, Bouchard P, Fauser BC. Human recombinant follicle-stimulating hormone induces growth of preovulatory follicles without concomitant increase in androgen and estrogen biosynthesis in a woman with isolated gonadotropin deficiency. *J Clin Endocrinol Metab* 1992;**74**(6):1471–3.

238. Shoham Z, Smith H, Yeko T, O'Brien F, Hemsey G, O'Dea L. Recombinant LH (lutropin alfa) for the treatment of hypogonadotrophic women with profound LH deficiency: a randomized, double-blind, placebo-controlled, proof-of-efficacy study. *Clin Endocrinol* 2008;**69**(3):471–8.

239. Kaufmann R, Dunn R, Vaughn T, Hughes G, O'Brien F, Hemsey G, et al. Recombinant human luteinizing hormone, lutropin alfa, for the induction of follicular development and pregnancy in profoundly gonadotrophin-deficient women. *Clin Endocrinol* 2007;**67**(4):563–9.

240. Castellano JM, Navarro VM, Fernandez-Fernandez R, Nogueiras R, Tovar S, Roa J, et al. Changes in hypothalamic KiSS-1 system and restoration of pubertal activation of the reproductive axis by kisspeptin in undernutrition. *Endocrinology* 2005;**146**(9):3917–25.

241. Abbara A, Jayasena CN, Christopoulos G, Narayanaswamy S, Izzi-Engbeaya C, Nijher GM, et al. Efficacy of kisspeptin-54 to trigger oocyte maturation in women at high risk of ovarian hyperstimulation syndrome (OHSS) during In vitro fertilization (IVF) therapy. *J Clin Endocrinol Metab* 2015;**100**(9):3322–31.

242. Jayasena CN, Nijher GM, Abbara A, Murphy KG, Lim A, Patel D, et al. Twice-weekly administration of kisspeptin-54 for 8 weeks stimulates release of reproductive hormones in women with hypothalamic amenorrhea. *Clin Pharmacol Ther* 2010;**88**(6):840–7.

243. Jayasena CN, Nijher GM, Chaudhri OB, Murphy KG, Ranger A, Lim A, et al. Subcutaneous injection of kisspeptin-54 acutely stimulates gonadotropin secretion in women with hypothalamic amenorrhea, but chronic administration causes tachyphylaxis. *J Clin Endocrinol Metab* 2009;**94** (11):4315–23.

244. Young J, George JT, Tello JA, Francou B, Bouligand J, Guiochon-Mantel A, et al. Kisspeptin restores pulsatile LH secretion in patients with neurokinin B signaling deficiencies: physiological, pathophysiological and therapeutic implications. *Neuroendocrinology* 2013;**97**(2):193–202.

245. Chan YM, Lippincott MF, Butler JP, Sidhoum VF, Li CX, Plummer L, et al. Exogenous kisspeptin administration as a probe of GnRH neuronal function in patients with idiopathic hypogonadotropic hypogonadism. *J Clin Endocrinol Metab* 2014;**99**(12):E2762–71.

246. Shimoda M, Iwayama H, Ishiyama M, Nakatani A, Yamashita M. Successful pregnancy by vitrified-warmed embryo transfer for a woman with Kallmann syndrome. *Reprod Med Biol* 2016;**15**(1):45–9.

247. Kuroda K, Ezoe K, Kato K, Yabuuchi A, Segawa T, Kobayashi T, et al. Infertility treatment strategy involving combined freeze-all embryos and single vitrified-warmed embryo transfer during hormonal replacement cycle for in vitro fertilization of women with hypogonadotropic hypogonadism. *J Obstet Gynaecol Res* 2018;**48**(5):922–8.

Chapter 17

Pineal Gland Disorders and Circadian Rhythm Alterations in Pregnancy and Lactation

Ana-Maria Zagrean*, Diana Maria Chitimus*, Francesca Gabriela Paslaru[†], Suzana Elena Voiculescu*, Corin Badiu[‡,§], Gheorghe Peltecu[¶] and Anca Maria Panaitescu[¶]

*Division of Physiology and Neuroscience, Department of Functional Sciences, "Carol Davila" University of Medicine and Pharmacy, Bucharest, Romania, [†]Department of Neurosurgery, "Bagdasar-Arseni" Clinical Emergency Hospital, Bucharest, Romania, [‡]National Institute of Endocrinology "C. I. Parhon", Bucharest, Romania, [§]Department of Endocrinology, "Carol Davila" University of Medicine and Pharmacy, Bucharest, Romania, [¶]Department of Obstetrics and Gynecology, "Carol Davila" University of Medicine and Pharmacy, Filantropia Clinical Hospital, Bucharest, Romania

Common Clinical Problems

- Lesions of the pineal gland are very rarely seen during pregnancy or lactation.
- Serum levels of melatonin are significantly reduced in women with preeclampsia and fetal growth restriction (FGR).
- Maternal chronodisruption and melatonin deficiency are linked to peripartum depression.
- Melatonin is currently being tested in clinical trials to determine if it reduces the incidence of preeclampsia, FGR, and birth asphyxia.

17.1 PINEAL GLAND PATHOLOGY IN PREGNANCY AND LACTATION

Lesions involving the pineal gland are uncommon in the general population and are very rarely seen during pregnancy or lactation. The main clinically relevant lesions of the pineal gland are tumors. However, glial benign cysts and (less frequently) ependymal benign cysts, calcifications, and vascular lesions can occur, resulting in both functional and morphological degradation of pineal tissue.[1, 2]

17.1.1 Pineal Tumors

Tumors of the pineal region are uncommon in adults, accounting for <1% of primary brain tumors[3]; however, they are more frequently encountered in children (3%–8% of cases).[4] The most common subtypes, accounting for 89% of tumors in the pineal region, are germ cell and parenchymal tumors.[5] Pineal gland tumors should be differentiated from tumors arising from adjacent structures, such as astrocytomas and meningiomas, metastases, and tumorlike conditions such as vascular malformations, cysts, and cysticercosis.

Of the pineal gland tumors, 65%–72% are germinomas and occur primarily in males; therefore, their impact on pregnancy is less well understood and investigated. Pineal region tumors can be classified as germ cell tumors (about 60%), parenchymal tumors (about 30%), and tumors of adjacent structures (about 10%), as well as rare forms of nonneoplastic conditions (<1%) and metastases (<0.1%).[6]

Malignant germ cell tumors can be germinomas and nongerminomas (i.e., choriocarcinoma, teratoma, yolk sac tumor, embryonal carcinoma). A classification based on the embryological origin and histological type of pineal tumors is shown in Table 17.1.

Clinical features of pineal tumors are related to their anatomic location and are caused by either direct invasion or compression during tumor enlargement. Parinaud's syndrome (upward gaze paralysis) is considered pathognomonic for pineal region lesions. Compression of the cerebral aqueduct can cause noncommunicating hydrocephalus (Figs. 17.1 and 17.2).[7] Growing masses in the pineal region can cause diminished melatonin secretion, with low serum melatonin levels and alterations of day/night variation.[7a]

Maternal-Fetal and Neonatal Endocrinology. https://doi.org/10.1016/B978-0-12-814823-5.00017-9

TABLE 17.1 Classification of pineal tumors

Classification	Subtypes
Pineal glandular tissue	Papillary tumor Pineocytoma Tumor of intermediate differentiation Pineoblastoma
Germ cell origin	Germinoma
	Nongerminomatous germ cell tumors (NGGCTs)[a] Embryonal carcinoma Teratoma Endodermal sinus tumor (yolk sac tumor) Choriocarcinoma
Glial	Astrocytoma Glioblastoma Oligodendroglioma Medulloepithelioma
Nonneoplastic	Pineal cysts Arachnoid cyst Cavernomas Aneurysms of the Galen vein Cysticercosis
Other	Meningioma Ependymoma Choroid plexus papilloma Chemodectoma Craniopharyngioma Hemangioma Hemangiopericytoma Hemangioblastoma Metastases

[a]*Also called nonseminomatous germ cell tumors (NSGCTs).*
Modified after Matula C. Tumors of the pineal region. In: Principles of neurological surgery. Elsevier; 2012. p. 565–84.

In pregnant women, pineal tumors tend to occur with a similar frequency as in age-matched, nonpregnant women.[8] The rate of tumor growth determines the symptoms that occur: headache (most frequent), nausea, vomiting, and visual changes, primarily due to mass effect. These symptoms are quite common in pregnancy, where they could indicate pregnancy-specific complications such as hyperemesis gravidarum or preeclampsia; hence, a correct diagnosis may be delayed. With severe, prolonged headaches, especially in association with visual disturbances or neurological signs, an intracranial mass can be suspected.

The recommended imaging technique in the case of suspicion of an intracranial mass is magnetic resonance imaging (MRI) because it does not utilize ionizing radiation and is considered safe for both mother and fetus. Gadolinium, which is frequently required when examining intracranial masses, crosses the placenta and can cause fetal kidney injury, but it is not associated with teratogenic effects. The use of gadolinium contrast with MRI should be limited but may be used as a contrast agent in a pregnant woman if it significantly improves diagnostic performance and is expected to improve fetal or maternal outcomes. Breastfeeding should not be interrupted after gadolinium administration.[9]

Pineal tumors can be locally invasive, and they can disseminate through the cerebrospinal fluid (CSF) on leptomeningeal membranes. Tumors arising from germ cells (particularly teratomas and germinomas) produce human chorionic gonadotropin (hCG), which is released into the CSF.[7] In rare cases, due to the identical structure of beta-hCG and beta-luteinizing hormone (beta-LH), the pineal tumor triggers central precocious puberty[10]; it is even more rare for this to happen in pregnancy.[7]

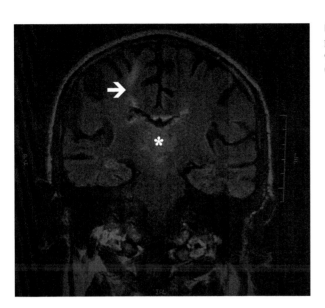

FIG. 17.1 Coronal T1-weighted MRI scan showing a mass situated in the pineal region *(asterisk)* that is compressing the cerebral aqueduct and causing obstructive hydrocephalus. It is treated using ventriculoperitoneal drainage *(arrow). (Courtesy of Professor Radu Mircea Gorgan.)*

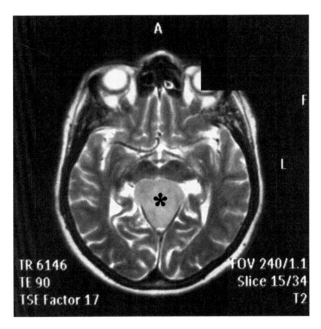

FIG. 17.2 Transverse T2-weighted MRI scan showing a pineal tumor *(asterisk)* that is causing noncommunicating hydrocephalus. *(Courtesy of Dr. George Vasilescu.)*

17.1.1.1 Pineal Parenchymal Tumors

Pineal parenchymal tumors can be pineocytomas, tumors of intermediate differentiation, pineoblastomas, or papillary tumors. Pineocytomas account for 45% of tumors originating in the pineal parenchyma. They are benign, are classified as grade I tumors by the World Health Organization (WHO), and usually occur between 25 and 35 years. They are rounded tumors that grow slowly, usually have a diameter under 3 cm, and are homogenous, less invasive, well delineated, and hypointense to isointense on T1 and hyperintense on T2 as shown via MRI. Clinically, they can present a hydrocephalus that progresses slowly as a result of the aqueduct obstruction. Within the tumor matrix, degenerative changes may be observed, such as calcifications, hemorrhagic areas, or cysts.

Pineoblastomas, classified as grade IV (WHO), are larger, highly malignant lesions representing a type of primitive neuroectodermal tumors. Dissemination through CSF has been reported as between 8% and 24%.[6]

17.1.1.2 Pineal Glial Tumors

Glial tumors arising from the tectal plate are characterized by a benign nature and a periaqueductal location. These lesions are found in patients younger than 25 years old and cause noncommunicating hydrocephalus by compressing the cerebral aqueduct.[11]

A staging workup includes a cerebral and spinal MRI scan, as well as assays of blood and CSF tumor markers: alpha fetoprotein for yolk sac tumors and hCG for choriocarcinoma. In pregnant patients, physiologically elevated levels of beta-hCG limit the use of this marker. Diagnosis of germ cell tumors can be established using only tumor markers.[12]

17.1.1.3 Therapeutic Approaches

A pineal gland tumor during pregnancy represents a challenge to both the neurosurgeon and obstetrician and requires a multidisciplinary care approach. Specific pregnancy care should be performed as usual; however, there should be a close collaboration among the surgeon, oncologist, and neurologist.

17.1.1.3.1 Surgical Therapeutic Intervention

Surgical treatment is rarely required during pregnancy, but when needed, it is best performed during the second trimester.[9] The neurosurgical approach is challenging because the pineal region is deeply located, with important vascular structures situated nearby. However, recent advances in microneurosurgery, anaesthesiology, stereotactic procedures, and neuroendoscopic techniques offer the opportunity to treat lesions in the pineal region with acceptable outcomes during the second trimester. After obtaining a tumor sample, immunocytochemistry can be used for identifying the tumor type, including the use of staining for alpha fetoprotein, beta subunit of hCG, and placental alkaline phosphatase. Gross tumor resection may be postponed according to the histological subtype until after delivery; therefore, biopsy should precede other treatments.

Surgical removal of pineal parenchyma, along with primary pineal tumors or tumors invading the pineal gland (pinealectomy), can cause low serum levels of melatonin and alterations of circadian rhythms, in addition to the already-diminished secretion of melatonin caused by the tumor.[7a] Stereotactic radiosurgery (using a gamma knife or cyberknife) can be used to treat pineal region tumors, either as the primary method or after conventional treatments have been used.

17.1.1.3.2 Chemotherapy

High-grade gliomas, pineoblastomas, and germ cell tumors require craniospinal irradiation and chemotherapy, either as the primary treatment option or as adjuvant therapy after surgical resection.[12] The administration of cytotoxic drugs during the first trimester is particularly dangerous because of its association with malformations, embryo death, and spontaneous abortion. The risk of malformations is cited as around 15% when a single-agent treatment is used and increases to 25% in cases of combination therapy. After 14 weeks of pregnancy, when organogenesis has finished, the influence of chemotherapy on fetal and child outcomes is significantly lower: the risk of malformations has not been explicitly demonstrated, but there is a higher risk of preterm birth and FGR. The relatively good tolerance of the fetus to maternal chemotherapy is partially explained by less exposure to the cytotoxic therapy compared to the mother. Also, no differences in growth and general development have been found between children of women who received chemotherapy during pregnancy and healthy controls.[13] Ideally, the last chemotherapy session in pregnancy should be planned 1–2 weeks before the expected time of delivery (labor induction or cesarean section).

17.1.1.4 Mode of Delivery in Patients with Pineal Tumors

While definitive therapy for pineal gland masses may be delayed until the postpartum period, the mode of delivery in affected patients must be considered. In healthy pregnant women, the intracranial pressure (ICP) increases with 33 cm of water (H_2O) in the first stage of labor, and with 70 cm H_2O in the second stage.[14] The accentuation during the second stage can be attributed not only to increasing Valsalva pressure with pushing, but also to spontaneous uterine contractions. An induced increase in intracranial pressure in a patient with an elevated baseline ICP can lead to rapid neurologic decline and cerebral herniation.[15] In patients with intracranial masses, delivery via cesarean section must be taken into consideration. Also, epidural anesthesia is generally considered risky, but it is not absolutely contraindicated[16] in patients with intracranial mass because of the associated morbidity from possible cerebral herniation due to a wet tap.

In summary, aggressive pineal area tumors rarely appear in women. The presence of a pineal region tumor is an even rarer event in pregnancy, but it requires a multidisciplinary approach with special restrictive management criteria (imaging and treatment) related to the fetus.

17.1.2 Pineal Cysts

In adults, pineal cysts are common neuroradiological findings via brain MRI (1%–10%),[17] and they are slightly more frequent in women. It is considered borderline between a normal anatomical variant and a pathological lesion. When viewed via MRI, a pineal cyst has low signal intensity on T1-weighted images compared to white matter, and has the same intensity as CSF on T2-weighted images, with round and smooth margins and a gadolinium-enhancing rim that is <2mm thick. Sometimes pineal cysts can be multilocular, with incomplete FLAIR signal suppression or septation of the internal structure, while cysts found in other organs tend to have a simpler structure.[18, 19] Most pineal cysts are asymptomatic and stable over time, with only 6% being reported to increase in size.[20] They can also present with nonspecific symptoms, such as headache, nausea, vertigo, and sleep disturbances, which are difficult to correlate to the presence of the cyst. Asymptomatic cysts do not need surgical treatment; the advised management is periodic clinical and radiological follow-up. Large cysts are very rarely encountered, but if causing mass effects, stenosis of the cerebral aqueduct with hydrocephalus, or compression of the tectum, causing Parinaud syndrome, then such patients should be straightforward candidates for resection. Also, surgery can be considered for cysts that are confirmed to be increasing in size.[21] Cysts smaller than 20mm in diameter are not likely to cause complications, and size alone should not be used as a reason to operate.[20]

The incidence of pineal cysts during pregnancy remains unknown, especially because these lesions are usually asymptomatic and rarely observed. Pineal cysts are an uncommon cause of complications during pregnancy or labor. Also, pregnancy does not seem to affect the naturally benign behavior of cysts found in the pineal gland[22] (Fig. 17.3).

17.1.3 Pineal Calcifications

Physiologic pineal gland calcifications, also called *brain sand, corpora arenacea,* or *acervuli,* are deposits of calcium and magnesium in the pineal gland, more frequently encountered in adults (Fig. 17.4). Benign calcifications should be differentiated from tumoral calcifications, pathologic metabolic calcifications, and hemorrhage. Isolated calcifications are

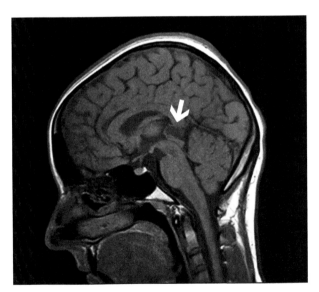

FIG. 17.3 Sagittal T1-weighted MRI scan showing a pineal cyst *(arrow)* discovered 4 months postpartum in a 28-year-old woman with an 8-year history of headache. *(Courtesy of Dr. Alexandru Papacocea.)*

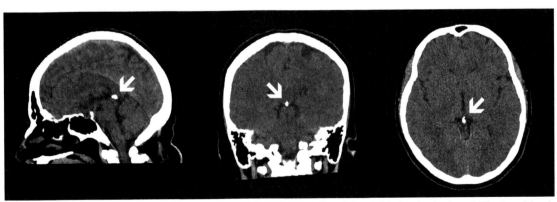

FIG. 17.4 Computed tomography (CT) scan in sagittal, coronal, and axial sections (from *left* to *right*), showing benign calcification of the pineal gland *(arrows). (Courtesy of Professor Radu Mircea Gorgan.)*

usually considered benign, while those associated with glandular enlargement can be suggestive of neoplasia.[19, 23] In younger patients, calcifications are found near pinealocytes and appear to be globular, while calcifications in older patients seem to be located near glial cells and to have a more concentric aspect.[24]

The available data in the literature suggest that calcification is more of an organized process than a passive phenomenon, but an association with dysfunction of the pineal gland has not been established.[23]

17.1.4 Pineal Vascular Lesions

Some infrequent nonneoplastic conditions that may appear in the pineal region are vascular malformations, such as cavernomas malformations of the vein of Galen, and arteriovenous malformations. These lesions are technically demanding to remove because of their deep location and risk of hemorrhage.

Cavernous malformations, also called *cavernous angiomas* or *cavernomas*, are clusters of capillarylike vascular channels, without intervening neural parenchyma, with sizes varying from 1 mm to a few centimeters in diameter. These benign lesions occur in the central nervous system, more frequently in the intracranial supratentorial area. The pineal region is a particularly rare location for cavernomas, with the risk of being misdiagnosed as germinoma, pineocytoma, pineoblastoma, or even being missed altogether. Signs and symptoms caused by cavernomas in the pineal region are usually due to the obstructive hydrocephalus, with increased intracranial pressure. Radical neurosurgical resection is the gold standard for treating these symptoms. Partial resection carries the risk of repeated subarachnoid hemorrhage. Considering the risks carried by general anesthesia and the complexity of the neurosurgical procedure, these lesions could be treated in pregnant patients using ventricular drainage until delivery.[25–27]

Malformations of the vein of Galen, usually diagnosed during childhood, are arteriovenous malformations with feeders from the choroidal system and drainage into the vein of Markowski (median prosencephalic vein). Clinical presentation can consist of headache, seizures, or subarachnoid hemorrhage. Asymptomatic lesions should also be treated because of the risk of cerebral sequelae, including subependymal atrophy and strokes with cortico-subcortical atrophy. Endovascular embolization techniques represent the gold standard in treating Galen's vein malformations.[28] In pregnant patients, treatment of asymptomatic lesions should be postponed until delivery, but associated risks should also be considered.

Arteriovenous malformations in the pineal region (Figs. 17.5 and 17.6) are rare vascular anomalies in the tectal region, with feeders such as tectal and circumferential arteries from the vertebrobasilar system, as well as drainage through tectal vein and superior cerebellar vein into the straight sinus. Because of the functional neural tissue related to the lesion, microsurgical resection requires a complex technique. A multimodal treatment can be used for pineal-region arteriovenous malformation and other deep-seated arteriovenous malformations involving microsurgery, embolization, and radiosurgery.[28] Due to the benign nature of the lesion and the complexity of the treatment strategies, treating arteriovenous malformations in the pineal region should be postponed until delivery.

FIG. 17.5 Coronal T1-weighted MRI scan showing a large arteriovenous malformation situated in the pineal region *(arrow). (Courtesy of Dr. George Vasilescu.)*

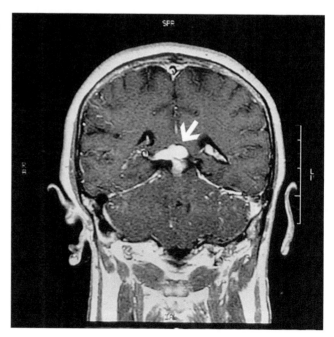

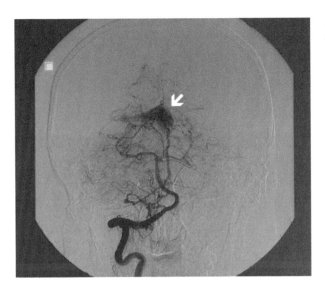

FIG. 17.6   Digital subtraction angiography (DSA) showing an arteriovenous malformation in the pineal region *(arrow). (Courtesy of Dr. George Vasilescu.)*

17.2   MELATONIN DEFICIENCY IN PREGNANCY AND LACTATION

17.2.1   Oxidative Stress

Oxidative stress is associated with various reproductive complications, among which miscarriage, preeclampsia, FGR, and preterm labor are of interest. Free radicals are classified according to the type of atom that is present in the radical center. The main species are reactive oxygen species (ROS), reactive nitrogen species (RNS), and reactive sulfur species (RSS). Consequently, the activity of each of these radicals depends on its chemical structure.[29] Their physiological function is related to cell signaling pathways; however, if present in excess concentrations, cellular proteins, lipids, and deoxyribonucleic acid (DNA) may be damaged by their actions. Antioxidants such as melatonin limit peroxidation reactions and thus cellular damage.[30]

Previously published studies support the importance of oxidative stress as a main stressor in placental disease.[31] During normal placental differentiation, the gene expression and activity of antioxidant enzymes increase in direct proportion with the oxygen tension,[31] while the loss of these antioxidant mechanisms[32] is correlated with the pathophysiology of early pregnancy loss.[33]

Aside from the increased miscarriage risk, preeclampsia has been associated with a significant increase in mitochondrial protein in placental samples compared to the normotensive controls,[34] which is relevant because of the role of the mitochondria in generating ROS. Lipid peroxides are formed in the placenta due to membrane disruption by ROS, and studies have shown significantly higher markers of lipid peroxidation in preeclampsia.[35, 36]

Up to 4% of the inhaled O_2 follows the path of the chemical reactions (Fig. 17.7) that lead to the formation of the free radicals and other compounds that can impair the reproductive system.[37]

Reduction of O_2 results in the formation of superoxide anion radical (O_2-), that either couples with nitric oxide to produce peroxynitrite anion ($ONOO^-$), or is metabolized by superoxide dismutase (SOD) to form hydrogen peroxide (H_2O_2). H_2O_2 is transformed to the hydroxyl radical ($\bullet OH$) in the presence of iron or other transition metals.

Another path that generates ROS is the conversion of O_2 to singlet oxygen ($^1O_2$), a less common but toxic species. Of all free radicals, OH and $ONOO^-$ create the greatest amount of cellular damage, while H_2O_2 is metabolized to nontoxic species.[37]

Access to the main sources of free radical generation, particularly the mitochondria and its speculated production inside the mitochondria,[38] supports melatonin potential to neutralize oxidative stress. Besides melatonin, several of its metabolites that result from the chemical interactions between melatonin and free radicals [i.e., cyclic 3-hydroxymelatonin, N^1-acetyl-N^2-formyl-5-methoxy-kynuramine (AFMK), N^1-acetyl-5-methoxykynuramine (AMK), etc.] can act as radical scavengers.[39, 40]

At physiological concentrations, melatonin has been shown to increase the messenger ribonucleic acid (mRNA) expression of both superoxide dismutase (SOD) and glutathione peroxidase (GPx). Its effect is supposedly mediated by a de novo synthesis of protein and involves the modulation of mRNA stability for Cu-Zn SOD and GPx in neuron cell cultures.[41] In humans, the ability of melatonin to prevent the downregulation of antioxidative enzymes was shown after exposing skin cells to ultraviolet (UV) radiation by Fisher et al.[42]

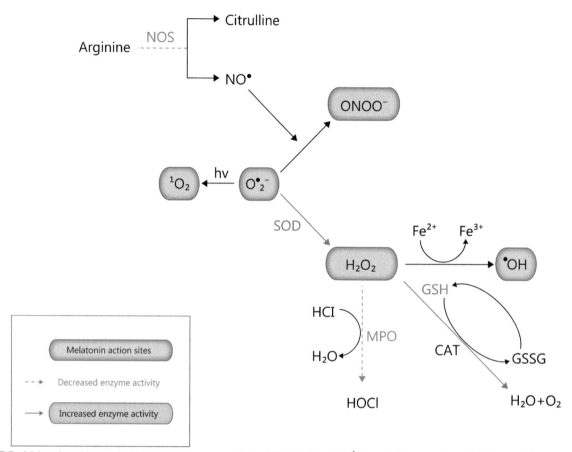

FIG. 17.7 Melatonin and its metabolites are useful scavengers for the $ONOO^-$, O_2^-, H_2O_2, $^1O_2$, and •OH. Its role in modulating oxidative-stress related enzymes is displayed as either stimulatory *(continuous arrows)* for SOD and the increased production of GSH or inhibitory for NOS and MPO. Abbreviations: *CAT*, catalase; *GSH*, glutathione; *GSSG*, glutathione disulfide; *HOCl*, hypochlorous acid; *MPO*, myeloperoxidase; *NOS*, nitric oxide synthase. *(Adapted after Reiter RJ, Tan DX, Korkmaz A, Rosales-Corral SA. Melatonin and stable circadian rhythms optimize maternal, placental and fetal physiology.* Hum Reprod Update *2014;20(2):293–307.)*

17.2.2 Chronodisruption

As Erren and Reiter suggested, defining chronodisruption can link disturbances in the circadian rhythm to a diversity of pathological conditions. Chronodisruption is a "relevant disturbance of the circadian organization of physiology, endocrinology, metabolism, and behavior, with melatonin being a key biological intermediary."[43] To better understand the ethology of chronodisruption, several agents have been identified as chronodisruptors: light exposure during nighttime, melatonin applied at unusual times, as well as nocturnal food intake and physical stress.[43]

The influence of the circadian timing system on hormonal fluctuations in human pregnancy and lactation has not been extensively investigated. Women who work in night shifts have a significantly lower melatonin peak level during the night, while also displaying lower prolactin levels.[44] These hormonal imbalances might contribute to the increased risk of preterm birth, low birth weight, and miscarriage in women who experience desynchronization of the sleep-wake cycle during pregnancy.[45]

17.2.2.1 Chronodisruption During Pregnancy

In rats, melatonin deprivation during gestation caused impaired behavior, with long-term effects on the cognitive functions of the fetus.[46] Exogenous administration of melatonin increased the levels of melatonin in the maternal circulation, which was shown to be neuroprotective for the fetal brain.[47]

Chronodisruption resulting from night-shift work and jet lag leads to a decrease in the nocturnal melatonin peak.[44] Abnormalities in circadian rhythms are associated with the development of mood disorders such as bipolar disorder, major depression, and seasonal affective disorder.[48, 49] Thus, these are strong indications that circadian rhythm alterations may contribute to mood disorders in pregnant women.

Depression during pregnancy is reported in up to 10% of pregnant women.[50] In addition to the abovementioned chronodisruptors, poor sleep quality is associated with increased risk of depression.[51]

During late pregnancy, sleep deprivation becomes chronic and insomnia can occur, contributing to disruptions in circadian rhythms and clinical depression.[52] Sleep deprivation is also associated[50] with prolonged labor duration and increased probability of cesarean section.[53]

Identifying a link between low melatonin concentrations due to chronodisruption and peripartum depression is important because it may point to alternative treatments for pregnant women who are not amenable to antidepressant medications or psychotherapy. Moreover, such treatments might prevent adverse birth outcomes in children who have been exposed to maternal depression during pregnancy, such as cognitive, emotional, and behavioral problems.[54]

Usually, plasma melatonin levels increase in late gestation[55]; by comparison, this pattern was not found in depressed pregnant women.[56] In addition, pregnant women with personal and family histories of depression displayed significantly lower levels and phased-advanced melatonin rhythms (shifted earlier) relative to women without a history of depression.[57]

Various therapeutic strategies were developed on the assumption that abnormal circadian rhythmicity and depression have a pathophysiological link. Protocols have been established to expose pregnant women with depression to morning bright-light therapy,[58] which should pose no risks for the unborn child.

Women who are at risk for antepartum depression are believed to be more prone to phase alterations in melatonin and cortisol timing during seasons with longer nights. Longer darkness is correlated with a shorter melatonin synthesis duration, compared to shorter periods of darkness exposure.[59] Studies have shown that depressed pregnant women respond anomalously to seasonal changes in darkness, and that antepartum depression is reduced in women exposed to morning light.[58, 60]

The cause for maternal depression is not known, but it has been linked to hypothalamus-pituitary-adrenal (HPA) axis malfunction, and more specifically to reduced inhibition by cortisol due to impaired glucocorticoid receptor function.[61] The suprachiasmatic nucleus (SCN; the biological clock) controls the HPA axis: decreased inhibitory control of the SCN on the HPA axis has been shown to be associated with HPA-axis hyperactivity.[62] Several studies have shown changes in melatonin secretion in psychiatric diseases such as depression.[63]

Another lead regarding a pathophysiological link between melatonin and depression through chronodisruption is the association between plasma tryptophan during pregnancy and poor sleep quality. Tryptophan is involved in both brain serotonin and melatonin availability, and it also influences sleep latency.[64] A lower risk of antenatal poor sleep quality was associated with higher plasma tryptophan concentrations measured at 26–28 weeks' gestation, particularly in subjects who also manifested anxiety.[65]

In addition to depression during pregnancy increasing the risk of severe outcomes on the fetus, there are risks for the depressive future mother. It has been shown that prepartum psychiatric illness itself is a risk factor for the development of postpartum mood disorders. Andersson et al. reported that depression, anxiety, or both were present in 29.2% of pregnant women, as opposed to 16.5% of postpartum women.[66] The factors that were most predictive for postpartum depression included antenatal depression and a previous positive history of postpartum depression.[67]

We speculate that low melatonin levels in depressed pregnant women might compromise their ability to regulate their circadian rhythms. After pregnancy, this may lead to ongoing desyncronization of circadian rhythms that may predispose to future depressive mood changes.[68]

17.2.2.2 *Chronodisruption During Lactation*

Human lactation is a complex phenomenon, and the process of initiation and duration is influenced by many variables. Depression or mood changes, night-eating syndrome, and sleep disturbances are known chronodisruptors that can lead to hormonal and metabolic alterations.[69]

In rodents, it has been shown that disruption of the circadian system decreases a dam's ability to initiate milk production. In humans, this could cause a delay in the onset of lactogenesis after delivery to >72h postpartum.

As discussed in more detail in Chapter 14, lactogenesis occurs in several stages. The first stage occurs during pregnancy and includes preparatory changes for synthesis in the mammary glands, while the second stage begins after delivery and is the time of initiation of the milk secretion. This stage is controlled by coordinated changes in hormones and metabolism so that the milk production starts properly in the early postpartum period. Thus, chronic disruption of the maternal circadian timing system during pregnancy and peripartum might alter hormones and metabolic adaptations, resulting in a delayed postpartum onset of lactogenesis.[69]

17.2.3 Impact on Fertility

Melatonin works in a variety of ways, as a circadian rhythm modulator, endocrine modulator, immunomodulator, direct free-radical scavenger, and indirect antioxidant and cytoprotective agent in human pregnancy. It may be essential for successful pregnancy.

Melatonin concentrations are increased in male infertility and hypogonadotrophic hypogonadism, but it increases in response to stress-induced amenorrhea as well.[70] In addition, exogenous melatonin administration suppresses LH levels in both men and women.

In female sheep, melatonin deficiency adversely affects follicle and corpus luteum growth, decreases the luteal cells' production of progesterone, and causes a low plasma antioxidant capacity,[71] with important effects on fertility and during pregnancy and lactation. In women, high melatonin levels are present in both primary and secondary hypothalamic amenorrhea, and these findings may reflect a causal relationship between high melatonin concentrations and hypothalamic-pituitary-gonadal (HPG) hypofunction.[72]

Infertility is defined as not being able to conceive after 1 year of a couple actively trying. It is a very common condition, affecting approximately 15% of reproductive-age women. Assisted reproductive technology (ART) is widely used to treat this condition.[73]

Oral administration of melatonin has been shown by some studies to improve fertilization rates in couples undertaking ART for conception, an effect potentially attributable to melatonin's oxygen-scavenging abilities that may reduce intrafollicular oxidative damage.[74] In interventional studies, oral supplementation of melatonin during the ovarian stimulation phase of in vitro fertilization (IVF) protocols has been shown to improve gamete and embryo quality.[75] However, in a recent systematic review and metaanalysis of five randomized controlled trials (RCTs) involving melatonin supplementation during controlled ovarian stimulation for women undergoing ART, the authors concluded that the potential benefits of melatonin on the most important reproductive outcomes (namely, live birth, miscarriage, ovarian hyperstimulation syndrome, and congenital abnormalities) remain uncertain. Melatonin supplementation during ovarian stimulation did not reduce the chances of clinical pregnancy and the number of oocytes retrieved; it was uncertain whether there was any benefit or no effect at all. Adding melatonin to myoinositol folic acid was considered unlikely to cause a relevant change in the number of oocytes retrieved. The authors concluded that larger studies investigating the role of melatonin in improving ART outcomes are required.[73]

The potential reproductive effects of melatonin also may extend to the male partner, with melatonin receptors being demonstrated in spermatozoa. Melatonin is considered to improve sperm quality and decrease sperm cell apoptosis.[76] Given the wide distribution of melatonin receptors in the testis (including in Leydig and Sertoli cells, prostate cells, and even spermatozoa), sperm quality and production may be modulated by melatonin. During the summer months, when the days are longer, sperm count and motility are significantly decreased,[77] which may indicate that melatonin improves spermatogenesis parameters. In vitro supplementation of embryo culture media with melatonin also has a significant impact on the development and quality of embryos, with lower concentrations of melatonin being more beneficial than higher levels.

17.2.4 Risk of Miscarriage and Preterm Birth

Some studies suggest that deficient pineal melatonin production in early pregnancy may be causally related to the development of spontaneous abortion. Spontaneous abortion before 20 weeks of gestation is estimated to occur in 15%–20% of identified pregnancies, and the frequency increases with age. The causes can be divided into two main categories: those arising from chromosomal anomalies, and those arising from abnormalities in the intrauterine environment. The proposition that melatonin could be involved is based on the findings that melatonin is a free-radical scavenger and antioxidant; plasma melatonin levels normally increase during pregnancy; pinealectomy increases the frequency of spontaneous abortions in pregnant rats;[78] melatonin has immunomodulatory effects; melatonin stimulates the secretion of progesterone, which reduces uterine contractility and prevents immunological rejection of the trophoblast; and melatonin inhibits the synthesis of prostaglandins, which are potent inducers of uterine contractility and labor. Melatonin prevented experimentally induced preterm labor and increased offspring survival in mice.[79] However, the potential clinical utility of melatonin to prevent preterm labor has not been studied.

17.2.5 Preeclampsia/Eclampsia and FGR

Melatonin levels are altered in women with abnormally functioning placentas during preeclampsia and FGR. Preeclampsia, defined by new-onset hypertension developing after 20 weeks' gestation alongside maternal end-organ dysfunction, is a condition specific to human pregnancy that can involve every organ or system.[80] It is one of the leading causes of maternal mortality and morbidity in pregnancy, and it is an important cause of fetal morbidity because of its need for iatrogenic preterm delivery. Currently, delivery is the only cure for preeclampsia.

The exact pathogenesis of preeclampsia is unknown, but it is likely multifactorial, involving a complex interplay between the mother, fetus, and the placenta. In preeclamspia, there is defective placentation, with abnormal invasion and remodeling of the spiral arteries.[81] Reduced perfusion of the placenta causes oxidative stress, which in turn triggers the release of trophoblast-derived factors (e.g., SFLT-1, soluble endoglin), which enter the maternal circulation to cause endothelial cell damage in the kidneys, liver, lungs, brain, and placenta, as well as an exaggerated inflammatory response with generalized endothelial dysfunction.[82] Serum levels of melatonin are significantly reduced in women with preeclampsia and FGR, and the reduction in melatonin is not associated with the severity or time onset of preeclampsia, or with seasonal variations.[55, 83] Also, the expression of the melatonin receptor MT1 is reduced in preeclamptic placentas.[83]

Melatonin's putative effects as an antioxidant and free-radical scavenger, as well as its perceived safety for administration during pregnancy, make it a candidate for the prevention and treatment of preeclamspia.[84] It easily crosses the placenta, which expresses receptors for melatonin. In a xanthine/xanthine oxidase (X/XO) placental explant model, melatonin was shown to reduce oxidative stress and enhance antioxidant markers, but it did not affect explant production of antiangiogenic factors (e.g., sFlt, soluble endoglin).[84] In primary trophoblast cell cultures, melatonin treatment increased the expression of antioxidant enzymes and reduced the production of sFLT-1.[85] In cultured human umbilical vein endothelial cells, melatonin mitigated tumor necrosis factor-alpha (TNF-α)-induced vascular cell adhesion molecule expression, and also rescued the subsequent disruption to endothelial monolayer integrity, but it did not affect other markers for endothelial activation and dysfunction.

One clinical trial has examined the utility of melatonin in the treatment of established preeclampsia.[84] In this trial, 20 pregnant women with a diagnosis of early preeclampsia received 10mg of melatonin three times daily from a median gestational age of 28 weeks until delivery was required for either fetal or maternal conditions. Compared to matched historical controls, in those treated with melatonin, there was a prolongation of pregnancy by about 6days, as well as a reduction in antihypertensive treatments needed by the mother.[84] These effects are promising, but more extensive, well-designed, randomized, double-blind, and placebo-controlled trials are required to confirm whether melatonin is beneficial for the treatment of preeclampsia.

Intrauterine FGR develops when there is chronic placental dysfunction. It is associated with increased risks of iatrogenic preterm birth and neurodevelopmental problems, including motor and sensory deficits, cognitive and learning difficulties, and cerebral palsy. Both placental metabolism and transport may be affected, thus modifying the normal supply of nutrients to the fetus. With chronic placental dysfunction, there is also intrauterine hypoxia and an increase in the oxidative stress within the placenta with ROS generation.[86]

The use of melatonin as an antenatal antioxidant agent to reduce oxidative stress within a dysfunctional placenta has been proposed and tested in animal studies. In human pregnancies, a pilot phase I clinical trial testing the safety and efficacy of melatonin was conducted by Miller et al. It included six pregnancies affected by severe early FGR with a median gestational age at study inclusion of 27 weeks. Melatonin was administered at a dose of 4mg twice daily in a prolonged release form. Compared to placentas from an historical control matched for diagnosis and gestational age, oxidative stress was significantly reduced in women treated with melatonin, as reflected by malondialdehyde levels.[87]

Intrauterine fetal growth retardation and prematurity in human infants have been associated with delay in melatonin secretion after the first 3months of life.[88, 89] Moreover, 6-sulfatoxymelatonin (6SaMT), a urinary melatonin metabolite, is reduced in adults who were either growth restricted prenatally or born after 40weeks of gestation.[88] Urinary excretion of 6SaMT suggests that there is a relationship between melatonin production and body size at birth.

Melatonin has been proposed to increase blood flow in umbilical arterial blood by increasing nitric oxide bioavailability[90] and stimulating a bradykinin-induced relaxation.[91] More insight will be gained on the effects of melatonin for intrauterine growth restriction after the results of the ongoing trials become available. These studies are summarized in the next section.

17.3 POTENTIAL CLINICAL UTILITY OF MELATONIN IN DISORDERS OF PREGNANCY AND LACTATION

17.3.1 Melatonin in Clinical Trials

Melatonin has been touted as a molecule with "virtual absence of toxicity"[92] and great potential for use in human medicine, due to its ability to contribute to improved cellular physiology. It has been used in clinical trials outside of pregnancy and has proved effective for reducing and preventing jet lag[93] and reducing specific behavioral disturbances associated with dementia (i.e., psychopathologic behaviors).[94] In studies on newborns, melatonin was shown to reduce indicators of oxidative stress and improve clinical outcomes in babies with septicemia.[95] Also, for newborns with birth asphyxia, melatonin has been shown to reduce the concentrations of products associated with oxidative stress and damage.[96] To date, there have been 12 registered clinical trials during pregnancy and lactation involving either exogenous administration of melatonin or the use of phototherapy to affect melatonin and circadian rhythms (Table 17.2). Most of the trials are ongoing and have no published results. As the trials will be completed and the results become available, more insight in the clinical utility of melatonin will be made available.

TABLE 17.2 Registered clinical trials involving melatonin during pregnancy and lactation

Study title (clinical trial registration number)	Study type	Conditions	Intervention	Primary outcome
Melatonin in Pregnancy Compared to Nonpregnant (NCT03014245)	Observational, prospective, case control	Transient hypertension of pregnancy		Change in melatonin and 6-hydroxymelatonin levels during pregnancy
Melatonin in Pregnancy (NCT03609086)	Observational, prospective, case-only	Pregnancy		6-hydroxymelatonin sulfate in serum 24 h after delivery
Melatonin Levels in Preterm and Term Newborn Infants (NCT01340417)	Observational	Preterm birth		Measurements of melatonin levels in urine, blood, milk in newborns (24–42 weeks old) and mothers
Effects of Light on Melatonin and Contractions in Pregnant Women (NCT01863446)	RCT	Pregnancy	Different lighting manipulations	Melatonin concentration in saliva and blood during experimental light exposure compared with nonlight exposure times
Blocking Blue Light in Pregnancy, Effects on Melatonin Profile and Sleep (NCT03114072)	RCT	Pregnancy	Glasses blocking blue light	Sleep diary; change in motor activity; melatonin levels
Melatonin to Prevent Brain Injury in Unborn Growth Restricted Babies (NCT01695070)	Open-label clinical trial	FGR	4 mg prolonged released (PR) melatonin twice daily	Oxidative stress in the umbilical artery at birth
Light Therapy for Depression During Pregnancy (NCT01043289)	RCT	Antenatal major depressive disorder	Specific light therapy	Change in depression ratings
Evaluation of Melatonin's Effect on Pain and Blood Loss After Cesarean Section (NCT01572805)		Postpartum hemorrhage in patients undergoing cesarean section	Melatonin 3 and 6 mg sublingually versus matched placebo before spinal of anesthesia	Time to first requirement of analgesic supplement; amount of blood loss after cesarean delivery
Therapeutic Effects of Maternal Melatonin Administration on Brain Injury and White Matter Disease (NCT02395783)		Premature birth	Melatonin 10 and 20 µg versus matched placebo	Analysis of white matter injury at 40 weeks corrected by brain MRI with diffusion tensor sequence
Melatonin as a Novel Neuroprotectant in Preterm Infants—Dosage Study (NCT00649961)	Single-dose, open-label escalation pharmacokinetic	Premature birth (<31 weeks); brain injury	Melatonin injections to achieve adult peak blood concentrations of melatonin (200–250 pmol/L)	Finding the dose of melatonin required to achieve physiological blood levels in preterm infants similar to that of their mothers

TABLE 17.2 Registered clinical trials involving melatonin during pregnancy and lactation—cont'd

Study title (clinical trial registration number)	Study type	Conditions	Intervention	Primary outcome
The Effects of Light Therapy on Circadian Rhythms, Sleep, and Mood in Postpartum Depression (NCT02769858)		Postpartum depression	Light therapy	
Integrated Chronotherapy for Perinatal Depression (NCT02053649)	Interventional, open-label	Depression/ major depressive disorder/ postpartum depression	Triple chronotherapy (special glasses) versus usual care	Change from baseline score of the Hamilton Depression Rating Scale-Seasonal Affective Version (SIGH-SAD) at 5 weeks

RCT, randomized control trial.

17.3.2 Safety and Pharmacokinetic Profile of Exogenous Melatonin

Melatonin supplementation has a good safety profile in humans. When administered in high doses intravenously, it does not induce sedation and has no reported adverse events[97] No adverse events have been reported for long-term use in human children and adults.[98] Supplementation with melatonin does not suppress endogenous secretion of the pineal hormone.[99]

In pregnant animal studies, there are no reported treatment-related side effects.[100] However, the data from human studies are more limited. It has been estimated that approximately 1% of women use melatonin during pregnancy.[101] Melatonin is not monitored by the US Food and Drug Administration (FDA), which means that the contents and doses of pills are not regulated. Moreover, exogenous doses are typically in quantities far greater than physiologic amounts.[102] However, despite these facts, melatonin is generally considered to be safe to use during human pregnancy, without teratogenic effects.[103]

The lack of definitive clinical trial data means that the plasma concentrations needed for clinical effectiveness and the best administration route for melatonin remain unproven. Melatonin has been administered in humans by intravenous, intranasal, transdermal, and transmucosal routes.[104] It is mainly metabolized by the liver and excreted into the urine, primarily as 6-sulfatoxymelatonin, which represents >60% of its metabolites.

Preclinical studies and emerging clinical data indicate that melatonin has the potential to be useful for the prevention of ischemic-hypoxic injuries in newborns with birth asphyxia, as well as preeclampsia and its related complications in mothers. There is evidence from animal studies that melatonin administration during pregnancy can confer neuroprotection against hypoxia/ischemia to the fetal and neonatal brain.[105] All these findings suggest that melatonin is a good candidate for preventing pregnancy-related complications, but clinical trials are needed to test these possibilities.

17.4 CONCLUSIONS

Lesions of the pineal gland are very rarely seen during pregnancy or lactation. Tumors of the pineal region are uncommon in adults and are only rarely seen during pregnancy. Growing lesions in the pineal region can be either pineal gland tumors, tumors arising from adjacent structures, metastases, or tumorlike conditions such as vascular malformations and cysts. Clinical symptoms can be caused either by compressing adjacent structures or by direct invasion. A pineal gland tumor during pregnancy represents a challenge to both the neurosurgeon and the obstetrician. Treatment options include surgical resection, stereotactic biopsy followed by radiation/chemotherapy, and stereotactic radiosurgery. Surgical treatment during pregnancy should best be performed during the second trimester. Chemotherapy should be performed after 14 weeks of gestation, when risks become significantly lower.

Pineal cysts are a common incidental neuroradiological finding, do not appear to be affected by pregnancy, and are unlikely to cause complications during pregnancy or labor. Pineal calcifications are benign deposits of calcium and magnesium; they are more frequent in adults and have not been associated with dysfunction of the pineal gland.

The hormonal imbalances that are generated by night-shift work or jet lag may contribute to the increased risk of preterm birth, low birth weight, and miscarriage in women who are exposed to a desynchronization of the sleep-wake cycle during pregnancy. Moreover, antepartum depression exposes the children to adverse birth outcomes such as cognitive, emotional, and behavioral problems. There are also risks for the depressive future mother because prepartum psychiatric illness is a risk factor for the development of postpartum mood disorders.

Melatonin is an antioxidant and free-radical scavenger with a good safety profile during pregnancy, with preclinical data suggesting that it is a candidate to prevent and treat preeclampsia and other pregnancy-related disorders. Deficient pineal melatonin production in early pregnancy in rodents has been associated with the development of spontaneous abortion, while the administration of melatonin reduced preterm delivery in mice. All these putative effects of exogenous melatonin require testing in clinical trials before it can be recommended as a treatment.

REFERENCES

1. Golzarian J, Balériaux D, Bank WO, Matos C, Flament-Durand J. Pineal cyst: normal or pathological? *Neuroradiology* 1993;**35**(4):251–3.
2. Tamaki N, Shirataki K, Lin T, Masumura M, Katayama S, Matsumoto S. Cysts of the pineal gland. *Childs Nerv Syst* 1989;**5**(3):172–6.
3. Mandera M, Marcol W, Kotulska K, Olakowska E, Gołka D, Malinowska I, et al. Childhood pineal parenchymal tumors: clinical and therapeutic aspects. *Neurosurg Rev* 2011;**34**(2):191–6.
4. Smith AB, Rushing EJ, Smirniotopoulos JG. From the archives of the AFIP: lesions of the pineal region: radiologic-pathologic correlation. *Radiographics* 2010;**30**(7):2001–20.
5. Al-Hussaini M, Sultan I, Abuirmileh N, Jaradat I, Qaddoumi I. Pineal gland tumors: experience from the SEER database. *J Neuro-Oncol* 2009;**94**(3):351–8.
6. Matula C. Tumors of the pineal region. In: *Principles of neurological surgery*. Elsevier; 2012. p. 565–84.
7. Rousselle C, des Portes V, Berlier P, Mottolese C. Pineal region tumors: clinical symptoms and syndromes. *Neurochirurgie* 2015;**61**(2–3):106–12.
7a. Leston J, Mottolese C, Champier J, Jouvet A, Brun J, Sindou M, Chazot G, Claustrat B, Fèvre-Montange M. Contribution of the daily melatonin profile to diagnosis of tumors of the pineal region. *J Neurooncol* 2009;**93**(3):387–94.
8. Ravindra VM, Braca JA, Jensen RL, Duckworth EAM, Duckworth EAM. Management of intracranial pathology during pregnancy: case example and review of management strategies. *Surg Neurol Int* 2015;**6**:43.
9. American College of Obstetricians and Gynecologists. ACOG committee opinion. Number 723, October 2017.
10. Dickerman RD, Stevens QE, Steide J-A, Schneider SJ. Precocious puberty associated with a pineal cyst: is it disinhibition of the hypothalamic-pituitary axis? *Neuro Endocrinol Lett* 2004;**25**(3):173–5.
11. Lensing FD, Abele TA, Sivakumar W, Taussky P, Shah LM, Salzman KL. Pineal region masses-imaging findings and surgical approaches. *Curr Probl Diagn Radiol* 2015;**44**(1):76–87.
12. Faure-Conter C. Tumoral markers in tumors of the pineal region. *Neurochirurgie* 2015;**61**(2–3):143–5.
13. Amant F, Vandenbroucke T, Verheecke M, Fumagalli M, Halaska MJ, Boere I, et al. Pediatric outcome after maternal cancer diagnosed during pregnancy. *N Engl J Med* 2015;**373**(19):1824–34.
14. Stevenson CB, Thompson RC. The clinical management of intracranial neoplasms in pregnancy. *Clin Obstet Gynecol* 2005;**48**(1):24–37.
15. Stevens RD, Shoykhet M, Cadena R. Emergency neurological life support: intracranial hypertension and herniation. *Neurocrit Care* 2015;**23**(Suppl 2):S76–82.
16. Korein J, Cravioto H, Leicach M. Reevaluation of lumbar puncture; a study of 129 patients with papilledema or intracranial hypertension. *Neurology* 1959;**9**(4):290–7.
17. Berhouma M, Ni H, Delabar V, Tahhan N, Memou Salem S, Mottolese C, et al. Update on the management of pineal cysts: case series and a review of the literature. *Neurochirurgie* 2015;**61**(2–3):201–7.
18. Májovský M, Netuka D, Beneš V. Conservative and surgical treatment of patients with pineal cysts: prospective case series of 110 patients. *World Neurosurg* 2017;**105**:199–205.
19. Whitehead MT, Oh CC, Choudhri AF. Incidental pineal cysts in children who undergo 3-T MRI. *Pediatr Radiol* 2013;**43**(12):1577–83.
20. Nevins EJ, Das K, Bhojak M, Pinto RS, Hoque MN, Jenkinson MD, et al. Incidental pineal cysts: is surveillance necessary? *World Neurosurg* 2016;**90**:96–102.
21. Májovský M, Netuka D, Beneš V. Clinical management of pineal cysts: a worldwide online survey. *Acta Neurochir* 2016;**158**(4):663–9.
22. Dede H, Ozdogan S, Dede SF. Pineal cyst during pregnancy and labor. *Ginecoro* 2011;(7):78–9.
23. Maślińska D, Laure-Kamionowska M, Deręgowski K, Maśliński S. Association of mast cells with calcification in the human pineal gland. *Folia Neuropathol* 2010;**48**(4):276–82.
24. Kim J, Kim H-W, Chang S, Kim JW, Je JH, Rhyu IJ. Growth patterns for acervuli in human pineal gland. *Sci Rep* 2012;**2**:984.
25. Figueiredo A, Maheshwari S, Goel A. Cavernoma in the pineal region. *J Clin Neurosci* 2010;**17**(5):652–3.
26. Ogura T, Kambe A, Sakamoto M, Shinohara Y, Ogawa T, Kurosaki M. Superficial siderosis associated with pineal cavernous malformation. *World Neurosurg* 2018;**109**:230–2.
27. Vishteh AG, Nadkarni T, Spetzler RF. Cavernous malformation of the pineal region: short report and review of the literature. *Br J Neurosurg* 2000;**14**(2):147–51.

28. Choque-Velasquez J, Resendiz-Nieves J, Colasanti R, Collan J, Hernesniemi J. *Microsurgical Management of Vascular Malformations of the Pineal Region*. [cited 1 Oct 2018]. Available from: https://www.google.ro/search?q=Choque-Velasquez+J%2C+Resendiz-Nieves+J%2C+Colasanti+R%2C+Collan+J%2C+Hernesniemi+J.+Microsurgical+Management+of+Vascular+Malformations+of+the+Pineal+Region&oq=Choque-Velasquez+J%2C+Resendiz-Nieves+J%2C+Colasanti+R%2C+Collan.

29. Reiter R, Tan D, Rosales-Corral S, Galano A, Zhou X, Xu B, et al. Mitochondria: central organelles for melatonin's antioxidant and anti-aging actions. *Molecules* 2018;**23**(2):509.

30. Duhig K, Chappell LC, Shennan AH. Oxidative stress in pregnancy and reproduction. *Obstet Med* 2016;**9**(3):113–6.

31. Jauniaux E, Watson AL, Hempstock J, Bao YP, Skepper JN, Burton GJ. Onset of maternal arterial blood flow and placental oxidative stress. A possible factor in human early pregnancy failure. *Am J Pathol* 2000;**157**(6):2111–22.

32. Simşek M, Naziroğlu M, Simşek H, Cay M, Aksakal M, Kumru S. Blood plasma levels of lipoperoxides, glutathione peroxidase, beta carotene, vitamin A and E in women with habitual abortion. *Cell Biochem Funct* 1998;**16**(4):227–31.

33. Toy H, Camuzcuoglu H, Camuzcuoglu A, Celik H, Aksoy N. Decreased serum prolidase activity and increased oxidative stress in early pregnancy loss. *Gynecol Obstet Investig* 2010;**69**(2):122–7.

34. Wang Y, Walsh SW. Placental mitochondria as a source of oxidative stress in pre-eclampsia. *Placenta* 1998;**19**(8):581–6.

35. Wu JJ. Lipid peroxidation in preeclamptic and eclamptic pregnancies. *Eur J Obstet Gynecol Reprod Biol* 1996;**64**(1):51–4.

36. Patil SB, Kodliwadmath MV, Kodliwadmath SM. Lipid peroxidation and antioxidant status in hypertensive pregnancies. *Clin Exp Obstet Gynecol* 2008;**35**(4):272–4.

37. Reiter RJ, Tan DX, Korkmaz A, Rosales-Corral SA. Melatonin and stable circadian rhythms optimize maternal, placental and fetal physiology. *Hum Reprod Update* 2014;**20**(2):293–307.

38. Reiter RJ, Rosales-Corral SA, Manchester LC, Tan D-X. Peripheral reproductive organ health and melatonin: ready for prime time. *Int J Mol Sci* 2013;**14**(4):7231–72.

39. Tan D-X, Manchester LC, Terron MP, Flores LJ, Reiter RJ. One molecule, many derivatives: a never-ending interaction of melatonin with reactive oxygen and nitrogen species? *J Pineal Res* 2007;**42**(1):28–42.

40. Hardeland R, Madrid JA, Tan D-X, Reiter RJ. Melatonin, the circadian multioscillator system and health: the need for detailed analyses of peripheral melatonin signaling. *J Pineal Res* 2012;**52**(2):139–66.

41. Mayo JC, Sainz RM, Antolín I, Herrera F, Martin V, Rodriguez C. Melatonin regulation of antioxidant enzyme gene expression. *Cell Mol Life Sci* 2002;**59**(10):1706–13.

42. Fischer TW, Kleszczyński K, Hardkop LH, Kruse N, Zillikens D. Melatonin enhances antioxidative enzyme gene expression (CAT, GPx, SOD), prevents their UVR-induced depletion, and protects against the formation of DNA damage (8-hydroxy-2′-deoxyguanosine) in ex vivo human skin. *J Pineal Res* 2013;**54**(3):303–12.

43. Erren TC, Reiter RJ. Defining chronodisruption. *J Pineal Res* 2009;**46**(3):245–7.

44. Miyauchi F, Nanjo K, Otsuka K. Effects of night shift on plasma concentrations of melatonin, LH, FSH and prolactin, and menstrual irregularity. *Sangyo Igaku* 1992;**34**(6):545–50.

45. Knutsson A. Health disorders of shift workers. *Occup Med (Lond)* 2003;**53**(2):103–8.

46. Voiculescu SE, Le Duc D, Roşca AE, Zeca V, Chiţimuş DM, Arsene AL, et al. Behavioral and molecular effects of prenatal continuous light exposure in the adult rat. *Brain Res* 2016;**1650**:51–9.

47. Motta-Teixeira LC, Machado-Nils AV, Battagello DS, Diniz GB, Andrade-Silva J, Silva S, et al. The absence of maternal pineal melatonin rhythm during pregnancy and lactation impairs offspring physical growth, neurodevelopment, and behavior. *Horm Behav* 2018;**105**:146–56.

48. McClung CA. Circadian genes, rhythms and the biology of mood disorders. *Pharmacol Ther* 2007;**114**(2):222–32.

49. Monteleone P, Maj M. The circadian basis of mood disorders: recent developments and treatment implications. *Eur Neuropsychopharmacol* 2008;**18**(10):701–11.

50. Colvin L, Slack-Smith L, Stanley FJ, Bower C. Are women with major depression in pregnancy identifiable in population health data? *BMC Pregnancy Childbirth* 2013;**13**(1):63.

51. Breslau N, Roth T, Rosenthal L, Andreski P. Sleep disturbance and psychiatric disorders: a longitudinal epidemiological study of young adults. *Biol Psychiatry* 1996;**39**(6):411–8.

52. Turek FW. From circadian rhythms to clock genes in depression. *Int Clin Psychopharmacol* 2007;**22**(Suppl. 2):S1–8.

53. Lee KA, Gay CL. Sleep in late pregnancy predicts length of labor and type of delivery. *Am J Obstet Gynecol* 2004;**191**(6):2041–6.

54. Bais B, Kamperman AM, van der Zwaag MD, Dieleman GC, van der Vliet-Torij HW H, Bijma HH, et al. Bright light therapy in pregnant women with major depressive disorder: study protocol for a randomized, double-blind, controlled clinical trial. *BMC Psychiatry* 2016;**16**(1):1–13.

55. Nakamura Y, Tamura H, Kashida S, Takayama H, Yamagata Y, Karube A, et al. Changes of serum melatonin level and its relationship to feto-placental unit during pregnancy. *J Pineal Res* 2001;**30**(1):29–33.

56. Parry BL, Meliska CJ, Fernando Martinez L, Maurer EL, Lopez AM, Sorenson DL. Neuroendocrine abnormalities in women with depression linked to the reproductive cycle. In: *Handbook of contemporary neuropharmacology*. Hoboken, NJ: John Wiley & Sons, Inc.; 2007.

57. Parry BL, Fernando Martínez L, Maurer EL, López AM, Sorenson D, Meliska CJ. Sleep, rhythms and women's mood. Part I. Menstrual cycle, pregnancy and postpartum. *Sleep Med Rev* 2006;**10**(2):129–44.

58. Oren DA, Wisner KL, Spinelli M, Epperson CN, Peindl KS, Terman JS, et al. An open trial of morning light therapy for treatment of antepartum depression. *Am J Psychiatry* 2002;**159**(4):666–9.

59. Meliska CJ, Martínez LF, López AM, Sorenson DL, Nowakowski S, Kripke DF, et al. Antepartum depression severity is increased during seasonally longer nights: relationship to melatonin and cortisol timing and quantity. *Chronobiol Int* 2013;**30**(9):1160–73.

60. Epperson CN, Terman M, Terman JS, Hanusa BH, Oren DA, Peindl KS, et al. Randomized clinical trial of bright light therapy for antepartum depression: preliminary findings. *J Clin Psychiatry* 2004;**65**(3):421–5.

61. Pariante CM, Lightman SL. The HPA axis in major depression: classical theories and new developments. *Trends Neurosci* 2008;**31**(9):464–8.

62. Deuschle M, Schweiger U, Weber B, Gotthardt U, Körner A, Schmider J, et al. Diurnal activity and pulsatility of the hypothalamus-pituitary-adrenal system in male depressed patients and healthy controls. *J Clin Endocrinol Metab* 1997;**82**(1):234–8.

63. Claustrat B, Brun J, Chazot G. The basic physiology and pathophysiology of melatonin. *Sleep Med Rev* 2005;**9**(1):11–24.

64. Silber BY, Schmitt JAJ. Effects of tryptophan loading on human cognition, mood, and sleep. *Neurosci Biobehav Rev* 2010;**34**(3):387–407.

65. van Lee L, Cai S, Loy SL, Tham EKH, Yap FKP, Godfrey KM, et al. Relation of plasma tryptophan concentrations during pregnancy to maternal sleep and mental well-being: the GUSTO cohort. *J Affect Disord* 2018;**225**:523–9.

66. Andersson L, Sundström-Poromaa I, Wulff M, Åström M, Bixo M. Depression and anxiety during pregnancy and six months postpartum: a follow-up study. *Acta Obstet Gynecol Scand* 2006;**85**(8):937–44.

67. Dennis C-L, Ross LE. The clinical utility of maternal self-reported personal and familial psychiatric history in identifying women at risk for postpartum depression. *Acta Obstet Gynecol Scand* 2006;**85**(10):1179–85.

68. Wehr TA, Wirz-Justice A, Goodwin FK, Duncan W, Gillin JC. Phase advance of the circadian sleep-wake cycle as an antidepressant. *Science* 1979;**206**(4419):710–3.

69. Fu M, Zhang L, Ahmed A, Plaut K, Haas DM, Szucs K, et al. Does circadian disruption play a role in the metabolic-hormonal link to delayed lactogenesis II? *Front Nutr* 2015;**2**:4.

70. Okatani Y, Sagara Y. Amplification of nocturnal melatonin secretion in women with functional secondary amenorrhoea: relation to endogenous oestrogen concentration. *Clin Endocrinol* 1994;**41**(6):763–70.

71. Manca ME, Manunta ML, Spezzigu A, Torres-Rovira L, Gonzalez-Bulnes A, Pasciu V, et al. Melatonin deprival modifies follicular and corpus luteal growth dynamics in a sheep model. *Reproduction* 2014;**147**(6):885–95.

72. Okatani Y, Okamoto K, Hayashi K, Wakatsuki A, Tamura S, Sagara Y. Maternal-fetal transfer of melatonin in pregnant women near term. *J Pineal Res* 1998;**25**(3):129–34.

73. Seko LMD, Moroni RM, Leitao VMS, Teixeira DM, Nastri CO, Martins WP. Melatonin supplementation during controlled ovarian stimulation for women undergoing assisted reproductive technology: systematic review and meta-analysis of randomized controlled trials. *Fertil Steril* 2014;**101**(1):154–161.e4.

74. Tamura H, Takasaki A, Taketani T, Tanabe M, Kizuka F, Lee L, et al. Melatonin as a free radical scavenger in the ovarian follicle. *Endocr J* 2013;**60**(1):1–13.

75. Tamura H, Takasaki A, Taketani T, Tanabe M, Kizuka F, Lee L, et al. The role of melatonin as an antioxidant in the follicle. *J Ovarian Res* 2012;**5**(1):5.

76. Espino J, Bejarano I, Ortiz Á, Lozano GM, García JF, Pariente JA, et al. Melatonin as a potential tool against oxidative damage and apoptosis in ejaculated human spermatozoa. *Fertil Steril* 2010;**94**(5):1915–7.

77. Levine RJ. Seasonal variation of semen quality and fertility. *Scand J Work Environ Health* 1999;**25**:34–7.

78. Tamura H, Nakamura Y, Terron MP, Flores LJ, Manchester LC, Tan DX, et al. Melatonin and pregnancy in the human. *Reprod Toxicol* 2008;**25**(3):291–303.

79. Domínguez Rubio AP, Sordelli MS, Salazar AI, Aisemberg J, Bariani MV, Cella M, et al. Melatonin prevents experimental preterm labor and increases offspring survival. *J Pineal Res* 2014;**56**(2):154–62.

80. Tranquilli AL, Brown MA, Zeeman GG, Dekker G, Sibai BM. The definition of severe and early-onset preeclampsia. Statements from the International Society for the Study of Hypertension in Pregnancy (ISSHP). *Pregnancy Hypertens* 2013;**3**:44–7.

81. Brosens I, Pijnenborg R, Vercruysse L, Romero R. The "Great Obstetrical Syndromes" are associated with disorders of deep placentation. *Am J Obstet Gynecol* 2011;**204**(3):193–201.

82. Karumanchi SA, Granger JP. Preeclampsia and pregnancy-related hypertensive disorders. *Hypertension* 2016;**67**(2):238–42.

83. Zeng K, Gao Y, Wan J, Tong M, Lee AC, Zhao M, et al. The reduction in circulating levels of melatonin may be associated with the development of preeclampsia. *J Hum Hypertens* 2016;**30**(11):666–71.

84. Hobson SR, Gurusinghe S, Lim R, Alers NO, Miller SL, Kingdom JC, et al. Melatonin improves endothelial function in vitro and prolongs pregnancy in women with early-onset preeclampsia. *J Pineal Res* 2018;**65**(3).

85. Hannan NJ, Binder NK, Beard S, Nguyen T-V, Kaitu'u-Lino TJ, Tong S. Melatonin enhances antioxidant molecules in the placenta, reduces secretion of soluble fms-like tyrosine kinase 1 (sFLT) from primary trophoblast but does not rescue endothelial dysfunction: an evaluation of its potential to treat preeclampsia. Hahn S, editor, *PLoS ONE* 2018;**13**(4).

86. Cetin I, Alvino G. Intrauterine growth restriction: implications for placental metabolism and transport. A review. *Placenta* 2009;**30**:77–82.

87. Miller SL, Yawno T, Alers NO, Castillo-Melendez M, Supramaniam VG, VanZyl N, et al. Antenatal antioxidant treatment with melatonin to decrease newborn neurodevelopmental deficits and brain injury caused by fetal growth restriction. *J Pineal Res* 2014;**56**(3):283–94.

88. Kennaway DJ. Potential safety issues in the use of the hormone melatonin in paediatrics. *J Paediatr Child Health* 2015;**51**(6):584–9.

89. Carloni S, Proietti F, Rocchi M, Longini M, Marseglia L, D'Angelo G, et al. Melatonin pharmacokinetics following oral administration in preterm neonates. *Molecules* 2017;**22**(12):2115.

90. Thakor AS, Herrera EA, Serón-Ferré M, Giussani DA. Melatonin and vitamin C increase umbilical blood flow via nitric oxide-dependent mechanisms. *J Pineal Res* 2010;**49**(4):399–406.

91. Shukla P, Lemley CO, Dubey N, Meyer AM, O'Rourke ST, Vonnahme KA. Effect of maternal nutrient restriction and melatonin supplementation from mid to late gestation on vascular reactivity of maternal and fetal placental arteries. *Placenta* 2014;**35**(7):461–6.

92. Reiter RJ, Tan D-X, Manchester LC, Paredes SD, Mayo JC, Sainz RM. Melatonin and reproduction revisited. *Biol Reprod* 2009;**81**(3):445–56.

93. Herxheimer A, Petrie KJ. Melatonin for the prevention and treatment of jet lag. *Cochrane Database Syst Rev* 2002;**2**:.

94. Jansen SL, Forbes D, Duncan V, Morgan DG, Malouf R. Melatonin for the treatment of dementia. *Cochrane Database Syst Rev* 2006;**1**:.

95. Gitto E, Karbownik M, Reiter RJ, Tan DX, Cuzzocrea S, Chiurazzi P, et al. Effects of melatonin treatment in septic newborns. *Pediatr Res* 2001;**50** (6):756–60.

96. Fulia F, Gitto E, Cuzzocrea S, Reiter RJ, Dugo L, Gitto P, et al. Increased levels of malondialdehyde and nitrite/nitrate in the blood of asphyxiated newborns: reduction by melatonin. *J Pineal Res* 2001;**31**(4):343–9.

97. Andersen LPH, Werner MU, Rosenkilde MM, Harpsøe NG, Fuglsang H, Rosenberg J, et al. Pharmacokinetics of oral and intravenous melatonin in healthy volunteers. *BMC Pharmacol Toxicol* 2016;**17**(1):8.

98. Jan JE, Wasdell MB, Freeman RD, Bax M. Evidence supporting the use of melatonin in short gestation infants. *J Pineal Res* 2007;**42**(1):22–7.

99. Palm L, Blennow G, Wetterberg L. Long-term melatonin treatment in blind children and young adults with circadian sleep-wake disturbances. *Dev Med Child Neurol* 1997;**39**(5):319–25.

100. Jahnke G, Marr M, Myers C, Wilson R, Travlos G, Price C. Maternal and developmental toxicity evaluation of melatonin administered orally to pregnant Sprague-Dawley rats. *Toxicol Sci* 1999;**50**(2):271–9.

101. Freeman MP, Sosinsky AZ, Moustafa D, Viguera AC, Cohen LS. Supplement use by women during pregnancy: data from the Massachusetts General Hospital National Pregnancy Registry for Atypical Antipsychotics. *Arch Womens Ment Health* 2016;**19**(3):437–41.

102. Prazinko BF, Sam JA, Caldwell JL, Townsend AT. *Dose uniformity of over-the-counter melatonin as determined by high-pressure liquid chromatography,* 2000.

103. Tamura H, Takasaki A, Taketani T, Tanabe M, Lee L, Tamura I, et al. Melatonin and female reproduction. *J Obstet Gynaecol Res* 2014;**40**(1):1–11.

104. Zetner D, Andersen L, Rosenberg J. Pharmacokinetics of alternative administration routes of melatonin: a systematic review. *Drug Res (Stuttg)* 2015;**66**(04):169–73.

105. Wilkinson D, Shepherd E, Wallace EM. Melatonin for women in pregnancy for neuroprotection of the fetus. *Cochrane Database Syst Rev* 2016;**3**.

Chapter 18

Pituitary Disorders During Pregnancy and Lactation

Raquel Soares Jallad*,†, Andrea Glezer*,†, Marcio Carlos Machado*,†,‡ and Marcello D. Bronstein*,†

*Neuroendocrine Unit, Division of Endocrinology and Metabolism, Hospital das Clinicas, University of São Paulo Medical School, São Paulo, Brazil, †Laboratory of Cellular and Molecular Endocrinology LIM-25, University of São Paulo Medical School, São Paulo, Brazil, ‡Endocrinology Service, AC Camargo Cancer Center, São Paulo, Brazil

Common Clinical Problems

- Pituitary disorders are uncommon to rare during pregnancy because the mass effect of a tumor or the underlying hormone disturbance can lead to hypogonadotropic hypogonadism and reduced fertility.
- The normal hormonal changes of pregnancy, lack of pregnancy-specific reference ranges for basal and dynamic hormone levels, and contraindication for use of gadolinium-enhanced magnetic resonance imaging (MRI) make it difficult to diagnose pituitary disorders in pregnant women.
- The physiological enlargement of the pituitary during normal pregnancy can provoke a mass effect of an underlying tumor.
- The increased vascularity, hyperplasia, and friability of normal and adenomatous pituitary cells during pregnancy increase the risk of hemorrhage (apoplexy) and hypotension-induced necrosis (Sheehan's syndrome).
- Prolactinomas are the most common pituitary tumors, with bromocripitine still the drug of choice in the scenario of pregnancy planning.
- Concerning hypopituitarism during pregnancy, the priority for hormonal replacement should be glucocorticoid, followed by thyroid hormone, with doses being adjusted as needed throughout pregnancy.

18.1 INTRODUCTION AND GENERAL APPROACH

Pituitary tumors represent 15.5% of all central nervous system (CNS) neoplasms.[1] The prevalence of pituitary adenomas in autopsy and radiological studies was found to be 16.7% and 22.5%, respectively.[2] In young adults (aged 20–34 years), more than 30% of CNS tumors are in fact pituitary adenomas.[3] The age-adjusted incidence rate of pituitary adenomas is estimated to be 3.4 cases per 100,000 inhabitants per year.[4–7] They are usually benign adenomas, with a peak incidence in young women of childbearing age.[3]

Pituitary tumors are divided into secreting (functional) and nonsecreting [or clinically nonfunctioning (CNF)], according to their hormone production.[7–9]

Most adenomas are functional (65%–70%), leading to phenotypes and clinical manifestations related to the hormonal hypersecretion.[3,8] Prolactin (PRL)-secreting adenomas (prolactinomas) are associated with hypogonadism, infertility, and galactorrhea and account for 32%–57% of pituitary tumors. Growth hormone (GH)-producing adenomas are associated with either gigantism (prior to epiphyseal plate closure) or acromegaly (after epiphyseal plate closure) and represent 8%–14% of pituitary tumors. Pituitary tumor secreting adrenocorticotropic hormone (ACTH secreting adenoma) account for 2%–6% and are associated with Cushing's syndrome (CS), which results from prolonged exposure to high levels of cortisol. TSH-producing tumors (which lead to secondary hyperthyroidism) and gonadotrophin-secreting tumors are rare, accounting for about 1% of all pituitary adenomas. In about 15%–54% of cases, the adenoma is clinically nonfunctioning, meaning that it does not secrete any appreciable hormones.[7,9]

With respect to morphology, pituitary tumors are typically divided into microadenomas (<10-mm diameter), and macroadenomas (≥10-mm diameter).[3] They may be confined to pituitary or expansive.[3] Pituitary adenomas may present because of effects caused by tumor growth, which compresses neighboring structures, thereby leading to visual changes (optic nerve compression), headache (compression of the dura), or pituitary hormone deficiencies (compression of the normal pituitary).[3,10] Such tumors may also present with symptoms and signs of pituitary hyperfunction (i.e., prolactinoma, acromegaly, Cushing's disease).[3,8] They may also be discovered incidentally, through imaging of the brain performed for other reasons.[7,9,11]

Hypogonadotropic hypogonadism is the most prevalent hormonal deficiency in pituitary disease.[3,7-9] It results from a variety of factors that can compromise the normal production of hypothalamic and gonadotrophic hormones, including compression by the tumor, hyperprolactinemia, treatment of the tumor (surgery, radiotherapy), stroke, comorbidities, and medications. In hypogonadotrophic hypogonadism, the ovaries have the capability of normal function but lack regulatory stimulation by pituitary gonadotrophins. Therefore, correction of disturbances in hypothalamic or pituitary function, or replacement of the relevant hormones, may allow normal ovulatory function (and subsequently conception) to occur.[12]

The presence of a pituitary adenoma may affect the course of pregnancy, as the hormonal changes related to these tumors may lead to early termination of pregnancy due to failure to implant or maintain the conceptus or early embryo.

Pregnancy itself may also affect the course of the pituitary tumor, causing a worsening the tumor's natural history, or unmasking a previously unknown diagnosis.[11] The high levels of estrogens present during pregnancy can stimulate normal and adenomatous cells to increase in size and number.[13] However, most microadenomas do not exhibit symptomatic growth during pregnancy.[14,15] There is significant concern in the realm of macroadenomas about tumor growth during pregnancy. The risk of symptomatic tumor growth is low (about 2.8%) in macroadenomas that were treated with surgery, radiotherapy, or both prior to pregnancy,[14-16] whereas in macroadenomas that have not yet been treated, the risk of symptomatic tumor growth increases to 31%.[17] This risk is greatest during the second and third trimesters.[14,15] Headaches and visual or ocular symptoms require visual fields and MRI evaluation to clarify if these symptoms result from increased volume of a macroadenoma that extends upward to compress the optic chiasm, or laterally to compress cranial nerves within the cavernous sinus, or whether they represent an effect of an enlarging pituitary within the limited intrasellar space already occupied by the adenoma.[16-22] Therefore, intensive prenatal surveillance of a pituitary adenoma is always recommended.[16-22] There is no evidence that pregnancy increases the incidence of adenomas per se. In an autopsy study performed on 69 pregnant women who died without having any symptoms of pituitary abnormalities, eight noninvasive microadenomas (12%) were found.[17] This number was not higher than that found in nonpregnant women or normal men of similar ages.[17]

During pregnancy, adenomas are at risk of pituitary apoplexy, which is rapid infarction from hemorrhage, caused by increased pituitary vascularity, edema, and estrogen-mediated hyperplasia.[18] Apoplexy is a rare event whose main symptoms are severe headache and retroorbital pain, accompanied by vomiting, rapid deterioration of vision or ocular motility (ophthalmoplegia), and reduced consciousness.[18,21] The emergency treatment is surgical in order to decompress the adjacent regions.[18,21]

Visual abnormalities such as bitemporal hemianopsia and ophthalmoplegias are caused by compression of the optic pathways and neurovascular structures within the cavernous sinuses.[10,19] The risk of these complications increases with the size of the tumor, as so patients with microadenomas have a significantly lower risk of developing visual loss than patients with macroadenomas.[10]

Additionally, pregnancy can also exacerbate headache[20-22] by causing stretching of the surrounding dura mater, hypertension, bradycardia, and respiratory irregularities. The endocrine evaluation of a pregnant woman with a pituitary tumor depends on whether the diagnosis was made prior to or during pregnancy.

Management of pituitary adenomas discovered during pregnancy in otherwise healthy women pose difficult challenges from various perspectives.[14-16,23-26] First, the normal physiological changes in the concentrations of pituitary hormones during pregnancy make it difficult to diagnose hypopituitarism or hypersecretion during pregnancy and postpartum. Second, results of the dynamic pituitary function tests in pregnancy are very difficult to interpret because there are no normal standards.[14-16,23-26] Preliminary hormonal assessments to determine the function of the anterior and posterior pituitary include GH, IGF-1, thyroid-stimulating hormone (TSH), free thyroxine (free T4), free triiodothyronine (free T3), PRL, gonadotrophins, morning serum cortisol (i.e., prior to 8 a.m.), urine volume, serum electrolytes, and serum osmolarity.[14-16,23-26] If clinical examination and laboratory tests reveal a specific endocrinopathy, then more targeted testing should be performed.

In patients in whom a pituitary adenoma was diagnosed before pregnancy, subsequent endocrine evaluation depends upon the type of tumor and also varies by trimester.[14-16,23-26]

18.1.1 Neuroimaging in Pregnancy

Imaging studies should be indicated only when used to answer the relevant clinical question or otherwise provide medical benefit to the patient. Therefore, magnetic resonance imaging of the pituitary gland will be indicated when there is a visual and/or neurological clinical picture secondary to tumor compression.[27,28]

MRI does not use ionizing radiation and is considered relatively safe for the fetus.[29,30] It should preferably be performed only after 4 months of pregnancy.[29,30] This recommendation aims to avoid fetal exposure to radiofrequency and acoustic noise fields.[29,30] The administration of gadolinium contrast enhances the diagnostic accuracy of MRI.[29,30] However, administration of this contrast is not indicated during pregnancy because of its potential teratogenicity in the first trimester.[29,30] In addition, gadolinium may cross the placenta in the second or third trimester,[31] be excreted by the fetal kidneys into the amniotic fluid, and then be recirculated by the fetus.[31] Therefore, there is a theoretical risk of nephrogenic systemic fibrosis developing as a result of fetal exposure to radiocontrast.[32] A recent Canadian study evaluated 1 424 105 deliveries beyond the 20th week of gestation to assess the risks associated with MRI performed with or without gadolinium.[33] The purpose of this study was to evaluate the long-term safety after exposure to MRI in the first trimester, in particular on the risk of death, fetal or neonatal death.[33] With regard to exposure to gadolinium, they assessed the risk of inflammatory rheumatic and/or skin or connective disorders or skin changes similar to nephrogenic systemic fibrosis, a condition also referred to as *nephrogenic fibrosing dermatopathy,* which is described in association with the use of gadolinium contrast in adult patients.[33] Compared with nonexposed pregnancies, pregnancies with exposure to gadolinium showed a higher frequency of intrauterine or neonatal death [relative risk (RR) 3.7, 95% confidence interval (CI) limits from 1.55 to 8.85, difference in absolute risk of 47.5 per 1000 pregnancies, 95% CI from 9.7 to 138.2] and rheumatologic, inflammatory, and cutaneous infiltrative pathologies (hazard ratio 1.36, 95% CI limits from 1.09 to 1,69, risk 45.3 per 1000 people/year, 95% CI limits from 11.3 to 86.8).[33] The risk of nephrogenic fibrosis was not increased. This study makes it clear for the first time that MRI is not such a dangerous investigation in pregnancy, even in the first trimester. However, it should be performed without gadolinium contrast.[33]

In patients with suprasellar expansion of pituitary adenomas, neuro-ophthalmological evaluation of visual fields and acuity is mandatory to assess the degree of compromise and to decide on the best therapeutic approach. Periodic assessment of visual fields and acuity allows monitoring of tumor size progression, independent of radiological imaging.

18.1.2 Pituitary Adenoma Treatment During Pregnancy

The management of pituitary adenomas during pregnancy depends on the clinical presentation and should be adapted to the individual case. The majority of pregnant women with pituitary adenomas can be safely observed with frequent neuro-ophthalmologic assessments and MRI, if needed.

18.1.3 Pharmacological Treatment

Due to issues related to embryonic, fetal, and postnatal child safety, the decision to maintain or initiate medication during pregnancy or breastfeeding should consider the relationship between potential gains and possible harm to mother and child. Food and Drug Administration (FDA) regulations on labeling for use during pregnancy, during labor and delivery, and by nursing mothers were originally issued in 1979 as part of a rule prescribing the content and format for labeling for human prescription drugs . The 1979 regulations also required that each product be classified under one of five pregnancy categories (A, B, C, D, or X) on the basis of risk of reproductive and developmental adverse effects or, for certain categories, on the basis of such risk weighed against potential benefit.[34–37] Based on this FDA criteria, dopamine agonists cabergoline (CAB) and bromocriptine (BRC), as well as the somastatin analog octreotide, are classified as category B (no fetal risks have been demonstrated in animal studies, but there are no adequate, well-controlled studies in pregnant women to date), while lanreotide and C (adverse fetal effects have been seen in animal studies but there are no adequate and well-controlled studies in pregnant women; nevertheless, potential benefits may warrant the use of the drug).[34–37]

The new FDA standards for the use of drugs in pregnancy and lactation have been in force since 2015.[34–37] They reformulate the content and format of the package inserts and, at the same time, remove any references to categories A, B, C, D, and X. These are replaced by a summary of the perinatal risks of the pertinent drug, discussion of the relevant evidence, and a summary of the most relevant data that affect making decisions on prescribing it. Also included in the new standards are essential information on identification of pregnancy, contraception, and infertility.[34–37] The ultimate goal of the new standards is to facilitate the prescribing process by offering a consistent and well-structured set of information regarding the use of medications during pregnancy and lactation.[34–37]

Due to the long half-lives of these drugs and limited data on the effects of in utero exposure, these drugs should ideally be discontinued prior to intended conception, CAB 1 month before, and long-acting somatostatin (SST) analogs or pegvisomant 2 months before. During pregnancy, it also is recommended that medical therapy should be withheld and administered only if necessary for control of tumor, headache, or both. This approach reduces the likelihood of an embryo being exposed to a drug, including residual exposure to a long-acting drug.[34–37]

18.1.4   Pituitary Surgery During Pregnancy

Surgical treatment should be considered in patients who demonstrate increased tumor volume, either clinically or on imaging studies, or when pituitary apoplexy occurs or is considered an imminent risk.[18] The best time for a neurosurgical intervention will depend on three basic factors: the severity of the compressive symptoms (neurological, visual, or both), gestational age, and tumor type.[38,39] Gestational age should be determined to evaluate how close to term the baby is and whether we can or should stop the pregnancy at the same time as, before, or after pituitary surgery. Preparations for possible delivery should be made in case any fetal distress develops in the perioperative period.[40]

A multidisciplinary approach, involving the neurosurgeon, endocrinologist, obstetrician, and anesthesiologist is necessary in order to determine the best plan.

18.1.5   Outcomes of Pregnancies of <20-week Gestation

During this time, the embryo or fetus is remote from being viable on its own, and as the hemodynamic changes in the mother have not yet peaked, the risks of intraoperative hemorrhage are less significant. If the woman is stable, the pregnancy may be permitted to advance into the early second trimester, when anesthesia and surgical management of the tumor can be undertaken more safely. If the patient is unstable, then urgent neurosurgery is indicated. The risks to the fetus at such a vulnerable stage should be made clear. An obstetrical assessment defines the risks associated with preterm birth, including respiratory distress, intraventricular hemorrhage, infection, and prolonged stay in the neonatal intensive care unit. Therefore, it can be a difficult challenge to prioritize tumor surgery versus continuing pregnancy.[8,38,41]

18.1.6   Outcomes of Pregnancies of 21–39 weeks' Gestation

Maternal intravascular volume peaks at the end of the second trimester, and tumor resection at this time poses risks for significant hemorrhage; consequently, delay of surgery until term is preferred. During this period, therapeutic decisions should take into account fetal viability and its prognosis.

In stable patients, gestational advancement may still be permitted, with close observation of the mother and fetus and possible hospitalization. If delivery is required, preferably one should wait until gestation reaches at least the 30th week, or the fetus reaches the weight of 1 kg as calculated by ultrasound, which corresponds to between the 26th and 30th weeks, because the chance of having a viable healthy infant is then above 90%. Around the 25th week, the chance of survival of the fetus is <50%, while before the 22nd week, only 5% of fetuses can survive. The delivery can be vaginal or cesarean, depending on obstetric criteria. Pituitary surgery for removal of the tumor can then be performed electively.

If visual and/or neurological symptoms worsen during the observational period in order to allow pregnancy advancement and fetal maturation, then pituitary surgery may need to be done as soon as possible. Cesarean section under general anesthesia is indicated immediately before or after surgery, depending on the stage of fetal maturation.

18.1.7   Outcomes of Full-Term Pregnancy

In full-term pregnancy around 40 weeks, a woman can be permitted to go into spontaneous labor or have an induced delivery.

In a stable patient, a cesarean section under general anesthesia is preferable because it is quick and safe and has minimal disadvantages to the fetus. However, spontaneous or induced vaginal delivery is an option. In fact, a cesarean section does not seem to provide any definitive advantage over vaginal delivery in protecting the mother from increased intracranial pressure. Therefore, most researchers indicate that cesarean section should be done only for obstetric and fetal indications. In an unstable patient, as mentioned previously, cesarean section under general anesthesia, followed immediately by surgical decompression of the tumor, is advised.

In cases of pituitary apoplexy, the surgical resection of the adenoma should preferably be done before delivery because delivery itself leads to increased risk of hemorrhage and rupture of vascular lesions. In the perioperative period, there can be large variations in blood volume. In pregnant patients, surgical resection of an adenoma increases the risk of perioperative compromised blood flow to the fetus and the risk of premature labor postoperatively. Therefore, care should be taken to avoid intraoperative blood loss, hypotension, hypovolemia, and hypoxia, all of which can significantly compromise the fetal circulation. In addition, delivery should be planned in case any evidence of fetal distress develops in the perioperative period.

The options for the pituitary surgical approach in pregnant women require some specific care regarding the following points:

(1) *Positioning of the patient*. During surgery, positioning is important in order to avoid mechanical compression of the inferior vena cava by the pregnant uterus. The reason for this is that this causes decreased venous return, leading to hypotension and shock. Conversely, a supine position increases both intrathoracic and intra-abdominal pressure and may decrease uterine blood flow. The supine patient may also be at increased risk for atelectasis. Gastric motility is decreased, leading to increased risk for vomiting and aspiration upon induction of anesthesia. A dorsal decubitus position, with rotation of the trunk to the left side, supported on a rigid roller, avoids compression of the inferior vena cava. When the pituitary lesion is located in the posterior fossa, a ventral decubitus is prohibited. In this situation, a lateral decubitus position is used.

(2) *Neuroanesthesia in pregnancy*. Pregnancy induces significant physiological changes that are largely the result of high levels of progesterone and estrogens, secreted initially by the corpus luteum (up to 12 weeks' gestation) and later by the placenta. Pregnancy leads to increased heart rate, systolic volume, and cardiac output, accompanied by a reduction in systemic vascular resistance. Hyperventilation is used to decrease cerebral blood volume and to facilitate the surgical approach. However, intense hyperventilation ($PaCO_2 < 28$ mmHg) should be avoided, as it may cause cerebral ischemia due to vasoconstriction and deviation of the maternal oxyhemoglobin dissociation curve to the left, with consequent decrease in the oxygen release for placental exchange. There may also be a decrease in maternal cardiac output due to increased intrathoracic pressure. A $PaCO_2$ between 28 and 30 mmHg is sufficient to maintain adequate surgical conditions without interfering with oxygenation of the fetus. Fetal monitoring detects suffering from hypoxia, while hemoglobin saturation at the jugular bulb monitors maternal cerebral oxygenation. If hypotension is induced with the objective of reducing tumor bleeding, it should be used with extreme caution and always accompanied by fetal monitoring. Because uterine blood flow depends on uterine blood pressure, uterine venous pressure, and uterine vascular resistance, lowering the perfusion blood pressure leads to decreased uterine flow. When fetal monitoring reveals the onset of fetal distress caused by hypotension, it also reveals the precise timing of systemic blood pressure readjustment. Aldosterone is elevated during pregnancy, with a concomitant increase in sodium, and especially body water. The plasma osmolarity guides the anesthetist with respect to fluid replacement during surgery.

Two anesthetic problems are relevant for pregnant patients with pituitary adenomas: (a) Anesthesia recommended for transsphenoidal surgery in pregnant women and (b) Anesthesia recommended for delivery in pregnant women with pituitary adenoma.[39,42,43]

(a) Anesthesia procedure recommended for transsphenoidal surgery in pregnant women.[39,42,43]

Multiple medications required during transsphenoidal surgery may increase the risk of fetal developmental abnormalities if administered during the first trimester. Surgery during pregnancy generally increases the risk of first- or second-trimester miscarriage, but it does not appear to increase the incidence of congenital anomalies, nor does it appear to induce preterm labor. Cardiac output is increased by 50%, and typically, anesthesia requirements are decreased by 30%.

(b) Anesthetic procedure recommended for delivery in pregnant women with pituitary adenoma.[39,42,43]

Gestational age is of primary importance for the baby's viability. In the past, delivery was postponed until 36–38 weeks of pregnancy to decrease the likelihood of respiratory distress syndrome. Currently, safe delivery can be performed at 32 weeks' gestation due to the use of glucocorticoid treatment to induce surfactant production.[44]

If the option is transesphenoidal surgery followed by delivery, anesthesia management should be what is necessary for transsphenoidal surgery. Rapid onset of general anesthesia with intravenous agents, endotracheal intubation, and mild hyperventilation do not appear to have an adverse effect on the fetus.

In the chosen option is delivery before neurosurgical treatment, the presence of an intracranial lesion requires a different strategy. A cesarean section under general anesthesia is preferable because it is quick, safe, and has minimal disadvantages to the fetus. Respiratory depression in the newborn, which is a potential problem associated with such delivery, is easily treated. In rare cases of patients who significant intracranial mass effect, regional anesthesia should be avoided because of the risk of cerebrospinal fluid loss and the consequent potential risk of herniation. In such instances, instrumented delivery should be encouraged.[39,42,43]

(3) *Medical treatment during pregnancy*. In some cases, the use of glucocorticoids is advised for the control of cerebral edema, intracranial hypertension, and to accelerate fetal lung maturity. However, prolonged use during pregnancy, especially in the third trimester, may cause suppression of the fetal pituitary-adrenal axis. Therefore, such use should be tailored to the pregnant patient, with consideration of the safety of the developing fetus.[39,42,43]

18.2 PROLACTINOMAS

The PRL-secreting pituitary adenomas (prolactinomas) are the most common pathological cause of hyperprolactinemia and the most common type of pituitary adenoma. Hyperprolactinemia can also be caused by physiological conditions (pregnancy and lactation), pharmacological agents (especially antipsychotics), systemic diseases (renal and hepatic failure), endocrine diseases (hypothyroidism, Cushing's disease), other pituitary or sellar region tumors causing pituitary stalk disconnection, and macroprolactinemia. Identifying the correct cause of hyperprolactinemia is crucial for its treatment.[45,46]

The prevalence of prolactinomas is 500 cases per million, with 60% of these being microadenomas. They affect preferentially women in their third and fourth decades of life, therefore being an important cause of hyperprolactinemia and infertility.[47] In this scenario, fertility and pregnancy are important issues among women harboring prolactinomas.

Hyperprolactinemia can cause galactorrhea and hypogonadism. The mechanisms involved in hypogonadism are the inhibition of gonadotropin-releasing hormone (GnRH) pulsatility, direct inhibition of the section of gonadotrophins, and inhibition of gonadal steroidogenesis.[48] Recently, it was reported in rodents that PRL directly acts on hypothalamic neurons by inhibiting the expression of the gene Kiss1 kisspeptin.[49] A spectrum of impairment in regular menses is described: short luteal phase, anovulatory cycles, oligomenorrhea, and amenorrhea.[50,51] In macroprolactinomas, which have a maximal tumor diameter of more than 1 cm, hypopituitarism can also result from pituitary stalk compression, compression of the anterior pituitary, or both.[45,46]

The gold standard treatment for prolactinomas is the use of dopamine agonists (DA), especially CAB and BRC. These drugs normalize serum PRL levels, leading to restoration of eugonadism and tumor shrinkage in more than 80% of the cases. CAB is currently the drug of choice due to its higher affinity to dopamine receptor type 2 (D2R) and better tolerance, as compared to BRC. A head-to-head study evaluating 459 women with hyperprolactinemia treated with CAB or BRC pointed to serum PRL normalization in 83% of patients on CAB and 59% of those on BRC. Ovulatory cycles were restored in 72% of patients on CAB and 52% on BRC.[52] Nevertheless, the use of CAB for induction of pregnancy is still a matter of debate, while only BRC is approved for this purpose to date.[53]

It is important to actively question the patient about her desire for pregnancy and the issues involved. Hyperestrogenism secondary to pregnancy can cause hypertrophy and hyperplasia of both normal and tumoral lactotrophs, leading to tumor increase and mass effect symptoms in untreated patients, such as headaches and visual impairment. Moreover, if the patient will be on DA to restore fertility, then withdrawal of DA will occur after a positive pregnancy test result is obtained, which means that there has been obligatory exposure of the embryo to the drug. Additionally, the question of whether the woman will want to breastfeed should be considered.

Molitch[54] reviewed the risk of tumor growth with symptoms during pregnancy, including 764 microprolactinomas, 238 macroprolactinomas without previous surgery or radiotherapy, and 148 macroprolactinomas in which these treatments have been already performed. Symptomatic tumor growth occurred in 2.4%, 21%, and 4.7% of cases, respectively. It is important to note that DA was withdrawn when pregnancy was confirmed, usually at 6 weeks' gestation, in the majority of the cases. Regarding the question as to whether prior DA treatment was reduced the risk of subsequent tumor growth in pregnant women, there is only one study showing reduced risk in women who used BRC for at least 12 months.[55]

BRC is the drug of choice for hyperprolactinemic women who desire pregnancy.[53] This is primarily due to the larger experience with BRC-induced pregnancies, as well as its shorter half-life compared to CAB.[56] Molitch[54] reviewed 938 CAB-induced pregnancies and 6239 BRC-induced pregnancies, and found no differences in the risks of premature labor, abortions, and fetal malformations.[54] After this review, four other case series were published, with additional data on 139 CAB-induced pregnancies,[14,15,24,57,58] bringing the worldwide published experience up to 1000 cases. Araujo described 32 pregnancies in 29 women, 6 induced by CAB and 26 induced by BRC, with one case of clubfoot among pregnancies induced by BRC Karaca reported 83 pregnancies in 60 women, 33 induced by BRC and 45 by CAB.[15] A total of 11% of pregnancies ended in abortion, 4% in fetal death, and 6% had malformations, including corpus callosum agenesis with abortion; Down syndrome in two cases induced by BRC; and microcefalia, cleft lip, and a fetal death with neural tube defect in three cases induced by CAB.[58] Finally, Rastogi described 48 pregnancies induced by CAB in 33 women, divided into two groups: one with 23 pregnancies in whom CAB was withdrawal after pregnancy confirmation, and another with 25 pregnancies in whom CAB was maintained throughout pregnancy due to tumor invasiveness.[59] There were three cases of neural tube defect only in the group which maintained CAB.[59] Therefore, although the number of reported CAB-induced pregnancies is increasing, and no clear differences in risks have been seen between CAB and BRC use prior to pregnancy, its safety in pregnancy is still a matter of debate.

The safety of using DA throughout pregnancy is also uncertain because there are few reports in the literature. There were two cases of malformations in 100 cases on BRC: one undescended testicle and another with a talipes deformity,[59,60] whereas there was one fetal death related to eclampsia in 15 pregnancies on CAB.[61] Use of DA throughout pregnancy may be considered for control of tumor growth.[62]

The neuropsychological developed of children exposed to BRC during embryogenesis has been assessed. Bronstein[45] reported one case of idiopathic hydrocephalus, one with tuberous sclerosis, and another with precocious puberty among 70 children, followed up during 12–240 months. In 2 other studies including 64 children (between the ages of 6 months and 9 years) and 988 children (4 months to 9 years-old), respectively,[63] no impaired physical development was observed. Regarding CAB, no abnormalities were described by Bronstein[45] and Ono[64] in 5 and 83 children, followed by 41 months and 12 years, respectively. However, Lebbe described two cases of slight delay in verbal fluency, and one case of difficulty in achieving complete continence, among 88 children.[65] Stalldecker[66] found 2 cases of seizures and 2 cases of pervasive developmental disorder among 61 children exposed to CAB in utero.[66] Due to the low numbers, it is unclear if there is any adverse effect of exposure to BRC or CAB in utero.

In microadenomas and enclosed macroadenomas that do not threaten the optic chiasm, DA discontinuation is recommended as soon as pregnancy is confirmed, while in expanding macroadeomas, tumor shrinkage so that it is within sellar boundaries is required before allowing elective pregnancy. For selective cases, DA can be maintained throughout pregnancy, depending on the specialists' recommendation. Because median serum PRL values of pregnant women with and without prolactinomas seem to be similar, routine measurement of serum PRL during pregnancy is not recommended.[45] For microprolactinomas, clinical evaluation in each trimester of pregnancy should be done, and sellar MRI without contrast and neuro-ophthalmologic evaluation should be performed if there is evidence of tumor size increase. For expanding macroprolactinomas, ophthalmologic evaluation should be performed in each trimester, and pituitary MRI without contrast is indicated if there is evidence of tumor growth. In the presence of mass effect symptoms, if there is no rapid improvement after DA introduction, then decompressive neurosurgery, especially in the second trimester, should be considered, or delivery if the pregnancy is near term (Fig. 18.1).[45]

After delivery, PRL levels and tumor size should be reassessed because reductions, or even normalizations of PRL levels after pregnancy, are well documented in literature. Some authors observed hemorrhagic zones in the tumor,

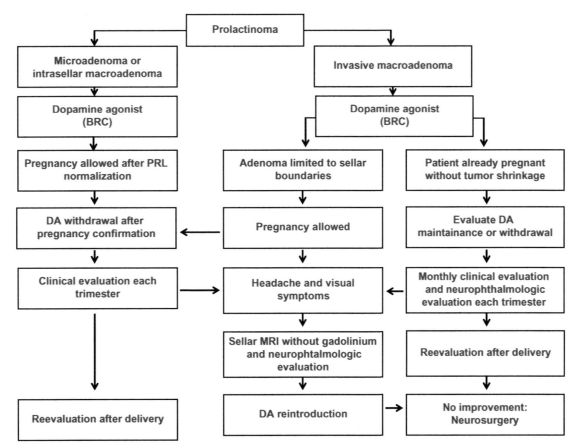

FIG. 18.1 Flowchart of management of pregnant women with prolactinoma. *DA*, dopaminergic agonist.

hypothesizing that hyperestrogenism during pregnancy can induce areas of tumor necrosis and microinfarction, leading to partial or complete tumor involution after pregnancy.[67] Spontaneous remission of hyperprolactinemia after pregnancy was 27% among eight studies and ranged from 10% to 68%.[45,65,68–74] In one of these studies, the authors found that small adenoma size and normal sellar appearance on MRI after pregnancy correlated with remission of hyperprolactinemia.[69]

In patients not requiring DA during pregnancy, serum PRL can be monitored although its utility is questionable, as mentioned previously. Breastfeeding is allowed, as it is not associated with increased risk of pituitary tumor growth per se. However, breastfeeding is contraindicated in patients receiving DA because such treatment inhibits lactation.[45,65,68–74]

18.3   ACROMEGALY

Acromegaly is a rare chronic disease, almost always caused by a pituitary GH-secreting adenoma, which leads to unrestrained secretion of GH and insulinlike growth factor-1 (IGF-1).[75] The average age at diagnosis is 40 years, with an equal number of men and women affected. Therefore, acromegaly is less frequent in women of childbearing age.

Women with acromegaly slowly develop coarse facial features, enlargement of hands and feet, and prognathism. The disease is associated with multiple significant comorbidities (particularly cardiovascular disease, diabetes, hypertension, sleep apnea, and arthropathy).[75] Therefore, patients with acromegaly require a coordinated approach involving many specialties (e.g., endocrinology, surgery, and cardiology). When clinical evidence exists, a glucose tolerance test is performed, and lack of suppression of GH below 1 ng/mL during this test (below 0.4 ng/mL according to other studies),[76] associated with high IGF-1, is in keeping with a diagnosis of acromegaly in nonpregnant patients. As the majority of GH effects are mediated through IGF-1, measurement of IGF-1 has been used to monitor the progression of the disease.[75]

18.3.1   Preconception Counseling and Prenatal Care

Clinical experience with pregnancies in patients with acromegaly has increased as a consequence of better diagnostic and therapeutic approaches.[2,77–83] This is evident from the volume of recent literature on this subject, including single-center case series[77–80] and multicenter retrospective[2,79–81,83] and prospective studies.[82,83] In addition, more information is available on the suggested management of these patients.[2,77–83] However, unplanned pregnancies are still the most prevalent among women with acromegaly.[2,77–83] Maternal and neonatal complications have been associated with acromegaly activity during pregnancy.[78] Therefore, preconception counseling has a positive role to play in evaluating the possibility of pregnancy and the ideal time for it. Such counseling is aimed at achieving adequate disease control before the onset of the pregnancy, thereby reducing the incidence of complications.[78]

Fertility can be an issue in acromegaly.[78–80,84] About 60% of patients with acromegaly have macroadenomas, which through their presence (mass effect) and prior treatment (surgery, radiotherapy) may compromise the normal production of hypothalamic and gonadotrophic hormones, thereby leading to hypogonadotrophic hypogonadism.[78–80,84] In addition, in acromegaly, other factors may compromise fertility, making gestation in a relatively rare event. These include high IGF-I levels, tumor-associated hyperprolactinemia in 30%–40% of patients, comorbidities (e.g., diabetes, heart disease), and other hormonal abnormalities (e.g., hypothyroidism, secondary adrenal insufficiency). Therefore, some patients will require fertility treatments in order to conceive.[78–80,84]

18.3.2   Impact of Pregnancy on Acromegaly

The clinical course of acromegaly during pregnancy may be quite varied. The literature reports a spectrum of improvement,[79–83,85,86] no changes,[79–83,85,87,88] or worsening during pregnancy.[79–83,85,87]

Normal pregnancy can lead to the development of hypertension, altered glucose metabolism, and dyslipidemia. Therefore, the physiological changes of pregnancy may mimic an exacerbation of acromegaly. Some studies support that pregnancy is not the cause of exacerbations of acromegaly and comorbidities,[81–83] while others show that during pregnancy, there was definite worsening of glycemic and blood pressure control.[82] These complications can be correlated with hormonal control before pregnancy.[79]

During pregnancy, pituitary GH(GH-N) levels includes both GH secreted by normal pituitary gland and by the adenoma.[89,90] In contrast with healthy pregnancy, GH-N evaluation by specific immunoassays that do not cross-react with placental GH shows that GH-N secretion remains stable in the presence of a GH-secreting pituitary adenoma.[82,89] Therefore, pregnancy seems not to have an important influence on GH secretion from somatotropinoma. As described in Chapter 3, there is a physiological decrease in IGF-I levels during the first semester, followed by an increase from the second to the third trimester.[91-94]

Tumor size is an important issue during pregnancies complicated by acromegaly. GH-secreting adenomas are slow growing and show variable behaviors during pregnancy. In some cases, they remained stable,[82,83,86] while in others, increased tumor size was evident,[77,83] some remained asymptomatic,[77,83] and others became symptomatic from the tumor mass effect.[77,83] The variability is based on the prepregnancy characteristics of the adenoma: tumor size, extension, and prior treatment. Compared to macroadenomas that have previously undergone surgery and radiotherapy, untreated macroadenomas are more likely to increase in size during pregnancy. The mechanism is multifactorial, including estrogenic stimulus in adenomatous cells and normal lactotrophic cells,[13] and withdrawal of medical therapy that was effectively controlling the tumor.

Jallad[83] reported two patients who became pregnant prior to primary treatment of acromegaly, and who underwent surgery during gestation.[83] Another patient had demonstrated enlargement of a previously resected tumor during pregnancy, which did not respond to CAB. That patient had repeat surgery, with resolution of symptoms and continued pregnancy without complications. Pregancy may be exacerbated by acromegaly, and abortion have been described in some patients.[87]

18.3.3 Impact of Acromegaly During Pregnancy

Maternal GH and IGF-1 do not cross the placental barrier and do not adversely affect fetal growth and development.[89,90,95] Therefore, high maternal GH and IGF-1 levels are not contraindications for pregnancy.[89,90,95] The development of macrosomia in these cases is a result of maternal diabetes mellitus induced by GH, rather than the GH directly.[89,95]

Due to the known insulin resistance and sodium-retaining effects of GH, impaired glucose tolerance, diabetes mellitus, and hypertension are common in patients with acromegaly.[88,89,96,97] In addition, pregnancy itself is an insulin-resistant state.[97] Therefore, compared with the general population, pregnant women with active acromegaly have an increased risk of developing those complications.[81] In a retrospective multicenter study of 59 pregnancies in 46 women with acromegaly, gestational diabetes was diagnosed in 4 of the 59 pregnancies (6.8%).[81] There is also an increased incidence of hypertension, preeclampsia, and coronary artery disease in pregnant women with acromegaly.[81]

Cheng et al. described 13 new cases and reviewed an additional 34 cases from the literature, and they concluded that pregnancy can proceed in treated acromegalic women without significant complications or teratogenicity.[86]

Jallad[83] reviewed 32 pregnancies in women with acromegaly and found that active or uncontrolled acromegaly may be associated with an increased risk of not only gestational diabetes, but also pregnancy-induced hypertension.[83] The altered IGF-axis in acromegaly also may be implicated in impaired glucose homeostasis.

18.3.4 GH-IGF-I Axis of Acromegaly During Pregnancy

During pregnancy, there is a decrease in the number of somatotroph cells. This results in decreased circulating GH levels, as measured by conventional radioimmunoassay (RIA) and immunoradiometric assay (IRMA) methods. Despite this, maternal levels of insulin like IGF-1 are slightly elevated.[91,93,94,98,99] Many clinicians are aware that pregnancy is associated with pseudoacromegaloid state.[100,101] As discussed in Chapter 3, this is because of production of placental GH (GHV), which indirectly decreases pituitary GH production by stimulating IGF1 production.[91,94,102] If GH-like activity is measured during pregnancy, only 3% of the activity is explained by maternal GH and 12% by placental lactogen.[16,103-105] In the presence of the increasing amount of estrogen during pregnancy, an enhanced GH response to provocative testing would be expected because estrogen facilitates GH secretion.[105] However, high levels of estrogen block the normal stimulation of IGF-1 production by GH (Fig. 18.2A).[106]

18.3.5 Hormonal Evaluation of Acromegaly During Pregnancy

It is difficult to establish a diagnosis of acromegaly during pregnancy for several reasons. There is a physiological increase of GH due to GH-V release from the placenta during normal pregnancy, while GH-N normally declines; however, current standard immunoassays cannot distinguish between GH-N and GH-V. Interference of circulating placental hormones with homology to pituitary GH can often lead to either falsely elevated[107] or suppressed GH values in GH assays.[108] The suppression of GH during an oral glucose tolerance test (OGTT) has not been properly assessed in pregnancy, so the usual reference ranges for both basal and postglucose GH cannot be applied to pregnant women. If they can be measured, GH-V levels should not be expected to change. Clues to the presence of a true increase in GH-N include documentation

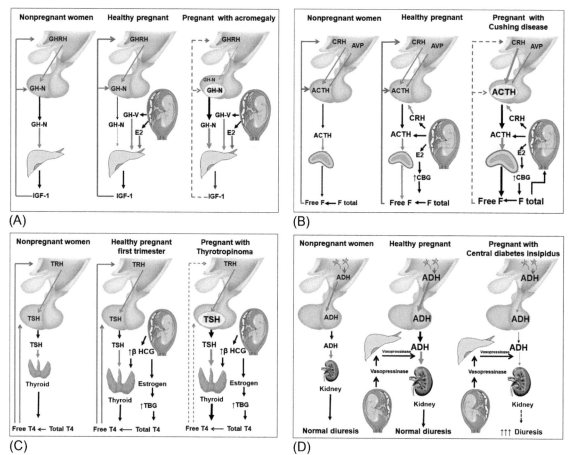

FIG. 18.2 Hypothalamic-pituitary axes in nonpregnant and pregnant women with or without a pituitary adenoma. (A) GH and IGF-1 axis in nonpregnant women compared with healthy pregnant women and pregnant women with acromegaly. *Left panel*: GH is secreted from the anterior pituitary (GH-N). Its biologic effects are mediated through IGF-1 and GH-N itself. *Middle panel*: Placental GH (GH-V) is the major hormone responsible for stimulating the hepatic production of maternal IGF-1, which inhibits maternal pituitary secretion of GH-N, thus replacing GH-N as the predominant form of GH by the second trimester. The pregnancy-associated increase in circulating estradiol leads to hepatic resistance to GH-N, decreasing IGF-I concentrations by 30% in early pregnancy. However, increasing levels of GH-V after midgestation overcome that blockade, leading to IGF-1 increasing by >40% after 24–27 weeks of pregnancy, and returning to prepregnancy levels after delivery. *Right panel*: GH-N secretion by the tumor is autonomous. Both GH-N and GH-V levels are persistently elevated and will drive IGF-1 secretion in opposition to the estrogen blockade. (B) HPA axis in nonpregnant women compared with healthy pregnant and in pregnant women with Cushing's disease. *Left panel*: The hypothalamic CRH stimulates pituitary adrenocortico-trophic hormone secretion (ACTH), with stimulation of cortisol synthesis on the adrenal cortex, which, by feedback, regulates CRH and ACTH secretion. *Middle panel*: A marked increase in estradiol due arising from the placenta in turn stimulates hepatic CBG production. This decreases free cortisol levels transiently, leading to an increase in pituitary ACTH secretion to maintain normal free cortisol levels. Free cortisol levels then rise by the 11th week of gestation, reaching a plateau in the third trimester, while plasma ACTH levels continue to increase throughout pregnancy. As a result, total cortisol levels increase and cortisol clearance decreases, resulting in a state of physiologic hypercortisolism that lacks specific clinical characteristics of CS. Despite hyperactivation of the HPA axis, the circadian rhythm is intact during gestation, with feedback mechanisms of cortisol being regulated at a higher set point. In contrast to the usual negative feedback of cortisol on hypothalamic CRH production, placental CRH production is increased in response to cortisol being the major stimulus for the HPA axis in the third trimester. *Right panel*: ACTH may not be suppressed in patients with cortisol-secreting adrenal adenomas, probably due to pituitary ACTH stimulation by placental CRH or by placental ACTH itself. (C) Hypothalamic-pituitary-thyroid (HPT) axis in nonpregnant women compared with healthy pregnant and in pregnant women with thyrotropinoma. *Left panel*: TRH, produced in the hypothalamus, acts upon thyrotrophs of the adenohypophysis to stimulate the synthesis and release of TSH, which stimulates the thyroid gland to secrete T4 and T3. The axis is controlled by negative feedback on the hypothalamus and pituitary, exerted by thyroid hormones. These hormones are transported in the blood noncovalently attached, mainly, to TBG. *Middle panel*: Beta-human chorionic gonadotropin (hCG) stimulates maternal thyroid function, resulting in an increase in the production of thyroid hormones. Through negative feedback, thyroid hormones reduce maternal TSH in the first semester. In most pregnant women, this effect is transient and has no clinical significance. After the 10th week of gestation, there is a reduction in hCG levels, and mean TSH levels increase. Additionally, at this time, increased TBG levels lead to decreased free T3 and free T4 levels, as well as an increase in TSH. Therefore, in the second half of pregnancy, TSH levels return to prepregnancy values. *Right panel*: TSH is not suppressed due to autonomous secretion by adenoma. (D). Hypothalamic-posterior-pituitary axis in nonpregnant women compared with healthy pregnancy and in pregnant with central DI. *Left panel*: ADH or AVP is secreted by the hypothalamic (supra-optic and paraventricular) nuclei and stored in the posterior pituitary. It is secreted in response to either increases in plasma osmolality or decreases in plasma volume. Its antidiuretic action results from effects on kidney-collecting ducts, consequently leading to water retention. *Middle panel*: Water metabolism is changed as characterized by increased total body water, expanded plasma volume, decreased serum osmolality, decreased thirst threshold, and reset of AVP secretion and thirst to a lower serum osmolality. There is a real increase in AVP production; however, plasma levels of AVP during pregnancy are similar to nonpregnant levels due to threefold-to-fourfold increased metabolic clearance caused by the placental enzyme vasopressinase, which degrades both AVP and oxytocin. Therefore, there is sufficient antidiuretic activity and water balance is maintained. *Right panel*: diuresis increases due to partial or total ADH deficiency. Women with overt or subclinical central DI that has previously been controlled by exogenous vasopressin or DDAVP (1-deamino-8-D-arginine vasopressin) may have increased dose requirements during pregnancy. *((A) Modified from Bronstein MD, Paraiba DB, Jallad RS. Management of pituitary tumors in pregnancy. Nat Rev Endocrinol 2011;7(5):301–10.)*

of pulsatility and/or a paradoxical GH release after TRH, which occurs with GH-N and is not seen with GH-V.[90] Pituitary GH-N levels are expected to decline to <1 mcg/L during the third trimester in normal pregnancy; therefore, higher GH levels by highly specific assays during that period would also be suggestive of acromegaly.[95,99,109]

IGF-1 levels increase during normal pregnancy.[93,109] However, normal adult reference references do not apply in pregnancy. The increased IGF-1 level usually occurs after midgestation.[94] Therefore, a high serum IGF-1 before midgestation is suggestive of acromegaly in pregnancy.

If a woman becomes pregnant prior to the diagnosis of acromegaly, confirmation may only be possible after delivery, due to the lack of normative data for both GH and IGF-1 levels during gestation. If there is a high degree of clinical suspicion of acromegaly, MRI without gadolinium is warranted during pregnancy to detect tumors.

18.3.6 Treatment of Acromegaly During Pregnancy

Surgery was performed during pregnancy in patients with visual and/or neurological symptoms of compression. The middle trimester is generally regarded as the most suitable period for elective surgery, and usually by the transsphenoidal approach (Fig. 18.3).

Medications used to treat acromegaly may pass through the placenta and may cause fetal damage. Therefore, the risks and benefits of treatment during pregnancy should be repeatedly considered against the risk of increased disease activity affecting mother and fetus. BRC, CAB, and octreotide cross the placenta.[54,110–114] The SST analogs (SAs) lanreotide and octreotide should be discontinued early in gestation, or ideally 2 months before trying to conceive. They cross the placental barrier and influence the fetus in the same way as human SST by decreasing the levels of insulin and IGF-1, among others.[54,110–114] SST receptors (SSTRs) are expressed in placenta and other tissues, including the fetal pituitary.[112,115] Therefore, SA could play a role in intrauterine[111,112] and postnatal growth. In addition, other investigators report a risk of severe fetal growth retardation and a likely association with neonatal necrotizing enterocolitis.[116–118]

However, some evidence supports that the placenta may spare the fetus from the effects of SA, allowing IGF-I levels that are sufficient for normal fetal development. First, Caron et al.[111,112] showed no changes in both maternal GH-V and IGF-I concentrations during octreotide treatment. Second, neonates of mothers treated with SA during pregnancy have been reported to have normal size.[118–120] In addition, Maffei[113] evaluated the impact of octreotide administration throughout pregnancy in a patient with acromegaly. The effects of octreotide on uterine artery blood flow, maternal and newborn octreotide concentrations, and SSTR expression and binding at the maternal-fetal barrier level were evaluated.[113] Following administration of subcutaneous octreotide, there was an acute decrease in blood flow from the uterine artery, which

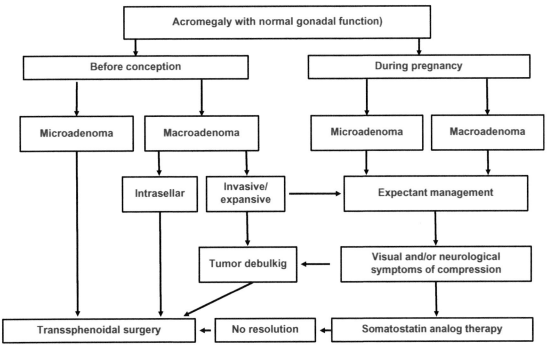

FIG. 18.3 Algorithm of therapeutic options for management of pregnancy in acromegaly.

had no effect on childbirth or fetal development.[113] Octreotide concentrations were high in maternal serum and colostrum and lower in umbilical cord serum, amniotic fluid, and newborn serum.[113] Placental tissue expressed all SST receptor subtypes, but the binding profile was weak in both the placenta and umbilical cord.[113] The child was born without incident, and his anthropometric, metabolic, and endocrine evaluations were normal. Therefore, the use of octreotide had no significant effect on mother or fetus.[113]

However, as there are no well-controlled studies on SA therapy used to treat acromegaly during pregnancy, these drugs should only be used if clearly needed.

A reduction in tumor size and normalization of GH and IGF-1 has also been reported in pregnant women with acromegaly who received treatment with DA drugs.[110,121–123] As discussed in Section 18.1.2 on prolactinomas, there is no evidence that these agents increase the risk of fetal malformations.

There are no adequate, well-controlled studies on the use of pegvisomant in pregnant women (placental passage, maternal and fetal serum levels) and lactating women (excretion of pegvisomant in human milk). Brian[124] reported on a patient with active acromegaly, in whom pegvisomant was maintained throughout gestation and during breastfeeding. This study showed that transplacental passage of pegvisomant is either absent or minimal, and so it does not affect fetal GH and IGF-I interactions.[124] The manufacturer has published data on 26 known cases of women who became pregnant with pegvisomant, and data on 8 pregnant women with partners who used the drug.[125] Most patients stopped pegvisomant when pregnancy was confirmed, and only three continued to take it during pregnancy; and no major problems were reported. However, these data are very limited and insufficient to determine the safety of using pegvisomant during pregnancy.[125]

18.3.7 Practical Approach

The approach to women with acromegaly who desire pregnancy includes laboratory, visual, and radiology assessments to confirm disease activity and the potential for tumor mass effect. This approach aims to minimize risks to the mother and both immediate and long-term consequences to the fetus. Transsphenoidal surgery is the preferred option for acromegalic women harboring a microadenoma, an intrasellar macroadenoma, and even invasive macroadenomas that can be debulked (Fig. 18.3).

If a woman with acromegaly has an unplanned pregnancy, a decision should be made as to whether the condition requires active treatment or if an expectant approach can be adopted. Definitive treatment can usually be delayed until after delivery. Drug treatment for acromegaly is currently not approved for use in pregnancy. Therefore, SA and DA should normally be stopped. Recurrence of GH hypersecretion, return of clinical signs of acromegaly, and reexpansion of the adenoma can occur. Therefore, close monitoring of visual fields is essential, with pituitary MRI done if there is evidence of tumor growth. In such cases, SA and DA have been effective in relieving symptoms. In cases not responsive to drug therapy during pregnancy, or if such therapy is declined, then surgery should be considered (Fig. 18.3).

18.4 CUSHING DISEASE AND PREGNANCY

Pregnancy in women with CS, including Cushing disease (CD), has become feasible due to advances in diagnosis and treatment. Nevertheless, in noncontrolled patients, the prevalence of maternal-fetal complications is high,[23,126] and so surgical and/or medical control of hypercortisolism is obligatory prior to conceiving. Due to similar clinical features and changes in the hypothalamic-pituitary-adrenal (HPA) axis during pregnancy, the diagnosis of CS during gestation can be difficult to make with certainty.[41]

There are substantial differences in the etiologies of CS that appears in pregnant versus nonpregnant women. During pregnancy, the prevalence of adrenal disorders (predominantly adenomas) is about 60%, whereas pituitary adenomas (CD) occur in about 33% of cases. On the other hand, nonpregnant patients have a higher prevalence of CD (70%) compared to adrenal adenomas (15%).[127] This disparity is probably related to CD causing mixed secretion of cortisol and androgens, which in turn can cause infertility due to hypogonadotrophic hypogonadism, as compared to adrenal adenomas that simply have autonomous cortisol production.[128,129] Lindsay[127] reviewed 136 pregnancies in 122 women with CS and found 56 adrenal adenomas, 40 cases of CD, 12 adrenal carcinomas, 4 ectopic ACTH-secreting (EAS) tumors, 4 cases of ACTH-independent hyperplasia (AIH) (possibly due to atypical receptor stimulation), and 1 patient with Carney's complex.[127]

The focus of this part of the chapter is on CD, but there is unavoidable overlap with discussing the diagnosis of CS. Chapter 25 should be consulted for more details about adrenal disorders during pregnancy, including CS.

18.4.1 CS Diagnosis During Pregnancy

The diagnosis of CS during pregnancy can be very challenging. It is possible to divide this situation into three scenarios: (1) pregnancy in a patient with known CS, (2) de novo development of CS during pregnancy, and (3) development of clinical signs and complications suggestive of CS during pregnancy (striae, arterial hypertension, and diabetes mellitus). Some features, such as muscular weakness, larger purple striae (especially outside of abdomen), and osteoporosis, are suspicious for CS. Hirsutism is uncommon in a de novo case of CS during pregnancy because most cases are due to benign adrenal adenomas without hyperandrogenism.[130] Despite these clinical clues, the diagnosis must be supported by hormonal and imaging procedures.

The laboratory diagnosis of CS during pregnancy is made challenging by alterations in serum and urinary cortisol levels, as well as abnormal dynamic testing, that can occur in normal pregnancy.[127] Characteristically, there is a rise of measured serum cortisol due to high levels of estrogen causing a marked increase in corticosteroid-binding globulin (CBG). This hormonal elevation causes false-positive results in low-dose dexamethasone suppression testing in normal pregnancies.[127] Urinary-free cortisol (UFC) can increase up to threefold the upper limit of the normal range during the second and third trimesters of pregnancy.[128–132] Therefore, UFC is more accurate for CS diagnosis when the value is more than three times the upper limit.[128–132] Evaluation of the circadian rhythm of cortisol secretion is recommended, as this is usually preserved during normal pregnancy. A recent study assessed nocturnal salivary cortisol (NSC) and identified the following limits: first trimester 0.25 μg/dL (6.9 nmol/L), second trimester 0.26 μg/dL (7.2 nmol/L), and third trimester 0.33 μg/dL (9.1 nmol/L)[133] (Fig. 18.4).

After this first step to confirm the diagnosis of hypercortisolism, the next phase is measuring ACTH levels to determine if the CS is ACTH-dependent or -independent. However, ACTH may not be suppressed in patients with cortisol-secreting adrenal adenomas, probably due to placental corticotrophin-releasing hormone (CRH) stimulating the production of pituitary ACTH, or because placental ACTH is detected by the assay[127] (Fig. 18.2B). Patients with CD diagnosed during pregnancy exhibit ACTH levels at or above the upper limit of normal.[127]

For the differential diagnosis of ACTH-dependent CS, the high-dose dexamethasone suppression test (HDDST) correctly identified virtually all reported cases of CD, using the cutoff of a 50% decrease in cortisol, while a stimulation test with 100 μg intravenous CRH induced the expected ACTH and cortisol responses in CD patients.[131] Bilateral and inferior petrosal sinus sampling has been performed in a few pregnant women with ACTH-dependent CS,[132] but they should be used cautiously to avoid unnecessary radiation and possible thromboembolic side effects.[127] MRI without galonium enhancement may not identify microadenomas, similar to nonpregnant CD patients.[127] Additionally, the physiological enlargement of the pituitary gland during pregnancy may mask small pituitary adenomas.[127] Imaging without gadolinium should be performed only if surgery is planned prior to term, while adrenal CT scans should be avoided due to radiation. Adrenal imaging by ultrasound is safe during pregnancy.

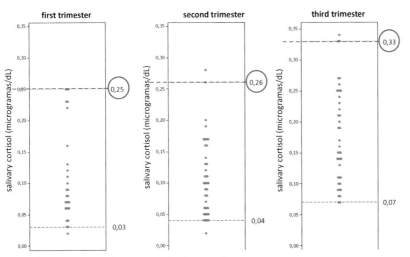

Individual values and reference limits using the percentile 2.5-97.5 for nocturnal salivary cortisol in the pregnant group, in the three trimesters of gestation

FIG. 18.4 Individual values of nighttime salivary cortisol in healthy pregnant groups (2.5th and 97.5th percentiles). To convert to nmol/L, multiply by 27.6. *T1*, first trimester of pregnancy; *T2*, second trimester of pregnancy; *T3*, third trimester of pregnancy. (*From Lopes LM, Francisco RP, Galletta MA, Bronstein MD. Determination of nighttime salivary cortisol during pregnancy: comparison with values in non-pregnancy and Cushing's disease. Pituitary 2016;19(1):30–8.*)

18.4.2 Materno-Fetal Complications

An important systematic review of published cases reported 214 cases of pregnancy that were complicated by active CS. However, this relevant study considered patients who delivered within the 12 months prior to CS diagnosis as having had active CS during the pregnancy.[134] The patients were categorized into two groups: active CS during pregnancy and patients with a history of CS, but treated and cured at the time of pregnancy.

In women with active CS during pregnancy, maternal complications were more prevalent. Among them are hypertension (40%–68%), diabetes or glucose intolerance (25%–37%), preeclampsia (14%–27%), osteoporosis and fractures (5%), psychiatric disorders (4%), cardiac failure (3%), wound infections (2%), and maternal death (2%).[127,134]

A trend for higher live birth rates was seen in women treated and cured before pregnancy. Women with active CS during pregnancy also showed increased risk of fetal morbidity. The most common fetal morbidity was prematurity, occurring in about 43%–66% of cases. Other described morbidities were intrauterine growth retardation (15%–21%), spontaneous abortion or intrauterine death (5%–24%), respiratory distress (14%), stillbirth (6%), and adrenal insufficiency (2%).[127,134]

18.4.3 Treatment of CS During Pregnancy

CS diagnosed near the end of pregnancy is generally treated conservatively, aiming to control comorbidities such as hypertension and diabetes mellitus.[135–143] Compared to nonpregnant women, surgery is the first treatment option in CS of any cause during pregnancy.[134,144,145] Radiotherapy and mitotane are contraindicated due to the delayed effect and potential harmful or teratogenic effects, respectively.

In published cases of pregnant patients with CD, 42.5% were not specifically treated to reduce cortisol levels.[134,144,145] Of those that were treated, the modalities included transsphenoidal pituitary surgery, medical treatment, and bilateral adrenalectomy. Pituitary surgery has been done in CD ideally between the end of the first and second trimesters (12–29 weeks' gestation), a period that correlates with a lower rate of maternal and fetal complications. The factors that influence the choice of surgical procedure are severity, trimester of gestation, and perceived therapeutic risk-benefit for the maternal-fetal consequences.[38]

Adrenalectomy for adrenal causes of CS, such as adrenal adenomas and carcinomas, was performed, with good results both for CS resolution and birth rate.[144,146] Bilateral adrenalectomy can be performed for other etiologies, such as non-controlled or refractory CD, and for severe CS due to ectopic ACTH production.

Medical therapy, initiated more frequently in the second or third trimester, is generally a secondary treatment choice. Of these, treatment with steroidogenesis inhibitors was the most frequent option reported, particularly with metyrapone (Table 18.1).[145] This drug was used in about half of the cases, with good control of CS achieved in the majority of them and one report of adrenal insufficiency.[127,147] The most wearisome side effect of metyrapone is the increase of precursors such as 11-deoxycorticosterone, which can aggravate arterial hypertension and increase the risk of preeclampsia. Although metyrapone crosses the placental membrane in animal studies, no neonatal abnormalities have been reported in human cases thus far.[148,149] Ketoconazole, one of the most used steroidogenesis inhibitors in nonpregnant CS patients, has been less utilized in pregnancy due to potential side effects, such as antiandrogenic effects and teratogenicity seen in animal studies.[127,135,136] Some recent case reports have shown good results (Table 18.1).[137,148]

Other adrenal steroidogenesis blockers, such as aminoglutethimide and mitotane, are rarely used because they can induce fetal masculinization and teratogenicity, respectively.[130] Of drugs that are potentially specific for pituitary tumors,

TABLE 18.1 Medications used in pregnancy by patients with active CS

Medication	n = 33	%	Dose	Obs
Metyrapone[127,138,145,147]	17	52	0.5–3.0 g/day	Hypertension worsening and preeclampsia increase
Ketoconazole[127]	7	21	0.6–1.0 g/day	Teratogenic (only in animals)
CAB[135,139]	4	12	2.0–3.5 mg/week	Only direct drug to tumor
Cyproheptadine[127]	3	9	–	Lack of efficacy
Aminoglutethimide[127]	1	3	2.5 g/day	Fetal masculinization
Mitotane[127]	1	3	–	Teratogenic

four patients were treated with CAB during pregnancy.[135,136,139] These women had good hormonal control and maternal-fetal outcomes after using 2.0–3.5 mg/week of CAB during pregnancy. There are no reports of the use of the SST analog pasireotide during pregnancy to control hypercortisolism.

18.5 CLINICALLY NONFUNCTIONING PITUITARY ADENOMAS

Clinically nonfunctioning adenomas are the second-most-common type of pituitary tumor; however, they usually affect older patients (between the fifth and ninth decades). Their prevalence is estimated in 70–90 cases per million. When they do occur in younger patients, they are more common among women.[3]

Hypogonadism and infertility occur with nonfunctioning tumors as a result of hyperprolactinemia from pituitary stalk disruption, and/or from compression of anterior pituitary gland, and ovulation induction by use of GnRH or gonadotropins can be indicated.[3] Overall, pregnancy in women harboring clinically nonfunctioning tumors is a rare event.

As noted in Chapter 3, hyperestrogenism during pregnancy causes physiological pituitary enlargement. When combined with a nonfunctioning tumor, this physiological enlargement can lead to symptomatic tumor mass effect. Table 18.2 summarizes 27 pregnancies in patients harboring clinically nonfunctioning adenomas, 10 with a diagnosis prior to pregnancy. Mass effect symptoms were reported in seven cases in the second and third trimesters, with visual disturbances and ptosis the most common complaints. In five of these seven symptomatic cases, dopaminergic therapy was introduced (BRC in three and CAB in two), and it was successful in four cases. It is speculated that the mass effect relief by DA may be related to normal lactotroph hyperplasia reduction.[140,141] There were 24 live births, including 2 premature deliveries, with no malformations reported. Surgery should be reserved for cases with no improvement after medical treatment, and preferably done during the second trimester.[26,142] Nevertheless, if pregnancy is near term and a patient has important mass effect symptoms, cesarean delivery should be performed, followed by pituitary surgery (Table 18.2).

TABLE 18.2 Pregnancy outcome in patients harboring nonfunctioning pituitary tumors

Ref.	Age (years)	N	Clinical picture	Sellar MRI	Treatment	Outcome and delivery
Masdig et al.[141]	29	1	Visual defect in left eye at 18 weeks' gestation	2.0 cm in vertical height	BRC 5 mg 3×/day	Vision improved after 5 days. Delivery at 39 weeks.
Lee et al.[143]	39	1	Headache and left ptosis for 1 week at 34 weeks' gestation	1.5 × 1.3 × 1 cm, expanding and invasive tumor	BRC 2.5 mg 3×/day	No improvement, Delivery at 39.3 weeks Improvement 2 days after delivery.
Lambert et al.[24]	31.6 ± 5	16	Tumor expansion in 4		CAB in 2 cases and surgery in 1	2 premature deliveries, 1 stillbirth among 16 pregnancies
Ennaifer[150]	43	1	Headache and left ptosis for 2 months, at 36 weeks' of gestation	1.35 × 2.9 × 1.2 cm	BRC 1.25 mg twice/day	Improved in 48 h Delivery at 38 weeks
Karaca[15]	–	8 pregnancies in 7 patients	No symptoms; 1 maintained CAB due to invasiveness			2 miscarriages. 6 live births, 1 macrosomic

BRC, bromocriptine; *CAB*, cabergoline.

18.6 TSH-SECRETING PITUITARY ADENOMAS

TSH-secreting pituitary adenomas (TSH-omas) are an unusual disorder, accounting for about 2% of all pituitary tumors.[3] Clinical manifestations are almost the same as those of ordinary hyperthyroidism. Hormonal evaluation shows high free T3 and free T4 levels and either a normal or a high level of TSH (Fig. 18.2C). Most of the tumors are macroadenomas and possess SSTRs, which are sensitive to SST and its analogs. The primary therapy for ectopic TSH-oma is surgery. Medical therapy with SST analogs is another option. It can be effective in both tumor size reduction and hormone control, leading to a decrease in TSH, and thereby lower free T3 and free T4 levels.[3,14]

The presence of macroadenoma (which causes hypogonadism from tumor mass effect) associated with hyperthyroidism (which also causes infertility) makes pregnancy a very rare event in this tumor.[15] Only four cases of pregnancy occurring in women with TSH-secreting tumors have been reported.[151–154] Hyperthyroidism should be controlled, and the first option is antithyroid drugs.[153] Due to the risk of teratogenicity, during the first trimester, the drug of choice is propylthiouracil. From the second trimester, methimazole is the drug of choice because it has lower hepatic toxicity. In cases of hyperthyroidism unresponsive to thionamides, the presence of tumor growth, or both, SST analogs may be introduced. In two patients, octreotide was administered during pregnancy.[151,152] Patients achieved hormonal control, without adverse events. In one patient, TSH-oma was diagnosed during pregnancy.[154]

The limited number of gestational cases in patients with TSH-omas is insufficient to draw any firm conclusions about treatment options.

18.7 PITUITARY INSUFFICIENCY

18.7.1 Hypopituitarism

Hypopituitarism is defined as the deficiency of one or more of the hormones secreted by the pituitary gland.[155] Depending on the cause, it can be divided into two types. Primary hypopituitarism is caused by disorders of the pituitary gland itself. The most common causes are pituitary adenoma and its treatment (surgery or radiation therapy). Secondary hypopituitarism is the result of dysfunction in the hypothalamus or pituitary stalk, which interrupts the nerve or vascular connections to the pituitary gland. Common causes of secondary hypopituitarism include craniopharyngioma (CP), germ cell tumor, traumatic brain injury (TBI), and subarachnoid hemorrhage.[155]

Hormonal deficiencies can be partial or total, involving one or more axes (gonadotrophic, somatotrophic, thyroidal, and adrenal).[155] GH-secreting cells are particularly vulnerable to pressure, which is why GH deficiency occurs first and most frequently among all pituitary hormones, followed by deficiencies of gonadotropins [luteinizing hormone (LH) and follicle-stimulating hormone (FSH)], thyroid-stimulating hormone (TSH), ACTH (or ACTH and then TSH), and finally PRL.[156]

In some cases, pituitary function was already compromised before pregnancy because of the presence of a pituitary tumor. In many other cases, the endocrine impairment is directly due to the sudden and rapid growth of pituitary tumors in pregnancy. There is an increase in intrasellar pressure, which compresses the portal circulation, pituitary stalk, and pituitary gland, resulting in further damage to normal residual tissue.[155] Causes of hypopituitarism that are most specific to pregnancy include lymphocytic hypophysitis and postpartum pituitary infarction (or Sheehan's syndrome).[155]

During pregnancy, the priority for hormonal replacement should be glucocorticoid, followed by thyroid hormone.[155] Doses should be adjusted throughout pregnancy based on the severity and nature of the condition. For this reason, it is necessary to follow these patients regularly and closely during pregnancy.

18.7.2 ACTH Deficiency

Patients with pituitary adenomas may present secondary adrenal insufficiency, isolated from or associated with other pituitary deficiencies.[155] Although there is impairment of CRH/ACTH secretion, with subsequent decrease in adrenal stimulation, the clinical picture is related only to glucocorticoid deficiency. Mineralocorticoid and adrenal androgens are preserved. Hyperpigmentation is not present (i.e., CRH secretion is not increased). The presence of hyponatremia and volume expansion can occur secondary to so-called inadequate increase in arginine vasopressin (AVP) secretion.[155]

Mineralocorticoid and androgen adrenal replacement should be started in patients with classic adrenal. The priority treatment for hormonal replacement should be glucocorticoid, followed by thyroid hormone.[155]

Hydrocortisone replacement (or cortisone acetate if hydrocortisone is not available) is the most physiological option for glucocorticoid replacement. The recommended daily hydrocortisone dose is 10–12 mg/m^2, which should be given in two to three doses, with administration of half to two-thirds of the total daily dose in the morning. Adrenal insufficiency requires lifelong replacement therapy, which should be tailored to such situations as stress and surgical procedures. The administration of hydrocortisone injections could and should be taught how and when to administer them.[157]

Pregnancy is a physiological state of glucocorticoid excess and is associated with high serum concentrations of cortisol-binding globulin (CBG), free cortisol, and progesterone, especially in the latter stages.[158,159] Patients with adrenal insufficiency in pregnancy should be treated with hydrocortisone (12–15 mg/m^2 daily), in three doses, with the largest one given in the morning. At the onset of labor, the daily hydrocortisone dose should be doubled or tripled, or the parenteral dose of 50–100 mg may be given during the second stage of labor.[157] If the patient undergoes cesarean section, hydrocortisone should be given intravenously at a dose of 100 mg every 6 h, and then tapered over the next 48 h.[157]

18.7.3 TSH Deficiency

Pregnancy is associated with an approximately 50% increase in demand for thyroid hormones, which is apparent within the first 16 weeks of gestation.[155] This increase is mainly attributed to the estrogen-driven doubling in thyroxine-binding globulin concentrations Hypothyroid mothers should be followed by using thyroid function tests (serum fT4) throughout pregnancy (4 weeks apart if test results are abnormal and 6–8 weeks apart if results are within reference intervals), and their thyroxine dosage must be altered when necessary.[155] The treatment of hypothyroidism during pregnancy should be adjusted so that fT4 levels remain within the established reference ranges for pregnant women.[155]

Several studies have documented that in the first-trimester of pregnancy 30%–50% of such women may be inadequately treated during this critical period for fetal development, when the fetal brain is entirely dependent on maternal thyroid hormones.[160,161] Inadequately treated hypothyroidism has been associated with spontaneous miscarriages. Low intelligent quotients (IQs) have been found in some of the children of women with suboptimally treated hypothyroxinemia during pregnancy.[160,161] The management of hypothyroidism in pregnancy is discussed in more detail in Chapter 19.

18.7.4 GH Deficiency

Normal production of GH is not a prerequisite for pregnancy success because a normal pregnancy is possible in women with Laron dwarfism, in which both the GH receptor and GH-binding protein (GHBP) are absent.[162,163] Therefore, GH replacement is usually not a consideration in women with hypopotuitarism who are contemplating pregnancy.[164,165]

18.7.5 PRL Deficiency

PRL deficiency is not a cause of infertility, so replacement is not required in women with hypopituitarism who are planning to conceive or who are pregnant. However, PRL deficiency can lead to failure of milk production in the postpartum period. In a retrospective study of 18 pregnancies in 9 hypopituitary patients, Overton[166] found that only one could breastfeed her baby. PRL deficiency causes only one clinical symptom, which is the inability to produce milk after childbirth.[13] Lack of PRL is more closely associated with difficulty synthesizing milk than producing milk.[167] Administration of exogenous PRL can be used to initiate and maintain breastfeeding, this also is discussed in Chapter 28, which addresses chest feeding in transgendered patients.

18.8 SHEEHAN'S SYNDROME

Sheehan's syndrome is a nontumoral cause of hypopituitarism, secondary to pituitary necrosis caused by hypovolemic shock from uterine bleeding during or after delivery. As perinatal care has improved in the last few decades, Sheehan's syndrome diminished considerably in incidence, falling to an estimated 1 in 10,000 deliveries.[168] In India, of 8730 parous females who were screened for Sheehan's syndrome, 98 (1.1%) were confirmed,[169] while in Iceland, the prevalence was estimated as 5.1 per 100,000 women in 2009.[6] Nevertheless, this diagnosis must be considered in cases with severe postpartum bleeding. Some authors considered massive uterine hemorrhage as being a loss of 3000 g or more of blood including amniotic fluid.[170]

The first case was described by Simmonds in 1913, as a consequence of hypopitutarism.[170,171] Nevertheless, the term *Sheehan syndrome* was coined in 1937 by the English pathologist Harold Leeming Sheehan on the basis of autopsy findings in patients with postpartum pituitary necrosis.[170–172]

The pathophysiology includes ischemia-induced pituitary dysfunction secondary to the arrest of blood flow to the adenohypophysis after postpartum hemorrhage. Those necrotized areas of the adenohypophysis undergo reorganization, leading to atrophic changes and chronically to an empty sella turcica, which can be clinically detected by MRI. During pregnancy, pituitary hyperplasia makes the gland more susceptible to ischemia which, when associated with other factors as small sella size, severe arterial hypotension, and autoimmunity, can culminate in the development of Sheehan's syndrome.[173,174]

The clinical picture varies from immediate postpartum circulatory collapse to mild symptoms of hypopituitarism. The most common presentation is the failure of postpartum lactation and menstruation, while acute adrenocortical insufficiency is rarely observed. The anatomic situation of GH and PRL cells within the lower lateral region of the adenohypophysis makes them more susceptible to be damaged by ischemic necrosis, thereby explaining the common deficiencies of GH and PRL.[175]

Symptoms of hypopituitarism are frequently insidious, so Sheehan's syndrome is rarely diagnosed in the acute phase.[176] It must be distinguished from pituitary apoplexy, which also can cause hypopituitarism.[177] Generally, the time between delivery and diagnosis of Sheehan's syndrome ranges from a few years to up to 30 years, with a mean of 14 years.[168,171,176,178]

The degree and severity of anterior pituitary deficiencies vary, with panhypopituitarism reported in 55%–86% of patients.[170] Sellar MRI usually reveals an empty sella of normal size in Sheehan's syndrome when performed months to years after delivery.[14] Anemia and other cytopenias, impairment in quality of life, hyperlipidemia, changes in body composition, sleep disorders, and osteoporosis have been observed in patients without a diagnosis and correct treatment of hormonal deficiencies.[168,179] The hormonal replacement required depends on identifying which anterior (and even posterior) pituitary deficiencies are present. Although ovulation induction can be necessary for subsequent pregnancies, spontaneous pregnancies have been reported, and pregnancy has even been associated with the recovery of some pituitary function.[168,179]

18.9 LYMPHOCITIC HYPOPHYSITIS

The first report of pituitary infiltration by inflammatory cells, or hypophysitis, was made by Brissaud in 1908.[180] However, its pathophysiology was only elucidated in 1962 by Goudie and Pinkerton,[181] who described, from an autopsy of a 22-year-old woman, inflammatory infiltration and atrophy of thyroid, adrenals, and pituitary. They attributed this to an autoimmune process related to pregnancy because she had delivered 14 months before her death.

Hypophysitis can be classified as primary or secondary. Primary hypophysitis includes lymphocytic, granulomatous, xanthomatous, IgG-4 related lymphoplasmacytic, necrotizing, and mixed forms (lymphogranulomatous, xanthogranulomatous). Secondary hypophysititis can develop in response to local lesions (rupture of Rathke's cleft cysts, germinoma),[182] systemic diseases (sarcoidosis, granulomatosis, vasculitis, tuberculosis, syphilis, hemochromatosis, histiocytosis), and immunomodulatory drugs (anti-CTLA-4 antibodies and IFN-α). More than 350 cases of hypophysitis have now been described in the literature.[183]

Lymphocytic hypophysitis (LyH) represents more than half the cases of primary hypophysitis. It is characterized by a predominantly lymphocytic infiltration, which may lead to pituitary tissue destruction and fibrotic reaction, with subsequent hypopituitarism.[182,183] Some authors pointed to an underestimation in diagnosis.[184] LyH, in its turn, can be classified according to the level of anatomical impairment within adenohypophysis (LAH), infundibuloneurohypophysitis (LINH), and panhypophysitis (LPH).[185]

LAH is about six times more common in women, with mean age at presentation of 35 years, and 57% presented during pregnancy or postpartum.[183–185] LINH and LPH have a mean age at presentation of 42 years and are not associated with pregnancy. In a review, Abe et al. described 26 histologically proven cases of LINH and 34 of LIPH. The female:male ratio was 4.3 for LAH, 1.3 for LINH, and 1.7 for LIPH. An association with late pregnancy and postpartum was described in 69% for LAH, 27% for LINH, and 18% for LIPH.[186] The association with pregnancy is not very well understood, although some authors hypothesized that with the molecular similarity between placental and pituitary antigenicity, increase in pituitary mass may lead to the release of pituitary antigens. Furthermore, hyperestrogenemia may modify circulating pituitary patterns, increasing the systemic circulation and rendering the pituitary more accessible to the immune system during pregnancy.[183]

In about 30% of cases, LH is associated with other autoimmune diseases, especially Hashimoto's thyroiditis.[187] Although considered an autoimmune disease, the causative antigens in LyH have not been identified to date. Antipituitary antibodies were described in research studies, but they cannot yet be used as a diagnostic tool.[186] Although these antibodies were found in patients previously diagnosed with idiopathic hypopituitarism of presumed autoimmune etiology (15% with ACTH deficiency, 26% with GH deficiency, and 21% with central hypogonadism),[173] these same antibodies were also described in other nonautoimmune pituitary disorders.[188]

The classical clinical picture of anterior LyH is related to mass effects, including headaches and visual impairment; and hormonal disturbances, especially ACTH deficiency and hyperprolactinemia.[183] It is interesting to note that in other series, classical ACTH deficiency was not so commonly found.[189] Diabetes insipidus (DI) is not as commonly found, and when isolated, it can occur in LINH, where gestational diabetes insipidus (GDI) is the main differential diagnosis. As in pregnancy, the posterior pituitary is pushed posteriorly by the increased size of the anterior pituitary, and there is a loss of the hypersignal in the posterior pituitary gland secondary to a decrease in AVP reserves. Therefore, the lack of a bright spot of the posterior pituitary on a T1-weighted sequence is a normal finding in pregnant women, and not always related to central DI. Pituitary stalk enlargement and antirabphilin-3A antibodies' positivity, are helpful tools for assessment of the infundibuloneurohypophysitis not always related to central DI during pregnancy.[190]

Classically, MRI imaging of LyH depicts a sellar mass with homogeneous enhancement by gadolinium, pituitary stalk thickening, and loss of spontaneous high signal intensity on T1-weighted imaging, corresponding to the posterior pituitary. A hypo signal in T2 sequences of sellar MRI was also described in some cases of hypophystis.[191] An empty sella may be found after years of continued disease. Nevertheless, pituitary imaging can be misleading, as a pituitary adenoma may be inaccurately diagnosed.[192]

The pathological analysis of pituitary tissue from a pituitary biopsy or surgery is necessary for the definitive diagnosis of LyH. Nevertheless, the development of hypopituitarism in young women, particularly with ACTH deficiency, a time course related to recent pregnancy and puerperium, a symmetrical sellar mass, and no history of peripartum hypovolemia, can point to a presumptive diagnosis of LyH.[193] Replacement of deficient hormones is required, especially for the adrenal axis. Spontaneous regression has been reported in some cases. Nevertheless, in cases with a central mass effect, immunosuppression with corticosteroids is recommended in an attempt to shrink the mass. If there is no improvement, neurosurgery is indicated.[193]

Caturelgi reviewed 210 women with anterior LyH and found that 120 (57%) presented during pregnancy or postpartum, with the majority doing so in the last month of pregnancy or the first 2 months after delivery.[183,194,195] In a recent Chinese cohort of 33 women with LyH, in 8 of them, the onset was related to pregnancy.[189] From Caturegli's review, anterior LyH cases during pregnancy were generally not complicated and typically conclude with spontaneous vaginal delivery at term, except for one patient who died during labor.[183,196]

Table 18.3 summarizes the clinical picture and outcome of reported cases in the literature found by searching for the terms "lympochytic hypophysitis" and "pregnancy" in PubMed. There were seven patients with an onset during pregnancy, with pathological confirmed diagnosis in five, and uneventful deliveries in all of them.

TABLE 18.3 Literature data on lymphocytic hypophysitis in pregnancy

Reference	Patient data	Outcome and delivery
Funazaki et al.[197]	33 years. Headache at 8 months of pregnancy. Diagnosis at 2 weeks after delivery: headache, visual impairment, and agalactia.	Prednisolone 60 mg/day. Treatment and tapering for 27 months.
Yaoita et al.[198]	27 years. Bitemporal hemianopsia was detected on the 28th week. Surgery at the 30th week and.glucocorticoid replacement therapy was required after surgery.	Delivery at 37th week.
Davies et al.[199]	30 years. Headache and visual impairment at 34th week. Intravenous glucocorticoids after pituitary biopsy.	Uneventful delivery.
Siddique et al.[200]	37 years. Headache and visual defects 5 weeks after delivery of her second child. Surgery.	Spontaneous pregnancy after 3 years.
Sinha et al.[201]	26 years. Headache and visual impairment at 38 weeks. No improvement with glucocorticoid therapy. Surgery after labor induction.	Spontaneous pregnancy after 1 year and mass effect symptoms at 16th week of pregnancy, controlled with medical therapy.
Kidd et al.[202]	31 years. Headache, visual defects at 22 weeks. Improvement after surgery.	Uneventful delivery at term.
Buckland and Popham[203]	23 years. Visual impairment at 36th week.	Delivery was indicated and visual improvement occurred in 48h.

18.10 DIABETES INSIPIDUS DURING PREGNANCY

DI is a syndrome characterized by excretion of abnormally large volumes (polyuria, >40–50 mL/kg of body weight) of diluted urine (osmolarity <300 mosm/L) and polydipsia.[155]

Other common clinical features include increased urinary frequency, incontinence, nocturia, enuresis, and craving for cold water. It should be differentiated from the polyuria and polydipsia of uncontrolled hyperglycemia and other forms of solute diuresis. Classically, DI may be caused by inadequate AVP production or secretion (central DI), renal AVP-signaling defects (nephrogenic DI), increased AVP degradation by placental vasopressinase during pregnancy (GDI), or suppression of AVP by excessive fluid intake (primary polydipsia).

Central DI is the more common subtype, caused by genetic or acquired hypothalamic or pituitary disease. Acquired forms include hypothalamic or pituitary lesions such as CPs, infiltrating or metastatic diseases, trauma, ischemia, or auto-immune disorders. Very rarely do pituitary adenomas present with DI at diagnosis.[204] On the contrary, DI occurs after pituitary surgery, usually transiently, or less commonly permanently. Genetic or familial forms of central DI are caused by mutations in the *AVP* gene, or rarely by mutations in the *WFS1* gene. Central X-linked DI has also been described in the literature, but the genetic cause has not been identified to date.[205]

Classically, DI during pregnancy can be divided into three categories according to AVP and desmopressin responses: AVP-resistant and desmopressin sensitive (typical and the main cause of GDI), AVP and desmopressin resistant (nephrogenic form), and AVP and desmopressin sensitive (central form).

18.10.1 Gestational Diabetes Insipidus

GDI is a rare complication of pregnancy, occurring in 2–3 cases/100,000 pregnancies.[206] Commonly, it develops near the end of the second or in the third trimester.[190] The more common explanation is excessive vasopressinase activity, a placental enzyme that degrades AVP and oxytocin, but not the synthetic form desmopressin.[207] In most cases, the clinical picture remits naturally 4–6 weeks after delivery.[208–210] These data are supported by the disappearance of vasopressinase in serum examined by Western blot analysis.[210]

Vasopressinase is metabolized in the liver, explaining the higher levels of this enzyme in patients with hepatic insufficiency. Therefore, another factor contributing to the pathophysiology of GDI is transient liver dysfunction in which degradation of vasopressinase in liver is reduced, explaining its association with acute fatty liver of pregnancy and HELLP syndrome.[211]

Other mechanisms may be involved in the establishment of GDI, such as enhanced AVP clearance by increased blood circulation in the liver and kidneys; renal resistance to AVP due to the increased prostaglandins; hyperplasia of the pituitary, which may compress the neurohypophysis; and possible AVP inhibition by increased levels of glucocorticoids, progesterone, and thyroxine.[208]

18.10.2 Diagnosis of GDI

Symptoms of GDI include hypotonic polyuria, polydipsia, fatigue, weight loss, decreased skin turgor, and nausea, which usually develop over a few days, and which may worsen in subsequent days if this condition is not properly identified and treated.[212] The differential diagnosis of polyuric and polydipsic states in pregnancy is extensive, and accurate diagnosis is difficult. Obtaining a detailed history is essential to making the differential diagnoses of DI. Primary polydipsia and head trauma should be excluded. Ingestion of drugs should be questioned such as lithium, mannitol, diuretics, and anticholinergic drugs. Because central DI or nephrogenic DI can also be observed during pregnancy, a precise differential diagnosis of DI is important.

This diagnosis is challenging because water metabolism changes during pregnancy. The water deprivation test usually is not recommended during pregnancy because it may lead to significant dehydration. Thus, the diagnosis is sometimes limited to assessment of urine and plasma osmolalities or after therapeutic testing with desmopressin administration.[213]

Pituitary MRI and measurements of plasma or urinary AVP are supported as useful methods in the differential diagnosis. MRI imaging during pregnancy without gadolinium can be safely performed. This imaging method is useful in excluding lesions of the hypophysis and hypothalamus. A key component of successful macroadenoma management during pregnancy is ongoing follow up and support to early detect hypothalamic dysfunction.

Measurements of plasma or urinary AVP are expensive, but they are needed when osmolality results are inconclusive. In a hypernatremic patient, a urine osmolality below that of the plasma suggests DI. Nephrogenic DI can be excluded if there is a normal response to desmopressin replacement.

Once the diagnosis is established, close monitoring of vital signs, fetal status, fluid balance, body weight, and renal function are essential. Fluid intake must approximate urine volume and other fluid losses (Fig. 18.2D).

18.10.3 Treatment

Many patients require parenteral treatment, which usually consists of dextrose and normal saline, but it is also essential to correct any electrolyte disturbances if present. Otherwise, hypernatremia and circulatory collapse may develop, especially if the patient has some thirst alterations (hypodipsia or adipsia).

The specific treatment of GDI requires 1-deamino-8-D-AVP (desmopressin), a synthetic form of AVP with a modified N-terminus and a second amino-acid change that renders it resistant to enzyme vasopressinase.[214] It may be used intravenously, intranasally, subcutaneously, or in oral form. Desmopressin has a prolonged antidiuretic activity; the antidiuretic effects last from 8 to 24 h depending on the route of administration. In the presence of an upper respiratory tract infection, nasal absorption can be reduced. In these cases, and in the postoperative period, the parenteral SC form is preferred. Lower-extremity edema and signs of water intoxication may develop in cases with excessive dosage.

Experience with the use of desmopressin during pregnancy is increasing; it is safe for both the mother and the fetus.[214] Plasma sodium should be closely monitored after the initiation of desmopressin treatment to avoid hyponatremia.

For labor and delivery, regional analgesia or anesthesia is the method of choice.[213] Because of increased urinary output and possible dehydration, attention to the potential hazard of hypovolemia is mandatory during regional techniques.

GDI may be associated with preeclampsia, acute fatty liver of pregnancy, or HELLP syndrome.[211] Consequently, evaluation for preeclampsia and HELLP syndrome is indicated in these patients.[206,210,215]

The absence of previous individual/familiar pituitary risk factors, absence of liver dysfunction, postpartum identification of the neurohypophyseal MRI bright T1-signal without gadolinium, resolution of symptoms, and normalization of the laboratory tests after delivery emphasize the diagnosis of transient gestational DI, most probably due to increased vasopressinase activity.[215]

18.11 DEFICIENCY OF OXYTOCIN

The contractile actions of oxytocin are observed not during pregnancy, but during labor and lactation.[216,217] During gestation, myometrial receptivity increases, especially in the last trimester, due to a high density of oxytocin receptors, which increase secondary to a decline in progesterone and an increase in estradiol.[218] The increase in the receptivity of the myometrium during late pregnancy favors the activity of oxytocin to generate vigorous and regular contractions until the fetus and placenta are expulsed. In association with PRL, oxytocin contributes to the control of lactation. While PRL stimulates milk synthesis, oxytocin acts on myoepithelial cells of the mammary glands to cause milk ejection.[217]

Therefore, pregnant patients with decreased oxytocin production and/or action (CP, central DI) might be expected to present with impaired labor and lactation.[219,220] However, studies in mice lacking the gene for oxytocin or the oxytocin receptor, as well as women with hypopituitarism of various etiologies, have shown successful spontaneous vaginal deliveries but the inability to eject milk in response to suckling.[219–222] Shinar[223] reported four cases of pan-hypopituitarism with spontaneous onset of labor. Therefore, maternal oxytocin does not seem to be necessary for labor.

Chard[224] suggested that fetal pituitary oxytocin, not maternal oxytocin, may play a role in childbirth based on higher concentrations of oxytocin and vasopressin observed in fetal umbilical plasma, suggesting that they originate from the fetal pituitary. It is possible that due to increased myometrial sensitivity to oxytocin, a small increase in oxytocin within the maternal circulation, even if oxytocin is of fetal origin, may be sufficient to induce contractions.[224] However, patients with hypopituitarism and likely significant oxytocin deficiency may show an increase in obstetric complications, including being small for gestational age, poor presentation, cesarean section, and postpartum hemorrhage.[220,223]

A large individual variation in oxytocin release in response to breastfeeding has been observed.[217,222] This variation can be explained by the increased sensitivity of the mammary glands to oxytocin during the establishment of lactation in the early postpartum period. There is increased sensitivity of the mammary gland to oxytocin as lactation is established, reaching maximum sensitivity on the fifth to the seventh day postpartum.[223,225] Patients with panhypopituitarism and deficiencies of PRL and oxytocin are incapable of lactation.[223,225]

Thus, patients with oxytocin deficiency may have normal vaginal delivery but potentially impaired lactation due to lack of oxytocin to enable milk letdown, or due to concurrent PRL deficiency. The oxytocin administration should be performed critically.

Oxytocin levels have also been shown to correlate with social and emotional behaviors, particularly empathic behavior.[226]

References

1. Ostrom QT, Gittleman H, Farah P, Ondracek A, Chen Y, Wolinsky Y, et al. CBTRUS statistical report: primary brain and central nervous system tumors diagnosed in the United States in 2006–2010. *Neuro-Oncology* 2013;**15**(Suppl. 2):ii1–56.
2. Cheng S, Grasso L, Martinez-Orozco JA, Al-Agha R, Pivonello R, Colao A, et al. Pregnancy in acromegaly: experience from two referral centers and systematic review of the literature. *Clin Endocrinol* 2012;**76**(2):264–71.
3. Molitch ME. Diagnosis and treatment of pituitary adenomas: a review. *JAMA* 2017;**317**(5):516–24.
4. Tjörnstrand A, Gunnarsson K, Evert M, Holmberg E, Ragnarsson O, Rosén T, et al. The incidence rate of pituitary adenomas in western Sweden for the period 2001–2011. *Eur J Endocrinol* 2014;**171**(4):519–26.
5. Raappana A, Koivukangas J, Ebeling T, Pirilä T. Incidence of pituitary adenomas in Northern Finland in 1992–2007. *J Clin Endocrinol Metab* 2010;**95**(9):4268–75.
6. Agustsson TT, Baldvinsdottir T, Jonasson JG, Olafsdottir E, Steinthorsdottir V, Sigurdsson G, et al. The epidemiology of pituitary adenomas in Iceland, 1955–2012: a nationwide population-based study. *Eur J Endocrinol* 2015;**173**(5):655–64.
7. Mercado M, Melgar V, Salame L, Cuenca D. Clinically non-functioning pituitary adenomas: pathogenic, diagnostic and therapeutic aspects. *Endocrinol Diabetes Nutr* 2017;**64**(7):384–95.
8. Mehta GU, Lonser RR. Management of hormone-secreting pituitary adenomas. *Neuro-Oncology* 2017;**19**(6):762–73.
9. Huang W, Molitch ME. Management of nonfunctioning pituitary adenomas (NFAs): observation. *Pituitary* 2018;**21**(2):162–7.
10. Kupersmith MJ, Rosenberg C, Kleinberg D. Visual loss in pregnant women with pituitary adenomas. *Ann Intern Med* 1994;**121**(7):473–7.
11. Vaninetti NM, Clarke DB, Zwicker DA, Yip CE, Tugwell B, Doucette S, et al. A comparative, population-based analysis of pituitary incidentalomas vs clinically manifesting sellar masses. *Endocr Connect* 2018;**7**(5):768–76.
12. Molitch ME, Findling JW, Clemmons DR. Excellence in the treatment of patients with pituitary tumors. *Pituitary* 2018;**21**(1):107.
13. Heaney AP, Fernando M, Melmed S. Functional role of estrogen in pituitary tumor pathogenesis. *J Clin Invest* 2002;**109**(2):277–83.
14. Karaca Z, Tanriverdi F, Unluhizarci K, Kelestimur F. Pregnancy and pituitary disorders. *Eur J Endocrinol* 2010;**162**(3):453–75.
15. Karaca Z, Yarman S, Ozbas I, Kadioglu P, Akturk M, Kilicli F, et al. How does pregnancy affect the patients with pituitary adenomas: a study on 113 pregnancies from Turkey. *J Endocrinol Investig* 2018;**41**(1):129–41.
16. Feldt-Rasmussen U, Mathiesen ER. Endocrine disorders in pregnancy: physiological and hormonal aspects of pregnancy. *Best Pract Res Clin Endocrinol Metab* 2011;**25**(6):875–84.
17. Scheithauer BW, Sano T, Kovacs KT, Young WF, Ryan N, Randall RV. The pituitary gland in pregnancy: a clinicopathologic and immunohistochemical study of 69 cases. *Mayo Clin Proc* 1990;**65**(4):461–74.
18. Grand'Maison S, Weber F, Bédard MJ, Mahone M, Godbout A. Pituitary apoplexy in pregnancy: a case series and literature review. *Obstet Med* 2015;**8**(4):177–83.
19. Inoue T, Hotta A, Awai M, Tanihara H. Loss of vision due to a physiologic pituitary enlargement during normal pregnancy. *Graefes Arch Clin Exp Ophthalmol* 2007;**245**(7):1049–51.
20. Bedford J, Dassan P, Harvie M, Mehta S. An unusual cause of headache in pregnancy. *BMJ* 2015;**351**:h4681.
21. Watson V. An unexpected headache: pituitary apoplexy in a pregnant woman on anticoagulation. *BMJ Case Rep* 2015;**2015**:1–4. https://doi.org/10.1136/bcr-2015-210198.
22. Negro A, Delaruelle Z, Ivanova TA, Khan S, Ornello R, Raffaelli B, et al. Headache and pregnancy: a systematic review. *J Headache Pain* 2017;**18**(1):106.
23. Caimari F, Corcoy R, Webb SM. Cushing's disease: major difficulties in diagnosis and management during pregnancy. *Minerva Endocrinol* 2018;**43**(4):435–45. https://doi.org/10.23736/S0391-1977.18.02803-1.
24. Lambert K, Rees K, Seed PT, Dhanjal MK, Knight M, McCance DR, et al. Macroprolactinomas and nonfunctioning pituitary adenomas and pregnancy outcomes. *Obstet Gynecol* 2017;**129**(1):185–94.
25. Glezer A, Jallad RS, Machado MC, Fragoso MC, Bronstein MD. Pregnancy and pituitary adenomas. *Minerva Endocrinol* 2016;**41**(3):341–50.
26. Bronstein MD, Paraiba DB, Jallad RS. Management of pituitary tumors in pregnancy. *Nat Rev Endocrinol* 2011;**7**(5):301–10.
27. Bulas D, Egloff A. Benefits and risks of MRI in pregnancy. *Semin Perinatol* 2013;**37**(5):301–4.
28. Patenaude Y, Pugash D, Lim K, Morin L, Bly S, Butt K, et al. The use of magnetic resonance imaging in the obstetric patient. *J Obstet Gynaecol Can* 2014;**36**(4):349–63.
29. De Santis M, Straface G, Cavaliere AF, Carducci B, Caruso A. Gadolinium periconceptional exposure: pregnancy and neonatal outcome. *Acta Obstet Gynecol Scand* 2007;**86**(1):99–101.
30. Hartwig V, Giovannetti G, Vanello N, Lombardi M, Landini L, Simi S. Biological effects and safety in magnetic resonance imaging: a review. *Int J Environ Res Public Health* 2009;**6**(6):1778–98.
31. Novak Z, Thurmond AS, Ross PL, Jones MK, Thornburg KL, Katzberg RW. Gadolinium-DTPA transplacental transfer and distribution in fetal tissue in rabbits. *Investig Radiol* 1993;**28**(9):828–30.
32. Cowper SE, Rabach M, Girardi M. Clinical and histological findings in nephrogenic systemic fibrosis. *Eur J Radiol* 2008;**66**(2):191–9.
33. Ray JG, Vermeulen MJ, Bharatha A, Montanera WJ, Park AL. Association between MRI exposure during pregnancy and fetal and childhood outcomes. *JAMA* 2016;**316**(9):952–61.
34. Food and Drug Administration HHS. Content and format of labeling for human prescription drug and biological products; requirements for pregnancy and lactation labeling. Final rule. *Fed Regist* 2014;**79**(233):72063–103.
35. Greene MF. FDA drug labeling for pregnancy and lactation drug safety monitoring systems. *Semin Perinatol* 2015;**39**(7):520–3.

36. Pernia S, DeMaagd G. The new pregnancy and lactation labeling rule. *P T* 2016;**41**(11):713–5.
37. Watkins EJ, Archambault M. Understanding the new pregnancy and lactation drug labeling. *JAAPA* 2016;**29**(2):50–2.
38. Abbassy M, Kshettry VR, Hamrahian AH, Johnston PC, Dobri GA, Avitsian R, et al. Surgical management of recurrent Cushing's disease in pregnancy: a case report. *Surg Neurol Int* 2015;**6**(Suppl. 25):S640–5.
39. Qaiser R, Black P. Neurosurgery in pregnancy. *Semin Neurol* 2007;**27**(5):476–81.
40. Witek P, Zieliński G, Maksymowicz M, Zgliczyński W. Transsphenoidal surgery for a life-threatening prolactinoma apoplexy during pregnancy. *Neuro Endocrinol Lett* 2012;**33**(5):483–8.
41. Brue T, Amodru V, Castinetti F. MANAGEMENT OF ENDOCRINE DISEASE: management of Cushing's syndrome during pregnancy: solved and unsolved questions. *Eur J Endocrinol* 2018;**178**(6):R259–66.
42. Cok OY, Akin S, Aribogan A, Acil M, Erdogan B, Bagis T. Anesthetic management of 29 week pregnant patient undergoing craniotomy for pituitary macroadenoma—a case report. *Middle East J Anaesthesiol* 2010;**20**(4):593–6.
43. Xia Y, Ma X, Griffiths BB, Luo Y. Neurosurgical anesthesia for a pregnant woman with macroprolactinoma: a case report. *Medicine (Baltimore)* 2018;**97**(37).
44. Kashanian M, Eshraghi N, Sheikhansari N, Bordbar A, Khatami E. Comparison between two doses of betamethasone administration with 12 hours vs. 24 hours intervals on prevention of respiratory distress syndrome: a randomised trial. *J Obstet Gynaecol* 2018;**38**(6):770–6.
45. Bronstein MD. Prolactinomas and pregnancy. *Pituitary* 2005;**8**(1):31–8.
46. Glezer A, Bronstein MD. Prolactinomas: how to handle prior to and during pregnancy? *Minerva Endocrinol* 2018;**43**(4):423–9. https://doi.org/10.23736/S0391-1977.17.02792-4.
47. Colao A, Sarno AD, Cappabianca P, Briganti F, Pivonello R, Somma CD, et al. Gender differences in the prevalence, clinical features and response to cabergoline in hyperprolactinemia. *Eur J Endocrinol* 2003;**148**(3):325–31.
48. Marshall JC, Dalkin AC, Haisenleder DJ, Griffin ML, Kelch RP. GnRH pulses—the regulators of human reproduction. *Trans Am Clin Climatol Assoc* 1993;**104**:31–46.
49. Sonigo C, Bouilly J, Carré N, Tolle V, Caraty A, Tello J, et al. Hyperprolactinemia-induced ovarian acyclicity is reversed by kisspeptin administration. *J Clin Invest* 2012;**122**(10):3791–5.
50. Franks S, Murray MA, Jequier AM, Steele SJ, Nabarro JD, Jacobs HS. Incidence and significance of hyperprolactinaemia in women with amenorrhea. *Clin Endocrinol* 1975;**4**(6):597–607.
51. Kleinberg DL, Noel GL, Frantz AG. Galactorrhea: a study of 235 cases, including 48 with pituitary tumors. *N Engl J Med* 1977;**296**(11):589–600.
52. Webster J, Piscitelli G, Polli A, Ferrari CI, Ismail I, Scanlon MF. A comparison of cabergoline and bromocriptine in the treatment of hyperprolactinemic amenorrhea. Cabergoline Comparative Study Group. *N Engl J Med* 1994;**331**(14):904–9.
53. Melmed S, Casanueva FF, Hoffman AR, Kleinberg DL, Montori VM, Schlechte JA, et al. Diagnosis and treatment of hyperprolactinemia: an Endocrine Society clinical practice guideline. *J Clin Endocrinol Metab* 2011;**96**(2):273–88.
54. Molitch ME. Endocrinology in pregnancy: management of the pregnant patient with a prolactinoma. *Eur J Endocrinol* 2015;**172**(5):R205–13.
55. Holmgren U, Bergstrand G, Hagenfeldt K, Werner S. Women with prolactinoma—effect of pregnancy and lactation on serum prolactin and on tumour growth. *Acta Endocrinol* 1986;**111**(4):452–9.
56. Persiani S, Sassolas G, Piscitelli G, Bizollon CA, Poggesi I, Pianezzola E, et al. Pharmacodynamics and relative bioavailability of cabergoline tablets vs solution in healthy volunteers. *J Pharm Sci* 1994;**83**(10):1421–4.
57. Araujo PB, Vieira Neto L, Gadelha MR. Pituitary tumor management in pregnancy. *Endocrinol Metab Clin N Am* 2015;**44**(1):181–97.
58. Araujo B, Belo S, Carvalho D. Pregnancy and tumor outcomes in women with prolactinoma. *Exp Clin Endocrinol Diabetes* 2017;**125**(10):642–8.
59. Rastogi A, Bhadada SK, Bhansali A. Pregnancy and tumor outcomes in infertile women with macroprolactinoma on cabergoline therapy. *Gynecol Endocrinol* 2017;**33**(4):270–3.
60. Canales ES, García IC, Ruíz JE, Zárate A. Bromocriptine as prophylactic therapy in prolactinoma during pregnancy. *Fertil Steril* 1981;**36**(4):524–6.
61. Glezer A, Bronstein MD. Prolactinomas, cabergoline, and pregnancy. *Endocrine* 2014;**47**(1):64–9.
62. Chen H, Fu J, Huang W. Dopamine agonists for preventing future miscarriage in women with idiopathic hyperprolactinemia and recurrent miscarriage history. *Cochrane Database Syst Rev* 2016;**7**:.
63. Raymond JP, Goldstein E, Konopka P, Leleu MF, Merceron RE, Loria Y. Follow-up of children born of bromocriptine-treated mothers. *Horm Res* 1985;**22**(3):239–46.
64. Ono M, Miki N, Amano K, Kawamata T, Seki T, Makino R, et al. Individualized high-dose cabergoline therapy for hyperprolactinemic infertility in women with micro- and macroprolactinomas. *J Clin Endocrinol Metab* 2010;**95**(6):2672–9.
65. Lebbe M, Hubinont C, Bernard P, Maiter D. Outcome of 100 pregnancies initiated under treatment with cabergoline in hyperprolactinaemic women. *Clin Endocrinol* 2010;**73**(2):236–42.
66. Stalldecker G, Mallea-Gil MS, Guitelman M, Alfieri A, Ballarino MC, Boero L, et al. Effects of cabergoline on pregnancy and embryo-fetal development: retrospective study on 103 pregnancies and a review of the literature. *Pituitary* 2010;**13**(4):345–50.
67. Peillon F, Racadot J, Olivier L, Racadot O, Vila-Porcile E. Proceedings: prolactin adenomas; a morphological study. Correlations between clinical and anatomical data in 91 cases (author's transl). *Ann Endocrinol (Paris)* 1975;**36**(5):277–8.
68. Auriemma RS, Perone Y, Di Sarno A, Grasso LF, Guerra E, Gasperi M, et al. Results of a single-center observational 10-year survey study on recurrence of hyperprolactinemia after pregnancy and lactation. *J Clin Endocrinol Metab* 2013;**98**(1):372–9.
69. Domingue ME, Devuyst F, Alexopoulou O, Corvilain B, Maiter D. Outcome of prolactinoma after pregnancy and lactation: a study on 73 patients. *Clin Endocrinol* 2014;**80**(5):642–8.

70. Rjosk HK, Fahlbusch R, von Werder K. Influence of pregnancies on prolactinomas. *Acta Endocrinol* 1982;**100**(3):337–46.

71. Crosignani PG, Mattei AM, Scarduelli C, Cavioni V, Boracchi P. Is pregnancy the best treatment for hyperprolactinaemia? *Hum Reprod* 1989;**4**(8):910–2.

72. Crosignani PG, Mattei AM, Severini V, Cavioni V, Maggioni P, Testa G. Long-term effects of time, medical treatment and pregnancy in 176 hyperprolactinemic women. *Eur J Obstet Gynecol Reprod Biol* 1992;**44**(3):175–80.

73. Jeffcoate WJ, Pound N, Sturrock ND, Lambourne J. Long-term follow-up of patients with hyperprolactinaemia. *Clin Endocrinol* 1996;**45**(3):299–303.

74. Huda MS, Athauda NB, Teh MM, Carroll PV, Powrie JK. Factors determining the remission of microprolactinomas after dopamine agonist withdrawal. *Clin Endocrinol* 2010;**72**(4):507–11.

75. Katznelson L, Laws ER, Melmed S, Molitch ME, Murad MH, Utz A, et al. Acromegaly: an endocrine society clinical practice guideline. *J Clin Endocrinol Metab* 2014;**99**(11):3933–51.

76. Giustina A, Chanson P, Bronstein MD, Klibanski A, Lamberts S, Casanueva FF, et al. A consensus on criteria for cure of acromegaly. *J Clin Endocrinol Metab* 2010;**95**(7):3141–8.

77. Cozzi R, Attanasio R, Barausse M. Pregnancy in acromegaly: a one-center experience. *Eur J Endocrinol* 2006;**155**(2):279–84.

78. Assal A, Malcolm J, Lochnan H, Keely E. Preconception counselling for women with acromegaly: more questions than answers. *Obstet Med* 2016;**9**(1):9–14.

79. Montini M, Pagani G, Gianola D, Pagani MD, Piolini R, Camboni MG. Acromegaly and primary amenorrhea: ovulation and pregnancy induced by SMS 201-995 and bromocriptine. *J Endocrinol Investig* 1990;**13**(2):193.

80. Muhammad A, Neggers SJ, van der Lely AJ. Pregnancy and acromegaly. *Pituitary* 2017;**20**(1):179–84.

81. Caron P, Broussaud S, Bertherat J, Borson-Chazot F, Brue T, Cortet-Rudelli C, et al. Acromegaly and pregnancy: a retrospective multicenter study of 59 pregnancies in 46 women. *J Clin Endocrinol Metab* 2010;**95**(10):4680–7.

82. Dias M, Boguszewski C, Gadelha M, Kasuki L, Musolino N, Vieira JG, et al. Acromegaly and pregnancy: a prospective study. *Eur J Endocrinol* 2014;**170**(2):301–10.

83. Jallad RS, Shimon I, Fraenkel M, Medvedovsky V, Akirov A, Duarte FH, et al. Outcome of pregnancies in a large cohort of women with acromegaly. *Clin Endocrinol* 2018;**88**(6):896–907.

84. Grynberg M, Salenave S, Young J, Chanson P. Female gonadal function before and after treatment of acromegaly. *J Clin Endocrinol Metab* 2010;**95**(10):4518–25.

85. Giustina A, Arnaldi G, Bogazzi F, Cannavò S, Colao A, De Marinis L, et al. Pegvisomant in acromegaly: an update. *J Endocrinol Investig* 2017;**40**(6):577–89.

86. Cheng V, Faiman C, Kennedy L, Khoury F, Hatipoglu B, Weil R, et al. Pregnancy and acromegaly: a review. *Pituitary* 2012;**15**(1):59–63.

87. Herman-Bonert V, Seliverstov M, Melmed S. Pregnancy in acromegaly: successful therapeutic outcome. *J Clin Endocrinol Metab* 1998;**83**(3):727–31.

88. Bétéa D, Valdes Socin H, Hansen I, Stevenaert A, Beckers A. Acromegaly and pregnancy. *Ann Endocrinol (Paris)* 2002;**63**(5):457–63.

89. Frankenne F, Closset J, Gomez F, Scippo ML, Smal J, Hennen G. The physiology of growth hormones (GHs) in pregnant women and partial characterization of the placental GH variant. *J Clin Endocrinol Metab* 1988;**66**(6):1171–80.

90. Beckers A, Stevenaert A, Foidart JM, Hennen G, Frankenne F. Placental and pituitary growth hormone secretion during pregnancy in acromegalic women. *J Clin Endocrinol Metab* 1990;**71**(3):725–31.

91. Caufriez A, Frankenne F, Englert Y, Golstein J, Cantraine F, Hennen G, et al. Placental growth hormone as a potential regulator of maternal IGF-I during human pregnancy. *Am J Phys* 1990;**258**(6 Pt 1):E1014–9.

92. de Zegher F, Vanderschueren-Lodeweyckx M, Spitz B, Faijerson Y, Blomberg F, Beckers A, et al. Perinatal growth hormone (GH) physiology: effect of GH-releasing factor on maternal and fetal secretion of pituitary and placental GH. *J Clin Endocrinol Metab* 1990;**71**(2):520–2.

93. Yang MJ, Tseng JY, Chen CY, Yeh CC. Changes in maternal serum insulin-like growth factor-I during pregnancy and its relationship to maternal anthropometry. *J Chin Med Assoc* 2013;**76**(11):635–9.

94. Chellakooty M, Vangsgaard K, Larsen T, Scheike T, Falck-Larsen J, Legarth J, et al. A longitudinal study of intrauterine growth and the placental growth hormone (GH)-insulin-like growth factor I axis in maternal circulation: association between placental GH and fetal growth. *J Clin Endocrinol Metab* 2004;**89**(1):384–91.

95. Persechini ML, Gennero I, Grunenwald S, Vezzosi D, Bennet A, Caron P. Decreased IGF-1 concentration during the first trimester of pregnancy in women with normal somatotroph function. *Pituitary* 2015;**18**(4):461–4.

96. Attanasio AF, Mo D, Erfurth EM, Tan M, Ho KY, Kleinberg D, et al. Prevalence of metabolic syndrome in adult hypopituitary growth hormone (GH)-deficient patients before and after GH replacement. *J Clin Endocrinol Metab* 2010;**95**(1):74–81.

97. Ryan EA, Enns L. Role of gestational hormones in the induction of insulin resistance. *J Clin Endocrinol Metab* 1988;**67**(2):341–7.

98. Hills FA, English J, Chard T. Circulating levels of IGF-I and IGF-binding protein-1 throughout pregnancy: relation to birthweight and maternal weight. *J Endocrinol* 1996;**148**(2):303–9.

99. Tennekoon KH, Pathmaperuma AN, Senanayake L, Karunanayake EH. Insulin-like growth factors-I and -II and insulin-like growth factor binding protein-1 during normal pregnancy: pattern of secretion and correlation with other placental hormones. *Ceylon Med J* 2007;**52**(1):8–13.

100. Daughaday WH, Trivedi B, Winn HN, Yan H. Hypersomatotropism in pregnant women, as measured by a human liver radioreceptor assay. *J Clin Endocrinol Metab* 1990;**70**(1):215–21.

101. Eriksson L, Frankenne F, Edén S, Hennen G, von Schoultz B. Growth hormone secretion during termination of pregnancy. Further evidence of a placental variant. *Acta Obstet Gynecol Scand* 1988;**67**(6):549–52.

102. McIntyre HD, Serek R, Crane DI, Veveris-Lowe T, Parry A, Johnson S, et al. Placental growth hormone (GH), GH-binding protein, and insulin-like growth factor axis in normal, growth-retarded, and diabetic pregnancies: correlations with fetal growth. *J Clin Endocrinol Metab* 2000; **85**(3):1143–50.

103. Eriksson L, Frankenne F, Edèn S, Hennen G, Von Schoultz B. Growth hormone 24-h serum profiles during pregnancy—lack of pulsatility for the secretion of the placental variant. *Br J Obstet Gynaecol* 1989;**96**(8):949–53.

104. Stone RT, Maurer RA, Gorski J. Effect of estradiol-17 beta on preprolactin messenger ribonucleic acid activity in the rat pituitary gland. *Biochemistry* 1977;**16**(22):4915–21.

105. Clemmons DR, Underwood LE, Ridgway EC, Kliman B, Kjellberg RN, Van Wyk JJ. Estradiol treatment of acromegaly. Reduction of immuno-reactive somatomedin-C and improvement in metabolic status. *Am J Med* 1980;**69**(4):571–5.

106. Attanasio AF, Jung H, Mo D, Chanson P, Bouillon R, Ho KK, et al. Prevalence and incidence of diabetes mellitus in adult patients on growth hormone replacement for growth hormone deficiency: a surveillance database analysis. *J Clin Endocrinol Metab* 2011;**96**(7):2255–61.

107. Obuobie K, Mullik V, Jones C, John R, Rees AE, Davies JS, et al. McCune-Albright syndrome: growth hormone dynamics in pregnancy. *J Clin Endocrinol Metab* 2001;**86**(6):2456–8.

108. Manolopoulou J, Alami Y, Petersenn S, Schopohl J, Wu Z, Strasburger CJ, et al. Automated 22-kD growth hormone-specific assay without interference from Pegvisomant. *Clin Chem* 2012;**58**(10):1446–56.

109. Fuglsang J, Skjaerbaek C, Espelund U, Frystyk J, Fisker S, Flyvbjerg A, et al. Ghrelin and its relationship to growth hormones during normal pregnancy. *Clin Endocrinol* 2005;**62**(5):554–9.

110. Bigazzi M, Ronga R, Lancranjan I, Ferraro S, Branconi F, Buzzoni P, et al. A pregnancy in an acromegalic woman during bromocriptine treatment: effects on growth hormone and prolactin in the maternal, fetal, and amniotic compartments. *J Clin Endocrinol Metab* 1979;**48**(1):9–12.

111. Caron P, Gerbeau C, Pradayrol L. Maternal-fetal transfer of octreotide. *N Engl J Med* 1995;**333**(9):601–2.

112. Caron P, Buscail L, Beckers A, Estève JP, Igout A, Hennen G, et al. Expression of somatostatin receptor SST4 in human placenta and absence of octreotide effect on human placental growth hormone concentration during pregnancy. *J Clin Endocrinol Metab* 1997;**82**(11):3771–6.

113. Maffei P, Tamagno G, Nardelli GB, Videau C, Menegazzo C, Milan G, et al. Effects of octreotide exposure during pregnancy in acromegaly. *Clin Endocrinol* 2010;**72**(5):668–77.

114. Fassnacht M, Capeller B, Arlt W, Steck T, Allolio B. Octreotide LAR treatment throughout pregnancy in an acromegalic woman. *Clin Endocrinol* 2001;**55**(3):411–5.

115. Tsalikian E, Foley TP, Becker DJ. Characterization of somatostatin specific binding in plasma cell membranes of human placenta. *Pediatr Res* 1984;**18**(10):953–7.

116. Boulanger C, Vezzosi D, Bennet A, Lorenzini F, Fauvel J, Caron P. Normal pregnancy in a woman with nesidioblastosis treated with somatostatin analog octreotide. *J Endocrinol Investig* 2004;**27**(5):465–70.

117. Skajaa GO, Mathiesen ER, Iyore E, Beck-Nielsen H, Jimenez-Solem E, Damm P. Poor pregnancy outcome after octreotide treatment during pregnancy for familial hyperinsulinemic hypoglycemia: a case report. *BMC Res Notes* 2014;**7**:804.

118. Reck-Burneo CA, Parekh A, Velcek FT. Is octreotide a risk factor in necrotizing enterocolitis? *J Pediatr Surg* 2008;**43**(6):1209–10.

119. Mozas J, Ocón E, López de la Torre M, Suárez AM, Miranda JA, Herruzo AJ. Successful pregnancy in a woman with acromegaly treated with somatostatin analog (octreotide) prior to surgical resection. *Int J Gynaecol Obstet* 1999;**65**(1):71–3.

120. Neal JM. Successful pregnancy in a woman with acromegaly treated with octreotide. *Endocr Pract* 2000;**6**(2):148–50.

121. Aono T, Shioji T, Kohno M, Ueda G, Kurachi K. Pregnancy following 2-bromo-alpha-ergocryptine (CB-154)-induced ovulation in an acromegalic patient with galactorrhea and amenorrhea. *Fertil Steril* 1976;**27**(3):341–4.

122. Espersen T, Ditzel J. Pregnancy and delivery under bromocriptine therapy. *Lancet* 1977;**2**(8045):985–6.

123. Luboshitzky R, Dickstein G, Barzilai D. Bromocriptine-induced pregnancy in an acromegalic patient. *JAMA* 1980;**244**(6):584–6.

124. Brian SR, Bidlingmaier M, Wajnrajch MP, Weinzimer SA, Inzucchi SE. Treatment of acromegaly with pegvisomant during pregnancy: maternal and fetal effects. *J Clin Endocrinol Metab* 2007;**92**(9):3374–7.

125. van der Lely AJ, Gomez R, Heissler JF, Åkerblad AC, Jönsson P, Camacho-Hübner C, et al. Pregnancy in acromegaly patients treated with pegvisomant. *Endocrine* 2015;**49**(3):769–73.

126. Machado MC, Fragoso MCBV, Bronstein MD. Pregnancy in patients with Cushing's syndrome. *Endocrinol Metab Clin N Am* 2018;**47**(2):441–9.

127. Lindsay JR, Jonklaas J, Oldfield EH, Nieman LK. Cushing's syndrome during pregnancy: personal experience and review of the literature. *J Clin Endocrinol Metab* 2005;**90**(5):3077–83.

128. Abdelmannan D, Aron DC. Adrenal disorders in pregnancy. *Endocrinol Metab Clin N Am* 2011;**40**(4):779–94.

129. Prebtani AP, Donat D, Ezzat S. Worrisome striae in pregnancy. *Lancet* 2000;**355**(9216):1692.

130. McClamrock HD, Adashi EY. Gestational hyperandrogenism. *Fertil Steril* 1992;**57**(2):257–74.

131. Nieman LK, Biller BM, Findling JW, Murad MH, Newell-Price J, Savage MO, et al. Treatment of Cushing's syndrome: an endocrine society clinical practice guideline. *J Clin Endocrinol Metab* 2015;**100**(8):2807–31.

132. Pinette MG, Pan YQ, Oppenheim D, Pinette SG, Blackstone J. Bilateral inferior petrosal sinus corticotropin sampling with corticotropin-releasing hormone stimulation in a pregnant patient with Cushing's syndrome. *Am J Obstet Gynecol* 1994;**171**(2):563–4.

133. Lopes LM, Francisco RP, Galletta MA, Bronstein MD. Determination of nighttime salivary cortisol during pregnancy: comparison with values in non-pregnancy and Cushing's disease. *Pituitary* 2016;**19**(1):30–8.

134. Caimari F, Valassi E, Garbayo P, Steffensen C, Santos A, Corcoy R, et al. Cushing's syndrome and pregnancy outcomes: a systematic review of published cases. *Endocrine* 2017;**55**(2):555–63.

135. Berwaerts J, Verhelst J, Mahler C, Abs R. Cushing's syndrome in pregnancy treated by ketoconazole: case report and review of the literature. *Gynecol Endocrinol* 1999;**13**(3):175–82.

136. Berwaerts J, Verhelst J, Abs R, Appel B, Mahler C. A giant prolactinoma presenting with unilateral exophthalmos: effect of cabergoline and review of the literature. *J Endocrinol Investig* 2000;**23**(6):393–8.

137. Zieleniewski W, Michalak R. A successful case of pregnancy in a woman with ACTH-independent Cushing's syndrome treated with ketoconazole and metyrapone. *Gynecol Endocrinol* 2017;**33**(5):349–52.

138. Boronat M, Marrero D, López-Plasencia Y, Barber M, Schamann Y, Nóvoa FJ. Successful outcome of pregnancy in a patient with Cushing's disease under treatment with ketoconazole during the first trimester of gestation. *Gynecol Endocrinol* 2011;**27**(9):675–7.

139. Woo I, Ehsanipoor RM. Cabergoline therapy for Cushing disease throughout pregnancy. *Obstet Gynecol* 2013;**122**(2 Pt 2):485–7.

140. Borgundvaag B, Kudlow JE, Mueller SG, George SR. Dopamine receptor activation inhibits estrogen-stimulated transforming growth factor-alpha gene expression and growth in anterior pituitary, but not in uterus. *Endocrinology* 1992;**130**(6):3453–8.

141. Masding MG, Lees PD, Gawne-Cain ML, Sandeman DD. Visual field compression by a non-secreting pituitary tumour during pregnancy. *J R Soc Med* 2003;**96**(1):27–8.

142. Flitsch J, Burkhardt T. Non-functioning pituitary tumors: any special considerations during pregnancy? *Minerva Endocrinol* 2018;**43**(4):430–4. https://doi.org/10.23736/S0391-1977.17.02784-5.

143. Lee HR, Song JE, Lee KY. Developed diplopia and ptosis due to a nonfunctioning pituitary macroadenoma during pregnancy. *Obstet Gynecol Sci* 2014;**57**(1):66–9.

144. Martínez García R, Martínez Pérez A, Domingo del Pozo C, Sospedra Ferrer R. Cushing's syndrome in pregnancy. Laparoscopic adrenalectomy during pregnancy: the mainstay treatment. *J Endocrinol Investig* 2016;**39**(3):273–6.

145. Lim WH, Torpy DJ, Jeffries WS. The medical management of Cushing's syndrome during pregnancy. *Eur J Obstet Gynecol Reprod Biol* 2013;**168**(1):1–6.

146. Andreescu CE, Alwani RA, Hofland J, Looijenga LHJ, de Herder WW, Hofland LJ, et al. Adrenal Cushing's syndrome during pregnancy. *Eur J Endocrinol* 2017;**177**(5):K13–20.

147. Blanco C, Maqueda E, Rubio JA, Rodriguez A. Cushing's syndrome during pregnancy secondary to adrenal adenoma: metyrapone treatment and laparoscopic adrenalectomy. *J Endocrinol Investig* 2006;**29**(2):164–7.

148. Hána V, Dokoupilová M, Marek J, Plavka R. Recurrent ACTH-independent Cushing's syndrome in multiple pregnancies and its treatment with metyrapone. *Clin Endocrinol* 2001;**54**(2):277–81.

149. Connell JM, Cordiner J, Davies DL, Fraser R, Frier BM, McPherson SG. Pregnancy complicated by Cushing's syndrome: potential hazard of metyrapone therapy. Case report. *Br J Obstet Gynaecol* 1985;**92**(11):1192–5.

150. Ennaifer H, Jemel M, Kandar H, Grira W, Kammoun I, Salem LB. Developed diplopia due to a pituitary macroadenoma during pregnancy. *Pan Afr Med J* 2018;**29**:39.

151. Caron P, Gerbeau C, Pradayrol L, Simonetta C, Bayard F. Successful pregnancy in an infertile woman with a thyrotropin-secreting macroadenoma treated with somatostatin analog (octreotide). *J Clin Endocrinol Metab* 1996;**81**(3):1164–8.

152. Blackhurst G, Strachan MW, Collie D, Gregor A, Statham PF, Seckl JE. The treatment of a thyrotropin-secreting pituitary macroadenoma with octreotide in twin pregnancy. *Clin Endocrinol* 2002;**57**(3):401–4.

153. Chaiamnuay S, Moster M, Katz MR, Kim YN. Successful management of a pregnant woman with a TSH secreting pituitary adenoma with surgical and medical therapy. *Pituitary* 2003;**6**(2):109–13.

154. Song M, Wang H, Song L, Tian H, Ge Q, Li J, et al. Ectopic TSH-secreting pituitary tumor: a case report and review of prior cases. *BMC Cancer* 2014;**14**:544.

155. Fleseriu M, Hashim IA, Karavitaki N, Melmed S, Murad MH, Salvatori R, et al. Hormonal replacement in hypopituitarism in adults: an endocrine society clinical practice guideline. *J Clin Endocrinol Metab* 2016;**101**(11):3888–921.

156. Toogood AA, Beardwell CG, Shalet SM. The severity of growth hormone deficiency in adults with pituitary disease is related to the degree of hypopituitarism. *Clin Endocrinol* 1994;**41**(4):511–6.

157. Charmandari E, Nicolaides NC, Chrousos GP. Adrenal insufficiency. *Lancet* 2014;**383**(9935):2152–67.

158. Yuen KC, Chong LE, Koch CA. Adrenal insufficiency in pregnancy: challenging issues in diagnosis and management. *Endocrine* 2013;**44**(2):283–92.

159. Lekarev O, New MI. Adrenal disease in pregnancy. *Best Pract Res Clin Endocrinol Metab* 2011;**25**(6):959–73.

160. Calvo RM, Jauniaux E, Gulbis B, Asunción M, Gervy C, Contempré B, et al. Fetal tissues are exposed to biologically relevant free thyroxine concentrations during early phases of development. *J Clin Endocrinol Metab* 2002;**87**(4):1768–77.

161. Thompson W, Russell G, Baragwanath G, Matthews J, Vaidya B, Thompson-Coon J. Maternal thyroid hormone insufficiency during pregnancy and risk of neurodevelopmental disorders in offspring: a systematic review and meta-analysis. *Clin Endocrinol* 2018;**88**(4):575–84.

162. Laron Z, Pertzelan A, Mannheimer S, Goldman J, Guttmann S. Lack of placental transfer of human growth hormone. *Acta Endocrinol* 1966;**53**(4):687–92.

163. Laron Z, Pertzelan A. Somatotrophin in antenatal and perinatal growth and development. *Lancet* 1969;**1**(7596):680–1.

164. Wirén L, Boguszewski CL, Johannsson G. Growth hormone (GH) replacement therapy in GH-deficient women during pregnancy. *Clin Endocrinol* 2002;**57**(2):235–9.

165. Vila G, Luger A. Growth hormone deficiency and pregnancy: any role for substitution? *Minerva Endocrinol* 2018;**43**(4):451–7. https://doi.org/10.23736/S0391-1977.18.02834-1.

166. Overton CE, Davis CJ, West C, Davies MC, Conway GS. High risk pregnancies in hypopituitary women. *Hum Reprod* 2002;**17**(6):1464–7.

167. Powe CE, Puopolo KM, Newburg DS, Lönnerdal B, Chen C, Allen M, et al. Effects of recombinant human prolactin on breast milk composition. *Pediatrics* 2011;**127**(2):e359–66.

168. Fatma M, Mouna E, Nabila R, Mouna M, Nadia C, Mohamed A. Sheehan's syndrome with pancytopenia: a case report and review of the literature. *J Med Case Rep* 2011;**5**:490.

169. Zargar AH, Singh B, Laway BA, Masoodi SR, Wani AI, Bashir MI. Epidemiologic aspects of postpartum pituitary hypofunction (Sheehan's syndrome). *Fertil Steril* 2005;**84**(2):523–8.

170. Matsuzaki S, Endo M, Ueda Y, Mimura K, Kakigano A, Egawa-Takata T, et al. A case of acute Sheehan's syndrome and literature review: a rare but life-threatening complication of postpartum hemorrhage. *BMC Pregnancy Childbirth* 2017;**17**(1):188.

171. Honegger J, Giese S. Acute pituitary disease in pregnancy: how to handle hypophysitis and Sheehan's syndrome? *Minerva Endocrinol* 2018;**43**(4):465–75. https://doi.org/10.23736/S0391-1977.

172. Kovacs K. Sheehan syndrome. *Lancet* 2003;**361**(9356):520–2.

173. De Bellis A, Pane E, Bellastella G, Sinisi AA, Colella C, Giordano R, et al. Detection of antipituitary and antihypothalamus antibodies to investigate the role of pituitary or hypothalamic autoimmunity in patients with selective idiopathic hypopituitarism. *Clin Endocrinol* 2011;**75**(3):361–6.

174. De Bellis A, Dello Iacovo A, Bellastella G, Savoia A, Cozzolino D, Sinisi AA, et al. Characterization of pituitary cells targeted by antipituitary antibodies in patients with isolated autoimmune diseases without pituitary insufficiency may help to foresee the kind of future hypopituitarism. *Pituitary* 2014;**17**(5):457–63.

175. Kilicli F, Dokmetas HS, Acibucu F. Sheehan's syndrome. *Gynecol Endocrinol* 2013;**29**(4):292–5.

176. Furnica RM, Gadisseux P, Fernandez C, Dechambre S, Maiter D, Oriot P. Early diagnosis of Sheehan's syndrome. *Anaesth Crit Care Pain Med* 2015;**34**(1):61–3.

177. Hale B, Habib AS. Sheehan syndrome: acute presentation with severe headache. *Int J Obstet Anesth* 2014;**23**(4):383–6.

178. Matsuwaki T, Khan KN, Inoue T, Yoshida A, Masuzaki H. Evaluation of obstetrical factors related to Sheehan syndrome. *J Obstet Gynaecol Res* 2014;**40**(1):46–52.

179. Motivala S, Gologorsky Y, Kostandinov J, Post KD. Pituitary disorders during pregnancy. *Endocrinol Metab Clin N Am* 2011;**40**(4):827–36.

180. Brissaud H, Gougerot H, Gy A. Nevrite localized avec troubles trophiques a la suitede coupure de pouce. Gougerot H, editor*Rev Neurol* 1908;645.

181. Goudie RB, Pinkerton PH. Anterior hypophysitis and Hashimoto's disease in a young woman. *J Pathol Bacteriol* 1962;**83**:584–5.

182. Guzzo MF, Bueno CB, Amancio TT, Rosemberg S, Bueno C, Arioli EL, et al. An intrasellar germinoma with normal tumor marker concentrations mimicking primary lymphocytic hypophysitis. *Arq Bras Endocrinol Metabol* 2013;**57**(7):566–70.

183. Caturegli P, Newschaffer C, Olivi A, Pomper MG, Burger PC, Rose NR. Autoimmune hypophysitis. *Endocr Rev* 2005;**26**(5):599–614.

184. Bellastella G, Maiorino MI, Bizzarro A, Giugliano D, Esposito K, Bellastella A, et al. Revisitation of autoimmune hypophysitis: knowledge and uncertainties on pathophysiological and clinical aspects. *Pituitary* 2016;**19**(6):625–42.

185. Joshi MN, Whitelaw BC, Carroll PV. MECHANISMS IN ENDOCRINOLOGY: hypophysitis: diagnosis and treatment. *Eur J Endocrinol* 2018;**179**(3):R151–63.

186. Guaraldi F, Giordano R, Grottoli S, Ghizzoni L, Arvat E, Ghigo E. Pituitary autoimmunity. *Front Horm Res* 2017;**48**:48–68.

187. Angelousi A, Cohen C, Sosa S, Danilowicz K, Papanastasiou L, Tsoli M, et al. Clinical, endocrine and imaging characteristics of patients with primary hypophysitis. *Horm Metab Res* 2018;**50**(4):296–302.

188. Glezer A, Bronstein MD. Pituitary autoimmune disease: nuances in clinical presentation. *Endocrine* 2012;**42**(1):74–9.

189. Wang S, Wang L, Yao Y, Feng F, Yang H, Liang Z, et al. Primary lymphocytic hypophysitis: clinical characteristics and treatment of 50 cases in a single centre in China over 18 years. *Clin Endocrinol* 2017;**87**(2):177–84.

190. Sakurai K, Yamashita R, Niituma S, Iwama S, Sugimura Y, Arihara Z, et al. Usefulness of anti-rabphilin-3A antibodies for diagnosing central diabetes insipidus in the third trimester of pregnancy. *Endocr J* 2017;**64**(6):645–50.

191. Nakata Y, Sato N, Masumoto T, Mori H, Akai H, Nobusawa H, et al. Parasellar T2 dark sign on MR imaging in patients with lymphocytic hypophysitis. *AJNR Am J Neuroradiol* 2010;**31**(10):1944–50.

192. Gutenberg A, Larsen J, Lupi I, Rohde V, Caturegli P. A radiologic score to distinguish autoimmune hypophysitis from nonsecreting pituitary adenoma preoperatively. *AJNR Am J Neuroradiol* 2009;**30**(9):1766–72.

193. Chiloiro S, Tartaglione T, Capoluongo ED, Angelini F, Arena V, Giampietro A, et al. Hypophysitis outcome and factors predicting responsiveness to glucocorticoid therapy: a prospective and double-arm study. *J Clin Endocrinol Metab* 2018;.

194. Caturegli P. Autoimmune hypophysitis: autoantigens and association with CTLA-4 blockade. *Ann Endocrinol (Paris)* 2012;**73**(2):78.

195. Caturegli P. Autoimmune hypophysitis: an underestimated disease in search of its autoantigen(s). *J Clin Endocrinol Metab* 2007;**92**(6):2038–40.

196. Gal R, Schwartz A, Gukovsky-Oren S, Peleg D, Goldman J, Kessler E. Lymphoid hypophysitis associated with sudden maternal death: report of a case review of the literature. *Obstet Gynecol Surv* 1986;**41**(10):619–21.

197. Funazaki S, Yamada H, Hara K, Ishikawa SE. Spontaneous pregnancy after full recovery from hypopituitarism caused by lymphocytic hypophysitis. *Endocrinol Diabetes Metab Case Rep* 2018;**2018**:https://doi.org/10.1530/EDM-18-0081.

198. Yaoita R, Ito M, Matsuda K, Kokubo Y, Sato S, Sonoda Y. A case of lymphocytic adenohypophysitis presenting visual disturbance in the third trimester of pregnancy. *No Shinkei Geka* 2017;**45**(2):161–5.

199. Davies EC, Jakobiec FA, Stagner AM, Rizzo JF. An atypical case of lymphocytic panhypophysitis in a pregnant woman. *J Neuroophthalmol* 2016; **36**(3):313–6.

200. Siddique H, Baskar V, Chakrabarty A, Clayton RN, Hanna FW. Spontaneous pregnancy after trans-sphenoidal surgery in a patient with lymphocytic hypophysitis. *Clin Endocrinol* 2007;**66**(3):454–5.

201. Sinha YN. Structural variants of prolactin: occurrence and physiological significance. *Endocr Rev* 1995;**16**(3):354–69.

202. Kidd D, Wilson P, Unwin B, Dorward N. Lymphocytic hypophysitis presenting early in pregnancy. *J Neurol* 2003;**250**(11):1385–7.

203. Buckland RH, Popham PA. Lymphocytic hypophysitis complicated by post-partum haemorrhage. *Int J Obstet Anesth* 1998;**7**(4):263–6.

204. Leroy C, Karrouz W, Douillard C, Do Cao C, Cortet C, Wémeau JL, et al. Diabetes insipidus. *Ann Endocrinol (Paris)* 2013;**74**(5–6):496–507.

205. Schernthaner-Reiter MH, Stratakis CA, Luger A. Genetics of diabetes insipidus. *Endocrinol Metab Clin N Am* 2017;**46**(2):305–34.

206. Ananthakrishnan S. Diabetes insipidus during pregnancy. *Best Pract Res Clin Endocrinol Metab* 2016;**30**(2):305–15.

207. Jin-no Y, Kamiya Y, Okada M, Watanabe O, Ogasawara M, Fujinami T. Pregnant woman with transient diabetes insipidus resistant to 1-desamino-8-D-arginine vasopressin. *Endocr J* 1998;**45**(5):693–6.

208. Bellastella A, Bizzarro A, Colella C, Bellastella G, Sinisi AA, De Bellis A. Subclinical diabetes insipidus. *Best Pract Res Clin Endocrinol Metab* 2012;**26**(4):471–83.

209. Wallia A, Bizhanova A, Huang W, Goldsmith SL, Gossett DR, Kopp P. Acute diabetes insipidus mediated by vasopressinase after placental abruption. *J Clin Endocrinol Metab* 2013;**98**(3):881–6.

210. Kondo T, Nakamura M, Kitano S, Kawashima J, Matsumura T, Ohba T, et al. The clinical course and pathophysiological investigation of adolescent gestational diabetes insipidus: a case report. *BMC Endocr Disord* 2018;**18**(1):4.

211. Yamanaka Y, Takeuchi K, Konda E, Samoto T, Satou A, Mizudori M, et al. Transient postpartum diabetes insipidus in twin pregnancy associated with HELLP syndrome. *J Perinat Med* 2002;**30**(3):273–5.

212. Gambito R, Chan M, Sheta M, Ramirez-Arao P, Gurm H, Tunkel A, et al. Gestational diabetes insipidus associated with HELLP syndrome: a case report. *Case Rep Nephrol* 2012;**2012**:.

213. Sherer DM, Cutler J, Santoso P, Angus S, Abulafia O. Severe hypernatremia after cesarean delivery secondary to transient diabetes insipidus of pregnancy. *Obstet Gynecol* 2003;**102**(5 Pt 2):1166–8.

214. Oiso Y, Robertson GL, Nørgaard JP, Juul KV. Clinical review: treatment of neurohypophyseal diabetes insipidus. *J Clin Endocrinol Metab* 2013; **98**(10):3958–67.

215. Marques P, Gunawardana K, Grossman A. Transient diabetes insipidus in pregnancy. *Endocrinol Diabetes Metab Case Rep* 2015;**2015**:.

216. Augustine RA, Seymour AJ, Campbell RE, Grattan DR, Brown CH. Integrative neuro-humoral regulation of oxytocin neuron activity in pregnancy and lactation. *J Neuroendocrinol* 2018;https://doi.org/10.1111/jne.12569.

217. Erickson EN, Emeis CL. Breastfeeding outcomes after oxytocin use during childbirth: an integrative review. *J Midwifery Womens Health* 2017; **62**(4):397–417.

218. Blanks AM, Shmygol A, Thornton S. Regulation of oxytocin receptors and oxytocin receptor signaling. *Semin Reprod Med* 2007;**25**(1):52–9.

219. Prevost M, Zelkowitz P, Tulandi T, Hayton B, Feeley N, Carter CS, et al. Oxytocin in pregnancy and the postpartum: relations to labor and its management. *Front Public Health* 2014;**2**:1.

220. Kübler K, Klingmüller D, Gembruch U, Merz WM. High-risk pregnancy management in women with hypopituitarism. *J Perinatol* 2009; **29**(2):89–95.

221. Daughters K, Manstead ASR, Rees DA. Hypopituitarism is associated with lower oxytocin concentrations and reduced empathic ability. *Endocrine* 2017;**57**(1):166–74.

222. Chatterton RT, Hill PD, Aldag JC, Hodges KR, Belknap SM, Zinaman MJ. Relation of plasma oxytocin and prolactin concentrations to milk production in mothers of preterm infants: influence of stress. *J Clin Endocrinol Metab* 2000;**85**(10):3661–8.

223. Shinar S, Many A, Maslovitz S. Questioning the role of pituitary oxytocin in parturition: spontaneous onset of labor in women with panhypopituitarism—a case series. *Eur J Obstet Gynecol Reprod Biol* 2016;**197**:83–5.

224. Chard T. Fetal and maternal oxytocin in human parturition. *Am J Perinatol* 1989;**6**(2):145–52.

225. Dawood MY, Khan-Dawood FS, Wahi RS, Fuchs F. Oxytocin release and plasma anterior pituitary and gonadal hormones in women during lactation. *J Clin Endocrinol Metab* 1981;**52**(4):678–83.

226. Krol KM, Grossmann T. Psychological effects of breastfeeding on children and mothers. *Bundesgesundheitsbl Gesundheitsforsch Gesundheitsschutz* 2018;**61**(8):977–85.

Chapter 19

Thyroid Disorders During Pregnancy, Postpartum, and Lactation

Zoe E. Quandt*, Kirsten E. Salmeen[†,‡] and Ingrid J. Block-Kurbisch[‡,§,¶]

*Department of Medicine, Division of Endocrinology and Metabolism, University of California, San Francisco, CA, United States, [†]Department of Obstetrics and Gynecology, Kaiser Permanente, San Francisco, CA, United States, [‡]Department of Obstetrics and Gynecology, University of California, San Francisco, CA, United States, [§]Department of Medicine, University of California, San Francisco, CA, United States, [¶]Department of Medicine, St. Mary's Medical Center, Dignity Health, San Francisco, CA, United States

---

Common Clinical Problems

- In women of childbearing age with preexisting primary hypothyroidism, LT4 replacement therapy should aim at maintaining a TSH value of <2.5 mIU/L.
- Thyroid hormone requirements increase between 30% and 50% in pregnancy; therefore, in preexisting hypothyroidism, the LT4 dose must be increased by 30%–50% in the early first trimester and then lowered to the prepregnancy dose postdelivery.
- Screening for the risk or presence of thyroid disorders should take place verbally in all women, while blood testing should be based on maternal risk factors.
- Women with Grave's hyperthyroidism must have preconception counseling regarding the risk of fetal congenital defects if ATD treatment is necessary in the first trimester.
- Gestational transient thyrotoxicosis requires clinical observation in most cases, but it should be differentiated from autoimmune hyperthyroidism if TSH is below 0.1 mIU/L, FT4 is elevated, or both.
- Thyroperoxidase antibody (TPO Ab)-positive women carry a 50% risk for postpartum thyroiditis (PPT), and up to 20% will become permanently hypothyroid within the first 12 months.

19.1 INTRODUCTION

Thyroid disease is the most prevalent endocrine disorder (next to hyperglycemia) in pregnancy worldwide. Hypothyroidism is more common; it affects women in both iodine-sufficient and -deficient areas. In areas of iodine sufficiency, autoimmune thyroid disease accounts for the majority of overt hypothyroidism, and thyroid antibodies have been found to be detectable in up to 60% of pregnant women with an elevated TSH. Subclinical hypothyroidism (SCH) remains a subject of controversy, as studies show variable outcomes. Hyperthyroidism due to Grave's disease (GD) affects about 0.2%–0.4% of pregnant women, followed by gestational hyperthyroidism and toxic adenomas. Postpartum thyroid disorders are important to recognize, given their prevalence and impact on maternal and neonatal health. This chapter reviews in depth the diagnosis and management of the continuum of thyroid disorders, including issues arising in the preconception and postpartum periods, and discusses the available evidence and clinical guidelines of thyroid disorders in pregnancy. Thyroid cancer is discussed separately in Chapter 20.

19.2 BIOMARKERS OF THYROID AUTOIMMUNITY

There are three markers of thyroid autoimmunity: anti-TPO Ab, antithyroglobulin antibody (TGAb), and thyroid-stimulating hormone receptor antibodies (TSHR Ab). These antibodies have varying degrees of disease-specific sensitivity, specificity, and pathogenicity (Table 19.1).

Maternal-Fetal and Neonatal Endocrinology. https://doi.org/10.1016/B978-0-12-814823-5.00019-2

TABLE 19.1 Comparison of thyroid autoantibodies

	TPO Ab	TGAb	TSHR Ab
Prevalence of Ab in			
Euthyroid adults	10%–15% (up to 9% of males and 26% of females)[2,3]	10%–27%[1–3]	Not present[3]
Hashimoto thyroiditis	90%–95%[2,3]	20%–90%[2,3]	~0%–20%[3]
GD	80%–85%[2,3]	30%–60%[2,3]	~90%[3]
Other autoimmune diseases	40% T1DM 12%–30% celiac disease 16%–37% rheumatoid arthritis[3]	30% T1DM 11%–32% celiac disease 12%–23% rheumatoid arthritis[3]	Usually none[3]
Action of antibodies	Stimulating, blocking, apoptosis[3]	Potentially pathogenic[3]	No defined action[3]
Transplacental passage	Possible[3]	Possible[3]	Possible[3]

19.2.1 Thyroperoxidase Antibody

Thyroperoxidase (TPO) is a membrane-bound protein located on thyrocytes, and it acts as the key enzyme in the synthesis of thyroid hormones. TPO Abs are polyclonal antibodies that form in response to thyroid injury but are also likely to contribute to disease pathogenicity.[1,2] TPO Abs may lead to autoimmune hypothyroidism through two mechanisms: (1) the ability to destroy thyrocytes through complement fixation and through antibody-dependent cytotoxicity and (2) inhibition of the enzymatic activity of TPO.[2,3] TPO Abs are very prevalent in people with autoimmune thyroid disease, present in over 90% of people with Hashimoto thyroiditis and about 80%–85% of people with GD.[2,3] They are also relatively prevalent in euthyroid, healthy adults, with estimated rates ranging from 10%–15% of all healthy adults to as high as 26% of healthy females.[2,3] TPO Ab positivity has been associated with increased risk for pregnancy loss and premature delivery in euthyroid women; however, within women with GD, there is no prognostic value for the fetus and newborn.[4] TPO Ab is the most sensitive test for predicting autoimmune hypothyroidism.[1]

19.2.2 Thyroglobulin Antibody

Thyroglobulin (Tg) is the major thyroid protein and is a precursor to thyroid hormones. Tg antibodies (Tg Abs) are polyclonal antibodies to Tg. Tg Abs are common in autoimmune thyroid disease, with a prevalence of 20%–90% in Hashimoto thyroiditis and 30%–60% in GD, but, like TPO Abs, they are also present in 10%–27% of healthy adults.[1–3] Unlike TPO Abs, a clear role in pathogenicity has not been found for TG Abs, although there is some evidence that the TG Abs present in patients with Hashimoto thyroiditis are biochemically distinct from the TG Abs found in healthy, euthyroid adults.[2,3]

19.2.3 Thyroid Stimulating Hormone Receptor Antibody

The thyroid-stimulating hormone receptor (TSHR) is an extracellular receptor that binds to TSH and drives the production of thyroid hormones and growth of thyroid follicular cells. TSHR antibodies (TSHR Abs) are oligoclonal antibodies that can be grouped into three categories: stimulating antibodies, blocking antibodies, and neutral antibodies. Different assays measure TSHR Abs in different ways, and the nomenclature varies, complicating our understanding of these tests. Bioassays measure the functional activity of TSHR Abs, while immunoassays measure TSHR Abs binding to TSHRs without functional discrimination.[3,5] To some, the term thyroid receptor antibody (TRAB) refers to the immunoassay measure that lacks functional discrimination,[3,5] but to others, TRAB is a catch-all term for any form of TSHR Ab.[4,6,7] In this discussion, we will use TRAB to refer to the immunoassay and *TSHR Ab* as the catch-all term. Thyrotropin-binding inhibitor immunoglobulin (TBII) is a competitive immunoassay that measures TSHR Ab; antibodies can be either stimulating or blocking.[3–5] On the other hand, thyroid-stimulating immunoglobulin (TSI) is a stimulating antibody measure of cyclic adenosine monophosphate (cAMP) by bioassay. Further, cAMP is part of the final pathway to hyperthyroidism in GD. Antibodies with different functional activities are not mutually exclusive and may coexist in the same patient.[5]

TSHR Abs, especially stimulating Abs such as TSI, are pathogenic for GD, and high levels of these antibodies predict relapse following antithyroid drug (ATD) treatments.[3,5] In pregnant women, these Abs can help predict fetal thyroid size and fetal hyperthyroidism.[6] Newer generations of both TSI and TBII assays have improved sensitivity and specificity relative to older generations.[7] TSHR Abs are present in 90% of GD patients, with stimulating Abs present in 73%–100% and blocking Ab present in 25%–75% of GD patients.[3] TBII alone has a 97% sensitivity and 99% specificity for GD.[4] TSHR Abs are also found in 0–20% of Hashimoto thyroiditis and 10%–75% of atrophic thyroiditis. In contrast to TPO Abs and Tg Abs, TSHR Abs are not found in the healthy population, and their presence in a euthyroid patient can be prognostic of later thyroid disease development and concurrent GD-related phenomenon such as orbitopathy.[1, 3]

19.3 PRIMARY SUBCLINICAL HYPOTHYROIDISM

19.3.1 Overview

Subclinical hypothyroidism (SCH) garners a great deal of attention in the obstetrical literature and causes a tremendous amount of maternal anxiety as a possible cause of subfertility, poor pregnancy outcomes, and decreased cognitive function in exposed offspring. These risks seem to be more dramatic among women who have antithyroid peroxidase antibodies. However, the literature regarding both pregnancy and neurocognitive outcomes varies widely, is heavily influenced by the retrospective and associational nature of the available studies with differing definitions of SCH, and is often inconsistent. Furthermore, data are not consistent with regard to the benefits of treating SCH during pregnancy. Nevertheless, given the benign nature of levothyroxine in pregnancy, treating SCH when identified is considered clinically appropriate, but mothers should be reassured that under most circumstances, outcomes are either entirely normal or only minimally affected.

19.3.2 Definition

SCH is defined by a maternal TSH exceeding trimester-specific concentrations while free T4 remains within the normal range. However, diagnosing and studying SCH are challenging because diagnosis depends on defining an upper limit of normal for TSH, and this varies by population and iodine status. The American Thyroid Association (ATA) recommends the use of population-specific and trimester-adjusted values for normal TSH, but suggests using an upper limit of 2.5 mU/L in the first trimester and 3.0 mU/L in the second and third trimesters if no population-specific range is available.[8] The available literature varies with regard to definitions of SCH, with the largest studies using a range of TSH >2.5 to >5.6 mU/L in the first trimester.[9, 10]

There is a normal, expected decline in TSH in the first trimester, which is related to the activity of human chorionic gonadotropin (hCG).[11] Thus, a slightly elevated TSH that would fall within the normal range for a nonpregnant woman likely represents slightly abnormal thyroid function in a pregnant woman in her first trimester.

Another potentially clinically important diagnosis during pregnancy is isolated hypothyroxinemia, which is defined as a TSH within the normal range but with reduced T4 levels.

19.3.3 Burden of Disease

When a TSH of 6.0 mU/L is used as the upper limit of normal, SCH is estimated to occur in approximately 2%–2.5% of screened women in the United States.[12, 13] Similar rates were identified (2.2%) from a general population of pregnant patients (testing done on stored serum obtained for another purpose) when a threshold TSH of >97.5% was utilized.[14] A study from the Netherlands demonstrated higher rates of SCH (approximately 9%) when a TSH of 2.5 mU/L in the first trimester and 3.0 mU/L in the second trimester was used to define SCH.[15] A study of over 100,000 American women undergoing screening for hypothyroidism demonstrated rates of SCH of close to 15% when an upper limit for TSH of 2.5 mU/L was utilized.[16]

Isolated hypothyroxinemia is also estimated to affect approximately 2% of pregnancies.[14]

19.3.4 Pathophysiology

During pregnancy, an increase from baseline thyroid hormone concentrations is necessary to produce appropriate physiologic changes in maternal cardiac output and blood volume, fat stores, cholesterol metabolism, and synthesis of pituitary hormones. Additionally, for the first 10–12 weeks of pregnancy until its own thyroid gland begins to function, the embryo/fetus is dependent upon maternal thyroid hormone to drive metabolic activity, most critically axonal growth, myelination, and cell differentiation within the brain and central nervous system (CNS).[17] If there are inadequate amounts of thyroid hormone, virtually all systems are affected, which can result in poor pregnancy outcomes and can prevent normal development of the fetal nervous system. While these complications are most pronounced when a mother has overt hypothyroidism, subtle deficiencies in thyroid hormone, particularly during critical windows of fetal development, may have a lasting impact.[18]

19.3.5 Pregnancy

19.3.5.1 Pregnancy Outcomes in SCH and Isolated Hypothyroxinemia

The impact of severe hypothyroidism during pregnancy on cognitive development for offspring was recognized as early as the late 1800s.[19] However, a number of studies published over the last 20 years have suggested an association between mild thyroid dysfunction during pregnancy and abnormal neurocognitive development in exposed fetuses. Additionally, SCH has been associated with pregnancy loss and other poor pregnancy outcomes, including increased rates of preeclampsia and preterm birth. Dozens of studies have been published exploring these associations, but they are limited by the variability in definition of SCH, variability in iodine status in different populations, measurement of antibody positivity which appears to affect outcomes, and the fact that screening for thyroid disease is not universal in pregnancy. However, the majority of these studies appear to support a conclusion that SCH somewhat increases pregnancy and neurodevelopmental risks.

The first studies exploring the possible association between abnormal neurocognitive development and SCH were published in the late 1990s. Haddow and colleagues studied the 7–9-year-old children of 62 women with either mild hypothyroidism or SCH (TSH levels $\geq$98%) and compared them to 124 matched women with normal thyroid values. (Controls were matched for maternal age, years of education, duration of serum storage, and sex of the child.) Children born to mothers with mild thyroid hypofunction performed slightly less well on 15 neurocognitive tests, including scoring 4 points lower on a full-scale IQ test.[20] In the same year, Pop and colleagues reported that 33 children born to women with low free T4 levels (hypothyroxinemia) in early pregnancy performed worse on psychomotor developmental tests than women with normal free T4 levels.[21] A more recent study from the Netherlands that included approximately 3600 children demonstrated an association between both mild and severe hypothyroxinemia and a higher risk of expressive language delay.[22] However, not all studies demonstrate an association, including a study from the United Kingdom of approximately 4600 children that did not demonstrate an association between SCH and poorer school performance.[23] These studies are all necessarily complicated by the lack of randomization and the extremely challenging nature of attempting to adjust for confounding by all potentially relevant cofactors pertaining to cognitive development. As such, it is very important that women who are found to have SCH in early pregnancy are counseled that while treatment is recommended, the potential impact on cognitive function for the child is uncertain at best.

Studies of pregnancy outcomes are also mixed with regard to an association between SCH and abnormal pregnancy outcomes. One large study included a population of women who underwent blood testing for other reasons and had TSH evaluated from banked serum. In that population, including approximately 500 women with TSH > 97.5%, there was no association with poor outcomes, including preterm labor, pregnancy loss, preeclampsia, or low birth weight.[14] Another study including 209 women with TSH > 6.0 who had it measured as part of routine prenatal care did demonstrate an association with fetal death (odds ratio (OR) 4.4, 95% confidence interval (CI) 1.9–9.5), but no other increased pregnancy risks (placental abruption, gestational hypertension, low Apgar, or low birth weight). Importantly, this study included 37 women with TSH $\geq$10, among whom the fetal death rate was 8.1%.[12] A prospective study of 3000 Chinese women suggested that women with SCH are at increased risk for miscarriage [adjusted odds ratio (aOR) 3.40, 95% CI 1.62–7.15].[24] Additionally, Negro and colleagues reported an increased rate of pregnancy loss (6.1% vs 3.6%) among women with mildly elevated TSH (2.5–5 mU/L).[25]

A recent systematic review and meta-analysis of 18 studies demonstrated an increased pooled risk for pregnancy loss [risk ratio (RR) 2.01, 95% CI 1.66–2.44], placental abruption (RR 2.14, 95% CI 1.23–3.70), premature rupture of membranes (RR 1.43, 95% CI 1.04–1.95), and neonatal death (RR 2.58, 95% CI 1.41–4.73) compared to women with normal thyroid function. This study did not show an increased risk for preeclampsia, gestational hypertension, gestational diabetes, or preterm birth.[26]

19.3.5.2 Thyroid Autoantibody Positivity

Common antithyroid antibodies include anti-TPO antibodies and antithyroglobulin antibodies, which are present in 2%–17% of unselected pregnant women.[8] TPO is responsible for oxidizing dietary iodide to iodine, as well as coupling the building blocks of T3 and T4. Women who are antithyroid antibody positive are at increased risk of developing clinically important hypothyroidism during pregnancy, despite having normal thyroid function prior to pregnancy.[27] Furthermore, some studies suggest that there may be an increased risk for pregnancy loss and other poor pregnancy outcomes among women who are positive for antithyroid antibodies, as compared to women with similar thyroid function who are antibody negative, including among euthyroid women.

A meta-analysis including 14 studies showed an OR of 2.31 (95% CI 1.90–2.82) for pregnancy loss in women with thyroid autoimmunity, as compared to women without antithyroid antibodies.[28] Additionally, although the data are mixed, several meta-analyses have demonstrated an association between thyroid autoimmunity and preterm delivery, with odds ranging from 1.4 to 2.9.[9, 29, 30] Other evidence suggests that antithyroid antibodies may also be associated with increased risk for fetal demise[31] as well as placental abruption,[32] although these data are not entirely consistent.

19.3.5.3 Diagnosis

SCH is diagnosed by blood testing, including TSH and typically free T4. Given variability in normal values by population and laboratory technique, the ATA recommends that when possible, population-based, trimester- and laboratory-specific reference ranges for thyroid function testing should be used. When these values are not available, an upper value of 2.5–3.0 for TSH is recommended.[8] Free T4 is expected to be within the normal range during pregnancy. Given the evidence suggesting that outcomes are worse among women who are antithyroid antibody positive, testing for TPO antibodies is recommended for women with a TSH >2.5 mU/L.

19.3.5.4 Treatment

The data regarding the benefits of treatment of SCH are somewhat limited; however, the available data suggest that there may be a benefit to reduce poor pregnancy outcomes, particularly among women who are antithyroid antibody positive. Studies are complicated by the fact that many do not start treatment until well into the first trimester, which may be later than would be beneficial. Based upon the available data, the ATA recommends levothyroxine treatment for anti-TPO antibody-positive women with a TSH above the pregnancy-specific reference range, as well as for anti-TPO antibody negative women whose TSH is >10.0 mU/L. They recommend considering treatment for women who are anti-TPO antibody positive with a TSH > 2.5 mU/L, but below the upper limit of the pregnancy-specific reference, as well as for women who are anti-TPO antibody negative with a TSH above the upper limit of the reference range.[8]

19.3.6 Postpartum and Lactation

Women who are diagnosed with SCH during pregnancy are at increased risk for clinical hypothyroidism after delivery; however, treatment that has been initiated during pregnancy for SCH can likely be discontinued postpartum, with close follow-up.

Some studies have suggested that clinical hypothyroidism may affect milk supply in lactating mothers; however, a wide range of TSH has been associated with normal breastfeeding.[33] Although there are no data based on randomized controlled trials (RCTs), given the low risk, it is reasonable to provide levothyroxine treatment for women with SCH who are having difficulty with milk supply.

19.3.7 Conclusion

Although the data are variable, there seems to be consistent evidence that SCH, particularly among women who are anti-TPO antibody positive, is associated with pregnancy loss, other poor pregnancy outcomes, and perhaps abnormal intellectual development in offspring. While treatment has not been established to have clear benefits, there are no known pregnancy risks associated with levothyroxine treatment. Thus, treatment is appropriate among women who are identified to have SCH, but mothers should be reassured that there is a high probability of a normal outcome, whether or not SCH is treated.

19.4 OVERT HYPOTHYROIDISM

19.4.1 Overview

Hypothyroidism in pregnancy is relatively common and affects women in both iodine sufficient and deficient areas. In areas of iodine sufficiency, autoimmune thyroid disease accounts for the majority of overt hypothyroidism. In the United States, approximately 0.3%–0.5% of pregnancies will be complicated by overt hypothyroidism,[34] most often from Hashimoto thyroiditis. Diagnosis and treatment of new onset hypothyroidism and appropriate dose adjustment of thyroid replacement hormone in known preconception hypothyroidism is crucial during early gestation as fetal neurodevelopment is dependent on maternal thyroid hormone until the fetal thyroid develops. There are no established adverse fetal or maternal outcomes if hypothyroidism is appropriately managed.

19.4.2 Definition

Overt hypothyroidism occurs when the level of thyroid hormone in the body is low, as opposed to SCH, in which the TSH may be elevated, but the thyroid hormone is not low. Due to maternal thyroid physiology, it is imperative to use reference ranges that reflect the gestational age to appropriately diagnose and treat overt hypothyroidism.

19.4.3 Pathophysiology

Overt hypothyroidism can be caused by iodine deficiency, autoimmune disease, thyroidectomy, radioablative therapy such as radioactive iodine (RAI), or pathology within the hypothalamus or pituitary gland. Table 19.10 provides a detailed list of causes of severe hypothyroidism. For many women, this pathology is known prior to pregnancy. For women without pre-existing hypothyroidism, the increased demand on the thyroid gland can reveal underlying thyroid pathology. In fact, some have described pregnancy as a stress test for the thyroid gland.[35] While hypothyroidism can impair fertility, 11% of women with overt hypothyroidism will be able to become pregnant without thyroid hormone replacement.[34] Before the fetal thyroid gland develops, fetal requirements of thyroid hormone are met by maternal production.

19.4.4 Causes

Worldwide, the most common cause of hypothyroidism is iodine deficiency.[34] Due to the changes in maternal physiology while pregnant that are described elsewhere in this chapter, iodine demand increases by approximately 50%, and these needs must be met through diet or supplements.[34] The Institute of Medicine recommended dietary allowance for iodine intake during pregnancy is 220 mcg, and during lactation it is 290 mcg.[35] Patients with iodine deficiency will often present with a goiter, and offspring of mothers with severe iodine deficiency can have multiple adverse outcomes.

Within iodine-sufficient countries such as the United States, autoimmune hypothyroidism is the main cause[34]. This can be distinguished by the presence of autoantibodies, with TPO Ab having the best sensitivity and specificity for autoimmune thyroid disease.

Less common causes of overt hypothyroidism include prior thyroid treatments, such as surgery and RAI, and dysfunction of the hypothalamus-pituitary axis. Women with a history of thyroid cancer, toxic thyroid nodules, or GD may have undergone treatment with either partial or complete thyroidectomy. These women may have also undergone RAI treatment. Some women with other disorders will have had head or neck surgery or external beam radiation therapy as treatment. These women will often already be on thyroid replacement at the time of conception, but some may be revealed to be hypothyroid during pregnancy. Alternatively, hypothyroidism can be caused by pathology in the hypothalamus or pituitary gland, called *secondary* or *central hypothyroidism*. Central hypothyroidism can occur suddenly during pregnancy or in the postpartum period due to inadequate blood flow (Sheehan syndrome), but it is also due to invasive or compressive lesions such as pituitary macroadenomas, prior head injuries, an autoimmune disease called *lymphocytic hypophysitis,* or infiltrative disease such as sarcoidosis.

19.4.5 Pregnancy

19.4.5.1 Preconception

In patients with known hypothyroidism on levothyroxine supplementation, preconception TSH should be targeted to <2.5,[8] with some arguing for a target of <1.2.[34] The lower threshold has been suggested because it has been shown that the majority of women on this dose will not become hypothyroid even if a dose change is not done.[35]

19.4.5.2 Diagnosis

Clinicians must maintain a high index of suspicion for hypothyroidism during pregnancy because many of the signs and symptoms are shared—namely, fatigue, constipation, and weight gain. The diagnosis is made based on lab results of TSH and free T4 or total T4 accounting for trimester-specific reference ranges and issues with interpreting assays during pregnancy. For the aforementioned causes, all but central hypothyroidism will present with an elevated TSH and a low free T4 or total T4. In central hypothyroidism, the free T4 and total T4 will be low, but the TSH will be low or inappropriately normal.

The presence of TPO Ab can be used to differentiate autoimmune hypothyroidism from other etiologies. While universal screening was not found to be effective, patients with particular conditions, including a history of TPO Abs, type 1 diabetes mellitus, head and neck irradiation, infertility, morbid obesity, and use of medications that can impair thyroid function, should be checked at preconception or in early pregnancy.

19.4.5.3 Treatment

If overt hypothyroidism is appropriately treated, there are no known adverse outcomes.[34] After ensuring adequate iodine intake (220 mcg/day during pregnancy, usually included in prenatal vitamins), the optimal treatment method is with T4 replacement (namely, levothyroxine).[8, 36] Because the fetal brain is relatively impermeable to T3, thyroid hormone replacement with desiccated thyroid or combined T4 and T3 medications should be avoided during pregnancy, as they have nonphysiologic T4:T3 ratios and the developing fetus would not be exposed to adequate T4.[8]

In women with known hypothyroidism, levels of T4 supplementation must be changed in order to meet the increased requirement. Over half of patients with known hypothyroidism would develop overt hypothyroidism in pregnancy if the doses were not changed.[8] The dose should immediately be increased by 30%–50% of the prepregnancy dose.[8, 34, 37] This can be accomplished by increasing from 7 to 9 doses per week.[8, 36] Dose adjustments can be further tailored based on TSH levels as described later in this chapter. Larger dose changes are usually needed in patients who have hypothyroidism due to surgery or RAI, as compared to autoimmune thyroid disease, as there is less residual thyroid reserve.[8, 34]

In women with a new diagnosis of overt hypothyroidism, weight-based dosing can be used to determine the initial dose. TSH levels should be monitored to make appropriate dose adjustments. In a nonpregnant woman, the replacement dose is 1.7–2.0 mcg/kg/day. Because of the increased need in a pregnant woman, full replacement dose for someone with overt hypothyroidism is 2.0–2.4 mcg/kg/day.[34, 37]

19.4.5.4 Monitoring

In patients already on thyroid hormone replacement, TSH should be checked with a missed period or at 8–12 weeks and at 20 weeks.[34] In select patients, monitoring of TSH and FT4 or total T4 as often as every 4 weeks may be needed when more than anticipated LT4 dose adjustment is required early in the first trimester or if adherence is a concern. While on thyroid hormone replacement, dose adjustments can be made based on the level of the TSH. For a TSH between 5 and 10 U/mL, the dose of the levothyroxine should be increased by 25–50 mcg/day; for TSH between 10 and 20 U/mL, the dose should be increased by 50–75 mcg/day and finally, for TSH over 20, the dose should be increased by 75–100 µg/day.[34, 38]

Treatment goals include maintaining a TSH in the low normal gestational age-specific reference range.[34] As mentioned, free T4 levels must be interpreted with caution, and total T4 levels should be multiplied by 1.5 if trimester-specific reference ranges are not available.[34] Caution should be paid to avoid overtreatment, which could lead to fetal hyperthyroidism.[36]

19.4.5.5 Pregnancy Outcomes

Pregnancy outcomes in women with overt hypothyroidism are dependent on appropriate thyroid hormone replacement. Trials of pregnancy outcomes are limited by ethical concerns, and therefore no RCTs have been done. Retrospective trials have not shown adverse outcomes as long as women are properly treated.[8] When pregnant women are not treated, there are a number of adverse maternal and fetal outcomes (Table 19.2). Adverse maternal outcomes include infertility, miscarriage, preterm delivery, anemia, preeclampsia, abruptio placenta, postpartum hemorrhage, and gestation hypertension.[34–36] Adverse fetal outcomes include fetal demise, preterm birth, intrauterine growth restriction (IUGR), low birth weight, impaired neurointellectual child development (including impaired cognition), attention deficit hyperactivity disorder (ADHD), and autism.[34–36] If maternal thyroid hormone concentrations are corrected by mid-to-late pregnancy (i.e., the 20th week or prior to the third trimester), many of these poor cognitive outcomes will be prevented.[34]

TABLE 19.2 Adverse maternal and fetal outcomes from overt hypothyroidism

Adverse maternal outcomes	Adverse fetal outcomes
Infertility	Fetal demise
Miscarriage	Preterm birth
Preterm delivery	Intrauterine growth restriction
Anemia	Low birth weight
Preeclampsia	Impaired neurointellectual child development
Abruptio placenta	ADHD
Postpartum hemorrhage	Autism
Gestation hypertension	

19.4.6 Postpartum and Lactation

In the postpartum period, dose changes are needed due to changes in thyroid physiology. In patients with known hypothyroidism prepregnancy, T4 supplementation should return to the prepregnancy dose.[8, 34] Many patients with autoimmune hypothyroidism will need to be on a higher dose postpartum, likely due to exacerbation of autoimmunity in the postpartum period.[8, 34] In patients who developed overt hypothyroidism during pregnancy, dose reduction will likely be needed postpartum. Patients who were TPO-Ab positive but euthyroid at the beginning of pregnancy should stop treatment. In any scenario, the TSH level should be rechecked in 6 weeks and continue to be monitored as needed based on these follow-up labs.

Overt hypothyroidism can impair lactation. A very small amount of LT4 transfers to breast milk.[8] Aside from their hormone replacement, mothers who are lactating should maintain adequate iodine levels, with the recommendation of ingesting 290 mcg/day.[35]

19.4.7 Isolated Hypothyroxinemia

Isolated hypothyroxinemia is diagnosed when the TSH is within the normal range but the woman has reduced T4 levels. It is estimated to affect approximately 2% of pregnancies.[14] It was initially thought to be driven by iodine deficiency, but it does not resolve with iodine supplementation and has been found in iodine-sufficient areas as well, suggesting that is not the true pathophysiology.[39] It is now thought to be a multifactorial and pregnancy-specific pathophysiology,[39] with risk factors including iodine deficiency, thyroid autoimmunity, assay techniques, and maternal characteristics such as age, body mass index, and coexistent diabetes.[40]

Pregnancy outcomes are described in detail within Section 19.3.5.1 In brief, hypothyroxinemia may have an association with adverse neurobehavioral outcomes in the child, but as of now, there is no evidence of adverse pregnancy outcomes.[8, 39] There is minimal evidence about treatment of isolated hypothyroxinemia, but thyroid hormone replacement seems to have had no benefit on the neurobehavioral outcomes that may be associated with hypothyroxinemia. Therefore, preconception treatment is generally not recommended, although some clinicians do consider treatment in early pregnancy.[8, 36, 40]

19.5 SECONDARY HYPOTHYROIDISM (CENTRAL HYPOTHYROIDISM)

Keywords
- Lymphocytic hypophysitis
- Pituitary apoplexy
- Sheehan Syndrome

Secondary hypothyroidism due to pituitary or hypothalamic disease is rare but important to be aware of, as interpretation of thyroid functions must take inadequate secretion of TSH into consideration. In many cases, maternal history of prior pituitary disease is known, but less commonly, acute pituitary pathology may complicate pregnancy. Etiologies of chronic pituitary insufficiency include prior pituitary surgery for a secreting or nonsecreting adenoma, a history of pituitary apoplexy, or in rare cases a history of Sheehan syndrome. Lymphocytic hypophysitis and pituitary apoplexy are rare but may be associated with acute pan-hypopituitarism in pregnancy. Patients usually present with a sudden, severe headache and severe pituitary dysfunction, including central hypothyroidism, as well as acute adrenal insufficiency. Hypothalamic and pituitary disorders are covered in detail in Chapters 16 and 18, respectively. Monitoring of chronic central hypothyroidism in pregnancy should focus on free T4 levels as TSH will be inappropriately low and cannot be used for accurate dose adjustment of L-thyroxine therapy. Serum free T4 levels should be kept at the trimester-specific physiologic ranges recommended for pregnancy, as outlined in table 1 in Chapter 4.

19.6 SYNDROMES OF REDUCED SENSITIVITY TO THYROID HORMONE

19.6.1 Overview

Keywords
- Resistance to thyroid hormone (RTH TH-receptor beta-gene defect)
- Thyroid hormone cell transporter defect (THCTD, MCT8 gene defect)
- Thyroid hormone metabolism defect (THMD, SBP2-gene defect)

Three syndromes of reduced end-organ sensitivity to thyroid hormone (TH) have been identified since Samuel Refetoff et al's original description of RTH in 1967. These rare disorders involve mutations of three of the six steps required to facilitate thyroid hormone action on target tissues.[41, 42] Although rare, these gene defects are not as uncommon as previously thought. In 95% of patients, the cause of RTH lies in a TH-receptor beta-gene mutation, whereas in 15% of these patients, the defect is unknown. Mutations in the cell-membrane transporter of TH (*MCT8*-gene) and in the intracellular metabolism of TH (*SBP2*-gene) are present in patients with THCTD and THMD syndromes.[42] In the latter, the mutation is associated with decreased synthesis of selenoproteins, including deiodinases.

A combination of an elevated FT4 or FT3 level (or both) with a nonsuppressed or slightly elevated TSH is the key laboratory finding in affected individuals. The focus of this section is on fetal/neonatal and maternal outcomes and the importance of preconception counseling in affected patients and those with a family history. Ongoing research is needed to gain further insight into the long-term implications of the two most recently discovered mutations and to better understand the observed outcomes of unaffected embryos and fetuses who are exposed to the excessive TH of an affected mother.

19.6.2   Incidence, Prevalence, and Inheritance

A retrospective study found the incidence of RTH to be 1/40,000 live births,[43] with autosomal-dominant inheritance in the majority of affected families. Among the three mutations, RTH is the most prevalent and is equally distributed between both sexes. The incidences of THCTD and THMD are unknown. Inheritance is X-chromosome-linked in THCTD and affects males phenotypically, while female carriers are asymptomatic in most cases. Ethnic and racial distribution is diverse in both RTH and THCTD. THMD is inherited recessively and has been found in Bedouins from Saudi Arabia, as well as in the Irish and Africans.[44]

19.6.3   Clinical Features and Maternal and Fetal Outcomes

Clinical manifestations are variable among patients with RTH, but up to 95% of individuals develop a goiter and a significant number will experience tachycardia and CNS symptoms, including ADHD, emotional disturbances, and hyperkinetic behavior. Recurrent ear and throat infections are found in 55%, whereas short stature and growth delay, as well as mental retardation and hearing loss, occur less commonly.[45–47]

In the retrospective study by Anselmo et al., obstetric outcomes tended to be poor in fetuses with RTH carried by normal mothers and in unaffected fetuses of mothers with RTH. In this study, affected mothers with RTH had a 23.7% miscarriage rate and there was a 6.7% rate in unaffected mothers who conceived from an affected father, compared to an 8.8% miscarriage rate in unaffected first-degree relatives and 8.1% in the general population.[48] Unaffected fetuses of mothers with RTH had a lower birth weight and lower TSH. The authors concluded that this likely due to exposure to supraphysiologic transplacental levels of maternal thyroxine. Adverse obstetric events, including preterm delivery, stillbirth, preeclampsia, and perinatal death were not increased in these children.[48] In a recent follow-up study of unaffected offspring of the same family, the authors demonstrated reduced TSH sensitivity to TH, with persistence of anterior pituitary TH inactivation in adulthood. Further research on these subjects to assess the long-term impact on peripheral tissues and on future generations is ongoing.[49]

Affected male offspring of asymptomatic female carriers of the *MCT8*-gene mutation present with severe psychomotor impairment, inability to walk, cognitive dysfunction, and inability to develop effective speech. This phenotype differs clinically from that described in fetuses exposed to global TH deficiency.[42] Offspring with the *SBP2* gene defect may have had a normal pregnancy course and birth, but can present later with short stature and delayed bone age. In general, the disease tends to be milder in them.

19.6.4   Treatment

Treatment of affected mothers with RTH in pregnancy should focus on maternal symptoms such as tachycardia, which can be controlled with a beta-adrenergic blocking agent such as propranolol. Because of the observed concern about the adverse effect of excessive fetal exposure to maternal T4, normalization of maternal TSH is not recommended and FT4 levels 20% above the upper range of normal are discouraged.[48, 50] In most patients with RTH, compensatory elevation of TSH and TH allows for adequate endogenous supply in pregnancy, unless a patient has undergone prior partial thyroidectomy or ablative therapy. Treatment of mothers with the *MCT8*-gene and *SBP2*-gene defects is unclear and currently under investigation.

Prenatal fetal diagnosis and counseling is recommended in patients with RTH, especially those whose affected family members display growth delay and mental retardation. Known asymptomatic female carries of the *MCT8*-gene mutation should be counseled on the risk of severe adverse outcomes of male offspring. In women affected by the *SBP2*-gene defect, the counseling should center around the need for future monitoring for growth delay in their offspring, even if pregnancy and birth were uncomplicated. Pregnant patients with a family or personal history of reduced sensitivity to TH may be best served by a collaborative effort of an interdisciplinary team that includes a genetic counselor, maternal-fetal medicine specialist, and adult and pediatric endocrinologists.

19.7 HYPERTHYROIDISM

Keywords
- GD
- Gestational transient thyrotoxicosis
- Toxic multinodular goiter (TMNG)
- Toxic adenoma (TA)
- Thyroid receptor antibody
- Antithyroid drug

19.7.1 Overview

Hyperthyroidism frequently affects women of childbearing age. Autoimmune hyperthyroidism due to GD is the most common cause of intrinsic thyroid disease and occurs in about 0.4%–1% of women before pregnancy and 0.2% during pregnancy. The incidence of GD increases with maternal age and may be up to 1.4% in women over 40 years old.[51] More often, biochemical thyroid function abnormalities suggestive of subclinical hyperthyroidism are the result of physiologic hCG-mediated stimulation of the thyroid gland in the first trimester and must be recognized as such.[52] Due to its structural homology with TSH, hCG shares an affinity to the TSH receptor, albeit much weaker than TSH and requiring high levels of hCG to achieve a significant supraphysiologic effect (see the discussion of thyroid physiology in Chapter 4). In iodine-deficient regions, TMNGs and adenomas are frequent, but because they occur more often in older women, they are still a relatively uncommon cause of hyperthyroidism in pregnancy.[53]

19.7.2 Differential Diagnosis of Hyperthyroidism in Pregnancy

Differentiating transient gestational hyperthyroidism from thyrotoxicosis due to intrinsic thyroid disease, especially Grave's hyperthyroidism, is important. It requires a comprehensive evaluation and exam (Table 19.3). Untreated overt hyperthyroidism due to GD carries a significant risk of adverse maternal and fetal outcomes, which are reviewed in detail in Section 19.7.3.5. In patients with a positive family history of thyroid disease, significant thyroid enlargement, or eye findings suggestive of thyroid-related orbitopathy such as proptosis, a full thyroid function panel with a TSH, TH, and TRAB should be obtained.[8] TSH concentrations <0.1 mIU/L also warrant the assessment of TH levels (FT4/FT3), as well as a TRAB evaluation.[54]

In a subset of patients with a preexisting history of GD that was in remission prior to conception, superimposed hCG-mediated stimulation of a large residual goiter may at times pose a diagnostic challenge, and the decision to treat with ATD therapy will depend on clinical judgment, guided by the patient's symptomatology, exam findings, and TRAB detectability.

Patients with overt TMNG or adenoma may present with symptoms of overt hyperthyroidism, including tachycardia, breathlessness, anxiety, and lack of weight gain. In addition, they may complain of difficulty with swallowing, and the physical exam should reveal an irregular, often asymmetrically enlarged thyroid gland. Aside from a lid lag, other eye findings such as proptosis and periorbital edema should be absent, but if present, they would suggest an underlying nodular form of autoimmune hyperthyroidism such as GD. Nonautoimmune autonomously functioning toxic goiters and adenomas will have a negative TRAB. There may be a family history of thyroid disease, especially in women who live in iodine-deficient regions.[52, 53] As with Grave's hyperthyroidism, overt symptomatic thyrotoxicosis due to a nodular goiter increases the risk of adverse obstetric outcomes if uncontrolled throughout pregnancy. The clinical course and treatment of GD will be reviewed in detail in Section 19.7.3.

TABLE 19.3 Causes of hyperthyroidism

Excessive TSH-receptor stimulation

- Graves' disease (TSH-receptor autoantibodies)
- Gestational-transient thyrotoxicosis (hCG-induced)
- Familial gestational hyperthyroidism TSH-receptor mutation[71]
- Trophoblastic disease (hCG-induced)
- TSH-producing pituitary adenoma [54a]

Autonomous thyroid hormone secretion

- Multinodular toxic goiter (TMNG)
- Solitary toxic thyroid adenoma (TA)
- Genomic-activating TSH-receptor mutation [54b]

Destruction of follicles with release of hormone

- Subacute (granulomatous, de Quervain's) thyroiditis (viral infection)
- Painless (silent) thyroiditis (autoimmunity)
- Acute thyroiditis (bacterial infection)

Extrathyroidal sources of thyroid hormone

- Overtreatment with thyroid hormone
- Factitious intake of thyroid hormone
- Functional thyroid cancer metastases
- Struma ovarii

hCG, human chorionic gonadotropin; TSH, thyroid-stimulating hormone.
(Reproduced with permission: Cooper DS, Laurberg P. Hyperthyroidism in pregnancy. *Lancet Diabetes Endocrinol* 2013;1: 238–249.)

19.7.3   Grave's Disease

19.7.3.1   Overview

GD is the most common cause of hyperthyroidism during pregnancy.[34] Approximately 0.4%–1.0% of women will have GD prior to pregnancy,[8] and 0.2% of women will develop GD during pregnancy.[4, 8] Of the women with active or prior history of GD, 1%–5% will have pregnancies complicated by fetal and neonatal hyperthyroidism.[4, 55]

GD is an autoimmune disease caused by autoantibodies that stimulate the thyroid gland to produce thyroid hormones. The immune responses in the pregnant woman affect the natural history of GD. In the initial stages of pregnancy, there is a small increase in the incidence of new onset GD and flares, likely due to TSH-receptor antibody levels or thyroid gland stimulation by hCG.[4, 8] Then, to allow continued immune tolerance of the fetus, there is an increase in regulatory T cells and a decrease in thyroid autoantibodies in mid-to-late pregnancy.[3, 8] This is followed by a rebound of the antibodies in the postpartum period, accompanied by an increase in disease incidence and flares.[3, 4, 8]

Clinical manifestations of GD include hyperthyroid signs and symptoms that are consistent across these diseases, including tachycardia, heat intolerance, weight loss or failure to gain weight appropriately through the pregnancy, anxiety, and tremor. There are also symptoms specific to GD, namely, Grave's orbitopathy and to some extent cosmetic and compressive effects related to thyroid enlargement.

TSH-receptor autoantibodies, including TSI and TBII, can help to distinguish GD from other causes of hyperthyroidism during pregnancy. Because of the acquired immune tolerance of pregnancy, the levels of these autoantibodies decline as pregnancy progresses, especially after 20 weeks.[56]

19.7.3.2   Preconception Counseling and Care for Women with a History of GD

Preconception counseling is imperative for women of child-bearing age with GD. The foremost recommendation is to postpone pregnancy until their disease is controlled.[4, 8, 34, 57, 58] Thyroid function tests should be stable for at least two tests, 1 month apart.[8]

These women have the usual three methods of treatment available to any nonpregnant individual (ATDs, RAI, and surgery), but the pregnancy alters the risk–benefit ratio for some of these treatment modalities.

Medical management with ATDs usually achieves a euthyroid state faster than treatment with RAI. Furthermore, there is a chance to go into remission, during which no medications will be necessary, and there is often a gradual reduction of the autoimmunity and antibody titers.[8] Despite these benefits, ATDs carry with them a risk of birth defects[8] and flare of the hyperthyroid state. Because of the higher rates of severe birth defects with methimazole (MMI) over propylthiouracil (PTU), some advocate a switch to PTU prior to conception[4] rather than at the time of confirmed pregnancy.

Two major factors complicate the use of RAI in women planning imminent pregnancy. The first is that conception must be delayed for 6 months following RAI treatment.[8, 34] The second is that TSH-receptor antibodies may increase and stay elevated for months (or even a year) following RAI treatments[4, 8, 34] and women with severe GD may take longer than a year to achieve normal, stable thyroid function.[8] Elevated TSH-receptor-antibody levels are prognostic of fetal thyroid dysfunction.[4] Additionally, most patients will need lifelong thyroid hormone replacement, and all patients will need a confirmed negative pregnancy test prior to RAI.[8, 34]

Surgical thyroidectomy offers definitive therapy of the hyperthyroid state and is often accompanied by gradual remission of the autoimmune state (perhaps most effectively of the three treatment modalities),[57] but it also carries a small risk of complication and requires lifelong thyroid hormone replacement.[8]

19.7.3.3 Treatment of GD During Pregnancy

Treatment of GD during pregnancy is limited to close monitoring of thyroid function tests, medical management, and surgical intervention. RAI is contraindicated.

19.7.3.3.1 ATDs

The mainstay of medical management are the ATDs MMI, PTU, and carbimazole. These medications cross the placenta and carry risks to both the mother and fetus; thus, in select patients, close monitoring of thyroid function will be chosen over the use of medical management. Carbimazole, which is rapidly metabolized to MMI after absorption, is used in some countries instead of MMI or PTU. The conversion is 10 mg of carbimazole for every 6 mg of PTU.[8]

Maternal side effects occur in 3%–5% of women treated with ATDs. The most common side effect is rash; but rare, serious side effects include agranulocytosis (0.15%) and liver failure (< 0.1%).[8] Side effects usually occur at initiation or reinitiation of treatment.[8] The severity of fetal congenital defects varies between the two drugs, but there is significant placental passage of both.[59]

In nonpregnant patients, MMI is the recommended first-line ATD. However, it is estimated that 2%–4% of pregnancies exposed to MMI will be complicated by fetal congenital defects, especially if that exposure is between weeks 6 and 10.[8] Serious teratogenic effects include aplasia cutis, dysmorphic facies, choanal and esophageal atresia, and abdominal wall defects.[8]

PTU was initially thought to be safe for the fetus during pregnancy,[8] but more recently, it has been associated with birth defects that are seen later in development. Approximately 2%–3% will have birth defects, which include cysts in the face and neck and urinary tract issues in males.[8] These side effects are usually less severe and often treatable through surgical intervention.[8] PTU has higher rates of liver failure than MMI and is therefore not preferred in the nonpregnant individual.

Because of the side-effect profile, PTU is recommended if medications are required in the first trimester of pregnancy.[8] The initial dose of PTU is 100–600 mg/day (usually 200–400 mg/day) split over two to three doses.[4, 8] The conversion from MMI to PTU is 1 mg of MMI for every 20 mg of PTU.[4, 8] Alternatively, a treatment holiday can be considered during the first trimester for women who have well-controlled GD while on ATD. This approach should be considered in women who are TSHR Ab negative, as only 5% of -TSHR Abnegative women will become hyperthyroid within 8 weeks of withdrawal of treatment.[8] Risk of disease relapse is higher if the woman has been on treatment for <6 months, is on a dose higher than 5–10 mg/day of MMI, continues to have a suppressed TSH, or has orbitopathy or goiter.[8]

At the second trimester, PTU should be switched to MMI. If the treatment holiday approach was elected, thyroid function should be assessed and a decision made around restarting MMI.[8]

In the third trimester, there is decreased autoimmunity, and many women are able to stop treatment (20%–40%).[4, 8] Having a low TSHR Ablevel increases the chance for successful medication cessation.[8] Fetal hypothyroidism would also be an indication to stop or decrease ATD.[4]

With these medication changes, thyroid function needs to be closely monitored. TFTs should be checked every 2–4 weeks after medication initiation or dose change, but can be spaced to every 4–6 weeks once a target is achieved.[4, 8] Fetal hypothyroidism can complicate either medication if doses are not appropriately tapered.[4, 8, 57]

19.7.3.3.2   Other agents

Beta-blockade is also used for symptom management while hyperthyroid. It is safe for short-term use, with propranolol being the preferred agent.[8] Long-term use is associated with IUGR, fetal bradycardia, and neonatal hypoglycemia.[4, 8]

Another medication not commonly used for treatment of GD during pregnancy in the United States is iodine. Management of GD with iodine has been tried, but with limited success. Many patients will achieve initial efficacy, followed by a return to hyperthyroidism. Additionally, there are reports of birth defects (likely in hyperthyroid mothers), as well as fetal hypothyroidism and fetal goiter.[58] It is not a recommended modality of treatment in the United States[8] but has been successfully used in Japan.[8] Other medications less often used for treatment of GD during pregnancy include cholestyramine, perchlorate, and rarely lithium[8] if hyperthyroidism cannot be controlled with the aforementioned agents.

19.7.3.3.3   Treatment targets

The lowest effective dose of ATD should be used to maintain the FT4 around the upper limit of normal and the TT4 at 1.5 times the upper limit of the nonpregnant reference range.[4, 8, 58] TSH may remain suppressed after T4 has normalized, and therefore it should not be the primary treatment end point.[4] If TSH goes from undetectable to detectable, the ATD dose should be lowered.[4, 58]

19.7.3.3.4   Radioactive iodine

RAI is contraindicated during pregnancy and in the lactating mother. While it is the standard of care to do a pregnancy test prior to administration of RAI, if a fetus is inadvertently exposed to RAI, the gestational age is quite important to the outcome. Prior to the 10–12th week, RAI is not taken up by the fetal thyroid; therefore, no fetal thyroid dysfunction or adverse outcomes should be expected.[34, 57] After 12 weeks of age, there will be uptake of RAI in the fetal thyroid, with destructive effect.[34] In this setting, adverse outcomes due to fetal thyroid destruction, in utero hypothyroidism, and subsequent neural damage are possible. RAI administration to postpartum woman is discussed in the section on monitoring and treatment of GD postpartum (Section 19.7.3.6).

19.7.3.3.5   Surgical management

There are a limited number of situations in which a thyroidectomy should be used to control GD during pregnancy. These situations include patients with allergies or contraindications to MMI or PTU, patients who are not adherent to ATDs, or patients in which a euthyroid state is not achievable with ATD.[8] If needed, surgery should be done in the second trimester.[8] Surgical preparation can be done with beta-blockade and high-dose iodine, such as saturated solution of potassium iodide (SSKI).[4, 8] Additionally, cholestyramine can be administered to decrease enterohepatic circulation of TH, and systemic glucocorticoids help decrease T4-to-T3 conversion. In severe cases of hyperthyroidism and in the setting of agranulocytosis, plasmapheresis has been used effectively in pregnancy.[60, 61] Postoperatively, the mother would need to be treated with thyroid hormone replacement, as described elsewhere in this chapter. If the patient is TSHR Ab positive, ongoing treatment with ATDs may prevent fetal hyperthyroidism and could be used concomitant with thyroid hormone replacement (known as *block and replace*).[8] The block-and-replace approach to treatment is in fact only indicated in situations such as this—where there is clear clinical evidence for fetal hyperthyroidism requiring ATD, but the mother would be hypothyroid without use of medication for thyroid hormone replacement.[8]

19.7.3.4   *Monitoring of the Mother and Fetus*

Aside from the need for monitoring of thyroid function to allow for medication dose changes, as previously described, maternal monitoring includes checking TSH-receptor antibodies. These antibodies can cross the placental barrier and stimulate the fetal thyroid gland, leading to fetal thyrotoxicosis[7] and are positive in 95% of people with active GD.[8]

TSH-receptor antibodies should be ordered if a patient has untreated hyperthyroidism, ATD treated hyperthyroidism, prior GD treated with RAI or total thyroidectomy, a history of thyroidectomy for treatment of hyperthyroidism during pregnancy, or delivery of a baby with hyperthyroidism.[8] If a patient has previously been treated for GD with ATDs and is now euthyroid, checking TSH-receptor antibodies can be deferred.[8]

TSH-receptor antibodies should be measured in early pregnancy. If low, they do not need to be repeated.[4, 6] If elevated and the patient is still requiring ATD in the second trimester, then the test should be repeated at 18–22 weeks' gestation,[4, 6, 8] and then if still elevated or the patient is still on ATD, again at 30–34 weeks' gestation.[4, 8]

In early pregnancy, a TRAB level that is >5 IU/L, or three times the upper limit of the reference range, indicates that the pregnancy should be closely monitored.[8] In late pregnancy, a TRAB level that is >5 IU/L is associated with increased risk of neonatal hyperthyroidism.[8] In fact, a maternal TRAB at this level in the second or third trimester predicted neonatal hyperthyroidism with 100% sensitivity and 43% specificity,[4, 8] and also can give information about fetal thyroid size.[6] On the other hand, if the TRAB is low, there is increased possibility that ATD therapy will be able to be discontinued.[8]

Indications for further monitoring of the fetus with fetal ultrasound include elevated TSH-receptor antibodies and signs of fetal hyperthyroidism such as fetal tachycardia or uncontrolled maternal hyperthyroidism in the second half of pregnancy.[4, 8] A TSHR Ab level >5 IU/L, or three times the upper limit of the reference range, is an indication of fetal ultrasound.[8] Fetal ultrasound can be used to assess gestational age, fetal viability, and amniotic fluid volume, as well as identify fetal anatomy and malformations.[8] In the case of elevated TSHR Abs, ultrasound could be used to identify or confirm a sustained fetal heart rate >170, IUGR, fetal goiter, accelerated bone maturation, fetal congestive heart failure, or fetal hydrops.[4, 8] Serial evaluation of fetal growth starting in the latter half of pregnancy and third trimester antenatal testing are recommended.[4, 8, 58]

Rarely, umbilical blood sampling, also known as *cordocentesis*, is needed for fetal monitoring to determine fetal hyperthyroidism or hypothyroidism.[4, 8] Because it carries with it a 1%–2% risk of fetal demise, it should be avoided unless absolutely necessary.[4, 8] Fetal monitoring with maternal GD is covered in more detail in Chapter 43.

19.7.3.5 Complications of Maternal GD in the Mother and Fetus

Controlled GD and subclinical hyperthyroidism are not associated with adverse pregnancy outcomes.[34, 62] Uncontrolled hyperthyroidism, especially severe hyperthyroidism, carries risks for both mother and fetus (Table 19.4), including pregnancy loss, gestational hypertension, preeclampsia, thyroid storm (TS), prematurity, low birth weight, and fetal and neonatal thyroid disease[4, 8, 34, 57, 58]:

Fetal thyroid development is discussed in Chapter 32, while the fetal and neonatal consequences of maternal GD during pregnancy are discussed in Chapter 43. Fetuses and neonates born to mothers with GD are at risk for hyperthyroidism and both primary and secondary hypothyroidism.[8, 58] Fetal and neonatal hyperthyroidism is caused by passage of TSHR Abs across the placenta in the second half of pregnancy. Fetal hyperthyroidism complicates 1%–2% of pregnancies in patients with active or prior GD.[4, 8, 59] Primary fetal and neonatal hypothyroidism can be caused by either excessive ATDs or passage of TSH-receptor-blocking antibodies, while secondary (central) neonatal hypothyroidism is caused by poor control of the maternal hyperthyroidism.[4, 8]

If a fetal goiter is seen on ultrasound, further workup is required to determine if fetal hyperthyroidism or hypothyroidism is causing it. Fetal goiter can cause both fetal/neonatal and obstetric complications, including polyhydramnios, cervical dystocia, and mechanical obstruction of the airway, and may be an indication for cesarean section.[4]

19.7.3.6 Treatment and Monitoring of GD in the Postpartum Period and During Lactation

The risk of new GD and disease flare increases in the postpartum period.[3, 4, 8] In addition, patients with GD are at significant risk for destructive PPT. The differential diagnosis and management of GD and PPT is discussed later in this chapter. TSH-receptor antibodies can help distinguish the two entities. Elevated TSHR Abs indicate a diagnosis of GD. Additionally, elevated TSHR Abs in the euthyroid woman with a history of GD increase the possibility of disease relapse in the postpartum period.[4] Radiographic studies during lactation are limited, but can be useful in differentiating GD from PPT and are discussed in the post-partum thyroid disorders Section 19.8.

Monitoring of thyroid function should be continued through the postpartum period. The highest risk for developing recurrent disease is between 4 and 12 months after delivery.[4] TSH and Free T4 should be checked starting at 6 weeks postdelivery.[4] While hypothyroidism can impair lactation, it is unclear if hyperthyroidism has that effect, as there have been no human studies.[8]

TABLE 19.4 Maternal and fetal adverse outcomes due to Grave's Disease

Maternal adverse outcomes	Fetal and neonatal adverse outcomes
Pregnancy loss	Prematurity
Gestational hypertension	Low birth weight
Preeclampsia	Intrauterine growth restriction
Preterm delivery	Stillbirth
Congestive heart failure	Fetal and neonatal thyroid disease
Placental abruption	Fetal distress
Thyroid storm	Subsequent seizure disorders or neurobehavioral disorders

Treatment modalities in the postpartum period include medical management, RAI, and surgical thyroidectomy. Medical management with ATDs should be continued if required during pregnancy.[4] ATDs are generally safe to be continued during lactation, with low quantities transferred in breast milk.[4, 8, 55] Studies have not shown adverse effects in babies of mothers who continue on ATDs.[8] As in pregnancy, the lowest effective dose should be used; doses of MMI should be limited to <20 mg/day, split into two to three doses and given after a feed.[4] PTU should be limited to less than 300 mg/day total.[4, 55]

Radioactive iodine is concentrated in breast milk and is contraindicated in the postpartum lactation period.[8] For the nonbreastfeeding woman, treatment should not be given until 6 weeks to 3 months after the last occurrence of breast-feeding, and even so the woman would have to be sequestered from her baby for a prolonged period, making this an illogical and impractical choice for management.[8, 57] Many women who need RAI ablation will delay treatment until they have had the opportunity to breastfeed. RAI should be delayed by 6 weeks to 3 months following the last occurrence of breastfeeding, and an ^{123}I scan can be done prior to an ^{131}I scan to verify that there is not sustained uptake in the breasts.[63] Surgical management can also be considered.

19.7.3.7 Euthyroid Women with a History of Previously Treated GD

Pregnant women who have a prior history of GD still require additional monitoring. Women who entered a remission through treatment with ATD are at risk for disease flare during pregnancy and in the postpartum period. Thyroid function and thyroid autoantibodies must continue to be monitored.[8] Women who achieved a euthyroid state through RAI or surgery will still need to undergo screening for TSHR Abs because the autoimmune process leading to these antibodies may persist when residual thyroid tissue is present and cause fetal hyperthyroidism. Furthermore, these women require thyroid function monitoring, as described in Section 19.4, as their treatments have most likely rendered them on lifelong thyroid hormone replacement.

19.7.4 Gestational Transient Thyrotoxicosis

In most cases of gestational transient thyrotoxicosis (GTT), women remain asymptomatic with a mildly suppressed TSH and normal or very mild elevation of FT4 and FT3 levels. GTT with overt hyperthyroxinemia occurs in about 1%–2% of pregnancies, and often no medical intervention is needed for this self-limited form of hyperthyroidism. In this subset of patients, thyroxine levels are mildly elevated in the first trimester, mirroring rising hCG levels and normalizing by 18–20 weeks. In regions of low dietary intake, women may develop a significant goiter in pregnancy,[52, 64] whereas the thyroid enlarges only by about 10%–20% in iodine-sufficient areas.[52, 65]

Overt symptomatic gestational thyrotoxicosis most commonly occurs in women with multiple gestations or severe hyperemesis gravidarum.[66–68] Both clinical scenarios are typically associated with very elevated levels of hCG, often well over 100,000 IU/L.[68] Less frequently, molar pregnancy and invasive trophoblastic tumors are the cause of hyperthyroidism and severe decompensated gestational thyrotoxicosis.[69, 70] A very rare familial form of gestational hyperthyroidism, caused by a mutant hypersensitive TSH-receptor, has been reported in Belgium.[71]

19.7.5 Toxic Adenomas and Toxic Multinodular Goiters

TA and TMNGs are more common in women over 50 years old and are most prevalent in iodine-deficient regions; thus, they tend to be quite rare in pregnancy.[72] When complicating pregnancy, this nonautoimmune, autonomous form of hyperthyroidism can be associated with the production of high levels of T3. In larger nodular goiters, compressive symptoms may be present and can complicate the clinical course. For example, dysphagia may interfere with the medication intake for thyrotoxicosis. Other uncommon etiologies of hyperthyroidism in pregnancy are listed in Table 19.3.[51]

19.7.5.1 Treatment of Nonautoimmune Hyperthyroidism

Most forms of GTT require no intervention other than close observation with monitoring of thyroid functions as indicated. A normalizing trend of TSH and TH levels can be anticipated over the course of the later second trimester in the majority of women. In cases of severe hyperemesis gravidarum (>5% weight loss), associated with persistent hCG-mediated thyrotoxicosis, treatment with beta-adrenergic blockade (and, in selected cases, with ATD therapy) may be necessary.[73] In patients with trophoblastic disease, definitive surgical treatment will result in resolution of the thyrotoxicosis, although preparatory treatment with ATD and beta-adrenergic blockade may be needed in cases of severe thyrotoxicosis.[70]

Treatment of overt thyrotoxicosis due to TMNG and TA can be challenging if high doses of ATD are necessary throughout pregnancy. Unlike autoimmune hyperthyroidism, this autonomous form of thyrotoxicosis will not remit in pregnancy. Furthermore, there is concern that a sudden increase of iodine supply in pregnancy could lead to excessive stimulation of nonaffected thyroid tissue, resulting in worsening hyperthyroidism.[8] The maternal and fetal effect of increased iodine supply in pregnant patients with TMGN/TA has not been well studied. The ATA recommends a lower iodine intake in these patients.[8, 74] Prospective studies are needed to address this concern.

Upper-airway compression and dysphagia may also complicate maternal health and well-being. Thus women who require 10–15 mg of MMI or an equivalent dose of PTU in the late second trimester should be considered to have a partial or total thyroidectomy to decrease the risk for thionamide induced fetal hypothyroidism.[74] The recommended timing for prenatal surgery is the end of the second trimester,[74] although it can be undertaken in the early third trimester if persistent severe, uncontrolled hyperthyroidism poses a serious risk for adverse maternal or fetal outcomes, and so long as the surgery takes place in a high-risk obstetric setting that allows for close fetal/maternal monitoring and consultative care by an experienced interdisciplinary team. Surgical removal is the treatment of choice for large toxic goiters and adenomas and is best planned and undertaken before pregnancy. Therefore, women with a toxic goiter or adenoma should be counseled prior to conception about this important surgical intervention. Smaller toxic nodules may be amenable to radioiodine ablation, which would need to be completed 6 months prior to conception.

19.8 POSTPARTUM THYROID DYSFUNCTION

Keywords
- Postpartum thyroid dysfunction (PPTD)
- Postpartum thyroiditis (PPT)
- Postpartum depression (PPD)

19.8.1 Definition

The spectrum of thyroid dysfunction occurring in the first 12 months postpartum includes destructive thyroiditis, de novo and recurrent GD, and (rarely) hypothalamic–pituitary disease.[75] Although PPT is traditionally defined as thyroid dysfunction in in a woman with no history of thyroid disease prior to and during pregnancy, there is evidence based on retrospective cohort data, that preexisting treated autoimmune hypothyroidism is associated with a significant risk of PPT.[76] PPT can also occur after spontaneous miscarriage or therapeutic abortion.[77]

19.8.2 Epidemiology

The worldwide reported prevalence of PPTD is highly variable due to the heterogeneous designs of available studies.[77] Nicholson et al. systematically reviewed the published literature (1975–2004) and conducted a pooled analysis to estimate the prevalence of PPTD. They identified 21 articles (8081 subjects) and reported a pooled prevalence of PPTD of 8.1% in the general population. Global prevalence ranged from 4.4% in Asia to 5.7% in the United States. Women with type 1 diabetes had a prevalence of 19.6%.[78] The study concluded that 1 out of 12 women in the general population worldwide and 1 of 17 women in the United States are affected by PPTD. Women with positive TPO-Abs are 5.7 times more likely to develop PPTD.[78]

19.8.3 Screening for PPTD

Women at significantly increased risk for PPT include those with positive TPO Abs in the early first trimester and the presence of a positive TPO Ab predicts a 33%–50% risk of PPT.[77] Women with a history of type 1 diabetes and other autoimmune disease and women with chronic viral hepatitis carry a risk up to 25% for the development of PPT.[54, 77] Other known risk factors include a family history of thyroid disease, smoking, and the presence of a goiter. The Endocrine Society and experts in the field recommend screening for the presence of a TPO Ab in the first trimester in all women at high risk for PPTD, and to measure a TSH at 3, 6, and 9–12 months and annually in euthyroid TPO Ab-positive women, and in those with a prior history of PPTD.[54, 77, 79]

Women with a history of GD who were in remission during pregnancy carry a risk of recurrence in the later postpartum period and should have follow-up for clinical and biochemical evaluation at 6 weeks and 3–6 months postpartum, or else they should undergo blood testing as soon as suggestive symptoms develop. It is also noteworthy that new-onset GD very commonly presents in the postpartum period; thus, it is important to maintain a high index of suspicion when symptoms of hyperthyroidism occur 3–6 months after delivery.

19.8.4   Pathophysiology and Clinical Course of PPTD

PPT presents as a painless and destructive thyroiditis caused by an underlying autoimmune process. Unlike GD, which tends to present de novo after 3–6 months, PPT typically manifests itself in the early postpartum period, usually within the first 3 months (Fig. 19.1). A TPO Ab-negative form also has been described.[80] Permanent hypothyroidism at 12 months postpartum has been reported to range from 2%–21% of cases, and up to 50% within 5 years after the initial diagnosis of PPT.[79]

The pathophysiology of GD is described in detail in Section 19.7.3.

Four clinical patterns of PPT have been recognized since its early description by Robertson in 1948,[79,79a] (Fig. 19.1):

(1) A classic triphasic course, with initial destructive thyrotoxicosis at 1–3 months, followed by a transient hypothyroid phase at 6–7 months and euthyroidism by 9–12 months
(2) A biphasic form of initial hypothyroid phase at 3–7 months, followed by euthyroidism
(3) A biphasic form with initial destructive thyrotoxicosis at 1–4 months, followed by euthyroidism
(4) A monophasic form, with permanent hypothyroidism after initial hypothyroid phase

About 80% of women experience a transient hypothyroid phase that may or may not be associated with symptoms of hypothyroidism.[78] There is also an overlap between destructive thyrotoxicosis and GD, and women with a history of GD frequently also can develop PPT.

19.8.5   Differential Diagnosis and Evaluation of PPTD

The onset of symptoms and the clinical course, as discussed previously (importantly, the temporal relationship between the thyrotoxic phase of PPT and Grave's hyperthyroidism, as well as the findings upon physical exam), are most helpful when differentiating between the two conditions. GD will invariably be associated with detectable TRAB, while the majority of women with PPT will have a positive TPO Ab. The thyroid gland tends to be more enlarged in GD.

Ide et al. assessed 42 patients with newly developed postpartum thyrotoxicosis using a rapid third-generation TRAB assay in conjunction with ultrasound-measured thyroid blood flow[81] and found that the combination of a positive TRAB with a thyroid blood flow of >4.0% was indicative of postpartum GD. As shown in previous studies, the large majority of the patients developed PPT, with onset in the first 3 months, while patients with GD developed thyrotoxicosis at 6.5 months. All women with PPT were TRAB negative.[81]

Although further studies are needed, the use of thyroid color Doppler ultrasonography may present a good alternative to distinguish GD from destructive thyroiditis.[8] Radiopharmaceuticals are generally contraindicated in lactating women. If a thyroid scan is needed for the diagnosis of GD vs PPT, the recommended test of choice in the lactating mother would be a Tc-99m pertechnetate scan, with the requirement that the patient pump and discard breast milk following the study. The length of time to pump and discard milk is unclear, but it should be over 4h,[82] and many experts advise 24h. A [123]iodine

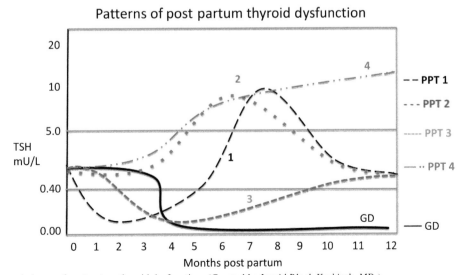

FIG. 19.1   Patterns and phases of postpartum thyroid dysfunction. *(Created by Ingrid Block-Kurbisch, MD.)*

scan is a less favorable alternative option, as its 8–13-h half-life necessitates pumping and discarding of breast milk for 3–5 days.[83] Also, [131]Iodine is absolutely contraindicated in breastfeeding women.[8].

19.8.6 Treatment of PPTD

Treatment for destructive thyroiditis is generally supportive. ATD treatment is not appropriate because there is no hyperfunction but rather hypofunction of the thyroid, which dumps stored hormone. In women who experience symptoms of thyrotoxicosis, beta-adrenergic blockade can be safely prescribed with propranolol or metoprolol in lactating women. Atenolol must be avoided, however, as it accumulates in breast milk and may affect the neonate with immature renal function.[84] Treatment of transient hypothyroidism is recommended in all symptomatic women and those whose TSH exceeds a level >10 mU/L.[74, 77] Discontinuation should be attempted at 12 months, although in women who plan to conceive, a TSH of <2.5 mU/L should be maintained and continuation of levothyroxine may be beneficial. Women should be counseled on their high risk for recurrent PPTD after the next pregnancy and that thyroiditis can also recur in response to other stressors.

19.8.7 Postpartum Depression and its Association with PPTD

The published literature on the possible causal relationship between PPT and PPD has been inconsistent. To date, there is no convincing evidence that PPTD is associated with a higher risk for PPD, nor did treatment of thyroid antibody-positive women with levothyroxine prevent the development of PPD.[85, 86] However, women who present with depression should have their thyroid function evaluated and be treated as appropriate if found to be hypothyroid.

19.8.7.1 Can PPTD be Prevented in Women with Positive TPO Abs?

Treatment with Levothyroxine or iodine during pregnancy has not been shown to decrease the incidence of PPT.[87, 88]

A reduction of the incidence of PPTD and hypothyroidism was suggested by a single, prospective, randomized, placebo-controlled study in which women with positive TPO-Abs were given 200 μg of selenium.[89] These results need further validation before a recommendation for routine supplementation can be endorsed.[8]

19.9 THYROID EMERGENCIES: THYROID STORM AND MYXEDEMA CRISIS

19.9.1 Overview

TS and myxedema coma represent the most extreme forms of decompensated hyperthyroidism and hypothyroidism, respectively. The pathogenesis remains to be fully understood, especially the exact mechanisms leading to thyrotoxic crisis. Both conditions are rare, but when present, they carry significant morbidity and mortality for mother and fetus. Because of the lack of prospective trials, available evidence for diagnostic tools and treatment relies on heterogeneous retrospective data and expert opinion.

This section provides a review of past and most current literature, lists causes known to precipitate these endocrine emergencies, and discusses diagnoses and treatments. The importance of early recognition of signs and symptoms of impending TS and severe myxedema, as well as the utility of both well established and newer diagnostic tools for TS that may help improve outcomes, will be highlighted.

19.9.2 Thyroid Storm

Key clinical findings
- Severe hyperthyroidism with known or unknown prior history
- Progressive weakness
- Agitation, restlessness
- Altered mentation
- Hyperthermia
- Hypertension
- Tachycardia
- Nausea, vomiting, abdominal pain
- Multiorgan decompensation

19.9.2.1 Thyroid Storm: Epidemiology, Precipitating Factors, and Clinical Outcomes

TS is estimated to complicate about 1% of all pregnancies with hyperthyroidism in the United States. GD accounts for the large majority of cases. Pregnancy itself carries a higher risk of TS than the nongestational state. Because TS is rare, its true incidence remains difficult to assess. In 2012, Akamizu et al. published results of their retrospective study, based on two nationwide reviews conducted between 2004 and 2008.[90] In this large case series, the 5-year incidence of TS was estimated to be 0.2 persons/100,000 Japanese/year, and about 0.22% of all thyrotoxic patients and 5.4% of all patients hospitalized with thyrotoxicosis.[90] In addition to epidemiologic data, the investigators evaluated diagnostic criteria, the prevalence of previously reported clinical manifestations,[91] mortality, and long-term outcomes of survivors of severe TS. The mortality rate was 10.9% in 282 patients with definite TS (grade 1 TS) and 9.9% in 74 patients with suspected TS (grade 2 TS). Multiple-organ failure and congestive heart failure were the most common causes of death. The landmark study of Akamizu et al. also brought attention to the irreversible long-term neurologic deficits observed in 9.9% of survivors of grade 1 TS and 3.3% of grade 2 TS.[92] Of the 282 patients with definite TS, 5 were pregnant with GD and had either untreated, uncontrolled thyrotoxicosis or TS prior to diagnosis of GD. Further, 1 patient was 4 months postpartum, and another presented with agranulocytosis and sepsis. These patients' Burch Wartofsky Severity Score (BWS), as defined and discussed next, ranged from 55 to 75, and they all recovered without complications.[90] The preceding discussion concerning the five pregnant patients includes unpublished data communicated to the senior author by Dr. Akamizu (personal correspondence in 2018).

Subsequently, a retrospective population-based cohort study of 4.2 million births in Canada conducted by Ngan et al. assessed the prevalence of TS and obstetrical and fetal outcomes, comparing women with and without TS in pregnancy between 2008 and 2012.[93] Using the Health Care Cost and Utilization Project–Nationwide Inpatient Sample database, this study identified 125 patients with TS that represented a prevalence of 2.97% per 1 million pregnancies. Patients with pre-existing hypertension, anemia of pregnancy, urinary tract infections, and pneumonia were more likely to develop TS. Table 19.5 details the precipitating factors for TS in pregnancy. In this study, black maternal race was associated with higher risk for TS, although the authors did not elaborate on possible reasons for this.

Maternal complications in the group with TS included congestive heart failure in 8.8% in patients without TS and respiratory failure requiring mechanical ventilation in 8% of patients, both of which are significantly higher than women without TS (Table 19.6). There were 9 cases of postpartum TS. No maternal death was reported in this study, which may reflect advances in perinatal and critical care management in recent years, and possibly less stringent inclusion criteria. Also, 44.8% of cases with TS were associated with the possible diagnosis of GD, which is significantly lower than previously reported. However, that also may reflect the difficulty of making a retrospective diagnosis.

Fetal outcomes included an increased risk of preterm birth and stillbirth (Table 19.7).

19.9.2.2 Pathogenesis and Clinical Presentation

TS presents as a constellation of symptoms and findings. Its onset tends to be abrupt, although signs of impending storm may precede the decompensated state. While the exact pathophysiologic mechanisms leading to TS remain incompletely understood, it is universally recognized that a superimposed severe physical or emotional event triggers the accelerated deterioration from a compensated thyrotoxic state to TS. In about 70% of patients, a precipitating event is discovered.[90] Of note, levels of FT4 and FT3 have not consistently been found to be higher than in patients with compensated

TABLE 19.5 Precipitating factors for thyroid storm in pregnancy

Undiagnosed or partly treated thyrotoxicosis
Infection
Diabetic ketoacidosis
Anemia of pregnancy
Pregestational hypertension
Congestive heart failure
Pulmonary embolism
Gestational trophoblastic disease
Hyperemesis gravidarum
Preeclampsia
Parturition or induction of labor
Emergent surgery and trauma
Psychosis or emotional stress

hyperthyroidism.[90, 91, 94] In fact, FT3 and even FT4 levels may be normal or low, reflecting the severity of an associated nonthyroidal illness. While studies have not demonstrated increased secretion of catecholamines,[95, 96] upregulated, tissue-specific beta-adrenergic receptors or modified postreceptor signaling pathways have been described.[91, 97, 98]

19.9.2.3 Maternal Signs and Symptoms Concerning for Impending or Established TS

- Fever with temp ≥38 °C
- CNS: agitation, restlessness, delirium, extreme lethargy, seizures, and coma
- Cardiovascular: tachycardia >130 bpm out of proportion to fever, congestive heart failure, atrial fibrillation, and pulmonary edema
- Gastrointestinal/hepatic: nausea, vomiting and abdominal pain, and unexplained jaundice with serum bilirubin >3 mg/dL

TABLE 19.6 Maternal complications in patients with thyroid storm in pregnancy, 2008–2012

Maternal complications[a]	Thyroid storm n = 125(%)	No thyroid storm n = 4,206,814 (%)	aOR (95% CI)	P-value
Hyperemesis gravidarum	15 (12.0)	38,935 (0.9)	11.71 (6.65–20.62.77)	<0.001
Mild preeclampsia	4 (3.2)	95,858 (2.3)	1.76 (0.53–5.81)	0.352
Severe preeclampsia	7 (5.6)	57,511 (1.4)	4.53 (1.90–10.82)	0.001
Abruptio placentae	5 (4.0)	45,061 (1.1)	3.14 (1.23–7.90)	0.016
PPROM	4 (3.2)	202,251 (4.8)	0.75 (0.27–2.41)	0.148
Labor induction	11 (8.8)	796,079 (18.9)	0.93 (0.89–0.99)	0.020
Cesarian section	28 (22.4)	1.306,081 (31.0)	0.55 (0.35–0.86)	0.009
Blood products transfusion	12 (9.6)	47,186 (1.1)	3.20 (1.51–2.71)	0.002
Elevated transaminases	2 (1.6)	3471 (0.1)	4.45 (1.02–19.60)	0.046
Acute kidney injury	3 (2.4)	2452 (0.1)	0.81 (0.19–3.32)	0.768
Cardiomyopathy	7 (5.6)	3679 (0.1)	1.03 (0.29–3.56)	0.961
Atrial fibrillation/flutter	5 (4.0)	1489 (0.04)	21.53 (7.14–64.95)	<0.0001
Congestive heart failure	11 (8.8)	3044 (0.03)	19.00 (6.14–58.82)	<0.0001
Mechanical ventilation	10 (8.0)	3.940 (0.12)	16.41 (6.55–41.11)	<0.0001
Post-partum Depression	3 (2.4)	6.247 (0.15)	11.19 (3.44–36.40)	<0.0001

[a]No cases of postpartum hemorrhage, deep vein thrombosis, cardiac arrest, or maternal death were identified.
(Adapted with permission from Ngan TYT, Faden M, El-Messidi, Brown R. Maternal and obstetric outcomes among women with TS in pregnancy: A population-based study of 4.2 million births. Am J Obstet Gynecol 2017;**216**(1):S460-S1, supplement to January 2017.)

TABLE 19.7 Fetal complications in patients with thyroid storm in pregnancy, 2008–2012

Fetal complications	Thyroid storm n = 125(%)	No thyroid storm n = 4,206,814 (%)	aOR (95% CI)	P-value
Preterm birth	7 (5.6)	283,926 (6.7)	5.26 (1.90–14.25)	0.001
Fetal growth restriction	3 (2.4)	93,127 (2.2)	1.01 (0.32–3.31)	0.981
Fetal anomalies	3 (2.4)	33,030 (0.8)	2.68 (0.84–8.56)	0.096
Stillbirth	3 (2.4)	24,641 (0.6)	3.75 (1.17–11.93)	0.025

(Adapted with permission from Ngan TYT, Faden M, El-Messidi, Brown R. Maternal and obstetric outcomes among women with TS in pregnancy: A population-based study of 4.2 million births. Am J Obstet Gynecol 2017;**216**(1):S460-S1, supplement to January 2017.)

- Psychiatric: anxiety, psychosis, and delirium
- Biochemical evidence of current or recent history of hyperthyroidism

19.9.2.4 Fetal Findings

- Tachycardia >180 bpm
- Fetal acidosis
- Changes in heart tracing, including late decelerations

If not treated aggressively, decompensated thyrotoxicosis with maternal multiorgan failure ensues. CNS dysfunction has been shown to be a key element of TS that portends a poor prognosis and should draw immediate clinical attention.[99, 100]

19.9.2.5 Diagnosis

The diagnosis of TS rests primarily on clinical judgment. Rapid diagnosis and timely aggressive multisystemic treatment of impending or fully established TS remains critical for maternal and fetal outcomes; therefore, maintaining a high clinical index of suspicion is most important. In pregnancy, clinical conditions that may mimic some manifestations of TS include toxemia, preeclampsia, and sepsis. Severe thyrotoxicosis or TS presenting in a patient without known prior history of hyperthyroidism in the first trimester should prompt an evaluation for gestational trophoblastic disease. Here, hCG levels will typically be disproportionally elevated, and levels may be extremely high.

Supporting diagnostic criteria, using a clinical scoring system, and more recently, a combination of similar categorical diagnostic criteria have been recommended to improve the positive and negative predictability of definitive TS vs compensated thyrotoxicosis.[90, 91, 99] Burch and Wartofsky introduced a semiquantitative scoring system (BWS; Table 19.8) in their landmark study in 1993[91]: a summative score defined by the presence and severity of five clinical manifestations (thermoregulatory, CNS, gastrointestinal/hepatic, cardiovascular dysfunction, and the presence or absence of a precipitating event) is applied as a predictor of the likelihood of TS or impending storm (Table 19.8). This scoring system has been widely used. Akamizu et al. proposed their own diagnostic criteria in 2012, which have been endorsed by the Japan Thyroid Association and are based on the results of two retrospective nationwide reviews, in which they assessed and validated combinations of similar clinical categories, correlating the BWS with thyrotoxicosis, suspected TS, and definite storm[90]. Although the BWS and the diagnostic criteria of Akamizu et al. assist in the diagnosis or exclusion of TS, their sensitivity and specificity will need further validation in prospective trials, and sound clinical judgment must continue to guide the decision to treat a patient for TS.[74]

19.9.2.6 Treatment

Effective treatment of TS is best achieved in an obstetric intensive care setting, allowing close maternal and fetal monitoring and providing care with a multispecialty team approach (Table 19.9). Depending on the patient's presentation and associated complications, the team should consist of a critical care and fetal maternal medicine specialist, an endocrinologist as well as other consultants needed to ensure stabilization of the mother prior to delivery. .

Treatment includes immediate administration of a high-loading dose of PTU to block synthesis and decrease release of thyroid hormone. PTU is the drug of choice, as it additionally decreases T4-to-T3 conversion and has been shown to lower T3 levels more effectively in the first 24 h compared to MMI.[101] Further, 1 h after PTU or MMI, potassium iodide is given to help block hormone synthesis and release. Beta-adrenergic blockade, to protect the patient from the peripheral effect of thyroid hormone, is achieved with propranolol orally or intravenously, which in high doses also decreases T4-to-T3 conversion and is the preferred drug in pregnancy. In the setting of severe congestive heart failure, intravenous esmolol administration is preferred. In patients with contraindication to beta-adrenergic antagonists, diltiazem can be substituted. Cholestyramine is useful as an adjunctive agent and enhances elimination of thyroid hormone by inhibiting its enterohepatic circulation. Glucocorticoids decrease T4-to-T3 conversion and add support in the setting of a stressful illness that may be associated with a high turnover of endogenous cortisol.[102]

Supportive therapy includes replacement of fluid loss in the setting of hyperthermia, antipyretic treatment with acetaminophen, and the cautious use of a cooling blanket to allow continued release of heat, while lowering core temperature. Aspirin must be avoided, as it displaces T4/T3 from thyroid-binding globulin, thereby worsening the thyrotoxicosis. Treatment directed at the underlying precipitating cause is important. If infection is suspected, broad coverage with antibiotic agents is initiated after blood and urine cultures are obtained. Phenobarbital can be administered for extreme agitation or restlessness. Management of multiple organ failure often requires treatment for congestive heart failure, respiratory failure, acute kidney injury, hepatic insufficiency, and coma. Obstetric complications such as preeclampsia, toxemia,

TABLE 19.8 Presence and severity of the most common signs and symptoms

Criteria	Score
Thermoregulatory dysfunction	
Temperature 37–37.7 °C	5
Temperature 37.8–38.2 °C	10
Temperature 38.3–38.8 °C	15
Temperature 38.9–39.3 °C	20
Temperature 39.4–39.9 °C	25
Temperature 40 °C or higher	30
Central nervous system effects	
Absent	0
Mild (agitation)	10
Moderate (delirium, psychosis, extreme lethargy)	20
Severe (seizure or coma)	30
Gastrointestinal and hepatic dysfunction	
Absent	0
Moderate (diarrhea, nausea, vomiting, abdominal pain)	10
Severe (unexplained jaundice)	20
Cardiovascular dysfunction (heart rate, beats/min)	
90–109	5
110–119	10
120–129	15
130–139	20
≥140	25
Congestive heart failure	
Absent	0
Mild (edema)	5
Moderate (bibasilar crackles)	10
Severe (pulmonary edema)	15
Atrial fibrillation	
Absent	0
Present	5
10	10
History of precipitating event	
Absent	0
Present	10

Based on the total score, the likelihood of the diagnosis of thyrotoxic storm is as follows: unlikely, <25; impending, 25–44; highly likely, >45.
(Adapted with permission from Burch HB, Wartofsky L. Life threatening thyrotoxicosis. Thyroid storm. *Endocrinol Metab Clin North Am* 1993;**22**:263–277.)

TABLE 19.9 Principles of treatment for TS

1. Reduction and blockage of T4/T3 synthesis with antithyroid drug therapy
   - *PTU* 600–800 mg loading dose, PO or via NGT, then 150–250 mg every 4–6 h (if needed, can be given in form of rectal enema) or
   - *MMI*: 60–80 mg PO daily or via NGT (available in IV form in Europe)
   - *Iodine* 1 h after PTU or MMI:
   Lugols 8–10 gtts every 8 h PO or
   Saturated solution of potassium iodide (SSKI) 2–5 gtt PO every 6 h in patients with contraindication to thionamides (agranulocytosis or hepatocellular injury) or if rapid preoperative reduction of T4/T3 is indicated

2. Block action of T4/T3 in the peripheral tissues
   - Propranolol 60–80 mg PO every 4–6 h, or 1–2 mg IV q 5 min, up to 6 mg, then 1–10 mg IV q 4 h or
   - Esmolol 0.25–0.5 mg/kg loading dose, 0.05–0.1 mg/kg/min IV continuous
   - Diltiazem q 6–8 h PO if patient is intolerant to propranolol

3. Decrease conversion of T4–T3
   - Propranolol (see above)
   - PTU (see above)
   - Dexamethasone 2 mg IV or IM every 6 h for 4 doses or
   - Hydrocortisone 100 mg IV every 8 h

4. Decrease enterohepatic circulation of thyroid hormone
   - Cholestyramine resin: 4 g every 6 h to enhance elimination of T4/T3

5. Supportive measures:
   - Fluid resuscitation and electrolyte management
   - Antipyretic acetaminophen and cooling
   - Avoid aspirin, as it displaces T4/T3 from thyroid-binding globulin
   - Phenobarbital 30–60 mg PO every 6–8 h as needed for extreme restlessness
   - Antiemetics as needed
   - Antiseizure therapy as needed
   - Reserpine 1–5 mg IM every 4–6 h for severe bronchospasm
   - Respiratory support, including mechanical ventilation if indicated
   - Initiate maternal and fetal monitoring

6. Evaluation and treatment of precipitating cause
   - Blood, urine, and sputum cultures
   - Empiric broad coverage antibiotics if infection is suspected

7. Treat multiple organ failure and obstetric complications

8. Plasmapheresis in selected patients

and preterm, premature rupture of the membranes pose a great clinical challenge and need careful weighing of the risk of early delivery against the risk of progressive maternal decompensation. Plasmapheresis and therapeutic plasma exchange have been used successfully and preoperatively in those patients with thionamide-induced agranulocytosis.[60, 61] This method allows for reduction of T4 and T3 levels within 36 h, but it only temporizes definitive treatment, as its effect lasts for 1–2 days.

In summary, TS is a rare endocrine emergency that requires rapid recognition and treatment, using a multidisciplinary approach in an intensive care setting.

19.9.3 Myxedema Crisis/Coma

Key clinical signs of myxedema crisis/coma include
- Lethargy and hypersomnolence
- Altered mentation, delirium, psychosis, and coma
- Hypothermia (temp <36 °C)
- Bradycardia and increased Q-T interval
- Generalized edema, pleural/pericardial effusions, and ascites
- Hypoventilation and respiratory acidosis

- Circulatory failure
- Anemia, hyponatremia, and hypoglycemia
- Multiorgan failure

19.9.3.1 Epidemiology, Pathogenesis, Precipitating Factors, and Clinical Course

Myxedema coma is an extremely rare complication in pregnancy, as overt hypothyroidism is a major cause of infertility. While the true incidence remains unknown, it has been reported to occur in the general population at a rate of 0.22 per million per year in one European study.[103] A literature review by Echt and Doss identified 29 cases of myxedema crisis (MC) in pregnancy between 1897 and 1963, including their own 3 patients. An additional seven reports were found from 1963 to 2001 by Turhan et al., including their own case.[104, 105] In 2016, Singh et al. published a case of myxedema in labor.[106]

Causes of the underlying hypothyroidism may include lack of prenatal care, self-discontinuation of LT4, or interference with oral hormone absorption, as well as undiagnosed primary or (much less often) secondary hypothyroidism in pregnancy (Table 19.10). Most major organizations recommend risk-based screening for hypothyroidism because overt untreated hypothyroidism tends to be uncommon. However, lack of access to prenatal care and low health literacy may increase the risk for severe undiagnosed hypothyroidism in vulnerable and underserved populations.[107]

MC represents the most severe decompensation of hypothyroidism. Its etiology and pathogenesis remain unclear, although a precipitating event is identified in many cases. Thyroid function tests will be abnormal, but levels of TSH, FT4, and FT3 do not always correlate well with the severity of illness. The term *myxedema coma* is misleading because patients may initially exhibit mild alteration in alertness and mentation, leading to a potential underrecognition of this serious endocrine emergency. Therefore, using the term *MC* has been proposed as more appropriate.[108]

In pregnancy, MC may present as a preeclampsialike picture, with symptoms and clinical findings such as hypertension, proteinuria, and encephalopathy mimicking this condition.[109] Fatigue and weight gain are common but nonspecific complaints in pregnancy. However, a high index of suspicion must be maintained in patients who present with some of the cardinal symptoms of severe progressive hypothyroidism. Changes in alertness and mood, increased sensitivity to cold, hypothermia, bradycardia, hypoventilation, generalized edema, and effusions should raise the concern for MC in patients with preexisting and uncontrolled hypothyroidism, or prompt an immediate evaluation in patients with no prior known history of thyroid disease. Hyponatremia due to impaired water clearance, hypoglycemia, acidosis, and anemia are commonly present. If untreated, progression to severe hypoventilation with carbon dioxide retention, hypothermia and cardiac arrhythmias, hypotension, and MC with multiorgan failure and coma will follow. Bleeding in the setting of a coagulopathy due to acquired van Willebrand syndrome (type 1), as well as disseminated intravascular coagulation (DIC) in septic patients, may further complicate the clinical course.[102]

Common precipitating factors include sepsis due to urinary or respiratory infection, preeclampsia, labor, surgery, exposure to cold temperature, and drugs, including codeine, sedatives, anesthetics, and lithium.[102] Medications commonly used in pregnancy that decrease absorption of LT4, such as ferrous sulfate and calcium supplements, also must be considered.

19.9.3.2 Diagnosis MC in Pregnancy

The diagnosis of MC in pregnancy is primarily based on clinical judgment, although diagnostic tools developed in a non-pregnant population also may help increase awareness and accuracy.[110] Advances in critical care management and results of studies of MC in nonpregnant populations, using GSC, APACHE II, and SOFA scores to predict severity and outcomes, may be effective in lowering maternal and fetal mortality of MC.[103, 111, 112] Prospective studies that include pregnant women are needed to validate these diagnostic and prediction tools. Management should take place in a critical care unit, using a multimodal and multidisciplinary approach similar to the treatment of TS. Collaboration between the fetal maternal medicine specialist, endocrinologist, and critical care specialist is critical, with additional consultations as needed from the infectious disease to other subspecialists.

19.9.3.3 Treatment

The treatment of MC must include the following:

(1) Supportive measures that address
   - Hypoventilation and airway protection in severely altered or comatose patients with mechanical ventilation.
   - Bleeding due to DIC or acquired coagulopathy.

TABLE 19.10 Causes of severe hypothyroidism

Primary thyroid failure (untreated or partially treated)

- Autoimmune hypothyroidism
- Postsurgical hypothyroidism
- Postablative hypothyroidism
- Iodine deficiency
- Thyroid agenesis
- Thyroid hormone resistance syndrome

Secondary thyroid failure

- Hypothalamic
- Pituitary
  - Infiltrative disease
  - Hemochromatosis, sarcoid, lymphoma, histiocytosis
  - Infection (TB, syphilis)
  - Macroadenoma
  - Lymphocytic hypophysitis
  - Malignancy (metastatic)

Decreased absorption of thyroid hormone

- Calcium supplements
- Ferrous sulfate
- Cholestyramine
- Sucralfate
- Aluminum hydroxide
- Proton pump inhibitors
- Soy products (including tube feeding)
- Postbariatric status
- Untreated celiac disease

- Hypothermia: Treatment with thyroid hormone to passively restore normal temperature in addition to using higher room temperature and blankets. Active warming can result in rapid vasodilation, hypotension, and shock and should be avoided. A normalizing trend should be expected within 36–48h.
- Multiorgan failure: address as appropriate.

(2) Replacement therapy:

LT4, starting with a loading dose of 250–300 mcg IV, followed by an initial maintenance dose of 50–100 mcg/day. If IV LT4 is not available, it can be administered via nasogastric tube, although absorption due to ileus and poor gastric motility may be less predictable. No prospective studies in pregnancy are available to validate the replacement doses used in pregnancy. A prospective study by Rodríguez et al. [103] compared LT4 500 mcg, followed by 100 mcg/day with patients who received a dose of 100 mcg/day LT4 without a high-loading dose. In this trial, which did not include pregnant women, mortality was lower in patients who received the high-loading dose of LT4 (16.7%) compared with those on a maintenance dose only (60%), although the difference was not statistically significant. Patients were significantly older (68 + − 19.5 years), and 10 out of 11 patients were female. Adding T3 intravenously has been recommended by some authors,[107] but this has not been endorsed by the ATA.[113] Further prospective studies are needed.

(3) Glucocorticoids: hydrocortisone 50–100 mg IV every 6–8h to all patients where the etiology of hypothyroidism is unknown. In the case of secondary hypothyroidism, or if there is concern about coexisting primary adrenal insufficiency, glucocorticoids should be administered prior to LT4 as turnover of cortisol increases with LT4 administration.

(4) Treat precipitating causes: sepsis, preeclampsia, labor, DKA, bleeding, or other.

(5) Hyponatremia, if severe and associated with seizures, should be cautiously treated with 3% sodium chloride until serum sodium is >120. Increase in serum sodium should be achieved per guidelines for treatment of severe symptomatic hyponatremia and with input from the fetal-maternal medicine specialist.

(6) Close fetal monitoring and careful timing of delivery after maternal stabilization is important.

In summary, MC is a very rare complication encountered in pregnancy. Its presentation deviates from that outside of pregnancy, in that it may mimic preeclampsia due to overlapping symptoms. A preexisting history of thyroid disease, hypothermia, bradycardia, generalized edema, and decreased mentation must raise the suspicion for MC and should prompt immediate evaluation and treatment in a critical care setting, using a multidisciplinary approach.

REFERENCES

1. Esfandiari NH, Papaleontiou M. Biochemical testing in thyroid disorders. *Endocrinol Metab Clin North Am* 2017;**46**(3):631–48.
2. Czarnocka B, Eschler DC, Godlewska M, Tomer Y. *Thyroid autoantibodies: thyroid peroxidase and thyroglobulin antibodies*. 3rd ed., Elsevier; 2013.
3. Fröhlich E, Wahl R. Thyroid autoimmunity: role of anti-thyroid antibodies in thyroid and extra-thyroidal diseases. *Front Immunol* 2017;**8**:521 May 9.
4. Nguyen CT, Sasso EB, Barton L, Mestman JH. Graves' hyperthyroidism in pregnancy: a clinical review. *Clin Diabetes Endocrinol* 2018;**4**:4.
5. Tozzoli R, Bagnasco M, Thyrotropin VD. *Receptor antibodies*. 3rd ed., Elsevier; 2013.
6. Winter WE, Jialal I, Devaraj S. Thyrotropin receptor antibody assays clinical utility. *Am J Clin Pathol* 2013;**139**(2):140–2.
7. Barbesino G, Tomer Y. Clinical Utility of TSH Receptor Antibodies. *J Clin Endocrinol Metabol* 2013;**98**(6):2247–55.
8. Alexander EK, Pearce EN, Brent GA, Brown RS, Chen H, Dosiou C, et al. 2017 Guidelines of the American Thyroid Association for the Diagnosis and Management of Thyroid Disease During Pregnancy and the Postpartum. *Thyroid* 2017;**27**(3):315–89.
9. Negro R. Re-thinking the definitions of subclinical thyroid disease in pregnancy. *J Endocrinol Invest* 2011;**34**(8):620–2.
10. Benhadi N, Wiersinga WM, Reitsma JB, Vrijkotte TGM, Bonsel GJ. Higher maternal TSH levels in pregnancy are associated with increased risk for miscarriage, fetal or neonatal death. *Eur J Endocrinol* 2009;**160**(6):985–91.
11. Glinoer D. What happens to the normal thyroid during pregnancy? *Thyroid* 1999;**9**(7):631–5.
12. Allan WC, Haddow JE, Palomaki GE, Williams JR, Mitchell ML. Maternal thyroid deficiency and pregnancy complications: implications for population screening. *J Med Screen* 2000;**7**(3):127–30.
13. Klein RZ, Haddow JE, Faix JD, Brown RS, Hermos RJ, Pulkkinen A, et al. Prevalence of thyroid deficiency in pregnant women. *Clin Endocrinol (Oxf)* 1991;**35**(1):41–6.
14. Cleary-Goldman J, Malone FD, Lambert-Messerlian G, Sullivan L, Canick J, Porter TF, et al. Maternal thyroid hypofunction and pregnancy outcome. *Obstet Gynecol* 2008;**112**(1):85–92.
15. Korevaar TIM, Schalekamp-Timmermans S, de Rijke YB, Visser WE, Visser W, de Muinck Keizer-Schrama SMPF. Hypothyroxinemia and TPO-antibody positivity are risk factors for premature delivery: the generation R study. *J Clin Endocrinol Metab* 2013;**98**(11):4382–90.
16. Blatt AJ, Nakamoto JM, Kaufman HW. National status of testing for hypothyroidism during pregnancy and postpartum. *J Clin Endocrinol Metab* 2012;**97**(3):777–84.
17. Oppenheimer JH, Schwartz HL. Molecular basis of thyroid hormone-dependent brain development. *Endocr Rev* 1997;**18**(4):462–75.
18. LaFranchi SH, Haddow JE, Hollowell JG. Is thyroid inadequacy during gestation a risk factor for adverse pregnancy and developmental outcomes? *Thyroid* 2005;**15**(1):60–71.
19. Ord WM. Report of a committee of the Clinical Society of London nominated December, to investigate the subject of myxedema. Transactions of the Clinical Society of London. *SRC—BaiduScholar* 1888;**14**:1–215.
20. Haddow JE, Palomaki GE, Allan WC, Williams JR, Knight GJ, Gagnon J, et al. Maternal thyroid deficiency during pregnancy and subsequent neuropsychological development of the child. *N Engl J Med* 1999;**341**(8):549–55.
21. Pop VJ, Kuijpens JL, van Baar AL, Verkerk G, van Son MM, de Vijlder JJ, et al. Low maternal free thyroxine concentrations during early pregnancy are associated with impaired psychomotor development in infancy. *Clin Endocrinol (Oxf)* 1999;**50**(2):149–55.
22. Henrichs J, Bongers-Schokking J, Schenk J, Ghassabian A, Schmidt HG, Visser TJ, et al. Maternal thyroid function during early pregnancy and cognitive functioning in early childhood: The generation R study. *J Clin Endocrinol Metab* 2010;**95**:4227–34.
23. Nelson S, Haig C, McConnachie A, Sattar N, Ring S, Smith G, et al. Maternal thyroid function and child educational attainment: prospective cohort study. *BMJ* 2018;**20**:360.
24. Liu H, Shan Z, Li C, Mao J, Xie X, Wang W, et al. Maternal subclinical hypothyroidism, thyroid autoimmunity, and the risk of miscarriage: a prospective cohort study. *Thyroid* 2014;**24**(11):1642–9.
25. Negro R, Schwartz A, Gismondi R, Tinelli A, Mangieri T, Stagnaro-Green A. Increased pregnancy loss rate in thyroid antibody negative women with TSH levels between 2.5 and 5.0 in the first trimester of pregnancy. *J Clin Endocrinol Metab* 2010;**95**(9):E44–8.
26. Maraka S, Ospina NMS, O'Keeffe DT, Espinosa De Ycaza AE, Gionfriddo MR, Erwin PJ, et al. Subclinical hypothyroidism in pregnancy: a systematic review and meta-analysis. *Thyroid* 2016;**26**(4):580–90.
27. Glinoer D, Riahi M, Grün JP, Kinthaert J. Risk of subclinical hypothyroidism in pregnant women with asymptomatic autoimmune thyroid disorders. *J Clin Endocrinol Metab* 1994;**79**(1):197–204.
28. Chen L, Hu R. Thyroid autoimmunity and miscarriage: a meta-analysis. *Clin Endocrinol (Oxf)* 2011;**74**(4):513–9.
29. Thangaratinam S, Tan A, Knox E, Kilby MD, Franklyn J, Coomarasamy A. Association between thyroid autoantibodies and miscarriage and preterm birth: meta-analysis of evidence. *BMJ* 2011;**342**:d2616.
30. He X, Wang P, Wang Z, Xu D, Wang B. Thyroid antibodies and risk of preterm delivery: a meta-analysis of prospective cohort studies. *Eur J Endocrinol* 2012;**167**(4):455–64.

31. Mannisto T, Vaarasmaki M, Pouta A, Hartikainen AL, Roukonen A, Surcel HM, et al. Perinatal outcome of children born to mothers with thyroid dysfunction or antibodies: a prospective population-based cohort study. *J Clin Endocrinol Metab* 2009;**94**:772–9.

32. Abbassi-Ghanavati M, Casey BM, Spong CY, McIntire DD, Halvorson LM, Cunningham FG. Pregnancy outcomes in women with thyroid peroxidase antibodies. *Obstet Gynecol* 2010;**116**(2 Pt 1):381–6.

33. Stuebe AM, Meltzer-Brody S, Pearson B, Pedersen C, Grewen K. Maternal neuroendocrine serum levels in exclusively breastfeeding mothers. *Breastfeed Med* 2015;**10**(4):197–202.

34. Lazarus J. CGDK DGL, et al. editors. *Thyroid regulation and dysfunction in the pregnant patient.* EndoText: South Dartmouth, MA; 2016.

35. Negro R, Stagnaro-Green A. Clinical aspects of hyperthyroidism, hypothyroidism, and thyroid screening in pregnancy. *Endocr Pract* 2014;**20** (6):597–607.

36. Kroopnick JM, Kim CS. Overview of hypothyroidism in pregnancy. *Semin Reprod Med* 2016;**34**(6):323–30.

37. Abalovich M, Vázquez A, Alcaraz G, Kitaigrodsky A, Szuman G, Calabrese C, et al. Adequate levothyroxine doses for the treatment of hypothyroidism newly discovered during pregnancy. *Thyroid* 2013;**23**(11):1479–83.

38. Abalovich M, Amino N, Barbour LA, Cobin RH, De Groot LJ, Glinoer D, et al. Management of thyroid dysfunction during pregnancy and postpartum: an Endocrine Society Clinical Practice Guideline. *J Clin Endocrinol Metab* 2007;**92**(8 Suppl):S1–47.

39. Korevaar TIM, Medici M, Visser TJ, Peeters RP. Thyroid disease in pregnancy: new insights in diagnosis and clinical management. *Nat Rev Endocrinol* 2017;**13**(10):610–22.

40. Okosieme OE, Khan I, Taylor PN. Preconception management of thyroid dysfunction. *Clin Endocrinol (Oxf)* 2018;(February):0–3.

41. Refetoff S, DeWind LT, DeGroot LJ. Familial syndrome combining deaf-mutism, stuppled epiphyses, goiter and abnormally high PBI: possible target organ refractoriness to thyroid hormone. *J Clin Endocrinol Metab* 1967;**27**(2):279–94.

42. Refetoff S, Dumitrescu AM. Syndromes of reduced sensitivity to thyroid hormone: genetic defects in hormone receptors, cell transporters and deiodination. *Best Pract Res Clin Endocrinol Metab* 2007;**21**(2):277–305.

43. LaFranchi SH, Snyder DB, Sesser DE, Skeels MR, Singh N, Brent GA, et al. Follow-up of newborns with elevated screening T4 concentrations. *J Pediatr* 2003;**143**(3):296–301.

44. Dumitrescu AM, Cosmo CD, Liao X-H, Weiss RE, Refetoff S. The syndrome of inherited partial SBP2 deficiency in humans. *Antioxid Redox Signal* 2010;**12**(7):905–20.

45. Refetoff S, Weiss RE, Usala SJ. The syndromes of resistance to thyroid hormone. *Endocr Rev* 1993;**14**(3):348–99.

46. Beck-Peccoz P, Chatterjee VK. The variable clinical phenotype in thyroid hormone resistance syndrome. *Thyroid* 1994;**4**(2):225–32.

47. Brucker-Davis F, Skarulis MC, Grace MB, Benichou J, Hauser P, Wiggs E, et al. Genetic and clinical features of 42 kindreds with resistance to thyroid hormone. The National Institutes of Health Prospective Study. *Ann Intern Med* 1995;**123**(8):572–83.

48. Anselmo J, Cao D, Karrison T, Weiss RE, Refetoff S. Fetal loss associated with excess thyroid hormone exposure. *JAMA* 2004;**292**(6):691–5.

49. Srichomkwun P, Anselmo J, Liao X-H, Hönes GS, Moeller LC, Alonso-Sampedro M, et al. Fetal exposure to high maternal thyroid hormone levels causes central resistance to thyroid hormone in adult humans and mice. *J Clin Endocrinol Metabol* 2017;**102**(9):3234–40.

50. Weiss RE, Refetoff S, Characteristic H. Editorial: treatment of resistance to thyroid hormone—primum non nocere. *J Clin Endocrinol Metabol* 1999;**84**(2):401–4.

51. Cooper DS, Laurberg P. Hyperthyroidism in pregnancy. *Lancet Diabetes Endocrinol* 2013;**1**(3):238–49.

52. Glinoer D. The regulation of thyroid function during normal pregnancy: Importance of the iodine nutrition status. *Best Pract Res Clin Endocrinol Metab* 2004;**18**(2):133–52.

53. Laurberg P, Cerqueira C, Ovesen L, Rasmussen LB, Perrild H, Andersen S, et al. Iodine intake as a determinant of thyroid disorders in populations. *Best Pract Res Clin Endocrinol Metab* 2010;**24**(1):13–27.

54. De Groot L, Abalovich M, Alexander EK, Amino N, Barbour L, Cobin RH, et al. Management of thyroid dysfunction during pregnancy and postpartum: an Endocrine Society clinical practice guideline. *J Clin Endocrinol Metab* 2012;**97**(8):2543–65.

54a. Bolz M, Körber S, Schober H-C. TSH secreting adenoma of pituitary gland (TSHom) – rare case of hyperthyroidism in pregnancy. *Dtsch Med Wochenschr* 2013;**138**:362–6.

54b. Paschke R, Niedziela M, Vaidya B, et al. 2012 European Thyroid Association guidelines for the management of familial and persistent and sporadic non-autoimmune hyperthyroidism caused by thyroid stimulating hormone receptor germline mutations. *Our Thyroid J* 2012;142–7.

55. Mallya M, Ogilvy-Stuart AL. Thyrotropic hormones. *Best Pract Res Clin Endocrinol Metab* 2018;**32**(1):17–25.

56. Hesarghatta Shyamasunder A, Abraham P. Measuring TSH receptor antibody to influence treatment choices in Graves' disease. *Clin Endocrinol (Oxf)* 2017;**86**(5):652–7.

57. Sarkar S, Bischoff LA. Management of hyperthyroidism during the preconception phase, pregnancy, and the postpartum period. *Semin Reprod Med* 2016;**34**(6):317–22.

58. Patil-Sisodia K, Mestman J. Graves hyperthyroidism and pregnancy: a clinical update. *Endocr Pract* 2010;**16**(1):118–29.

59. Luton D, Le Gac I, Vuillard E, Castanet M, Guibourdenche J, Noel M, et al. Management of Graves' disease during pregnancy: The key role of fetal thyroid gland monitoring. *J Clin Endocrinol Metabol* 2005;**90**(11):6093–8.

60. Adali E, Yildizhan R, Kolusari A, Kurdoglu M, Turan N. The use of plasmapheresis for rapid hormonal control in severe hyperthyroidism caused by a partial molar pregnancy. *Arch Gynecol Obstet* 2009;**279**(4):569–71.

61. Vyas AA, Vyas P, Fillipon NL, Vijayakrishnan R, Trivedi N. Successful treatment of thyroid storm with plasmapheresis in a patient with methimazole-induced agranulocytosis. *Endocr Pract* 2010;**16**(4):673–6.

62. Casey BM, Dashe JS, Wells CE, McIntire DD, Leveno KJ, Cunningham FG. Subclinical hyperthyroidism and pregnancy outcomes. *Obstet Gynecol* 2006;**107**(2 Pt 1):337–41.

63. Nathan N, Sullivan SD. Thyroid disorders during pregnancy. *Endocrinol Metab Clin North Am* 2014;**43**(2):573–97.

64. Rasmussen NG, Hornnes PJ, Hegedüs L. Ultrasonographically determined thyroid size in pregnancy and post partum: the goitrogenic effect of pregnancy. *Am J Obstet Gynecol* 1989;**160**(5 Pt 1):1216–20.

65. Nelson M, Wickus GG, Caplan RH, Beguin EA. Thyroid gland size in pregnancy. An ultrasound and clinical study. *J Reprod Med* 1987;**32**(12):888–90.

66. Goodwin TM, Montoro M, Mestman JH. Transient hyperthyroidism and hyperemesis gravidarum: clinical aspects. *Am J Obstet Gynecol* 1992;**167**(3):648–52.

67. Grun JP, Meuris S, De Nayer P, Glinoer D. The thyrotropic role of human chorionic gonadotropin in the early stages of twin versus single pregnancies. *Clin Endocrinol Oxf Jun* 1997;**46**(6 SRC—BaiduScholar):719–25.

68. Lockwood CM, Grenache DG, Gronowski AM. Serum human chorionic gonadotropin concentrations >400,000 IU/L are invariably associated with suppressed serum thyrotropin concentrations. *Thyroid* 2009;**19**(8):863–8.

69. Walkington L, Webster J, Hancock BW, Everard J, Coleman RE. Hyperthyroidism and human chorionic gonadotrophin production in gestational trophoblastic disease. *Br J Cancer* 2011;**104**(11):1665–9.

70. Moskovitz JB, Bond MC. Molar pregnancy-induced thyroid storm. *J Emerg Med* 2010;**38**(5):e71–6.

71. Rodien P, Brémont C, Sanson ML, Parma J, Van Sande J, Costagliola S, et al. Familial gestational hyperthyroidism caused by a mutant thyrotropin receptor hypersensitive to human chorionic gonadotropin. *N Engl J Med* 1998;**339**(25):1823–6.

72. Carlé A, Pedersen IB, Knudsen N, Perrild H, Ovesen L, Rasmussen LB, et al. Epidemiology of subtypes of hyperthyroidism in Denmark: a population-based study. *Eur J Endocrinol* 2011;**164**(5):801–9.

73. Hershman JM. Physiological and pathological aspects of the effect of human chorionic gonadotropin on the thyroid. *Best Pract Res Clin Endocrinol Metab* 2004;**18**(2):249–65.

74. Ross DS, Burch HB, Cooper DS, Greenlee MC, Laurberg P, Maia AL, et al. 2016 American Thyroid Association Guidelines for Diagnosis and Management of hyperthyroidism and other causes of thyrotoxicosis. *Thyroid* 2016;**26**(10):1343–421.

75. Mestman JH. Endocrine disease in pregnancy. In: Sciarra JJ, editor. *Gynecology and obstetrics*. Philadelphia: Lipincott Raven; 1997 34 pp.

76. Sergi M, Tomlinson G, Feig DS. Changes suggestive of post-partum thyroiditis in women with established hypothyroidism: incidence and predictors. *Clin Endocrinol (Oxf)* 2015;**83**(3):389–93.

77. Stagnaro-Green A. Approach to the patient with postpartum thyroiditis. *J Clin Endocrinol Metabol* 2012;**97**(2):334–42.

78. Nicholson WK, Robinson KA, Smallridge RC, Ladenson PW, Powe NR. Prevalence of postpartum thyroid dysfunction: a quantitative review. *Thyroid* 2006;**16**(6):573–82.

79. Mestman JH. Thyroid and parathyroid diseases in pregnancy. In: Gabbe Steven G, et al. editors. *Obstetrics: normal and problem pregnancies* 7th ed., ; 2017. p. 910–37 Chapter 42.

79a. Robertson HE. Lassitude, coldness, and hair changes following pregnancy, and their response to treatment with thyroid extract. *Br Med J* 1948;**2**:93.

80. Stagnaro-Green A, Schwartz A, Gismondi R, Tinelli A, Mangieri T, Negro R. High rate of persistent hypothyroidism in a large-scale prospective study of postpartum thyroiditis in Southern Italy. *J Clin Endocrinol Metabol* 2011;**96**(3):652–7.

81. Ide A, Amino N, Kang S, Yoshioka W, Kudo T, Nishihara E, et al. Differentiation of postpartum graves' thyrotoxicosis from postpartum destructive thyrotoxicosis using antithyrotropin receptor antibodies and thyroid blood flow. *Thyroid* 2014;**24**(6):1027–31.

82. Protection ICR. Pregnancy and medical radiation. *Ann ICRP* 2000;**30**(1):1–43 iii–viii.

83. Stabin MG, Breitz HB. Breast milk excretion of radiopharmaceuticals: mechanisms, findings, and radiation dosimetry. *J Nucl Med* 2000;**41**:863–73.

84. Eidelman AI, Schimmel MS. Drugs and breast milk. *Pediatrics* 1995;**95**(6):956–7 author reply 7–8.

85. Lucas A, Pizarro E, Granada ML, Salinas I, Sanmarti A. Postpartum thyroid dysfunction and postpartum depression: are they two linked disorders? *Clin Endocrinol (Oxf)* 2001;**55**(6):809–14.

86. Harris B, Oretti R, Lazarus J, Parkes A, John R, Richards C, et al. Randomized trial of thyroxine to prevent postnatal depression in thyroid-antibody-positive women. *Br J Psychiatry* 2002;**180**(APR.):327–30.

87. Kämpe O, Jansson R, Karlsson FA. Effects of L-thyroxine and iodide on the development of autoimmune postpartum thyroiditis. *J Clin Endocrinol Metabol* 1990;**70**(4):1014–8.

88. Nøhr SB, Jørgensen A, Pedersen KM, Laurberg P. Postpartum thyroid dysfunction in pregnant thyroid peroxidase antibody-positive women living in an area with mild to moderate iodine deficiency: is iodine supplementation safe? *J Clin Endocrinol Metabol* 2000;**85**(9):3191–8.

89. Negro R, Greco G, Mangieri T, Pezzarossa A, Dazzi D, Hassan H. The influence of selenium supplementation on postpartum thyroid status in pregnant women with thyroid peroxidase autoantibodies. *J Clin Endocrinol Metabol* 2007;**92**(4):1263–8.

90. Akamizu T, Satoh T, Isozaki O, Suzuki A, Wakino S, Iburi T, et al. Diagnostic criteria, clinical features, and incidence of thyroid storm based on nationwide surveys. *Thyroid* 2012;**22**(7):661–79.

91. Burch HB, Wartofsky L. Life-threatening thyrotoxicosis. Thyroid storm. *Endocrinol Metab Clin North Am* 1993;**22**(2):263–77.

92. Feldt-Rasmussen U, Emerson CH. Further thoughts on the diagnosis and diagnostic criteria for thyroid storm. *Thyroid* 2012;**22**(11):1094–5.

93. Ngan TYT, Faden M, El-Messidi A, Brown R. Maternal and obstetric outcomes among women with thyroid storm in pregnancy: a population-based study of 4.2 million births. *Am J Obstet Gynecol* 2017;**216**(1) S460-S1.

94. Angell TE, Lechner MG, Nguyen CT, Salvato VL, Nicoloff JT, LoPresti JS. Clinical features and hospital outcomes in thyroid storm: a retrospective cohort study. *J Clin Endocrinol Metab* 2015;**100**(2):451–9.

95. Coulombe P, Dussault JH, Letarte J, Simmard SJ. Catecholamines metabolism in thyroid diseases. I. Epinephrine secretion rate in hyperthyroidism and hypothyroidism. *J Clin Endocrinol Metab* 1976;**42**(1):125–31.
96. Coulombe P, Dussault JH, Walker P. Catecholamine metabolism in thyroid disease. II. Norepinephrine secretion rate in hyperthyroidism and hypothyroidism. *J Clin Endocrinol Metab* 1977;**44**(6):1185–9.
97. Bilezikian JP, Loeb JN. The influence of hyperthyroidism and hypothyroidism on alpha- and beta-adrenergic receptor systems and adrenergic responsiveness. *Endocr Rev* 1983;**4**(4):378–88.
98. Silva JE, Bianco SDC. Thyroid-adrenergic interactions: physiological and clinical implications. *Thyroid* 2008;**18**(2):157–65.
99. Akamizu T. Thyroid storm: a Japanese perspective. *Thyroid* 2018;**28**(1):32–40.
100. Kofinas JD, Kruczek A, Sample J, Eglinton GS. Thyroid storm-induced multi-organ failure in the setting of gestational trophoblastic disease. *J Emerg Med* 2015;**48**(1):35–8.
101. Abuid J, Larsen PR. Triiodothyronine and thyroxine in hyperthyroidism. Comparison of the acute changes during therapy with antithyroid agents. *J Clin Invest* 1974;**54**(1):201–8.
102. Klubo-Gwiezdzinska J, Wartofsky L. Thyroid emergencies. *Med Clin North Am* 2012;**96**(2):385–403.
103. Rodríguez I, Fluiters E, Pérez-Méndez LF, Luna R, Páramo C, García-Mayor RV. Factors associated with mortality of patients with myxoedema coma: prospective study in 11 cases treated in a single institution. *J Endocrinol* 2004;**180**(2):347–50.
104. Echt CR, Doss JF. Myxedema in pregnancy. Report of 3 cases. *Obstet Gynecol* 1963;**22**:615–20.
105. Turhan NO, Koçkar MC, Inegöl I. Myxedematous coma in a laboring woman suggested a pre-eclamptic coma: a case report. *Acta Obstet Gynecol Scand* 2004;**83**(11):1089–91.
106. Singh N, Tripathi R. Undiagnosed hypothyroidism in pregnancy leading to myxedema coma in labor: diagnosing and managing this rare emergency. *J Pregn Child Health* 2016;**03**(02):247.
107. Kwaku MP, Burman KD. Myxedema coma. *J Intensive Care Med* 2007;**22**(4):224–31.
108. Mathew V, Misgar RA, Ghosh S, Mukhopadhyay P, Roychowdhury P, Pandit K, et al. Myxedema coma: a new look into an old crisis. *J Thyroid Res* 2011;**2011**:493462.
109. Patel S, Robinson S, Bidgood RJ, Edmonds CJ. A pre-eclamptic-like syndrome associated with hypothyroidism during pregnancy. *Q J Med* 1991;**79** (289):435–41.
110. Chiong YV, Bammerlin E, Mariash CN. Development of an objective tool for the diagnosis of myxedema coma. *Transl Res* 2015;**166**(3):233–43.
111. Dutta P, Bhansali A, Masoodi S, Bhadada S, Sharma N, Rajput R. Predictors of outcome in myxoedema coma: a study from a tertiary care centre. *Crit Care* 2008;**12**(1).
112. Ono Y, Ono S, Yasunaga H, Matsui H, Fushimi K, Tanaka Y. Clinical characteristics and outcomes of myxedema coma: analysis of a national inpatient database in Japan. *J Epidemiol* 2017;**27**(3):117–22.
113. Jonklaas J, Bianco AC, Bauer AJ, Burman KD, Cappola AR, Celi FS, et al. Guidelines for the treatment of hypothyroidism: prepared by the American thyroid association task force on thyroid hormone replacement. *Thyroid* 2014;**24**(12):1670–751.

Chapter 20

Thyroid Cancer During Pregnancy and Lactation

Christopher W. Rowe*,†, Kristien Boelaert‡ and Roger Smith*,†

*Department of Endocrinology, John Hunter Hospital, Newcastle, NSW, Australia, †School of Medicine and Public Health, University of Newcastle, Newcastle, NSW, Australia, ‡Institute of Metabolism and Systems Research, College of Medical and Dental Sciences, University of Birmingham, Birmingham, United Kingdom

Common Clinical Problems

- Thyroid nodules detected in pregnancy are common and require structured assessment, accounting for the unique circumstances of pregnancy.
- Survival from thyroid cancers diagnosed in pregnancy is similar to the nonpregnant population, although observational data may suggest an increased rate of locoregional recurrence.
- The timing of investigation of thyroid nodules, as well as consideration of surgery for thyroid cancer in pregnancy, should account for the stage of pregnancy and disease aggressiveness.
- A newly diagnosed differentiated thyroid cancer presenting during pregnancy, and without high risk features, may often be managed conservatively during pregnancy with surgery in the postpartum period.
- Active surveillance of papillary microcarcinomas in pregnancy is increasingly reported, but long-term-outcome data are lacking.
- Survivors of thyroid cancer should have specific prepregnancy counseling and intrapartum monitoring according to disease status, but they generally see favorable obstetric and oncologic outcomes.

20.1 INTRODUCTION

The detection of a thyroid nodule during pregnancy is a common clinical scenario, usually resulting in anxiety in both the woman and her physician. Two factors need to be considered in the assessment of a thyroid nodule: the presence of local symptoms due to mass effect, which occasionally necessitates removal if it compresses vital structures such as the trachea or great vessels; and the risk of malignancy. A third important factor—namely, whether the nodule is autonomously producing thyroid hormone—is unable to be assessed until the postpartum period due to the contraindication of scintigraphy during pregnancy. Any proposed treatment for a thyroid nodule must carefully balance the potential risks and benefits to both mother and developing fetus. We concur with the conclusions of Oduncu and colleagues that there is inevitable "maternal-fetal conflict" between the best care for the two patients, and thoughtful, patient-centered clinical reasoning is essential.[1]

Malignancy of the thyroid gland usually arises from follicular epithelial cells, occurring in either a papillary thyroid cancer (PTC) or follicular thyroid cancer (FTC) pattern, and together, these are termed *differentiated thyroid cancer (DTC)*. The rare, undifferentiated anaplastic thyroid cancer (ATC) is a highly aggressive subtype. Malignancy can also arise from the parafollicular, neuro-endocrine derived C-cells, termed *medullary thyroid cancer (MTC)*. Infiltration of the thyroid due to lymphoma or solid organ metastases is rare. In the absence of distant metastases, DTC has an excellent prognosis in women of childbearing age, with greater than 98% experiencing greater than 10-year survival.[2]

Maternal-Fetal and Neonatal Endocrinology. https://doi.org/10.1016/B978-0-12-814823-5.00020-9

20.2 EPIDEMIOLOGY OF NODULAR THYROID DISEASE AND THYROID CANCER

20.2.1 Nodular Thyroid Disease

For reasons that are still not well understood, thyroid nodules are more common in women and increase with age,[3] a pattern that is observed across ethnicities and iodine-availability states.[4–6] Increased exposure to female reproductive hormones is associated with increased nodularity. For example, later menopause, longer reproductive life, and multiparity are associated with increased thyroid nodules in a large community-based study from China.[7] Multiparity is again associated with increased thyroid nodularity according to a study from Germany,[8] and it may be exacerbated by iodine deficiency.[6] Thyroid nodularity has also been associated with the presence of uterine fibroids.[9, 10] Current or previous oral contraceptive pill usage has been associated with reduced thyroid volume in a single study, although no difference in thyroid nodularity was found.[11]

20.2.2 Thyroid Cancer

Correlating with this pattern of increased thyroid nodularity, there is a strong female preponderance of thyroid cancer. Data from the U.S. National Cancer Institute Surveillance, Epidemiology, and End Results (SEER) Database shows an incidence of 21 cases per 100,000 females, compared to 7.1 per 100,000 males.[12] SEER data (Fig. 20.1) also show that female preponderance is evident at puberty and that the female peak in incidence (ages 35–59 years) precedes the male peak in incidence (ages 65–75 years), corresponding with exposure to female reproductive hormones. There is no gender difference in incidence for ATC or MTC.

Despite these compelling epidemiological data, evidence linking reproductive-hormone exposure to thyroid cancer risk, examining factors such as age or pattern of menstrual cycle, menopause, or exogenous hormone therapy, is generally weak and heterogenous.[13] However, reproductive history has a stronger link with DTC, particularly PTC risk, with some (but not all) studies finding a small or transient increase in risk of DTC following pregnancy compared to nulliparous women.[13] Prolonged breastfeeding is associated with significant reductions in circulating estradiol levels and has been associated with reduced thyroid cancer risk in several studies.[14, 15]

20.2.3 Incidence of Thyroid Cancer in Pregnancy

Thyroid cancer is the second-most-common solid organ malignancy complicating pregnancy (behind breast cancer), occurring in 14 in 100,000 births.[16] Most of these cases represent a new diagnosis, usually of disease localized in the neck. Due to the increasing incidence of thyroid cancer and excellent prognosis,[17] more survivors of thyroid cancer are presenting for obstetric management. For example, the prevalence of thyroid cancer among women in Taiwan (175 cases per 100,000 women) is approximately ninefold higher than the incidence (18 cases per 100,000 women).[18] Pregnancy in the setting of persistent structural disease is uncommon.

FIG. 20.1 Histogram showing age- and gender-specific incidence of thyroid cancer in the United States. *Data source: SEER 18 (2010–2014). https://seer.cancer.gov/faststats.*

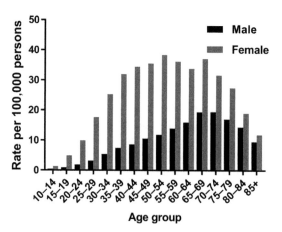

20.3 EFFECTS OF PREGNANCY ON THYROID NODULES

20.3.1 Effects of Pregnancy Hormones on Thyroid Follicular Epithelium

Fig. 20.2 illustrates the known pregnancy-associated stimuli to the thyroid follicular cells.

The glycoprotein hormone human chorionic gonadotropin (hCG) is a heterodimer comprised of a common alpha-subunit shared with luteinizing hormone (LH), follicle-stimulating hormone (FSH), and thyroid-stimulating hormone (TSH), as well as a unique beta-subunit. This structural homology results in cross-stimulation of the seven-transmembrane domain G protein-coupled TSH receptor and contributes to the physiological suppression of endogenous TSH during the first trimester, gestational transient thyrotoxicosis, and stimulus for TSH receptor-mediated thyroid growth.[19] An association between prolonged increase in TSH receptor-mediated signaling and subsequent risk of thyroid cancer has been demonstrated in several large observational studies, although the impact of shorter periods of increased TSH-receptor signaling is not known.[20]

Driven by the strong epidemiological data linking female sex and nodular thyroid disease, the effect of estrogen on benign and malignant thyrocytes has been extensively studied in vitro and in animal models. Both benign and malignant thyrocytes express the estrogen receptors alpha and beta, and estrogen acts to stimulate growth of thyroid cells in culture.[21] The G protein-coupled estrogen receptor 1 (GPER1), located on the endoplasmic reticulum, is overexpressed in thyroid cancers and may correlate with nodal metastases.[22] Although less studied, progesterone receptors are also found in benign and malignant thryocytes and may contribute to cell growth and gene transcription, although the magnitude of progesterone increase in pregnancy is around 10-fold lower than that of estradiol (Chapter 9).[23, 24]

Although not a pregnancy hormone, the trace element iodine is essential for maternal and fetal thyroid function, and metabolic demands for iodine increase during pregnancy. Both conditions of iodine excess and iodine deficiency are associated with increased thyroid nodule formation.[4, 25] Iodine requirements in pregnancy are approximately 250–300 mcg/day.[26]

20.3.2 Physiology of Thyroid Nodules During Pregnancy

Thyroid nodules are detected by ultrasound screening in 3%–21% of healthy pregnant women,[8, 25, 27] although the majority are less than 1 cm in size.[25] Pregnancy has a small but significant effect on thyroid size and thyroid nodule growth. A prospective study of 221 Chinese women using serial thyroid ultrasound in pregnancy found that of the 34 women with nodules at baseline, 25/34 (74%) developed new nodules during pregnancy. Of women without nodules at baseline, 25/187 (11%) developed new nodules during pregnancy.[25] No nodule was suspicious for malignancy. A prospective study of 726 pregnant Belgian women found 20 of 726 women (3%) with nodules at baseline (identified using two-stage screening of palpation, and then ultrasound), with 12/20 having nodules double in size during pregnancy, and 4/20 women developing new nodules during pregnancy.[27]

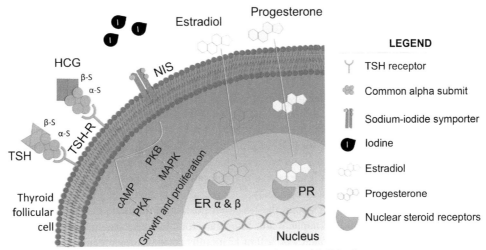

FIG. 20.2 Stimulatory signaling of pregnancy-associated factors on thyroid follicular epithelial cells.

20.4 EVALUATION OF A NEWLY DISCOVERED THYROID NODULE IN PREGNANCY

As in the nonpregnant population, ultrasound-based screening for thyroid nodules in pregnancy is not recommended.[28] Hence, any thyroid nodule newly discovered in pregnancy should present either as an incidental finding or as a symptomatic/palpable lump.

The initial assessment of a thyroid lump should proceed as in a nonpregnant woman, with a goal of identifying lesions at high risk for malignancy. This assessment should include a thorough history, including risk factors for thyroid cancer, such as

- Familial syndromes of multiple endocrine neoplasia 2 (MEN2), familial PTC, Cowden's syndrome, familial adenomatosis polyposis, and Carney complex
- Childhood neck irradiation, such as in treatment for prior head and neck cancers
- Early life exposure (<18 years) to ionizing radiation

Clinical examination of the neck should characterize the lump, assess for symptoms due to mass-effect, and determine any cervical lymphadenopathy.

Although TSH and free thyroid hormones should be measured, their utility for risk stratification of thyroid nodules in pregnancy is limited by the contraindication of thyroid scintigraphy during pregnancy. Radioactive iodine readily crosses the placenta and can cause fetal hypothyroidism due to gland destruction if administered after fetal thyrogenesis in the 12th week of gestation. Further, exposure to gamma emissions from radioiodine being concentrated in the maternal bladder should be avoided. Thus, it is not possible to determine conclusively if a thyroid nodule is functional (and hence at very low risk of malignancy), or nonfunctional during pregnancy. Calcitonin is a sensitive serum biomarker for MTC,[29] although it has not been specifically validated in pregnant women and is generally not a recommended screening test in patients with thyroid nodules, either during or outside pregnancy. Further, calcitonin levels increase during normal pregnancy (see Chapter 5). CEA, also a sensitive biomarker of MTC, may rise slightly in normal pregnancy and should be interpreted cautiously.[30]

The definitive risk stratification of a thyroid nodule uses thyroid/neck ultrasound using a high-frequency linear transducer, including detailed sonographic characterization of the nodule, and an assessment of the lateral neck for pathologically enlarged lymph nodes. Ultrasound-based risk-stratification systems for thyroid nodules have been published by the American Thyroid Association (ATA)[31] and the American College of Radiology.[32] Neck ultrasound is safe in pregnancy.

Based on this information, an initial risk stratification of malignancy risk can be performed, and the need for fine-needle aspiration biopsy (FNAB) determined. Indications for FNAB are identical to those in the nonpregnant population.[31] Although FNAB is safe in all trimesters of pregnancy, careful consideration should be given to how this knowledge will be used. Several studies (reviewed next) have concluded that there is no impact on overall survival if surgery for a newly diagnosed DTC is deferred to the postpartum period, so a PTC with a typical ultrasound appearance and no pathological lymphadenopathy could be considered for deferred biopsy and surgery in the postpartum period. While the impact of pregnancy on MTC or ATC is unknown, given the more aggressive nature of these tumors earlier surgery may be warranted, and cytological assessment of a sonographically concerning lesion during pregnancy may be useful. Patient preference is an important factor. This approach is consistent with published guidelines.[33]

20.5 EFFECT OF PREGNANCY ON NEWLY DIAGNOSED THYROID CANCER

20.5.1 Impact on Prognosis

Historically, outcome data for thyroid cancers diagnosed in pregnancy has been similar to the nonpregnant population, both in terms of recurrence and overall survival. These conclusions are based on data from retrospective studies from the United States over the period 1962–1999,[34–36] with the most recent study (1991–1999) examining mortality only. Timing of surgery in these studies, either during pregnancy or postpartum, did not affect survival. While these studies draw on long follow-up periods, they are retrospective in nature and were conducted prior to the availability of now-standard tools for monitoring and detecting recurrences, such as ultrasensitive thyroglobulin assays and high-resolution neck ultrasound.[33]

Contrastingly, two recent retrospective studies from Italy,[37, 38] recruiting patients diagnosed between 1995 and 2011, found that DTC diagnosed during pregnancy or within the first year postpartum may be associated with a higher risk of residual or recurrent disease. In the first study, Vannuchi and colleagues found that persistence/recurrence rates for women who were diagnosed with thyroid cancer in pregnancy or within 12 months postpartum were higher (Group 2, 9/15, or 60%) than women with thyroid cancer diagnosed more than 12 months following pregnancy (Group 1, 2/47, about 4%) or never pregnant (Group 3, 8/61, about 13%).[37] However, an important confounder is that 11 of the 15 patients in Group 2 underwent surgery in the second trimester, and it is possible that a more cautious surgical approach prompted by pregnancy may have resulted in incomplete nodal clearance. In the second, larger study, Messuti and colleagues retrospectively stratified women less than 45 years into three groups: thyroid cancer diagnosed more than 2 years postpartum (Group 1, $n = 152$), thyroid cancer diagnosed during pregnancy or within 2 years (Group 2, $n = 38$), and nulliparous women (Group 3, $n = 150$).[38] Group 2 again had a higher incidence of persistent/recurrent disease in univariate analysis (11%, as opposed to 1% for Group 1 and 5% for Group 3, $p = 0.02$), although this difference was not observed in a multivariate model. The number of Group 2 patients who underwent thyroidectomy during pregnancy was not reported.

An Australian study over a similar period noted that DTC diagnosed in pregnancy or within 12 months postpartum had a larger size and a greater number of positive neck nodes than age- and sex-matched nonpregnant controls, although no difference in tumor micro-ribonucleic acid (microRNA) expression profiles between the two groups was noted.[39]

A retrospective ultrasound study followed 19 patients with PTC diagnosed just prior to or in the early stages of pregnancy.[40] Among the findings, 13/19 tumors were <1 cm in diameter and 3/19 showed evidence of involved lymph nodes. Over the course of pregnancy, increase in the tumor maximal diameter was noted in 16% of cases (3/19), and increase in tumor volume in 26% (5/19). Of the 3 patients with sonographically detected lymph nodes at diagnosis, 2 showed an increase in nodal size, although no new lymph nodes were observed and the extent of surgery was not altered. Further, 16/19 patients were managed surgically at a mean duration of 12 months following diagnosis, with either an ATA Excellent or ATA Indeterminate response to therapy after median follow-up of 54 months.

Overall, the available evidence suggests that DTC diagnosed in pregnancy has comparable overall survival to nonpregnant cohorts, whether surgery occurs during or after pregnancy. These data should reassure clinicians and patients that deferring surgery for a low-risk DTC until the postpartum period is a reasonable strategy. While it is possible that DTC diagnosed during pregnancy may be more likely to have local persistence or recurrence, appropriate surveillance will facilitate timely detection and management. Tumors with suspected high-risk features should be discussed in the context of an experienced multidisciplinary team for individualized management.

20.5.2   Timing of Surgery

The decision of whether to proceed to thyroidectomy during pregnancy or to defer surgery until the postpartum period is largely based on expert opinion, as summarized in recent guidelines of the ATA.[33] In general, the presence of clinically aggressive features would prompt strong consideration of surgery during pregnancy, while their absence would lend support for a surveillance strategy, with surgery in the postpartum period. At present, specialized thyroid and neck ultrasound is the most useful tool to predict clinically aggressive DTC, and this should be performed at the initial assessment, and again by 24 weeks. Sonographic detection of lymph node metastases, or definite growth of the primary tumor, favor early surgery. MTC and ATC are considered more aggressive lesions by definition and early surgery should be strongly considered.

Repeat clinical and sonographic assessment of a suspicious thyroid nodule should occur prior to 24 weeks' gestation, to allow planning for thyroidectomy in the second trimester if required.

There is no optimal time for surgical management in the peripartum period. Surgery and anesthesia during pregnancy carry small but definite risks for the mother and fetus, which are minimized by elective operations in the second trimester. Conversely, surgery in the postpartum period may disrupt mother-child attachment and the establishment of breastfeeding, as well as placing increased stress on the family unit. Given the absence of evidence, patient-centered care that includes balanced discussion of various treatment options is appropriate.

20.5.3   Supportive Management in Pregnancy

TSH is an established growth factor for benign and malignant thyrocytes.[19] While there are no studies examining the effect of supplemental levothyroxine to target lower TSH levels in thyroid cancers diagnosed during pregnancy, it is reasonable to establish a TSH target of the lower half of the pregnancy-specific reference range and administer levothyroxine if required to achieve this target.

We do not recommend restricting dietary iodine. Iodine is essential for fetal thyroid development, and maternal iodine requirements rise in pregnancy. Iodine deficiency in pregnancy is associated with development of maternal goiter, presumably in part through TSH-mediated stimulation of thyrocyte growth, and may contribute to increased nodularity as well.

20.5.4 Planning for Radioiodine Therapy

Serum thyroglobulin values in pregnancy may rise compared to prepregnancy levels, possibly due to maternal thyroid stimulation from hCG and estrogen, but they return to baseline levels within 1–6 months postpartum.[41-43] We recommend waiting at least 6 weeks postpartum before assessing thyroglobulin status following pregnancy.

The indications for radioiodine therapy for either remnant ablation and adjuvant therapy have narrowed recently, such that fewer patients are requiring this treatment. This simplifies the initial management of the majority of women; however, a subset still will require radioiodine therapy based on risk stratification from recent guidelines.[31]

Radioiodine administration in the postpartum period presents unique medical and social challenges. Close contact with infants and children should be avoided for a minimum of 7 days after radioiodine therapy (the specific interval is determined by the administered dose and by the recommendations of the nuclear medicine physician).[44] Lactating mammary tissue overexpresses the sodium-iodide symporter and concentrates iodine,[45] and so to minimize radiation exposure to breast tissue, it is recommended that breastfeeding ceases at least 8 weeks prior to treatment with radioiodine therapy (ideally 3 months), and not be resumed for the current child to avoid radiation exposure to the child through breast milk.

If radioiodine therapy is required, the timing of therapy should be carefully considered, taking into account the risk of DTC progression, establishment of breastfeeding, and maternal-child bonding. A recent retrospective database study of over 9,000 patients with high-risk PTC (>4 cm, nodal disease or grossly positive margins) found no impact on mortality (median survival 75 months) when radioiodine was administered early (within 3 months of surgery) compared to late (within 3–12 months), after adjustment for confounders.[46] In contrast, a smaller retrospective study of 235 ATA Low- and Intermediate-risk patients found a higher rate of persisting biochemical or structural disease (18.8% vs 4.3%) in patients with radioiodine therapy deferred longer than 3 months.[47]

20.6 PRECONCEPTION COUNSELING OF WOMEN WITH A PRIOR HISTORY OF THYROID CANCER

Women of childbearing age with a prior history of thyroid cancer should be advised to seek preconception counseling. Periconception issues should be opportunistically addressed at regular follow-up appointments, both in primary and tertiary care.

Issues in preconception care for women with a past history of thyroid cancer

- Assessment of disease status: structural and biochemical
- Potential impact of pregnancy on disease progress
- Thyroxine dosing prior to, and following, conception
- Impact of prior radioiodine therapy on timing of conception and future fertility
- Use of pregnancy supplements that may interfere with thyroxine absorption

---

20.6.1 Establishment of Disease Status

The 2015 ATA guidelines for DTC provide a helpful framework for evaluating disease status in the period following initial treatment, accounting for the patient's response to therapy (Table 20.1).[31] Different management considerations are relevant depending on a woman's prior treatment (total or hemithyroidectomy and whether radioiodine was administered), level of functional thyroid reserve (if hemithyroidectomy), and presence of any residual cancer. The presence of a microPTC under active surveillance represents a separate issue which is discussed in the following section.

In patients with a past history of MTC, serum calcitonin and CEA are sensitive tumor markers and allow risk stratification of likelihood of structural disease.[48] No studies examine the impact of pregnancy on MTC.

20.6.2 Risk of Recurrence

There is a theoretical risk that pregnancy may accelerate the recurrence or progression of previously treated DTC. Four key retrospective studies performed during the last 30 years are presented.

Leboeuf and colleagues[43] evaluated 36 women with one or more pregnancies following therapy for DTC between 1997 and 2006, with pregnancy occurring a median of 4.3 years after DTC treatment. Only 44% of the cohort had neck imaging both before and after delivery, limiting the comparability of prepartum and postpartum assessments. Of the 3 women with

TABLE 20.1 2015 ATA risk stratification for DTC

2015 ATA response-to-therapy classification	Description
Excellent response	No clinical, biochemical, or structural evidence of persistent or recurrent thyroid cancer
Biochemical-incomplete response	Elevated serum thyroglobulin, or rising antithyroglobulin antibodies, in the absence of structural disease identifiable on imaging
Structural-incomplete response	Persistent or recurrent thyroid cancer visible upon imaging, either in neck or distant metastases
Indeterminate response	Nonspecific biochemical or structural findings that are not able to be classified as benign or malignant (includes stable/declining antithyroglobulin antibody levels without evidence of structural disease)

Note: Refer to ATA Guideline[31] for full discussion of each class and qualifying criteria (table 13).
Tabulated from Haugen BR, Alexander EK, Bible KC, Doherty GM, Mandel SJ, Nikiforov YE, et al. 2015 American Thyroid Association Management Guidelines for adult patients with thyroid nodules and differentiated thyroid cancer: the American Thyroid Association Guidelines task force on thyroid nodules and differentiated thyroid cancer. *Thyroid* 2016;**26**(1):1–133.

structural disease prepartum, 1 had evidence of growth of a cervical lymph node metastasis during pregnancy. The 2 other women were noted to have new structural disease postpartum upon *imaging* that was not detected on *physical examination* prepartum. Further, 8/36 women had a >20% rise in serum thyroglobulin following pregnancy, including 2 women with known structural disease, 1 with a new cervical lymphadenopathy, 3 with negative neck US, and 2 with negative physical examination.

Rosario and colleagues[49] reviewed 64 pregnancies following DTC, managed prior to 2006, with median time from treatment to conception being 2.4 years. All patients had no structural evidence of disease by neck ultrasound, either before or after pregnancy. The 49 patients with negative prepregnancy thyroglobulin remained negative postpartum. Eight patients with thyroglobulin 1–2 ng/mL did not show a rise in thyroglobulin postpartum.

Hirsch and colleagues[50] reviewed 63 women between 1992 and 2009 with pregnancy following PTC, with conception occurring a median of 5.1 years after initial treatment. They found that 5 of 6 women with documented structural disease prior to pregnancy demonstrated progression within 12 months postpartum (3 structural progressions and 2 biochemical progressions). All 5 women with biochemical-incomplete disease prior to conception did not have a rise in thyroglobulin postpartum. In 39 women with thyroglobulin <0.9 ng/mL prior to pregnancy, no change was observed in thyroglobulin.

Rakhlin and colleagues reviewed 235 women between 1997 and 2015 with a term pregnancy following treatment for DTC, retrospectively stratified according to the 2015 "ATA Response to Therapy" criteria (Table 20.1).[51] Of the 197 women without evidence of structural disease prepregnancy (comprising 148 ATA Excellent Response, 29 ATA Indeterminate, and 20 ATA Biochemical Incomplete), no structural disease was detected postpartum. However, 16/197 (8%) had a higher postpregnancy thyroglobulin than the prepregnancy value.

These data support the conclusion that women with an ATA Excellent response to therapy classification (that is, no evidence of disease structurally or biochemically) have minimal increased risk of DTC recurrence or progression in pregnancy and do not require additional monitoring during pregnancy.[33]

Women with ATA Biochemical Incomplete or ATA Structural Incomplete disease may be at increased risk of disease progression from pregnancy. Risk and benefit discussions should involve the patient and be individualized. Women with known structural disease are discussed in further detail below.

20.6.3 Mitigating Pregnancy-Impacts of Prior Thyroid Cancer Treatment

20.6.3.1 Levothyroxine Supplementation

All women require written advice for management of thyroid hormone replacement in the periconception period. Pregnancy increases requirements for thyroid hormone production, due in part to a rise in thyroid-binding globulin (see also Chapter 4). Additionally, adequate thyroid hormone is essential for fetal development and may reduce risk of early pregnancy loss. Women who were euthyroid in the nonpregnant state from a remaining hemithyroid may require supplemental levothyroxine due to insufficient functional thyroid reserve. Women dependent on exogenous levothyroxine due to total thyroidectomy should be instructed to increase their dose by 20%–40% as soon as conception occurs (our practice is to "double the dose" on 2 days of the week), with further adjustments based on monthly thyroid function testing for the first two trimesters.[33, 52] Pregnancy multivitamins containing calcium or iron may inhibit absorption of levothyroxine, and patients should be instructed to take these at a time well away from levothyroxine (usually at night).[53] Women should be reassured that levothyroxine is safe to take in pregnancy to reduce risk of misinformed discontinuation at conception.[54]

For most women, the individualized TSH target established prior to pregnancy will remain appropriate in the pregnant state, which is usually the lower half of the nonpregnant reference range. TSH suppression for women with persistent structural disease should be maintained in the pregnant state, as mild hyperthyroidism has not been shown to result in maternal or fetal complications.[33, 55] However, overt thyrotoxicosis increases pregnancy risk.[56]

20.6.3.2 Radioiodine

It is recommended that women avoid conception for 6 months following radioiodine therapy. This period is longer than the time required for radioiodine to totally decay (about 10 weeks, thus preventing fetal exposure to gamma emissions) and is recommended to allow the assessment of response to therapy and ensure that further treatments are not required in the following 15 months.[57] A longitudinal study enrolling 2,673 pregnancies did not show any increase in risk of pregnancy or neonatal complications in women treated with radioiodine.[58] A systematic review from 2008 confirmed these findings and reported no impact of radioiodine on fertility.[59] However, a recent prospective observational study of 30 premenopausal women receiving radioactive iodine (30–150 mCi) found a persistent decline in anti-Mullerian hormone (AMH) levels in 82% of women at 12 months following radioiodine therapy, which was associated with age, but not with dose of radioiodine.[60] There is some evidence of impaired testicular germ cell function following radioiodine, and men should be advised to avoid fathering children for 3–6 months after treatment.[61]

20.6.3.3 Hypoparathyroidism

Permanent surgical hypoparathyroidism is an uncommon long-term complication of neck surgery which requires active management during pregnancy. This condition is addressed in more detail in Chapter 21.

20.6.4 Surveillance and Monitoring

Women with an ATA Excellent response to therapy do not require DTC-specific monitoring during pregnancy, but they should have a repeat thyroglobulin and thyroglobulin-antibody measurement at least 6 months postpartum as part of ongoing surveillance.

Women with ATA Biochemical Incomplete or ATA Indeterminate disease should have periodic monitoring during pregnancy, using thyroglobulin, thyroglobulin antibody, and neck ultrasound. Evidence of disease progression may prompt an increase in the level of TSH suppression, or in rare cases, could prompt expedited delivery. However there is no evidence to guide practice, and multidisciplinary decision-making is recommended.

20.6.4.1 Papillary Thyroid Microcarcinoma

Active surveillance of biopsy-proven papillary thyroid microcarcinoma (PMC; <1 cm, no high-risk features) is an emerging management strategy, and three recent studies have evaluated the impact of pregnancy on its course. Shindo and colleagues followed 9 patients with PMC through pregnancy, noting that there was growth in size in 4/11 PMC (36%), compared to growth in 3/27 (11%) of nonpregnant controls.[62] Ito and colleagues followed 50 pregnant patients with PMC and found growth of >1 mm in 4 (8%), reduction in size in 1 (2%), and stable disease in the remaining 45 (90%). No lymph node metastases were observed.[63] Oh and colleagues followed 13 PMC patients through pregnancy, with 1 lesion showing significant growth.[40] Based on these studies, it appears reasonable to continue a strategy of active surveillance through pregnancy, monitored with serial maternal neck ultrasound; however, note that some microcarcinomas will grow during this period, and this may result in anxiety for the patient and clinicians. Further long-term follow-up data are required to guide practice in this area, as this remains an investigational strategy outside pregnancy, although supported by some recent guidelines.[31]

20.6.5 Germline RET Mutations

Women either with syndromic MEN2 or known germline carriers of mutations in the REarranged during Transfection (RET) proto-oncogene should be offered prenatal counseling, regardless of a prior history of MTC, pheochromocytoma, or hyperparathyroidism. Mutations in RET in the mother, as well as in the fetus or child, can be stratified according to risk of early-onset MTC, which can inform management, including prophylactic thyroidectomy in early childhood for the most aggressive mutations.[48] Pheochromocytoma and hyperparathyroidism should be excluded prior to pregnancy in women with MEN2.

20.7 MANAGEMENT OF KNOWN RESIDUAL STRUCTURAL DISEASE IN PREGNANCY

A study of women with pregnancy in the setting of known structural disease retrospectively followed 38 women from a tertiary cancer center in the United States.[51] They showed that 11/38 (29%) women demonstrated progression of known structural disease during pregnancy (5 with an increase in size of known abnormal lymph nodes, 3 with newly detected abnormal lymph nodes, and 1 with progression of known distant metastases). The authors subclassified 3 of these progressions as "clinically significant," resulting in additional treatment within 12 months postpartum. The cohort included 10 women who had pulmonary metastases at diagnosis, 7 of whom had persistent structural disease prior to pregnancy. Disease progression was documented in 1 of these 10 cases.

These data suggest that pregnancy is a stimulatory environment for thyroid cancer, in keeping with epidemiological and in vitro data. However, the absolute magnitude of these effects appears small, and the majority of women with known structural disease can have a successful pregnancy without demonstrable impact on thyroid cancer status.

TSH suppression should be maintained in such cases, in keeping with prepregnancy targets. The effect of mild hyperthyroidism on pregnancy appears to be negligible. Anticipatory increases in levothyroxine in the first trimester, with monthly thyroid function tests, are required.

It is appropriate to monitor known neck disease with serial neck ultrasounds during pregnancy. Structural chest imaging with ionizing radiation should be avoided in pregnancy. If there are concerns regarding pulmonary function due to prior radioiodine exposure or widespread pulmonary metastases, serial lung function testing may provide some reassurance.

There are three tyrosine kinase inhibitors currently approved for the treatment of progressive or symptomatic metastatic thyroid cancer (lenvatanib, sorafenib, and cabozatenib). In animal studies using less than 10% of the recommended human dose, lenvatinib and sorafenib resulted in embryotoxicity, fetotoxicity, and teratogenicity in rats and rabbits.[64, 65] No specific advice was provided for cabozatenib. Women of childbearing age should be advised to avoid pregnancy while on treatment with these agents. A single case of a woman with MEN2 and MTC treated with vandetanib up until 6 weeks gestation reported no adverse fetal outcomes.[66]

20.8 CONCLUSION

Despite the conundrum of female preponderance of DTC remaining largely unexplained, effective treatment for thyroid cancer results in minimal long-term sequelae for the vast majority of women, including those who are pregnant or contemplating pregnancy. The increasing survivorship of young thyroid cancer patients, as well as the increased detection of thyroid nodules, mandates that pregnancy physicians are competent with the assessment and management of these conditions.

REFERENCES

1. Oduncu FS, Kimmig R, Hepp H, Emmerich B. Cancer in pregnancy: maternal-fetal conflict. *J Cancer Res Clin Oncol* 2003;**129**(3):133–46.
2. Tuttle RM, Haugen B, Perrier ND. Updated American Joint Committee on cancer/tumor-node-metastasis staging system for differentiated and anaplastic thyroid cancer (eighth edition): what changed and why? *Thyroid* 2017;**27**(6):751–6.
3. Reiners C, Wegscheider K, Schicha H, Theissen P, Vaupel R, Wrbitzky R, et al. Prevalence of thyroid disorders in the working population of Germany: ultrasonography screening in 96,278 unselected employees. *Thyroid* 2004;**14**(11):926–32.
4. Song J, Zou SR, Guo CY, Zang JJ, Zhu ZN, Mi M, et al. Prevalence of thyroid nodules and its relationship with iodine status in shanghai: a population-based study. *Biomed Environ Sci* 2016;**29**(6):398–407.
5. Moifo B, Moulion Tapouh JR, Dongmo Fomekong S, Djomou F, Manka'a Wankie E. Ultrasonographic prevalence and characteristics of non-palpable thyroid incidentalomas in a hospital-based population in a sub-Saharan country. *BMC Med Imaging* 2017;**17**(1):21.
6. Knudsen N, Laurberg P, Perrild H, Bulow I, Ovesen L, Jorgensen T. Risk factors for goiter and thyroid nodules. *Thyroid* 2002;**12**(10):879–88.
7. Wang K, Yang Y, Wu Y, Chen J, Zhang D, Liu C. The association of menstrual and reproductive factors with thyroid nodules in Chinese women older than 40 years of age. *Endocrine* 2015;**48**(2):603–14.
8. Struve CW, Haupt S, Ohlen S. Influence of frequency of previous pregnancies on the prevalence of thyroid nodules in women without clinical evidence of thyroid disease. *Thyroid* 1993;**3**(1):7–9.
9. Spinos N, Terzis G, Crysanthopoulou A, Adonakis G, Markou KB, Vervita V, et al. Increased frequency of thyroid nodules and breast fibroadenomas in women with uterine fibroids. *Thyroid* 2007;**17**(12):1257–9.

10. Kim MH, Park YR, Lim DJ, Yoon KH, Kang MI, Cha BY, et al. The relationship between thyroid nodules and uterine fibroids. *Endocr J* 2010;**57**(7):615–21.

11. Knudsen N, Bulow I, Laurberg P, Perrild H, Ovesen L, Jorgensen T. Low goitre prevalence among users of oral contraceptives in a population sample of 3712 women. *Clin Endocrinol* 2002;**57**(1):71–6.

12. *Thyroid cancer*. Bethesda, MD: National Cancer Institute; 2016. [cited 2016 05/10/2016]; Available from: http://seer.cancer.gov/statfacts/html/thyro.html.

13. Moleti M, Sturniolo G, Di Mauro M, Russo M, Vermiglio F. Female reproductive factors and differentiated thyroid cancer. *Front Endocrinol* 2017;**8**:111.

14. Yi X, Zhu J, Zhu X, Liu GJ, Wu L. Breastfeeding and thyroid cancer risk in women: a dose-response meta-analysis of epidemiological studies. *Clin Nutr* 2016;**35**(5):1039–46.

15. Kim H, Kim KY, Baek JH, Jung J. Are pregnancy, parity, menstruation and breastfeeding risk factors for thyroid cancer? Results from the Korea National Health and Nutrition Examination Survey, 2010–2015. *Clin Endocrinol* 2018;**89**(2):233–9.

16. Smith LH, Danielsen B, Allen ME, Cress R. Cancer associated with obstetric delivery: results of linkage with the California cancer registry. *Am J Obstet Gynecol* 2003;**189**(4):1128–35.

17. Lim H, Devesa SS, Sosa JA, Check D, Kitahara CM. Trends in thyroid cancer incidence and mortality in the United States, 1974–2013. *JAMA* 2017;**317**(13):1338–48.

18. Liu F-C, Lin H-T, Lin S-F, Kuo C-F, Chung T-T, Yu H-P. Nationwide cohort study on the epidemiology and survival outcomes of thyroid cancer. *Oncotarget* 2017;**8**(45):78429–51.

19. Rowe CW, Paul J, Geyde C, Tolosa J, Bendinelli C, McGrath S, et al. Targeting the TSH receptor in thyroid cancer. *Endocr Relat Cancer* 2017;**24**:R191–202.

20. Nieto HR, Boelaert K. Thyroid stimulating hormone in thyroid cancer: does it matter? *Endocr Relat Cancer* 2016;.

21. Derwahl M, Nicula D. Estrogen and its role in thyroid cancer. *Endocr Relat Cancer* 2014;**21**(5):T273–83.

22. Zhao L, Zhu X-Y, Jiang R, Xu M, Wang N, Chen GG, et al. Role of GPER1, EGFR and CXCR1 in differentiating between malignant follicular thyroid carcinoma and benign follicular thyroid adenoma. *Int J Clin Exp Pathol* 2015;**8**(9):11236–47.

23. Vannucchi G, De Leo S, Perrino M, Rossi S, Tosi D, Cirello V, et al. Impact of estrogen and progesterone receptor expression on the clinical and molecular features of papillary thyroid cancer. *Eur J Endocrinol* 2015;**173**(1):29–36.

24. Bertoni APS, Brum IS, Hillebrand AC, Furlanetto TW. Progesterone upregulates gene expression in normal human thyroid follicular cells. *Int J Endocrinol* 2015;**2015**.

25. Kung AW, Chau MT, Lao TT, Tam SC, Low LC. The effect of pregnancy on thyroid nodule formation. *J Clin Endocrinol Metab* 2002;**87**(3):1010–4.

26. Delange F. Iodine requirements during pregnancy, lactation and the neonatal period and indicators of optimal iodine nutrition. *Public Health Nutr* 2007;**10**(12a):1571–80 (discussion 81-3).

27. Glinoer D, Soto MF, Bourdoux P, Lejeune B, Delange F, Lemone M, et al. Pregnancy in patients with mild thyroid abnormalities: maternal and neonatal repercussions. *J Clin Endocrinol Metab* 1991;**73**(2):421–7.

28. US Preventative Services Task Force. Screening for thyroid cancer: US preventive services task force recommendation statement. *JAMA* 2017;**317**(18):1882–7.

29. Costante G, Meringolo D, Durante C, Bianchi D, Nocera M, Tumino S, et al. Predictive value of serum calcitonin levels for preoperative diagnosis of medullary thyroid carcinoma in a cohort of 5817 consecutive patients with thyroid nodules. *J Clin Endocrinol Metab* 2007;**92**(2):450–5.

30. Ercan S, Kaymaz O, Yucel N, Orcun A. Serum concentrations of CA 125, CA 15-3, CA 19-9 and CEA in normal pregnancy: a longitudinal study. *Arch Gynecol Obstet* 2012;**285**(3):579–84.

31. Haugen BR, Alexander EK, Bible KC, Doherty GM, Mandel SJ, Nikiforov YE, et al. 2015 American Thyroid Association Management Guidelines for adult patients with thyroid nodules and differentiated thyroid cancer: the american thyroid association guidelines task force on thyroid nodules and differentiated thyroid cancer. *Thyroid* 2016;**26**(1):1–133.

32. Tessler FN, Middleton WD, Grant EG, Hoang JK, Berland LL, Teefey SA, et al. ACR thyroid imaging, reporting and data system (TI-RADS): white paper of the ACR TI-RADS committee. *J Am Coll Radiol* 2017;**14**(5):587–95.

33. Alexander EK, Pearce EN, Brent GA, Brown RS, Chen H, Dosiou C, et al. 2017 Guidelines of the american thyroid association for the diagnosis and management of thyroid disease during pregnancy and the postpartum. *Thyroid* 2017;**27**(3):315–89.

34. Moosa M, Mazzaferri EL. Outcome of differentiated thyroid cancer diagnosed in pregnant women. *J Clin Endocrinol Metab* 1997;**82**(9):2862–6.

35. Yasmeen S, Cress R, Romano PS, Xing G, Berger-Chen S, Danielsen B, et al. Thyroid cancer in pregnancy. *Int J Gynaecol Obstet* 2005;**91**(1):15–20.

36. Herzon FS, Morris DM, Segal MN, Rauch G, Parnell T. Coexistent thyroid cancer and pregnancy. *Arch Otolaryngol Head Neck Surg* 1994;**120**(11):1191–3.

37. Vannucchi G, Perrino M, Rossi S, Colombo C, Vicentini L, Dazzi D, et al. Clinical and molecular features of differentiated thyroid cancer diagnosed during pregnancy. *Eur J Endocrinol* 2010;**162**(1):145–51.

38. Messuti I, Corvisieri S, Bardesono F, Rapa I, Giorcelli J, Pellerito R, et al. Impact of pregnancy on prognosis of differentiated thyroid cancer: clinical and molecular features. *Eur J Endocrinol* 2014;**170**(5):659–66.

39. Lee JC, Zhao JT, Clifton-Bligh RJ, Gill AJ, Gundara JS, Ip J, et al. Papillary thyroid carcinoma in pregnancy: a variant of the disease? *Ann Surg Oncol* 2012;**19**(13):4210–6.

40. Oh H-S, Kim WG, Park S, Kim M, Kwon H, Jeon MJ, et al. Serial neck ultrasonographic evaluation of changes in papillary thyroid carcinoma during pregnancy. *Thyroid* 2017;**27**(6):773–7.

41. Nakamura S, Sakata S, Komaki T, Kojima N, Kamikubo K, Miyazaki S, et al. Serum thyroglobulin concentration in normal pregnancy. *Endocrinol Jpn* 1984;**31**(6):675–9.

42. Rasmussen NG, Hornnes PJ, Hegedüs L, Feldt-Rasmussen U. Serum thyroglobulin during the menstrual cycle, during pregnancy, and post partum. *Acta Endocrinol* 1989;**121**(2):168–73.

43. Leboeuf R, Emerick LE, Martorella AJ, Tuttle RM. Impact of pregnancy on serum thyroglobulin and detection of recurrent disease shortly after delivery in thyroid cancer survivors. *Thyroid* 2007;**17**(6):543–7.

44. Sisson JC, Freitas J, McDougall IR, Dauer LT, Hurley JR, Brierley JD, et al. Radiation safety in the treatment of patients with thyroid diseases by radioiodine 131I: practice recommendations of the American Thyroid Association. *Thyroid* 2011;**21**(4):335–46.

45. Azizi F, Smyth P. Breastfeeding and maternal and infant iodine nutrition. *Clin Endocrinol* 2009;**70**(5):803–9.

46. Suman P, Wang CH, Abadin SS, Block R, Raghavan V, Moo-Young TA, et al. Timing of radioactive iodine therapy does not impact overall survival in high-risk papillary thyroid carcinoma. *Endocr Pract* 2016;**22**(7):822–31.

47. Li H, Zhang YQ, Wang C, Zhang X, Li X, Lin YS. Delayed initial radioiodine therapy related to incomplete response in low- to intermediate-risk differentiated thyroid cancer. *Clin Endocrinol* 2018;**88**(4):601–6.

48. Wells Jr SA, Asa SL, Dralle H, Elisei R, Evans DB, Gagel RF, et al. Revised American Thyroid Association Guidelines for the management of medullary thyroid carcinoma. *Thyroid* 2015;**25**(6):567–610.

49. Rosario PW, Barroso AL, Purisch S. The effect of subsequent pregnancy on patients with thyroid carcinoma apparently free of the disease. *Thyroid* 2007;**17**(11):1175–6.

50. Hirsch D, Levy S, Tsvetov G, Weinstein R, Lifshitz A, Singer J, et al. Impact of pregnancy on outcome and prognosis of survivors of papillary thyroid cancer. *Thyroid* 2010;**20**(10):1179–85.

51. Rakhlin L, Fish S, Tuttle RM. Response to therapy status is an excellent predictor of pregnancy-associated structural disease progression in patients previously treated for differentiated thyroid cancer. *Thyroid* 2017;**27**(3):396–401.

52. Alexander EK, Marqusee E, Lawrence J, Jarolim P, Fischer GA, Larsen PR. Timing and magnitude of increases in levothyroxine requirements during pregnancy in women with hypothyroidism. *N Engl J Med* 2004;**351**(3):241–9.

53. Zamfirescu I, Carlson HE. Absorption of levothyroxine when coadministered with various calcium formulations. *Thyroid* 2011;**21**(5):483–6.

54. Rowe C, Murray K, Woods A, Gupta S, Smith R, Wynne K. Metastatic thyroid cancer in pregnancy: risk and uncertainty. *Endocrinol Diabetes Metab Case Rep* 2016;**2016**(1).

55. Casey BM, Dashe JS, Wells CE, McIntire DD, Leveno KJ, Cunningham FG. Subclinical hyperthyroidism and pregnancy outcomes. *Obstet Gynecol* 2006;**107**(2 Pt 1):337–41.

56. Millar LK, Wing DA, Leung AS, Koonings PP, Montoro MN, Mestman JH. Low birth weight and preeclampsia in pregnancies complicated by hyperthyroidism. *Obstet Gynecol* 1994;**84**(6):946–9.

57. International Atomic Energy Agency. *Radiation protection of pregnant women in nuclear medicine*. International Atomic Energy Agency; 2018. [cited 2018 January]; Available from: https://www.iaea.org/resources/rpop/health-professionals/nuclear-medicine/pregnant-women.

58. Garsi JP, Schlumberger M, Rubino C, Ricard M, Labbe M, Ceccarelli C, et al. Therapeutic administration of 131I for differentiated thyroid cancer: radiation dose to ovaries and outcome of pregnancies. *J Nucl Med* 2008;**49**(5):845–52.

59. Sawka AM, Lakra DC, Lea J, Alshehri B, Tsang RW, Brierley JD, et al. A systematic review examining the effects of therapeutic radioactive iodine on ovarian function and future pregnancy in female thyroid cancer survivors. *Clin Endocrinol* 2008;**69**(3):479–90.

60. Yaish I, Azem F, Gutfeld O, Silman Z, Serebro M, Sharon O, et al. A single radioactive iodine treatment has a deleterious effect on ovarian reserve in women with thyroid cancer: results of a prospective pilot study. *Thyroid* 2018;**28**(4):522–7.

61. Pacini F, Gasperi M, Fugazzola L, Ceccarelli C, Lippi F, Centoni R, et al. Testicular function in patients with differentiated thyroid carcinoma treated with radioiodine. *J Nucl Med* 1994;**35**(9):1418–22.

62. Shindo H, Amino N, Ito Y, Kihara M, Kobayashi K, Miya A, et al. Papillary thyroid microcarcinoma might progress during pregnancy. *Thyroid* 2014;**24**(5):840–4.

63. Ito Y, Miyauchi A, Kudo T, Ota H, Yoshioka K, Oda H, et al. Effects of pregnancy on papillary microcarcinomas of the thyroid re-evaluated in the entire patient series at Kuma Hospital. *Thyroid* 2015;**26**(1):156–60.

64. U.S Food & Drug Administration. *Lenvima prescribing information*. FDA; 2015. Available from: https://www.accessdata.fda.gov/drugsatfda_docs/label/2016/208692s000lbl.pdf. Accessed 22 January 2018.

65. U.S Food & Drug Administration. *Nexavar prescribing information*. FDA; 2013. Available from: https://www.accessdata.fda.gov/drugsatfda_docs/label/2013/021923s016lbl.pdf. Accessed 22 January 2018.

66. Thomas N, Glod J, Derse-Anthony C, Baple EL, Obsborne N, Sturley R, et al. Pregnancy on vandetanib in metastatic medullary thyroid carcinoma associated with multiple endocrine neoplasia type 2B. *Clin Endocrinol* 2018;**88**(5):754–6.

Chapter 21

Disorders of Mineral and Bone Metabolism During Pregnancy and Lactation

Christopher S. Kovacs*, Marlene Chakhtoura[†] and Ghada El-Hajj Fuleihan[†]

*Faculty of Medicine, Endocrinology, Memorial University of Newfoundland, St. John's, NL, Canada, [†]Calcium Metabolism and Osteoporosis Program, WHO Collaborating Center for Metabolic Bone Disorders, Faculty of Medicine, American University of Beirut—Medical Center, Beirut, Lebanon

---

Common Clinical Problems

- Multiple vertebral crush fractures can occur in association with pregnancy, especially with lactation; pharmacotherapy has an uncertain benefit in these cases.
- Physiological hypercalciuria during pregnancy will mask the diagnosis of familial hypocalciuric hypercalcemia (FHH), while physiological hypocalciuria during lactation can mask the diagnosis of primary hyperparathyroidism.
- Mild primary hyperparathyroidism can cause a sudden hypercalcemic crisis in the third trimester or puerperium, as well as fetal parathyroid suppression that leads to prolonged neonatal hypocalcemia.
- Hypercalcemia can also occur during pregnancy due to excess calcitriol (from 24-hydroxylase deficiency) or excess parathyroid hormone-related protein (PTHrP) arising from the breasts, placenta, or both.
- Hypoparathyroidism can improve during pregnancy (requiring less supplemental calcium or calcitriol), but in some instances the condition can worsen (requiring increased doses of supplements).
- Lactation improves or normalizes mineral homeostasis in hypoparathyroidism, such that severe hypercalcemia can ensue if supplemental calcium and calcitriol are not reduced or stopped.

21.1 INTRODUCTION

As discussed in Chapter 5, specific adaptations are invoked to meet the increased mineral requirements of the developing fetus and neonate. Increased intestinal absorption of calcium and phosphorus is the main adaptation during pregnancy, while increased skeletal resorption of minerals predominates during lactation. In turn, these adaptations can influence the presentation, diagnosis, and management of disorders of bone and mineral metabolism that may predate pregnancy or onset for the first time during a reproductive cycle.

For more detailed citation of more than 1000 papers of primary animal and human data relevant to this subject, the reader is referred to a recent comprehensive review.[1] We have updated the results of this review with a systematic search conducted in PubMed and Medline current to April 2018. Due to restrictions on the length of the reference list, only selected recent papers will be cited herein.

21.2 DISORDERS OF BONE AND MINERAL METABOLISM DURING PREGNANCY

21.2.1 Osteoporosis in Pregnancy

The first description of osteoporosis occurring in association with pregnancy is often attributed to Albright and Reifenstein in 1948,[2] although low bone mineral density (BMD) and vertebral fractures have been recognized in Egyptian mummies and other archaeological remains of women who were 16–30 years of age at the time of their deaths several millennia ago.[3] Fragility fractures rarely occur during pregnancy, but they are somewhat more common during lactation, as described in Section 21.3. Although fragility fractures may occur at any skeletal site, two presentations have generally been reported in association with pregnancy: vertebral compression fractures and transient osteoporosis of the hip.[4]

Maternal-Fetal and Neonatal Endocrinology. https://doi.org/10.1016/B978-0-12-814823-5.00021-0

21.2.1.1 Vertebral and Appendicular Fractures in Pregnancy

Fragility fractures during pregnancy are rare, but among them, vertebral compression fractures have been described most often. The condition may be underrecognized and underreported, given how often back pain is reported with pregnancy. In general, case reports and series have emphasized women who presented with a cascade of multiple compression fractures.[4,5] However, one recent retrospective study spanning 17 years suggested that ankle and other lower limb fractures (67%) may be more common during pregnancy, usually occurring with falls, whereas vertebral fractures occur without much trauma.[6]

Pregnancy-related fractures typically occur in women not previously known to have any abnormality of bone or mineral metabolism.[1,7,8] Consequently, a BMD reading prior to pregnancy is usually unavailable. Investigations typically reveal normal serum chemistries and bone-relevant hormones. However, BMD is usually low at diagnosis and shows spontaneous improvement afterward, thereby implicating that transient bone loss occurred during pregnancy. Of the small number of bone biopsies that have been reported, the methodology was not detailed, publication preceded the standardized histomorphometry nomenclature for reporting,[9] the timing since delivery varied, some had no tetracycline label uptake, and a few reported findings consistent with mild osteoporosis.[10–12]

Fractures may occur because skeletal fragility preceded pregnancy or significant bone loss occurred during pregnancy. Table 21.1 lists the conditions that have been reported among women with pregnancy- or lactation-associated osteoporosis.

Insufficient calcium absorption can cause substantially increased skeletal resorption in order to meet the fetal and maternal requirements for calcium. Poor dietary calcium intake, lactose intolerance, vitamin D deficiency, celiac disease, and other malabsorptive disorders can all lead to the same outcome. For example, a woman's habitual intake of only 229 mg of calcium was likely a substantial factor resulting in high skeletal resorption, especially during the third trimester, to meet her own calcium needs and those of her baby, and thus leading to the cascade of vertebral compression fractures experienced during pregnancy.[4]

Parathyroid hormone-related protein (PTHrP) concentrations rise progressively in the maternal circulation during pregnancy. In some women, the release of PTHrP has been excessive, leading to high circulating levels, hypercalcemia, and even fractures (a condition called pseudohyperparathyroidism; see Section 21.2.6). While this is a relatively extreme situation, it is conceivable that less marked elevations in PTHrP may also occur, thereby inducing bone loss without causing symptomatic hypercalcemia.

The available data come largely from individual case reports, and mostly from small retrospective case, or case control, series.[4,5] Fractures typically occur in a first pregnancy, during the third trimester or the first few months in the postpartum period; are not necessarily associated with higher parity; and have a low risk of recurrence with future pregnancies.[4,13–17] For example, in a retrospective series of 52 patients with pregnancy-associated osteoporotic fractures, only 2 saw recurrence of a fracture during a second pregnancy.[5] The low risk of recurrence may imply that treatable factors (such as nutritional deficiencies) were corrected after the first pregnancy.

21.2.1.2 Transient Osteoporosis of the Hip

Transient osteoporosis of the hip is a rare condition causing skeletal fragility localized to one or both hips.[4,18] It may be a form of chronic regional pain syndrome 1 or reflex sympathetic dystrophy. Risk factors include pregnancy, alcohol, nicotine, corticosteroid, abnormal vascularity, drugs, inflammation, metabolic derangement, mechanical injury, neurologic deficit, and osteogenesis imperfecta.[4,18] Although the condition is more common in men, in women, it often onsets during the third trimester or puerperium with unilateral hip pain, limping, or a hip fracture; it may be bilateral at presentation or become so later. The femoral head and neck are osteopenic and radiolucent, while the hip BMD is usually quite low and out of keeping with the lumbar spine measurement. Magnetic resonance imaging (MRI) studies have revealed an edematous femoral head and neck. Prophylactic arthroplasties have been carried out in some cases. In women who were not operated on and did not fracture, the MRI and BMD abnormalities typically resolved within 3–12 months, accompanied by 20%–40% increases in femoral neck BMD. The question of whether these changes in BMD represent real changes in mineralization or artifacts resulting from changes in the marrow remains uncertain.

Several theories have been advanced to explain why pregnancy might increase the risk, including femoral venous stasis caused by pressure from the pregnant uterus, reduced activity or bed rest, and fetal pressure on the obturator nerve. It is not associated with systemic skeletal resorption, and thereby it appears to be distinct from the form of osteoporosis described previously, which leads to vertebral compression fractures. It may appear in any pregnancy and can recur in the opposite hip in a subsequent pregnancy. A few reported cases have involved women who had both vertebral compression fractures and transient osteoporosis of the hip, and thus the two conditions may share some pathophysiology or risk factors.[19–22]

TABLE 21.1 Conditions contributing to pregnancy- and lactation-related osteoporosis

Hormonal and endocrine disorders

Excess PTHrP-mediated bone resorption during pregnancy

Excess PTHrP- and low-estradiol-mediated resorption during lactation

Primary hyperparathyroidism

Hyperthyroidism

Cushing's syndrome

Chronic oligoamenorrhea

Hypothalamic amenorrhea

Pituitary disorders leading to sex steroid deficiency

Premature ovarian failure

Prolonged lactation

Diabetes (type 1 and 2)

Hypophosphatemic rickets

Nutritional

Low dietary calcium intake

Dairy avoidance

Lactose intolerance

Low vitamin D intake/vitamin D deficiency

Anorexia nervosa

Mechanical

Petite frame

Low body weight

Low peak bone mass

Excess exercise

Increased weight-bearing of pregnancy

Lordotic posture of pregnancy

Bed rest

Carrying child

Prolonged lactation with insufficient skeletal recovery afterward

Pharmacological

GnRH analog treatment

Depo-Provera

Glucocorticoids

Calcineurin inhibitors

Proton pump inhibitors

Certain antiseizure medications (phenytoin, carbamazepine)

Cancer chemotherapy

Alcohol

High-dose thyroxine

Continued

TABLE 21.1 Conditions contributing to pregnancy- and lactation-related osteoporosis—cont'd

Cyclosporine
Heparin (long term)
Highly active antiretroviral therapy
Antidepressants (particularly selective serotonin reuptake inhibitors)
Excess vitamin A intake
Thiazolidinediones
Gastrointestinal
Celiac disease
Crohn's disease
Cystic fibrosis
Other malabsorptive disorders
Renal
Hypercalciuria/renal calcium leak
Chronic renal insufficiency
Renal tubular acidosis
Primary disorders of bone quality
Osteogenesis imperfecta
Osteopetrosis and other sclerosing bone disorders
LRP5-inactivating mutations
Hypophosphatasia
Hematologic disorders
Thalassemia
Sickle cell disease
Leukemia
Connective tissue disorders
Ehlers-Danlos syndrome
Marfan syndrome
Rheumatological disorders
Rheumatoid arthritis
Systemic lupus erythematosus
Mastocytosis
Other nonspecified genetic disorders
Family history of osteoporosis or skeletal fragility
Idiopathic osteoporosis
Other
Hereditary hemochromatosis
Gaucher's disease
Malignancy: breast cancer

21.2.1.3 Investigations and Overall Management Considerations

Table 21.2 lists suggested investigations for women who present with low trauma fractures during pregnancy (or lactation), while Table 21.3 lists additional suggested investigations for women who present with multiple vertebral compression fractures.[4,7,8]

Because fragility fractures occur rarely during or after pregnancy, there are no randomized trials of management approaches. Sound clinical judgment must be used to balance the potential benefit and risks of treatments, which are delineated in Table 21.4. With both vertebral compression fractures and transient osteoporosis of the hip, spontaneous recovery of bone mass and strength typically occurs (even when there were fractures), so watchful waiting may be the first approach. Pharmacological therapy in the postpartum period and surgical intervention should be reserved for more severe or recalcitrant cases, such as those who experience multiple vertebral fractures or persistent disabling pain or who do not achieve a satisfactory spontaneous increase in BMD. The evidence regarding the safety and efficacy of drugs used during pregnancy is quite limited and mostly based on experience from case reports and series.[4,23]

21.2.1.4 Nonpharmacological Treatment

Calcium and vitamin D intake should be optimized for all women. For calcium, this is a total intake of 1200 mg/day elemental calcium from all sources, whereas for vitamin D, it is whatever intake is required to achieve a 25-hydroxyvitamin D (25OHD) level of at least >50–75 nmol/L (see the discussion of vitamin D replacement guidelines during pregnancy later in Section 21.2.7.4).[24] Reasonable weight-bearing physical activity should be encouraged, nutritional deficiencies should be corrected, and reversible causes of bone loss or fragility discovered during the workup should be treated wherever possible. Women who experienced compression fractures should avoid lifting heavy objects or other activities that may precipitate a fracture. A supportive corset may be helpful for short-term pain relief. Breastfeeding for the first few weeks postpartum may be allowed in order to optimize neonatal immunity through the transfer of maternal immunoglobulins. However, this must be balanced against the progressive loss in BMD and transient increase in fracture risk that may occur with prolonged breastfeeding, as explained in Chapter 5.

21.2.1.5 Pharmacological Therapy

It is tempting to prescribe antiosteoporosis medications immediately for women who fractured during pregnancy, but this enthusiasm should be tempered by the realization that BMD normally increases during the subsequent 6–12 months in women who fractured, without any interventions. Indeed, BMD by dual X-ray absorptiometry (DXA) or quantitative computed tomography (qCT) was shown to increase spontaneously by means of 20%–70% in such cases.[15,17,25–29] Furthermore, the common antiresorptive treatments lead to a secondary reduction in osteoblast activity, which raises the concern that such treatments could impair spontaneous skeletal recovery. Therefore, it would be prudent to delay the use of pharmacological therapy for 12–18 months until the extent of spontaneous recovery has been assessed.

Pharmacological therapy has been used in many women who presented with clinical fractures associated with pregnancy. This includes nasal calcitonin, bisphosphonates, denosumab, strontium ranelate, and teriparatide (see Refs. 1 and 4 for an extensive list of studies). The doses were typically the same as those for postmenopausal osteoporosis. Treatment duration varied between 6 months and 2–3 years, and can extend to as much as 10 years.[1,4,5,30–35] Breastfeeding was usually stopped during treatment, while subsequent pregnancies occurred as early as 3 months after pharmacological therapy ended. All these reports are observational and lacked controls to determine whether the BMD changes exceeded the substantial (20%–70%) increments that would have been observed with spontaneous recovery. These agents are generally not indicated for premenopausal women, so any use is off-label.[4,7,23] In postmenopausal women, there are concerns about potential long-term skeletal and nonskeletal adverse effects of bisphosphonates, denosumab, and strontium ranelate.[4] Calcitonin is available now only in injectable form for short-term use. Given the safety concerns, clinicians should carefully consider whether a young woman should be committed to long-term treatment and what the end point might be.

Additional concerns are that bisphosphonates cross the placenta and theoretically could interfere with fetal endochondral bone development. However, in a review of 78 patients in whom bisphosphonates were used during pregnancy, no obvious problems were reported in most cases, with the possible exception of transient hypocalcemia in the infant with bisphosphonate use during lactation.[23] The number of pregnancies involving bisphosphonate use is too small to be completely reassured about its safety. Denosumab should be avoided because it crosses the placenta and caused an osteopetrotic-like disorder in cynomolgus monkeys and mice.[36,37] Teriparatide and abaloparatide are limited to 24 months of lifetime exposure, and their use might be best reserved for older people, when fracture risk can be expected to be substantially higher.

TABLE 21.2 Suggested initial investigations

Anthropometric

Height by stadiometer

Weight

Body mass index (BMI)

Comparison to best recalled height or prior documented height

Radiological

Areal BMD by DXA (preferred use of *z*-scores)

Plain radiographs of thoracic and lumbar spine to assess for compression fractures

Radiographs of both hips (when presenting with hip pain or fracture)

MRI of affected hips (when presenting with hip pain or fracture)

Dietary assessment for nutritional deficiencies

Calcium intake

Vitamin D intake

Other nutritional deficiencies

Hematological

Complete blood count

Erythrocyte sedimentation rate (ESR)

Serum protein electrophoresis/myeloma screen

Biochemical

Electrolytes

Epidermal growth factor receptor (EGFR)

Ionized calcium or albumin-corrected serum calcium

Serum phosphate

Serum magnesium

Alkaline phosphatase

25-Hydroxyvitamin D

TTG and antiendomesial antibodies

Hormonal

PTH

PTHrP

Thyroid-stimulating hormone (TSH)

Luteinizing hormone (LH), follicle-stimulating hormone (FSH), estradiol (off hormonal contraceptives)

Prolactin

Urine

24-h urine calcium, creatinine, and sodium[a]

[a]Note that 24-h urine calcium may be high (hypercalciuric) during pregnancy and low (hypocalciuric) during lactation; see Chapter 5.

TABLE 21.3 Additional secondary investigations in severe cases

Radiological

Skeletal survey for evidence of sclerosing bone disorders

Radionuclide bone scan for evidence of myeloma or other pathology

Biochemical

Bone formation markers[a]—e.g., bone-specific alkaline phosphatase, P1NP, or osteocalcin

Bone resorption markers[a]—e.g., C-telopeptide (CTX), N-telopeptide (NTX), or deoxypyridinoline/creatinine

Ferritin or serum iron measurements

Tryptase, IgE levels

Glucocerebrosidase

Hormonal

Calcitriol

24-h urine-free cortisol

Late-night salivary cortisol

Other

Bone biopsy at hip fracture site

Tetracycline-labeled, transiliac bone biopsy

Genetic referral when family history of early or severe fragility present (low BMD and/or vertebral fracture, and/or multiple fractures) in the absence of secondary causes, constitutional leanness, and late puberty

Gastroenterology referral for small bowel biopsy in those who have abdominal symptoms but negative celiac antibodies

[a]Note that there are confounding considerations if these are measured during pregnancy or lactation; see Chapter 5.

21.2.1.6 Surgical Therapy

Vertebroplasty and kyphoplasty introduce cement into a crushed vertebral body to treat painful vertebral fractures during the postpartum period. The overall efficacy of these methods is uncertain, given that blind, randomized trials have found no superiority over sham surgery or medical approaches in older subjects.[38, 38a] Another concern is that the cement may increase mechanical strain on adjacent vertebrae, thereby predisposing to more crush fractures.

For transient osteoporosis of the hip, the main consideration is whether to rod the affected femur or femurs prophylactically or only to observe, expecting spontaneous recovery without fracture.

21.2.2 Primary Hyperparathyroidism

21.2.2.1 Incidence and Epidemiology

Hypercalcemia, which presumably and in large part represents primary hyperparathyroidism, has been found in 0.03% of routinely screened, reproductive age women, but how often it is present during pregnancy is uncertain.[1] There are at least several hundred cases in English-language medical journals, while the first author's advice has been sought for several cases each year by clinicians across North America. Two case series found that approximately 1% of all parathyroidectomies were done during pregnancy,[39,40] so the condition may not be as rare as previously thought. Similar to nonpregnant cases, single adenomas are the most common pathology, followed by four-gland hyperplasia.

The dilutional fall in serum albumin and calcium that occur during normal pregnancy (see Chapter 5) may mask hypercalcemia, delay the diagnosis, and contribute to it being underrecognized. The albumin-corrected calcium or ionized calcium should be used, combined with a nonsuppressed parathyroid hormone (PTH) level, to diagnose primary hyperparathyroidism during pregnancy.[1,41,42]

TABLE 21.4 Suggested treatment strategy

For all women

Optimize calcium and vitamin D intake

Early mobilization; avoid bed rest

Encourage weight-bearing and muscle-strengthening physical activity

Consider shortening the duration of lactation (with pregnancy fractures) or weaning the baby (with lactation fractures)

Avoid lifting heavy objects

Avoid high-risk activities that include flexion, twisting, sudden loads, or risk of falls

Supportive corset (temporary) for vertebral fracture pain

Cane or crutches for transient osteoporosis of the hip without fracture

Assess spontaneous recovery of vertebral BMD at 12–18 months and reassess

Assess spontaneous recovery of hip edema (MRI) and BMD (DXA) at 12–18 months

For severe cases (Recurrent fractures, disabling pain, insufficient spontaneous regain of vertebral BMD)

Analgesia

Paracetamol/Acetaminophen

NSAID

Opioids

Antineuropathic drugs

Bone-specific therapy[a]

Estrogen replacement for oligoamenorrheic women

Bisphosphonate (e.g., alendronate, risedronate, zoledronic acid)

Denosumab

Teriparatide

Parenteral calcitonin—only short-term use for vertebral fracture pain relief, if at all

Surgical treatment[a]

Kyphoplasty

Vertebroplasty

Spinal fusion

For transient osteoporosis of the hip

Analgesia

Paracetamol/acetaminophen

Nonsteroidal antiinflammatory drug (NSAID)

Opioids

Surgical treatment[a]

Hip replacement/arthroplasty for fracture

Consider prophylactic arthroplasty or rodding for opposite hip if radiological features indicate low BMD with increased water content

[a]*Drugs or surgical intervention should be considered only in severe refractory cases that do not improve with conservative measures because the safety and efficacy of these approaches is not well established in these conditions.*

On the other hand, pregnancy can also worsen primary hyperparathyroidism because the physiological changes of pregnancy have their own effects to increase intestinal calcium absorption, hypercalciuria, and bone resorption. Indeed, primary hyperparathyroidism during pregnancy is perceived to confer higher risks of severe hypercalcemia, pancreatitis, and kidney stones. On balance, the transfer of calcium across the placenta and into the developing fetus should protect somewhat against severe maternal hypercalcemia by creating an outflow for excess calcium. This likely explains why sudden hypercalcemic crises have occurred after delivery. Physical inactivity and bed rest during late pregnancy and the puerperium will also increase skeletal resorption, which in turn aggravates hypercalcemia.

Maternal hypercalcemia has been shown in animal models to increase the flow of calcium across the placenta and suppress the fetal parathyroids. Fetal hypercalcemia in turn causes increased renal water excretion and polyhydramnios.

21.2.2.2   Clinical Presentation

Maternal hypercalcemia causes nonspecific, constitutional symptoms (e.g., nausea, constipation, fatigue, weakness, and mental symptoms), which are difficult to distinguish from those of normal pregnancy. More severe hypercalcemia has been associated with hyperemesis, weight loss, seizures, and preeclampsia. Additional maternal signs may include nephrocalcinosis, nephrolithiasis, urinary tract infection, acute pancreatitis, bone loss, and fractures. It can rarely present as brown tumors of the jaw.[43] The serum calcium may be somewhat reduced initially due to the dilutional fall in serum albumin, but the calcium may rise higher under the influence of the pregnancy-related increase in intestinal calcium absorption. A hypercalcemic crisis can occur during the third trimester or puerperium.

Risks to the fetus and neonate include miscarriage, stillbirth, intrauterine growth retardation, premature birth, transient hypocalcemia, and rarely permanent hypoparathyroidism. These are discussed in Chapter 44.

21.2.2.3   Approach and Management

There have been four international consensus conferences on the management of primary hyperparathyroidism, but none have addressed pregnancy.[44]

Localizing an adenoma preoperatively is difficult because radioisotope-based parathyroid scans must be avoided, ultrasound has limited sensitivity, 10%–20% of cases may involve hyperplasia of all four glands, and ectopic parathyroids occur.

Traditionally, parathyroidectomy has been done during the second trimester to avoid fetal and neonatal morbidity and mortality, as well as maternal hypercalcemic crisis during the third trimester or postpartum period. Due to the rarity of this condition, there are no randomized trials comparing medical vs surgical approaches. In a 1991 review of 109 cases, neonatal deaths and morbidity were lower in surgically treated mothers than medically treated mothers, but the analysis was confounded by the undeclared circumstances that led clinicians to choose a particular modality in each case.[40] If surgery is to be performed, the second trimester is preferred for the lower risks of anesthetic or surgical complications, precipitated delivery, and neonatal death, although other reports have defended the apparent safety of intervening during the third trimester.

Modern cases of primary hyperparathyroidism are, for the most part, milder than the older cases in the literature. This has led to the impression that the adverse effects of primary hyperparathyroidism may be lower for the mother and baby, and that surgery may be safely delayed until postpartum. Analysis of a database registry found 1057 reproductive-age women with primary hyperparathyroidism (60% had been pregnant before the diagnosis, while 15% had been pregnant after it) who were compared to 3171 age-matched women. The rate of cesarean sections was doubled in women with primary hyperparathyroidism, there was no difference in the incidence of spontaneous abortions, and no data were available on other pregnancy outcomes or neonatal complications.[45] In another study, 134 pregnancies in 74 women with primary hyperparathyroidism were compared to 431 pregnancies in 175 normocalcemic women.[41] There were no differences in the rates of spontaneous abortions or pregnancy-related complications; however, neonatal complications were not reported.[41]

Other recent cases appear to confirm lower rates of stillbirth, neonatal death, and neonatal tetany than shown in older research. Yet fetal death still occurred in 30 out of 62 medically managed cases (maternal serum calcium correlated with the risk), but in none of 15 cases that were operated on during the second trimester.[46] Mild primary hyperparathyroidism in the mother can still result in a third-trimester hypercalcemic crisis, neonatal hypocalcemia, and even permanent neonatal hypoparathyroidism.[1] The variability of outcomes is probably related to other maternal and fetal risk factors for adverse obstetrical outcomes, as emphasized by a twin pregnancy in which one neonate had hypocalcemic seizures while the other remained normocalcemic.[47]

Medical management includes the first-line approach of hydration and correction of electrolyte abnormalities. Pharmacotherapy has not been systematically studied in pregnancy, but available medications have been used in individual case reports, with the same doses as those administered in nonpregnant women. Calcitonin is a Category B medication for pregnancy because it does not cross the placenta, and it has been used safely (4–8 IU/kg every 12 h) to suppress bone resorption and promote urine calcium excretion in pregnant women. Oral phosphate is Category C, with modest efficacy to bind calcium, but its use is limited by diarrhea, hypokalemia, and the potential risk of ectopic calcifications. Furosemide is a Category C medication that promotes renal calcium excretion. As mentioned previously, bisphosphonates (also Category C) cross the placenta, but no overt adverse skeletal effects have been seen; there may be an increased risk of neonatal hypocalcemia. Denosumab should be avoided because its transplacental passage has led to an osteopetrotic-like disorder in monkeys and mice.[36,37]

Cinacalcet is Category C, but it has been used during pregnancy in several cases, in doses ranging from 30 to 360 mg/day.[1] It suppresses PTH synthesis and release and stimulates calcitonin through its actions on the calcium receptor in the parathyroids and C-cells, respectively. The calcium receptor is also expressed in placenta, fetal parathyroids, and C-cells, which raises the concern that the drug may suppress the fetal parathyroids, stimulate fetal calcitonin, and alter placental calcium transfer. High-dose magnesium can be useful because it binds to the calcium receptor and lowers PTH and calcium. Heparin-free hemodialysis has been used to lower serum calcium before surgery.[48]

The relative benefits and risks of each option are uncertain, given that the data come from case reports and follow-up on the children has been very brief. Given that these women are young, genetic disorders that cause hypercalcemia should be ruled out through selective mutation analysis.

21.2.2.4 Conclusion: Surgical vs Medical Management?

Overall, maternal and fetal complications appear less likely to occur with the milder forms of primary hyperparathyroidism that are encountered in the modern era; however, risks are not completely absent.[1] Surgery is still preferred; ideally, it should be carried out during the second trimester if medical management fails or symptoms worsen. There is some consensus that a serum calcium level that persists at >2.80 mmol/L (11.1 mg/dL), or an ionized calcium >1.4 mmol/L (5.6 mg/dL), are indications for surgery.[49,50] A bilateral approach is often warranted because of the lack of preoperative imaging to localize the adenoma. If medical observation is undertaken for seemingly mild hypercalcemia, the clinician must beware of the potential for a hypercalcemic crisis to occur during the third trimester, and even more abruptly after delivery. Newborns must be watched for neonatal hypocalcemia that may have an immediate or delayed presentation.

21.2.3 Familial Hypocalciuric Hypercalcemia

Autosomal-dominant, inactivating mutations of the calcium receptor gene (*CASR*) account for the majority of cases of FHH. It is characterized by hypercalcemia, hypocalciuria [with a calcium/creatinine (Ca/Cr) clearance ratio of <0.01], and nonsuppressed PTH.[51] It is asymptomatic, probably because its origin in utero[52] results in full adaptation of the brain and other tissues to hypercalcemia, while the hypocalciuria protects against nephrocalcinosis and stones.

A pregnant woman with known FHH will have persistent hypercalcemia with nonsuppressed PTH; the serum calcium may rise even higher during the second and third trimesters. Importantly, the normal diagnostic criteria of FHH cannot be used because the pregnancy-related increase in intestinal calcium absorption results in absorptive hypercalciuria and a Ca/Cr clearance of well over 0.01.[53,54] Consequently, FHH presenting during pregnancy can be easily mistaken for primary hyperparathyroidism.

FHH does not pose any maternal risks; however, the fetal parathyroids can become suppressed by even mild maternal hypercalcemia. Consequently, women have been diagnosed with FHH in the puerperium after their newborns presented with neonatal hypocalcemia or seizures. With the mother having FHH, neonates are also at increased risk not only for inheriting FHH, but also for developing neonatal severe hypercalcemia (see Chapter 44).

21.2.3.1 Clinical Management

The key approach to FHH is to consider the diagnosis whenever a woman presents with hypercalcemia during pregnancy, and also to be wary that fractional urine calcium excretion will not be suppressed. A genetic test may be needed to confirm the diagnosis. Above all else, FHH must not be mistaken for primary hyperparathyroidism. Surgery is never indicated for FHH; moreover, a seemingly normal serum calcium level will be experienced as symptomatic hypocalcemia by someone with FHH. Unfortunately, at least one woman with FHH underwent a three-and-a-half-gland parathyroidectomy during the second trimester when she presented with marked hypercalcemia and hypercalciuria in pregnancy. FHH was only considered and recognized after maternal hypercalcemia persisted and her neonate developed hypercalcemia.[53] When pregnant women were recognized to have FHH, the serum calcium was not treated; however, close monitoring of the neonate for hypocalcemia is recommended.

21.2.4 Hypoparathyroidism

Studies in genetic and surgical animal models of hypoparathyroidism have shown that maternal hypocalcemia is hazardous for the fetus, with increased likelihood of the development of secondary hyperparathyroidism, skeletal demineralization, and fragility fractures occurring in utero or during and after delivery.[1] These adverse outcomes do not occur if the mother is normocalcemic or has mild hypocalcemia. Moreover, these models also have shown that maternal hypocalcemia can spontaneously improve during pregnancy, whereas it worsens in other models.[1] A physiological increase in calcitriol synthesis and intestinal calcium absorption still occur during pregnancy without PTH, but with varying effectiveness.[1]

The same divergent outcomes have been documented in women in whom hypoparathyroidism was known to be present prior to pregnancy. But longstanding hypoparathyroidism can also be asymptomatic, and some affected women have not been diagnosed until their newborns presented with severe secondary hyperparathyroidism, hypercalcemia, increased bone resorption, and fractures. As in the animal models, maternal hypocalcemia can have serious effects on the fetus and neonate (see Chapter 44).

Multiple published cases have shown that hypoparathyroidism can improve during pregnancy, as seen by fewer hypocalcemic symptoms and reduced need for supplemental calcium or treatment with calcitriol, 1α-cholecalciferol, or vitamin D.[1] In a well-documented case, calcitriol was stopped and the woman required only 1.2 g of calcium intake daily during the third trimester.[55] In a group of 10 cases of hypoparathyroidism, serum calcium declined due to the pregnancy-related fall in serum albumin, but the ionized calcium remained normal during pregnancy, with no need for calcitriol.[56] The author is aware of other unpublished cases in which hypoparathyroidism improved during pregnancy, and the dose of calcitriol was significantly decreased or stopped. When hypoparathyroidism improves during pregnancy, that may imply that upregulation of calcitriol synthesis, intestinal calcium absorption, or both have occurred without PTH, but they may possibly be due to PTHrP, consistent with what has been seen in rodent models.[1] However, in 1 case where maternal symptoms were subjectively improved but serum calcium measurements were not taken, the fetus had secondary hyperparathyroidism, which suggests that maternal hypocalcemia must have been present.[57]

Other reports have documented no change in serum calcium during pregnancy while on stable replacement doses of calcium and calcitriol/vitamin D; however, in some of these cases, serum calcium even increased in the last week or two before delivery.[1] In all these cases, serum calcium was not adjusted for the declining serum albumin, so the lack of a drop in unadjusted serum calcium during pregnancy may imply that ionized calcium had increased. Two reports on hypoparathyroid women found that ionized calcium did not change during pregnancy,[58,59] but in one case, the ionized calcium abruptly fell during labor, perhaps due to hyperventilation-induced alkalosis.[58]

However, other reports have found significant worsening of calcium metabolism during pregnancy. The evidence for this includes a decline in serum calcium, hypocalcemic symptoms that may increase, and increases in the prescribed doses of supplemental calcium and vitamin D, 1α-cholecalciferol, or calcitriol.[1] In most cases, calcitriol levels were not done or cannot be interpreted because of concurrent treatment with calcitriol or 1α-cholecalciferol (endogenous and exogenous calcitriol are indistinguishable).

However, in some of the reports in which hypoparathyroidism appeared to worsen during pregnancy, the normal dilutional decrease in serum calcium during pregnancy appears to have prompted an increase in the prescribed doses of calcium, vitamin D, or calcitriol.[1] In other words, the artifactual decline in total serum calcium, which is physiologically irrelevant, was misinterpreted to mean that an intervention was required. For example, in 1 case, the serum albumin had fallen from 4.2 to 2.0 g/dL, and the resulting change in serum calcium prompted increases in the doses of calcium and calcitriol.[60] But when the data in that report are reviewed, it is clear that the albumin-corrected serum calcium rose from 9.5 mg/dL (normal) in early pregnancy to 10.2 mg/dL (also normal) by 2 weeks before delivery; it had not decreased. Similarly, treatment of the albumin-related drop in unadjusted serum calcium resulted in women becoming hypercalcemic,[61,62] which confers fetal risks, as described earlier. In another case, an increase in urine calcium excretion was misinterpreted as worsening hypoparathyroidism when it represented the consequence of the pregnancy-related physiological increase in intestinal calcium absorption.[63] In yet another case, hypoparathyroidism did objectively worsen during pregnancy, but it was in a woman who took high-dose prednisone and azathioprine for a kidney transplant;[64] the high-dose prednisone would have reduced intestinal calcium absorption and likely played a role in what occurred during that pregnancy.

In summary, the available evidence indicates that many hypoparathyroid women have improvements in calcium metabolism during pregnancy, whereas some have objective evidence of worsening. In still other cases, the artifactual fall in total serum calcium or the physiological increase in urine calcium excretion was misinterpreted as evidence of worsening of hypoparathyroidism. A recent study of 10 cases by one group of investigators similarly found that some pregnant hypoparathyroid women improved, while others worsened.[65]

Why does hypoparathyroidism improve during pregnancy in some women and yet appear to worsen in others? It may be due to variability in the adaptive responses to pregnancy or in the achieved concentrations of hormones that stimulate intestinal calcium absorption or calcitriol synthesis. For example, high estradiol concentrations occur in pregnancy and have somewhat opposing effects of suppressing bone turnover and stimulating Cyp27b1 activity to synthesize calcitriol. If the greatest effect is on stimulating Cyp27b1, that may lead to overall improvements in pregnancy, as opposed to a potential worsening in women in whom the suppression of bone turnover may be more dominant. There also may be variations in how much PTHrP is released from the breasts and placenta, or in the increases in other pregnancy hormones (placental lactogen, oxytocin, etc.) that are thought to contribute to maternal mineral homeostasis during pregnancy. Calcium intake is critical, with Institute of Medicine guidelines suggesting a daily requirement of 1200 mg of calcium during pregnancy.[24] Yet in half of the reports in which hypoparathyroidism appeared to worsen during pregnancy, either no supplemental calcium or at most 300 mg/day was consumed, and the dietary intake of calcium was not determined.[1] Lack of adequate calcium intake in the first half of pregnancy will prevent the net positive calcium balance that is normally achieved, and it also may increase the likelihood of inadequate calcium delivery to the fetus in the third trimester.

21.2.4.1 Clinical Management

The available animal and human data, summarized previously, indicate two polar opposite extremes can occur when hypoparathyroid women become pregnant: there may be substantial improvement (normalization of serum calcium and phosphorus with reduced need for supplemental calcium and calcitriol) or worsening (more marked hypocalcemia requiring significant increases in supplemental calcium and calcitriol). There also will be women who exhibit no significant changes during pregnancy. These differences reflect such factors as variability in the adaptive response to increase intestinal calcium absorption during pregnancy despite the absence of PTH, as well as in the baseline calcium intake.

The ionized calcium or albumin-corrected calcium must be followed every 2–4 weeks during pregnancy, while changes in the unadjusted serum calcium should not be acted on. The prescribed doses of calcium and calcitriol (or other vitamin D analogs) need to be adjusted according to each individual's response to pregnancy. The doses will need to decrease in some women, others will require progressive increases, and still others may require no changes. PTH analogs are generally too expensive to use for physiological replacement and have not been formally studied during pregnancy, but a continuous infusion of teriparatide normalized calcium homeostasis during 1 pregnancy.[66]

In nonpregnant adults treated with calcium and calcitriol, the goal is to maintain the albumin-adjusted calcium or ionized calcium at or just below the lower end of normal. This minimizes hypocalcemic symptoms, while protecting the kidneys from an increased filtered load of calcium. However, during the 9 months of pregnancy, the ionized or albumin-corrected calcium should be preferably maintained within the normal range, in order to minimize the risk of fetal and neonatal complications from maternal hypocalcemia. Hypercalcemia also must be avoided because of the adverse effects that it has on fetal development. Thiazides are commonly used in the management of hypoparathyroidism, but they should be discontinued during pregnancy, as they are Category C medications.

21.2.5 Pseudohypoparathyroidism

Resistance to the actions of PTH is termed *pseudohypoparathyroidism*. This condition results not from absence of the PTH receptor, but from postreceptor defects in Gs-α that create end-organ resistance. Affected individuals have hypocalcemia, hyperphosphatemia, blunted phosphaturic response to PTH, and increased circulating concentrations of PTH. There are two main subtypes: Type I has blunted PTH-induced phosphaturia and renal production of cyclic adenosine monophosphate (cAMP), while Type II has just blunting of PTH-induced phosphaturia. They are managed similarly to hypoparathyroidism, with calcium, vitamin D, and calcitriol (or other analogs).

Type I pseudohypoparathyroidism improved during four pregnancies in women who maintained 1 g/day of supplemental calcium intake. Hypocalcemic symptoms lessened, normocalcemia was achieved, PTH levels lowered to near normal, endogenous calcitriol increased threefold to fourfold, urinary excretion of calcium normalized, and supplemental vitamin D, calcitriol, or analogs were no longer required.[67] Hypocalcemia and the need for supplemental calcium and calcitriol recurred within 3 weeks after delivery (none of the women breastfed). These reports are consistent with PTH-independent increases in intestinal calcium absorption and calcitriol synthesis occurring during pregnancy. In contrast, seven other pregnancies in women with Types I and II pseudohypoparathyroidism (described in detail in Ref. 1) resulted in subjective worsening of hypocalcemia-like symptoms or the need to increase the prescribed doses of calcium, calcitriol, or 1α-cholecalciferol.[1]

Overall, the clinical experience with pseudohypoparathyroidism appears to be similar to that of hypoparathyroidism, ranging from improvement to worsening, as described in Section 21.2.5. PTH-independent upregulation of calcitriol synthesis and intestinal calcium absorption could explain improved mineral metabolism in women with pseudohypoparathyroidism during pregnancy. Indeed, there is evidence of this from several pregnancies. Serum calcitriol doubled during the second and third trimesters in 2 women in whom supplemental calcitriol was discontinued. Another woman had increases in endogenous serum calcitriol during the first two trimesters, accompanied by stable serum calcium, but then serum calcitriol declined to the prepregnancy value in the third trimester, accompanied by reemergence of hypocalcemia. These changes in serum calcitriol among these women may indicate that a sustained increase in endogenous serum calcitriol during the third trimester predicts whether pseudohypoparathyroidism remains improved by pregnancy.

Placental production of calcitriol has previously been touted as a possible explanation for improvements in pseudohypoparathyroidism during pregnancy, but this is unlikely because the placenta contributes little calcitriol to the maternal circulation.[1] Analysis of placentas from 4 pseudohypoparathyroid women also confirmed that calcitriol production was no different than in placentas from normal women.[1]

As noted in Chapter 5, as well as in Section 21.2.4, evidence from animal models indicates that independent of PTH, other hormones of pregnancy may stimulate intestinal calcium absorption and the activity of Cyp27b1 to produce calcitriol. These considerations also apply to pseudohypoparathyroidism. It is also possible that hormonal changes during pregnancy (such as 100-fold higher estradiol) could improve postreceptor PTH signaling.

The intake of calcium is an important consideration. In four pregnancies in which pseudohypoparathyroidism objectively improved, the women took 1 g daily of supplemental calcium throughout.[67] In contrast, in pregnancies where pseudohypoparathyroidism appears to worsen, either no supplemental calcium was consumed, or at most 250–500 mg/day.[1] In none of these pregnancies was dietary intake of calcium assessed.

An intake of 1200 mg/day of calcium, combined with the doubling of efficiency of intestinal calcium absorption that occurs during normal pregnancy, should be more than sufficient to meet the combined needs of mother and fetus during a normal pregnancy. But if calcium intake is below this amount, then secondary hyperparathyroidism will be invoked to provide additional mineral from the mother's skeleton. Consequently, pseudohypoparathyroidism can be expected to worsen during pregnancy if oral calcium intake is insufficient.

21.2.5.1 Clinical Management

As is the case with hypoparathyroidism, women with pseudohypoparathyroidism can have polar opposite outcomes during pregnancy: an improved or worsened condition, as well as unchanged. Furthermore, the dilutional drop in total serum calcium that occurs during normal pregnancy—and which is physiologically unimportant—can be mistaken for evidence of clinical worsening.

Dietary calcium intake should be formally assessed and adjusted with supplements as needed to provide a total intake of 1200 mg/day. If dietary intake cannot be assessed, then a 1-g supplement may reasonably be prescribed to meet the combined maternal and fetal requirements. Variability in the responses of women with pseudohypoparathyroidism to the demands of pregnancy may be due to relative contributions of pregnancy-related hormones to regulating maternal mineral homeostasis, genetic or ethnic differences that influence these pregnancy-related adaptations, and the phenotypes of Type 1 or 2 pseudohypoparathyroidism. The progressive rise of PTHrP in the maternal circulation may have effects on maternal mineral metabolism, but this should not increase renal Cyp27b1 activity in women with pseudohypoparathyroidism because of the absence of Gs-α activity in the proximal tubules.

The goal of management should be to monitor and maintain normal ionized or albumin-corrected serum calcium in pregnant women with pseudohypoparathyroidism, thereby minimizing the risk of fetal and neonatal complications from maternal hypocalcemia or hypercalcemia. As with hypoparathyroidism, this means expectant management with adjustments to oral calcium and calcitriol doses as required during pregnancy. It should be anticipated that some women will require decreases in their doses to avoid hypercalcemia, while others will need increases to avoid hypocalcemia.

21.2.6 Pseudohyperparathyroidism

The breasts and placenta are sources of PTHrP in the maternal circulation during pregnancy.[1] It appears as if this increase in PTHrP results from autonomous production, or at least through mechanisms that are not responsive to maternal serum calcium. The production of PTHrP by the breasts during pregnancy may correlate with the amount of mammary tissue.

Pseudohyperparathyroidism is the condition of PTHrP-mediated hypercalcemia that occurs for physiological reasons, as opposed to hypercalcemia of malignancy, in which PTHrP is overproduced due to production by a tumor.

The development of this condition during pregnancy confirms that production of PTHrP by the breasts and placenta can alter the regulation of maternal mineral homeostasis. While this section discusses the onset of hypercalcemia as a result of PTHrP production during pregnancy, it is likely that the systemic release of PTHrP during normal pregnancy plays a role in maternal calcium and bone metabolism.

Hypercalcemia has developed as a consequence of very high circulating concentrations of PTHrP that have arisen from the breasts or placenta. The culprit is evident after reviewing the clinical course: hypercalcemia and PTHrP production persist after delivery, when the breasts are the source of PTHrP, whereas the serum calcium and PTHrP concentration plummet within a few hours when the placenta is the source.[1]

The breasts have been implicated in several cases of PTHrP-mediated hypercalcemia, including women with massive mammary hyperplasia (pregnant or nonpregnant), as well as in pregnant women with normal-sized breasts.[1] In several cases of hypercalcemia during pregnancy, serum PTH was undetectable, PTHrP circulated at a high concentration or its expression was markedly increased in breast tissue, and the hypercalcemia resolved only after weaning, bilateral mastectomy, or use of a dopamine agonist (bromocriptine or cabergoline). When PTHrP-mediated hypercalcemia persists after delivery, it confirms that breasts are the source of PTHrP because placental PTHrP should disappear from the circulation within minutes of the afterbirth. In a woman with marked hypercalcemia and an elevated PTHrP of 34.9 pmol/L during pregnancy, and who did not breastfeed, the hypercalcemia resolved slowly, while the elevated circulating PTHrP concentration persisted for 3 months.[68] This was evidently due to sustained production of PTHrP in the breasts, despite refraining from breastfeeding.

Release of PTHrP from the breasts occurs physiologically during lactation and partially or completely normalizes mineral homeostasis in women with hypoparathyroidism; this was discussed in Section 21.2.4. Pseudohyperparathyroidism also occurs from overproduction of PTHrP by the placenta. A clear-cut case involved a woman with normal-sized breasts who had severe hypercalcemia (21 mg/dL or 5.25 mmol/L), undetectable PTH, and a serum PTHrP of 21 pmol/L in the third trimester.[69] So, 6 h after an urgent cesarean section, she was profoundly hypocalcemic, with undetectable PTHrP and elevated PTH. The rapid reversal toward low PTHrP, high PTH, and hypocalcemia can be explained only by the abrupt loss of placental-derived PTHrP.

21.2.6.1 Clinical Management

It will be difficult to be certain of the source of excess PTHrP until after delivery. When the placenta is the cause, the hypercalcemia should self-correct within hours after delivery, whereas overproduction of PTHrP by the breasts is more likely to lead to hypercalcemia that persists and may worsen after delivery due to loss of the placental efflux of calcium and the onset of lactation. Prior to delivery, hypercalcemia may be addressed with fluid resuscitation and correction of electrolyte abnormalities, and the measures discussed previously with respect to primary hyperparathyroidism (loop diuretic, calcitonin, and bisphosphonate; denosumab should be avoided due to a transplacental passage). A more specific treatment that addresses the cause is bromocriptine or cabergoline, which can be expected to suppress both placental and mammary production of PTHrP.[70] A reduction mammoplasty is also a consideration if it is clear that the breasts are the cause, such as in massive mammary hyperplasia.

21.2.7 Vitamin D Deficiency, Genetic Vitamin D Resistance, and 24-Hydroxylase Deficiency

21.2.7.1 Animal Data: Vitamin D Deficiency and Genetic Vitamin D Resistance

Calcitriol's role in reproductive physiology has been examined through several approaches, including studying severely vitamin D-deficient rats, *Cyp27b1*-null mice that cannot make calcitriol, and *Vdr*-null mice that lack the receptor for calcitriol.[1] In all these instances, females conceive less frequently and bear fewer pups per litter. However, fertility is unaffected in *Cyp27b1*-null (Hannover) pigs, which bear only singletons or twins. In the rodent examples, both the reduced fertility and smaller litter sizes are fully treated by providing a high-calcium diet that is also enriched in lactose to enhance calcium absorption.[1] Therefore, it is not lack of calcitriol, but calcium itself, that causes these fertility problems.

Studies have also been carried out in severely vitamin D-deficient rats, *Cyp27b1*-null pigs, *Cyp27b1*-null mice, and *Vdr*-null mice, to determine if loss of calcitriol or its receptor causes any disruption of normal pregnancy.[1,71] In each study, occasional sudden deaths, presumably from hypocalcemia, occurred during late pregnancy in response to anesthesia or exposure to colder temperatures. This may indicate that rapid transfer of calcium across the placenta, which is at its highest rate during late pregnancy, can overwhelm maternal regulation of the ionized calcium. But as noted in Chapter 44, the fetuses of each of these models exhibit normal mineral homeostasis and skeletal development. This includes that *Vdr*-null fetuses and their WT littermates, and *Cyp27b1*-null fetuses and their WT littermates, which were indistinguishable from each other when born of their respective heterozygous-deleted mothers. However, all offspring of *Vdr*-null females were proportionately smaller than offspring of their WT and *Vdr*$^{+/-}$ sisters, a difference that was not seen between fetuses born of vitamin D-deficient and replete rats, or born of *Cyp27b1*-null vs WT mice.[72] The smaller sizes of offspring of *Vdr*-null mothers may indicate that maternal expression of VDR affects offspring growth, independent of the fetal genotypes and calcitriol.

Pregnancy in severely vitamin D-deficient rats, *Vdr*-null mice, and *Cyp27b1*-null mice results in increases in maternal serum calcium and phosphorus, suppression of secondary hyperparathyroidism, increased mineralization of osteoid, and significant gains in skeletal mineral content.[1,71] These improvements result from a calcitriol-independent increase in intestinal calcium absorption that has been confirmed in severely vitamin D-deficient rats and *Vdr*-null mice, and inferred to be present in *Cyp27b1*-null mice.[71] In these studies, it was the onset of pregnancy that invoked improvements in intestinal calcium absorption and mineral homeostasis, without requiring vitamin D, calcitriol, and VDR. What factors regulate the increase in intestinal calcium absorption during pregnancy in the absence of calcitriol remain unknown.[1] The apical calcium channels (Trpv6, Trpv5), the Ca2+-ATPase, and the sodium-calcium exchanger Ncx1, are upregulated within the enterocytes of normal mice during pregnancy,[1] whereas in *Vdr*-null mice, a further upregulation of Trpv6 and PTHrP has been seen compared to normal pregnant, related controls.[73,74]

Vitamin D/calcitriol has been proposed to play diverse, nonskeletal roles during pregnancy, but these have not been extensively examined in these animal studies. Pregnant vitamin D-deficient mice had higher systolic and diastolic blood pressure and upregulation of renal expression of renin and angiotensin II receptor messenger ribonucleic acid (mRNA) compared to pregnant vitamin D-sufficient mice.[75] These data are consistent with the possibility that vitamin D deficiency could increase the risk of pregnancy-induced hypertension.

21.2.7.2 Animal Data: 24-Hydroxylase Deficiency

Mice with 24-hydroxylase deficiency are fertile. During the last 5 days of gestation, they develop a marked elevation in calcitriol, severe hypercalcemia, and hypercalciuria.[76]

21.2.7.3 Human Data: Vitamin D Deficiency and Genetic Vitamin D Resistance

Calcitriol-dependent active absorption of calcium represents about 20% of net calcium absorption, and this route of delivery is especially important when dietary intake of calcium is low. The remaining 80% of calcium is absorbed through passive, nonsaturable mechanisms, which are also stimulated in part by calcitriol. Because pregnancy represents a time of increased need for calcium delivery and many women do not meet the recommended daily intake for calcium, calcitriol's role in regulating intestinal calcium absorption should become critical during pregnancy. But the animal models described previously have displayed normal pregnancies and fetal development, which suggests that calcitriol is not required.

Therefore, is there any clinical evidence that vitamin D deficiency, or genetic disorders causing loss of calcitriol or VDR, will affect maternal mineral metabolism and obstetrical or fetal outcomes?

No clinical study has measured intestinal calcium absorption during pregnancy in vitamin D-deficient compared to vitamin D-sufficient women, or in women with genetic disorders of vitamin D physiology. Consequently, it remains unknown whether a doubling of intestinal calcium absorption occurs during pregnancy when calcitriol or its receptor is absent.

Definitive evidence of calcitriol's role in human pregnancy (and fetal/neonatal development) would come from large, randomized, blind clinical trials that enrolled vitamin D-deficient women and randomized them to supplementation or placebo. Such studies would control for confounding, including any factors that led to the women being vitamin D deficient. However, no such large studies have been carried out for ethical and logistical considerations.

Instead, numerous small to modestly sized clinical trials of vitamin D supplementation have been done.[1] Only a few of these compared truly vitamin D-deficient to -sufficient women, while more recent larger studies have compared varying degrees of vitamin D sufficiency without having a group with clear-cut vitamin D deficiency.

The fetal and neonatal outcomes of these studies are described in Chapter 44, as well as in a comprehensive review article.[72] In brief, no changes in cord blood calcium, phosphorus, PTH, birth weight, or anthropometric measurements were observed when babies of vitamin D-supplemented mothers were compared to babies of placebo-treated mothers. However, the incidence of neonatal hypocalcemia after 48 h was reduced by vitamin D supplementation in several studies when the babies of placebo-treated mothers had cord blood 25OHD below 20 nmol/L.[72] This is consistent with the postnatal role that calcitriol has in the regulation of intestinal calcium absorption.

Due to considerations of space and limits on the reference list, all of the abovementioned studies cannot be described in detail. Instead, a recent comprehensive review can be consulted for more details and a review of many studies.[1] We will not discuss associational studies, as they are confounded by factors that predict a lower 25OHD level and the outcome analyzed, including race/ethnicity, maternal overweight/obesity, lower socioeconomic status, poor nutrition, and others. For example, maternal overweight/obesity is well established to confer substantial risks of preterm delivery, cesarean sections, low birth weight, preeclampsia/pregnancy-induced hypertension, vaginal infections, and other adverse obstetrical outcomes.[77] Furthermore, associations do not prove causation; instead, they should suggest the need for large randomized controlled trials (RCTs) that compare vitamin D-deficient and -sufficient mothers to test the outcome of interest.

This chapter will focus on obstetrical outcomes from a few RCTs that included over 100 participants per study who were vitamin D deficient at entry, and some recent studies that gained press attention over the last few years but which did not include many vitamin D-deficient subjects (see Table 21.5). Fetal and neonatal outcomes from these studies are addressed in more detail in Chapter 44.

There were two trials each in Bangladesh, the United States, and the United Kingdom, and one each in New Zealand, Iran, and the United Arab Emirates.[78–86] The largest studies were in Bangladesh and the United Kingdom, with over 1000 participants.[85,86] Baseline maternal 25OHD levels were lowest (20–29 nmol/L) in the trials from Bangladesh, the United Kingdom, Iran, and UAE, and they were in the 40–60 nmol/L range in the others. The interventions consisted of placebo or low-dose (400 IU/day) or high-dose vitamin D (1000–5000 IU/day equivalent), which were started between the end of the first trimester and the mid-second trimester, and maintained until delivery. For almost all trials, the primary outcomes were simply maternal and neonatal-cord blood 25OHD and calcium (Table 21.5).

The most recent, and largest, study from Bangladesh administered prenatal vitamin D, and in one of the treatment arms, it was continued for 26 weeks postpartum, and prespecified infants' length for age z-scores at 1 year of age as the primary outcome.[86] In the remaining studies, offspring anthropometric parameters, bone mineral content (BMC), or both were prespecified in a limited number of studies.[82,84,85]

In all these studies, the administration of vitamin D increased maternal serum and cord blood 25OHD, while there was no overall effect on cord blood calcium. Maternal serum 25OHD reached a mean between 60 and 165 nmol/L at delivery, depending on the baseline level and the dose administered (Table 21.5). The largest difference achieved in a single study was 16 nmol/L (6.4 ng/mL) in the placebo-treated and 168 nmol/L (67 ng/mL) in vitamin D-supplemented mothers at term; however, there was no obstetrical benefit.[78] There was a benefit in reducing the incidence of neonatal hypocalcemia, which is discussed in Chapter 44.

In the recent study from Bangladesh, there was no significant difference in infant length, or any other clinical or anthropometric neonatal or maternal outcome, between treatment arms.[86] In one US-based study, there was no benefit to mode of delivery, gestational age at delivery, and preterm birth,[79] while in the other, there was no benefit in terms of mode of delivery, cesarean section rates, adverse events, hypertension, infection, gestational diabetes, stillbirth, gestational age at delivery, or combinations of these outcomes.[81]

The UK MAVIDOS trial reported no obstetrical benefit, and no benefit to any of the neonatal primary (neonatal bone area, BMC, and BMD within the first 10–14 days after birth) and secondary outcomes (anthropometric and body composition parameters within 48 h of birth). However, it was well publicized for a demonstrated increase in BMC and BMD in winter-born neonates of vitamin D-supplemented vs placebo-treated mothers.[85] Due to the normal rapid (100 mg/day) accumulation of skeletal mineral content after birth, this result may reflect improved intestinal mineral delivery over 14 days after birth, rather than a prenatal effect on skeletal mineralization. Curiously, autumn-born neonates of vitamin D-supplemented vs placebo-treated mothers showed an adverse trend of similar magnitude on BMC and BMD, which suggests possible harm from vitamin D supplementation. These results were based on significant findings from subgroup analyses of treatment by season interaction, which were not specified outcomes in the trial registries (ISRCTN 82927713 and EUDRACT 2007-001716-23). In the UK study that consisted mostly of vitamin D-deficient, subjects from India, there was a trend for a lower proportion of neonates being born small for gestational age (SGA) to mothers in the vitamin D-supplemented group (15% vs 28%, $0.05 < P < 0.1$), but the study was not powered for this outcome, which was also not prespecified.[78] In the studies from the UAE and Iran, there was also no benefit to obstetrical outcomes (variably, mode of delivery, cesarean section rates, adverse events, stillbirths, gestational age at delivery) or neonatal anthropometric measurements and bone mass measurements.[80,82,84]

The lack of any beneficial effect on maternal, immediate fetal/neonatal, and neonatal outcomes (anthropometrics and cord blood calcium), even in studies that included mothers with some of the lowest 25OHD levels,[78,82,84,86] may suggest that vitamin D supplementation during pregnancy confers no benefit to neonates. In contrast to almost all previous trials that were not sufficiently powered for obstetrical or neonatal outcomes, the most recent one was well powered to demonstrate a beneficial effect on infant length, but it still did not yield any significant results, despite low vitamin D levels in the mothers at the start of the study.[86]

Hollis and Wagner subsequently carried out multiple posthoc analyses of their two trials, including analyses in which selective data from both studies were pooled and analyses were done by achieved 25OHD level.[79,87–89] They reported

TABLE 21.5 Summary of large RCTs of vitamin D supplementation during pregnancy

Author Journal Year Country	N Age (years) Mean ± SD or median (range)	Study design	Gestational age (weeks) at entry Mean ± SD or median (range)	Baseline maternal 25OHD (nmol/L) Mean ± SD or median (range) 25OHD assay type	Prespecified outcomes as reported in paper and trial register	Results
Brooke et al. *BMJ* 1980 United Kingdom	C N=67 23.7 ± 3.1 I N=59 23.9 ± 4.8	Double-blind trial *Intervention:* C: No intervention I: Calciferol: 1000 IU/day *Inclusion criteria:* • Pregnant Asian women • 28–32 weeks' gestation *Exclusion criteria:* • Preterm deliveries • Congenital malformations • Maternal illnesses likely to affect fetal growth (such as diabetes) *Ethnicity:* Asian (70% Indian)	28	20.1 ± 1.9 Competitive protein-binding	*Paper* **Outcomes:** • Maternal and infant calcium homoeostasis and fetal growth *Trial register not available*	*Maternal daily weight gain (g)* Mean±SD: C: 46.4 ± 3.6 I: 63.3 ± 2.6 (P<0.001) *Maternal 25OHD at delivery (nmol/L)* Mean±SD: C: 16.2 ± 27 I: 168 ± 12.5 *Neonatal 25OHD at delivery (nmol/L)* Mean±SD: C: 10.2 ± 2 I: 137.9 ± 10.8 *Maternal calcium at delivery (mmol/L)* Mean±SD: C: 2.51 ± 0.01 I: 2.58 ± 0.02 (P<0.001) *Maternal alkaline phosphatase at delivery (IU/l)* Mean±SD: C: 136.1 ± 7.9 I: 114.3 ± 6.5 *Infant plasma calcium at day 6 (mmol/l)* Mean±SD: C: 2.29 ± 0.02

Continued

TABLE 21.5 Summary of large RCTs of vitamin D supplementation during pregnancy—cont'd

Author Journal Year Country	N Age (years) Mean ± SD or median (range)	Study design	Gestational age (weeks) at entry Mean ± SD or median (range)	Baseline maternal 25OHD (nmol/L) Mean ± SD or median (range) 25OHD assay type	Prespecified outcomes as reported in paper and trial register	Results
						I: 2.49 ± 0.04 ($P < 0.05$) Five infants developed symptomatic hypocalcemia in the control group and none in the treatment group
						Neonatal fontanelle area measurement (cm^2): Mean ± SD: C: 6.1 ± 0.7 I: 4.1 ± 0.4 ($P < 0.05$)
						Infants small for gestational age (%): C: 28.6% I: 15.3%, $0.05 < P < 0.1$
Hollis et al. *JBMR* 2011 United States	C N=111 27.0 ± 5.6 I1 N=122 27.4 ± 5.7 I2 N=117 26.6 ± 5.4	Single-center, randomized, controlled, double-blind study *Intervention:* C: 400IU vitamin D3/day I1: 2000IU vitamin D3/day I2: 4000IU vitamin D3/day *Inclusion criteria:* • Age ≥16 years • Confirmed singleton pregnancy • <16 completed weeks' gestation at the time of consent	C 12.5 ± 1.9 I1 12.6 ± 1.6 I2 12.4 ± 2.0	C 61.6 ± 27.1 I1 58.3 ± 22.3 I2 58.2 ± 21.8 Direct ultraviolet detection preceded by organic extraction and high-performance liquid chromatography	*Paper* *Primary outcomes:* • Maternal 25OHD^a at delivery • Neonatal 25OHD at delivery *Secondary outcomes:* • 25OHD concentration of 80 nmol/L or greater achieved • 25OHD concentration required to achieve maximal 1,25OH$_2$D$_3$ production	*Maternal 25OHD 1 month before delivery (nmol/L)* Mean ± SD: C: 79.4 ± 34.3 I1: 105.4 ± 35.7 I2: 118.5 ± 34.9 ($P < 0.0001$) *Maternal 25OHD at delivery (nmol/L)* Mean ± SD: C: 78.9 ± 36 I1: 98 ± 34 I2: 111 ± 40 ($P < 0.0001$)

Source	Sample		Study design / Intervention			Outcomes
		Exclusion criteria: • Preexisting calcium or para-thyroid conditions • Chronic diuretic or cardiac medication therapy, including calcium channel blockers • Active thyroid disease (e.g., Grave's disease, Hashimoto's thyroiditis, or thyroiditis) *Ethnicity:* African American (28%–33%), Hispanic (44%–48%), Caucasian (37%–40%)			*Register/NCT00292591* *Primary outcome measures:* • 25OHD Concentration [Time frame: 7 months]. Circulating total 25OHD concentration measured in serum at visit 7, 1 month prior to delivery • BMD of both mother and infant 1.5 years[b]	*RR for achieving a 25OHD ≥80 nmol/L within 1 month of delivery* *RR (95% CI):* RR=1.52 (95% CI 1.24–1.86) between I1 and I2 RR=1.60 (95% CI 1.32–1.95) between C and I2 *Maternal PTH 1 month prior to delivery (pmol/L)* Mean±SD: C: 2.2±1.3 I1: 2.1±1.1 I2: 1.9±1.1 PTH not significantly different by treatment groups; significance was obtained when PTH was stratified by race *Maternal circulating 25OHD required to achieve maximal 1,25OH₂D3 production during pregnancy (nmol/L):* At least 100 ($P<0.0001$) *No effect on any obstetrical outcome:* • Preterm birth • Mode of delivery • Gestational age
Roth et al. *Nutrition Journal* 2013 Bangladesh	C N=80 22.4±3.4 I N=80 22.4±3.5		Double-blind, placebo-controlled, randomized trial *Intervention:* C: No intervention I: 35,000IU vitamin D3/week	C 27.9±1.0 I 27.6±1.1	C 44.0±20.9 I 45.4±18.4	*Paper* *Primary outcomes:* • 25OHD in mother[a] and infant at delivery (primary bio-chemical efficacy outcome) *Maternal 25OHD at delivery (nmol/L)* Mean±SD: C: 38.4±18.1 I: 134.4±30.7 ($P<0.001$)

Continued

TABLE 21.5 Summary of large RCTs of vitamin D supplementation during pregnancy—cont'd

Author Journal Year Country	N Age (years) Mean ± SD or median (range)	Study design	Gestational age (weeks) at entry Mean ± SD or median (range)	Baseline maternal 25OHD (nmol/L) Mean ± SD or median (range) 25OHD assay type	Prespecified outcomes as reported in paper and trial register	Results
		Inclusion criteria: • Age 18 to <35 years • GA 26–30 weeks *Exclusion criteria:* • D supplement 400 IU/day within the month prior to enrolment • Refusal to stop supplemental vitamin D after enrollment • Current use of anticonvulsant or antimycobacterial drugs • Severe anemia (hemoglobin <70 g/L) • Systolic blood pressure ≥140 mmHg or diastolic blood pressure ≥90 mmHg • Proteinuria or glycosuria • Complicated medical or obstetric history • History of delivery of an infant with a major congenital anomaly • Birth asphyxia • Perinatal death *Ethnicity:* Not described		Chemiluminescent microparticle immune assay	Maternal serum calcium concentration at delivery (primary safety measure) *Register/NCT01126528* *Primary outcome measures:* • Serum 25OHD concentration [Time frame: Maternal: during third trimester; Neonatal (cord blood)]. Biomarker of vitamin D status *Secondary outcome measures:* • Serum calcium concentration [Time frame: Maternal: third trimester; cord blood] • Urine Ca:Cr ratio [Time frame: Maternal: third trimester] • Neonatal immune function [Time frame: cord blood]. Selected markers of innate and adaptive immunity • Infant growth [Time frame: Postnatal observational follow-up phase]. Infant growth parameters during postnatal follow-up, up to 12 months of age • Infant and maternal postnatal vitamin D status [Time frame: Postnatal observational follow-up phase] • Neonatal serum calcium [Time frame: First week postnatal].	*Neonatal 25OHD (nmol/L)* Mean ± SD: C: 39.0 ± 18.7 I: 102.8 ± 28.6 (P < 0.001) *Maternal serum calcium at delivery (mmol/L)* Mean ± SD: C: 2.31 ± 0.11 I: 2.32 ± 0.10 *Maternal albumin-adjusted calcium at delivery (mmol/L)* Mean ± SD: C: 2.40 ± 0.08 I: 2.43 ± 0.09 (P < 0.05) *Maternal urine Ca: Cr ratio at delivery (mmol/mmol)* Median (Range): C: 0.13 (0.0, 1.26) I: 0.20 (0.0, 2.26) *Maternal PTH at delivery (pmol/L)* Median (Range): C: 3.9 (0.3, 20.5) I: 2.3 (0.3, 9.8) (P < 0.001) There was no effect on obstetrical outcomes: • Mode of delivery

Continued

Study	N / Age			Methods	Outcomes	Results
Wagner et al. AJOG 2013 United States	I1 N=130 24.5±5.3 I2 N=127 25.4±5.0	12.4±1.8	56.6±24.2 Direct RIA developed in another laboratory	Two-center, randomized, double-blind study *Intervention:* I1: 2000IU/day I2: 4000IU/day *Inclusion criteria:* • Age ≥16 years • Confirmed singleton pregnancy of <16 completed weeks' gestation *Exclusion criteria:* • Preexisting calcium or parathyroid conditions • Chronic diuretic or cardiac medication therapy including calcium channel blockers • Active thyroid disease (e.g., Graves, Hashimoto's thyroiditis) *Ethnicity:* African American (47%—50%), Caucasian (9%—10%), Hispanic (36%—42%), other (2%—4%)	Infant serum calcium during the first week postnatal; Last three outcomes were added in the latest version of the protocol in Aug 2012 — *Paper Coprimary outcomes:* • Change in circulating maternal 25OHD[a] concentration from baseline to the completion of pregnancy • Neonate's 25OHD concentration at birth — *Register/NCT00412087 Primary outcome measures:* • 25OHD at Visit 7 [Time frame: 7 months] 25OHD at Visit 7, 1 month prior to delivery *Secondary outcome measure:* • Parathyroid hormone at Visit 7 [Time frame: 7 months] Intact parathyroid hormone at Visit 7, 1 month prior to delivery V1 and V2 of trial register do not specify timing to measure outcomes, V3, 4, 5 specify 9 months, and V6 states 7 months and 1 month prior to delivery	• Cesarean section rates • Adverse events • Stillbirths or gestational age at delivery • Neonatal anthropometry (birth weight, length at birth, head circumference) — *Maternal 25OHD at delivery (nmol/L)* Mean±SD: I1: 90±24 I2: 94±33 — *Neonatal 25OHD at delivery (nmol/L)* Mean±SD: I1: 55±26 I2: 67±33 — *Maternal iPTH 1 month prior to delivery (pg/ml)* Mean±SD: I1: 17.5±8.2 I2: 15.2±9.3 — *Preterm labor* N (%): I1: 24 (28.9%) I2: 13 (16.7%) (P=0.091) — *Fenton weight percentile:* I2 had 2.40 (95% CI 1.26—4.61) times the odds of having an infant in the 50th percentile, compared to I1 — *There was no effect on obstetrical outcomes:* • Mode of delivery • Cesarean section rates

TABLE 21.5 Summary of large RCTs of vitamin D supplementation during pregnancy—cont'd

Author Journal Year Country	N Age (years) Mean ± SD or median (range)	Study design	Gestational age (weeks) at entry Mean ± SD or median (range)	Baseline maternal 25OHD (nmol/L) Mean ± SD or median (range) 25OHD assay type	Prespecified outcomes as reported in paper and trial register	Results
Dawodu et al. JCEM 2013 UAE	I1 N=64 27.5±5.5 I2 N=65 27.3±4.9 I3 N=63 25.6±5.5	Randomized, controlled, double-blind study Intervention: I1: 400IU vitamin D3/day I2: 2000IU vitamin D3/day I3: 4000IU vitamin D3/day Inclusion criteria: • 12–16 weeks' gestation • Singleton pregnancy Exclusion criteria: • Preexisting calcium and parathyroid conditions • Active thyroid disease, liver or kidney disease • Type 1 diabetes, which is likely to affect vitamin D and calcium status Ethnicity: Gulf Arab (92%–94%), non-Gulf Arab (6%–8%)	I1: 12.2±0.9 I2: 12.5±1.1 I3: 12.6±1.1	I1: 21.5±13.0 I2: 20.5±11.9 I3: 19.6±7.7 RIA (DiaSorin, Stillwater, MN)	Paper Primary outcomes: • Maternal serum 25OHDᵃ concentrations at delivery Secondary outcomes: • Proportion of mothers who achieved serum 25OHD 32ng/mL or greater (≥80nmol/L) defined as vitamin D sufficiency at the time of delivery Register/NCT00610688 Primary outcome measures: • Serum maternal and neonatal 25OHD measurement [Time frame: 29 weeks] Maternal serum 25OHD measurement at 12, 16, and 28 weeks during pregnancy and at delivery and cord blood or neonatal serum 25OHD measurement Secondary outcome measures:	• Adverse events • Hypertension • Infection • Stillbirths or gestational age at delivery Maternal 25OHD at delivery (nmol/L) Mean ± SD: I1: 48 I2: 65 I1: 90 (P<0.0001) Mothers achieving 25 (OH)D >80 (nmol/L)(%): I1: 9.5% I2: 24.4% I3: 65.1% (P<0.0001) PTH concentration at delivery: Reduced in high-dose group Maternal serum calcium and urine calcium/creatinine: No differences were detected No effect on: • Mean birth weight • Length • Head circumference

Grant et al. *Pediatrics* 2014 New Zealand	C N=87 28±6 I1 N=87 27±6 I2 N=86 26±7	Randomized, double-blind, placebo-controlled trial *Intervention:* C: No intervention I1: 1000IU vitamin D3/day I2: 2000IU vitamin D3/day *Inclusion criteria:* • GA 26–30 weeks • Singleton pregnancy *Exclusion criteria:* • Vitamin D supplementation > 200IU/day • History of renal stones or hypercalcemia • Any serious pregnancy complication at enrollment *Ethnicity:* 34% European, 24% Maori, 49% Pacific, and other 25%. Ethnicity was defined by the participants. More than 1 ethnic group could be identified; therefore, percentages do not add up to 100	*C:* 27 (26, 29) *I1:* 28 (26, 29) *I2:* 27 (26, 29) *C:* 55 (32, 80) *I1:* 57 (40, 90) *I2:* 55 (32, 87) Isotope-dilution liquid chromatography–tandem mass spectrometry	*Paper* *Primary outcomes:* • The proportion of infants[a] achieving a serum 25OHD ≥ 75 nmol/L during the first 6 months of infancy • Number of mothers and infants with hypercalcemia at any measurement point *Register/ACTRN12610000483055* *Primary outcome:* • The proportion of infants achieving a serum 25OHD concentration >75 nmol/L at 6 months of age. • The number of mothers and infants with hypercalcemia at any measurement point *Secondary outcome:* • The proportion of mothers achieving a serum 25[OH] vitamin D concentration >75 nmol/L at 36 weeks' gestation	• Growth of the newborn infant as measured by crown-heel length and head circumference at birth [Time frame: At delivery] • Birthweight of newborn infant [Time frame: Measured at birth] Growth of the newborn infant as measured by birth weight in gramsOnly V4 of trial register specifies all time points to measure the primary outcome • Gestational age	*Maternal 25OHD at delivery (nmol/L)* Mean (25th, 75th centile): C: 50 (30, 75) I1: 97 (80, 115) I2: 102 (72, 125) (P<0.001) *Maternal serum 25OHD concentration > 75 (nmol/L) at 36 wks gestation (%):* C: 27% I1: 79% I2: 71% (P<0.001) *Maternal serum calcium Concentration at 36 wks gestation (mg/dL)* Mean±SD: C: 10.31±0.53 I1: 9.04±0.37 I2: 9.02±0.29 (P=0.09) *Neonatal 25OHD at delivery (nmol/L)* Mean (25th, 75th centile): C: 32.4 (22.5, 44.9) I1:59.9 (44.9, 74.9) I2: 64.9 (44.9, 87.4) (P<0.001) *Infant serum 25OHD*

Continued

TABLE 21.5 Summary of large RCTs of vitamin D supplementation during pregnancy—cont'd

Author Journal Year Country	N Age (years) Mean ± SD or median (range)	Study design	Gestational age (weeks) at entry Mean ± SD or median (range)	Baseline maternal 25OHD (nmol/L) Mean ± SD or median (range) 25OHD assay type	Prespecified outcomes as reported in paper and trial register	Results
						concentration > 50 (nmol/L) at 6 months, (%): C: 74% I1:82% I2:89% (P < 0.07)
Vaziri et al. *Early Human Development* 2016 Iran	C N = 65 26.0 ± 4.34 I N = 62 26.8 ± 4.92	Randomized clinical trial *Intervention:* C: Placebo (no intervention) I: 2000IU/day vitamin D3 *Inclusion criteria:* • Age > 18 years • No history of mental illness and internal diseases such as hyperthyroidism/hypothyroidism • No addiction to any kind of narcotic drugs or alcohol • Not divorced or widowed • No pregnancy complications such as preeclampsia, gestational diabetes, ruptured membranes, and suspicion of preterm birth • No previous cesarean sections, with a live fetus singleton pregnancy • GA 26–28 weeks	26–28	C: 31.8 ± 20.9 I: 29 ± 13.9 CLIA	*Paper outcomes:* • Maternal 25OHD at delivery[a] • Infants' anthropometric measurements (at birth, 4th and 8th weeks postnatal) • Maternal and infant bone mass parameters were examined during first 2 months after birth *Register/IRCT2015040910327N13 Primary outcomes* • Description: Blood cord vitamin D concentration Time point: After delivery • Description: Bone densitometry Time point: During first 2 months after birth • 3.Description: Antropometric	Maternal 25OHD at delivery (nmol/L) Mean ± SD: C: 30 ± 14.5 I: 45 ± 23.9 (P < 0.001) *No significant differences between C and I:* • Birth weight • Height • Head circumference *No significant differences between C and I:* Bone mass measurements of the mothers: • BMD • BMC • BA

Continued

		Exclusion criteria: • Unwillingness to cooperate during the study • Consumption of <8 weeks of vitamin D3 supplements Gross congenital malformations and chromosomal disorders in infants *Ethnicity:* Not described		measurments (height, weight, and head circumference) Time point: At birth and 4 and 8 weeks later *Secondary outcomes:* None described	*No significant differences between C and I:* Bone mass measurements of the infants at birth and 4th and 8th weeks after birth: • BMD • BMC • BA
Cooper et al. *Lancet Diabetes Endocrinol* 2016 United Kingdom	C N=569 30.5±5.2 I N=565 30.5±5.2	Multicenter, double-blind, randomized, placebo-controlled trial *Intervention:* C: No intervention I: 1000 IU/day cholecalciferol *Inclusion criteria:* • Age >18 years • Singleton pregnancy • GA <17 weeks *Exclusion criteria:* • Women with known metabolic bone disease • Renal stones • Hyperparathyroidism • Hypercalciuria • Diagnosis of cancer in the last 10 years • Unable to give informed consent or comply with the protocol • Taking medication known to interfere with fetal growth • Fetal anomalies on ultrasonography	14	C: 46±17 I: 47±18 Liaison RIA automated platform	*Paper* *Primary outcomes:* • Neonatal whole BMC[a], assessed within 2 weeks after birth by DXA *Secondary outcomes:* • Maternal 25OHD concentration at 34 weeks' gestation • Change in 25OHD between 14 and 34 weeks' gestation • Neonatal whole-body bone area and BMD within 2 weeks after birth • Neonatal bone indexes at the spine *Register/ISRCTN82927713* *Primary outcome measures:* • Neonatal whole-body bone area, BMC, and BMD assessed by DXA within 10 days of birth.	*Maternal 25OHD at 34 weeks' gestation (nmol/L)* Mean±SD: C: 43±22 I: 68±22 (P<0.001) *No significant differences between C and I:* Bone mass measurements of the infants: • BMD • BMC • BA • Lean mass • Median fat mass • Birth weight • Length • Head circumference • Abdominal circumference

TABLE 21.5 Summary of large RCTs of vitamin D supplementation during pregnancy—cont'd

Author Journal Year Country	N, Age (years) Mean ± SD or median (range)	Study design	Gestational age (weeks) at entry Mean ± SD or median (range)	Baseline maternal 25OHD (nmol/L) Mean ± SD or median (range); 25OHD assay type	Prespecified outcomes as reported in paper and trial register	Results
		Women already using >400 IU/day vitamin D supplementation. Ethnicity: White 94%			Secondary outcome measures: • Neonatal and childhood anthropometry and body composition (weight, length and skinfold thickness measurements), assessed within 48 h of birth. Women's attitude to pregnancy vitamin D supplementation (qualitative study; assessed in main study only). Methodology and time points of assessment not yet defined as of March 3, 2008 Childhood bone mass at 4 years	
Roth et al. NEJM 2018 Bangladesh	C: N=259 Median (range) 23 (18–38); I1: N=260 Median (range) 22.5 (18–40); I2: N=259 Median (range) 22 (18–35); I3: N=260 Median	Randomized, double-blind, placebo-controlled, dose-ranging trial. Intervention: C: Placebo; I1: 4200 IU vitamin D3/week; I2:16,800 vitamin IU D3/week; I3: 28,000 IU vitamin D3/week; I4: 28,000 IU vitamin D3/week (prenatal and postpartum until week 26). Inclusion criteria: • Age ≥18 years • GA 17–24 weeks	C: Median (range) 20.4 (17–24); I1: Median (range) 20.1 (17–24); I2: Median (range) 20.3 (17–24); I3: Median (range) 20.4 (17–24)	C: 27.7 ± 13.8; I1: 27.4 ± 14.3; I2: 28.7 ± 14.0; I3: 27 ± 14.7; I4: 26.6 ± 13.2. LC-MS/MS using an Agilent 1290 HPLC interfaced with an AB Sciex 5500 Q-Trap mass spectrometer	Paper Primary outcomes: • Length-for-age z-score at 1 year (364–420 days). Secondary outcomes: • Infant anthropometric variables • Preterm birth (<37 weeks' gestation) • Gestational hypertension • Delivery characteristics • Stillbirth • Mother and infant symptoms, clinical encounters, and hospitalizations • Deaths • Congenital anomalies	No significant differences across groups: Infants mean length-for-age z-scores. Other anthropometric measures, birth outcomes, and morbidity did not differ significantly across groups. Maternal 25OHD at or near delivery (nmol/L) Mean ± SD: C: 23.8 ± 13.9; I1: 69.7 ± 19.5; I2: 109 ± 23.6

(range) 22 (18–38) *I4* N=260 Median (range) 23 (18–38)	*Exclusion criteria:* • History of any medical condition or medications that may predispose to vitamin D sensitivity, altered vitamin D metabolism, and/or hypercalcemia (tuberculosis sarcoidosis, history of renal/ureteral stones, parathyroid disease, renal or liver failure, or current use of anticonvulsants) • High-risk pregnancy based on one or more of the following findings by point-of-care testing: • Severe anemia • Moderate-severe proteinuria • Hypertension • Multiple gestation • Major congenital anomaly +Severe oligohydramnios • Unwillingness to stop taking nonstudy vitamin D or calcium supplements or a multivitamin containing calcium and/or vitamin D • Previous enrolment in the trial during a previous pregnancy *Ethnicity: not described*	• Infant neurologic disabilities • Infant rickets • Other secondary biochemical, anthropometric and clinical outcomes listed in the paper supplementary material) *Register/NCT01924013* *Primary outcomes:* • Infant length for age z-scores with prenatal supplementation • Infant length for age z-scores with postpartum supplementation *Secondary outcomes:* • Serum calcium In addition to outcomes listed under *"Other outcome measures"*	*I3* 110.7±28 *I4* 113.6±25.7 (*P*<0.001)

[a] Denotes the primary outcome on which the sample size was calculated in each trial, as reported in the paper.
[b] Outcome removed from the latest version of trial protocol in 2016. P-Values only reported when <0.1.
Primary and secondary outcomes as reported under "Methods" in the respective trial published papers and trial registers.1,25OH₂D₃: 1,25-dihydroxyvitamin D3; 25OHD: 25-hydroxyvitamin D; BA: bone area; C: control; Ca: calcium; CLIA: chemiluminescence immunoassay; Crea: creatinine; I: intervention; iPTH: intact parathyroid hormone; NA: Not available; RIA: direct radioimmunoassay; RR: relative risk; SD: standard deviation; V: version.

that mothers with serum 25OHD reaching above 100 nmol/L had a 47% reduction in preterm birth; however, these results must be viewed with skepticism. The analyses suffer from being associational (thereby removing the protection against confounding achieved by randomization into groups), lack of adjustment for multiple comparisons, arbitrary grouping of outcomes, and arbitrary exclusion of some ethnicities from the analysis. Noteworthy, these were not prespecified analyses. Overall, therefore, it is unclear that these posthoc analyses provide meaningful data on the beneficial effect of vitamin D supplementation during pregnancy. A recent follow-up report on one of these trials revealed that there were no differences between groups in BMD or BMC of the spine and femoral neck at the gestational or postpartum measurements.[90]

We identified six recent systematic reviews that specifically assessed the effect of vitamin D supplementation during pregnancy.[91–96] The studies discussed in detail earlier in this chapter were sometimes included among these reviews. For example, data from the UK trial by Brooke et al., which had the largest achieved difference in 25OHD between placebo-treated and vitamin D-supplemented mothers, was included in four systematic reviews,[92,94–96] while data from the trial of Hollis et al. was included in three of them.[94,95] All the reviews assessed the effect of vitamin D supplementation on maternal and neonatal extraskeletal outcomes, but they differed in their methodology, inclusion/exclusion criteria, whether combined calcium and vitamin D data could be included, and whether the review was explicitly stated.

Among these six systematic reviews, vitamin D supplementation had no significant effect on preeclampsia in four,[92,94–96] and a positive effect in two reviews,[91,93] while combined vitamin D and calcium supplementation reduced the incidence of preeclampsia by 34%–53% in three systematic reviews.[91–93] No consistent effect was seen on other outcomes, such as preterm birth, low birth weight, SGA infants, infections, cesarean section rate, and newborn anthropometrics. Overall, available data are insufficient within these systematic reviews to conclude that vitamin D supplementation during pregnancy confers any proven obstetrical benefits.

In summary, the few large RCTs reported today do not provide evidence of a beneficial effect of high-dose vitamin D supplementation (1000–5000 IU/day), on maternal and neonatal outcomes. The most recent large trial seems to make it unlikely that vitamin D supplementation in deficient women would yield any beneficial effect on infant length.[86] The other studies were limited by low power, baseline maternal serum 25 OHD levels that were often not low, and lack of prespecification of obstetrical and neonatal outcomes. The potential protective effect of vitamin D on neonatal BMC in the MAVIDOS trial makes physiological sense because the intestines become the route of calcium delivery after birth, and this finding is consistent with the benefit observed in some RCTs of prenatal vitamin D supplementation reducing the incidence of neonatal hypocalcemia; these issues are discussed further in Chapter 44. Systematic reviews and meta-analyses of vitamin D RCTs suggest that combined calcium and vitamin D administration may reduce the risk of pre-eclampsia, but whether this is driven by the proven benefit of calcium alone is unknown. In contrast, there are suggestive but no consistent results among the meta-analyses as to whether vitamin D alone confers any obstetrical or neonatal benefits.

Any putative protective effects of vitamin D on maternal or neonatal outcomes are worthy of further study in adequately powered and designed trials, which also must enroll a significant number of women with low 25OHD. This is particularly relevant in view of their potential public health implications, especially in developing countries where some of the lowest maternal 25OHD levels are reported. However, ethical considerations (in particular, fear that vitamin D deficiency may be harmful to either mother or fetus) makes it difficult for such studies to be carried out.

With the genetic disorders of vitamin physiology, available data come from case reports and series. Pregnancies have been unremarkable in women with vitamin D-dependent rickets type 1 (VDDR-I) which is due to the absence of Cyp27b1, and in women with VDDR-II that is due to absence of functional VDRs.[97–99] In one published VDR-II case, pregnancy was unremarkable in a woman who maintained her prepregnancy intake of supplemental calcium (800 mg) and high-dose calcitriol.[98] The clinicians increased her calcitriol later in the pregnancy "because of the knowledge that the circulating 1,25-(OH)$_2$D concentration normally rises during pregnancy," but not because of any change in albumin-adjusted serum calcium.[98] Consequently, it is unclear that any change was needed. In pregnant women with VDDR-I, the dose of calcitriol was unchanged in one-third of pregnancies and increased 1.5-fold to twofold in others.[97]

Overall, and in summary, the previously discussed animal data (severe vitamin D deficiency and genetic loss of VDR or *Cyp27b1*) demonstrated that maternal mineral homeostasis and intestinal calcium absorption improve during pregnancy, resulting in normalization or near-normalization of mineral and bone metabolism. Such findings suggest that calcitriol is not required for the adaptations that are invoked during pregnancy or that unknown mechanisms compensate for its absence. Human data are less extensive or robust, but available clinical trials do not show a clear benefit of high-dose vitamin D supplementation on maternal mineral or skeletal homeostasis, or obstetrical and fetal outcomes. Many of the clinical trials did not enroll women who were truly vitamin D deficient and did not prespecify obstetrical and neonatal outcomes, and thus they had reduced power to be able to detect a benefit from vitamin D supplementation.

21.2.7.4   Clinical Management: Vitamin D Deficiency and Genetic Vitamin D Resistance

Pregnant women appear to require the same intake of vitamin D as nonpregnant women to maintain a certain 25OHD level. No data suggest that pregnant women need a higher 25OHD level than nonpregnant women.[24] Therefore, whatever intake maintains a sufficient level of 25OHD in an individual woman should be maintained during pregnancy.

The desirable 25OHD level in pregnant women is still a matter of debate. While the Institute of Medicine and the American College of Obstetricians and Gynecologists (ACOG) recommend a minimum of 50nmol/L (20ng/mL),[100,101] the Endocrine Society recommends ≥75 nmol/L (30ng/mL).[102] The doses needed to reach such targets also vary, ranging from 600 to as much as 2000 IU/day.[100,102] The World Health Organization (WHO) does not recommend supplementation of pregnant women unless they are from poor countries, have a darker skin color, and come from populations with a high prevalence of hypovitaminosis D or inadequate exposure to sunshine.[103]

If a woman presents with vitamin D deficiency while pregnant, then supplementation should be prescribed immediately, with loading doses considered to replenish maternal vitamin D stores more rapidly. The preceding discussion of animal and human data revealed that vitamin D deficiency does not clearly have adverse effects on obstetrical outcomes, and so vitamin D insufficiency is even more unlikely to have adverse consequences.

The review of evidence is not intended to suggest that a woman should be left vitamin D deficient during pregnancy. Instead, these data should reassure the clinician that if a woman presents late in pregnancy with vitamin D deficiency, it is unlikely to be associated with adverse maternal or fetal outcomes unless there is global maternal (and, thereby, fetal) malnutrition. It is still prudent to correct and avoid a vitamin D-deficient state wherever possible.

In the genetic disorders, calcium and calcitriol or 1α-cholecalciferol should be adjusted as needed to maintain a normal level of ionized or albumin-corrected serum calcium. It is possible that the doses will remain the same or that they might need to increase, and this can be determined only on an individual basis.

21.2.7.5   Human Data: 24-Hydroxylase Deficiency

More recently, 24-hydroxylase deficiency has been identified as a cause of significant gestational hypercalcemia. Loss of the catabolic effects of 24-hydroxylase in nonpregnant adults leads to persistently high calcitriol and mild hypercalcemia that may be asymptomatic and go unnoticed.[104] But during pregnancy, the physiological increase in calcitriol is unopposed by catabolism and appears to lead to an exaggerated increase in calcitriol, with resulting symptomatic hypercalcemia. Presenting patients will have hypercalcemia (sometimes quite marked), suppressed or undetectable PTH, and calcitriol concentrations that exceed what is expected for pregnancy.[105–107] In addition to symptoms of hypercalcemia, complications have included nephrolithiasis and acute pancreatitis.[107,108]

21.2.7.6   Clinical Management: 24-Hydroxylase Deficiency

Treatment of the hypercalcemia is complicated by the pathophysiology of 24-hydroxylase deficiency and that all agents that could be used are not approved for pregnancy. The main mechanism for the hypercalcemia is likely through increased intestinal calcium absorption, and thus the use of increased hydration and a modestly restricted calcium diet, combined with phosphate supplementation to bind dietary calcium, is a relatively safe approach that addresses the mechanism of the hypercalcemia. If PTH rises above normal, that would suggest that the dietary calcium restriction is too severe and should be lessened to prevent maternal bone resorption and fetal secondary hyperparathyroidism. Other pharmacologic therapies should be reserved for the most severe cases and used with caution. Oral glucocorticoids (Category C or D) could conceivably be used to suppress intestinal calcium absorption, but at the lowest doses to minimize any adverse effects on maternal glucose, blood pressure, risk of avascular necrosis of the hip, and the fetus (prednisone is converted in the liver to prednisolone and crosses the placenta, where it gets converted back to prednisone). Additional options include the use of a loop diuretic to promote urinary calcium excretion and a bisphosphonate to reduce bone resorption. However, because the main action of calcitriol is on intestinal calcium absorption, a bisphosphonate would be of limited efficacy at best. Cinacalcet will not be useful because PTH will be suppressed due to the combined effects of pregnancy and hypercalcemia.

21.2.8   Calcitonin Deficiency

Calcitonin circulates at higher levels during pregnancy and has been theorized to protect the maternal skeleton from excessive resorption. *Ctcgrp*-null mice lack both calcitonin and calcitonin gene-related peptide-α, but they displayed no disturbance in calcium metabolism during pregnancy, nor was there any alteration in skeletal mineral content or structure by the end of pregnancy.[109,110] These studies indicate that calcitonin is not required during pregnancy in mice.

No women with genetic loss of calcitonin or its receptor have been identified or studied during pregnancy. The closest thing to subjects with an absence of calcitonin are totally thyroidectomized women, but it is not deficient during pregnancy due to the production of calcitonin by the breasts and placenta.[1] No studies have specifically examined whether thyroid-ectomized women have disturbances in calcium metabolism or BMD while pregnant. Several studies have examined whether total thyroidectomy increases BMD loss and fracture risk over the long term in both men and women, with just as many reporting adverse effects as those that reported no effects.[1]

Overall, the available evidence suggests that loss of calcitonin should have no adverse effects on maternal calcium and bone metabolism during pregnancy.

21.2.9 Low or High Calcium Intake

It is very clear from multiple animal studies that a calcium-restricted diet can lead to marked hypocalcemia and secondary hyperparathyroidism during pregnancy, with the potential for sudden hypocalcemic death near term.[1] Placental calcium transport must be impaired because a low-calcium diet also leads to secondary hyperparathyroidism and skeletal resorption in the fetus.[1] Conversely, high calcium intake prevents any resorption of the maternal skeleton by enabling all or most of the calcium transported to the fetus to come from the maternal diet.[1]

In women, pregnancy normally results in absorptive hypercalciuria with suppressed PTH, which implies that calcium intake and absorption exceed maternal requirements. But in women with low dietary calcium intake, or high intake of phytate that blocks calcium absorption, PTH does not fall and indeed actually may rise above normal, consistent with sec-ondary hyperparathyroidism.[1] Intestinal calcium absorption may increase further in pregnant women with low calcium intake, as suggested by women who were estimated to be in a positive calcium balance during all three trimesters despite a total intake of <420 mg of calcium.[111] However, low calcium intake should be anticipated to provoke bone loss during pregnancy (especially the third trimester) and to increase the risk of osteoporosis.[1] If maternal hypocalcemia occurs, that reduces calcium delivery to the fetus, which may develop secondary hyperparathyroidism, skeletal demineralization, and fractures.[1] The lowest quintile of maternal calcium intake is also associated with increased risk of preeclampsia, whereas calcium supplementation reduces that risk.[1]

High calcium intake can have effects that are similar to primary hyperparathyroidism, including increased intestinal calcium absorption, maternal hypercalcemia, increased flow of calcium across the placenta to the fetus, and suppression of the fetal parathyroids. Cases of neonatal hypoparathyroidism have been reported in which women consumed 3–6 g of elemental calcium daily to treat nausea.[1]

Overall, it is clear that extremes of calcium intake should be avoided during pregnancy because both low and high calcium can have adverse effects on the mother and fetus.

21.2.10 Hypercalcemia of Malignancy

More than a dozen cases have been published of hypercalcemia of malignancy during pregnancy.[1] It is often (but not always) a terminal condition. Treatment options include surgery, hydration, diuresis, pharmacotherapy for the hypercal-cemia (calcitonin, bisphosphonates, or denosumab), and chemotherapy. The potential teratogenic effects and other con-cerns about pharmacotherapy were discussed in Section 21.2.2. At the earliest opportunity, a decision needs to be made about whether to terminate or continue the pregnancy, as well as whether chemotherapy will be administered during pregnancy or deferred until the baby is born. In some cases, chemotherapy was given during pregnancy regardless of its potential teratogenic effects. The fetus can be expected to have hypercalcemia with suppression of the parathyroids and a high risk for neonatal hypocalcemia. In over half the reported cases, the fate of the baby wasn't mentioned.[1]

21.2.11 Fibroblast Growth Factor 23 (FGF23)-Related Disorders

The most common disorder of fibroblast growth factor 23 (FGF23) is X-linked hypophosphatemic rickets, in which inac-tivating mutations in the *PHEX* gene lead to high circulating levels of FGF23, hypophosphatemia, and rickets or osteo-malacia. In a mouse model of XLH, pregnancies were uneventful. In particular, despite very high circulating levels of FGF23, which normally downregulate calcitriol synthesis and increase its catabolism, maternal serum calcitriol increased to the high levels normally seen during pregnancy.[112,113] In turn, this rise in calcitriol should improve intestinal calcium and phosphorus absorption.

Several case reports of women with XLH reported persistent hypophosphatemia during pregnancy, without obvious adverse outcomes.[114,115] It is advisable to maintain calcitriol and phosphorus supplementation as need to keep the serum phosphorus close to normal throughout pregnancy.

Hyperphosphatemic disorders due to loss of FGF23 action have not been studied during pregnancy. In the animal models, the conditions are lethal prior to reproductive maturity. There have been no case reports of pregnancies in women with hyperphosphatemic disorders caused by deficiency of FGF23 or its coreceptor. Animal and human data from renal insufficiency or failure, which cause hyperphosphatemia, indicate increased obstetrical risks of gestational hypertension, preeclampsia, eclampsia, and maternal mortality. However, the extent to which the hyperphosphatemia contributes to these risks, beyond that of the renal failure, is unknown.

21.2.12   Tocolytic Therapy with Magnesium Sulfate

Magnesium sulfate infusions are typically used for 24–72 h to treat preterm labor, preeclampsia, and eclampsia. Magnesium is a natural ligand for the calcium-sensing receptor; therefore, prolonged tocolytic therapy can suppress PTH and cause hypocalcemia.[116–118] PTH drops within the first hour, and the total and ionized serum calcium levels remain suppressed several hours later.[117,118] These findings are in keeping with hypoparathyroidism induced by the magnesium acting on the calcium receptor. Most cases are asymptomatic, but symptomatic hypocalcemia has been reported with positive Chvostek and Trousseau signs, and even tetany.[119]

If the magnesium infusion is maintained for several weeks, PTH can rise above normal. This is probably secondary hyperparathyroidism in response to the hypocalcemia, which increases the loss of calcium in the urine.[120] In a series of 20 women treated for weeks with magnesium for premature labor, serum magnesium and phosphorus increased, serum calcium decreased, serum PTH increased, and urinary excretion of magnesium and calcium increased twofold-to-threefold.[120] This will contribute to loss of BMC and strength, and it explains why prolonged magnesium infusions have been associated with postpartum loss of BMD and calcaneal stress fractures.[120–122] There are also potential effects on the fetus and neonate, which are discussed in Chapter 44.

21.2.12.1   Clinical Management

Maternal serum and cord blood magnesium are usually not monitored during tocolytic therapy. However, this should be done if the infusion is given for 2 or more days because hypermagnesemia can cause hypotonia, respiratory depression, and bone abnormalities.[116,123–125] Fetal movements should also be assessed by ultrasound to detect evidence of hypotonia.

21.3   DISORDERS OF BONE AND MINERAL METABOLISM DURING LACTATION

21.3.1   Osteoporosis of Lactation

Osteoporotic fractures occur rarely in breastfeeding women, but more often than during pregnancy.[4] These are most often vertebral compression fractures, with many reports describing extreme cases of women who experienced 6–10 crush fractures within a short interval.

As noted in Section 21.2.1, skeletal fragility may precede pregnancy and multiple factors can contribute to bone loss during pregnancy and lactation (Table 21.1). All these causes need to be considered in a woman who presents with fragility fractures while breastfeeding. Lactation introduces an added physiological cause of bone resorption that is stimulated by PTHrP (produced by the breasts) and systemic low estradiol concentrations.

As described in Chapter 5, lumbar spine BMD normally declines 5%–10% during lactation and can reach values well below normal for healthy women, including z-scores of −3 or lower. In addition, it is conceivable that in some women, release of PTHrP by the breasts may be more excessive than normal, or there may be increased sensitivity to high PTHrP or low estradiol, each of which could contribute to enhanced bone loss. The idea that excess PTHrP-mediated bone resorption can cause fragility fractures has been suggested by several published cases in which women presented with hypercalcemia, increased plasma PTHrP, and vertebral compression fractures.[1] After weaning, serum calcium and plasma PTHrP normalized.

21.3.1.1   Clinical Management

Diagnostic and management strategies are summarized in Tables 21.2–21.4.

If a woman is known to have skeletal fragility or very low bone mass, it may be reasonable to advise against breastfeeding or limit its duration because the progressive physiological bone loss that occurs over the first 6 months of lactation may lead to structural compromise of that woman's skeleton.[4] This must be balanced against other benefits of breast-feeding, including bonding and immune function. Furthermore, whenever fractures occur during lactation, it may also be reasonable to advise that breastfeeding stop in order to prevent further bone loss and initiate postweaning skeletal recovery.

Case series have shown that bone density spontaneously increases by 20%–70% in women who fractured while breast-feeding.[43] Therefore, as with pregnancy-associated fractures (as discussed previously), it may be prudent to withhold pharmacological therapy for 12–18 months to allow spontaneous recovery to occur, and then assess the need for additional treatment.[4] It is also a concern that antiremodeling agents such as a bisphosphonate or denosumab might blunt the spontaneous bone recovery that is expected during the postweaning interval.

Furthermore, all of the issues discussed earlier about pharmacotherapy (safety of individual agents, end-point to treatment) apply to breastfeeding women. Although individual case reports have described marked increases in bone mass associated with a variety of osteoporosis therapies, in each of these cases, the observed increase in bone mass was within the expected range that occurs with spontaneous postweaning recovery. Consequently, it is unclear that the use of pharmacotherapy in these studies achieved an added benefit. It is also unresolved as to whether an agent with a 2-year lifetime restriction on duration of use (i.e., teriparatide) should be used at a reproductive age when fracture risk should be inherently lower than it will be at older and postmenopausal ages, when pharmacotherapy might be more acutely needed.

21.3.2 Primary Hyperparathyroidism

If primary hyperparathyroidism was monitored rather than surgically treated during pregnancy, the postpartum period may remain uneventful. However, severe hypercalcemia from a parathyroid crisis can occur during the puerperium. This results from a combination of factors: Calcium is no longer being lost across the placenta, physiological bone resorption will occur from physical inactivity and bed rest, the onset of milk production will induce marked bone resorption (stimulated by low estradiol and increased PTHrP), and the systemic low estradiol levels of lactation will enhance skeletal responsiveness to the high circulating concentration of PTH. Consequently, significant worsening of hypercalcemia can occur in women with primary hyperparathyroidism who choose to breastfeed. However, a parathyroid crisis is not inevitable. In one published case, breastfeeding lessened hypercalcemia,[126] likely because production of breast milk also represents a new route for excess calcium to be drained from the circulation, thereby reducing the risk of severe hypercalcemia.

21.3.2.1 Clinical Management

Primary hyperparathyroidism can worsen significantly during the postpartum interval, with potential for more marked hypercalcemia in women who breastfeed. The clinician should reevaluate whether parathyroidectomy or medical therapy with cinacalcet is warranted at this time. Because the physiological hypercalciuria of pregnancy will have obscured the diagnosis of FHH, the possibility of this diagnosis should be reconsidered during the postpartum period. However, the physiological hypocalciuria of lactation will continue to make the calcium/creatinine clearance in urine to be invalid for diagnostic purposes. According to consensus guidelines for management of asymptomatic primary hyperparathyroidism, age <50 is an indication for surgery.[44] Therefore, postpartum women with primary hyperparathyroidism should be candidates for parathyroidectomy.

21.3.3 Familial Hypocalciuric Hypercalcemia

The calcium receptor not only controls the release of PTH by the parathyroids, but also the production of PTHrP by mammary tissue and the calcium content of milk.[1] When the *Casr* gene is ablated globally in mice, or selectively in mammary tissue, the consequences include reduced milk calcium content, increased mammary expression of PTHrP, greater bone loss during lactation, and urinary calcium excretion that exceeds that in normal controls.[127] Conversely, treatment with a calcimimetic drug such as cinacalcet results in increased milk calcium content and reduced mammary PTHrP production.[128,129]

These animal data predict that women with FHH will produce milk with reduced calcium content, accompanied by increased PTHrP, greater lactational bone loss, and increased renal calcium excretion. However, no such studies in lactating women with FHH have been done.

21.3.3.1   Clinical Management

FHH requires no management, apart from making certain that the affected women are not mistaken for having primary hyperparathyroidism and vice versa. During pregnancy, there is physiological hypercalciuria that can obscure the diagnosis of FHH, while during lactation, the resulting physiological hypocalciuria can obscure the diagnosis of primary hyperparathyroidism.[43] These considerations may require biochemical and genetic testing of relatives to determine if a mutation in *CASR* or other relevant genes are present, or waiting until the postweaning interval to determine if the biochemical picture is more in keeping with FHH vs primary hyperparathyroidism.

21.3.4   Hypoparathyroidism

For decades, hypoparathyroidism has been appreciated to improve during lactation, such that supplemental calcium and vitamin D analogs often are no longer required.[1] Some women with autoimmune hypoparathyroidism have been diagnosed when hypocalcemia abruptly occurs after weaning. The time of onset is consistent with a postpartum onset (typical of autoimmune endocrinopathies), but with a delay in clinical manifestation because of the effects that normal lactation has on bone and mineral metabolism. These observations led to the astute deduction that lactating breasts must produce a PTH-like hormone, which later proved to be PTHrP.

Animal studies have confirmed the physiological role that PTHrP plays in altering mineral and bone homeostasis during lactation, and that lactation can reverse the abnormalities created by absence of PTH.[1] In women, PTHrP has been confirmed to be expressed at high levels in lactating mammary tissue and milk, as well as being detectable in the circulation. PTHrP reaches the maternal circulation from the breasts, stimulates bone turnover, enhances renal tubular calcium reabsorption, and stimulates production of calcitriol.[60,130,131] Calcitriol increases in hypoparathyroid women from low levels, but it does not increase above normal, likely because PTHrP is less potent than PTH at stimulating the enzyme Cyp27b1 to produce calcitriol. The high prolactin and low estradiol of lactation may also alter the activity of Cyp27b1.[1]

Occasionally during the first 2 days postpartum, hypoparathyroid women have experienced transient hypocalcemia, presumably from the sudden loss of placental PTHrP.[55] This will resolve as lactation forces increased production of PTHrP by the breasts. In most cases, there has been no worsening in the early postpartum period. Instead, there has been a progressive lowering of the requirement for supplemental calcium and calcitriol as milk production upregulates. If this physiological response to lactation is not anticipated or recognized, the consequences have included severe hypercalcemia and even vertebral compression fractures.[28,60,131–135] In some women, all supplements need to be stopped, whereas in others, reduced doses are still required.

The rise and subsequent decline in plasma PTHrP has been shown to correspond to the rise and decline in serum calcium, calcitriol, and bone turnover markers in hypoparathyroid women.[28,60,130] In these cases, the improvement in mineral homeostasis correlates with the increasing intensity of lactation, while the subsequent decline correlates with reduced breastfeeding, and especially weaning. The less intensive or exclusive the breastfeeding, the more likely it is that hypoparathyroid women require some supplemental calcium and calcitriol to be maintained.

The rapidity with which the influence of PTHrP declines will vary, with some women requiring supplemental calcium and calcitriol to be restored before weaning, while others have not required this for weeks or months after weaning. In the latter cases, it is inferred that PTHrP production by the breasts has continued autonomously for months after weaning, which has been demonstrated in some women.[136] In one case described in the essay by Krista Rideout that introduces this textbook, a hypoparathyroid woman previously dependent on supplemental calcium and calcitriol has not required either for more than 6 years after weaning her child.

21.3.4.1   Clinical Management

The clinician should anticipate that lactation will cause normalization or near-normalization of mineral and skeletal homeostasis in hypoparathyroid women. Calcium monitoring should be done once or twice within 1 week after delivery in women who breastfeed, and every 2–4 weeks thereafter. The doses of supplemental calcium and calcitriol will need to be decreased as lactation becomes fully established, guided by measurements of the albumin-adjusted calcium or ionized calcium over the first several postpartum weeks. This should be followed by an interval of stability. But as lactation lessens, and especially after weaning, the need for supplemental calcium and calcitriol will gradually (or even abruptly) revert to prepregnancy levels.

21.3.5 Pseudohypoparathyroidism

The effect of breastfeeding on women with pseudohypoparathyroidism has not been described, and no animal model has been studied during lactation. Lactation can be anticipated to lead to an overall improvement in bone and mineral homeostasis due to the release of PTHrP from the breasts, akin to the clinical course of hypoparathyroidism. There is renal but not skeletal resistance to PTH in pseudohypoparathyroidism, and so it is possible that skeletal resorption may even be greater than normal during lactation, as the high levels of PTH and PTHrP combine to affect bone turnover.

21.3.5.1 Clinical Management

In the absence of any data to indicate otherwise, clinicians should consider that pseudohypoparathyroidism may improve during lactation (as does hypoparathyroidism), resulting in the need for decreased doses of calcium and calcitriol during lactation. If this occurs, it will be followed by a return of the need for the prior doses during or after weaning.

21.3.6 Pseudohyperparathyroidism

As noted earlier in Chapter 5, the physiological release of PTHrP from the breasts will contribute to a small increase in serum calcium and phosphorus, suppression of PTH, increased bone resorption, and reduced renal calcium excretion. This is a silent aspect of lactational physiology that most women are unaware of unless they have hypoparathyroidism and find that they no longer need supplemental calcium and calcitriol while breastfeeding.

However, the effects of breast-derived PTHrP occasionally cause symptomatic hypercalcemia in otherwise-normal breastfeeding women. Such PTHrP-mediated hypercalcemia is called *pseudohyperparathyroidism* because it mimics primary hyperparathyroidism but is not due to PTH. It can develop during normal lactation, in women who deliver but are unable to breastfeed, and in nonlactating women with unduly large breasts.[1] The main pathophysiology is that high levels of PTHrP induce skeletal resorption accompanied by increased renal reabsorption of calcium. If PTHrP also causes increased calcitriol, then intestinal calcium absorption may be increased. Vertebral compression fractures have occurred in some women.

The published cases have emphasized extremes in which women developed symptomatic hypercalcemia while breastfeeding. Some cases may not be recognized because the symptoms of hypercalcemia are nonspecific and not readily distinguishable from the constitutional symptoms that any woman may experience when she is feeding a baby on demand. Furthermore, considering that serum calcium and ionized calcium rise modestly during normal lactation,[1] it is possible that asymptomatic hypercalcemia is more common during lactation than the case reports would suggest.

21.3.6.1 Clinical Management

If severe hypercalcemia occurs, the condition can be reversed rapidly by weaning the baby, combined with judicious use of breast binders and dopaminergic medications (cabergoline or bromocriptine) to suppress prolactin and shut off the production of PTHrP. This is likely a safer approach than using other drugs in the presence of continued breastfeeding. Indeed, there is limited evidence that bisphosphonates likely do not enter breast milk, but this has not been determined for denosumab.

Excess production of PTHrP has occasionally persisted long after weaning and has rarely required reduction mammoplasty or bilateral mastectomy to correct the disorder.[137]

21.3.7 Vitamin D Deficiency, Genetic Vitamin D Resistance, and 24-Hydroxylase Deficiency

21.3.7.1 Vitamin D Deficiency and Genetic Vitamin D Resistance

The effect of disrupted vitamin D physiology on lactation has been studied in *Vdr*-null and *Cyp27b1*-null mice, and vitamin D-deficient mice and rats.[1] The findings have been generally consistent among the various models, including that the calcium content of milk is normal, mineral metabolism improves to normalize the serum calcium, intestinal calcium absorption increases, lactational bone loss occurs that may be equal to or greater than normal, and during postweaning, there is increased bone formation with complete or near-complete recovery of skeletal microarchitecture and bone mass.[1] Occasional deaths occur during lactation, which are presumed to result from hypocalcemia, precipitated by milk production overwhelming the mother's ability to maintain her blood calcium. The overall findings suggest that calcitriol is not required for lactation to proceed normally or for the skeleton to restore itself after weaning.

Clinical data come from observational cohort studies and randomized interventional trials of vitamin D supplementation.[1] These have not shown any effect of higher 25OHD concentrations or vitamin D intake on maternal mineral or skeletal homeostasis in otherwise-healthy, lactating women. Vitamin D supplementation increases maternal 25OHD levels with similar efficacy as in nonpregnant or nonlactating women.

No studies have directly compared severely vitamin D-deficient and -sufficient women. However, the data discussed next support the proposition that vitamin D deficiency, VDDR-I, and VDDR-II are unlikely to affect lactation or milk production adversely.

Milk normally contains little vitamin D or 25OHD (approximately 30–40 IU/L combined), with very low to undetectable amounts of calcitriol. Consequently, milk production does not drain maternal vitamin D stores, and maternal 25OHD remains unchanged during lactation unless there are changes in dietary intake of vitamin D or exposure to sunlight. Randomized interventional studies have found that maternal vitamin D doses of 400–1000 IU/day do not consistently increase the breast milk content of vitamin D or 25OHD, whereas with doses of 2000 IU/day or higher, the milk content of vitamin D and 25OHD demonstrably improve and lead to an increase in neonatal 25OHD.[138–145]

The calcium content of breast milk calcium is unaffected by maternal 25OHD concentrations ranging from low [25 nmol/L (10 ng/mL)] to high [160 nmol/L (64 ng/mL)].[145,146] These data come from cohort studies[146] and randomized interventions that administered up to 6400 IU/day of vitamin D.[138,143,145] However, there have been a few cases from India in which milk calcium content was low in mothers with severe vitamin D deficiency [mean 25OHD of 6 nmol/L (2.5 ng/mL)]; they also had severe hypocalcemia, hypophosphatemia, and markedly elevated PTH.[147] Overall, these results indicate that calcitriol does not play a substantial role in stimulating calcium to enter milk. But in very severe vitamin D-deficient women, it may be the marked hypocalcemia, rather than a direct effect of loss of calcitriol, that leads to reduced milk calcium content.

In regions where severe vitamin D-deficiency rickets is endemic, such as India, affected neonates have been treated with breast milk as their only form of nutrition, while their mothers were receiving the equivalent of 1800 IU of vitamin D per day.[147,148] Mothers and babies were protected from sun exposure and had negligible amounts of vitamin D in the diet, and so the maternal supplement was the principal source of vitamin D for both. The mean 25OHD rose from 6 nmol/L (2 ng/mL) or below in mothers and babies to approximately 50 nmol/L (20 ng/mL) in the mothers and 40 nmol/L (16 ng/mL) in their babies. This finding indicates that more vitamin D enters breast milk than has been appreciated by the previously cited studies. Moreover, the normal calcium content of breast milk is very relevant because providing sufficient calcium alone will heal rickets due to vitamin D deficiency or VDDR-II.[72]

No clinical studies have explicitly examined whether vitamin D deficiency, VDDR-I, or VDDR-II affects the ability of the skeleton to acutely recover bone mass and architecture after weaning. As discussed in Chapter 5, dozens of large epidemiological studies have found neutral or protective associations of lactation on BMD and fracture risk in the long term, with many of the women in those studies being vitamin D insufficient or deficient by modern criteria.[1] Despite the limitations of associational studies, these consistent findings suggest that skeletal recovery after weaning is not impaired by vitamin D insufficiency either.

21.3.7.2 24-Hydroxylase Deficiency

As noted earlier, hereditary absence of Cyp24a1 reduces calcitriol catabolism and can lead to marked maternal hypercalcemia during pregnancy, accompanied by very high calcitriol concentrations. But calcitriol production falls to nonpregnant levels during normal lactation, and the same should be true in women with 24-hydroxylase deficiency. Consistent with this, in one affected woman who breastfed, hypercalcemia was milder compared to pregnancy and serum calcitriol was normal.[105]

21.3.7.3 Clinical Management: Vitamin D Deficiency and Genetic Vitamin D Resistance

Animal data consistently indicate that milk calcium content, skeletal resorption during lactation, and postweaning skeletal recovery may be unaffected by extremes of vitamin D physiology, including absence of VDR, calcitriol, and vitamin D. The more limited clinical data are similar, indicating that maternal vitamin D stores are not adversely affected by lactation, milk calcium content is unaffected by vitamin D deficiency (unless significant hypocalcemia is present), and lactational bone loss and recovery also may be unaffected by the absence of calcitriol's actions. There is no evidence that the requirement for vitamin D increases during lactation to meet maternal or neonatal needs.

Nevertheless, it remains prudent to correct vitamin D deficiency promptly whenever it is recognized. The available data suggest that the amount of vitamin D intake required to replenish total body stores and maintain a set level of 25OHD should be unaffected by lactation. Similarly, management of VDDR-I and VDDR-II should be unaffected by lactation.

Because milk normally contains low amounts of vitamin D or 25OHD, high-dose vitamin D supplementation has the possible benefit of enabling all of a baby's nutrition to come from breast milk rather than requiring that oral vitamin D supplements be given to breastfed babies. However, the high doses used in the studies cited previously are not needed if the goal is a 25OHD level of 50 nmol/L, as the Institute of Medicine and pediatric societies have suggested.[24]

21.3.7.4 Clinical Management: 24-Hydroxylase Deficiency

Lactation could conceivably worsen hypercalcemia in women with 24-hydroxylase deficiency by introducing the physiological bone resorption stimulated by PTHrP and low estradiol. However, because calcitriol production is normal during lactation, hypercalcemia is much less likely to occur than during pregnancy, and breastfeeding can be encouraged.

21.3.8 Calcitonin Deficiency

Calcitonin has been theorized to protect the maternal skeleton against excessive resorption during lactation. Earlier studies in thyroidectomized rats and goats yielded inconsistent results, likely because it is now recognized that lactating mammary tissue produces substantial calcitonin. Consequently, a thyroidectomized animal is not calcitonin deficient while lactating.[1] More recent studies examined *Ctcgrp*-null mice, which lack calcitonin and calcitonin gene-related peptide-α but retain calcitonin gene-related peptide-B.[149] This global calcitonin deficiency resulted in lactating mice losing twice the bone mass as their normal sisters during lactation—an effect that was prevented by treating with calcitonin injections at the onset of lactation.[110] The lactating calcitonin-ablated mice have increased expression of PTHrP, a doubling of milk calcium content, doubling of osteoclast numbers and surface, and half the osteoblast numbers and surface compared to normal sister mice.[109,110,150] Remarkably, the skeleton recovers from these marked deficits within 18 days of weaning, accompanied by a substantial fall in osteoclast numbers and a surge in osteoblast numbers and activity.[110,150] Overall, the *Ctcgrp*-null model confirms that calcitonin protects the rodent skeleton from excessive resorption during lactation, but whether the same is true for women has not been determined.

No clinical studies have specifically tested whether calcitonin deficiency causes increased bone loss during lactation. This is mainly because inactivating mutations of calcitonin or its receptor have not been identified in humans. A thyroidectomized woman nursing twins experienced multiple vertebral compression fractures and had marked bone loss confirmed by DXA; the authors speculated that calcitonin deficiency was to blame.[28] But thyroidectomized women are not expected to be calcitonin deficient while breastfeeding because lactating breast tissue produces normal circulating calcitonin levels.[1]

21.3.8.1 Clinical Management

There are no human data on clinical management, and so firm recommendations cannot be offered. However, the available animal data suggest that lactation leads to excessive skeletal losses, and so it may be prudent to recommend against breastfeeding in lactating women. Treatment with calcitonin conceivably could prevent excessive bone loss and allow lactation to continue, but there are no reports to validate this speculation.

21.3.9 Low or High Calcium Intake

Lactating rodents have a proportionately very high demand for calcium, given their large litter sizes (8–12 pups) and short duration of lactation (3 weeks). They rely on the combined effects of increased intestinal calcium absorption, skeletal resorption, and renal tubal calcium reabsorption. The rodent is capable to some extent of extracting more calcium from the skeleton when the diet is deficient, or more from the diet when the skeleton cannot be resorbed. Consequently, a calcium-restricted diet increases skeletal losses but also can lead to hypocalcemia and sudden death from tetany; conversely, a high-calcium diet reduces skeletal losses.[1] During postweaning, a low calcium intake impairs skeletal recovery in rats, but full recovery in the same rats was achieved when a normal-calcium diet was administered later.[151]

In contrast to the animal data, the calcium content of human milk appears to be largely derived from skeletal resorption. Consequently, low calcium intake does not reduce breast-milk calcium, nor does it cause increased skeletal resorption.[146,152-156] Conversely, high calcium intake neither increases breast-milk calcium nor reduces the amount of skeletal resorption that occurs during lactation.[153-161] These data come from well-designed randomized clinical trials and cohort studies and indicate that maternal calcium intake may be irrelevant during lactation because skeletal resorption is hormonally programmed to supply the needed amount of calcium. There is no evidence that women require a higher intake of calcium while breastfeeding.

No clinical studies have examined calcium intake during postweaning, which may be a more critical time to ensure adequate calcium intake. However, adolescents recovering from lactation experienced a substantial increment in bone mass despite a habitual intake of <500 mg/day of calcium.[162] Randomization to a 1-g calcium supplement daily resulted in a small gain in bone mass gain during 6 months of recovery.[159]

21.3.9.1 Clinical Management

The available data indicate that women do not require increased calcium intake during lactation or postweaning recovery. Instead, for all women, the recommended calcium intake remains the same as that of nonpregnant women, which is 1200 mg/day of calcium.[24]

21.3.10 FGF23-Related Disorders

Phex[+/−] females are the murine equivalent of XLH. The affected mice remain hypophosphatemic during lactation; produce milk with normal phosphorus, calcium, and protein content; and have pups that grow normally.[163] Hyperphosphatemic disorders due to loss of FGF23 of its coreceptor Klotho have not been studied during lactation because the mice die before reaching reproductive maturity.

In one case report, serum phosphorus normalized during lactation in a woman with XLH, whereas it was low during pregnancy and equivalent to expected nonpregnant values.[114] Serum phosphorus likely normalizes because of the increased skeletal resorption during lactation, which brings calcium and phosphorus into the circulation. However, despite normalization of serum phosphorus in the mother during lactation, the phosphorus content of expressed milk was reduced to 50% of normal in two cases, whereas the calcium content was modestly reduced in one but normal in the other.[114,115] It is unclear why milk from women with XLH had low phosphorus, while the content was normal in the animal model. Oral phosphorus supplementation normalized the milk composition.[114] In both cases, the babies inherited XLH, so the development of hypophosphatemia and rickets was likely due to the combined effects of the mutation and the low phosphorus content of milk.[114,115]

No studies have examined lactation in hyperphosphatemic disorders from the loss of FGF23 or its coreceptor, but it is conceivable that phosphorus content of milk will be increased.

21.3.10.1 Clinical Management

Women with XLH may require phosphorus supplementation to maintain normal phosphorus content in milk. If the calcium content is also reduced, this cannot be fixed by oral calcium supplementation. If a baby born of a woman with XLH develops hypophosphatemia, this could indicate that milk is deficient in phosphorus or that the baby inherited the mutation.

21.4 CONCLUSIONS

Doubling of intestinal calcium and phosphorus absorption during pregnancy meets the fetal demand for these minerals, while an increase in skeletal resorption provides the required mineral content of milk during lactation. These adaptations during pregnancy and lactation have important effects on preexisting disorders of bone and mineral metabolism. The symptoms, signs, diagnostic indexes, and treatment strategies may be altered. This is best exemplified by how lactation can normalize mineral homeostasis in hypoparathyroid women, but when this is overlooked, it has led to iatrogenic and life-threatening hypercalcemia.

REFERENCES

1. Kovacs CS. Maternal mineral and bone metabolism during pregnancy, lactation, and post-weaning recovery. *Physiol Rev* 2016;**96**(2):449–547.
2. Albright F, Reifenstein EC. *Parathyroid glands and metabolic bone disease*. Baltimore: Williams & Wilkins; 1948.
3. Stride PJ, Patel N, Kingston D. The history of osteoporosis: why do Egyptian mummies have porotic bones? *J R Coll Physicians Edinb* 2013; **43**(3):254–61.
4. Kovacs CS, Ralston SH. Presentation and management of osteoporosis presenting in association with pregnancy or lactation. *Osteoporos Int* 2015; **26**(9):2223–41.
5. Laroche M, Talibart M, Cormier C, Roux C, Guggenbuhl P, Degboe Y. Pregnancy-related fractures: a retrospective study of a French cohort of 52 patients and review of the literature. *Osteoporos Int* 2017;**28**(11):3135–42.
6. Herath M, Wong P, Trinh A, Allan CA, Wallace EM, Ebeling PR, et al. Minimal-trauma ankle fractures predominate during pregnancy: a 17-year retrospective study. *Arch Osteoporos* 2017;**12**(1):86.

7. Ferrari S, Bianchi ML, Eisman JA, Foldes AJ, Adami S, Wahl DA, et al. Osteoporosis in young adults: pathophysiology, diagnosis, and management. *Osteoporos Int* 2012;**23**(12):2735–48.

8. Abraham A, Cohen A, Shane E. *Clin Obstet Gynecol* 2013;**56**(4):722–9.

9. Dempster DW, Compston JE, Drezner MK, Glorieux FH, Kanis JA, Malluche H, et al. Standardized nomenclature, symbols, and units for bone histomorphometry: a 2012 update of the report of the ASBMR Histomorphometry Nomenclature Committee. *J Bone Miner Res* 2013;**28**(1):2–17.

10. Smith R, Stevenson JC, Winearls CG, Woods CG, Wordsworth BP. Osteoporosis of pregnancy. *Lancet* 1985;**1**(8439):1178–80.

11. Smith R, Athanasou NA, Ostlere SJ, Vipond SE. Pregnancy-associated osteoporosis. *Q J Med* 1995;**88**(12):865–78.

12. Yamamoto N, Takahashi HE, Tanizawa T, Kawashima T, Endo N. Bone mineral density and bone histomorphometric assessments of postpregnancy osteoporosis: a report of five patients. *Calcif Tissue Int* 1994;**54**(1):20–5.

13. Dent CE, Friedman M. Pregnancy and idiopathic osteoporosis. *Q J Med* 1965;**34**(135):341–57.

14. Nordin BE, Roper A. Post-pregnancy osteoporosis; a syndrome? *Lancet* 1955;**268**(6861):431–4.

15. Dunne F, Walters B, Marshall T, Heath DA. Pregnancy associated osteoporosis. *Clin Endocrinol (Oxf)* 1993;**39**(4):487–90.

16. Khovidhunkit W, Epstein S. Osteoporosis in pregnancy. *Osteoporos Int* 1996;**6**(5):345–54.

17. Phillips AJ, Ostlere SJ, Smith R. Pregnancy-associated osteoporosis: does the skeleton recover? *Osteoporos Int* 2000;**11**(5):449–54.

18. Asadipooya K, Graves L, Greene LW. Transient osteoporosis of the hip: review of the literature. *Osteoporos Int* 2017;**28**(6):1805–16.

19. Baki ME, Uygun H, Ari B, Aydin H. Bilateral femoral neck insufficiency fractures in pregnancy. *Eklem Hastalik Cerrahisi* 2014;**25**(1):60–2.

20. Aynaci O, Kerimoglu S, Ozturk C, Saracoglu M. Bilateral non-traumatic acetabular and femoral neck fractures due to pregnancy-associated osteoporosis. *Arch Orthop Trauma Surg* 2008;**128**(3):313–6.

21. Bonacker J, Janousek M, Krober M. Pregnancy-associated osteoporosis with eight fractures in the vertebral column treated with kyphoplasty and bracing: a case report. *Arch Orthop Trauma Surg* 2014;**134**(2):173–9.

22. Pallavi P, Padma S, Vanitha Anna Selvi D. Transient osteoporosis of hip and lumbar spine in pregnancy. *J Obstet Gynaecol India* 2012;**62**(Suppl 1):8–9.

23. Stathopoulos IP, Liakou CG, Katsalira A, Trovas G, Lyritis GG, Papaioannou NA, et al. The use of bisphosphonates in women prior to or during pregnancy and lactation. *Hormones (Athens)* 2011;**10**(4):280–91.

24. Ross AC, Abrams SA, Aloia JF, Brannon PM, Clinton SK, Durazo-Arvizu RA, et al. Ross AC, Taylor CL, YA L, Del Valle HB, editors. *Dietary reference intakes for calcium and vitamin D*. Washington, DC: Institute of Medicine; 2011.

25. Iwamoto J, Sato Y, Uzawa M, Matsumoto H. Five-year follow-up of a woman with pregnancy and lactation-associated osteoporosis and vertebral fractures. *Ther Clin Risk Manag* 2012;**8**:195–9.

26. Anai T, Tomiyasu T, Arima K, Miyakawa I. Pregnancy-associated osteoporosis with elevated levels of circulating parathyroid hormone-related protein: a report of two cases. *J Obstet Gynaecol Res* 1999;**25**(1):63–7.

27. Tran HA, Petrovsky N. Pregnancy-associated osteoporosis with hypercalcaemia. *Intern Med J* 2002;**32**(9–10):481–5.

28. Segal E, Hochberg I, Weisman Y, Ish-Shalom S. Severe postpartum osteoporosis with increased PTHrP during lactation in a patient after total thyroidectomy and parathyroidectomy. *Osteoporos Int* 2011;**22**(11):2907–11.

29. Liel Y, Atar D, Ohana N. Pregnancy-associated osteoporosis: preliminary densitometric evidence of extremely rapid recovery of bone mineral density. *South Med J* 1998;**91**(1):33–5.

30. Ijuin A, Yoshikata H, Asano R, Tsuburai T, Kikuchi R, Sakakibara H. Teriparatide and denosumab treatment for pregnancy and lactation-associated osteoporosis with multiple vertebral fractures: a case study. *Taiwan J Obstet Gynecol* 2017;**56**(6):863–6.

31. Hong N, Kim JE, Lee SJ, Kim SH, Rhee Y. Changes in bone mineral density and bone turnover markers during treatment with teriparatide in pregnancy- and lactation-associated osteoporosis. *Clin Endocrinol (Oxf)* 2018;**88**(5):652–8.

32. Campos-Obando N, Oei L, Hoefsloot LH, Kiewiet RM, Klaver CC, Simon ME, et al. Osteoporotic vertebral fractures during pregnancy: be aware of a potential underlying genetic cause. *J Clin Endocrinol Metab* 2014;**99**(4):1107–11.

33. Grizzo FM, da Silva MJ, Pinheiro MM, Jorgetti V, Carvalho MD, Pelloso SM. Pregnancy and lactation-associated osteoporosis: bone histomorphometric analysis and response to treatment with zoledronic acid. *Calcif Tissue Int* 2015;**97**(4):421–5.

34. Chan B, Zacharin M. Maternal and infant outcome after pamidronate treatment of polyostotic fibrous dysplasia and osteogenesis imperfecta before conception: a report of four cases. *J Clin Endocrinol Metab* 2006;**91**(6):2017–20.

35. Tanriover MD, Oz SG, Sozen T. Ten-year follow-up in pregnancy and lactation-associated osteoporosis: sequential therapy with strontium ranelate and ibandronate. *Spine J* 2015;**15**(5):1164–5.

36. Boyce RW, Varela A, Chouinard L, Bussiere JL, Chellman GJ, Ominsky MS, et al. Infant cynomolgus monkeys exposed to denosumab in utero exhibit an osteoclast-poor osteopetrotic-like skeletal phenotype at birth and in the early postnatal period. *Bone* 2014;**64**:314–25.

37. Okamatsu N, Sakai N, Karakawa A, Kouyama N, Sato Y, Inagaki K, et al. Biological effects of anti-RANKL antibody administration in pregnant mice and their newborns. *Biochem Biophys Res Commun* 2017;**491**(3):614–21.

38. Rodriguez AJ, Fink HA, Mirigian L, Guanabens N, Eastell R, Akesson K, et al. Pain, quality of life, and safety outcomes of kyphoplasty for vertebral compression fractures: report of a task force of the American Society for Bone and Mineral Research. *J Bone Miner Res* 2017;**32**(9):1935–44.

38a. Ebeling PR, Akesson K, Bauer DC, Buchbinder R, Eastell R, Fink HA, Giangregorio L, Guanabens N, Kado D, Kallmes D, Katzman W, Rodriguez A, Wermers R, Wilson HA, Bouxsein ML. The Efficacy and Safety of Vertebral Augmentation: A Second ASBMR Task Force Report. *J Bone Miner Res* 2019;**3**(1):3–21.

39. Kort KC, Schiller HJ, Numann PJ. Hyperparathyroidism and pregnancy. *Am J Surg* 1999;**177**(1):66–8.

40. Kelly TR. Primary hyperparathyroidism during pregnancy. *Surgery* 1991;**110**(6):1028–33. discussion 33-34.

41. Hirsch D, Kopel V, Nadler V, Levy S, Toledano Y, Tsvetov G. Pregnancy outcomes in women with primary hyperparathyroidism. *J Clin Endocrinol Metab* 2015;**100**(5):2115–22.

42. Dochez V, Ducarme G. Primary hyperparathyroidism during pregnancy. *Arch Gynecol Obstet* 2015;**291**(2):259–63.

43. Ghaznavi SA, Saad NM, Donovan LE. The biochemical profile of familial hypocalciuric hypercalcemia and primary hyperparathyroidism during pregnancy and lactation: two case reports and review of the literature. *Case Rep Endocrinol* 2016;**2016**:2725486.

44. Bilezikian JP, Brandi ML, Eastell R, Silverberg SJ, Udelsman R, Marcocci C, et al. Guidelines for the management of asymptomatic primary hyperparathyroidism: summary statement from the Fourth International Workshop. *J Clin Endocrinol Metab* 2014;**99**(10):3561–9.

45. Abood A, Vestergaard P. Pregnancy outcomes in women with primary hyperparathyroidism. *Eur J Endocrinol* 2014;**171**(1):69–76.

46. Norman J, Politz D, Politz L. Hyperparathyroidism during pregnancy and the effect of rising calcium on pregnancy loss: a call for earlier intervention. *Clin Endocrinol (Oxf)* 2009;**71**(1):104–9.

47. McDonnell CM, Zacharin MR. Maternal primary hyperparathyroidism: discordant outcomes in a twin pregnancy. *J Paediatr Child Health* 2006;**42**(1–2):70–1.

48. Zeng H, Li Z, Zhang X, Wang N, Tian Y, Wang J. Anesthetic management of primary hyperparathyroidism during pregnancy: a case report. *Medicine (Baltimore)* 2017;**96**(51).

49. Han ES, Fritton K, Bacon P, Slodzinski MK, Argani C. Preterm parturient with polyhydramnios and pancreatitis: primary presentation of hyperparathyroidism. *Case Rep Obstet Gynecol* 2018;**2018**:2091082.

50. Herrera-Martinez AD, Bahamondes-Opazo R, Palomares-Ortega R, Munoz-Jimenez C, Galvez-Moreno MA, Quesada Gomez JM. Primary hyperparathyroidism in pregnancy: a two-case report and literature review. *Case Rep Obstet Gynecol* 2015;**2015**:171828.

51. Brown EM. The calcium-sensing receptor: physiology, pathophysiology and CaR-based therapeutics. *Subcell Biochem* 2007;**45**:139–67.

52. Kovacs CS, Ho-Pao CL, Hunzelman JL, Lanske B, Fox J, Seidman JG, et al. Regulation of murine fetal-placental calcium metabolism by the calcium-sensing receptor. *J Clin Invest* 1998;**101**:2812–20.

53. Walker A, Fraile JJ, Hubbard JG. "Parathyroidectomy in pregnancy"—a single centre experience with review of evidence and proposal for treatment algorithim. *Gland Surg* 2014;**3**(3):158–64.

54. Morton A. Altered calcium homeostasis during pregnancy may affect biochemical differentiation of hypercalcaemia. *Intern Med J* 2004;**34**(11):655–6 author reply 6-7.

55. Sweeney LL, Malabanan AO, Rosen H. Decreased calcitriol requirement during pregnancy and lactation with a window of increased requirement immediately post partum. *Endocr Pract* 2010;**16**(3):459–62.

56. Graham III WP, Gordon CS, Loken HF, Blum A, Halden A. Effect of pregnancy and of the menstrual cycle on hypoparathyroidism. *J Clin Endocrinol Metab* 1964;**24**:512–6.

57. Bronsky D, Kiamko RT, Moncada R, Rosenthal IM. Intra-uterine hyperparathyroidism secondary to maternal hypoparathyroidism. *Pediatrics* 1968;**42**:606–13.

58. Furui T, Imai A, Tamaya T. Successful outcome of pregnancy complicated with thyroidectomy-induced hypoparathyroidism and sudden dyspnea. A case report. *Gynecol Obstet Invest* 1993;**35**:57–9.

59. Anai T, Tomiyasu T, Takai N, Miyakawa I. Remission of idiopathic hypoparathyroidism during lactation: a case report. *J Obstet Gynaecol Res* 1999;**25**(4):271–3.

60. Shomali ME, Ross DS. Hypercalcemia in a woman with hypoparathyroidism associated with increased parathyroid hormone-related protein during lactation. *Endocr Pract* 1999;**5**(4):198–200.

61. Markestad T, Ulstein M, Bassoe HH, Aksnes L, Aarskog D. Vitamin D metabolism in normal and hypoparathyroid pregnancy and lactation. Case report. *Br J Obstet Gynaecol* 1983;**90**:971–6.

62. Hoper K, Pavel M, Dorr HG, Kandler C, Kruse K, Wildt L, et al. Calcitriol administration during pregnancy in a partial DiGeorge anomaly. *Dtsch Med Wochenschr* 1994;**119**(51–52):1776–80.

63. Kurzel RB, Hagen GA. Use of thiazide diuretics to reduce the hypercalciuria of hypoparathyroidism during pregnancy. *Am J Perinatol* 1990;**7**:333–6.

64. Rabau-Friedman E, Mashiach S, Cantor E, Jacob ET. Association of hypoparathyroidism and successful pregnancy in kidney transplant recipient. *Obstet Gynecol* 1982;**59**:126–8.

65. Hatswell BL, Allan CA, Teng J, Wong P, Ebeling PR, Wallace EM, et al. Management of hypoparathyroidism in pregnancy and lactation—a report of 10 cases. *Bone Rep* 2015;**3**:15–9.

66. Ilany J, Vered I, Cohen O. The effect of continuous subcutaneous recombinant PTH (1-34) infusion during pregnancy on calcium homeostasis—a case report. *Gynecol Endocrinol* 2013;**29**(9):807–10.

67. Breslau NA, Zerwekh JE. Relationship of estrogen and pregnancy to calcium homeostasis in pseudohypoparathyroidism. *J Clin Endocrinol Metab* 1986;**62**:45–51.

68. Morton A. Milk-alkali syndrome in pregnancy, associated with elevated levels of parathyroid hormone-related protein. *Intern Med J* 2002;**32**(9–10):492–3.

69. Eller-Vainicher C, Ossola MW, Beck-Peccoz P, Chiodini I. PTHrP-associated hypercalcemia of pregnancy resolved after delivery: a case report. *Eur J Endocrinol* 2012;**166**(4):753–6.

70. Winter EM, Appelman-Dijkstra NM. Parathyroid hormone-related protein-induced hypercalcemia of pregnancy successfully reversed by a dopamine agonist. *J Clin Endocrinol Metab* 2017;**102**(12):4417–20.

71. Gillies BR, Ryan BA, Tonkin BA, Poulton IJ, Ma Y, Kirby BJ, et al. Absence of calcitriol causes increased lactational bone loss and lower milk calcium but does not impair post-lactation bone recovery in Cyp27b1 null mice. *J Bone Miner Res* 2018;**33**(1):16–26.

72. Kovacs CS. Bone development and mineral homeostasis in the fetus and neonate: roles of the calciotropic and phosphotropic hormones. *Physiol Rev* 2014;**94**(4):1143–218.

73. Fudge NJ, Kovacs CS. Pregnancy up-regulates intestinal calcium absorption and skeletal mineralization independently of the vitamin D receptor. *Endocrinology* 2010;**151**(3):886–95.

74. Lieben L, Stockmans I, Moermans K, Carmeliet G. Maternal hypervitaminosis D reduces fetal bone mass and mineral acquisition and leads to neonatal lethality. *Bone* 2013;**57**(1):123–31.

75. Liu NQ, Ouyang Y, Bulut Y, Lagishetty V, Chan SY, Hollis BW, et al. Dietary vitamin D restriction in pregnant female mice is associated with maternal hypertension and altered placental and fetal development. *Endocrinology* 2013;**154**(7):2270–80.

76. St-Arnaud R, Arabian A, Travers R, Barletta F, Raval-Pandya M, Chapin K, et al. Deficient mineralization of intramembranous bone in vitamin D-24-hydroxylase-ablated mice is due to elevated 1,25-dihydroxyvitamin D and not to the absence of 24,25-dihydroxyvitamin D. *Endocrinology* 2000;**141**(7):2658–66.

77. Lee CY, Koren G. Maternal obesity: effects on pregnancy and the role of pre-conception counselling. *J Obstet Gynaecol* 2010;**30**(2):101–6.

78. Brooke OG, Brown IR, Bone CD, Carter ND, Cleeve HJ, Maxwell JD, et al. Vitamin D supplements in pregnant Asian women: effects on calcium status and fetal growth. *Br Med J* 1980;**280**:751–4.

79. Hollis BW, Johnson D, Hulsey TC, Ebeling M, Wagner CL. Vitamin D supplementation during pregnancy: double-blind, randomized clinical trial of safety and effectiveness. *J Bone Miner Res* 2011;**26**(10):2341–57.

80. Roth DE, Al Mahmud A, Raqib R, Akhtar E, Perumal N, Pezzack B, et al. Randomized placebo-controlled trial of high-dose prenatal third-trimester vitamin D3 supplementation in Bangladesh: the AViDD trial. *Nutr J* 2013;**12**(1):47.

81. Wagner CL, McNeil R, Hamilton SA, Winkler J, Rodriguez Cook C, Warner G, et al. A randomized trial of vitamin D supplementation in 2 community health center networks in South Carolina. *Am J Obstet Gynecol* 2013;**208**(2) 137.e1-13.

82. Dawodu A, Saadi HF, Bekdache G, Javed Y, Altaye M, Hollis BW. Randomized controlled trial (RCT) of vitamin D supplementation in pregnancy in a population with endemic vitamin D deficiency. *J Clin Endocrinol Metab* 2013;**98**(6):2337–46.

83. Grant CC, Stewart AW, Scragg R, Milne T, Rowden J, Ekeroma A, et al. Vitamin D during pregnancy and infancy and infant serum 25-hydroxyvitamin D concentration. *Pediatrics* 2014;**133**(1):e143–53.

84. Vaziri F, Dabbaghmanesh MH, Samsami A, Nasiri S, Shirazi PT. Vitamin D supplementation during pregnancy on infant anthropometric measurements and bone mass of mother-infant pairs: A randomized placebo clinical trial. *Early Hum Dev* 2016;**103**:61–8.

85. Cooper C, Harvey NC, Bishop NJ, Kennedy S, Papageorghiou AT, Schoenmakers I, et al. Maternal gestational vitamin D supplementation and offspring bone health (MAVIDOS): a multicentre, double-blind, randomised placebo-controlled trial. *Lancet Diabetes Endocrinol* 2016;**4**(5):393–402.

86. Roth DE, Morris SK, Zlotkin S, Gernand AD, Ahmed T, Shanta SS, et al. Vitamin D Supplementation in pregnancy and lactation and infant growth. *N Engl J Med* 2018;**379**(6):535–46.

87. Hollis BW, Wagner CL. Vitamin D and pregnancy: skeletal effects, nonskeletal effects, and birth outcomes. *Calcif Tissue Int* 2013;**92**(2):128–39.

88. Wagner CL, McNeil RB, Johnson DD, Hulsey TC, Ebeling M, Robinson C, et al. Health characteristics and outcomes of two randomized vitamin D supplementation trials during pregnancy: a combined analysis. *J Steroid Biochem Mol Biol* 2013;**136**:313–20.

89. Wagner CL, Baggerly C, McDonnell SL, Baggerly L, Hamilton SA, Winkler J, et al. Post-hoc comparison of vitamin D status at three timepoints during pregnancy demonstrates lower risk of preterm birth with higher vitamin D closer to delivery. *J Steroid Biochem Mol Biol* 2015;**148**:256–60.

90. Wei W, Shary JR, Garrett-Mayer E, Anderson B, Forestieri NE, Hollis BW, et al. Bone mineral density during pregnancy in women participating in a randomized controlled trial of vitamin D supplementation. *Am J Clin Nutr* 2017;**106**(6):1422–30.

91. Khaing W, Vallibhakara SA, Tantrakul V, Vallibhakara O, Rattanasiri S, McEvoy M, et al. Calcium and Vitamin D Supplementation for Prevention of Preeclampsia: A Systematic Review and Network Meta-Analysis. *Nutrients* 2017;**9**(10). https://doi.org/10.3390/nu9101141.

92. De-Regil LM, Palacios C, Lombardo LK, Pena-Rosas JP. Vitamin D supplementation for women during pregnancy. *Cochrane Database Syst Rev* 2016;**1**.

93. Hypponen E, Cavadino A, Williams D, Fraser A, Vereczkey A, Fraser WD, et al. Vitamin D and pre-eclampsia: original data, systematic review and meta-analysis. *Ann Nutr Metab* 2013;**63**(4):331–40.

94. Thorne-Lyman A, Fawzi WW. Vitamin D during pregnancy and maternal, neonatal and infant health outcomes: a systematic review and meta-analysis. *Paediatr Perinat Epidemiol* 2012;**26**(Suppl 1):75–90.

95. Roth DE, Leung M, Mesfin E, Qamar H, Watterworth J, Papp E. Vitamin D supplementation during pregnancy: state of the evidence from a systematic review of randomised trials. *BMJ* 2017;**359**:j5237.

96. Harvey NC, Holroyd C, Ntani G, Javaid K, Cooper P, Moon R, et al. Vitamin D supplementation in pregnancy: a systematic review. *Health Technol Assess* 2014;**18**(45):1–190.

97. Edouard T, Alos N, Chabot G, Roughley P, Glorieux FH, Rauch F. Short- and long-term outcome of patients with pseudo-vitamin D deficiency rickets treated with calcitriol. *J Clin Endocrinol Metab* 2011;**96**(1):82–9.

98. Marx SJ, Swart Jr EG, Hamstra AJ, DeLuca HF. Normal intrauterine development of the fetus of a woman receiving extraordinarily high doses of 1,25-dihydroxyvitamin D3. *J Clin Endocrinol Metab* 1980;**51**(5):1138–42.

99. Malloy PJ, Tiosano D, Feldman D. Hereditary 1,25-dihydroxyvitamin-D-resistant rickets. In: Feldman D, Pike JW, Adams JS, editors. *Vitamin D*. 3rd ed. San Diego, CA: Academic Press; 2011. p. 1197–232.

100. Institute of Medicine. *Dietary reference intakes for calcium and vitamin D*. Washington, DC: The National Academies Press; 2011.

101. American College of Obstetricians and Gynecologists. ACOG Committee Opinion No. 495: Vitamin D: Screening and supplementation during pregnancy. *Obstet Gynecol* 2011;**118**(1):197–8.

102. Holick MF, Binkley NC, Bischoff-Ferrari HA, Gordon CM, Hanley DA, Heaney RP, et al. Evaluation, treatment, and prevention of vitamin D deficiency: an Endocrine Society clinical practice guideline. *J Clin Endocrinol Metab* 2011;**96**(7):1911–30.

103. WHO. *Guideline: Vitamin D supplementation in pregnant women.* Geneva: World Health Organization; 2012.

104. Carpenter TO. CYP24A1 loss of function: Clinical phenotype of monoallelic and biallelic mutations. *J Steroid Biochem Mol Biol* 2017;**173**:337–40.

105. Shah AD, Hsiao EC, O'Donnell B, Salmeen K, Nussbaum R, Krebs M, et al. Maternal hypercalcemia due to failure of 1,25-dihydroxyvitamin-D3 catabolism in a patient with CYP24A1 mutations. *J Clin Endocrinol Metab* 2015;**100**(8):2832–6.

106. Dinour D, Davidovits M, Aviner S, Ganon L, Michael L, Modan-Moses D, et al. Maternal and infantile hypercalcemia caused by vitamin-D-hydroxylase mutations and vitamin D intake. *Pediatr Nephrol* 2015;**30**(1):145–52.

107. Woods GN, Saitman A, Gao H, Clarke NJ, Fitzgerald RL, Chi NW. A young woman with recurrent gestational hypercalcemia and acute pancreatitis caused by CYP24A1 deficiency. *J Bone Miner Res* 2016;**31**(10):1841–4.

108. Kwong WT, Fehmi SM. Hypercalcemic pancreatitis triggered by pregnancy with a CYP24A1 mutation. *Pancreas* 2016;**45**(6):e31–2.

109. Woodrow JP. *Calcitonin modulates skeletal mineral loss during lactation through interactions in mammary tissue and directly though osteoclasts in bone.* [PhD thesis] [PhD]. St. John's, NL: Memorial University of Newfoundland; 2009.

110. Woodrow JP, Sharpe CJ, Fudge NJ, Hoff AO, Gagel RF, Kovacs CS. Calcitonin plays a critical role in regulating skeletal mineral metabolism during lactation. *Endocrinology* 2006;**147**(9):4010–21.

111. Shenolikar IS. Absorption of dietary calcium in pregnancy. *Am J Clin Nutr* 1970;**23**(1):63–7.

112. Ma Y, Samaraweera M, Cooke-Hubley S, Kirby BJ, Karaplis AC, Lanske B, et al. Neither absence nor excess of FGF23 disturbs murine fetal-placental phosphorus homeostasis or prenatal skeletal development and mineralization. *Endocrinology* 2014;**155**(5):1596–605.

113. Ohata Y, Yamazaki M, Kawai M, Tsugawa N, Tachikawa K, Koinuma T, et al. Elevated fibroblast growth factor 23 exerts its effects on placenta and regulates vitamin d metabolism in pregnancy of hyp mice. *J Bone Miner Res* 2014;**29**(7):1627–38.

114. Jonas AJ, Dominguez B. Low breast milk phosphorus concentration in familial hypophosphatemia. *J Pediatr Gastroenterol Nutr* 1989;**8**(4):541–3.

115. Reade TM, Scriver CR. Hypophosphatemic rickets and breast milk. *N Engl J Med* 1979;**300**(24):1397.

116. Donovan EF, Tsang RC, Steichen JJ, Strub RJ, Chen IW, Chen M. Neonatal hypermagnesemia: effect on parathyroid hormone and calcium homeostasis. *J Pediatr* 1980;**96**(2):305–10.

117. Cholst IN, Steinberg SF, Tropper PJ, Fox HE, Segre GV, Bilezikian JP. The influence of hypermagnesemia on serum calcium and parathyroid hormone levels in human subjects. *N Engl J Med* 1984;**310**(19):1221–5.

118. Cruikshank DP, Pitkin RM, Reynolds WA, Williams GA, Hargis GK. Effects of magnesium sulfate treatment on perinatal calcium metabolism. I. Maternal and fetal responses. *Am J Obstet Gynecol* 1979;**134**(3):243–9.

119. Koontz SL, Friedman SA, Schwartz ML. Symptomatic hypocalcemia after tocolytic therapy with magnesium sulfate and nifedipine. *Am J Obstet Gynecol* 2004;**190**(6):1773–6.

120. Smith Jr LG, Burns PA, Schanler RJ. Calcium homeostasis in pregnant women receiving long-term magnesium sulfate therapy for preterm labor. *Am J Obstet Gynecol* 1992;**167**:45–51.

121. Hung JW, Tsai MY, Yang BY, Chen JF. Maternal osteoporosis after prolonged magnesium sulfate tocolysis therapy: a case report. *Arch Phys Med Rehabil* 2005;**86**(1):146–9.

122. Levav AL, Chan L, Wapner RJ. Long-term magnesium sulfate tocolysis and maternal osteoporosis in a triplet pregnancy: a case report. *Am J Perinatol* 1998;**15**(1):43–6.

123. Savory J, Monif GR. Serum calcium levels in cord sera of the progeny of mothers treated with magnesium sulfate for toxemia of pregnancy. *Am J Obstet Gynecol* 1971;**110**(4):556–9.

124. Lipsitz PJ. The clinical and biochemical effects of excess magnesium in the newborn. *Pediatrics* 1971;**47**(3):501–9.

125. Malaeb SN, Rassi AI, Haddad MC, Seoud MA, Yunis KA. Bone mineralization in newborns whose mothers received magnesium sulphate for tocolysis of premature labour. *Pediatr Radiol* 2004;**34**(5):384–6.

126. Krysiak R, Wilk M, Okopien B. Recurrent pancreatitis induced by hyperparathyroidism in pregnancy. *Arch Gynecol Obstet* 2011;**284**(3):531–4.

127. Mamillapalli R, VanHouten J, Dann P, Bikle D, Chang W, Brown E, et al. Mammary-specific ablation of the calcium-sensing receptor during lactation alters maternal calcium metabolism, milk calcium transport, and neonatal calcium accrual. *Endocrinology* 2013;**154**(9):3031–42.

128. Ardeshirpour L, Dann P, Pollak M, Wysolmerski J, VanHouten J. The calcium-sensing receptor regulates PTHrP production and calcium transport in the lactating mammary gland. *Bone* 2006;**38**(6):787–93.

129. VanHouten J, Dann P, McGeoch G, Brown EM, Krapcho K, Neville M, et al. The calcium-sensing receptor regulates mammary gland parathyroid hormone-related protein production and calcium transport. *J Clin Invest* 2004;**113**(4):598–608.

130. Mather KJ, Chik CL, Corenblum B. Maintenance of serum calcium by parathyroid hormone-related peptide during lactation in a hypoparathyroid patient. *J Clin Endocrinol Metab* 1999;**84**(2):424–7.

131. Caplan RH, Beguin EA. Hypercalcemia in a calcitriol-treated hypoparathyroid woman during lactation. *Obstet Gynecol* 1990;**76**(3 Pt 2):485–9.

132. Salle BL, Berthezene F, Glorieux FH, Delvin EE, Berland M, David L, et al. Hypoparathyroidism during pregnancy: treatment with calcitriol. *J Clin Endocrinol Metab* 1981;**52**(4):810–3.

133. Sadeghi-Nejad A, Wolfsdorf JI, Senior B. Hypoparathyroidism and pregnancy. Treatment with calcitriol. *JAMA* 1980;**243**(3):254–5.

134. Cathebras P, Cartry O, Sassolas G, Rousset H. Hypercalcemia induced by lactation in 2 patients with treated hypoparathyroidism. *Rev Med Interne* 1996;**17**(8):675–6.

135. Yasumatsu R, Nakashima T, Kuratomi Y, Komiyama S. Postpartum hypercalcemia in a patient with previous thyroid carcinoma: a report of 2 cases. *Nihon Jibiinkoka Gakkai Kaiho* 2002;**105**(8):897–900.

136. Reid IR, Wattie DJ, Evans MC, Budayr AA. Post-pregnancy osteoporosis associated with hypercalcaemia. *Clin Endocrinol (Oxf)* 1992;**37**(3):298–303.

137. Khosla S, van Heerden JA, Gharib H, Jackson IT, Danks J, Hayman JA, et al. Parathyroid hormone-related protein and hypercalcemia secondary to massive mammary hyperplasia. *N Engl J Med* 1990;**322**(16):1157.

138. Hollis BW, Wagner CL. Vitamin D requirements during lactation: high-dose maternal supplementation as therapy to prevent hypovitaminosis D for both the mother and the nursing infant. *Am J Clin Nutr* 2004;**80**(6 Suppl):1752S–8S.

139. Rothberg AD, Pettifor JM, Cohen DF, Sonnendecker EW, Ross FP. Maternal-infant vitamin D relationships during breast-feeding. *J Pediatr* 1982;**101**(4):500–3.

140. Ala-Houhala M, Koskinen T, Parviainen MT, Visakorpi JK. 25-Hydroxyvitamin D and vitamin D in human milk: effects of supplementation and season. *Am J Clin Nutr* 1988;**48**(4):1057–60.

141. Ala-Houhala M. 25-Hydroxyvitamin D levels during breast-feeding with or without maternal or infantile supplementation of vitamin D. *J Pediatr Gastroenterol Nutr* 1985;**4**(2):220–6.

142. Oberhelman SS, Meekins ME, Fischer PR, Lee BR, Singh RJ, Cha SS, et al. Maternal vitamin D supplementation to improve the vitamin D status of breast-fed infants: a randomized controlled trial. *Mayo Clin Proc* 2013;**88**(12):1378–87.

143. Wagner CL, Hulsey TC, Fanning D, Ebeling M, Hollis BW. High-dose vitamin D3 supplementation in a cohort of breastfeeding mothers and their infants: a 6-month follow-up pilot study. *Breastfeed Med* 2006;**1**(2):59–70.

144. Saadi HF, Dawodu A, Afandi B, Zayed R, Benedict S, Nagelkerke N, et al. Effect of combined maternal and infant vitamin D supplementation on vitamin D status of exclusively breastfed infants. *Matern Child Nutr* 2009;**5**(1):25–32.

145. Basile LA, Taylor SN, Wagner CL, Horst RL, Hollis BW. The effect of high-dose vitamin D supplementation on serum vitamin D levels and milk calcium concentration in lactating women and their infants. *Breastfeed Med* 2006;**1**(1):27–35.

146. Prentice A, Yan L, Jarjou LM, Dibba B, Laskey MA, Stirling DM, et al. Vitamin D status does not influence the breast-milk calcium concentration of lactating mothers accustomed to a low calcium intake. *Acta Paediatr* 1997;**86**(9):1006–8.

147. Teotia M, Teotia SP, Nath M. Metabolic studies in congenital vitamin D deficiency rickets. *Indian J Pediatr* 1995;**62**(1):55–61.

148. Teotia M, Teotia SP. Nutritional and metabolic rickets. *Indian J Pediatr* 1997;**64**(2):153–7.

149. Ho C, Conner DA, Pollak MR, Ladd DJ, Kifor O, Warren HB, et al. A mouse model of human familial hypocalciuric hypercalcemia and neonatal severe hyperparathyroidism. *Nat Genet* 1995;**11**:389–94.

150. Collins JN, Kirby BJ, Woodrow JP, Gagel RF, Rosen CJ, Sims NA, et al. Lactating Ctcgrp nulls lose twice the normal bone mineral content due to fewer osteoblasts and more osteoclasts, whereas bone mass is fully restored after weaning in association with up-regulation of Wnt signaling and other novel genes. *Endocrinology* 2013;**154**(4):1400–13.

151. Hagaman JR, Ambrose WW, Hirsch PF. A scanning electron microscopic and photon absorptiometric study of the development, prolongation, and pattern of recovery from lactation-induced osteopenia in rats. *J Bone Miner Res* 1990;**5**:123–32.

152. Prentice A. Calcium in pregnancy and lactation. *Annu Rev Nutr* 2000;**20**:249–72.

153. Prentice A, Jarjou LM, Cole TJ, Stirling DM, Dibba B, Fairweather-Tait S. Calcium requirements of lactating Gambian mothers: effects of a calcium supplement on breast-milk calcium concentration, maternal bone mineral content, and urinary calcium excretion. *Am J Clin Nutr* 1995;**62**(1):58–67.

154. Prentice A, Jarjou LM, Stirling DM, Buffenstein R, Fairweather-Tait S. Biochemical markers of calcium and bone metabolism during 18 months of lactation in Gambian women accustomed to a low calcium intake and in those consuming a calcium supplement. *J Clin Endocrinol Metab* 1998;**83**(4):1059–66.

155. Laskey MA, Prentice A, Hanratty LA, Jarjou LM, Dibba B, Beavan SR, et al. Bone changes after 3 mo of lactation: influence of calcium intake, breast-milk output, and vitamin D-receptor genotype. *Am J Clin Nutr* 1998;**67**(4):685–92.

156. Jarjou LM, Prentice A, Sawo Y, Laskey MA, Bennett J, Goldberg GR, et al. Randomized, placebo-controlled, calcium supplementation study in pregnant Gambian women: effects on breast-milk calcium concentrations and infant birth weight, growth, and bone mineral accretion in the first year of life. *Am J Clin Nutr* 2006;**83**(3):657–66.

157. Kolthoff N, Eiken P, Kristensen B, Nielsen SP. Bone mineral changes during pregnancy and lactation: a longitudinal cohort study. *Clin Sci (Lond)* 1998;**94**(4):405–12.

158. Polatti F, Capuzzo E, Viazzo F, Colleoni R, Klersy C. Bone mineral changes during and after lactation. *Obstet Gynecol* 1999;**94**(1):52–6.

159. Kalkwarf HJ, Specker BL, Bianchi DC, Ranz J, Ho M. The effect of calcium supplementation on bone density during lactation and after weaning. *N Engl J Med* 1997;**337**(8):523–8.

160. Cross NA, Hillman LS, Allen SH, Krause GF. Changes in bone mineral density and markers of bone remodeling during lactation and postweaning in women consuming high amounts of calcium. *J Bone Miner Res* 1995;**10**(9):1312–20.

161. Fairweather-Tait S, Prentice A, Heumann KG, Jarjou LM, Stirling DM, Wharf SG, et al. Effect of calcium supplements and stage of lactation on the calcium absorption efficiency of lactating women accustomed to low calcium intakes. *Am J Clin Nutr* 1995;**62**:1188–92.

162. Bezerra FF, Mendonca LM, Lobato EC, O'Brien KO, Donangelo CM. Bone mass is recovered from lactation to postweaning in adolescent mothers with low calcium intakes. *Am J Clin Nutr* 2004;**80**(5):1322–6.

163. Delzer PR, Meyer Jr RA. Normal milk composition in lactating X-linked hypophosphatemic mice despite continued hypophosphatemia. *Calcif Tissue Int* 1983;**35**(6):750–4.

Chapter 22

Gestational Diabetes and Type 2 Diabetes During Pregnancy

Geetha Mukerji*,†, Sioban Bacon*,‡ and Denice S. Feig*,‡

*Department of Medicine, Division of Endocrinology and Metabolism, University of Toronto, Toronto, ON, Canada, †Division of Endocrinology, Women's College Hospital, Toronto, ON, Canada, ‡Division of Endocrinology, Mt. Sinai Hospital, Toronto, ON, Canada

Common Clinical Problems

- Incidence rates of gestational diabetes mellitus (GDM) and Type 2 diabetes mellitus (T2DM) have doubled over the last two decades and continue to rise.
- Women with GDM are at higher risk of preeclampsia and gestational hypertension, and their infants are at higher risk of adverse neonatal outcomes.
- There is a continuous relationship between increasing hyperglycemia and the rate of adverse outcomes in women with GDM.
- Higher lactation intensity and longer duration have been associated with lower incidences of maternal diabetes after GDM pregnancy.
- Women with T2DM have increased rates of perinatal mortality and similar rates of congenital anomalies compared to women with Type 1 diabetes mellitus (T1DM).
- Metformin and glyburide are not teratogenic and can be used when planning pregnancy; however, other medications, such as angiotensin-converting enzyme inhibitors, angiotensin-receptor blockers, and statins, should be discontinued prepregnancy.
- To lower the risk of preeclampsia, aspirin should be given to women with T2DM before 17 weeks' gestation.

22.1 GESTATIONAL DIABETES

22.1.1 Epidemiology

GDM is a medical condition in which carbohydrate intolerance develops or is first recognized in pregnancy.[1] The incidence of GDM is rising worldwide. In a recent population-based study in Ontario, the incidence doubled over the 14 years between 1996 and 2010.[2] There may be several reasons contributing to this, including increasing maternal age, higher rates of obesity, changes in diet and lifestyle, screening practices, and changes in diagnostic criteria. The incidence of GDM in the United States ranges from 6% to 16%, depending on screening and diagnostic criteria used and ethnic distribution of the population.[3] In a study from Germany, the prevalence of GDM was 13%, but it rose to 26% in women 45 years of age or older.[4] In a study of obese women in Europe [body mass index (BMI) ≥29] using criteria from the International Association of Diabetes and Pregnancy Study Groups (IADPSG), the prevalence of GDM was 39%.[5] There is higher prevalence of GDM among Hispanic, African American, Native American, Pacific Islander, Aboriginal, Middle Eastern, and East and South Asian women compared to Caucasians.[6, 7]

22.1.2 Pathophysiology

Women who develop GDM have a beta-cell defect that is unable to compensate for the rising insulin resistance of pregnancy.[8] There is evidence that this defect likely predates the pregnancy but is manifested during pregnancy with rising insulin resistance.[9] This defect results in the inability to produce sufficient insulin to maintain glucose levels, resulting in maternal hyperglycemia. Maternal glucose is then transferred via the placenta to the fetus and stimulates fetal hyperinsulinemia and excess fetal growth, resulting in neonatal hypoglycemia and macrosomia, respectively. The beta-cell defect worsens over time, predisposing these women to an increased risk of developing T2DM postpartum.[10] Along with pregnancy itself, factors contributing to this beta-cell defect include obesity, inflammation, overeating, sedentary lifestyle, genetic susceptibility, epigenetic changes, endocrine-disrupting chemicals, and aging.[11]

22.1.3 Adverse Pregnancy Outcomes Associated with GDM

The Hyperglycemia and Adverse Pregnancy Outcome (HAPO) study, a large, multicenter study, demonstrated a continuous relationship between maternal glucose levels and four primary outcomes: cesarean delivery, birth weight greater than the 90th percentile, clinical neonatal hypoglycemia, and fetal hyperinsulinemia.[12] Women with GDM are at higher risk of hypertensive disorders, including preeclampsia and gestational hypertension. In the HAPO study, 5.9% of women with GDM had gestational hypertension and 4.8% had preeclampsia.[12] Other adverse neonatal outcomes among women with untreated GDM include macrosomia, shoulder dystocia, birth trauma, respiratory distress syndrome, and hyperbilirubinemia. Maternal obesity and GDM are additive in their effects on neonatal outcomes. In the HAPO study, both maternal GDM and obesity were independently associated with birth weight >90th percentile, primary cesarean section, preeclampsia, cord c-peptide, and newborn percentage of body fat >90th percentile. However, the combination of maternal GDM and obesity increased the risk over and above each alone.[13]

22.1.4 Screening for GDM

There are two types of screening approaches for GDM: risk factor based and universal screening. Risk factors for GDM include family history of T2DM, maternal age, prepregnancy elevated BMI, previous GDM, previous large-for-gestational-age (LGA) baby, high maternal age, and excessive gestational weight gain (GWG).[14] The main concern with the use of a risk factor-based approach is the inability to identify all women with GDM, as up to half of women with GDM will be missed depending on which set of risk factors are used.[15] Most international guidelines recommend universal screening for GDM that includes all pregnant women at or beyond 24 weeks' gestational age.[16, 17]

22.1.5 Early Screening for GDM/T2DM in Pregnancy

To date, there is no good evidence to dictate which criteria to use to screen or diagnose GDM prior to the usual time of 24 weeks' gestation. While the measurement of hemoglobin A1C (HbA1c) can be used to detect dysglycemia, it may not be suitable for use alone to detect GDM because of its decreased sensitivity for the detection of GDM compared with the oral glucose tolerance test (OGTT).[18] However, it has a high specificity (94%) for predicting second-trimester GDM.[19] Studies are underway to try to identify suitable criteria for the diagnosis of GDM early in pregnancy. The Treatment of Booking Gestational diabetes Mellitus (ToBOGOM) Study is a randomized controlled trial (RCT) aimed at determining whether the criteria used to diagnose and treat GDM at 24 weeks can be used at booking appointments to reduce pregnancy complications.[20] In their recently published pilot study, they found that early treatment led to reduced LGA infants, but there were more small-for-gestational-age (SGA) infants.[21] The full study is ongoing.

However, similar to the criteria used outside of pregnancy, an early HbA1c of ≥6.5% or fasting glucose of ≥7.0 mmol/L can be used to identify women with an elevated risk of undiagnosed T2DM and to treat them accordingly.[1] The diagnosis should be confirmed postpartum, as one study showed that only 21% of women with these criteria early in pregnancy continued to have diabetes, and 37% had prediabetes when tested at 6–8 weeks postpartum.[22]

An early HbA1c can also be used to identify women with an increased risk of adverse outcomes. In a study of 16,122 women screened with an early HbA1c at a median of 47 days gestation, excluding women referred for GDM, women with an early HbA1c of 5.9%–6.4% had worse pregnancy outcomes than women with HbA1c <5.9%, including an increase in major congenital anomalies, preeclampsia, shoulder dystocia, and perinatal death.[23] There are no data, however, on the benefits of treatment in this group. Further research is needed.

22.1.6 Diagnosis of GDM: One Step vs Two Step

The HAPO study demonstrated a continuous relationship between the risk of adverse outcomes and maternal glycemia at 24–28 weeks, with no clear threshold.[12] For this reason, societies have chosen different thresholds for the diagnosis of GDM, depending on the level of risk that one wants to detect. Also, some societies continue to advocate the use of the glucose screening test (the two-step approach), while others advocate going straight to a 2-h OGTT (the one-step approach).

The one-step screening approach recommends that pregnant women undergo a 75-g OGTT at 24–28 weeks of gestation, without a glucose challenge test (used as a screening). The IADPSG recommends a one-step approach (see Table 22.1).[24]

TABLE 22.1 Screening and diagnostic recommendations

	Screen	Diagnosis
IADPSG[24]	None	2h 75g OGTT Diagnosis if 1 or more glucose $\geq$: Fasting 5.1 mmol/L (92 mg/dL), 1h 10.0 mmol/L (180 mg/dL), 2h 8.5 mmol/L (153 mg/dL)
ACOG[16]	50g glucose challenge test Abnormal: can choose from 7.2 mmol/L (130 mg/dL), 7.4 mmol/L (133 mg/dL), or 7.8 mmol/L (140 mg/dL)	3h 100g OGTT Diagnosis if 2 or more $\geq$: Fasting 5.3 mmol/L (95 mg/dL), 1h 10.0 mmol/L (180 mg/dL), 2h 8.6 mmol/L (155 mg/dL), 3h 7.8 mmol/L (140 mg/dL) or Fasting 5.8 mmol/L (105 mg/dL), 1h 10.6 mmol/L (190 mg/dL), 2h 9.2 mmol/L (165 mg/dL), 3h 8.0 mmol/L (144 mg/dL)
ADA[1]	One-step: none or Two-step: see ACOG	One-step: see IADPSG or Two-step: see ACOG
Diabetes Canada[17]	Preferred approach: 50g Glucose challenge test Abnormal if $\geq$7.8 mmol/L (140 mg/dL) Diagnostic if $\geq$11.1 mmol/L (200 mg/dL) Alternative approach: None	Preferred approach: 2h 75g OGTT Diagnosis if 1 or more $\geq$: Fasting 5.3 mmol/L (95 mg/dL), 1h 10.6 mmol/L (190 mg/dL), 2h 9.0 mmol/L (162 mg/dL) Alternative approach: See IADPSG
WHO[25]	None	—[a]

[a]As of March 8, 2018, this statement has been added: "WHO currently does not have a recommendation on whether or how to screen for GDM, and screening strategies for GDM are considered a priority area for research, particularly in LMICs."

The IADPSG defined GDM cut points as being set where the risk of the four adverse outcomes (LGA baby, cesarean section, neonatal hypoglycemia, and fetal hyperinsulinemia) is 1.75 times the risk of the general population. A diagnosis of GDM is made if one plasma glucose value is abnormal (i.e., fasting $\geq$5.1 mmol/L (92 mg/dL), 1h $\geq$10.0 mmol/L (180 mg/dL), 2h $\geq$8.5 mmol/L (153 mg/dL)).

In the two-step approach, an initial 50-g glucose challenge test is done as a screening, followed, if abnormal, with a 75-g OGTT. Several societies continue to advocate this two-step approach but use various thresholds for going on to a diagnostic test (Table 22.1). In addition, the thresholds for diagnosis vary. The American College of Physicians and Surgeons recommends a 50-g glucose challenge test, followed by a 3-h, 100-g OGTT (Table 22.1).[16] The American Diabetes Association gives a choice of either the one-step or two-step approach. In the "preferred" Canadian approach (named as such by Diabetes Canada), the 50-g screen is considered abnormal if it is $\geq$7.8 mmol/L and diagnostic if it is $\geq$11.1 mmol/L (200 mg/dL).[17] If the screen is between 7.8 mmol/L (140 mg/dL) and 11.0 mmol/L (199 mg/dL), then a 75-g OGTT is done. The diagnostic cut points are set where the risk of the four outcomes in the HAPO study is 2.0 times the risk of the general population. The diagnosis of GDM is made if one plasma glucose value is abnormal (i.e., fasting $\geq$5.3 mmol/L (95 mg/dL), 1-h $\geq$10.6 mmol/L (190 mg/dL), 2h $\geq$9.0 mmol/L (162 mg/dL)).

The additional women in whom GDM would be diagnosed with the one-step approach may not derive similar benefits from treatment as women in whom GDM was diagnosed by the two-step approach.[26] Up until 2018, the World Health Organization (WHO) recommended the IADPSG approach. As of March 2018, they have no recommendation and consider this area a priority for research (Table 22.1).[25] There is a need for adequately powered studies to compare these approaches.

22.1.7   Management

22.1.7.1   During Pregnancy

There have been two trials to date that have given clear evidence of the treatment benefit of GDM. The Australian Carbohydrate Intolerance Study in Pregnant Women (ACHOIS) trial randomized 1000 women with GDM to diet, monitoring, and insulin as necessary vs usual care. ACHOIS demonstrated a significant reduction of a composite outcome of serious pregnancy and neonatal complications (e.g., death, birth trauma, shoulder dystocia) with improved glycemic control of GDM.[27] In another randomized trial, 958 women with mild GDM received diet, monitoring, and insulin as necessary vs usual prenatal care.[28] Although they did not find a significant difference in the primary outcome (the neonatal composite outcome), the intervention resulted in a reduction of fetal overgrowth, shoulder dystocia, cesarean delivery, and hypertensive disorders. Subsequent systematic reviews and meta-analyses have supported the benefits of treatment of GDM, including reductions in fetal overgrowth, shoulder dystocia, and preeclampsia.[29, 30]

22.1.7.1.1 Self-Management

Frequency of monitoring and targets Self-monitoring of blood glucose (SMBG) is required to guide therapy for GDM. There is insufficient evidence to outline the optimal frequency of SMBG among women with GDM. The general recommendations are to test blood glucose four times a day to include both fasting and either 1- or 2-h postprandial blood glucose readings.[16] Although the evidence for these targets is insufficient, many societies aim for target blood glucose readings of a fasting and preprandial reading of <5.3 mmol/L (95 mg/dL), 1-h postprandial reading <7.8 mmol/L (140 mg/dL), and/or 2 h postprandial reading of <6.7 mmol/L (120 mg/dL). These thresholds are considerably higher than glucose values in normoglycemic women, and therefore have been postulated to be too lenient. In a recent meta-analysis of 26 studies in women with GDM, a fasting glucose of <5 mmol/L (90 mg/dL) resulted in a decrease in macrosomia, LGA, neonatal hypoglycemia, and preeclampsia.[31] Further research is needed to confirm the optimal treatment targets during pregnancy. Once glycemic targets are met with intensive lifestyle modification, the frequency of glucose monitoring may be modified.[32]

Lifestyle management Women with GDM should receive nutrition and exercise counseling as part of intensive lifestyle management. Nutrition therapy in the context of GDM should promote adequate dietary intake without resulting in ketosis to achieve glycemic targets, maternal weight gain, and appropriate fetal growth.[33] Generally, meal planning among women with GDM can focus on promoting intake of three moderate-sized meals with two or more snacks to distribute carbohydrates throughout the day and minimize postprandial excursions. In recent meta-analyses, the low-glycemic index diet has been associated with a lower rate of LGA infants and less frequent need for insulin therapy.[34, 35] Physical activity should be encouraged among women with GDM unless contraindicated for the pregnancy.[36] Women with GDM are suggested to follow GWG recommendations from the 2009 Institute of Medicine guidelines,[37] as prevention of excessive GWG can reduce the potential of LGA during pregnancy.[38]

22.1.7.1.2 Pharmacological Treatment

If women with GDM do not achieve glycemic targets within 1–2 weeks with intensive lifestyle management, pharmacological therapy should be initiated.

Insulin Insulin as subcutaneous injection therapy has been traditionally used as first-line therapy among women with GDM if glycemic targets are not met. Insulin does not cross the placenta due to its large molecular size, except at very high doses.[39] The use of insulin to achieve glycemic targets has been shown to reduce fetal and maternal morbidity.[27, 28, 40] The type of insulin, timing, and frequency needs to be individualized based on the SMBG values.

Rapid-acting insulin analogs, such as aspart/lispro/glulisine, can be given before meals and can used over regular insulin for better postprandial control of blood glucose, although fetal outcomes have been similar.[41–44]They peak sooner than regular insulin and can be given 5–10 min before a meal, and their duration of action is shorter (3–5 h) than regular insulin.

Intermediate-acting (neutral protamine hagedorn, NPH) and long-acting insulin (detemir, glargine, and degludec), also termed *basal insulin,* is primarily used to provide a continuous supply of lesser amounts of insulin to regulate lipolysis and prevent hepatic gluconeogenesis, independent of food intake, and is generally given at bedtime or in the morning. Detemir can be used as an alternative basal insulin compared to NPH. An RCT of 87 pregnant women with T2DM and GDM treated with either detemir ($n = 42$) or insulin NPH ($n = 45$) with short-acting insulin aspart as add on therapy as needed noted a similar efficacy in glycemic control in both treatment arms, but hypoglycemic episodes were significantly lower in the detemir arm.[45] Glargine may be considered as an alternative to NPH, but there are theoretical risks with use among women with GDM, as glargine has a 6.5-fold increased affinity to the type 1 insulin-like growth factor receptor. Such binding may have the potential to increase fetal growth, but this has not been demonstrated in clinical studies.[46] Unlike detemir, glargine has not been tested in randomized trials during pregnancy but has gradually become accepted for use by clinicians. Degludec is a newer, ultra-long-acting insulin; it is described in more detail in Section 22.2.

Noninsulin antihyperglycemic agents

   Metformin. Metformin is a biguanide that decreases hepatic glucose output, increases peripheral glucose uptake in muscles and adipocyte cells, increases secretion of glucagon-like peptide 1 (GLP-1), and decreases intestinal glucose absorption.[47] Metformin freely crosses the placenta and cord blood levels detected can be as high as 50%–100% of maternal blood levels.[48]

The largest study of metformin use in GDM was in the MiG (Metformin use in GDM) trial, where 751 women with GDM were randomly treated with metformin (titrated to a maximum of 2500 mg as necessary, with insulin added if glycemic targets were not achieved) as opposed to insulin alone.[49] In this study, there was no difference in the primary composite neonatal outcome (neonatal hypoglycemia, respiratory distress, need for phototherapy, birth trauma, 5-min Apgar score <7, and prematurity) among women with GDM treated with metformin compared to insulin. Severe neonatal hypoglycemia (<1.6 mmol/L [<28.8 mg/dL]) was significantly lower in the metformin arm, but preterm birth was more common (12.1% vs 7.6%; P = 0.04). A total of 46% of women in the metformin group required supplemental insulin to maintain adequate glycemic control, and 1.9% of women discontinued metformin due to gastrointestinal side effects.

In a systematic review and meta-analysis of six open-label studies comparing metformin to insulin for GDM that included the MiG trial, metformin was associated with less maternal weight gain, lower gestational age at delivery, and more preterm birth.[50] Subsequent meta-analyses have not demonstrated an increase in preterm birth with metformin use vs insulin,[51] but have demonstrated less maternal weight gain, less pregnancy-induced hypertension in mothers, and less neonatal hypoglycemia in infants of mothers taking metformin compared to insulin. Of note, treatment failure was 33.8% with metformin use, necessitating the addition of insulin to maintain adequate glycemic control.

In terms of long-term follow-up, children at 2 years whose mothers were treated with metformin from the MiG study demonstrated higher mid-upper-arm circumferences and subscapular and biceps skinfolds as compared to infants whose mothers were treated with insulin.[52] In this follow-up study, however, total fat mass, waist circumference, and percentage body fat assessed by bioimpedance and DEXA were not different in the two arms of the study. The authors postulated that metformin resulted in a more favorable redistribution of peripheral fat relative to visceral fat; however, visceral fat could not be directly measured.[52] In a more recent publication of these infants, looking at anthropometrics at 7–9 years of age, the authors reported the results of the children by center, in an unusual approach.[53]

In Adelaide, mothers randomized to metformin had higher blood glucose readings during pregnancy, and more infants were born at >90th percentile. At 7 years, there were no differences in offspring anthropometrics. The authors hypothesized that metformin was protective in the offspring of mothers exposed in utero to metformin. In Auckland, however, glycemic control and birth weights were similar, but at 9 years, children exposed to metformin in utero were larger, with larger volumes of fat but similar percentages of fat. The authors hypothesized that metformin may lead to different outcomes depending on other fetal environmental factors, and epigenetics may play a role. In another study, infants of women with polycystic ovarian syndrome (PCOS) exposed to metformin were also found to be larger, with higher BMI z-score, and more infants are overweight/obese compared to infants not exposed to metformin at 4 years of age.[54] Clearly, longer follow-up is necessary. The 2-year follow-up of metformin-exposed infants for neurodevelopmental outcomes have shown no differences compared to controls.[55, 56]

Glyburide. Glyburide (glibenclamide) is a sulfonylurea that binds to pancreatic beta cell receptors and stimulates insulin secretion.[57] Glyburide crosses the placenta, and drug concentrations in cord blood have been demonstrated to be 50%–70% of maternal concentrations.[58]

In a large RCT among 404 women with GDM, who received either insulin or glibenclamide therapy, there were no significant differences in glycemic control or neonatal outcomes (i.e., LGA, macrosomia, birth weight, neonatal hypoglycemia, pulmonary complications, admission to the neonatal intensive care unit, congenital anomalies, or perinatal mortality) between each treatment arm.[59] However, in a large meta-analysis of RCTs examining perinatal outcomes among GDM women randomized to receive glibenclamide or insulin, higher birth weight, more macrosomia, and more neonatal hypoglycemia were found among neonates of mothers receiving glibenclamide compared to those women with GDM treated with insulin.[50] In the same meta-analysis, two studies compared glibenclamide to metformin directly and noted that metformin was associated with less maternal weight gain, lower birth weight, less macrosomia, and fewer LGA newborns. The average treatment failure among these studies was 26.8% with metformin, as opposed to 23.5% with glibenclamide.

Alpha-glucosidase inhibitors. Two alpha-glucosidase inhibitors, acarbose and voglibose, slow carbohydrate absorption and reduce postprandial glucose levels by inhibiting the alpha-glucosidase enzymes on the brush border of the small intestine. Acarbose may be considered for adjunctive use among women with GDM. In a small case series of 6 women with GDM, the use of acarbose three times a day normalized blood glucose and infants were healthy, but acarbose was associated with intenstinal discomfort.[60] There is a small RCT demonstrating no difference in adverse pregnancy outcomes compared to insulin among women with GDM.[61] However, the gastrointestinal side effects of acarbose may limit the use of acarbose in pregnancy.

Other oral-antidiabetic agents. Peroxisome proliferator-activated receptor (PPAR)-gamma agonists (thiazolidine-diones) cross the placenta and should be avoided in pregnancy until more safety data are available.[62, 63] Meglitinides cross the placenta, and their use among women with GDM has not been evaluated.[64] Dipeptidyl peptidase-4 (DPP4) inhibitors, GLP-1 receptor agonists, or sodium-glucose cotransporter (SGLT2) inhibitors have not been studied among women with GDM and are therefore not recommended.

22.1.7.2 Intrapartum

Women with GDM need to be monitored during labor and delivery. Levels of blood glucose are generally kept between 4.0 and 7.0 mmol/L to minimize the risk of neonatal hypoglycemia, although evidence for the ideal target range is weak, and more evidence is needed.

22.1.7.3 Postpartum

22.1.7.3.1 Breastfeeding

Women with GDM should be encouraged to breastfeed. Higher lactation intensity and longer duration has been associated with lower incidences of maternal diabetes after pregnancies complicated by GDM.[65]

22.1.7.3.2 Fetal and Maternal Risks

There is increasing evidence that maternal hyperglycemia can result in metabolic imprinting on the fetus, leading to an increased risk of negative metabolic outcomes. In utero exposure to maternal diabetes results in a higher risk of childhood and adult obesity and T2DM.[66] Breastfeeding may lower the risk of obesity and diabetes in infants of mothers with diabetes. Women with GDM also have an increased long-term risk of developing diabetes[67] and cardiovascular disease.[68] To screen for dysglycemia postpartum, various international bodies recommend a postpartum 75-g OGTT anywhere from 4 weeks to 6 months postpartum.[16, 17] Women with a history of GDM who have prediabetes postpartum should receive intensive life-style intervention or metformin to prevent diabetes.[69, 70]

22.1.7.3.3 Considerations for future pregnancy planning

Women with a history of GDM should be screened for diabetes prior to conception to detect undiagnosed diabetes or pre-diabetes. The recurrence rate of GDM is high, from 30% to 85% in subsequent pregnancies, which requires early screening and management.[71, 72]

22.2 TYPE 2 DIABETES

22.2.1 Epidemiology of T2DM in Pregnancy

The prevalence of preexisting diabetes complicating pregnancy has been increasing globally for the last four decades. In Ontario, Canada, the incidence of women with preexisting diabetes during pregnancy and GDM has doubled between 1996 and 2010.[2] National registries from the United Kingdom and Nordic countries have demonstrated an increase in all forms of diabetes in pregnancy. In particular regions, the incidence of T2DM surpasses T1DM among women of reproductive age with preexisting diabetes.[73] The Swedes have identified a 111% increase in the number of pregnant women with T2DM over a 15-year period.[74] Over a similar time, the Scottish registries have reported a 90% increase in women with T2DM attending their maternity services.[75]

The increasing prevalence in T2DM among women of reproductive age is largely thought to reflect the ongoing obesity epidemic. Women with T2DM tend to be older, have a higher BMI, and have additional risk factors such as chronic hypertension, which contribute to poor obstetrical outcomes.

22.2.2 Prepregnancy Counseling

Congenital anomalies associated with maternal diabetes occur very early in embryogenesis, as most affected organs are formed by 6–8 weeks' gestation. The importance of improving glucose control preconception is essential, as these organs have often already formed by the time women know they are pregnant. Prepregnancy counseling involves providing education to women with preexisting diabetes regarding the risks of poor glycemic control, how one can improve outcomes with weight management, folic acid supplementation, avoidance of teratogenic medication, and monitoring for existing microvascular complications. Multiple studies have highlighted the benefits of attendance at prepregnancy clinics.[76]

Meta-analyses of studies of prepregnancy counseling showed that the *absence* of prepregnancy counseling is associated with a threefold-to-fourfold increase in the risk of major malformations. In women with T2DM, attendance at prepregnancy counseling appointments has been demonstrated to achieve a reduction in HbA1c in the first trimester of 1.9%.[77]

Several professional bodies [including the National Institute for Clinical Excellence (NICE), American Diabetes Association (ADA), and Diabetes Canada] strongly recommend preconception optimization for women with preexisting diabetes. Multifaceted diabetes in pregnancy programs incorporating preconception care, centralized clinics, electronic patient records, and patient-friendly resources result in significant improvements in perinatal outcomes. For example, the Atlantic Diabetes in Pregnancy program was founded in 2005 with the aim of providing coordinated central care to women with diabetes in pregnancy. One study that emerged from this program analyzed 445 women, of which 39% had T2DM. It demonstrated that implementation of the program resulted in a significant increase in the number of women entering into a pregnancy with optimal HbA1c < 6.5%, with a significant reduction in miscarriage rate (2.6 vs 17%, $P < 0.0001$), and a trend toward fewer congenital malformations (3.6 vs 7.4%, $P = 0.16$).[76]

Unfortunately, fewer women with T2DM attend preconception counseling. There are multiple factors contributing to the lower reported attendance rate. Women with T2DM are more likely to be from areas of deprivation or from marginalized socioeconomic groups. Women with T2DM cited perceived lower expected fertility, negative experiences with healthcare professionals, and logistics as principal reasons for nonattendance.[78–80]

In an attempt to address the challenge of improving access to women with T2DM in pregnancy, a group in the United Kingdom developed a pragmatic, community-based, preconception care program.[81] Women with T2DM, unlike T1DM, tend to receive their care outside of pregnancy, in the general community. This preconception program was unique, in that it focused care in the community, targeting primary care practitioners as opposed to specialized, hospital-based prepregnancy care. They recently reported a significant improvement in pregnancy preparation among women with T2DM attending the program. The number achieving target HbA1c prepregnancy increased by 60%, and there was an increase in folic acid intake to 50% of participants. The intervention was conducted over 17 months, at a cost of approximately £50,000. This is equivalent to the cost of one cleft lip and palate repair, and significantly lower than the quoted National Reference Costs in the United Kingdom for a single major congenital anomaly.[81]

22.2.3 Prepregnancy Counseling: BMI

Women with T2DM are often obese. Obesity, independent of dysglycemia, is associated with higher adverse maternal and perinatal outcomes. From a maternal aspect, there is a higher risk of venous thromboembolic disease, postpartum hemorrhage, cesarean delivery, postpartum wound infection, postpartum depression, and lower rates of long-term breastfeeding. Perinatal complications include higher miscarriage rate, more congenital anomalies, higher stillbirth rate, and higher rates of SGA and LGA infants.[82, 83] Ideally, nutritional consultation should be offered prepregnancy to all women who are overweight or obese to reduce these complications. Bariatric surgery should be suggested as a potential treatment in significantly obese women who are contemplating pregnancy. A recent systematic review and meta-analysis, however, found that there are both benefits and risks to bariatric surgery done before pregnancy.[84] The meta-analysis of over 8000 patients postbariatric surgery demonstrated a reduction in the rate of LGA [odds ratio (OR) 0.31; number needed to benefit: 6], gestational hypertension (OR 0.38; number needed to benefit: 11), cesarean delivery rates (OR 0.5; number needed to benefit: 9) and postpartum hemorrhage (OR 0.32; number needed to benefit: 21), when compared to subjects matched for prebariatric surgery BMI. Despite the important benefits of bariatric surgery there were associated risks. The same study reported an increase in preterm delivery (OR 1.35; number needed to harm: 35) and an increase in SGA (OR 2.16; number needed to harm: 66), some of which may be due to micronutrient deficiency.

The European Association for the Study of Obesity has published practical recommendations for the management of postbariatric surgical patients and recommend that patients wait at least 12–18 months' postbariatric surgery before planning pregnancy.[85] The principal reason for the delay is to try to reduce the effect of the immediate catabolic changes associated with rapid weight loss and maternal micronutrient depletion on the fetus. Antenatal care should be delivered at a specialized center with obstetricians, midwives, and physicians who are familiar with the management of such patients. Nutrition counseling should ensure adequate protein intake (up to 60 g/day, particularly in the initial postoperative period) and micronutrient supplementation. Micronutrient deficiency is present in approximately 80% of patients postbariatric surgery. Adequate replacement of B vitamins and fat-soluble vitamins (in some cases, parenteral supplementation may be necessary), vitamin D, calcium, and other minerals such as zinc and copper should be considered. Micronutrient deficiencies can adversely affect the fetus, causing preterm delivery (PTD) and SGA, among other concerns.[86] The biological availability of drugs, including metformin, is altered postsurgery, and amendments in dosing and schedules may be required. Malabsorptive surgeries such as Roux-on-Y gastric bypass are associated with both early- and late-dumping syndromes in 40% of patients.[87] Nutrient manipulation, such as eating food with different glycemic indexes and having small, frequent meals, can be used to treat this phenomenon. In addition, technologies such as a continuous glucose monitoring system (CGMS) can be used to monitor fluctuations in glucose levels.

22.2.4 Antenatal Screening of Microvascular and Macrovascular Complications in T2DM

Pregnancies in women with known microvascular complications tend to have worse outcomes than those without complications. Antenatal screening of women with T2DM should include testing for nephropathy and retinopathy. Other potential complications to consider, particularly in women with a high BMI and T2DM, are obstructive sleep apnea (OSA) and acute nonalcoholic fatty liver disease.

22.2.4.1 Nephropathy

At the diagnosis of diabetes, 6%–7% of women with T2DM have microalbuminuria. The progression through the stages of kidney disease to macroalbuminuria and ultimately elevated creatinine occurs at a rate of 2%–3% per annum. In a meta-analysis of 33 studies, 2.9% of pregnant women with T2DM had micro/macroalbuminuria. This figure was significantly less than that reported among the T1DM population (6.8%).[88] In contrast, Damm et al. demonstrated equivalent rates of diabetic nephropathy and microalbuminuria among pregnant women with T2DM and T1DM (6.8% vs 5.8%, $P = 0.62$). In the same study, those with T1DM with renal involvement were more likely to be on antihypertensive treatment (62%, compared to none of the women with T2DM).[89]

A urinary albumin:creatinine ratio (ACR) and serum creatinine should be measured, ideally at the prepregnancy counseling visit, but if not, at the first antenatal visit and followed throughout pregnancy. Women with diabetic nephropathy are at increased risk of gestational hypertension and preeclampsia, and the patient should be monitored for these conditions. At the booking visit, a referral to nephrology should be made if creatinine is >120 μmol, as there is an increased risk of an increase in creatinine and fall in glomerular filtration rate with this degree of kidney disease.[90]

22.2.4.2 Retinopathy

A total of 20% of patients with preexisting T2DM have retinopathy at diagnosis. NICE guidelines state that a retinal screen should be performed, ideally at prepregnancy and again in the first and third trimesters. If there is proliferative disease, further antenatal ophthalmological assessment may be required. A postpartum retinal screen is also advised. The reason for this vigilance is that retinopathy can progress during pregnancy. Risk factors for progression include poor glycemic control, but also rapid improvement in glucose control in pregnancy, hypertension, and pregnancy itself.[91]

22.2.4.3 Ischemic Heart Disease

Cardiovascular disease (CVD) complicates approximately 0.4%–4% of all pregnancies. Although rare, pregnancy results in a threefold-to-fourfold increased risk of myocardial infarction.[92] The risk factors for CVD in pregnancy are similar to the traditional risk factors (familial history, hypertension, dyslipidemia, and diabetes). Hypertensive disorders of pregnancy, including preeclampsia, complicate 41% of pregnancies with T2DM. Dyslipidemia, with high low-density lipoprotein (LDL) and low high-density lipoprotein (HDL) levels, is common in T2DM. In pregnancy, HDL decreases further and LDL increases secondary to altered hepatic metabolism, with an increase in hepatic lipase, particularly in the second and third trimesters. In women who present with active ischemic coronary disease, definitive therapy is recommended. The use of statin therapy and ACE inhibitors is discussed in Section 22.2.9.2.1.

22.2.5 Obstructive Sleep Apnea

OSA and obesity commonly coexist. In women with T2DM who are obese, pregnancy can unmask symptoms of OSA. Women with suspected OSA should ideally be screened, as it is a risk factor for hypertensive disorders in pregnancy, and hence maternal and perinatal morbidity. A recent meta-analyses and systematic review of pregnancy outcomes in women with OSA reiterated the association between gestational sleeping disturbance and hypertensive disorders of pregnancy and preterm delivery.[93] The OR of preterm delivery in those with OSA was 1.75 (95% CI = 1.21–2.55). If sleep apnea is suspected, referral to a sleep specialist is advised, as treatment with a nasal continuous positive airway pressure (CPAP) machine has been shown to improve hypertension and perinatal outcomes.[94]

22.2.6   Nonalcoholic Fatty Liver Disease

Nonalcoholic fatty liver disease (NAFLD) is a leading cause of liver disease in the Western world. The risk factors for NAFLD in pregnancy are advanced maternal age, obesity, and diabetes. The studies to date in pregnancy have focused on NAFLD in those with a diagnosis of GDM. There are no studies conducted on NAFLD in pregnant women with T2DM. Women with NAFLD have increased risk of adverse perinatal outcomes, including a higher incidence of low birth weight and instrumental and preterm delivery.[95] It is difficult to extrapolate the effects of NAFLD on maternal and perinatal outcomes from those of obesity. Liver enzymes are not typically altered in NAFLD, and noninvasive testing such as fibrosis-4 scoring are inaccurate during pregnancy.[96] If mild disease is diagnosed, lifestyle modifications are typically sufficient. If moderate-to-severe disease is discovered, then further investigation with a hepatologist is warranted.

22.2.7   Maternal Outcomes with T2DM

Severe maternal complications are considerably increased in women with T2DM. These include preeclampsia, preterm delivery, and the sequelae of delivering an LGA offspring.

22.2.7.1   Preeclampsia

A total of 4 out of 10 women with preexisting diabetes are diagnosed with hypertension in pregnancy. Hypertension is a significant risk factor for the development of preeclampsia. Preeclampsia is defined classically as hypertension developing after 20 weeks' gestation associated with proteinuria, evidence of end organ damage, or both. A recent Swedish study demonstrated that the rate of PET among women with T2DM was 2.5-fold higher than in the general population.[97] Preeclampsia is associated with both maternal and fetal morbidities, such as pulmonary edema, multiorgan failure, cardiomyopathy, intrauterine growth restriction (IUGR), and stillbirth. In T1DM, clearly defined risk factors for an increase in preeclampsia include glycemic control in the first trimester, duration of diabetes, and microangiopathies such as nephropathy. In T2DM, however, increased risk factors for the development of preeclampsia are less well studied. It is known that increased BMI, independent of glycemic control, is a risk factor for PET, and it may be playing an added role in women with T2DM. Obesity and preeclampsia share several features, including subclinical inflammation, a reduction in nitrous oxide production, and lipotoxicity. These features result in maternal vascular dysfunction and reduced trophoblastic placental invasion.

22.2.8   Obstetric Intervention

T1DM pregnancies are associated with the highest rate of obstetric intervention, followed closely by T2DM and GDM. The same large Canadian cross-sectional study mentioned previously demonstrated increased rates of induction of labor (IOL) in pregnancies complicated by T2DM, at 43.6%, and just over 50% were delivered by cesarean section.[22] The maternal length of hospital stay was prolonged in 38% of women with T2DM.

22.2.9   Fetal/Perinatal Complications

Preexisting T2DM transforms a gestation into a high-risk pregnancy.[98] Despite significant improvements in the management of preexisting diabetes, there remains a higher incidence of fetal and perinatal complications compared to the background population.

22.2.9.1   Pregnancy Loss

Pregestational diabetes is associated with a threefold increase in both miscarriage and perinatal mortality rate. There is also a fivefold increase in the incidence of stillbirth.[99] In the past, investigators hypothesized that pregnancy outcomes would be better in women with T2DM compared to women with T1DM. However, studies have found similarly poor, or sometimes even worse, outcomes.[88] A systematic review of 33 observational studies comparing T1DM to T2DM in pregnancy over a 20-year period demonstrated higher perinatal mortality rates in women with T2DM compared to T1DM. Obesity and advanced maternal age among women with T2DM are contributing factors to the higher perinatal mortality rate.

22.2.9.2 Congenital Anomalies

The excessive incidence of congenital anomalies in the offspring of women with diabetes was first described in the 1960s by Molsted-Pedersen. The background population risk of any congenital anomaly is 2%–3%. There is a three- to tenfold increase in the rate of major congenital anomalies in pregnancies complicated by preexisting diabetes,[88, 99] with similar rates in women with T2DM and T1DM.[12]

22.2.9.2.1 Factors Contributing to Congenital Anomalies in Women with T2DM

The pathogenesis for anomalies in offspring of women with T2DM is multifactorial. Proposed contributing factors include glycemic control, obesity, and medication. We will discuss each in detail next.

Glycemic control Hyperglycemia per se is accepted as playing the principal role in the occurrence of congenital anomalies. The risk of a congenital anomaly when HbA1c >10% is approximately 16% in women with preexisting diabetes.[100] This risk drops to almost that of the background population when the HbA1c is <6.3%. A reduction in HbA1c, even by 1%, reduces the risk of an anomaly by 30%.[101]

Obesity The burden of obesity is increasing in prevalence among women of reproductive age. The increase in numbers with T2DM in pregnancy is undoubtedly linked to the obesity epidemic. In Europe, a maternity tertiary referral center reported a 48.5% increase in severe obesity (BMI $> 40 \text{kg/m}^2$) over a 5-year period.[102] A recently published study reported a high BMI among 63% of those women aged between 15 and 49 years old.[103] In the United States, two-thirds of women of reproductive age are obese.[104] There is an association between increased BMI (without diabetes) and congenital anomalies, and the risk increases based on the category of obesity. A meta-analysis reported that the offspring of obese mothers are at increased risk of a wide range of congenital malformations, including neural tube defects, cardiovascular anomalies, cleft lip and palate, anorectal atresia, and limb reduction anomalies.[105] The pathogenesis for the increased incidence of congenital anomalies in the absence of dysglycemia remains unclear. Obesity results in metabolic derangements such as hyperlipidemia and inflammation, which may play a teratogenic role.[106]

Drugs Angiotensin-converting enzyme (ACE) inhibitors and angiotensin-receptor blockers (ARBSs): These drugs are commonly prescribed to women with preexisting diabetes, including women with T2DM. The study that prompted concern regarding these agents found an increase in congenital anomalies in women without diabetes receiving ACE inhibitors, compared to those not exposed to antihypertensives in the first trimester.[32] The relative risk (RR) of an anomaly was 2.71. However, subsequent studies have shown that not only do women exposed to ACE inhibitors/ARBSs have an increased risk of anomalies, but also women exposed to other antihypertensive agents, suggesting that it may be the hypertension per se, or something about the women with hypertension, that is increasing the risk of anomalies, as opposed to the agent used. For women with overt proteinuria, a discussion should be had regarding the risks and benefits of stopping the medication while trying for pregnancy, or stopping as soon as pregnancy is diagnosed, given the often rapid return of proteinuria when these medications are discontinued. These medications should not be used in the second or third trimester, where they are associated with oligohydramnios and its consequences, including anuria and fetal death. Little is known about dipeptidyl peptidase 4 (DPP-4) inhibitors, sodium-glucose cotransporter 2 (SGLT2) inhibitors, or glucagon-like peptide-1 (GLP-1) receptor agonists, and they should not be used during pregnancy or when planning pregnancy.

Statins: Cholesterol is an activator of sonic hedgehog proteins, which are essential for morphogenesis in vertebrates. Based on animal data and case reports, the U.S. Food and Drug Administration (FDA) has given statin therapy a Category X in pregnancy, meaning it should not be used. The clinical literature, however, has been conflicting, with a recent meta-analysis failing to show an increased risk of anomalies.[107]

22.2.9.3 Preterm Delivery

There is an increased rate of preterm delivery in pregnancies complicated by T2DM. Preterm delivery for maternal or fetal concerns, either spontaneous or iatrogenic, can result in significant neonatal morbidities. Early preterm (i.e., <34 weeks) is associated with a higher perinatal mortality rate, as well as respiratory, neurological, and gastrointestinal neonatal morbidities. In the Canadian cross-sectional study conducted between 2004 and 2015, preterm delivery (i.e., <37/40 weeks) occurred in 23% of the offspring of women with T2DM, and early preterm (i.e., <34/40) in 6% of the offspring. As a result, there was a prolonged neonatal length of stay in 34% of the offspring.[108]

22.2.9.4 Birth Weight and Peripartum Consequences

The offspring of women with T2DM are more likely to be LGA.[109] An Australian review that compared 138 pregnancies in women with T2DM to 27,075 pregnancies in women without diabetes demonstrated an OR of 2.13 [95% confidence interval (CI) 1.37–3.32] for LGA. There was also an increased rate of neonatal hypoglycemia (OR 4.9 (95% CI 2.79–8.61), jaundice (OR 2.58 (95% CI 1.61–4.13), and shoulder dystocia (OR 2.72 (95% CI 1.09–6.78).

22.2.10 Management

22.2.10.1 What is expected at the first diabetes clinic visit in pregnancy for women with T2DM?

As soon as a woman discovers that she is pregnant, she should contact the diabetes antenatal clinic. This clinic ideally should be a combined practice with the obstetric team. Close surveillance with a clinic review every 1–2 weeks antenatally is recommended. The booking visit should occur as early as possible in the pregnancy.

The first visit should be comprehensive covering the topics described next.

22.2.10.2 Glucose Control and Glucose Monitoring

Capillary blood glucose monitoring (fasting and either 1 or 2 h postprandial) is advised. Glucose targets, as recommended by the international professional bodies, are highlighted in Table 22.2. Women should be counseled regarding the risk of hypoglycemia. If the patient is on insulin, the requirements may decrease toward the end of the first trimester, but then they typically escalate with the increasing insulin resistance of pregnancy. Requirements typically rise to double prepregnancy levels at 30 weeks' gestation.[110] There are limited studies on CGMS usage in T2DM. CGMS can be beneficial, as it records glucose levels every 5 min. This can be of use in patients prone to hypoglycemia, particularly nocturnal hypoglycemia. The NICE guidelines in 2015 state that CGMS is not to be offered routinely to patients with diabetes in pregnancy, but it can be considered in certain cases, such as significant hypoglycemia. One study found, surprisingly, that the T2DM population in pregnancy experiences a similar rate of nocturnal hypoglycemia as the T1DM group, despite a shorter duration of diabetes.[111]

22.2.10.3 Dietary Advice and Weight Gain

A dietician specializing in pregnancy should consult with the patient. Sugar and simple carbohydrates should be eliminated and replaced by complex carbohydrates. One choice includes 15 g of carbohydrate. A daily minimum of 175 g or 12 carbohydrate choices is recommended. A basic dietary plan should consist of three main meals with two to three snacks per day. In 2009, the U.S. Institute of Medicine published the guidelines for appropriate GWG in pregnancy, which depend upon prepregnancy BMI category (as discussed in the section on GDM earlier in this chapter). Excess maternal weight gain, independent of glycemic control, can have adverse effects on the fetus in a woman with T2DM in pregnancy. An observational study by Egan et al. demonstrated that despite dietary advice, excessive GWG occurred in over 50% of the women studied with T2DM.[112] Excessive weight gain was an independent risk factor for gestational hypertension, LGA offspring, and macrosomia in these women.

TABLE 22.2 Glucose targets as recommend by professional bodies in pregnancy

Organization	FPG	1 h Postprandial	2 h Postprandial
ADA (American Diabetes Association)	≤5.3 (≤95 mg/dL)	≤7.8 (≤140 mg/dL)	≤6.7 (≤120 mg/dL)
ACOG (American College of Obstetrics & Gynecology)	≤5.3 (≤95 mg/dL)	≤7.8 (≤140 mg/dL)	≤6.7 (≤120 mg/dL)
CDA (Diabetes Canada)	≤5.3 (≤95 mg/dL)	≤7.8 (≤140 mg/dL)	≤6.7 (≤120 mg/dL)
Endocrine Society	≤5.0 (≤90 mg/dL)	≤7.8 (≤140 mg/dL)	≤6.7 (≤120 mg/dL)
NICE (National Institute for Clinical Excellence)	<5.3 (<95 mg/dL)	<7.8 (≤140 mg/dL)	<6.4 (≤115 mg/dL)
AIDPS (Australian Diabetes in Pregnancy Society)	≤5.0 (≤90 mg/dL)	≤7.4 (≤133 mg/dL)	≤6.7 (≤120 mg/dL)

22.2.10.4 Drugs/vitamin Supplementation

It is important to review the medications that the woman is prescribed. If on ACE inhibitors/ARBs or statins, the recommendation is to discontinue. Ensure that folic acid (1 mg) is being taken at least up to 12 weeks' gestation, but ideally throughout pregnancy until breastfeeding is completed.[113] Calcium and vitamin D supplementation is advised. Calcium supplementation reduces the risk of PET and PTD compared to placebo.[114] The benefit is most marked in the setting of a low-calcium diet. Vitamin D deficiency is common in pregnancy. Vitamin D sufficiency is believed to play a beneficial role in the prevention of adverse pregnancy outcomes primarily preeclampsia. A Cochrane meta-analysis of two trials involving 219 women suggested a lower risk of preeclampsia in those receiving vitamin D supplementation compared to no intervention or placebo (8.9% versus 15.5%, RR 0.52; 95% CI 0.25–1.05).[115] Other meta-analyses, however, have shown no effect on maternal or fetal outcomes except for a reduction in childhood wheezing at 3 years.[116]

22.2.10.5 Pharmacological Management of Pregnancy in Women with T2DM

22.2.10.5.1 Aspirin

Women with T2DM are at higher risk of preeclampsia, and thus they all should be advised to take aspirin for the prevention of early preeclampsia. The dosing and timing of aspirin initiation remain the subject of much debate. A meta-analysis by Bujold et al. demonstrated a halving in the rate of PET, IUGR, and perinatal death if aspirin is initiated before 16 weeks' gestation in women at high risk of PET, with no effect if administered after this gestation.[117] A study by Roberge et al. reported that a dose of 100 mg aspirin was more effective than a low dose (75 mg) at preventing preeclampsia.[118] The large Aspirin for Evidence-Based Preeclampsia Prevention (ASPRE) trial used a higher dose of aspirin (150 mg) (commenced between 11 and 14 weeks' gestation) compared to a placebo group among a cohort at high risk for preterm preeclampsia. In the treated group, 1.6% of women developed severe PET compared to 4.3% (P = 0.004) in the placebo group.[119] Although these studies did not include many women with T2DM per se, given their increased risk of preeclampsia, the evidence for aspirin has been extrapolated to women with both T1DM and T2DM during pregnancy.

22.2.10.5.2 Oral Hypoglycemic Agents

What about using or continuing oral hypoglycemic agents in pregnancy in women with T2DM?

Metformin and glyburide (glibenclamide), as discussed in Section 22.1.7.1.2, are both used in pregnancy. The following section discusses metformin usage only in women with T2DM.

Metformin The evidence for the use of metformin in T2DM in pregnancy is sparse in comparison to its use in women with PCOS and GDM. A recent large US study of birth defects failed to demonstrate an association between metformin and the risk of congenital malformation.[120]

Metformin as an insulin-sparing agent and is an attractive option as an adjunct to insulin therapy. A 2006 report of 93 women with T2DM using metformin concluded that no adverse fetal affects were noted.[121] In an Egyptian study of 90 women with GDM or T2DM and insulin resistance (defined as poor glycemic control on >1.12 units/kg of insulin), women were randomized to add metformin to their insulin or increase their insulin alone as needed.[122] They reported significant benefits (both maternal and neonatal) in the metformin group. There was also a reduction in hospital admissions for extremes in maternal glucose control, and reduced admission to the neonatal intensive care unit, neonatal hypoglycemia, and rate of respiratory distress syndrome. All of these developments caused significant cost savings to the center.[122] These results are encouraging. However, this study had several methodological problems, including small sample size, failure to employ an intention to treat analysis, and recruitment of women with both T2DM and GDM, resulting in recruitment for up to 34 weeks' gestation.

There is a need for additional large-scale studies to ascertain the potential benefits and adverse effects of metformin usage among women with T2DM. The MiTy is a large multicenter randomized trial that is attempting to answer these questions.[123] Women in the treatment arm will receive metformin 1000 mg bid in addition to insulin therapy. The primary outcome is a composite that includes pregnancy loss, preterm birth, and neonatal hypoglycemia. The secondary outcomes will include LGA and maternal outcomes such as GWG and hypertension.

What is the effect of metformin on offspring outcomes in women with T2DM?

To date, there is no long-term follow-up data on the offspring of mothers with T2DM taking metformin during pregnancy. MiTy Kids is a follow-up cohort study of infants of mothers in the MiTy trial.[123] It will study the neonatal and early childhood outcomes in those exposed to metformin antenatally in women with T2DM, and determine whether treatment with metformin during pregnancy leads to a reduction in adiposity and improvement in insulin resistance at 2 years of age.

The usage of OHAs in pregnancies complicated by T2DM remains controversial. There is little agreement between the international professional diabetes bodies. The American Diabetes Association (ADA) and the Australian guidelines state that insulin is the preferred agent, as it does not cross the placenta. Diabetes Canada states that women with T2DM who conceive on metformin can continue until insulin is initiated. The NICE guidance states that women with diabetes may be advised to use metformin as an adjunct or an alternative to insulin during pregnancy, when the benefits from improved glucose control outweighs potential harm. All other oral blood-glucose-lowering agents should be discontinued.

22.2.10.5.3 Insulin Therapy in T2DM Pregnancy

Professional guidelines generally recommend the use of insulin, particularly insulin analogs in the management of T2DM in pregnancy. A concern with all drugs used in pregnancy is their ability to traverse the placenta. Insulin, however, which has a large molecular size and as such should not cross the placenta, is deemed to be safe. For the purpose of this section on T2DM in pregnancy, we will focus on concentrated and longer-acting basal insulin analogs.

Concentrated basal insulin analogs Pregnancy is a period of weight gain and increasing insulin resistance. Doses of insulin, therefore, typically escalate during pregnancy. The dose of insulin increases the volume of insulin injected subcutaneously. Concentrated basal insulin can offer several advantages outside of pregnancy: There is a lower volume required, less hypoglycemia, less weight gain, and increased adherence. For decades, U500 R insulin was the only available concentrated insulin on the market.[124] Glargine U300 is a new, concentrated insulin, with a duration of action of over 30 h. A steady state is typically reached in 5 days. There have been no reported cases of U300 insulin use in pregnancy. Lispro U200 is the first bolus concentrated insulin analog to receive FDA approval. This approval is based on the bioequivalence of lispro U-200 relative to lispro U-100 from a pharmacokinetic/pharmacodynamic aspect. Lispro U200, as for U100, has a FDA Category B in pregnancy.

To conclude, concentrated insulin may be useful, particularly in a pregnancy complicated by T2DM. However, to date, there has been insufficient information to support their use in pregnancy. The new concentrated types of insulin are also costly, and none can be used in combination with insulin-pump therapy as yet.

Ultralong-acting basal insulin analogs Degludec is an ultralong-acting basal analog with a half-life of 25 h. A steady state is achieved between 48 and 72 h postinjection. A recent meta-analysis was conducted of studies in the nonpregnant population with diabetes to determine the safety and efficacy of insulin degludec compared to glargine. The analysis included 18 RCTs and over 16,000 patients. Insulin degludec was associated with a slightly higher HbA1c compared to glargine. Favoring insulin degludec was a significant reduction in severe hypoglycemia in the T2DM population.[125] There are three case reports on four women using insulin degludec in pregnancy, with good glycemic response and neonatal outcomes. Guidelines for the use of degludec in the nonpregnant population suggest that dose adjustments be made every 2–5 days to achieve a steady state. Given that pregnancy is a dynamic environment requiring sufficient flexibility, this kind of dose adjustment may be less advantageous for pregnancy.

Currently, there is an ongoing randomized trial of degludec in women with T1DM. Animal reproduction studies have not demonstrated embryotoxicity compared to NPH; however, additional human safety data is required prior to general consideration in pregnancy.

22.2.11 Peripartum Monitoring: Maternal and Neonatal

The timing and mode of delivery depend upon a number of factors not limited to fetal size, presence of medical comorbidities, and signs of placental insufficiency, including decreasing insulin requirements. The rationale for delivery by either induction of labor or cesarean section between 37 + 0 and 38 + 6 weeks' gestation is largely the feared complication of intrauterine death, which is increased in women with T2DM. The presence of diabetes alone is not a clear indication for cesarean section.

Maternal hyperglycemia is associated with neonatal hypoglycemia; therefore, tight glycemic control is recommended during delivery. The aim is to maintain glucose levels between 4 and 7 mmoL/L, although evidence for the ideal target range is lacking.

22.2.12 Postpartum: Insulin Doses and Breastfeeding

Once the patient is eating, approximately 30% of the patient's prepregnancy dose is given to avoid hypoglycemia in an environment of increased insulin sensitivity in the immediate postpartum period. Metformin and glyburide are deemed to be safe in breastfeeding and should be begun again postpartum. There are no safety data for the use of dipeptidyl peptidase IV inhibitors, the SGLT2 inhibitors or GLP-1 agonists during breastfeeding. Therefore, their use during breastfeeding is not recommended.

22.2.13 Future Pregnancies

The importance of preconception counseling for the next pregnancy should be emphasized. Ideally, encourage interpregnancy weight loss to reduce the incidence of obesity-related conditions. Contraception should be discussed, with the choice being based on patient preference and the presence of comorbidities such as hypertension.

22.2.14 Risk for Offspring

The exposure of the fetus to maternal metabolic derangements in utero can result in short- and long-term consequences. The short-term consequences have been discussed. The long-term sequelae of T2DM to the offspring include dysglycemia, obesity, hyperlipidemia, and cardiovascular disease. A study of 9439 mother-child pairs found that increased glucose levels during pregnancy (GDM) were associated with childhood obesity at 5–7 years.[126] In a study of 467,850 First Nation and non-First Nation offspring of women in Manitoba, Canada (mean follow-up 17 years), T2DM exposure in utero conferred a greater risk of diabetes in offspring than did GDM. Any diabetes exposure accelerated the time to development of T2DM in the offspring.[127] Mothers should be advised regarding the benefits of a healthy lifestyle, not only for themselves but for their children.

REFERENCES

1. American Diabetes Association. 2. Classification and diagnosis of diabetes: standards of medical care in diabetes-2018. *Diabetes Care* 2018;**41** (Suppl 1):S13–27.
2. Feig DS, Hwee J, Shah BR, Booth GL, Bierman AS, Lipscombe LL. Trends in incidence of diabetes in pregnancy and serious perinatal outcomes: a large, population-based study in Ontario, Canada, 1996–2010. *Diabetes Care* 2014;**37**(6):1590–6.
3. Correa A, Bardenheier B, Elixhauser A, Geiss LS, Gregg E. Trends in prevalence of diabetes among delivery hospitalizations, United States, 1993–2009. *Matern Child Health J* 2015;**19**(3):635–42.
4. Melchior H, Kurch-Bek D, Mund M. The prevalence of gestational diabetes. *Dtsch Arztebl Int* 2017;**114**(24):412–8.
5. Egan AM, Vellinga A, Harreiter J, Simmons D, Desoye G, Corcoy R, Adelantado JM, Devlieger R, Van Assche A, Galjaard S, Damm P, Mathiesen ER, Jensen DM, Andersen L, Lapolla A, Dalfra MG, Bertolotto A, Mantaj U, Wender-Ozegowska E, Zawiejska A, Hill D, Jelsma JGM, Snoek FJ, Worda C, Bancher-Todesca D, Van Poppel MNM, Kautzky-Willer A, Dunne FP, DALI Core Investigator Group. Epidemiology of gestational diabetes mellitus according to IADPSG/WHO 2013 criteria among obese pregnant women in Europe. *Diabetologia* 2017;**60** (10):1913–21.
6. Mukerji G, Chiu M, Shah BR. Impact of gestational diabetes on the risk of diabetes following pregnancy among Chinese and South Asian women. *Diabetologia* 2012;**55**(8):2148–53.
7. Zhu Y, Zhang C. Prevalence of gestational diabetes and risk of progression to type 2 diabetes: a global perspective. *Curr Diab Rep* 2016;**16**(1):7.
8. Buchanan TA. Pancreatic B-cell defects in gestational diabetes: implications for the pathogenesis and prevention of type 2 diabetes. *J Clin Endocrinol Metab* 2001;**86**(3):989–93.
9. Catalano PM, Huston L, Amini SB, Kalhan SC. Longitudinal changes in glucose metabolism during pregnancy in obese women with normal glucose tolerance and gestational diabetes mellitus. *Am J Obstet Gynecol* 1999;**180**(4):903–16.
10. Feig DS, Zinman B, Wang X, Hux JE. Risk of development of diabetes mellitus after diagnosis of gestational diabetes. *CMAJ* 2008;**179**(3):229–34.
11. Chiefari E, Arcidiacono B, Foti D, Brunetti A. Gestational diabetes mellitus: an updated overview. *J Endocrinol Invest* 2017;**40**(9):899–909.
12. HAPO Study Cooperative Research Group, Metzger BE, Lowe LP, Dyer AR, Trimble ER, Chaovarindr U, Coustan DR, Hadden DR, McCance DR, Hod M, McIntyre HD, Oats JJ, Persson B, Rogers MS, Sacks DA. Hyperglycemia and adverse pregnancy outcomes. *N Engl J Med* 2008;**358** (19):1991–2002.
13. Catalano PM, McIntyre HD, Cruickshank JK, McCance DR, Dyer AR, Metzger BE, Lowe LP, Trimble ER, Coustan DR, Hadden DR, Persson B, Hod M, Oats JJ, HAPO Study Cooperative Research Group. The hyperglycemia and adverse pregnancy outcome study: associations of GDM and obesity with pregnancy outcomes. *Diabetes Care* 2012;**35**(4):780–6.
14. Mendoza LC, Harreiter J, Simmons D, Desoye G, Adelantado JM, Juarez F, Chico A, Devlieger R, van Assche A, Galjaard S, Damm P, Mathiesen ER, Jensen DM, Andersen LLT, Tanvig M, Lapolla A, Dalfra MG, Bertolotto A, Mantaj U, Wender-Ozegowska E, Zawiejska A, Hill D, Jelsma JG, Snoek FJ, Van Poppel MNM, Worda C, Bancher-Todesca D, Kautzky-Willer A, Dunne FP, Corcoy R, HAPO Study

Cooperative Research Group. Risk factors for hyperglycemia in pregnancy in the DALI study differ by period of pregnancy and OGTT time point. *Eur J Endocrinol* 2018;**179**(1):39–49.

15. Avalos GE, Owens LA, Dunne F. Atlantic DIP Collaborators. Applying current screening tools for gestational diabetes mellitus to a European population: is it time for change? *Diabetes Care* 2013;**36**(10):3040–4.

16. Committee on Practice Bulletins—Obstetrics. ACOG practice bulletin No. 190: gestational diabetes mellitus. *Obstet Gynecol* 2018;**131**(2):e49–64.

17. Diabetes Canada Clinical Practice Guidelines Expert Committee, Feig DS, Berger H, Donovan L, Godbout A, Kader T, Keely E, Sanghera R. Diabetes and pregnancy. *Can J Diabetes* 2018;**42**(Suppl 1) S255–S82.

18. Benaiges D, Flores-Le Roux JA, Marcelo I, Mane L, Rodriguez M, Navarro X, Chillaron JJ, Llaurado G, Gortazar L, Pedro-Botet J, Paya A. Is first-trimester HbA1c useful in the diagnosis of gestational diabetes? *Diabetes Res Clin Pract* 2017;**133**:85–91.

19. Osmundson SS, Zhao BS, Kunz L, Wang E, Popat R, Nimbal VC, Palaniappan LP. First trimester hemoglobin A1c prediction of gestational diabetes. *Am J Perinatol* 2016;**33**(10):977–82.

20. Simmons D, Hague WM, Teede HJ, Cheung NW, Hibbert EJ, Nolan CJ, Peek MJ, Girosi F, Cowell CT, Wong VW, Flack JR, McLean M, Dalal R, Robertson A, Rajagopal R. Hyperglycaemia in early pregnancy: the treatment of booking gestational diabetes mellitus (TOBOGM) study. A randomised controlled trial. *Med J Aust* 2018, 405.e1-6.

21. Simmons D, Nema J, Parton C, Vizza L, Robertson A, Rajagopal R, Ussher J, Perz J. The treatment of booking gestational diabetes mellitus (TOBOGM) pilot randomised controlled trial. *BMC Pregnancy Childbirth* 2018;**18**(1):151.

22. Wong T, Ross GP, Jalaludin BB, Flack JR. The clinical significance of overt diabetes in pregnancy. *Diabet Med* 2013;**30**(4):468–74.

23. Hughes RC, Moore MP, Gullam JE, Mohamed K, Rowan J. An early pregnancy HbA1c ≥5.9% (41 mmol/mol) is optimal for detecting diabetes and identifies women at increased risk of adverse pregnancy outcomes. *Diabetes Care* 2014;**37**(11):2953–9.

24. International Association of Diabetes and Pregnancy Study Groups Consensus Panel, Metzger BE, Gabbe SG, Persson B, Buchanan TA, Catalano PA, Damm P, Dyer AR, Leiva A, Hod M, Kitzmiler JL, Lowe LP, McIntyre HD, Oats JJ, Omori Y, Schmidt MI. International association of diabetes and pregnancy study groups recommendations on the diagnosis and classification of hyperglycemia in pregnancy. *Diabetes Care* 2010;**33**(3):676–82.

25. Diagnostic criteria and classification of hyperglycaemia first detected in pregnancy. Available from: http://www.who.int/diabetes/publications/Hyperglycaemia_In_Pregnancy; 2013, WHO/NMH/MND/13.2.

26. Vandorsten JP, Dodson WC, Espeland MA, Grobman WA, Guise JM, Mercer BM, Minkoff HL, Poindexter B, Prosser LA, Sawaya GF, Scott JR, Silver RM, Smith L, Thomas A, Tita AT. NIH consensus development conference: diagnosing gestational diabetes mellitus. *NIH Consens State Sci Statements* 2013;**29**(1):1–31.

27. Crowther CA, Hiller JE, Moss JR, McPhee AJ, Jeffries WS, Robinson JS. Australian carbohydrate intolerance study in pregnant women trial G. Effect of treatment of gestational diabetes mellitus on pregnancy outcomes. *N Engl J Med* 2005;**352**(24):2477–86.

28. Landon MB, Spong CY, Thom E, Carpenter MW, Ramin SM, Casey B, Wapner RJ, Varner MW, Rouse DJ, Thorp Jr. JM, Sciscione A, Catalano P, Harper M, Saade G, Lain KY, Sorokin Y, Peaceman AM, Tolosa JE, Anderson GB, Eunice Kennedy Shriver National Institute of Child Health and Human Development Maternal–Fetal Medicine Units Network. A multicenter, randomized trial of treatment for mild gestational diabetes. *N Engl J Med* 2009;**361**(14):1339–48.

29. Horvath K, Koch K, Jeitler K, Matyas E, Bender R, Bastian H, Lange S, Siebenhofer A. Effects of treatment in women with gestational diabetes mellitus: systematic review and meta-analysis. *BMJ* 2010;**340**:c1395.

30. Hartling L, Dryden DM, Guthrie A, Muise M, Vandermeer B, Donovan L. Benefits and harms of treating gestational diabetes mellitus: a systematic review and meta-analysis for the U.S. Preventive Services Task Force and the National Institutes of Health Office of Medical Applications of Research. *Ann Intern Med* 2013;**159**(2):123–9.

31. Prutsky GJ, Domecq JP, Wang Z, Carranza Leon BG, Elraiyah T, Nabhan M, Sundaresh V, Vella A, Montori VM, Murad MH. Glucose targets in pregnant women with diabetes: a systematic review and meta-analysis. *J Clin Endocrinol Metab* 2013;**98**(11):4319–24.

32. Mendez-Figueroa H, Daley J, Lopes VV, Coustan DR. Comparing daily versus less frequent blood glucose monitoring in patients with mild gestational diabetes. *J Matern Fetal Neonatal Med* 2013;**26**(13):1268–72.

33. Moreno-Castilla C, Mauricio D, Hernandez M. Role of medical nutrition therapy in the management of gestational diabetes mellitus. *Curr Diab Rep* 2016;**16**(4):22.

34. Wei J, Heng W, Gao J. Effects of low glycemic index diets on gestational diabetes mellitus: a meta-analysis of randomized controlled clinical trials. *Medicine (Baltimore)* 2016;**95**(22).

35. Viana LV, Gross JL, Azevedo MJ. Dietary intervention in patients with gestational diabetes mellitus: a systematic review and meta-analysis of randomized clinical trials on maternal and newborn outcomes. *Diabetes Care* 2014;**37**(12):3345–55.

36. Ruchat SM, Mottola MF. The important role of physical activity in the prevention and management of gestational diabetes mellitus. *Diabetes Metab Res Rev* 2013;**29**(5):334–46.

37. Rasmussen KM. *Weight gain during pregnancy: reexamining the guidelines*. The National Academies Collection: Reports Funded by National Institutes of Health; 2009. [cited 2009]; Available from, *https://www.ncbi.nlm.nih.gov/pubmed/20669500*.

38. Kim SY, Sharma AJ, Sappenfield W, Wilson HG, Salihu HM. Association of maternal body mass index, excessive weight gain, and gestational diabetes mellitus with large-for-gestational-age births. *Obstet Gynecol* 2014;**123**(4):737–44.

39. Challier JC, Hauguel S, Desmaizieres V. Effect of insulin on glucose uptake and metabolism in the human placenta. *J Clin Endocrinol Metab* 1986;**62**(5):803–7.

40. Kjos SL, Schaefer-Graf U, Sardesi S, Peters RK, Buley A, Xiang AH, Bryne JD, Sutherland C, Montoro MN, Buchanan TA. A randomized controlled trial using glycemic plus fetal ultrasound parameters versus glycemic parameters to determine insulin therapy in gestational diabetes with fasting hyperglycemia. *Diabetes Care* 2001;**24**(11):1904–10.

41. Di Cianni G, Volpe L, Ghio A, Lencioni C, Cuccuru I, Benzi L, Del Prato S. Maternal metabolic control and perinatal outcome in women with gestational diabetes mellitus treated with lispro or aspart insulin: comparison with regular insulin. *Diabetes Care* 2007;**30**(4).

42. Jovanovic L, Ilic S, Pettitt DJ, Hugo K, Gutierrez M, Bowsher RR, Bastyr 3rd EJ. Metabolic and immunologic effects of insulin lispro in gestational diabetes. *Diabetes Care* 1999;**22**(9):1422–7.

43. Pettitt DJ, Ospina P, Kolaczynski JW, Jovanovic L. Comparison of an insulin analog, insulin aspart, and regular human insulin with no insulin in gestational diabetes mellitus. *Diabetes Care* 2003;**26**(1):183–6.

44. Toledano Y, Hadar E, Hod M. Safety of insulin analogues as compared with human insulin in pregnancy. *Expert Opin Drug Saf* 2016;**15**(7):963–73.

45. Herrera KM, Rosenn BM, Foroutan J, Bimson BE, Al Ibraheemi Z, Moshier EL, Brustman LE. Randomized controlled trial of insulin detemir versus NPH for the treatment of pregnant women with diabetes. *Am J Obstet Gynecol* 2015;**213**(3). 426 e1–7.

46. Lv S, Wang J, Xu Y. Safety of insulin analogs during pregnancy: a meta-analysis. *Arch Gynecol Obstet* 2015;**292**(4):749–56.

47. Markowicz-Piasecka M, Huttunen KM, Mateusiak L, Mikiciuk-Olasik E, Sikora J. Is metformin a perfect drug? Updates in pharmacokinetics and pharmacodynamics. *Curr Pharm Des* 2017;**23**(17):2532–50.

48. Vanky E, Zahlsen K, Spigset O, Carlsen SM. Placental passage of metformin in women with polycystic ovary syndrome. *Fertil Steril* 2005;**83**(5):1575–8.

49. Rowan JA, Hague WM, Gao W, Battin MR, Moore MP, Mi GTI. Metformin versus insulin for the treatment of gestational diabetes. *N Engl J Med* 2008;**358**(19):2003–15.

50. Balsells M, Garcia-Patterson A, Sola I, Roque M, Gich I, Corcoy R. Glibenclamide, metformin, and insulin for the treatment of gestational diabetes: a systematic review and meta-analysis. *BMJ* 2015;**350**:h102.

51. Farrar D, Simmonds M, Bryant M, Sheldon TA, Tuffnell D, Golder S, Lawlor DA. Treatments for gestational diabetes: a systematic review and meta-analysis. *BMJ Open* 2017;**7**(6).

52. Rowan JA, Rush EC, Obolonkin V, Battin M, Wouldes T, Hague WM. Metformin in gestational diabetes: the offspring follow-up (MiG TOFU): body composition at 2 years of age. *Diabetes Care* 2011;**34**(10):2279–84.

53. Rowan JA, Rush EC, Plank LD, Lu J, Obolonkin V, Coat S, Hague WM. Metformin in gestational diabetes: the offspring follow-up (MiG TOFU): body composition and metabolic outcomes at 7–9 years of age. *BMJ Open Diabetes Res Care* 2018;**6**(1).

54. Hanem LGE, Stridsklev S, Juliusson PB, Salvesen O, Roelants M, Carlsen SM, Odegard R, Vanky E. Metformin use in PCOS pregnancies increases the risk of offspring overweight at 4 years of age: follow-up of two RCTs. *J Clin Endocrinol Metab* 2018;**103**(4):1612–21.

55. Wouldes TA, Battin M, Coat S, Rush EC, Hague WM, Rowan JA. Neurodevelopmental outcome at 2 years in offspring of women randomised to metformin or insulin treatment for gestational diabetes. *Arch Dis Child Fetal Neonatal Ed* 2016;**101**:F488–93.

56. Tertti K, Eskola E, Ronnemaa T, Haataja L. Neurodevelopment of two-year-old children exposed to metformin and insulin in gestational diabetes mellitus. *J Dev Behav Pediatr* 2015;**36**(9):752–7.

57. Malek R, Davis SN. Pharmacokinetics, efficacy and safety of glyburide for treatment of gestational diabetes mellitus. *Expert Opin Drug Metab Toxicol* 2016;**12**(6):691–9.

58. Hebert MF, Ma X, Naraharisetti SB, Krudys KM, Umans JG, Hankins GD, Caritis SN, Miodovnik M, Mattison DR, Unadkat JD, Kelly EJ, Blough D, Cobelli C, Ahmed MS, Snodgrass WR, Carr DB, Easterling TR, Vicini P, Obstetric-Fetal Pharmacology Research Unit Network. Are we optimizing gestational diabetes treatment with glyburide? The pharmacologic basis for better clinical practice. *Clin Pharmacol Ther* 2009;**85**(6):607–14.

59. Langer O, Conway DL, Berkus MD, Xenakis EM, Gonzales O. A comparison of glyburide and insulin in women with gestational diabetes mellitus. *N Engl J Med* 2000;**343**(16):1134–8.

60. Zarate A, Ochoa R, Hernandez M, Basurto L. Effectiveness of acarbose in the control of glucose tolerance worsening in pregnancy. *Ginecol Obstet Mex* 2000;**68**:42–5.

61. Bertini AM, Silva JC, Taborda W, Becker F, Lemos Bebber FR, Zucco Viesi JM, Aquim G, Engel Ribeiro T. Perinatal outcomes and the use of oral hypoglycemic agents. *J Perinat Med* 2005;**33**(6):519–23.

62. Chan LY, Yeung JH, Lau TK. Placental transfer of rosiglitazone in the first trimester of human pregnancy. *Fertil Steril* 2005;**83**(4):955–8.

63. Holmes HJ, Casey BM, Bawdon RE. Placental transfer of rosiglitazone in the ex vivo human perfusion model. *Am J Obstet Gynecol* 2006;**195**(6):1715–9.

64. Tertti K, Petsalo A, Niemi M, Ekblad U, Tolonen A, Ronnemaa T, Turpeinen M, Heikkinen T, Laine K. Transfer of repaglinide in the dually perfused human placenta and the role of organic anion transporting polypeptides (OATPs). *Eur J Pharm Sci* 2011;**44**(3):181–6.

65. Gunderson EP, Hurston SR, Ning X, Lo JC, Crites Y, Walton D, Dewey KG, Azevedo RA, Young S, Fox G, Elmasian CC, Salvador N, Lum M, Sternfeld B, Quesenberry Jr. CP, Study of Women, Infant Feeding and Type 2 Diabetes After GDM Pregnancy Investigators. Lactation and progression to type 2 diabetes mellitus after gestational diabetes mellitus: a prospective cohort study. *Ann Intern Med* 2015;**163**(12):889–98.

66. Burlina S, Dalfra MG, Lapolla A. Short- and long-term consequences for offspring exposed to maternal diabetes: a review. *J Matern Fetal Neonatal Med* 2017;**32**:1–8.

67. Dabelea D, Hanson RL, Lindsay RS, Pettitt DJ, Imperatore G, Gabir MM, Roumain J, Bennett PH, Knowler WC. Intrauterine exposure to diabetes conveys risks for type 2 diabetes and obesity: a study of discordant sibships. *Diabetes* 2000;**49**(12):2208–11.

68. McKenzie-Sampson S, Paradis G, Healy-Profitos J, St-Pierre F, Auger N. Gestational diabetes and risk of cardiovascular disease up to 25 years after pregnancy: a retrospective cohort study. *Acta Diabetol* 2018;**55**(4):315–22.

69. Aroda VR, Christophi CA, Edelstein SL, Zhang P, Herman WH, Barrett-Connor E, Delahanty LM, Montez MG, Ackermann RT, Zhuo X, Knowler WC, Ratner RE, Diabetes Prevention Program Research Group. The effect of lifestyle intervention and metformin on preventing or delaying diabetes among women with and without gestational diabetes: the diabetes prevention program outcomes study 10-year follow-up. *J Clin Endocrinol Metab* 2015;**100**(4):1646–53.

70. Hemmingsen B, Gimenez-Perez G, Mauricio D, Roque IFM, Metzendorf MI, Richter B. Diet, physical activity or both for prevention or delay of type 2 diabetes mellitus and its associated complications in people at increased risk of developing type 2 diabetes mellitus. *Cochrane Database Syst Rev* 2017;**12**.

71. Nohira T, Kim S, Nakai H, Okabe K, Nohira T, Yoneyama K. Recurrence of gestational diabetes mellitus: rates and risk factors from initial GDM and one abnormal GTT value. *Diabetes Res Clin Pract* 2006;**71**(1):75–81.

72. Kim C, Berger DK, Chamany S. Recurrence of gestational diabetes mellitus: a systematic review. *Diabetes Care* 2007;**30**(5):1314–9.

73. Murphy HR, Bell R, Dornhorst A, Forde R, Lewis-Barned N. Pregnancy in diabetes: challenges and opportunities for improving pregnancy outcomes. *Diabet Med* 2018;**35**(3):292–9.

74. Fadl HE, Simmons D. Trends in diabetes in pregnancy in Sweden 1998–2012. *BMJ Open Diabetes Res Care* 2016;**4**(1).

75. Mackin ST, Nelson SM, Kerssens JJ, Wood R, Wild S, Colhoun HM, Leese GP, Philip S, Lindsay RS, SDRN Epidemiology Group. Diabetes and pregnancy: national trends over a 15 year period. *Diabetologia* 2018;**61**(5):1081–8.

76. Owens LA, Egan AM, Carmody L, Dunne F. Ten years of optimizing outcomes for women with type 1 and type 2 diabetes in pregnancy-the Atlantic DIP experience. *J Clin Endocrinol Metab* 2016;**101**(4):1598–605.

77. Wahabi HA, Alzeidan RA, Esmaeil SA. Pre-pregnancy care for women with pre-gestational diabetes mellitus: a systematic review and meta-analysis. *BMC Public Health* 2012;**12**:792.

78. Forde R, Patelarou EE, Forbes A. The experiences of prepregnancy care for women with type 2 diabetes mellitus: a meta-synthesis. *Int J Womens Health* 2016;**8**:691–703.

79. Klein J, Boyle JA, Kirkham R, Connors C, Whitbread C, Oats J, Barzi F, McIntyre D, Lee I, Luey M, Shaw J, Brown ADH, Maple-Brown LJ. Preconception care for women with type 2 diabetes mellitus: a mixed-methods study of provider knowledge and practice. *Diabetes Res Clin Pract* 2017;**129**:105–15.

80. Murphy HR, Steel SA, Roland JM, Morris D, Ball V, Campbell PJ, Temple RC, East Anglia Study Group for Improving Pregnancy Outcomes in Women With Diabetes (EASIPOD). Obstetric and perinatal outcomes in pregnancies complicated by type 1 and type 2 diabetes: influences of glycaemic control, obesity and social disadvantage. *Diabet Med* 2011;**28**(9):1060–7.

81. Yamamoto JM, Hughes DJF, Evans ML, Karunakaran V, Clark JDA, Morrish NJ, Rayman GA, Winocour PH, Hambling C, Harries AW, Sampson MJ, Murphy HR. Community-based pre-pregnancy care programme improves pregnancy preparation in women with pregestational diabetes. *Diabetologia* 2018;**61**(7):1528–37.

82. Vitner D, Harris K, Maxwell C, Farine D. Obesity in pregnancy: a comparison of four national guidelines. *J Matern Fetal Neonatal Med* 2018;1–11.

83. Scott-Pillai R, Spence D, Cardwell CR, Hunter A, Holmes VA. The impact of body mass index on maternal and neonatal outcomes: a retrospective study in a UK obstetric population, 2004–2011. *BJOG* 2013;**120**(8):932–9.

84. Kwong W, Tomlinson G, Feig DS. Maternal and neonatal outcomes after bariatric surgery; a systematic review and meta-analysis: do the benefits outweigh the risks? *Am J Obstet Gynecol* 2018;**218**(6):573–80.

85. Busetto L, Dicker D, Azran C, Batterham RL, Farpour-Lambert N, Fried M, Hjelmesaeth J, Kinzl J, Leitner DR, Makaronidis JM, Schindler K, Toplak H, Yumuk V. Practical recommendations of the obesity management task force of the European Association for the Study of obesity for the post-bariatric surgery medical management. *Obes Facts* 2017;**10**(6):597–632.

86. Gascoin G, Gerard M, Salle A, Becouarn G, Rouleau S, Sentilhes L, Coutant R. Risk of low birth weight and micronutrient deficiencies in neonates from mothers after gastric bypass: a case control study. *Surg Obes Relat Dis* 2017;**13**(8):1384–91.

87. Ramadan M, Loureiro M, Laughlan K, Caiazzo R, Iannelli A, Brunaud L, Czernichow S, Nedelcu M, Nocca D. Risk of dumping syndrome after sleeve gastrectomy and Roux-en-Y gastric bypass: early results of a multicentre prospective study. *Gastroenterol Res Pract* 2016;**2016**:2570237.

88. Balsells M, Garcia-Patterson A, Gich I, Corcoy R. Maternal and fetal outcome in women with type 2 versus type 1 diabetes mellitus: a systematic review and metaanalysis. *J Clin Endocrinol Metab* 2009;**94**(11):4284–91.

89. Damm JA, Asbjornsdottir B, Callesen NF, Mathiesen JM, Ringholm L, Pedersen BW, Mathiesen ER. Diabetic nephropathy and microalbuminuria in pregnant women with type 1 and type 2 diabetes: prevalence, antihypertensive strategy, and pregnancy outcome. *Diabetes Care* 2013;**36** (11):3489–94.

90. Egan AM, Murphy HR, Dunne FP. The management of type 1 and type 2 diabetes in pregnancy. *QJM* 2015;**108**(12):923–7.

91. The Diabetes Control and Complications Trial Research Group. Early worsening of diabetic retinopathy in the diabetes control and complications trial. *Arch Ophthalmol* 1998;**116**(7):874–86.

92. James AH, Jamison MG, Biswas MS, Brancazio LR, Swamy GK, Myers ER. Acute myocardial infarction in pregnancy: a United States population-based study. *Circulation* 2006;**113**(12):1564–71.

93. Li L, Zhao K, Hua J, Li S. Association between sleep-disordered breathing during pregnancy and maternal and fetal outcomes: an updated systematic review and meta-analysis. *Front Neurol* 2018;**9**:91.

94. Poyares D, Guilleminault C, Hachul H, Fujita L, Takaoka S, Tufik S, Sass N. Pre-eclampsia and nasal CPAP: part 2. Hypertension during pregnancy, chronic snoring, and early nasal CPAP intervention. *Sleep Med* 2007;**9**(1):15–21.

95. Hagstrom H, Hoijer J, Ludvigsson JF, Bottai M, Ekbom A, Hultcrantz R, Stephansson O, Stokkeland K. Adverse outcomes of pregnancy in women with non-alcoholic fatty liver disease. *Liver Int* 2016;**36**(2):268–74.

96. Page LM, Girling JC. A novel cause for abnormal liver function tests in pregnancy and the puerperium: non-alcoholic fatty liver disease. *BJOG* 2011;**118**(12):1532–5.

97. Persson M, Cnattingius S, Wikstrom AK, Johansson S. Maternal overweight and obesity and risk of pre-eclampsia in women with type 1 diabetes or type 2 diabetes. *Diabetologia* 2016;**59**(10):2099–105.

98. Feig DS, Palda VA. Type 2 diabetes in pregnancy: a growing concern. *Lancet* 2002;**359**(9318):1690–2.

99. Inkster ME, Fahey TP, Donnan PT, Leese GP, Mires GJ, Murphy DJ. Poor glycated haemoglobin control and adverse pregnancy outcomes in type 1 and type 2 diabetes mellitus: systematic review of observational studies. *BMC Pregnancy Childbirth* 2006;**6**:30.

100. Jensen DM, Korsholm L, Ovesen P, Beck-Nielsen H, Moelsted-Pedersen L, Westergaard JG, Moeller M, Damm P. Peri-conceptional A1C and risk of serious adverse pregnancy outcome in 933 women with type 1 diabetes. *Diabetes Care* 2009;**32**(6):1046–8.

101. Guerin A, Nisenbaum R, Ray JG. Use of maternal GHb concentration to estimate the risk of congenital anomalies in the offspring of women with prepregnancy diabetes. *Diabetes Care* 2007;**30**(7):1920–5.

102. McKeating A, Maguire PJ, Daly N, Farren M, McMahon L, Turner MJ. Trends in maternal obesity in a large university hospital 2009–2013. *Acta Obstet Gynecol Scand* 2015;**94**(9):969–75.

103. Kanguru L, McCaw-Binns A, Bell J, Yonger-Coleman N, Wilks R, Hussein J. The burden of obesity in women of reproductive age and in pregnancy in a middle-income setting: a population based study from Jamaica. *PLoS One* 2017;**12**(12).

104. Hillemeier MM, Weisman CS, Chuang C, Downs DS, McCall-Hosenfeld J, Camacho F. Transition to overweight or obesity among women of reproductive age. *J Womens Health (Larchmt)* 2011;**20**(5):703–10.

105. Stothard KJ, Tennant PW, Bell R, Rankin J. Maternal overweight and obesity and the risk of congenital anomalies: a systematic review and meta-analysis. *JAMA* 2009;**301**(6):636–50.

106. Persson M, Cnattingius S, Villamor E, Soderling J, Pasternak B, Stephansson O, Neovius M. Risk of major congenital malformations in relation to maternal overweight and obesity severity: cohort study of 1.2 million singletons. *BMJ* 2017;**357**:j2563.

107. Zarek J, Koren G. The fetal safety of statins: a systematic review and meta-analysis. *J Obstet Gynaecol Can* 2014;**36**(6):506–9.

108. Metcalfe A, Sabr Y, Hutcheon JA, Donovan L, Lyons J, Burrows J, Joseph KS. Trends in obstetric intervention and pregnancy outcomes of Canadian women with diabetes in pregnancy from 2004 to 2015. *J Endocr Soc* 2017;**1**(12):1540–9.

109. Glinianaia SV, Tennant PW, Bilous RW, Rankin J, Bell R. HbA(1c) and birthweight in women with pre-conception type 1 and type 2 diabetes: a population-based cohort study. *Diabetologia* 2012;**55**(12):3193–203.

110. Hadden DR. The management of diabetes in pregnancy. *Postgrad Med J* 1996;**72**(851):525–31.

111. Murphy HR, Rayman G, Duffield K, Lewis KS, Kelly S, Johal B, Fowler D, Temple RC. Changes in the glycemic profiles of women with type 1 and type 2 diabetes during pregnancy. *Diabetes Care* 2007;**30**(11):2785–91.

112. Egan AM, Dennedy MC, Al-Ramli W, Heerey A, Avalos G, Dunne F. ATLANTIC-DIP: excessive gestational weight gain and pregnancy outcomes in women with gestational or pregestational diabetes mellitus. *J Clin Endocrinol Metab* 2014;**99**(1):212–9.

113. Wilson RD, Genetics C, Wilson RD, Audibert F, Brock JA, Carroll J, Cartier L, Gagnon A, Johnson JA, Langlois S, Murphy-Kaulbeck L, Okun N, Pastuck M, Special C, Deb-Rinker P, Dodds L, Leon JA, Lowel HL, Luo W, MacFarlane A, McMillan R, Moore A, Mundle W, O'Connor D, Ray J, Van den Hof M. Pre-conception folic acid and multivitamin supplementation for the primary and secondary prevention of neural tube defects and other folic acid-sensitive congenital anomalies. *J Obstet Gynaecol Can* 2015;**37**(6):534–52.

114. Kumar A, Devi SG, Batra S, Singh C, Shukla DK. Calcium supplementation for the prevention of pre-eclampsia. *Int J Gynaecol Obstet* 2009;**104**(1):32–6.

115. De-Regil LM, Palacios C, Lombardo LK, Pena-Rosas JP. Vitamin D supplementation for women during pregnancy. *Cochrane Database Syst Rev* 2016;**1**.

116. Roth DE, Leung M, Mesfin E, et al. Vitamin D supplementation during pregnancy: state of the evidence from a systematic review of randomised trials. *BMJ* 2017;**359**:j5237.

117. Bujold E, Roberge S, Lacasse Y, Bureau M, Audibert F, Marcoux S, Forest JC, Giguere Y. Prevention of preeclampsia and intrauterine growth restriction with aspirin started in early pregnancy: a meta-analysis. *Obstet Gynecol* 2010;**116**(2 Pt 1):402–14.

118. Roberge S, Bujold E, Nicolaides KH. Aspirin for the prevention of preterm and term preeclampsia: systematic review and metaanalysis. *Am J Obstet Gynecol* 2018;**218**(3). 287–93.e1.

119. Rolnik DL, Wright D, Poon LC, O'Gorman N, Syngelaki A, de Paco Matallana C, Akolekar R, Cicero S, Janga D, Singh M, Molina FS, Persico N, Jani JC, Plasencia W, Papaioannou G, Tenenbaum-Gavish K, Meiri H, Gizurarson S, Maclagan K, Nicolaides KH. Aspirin versus placebo in pregnancies at high risk for preterm preeclampsia. *N Engl J Med* 2017;**377**(7):613–22.

120. Dukhovny S, Van Bennekom CM, Gagnon DR, Hernandez Diaz S, Parker SE, Anderka M, Werler MM, Mitchell AA. Metformin in the first trimester and risks for specific birth defects in the National Birth Defects Prevention Study. *Birth Defects Res* 2018;**110**(7):579–86.

121. Hughes RC, Rowan JA. Pregnancy in women with type 2 diabetes: who takes metformin and what is the outcome? *Diabet Med* 2006;**23**(3):318–22.

122. Ibrahim MI, Hamdy A, Shafik A, Taha S, Anwar M, Faris M. The role of adding metformin in insulin-resistant diabetic pregnant women: a randomized controlled trial. *Arch Gynecol Obstet* 2014;**289**(5):959–65.

123. Feig DS, Murphy K, Asztalos E, Tomlinson G, Sanchez J, Zinman B, Ohlsson A, Ryan EA, Fantus IG, Armson AB, Lipscombe LL, Barrett JF. MiTy Collaborative Group. Metformin in women with type 2 diabetes in pregnancy (MiTy): a multi-center randomized controlled trial. *BMC Pregnancy Childbirth* 2016;**16**(1):173.

124. Okeigwe I, Yeaton-Massey A, Kim S, Vargas JE, Murphy EJ. U-500R and aspart insulin for the treatment of severe insulin resistance in pregnancy associated with pregestational diabetes. *J Perinatol* 2013;**33**(3):235–8.

125. Zhang XW, Zhang XL, Xu B, Kang LN. Comparative safety and efficacy of insulin degludec with insulin glargine in type 2 and type 1 diabetes: a meta-analysis of randomized controlled trials. *Acta Diabetol* 2018;**55**(5):429–41.

126. Hillier TA, Pedula KL, Schmidt MM, Mullen JA, Charles MA, Pettitt DJ. Childhood obesity and metabolic imprinting: the ongoing effects of maternal hyperglycemia. *Diabetes Care* 2007;**30**(9):2287–92.

127. Kuciene R, Dulskiene V, Medzioniene J. Associations between high birth weight, being large for gestational age, and high blood pressure among adolescents: a cross-sectional study. *Eur J Nutr* 2018;**57**(1):373–81.

Chapter 23

Type 1 Diabetes: During Preconception, Pregnancy, Postpartum, and Breastfeeding

Jennifer M. Yamamoto[*,†] and Lois E. Donovan[*,†]

[*]Division of Endocrinology and Metabolism, Department of Medicine, Cumming School of Medicine, University of Calgary, Calgary, AB, Canada,
[†]Department of Obstetrics and Gynaecology, Cumming School of Medicine, University of Calgary, Calgary, AB, Canada

---

Common Clinical Problems

- Women with Type 1 diabetes require safe effective contraception until glycemic control is optimized prior to pregnancy. This reduces risk of congenital malformation in their offspring and stillbirth.
- Retinal screening should be performed preconception so that active retinal disease that requires therapy can be optimally treated and stabilized preconception, reducing the risk of progression of retinopathy.
- Familiarity with expected changes in insulin dosing during pregnancy and postpartum aids in appropriate insulin dose adjustment to maintain excellent glycemic control and reduces the risk of severe hypoglycemia.

23.1 PREPREGNANCY

23.1.1 Prepregnancy Care

Prepregnancy care (PPC) is the additional support of women who may become pregnant. It takes the form of targeted care that provides advice and assistance regarding contraception and pregnancy preparation. It is an essential part of the optimal care of women with Type 1 diabetes who could become pregnant.

23.1.1.1 Importance of PPC in Women with Type 1 Diabetes

Hyperglycemia is an established teratogen that modulates the expression of apoptosis regulatory genes even prior to implantation. Because the fetal neural tube and heart are developing at 4 weeks' gestation, often prior to women being aware that they are pregnant, prepregnancy optimization of glycemic control is imperative.[1] PPC has been associated with improved pregnancy preparation and neonatal outcomes. Specifically, women who receive PPC are more likely to have a lower HbA1c early in pregnancy and take folic acid and are less likely to be on potentially harmful medications.[2–5] Furthermore, PPC is associated with fewer serious adverse pregnancy outcomes.[2,4] PPC also has the potential to be cost saving because the cost is offset by the saved costs in treating adverse pregnancy outcomes.[4]

A large cohort study in the United Kingdom found that less than half of women with Type 1 diabetes were on recommended folic acid dosing, and only 14% of women with Type 1 diabetes met guideline-recommended HbA1c targets in early pregnancy.[6] Another study found that less than half of women with Type 1 and Type 2 diabetes taking medications not recommended for pregnancy were using contraception.[7] All these measures may be improved by PPC attendance.

Despite its importance, the rates of PPC continue to be low, with less than half of women receiving PPC. This is true even in areas with established PPC programs.[2,5] The reason for the low rates of participation in PPC programs is likely multifactorial. Some barriers to participating in PPC may include lack of knowledge regarding its importance and how to access it; difficulty arranging childcare, time off work, or both; and patient concerns that practitioners will focus on risks rather than the more positive aspects of pregnancy.[8]

Maternal-Fetal and Neonatal Endocrinology. https://doi.org/10.1016/B978-0-12-814823-5.00023-4

23.1.1.2 Elements of PPC

Women who wish to prepare for pregnancy typically attend interdisciplinary diabetes clinics, where they should receive counseling and PPC. Elements of pregnancy preparation include (1) discussion of the risks associated with pregnancies complicated by diabetes and how those may be attenuated; (2) discussion of the role and importance of preconception counseling; (3) education and tools for achieving target glycemic control (typically a HbA1c <6.5%–7% [48–53 mmol/mol]); (4) folic acid supplementation; (5) discussion of the timing of discontinuing potentially harmful medication; (6) smoking cessation; (7) screening for and management of diabetes-related compilations (for more details, see the discussion of this topic later in this chapter); (8) discussion of healthy weight and support to achieve this preconception; and (9) reliable contraception until the other points are achieved. Table 23.1 presents a checklist of things to consider before contraception is discontinued. While it is essential to discuss the risks associated with pregnancy, PPC is also an opportunity to empower women to optimize their health and facilitate a positive pregnancy experience.

23.1.1.3 Optimization of Glycemic Control: Goals and Strategies

The risk of congenital anomalies and fetal death following pregnancies complicated by preexisting diabetes is two to four times that of the general population.[9, 10] There is a linear increase in the risk of congenital anomalies with every 1% increase in HbA1c above 6.3% (45 mmol/mol).[11] For example, the risk of congenital anomalies for women with a HbA1c of 6.5% (48 mmol/mol) is 1 in 33, as opposed to 1 in 20 for those with a HbA1c of 7.5% (59 mmol/mol) and 1 in 6 with those with a HbA1c above 12.5% (113 mmol/mol).[11] Optimizing glycemic control prior to pregnancy can decrease the risk of congenital anomalies, miscarriage, stillbirth, and neonatal death. Thus, this period offers a great opportunity to improve pregnancy outcomes.[9, 11]

The interdisciplinary or multidisciplinary health-care team should review glucose monitoring, insulin regimen, current activity level, and dietary intake in women with Type 1 diabetes who hope to become pregnant, as detailed in the next sections.

23.1.1.3.1 Glucose Monitoring

All women should perform frequent capillary blood glucose testing. Specifically, women should be testing their blood glucose at least four times a day (prior to meals and before bed); however, most women will require more frequent testing

TABLE 23.1 Checklist of PPC goals

☐	Discuss risks associated with pregnancy
☐	Review the importance of preconception counselling
☐	Reviewing the risk of hypoglycemia and impaired awareness
☐	Achieving target glycemic control
☐	Ensure folic acid supplementation
☐	Discontinue potentially harmful medication
☐	Advise smoking cessation
☐	Screen for and manage of diabetes-related compilations
	Retinopathy screening, management as required, and stabilization
	Check the albumin:creatinine ratio and estimated glomerular filtration rate (EGFR)
	Hypertension
☐	Discuss healthy weight and support to achieve this preconception
☐	Psychological support to address the demands of optimum glycemic management
☐	Review immunization status, i.e., rubella, influenza
☐	Ensure that TSH is normal prior to conception

If any of these points cannot be achieved, a discussion of the risks and benefits should take place.

to achieve tight control and avoid excess hypoglycemia. Postprandial glucose testing is often important to optimize not only insulin dosing, but also dietary strategies. Women should be targeting glucose as close to euglycemia as possible without excess or severe hypoglycemia.[1,12,13]

HbA1c should also be monitored frequently prior to pregnancy. The target HbA1c is as close to normal as safely possible. Guidelines suggest a target of <6.5%–7% (48–53 mmol/mol) (Table 23.3); however, it is important to note that some women with Type 1 diabetes may not be able to achieve these targets without frequent or severe hypoglycemia.[1,12,13]

In some cases, clinicians should consider continuous glucose monitoring (CGM) in women planning pregnancy. The largest ($n = 110$) prepregnancy trial of CGM in women with Type 1 diabetes to date (CONCEPTT) found no significant difference in HbA1c between women randomized to CGM vs controls; however, it may have lacked the power to demonstrate a difference.[14] CGM still may play an important role in PPC in women who have a history of severe or frequent lows, women unable to meet targets with capillary glucose testing, women who have labile capillary glucose, women who find the demands of frequent capillary glucose testing and recording challenging to achieve, and women in whom a more detailed assessment of glycemic excursions is desired.

23.1.1.3.2 Insulin Dosing

PPC is the ideal time to optimize insulin. This includes an assessment of basal insulin doses, insulin-to-carbohydrate ratios, and insulin sensitivity factors. Women on multiple daily insulin injections who wish to switch to the insulin pump should ideally be transitioned during the prepregnancy period so they establish comfort and safety with subcutaneous insulin pump use prior to pregnancy.

While it is less common for women with Type 1 diabetes to be on oral diabetes medications, some women may be taking medications such as metformin, GLP-1 inhibitors, or SGLT-2 inhibitors. It is important to discontinue all oral diabetes medications other than metformin. If women or their diabetes team wish to continue metformin therapy, its risks and benefits should be discussed.[15] Metformin is not approved for use in pregnancy in all countries. See Chapter 22 for a review of the safety of metformin use in pregnancy.

When tight glycemic control results in frequent hypoglycemia, the risk of unrecognized hypoglycemia increases. It is important to review the risk of hypoglycemia, as well as strategies to avoid and treat it. This education is of particular importance to prepare women for early pregnancy, when the risk of severe hypoglycemia is highest.[16]

23.1.1.3.3 Nutrition and Physical Activity

Ensuring adequate nutrition prior to pregnancy is an essential part of pregnancy preparation for all women. Women with Type 1 diabetes should receive individualized dietary advice as part of PPC. This includes (1) a diet that ensures adequate nutrition, (2) advice regarding the avoidance of excess carbohydrate at meals and ensuring proficient carbohydrate counting, (3) folic acid and other nutritional supplements, and (4) advice regarding weight management strategies if indicated. Physical activity is part of a healthy lifestyle, so it is important to discuss the role of exercise in overall health and pregnancy, as well as the influence of physical activity on blood glucose and effective ways to adjust insulin and food for exercise or other physical activity.

Obesity is becoming increasingly common in the general population, and the same is true for women with Type 1 diabetes. Up to half of women with Type 1 diabetes in pregnancy are overweight or obese, which are known risk factors for a variety of pregnancy complications.[14] Before pregnancy is the ideal time to discuss risks associated with obesity, as well as weight management strategies when appropriate. Obesity is associated with an increase in all negative pregnancy outcomes. Target weight should be identified and sought prior to conception. See Chapter 27 for a discussion on the impact of overweight and obesity on reproductive health.

23.1.1.4 Prepregnancy Management of Diabetes Complications and Risk Assessment

Assessment of diabetes complications prior to pregnancy is an essential component of PPC.[1] Women with Type 1 diabetes need to understand the additional risks that diabetes complications may pose to their fetus and to their personal health in pregnancy, as well as the risk that pregnancy may or may not pose for the progression of diabetes complications. They also require a good understanding of what therapeutic strategies used to treat diabetes complications outside of pregnancy must be discontinued or avoided when they become pregnant or are attempting to conceive.

23.1.1.4.1 Diabetic Retinopathy

Preconception optimization of glycemic control is strongly advised not only for better pregnancy outcomes, but also because a greater decrease in HbA1c between the first and third trimesters of pregnancy is a risk for the progression of retinopathy.[17] Furthermore, women with poorer glycemic control before conception experience more retinopathy progression in pregnancy and postpartum than those with better glycemic control before pregnancy.[18]

The Diabetes Control and Complications Trial (DCCT) showed that in the short term, pregnancy is associated with an increase in retinopathy progression that persists into the first postpartum year.[18] Pregnancy may promote the onset of diabetic retinopathy in about 10% of women, as well as contributing to its worsening when already present. The presence of proliferative and moderate to severe nonproliferative diabetic retinopathy is a strong predictor of progressive retinal disease during pregnancy.[19] Reassuringly, at the end of DCCT (6.5-year mean follow-up), pregnancy had no influence on the prevalence of retinopathy. Preeclampsia has been associated with increased risk for severe diabetic retinopathy after a median 16 years of follow-up.[20] Women without retinopathy preconception can be reassured that the development of retinopathy during pregnancy is usually only in the form of background retinopathy, even with a duration of diabetes of >20 years.[19,21] When no diabetic retinopathy is present, preconception progression to vision-threatening retinopathy has never been documented.[17]

Screening and treatment for diabetic retinopathy preconception has become increasingly important with the demonstrated success of intravitreal antivascular endothelial growth factor (anti-VEGF) injections for stabilization and reversal of diabetic macular edema or proliferative retinopathy. The safety of anti-VEGF therapies in pregnancy is currently unknown. This results in the reluctance to use these very effective therapeutic options during pregnancy and emphasizes the need to delay conception if therapy with these agents is being considered or is being used actively preconception. Further study is required to assess the safety of intravitreal anti-VEGF therapy in pregnancy. Until such time, we recommend that contraception be used during intravitreal anti-VEGF therapy, conception be delayed until 3 months after the last intravitreal anti-VEGF treatment, and stabilization of retinal disease be established prior to conception.[22,23]

23.1.1.4.2 Hypertension

The presence of hypertension prior to or at any time during pregnancy or preeclampsia increases mortality among mothers with Type 1 diabetes in pregnancy in the two decades following childbirth.[24] Women with preexisting hypertension need to be switched either preconception or upon pregnancy confirmation to antihypertensive options that are safe for use in pregnancy.[1] These include calcium channel blockers, labetalol, and methyldopa. Angiotensin-converting enzyme inhibitors and angiotensin-receptor blockers are well established second-trimester teratogens that should be stopped either preconception or at the time pregnancy is confirmed. Type 1 diabetes in pregnancy is associated with an increased risk of preeclampsia that fails to decrease after the first pregnancy.[25]

23.1.1.4.3 Diabetic Nephropathy

It is important to screen for diabetic nephropathy (eGFR and urinary albumin) preconception in order to provide appropriate counseling of pregnancy risk and to document baseline renal function, which may aid in differentiating preexisting diabetic nephropathy from preeclampsia during pregnancy.[24] Progressive increases in protein excretion within the range of microalbuminuria (spot urine albumin-to-creatinine ratio of 30–300 μg/mg), or overt diabetic nephropathy (albumin excretion >300 mg/24 h), are both associated with increasing maternal mortality and morbidities in the two decades following childbirth.[24] Preconception albuminuria and overt nephropathy are also associated with an increased risk of impaired placental development, which often leads to preeclampsia, preterm delivery, fetal intrauterine growth restriction, and higher risk of stillbirth.[26] Pregnancy outcomes are more favorable in women with normal blood pressure and minor elevations in serum creatinine and urine protein (i.e., <124 μmol/L and <1 g/24 h, respectively).[27] Poor pregnancy outcomes are more commonly seen in women with hypertension and greater elevations in creatinine and urine protein (i.e., >176 μmol/L and >3 g/24 h, respectively).[27] The best predictor of pregnancy-induced end-stage kidney disease during or shortly after pregnancy is serum creatinine >176 μmol/L and reduced preconception GFR; it is influenced by hypertension during pregnancy, especially in the third trimester.[27,28] The rate of GFR decline was similar among a group of women with diabetic nephropathy who had been pregnant or had not been pregnant up to 16 years later.[29]

Women who are taking angiotensin-converting enzyme inhibitors or angiotensin-receptor blockers for nephropathy prevention prior to pregnancy require a discussion of the best time to discontinue these medications (i.e., during attempted conception or upon pregnancy confirmation). This needs to be individualized for each woman based on the severity of her diabetic nephropathy, fertility, menstrual pattern, and likelihood of early pregnancy confirmation. Women who remain on angiotensin-converting enzyme inhibitors or angiotensin-receptor blockers as they attempt to conceive should be instructed to perform a pregnancy test within 2 days of a missed menstrual withdrawal bleed, so that the use of these medications is promptly discontinued once pregnancy is achieved.

23.1.1.4.4 Diabetic Neuropathy

Diabetic neuropathy has not been well studied in pregnancy. If painful peripheral diabetic neuropathy is present and requires medication for pain control, a discussion of the safety of the pain medication in use in pregnancy should occur. If diabetic gastroparesis is present, it can greatly impair the achievement of optimal glycemic control. Should a woman with diabetic gastroparesis be interested in pregnancy, it is imperative to assess her for ischemic cardiac disease because these end-stage complications of diabetes often coexist.

23.1.1.4.5 Cardiovascular Disease

Cardiovascular disease may be present in reproductive-age women with Type 1 diabetes. Women with a history of long-standing, poorly controlled diabetes or evidence of other end-stage diabetes complications should be screened. Should cardiovascular disease be present, women need to be counseled on the significant risk that a pregnancy could pose to their personal health. Statin and fibrates should be discontinued prior to pregnancy.

23.1.1.4.6 Smoking Cessation

Smoking cessation is especially important for women with Type 1 diabetes contemplating pregnancy and should be supported preconception.

23.1.1.4.7 Thyroid Function

Thyroid dysfunction is common in women with Type 1 diabetes. Euthyroid status should be confirmed with a screening of thyroid-stimulating hormone (TSH) prior to preconception. For women with preexisting thyroid dysfunction requiring medical management, the pregnancy safety of the agents in use should be reviewed. Specifically, if women are treated with liothyronine-containing products, they should be switched to levothyroxine to avoid concerns of inadequate fetal central nervous system transfer of levothyroxine.

23.1.1.4.8 Immunization

Rubella immunization status should be confirmed preconception and addressed if required.

23.1.1.4.9 Psychological Support

The demands of achieving optimal glycemic control prior to and during pregnancy can be considerable. Social support for an individual's personal agency for diabetes management from family and friends reduces the negative impact of diabetes distress on glycemic control.[30] Trained psychologists or social workers may assist with addressing concerns of the woman with diabetes and/or her family and friends that could impair her achievement of glycemic targets such as hypoglycemia phobia or financial barriers for obtaining diabetes management supplies. Establishing trusted relationships preconception with educators about diabetes in pregnancy and physicians that assist with diabetes care during pregnancy may help to alleviate the fears of women preparing for pregnancy. Mental illness can affect diabetes self-management practices profoundly and negatively. It is important to assess women for such concerns and initiate appropriate referrals preconception in order to aid in preventing poor diabetes self-management skills during pregnancy.

23.1.1.5 Neonatal Complications

Preconception is a good time to ensure that women with Type 1 diabetes understand the potential impact of Type 1 diabetes on their fetus/neonate/child. The specific congenital anomalies and complications common to pregnancies of women with Type 1 diabetes and pathophysiology behind these are reviewed in Chapter 45. Briefly, this includes heart and neural tube defects, macrosomia, neonatal hypoglycemia, hyperbilirubinemia, complications of preterm delivery, stillbirth, and neonatal death.[10,11,31] Many of these complications are believed to be the result of high maternal glucose resulting in elevated fetal glucose causing fetal hyperinsulinemia and promoting excess nutrient storage, thus culminating in a big fetus. The energy associated with conversion of excess glucose into fat causes depletion in fetal oxygen levels and relative fetal hypoxia. Relative fetal hypoxia results in surges in adrenal catecholamines that cause hypertension, cardiac remodeling and hypertrophy stimulation of erythropoietin, red cell hyperplasia, and polycythemia. High hematocrit leads to vascular sludging, poor circulation, and postnatal hyperbilirubinemia.

Unfortunately, consistent achievement of ideal glycemic control with current technologies is an unrealistic expectation for most women with Type 1 diabetes. Complication rates in pregnancies of women with Type 1 diabetes remain high. Fortunately, in recent decades, there has been a dramatic decline in the most serious pregnancy complications (i.e., congenital malformations and intrauterine fetal death); however, macrosomia and neonatal hypoglycemia remain common. The relationships among macrosomia, neonatal hypoglycemia, and maternal glycemic control are complex, and other factors such as lipid metabolism and cytokines are suspected to contribute to the ongoing high rate of morbidity among neonates of women with Type 1 diabetes as well.[32,33]

23.2 PREGNANCY

23.2.1 Glycemic Management Throughout Pregnancy

23.2.1.1 The Role of Physiologic Changes in Developing Management Strategies

Familiarity with expected physiologic changes in glucose metabolism that occur during pregnancy and postpartum aids in appropriate insulin dose and dietary adjustments. Fig. 23.1 demonstrates the expected gestational changes in insulin requirements during pregnancy.

Hypoglycemia risk increases in early pregnancy for several reasons, including alterations in oral intake in response to pregnancy-associated nausea and vomiting, as well as facilitated diffusion of glucose across the placenta by placental glucose transporters to meet fetal demands for glucose. In early pregnancy, a double peak in serum glucose that lasts for up to 5 h after supper has been demonstrated.[34] Possible management strategies to address this issue include more frequent glucose testing after supper or CGM to assess whether this is occurring, dual- or square-wave meal bolus at supper if on an insulin pump, and postprandial exercise.

By 20 weeks' gestation, insulin resistance increases as a result of increasing placental size and secretion of human placental growth hormone (previously known as *human placental lactogen*), tumor necrosis factor alpha (TNF-α), and progesterone. As a result, progressive increments in insulin dosing are required, usually after 18 weeks' gestation, as outlined in Fig. 23.1.

As pregnancy progresses, postprandial glucose disposal becomes more delayed.[34] This appears to result from a delay in insulin absorption and increasing peripheral insulin resistance with advancing gestational age.[34,35] This results in an approximately 50% slower rate of insulin absorption at 38 weeks' gestation, compared to 8 weeks' gestation.[35] In practical terms, this requires premeal insulin bolusing that is progressively longer in advance of the meal as the pregnancy progresses (up to 60 min prior to the meal at advanced gestation) to maintain tight glycemic control during pregnancy.[34]

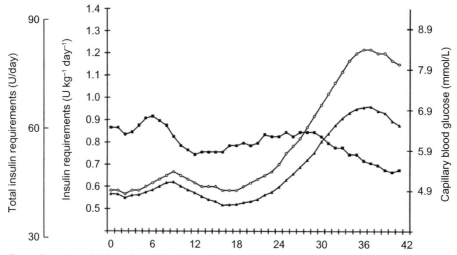

FIG. 23.1 Mean insulin requirements and self-monitored blood glucose in Type 1 diabetic pregnant women. *Square*, capillary blood glucose; *circle*, total insulin requirement (units/day); *triangle*, insulin requirements (unit/kg/day). *From Garcia-Paterson et al.* Diabetologia *2010;53:446–451—permission from Diabetologia granted.*

Antenatal glucocorticoid administrations for fetal lung maturity results in a need for substantial insulin increments (sometimes two to three times baseline insulin requirements). Anticipatory insulin-dosing adjustment should occur with antenatal steroid administration, as well as careful monitoring and frequent adjustment of insulin dosing in the week during and following antenatal glucocorticoid adjustment, in order to prevent marked maternal hyperglycemia and hypoglycemia.

Mild reductions in insulin requirements ($<15\%$) near term are common in women with well-controlled Type 1 diabetes in pregnancy.[36] The cause of declining insulin requirements in the third trimester of pregnancy is not known for certain, but possibilities may include increased fetal activity, reduced maternal oral intake, increasing glucose demands of a growing fetus, and possibly pregnancy-induced improvement in beta cell function,[37] reduction in placental counterregulatory hormones, decline in placental insulinase, and altered endogenous glucose production. There are theoretical concerns that more marked decline in insulin requirements in the third trimester of pregnancy, not explained by increased activity, reduced carbohydrate intake or overaggressive insulin increments, is an indicator of declining placental function and a harbinger of fetal demise.

Six studies that have examined the relationship between reduced insulin requirements and pregnancy outcomes among women with Type 1, Type 2, or gestational diabetes ($n = 943$)[38–43] report only three stillbirths: two that occurred in women who had $<15\%$ decline in insulin requirements[38,42] and one that occurred in a woman with $>15\%$ decline in insulin requirements.[38] Women with greater declines in insulin requirements were more likely to be delivered earlier (by approximately half a week).[38,42] Therefore, it cannot be determined if earlier delivery among women with larger decline in insulin requirements, resulted in the avoidance of fetal demise. A $>15\%$ drop in third-trimester insulin requirements was associated with more frequent admission to neonatal intensive care unit,[38,42] which is likely a result of earlier gestational age at delivery. A drop in insulin requirements of greater than or equal to 15% was associated with more preeclampsia in two studies,[38,42] and more small-for-gestational-age neonates in one study[38]; both of these outcomes are indicators of placental insufficiency. The one prospective study that examined placental hormones longitudinally failed to demonstrate a difference in placental hormones (human placental lactogen, progesterone, and TNF-α) in women whose insulin requirements fell more than or less than 15% in the third trimester of pregnancy.[42] Other studies have found no association between large declines in insulin requirements and adverse obstetrical and fetal outcomes.[39–41]

Given the inconsistency among studies, when large declines in insulin requirements occur, an individualized approach is required. Management considerations such as more frequent fetal surveillance and timing of delivery need to be reviewed carefully, along with the established risk factors for intrauterine fetal demise, such as poor periconception and pregnancy glycemic control, smoking history, presence of retinopathy, previous stillbirth, maternal age, gestational age, and obesity (Table 23.2).[9] After delivery, insulin requirements drop precipitously.

23.2.1.2 The Role of Dietary Strategies and Exercise in Glycemic Control

In the management of Type 1 diabetes, women and clinicians must use all available strategies; diet and exercise are important tools in achieving optimal glycemic control in women with Type 1 diabetes in pregnancy. Unfortunately, there is little high-quality evidence to inform clinical practice. Outside pregnancy, the importance of accurate carbohydrate

TABLE 23.2 Physiologic changes in pregnancy and suggested management strategies

Physiologic change	Possible management strategy
Hypoglycemia risk	Insulin-dosing reductions often required from 7 to 13 weeks' gestation. Review driving safety and hypoglycemia treatment
Increasing insulin resistance	Progressive increments in insulin-dosing requirements usually begin at 18 weeks' gestation
Increased speed of glucose absorption on an empty stomach	Premeal insulin dosing
Second-wave glucose absorption after dinner extended in early pregnancy	Square- or dual-wave insulin bolusing with supper, postprandial physical activity
Antenatal steroid administration	Marked insulin increments and frequent glucose monitoring is required
Unexplained 15% decrease in insulin requirements	Reduced overnight insulin dosing commonly required. Consider increased fetal surveillance vs delivery based on gestational age and risk factors for stillbirth

counting, as well as both carbohydrate quantity and quality, have been documented to affect glycemic control. In pregnancy, observational studies have demonstrated that high HbA1c is associated with high carbohydrate intake, and excessive weight gain has been associated with birth weight independent of glycemic control.[44,45]

Both the quality and quantity of carbohydrates are likely important in pregnancy. Excessive carbohydrate intake can make achieving postprandial glucose targets exceptionally difficult. Thus, some centers recommend a moderately low carbohydrate diet (150 g/day) and a preference for low glycemic index carbohydrates.[46] The recommended carbohydrate breakdown throughout the day, therefore, is 20 g with breakfast, 40 g with lunch, 40 g with dinner, and the remainder as snacks.[46] Due to increased insulin resistance in the morning, limiting the amount of carbohydrate intake and choosing low-glycemic-index options are of particular importance.

Consensus guidelines recommend exercise for all pregnant women without contraindications, with the goal of three or more 30-min sessions per week.[47-49] Benefits of exercise may include preventing excessive gestational weight gain, improving fitness for labor and delivery, and reducing delivery-related complications.[50] Exercise in women with Type 1 diabetes may also have specific benefits to glycemic control, such as the attenuation of insulin resistance in pregnancy. Structured physical activity programs combined with diet may help improve glycemic control in women with Type 1 diabetes in pregnancy.[51] Thus, diabetes teams should discuss the importance of safe exercise as an important part of a healthy pregnancy.

23.2.1.3 Mode of Insulin Delivery

Tight glycemic control in pregnancies complicated by Type 1 diabetes is essential to decrease the risks of potentially serious complications. The physiologic changes throughout pregnancy discussed previously further complicate the challenge of achieving target glycemic control. There are varying modalities of insulin delivery that help women and their diabetes teams to achieve these goals. At present, the main modalities of insulin delivery include multiple daily insulin (MDI) injections and the insulin pump.

23.2.1.3.1 MDI Injections

MDI injections consist of a basal insulin (e.g., detemir, NPH, or N) given once or twice daily, as well as multiple bolus injections given with meals and as correction doses when necessary. Although the use of MDI vs pump varies by center, MDI continues to be the most common modality of insulin delivery in women with preexisting diabetes in pregnancy.[52]

23.2.1.3.2 The Insulin Pump

The insulin pump, also known as *continuous subcutaneous insulin infusion,* delivers insulin via a cannula inserted subcutaneously. Basal insulin delivery is accomplished by giving small amounts of rapid-acting insulin every few minutes, and bolus insulin is delivered with meals or as corrections by the pump user. Basal settings can be easily customized, and subtle changes in basal insulin delivery can be accomplished. Insulin pumps also have built-in bolus calculators that help determine bolus and correction insulin doses based on insulin-to-carbohydrate and insulin-sensitivity factors that are inputted by the user. It can be used on its own or with CGM.[53]

Given the changing insulin resistance and need for frequent insulin adjustments throughout pregnancy, the insulin pump seems ideally suited. It allows clinicians to vary basal rates throughout the day. This can be particularly important late in pregnancy, where women tend to need more basal insulin in the morning relative to later in the day. It can also allow different bolus administration patterns that may help avoid postprandial glycemic excursions. As with MDI, the physiologic changes in glucose disposal, and insulin absorption in pregnancy, care must be taken with regard to carbohydrate intake, and insulin doses should usually be given 15–60 min prior to eating. It should be noted that the cost of the insulin pump (about 7000 Canadian dollars or US$4500–6500 upfront, plus the cost of ongoing pump supplies, which is 2000 Canadian dollars or US$1500 per year) may be prohibitive for many women in pregnancy if it is not covered by insurance or local insulin pump programs.

23.2.1.3.3 MDIs vs the Insulin Pump

While there are many theoretic advantages to the use of the insulin pump during pregnancies, it remains unclear if it can achieve superior glycemic control compared to MDI. The research literature consists primarily of observational studies, which are limited by bias introduced from baseline differences in women on the insulin pump compared to MDI.[54] The largest cohort study to date found that the insulin pump was associated with lower HbA1c but did not result in improved pregnancy outcomes.[52] However, the research as a whole is discordant.[54]

Despite the uncertainty in its benefits over MDI, the pump appears to be safe in pregnancy, as it has not been associated with severe hypoglycemia or diabetic ketoacidosis (DKA).[52,54] Because these are uncommon events in pregnancies, studies would be underpowered to show a significant difference in these serious complications. Therefore, caution still must be taken throughout pregnancy, including frequent glucose testing, as well as urgent testing for ketones if a pregnant woman has hyperglycemia or is unwell. It is important to note that euglycemic DKA is more common in pregnancy due to accelerated starvation. Caution should be taken to avoid pump failure overnight, and thereby prolonged ketosis, with strategies such as overnight testing, avoidance of infusion site changes prior to bed, and if necessary, injection of a long-acting insulin prior to bed.

23.2.1.3.4 Closed-Loop Insulin Delivery

Despite the substantial amount of time and effort that women with Type 1 diabetes can spend on improving and maintaining their glycemic control during preconception and throughout pregnancy, the current insulin-delivery modalities still fall short, with less than half of women achieving glycemic targets.[52] Closed-loop insulin delivery, also known as *sensor-integrated insulin delivery* or the *artificial pancreas,* may help women to achieve the tight glycemic control required in pregnancy, which remains elusive for so many. Closed-loop insulin delivery consists of a hormone pump, CGM, and an external device (typically a smart phone or tablet) that has an algorithm capable of adjusting insulin in real time.

In pregnancy, closed-loop insulin delivery has been shown to improve overnight control.[55] It is also able to adapt to the many challenges of pregnancy, including antenatal steroid administration, labor and delivery, and the postpartum period.[55,56] While the device used in the abovementioned clinical trials is available only as part of clinical trials in pregnancy, it is an exciting technology that has the potential to not only improve glycemic control, but also decrease the workload carried by women with diabetes.[57] Hybrid closed-loop systems now commercially available in the United States have yet to be formally tested in pregnancy and currently have preset glucose targets that are above those recommended for pregnancy.

23.2.1.4 Types of Insulins and Oral Agents

The types of basal and bolus insulins available for use continue to expand. A retrospective study showed that first-trimester exposure to insulin analogs in use prior to 2013 was not associated with increased risk of major congenital anomalies compared with exposure to human insulin.[58] However, the risk of each individual insulin analog could not be evaluated separately in this study due to the low number of anomalies. This limits extrapolation of these results because biological effects vary according to the type of insulin analog. Thus, this study does not provide definitive evidence of safety in pregnancy of all insulin analogs; further research is merited. Currently available evidence is discussed next.

23.2.1.4.1 Bolus Insulins

Bolus insulins currently available for use include human regular insulin, lispro, aspart, fast insulin aspart, and glulisine. Like human insulin, lispro insulin does not cross the placenta except at very high doses.[59] A randomized control trial (RCT) of human regular insulin vs insulin aspart demonstrated similar pregnancy outcomes and HbA1c measurement between women randomized to these types of insulin and less postprandial hyperglycemia with aspart.[60] There are no data on the safety of fast-acting insulin aspart in pregnancy. A case series of glulisine insulin use during pregnancy in a study of 170 exposed pregnancies with known outcomes, failed to show any pattern of congenital anomalies that would suggest teratogenicity.[61] The 2018 Diabetes Canada pregnancy guidelines indicate that aspart, lispro, or glulisine may be used in pregnancy,[1] whereas the National Institute of Health and Clinical Excellence (NICE) pregnancy guidelines indicate that aspart or lispro may be used.[13]

23.2.1.4.2 Intermediate and Long-Acting Basal Insulins

The options for basal insulin for MDI users continues to expand and includes NPH, detemir, glargine, glargine insulin U-300, and degludec insulin U-100 and U-200. NPH is still commonly used in pregnancy because unlike the flatter profile of other basal insulins, the 6–8-h peak in the action of NPH can effectively control the dawn effect when administered at bedtime. At usual therapeutic dosages, detemir and glargine do not cross the placenta.[62] Detemir use has been compared to NPH use in pregnancy in one RCT in women with Type 1 diabetes, as well as another small RCT in women with gestational or Type 2 diabetes in pregnancy.[63,64] There were no differences in maternal and fetal outcomes between these two insulins other than the following: (1) a lower fasting blood glucose with detemir, but similar HbA1c in the trial in women with Type 1 diabetes; and (2) less hypoglycemia, but frequent allergic reaction with detemir in the trial in women with gestational diabetes or Type 2 diabetes in pregnancy.[63,64]

Detemir insulin is approved for use in pregnancy. In the authors' experience, the potency of detemir insulin appears to wane considerably when dosages of >20 units are required. Glargine use in pregnancy has not been evaluated in any RCTs in pregnancy, and it is currently not approved for use in pregnancy. Because glargine binds to the IGF-1 receptor with increased affinity compared to other insulins, there have been concerns about the mitogenic potential and risk for large-for-gestational-age neonates with the use of glargine in pregnancy.[65] However, a meta-analysis of cohort studies of glargine use in pregnancy compared with NPH demonstrated similar maternal and fetal outcomes.[66] There are no data in pregnancy about the safety of glargine insulin U-300 and degludec insulin U-100 and U-200. A trial comparing the effects and safety of degludec insulin vs detemir insulin in women with Type 1 diabetes in pregnancy is currently underway (NCTT03377677). Glargine insulin U-300 is a concentrated preparation of glargine U-100, with a flatter profile of action. Thus, it appears to be a reasonable choice for use in pregnancy in women with Type 1 diabetes who experience glycemic improvements with its use. The 2018 Diabetes Canada and NICE pregnancy guidelines indicate that detemir or glargine insulin may be used as alternatives to NPH insulin in pregnancy.[1, 13]

23.2.1.4.3 Oral Agents

The risk and benefits of adding metformin to insulin therapy is currently unknown for women with Type 1 diabetes during pregnancy. In women with Type 2 diabetes in pregnancy, this is being investigated in an ongoing RCT.[67] The risks and benefits of metformin use in pregnancy are discussed in detail in Chapter 22. The safety of SGLT-2 inhibitors in pregnancy is unknown, so their use should be discontinued in pregnancy if women with Type 1 diabetes were on these medications prior to pregnancy.

23.2.2 Glycemic Measurements and Targets in Pregnancy

23.2.2.1 Capillary Blood Glucose Monitoring

Capillary blood glucose monitoring, also referred to as *point-of-care testing,* and self-monitoring of blood glucose form the backbone of glycemic measurements throughout pregnancy. Women are instructed to self-test at least four times per day (before meals and before bed); however, most women with Type 1 diabetes require more testing to achieve target control safely. Additional capillary blood glucose monitoring should be done 1–2h postprandial to help tailor insulin dose, timing, and diet to avoid significant postprandial glycemic excursions. Women must also test with any symptomatic low or high glucose. See Table 23.3 for glucose targets (Table 23.3).

TABLE 23.3 Glucose levels for women to aim for as per guidelines[1,12,13]

	Diabetes Canada 2018	American diabetes association 2018	NICE
	Preconception—all say as close to normal as safely possible		
HbA1c	≤7.0% (<53 mmol/mol) (ideally ≤6.5% if possible [48 mmol/mol])	Ideally <6.5% (48 mmol/mol)	<6.5% (48 mmol/mol)
	During pregnancy		
HbA1c	≤6.5% (48 mmol/mol) ≤6.1% [43 mmol/mol] (ideally if possible)	<6% (42 mmol/mol) may be optimal 6%–6.5% (42–48 mmol/mol) but may be relaxed to <7% (53 mmol/L) if necessary to prevent hypoglycemia	
Fasting	<5.3 mmol/L (<95 mg/dL)	<5.3 mmol/L (<95 mg/dL)	<5.3 mmol/L (<95 mg/dL)
1-h postprandial	<7.8 mmol/L (<140 mg/dL)	<7.8 mmol/L (<140 mg/dL)	<7.8 mmol/L (<140 mg/dL)
2-h postprandial	<6.7 mmol/L (<120 mg/dL)	<6.7 mmol/L (<120 mg/dL)	<6.4 mmol/L (<115 mg/dL)

23.2.2.2   Hemoglobin A1c in Pregnancy

Hemoglobin A1c remains an important tool in the management of diabetes in pregnancy. It is an easy, inexpensive blood test that can be taken in the nonfasting state. More important, it has been associated with important pregnancy outcomes across many studies.

23.2.2.2.1   Limits of HbA1c in Pregnancy

While it is an important measure of glycemic control, HbA1c has limitations for its use in pregnancy. There are many physiologic changes in pregnancy that influence HbA1c reference ranges, such as increased red blood cell turnover, as well as lower fasting glucose in early pregnancy. In women without diabetes, HbA1c has been shown to have different reference ranges in pregnancy compared to outside pregnancy. Specifically, HbA1c tends to be lower in early to middle gestation; this can falsely reassure women and clinicians regarding glycemic control during this time if pregnancy-adjusted references ranges are not considered.[68–70]

HbA1c also has some general limitations. It is influenced by iron-deficiency anemia, which is common in pregnancy; the prolonged survival of red blood cells can lead to an increased HbA1c.[71] It also has limited use in women with hemoglobinopathies. The reference ranges for HbA1c may also have ethnic variations. Perhaps most important, HbA1c is a measure of average glycemic control and does not give information regarding glycemic variability. This can be especially important in pregnancy, where it can be especially important to avoid hypoglycemia and hyperglycemia. Interestingly, the relationship between HbA1c and estimated average glucose differs during pregnancy when compared to outside of pregnancy.[72] Using CGM data, Law et al. demonstrated that a change in HbA1c in pregnancy represents a smaller change in estimated average glucose when compared to outside pregnancy. Using the NICE guideline target of 6.5% HbA1c (48 mmol/mol), these authors recommend targeting an estimated average glucose of 6.4–6.7 mmol/L (115–121 mg/dL) during pregnancy. The limitations of HbA1c are highlighted in Table 23.4.

23.2.2.2.2   Targets for Women with Type 1 Diabetes

In general, HbA1c should be checked on a monthly basis throughout pregnancy. The physiologic changes associated with pregnancy, as detailed previously, must be considered when interpreting HbA1c testing. The exact targets for HbA1c differ in various guidelines. The most recent Diabetes Canada guidelines (2018) recommend targets of ≤6.5% (48 mmol/mol) [ideally ≤6.1% (43 mmol/mol), if safely possible] during pregnancy.[1] It should be noted that not all guidelines recommend HbA1c targets during pregnancy. The NICE guidelines recommend against the routine measurement of HbA1c in the second and third trimesters of pregnancy and instead recommend capillary glucose monitoring to assess targets later in pregnancy.[13] In this case, the measurement of HbA1c in the second and third trimesters is done primarily for risk assessment.

23.2.2.3   Continuous Glucose Monitoring

CGM should be considered for all pregnant women with Type 1 diabetes in pregnancy, regardless of their form of insulin delivery (i.e., MDI or subcutaneous insulin pump therapy) because initiation of CGM in pregnancy has been shown to

TABLE 23.4 Limitations of HbA1c in pregnancy

Limitation	Effect on clinical care
Increased red cell turnover	Decreased HbA1c
Lower fasting glucose	Decreased HbA1c
Iron-deficiency anemia	Increased HbA1c
Hemoglobinopathies	Unreliable HbA1c
Lower reference range	False reassurance
Does not measure variability	Must be supplemented with additional information
A different relationship with estimated average glucose	Use an estimated average glucose target of 6.4–6.7 mmol/L (115–121 mg/dL) in pregnancy

reduce neonatal complications, including being large for gestational age, neonatal hypoglycemia, neonatal intensive care unit admissions longer than 24 h, and infant length of hospital stay.[14] These better neonatal outcomes are felt to be mediated through the longer time spent within glycemic targets for women with Type 1 diabetes who were randomized to CGM during pregnancy. Benefits of CGM were evident both for MDI and insulin pump users.

23.2.2.4 Other Measurements of Glycemic Control

There are several other methods of assessing glycemic control in persons with Type 1 diabetes, including fructosamine, glycated albumin, plasma glycated CD 59, and 1,5-anhydroglucitol (1,5-AG). However, there have been limited studies of the use of these tests in the setting of pregnancy.

Fructosamine is a test used to assess the glycation of other proteins. Unlike HbA1c, fructosamine is not affected by iron-deficiency anemia and hemoglobinopathies.[73] It is primarily made up of glycated albumin; therefore, due to the faster turnover time of albumin compared to hemoglobin, it offers a much shorter period of glucose control than HbA1c (about 2 weeks). Further, its high intraindividual variability, as well as its sensitivity to dilutional anemia, make it a limited tool in pregnancy. Glycated albumin, the primary constituent measure of fructosamine, also offers a shorter period of glycemic control.[73] Its limited availability and the lack of pregnancy outcome studies in Type 1 diabetes also limit its use in practice. Either of these measures, fructosamine or albumin, may have a role in the clinical care of pregnant women for which HbA1c is not reliable.

Plasma glycated CD59 and 1,5-anhydroglucitol are novel glucose markers that have the potential for use in pregnancy.[74,75] The latter has been shown to more closely reflect glycemic excursions, such as postprandial hyperglycemia, than HbA1c.[76] As for plasma glycated CD59, it has been shown to identify women at high risk of gestational diabetes and may help predict the risk of macrosomia in women with Type 1 diabetes.[74,75] While promising, it is unclear whether these markers will play an important role in the future care of women with Type 1 diabetes in pregnancy.

23.2.3 The Prevention and Management of Diabetes Complications

23.2.3.1 Retinopathy

The exact surveillance interval for diabetic retinopathy screening and follow-up during pregnancy and postpartum requires individualization for each woman. It should be based on existing retinal pathology, as well the presence of other known risk factors for retinopathy progression, such as chronic hypertension, poor glycemic control preconception, a marked rapid improvement in glycemic control during pregnancy, and duration of diabetes. It is appropriate to ensure retinal stability prior to delivery. This allows an alternative plan for a "no-push" delivery in situations when fragile retinal vessels are present. Laser therapy for the management of proliferative retinopathy in pregnancy is safe and should be used as indicated during pregnancy.

There are several theoretical concerns regarding the use of intraocular anti-VEGF therapy, particularly in the first trimester of pregnancy. These include concerns that anti-VEGF therapy may be associated with defective embryogenesis, fetal loss, hypertension, and proteinuria.[22,23] It is currently unknown if anti-VEGF agents cross the placenta or are secreted in breast milk; however, it is likely that, when given as an intravitreal injection, systemic absorption is minimal. Further study is required to assess the safety of intravitreal anti-VEGF therapy in pregnancy. Until this information becomes available, we recommend avoidance of intravitreal anti-VEGF therapy in the first trimester, and limited use in the second and third trimesters. Even then, it should be used only when alternative therapies and the potential benefits of intravitreal anti-VEGF therapy are considered carefully and are believed to outweigh the unknown risks.

Pregnancy can cause macular edema, and data to guide its management during pregnancy is lacking. Spontaneous regression of macular edema postpartum is frequently observed, indicating that diabetic macular edema does not always require immediate treatment. Delivery of the fetus (when appropriate) can be an effective way to reverse macular edema.

23.2.3.2 Hypertension and Nephropathy

Preeclampsia occurs in 5%–20% of women with Type 1 diabetes in pregnancy,[52,77] which is two to four times the occurrence rate in pregnant women without Type 1 diabetes.[78] Poor glycemic control prior to and during pregnancy, as well as preexisting albuminuria and nephropathy, increase the risk of preeclampsia. Preeclampsia in women with Type 1 diabetes is a common cause of preterm delivery. For women with Type 1 diabetes, intervening with pregnancy-safe antihypertensive therapy (as discussed previously) to target a blood pressure of 135/85, as well as urinary albumin excretion to <300 mg/24 h, has been reported to reduce the prevalence of preeclampsia and preterm delivery.[79] ASA prophylaxis started prior to 16 weeks' gestation for preeclampsia prevention, although not specifically studied in women with Type 1 diabetes, is recommended because it does little harm and is likely beneficial.[80]

Among women with overt nephropathy, proteinuria increases during pregnancy, sometimes quite steeply. This makes it difficult to distinguish the natural history of overt diabetic nephropathy in pregnancy from preeclampsia. Intermittent quantification of protein excretion is needed in pregnancy so that once protein excretion is in excess of 3 g/24 h, deep vein thrombosis prophylaxis is considered. In these cases, thyroid function also should be rescreened because some of the urinary protein losses will include antithrombin-3 and thyroid-binding globulin. Such losses contribute to a prothrombotic state, as well as transient hypothyroidism that requires levothyroxine for the remainder of the pregnancy.

23.2.3.3 Neuropathy

Low-dose gabapentin for control of painful peripheral neuropathy in pregnancy is safe, but dosages of 600 mg three times per day has caused neonatal gabapentin withdrawal.[81]

23.2.3.4 Hypoglycemia

A history of severe hypoglycemia prior to pregnancy is a predictor of severe hypoglycemia in pregnancy.[82] It is the main obstacle to tight glycemic control in pregnancy and often results in the need to relax glycemic targets. Severe hypoglycemic events are more common prior to 20 weeks' gestation, and the most frequent gestational age for maternal severe hypoglycemia is 9 weeks' gestation.[82] Hence, accurate gestational-age dating may be helpful in making anticipatory adjustments in insulin dosing to avoid severe hypoglycemia. Driving safety and avoidance when indicated should be reviewed frequently with women who have Type 1 diabetes in pregnancy. Animal studies have suggested that maternal hypoglycemia may be harmful to the developing fetus; however, the limited data on this topic in human studies suggest maternal hypoglycemia has no adverse effects on the fetus.[83]

23.2.3.5 Diabetic Ketoacidosis

The accelerated starvation of pregnancy often worsened by nausea and vomiting of pregnancy may trigger glucagon-mediated ketogenesis, dehydration, acidosis, and release of other counterregulatory hormones including cortisol and catecholamines. Increased renal excretion of bicarbonate is a compensatory response to respiratory alkalosis, which results from increased alveolar ventilation in pregnancy. This reduces buffering capacity in pregnant women, which contributes to pregnant women with Type 1 diabetes being more prone to develop DKA at lower glycemic thresholds. Neonatal morbidity and mortality are high in pregnancies complicated by DKA. Maternal hypokalemia and fetal hyperinsulinemia in response to high glucose from maternal transfer may lead to fatal fetal arrhythmias. The fetus should be monitored closely in the setting of DKA that occurs after 24 gestational weeks. A nonreassuring fetal status does not always indicate the need for urgent delivery because the situation can improve with metabolic management of DKA.[84]

23.2.4 Fetal Surveillance and Timing of Delivery

Poor glycemic control both periconception and during pregnancy is an established risk factor for stillbirth among women with Type 1 diabetes in pregnancy.[9] Although fetal surveillance can provide reassurance of fetal health in women with diabetes, it may not be as good a predictor of fetal health as it is for women without diabetes in pregnancy. A team approach to determine the timing of delivery, including the obstetrician, ophthalmologist, neonatologist, and endocrinologist or internist, is recommended to ensure that glycemic control and retinal health of the women are factored into this important decision. The stillbirth risk of pregnancy progressing beyond 37 weeks' gestation needs to be carefully weighed against the risk of early-term delivery. Table 23.5 provides the estimated risk of stillbirth per 1000 pregnancies in women with pre-existing diabetes based on glycemic control.

23.2.5 Management During Labour and Delivery

Labor and delivery are especially challenging aspects of pregnancies complicated by Type 1 diabetes. Dynamic changes in glucose utilization, as well as the often-unpredictable nature of the labor and delivery period, make achieving tight glucose control (4–7 mmol/L) (72–126 mg/dL) difficult. Tight glucose control is generally recommended, as hyperglycemia in labor has been associated with neonatal hypoglycemia in some studies.[1,85]

TABLE 23.5 Absolute risk/1000 of fetal death in normally formed singleton fetuses in women with preexisting diabetes

Third-trimester HbA1c	Periconception HbA1c				
	HbA1c % (mmol/mol)	5.8–6.6 (40–49)	6.7–7.5 (50–59)	7.6–8.5 (60–69)	8.6–9.4 (70–79)
	5.4–6.2 (35–44)	7	6	8	10
	6.3–7.1 (45–54)	9	8	10	13
	7.2–8.0 (55–64)	16	15	18	23
	8.1–8.9 (65–74)	29	26	33	42
	9.0–9.8 (75–84)	54	49	62	78

Adapted from Tennant PW, Glinianaia SV, Bilous RW, Rankin J, Bell R. Pre-existing diabetes, maternal glycated haemoglobin, and the risks of fetal and infant death: a population-based study. *Diabetologia* 2014;**57**(2):285–94.

23.2.5.1 Prior to Delivery

Peripartum considerations should be discussed with women prior to labor. From a diabetes team perspective, these include the method and goals of insulin delivery, common complications such as high rates of cesarean section, admission to neonatal intensive care, neonatal hypoglycemia, and postpartum insulin doses. Additionally, women should be instructed about which diabetes supplies to bring to the hospital; this is of particular importance for women on the insulin pump, who will need to bring extra batteries, pump cartridges, and infusion sets.

The management plan for insulin in the peripartum period often will depend on the plan for delivery (i.e., induction of labor, vaginal delivery, or elective cesarean section); thus, close communication with the obstetrical team is essential. The location of the delivery also must be considered as women with Type 1 diabetes should ideally be delivered at a tertiary care center from both a maternal and neonatal perspective.

23.2.5.2 Strategies for Insulin Delivery

The main options for achieving target glycemic control in labor and delivery are subcutaneous insulin, an intravenous (IV) insulin/dextrose infusion, and the insulin pump. Women who are on MDIs are generally switched to IV insulin at the onset of labor. Women who are on the insulin pump during pregnancy can be switched to an IV insulin/dextrose infusion or can continue to use their insulin pump safely, provided that medication used for pain control during delivery or maternal exhaustion does not impair her ability to manage her pump effectively.[86, 87]

Regardless of the method of insulin delivery, some principles are the same. Capillary blood glucoses should be checked every hour at the onset of labor, or sooner if there are concerns. A target glucose of 4–7 mmol/L (72–126 mg/dL) should be maintained until delivery.[1, 13, 87] Hypoglycemia is common during this time, with up to half of women having at least one episode; therefore, treatment of hypoglycemia should be readily available.[85] Regardless of the protocol or method of insulin delivery, treatment should be individually tailored to both the women with diabetes and the clinical situation.

23.2.5.3 Management of IV Insulin Infusion During Labor and Delivery
23.2.5.3.1 Vaginal Delivery

The exact protocol used to guide the administration of IV insulin tends to vary from center to center. However, most protocols will have a variable-rate IV insulin infusion-dosing algorithm that is based on total daily insulin requirements late in pregnancy and changes depending on capillary blood glucose testing. Also, fluids containing a 5% dextrose infusion are administered with insulin infusion to avoid hypoglycemia. Immediately after the delivery, the IV insulin infusion should generally be decreased by about 50%.

23.2.5.3.2 Cesarean Section

Women with Type 1 diabetes should be put first on the elective list. The night prior to cesarean section, women can take their normal evening long-acting insulin dose or decrease it by 20%, depending on the clinical scenario and type of long-acting insulin. The IV insulin infusion, if required, can be started at 6 a.m. on the day of the cesarean section and adjusted accordingly. After delivery, the IV insulin infusion can be decreased by 50%, and women can be transitioned to subcutaneous insulin when it is safe to do so with a 2-h overlap.

23.2.5.4 Management of the Insulin Pump During Labor and Delivery

The decision to continue to use the insulin pump during labor and delivery should be made by the woman and her diabetes team prior to admission. Many women can safely pump throughout labor and delivery; however, the reasons to change to IV insulin during this time should be thoroughly discussed. These include severe or frequent hypoglycemia, persistent hyperglycemia (i.e., above target for two consecutive measurements), or if the woman becomes unable or unwilling to manage her pump actively for any reason. The delivery team should have explicit instructions regarding these elements and the capability to change quickly to IV insulin should the need arise. Regardless of whether women on the insulin pump choose to continue to use it during labor and delivery, postpartum insulin doses should be programmed into the pump beforehand.

23.2.5.4.1 Vaginal Delivery

Women should be instructed to maintain a glucose level of 4–7 mmol/L (72–126 mg/dL). If a woman falls below target, she should treat her low rate as per the hospital hypoglycemia protocol and decrease her basal rate by 30%–50%, depending on the glucose value. If she goes >7 mmol/L (126 mg/dL), she should be instructed to give a correction bolus.[86] At the time of pushing, women should decrease their basal rate by about 50% to avoid hypoglycemia. Finally, after the delivery of the placenta, women should change to their preprogrammed postpartum insulin-pump settings.

23.2.5.4.2 Elective Cesarean Section

Because cesarean sections tend to be fairly short, women on the insulin pump who have a scheduled cesarean section can be instructed to continue their pump and change to the postpartum settings 1–2 h prior to the planned event. Capillary glucose should be checked every 30 min. Again, if women have severe or frequent hypoglycemia or persistent hyperglycemia, or she becomes unstable, an IV insulin infusion should be started and the insulin pump discontinued.

23.2.5.5 Conclusions on Labor and Delivery

The peripartum period is a unique challenge in the management of diabetes in pregnancy. While protocols should be in place to guide the health-care team, every woman and clinical scenario must be individualized. Women who are able and willing can continue the insulin pump safely during labor and delivery, but IV insulin therapy must be discussed and used if necessary. Immediately following the delivery of the placenta, there is a steep reduction in insulin resistance, and thus postpartum dosing must be considered prior to the onset of labor. The detailed considerations with regard to this will be discussed in the following section.

23.3 POSTPARTUM

23.3.1 Physiological Changes and their Impact on Diabetes Management

There is a dramatic decrease in insulin resistance following the delivery of the placenta; this requires a concomitant decrease in insulin. Women will often require about 50%–60% of their prepregnancy insulin dose in the immediate postpartum period. Predicting postpartum insulin doses for individuals with Type 1 diabetes can be very challenging, and during this period, women are at high risk of hypoglycemia. Postpartum insulin doses should be determined through a discussion between women and their primary diabetes team prior to delivery. Ideally, a copy of this plan should be provided to the on-call team and for the woman to bring to the hospital.

23.3.1.1 For Women on An IV Insulin Infusion for Labor and Delivery

Prior to labor and delivery, postpartum insulin doses (basal rates, insulin-to-carbohydrate ratios, and insulin sensitivity factors) should be programmed into the pump. Immediately after delivery, the insulin-pump settings should be changed to the recommended or preprogrammed postpartum doses. It is important to remember to change the target glucose level in the pump, as this cannot be preprogrammed into the pump prior to delivery.

23.3.1.2 For Women on an IV Insulin Infusion for Labor and Delivery

Following the delivery of the placenta, the IV insulin infusion should be reduced by half to avoid hypoglycemia. However if IV insulin has already been reduced because of the effects of labor or lingering effects of basal insulin administered prior to labor, it may not need to be reduced this aggressively following delivery. Women on an IV insulin infusion should continue it until it is safe to transition to either MDIs or the insulin pump. This should be clearly indicated in the postpartum hospital insulin orders.

23.3.1.3 Insulin-Dosing Postpartum Recommendations

Immediately after delivery, the overall glucose targets are less stringent. We recommend aiming for initial glucose targets of 6–10 mmol/L (108.0–180 mg/dL) after delivery. Women should be counseled on this point, as well of the importance of relaxed targets to decrease the risk of hypoglycemia. While insulin orders and instructions should be individualized where possible, in general, most women should avoid bolusing for their first light meal, and instead take a correction doses of bolus insulin for glucose readings >12 mmol/L (216 mg/dL).

Deciding on exact and individualized postpartum insulin doses is challenging, as doses vary significantly and are often unpredictable.[55] It is essential, therefore, that women continue to test their glucose frequently and make appropriate adjustments. Most women will generally require about half of their late pregnancy basal insulin, although this may depend on factors such as the level of glycemic control achieved with their late-pregnancy insulin doses. For those on an insulin pump, we generally give a flat basal insulin rate because the finely tuned varying basal rates during pregnancy are not applicable during the significantly altered sleep–wake cycle that will occur postpartum. A starting point for insulin doses that may work for most women would be an insulin-to-carbohydrate ratio of 1:15 g, a basal rate of 0.5 units/h, and a halving of the insulin sensitivity factor. Women who require larger insulin doses may require more aggressive insulin dosing. The elements to include in postpartum insulin orders are itemized in Table 23.6.

23.3.2 Contraception

Safe, effective contraception should be discussed with all women with Type 1 diabetes at risk of unintended pregnancy; this is especially important in the postpartum period. Ideally, contraceptive planning should be discussed prior to delivery, and again prior to discharge from the hospital. A contraceptive plan prior to discharge is important, as half of women have intercourse prior to their first visit postpartum, and many women do not attend their first postpartum visit.[88] As previously discussed, glycemic targets in the postpartum period are more relaxed. If another pregnancy is desired, women need adequate interpregnancy time to achieve tight glycemic control, take folic acid, and receive appropriate complication-related screening prior to conceiving.

Many factors need to be considered in choosing the best individualized contraceptive option. These include typical use failure rates, decision to breastfeed, time postpartum, convenience/likelihood of adherence, and cardiovascular safety. The risks associated with each contraception option should be weighed against the risks associated with pregnancies complicated by diabetes. Uncomplicated Type 1 diabetes should not limit contraceptive choice, although data suggest that women with diabetes are less likely to use contraception.[89] In those women with a history of microvascular complications (nephropathy, retinopathy, or neuropathy), history of vascular disease, or diabetes duration >20 years, medical eligibility for contraception is more limited.

Contraceptive methods compatible with breastfeeding include the intrauterine device and progesterone-only contraceptives. The following factors may influence contraceptive choice: (1) depot medroxyprogesterone acetate has been associated with weight gain, (2) the progesterone-only pill has high rates of user error because full efficacy requires

TABLE 23.6 Elements to include in postpartum insulin orders
When to discontinue IV insulin
Insulin doses
Parameters of when to call the diabetes team
Frequency of capillary glucose monitoring

ingestion within the same hour of each day; and (3) relative and absolute contraindications for estrogen-containing contraceptive use include hypertension, breastfeeding, cardiovascular disease, and microvascular complications.

23.3.3 Screening for Diabetes Complications Postpartum

Retinal assessment during the postpartum interval is important for women with Type 1 diabetes because the risk of progressive retinal changes continue to be increased in the first year after delivery.

Women who experience preeclampsia during pregnancy require close follow-up of antihypertensive management. Eclampsia can first occur postpartum; thus, women with Type 1 diabetes need to be counseled to seek medical attention should they experience new onset hypertension postpartum or signs and symptoms of eclampsia. Antihypertensive medications considered to be safe during lactation include calcium channel blockers, short-acting angiotensin-converting enzyme inhibitors (e.g., captopril and enalapril), and spironolactone.[90] Methyldopa is safe for breastfeeding; however, because of the side effect of fatigue, it is not the preferred medication for lactating mothers. Although beta-blockers that have a high degree of protein binding and are considered safe for lactation, their use in women with Type 1 diabetes postpartum is discouraged. Their use can mask symptoms of hypoglycemia at a time when women are at increased risk for hypoglycemia as they adjust to new insulin dosing postpartum, breastfeeding, and the demands of caring for a newborn. Lactation may be suppressed by diuretics. The safety of angiotensin-receptor blockers during lactation remains unknown.

Women with Type 1 diabetes who experience hypertension prior to or during pregnancy, kidney dysfunction preconception, or both have increased mortality in the two decades following childbirth.[24] Close follow-up is merited to ensure that such women receive appropriate management to prevent progressive kidney dysfunction and reduce the risk of cardiovascular disease. The risk for future pregnancies requires reassessment postpartum. Women with Type 1 diabetes do not experience lower rates of preeclampsia when they are multiparous.[25] They need to be counseled that preeclampsia is likely to recur in future pregnancies if it occurred in any of their previous pregnancies.

23.3.3.1 Thyroid Function

The prevalence of postpartum thyroiditis is increased in women with Type 1 diabetes. Especially when women with Type 1 diabetes are symptomatic of thyroid dysfunction postpartum, they should be screened for postpartum thyroiditis. Thyroid disorders are common in women with Type 1 diabetes. Management of thyroid disorders in pregnancy and postpartum is covered in Chapter 19.

23.3.4 Breastfeeding

The importance of breastfeeding for mothers and infants is well established across many populations. Consensus guidelines recommend breastfeeding for women with diabetes.[1, 12, 13, 91] Despite this, some studies suggest that diabetes in pregnancy has been associated with decreased rates of breastfeeding initiation when compared to mothers without diabetes.[92] The reason for this may be multifactorial and include both pathophysiologic causes, as well as other mechanisms, as discussed next.

23.3.4.1 Challenges in Breastfeeding and Type 1 Diabetes

23.3.4.1.1 Delayed Lactogenesis

Studies of women with diabetes in pregnancy have consistently found an association between diabetes and delayed onset of lactogenesis (also referred to as the *second stage of lactogenesis*).[93] It should be noted that there are many potential confounders when examining this relationship, such as differences in maternal–infant separation, neonatal intensive care unit admission, mode of delivery, and treatment for neonatal hypoglycemia.[93] Suboptimal glycemic control itself has been associated with delayed onset of lactogenesis; however, it is less clear if hyperglycemia is directly on the causal pathway. Specifically, it is unknown whether poor glycemic control induces new gene expression directly, or if the poor glycemic control is associated with large-for-gestational-age infants and neonatal hypoglycemia that may affect the onset of lactogenesis.[93]

23.3.4.1.2 Impact of Dysglycemia on Milk Supply, Milk Content, and Infant

The content of the breast milk of mothers with and without diabetes may differ. Small studies have suggested that the ingestion of hyperglycemic breast milk may be associated with adverse infant outcomes, such as obesity and delayed language development; however, these studies have not been replicated.[94] Studies are discordant as to the glucose content in the breast milk of women with diabetes. However, if a difference exists between the glucose concentration in the breast milk of women and without diabetes, it is small. Milk supply may also vary with maternal hypoglycemia and hyperglycemia; both have been associated with a change in milk production.[94]

23.3.4.2 Strategies to Help Establish and Maintain Breastfeeding

A recent large trial of women with preexisting and gestational diabetes suggests that women can begin to express breast milk safely in late pregnancy.[95] Although it remains to be seen if this will improve breastfeeding rates postpartum, this study offers important data that may address the concerns that expressing breast milk may lead to early onset of labor.

As much as possible, it is important to reduce maternal–infant separation, encourage early skin-to-skin contact, and have mother and infant in the same room.[93] Unfortunately, this cannot always happen, as half of infants of mothers with diabetes will be admitted to neonatal intensive care or be diagnosed with neonatal hypoglycemia.

23.3.4.3 Impact of Breastfeeding on Glycemic Control and Insulin Requirements

The evidence regarding the impact of breastfeeding on glycemic control and insulin requirements is discordant.[94] Some studies suggest an increased risk of hypoglycemia and lower insulin requirements, while others suggest more stable glycemic patterns in women who breastfeed when compared to women who bottle-feed, and still others find no difference at all. Outside diabetes, breastfeeding is associated with faster postpartum weight loss, which also may affect insulin requirements.

Overall, women should be advised that it is safe to breastfeed, and there is no clear evidence that breastfeeding is associated with an increased risk of severe hypoglycemia. Nonetheless, they should be counseled that breastfeeding may affect insulin requirements; therefore, it is important that women should continue to monitor their blood glucose frequently and adjust their insulin doses accordingly.

23.3.5 Risks to Offspring

Observational studies have examined the relationship between exposure to maternal Type 1 diabetes in utero and the health of future offspring, including metabolic and neurocognitive outcomes. Metabolic outcomes including being overweight, obesity, insulin sensitivity and secretion, metabolic syndrome, and development of impaired glucose tolerance and diabetes have been studied. Conflicting results have been found. In utero maternal Type 1 diabetes exposure may increase risk of Type 2 or impaired glucose tolerance in offspring, as well as overweight and metabolic syndrome compared to nondiabetic mothers.[96, 97] However, adjustments for maternal family history of diabetes, maternal overweight, and offspring age, attenuated or eliminated these associations. Studies have also yielded conflicting results as to whether there is an association between maternal glycemic control in pregnancy for mothers with Type 1 diabetes and the future metabolic risk of their offspring.[97, 98]

Children of mothers of Type 1 diabetes aged 1–15 years compared to controls have been shown to have similar mortality but greater morbidity, reflected by more hospitalizations and higher overall medication use.[99] Childhood hospital admissions were directly associated with maternal HbA1c (preconception and during pregnancy).

Reassuringly, children of women with Type 1 diabetes during pregnancy have been found to have similar average grades at the end of primary school compared with matched control offspring.[99] But an inverse relationship was observed between primary-school grades and maternal HbA1c (preconception and during pregnancy). It remains unclear if these associations are the result of a causal influence of maternal glycemic control during pregnancy on future childhood health and neurological development, or if maternal glycemic control is just a reflection of other confounders such as mode and gestational timing of delivery or parental factors or habits that influence offspring health and neurocognition.[99] However, another study at 13–19 years of age found slightly lower scores in intelligence indexes compared to a control background population, and no direct association between maternal HbA1c and cognitive function in offspring exposed to Type 1 diabetes during gestation.[100] Further studies with more precise measures of maternal glycemic control, such as from CGM, are needed to help clarify these associations.

CONFLICT OF INTEREST

Authors report no conflicts.

REFERENCES

1. Diabetes Canada Clinical Practice Guidelines Expert Committee, Feig DS, Berger H, Donovan L, Godbout A, Kader T, et al. Diabetes and pregnancy. *Can J Diabetes* 2018;**42**(Suppl 1):S255–82.
2. Murphy HR, Roland JM, Skinner TC, Simmons D, Gurnell E, Morrish NJ, et al. Effectiveness of a regional prepregnancy care program in women with type 1 and type 2 diabetes: benefits beyond glycemic control. *Diabetes Care* 2010;**33**(12):2514–20.
3. Yamamoto JM, Hughes DJF, Evans ML, Karunakaran V, Clark JDA, Morrish NJ, et al. Community-based pre-pregnancy care programme improves pregnancy preparation in women with pregestational diabetes. *Diabetologia* 2018; https://doi.org/10.1007/s00125-018-4613-3.
4. Egan AM, Danyliv A, Carmody L, Kirwan B, Dunne FP. A Prepregnancy care program for women with diabetes: effective and cost saving. *J Clin Endocrinol Metab* 2016;**101**(4):1807–15.
5. Kallas-Koeman MM, Khandwala F, Donovan L. Rate of preconception care in women with type 2 diabetes still lags behind that of women with type 1 diabetes. *Can J Diabetes* 2012;**36**(2012):170–4.
6. Murphy HR, Bell R, Cartwright C, Curnow P, Maresh M, Morgan M, et al. Improved pregnancy outcomes in women with type 1 and type 2 diabetes but substantial clinic-to-clinic variations: a prospective nationwide study. *Diabetologia* 2017;**60**(9):1668–77.
7. Makda SI, Davies MJ, Wilmot E, Bankart J, Yates T, Varghese EM, et al. Prescribing in pregnancy for women with diabetes: use of potential teratogenic drugs and contraception. *Diabet Med* 2013;**30**(4):457–63.
8. O'Higgins S, McGuire BE, Mustafa E, Dunne F. Barriers and facilitators to attending pre-pregnancy care services: the Atlantic-dip experience. *Diabet Med* 2014;**31**(3):366–74.
9. Tennant PW, Glinianaia SV, Bilous RW, Rankin J, Bell R. Pre-existing diabetes, maternal glycated haemoglobin, and the risks of fetal and infant death: a population-based study. *Diabetologia* 2014;**57**(2):285–94.
10. Macintosh MC, Fleming KM, Bailey JA, Doyle P, Modder J, Acolet D, et al. Perinatal mortality and congenital anomalies in babies of women with type 1 or type 2 diabetes in England, Wales, and Northern Ireland: population based study. *BMJ* 2006;**333**(7560):177.
11. Bell R, Glinianaia SV, Tennant PW, Bilous RW, Rankin J. Peri-conception hyperglycaemia and nephropathy are associated with risk of congenital anomaly in women with pre-existing diabetes: a population-based cohort study. *Diabetologia* 2012;**2012**(55):936–47.
12. American Diabetes Association. 13. Management of diabetes in pregnancy: standards of medical care in diabetes-2018. *Diabetes Care* 2018;**41**(Suppl 1):S137–43.
13. National Instutite of Health and Care Excellence. *Diabetes in pregnancy: management from preconception to the postnatal period.* Available from: https://www.nice.org.uk/guidance/ng3; 2015 [Accessed 11 May 2018].
14. Feig DS, Donovan LE, Corcoy R, Murphy KE, Amiel SA, Hunt KF, et al. Continuous glucose monitoring in pregnant women with type 1 diabetes (CONCEPTT): a multicentre international randomised controlled trial. *Lancet* 2017;**390**(10110):2347–59.
15. Butalia S, Gutierrez L, Lodha A, Aitken E, Zakariasen A, Donovan L. Short- and long-term outcomes of metformin compared with insulin alone in pregnancy: a systematic review and meta-analysis. *Diabet Med* 2017;**34**(1):27–36.
16. Ringholm L, Secher AL, Pedersen-Bjergaard U, Thorsteinsson B, Andersen HU, Damm P, et al. The incidence of severe hypoglycaemia in pregnant women with type 1 diabetes mellitus can be reduced with unchanged HbA1c levels and pregnancy outcomes in a routine care setting. *Diabetes Res Clin Pract* 2013;**101**(2):123–30.
17. Egan AM, McVicker L, Heerey A, Carmody L, Harney F, Dunne FP. Diabetic retinopathy in pregnancy: a population-based study of women with pregestational diabetes. *J Diabetes Res* 2015;**2015**:310239.
18. Diabetes Control and Complications Trial Research Group. Effect of pregnancy on microvascular complications in the diabetes control and complications trial. The Diabetes Control and Complications Trial Research Group. *Diabetes Care* 2000;**23**(8):1084–91.
19. Chew EY, Mills JL, Metzger BE, Remaley NA, Jovanovic-Peterson L, Knopp RH, et al. Metabolic control and progression of retinopathy. The Diabetes in Early Pregnancy Study. National Institute of Child Health and Human Development Diabetes in Early Pregnancy Study. *Diabetes Care* 1995;**18**(5):631–7.
20. Gordin D, Kaaja R, Forsblom C, Hiilesmaa V, Teramo K, Groop PH. Pre-eclampsia and pregnancy-induced hypertension are associated with severe diabetic retinopathy in type 1 diabetes later in life. *Acta Diabetol* 2013;**50**(5):781–7.
21. Temple RC, Aldridge VA, Sampson MJ, Greenwood RH, Heyburn PJ, Glenn A. Impact of pregnancy on the progression of diabetic retinopathy in Type 1 diabetes. *Diabet Med* 2001;**18**(7):573–7.
22. Galazios G, Papazoglou D, Tsikouras P, Kolios G. Vascular endothelial growth factor gene polymorphisms and pregnancy. *J Matern Fetal Neonatal Med* 2009;**22**(5):371–8.
23. Peracha ZH, Rosenfeld PJ. Anti-vascular endothelial growth factor therapy in pregnancy: what we know, what we don't know, and what we don't know we don't know. *Retina* 2016;**36**(8):1413–7.
24. Knorr S, Juul S, Bytoft B, Lohse Z, Clausen TD, Jensen RB, et al. Impact of type 1 diabetes on maternal long-term risk of hospitalisation and mortality: a nationwide combined clinical and register-based cohort study (the EPICOM Study). *Diabetologia* 2018;**61**(5):1071–80.
25. Castiglioni MT, Valsecchi L, Cavoretto P, Pirola S, Di Piazza L, Maggio L, et al. The risk of preeclampsia beyond the first pregnancy among women with type 1 diabetes parity and preeclampsia in type 1 diabetes. *Pregnancy Hypertens* 2014;**4**(1):34–40.
26. Jensen DM, Damm P, Ovesen P, Molsted-Pedersen L, Beck-Nielsen H, Westergaard JG, et al. Microalbuminuria, preeclampsia, and preterm delivery in pregnant women with type 1 diabetes: results from a Nationwide Danish Study. *Diabetes Care* 2010;**33**(1):90–4.
27. Ringholm L, Mathiesen ER, Kelstrup L, Damm P. Managing type 1 diabetes mellitus in pregnancy—from planning to breastfeeding. *Nat Rev Endocrinol* 2012;**8**(11):659–67.

28. Biesenbach G, Stoger H, Zazgornik J. Influence of pregnancy on progression of diabetic nephropathy and subsequent requirement of renal replacement therapy in female type I diabetic patients with impaired renal function. *Nephrol Dial Transplant* 1992;**7**(2):105–9.

29. Rossing K, Jacobsen P, Hommel E, Mathiesen E, Svenningsen A, Rossing P, et al. Pregnancy and progression of diabetic nephropathy. *Diabetologia* 2002;**45**(1):36–41.

30. Lee AA, Piette JD, Heisler M, Rosland AM. Diabetes distress and glycemic control: the buffering effect of autonomy support from important family members and friends. *Diabetes Care* 2018;**41**(6):1157–63.

31. Evers IM, de Valk HW, Visser GH. Risk of complications of pregnancy in women with type 1 diabetes: nationwide prospective study in the Netherlands. *BMJ* 2004;**328**(7445):915.

32. Law GR, Ellison GT, Secher AL, Damm P, Mathiesen ER, Temple R, et al. Analysis of continuous glucose monitoring in pregnant women with diabetes: distinct temporal patterns of glucose associated with large-for-gestational-age infants. *Diabetes Care* 2015;**38**(7):1319–25.

33. Yamamoto JM, Kallas-Koeman MM, Butalia S, Lodha AK, Donovan LE. Large-for-gestational-age (LGA) neonate predicts a 2.5-fold increased odds of neonatal hypoglycaemia in women with type 1 diabetes. *Diabetes Metab Res Rev* 2017;**33**(1): e2824.

34. Murphy HR, Elleri D, Allen JM, Harris J, Simmons D, Rayman G, et al. Pathophysiology of postprandial hyperglycaemia in women with type 1 diabetes during pregnancy. *Diabetologia* 2012;**55**(2):282–93.

35. Goudie RJ, Lunn D, Hovorka R, Murphy HR. Pharmacokinetics of insulin aspart in pregnant women with type 1 diabetes: every day is different. *Diabetes Care* 2014;**37**(6):e121–2.

36. Garcia-Patterson A, Gich I, Amini SB, Catalano PM, de Leiva A, Corcoy R. Insulin requirements throughout pregnancy in women with type 1 diabetes mellitus: three changes of direction. *Diabetologia* 2010;**53**(3):446–51.

37. Nielsen LR, Rehfeld JF, Pedersen-Bjergaard U, Damm P, Mathiesen ER. Pregnancy-induced rise in serum C-peptide concentrations in women with type 1 diabetes. *Diabetes Care* 2009;**32**(6):1052–7.

38. Padmanabhan S, McLean M, Cheung NW. Falling insulin requirements are associated with adverse obstetric outcomes in women with preexisting diabetes. *Diabetes Care* 2014;**37**(10):2685–92.

39. Achong N, Callaway L, d'Emden M, McIntyre HD, Lust K, Barrett HL. Insulin requirements in late pregnancy in women with type 1 diabetes mellitus: a retrospective review. *Diabetes Res Clin Pract* 2012;**98**(3):414–21.

40. McManus RM, Ryan EA. Insulin requirements in insulin-dependent and insulin-requiring GDM women during final month of pregnancy. *Diabetes Care* 1992;**15**(10):1323–7.

41. Steel JM, Johnstone FD, Hume R, Mao JH. Insulin requirements during pregnancy in women with type I diabetes. *Obstet Gynecol* 1994;**83**(2):253–8.

42. Padmanabhan S, Lee VW, McLean M, Athayde N, Lanzarone V, Khoshnow Q, et al. The association of falling insulin requirements with maternal biomarkers and placental dysfunction: a prospective study of women with preexisting diabetes in pregnancy. *Diabetes Care* 2017;**40**(10):1323–30.

43. Ram M, Feinmesser L, Shinar S, Maslovitz S. The importance of declining insulin requirements during pregnancy in patients with pre-gestational gestational diabetes mellitus. *Eur J Obstet Gynecol Reprod Biol* 2017;**215**:148–52.

44. Asbjornsdottir B, Akueson CE, Ronneby H, Rytter A, Andersen JR, Damm P, et al. The influence of carbohydrate consumption on glycemic control in pregnant women with type 1 diabetes. *Diabetes Res Clin Pract* 2017;**127**:97–104.

45. Secher AL, Parellada CB, Ringholm L, Asbjornsdottir B, Damm P, Mathiesen ER. Higher gestational weight gain is associated with increasing offspring birth weight independent of maternal glycemic control in women with type 1 diabetes. *Diabetes Care* 2014;**37**(10):2677–84.

46. Roskjaer AB, Andersen JR, Ronneby H, Damm P, Mathiesen ER. Dietary advices on carbohydrate intake for pregnant women with type 1 diabetes. *J Matern Fetal Neonatal Med* 2015;**28**(2):229–33.

47. Davies GAL, Wolfe LA, Mottola MF, MacKinnon C. No. 129-exercise in pregnancy and the postpartum period. *J Obstet Gynaecol Can* 2018;**40**(2): e58–65.

48. Practice ACOG. ACOG Committee opinion. Number 267, January 2002: exercise during pregnancy and the postpartum period. *Obstet Gynecol* 2002;**99**(1):171–3.

49. National Instutitue of Health and Care Excellence. *Weight management before, during and after pregnancy*. Available from: https://www.nice.org.uk/guidance/ph27/chapter/1-Recommendations-recommendation-2-pregnant-women; 2010 [Accessed 10 June 2018].

50. Melzer K, Schutz Y, Boulvain M, Kayser B. Physical activity and pregnancy: cardiovascular adaptations, recommendations and pregnancy outcomes. *Sports Med* 2010;**40**(6):493–507.

51. Kumareswaran K, Elleri D, Allen JM, Caldwell K, Westgate K, Brage S, et al. Physical activity energy expenditure and glucose control in pregnant women with type 1 diabetes: is 30 minutes of daily exercise enough? *Diabetes Care* 2013;**36**(5):1095–101.

52. Kallas-Koeman MM, Kong JM, Klinke JA, Butalia S, Lodha AK, Lim KI, et al. Insulin pump use in pregnancy is associated with lower HbA1c without increasing the rate of severe hypoglycaemia or diabetic ketoacidosis in women with type 1 diabetes. *Diabetologia* 2014;**57**(4):681–9.

53. Cohen O, Vigersky RA, Lee SW, Cordero TL, Kaufman FR. Automated insulin delivery system nomenclature. *Diabetes Technol Ther* 2017;**19**(6):379–80.

54. Yamamoto JM, Murphy HR. Emerging technologies for the management of type 1 diabetes in pregnancy. *Curr Diab Rep* 2018;**18**(1):4.

55. Stewart ZA, Wilinska ME, Hartnell S, Temple RC, Rayman G, Stanley KP, et al. Closed-loop insulin delivery during pregnancy in women with type 1 diabetes. *N Engl J Med* 2016;**375**(7):644–54.

56. Stewart ZA, Yamamoto J, Wilinska ME, Hartnell S, Farrington C, Hovorka R, et al. Adaptability of closed-loop during labour, delivery and postpartum: a secondary analysis of data from two randomized crossover trials in type 1 diabetes pregnancy. *Diabetes Technol Ther* 2018;**20**(7):501–5.

57. Farrington C, Stewart ZA, Barnard K, Hovorka R, Murphy HR. Experiences of closed-loop insulin delivery among pregnant women with Type 1 diabetes. *Diabet Med* 2017;**34**(10):1461–9.

58. Wang H, Wender-Ozegowska E, Garne E, Morgan M, Loane M, Morris JK, et al. Insulin analogues use in pregnancy among women with pregestational diabetes mellitus and risk of congenital anomaly: a retrospective population-based cohort study. *BMJ Open* 2018;**8**(2).

59. Boskovic R, Feig DS, Derewlany L, Knie B, Portnoi G, Koren G. Transfer of insulin lispro across the human placenta: in vitro perfusion studies. *Diabetes Care* 2003;**26**(5):1390–4.

60. Mathiesen ER, Kinsley B, Amiel SA, Heller S, McCance D, Duran S, et al. Maternal glycemic control and hypoglycemia in type 1 diabetic pregnancy: a randomized trial of insulin aspart versus human insulin in 322 pregnant women. *Diabetes Care* 2007;**30**(4):771–6.

61. Doder Z, Vanechanos D, Oster M, Landgraf W, Lin S. Insulin glulisine in pregnancy—experience from clinical trials and post-marketing surveillance. *Eur Endocrinol* 2015;**11**(1):17–20.

62. McCance DR, Damm P, Mathiesen ER, Hod M, Kaaja R, Dunne F, et al. Evaluation of insulin antibodies and placental transfer of insulin aspart in pregnant women with type 1 diabetes mellitus. *Diabetologia* 2008;**51**(11):2141–3.

63. Mathiesen ER, Hod M, Ivanisevic M, Duran Garcia S, Brondsted L, Jovanovic L, et al. Maternal efficacy and safety outcomes in a randomized, controlled trial comparing insulin detemir with NPH insulin in 310 pregnant women with type 1 diabetes. *Diabetes Care* 2012;**35**(10):2012–7.

64. Herrera KM, Rosenn BM, Foroutan J, Bimson BE, Al Ibraheemi Z, Moshier EL, et al. Randomized controlled trial of insulin detemir versus NPH for the treatment of pregnant women with diabetes. *Am J Obstet Gynecol* 2015;**213**(3). 426 e1–7.

65. Kurtzhals P, Schaffer L, Sorensen A, Kristensen C, Jonassen I, Schmid C, et al. Correlations of receptor binding and metabolic and mitogenic potencies of insulin analogs designed for clinical use. *Diabetes* 2000;**49**(6):999–1005.

66. Pollex E, Moretti ME, Koren G, Feig DS. Safety of insulin glargine use in pregnancy: a systematic review and meta-analysis. *Ann Pharmacother* 2011;**45**(1):9–16.

67. Feig DS, Murphy K, Asztalos E, Tomlinson G, Sanchez J, Zinman B, et al. Metformin in women with type 2 diabetes in pregnancy (MiTy): a multicenter randomized controlled trial. *BMC Pregnancy Childbirth* 2016;**16**(1):173.

68. Radder JK, van Roosmalen J. HbA1c in healthy, pregnant women. *Neth J Med* 2005;**63**(7):256–9.

69. Hiramatsu Y, Shimizu I, Omori Y, Nakabayashi M, Group JGAS. Determination of reference intervals of glycated albumin and hemoglobin A1c in healthy pregnant Japanese women and analysis of their time courses and influencing factors during pregnancy. *Endocr J* 2012;**59**(2):145–51.

70. Versantvoort AR, van Roosmalen J, Radder JK. Course of HbA1c in non-diabetic pregnancy related to birth weight. *Neth J Med* 2013;**71**(1):22–5.

71. Rafat D, Rabbani TK, Ahmad J, Ansari MA. Influence of iron metabolism indices on HbA1c in non-diabetic pregnant women with and without iron-deficiency anemia: effect of iron supplementation. *Diabetes Metab Syndr* 2012;**6**(2):102–5.

72. Law GR, Gilthorpe MS, Secher AL, Temple R, Bilous R, Mathiesen ER, et al. Translating HbA1c measurements into estimated average glucose values in pregnant women with diabetes. *Diabetologia* 2017;**60**(4):618–24.

73. Hashimoto K, Koga M. Indicators of glycemic control in patients with gestational diabetes mellitus and pregnant women with diabetes mellitus. *World J Diabetes* 2015;**6**(8):1045–56.

74. Nowak N, Skupien J, Cyganek K, Matejko B, Malecki MT. 1,5-Anhydroglucitol as a marker of maternal glycaemic control and predictor of neonatal birthweight in pregnancies complicated by type 1 diabetes mellitus. *Diabetologia* 2013;**56**(4):709–13.

75. Ghosh P, Luque-Fernandez MA, Vaidya A, Ma D, Sahoo R, Chorev M, et al. Plasma glycated CD59, a novel biomarker for detection of pregnancy-induced glucose intolerance. *Diabetes Care* 2017;**40**(7):981–4.

76. Dungan KM, Buse JB, Largay J, Kelly MM, Button EA, Kato S, et al. 1,5-anhydroglucitol and postprandial hyperglycemia as measured by continuous glucose monitoring system in moderately controlled patients with diabetes. *Diabetes Care* 2006;**29**(6):1214–9.

77. Holmes VA, Young IS, Patterson CC, Pearson DW, Walker JD, Maresh MJ, et al. Optimal glycemic control, pre-eclampsia, and gestational hypertension in women with type 1 diabetes in the diabetes and pre-eclampsia intervention trial. *Diabetes Care* 2011;**34**(8):1683–8.

78. Persson M, Norman M, Hanson U. Obstetric and perinatal outcomes in type 1 diabetic pregnancies: a large, population-based study. *Diabetes Care* 2009;**32**(11):2005–9.

79. Nielsen LR, Damm P, Mathiesen ER. Improved pregnancy outcome in type 1 diabetic women with microalbuminuria or diabetic nephropathy: effect of intensified antihypertensive therapy? *Diabetes Care* 2009;**32**(1):38–44.

80. LeFevre ML. Force USPST. Low-dose aspirin use for the prevention of morbidity and mortality from preeclampsia: U.S. Preventive Services Task Force recommendation statement. *Ann Intern Med* 2014;**161**(11):819–26.

81. Carrasco M, Rao SC, Bearer CF, Sundararajan S. Neonatal gabapentin withdrawal syndrome. *Pediatr Neurol* 2015;**53**(5):445–7.

82. Nielsen LR, Pedersen-Bjergaard U, Thorsteinsson B, Johansen M, Damm P, Mathiesen ER. Hypoglycemia in pregnant women with type 1 diabetes: predictors and role of metabolic control. *Diabetes Care* 2008;**31**(1):9–14.

83. Kawaguchi M, Tanigawa K, Tanaka O, Kato Y. Embryonic growth impaired by maternal hypoglycemia during early organogenesis in normal and diabetic rats. *Acta Diabetol* 1994;**31**(3):141–6.

84. Sibai BM, Viteri OA. Diabetic ketoacidosis in pregnancy. *Obstet Gynecol* 2014;**123**(1):167–78.

85. Yamamoto JM, Benham J, Mohammad K, Donovan LE, Wood S. Intrapartum glycaemic control and neonatal hypoglycaemia in pregnancies complicated by diabetes mellitus: a systematic review. *Diabet Med* 2018;**35**(2):173–83.

86. Drever E, Tomlinson G, Bai AD, Feig DS. Insulin pump use compared with intravenous insulin during labour and delivery: the inspired observational cohort study. *Diabet Med* 2016;**33**(9):1253–9.

87. Dashora U, Temple R, Murphy H. *Joint british diabetes societies for inpatient care: management of glycaemic control in pregnant women with diabetes on obstetric wards and delivery units.* Available from http://www.diabetologists-abcd.org.uk/JBDS/JBDS_Pregnancy_final_18082017.pdf; 2017 [Accessed 10 June 2018].

88. Speroff L, Mishell Jr DR. The postpartum visit: it's time for a change in order to optimally initiate contraception. *Contraception* 2008;**78**(2):90–8.

89. Vahratian A, Barber JS, Lawrence JM, Kim C. Family-planning practices among women with diabetes and overweight and obese women in the 2002 national survey for family growth. *Diabetes Care* 2009;**32**(6):1026–31.

90. Beardmore KS, Morris JM, Gallery ED. Excretion of antihypertensive medication into human breast milk: a systematic review. *Hypertens Pregnancy* 2002;**21**(1):85–95.

91. Organization WH, editor. *Indicators for assessing infant and young child feeding practices: conclusion of a consensus meeting held 6–8 November 2007 in Washinton DC, USA 2008. Geneva, Switzerland*; 2008.

92. Finkelstein SA, Keely E, Feig DS, Tu X, Yasseen 3rd AS, Walker M. Breastfeeding in women with diabetes: lower rates despite greater rewards. A population-based study. *Diabet Med* 2013;**30**(9):1094–101.

93. De Bortoli J, Amir LH. Is onset of lactation delayed in women with diabetes in pregnancy? A systematic review. *Diabet Med* 2016;**33**(1):17–24.

94. Achong N, Duncan EL, McIntyre HD, Callaway L. The physiological and glycaemic changes in breastfeeding women with type 1 diabetes mellitus. *Diabetes Res Clin Pract* 2018;**135**:93–101.

95. Forster DA, Moorhead AM, Jacobs SE, Davis PG, Walker SP, McEgan KM, et al. Advising women with diabetes in pregnancy to express breastmilk in late pregnancy (diabetes and antenatal milk expressing [DAME]): a multicentre, unblinded, randomised controlled trial. *Lancet* 2017;**389**(10085):2204–13.

96. Clausen TD, Mathiesen ER, Hansen T, Pedersen O, Jensen DM, Lauenborg J, et al. Overweight and the metabolic syndrome in adult offspring of women with diet-treated gestational diabetes mellitus or type 1 diabetes. *J Clin Endocrinol Metab* 2009;**94**(7):2464–70.

97. Clausen TD, Mathiesen ER, Hansen T, Pedersen O, Jensen DM, Lauenborg J, et al. High prevalence of type 2 diabetes and pre-diabetes in adult offspring of women with gestational diabetes mellitus or type 1 diabetes: the role of intrauterine hyperglycemia. *Diabetes Care* 2008;**31**(2):340–6.

98. Vlachova Z, Bytoft B, Knorr S, Clausen TD, Jensen RB, Mathiesen ER, et al. Increased metabolic risk in adolescent offspring of mothers with type 1 diabetes: the EPICOM study. *Diabetologia* 2015;**58**(7):1454–63.

99. Knorr S, Clausen TD, Vlachova Z, Bytoft B, Damm P, Beck-Nielsen H, et al. Academic achievement in primary school in offspring born to mothers with type 1 diabetes (the EPICOM Study): a Register-Based Prospective Cohort Study. *Diabetes Care* 2015;**38**(7):1238–44.

100. Bytoft B, Knorr S, Vlachova Z, Jensen RB, Mathiesen ER, Beck-Nielsen H, et al. Long-term cognitive implications of intrauterine hyperglycemia in adolescent offspring of women with type 1 diabetes (the EPICOM Study). *Diabetes Care* 2016;**39**(8):1356–63.

Chapter 24

Gut and Pancreatic Neuroendocrine Tumors in Pregnancy and Lactation

Sahar Sherf and Run Yu

Division of Endocrinology, UCLA David Geffen School of Medicine, Los Angeles, CA, United States

Common Clinical Problems

- Neuroendocrine tumors (NETs) of the gut and pancreas are heterogeneous tumors with distinct clinical and pathologic features.
- Appendiceal carcinoid and pancreatic NETs are relatively more common in young women.
- Women with history of appendiceal carcinoids with benign features, or benign insulinoma, are assumed to have unchanged baseline fertility after surgical removal of the tumors.
- Most women with active gut or pancreatic NETs that require treatment are advised against pregnancy, with some exceptions.
- Management of NETs in pregnancy should be multidisciplinary; medical therapy with somatostatin analog is the mainstay of treatment.

24.1 INTRODUCTION

Neuroendocrine tumors (NETs) can arise from most organs, but those from the gut and pancreas are most common and include heterogeneous tumors with distinct clinical and pathologic features.[1–4] The incidence of gut NETs is 2.5 cases per 100,000 per year.[5, 6] Gut NETs are solid masses of neuroendocrine cells containing secretory granules that release various peptide hormones, including serotonin, kinins, histamine, and kallikreins. Gut NETs include gastrin-producing duodenal NETs, somatostatin-producing ampullary NETs, somatostatin-producing gangliocytic paragangliomas, serotonin-producing jejunal and ileal NETs, appendiceal NETs, and colorectal NETs.[1, 2]

According to the Surveillance Epidemiology End Results database, gut NETs in the United States are most commonly found in the small intestine (at 38%).[5, 6] Appendiceal NETs can be classified into typical carcinoids and goblet cell carcinoids, and they comprise only about 5% of gut NETs.[7, 8] Pancreatic NETs (incidence of 0.32 cases per 100,000 per year[5]) are classified in multiple ways.[4, 9] Pancreatic NETs are classified as functioning or nonfunctioning based on whether they cause hormonal hypersecretion syndromes or not. Most functioning pancreatic NETs secrete insulin, gastrin, vasoactive intestinal peptide (VIP), glucagon, or somatostatin. In addition, both gut and pancreatic NETs are divided into subgroups according to tumor grade and stage.[1–4] Although most gut and pancreatic NETs exhibit indolent behaviors, some of them can metastasize to the lymph nodes, liver, and other organs.

In both women and men, gut and pancreatic NETs are usually diseases that strike in late middle age; thus, in women, most gut and pancreatic NETs are diagnosed at postreproductive age.[5, 9] Appendiceal carcinoid and some pancreatic NETs can occur during childhood and young adulthood. Appendiceal carcinoids are usually an incidental finding in young women with a clinical diagnosis of appendicitis who undergo appendectomy.[7, 8, 10] Most appendiceal carcinoids are small (<1 cm) and noninvasive in otherwise healthy young women; appendiceal carcinoids with those benign features have an excellent prognosis and do not require further surgical intervention or surveillance. Rarely, appendiceal carcinoids can be large (>2 cm), invasive, or metastatic to lymph nodes or remote organs. Appendiceal carcinoids with those unfavorable features require right hemicolectomy, lymph node dissection, liver-directed therapies, and systemic therapies.

Pancreatic NETs affect a significant number of young people, including women.[4, 9] In a large series of pancreatic NETs, of the 539 female participants, 143 (26.5%) were under 40 years old at diagnosis of pancreatic NET, including 14 (2.6%) under 20, 48 (8.9%) between 20 and 29, and 81 (15.0%) between 30 and 39.[9] Insulinoma is the most common (38.9%), and gastrinoma the second most common (7.4%) functioning pancreatic NET in female patients younger than 40, whereas nonfunctioning tumors are as common as insulinomas.[9] Benign insulinoma carries an excellent prognosis after surgical resection in general, and in young women in particular.[3, 4, 9] Other pancreatic NETs carry various prognoses depending on the tumor grade and stage, and they may require abdominal surgery, liver-directed therapy, somatostatin analog treatment, and other systemic therapies, which may decrease female fertility.[3, 4, 9]

It needs to be emphasized that due to the low prevalence of gut and pancreatic NETs, there have been no systematic studies on the consequences of those tumors on pregnancy and lactation, or vice versa. Relatively more cases are reported on appendiceal carcinoid and insulinoma before or during pregnancy. The following sections are based on the relationship between pregnancy and lactation and other more common cancers or tumors, case reports, and the authors' clinical experience. General guidelines and reviews on managing cancers in general, and endocrine tumors in particular, related to pregnancy are available.[11, 12]

24.2 PREGNANCY PLANNING AND PROSPECTIVE MANAGEMENT OF GUT AND PANCREATIC NETs IN WOMEN WITH HISTORY OF SUCH TUMORS

24.2.1 Women with no Current Evidence of NETs

Although the topic has never been directly addressed, there has been no clinical or experimental evidence that hormones secreted by gut and pancreatic NETs have specific, long-lasting effects on female fertility. Once the functioning NETs are completely removed surgically, female patients gradually resume their baseline health status. Women with a history of appendiceal carcinoids with benign features are usually assumed to have preserved baseline fertility and general health. Anecdotally, spontaneous pregnancy may happen soon after the removal of appendiceal carcinoids.[13] A successful pregnancy has been reported in a young woman with aggressive appendiceal carcinoids; several years after tumor debulking and intraperitoneal chemotherapy, she became pregnant twice through assisted reproductive methods and delivered a healthy term baby each time.[14] In the authors' clinical experience, most young female patients with benign insulinomas can be fertile after tumor removal. In patients with history of NETs of higher grade and stage, extensive abdominal surgical operation may result in adhesions, and systemic targeted therapy or chemotherapy may result in irregular menstruation or even secondary amenorrhea, resulting in decreased fertility.

There are also no systematic studies on the effects of pregnancy on the recurrence of gut or pancreatic NETs. In our clinical experience, recurrence of gut or pancreatic NETs during or right after pregnancy is exceedingly rare, if it happens at all.

Thus, women with a history of appendiceal carcinoids with benign features or benign insulinomas are assumed to have unchanged baseline fertility after surgical removal of the tumors. There are no specific precautions to be taken before, during, or after pregnancy. If a woman with a history of NET of higher grade and stage wants to become pregnant, she needs to be counseled on her current fertility status and the uncertainty of pregnancy on the risk of recurrence of her previous NETs. In the absence of evidence of higher risk of NET recurrence during pregnancy, we believe that having a history of NET itself is not a contraindication of pregnancy.

24.2.2 Women with Active Gut or Pancreatic NETs

Female patients with small, nonfunctioning pancreatic NETs, often in the background of multiple endocrine neoplasia syndrome type 1 (MEN1)[15] may require only surveillance and do not require any active treatment, especially after the removal of hyperplastic parathyroid glands or parathyroid adenomas and treatment of pituitary tumors if they have MEN1.[16] There are no clear contraindications of pregnancy in those women. If the female MEN1 patients have active pituitary tumors or primary hyperparathyroidism, these issues need to be addressed before considering pregnancy (see Chapters 18 and 21, respectively, for further discussion).[16]

In our experience, most women with active gut or pancreatic NETs that require ongoing treatment don't desire pregnancy due to the burden of the disease, may have irregular menstruation due to their treatments, and are generally advised against pregnancy by their physicians. Several factors make pregnancy a challenging issue. Surgical debulking may cause miscarriages, liver-directed therapies often use radioactive pharmaceuticals or chemotherapeutic agents, systemic therapies with targeted agents such as everolimus and sunitinib may be teratogenic, and peptide receptor radionuclide therapy (PRRT) also uses radiopharmaceuticals.[1–4] Monitoring response to therapies by imaging may be limited in pregnancy, as computed tomography (CT) and nuclear imaging should be used with caution during pregnancy.[17] The only exceptions may be patients with stable gut or pancreatic NETs who require only somatostatin analog or proton pump inhibitor treatments. We are not aware of any case reports on conception while on somatostatin analog treatment for gut or pancreatic NETs, but females treated with somatostatin analog for acromegaly can be pregnant with no adverse fetal consequences.[18, 19]

There are two case reports of pregnancy in women with known and active gastrinomas treated with proton pump inhibitors; a healthy baby was delivered in each case.[20, 21]

If a patient with active gut or pancreatic NETs exhibits a satisfactory treatment response but still has a clear disease burden, and she strongly desires pregnancy, then pausing treatment may be tried to see if the tumor burden remains stable. If the tumor is stable, pregnancy should be possible. A case report describes such a scenario.[22] A young woman with pancreatic NETs with liver metastases was diagnosed 6 years prior to pregnancy. The patient received multiple treatment modalities with a stable disease burden. Pregnancy ensued after pausing all treatment for a year. She underwent induced labor at 38 weeks' gestation; octreotide was not needed. She delivered a healthy baby via uncomplicated vaginal delivery.

There is no clear evidence that gut or pancreatic NETs progress more rapidly in pregnancy. Instead, case reports generally show no tumor progression during pregnancy,[20–22] while other case reports show spontaneous regression of pelvic NETs and bronchial carcinoids after pregnancy in the absence of any treatment.[23–25] It is postulated that pregnancy contributes to tumor regression by immunological response and activation of proapoptotic pathways, cytokines, T and B cells, and growth factors in pregnancy.

The presence of metastatic carcinoid disease in pregnancy, particularly with carcinoid syndrome, may increase the risk of fetal demise. In a review of pregnant patients with carcinoid tumor in 1983, 4 of 18 patients developed carcinoid syndrome; 2 of these patients had successful pregnancies, but the others resulted in fetal death.[26] Hypoglycemia caused by insulinoma during pregnancy may also cause fetal demise.[27]

24.3   GUT AND PANCREATIC NETs FOUND DE NOVO DURING PREGNANCY

It is exceedingly rare that gut or pancreatic NETs are diagnosed de novo during pregnancy. Functioning NETs are usually diagnosed during pregnancy via severe hormonal hypersecretion syndromes, but diagnosis can be particularly challenging because the symptoms of functioning NETs can mimic the physiologic changes or complications of pregnancy.

Carcinoid syndrome is seen in patients with small bowel NET with metastases to the liver as a result of bypassing the hepatic clearance of serotonin from the portal circulation.[1, 2] Carcinoid syndrome is characterized by flushing, diarrhea, abdominal cramps, and (less commonly) right heart valvular lesions (i.e., carcinoid heart disease). Carcinoid crisis is characterized by hemodynamic instability due to the sudden release of large amounts of vasoactive peptides in the circulation, often elicited by anesthesia or invasive procedures. We are not aware of cases of de novo diagnosis of carcinoid syndrome in pregnancy.

Insulinoma is a relatively common functioning NET in pregnancy, and it causes hypoglycemia.[27–30] Pancreatic NET may also secrete parathyroid hormone (PTH)-related protein (PTHrp), which causes hypercalcemia.[31] We are not aware of other functioning pancreatic NETs diagnosed de novo during pregnancy. Nonfunctioning gut and pancreatic NETs present with mass effects, such as gastrointestinal bleeding, abdominal pain, vomiting, or incidental findings.[32–35] The most common nonfunctioning NETs diagnosed de novo in pregnancy is appendiceal carcinoids.[33, 34, 36, 37]

Diagnosis of gut and pancreatic NETs in pregnancy requires a high index of suspicion. As blood glucose levels are often lower during pregnancy and insulinoma is a rare cause of hypoglycemia, hypoglycemia caused by insulinoma is often missed until a profound level is reached.[27–30] It is key to document insulin and proinsulin levels at the time of hypoglycemia to ascertain whether hypoglycemia is caused by insulinoma. High proinsulin levels suggest malignant insulinoma.[30] Magnetic resonance imaging (MRI) usually localizes an insulinoma in the pancreas. Appendiceal carcinoids most commonly present as appendiceal masses found by imaging for abdominal pain in pregnancy, presumably caused by appendicitis; carcinoids are then found in the surgical specimen.[33, 34, 36, 37]

24.4   MANAGEMENT OF GUT AND PANCREATIC NETs DURING PREGNANCY AND PERIPARTUM

The management of gut and pancreatic NETs in pregnancy and peripartum should be individualized based on the tumor grade, stage, hormonal secretion status, and comorbidities. As the care of pregnant patients with NETs is complicated, they should seek care at an institution with a multidisciplinary team of specialists on NETs, including obstetricians and anesthesiologists.[38] We agree with the conclusions of a recent review on management of NETs in pregnancy.[39] Asymptomatic NETs may be best monitored closely, with no intervention. Given the procedural risk and the possibility of disease regression, surgical resection of NETs, which is recommended in nonpregnant patients with localized disease, should be postponed until after delivery if possible. While hepatic artery embolization and radiofrequency ablation have been used in pregnancy, they too should be avoided during organogenesis. Finally, medical therapy with somatostatin analogs also should be deferred in asymptomatic disease or in the absence of carcinoid syndrome, hypoglycemia, other hormonal hypersecretion syndromes, and disease progression.[39] Other systemic therapies such as everolimus, sunitinib, telotristat, and PRRT should mostly be deferred until after pregnancy for their potential fetal risk. Close monitoring for development of symptoms and evidence of tumor progression is nevertheless necessary.

24.4.1 Management of Carcinoid Syndrome in Pregnancy and Peripartum

Although carcinoid syndrome is exceedingly rare in pregnancy, it poses a unique challenge to the treatment team.[22, 26, 39] Contrast studies and biopsies are limited during pregnancy due to iodine exposure and procedural risks; therefore, laboratory testing and ultrasound surveillance are of paramount importance. We recommend frequent laboratory and diagnostic monitoring with serum chromogranin A and serotonin levels, liver function tests, urinary 5-hydroxyindoleacetic acid (5HIAA) level, transthoracic echocardiogram, and abdominal ultrasound every 3 months. Serial abdominal ultrasounds should assess for fetal anomalies and growth, particularly in symptomatic patients treated with octreotide.

It is reasonable to increase the frequency of monitoring in patients with high-grade tumors, secretory tumors, and larger tumors, as well as in symptomatic patients. It should be noted, however, that chromogranin A levels can rise in pregnancy partly due to contributions from the placenta, which has neuroendocrine activity, as well as from stress, so that does not necessarily implicate an increase in tumor size.[40, 41] As such, urinary 5HIAA and serotonin levels may be better indicators of disease stability or progression during pregnancy. In those patients with elevated prepregnancy urinary 5HIAA or evidence of carcinoid heart disease, extra precaution is warranted, as they are at higher risk of complications during labor and delivery.

In contrast to asymptomatic tumors, pregnancies affected by carcinoid syndrome could place patients at higher risk for fetal demise.[26] The management of carcinoid syndrome focuses on blocking the production and release of vasoactive mediators. Octreotide is a synthetic somatostatin analog used to treat carcinoid syndrome during pregnancy.[39] Most circulating octreotide is bound by maternal proteins; the unbound fraction is thought to cross the placenta by passive diffusion and to bind to the placenta and umbilical cord tissues, albeit with low affinity.[42–45] Both the long- and short-acting forms cross the placental barrier, although data indicate that short-acting octreotide is found in lower concentrations in umbilical cord serum, amniotic fluid, and newborn serum.

Octreotide use in pregnancy remains somewhat controversial. Its use during pregnancy has been limited to a small population, most of whom had acromegaly, which showed that octreotide use appears to be largely safe in pregnancy.[45] Fetal weight is normal, and no malformations or cases of abnormal development are noted in pregnancies with octreotide exposure. Over the course of 6 years, linear growth, weight, neuropsychological development, and pituitary function of the children exposed to octreotide in utero remained normal. In one patient, an acute decrease in uterine artery blood flow was seen after octreotide injections, with no effect on pregnancy course, delivery, or fetal development. Octreotide concentrations were high in maternal serum and colostrum, and lower in umbilical cord serum, amniotic fluid, and newborn serum.[44, 45]

We recommend the use of short-acting, subcutaneous octreotide injections for symptomatic carcinoid patients.[22, 39, 42] Intravenous octreotide infusions should be available when anesthesia and surgery are planned or if any signs of carcinoid crisis develop, but they should be used only if truly warranted. In active carcinoid syndrome, an intravenous bolus of octreotide should be given 1–2h before surgery. In the case of an operative carcinoid crisis, an intravenous bolus and infusion of octreotide should be administered.

Appropriate anesthetic management is vital during labor and delivery to avoid a carcinoid crisis.[22, 39, 42] Analgesics should be provided to blunt a hyperadrenergic stress response, and euvolemia should be maintained. If abdominal delivery becomes necessary, both neuraxial and general anesthesia should be given.[22, 42] General anesthesia should avoid drug triggers of carcinoid crisis, and it should help to blunt the stress response. Some suggest epidural over spinal anesthesia for patients with carcinoid syndrome because spinal anesthesia is thought to have more profound effects on sympathetic innervation. However, this is controversial. Furthermore, epidural analgesia should be started before the induction of labor to minimize pain-induced catecholamine release and allow controlled hemodynamic stability.

24.4.2 Management of Insulinoma During Pregnancy and Peripartum

Surgical resection of insulinoma generally should be avoided during pregnancy.[27–30] Medical therapies should be emphasized, including frequent feeding, diazoxide, calcium channel blockers, and subcutaneous octreotide. In patients with recalcitrant and dangerous hypoglycemia, surgical resection or mammalian target of rapamycin (mTOR) inhibitors such as everolimus may have to be used. Early induction of labor can be attempted if the fetus is already mature. Intravenous infusions of octreotide and glucose are important during labor to minimize the risk of severe hypoglycemia.[30]

24.5   LACTATION IN WOMEN WITH GUT AND PANCREATIC NETs

In women with no evidence of disease or with stable NET disease not requiring active treatments, there are no contraindications to breastfeeding. In patients with progressive disease requiring active treatments, breastfeeding is generally challenging due to concern about drug excretion into breast milk, radioactivity exposure, and logistics. Patients requiring only somatostatin analog treatment may breastfeed safely.[19]

24.6   CONCLUSIONS

While gut and pancreatic NETs before or during pregnancy are rare, they present unique challenges to the patient and treatment team. In the absence of objective evidence from systematic studies, we have provided our opinion on the management of these tumors during pregnancy and in prepregnancy planning in patients with known tumors. We drew heavily on experience with other more common cancers or tumors during pregnancy and lactation, case reports, and our own clinical experience.

Our main opinions are that (1) women with a history of appendiceal carcinoids with benign features or benign insulinomas are assumed to have unchanged baseline fertility after surgical removal of the tumor; (2) most women with active gut or pancreatic NETs are advised against pregnancy, with a few exceptions; (3) management of NETs in pregnancy should be multidisciplinary; and (4) medical therapy with somatostatin analog is the mainstay of treatment.

REFERENCES

1. Kunz PL. Carcinoid and neuroendocrine tumors: building on success. *J Clin Oncol* 2015;**33**:1855–63.
2. Kim JY, Hong SM. Recent updates on neuroendocrine tumors from the gastrointestinal and pancreatobiliary tracts. *Arch Pathol Lab Med* 2016;**140**:437–48.
3. Öberg K. Management of functional neuroendocrine tumors of the pancreas. *Gland Surg* 2018;**7**:20–7.
4. Ro C, Chai W, Yu VE, et al. Pancreatic neuroendocrine tumors: biology, diagnosis, and treatment. *Chin J Cancer* 2013;**326**:312–24.
5. Yao JC, Hassan M, Phan A, et al. One hundred years after "carcinoid": epidemiology of and prognostic factors for neuroendocrine tumors in 35,825 cases in the United States. *J Clin Oncol* 2008;**26**:3063–72.
6. Mocellin S, Nitti D. Gastrointestinal carcinoid: epidemiological and survival evidence from a large population-based study. *Ann Oncol* 2013;**24**:3040–4.
7. Tchana-Sato V, Detry O, Polus M, et al. Carcinoid tumor of the appendix: a consecutive series from 1237 appendectomies. *World J Gastroenterol* 2006;**12**:6699–701.
8. Tang LH. Epithelial neoplasms of the appendix. *Arch Pathol Lab Med* 2010;**134**:1612–20.
9. Zhu LM, Tang L, Qiao XW, et al. Differences and similarities in the clinicopathological features of pancreatic neuroendocrine tumors in China and the United States: a multicenter study. *Medicine (Baltimore)* 2016;**95**.
10. Anastasiadis K, Kepertis C, Lampropoulos V, et al. Carcinoid tumors of the appendix-last decade experience. *J Clin Diagn Res* 2014;**8**:NC01–2.
11. Peccatori FA, Azim Jr HA, Orecchia R, et al. Cancer, pregnancy and fertility: ESMO clinical practice guidelines for diagnosis, treatment and follow-up. *Ann Oncol* 2013;**24**(Suppl 6):vi160–170.
12. Lansdown A, Rees DA. Endocrine oncology in pregnancy. *Best Pract Res Clin Endocrinol Metab* 2011;**25**:911–26.
13. Swelstad BB, Brezina PR, Johnson CT. Primary infertility associated with neuroendocrine tumor (Carcinoid) of the appendix. *Asian Pac J Reprod* 2012;**1**:152–4.
14. Smaldone GM, Richard SD, Krivak TC, et al. Pregnancy after tumor debulking and intraperitoneal cisplatin for appendiceal carcinoid tumor. *Obstet Gynecol* 2007;**110**(2 Pt 2):477–9.
15. Thompson NW, Lloyd RV, Nishiyama RH, et al. MEN I pancreas: a histological and immunohistochemical study. *World J Surg* 1984;**8**:561–74.
16. Thakker RV, Newey PJ, Walls GV, et al. Clinical practice guidelines for multiple endocrine neoplasia type 1 (MEN1). *J Clin Endocrinol Metab* 2012;**97**:2990–3011.
17. Committee on Obstetric Practice. Guidelines for diagnostic imaging during pregnancy and lactation. *Obstet Gynecol* 2017;**130**:e210–6.
18. Caron P, Broussaud S, Bertherat J, et al. Acromegaly and pregnancy: a retrospective multicenter study of 59 pregnancies in 46 women. *J Clin Endocrinol Metab* 2010;**95**:4680–7.
19. Assal A, Malcolm J, Lochnan H, et al. Preconception counselling for women with acromegaly: more questions than answers. *Obstet Med* 2016;**9**:9–14.
20. Mayer A, Sheiner E, Holcberg G. Zollinger Ellison syndrome, treated with lansoprazole, during pregnancy. *Arch Gynecol Obstet* 2007;**276**:171–3.
21. Mistry M, Gupta M, Kaler M. Pregnancy in multiple endocrine neoplasia type 1 equals multiple complications. *Obstet Med* 2014;**7**:123–5.
22. Woo KM, Imasogie NN, Bruni I, et al. Anaesthetic management of a pregnant woman with carcinoid disease. *Int J Obstet Anesth* 2009;**18**:272–5.
23. Luosto R, Koikkalainen K, Sipponen P. Spontaneous regression of a bronchial carcinoid tumour following pregnancy. *Ann Chir Gynaecol Fenn* 1974;**63**:342–5.
24. Venkatram S, Sinha N, Hashmi H, et al. Spontaneous regression of endobronchial carcinoid tumor. *J Bronchol Interv Pulmonol* 2017;**24**:70–4.
25. Sewpaul A, Bargiela D, James A, et al. Spontaneous regression of a carcinoid tumor following pregnancy. *Case Rep Endocrinol* 2014;**2014**:481823.

26. Durkin JW. Carcinoid tumor and pregnancy. *Am J Obstet Gynecol* 1983;**145**:757–61.

27. Besemer B, Müssig K. Insulinoma in pregnancy. *Exp Clin Endocrinol Diabetes* 2010;**118**:9–18.

28. Takacs CA, Krivak TC, Napolitano PG. Insulinoma in pregnancy: a case report and review of the literature. *Obstet Gynecol Surv* 2002;**57**:229–35.

29. Diaz AG, Herrera J, López M, et al. Insulinoma associated with pregnancy. *Fertil Steril* 2008;**90**: 199.e1-4.

30. Yu R, Nissen NN, Hendifar A, et al. A clinicopathological study of malignant insulinoma in a contemporary series. *Pancreas* 2017;**46**:48–56.

31. Abraham P, Ralston SH, Hewison M, et al. Presentation of a PTHrP-secreting pancreatic neuroendocrine tumour, with hypercalcaemic crisis, preeclampsia, and renal failure. *Postgrad Med J* 2002;**78**:752–3.

32. Hogan RB, Ahmad N, Hogan 3rd RB, et al. Video capsule endoscopy detection of jejunal carcinoid in life-threatening hemorrhage, first trimester pregnancy. *Gastrointest Endosc* 2007;**66**:205–7.

33. Gilboa Y, Fridman E, Ofir K, et al. Carcinoid tumor of the appendix: ultrasound findings in early pregnancy. *Ultrasound Obstet Gynecol* 2008;**31**:576–8.

34. Korkontzelos I, Papanicolaou S, Tsimoyiannis I, et al. Large carcinoid tumor of the appendix during pregnancy. *Eur J Obstet Gynecol Reprod Biol* 2005;**118**:255–7.

35. CH1 K, Röcken C, Neuhaus P, et al. Non-functioning, malignant pancreatic neuroendocrine tumour (PNET): a rare entity during pregnancy. *Langenbeck's Arch Surg* 2009;**394**:387–91.

36. Pitiakoudis M, Kirmanidis M, Tsaroucha A, et al. Carcinoid tumor of the appendix during pregnancy. A rare case and a review of the literature. *J BUON* 2008;**13**:271–5.

37. Piatek S, Gajewska M, Panek G, et al. Carcionoid of the appendix in pregnant woman-case report and literature review. *Neuro Endocrinol Lett* 2017;**37**:535–9.

38. Metz DC, Choi J, Strosberg J, et al. A rationale for multidisciplinary care in treating neuroendocrine tumours. *Curr Opin Endocrinol Diabetes Obes* 2012;**19**:306–13.

39. Kevat D, Chen M, Wyld D, et al. A case of pulmonary carcinoid in pregnancy and review of carcinoid tumours in pregnancy. *Obstet Med* 2017;**10**:142–9.

40. Florio P, Mezzesimi A, Turchetti V, et al. High levels of human chromogranin A in umbilical cord plasma and amniotic fluid at parturition. *J Soc Gynecol Investig* 2002;**9**:32–6.

41. Syversen U, Opsjøn SL, Stridsberg M, et al. Chromogranin A and pancreastatin-like immunoreactivity in normal pregnancies. *J Clin Endocrinol Metab* 1996;**81**:4470–5.

42. Le BT, Bharadwaj S, Malinow AM. Carcinoid tumor and intravenous octreotide infusion during labor and delivery. *Int J Obstet Anesth* 2009;**18**:182–5.

43. McLean LK, Roussis P, Bradley B, et al. Carcinoid tumors and pregnancy: case report and review of the literature. *J Matern Fet Med* 1994;**3**:139–41.

44. Pistilli B, Grana C, Fazio N. Pregnant with metastatic neuroendocrine tumour of the ovary: what now? *Ecancermedicalscience* 2012;**6**:240.

45. Maffei P, Tamango G, Nardelli GB, et al. Effects of octreotide exposure during pregnancy in acromegaly. *Clin Endocrinol* 2010;**72**:668–77.

Chapter 25

Adrenal Pathologies During Pregnancy and Postpartum

Matthieu St-Jean, Isabelle Bourdeau and André Lacroix

Division of Endocrinology, Department of Medicine and Research Center, Centre hospitalier de l'Université de Montréal (CHUM), Montréal, QC, Canada

---

Common Clinical Problems

- Primary adrenal insufficiency is rarely diagnosed during pregnancy, but its diagnosis must be suspected in the context of persistent and severe hyperemesis gravidarum.
- Cushing's syndrome during pregnancy is caused by adrenal disease in 50%–60% of cases.
- Adrenocortical carcinoma diagnosed during pregnancy is associated with a poorer survival than if diagnosed in nonpregnant patients.
- Primay aldosteronism is probably underdiagnosed during pregnancy and uncontrolled hypertension seems to be the main contributor to materno-fetal morbidity.
- Pheochromocytoma and paraganglioma are associated with poorer maternal and fetal outcomes if undiagnosed in the antenatal period.
- Prenatal treatment for the prevention of female genital virilization in the context of congenital adrenal hyperplasia remains controversial because of the concerns for long-term safety on the cognition and behavior of the in utero exposed child to glucocorticoids.

25.1 INTRODUCTION

In this chapter, we will review the diagnostic approach and management of the most common adrenal disorders during pregnancy. Their diagnosis can be particularly difficult because of overlap between their nonspecific symptoms and those physiologic impacts of pregnancy on endocrine systems. It is primordial to diagnose and treat those diseases appropriately in pregnancy because of their significant morbidity and mortality for both mother and fetus.

25.1.1 Adrenal Insufficiency

Adrenal insufficiency (AI) is characterized by inability of the adrenal cortex to produce sufficient amounts of glucocorticoids or mineralocorticoids.[13] AI can be caused by impairment of the adrenal cortex, known as *primary adrenal insufficiency* (PAI); pituitary adrenocorticotropic hormone (ACTH) secretion (secondary); or hypothalamic corticotropin-releasing hormone (CRH) secretion (tertiary).[14] In primary AI, the adrenal cortex is unable to produce sufficient glucocorticoids, mineralocorticoids, or androgens.[11] In secondary and tertiary AI, mineralocorticoid production is maintained because aldosterone production is mainly regulated by angiotensin II (ANG II) and potassium[11] (Table 25.1). In this chapter, we will focus on primary AI and only briefly describe secondary and tertiary AI, which are discussed more extensively in Chapter 18.

25.1.2 Epidemiology

In the general population, secondary and tertiary AI are more common than PAI.[15] The prevalence of secondary AI is estimated to be between 150 and 280/million. The prevalence of PAI is estimated to be between 100 and 140/million and its

Maternal-Fetal and Neonatal Endocrinology. https://doi.org/10.1016/B978-0-12-814823-5.00025-8

TABLE 25.1 Most common etiologies of adrenal insufficiency in the general population in developed countries

Primary adrenal insufficiency

Autoimmune adrenalitis (Addison's disease): 80%–90%
  Isolated (40%)
  Autoimmune polyglandular syndrome (APS) (60%)
    APS 1 (hypoparathyroidism and mucocutaneous candidiasis)
    APS 2 (hypothyroidism and Type 1 diabetes)
    APS 4 (vitiligo, celiac disease, alopecia, and autoimmune gastritis)

Infectious adrenalitis:
  Tuberculosis
  HIV/AIDS
  Fungal: histoplasmosis, cryptococcosis, and coccidiomycosis

Bilateral adrenal hemorrhage
  Antiphospholipid syndrome
  Meningococcemia
  Anticoagulants
  Abdominal surgery

Bilateral adrenal metastasis

Bilateral adrenal infiltration
  Primary adrenal lymphoma
  Amyloidosis
  Hemochromatosis

Genetic disorder:
  Adrenoleukodystrophy (X-linked disorder)
  Congenital adrenal hyperplasia:
    21-hydroxylase deficiency, 3β-hydroxysteroid dehydrogenase Type 2 deficiency, 11β-hydroxylase deficiency, 17α-hydroxylase
      deficiency, CYP450scc, congenital lipoid adrenal hyperplasia (STAR deficiency)
  Familial glucocorticoid deficiency
  Triple A syndrome

Drugs:
  Ketoconazole, fluconazole, and etomidate
  Trilostane
  Mifepristone
  Phenobarbital, phenytoin, rifampicin

Bilateral adrenalectomy

Secondary and tertiary adrenal insufficiency

Excess of exogenous glucocorticoids or endogenous glucocorticoids (CS)

Pituitary or hypothalamic tumor:
  Craniopharyngioma
  Adenoma
  Meningioma
  Cyst
  Metastasis

Pituitary stalk trauma

Pituitary or hypothalamic surgery/irradiation

Infiltrative process or infectious of the pituitary, hypothalamus, or both:
  Hemochromatosis
  Tuberculosis
  Meningitis
  Sarcoidosis
  Histiocytosis X
  Wegener granulomatosis
  Lymphocytic hypophysitis

Pituitary apoplexy

Sheehan syndrome

Genetic: POMC mutation, HESX1, ...

Modified from Charmandari E, Nicolaides NC, Chrousos GP. Adrenal insufficiency. *Lancet* 2014;**383**(9935):2152–2167.

incidence around four new cases per million per year.[13] However, during pregnancy, the causes of AI are evenly distributed between PAI (44%) and secondary AI (45%).[14] PAI was found to affect mostly women in one study but other studies have found it affects men and women equally.[11] PAI can occur at any age, but the peak age at diagnosis is 30–40 years.[16] PAI is very rare in pregnancy, despite affecting mostly women of reproductive age, possibly because decreased fertility rate can also occur, secondary to chronic anovulation or autoimmune oophoritis.[14,17,18] A recent U.S. population-based retrospective cohort study (2003–11) reported a prevalence of 5.5 cases/100,000 pregnant women[16]; the prevalence of PAI in pregnancy increased from 5.6 to 9.6 cases/100,000 over the 9-year study period.[16] Most cases of AI are already diagnosed before pregnancy.[14,15] The incidence of new cases of autoimmune PAI during pregnancy is very rare, probably because of the pregnancy-induced immunotolerance.[19] Between 1950 and 2017, there were only 10 published cases of autoimmune PAI diagnosed during pregnancy[1–9,14]; diagnosis of these new-onset PAI cases was evenly distributed between trimesters.[14] Few cases were diagnosed in the early postpartum period.[14] The prevalence of secondary AI in the context of pregnancy is unknown.[11]

25.1.3 Etiologies

Autoimmune destruction of the adrenal cortex is the most common cause of PAI in developed countries, whereas tuberculosis is the main cause worldwide.[11,14] Frequently, there are other autoimmune diseases associated with Addison's disease during pregnancy (Table 25.1). In a recent review, 41.7% of patients with PAI were reported to also have autoimmune hypothyroidism, and 8% had Type 1 diabetes.[14] Others causes of PAI include infectious adrenalitis, bilateral adrenal hemorrhage or infiltration or metastasis, bilateral adrenalectomy (Cushing's disease (CD), genetic bilateral pheochromocytomas), drugs, and genetic disorders such as congenital adrenal hyperplasia (discussed later in this chapter). Rare cases of bilateral adrenal hemorrhage that occur during pregnancy or in the puerperium were reported in the research literature.[20] AI is found in 50% of nonpregnant patients following bilateral adrenal hemorrhage.[21] However, the incidence of PAI in pregnant patients with bilateral adrenal hemorrhage is unknown, as they were only case reports. Bilateral adrenal hemorrhage during pregnancy can be caused by pregnancy-induced hypercoagulability, which may trigger adrenal vein thrombosis in women with preexisting thrombophilic disorder.[19]

The most common cause of secondary and tertiary AI in the general population is secondary to exogenous glucocorticoid therapy for inflammatory diseases.[11,17] However, the prevalence of AI secondary to exogenous glucocorticoid use is unknown in pregnancy.[11] Hypothalamic-pituitary-adrenal (HPA) axis suppression should be suspected if a patient recently received ≥5 mg of prednisone equivalent for ≥3 weeks .[11,19] Interestingly, repeat courses (2 days weekly repeated for ≥2 times) of short-term betamethasone for preterm delivery induced maternal HPA axis suppression[11,22]; in contrast, a single short-term course (2 days) of betamethasone did not induce maternal HPA axis suppression.[23] Pregnancy is a period of stress, and patients with chronic exposure to exogenous glucocorticoids are at particular risk of decompensation; however, only isolated cases of pregnant patients presenting in secondary adrenal crisis have been reported.[11] Others causes of secondary or tertiary AI include pituitary or hypothalamic tumors, their surgery, infiltrative diseases, trauma, or necrosis of the pituitary, hypothalamus, or both.[24] There are frequently other pituitary or hypothalamic hormone deficits in these patients that need to be remedied.[25] Usually, cases of secondary or tertiary AI are already known and treated before conception.[14] However, pregnancy in the context of hypopituitarism is associated with higher rates of obstetrical complications.[25]

There are two causes of secondary/tertiary AI that are specifically related to pregnancy or the early puerperium: postpartum pituitary necrosis (Sheehan syndrome) and lymphocytic hypophysitis.[11,14,17] Sheehan syndrome is a pituitary (and sometimes also hypothalamic) infarction and necrosis that results from blood flow interruption to the adenohypophysis.[26] The main risk factors are postpartum hemorrhage, anemia, or hypotension occurring in a gland that is richly vascularized and in the physiological hyperplastic stage, with increased secretion of oxytocin at time of delivery.[26,27] The degree of hypopituitarism (secondary or tertiary) that develops depends on the extent of the necrosis in the pituitary and hypothalamus.[26] With improved obstetrical care, the incidence of Sheehan syndrome has decreased over time.[11,27] It can present with failure to lactate or to resume normal menses, but the diagnosis also must be considered in postpartum women with seizure, hypoglycemia, or coma.[11,27] A certain degree of ACTH deficiency is frequent in Sheehan syndrome, as has been demonstrated by an abnormal insulin tolerance test response in 92% of patients in a case series.[26] Also, secondary AI was the presenting sign in 57% (12/21) of patients with acute severe Sheehan syndrome.[27] However, most cases of Sheehan are mild, with a delay of several years before diagnosis.[26]

Lymphocytic hypophysitis can affect only the anterior pituitary, but it can also affect the infundibulo-hypophysis.[28] The process underlying the development of lymphocytic hypophysis is unknown, but speculated to be autoimmune.[28] This is supported by the fact that almost 30% of patients with lymphocytic hypophysitis also have coexisting autoimmune disease, such as Type 1 diabetes, Addison's disease, Hashimoto thyroiditis, and pernicious anemia.[28] Lymphocytic hypophysitis is more frequently diagnosed in the last trimester of pregnancy or the first postpartum year, but it also is described in non-pregnant women and men.[28] In 65% of cases, lymphocytic hypophysitis is associated with secondary AI.[28]

25.1.4 Clinical Presentation

The clinical presentation of AI differs between primary and secondary-tertiary etiologies, and this fact should guide clinicians in narrowing the differential diagnosis.

25.1.4.1 Primary AI

The most frequent symptoms reported in the 10 new-onset cases of autoimmune PAI during pregnancy were the classic symptoms, such as nausea, vomiting, extreme fatigue, weight loss, dizziness, muscle weakness, and anorexia (Table 25.2).[1–9] However, these symptoms also occur frequently in normal pregnancy, making the diagnosis of mild PAI challenging.[29] New-onset PAI can mimic hyperemesis gravidarum during pregnancy, and five cases of hyperemesis gravidarum-like secondary to PAI were reported.[2–4,7,8,11] AI may also present during pregnancy with neuropsychiatric symptoms such as psychosis.[11] Skin hyperpigmentation is a frequently encountered sign, being noted in 80% of PAI patients diagnosed during pregnancy[1–9]; it results from stimulation of the skin melanocortin receptor 1 by the elevated ACTH.[30] It can be mistaken for physiologic chloasma of pregnancy, a skin hyperpigmentation restricted to sun-exposed areas; hyperpigmentation driven by ACTH is more commonly encountered in areas of mechanical friction such as scars, nipples, knuckles, toes, and oral mucosa.[29,30]

TABLE 25.2 Incidence of symptoms and signs in the 10 cases of autoimmune primary adrenal insufficiency diagnosed during pregnancy reported in the literature[1–9]

Symptoms
Hyperemesis gravidarum or nausea/vomiting: 8/10 (80%)
Fatigue: 6/10 (60%)
Weight loss: 5/10 (50%)
Dizziness: 5/10 (50%)
Headache: 4/10 (40%)
Muscle weakness or aches: 4/10 (40%)
Anorexia: 3/10 (30%)
Signs
Dark pigmentation of the skin: 8/10 (80%)
Orthostatic hypotension: 4/10 (40%)
Laboratory findings
Hyponatremia (> 5 mmol/L from N): 9/10 (90%)
Adrenal antibodies: 5/6 (83%)[a]
Metabolic acidosis: 3/10 (30%)
Hypoglycemia: 1/10 (10%)
Hyperkaliemia: 1/10 (10%)[b]
Others
Other autoimmune endocrinopathies: 7/10 (70%)
Familial history of autoimmune disease: 2/10 (20%)

Note: The symptoms, signs, and other elements are not always mentioned if they were verified.
[a]*Measured in only six cases.*
[b]*Potassium measured after spontaneous abruption at 31 weeks' gestation.*[9]

Mineralocorticoid deficiency of PAI causes dizziness and orthostatic hypotension.[30] Normal pregnancy is associated with a small reduction in serum sodium of <5 mmol/L.[11] AI must be excluded if hyponatremia is more severe than this; hyponatremia was found in almost every case of new-onset autoimmune PAI during pregnancy[11] (Table 25.2). Mineralocorticoid deficiency may also cause a metabolic acidosis and hyperkalemia.[30]

In autoimmune adrenalitis, there is frequently a history of other autoimmune disease in the patient or family (Table 25.2).[11,30] In 50% of bilateral adrenal hemorrhage, there are symptoms and signs compatible with AI, and the majority of patients complain of constant upper abdominal pain or tenderness.[20] Therefore, bilateral adrenal hemorrhage must be excluded in the context of PAI with constant upper abdominal pain.[11,17]

PAI during pregnancy also may present in acute adrenal crisis, precipitated by stressful situations that usually necessitate a marked increase in cortisol level. These include hyperemesis gravidarum, infections during pregnancy or postpartum, new-onset hypothyroidism, new supplementation of hypothyroidism (which increases cortisol clearance), hyperthyroidism, labor, delivery, surgery, or with noncompliance to therapy.[11,14,19,30] Adrenal crisis is a life-threatening condition presenting with hypotension or hypovolaemic shock, severe weakness, hypoglycemia, confusion or reduced consciousness, acute abdominal pain, vomiting, and often fever.[13,30] In acute adrenal crisis, treatment must be started immediately to avoid a high mortality risk.[14]

25.1.4.2 Secondary and Tertiary AI

Patients with secondary or tertiary AI rarely exhibit orthostasis and hypotension or hyperkalemia because they conserve normal mineralocorticoid physiology under the regulation of ANG II and potassium.[11] However, despite normal aldosterone levels, cortisol deficiency will present with relatively hypervolemic hyponatremia secondary to increased levels of vasopressin (decreased cortisol feedback on vasopressin secretion).[24] Secondary or tertiary AI is not associated with skin hyperpigmentation because ACTH levels are not increased. Symptoms and signs secondary to the local effects of space-occupying lesions in or above the sella turcica, such as headache, visual fields disturbance, or associated hypopituitarism, may be present.[11,17] Corticotrope deficit is usually a late presentation of pituitary lesions, and the patients usually have other pituitary deficits.[11]

Typical signs of postpartum hypopituitarism that can be due to Sheehan syndrome or lymphocytic hypophysitis include failure of lactation or resumption of menses.[11,17] In Sheehan syndrome, the majority of the symptoms and signs are those of pituitary hormone deficit.[27] In a recent case series of acute Sheehan syndrome, only 6/21 (29%) women reported severe headache during delivery, and there was no correlation between headache and pituitary deficits.[27] In lymphocytic hypophysitis, partial or panhypopituitarism occur in approximatively 80% of the cases, with a predilection for corticotrope and thyrotrope involvement.[28] Multiple hormone deficiencies are found in 75% of cases.[28] Patients with lymphocytic hypophysitis frequently reported mass effect symptoms such as headache in 60% and visual disturbance in 40% of cases.[28]

25.1.5 Diagnosis

The diagnosis of AI in pregnancy is challenging because of the physiologic hypercortisolism that is present during pregnancy. As reported in Chapter 8, total and free cortisol increase progressively during pregnancy to reach levels that are two to three times higher than in nonpregnant women during the third trimester.[11] Also, the regulation of the HPA axis is modified during pregnancy. One pertinent point in the investigation of AI is that the adrenal response to ACTH is increased by 60%–80% in pregnant women compared to nonpregnant patients.[17]

The diagnostic approach of possible AI depends on the degree of clinical suspicion and pretest probability (Fig. 25.1). In fact, in the context of high clinical suspicion such as in acute adrenal crisis, the treatment must be instituted rapidly after drawing a blood sample to measure cortisol, aldosterone, ACTH, and renin if possible, or testing should be postponed until after patient stabilization.[14] The diagnostic approach can be divided into three principal objectives: (1) evaluation of cortisol levels and the functional integrity of the HPA axis, (2) determination of the subcategory (primary or secondary/tertiary) of the AI by measuring the ACTH levels, and (3) identifying the cause of the AI (e.g., autoimmune, tuberculosis, pituitary adenoma).[11,17]

25.1.5.1 Random or Morning Cortisol Levels

In the nonpregnant and pregnant population, a morning cortisol <83 nmol/L usually confirms the diagnosis of AI in the setting of a suggestive clinical presentation.[11,19,31] Also, the most recent Endocrine Society clinical guidelines on PAI indicate that a morning cortisol <140 nmol/L with an elevated ACTH (≥2 times the upper limit of normal) are sufficient to diagnose PAI.[13] In a recent review, Anand and Beuschlein support the utilization of this cutoff in the pregnant population

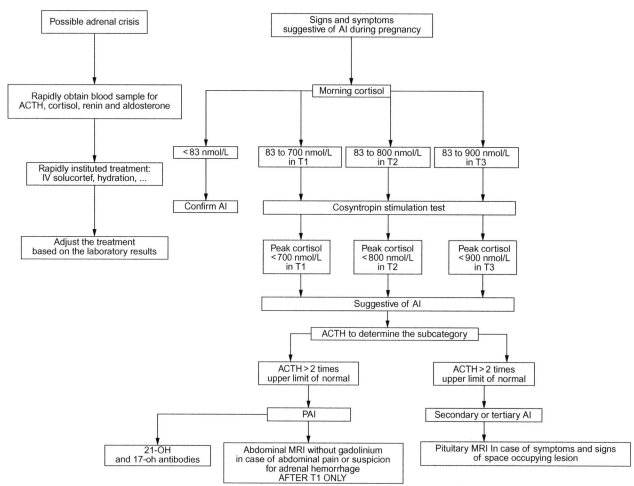

FIG. 25.1 Proposed algorithm for diagnosis of AI during pregnancy.

as well.[14] Some authors suggest that AI can be excluded in the first and early second trimesters when the morning cortisol is >525 nmol/L in clinically stable pregnant women.[11,15]

However, caution is needed when interpreting the morning cortisol value in pregnant women during the second and third trimesters of pregnancy, given the fact that cortisol may appear falsely normal in patients with AI, particularly with partial AI.[11,19] In two recent studies that included healthy pregnant women, the mean morning cortisol levels were 833.1 and 878 nmol/L in the second trimester and 973.5 and 1043 nmol/L in the third trimester, respectively.[32,33] Therefore, it seems appropriate to suggest that pregnant women suspected of having AI who have morning cortisol between 83 and 700–900 nmol/L, depending on the trimester, should undergo a stimulation test to evaluate the adrenal reserve.[19] The only stimulation testing that is approved in the context of pregnancy is the cosyntropin stimulation test; the insulin-induced hypoglycemia test and the metyrapone stimulation test are contraindicated during pregnancy for safety reasons.[11,14]

25.1.5.2 Cosyntropin Stimulation Test

Cosyntropin (1–24 corticotropin) is defined by the U.S. Food and Drug Administration (FDA) as a Category C drug for administration during pregnancy, but a single dose used during a stimulation test is unlikely to have significant adverse effects.[11,13] The test consists of administering 250 mcg of cosyntropin as an intravenous (IV) or intramuscular bolus and measuring cortisol levels before the administration and again 30 and 60 min after it.[11] It can be performed at any time during the day.[13] In the Endocrine Society clinical guidelines on PAI, the standard dose of 250 mcg was proposed as the test to use in the diagnosis of PAI because it is well validated, and the low-dose (1 mcg) cosyntropin test does not provide best diagnostic accuracy.[13] The standard-dose cosyntropin test provides a sensitivity of 92% in the diagnosis of PAI.[34] In the investigation of secondary AI, the guidelines of the Endocrine Society on the hormonal replacement in hypopituitarism of 2017 do not suggest one dosage over the other, given the fact that in one meta-analysis including 30 studies,[34] the diagnostic performance of both tests were similar for the investigation of hypopituitarism.[31] The sensitivity of both the standard and low-dose cosyntropin tests is less in the context of secondary AI than PAI, but the sensitivity for the low-dose test seems a little bit higher (83%) than the standard-dose test (64%).[34] It should also be noted that in recent onsets of secondary AI, the cosyntropin test may be normal because the adrenal still responds to exogenous ACTH.[14]

In nonpregnant patients, the cosyntropin test is considered normal when the peak cortisol value is more than 500 or 550 nmol/L, depending on the studies, and the normal values tend to be lower with more precise LC-MS assays.[34] However, this threshold cannot be used during pregnancy because of the increases in cortisol-binding globulin (CBG) and total cortisol and increased adrenal responsiveness to ACTH during pregnancy. Suri et al.[35] have evaluated the response of total serum cortisol to a standard-dose cosyntropin test in 36 healthy pregnant women throughout pregnancy, and they reported median levels up to 1000 nmol/L during the second and third trimesters of pregnancy. These levels were higher than the response in the postpartum state.[35] The mean (±SD) plasma total cortisol after cosyntropin stimulation was 813.9 ± 154.5 nmol/L in the first trimester, 1045.7 ± 248.3 nmol/L in the second trimester, and 957.4 ± 206.9 nmol/L in the third trimester.[35] However, in this study including healthy pregnant women, the range of stimulated peak total cortisol is large, with the lower values being 331.2 nmol/L in the first trimester, 662.2 nmol/L in the second trimester, and 552 nmol/L in the third trimester.[35]

Based on these findings, as well as the increased level of total cortisol during pregnancy, it is suggested to use higher-than-normal diagnostic thresholds for poststimulation cortisol levels during pregnancy. Many authors have suggested the following cutoffs of poststimulation total cortisol: 700 nmol/L in the first trimester, 800 nmol/L in the second trimester, and 900 nmol/L in the third trimester.[13,14,19,30] These thresholds err on the side of safety, and the diagnostic performance of these suggested thresholds is still unknown.[30] Therefore, these thresholds probably include many normal pregnant women, and clinical judgment must be exerted before diagnosing AI in a pregnant woman based on these cutoffs. In the postpartum period, the threshold of 500 nmol/L use in the nonpregnant patient can be used.[19]

Only two studies reported stimulated total cortisol values with the low-dose cosyntropin test. The two studies were conducted to evaluate the incidence of secondary AI after a single or repeated course of betamethasone for preterm delivery in the third trimester of pregnancy.[22,23] Both have demonstrated that all control pregnant patients had peak serum total cortisol levels over 828 nmol/L.[22,23] In the study with repeated doses of betamethasone, the 18 pregnant women who received the betamethasone developed secondary AI, and their mean peak-stimulated cortisol levels were 298 ± 38.6 nmol/L.[22] In that study, the diagnosis could be predicted in most patients by a morning cortisol value <83 nmol/L; in fact, only 17% of patients with a subnormal cortisol peak during the low-dose cosyntropin test had a morning cortisol >83 nmol/L.[22] However, there are no existing data for the use of the low-dose cosyntropin stimulation test in the other trimesters of pregnancy.

25.1.5.3 Differentiation Between Primary and Secondary-Tertiary AI

The ACTH levels are useful to determine if the AI is of primary versus secondary or tertiary origin.[13] An ACTH level that is twice the upper limit of normal is consistent with PAI in both nonpregnant and pregnant patients.[13,14] An ACTH value >66 pmol/L provides maximal stimulation of the adrenal cortex for cortisol secretion.[13] In PAI cases diagnosed during pregnancy, ACTH levels were elevated, with values between 18.56 and 330 pmol/L.[2–4] As ACTH levels fluctuate from day to day, a single value may not be sufficient for the diagnosis of either primary or secondary AI, and the test may need to be repeated.[11,31] A falsely low result can be obtained if the sample is not placed in an ice bath immediately and then promptly centrifuged and refrigerated in the laboratory.[11]

Another suggestive element of PAI is the presence of mineralocorticoid deficiency.[11] However, during pregnancy, there is a physiological upregulation of the renin-angiotensin-aldosterone system,[36] and the cutoff for abnormal levels during pregnancy in the context of PAI has not been established.[11] To our knowledge, aldosterone and renin levels were reported in only one case report of PAI during pregnancy. In this case of a pregnant woman with previously known Addison's disease that was not compliant to therapy, her supine and standing aldosterone were suppressed, and renin was grossly elevated.[37] Also, as mentioned previously, hyperkalemia is rarely noted in the context of PAI diagnosed during pregnancy.[30]

In the context of secondary AI, the other pituitary hormones need to be assessed.[11,17] However, it is important to take into consideration the physiologic changes in pituitary hormone levels during pregnancy that are discussed in Chapter 3.

25.1.5.4 Determining the Etiology of Primary or Secondary/Tertiary AI

Most of the case of PAI in Western countries are due to autoimmune adrenalitis.[14] In a cohort of nonpregnant patients, 90% of primary AI cases were positive for 21-hydroxylase antibodies and 30% were positive for 17-hydroxylase or side-chain cleavage enzymes.[11] When measured, adrenal antibodies were reported to be positive in most cases of PAI that were newly diagnosed during pregnancy.[2–5,7] The presence of positive antibodies should raise the suspicion for other autoimmune endocrinopathies, and a workup for other endocrine autoimmune diseases, such as thyroid disease and Type 1 diabetes, is recommended.[17] Imaging may be useful in the context of negative adrenal antibodies to diagnose other causes of PAI.[17] It can identify large adrenal glands associated with tuberculosis or other fungal infections, bilateral adrenal metastasis, hemorrhage, or infarction.[17] If possible, it is preferable to delay imaging until the postpartum period, but if needed during pregnancy, magnetic resonance imaging (MRI) without gadolinium injection is the technique of choice.[17] MRI is contraindicated during the first trimester of pregnancy because of the risk for teratogenic unproven effect, so it is preferable to do it after the 32nd week of pregnancy.[38]

In the context of secondary AI, pituitary MRI without gadolinium injection can be used safely in the third trimester, particularly in patients with mass effect symptoms, to identify the presence of a pituitary tumor, lymphocytic hypophysitis, or pituitary apoplexy.[14,17,39] If there are no mass effect symptoms, the pituitary MRI can be delayed until the postpartum period.[14,17]

25.1.6 Morbidity and Complications Associated with AI in Pregnancy

Before the availability of hormonal replacement therapy, AI was associated with high maternal mortality. Before 1930, the mortality rate from AI among women during pregnancy was 35%.[17] Since 1950, though, maternal death associated with AI has rarely been reported.[15–17] However, Addison's disease during pregnancy is associated with significant fetal morbidity. A recent population-based cohort study reported that women with Addison's disease who gave birth <3 years after diagnosis have an increased risk of preterm delivery (odds ratio (OR) 2.40; 95% confidence interval (CI) 1.27–4.53), and of having a low-birth-weight infant (OR 3.50; 95% CI 1.83–6.67) when compared to controls.[18] Low-birth-weight risk was much higher if the mother was diagnosed <1 year before giving birth (OR 4.52; 95% CI 1.53–13.33).[18]

Another recent, retrospective, population-based cohort study reported that women with Addison's disease were more likely to deliver preterm (OR 1.50; 95% CI 1.16–1.95), have small-for-gestational-age infants (OR 1.78; 95% CI 1.15–2.75), have impaired wound healing (OR 4.28; 95% CI 2.55–7.18), develop intrapartum or postpartum infections (OR 2.44; 95% CI 1.66–3.58), develop thromboembolism (OR 5.21; 95% CI 2.15–12.63), require transfusion (OR 6.69; 95% CI 4.69–9.54), and have prolonged postpartum hospital admissions (OR 5.71; 95% CI 4.37–7.47) compared to controls.[16] Maternal mortality was also significantly increased in pregnant women with Addison's disease (OR 22.30; 95% CI 6.82–72.96).[16]

The data on congenital malformation risks are conflicting.[16,18] There are case reports of fetal distress, oligohydramnios, intrauterine death, and neonatal death linked to autoimmune adrenalitis during pregnancy.[4,6,7,9,17]

The maternal side effects of excessive glucocorticoid treatment include hypertension, edema, easy bruising, and exacerbation of preeclampsia.[17] Excessive glucocorticoid replacement can provoke adverse effects on the fetus, such as low birth weight and premature delivery, long-term impact on the HPA axis, and possible susceptibility to cardiometabolic disorders.[19]

25.1.7 Therapy

The management of AI during pregnancy is preferably done by a multidisciplinary team that includes an endocrinologist, an obstetrician, and, in cases of secondary AI associated with a pituitary tumor, an experienced pituitary surgeon.[11] The roles of the endocrinologist are to diagnose, supplement, and monitor glucocorticoid and mineralocorticoid deficiency during pregnancy, labor, and puerperium.[11,14] The main goals of replacement hormonal therapy are to avoid adrenal crisis, as well as underreplacement and overreplacement because they are associated with increased risk of maternal and fetal complications.[14] In the case of secondary/tertiary AI associated with a large pituitary tumor that produces mass effect symptoms, the team must decide on the optimal timing of surgery, which is usually the second trimester. In cases where there is no indication for emergency surgery, it is better to delay it until the postpartum period.[11,17]

25.1.7.1 Glucocorticoid Replacement

Hydrocortisone is the glucocorticoid substitution of choice, as it is metabolized by the placental 11β-hydroxysteroid dehydrogenase Type 2 (11β-HSD 2).[14,19] Dexamethasone is contraindicated during pregnancy because it is not inactivated by the placental 11β-HSD 2 and can readily cross the placenta.[11,13,19,31] In the majority of cases of AI treated during pregnancy, hydrocortisone was used with or without mineralocorticoids .[14] Hydrocortisone should be divided into two or three oral doses during the day—the first and highest dose rapidly at awakening and the second dose 2 h after lunch if the two-dose regimen is used, or the second dose at lunch and the third in the afternoon if the three-dose regimen is used.[13] The best regimen of glucocorticoid replacement during pregnancy is not well established.[31] In clinical practice, women with AI who are taking oral contraceptive pills, which increase CBG and total cortisol similar to the way pregnancy does, do not have increased glucocorticoid requirements.[11,19]

There are two suggested approaches to optimize the glucocorticoid replacement regimen during pregnancy. The first is to follow the patient frequently and adjust the glucocorticoids based on clinical evaluation; the second is to increase by 20%–40% the daily glucocorticoid dosage at 24 weeks' gestation to reflect the physiologic increase in free cortisol associated with pregnancy.[13,31] Close clinical evaluation is recommended at least once every trimester to monitor for signs of underreplacement or overreplacement, including weight gain, fatigue, blood pressure (BP), and glycemic control.[13]

During labor and delivery, a stress dose of 100 mg hydrocortisone given intravenously is suggested during the second stage of labor, followed by a continuous infusion of hydrocortisone at a rate of 100–200 mg/24 h.[13,14] Similar hydrocortisone dosage can be given for cesarean section.[14,31] After delivery, the hydrocortisone can be rapidly decreased to the prepregnancy dosage over a period of 24–72 h to a week, based on the postpartum clinical evolution.[13,14,17,19]

Lactation is not contraindicated in women with AI receiving physiological doses of hydrocortisone replacement, given that even at a dose of 80 mg/day of prednisolone, the infant will ingest <0.1% of the dose.[14]

25.1.7.2 Mineralocorticoid Replacement

Mineralocorticoid replacement therapy is only necessary in PAI[11]; however, not all patients with PAI need this treatment because hydrocortisone may rarely provide sufficient mineralocorticoid activity.[11] The usual daily doses of oral fludrocortisone in nonpregnant patients range from 0.05 to 0.2 mg/day.[13] During normal pregnancy, there is an increase in aldosterone secretion to counteract the antimineralocorticoid effect of the increasing progesterone and to maintain the hemodynamic equilibrium.[13] However, the daily requirement of fludrocortisone during pregnancy is more variable; some will need an increase in their total daily dose, but others will not.[19] The fludrocortisone changes should be based on BP, orthostatic symptoms, and potassium. An increase of fludrocortisone might be necessary in cases of hypotension, postural hypotension, and hyperkalemia. Sometimes it is necessary to decrease the fludrocortisone dosage if hypertension or hypokalemia develops, and even eliminate it entirely in cases of preeclampsia.[11,14] The measurement of renin is useless during pregnancy because there is a physiological twofold to threefold increase in renin during pregnancy.[14,19] In most patients in which the glucocorticoid dosage is increased in the second or third trimester of pregnancy, an increased dosage of fludrocortisone is not necessary, as the glucocorticoid increase will cover the increased mineralocorticoid requirement.[11,14]

25.1.7.3 Adrenal Crisis Management

Adrenal crisis was reported in 1/54 (1.9%) of pregnancies in patients with autoimmune adrenalitis.[40] However, even if the occurrence of adrenal crisis has been rarely reported in recent years, pregnancy is associated with an increased adrenal crisis risk, as shown by the high maternal mortality rate observed prior to the availability of hormonal replacement therapy.[17] It is of paramount importance to educate the patient, partner, and family about wearing a medical alert bracelet; appropriate sick-day dosing adjustment in case of infections, fever, or other stresses; and the indications for emergency parenteral glucocorticoids, such as intractable vomiting in the first trimester.[13,14,19] The management of adrenal crisis in pregnancy is the same than in nonpregnant patients, but the additional requirement is fetal monitoring by the obstetrical team.[14] As suggested in the Endocrine Society guidelines, the treatment of adrenal crisis necessitates an aggressive volume repletion, high-dose IV hydrocortisone (a bolus of 100 mg of IV hydrocortisone, followed by an IV infusion of 200 mg/24 h), and treatment of hypoglycemia with IV dextrose bolus and perfusion.[13]

25.2 CUSHING'S SYNDROME

Cushing's syndrome (CS) is defined as a state of pathological hypercortisolism.[41] The incidence of CS in the general population is about 0.2–5 per million/year, and its prevalence is around 39–79 per million.[42] CS affect mostly women, as reflected by a female-to-male ratio of 3:1.[42] However, CS rarely occurs during pregnancy, probably because hypercortisolism induces ovulatory dysfunction and relative infertility.[29] In a literature review, 214 cases of active and 49 cases of cured CS were reported during pregnancy.[43] In the group of active CS during pregnancy, the diagnosis was made prior to pregnancy in 14% (n=30), during gestation in 64.5% (n=138), and after pregnancy in 21.5% (n=46).[43]

25.2.1 Etiologies of CS

The causes of CS are typically divided into ACTH-dependent causes and ACTH-independent causes.[11] The ACTH-dependent etiologies are either a pituitary tumor that produces excessive amount of ACTH, also termed Cushing's disease (CD), or an ectopic tumor, such as a carcinoid or solid tumor, that secretes excessive amounts of ACTH (or rarely CRH).[11] The ACTH-independent causes are either an iatrogenic exogenous glucocorticoid excess or a primary adrenal lesion, such as an adrenocortical adenoma, adrenocortical carcinoma (ACC), bilateral macronodular adrenal hyperplasia (BMAH), or a primary, pigmented, nodular, adrenocortical disease [i.e., primary pigmented adrenal disease (PPNAD)], which produces excessive amounts of cortisol.[11,43]

In nonpregnant patients, CD is the most frequent cause of CS, representing 70% of the cases.[43] However, during pregnancy, adrenal etiologies represent 50%–60% of the cases of active CS, and CD represents approximatively 30% of the cases.[11,43] The reasons for this difference of etiology in pregnancy are unknown. However, it has been suggested that CD is associated with cortisol and androgen excess and that hyperandrogenism suppresses ovulation more efficiently, resulting in infertility compared to primary adrenal lesions (apart from carcinomas) that produce minimal androgens.[11,43] Another possible explanation for this finding is that some adrenal adenomas or BMAHs expressed aberrant luteinizing hormone (LH)/human chorionic gonadotropin (hCG) receptors that can be stimulated during early pregnancy by the increasing levels of hCG, thereby resulting in tumor proliferation and increased steroidogenesis.[44] A total of seven cases of transient CS during sequential pregnancies with spontaneous resolution following delivery have been reported.[44] In three cases, CS became apparent during pregnancy but did not regress after pregnancy.[45] The aberrant expression of LH/HCG receptors was demonstrated in some of these cases of transient and persistent CS.[44–46] In vitro stimulation of cortisol production by LH and hCG was demonstrated in dispersed adrenal cells from 1 woman with BMAH and very severe transient adrenal CS, which normalized after delivery; aberrant LH/CGR remained expressed in BMAH cells, which regressed in size between pregnancies.[46]

ACC is a rare cause of CS during pregnancy; only 30 cases have been reported.[47,48] Carney complex is a rare autosomal dominant syndrome that includes endocrine overactivity such as PPNAD, somatotroph pituitary adenoma, testicular tumors, and benign and malignant tumors of the thyroid gland, in addition to myxomas and cutaneous pigmented lesions.[10] PPNAD is present in up to 60% of patients with Carney complex.[10] Carney complex is due to a disease-causing germline mutation in the *PRKAR1A* gene in more than two-thirds of cases.[49] One case of Carney complex with PPNAD diagnosed during pregnancy was described previously.[10] Another patient with PPNAD demonstrated increased cortisol secretion during pregnancy and with oral contraceptive use; β-estradiol (E2) was subsequently shown in her cultured adrenal cells to stimulate cortisol secretion in a dose-responsive manner in the absence of ACTH.[50] Ectopic ACTH tumors are rare during pregnancy, probably because the hypercortisolism is severe and associated with amenorrhea in most cases.[11] Rare case reports of ectopic ACTH production by a pheochromocytoma were reported during pregnancy or the early postpartum period.[11,12] The reported causes of CS during pregnancy are presented in Table 25.3.

TABLE 25.3 Etiologies of CS in pregnancy

ACTH-independent CS: ≈ *70%*
Adrenal adenoma: 44.1%
Adrenal carcinoma: 9.4%
Pregnancy-induced Cushing's (LH or hCG receptor): 13.2%
Bilateral adrenal hyperplasia: <1%
Carney complex/PPNAD: <1%[10]
ACTH-dependent CS ≈ *30%*
Cushing's disease: 28.2%
Ectopic tumor: 3.8%
Pheochromocytoma with ectopic ACTH: <1%[11,12]

Note: Percentages may be misleading considering the small sample size.
Modified from Caimari F, Valassi E, Garbayo P, Steffensen C, Santos A, Corcoy R, et al. Cushing's syndrome and pregnancy outcomes: a systematic review of published cases. *Endocrine* 2017;**55**(2):555–563.

25.2.2 Clinical Presentation

CS usually presents with an association of symptoms and signs that are secondary to the sustained hypercortisolism.[51] When the syndrome has become severe over time, the diagnosis is usually evident, but the spectrum of clinical presentation is wide. It includes very mild-to-severe syndromes, and it also can be cyclical, with periods of eucortisolism and hypercortisolism.[42,51] The nonspecific symptoms associated with CS in adults include weight gain, fatigue, decreased concentration and memory, insomnia, irritability, depression, menstrual irregularities, decreased libido, and changes in appetite.[51] The signs that discriminate better CS include easy bruising, skin thinning, facial plethora, proximal muscle weakness, and wide (0.5–2-cm) purple striae on the abdomen and proximal thigh.[51] However, these signs do not have high sensitivity for the diagnosis of CS because they are usually present in the most severe cases.[42,51]

Other signs that are associated with CS and that are also found in high proportion in the general population are buffalo hump, facial fullness, obesity, supraclavicular fullness, thin skin, peripheral edema, acne, hirsutism, and poor skin healing.[51] CS can also present with hypertension, osteoporosis, Type 2 diabetes, hypokalemia, kidney stones, and unusual infections.[51] These symptoms and signs overlap with many of those associated with normal pregnancy, such as weight gain, striae, hirsutism, acne, fatigue, obesity, and emotional lability.[52] The striae associated with pregnancy are usually white and localized on the abdomen.[53] Normal pregnancy can be complicated by hypertension or glucose intolerance and gestational diabetes.[52] However, features such as muscle weakness, severe hypokalemia, large purple striae, and osteoporosis are important clues that suggest CS because they are not usually associated with pregnancy.[54,55] In summary, the diagnosis of CS in pregnancy is not easy and requires a high level of suspicion.

25.2.3 Morbidity Associated with CS in Pregnancy

CS during pregnancy is associated with significant morbidity and mortality for both mother and fetus.[38,43] Active CS during pregnancy is associated with high prevalence of gestational diabetes or glucose intolerance (25%–37%), gestational hypertension (41%–68%), and preeclampsia (14%–26.5%).[38,43,53] These rates are higher than in CS cases that were cured before pregnancy, in which the prevalence of gestational diabetes, hypertension, and preeclampsia are similar to the general population.[43] CS in pregnancy was also associated with osteoporosis, fracture, psychiatric disorder, cardiac failure, and wound infections.[38] Maternal death was reported in three pregnant women with CS during the first month after delivery.[38,43] Therefore, the maternal mortality ratio in active CS during pregnancy is higher than in normal pregnancy, and even higher than in countries with the worst maternal mortality ratio worldwide.[43] Furthermore, it is associated with fetal complications such as fetal loss (11%–24%), preterm birth (43%–65.8%), low birth weight (71.1%), and intrauterine growth restriction (IUGR; 15%–21%).[38,43] Less frequent fetal morbidity with active CS during pregnancy includes respiratory distress (13.77%), fetal distress (9.66%), jaundice (6.47%), fetal hypoadrenalism (2%–5.6%), and sepsis (2.82%).[38,43]

During pregnancy, the fetus is partially protected from maternal hypercortisolism by placental 11-β-HSD2. Consequently, the adverse fetal effects are probably related to placental and maternal changes associated with CS, and potentially to the enzyme capacity being oversaturated by the very high levels of cortisol that can be observed in CS.[52] The risk for these fetal complications are higher in women with active CS during pregnancy compared to those in remission.[43] In fact, women in remission before pregnancy have fetal loss rates similar to those expected in healthy women, and three times less than in active CS.[43] Moreover, CS diagnosed during pregnancy is associated with a sevenfold-higher risk of low birth weight and fivefold increase in the overall fetal morbidity and mortality compared to women diagnosed prior to pregnancy.[43] This suggests that a delay in diagnosis during pregnancy is associated with poorer fetal outcomes.

25.2.4 Diagnosis of CS During Pregnancy

Diagnosis of CS should be suspected in pregnant women with unusual features for age and pregnancy and in patients with multiple features of the syndrome, especially if the more predictive ones are present.[42,51] It is primordial to have a high suspicion level because CS causes significant morbidity and mortality for both mother and fetus. The diagnosis of CS during pregnancy is challenging because of the physiological changes that occur in the regulation of the HPA axis during pregnancy (see Chapter 8).[11]

25.2.4.1 Biochemical Screening and Diagnosis of CS

Important factors need to be taken into account for the diagnosis of CS during pregnancy. First, there is a progressive increase in the plasma total and free cortisol levels, as well as urinary free cortisol (UFC) excretion, by two to three times toward the end of the third trimester. Second, the plasma cortisol suppressibility by 1 mg dexamethasone is blunted during pregnancy.[11] In the nonpregnant population, after excluding exogenous glucocorticoid use, screening tests can include the 1-mg dexamethasone suppression test (or 2 mg over 48 h), 24-h UFC collection done twice, or the late-night salivary free cortisol (LNSC) (also done twice).[42,51] If one test is abnormal, one or two additional tests should be performed to confirm the diagnosis after excluding pseudo-CS.[51]

However, this diagnostic approach cannot be followed in the pregnant population because of the physiological hypercorticism and the changes in the HPA regulation mentioned previously. The Endocrine Society guidelines for the diagnosis of CS indicate that the 1-mg suppression dexamethasone test (1-mg DST) is not useful during pregnancy, and that a value of more than three times the upper limit of nonpregnant normal 24-h UFC values during the second and third trimesters strongly supports the diagnosis of CS during pregnancy.[51] In healthy pregnant women, the 1-mg DST results in false positive results in 80% of women, and this lack of suppressibility persists for up to 5 weeks postpartum.[52] However, if the 1-mg DST provided a normal suppression (cortisol < 50 nmol/L), CS can probably be excluded.[53] In 34 cases of CS during pregnancy, a mean eightfold elevation in UFC levels (with a range of 2–22-fold) was reported.[38]

Lindsay et al. pointed out that the diagnostic performance of 24-h UFC using the cutoff of three times the upper limit of normal is not specific because some pregnant women with CS had 24-h UFC of only twice the upper limit of normal.[11,38] Recently, Jung et al. established trimester-specific normal values for 24-h UFC measures by liquid chromatography-tandem mass spectrometry (LC-MS/MS) in 20 healthy pregnant patients compared to nonpregnant patients.[33] The mean level with standard deviations are reported to be 135 ± 10 nmol/24 h in the first trimester, 187 ± 13 nmol/24 h in the second trimester, and 242 ± 15 nmol/24 h in the last trimester, compared to 78 ± 12 nmol/24 h in the nonpregnant state.[33]

During normal pregnancy, the circadian rhythm in blood cortisol is maintained even if it is sometimes partially blunted with higher nighttime values. In cases of CS diagnosed during pregnancy, there were no diurnal variations of cortisol.[38,53,54] Salivary cortisol is an easy way to assess circadian rhythms by measuring the morning peak and midnight nadir. Manetti et al. reported a sensitivity of 100% and a specificity of 83.3%, using a cutoff of 7.64 nmol/L for LNSC to differentiate untreated nonpregnant CD patients from normal pregnant patients in the second and third trimesters of pregnancy.[56] However, it must be taken into account that 3/18 (16.7%) of the healthy pregnant women had LNSC over 7.64 nmol/L, with the highest value being 18.8 nmol/L.[56]

In a recent, larger cohort studied by Lopes et al. using an enzyme-linked immunoabsorbent assay (ELISA), a ROC curve was used to identify the best cutoff to improve sensitivity and specificity for LNSC in each trimester of pregnancy[57]: they were 7.0 nmol/L in the first trimester, 7.2 nmol/L in the second trimester, and 7.9 nmol/L in the last trimester. The associated sensitivity and specificity for each cutoff are 92% and 100% in the first trimester, 84% and 98% in the second trimester, and 80% and 93% in the last trimester, respectively.[57] This remains to be confirmed in larger cohorts, but the lack of a diurnal variation in serum or salivary cortisol strongly supports the diagnosis of CS during pregnancy, and salivary cortisol is probably easier to do because it can be done at home.[38,53]

In conclusion, the preferred tests for the diagnosis of CS in pregnancy are the 24-h UFC and assessment of the diurnal variation of salivary or serum cortisol.[53] However, it is important to take into account that these tests have limitations in the context of pregnancy, particularly to diagnose milder cases of CS, because of the significant overlap between levels found in mild CS and those found in the second and third trimesters of normal pregnancy.

25.2.4.2 Establishing the Cause of the CS

After biochemical confirmation of CS diagnosis, the next objective is to identify its cause. The first step is to differentiate ACTH-dependent or -independent causes by measuring plasma ACTH levels.[42] In primary adrenal etiologies, excess cortisol suppresses ACTH release by the normal pituitary corticotroph cells.[42] In nonpregnant patients, an ACTH level < 2.2 pmol/L indicates an ACTH-independent cause, while an ACTH level > 4.4 pmol/L shows an ACTH-dependent cause. When ACTH levels are between 2.2 and 4.4 pmol/L, a CRH test is recommended to clarify ACTH responsiveness.[42] However, in the context of pregnancy, the diagnostic performance of ACTH is reduced.[38] A total of 8/16 (50%) patients with adrenal adenomas or BMAHs had ACTH values > 2.2 pmol/L, and 2/18 (11%) with CD had ACTH values < 2.2 pmol/L.[38] This lack of ACTH suppression during pregnancy in cases of adrenal CS can possibly be explained by placental ACTH secretion and the pituitary response to chronically elevated plasma levels of placental CRH.[54]

The high-dose dexamethasone suppression test (HDDST) facilitates the differentiation of CD from ectopic ACTH secretion, as more pituitary adenomas than ectopic CS tumors retain a certain degree of suppressibility by dexamethasone.[58] The classic HDDST test consists of the determination of serum cortisol or UFC after the administration of 2 mg of oral dexamethasone every 6 h for 48 h. An easier approach is to measure serum cortisol in the morning and administer 8 mg of oral dexamethasone (8-mg DST) at 11 p.m. the same day, followed by the measure of the plasma cortisol the next day at 8 a.m. A suppression cutoff of more than 80% is associated with sensitivity ranging from 60% to 80% and specificity >80% to differentiate CD from ectopic ACTH secretion.[11] The ability of HDDST to differentiate CD from ectopic ACTH secretion during pregnancy is unknown.[11] The 8-mg DST or the classic HDDST was done in 14 pregnant patients with CS to differentiate adrenal causes from CD.[38] Using a cutoff of 80% suppression, all the patients with ACTH-independent CS were correctly identified, but 3/7 (≈43%) of the patients with CD did not suppress.[38] Therefore, HDDST has a limited capacity to differentiate CD from adrenal causes of CS during pregnancy.

In the diagnostic approach of CS, the CRH stimulation test can help to differentiate CD from ectopic ACTH secretion and adrenal disease. In fact, in CD, the tumor retains the capacity to respond to CRH by increasing ACTH and cortisol compared to most of the malignant ectopic ACTH-secreting tumors that do not respond to exogenous CRH.[11] However, up to 50% of benign ectopic ACTH-secreting neuroendocrine tumors can respond to CRH, desmopressin, or dexamethasone, similar to CD patients. In the two largest studies on CRH testing in the nonpregnant population, the ACTH response to CRH (defined as an ACTH increase >35% or 50% compared to basal levels, depending on the study) had a sensitivity of 70% and 93% and a 100% specificity to differentiate CD from ectopic ACTH secretion.[42] For the cortisol response (defined as an increase over baseline of 18%–20% at 30min), the sensitivity was 85%–91% and the specificity was 88%–100% to detect CD.[42]

Ovine CRH is classified by the FDA as a Category C drug for use in pregnancy; therefore, it must be used only when absolutely clinically indicated.[11] In one study, the ACTH and cortisol response to an IV bolus of CRH 1mcg/kg was demonstrated to be decreased in late normal pregnancy.[59] It also should be noted that plasma ACTH response to IV CRH is abnormally low at 3 and 6 weeks, but normal at 12 weeks postpartum, and the cortisol response to CRH is at the upper limit of normal at all three time periods.[53] However, the CRH stimulation test was used in five cases of CS during pregnancy, and there was a substantial rise in plasma cortisol levels (44%–130%) that was consistent with surgically confirmed CD in these patients.[38,58] There were no adverse events associated with the CRH testing in these five cases.[58]

Once the differentiation between ACTH-dependent and ACTH-independent etiologies is established with biochemical testing, the appropriate imaging is suggested in nonpregnant women in order to localize the tumor.[42] In nonpregnant patients with ACTH-independent CS, computed tomography (CT) of the adrenal glands usually identifies the responsible lesions.[42] In nonpregnant patients with ACTH-dependent CS, imaging of the pituitary by MRI with gadolinium is indicated.[42]

During pregnancy, imaging should be done only if a surgery is planned to be performed during pregnancy; if not, it can be postponed until postpartum.[53,54] During pregnancy, adrenal imaging with ultrasound was done in 15 patients with CS, and it correctly identified the adrenal lesion in 11 (73%) of these patients.[38] Thus, adrenal ultrasound is considered the imaging technique of choice to identify adrenal lesions during pregnancy because of its safety, despite reduced sensitivity for small tumors.[53] Adrenal MRI without gadolinium contrast is reserved for cases in which no adrenal lesions were identified with abdominal ultrasound.[38,53] Gadolinium is an FDA Category C drug, and thus it is not utilized during pregnancy.[38] MRI is considered contraindicated in the first trimester of pregnancy because of potential unproven teratogenic effects, but it is considered safe after 32 weeks' gestation. Between 12 and 32 weeks' gestation, the unknown risk must be balanced against the potential benefits.[38]

In nonpregnant patients, T1-weighted spin echo pituitary MRI with gadolinium identified a pituitary adenoma in only 50% of the patients with CD.[42] At least 10% of the normal population have incidental lesions of up to 6mm on MRI,[42] and so a pituitary lesion of that size or less in the nonpregnant population is not reliable to confirm the pituitary as the source of excess ACTH.[42] In nonpregnant patients, noncontrast pituitary MRI had reduced sensitivity to detect CD compared to pituitary MRI with gadolinium (38% versus 52).[38] The utilization and performance of MRI during pregnancy are limited by pregnancy-associated pituitary hyperplasia, which may be associated with an increased rate of incidentaloma and a risk of missing small lesions.[38,54] Pituitary MRI correctly identified an adenoma in 5/8 (63%) pregnant patients with CD. In these five cases, three had macroadenomas, which suggested that pituitary MRI during pregnancy is not sufficiently sensitive for the detection of microadenomas.[11] Overall, more than 50% of those adenomas associated with CD that were studied by MRI were macroadenomas—a higher proportion than in nonpregnant CD cases, in which microadenomas predominate.[38,53] Of course, the numbers studied to date remain limited, and more data will be welcome.

During pregnancy, in cases with ACTH-dependent CS, an identified pituitary lesion >6mm, and with CRH or desmopressin and HDDST responses that are consistent with CD, no additional testing is usually necessary, similar to the nonpregnant population.[58] However, for other cases, such as where to pituitary lesions were identified, bilateral inferior petrosal sinus sampling (BIPSS) may be necessary to confirm the pituitary origin of ACTH-dependent CS.[11,58] In the nonpregnant population, BIPSS is the gold standard to differentiate CD from ectopic ACTH secretion in ACTH-dependent CS, with sensitivity and specificity around 95%.[42] A central-to-peripheral ACTH gradient >2 (basal) or 3 (after CRH or desmopressin bolus) is consistent with CD.[42] False positive results can occur in the rare case of ectopic ACTH with cyclic or mild hypercortisolism, without suppression of normal corticotropes and CRH-producing tumors.[42] Successful catheterization can be confirmed by the measurement of prolactin during BIPSS.[42] However, BIPSS has rarely been done during pregnancy, likely because of safety concerns about radiation.[38] It is suggested to consider BIPSS only if the non-invasive tests (HDDST, CRH test, and pituitary MRI) were not consistent and doubt persists about the origin of ACTH-dependent CS.[38] However, BIPSS should be done only in cases in which surgery will be necessary during pregnancy.[53] Thus, it should be done only in experienced centers. Specific precautions are necessary during pregnancy, such as using a jugular approach instead of a femoral approach and using additional lead barrier protection to limit fetal exposure to radiation.[38] Also, considering the variability of ACTH levels in cases of adrenal CS during pregnancy, the usual criteria used in the nonpregnant population might not be appropriate during pregnancy, and there is a valid concern that adrenal CS might be falsely diagnosed as CD.[38,58]

In nonpregnant patients with CS caused by ectopic ACTH secretion, thin-cut CT or MRI of the thorax and abdomen, as well as scintigraphic studies [i.e., 111-In-pentreotide (octreoscan)], localize the tumor in 70%–90% of cases.[42] However, in the context of pregnancy, most cases of ectopic ACTH secretion were diagnosed in the postpartum period with CT.[12,60–62] Further, 111-In-pentreotide is a FDA Category C drug that should not be used in pregnancy and lactation because of potential risks for the fetus and newborn.[63] Therefore, in cases of suspected ectopic ACTH tumor that necessitate localization during pregnancy, noncontrasted MRI of the thorax and the abdomen probably would be preferable.

25.2.4.3 Therapy of CS During Pregnancy

As mentioned previously, active CS during pregnancy is associated with significant morbidity and mortality for mother and fetus.[38,43,64] Fetal loss, preterm birth, and low birth weight were more frequent in patients with active CS compared to CS cured before pregnancy.[38,43] It is clearly preferable to treat and cure the disease before conception. Medical and surgical treatment of CS during pregnancy was associated with reduced risk of fetal loss, whereas the risk of preterm birth or low birth weight remained unchanged.[38,43] The impact of treatment during pregnancy on maternal outcomes such as gestational diabetes, gestational hypertension, and preeclampsia has not been reported. In the context of CS diagnosed during pregnancy, surgical treatment is the preferred option when it can be done, but medical therapy is an alternative.[38,53] Radiosurgery during pregnancy is contraindicated, but normal pregnancy outcome can be obtained if pregnancy occurs shortly after radiosurgery treatment for CD.[54,65]

25.2.4.4 Surgical Therapy of CD

In the nonpregnant situation, resection of the pituitary adenoma by transphenoidal surgery (TSS) is the initial treatment of choice unless surgery is not feasible, such as with high anesthesia risk or invasive macroadenomas.[41,42] Complications associated with TSS include hypopituitarism, diabetes insipidus (DI), syndrome of inappropriate antidiuretic hormone secretion, and visual loss; they are more common with macroadenomas or extensive pituitary exploration.[42] In the nonpregnant population, remission is generally defined by a cortisol concentration <50 nmol/L or 24-h UFC <28–56 nmol/day within 7 days postoperatively, based on multiple studies that showed prolonged remission with these cutoffs.[41,42] Also, in the nonpregnant population, the remission rate for selectively resected microadenomas is 73%–76%, as opposed to $\approx$43% for macroadenomas.[41]

During pregnancy, patients with CD were not submitted to any treatment in almost half of reported cases.[54] TSS was performed in 13 pregnant patients with CD.[66,67] It has been done between 12 and 29 weeks' gestation, a period associated with a lower rate of maternal and fetal complication.[54] Remission, defined by variable cutoffs, was reported in 8/13 cases (62%) and associated with significant clinical improvement (physical appearance, BP, and diabetes).[38,66,68–74] As in the nonpregnant population, macroadenomas were less likely to achieve remission with TSS; however, biochemical improvement was obtained with surgery in these cases.[38,67,72] However, even when remission and clinical improvement were obtained after surgery, gestational hypertension and preeclampsia complicated 5/8 (62.5%) of these pregnancies.[38,68,69,73,74] Complications associated with TSS performed during pregnancy included 1 (8%) patient with transient DI, 2 (17%) patients who had persistent DI, and 2 (17%) patients with transient SIADH.[38,66,68–74] These complications were mostly associated (4/5: 80%) with macroadenomas.[38,66,69,73] After successful TSS for CD, glucocorticoid replacement should be given to the patient until the HPA axis recovers, which may take a year or more.[42]

In cases of severe CD not cured by TSS or uncontrolled with medical therapy, bilateral adrenalectomy can be performed during the second trimester to control hypercortisolism.[42,54] However, patients undergoing bilateral adrenalectomy need lifelong replacement therapy with glucocorticoids and mineralocorticoids.[42] Also, after bilateral adrenalectomy for CD, there is a 8%–25% risk of corticotrope tumor progression; therefore, regular follow-up pituitary MRI, and measurements of ACTH should be done in these patients after pregnancy.[42]

25.2.4.5 Surgical Therapy of Adrenal CS

In patients with CS caused by an unilateral adrenal adenoma, unilateral adrenalectomy is curative in nearly 100% of cases if performed by an experienced surgeon.[41] During pregnancy, 44 cases of unilateral adrenalectomy were performed and reported in the literature.[43] In 35/38 (92%) of the cases with postoperative available data, the patient achieved remission.[43] Most unilateral adrenalectomies were performed during the second trimester, but nine cases were conducted during the early third trimester.[43,75] The latest gestational age reported at surgery was 32 weeks.[75]

Since 2000, laparoscopic adrenalectomy has been the most widely used method for unilateral adrenalectomy, even during pregnancy.[76] In nonpregnant patients, the laparoscopic approach is the method of choice for adrenal adenomas because of its reduced morbidity and hospital stay when compared to an open approach.[76] During pregnancy, in cases that underwent a unilateral adrenalectomy, intraoperative and postoperative complications were rarely reported.[76] Only one case of late fetal abortion was described 3 weeks following adrenalectomy[76]; however, CS was severe, and it is difficult to conclude if surgery is responsible for the late abortion.[76]

The risks associated with surgery are higher during the third trimester because of technical difficulties associated with the enlarged uterus.[75] Where unilateral adrenalectomy was performed during the third trimester, 11% (1/9 cases) were complicated by signs of fetal distress 12 h after the surgery.[75] In that same review, unilateral adrenalectomy during the early third trimester for adrenal CS was associated with better maternal and fetal outcomes than was conservative management.[75] Unilateral adrenalectomy is an efficient and safe treatment for CS if it is performed during the second trimester or early third trimester (i.e., before 32 weeks' gestation). After successful unilateral adrenalectomy, glucocorticoid replacement should be administered to the patient until the recovery of the HPA axis, which may take several months or years.[42,76]

During pregnancy, bilateral adrenalectomy was reported in six cases of CS, mostly due to BMAH.[43,64,77] In the recent review by Caimari et al. the remission rate was 100% for bilateral adrenalectomy. These patients need lifelong replacement therapy with glucocorticoids and mineralocorticoids after the surgery.[42]

The live birth rate associated with unilateral and bilateral adrenalectomy is 87%.[11] Among women with CS during pregnancy who underwent some surgery (mostly unilateral adrenalectomy, but also TSS and bilateral adrenalectomy), those who achieved remission had better pregnancy outcomes than those who did not: 6.7% of the former resulted in fetal loss, compared to 28.6% of the latter (*P* 0.067); 56.1% versus 80% had preterm birth (*P* not significant); and 70.6% versus 100% had low birth weight (*P* not significant).[43]

25.2.4.6 Medical Treatment of CS

Medical therapy should be used to control hypercortisolism in cases of severe hypercortisolism that require improvement before surgery, or when surgery is contraindicated, fails, or the patient refuses it.[54] Medical options during pregnancy include steroidogenesis inhibitors and pituitary tumor-directed drugs.[54] The glucocorticoid receptor antagonist mifepristone is contraindicated in pregnancy because its use can result in termination of pregnancy.[78] The most commonly used steroidogenesis inhibitor during pregnancy is metyrapone,[54] which mainly inhibits 11β-hydroxylase.[42] This drug was used in 16 pregnant patients with CS and showed good control of hypercortisolism in most of them, with one report of AI.[54] The majority of these patients were treated during the second and third trimesters of pregnancy.[79] The doses that were used during pregnancy range from 250 mg to 3 g daily.[79] The most common reported side effects are hypertension, hypokalemia, hirsutism, and edema, and they are related to an increase in ACTH and steroidogenic precursors.[42]

In pregnancy, the most worrisome side effect is the worsening of hypertension and the progression to preeclampsia that has been reported in some cases.[11,54] Although metyrapone crosses the placental barrier in animal studies, no congenital abnormalities were reported in humans.[54] Ketoconazole is another steroidogenesis inhibitor that is mostly used in nonpregnant patients because of its potential for teratogenicity, which was shown only in animal studies, and its antiandrogenic effect.[54] Ketoconazole use was reported in four patients with CS during pregnancy, and no congenital malformations were reported.[54] A population-based case-control study of congenital anomalies in Hungary did not report a higher rate of congenital abnormalities in children born from mothers that received ketoconazole during pregnancy for fungal infections.[67] However, it is probably prudent to avoid its use in pregnancy and instead to use metyrapone, with which there is more experience in pregnancy.[67] Other adrenal steroidogenesis blockers, such as aminoglutethimide and mitotane, are contraindicated during pregnancy because of the risk for fetal masculinization and teratogenicity, respectively.[67]

Concerning pituitary tumor-directed drugs, there are two drugs that can be used in nonpregnant patients: pasireotide and cabergoline.[42] Pasireotide is a somatostatin receptor (SSTR) analog that has affinity mostly for the SST5R subtypes, but also has affinity for SST1R, SST2R, and SST3R. Corticotroph tumor cells express mainly SST5R and SST2R.[42] A trial including 162 nonpregnant patients showed that subcutaneous pasireotide normalized UFC at 6 months in 15% of subjects receiving 600 mcg twice daily, and 26% of subjects receiving 900 mcg twice daily.[80] At 12 months, UFC was normalized in 13% of subjects taking 600 mcg twice daily and in 25% with 900 mcg twice daily.[80] The normalization of UFC was associated with clinical improvement.[80] Patients with favorable responses usually show UFC improvement in the first 2 months.[80] However, hyperglycemia occurred in 73% of the patients.[80] A 60-month extension of the study demonstrated that in the small number of patients who continued the treatment, the beneficial effects persisted in most patients who had an initial response.[81] A recent study in nonpregnant patients using long-acting pasireotide at a dose of 10 mg or 30 mg every 28 days demonstrated normalization of UFC in approximatively 40% of patients with either dose, and with a similar safety profile as taking pasireotide twice daily.[82]

However, the somatostatin analogs (SAs) can cross the placental barrier and thus are not recommended for use during pregnancy because of safety concerns.[83] Large retrospective studies and a few case reports that have used SA for the treatment of acromegaly showed a possible increase in low birth weight.[83] In nearly 50 cases of transient exposure (mostly in the first trimester) to octreotide (another SA) in acromegaly, no serious adverse fetal outcomes were detected.[83] In the research literature, there is no reported patient with CD that was treated with pasireotide during pregnancy. Therefore, because of the potential risk associated with SA use during pregnancy and the lack of data concerning it, it is preferable to stop using pasireotide before or in early pregnancy and avoid this treatment throughout pregnancy.

The other pituitary tumor-directed drug is cabergoline.[42] Functional dopamine D2 receptors are expressed in about 60%–80% of corticotroph pituitary adenomas.[84] Cabergoline induces long-term remission in about 30% of the patients, but escapes can occur.[42] The most common side effects are nausea, headache, and dizziness.[42] The usual maximal suggested dose is 7 mg/week.[42] Cabergoline has not demonstrated fetal risk in animals and is a FDA Category B drug for its use during pregnancy.[84] Four women treated with cabergoline during pregnancy are reported in the literature; one treated with a combination of ketoconazole and cabergoline[85] and three with cabergoline alone.[84,86] The doses that were used in these patients were 0.875–1.75 mg/week in combination with ketoconazole[85] and 0.5–10 mg/week when used alone.[84,86,87] The patient that received only 0.5 mg/week of cabergoline had been treated by gamma-knife radiosurgery 7 years earlier, and this potentially can explain the lower required dose.[87] No congenital abnormalities and neonatal complications were noted in these patients, even in one case where the weekly dose was over the maximal suggested dose.[84–87] Cabergoline was used throughout pregnancy in approximatively 10 cases of prolactinoma, although at lower doses, and was not associated with any adverse fetal outcomes.[88]

Therefore, in cases of CS during pregnancy, surgery during the second trimester represents the best treatment option.[54] If surgery is not feasible or refused by the patient, the second option is medical treatment with metyrapone, cabergoline, or both, depending on the cause of CS.[54] Conservative management is not as good an option because it is associated with an increase in maternal and fetal morbidity and mortality.[43]

25.2.4.7 Medical Treatment During Breastfeeding

The data on safety of medical treatments for CS during breastfeeding are sparse and based mostly on case reports. In one case of 1 nursing mother, the baby had been exposed in utero to metyrapone for 9 weeks and was breastfed for 1 week, but did not show any signs of AI.[89] The total relative infant dose of metyrapone and rac-metylrapol, its major metabolite, is 0.1% of the weight-adjusted maternal dose, so it is below the 10% level of concern for safety during breastfeeding.[89] The authors of this study suggested that maternal metyrapone use during breastfeeding is unlikely to represent a significant risk for the breastfed infant.[89] However, if there is concern about potential hypoadrenalism in a breastfed infant of a mother taking metyrapone, the baby's adrenocortical function should be verified.[89]

There are no data on the passage of cabergoline into breast milk, and the manufacturer recommends not to breastfeed during cabergoline treatment because of the potential for serious adverse effects in the nursing infant.[90] Cabergoline impairs prolactin elevation, interferes with lactation, and can be used to stop lactation in women who do not wish to breastfeed.[55]

Ketoconazole excretion into breast milk was studied in 1 woman treated for a fungal infection with a dose of 200 mg daily of ketoconazole.[91] The maximum exposure of the baby was calculated to be 1.4% of the total mother-dose per body weight, which is considered to be safe.[91] However, the dose used for the treatment of CS is usually >200 mg daily,[41] and the concentration that will be reached in breast milk with such higher doses is unknown. Therefore, breastfeeding is not recommended by the manufacturer. Based on sparse data, if a woman with CS absolutely wants to breastfeed, metyrapone seems to be the most secure drug to employ, but close follow-up of the infant for signs of hypoadrenalism is recommended.

25.2.4.8 Treatment of Iatrogenic CS During Pregnancy

The prolonged use of supraphysiological doses of synthetic glucocorticoids for the treatment of inflammatory diseases such as asthma, inflammatory bowel disease, and rheumatologic diseases results in exogenous CS.[92] The fetus is partially protected against maternal glucocorticoids by placental 11-βHSD 2, which catalyzes the conversion of cortisol to its inactive metabolite cortisone.[14] However, the inactivation of synthetic glucocorticoids by placental 11-βHSD 2 depends on the particular molecule administered. In fact, of the total dose of synthetic glucocorticoids administered to the mother, 10% of the prednisolone-related drugs, 33% of betamethasone, and 50% of dexamethasone will reach the fetal circulation.[92] High concentrations of prednisolone-related drugs can saturate the placental enzyme and enter in the fetal circulation at significant concentrations.[92]

The fetal HPA axis can be suppressed by synthetic glucocorticoids that reach the fetal circulation.[93] Several cases of AI presenting with hyponatremia, hypoglycemia, or seizure were reported in neonates of pregnant women treated with synthetic glucocorticoids through pregnancy.[92,94,95] In a recent case series of 16 pregnant women treated with prednisolone for a mean duration of 18.4 ± 15.4 weeks, with a mean dose of 29.7 ± 16.1 mg/day, there were no case of neonatal AI.[96] However, one case of neonatal AI was reported in a newborn of a mother who had received the equivalent of 11 mg of prednisone daily, combined with inhaled corticosteroids throughout her pregnancy.[97] Thus, the maternal daily dose that is necessary to suppress the fetal HPA with various subtypes and routes of administration of synthetic glucocorticoids is unknown. Therefore, neonates of mothers who were treated with systemic glucocorticoids during pregnancy should be followed postnatally for signs of neonatal AI.[92]

There are no existing data in the literature that address the management of iatrogenic CS or glucocorticoid weaning during pregnancy. However, for the management of inflammatory disease during pregnancy, it is suggested to use the lowest possible dose of prednisone or prednisolone for control of the disease.[98] In cases in which the glucocorticoids are not necessary to control an inflammatory disease, hydrocortisone at the physiologic replacement dose is probably sufficient to protect mother and fetus from AI, as described in the section entitled "Primary Adrenal Insufficiency," earlier in this chapter. In fact, 95% of fetal glucocorticoids originate from the maternal circulation until the 33rd week of gestation; thereafter, the fetal adrenal contribution increases.[14] There are no reported adverse effects on the fetus from the administration of physiological replacement doses of hydrocortisone that are used for AI in pregnant women.

25.3 ADRENOCORTICAL CARCINOMA

In the general population, ACC has an annual incidence of 1–2 cases per million, and 60% of these patients are women.[47,52,99] ACC is associated with a 5-year overall survival rate of <30%.[52] ACC cases have been rarely reported during pregnancy, not only because it is a rare disease but because the high levels of cortisol and androgens will reduce fertility.[47] In CS cases diagnosed during pregnancy, approximately 10% are caused by ACC.[53] A total of 30 cases of ACC during pregnancy or early postpartum (<6 months) were reported in the literature.[47,48,100–105] In the most recent case series of 12 women diagnosed during pregnancy or early postpartum, only 3 were diagnosed during pregnancy, despite the fact that retrospectively, they were all symptomatic during pregnancy.[106]

25.3.1 Clinical Presentation

In nonpregnant patients with ACC, clinical manifestations of excessive hormone production are found in approximatively 60%,[47,99] with cortisol excess (CS) in 45%, combined with androgen excess in 25%, and androgen excess (virilization and hirsutism) alone in 10%.[99] Manifestations of estrogen or mineralocorticoid excess are present in <10%.[99] In nonsecreting tumors, patients may present with abdominal pain only or as an incidental mass on abdominal imaging.[99]

In the series of Abiven-Lepage et al. of ACC diagnosed during pregnancy or early postpartum, the presenting features were signs and symptoms of CS and/or androgen excess in 75% (9/12), and regional manifestation in 17% (2/12) of cases.[106] Also, one patient presented with symptomatic hypoglycemia that was possibly related to insulin-like growth factor 2 (IGF-2) hypersecretion.[106] All cases of this series were eventually shown to produce excess steroids: 25% (3/12) were secreting cortisol only and 75% were cosecreting cortisol and androgens.[106] Cortisol excess alone[101,104] or combined with androgen excess[48,100,102,103] was found in almost every ACC case reported during pregnancy.

25.3.2 Maternal and Fetal Morbidity

In the series of Abiven-Lepage et al., only four ACC cases were diagnosed in the early postpartum period after an uncomplicated pregnancy. ACC diagnosed during pregnancy or early postpartum was associated with significant fetal and neonatal complications, such as premature birth,[48,100,101,104] intrauterine growth retardation or low birth weight,[101,104] intrauterine fetal death,[103] and neonatal hypoglycemia.[102,106]

The fetus is protected against maternal androgens by the placental aromatase complex, which rapidly converts testosterone or androstenedione to estrone and estradiol, respectively, and by the elevation of sex hormone-binding globulin (SHBG), which binds circulating androgens, resulting in diminished free concentrations.[107] However, virilization of the fetus still can occur in cases of severe maternal hyperandrogenism.[107] One case of partial virilization of a female fetus was described in an ACC case with cortisol and androgen secretion during pregnancy, despite absence of virilizing signs in the woman[102]; this ACC was shown to overexpress the LH/hCG receptor.[102]

In a case of adrenal adenoma associated with fetal virilization, hCG injection (5000 IU) resulted in a ninefold increase in dehydroepiandrosterone sulfate (DHEAS) levels over baseline before surgery, and there was no response to the same test repeated 6 months after adrenalectomy.[102] The authors suggested that the increase of hCG in early pregnancy triggered the elevation of androgens and virilization of the fetus, without being associated with significant maternal virilization, because hCG decreases in the second half of pregnancy.[102]

The most frequently reported maternal complications of ACC were gestational hypertension or preeclampsia,[48,100–104,106] diabetes,[43,100,101,103,106] and severe hypokalemia.[48,100,101,103] HELLP syndrome was also reported in a single case.[106] In the case series of Abiven-Lepage et al., they compared ACC in pregnant and nonpregnant women aged <50 years old. ACC that were diagnosed during pregnancy or in the early postpartum period were associated with a more advanced stage (66% were ENSAT stage 3 or 4, compared to 39% of nonpregnant cases), were larger at diagnosis, and were associated with a poorer prognosis.[106] In fact, the survival rate of ACC diagnosed during pregnancy or in the early postpartum period is poorer than that in nonpregnant patients with a hazard ratio for death of 3.98.[106] In the largest case series, survival rates were only 50% at 1 year, 28% at 3 years, 13% at 5 years, and 0% at 8 years.[106]

The higher level of cortisol excess in the pregnant group does not appear to explain the survival difference.[106] Diagnostic delay may explain this, but the contribution of more rapid tumor growth during pregnancy could not be excluded.[47] Recently, it is suggested that pregnancy might contribute to proliferation of adrenal tumors.[108] In vitro studies have showed that some ACCs express LH/hCG receptors,[102,109] and that stimulation of LH/hCG receptors can induce tumor proliferation.[108] It was also demonstrated that benign and malignant adrenal cells express estradiol and progesterone receptors at levels similar to hormone-dependent breast tumors, and that estradiol has a mitogenic effect on adrenal H295R cell lines.[108]

25.3.3 Diagnosis

Given that most ACC cases are associated with some degree of steroid secretion, a thorough hormonal evaluation is suggested.[99] The diagnostic approach to CS during pregnancy was detailed earlier in this chapter. For androgens, the ENSAT group recommends measuring DHEAS, androstenedione, testosterone, and 17-OH-progesterone.[99] However, the results of these tests must be interpreted while taking into account the physiological changes occurring during pregnancy. During normal pregnancy, DHEAS usually decreases by 50% compared to nonpregnant values during the second trimester.[107] Androstenedione levels are highly variable in pregnancy.[110,111] Total testosterone increases especially during the second half of pregnancy because of the increase in SHBG, but free testosterone increases only slightly.[107] The mean levels of 17-OH-progesterone were shown to increase by ninefold during pregnancy.[111] Thus, elevated DHEAS and highly elevated levels of testosterone (especially free testosterone) and androstenedione are suggestive of androgen secretion by the tumor. However, 17-OH-progesterone might be difficult to interpret if it is the only elevated androgen, especially if it is only slightly elevated.

In the nonpregnant population, CT is the initial imaging of choice for ACTH-independent CS.[11] The risk for malignancy in cases of adrenal tumors increases with tumor size and increasing density and heterogeneity on CT.[99] A nonlipid-rich adrenal tumor >4 cm is associated with a sensitivity of 97% and specificity of 52%, and a tumor >6 cm is associated with a sensitivity of 91% and a specificity of 80% to identify malignancy.[112] In CT scans, a threshold of ≤ 10 Hounsfield units (HU) on noncontrast CT is diagnostic of benign lesions.[99,112] When the noncontrast density is >10 HU, an absolute contrast media washout >50% helps to identify benign lesions.[112] Other features suggestive of ACC are heterogeneity, irregular borders, calcifications, local invasion, and lymphadenopathy.[99,112] However, for the investigation of ACTH-independent CS during pregnancy, abdominal ultrasound is the first choice, given that it identifies 73% of the lesions, it is safer, and abdominal CT is contraindicated because of the potential risks associated with radiation.[38]

When an ACC is suspected based on abdominal ultrasound, an abdominal MRI without gadolinium is suggested to better evaluate the risk of malignancy based on the size and other characteristics of the lesion.[52,108] Major characteristics suggestive of malignancy on MRI are the presence of isointense-to-hypointense signals on T1-weighted images, a hyperintense signal on T2-weighted images, and a heterogeneous signal drop in chemical shift.[112] Abdominal MRI can also identify local and vena cava invasion.[99] For the staging of ACC, it is recommended to perform a CT scan of the thorax in all patients.[112] However, no strategy for the staging of ACC diagnosed during pregnancy is suggested, given that CT is contraindicated in pregnancy; indeed, in most cases, staging was not done during pregnancy.[101,103,104,109] It may be adequate to postpone staging with chest CT until the postpartum period because complementary treatments, such as chemotherapy and mitotane, are usually contraindicated during pregnancy.[52]

25.3.4 Treatment

The only potentially curative treatment for ACC is complete tumor resection[112], which must be done as quickly as possible after the diagnosis, even during pregnancy. It is indicated in every case of localized ACCs (ENSAT stage I–II–III).[112] If pregnancy is in the first 12 weeks and the tumor seems clearly aggressive, an informed discussion must be conducted with the patient and family on the prognosis and risks of ACC and related therapy. In cases of metastatic ACC at diagnosis, debulking surgery is beneficial only in patients with a large tumoral mass with absent or slow progression in two or more affected organs, and where there is severe hormone excess that cannot be otherwise controlled.[112] In a recent review, six cases of ACC that underwent adrenalectomy during pregnancy are reported.[108] The surgery was done between 20 and 29 weeks' gestation by open surgery in most cases, as is suggested for most tumors >5 cm.[112] Only one surgery was complicated by a lymphocele.[108] In 4/6 cases (67%), there was an early recurrence in the surgical bed, suggesting incomplete resection[108] or highly aggressive disease. Also, there were cases of premature labor, fetal death, and fetal distress happening a few days or weeks following surgery, which necessitated an emergency cesarean section.[108] Medical treatment to control hypercortisolism can be used before surgery, or after surgery if persistent hypercortisolism is noted.[47] As discussed previously, the best medical option is metyrapone.

After performing a resection of presumed localized disease (ENSAT stage I–II–III), the final staging (Table 25.4) and pathology guide the indications for adjuvant therapy.[112] In nonpregnant cases of complete resection (R0) of adrenal carcinoma with an ENSAT stage I–II and a Ki-67 < 10%, close follow-up (or inclusion in ADUVIO study, which is an international, prospective, open-label, controlled phase III trial of mitotane therapy versus observation in patients with ACC after R0 resection and in the absence of metastasis and Ki-67 < 10%) is recommended at 3 months interval with complete physical examination, hormonal investigations, and imaging workup; imaging by chest and abdominal CT should be done in the postpartum period.[112] In cases of complete resection, but with high risk of recurrence (ENSAT stage III and Ki-67 > 10%), adjuvant therapy with mitotane with or without local radiotherapy is indicated.[112]

Mitotane or radiotherapy is contraindicated during pregnancy and should be used only in the postpartum period. Mitotane improved recurrence-free survival in patients with localized ACC.[112] It has adrenolytic and cytotoxic activity and also inhibits several enzymes of steroidogenesis.[112] It is usually introduced progressively to reach the target mitotane plasma levels of 14–20 mcg/mL.[99] Significant toxicities are associated with mitotane therapy, such as vertigo, central nervous system disturbance, and gastrointestinal symptoms.[112] Also, given the adrenolytic activity, steroidogenesis inhibition, and increased hepatic steroid metabolism connected with it, all patients receiving mitotane therapy are adrenal insufficient and require hydrocortisone replacement. The necessary dose is higher than usually prescribed for physiological replacement.[112]

TABLE 25.4 ENS@T staging system

Stage	TNM classification
I	T1, N0, M0
II	T2, N0, M0
III	T3–T4, N1
IV	T1–T4, N0–N1, M1

T1: tumor ≤5 cm; T2: tumor ≥5 cm, T3: histologically proven tumor invasion of surrounding tissue; T4: tumor invasion of adjacent organs or venous tumor thrombus in vena cava or renal vein.
N0: negative lymph nodes; N1: positive lymph nodes.
M0: absence of distant metastases; M1: presence of distant metastases.

A few cases of women who were treated with mitotane before pregnancy and became pregnant during treatment have been described.[113] In these cases, no fetal AI or teratogenic effects were reported.[113] However, because of the potential risk of teratogenicity associated with mitotane transfer to the fetus, treatment should be delayed until the postpartum period.[47,52,113] It should be initiated as soon as possible in the postpartum period, and breastfeeding is not recommended during mitotane treatment.[47]

In cases of locally invasive or distant metastatic ACC at diagnosis, mitotane is recommended in every patient.[112] Loco-regional therapy for metastases, such as radiofrequency ablation or transarterial chemoembolization, are nonsurgical options that can be used to control the disease.[112] Also, in cases of progressive metastatic disease despite mitotane treatment, chemotherapy with etoposide-cisplatin-doxorubicin can be added.[112] However, these treatments are not recommended during pregnancy because of their potential toxicity for the fetus.

Because of the scarcity of data regarding management of ACC during pregnancy, it is difficult to establish recommendations on how to manage these patients. Therefore, in cases of newly diagnosed ACCs during pregnancy, the possibility of termination of pregnancy for medical reasons should be discussed with the patient, especially for ACCs in stage 3 or 4 discovered in the first trimester.[106] In cases of localized disease and desire for continuation of pregnancy, the surgery must be done as soon as possible, and the potential risk and benefits of doing so must be explained to the patient. In cases of metastatic disease, the absence of treatment options during pregnancy besides debulking surgery, as well as the risk to postponed treatment, need to be fully discussed.

25.4 PRIMARY ALDOSTERONISM

In the nonpregnant population, primary aldosteronism (PA) has an estimated prevalence of $\approx 10\%$ in overall hypertensive patients[114]; however, this prevalence concerns a population that is quite different than young women of reproductive age.

Hypertensive disorders complicate 6%–8% of pregnancies. By assuming that the similar range of prevalence of PA was present in hypertensive women of reproductive age, it could be expected that 0.6%–0.8% of pregnant women could have PA.[115] However, only 40 cases of nonfamilial PA during pregnancy have been reported.[114,116–118] In these cases, 33 were newly diagnosed during pregnancy.[114,116] PA in pregnancy is probably underdiagnosed, given that the number of reported cases are lower than those of CS and pheochromocytoma in pregnancy, but CS and pheochromocytoma have a much lower prevalence than PA in the general population.[118]

25.4.1 Etiologies of Hyperaldosteronism

PA is a condition of increased secretion of aldosterone which is relatively independent from renin, angiotensin II, and potassium levels.[119] Secondary hyperaldosteronism is a state of increased aldosterone secretion in response to increased activity of the renin-angiotensin-aldosterone system (RAAS), such as in renal artery stenosis, or an excessive production of renin by a tumor.

In the general population, 50%–70% of PA are caused by bilateral adrenal hyperplasia (BAH), and 30%–50% are caused by a unilateral adenoma (APA); however, nodular zona glomerulosa hyperplasia is often found adjacent to the functioning adenoma.[44] Approximately 1% of patients with PA present with one of the few familial forms (types I, II, III, and IV).[115]

Familial hyperaldosteronism type I (FH I), also known as *glucocorticoid remediable aldosteronism* (GRA), occurs due to a hybrid gene caused by unequal crossing of the genes that encode CYP11B1 and aldosterone synthase (CYP11B2).[120] Consequently, the expression of aldosterone synthase is regulated by ACTH instead of ANG II.[115] To date, 65 pregnancies in 25 women with FH I have been reported.[115,120]

In familial hyperaldosteronism type III (FH III), germline mutations have been identified in *KCNJ5*, a potassium channel gene that promotes aldosterone production and cell proliferation.[121] It usually presents as a severe form of hyperaldosteronism associated with massive bilateral hyperplasia, but in some cases, it presents as a mild form of the disease without massive adrenals.[121]

Germline mutation in *CACNA1D*, encoding a voltage-gated calcium channel (CaV3.2), has been reported as a cause of a new familial hyperaldosteronism, called *familial hyperaldosteronism type IV* (FH IV).[121] FH IV is associated in some cases with a developmental disorder.[121]

Familial hyperaldosteronism type II (FH II) is clinically similar to nonfamilial PA and is usually only diagnosed based on the fact that two or more individuals are affected in the same family.[121] FH II can present as APA or BAH. Germline mutation in the *CACNA1D*, *KCNJ5*, and *CACNA1D* genes has been identified in patients diagnosed as FH II.[121] Recently, activating mutations in chloride channel CLCN2 were also identified in multiple probands of families diagnosed with FH II, with some being germline and some being de novo mutations.[122]

Somatic mutations in the *KCNJ5, CACNA1D*, and *ATP1A1* genes (encoding the Na+/K+ ATPase-α subunit) and ATP2B3 (encoding the plasma membrane Ca2-β ATPase) have also been found in APA.[44,121] Mutations in these genes impair pathways involved in maintaining intracellular ionic homeostasis and cell membrane potential that ultimately lead to increased calcium signaling, which is the main trigger for aldosterone production.[121] No ionic channel mutation are found in BAH or zona glomerulosa hyperplasia adjacent to an APA.[44] In BAH, activation of the Wnt/β-catenin, associated with increased cellular proliferation, have been identified.[44] Other rare causes of PA include adrenal carcinoma and ectopic aldosterone secretion.[52]

In PA, the aldosterone production is not really autonomous, despite suppression of renin and ANG II levels, and is regulated by multiple autocrine and paracrine actions of hormones and regulatory mechanisms that activate variable levels of eutopic or ectopic G protein-coupled receptors in APA and BAH.[44] In vivo and in vitro studies demonstrated the presence of aberrant receptors for serotonin (5-HT4R), gastric inhibitory polypeptide (GIPR), vasopressin (V1aR, V2R), glucagon, gonadotropin-releasing hormone (GnRHR), and LH/hCG (LHCGR). LHCGR and GnRHR can be expressed in normal adrenal tissue, but only fetal adrenal cells exhibit DHEAS secretion stimulated by LH/hCG.[44] LHCGR and/or GnRHR protein and messenger ribonucleic acid (mRNA) were shown to be overexpressed in certain cases of PA.[44]

Three cases of PA associated with aberrant expression of LHCGR and GnRHR were reported. The first is a 32-year-old woman with APA diagnosed during pregnancy that was studied after delivery. In vivo experimentation in this patient demonstrated that a long-acting GnRH analog triptorelin, which inhibits endogenous LH, stimulates aldosterone secretion. This was confirmed by the demonstration of GnRHR and LHCGR in APA tissues.[123] In the two other women with APA diagnosed during pregnancy, the expression of LHCGR and GnRHR was at levels 100-fold higher than those of other APAs, but no in vivo studies were done with these patients.[116] The APAs of these two patients were found to harbor an activating somatic *CTNNB1* (β-catenin) mutation, which led to the activation of the WNT pathway in vitro, as well as the overexpression of GnRHR and LHCGR in transfected cells. Therefore, it was suggested that *CTNNB1* mutations caused dedifferentiation of gonadal progenitor cells, which leads to the overexpression of gonadal receptors.[116] However, other investigators did not find *CTNNB1* mutations in several patients with APA having aberrant LHCGR or GnRHR.[124] Therefore, the link between CTNNB1 and aberrant LHCGR and GnRHR has not been confirmed.[44]

25.4.2 Clinical Presentation of PA in Pregnancy

During pregnancy, the diagnosis of PA was identified either by high blood pressure (HBP) that first presented during pregnancy (80%) or that was already known before pregnancy (20%).[114] Moderate-to-severe hypokalemia was found in 68% of the patients diagnosed with PA.[118] Proteinuria was also reported in several cases.[29] Other reported symptoms include headache, malaise, and muscle cramps.[29]

In patients already known to have PA before pregnancy, the course of HBP during pregnancy appears to be highly variable, with some patients having worsened hypertension and hypokalemia, and others having spontaneous improvement, or even normotension.[114,115,118] Therefore, it was suggested that clinical consequences of PA, hypertension, and hypokalemia develop during pregnancy only if the amount of progesterone, a physiological mineralocorticoid antagonist, is unable to compensate for the aldosterone excess.[115]

Because pregnancy is associated with an elevation in ACTH levels, it was thought that hypertension and hypokalemia would worsen in patients with FH I, in whom aldosterone secretion is driven by ACTH.[115] However, only 39% of the women saw aggravated hypertension, and 23% needed antihypertensive drugs during pregnancy.[125] Moreover, potassium levels were normal in most pregnant patients with FH I.[120,126]

25.4.3 Maternal and Fetal Morbidity Associated with PA During Pregnancy

In cases of PA diagnosed during pregnancy, BP was > 140/90 mmHg in 80%–85% of pregnant women with PA, and more than 50% had associated proteinuria.[52,114] In a recent review, preeclampsia complicated almost 25% of pregnancies in women with newly diagnosed PA.[114] The prevalence of cesarean section was 44.4%, while 61.2% had induced labor.[114] Fetal complications included preterm birth, intrauterine growth retardation or being small for gestational age, and stillbirth.[114] The mean gestational age at delivery was 33.7 weeks.[114] Three cases of stillbirth were reported, and they happened in women with uncontrolled hypertension.[114] In women previously diagnosed with PA who became pregnant, BP was controlled in 5/7 (71%).[114] The majority of women with previously known PA gave birth between 36 and 39 weeks' gestation, with 1 giving birth at 26 weeks because of fetal bradycardia associated with uncontrolled hypertension.[114] Therefore, uncontrolled hypertension is an important determinant of the maternal and fetal complications associated with PA during pregnancy. PA diagnosed before pregnancy usually maintains better BP control during pregnancy than PA diagnosed during pregnancy.[114,115]

In the few reports of pregnancies in FH I, 75% of those patients have hypertension during pregnancy, but there was no increased prevalence of preeclampsia (6%) compared to the general population (2.5%–10%).[115,125] In one series of FH I during pregnancy, 32% of the deliveries were by primary cesarean section.[125] Premature delivery occurred in 11.4% of pregnancies.[125] There were no fetal malformations, prolonged neonatal hospitalization, or neonatal death, and the mean birth weight was 3124 kg.[125] However, in the 39% of patients with worsening hypertension during pregnancy, there was an increased risk for cesarean section and a trend toward lower birth weight.[52,125] In another series of a four-generation Italian pedigree, there was no pregnancy-aggravated hypertension, no preeclampsia, and no cesarean delivery.[126] Another case report of FH I during pregnancy with normotension was reported.[120] The outcomes of pregnancy in the context of FH I seem to be better than in nonfamilial PA, but it varies among the few reported patients.

25.4.4 Diagnosis of PA During Pregnancy

The diagnostic approach of PA during pregnancy is complicated by the physiological changes that happen in the RAAS (see Chapters 8 and 10).[118] Pregnancy is a state of hyperreninemic hyperaldosteronism that counteracts the increased production of progesterone and its mineralocorticoid antagonist activity.[114] Plasma renin activity increases by three to seven times in the first 20 weeks of gestation and plateaus afterward.[11] Plasma aldosterone increases in parallel with progesterone. Aldosterone increases by 5–7 times during the first trimester and by 10–20 times by the end of the third trimester.[11]

Given that PA during pregnancy is associated with significant maternal and fetal morbidity, it is essential to suspect this diagnosis in cases of severe hypertension, hypokalemia, or both during pregnancy, especially if it manifests before 20 weeks' gestation.[115]

In the general population, the aldosterone-renin ratio (ARR) is the screening procedure used to identify the patient suspected of PA.[127] However, the physiological increase in renin levels may cause a fall in ARR during pregnancy, and false-negative results in pregnant women with PA.[118] In a review, elevated ARR with suppressed plasma renin activity was demonstrated in 14/33 (61%) of PA during pregnancy.[118] There is one case published of PA during pregnancy with normal renin levels.[114] Therefore, an elevated ARR is suggestive of PA in pregnancy, but a normal ARR does not rule out PA.[118,119] Therefore, it will be important in the future to establish normal values for ARR during pregnancy.[114] After a positive screening test, in the general population, there is a need to do a confirmatory test, such as saline infusion test, oral sodium-loading test, captopril challenge test, or fludrocortisone suppression test.[127] These tests result in a volume expansion, but they have not been validated during pregnancy, nor are they recommended during pregnancy.[114,115]

During pregnancy, when surgery is considered because of poorly controlled hypertension or hypokalemia despite medical therapy, an evaluation of subtype needs to be done.[115] In the general population, it is recommended that all patients undergo an adrenal CT to identify the presence of unilateral or bilateral adrenal lesions, despite their lack of specificity.[127] However, during pregnancy, CT is contraindicated, and adrenal ultrasonography or MRI without contrast should be used.[115] In the general population, adrenal vein sampling (AVS) is required in most patients that are eligible to have surgery if a unilateral source of aldosterone is found; adrenal CT is not predictive of lateralization status in almost 50% of patients >35 years old.[127] In younger patients (<35 years old) with spontaneous hypokalemia and marked aldosterone excess, the finding of a unilateral adrenal adenoma on imaging is usually sufficient to subtype a PA because nonsecreting adrenal adenomas are rare in that subgroup of patients.[127] During pregnancy, AVS is contraindicated because it is associated with significant radiation exposure that represents a risk for the fetus.[115] However, given that most pregnant women are <35 years old, and that hypokalemia is reported frequently in pregnant patients with PA, the finding of an unilateral adenoma on abdominal imaging might be sufficient to subtype PA.[115]

25.4.5 Treatment of PA During Pregnancy and Breastfeeding

Efficient therapy of PA during pregnancy is important because it is associated with significant morbidity for mother and fetus, and uncontrolled hypertension is a major contributor to these complications.[114,115] In the nonpregnant population, where there is a unilateral source of PA, the suggested therapy is unilateral adrenalectomy, or use of a mineralocorticoid receptor antagonist (MRA) when the patient refuses surgery.[127] In patients with PA due to bilateral disease, MRA is the recommended treatment, with spironolactone being the first choice and eplerenone suggested as an alternative.[127]

No consensus guideline recommendations for the management of PA during pregnancy exist.[114] In the most recent guidelines from the Society of the Obstetrician and Gynecologist of Canada (SOGC), the goal of treatment of hypertension during pregnancy is to lower the BP to <160/110 mmHg in cases of severe hypertension (systolic BP ≥160 or diastolic

BP≥110 mmHg), between 130–155/80–105 mmHg in nonsevere hypertension (BP 140–159/90–109 mmHg) without comorbid conditions, and <140/90 mmHg in patients with nonsevere hypertension with comorbid conditions.[128]

Methyldopa is the first-line drug for the management of hypertension during pregnancy in the majority of guidelines.[114] It has been prescribed for decades, and no teratogenic effect have been described with its use.[114] Labetalol is the most widely used combined alpha- and beta-blocker during pregnancy. Data published on women using labetalol during the second and third trimesters of pregnancy are numerous, and no fetal toxicity was reported.[114] The dihydropyridine calcium channel blockers that can be used during pregnancy include nifedipine and nicardipine. In animal models, nifedipine was associated with a risk of fetal toxicity and teratogenicity, but in human data, no adverse effects have been described.[114] There are insufficient data to support the use of amlodipine during pregnancy.[114] Diuretics are usually not suggested because of the potential risk for hypovolemia, but reassuring data on their use during pregnancy are reported.[114]

When the diagnosis is made before conception, it is preferable to treat the disease before a woman attempts to become pregnant.[115] In cases of unilateral disease, unilateral adrenalectomy should be done before conception.[115] The management is more complex in cases of confirmed bilateral disease.[115] In these patients, it is preferable to achieve normal BP before conception, and there are different suggested approaches for treatment.

The first strategy is to stop MRA in the preconception period and adjust treatment of BP with drugs that are known to be safe during pregnancy (such as methyldopa, labetalol, and nifedipine or nicardipine), and potassium supplements.[114] In cases in which the BP is still uncontrolled after 1 month, addition of a diuretic such as thiazide or amiloride can be proposed depending on potassium levels.[114]

The second approach is to switch in the preconception period to the previously mentioned antihypertensive drugs that are known to be safe during pregnancy only in normokalemic, mild cases of PA.[115] In moderate and severe cases, it is probably safer to keep the MRA in the preconception period and to switch to the safer antihypertensive drugs once the pregnancy is confirmed, or else switch to eplerenone if the MRA was spironolactone.[115] In cases where the other antihypertensive drugs do not achieve BP and potassium control, eplerenone can be added.[115]

These strategies were not evaluated head to head, and it is currently impossible to support one over the other.

Angiotensin-converting enzyme inhibitors and angiotensin-receptor blockers should not be used during pregnancy because of their frequent associated teratogenicities.[128,129] The congenital anomalies that were associated with their use include renal failure, anuria, skull and lung hypoplasia, craniofacial deformation, and death.[129]

When the diagnosis of PA is made during pregnancy, the most common suggested approach is to manage BP and potassium with medical therapy. In cases in which BP and potassium control cannot be achieved with the usual antihypertensive drugs of pregnancy, eplerenone might be added.[115] Eplerenone, a selective MRA without antiandrogenic activity, is a Category B FDA drug for use during pregnancy. No teratogenic effects were observed in animal models.[115] It was used in one case of APA during pregnancy from 27 weeks' gestation.[115,118] There was no fetal adverse effects associated with eplerenone use in that case for up to 2 years of follow-up of the male newborn.[115] Two other cases of eplerenone use during pregnancy are reported, one for Gitelman syndrome and one for diastolic heart failure, with no adverse effects.[115,118] Despite insufficient data to recommend the use of eplerenone for the treatment of PA during pregnancy, it seems to be safe.[114]

Amiloride, a potassium-sparing diuretic, has been used in three pregnancies of women with PA and is associated with favorable outcomes.[118] It was also used in 17 pregnancies in women with severe hypertension, Liddle, Bartter, and Gitelman syndromes without any adverse effects.[118] It should not be considered a first-line therapy for PA during pregnancy, but it can be considered in cases where BP and potassium have been difficult to control with conventional drugs.

Spironolactone, which is the first recommended drug in nonpregnant patients, is not recommended during pregnancy.[114] It is an MRA that also has antiandrogenic activity.[114] It is a FDA Category C drug in pregnancy because it crosses the placenta and has been demonstrated to cause feminization in male rats.[52] The most important steps of sex differentiation occur during the first trimester of pregnancy.[114] In humans, only 1 case of ambiguous genitalia in a newborn of a mother treated with spironolactone until the fifth week of gestation for polycystic ovarian syndrome (PCOS) is reported.[115] Around 20 cases of pregnant women treated with spironolactone at various times during pregnancy for Bartter syndrome, PA, pregnancy edema, or Gitelman syndrome are reported, and no cases of ambiguous genitalia were described in male newborns.[115] Another feared side effect of spironolactone in pregnancy is the natriuretic effect of the drugs that might result in a higher risk of intrauterine growth retardation.[115]

Unilateral adrenalectomy may be considered in cases of unilateral disease that remain uncontrolled despite optimal medical treatment.[52,115,118] There are nine cases of unilateral adrenalectomy for PA that were performed during pregnancy.[118] Biochemical cures and BP improvement mostly were achieved after the surgery, but significant fetal morbidity and mortality still took place in 44% of cases.[118] There is one case of intrauterine fetal death at 26 weeks' gestation, two deliveries at 26 weeks' gestation because of intrauterine growth retardation and fetal distress, and one preterm birth at 34 weeks' gestation.[118] However, the outcome obtained with surgery was not compared to those obtained with medical treatment, so it is impossible to conclude which option is the best.[118]

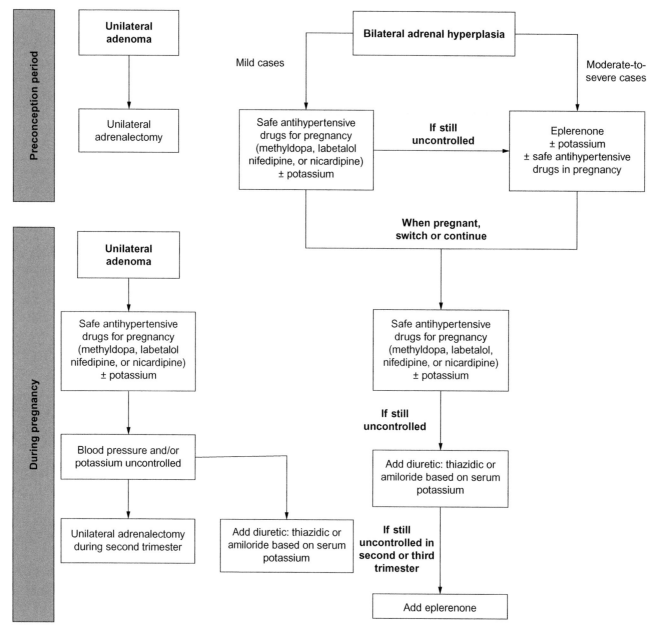

FIG. 25.2 Management of primary hyperaldosteronism in the context of the preconceptional period and during pregnancy.

Overall, in cases of PA diagnosed during pregnancy, we suggest, based on safety issues, using the antihypertensive drugs that are known to be safe during pregnancy, with or without potassium supplementation, as the first step of treatment (Fig. 25.2). In cases of uncontrolled BP or potassium, despite the optimal usual medical treatment of BP during pregnancy, eplerenone might be added to the treatment to achieve BP and potassium control. In cases of unilateral PA where BP or potassium control cannot be achieved with medical therapy, unilateral adrenalectomy can be suggested, but doing so may not prevent fetal morbidity and mortality, as mentioned previously. In cases of bilateral disease uncontrolled with the abovementioned treatment, amiloride or eplerenone might be added.

Breastfeeding is not contraindicated in patients with PA. The antihypertensive agents that are acceptable for use during breastfeeding include nifedipine, labetalol, methyldopa, captopril, and enalapril.[128] No case reports of treatment of PA with MRA during breastfeeding are available.[115] The major and active metabolite of spironolactone, canrenone, appears in human breast milk, but the relative dose for the newborn is 1.2% of the daily dose of the nursing mother.[115] An impact on the newborn is not expected, given that it is <10% of the maternal daily dose, which is the level of concern for safety in breastfeeding.[115] Therefore, spironolactone is considered safe in breastfeeding.[118] For eplerenone, there are no published data on human breast milk, but it was detectable in rat breast milk.[115] Morton mentioned 1 unpublished case of a mother using eplerenone during breastfeeding of two infants, without adverse effects.[118] Therefore, if an MRA is necessary during breastfeeding, spironolactone seems the one to use.[115,118] There are no published data on amiloride use in humans during breastfeeding, so it is impossible to recommend its use.[118]

25.5 PHEOCHROMOCYTOMA AND PARAGANGLIOMA (PPGL)

Catecholamine-secreting tumors are derived from the neural-crest chromaffin cells located in the adrenal medulla in cases of pheochromocytoma, or in extraadrenal autonomic ganglia in cases of paraganglioma.[130] The most frequent catecholamine-secreting tumors are pheochromocytomas, in one or both adrenal glands, representing 85% of cases.[131,132] In this chapter, all catecholamine-secreting tumors will be referred to as *pheochromocytoma and paraganglioma* (PPGL). They usually produce one or more catecholamines, including norepinephrine, epinephrine, and dopamine.[132] In rare cases, they can be silent.[132] The prevalence of PPGL in the population of hypertensive patients is 0.1%–0.6%.[132] PPGL is rare during pregnancy; the reported incidence, in a case series of 30,246 pregnancies over a period of 22 years, is 0.007%.[133]

25.5.1 Genetic Susceptibility to PPGL

In the general population, 30%–40% of PPGL have a disease-causing germline mutation.[132] A similar prevalence of 30%–40% for genetic susceptibility genes is reported in PPGL diagnosed during pregnancy.[134,135] In the general population, 14 susceptibility genes for PPGL have been reported: *NF1, RET, VHL, SDHD, SDHB, EGLN1/PHD2, KIF1β, SDH5/SDHAF2, IDH1, TMEM127, SDHA, MAX*, and *HIF2α*.[132] The genetic susceptibility genes that were identified in cases of PPGL diagnosed during pregnancy include *RET*, associated with multiple endocrine neoplasia (MEN) 2A and 2B[134]; *VHL* (Von-Hippel Lindau)[134]; *SDHB*[134]; and *NF1* (neurofibromatosis Type 1)[136] (Table 25.5) Given the high prevalence of genetic susceptibility genes in PPGL, the diagnostic screening should be offered to every patient. It allows for identifying the susceptibility to other diseases associated with syndromic PPGL in the patient, and it also allows relatives to be screened and diagnosed earlier.[130,132]

25.5.2 Clinical Manifestations of PPGL During Pregnancy

Symptoms of PPGL in pregnancy are no different from those of PPGL in nonpregnant patients.[137] In fact, in multiple case series, 60%–85% of the pregnant women with PPGL present with hypertension.[135] In pregnant women, hypertensive crisis as the first presentation is reported in 15%–40% of cases.[135] Hypertension in PPGL is paroxysmal in 25%–45% of PPGL cases during pregnancy.[130] Also, ≈50% of pregnant women with PPGL have episodes of hypotension.[130,137] Given that PPGL during pregnancy presents with hypertension in most cases, it can be misdiagnosed initially as gestational hypertension or preeclampsia.[131] However, it is of prime importance to make the correct diagnosis because if undiagnosed during pregnancy, PPGL is associated with ≈40%–50% mortality for both mother and fetus.[131,134]

Some items can help to differentiate PPGL from gestational hypertension and preeclampsia, which usually develop after 20 weeks' gestation and are usually not associated with episodes of hypotension.[130] In cases of PPGL, hypertension can appear anytime during pregnancy.[137] Therefore, pregnant patients presenting with hypertension before 20 weeks' gestation, paroxysmal hypertension and/or episodes of hypotension, or both should be screened for PPGL.[137] Proteinuria and edema are more suggestive of gestational hypertension or preeclampsia, given that it is usually absent in the context of PPGL.[130,137] Also, pregnant patients with PPGL frequently reported other signs and symptoms associated with catecholamine excess. The classic triad of headache, palpitations, and hyperhidrosis is reported by ≈50% of pregnant patients with PPGL.[130] Hyperglycemia is reported in a significant proportion of PPGL diagnosed during pregnancy.[130,137] Other symptoms, such as pallor, weight loss, dyspnea, nausea, and anxiety, are found in some pregnant women with PPGL, but they are less frequently reported.[52,130,131] Rarely, PPGL during pregnancy were complicated by Takotsubo-like cardiomyopathy[138] or myocardial infarction.[139] Takotsubo-like cardiomyopathy occurs mostly in the peripartum period and is potentially reversible after tumor removal.[130] PPGL also can secrete ACTH in some cases, resulting in associated ectopic ACTH-dependent severe CS.[12,60]

Symptoms associated with PPGL may worsen during pregnancy because of the increasing pressure exerted on the tumor by the gravid uterus, fetal movement, uterine contractions, or abdominal palpation.[52,131,137] During the evaluation, a personal or family history of PPGL and the findings of signs and symptoms associated with syndromic PPGL should raise suspicions for the condition (Table 25.5).[130]

TABLE 25.5 Clinical manifestations associated with the syndromic PPGL reported in pregnancy

Syndromes	Clinical manifestations

MEN 2A (AD: *RET* gene)	• Pheochromocytoma ≈25%–50%ᵃ (bilateral≈60%), rarely malignant
	  o High-risk codon for pheochromocytoma (50%): D631Y, C634F/G/R/S/W/Y
	• Medullary thyroid cancer (≈100%)
	• Primary hyperparathyroidism (PHPT) (≈10%–30%)
	  o High-risk codon for PHPT: C634F/G/R/S/W/Y
	• Hirschsprung's disease (codons 618 or 620) (7%)
	• Cutaneous lichen amyloidosis (rare)

MEN 2B (AD: *RET* gene) Codons M918T and A883F	• Pheochromocytoma ≈50% (bilateral≈60%), rarely malignant • Medullary thyroid cancer (≈100%) • Skeletal malformations: marfanoid body habitus, narrow long facies, pes cavus, pectus excavatum, high-arched palate, scoliosis, and slipped capital femoral epiphyses • Generalized ganglioneuromatosis throughout the lips, tongue, and aerodigestive tract • Ophthalmologic abnormalities: myelinated corneal nerves, mild ptosis, thickened and everted eyelids, and inability to make tears in infancy
Von-Hippel Lindau (AD: *VHL* gene)	• Pheochromocytoma: 10%–20% (bilateral≈40%), sometimes malignant • Associated conditions: hemangioblastoma (cerebellum, spinal cord, or brain stem), retinal angioma, clear-cell renal carcinoma, pancreatic neuroendocrine tumors, serous cystadenomas, endolymphatic sac tumors of the middle ear, papillary cystadenomas of the epididymis, and broad ligament
Neurofibromatosis Type 1 (AD: *NF1* gene)	• Pheochromocytoma: 0.1%–6% (bilateral≈15%), 3%–12% malignancy risk • Associated conditions: neurofibromas, café-au-lait spots, axillary and inguinal freckling, Lisch nodules, bone abnormalities, central nervous system gliomas, cognitive deficits, and macrocephaly
Paraganglioma syndrome type 4 (AD: *SDHB* gene)	• Paragangliomas: sympathetic≈50% (sometimes multiple: ≈20%), parasympathetic 20%–30% (sometimes multiple) • Pheochromocytomas: 20%–25% (sometimes bilateral) • Metastatic disease in up to 40% • Associated conditions; renal cell cancer

AD: autosomal dominant.
ᵃ*For MEN2A, depend on the codon mutated for pheochromocytoma and PHPT.*
Modified from Prete A, Paragliola RM, Salvatori R, Corsello SM. Management of catecholamine-secreting tumors in pregnancy: a review. *Endocr Pract* 2016;22(3):357–370.

25.5.3 Morbidity and Mortality Associated with PPGL During Pregnancy

PPGL during pregnancy is associated with significant mortality and morbidity for mother and fetus. Maternal death was reported to be caused by the consequences of pulmonary edema, myocardial infarction, cerebral hemorrhage, respiratory distress syndrome, and disseminated intravascular coagulation, all of which are precipitated by an abrupt discharge of catecholamines.[140] The fetal risks are due to the vasoconstrictor effects of catecholamines on the uteroplacental unit rather than to direct effects of catecholamines on the fetus, given that the placenta possesses high enzymatic activity that protects the fetus against maternal catecholamines.[130,140] The maternal and fetal death rates were 48% and 55%, respectively, before 1969, but fell to 8% and 17% respectively between 2000 to 2011.[134,140] The peripartum period represent a high-risk period for catecholamine excess because of abdominal palpation, labor, delivery, anesthesia (associated with the use of thiopenthal, ketamine, halothane, desflurane, atropine, ephedrine, and muscle relaxants), and the use of certain medications (metoclopramide, corticosteroids, and opioids) that can trigger catecholamine release.[130,137] Therefore, the outcomes are better for both mother and fetus when the diagnosis is made in the antenatal period.[134]

Between 2000 and 2011, the reported rate for maternal death was 0% when the diagnosis of PPGL was made in the antenatal period, and 29% when the diagnosis was made in the postnatal period.[134] In cases of hypertensive crisis, the maternal mortality rate remains high (55%) and occurred in every maternal mortality reported between 2000 to 2011.[134] During the same period, fetal death was 12% if the diagnosis was antenatal and 29% if it was postnatal.[134] Also,

PPGL during pregnancy can be associated with other fetal complications, such as IUGR, prematurity, and fetal hypoxia.[130,131,140] Therefore, it is primordial to diagnose PPGL in the antenatal period to diminish the maternal and fetal mortality rates associated with PPGL during pregnancy.

25.5.4 Diagnosis of PPGL During Pregnancy

The first steps in the diagnostic approach of PPGL are to confirm the biochemical diagnosis and then to localize the tumor.

25.5.4.1 Biochemical Diagnosis

When PPGL is suspected during pregnancy, the first step is to measure the plasma-free metanephrines or the fractionated urinary metanephrines by LC/MSMS or liquid chromatography with electrochemical determination (LC-ECD), which are the most sensitive tests (sensitivity >95%). Also, they are associated with a high negative predictive value, so they are good to exclude the disease in cases where normal results are obtained.[131,132,137] The excellent sensitivity of metanephrines is explained by the intratumoral O-methylation of catecholamines, which is the dominant metabolism pathway of catecholamines, and by the continuous release of metanephrines in the circulation by the tumor, independent of the episodic and variable release of catecholamines.[131] The measurement of catecholamines and VMA is associated with a risk of false negatives, and therefore it is less sensitive than that of metanephrines.[132]

Extraadrenal PPGL produce almost exclusively norepinephrine and normetanephrine because they lack appreciable expression of phenylethanolamine N-methyltransferase (PNMT), the enzyme responsible for the conversion of norepinephrine to epinephrine. The expression of PNMT is induced by glucocorticoids. Thus, the production of epinephrine is almost completely confined to the adrenal medulla, which receives blood flow containing very high concentrations of glucocorticoids produced in the adjacent adrenal cortex. Therefore, PPGL that produce epinephrine and metanephrines originate from adrenal medulla and are called *pheochromocytomas*.[141]

During pregnancy, the metabolism of the catecholamines is unaltered, and even in cases of gestational hypertension or preeclampsia, the plasma levels of catecholamines are only slightly elevated, while the levels of metanephrines are usually normal.[130,137] In the case of a slightly elevated level (i.e., less than two to three times normal value), the presence of false positives due to the sampling method, medications or medical conditions must be excluded.[130,132,137] For plasma-free metanephrines, false positives can be obtained if the sampling is done while the patient is upright.[132] In the cases in which this interference is suspected, the test must be repeated after the patient is supine for 30 min.[132]

Some medications (labetalol, α-methyldopa, sotalol, acetaminophen, buspirone, and sulfasalazine) may cause false positives by interfering with the measurement of the metanephrines by LC-ECD methods.[132] Other medications, such as tricyclic antidepressants, monoamine oxydase (MAO) inhibitors, sympathomimetic, cocaine, and phenoxybenzamine, interfere with the disposition of the catecholamines, and therefore lead to elevated levels of catecholamines and metanephrines in all methods.[132] Levodopa causes a false elevation of 3-methoxytyramine, the metabolite of dopamine.[132] Medical conditions such as congestive heart failure, acute myocardial infarction, alcohol or clonidine withdrawal, panic attacks, brain tumors, and subarachnoid bleeding can be associated with increased circulating levels of metanephrines and catecholamines.[130] In the general population, in cases of persistent elevation of plasma metanephrines after the exclusion of sampling method error or artifactual medications/medical conditions, clonidine suppression can be achieved.[132] However, clonidine suppression testing is not recommended during pregnancy because it is potentially associated with significant adverse side effects.[131]

25.5.4.2 Localization of the Tumor

Once the biochemical diagnosis of PPGL is done, imaging studies must be done to localize the tumor.[132] In the general population, abdominal CT scan with contrast is the first choice of imaging for PPGL localization because it has a sensitivity of 88%–100% and most tumors are located in the abdomen.[132] PPGL may be homogenous or heterogeneous, with cystic and solid portions, necrosis, and calcifications.[132] From 87% to 100% of PPGL exhibit a mean attenuation of >10 HU on unenhanced CT scan, but sometimes they have a washout of contrast >60% on 15-min delayed scanning.[132] In cases of extraadrenal or metastatic tumor, the sensitivity of CT was reported to be as low as 57%.[132] MRI is associated with a higher sensitivity, with the exception of lung metastasis.[132] In a recent review of PPGL in pregnancy, 80% were located in the adrenal, with 15% being bilateral and 20% were extraadrenal.[134]

In the context of pregnancy, CT scan is not recommended because of the potential hazards associated with radiation.[131] Therefore, abdominal ultrasound or MRI without contrast are the preferred techniques for localization of PPGL during pregnancy.[52,134,137] Ultrasound has a limited sensitivity for small tumors; thus, a negative test does not exclude the presence of PPGL.[131] Abdominal MRI without gadolinium is the preferred option to localize PPGL during pregnancy, but its sensitivity is unknown.[130] Further, ^{123}I-MIBG is a functional imaging that can be used to localize PPGL, but its sensitivity (85%–88% for pheochromocytoma and 56%–75% for paraganglioma) is less than for CT scan, and 50% of normal adrenal glands demonstrate a physiological uptake of the isotope, which can be associated with false positives.[132] The diagnostic performance of ^{123}I-MIBG is less in cases of metastatic PPGL or SDHx mutation-associated PPGL.[132] However, it can be useful in the context of metastatic disease with positive ^{123}I-MIBG because treatment with ^{131}I-MIBG may be considered.[132] Also, ^{18}F-fluorodeoxyglucose (^{18}F-FDG) positron emission tomography (PET)/CT scanning has a sensitivity from 74% to 100% and a higher diagnostic performance with metastatic or *SDHB*-related disease.[132]

Recently, ^{68}Ga-labeled SAs (^{68}Ga-DOTA-SSAs) PET/CT imaging was reported to be more sensitive than ^{18}F-FDG PET/CT in SDHx, metastatic, and head-and-neck PPGL.[142] Also, labeled SAs can be used in the radioactive treatment of these tumors.[142] However, during pregnancy, ^{123}I-MIBG, ^{18}F-FDG PET/CT, and ^{68}Ga-DOTA-SSAs scanning are contraindicated because of the placental transfer of those isotopes, resulting in significant radiation of the fetus.[47,137] In case of suspected extraabdominal disease, MRI of the thorax and neck might be considered. Functional imaging with ^{123}I-MIBG and ^{18}F-FDG PET/CT scanning can be used in the postpartum period to confirm the absence of other lesions, but consulting with the nuclear medicine specialist should be obtained for a nursing mother to determine the period for which breastfeeding should be interrupted to ensure the security of the newborn.[132,135,143]

25.5.5 Treatment of Pheochromocytoma During Pregnancy

The optimal treatment of PPGL is the removal of the tumor by surgery after an adequate medical preparation of the patient.[132,137]

25.5.5.1 Preoperative Medical Treatment

Adequate medical preoperative treatment with α-adrenoreceptor blockade is one of the main reasons that explain the decrease in surgical mortality to <3% during the last 30 years.[131] It is imperative to start the α-adrenoreceptor blockade as soon as the diagnosis of PPGL is made, and it should be administered to the patient for at least 10–14 days before surgery to achieve proper control of the BP, avoid paroxysms, and restore normal blood volume.[130] The usual target of BP in nonpregnant patients is <130/80 mmHg while in a seated position and a systolic BP > 90 mmHg while standing, with a target heart rate of 60–70 bpm while seated and 70–80 bpm while standing.[132] However, the target BP in pregnant women with PPGL is unknown.[137]

The BP targets for the management of gestational hypertension or chronic hypertension during pregnancy, according to the latest SOGC guidelines, are <160/110 mmHg for severe hypertension (systolic BP ≥ 160 or diastolic BP ≥ 110 mmHg), between 130–155/80–105 mmHg for nonsevere hypertension (BP 140–159/90–109 mmHg) without comorbid conditions, and to <140/90 mmHg for nonsevere hypertension with comorbid conditions.[128] However, it is unknown if the catecholamine blockade is sufficiently achieved with these targets in most pregnant patients with PPGL. It should also be taken into account that excessive treatment can result in hypotension, which in turn can reduce uteroplacental circulation, which is not subject to autoregulation.[137] Therefore, the dosing of α-adrenoreceptor blockade during pregnancy is a delicate balance between treating the consequence of the catecholamines excess, such as hypertension and uteroplacental vasoconstriction, while maintaining adequate uteroplacental perfusion.[137]

Even normotensive pregnant women with PPGL should be treated with low-dose α-adrenergic receptor blockers to prevent an acute hypertensive crisis that is associated with high mortality.[137] Actually, there are insufficient data to support the use of α1-selective adrenoreceptor blockers (doxazosin or prazosin) rather than nonselective α-adrenoreceptor blockers (phenoxybenzamine).[132] All α-adrenoreceptor blockers are FDA Category C drugs for use in pregnancy, which indicates that risk for the fetus cannot be ruled out.[130]

Phenoxybenzamine, a noncompetitive α1- and α2-adrenoreceptor antagonist, remains the α-adrenoreceptor antagonist most widely used to treat PPGL diagnosed during pregnancy.[130,134,137] However, it crosses the placenta and has been associated in some cases with neonatal hypotension and respiratory depression; if phenoxybenzamine is used during pregnancy, the newborn must be carefully monitored for the first days of life.[137] It also blocks the presynaptic α2-adrenergic receptor, which enhances norepinephrine release from the presynaptic nerve and then can cause a reflex tachycardia in the mother.[130,137] Other disadvantages of phenoxybenzamine are its prolonged half-life and the irreversible blockade of α-adrenoreceptors, which can cause hypotension in postoperative periods that can last for 14 to longer than 48 h.[137] If used, the suggested starting dose of phenoxybenzamine is 10 mg PO twice daily, and the final dose is usually around 1 mg/kg/day.[132] The most frequent maternal side effects are tachycardia, nasal congestion, and orthostatic hypotension.[130,131]

Doxazosin is a competitive α1-selective adrenoreceptor blocker, and it is associated with less reflex tachycardia than phenoxybenzamine,[130,131] which could make the use of concomitant β-blocker unnecessary.[130] Also, its half-life (22 h) is shorter than phenoxybenzamine, and it is associated with less postoperative hypotension.[130,131] Patients pretreated with doxazosin or other α1-selective adrenoreceptor blockers showed higher maximal systolic BP than those pretreated with phenoxybenzamine, but the surgical outcome was reported to be the same in both groups.[131] The starting dose of doxazosin is 2 mg/day in one or divided doses, and usually the maximal dose is 32 mg/day.[132] So far, the neonatal outcomes associated with the use of doxazosin during pregnancy are good, and even if it can cross the placenta, but no adverse effects were reported in newborns.[137,144]

Prazosin is also associated with a low incidence of reflex tachycardia and postoperative hypotension.[130] In fact, it has a short half-life of 2–3 h, and it must be administered twice or thrice daily.[130] Because of this short half-life, it is possible that at the time of the surgery, the plasmatic level of prazosin may be low and ineffective.[130] The most frequent side effects associated with doxazosin and prazosin are dizziness, malaise, fatigue, and headache.[130] The medical treatment also should include a high-sodium diet and continuous IV fluid intake, which needs to be started a few days after the α-adrenergic blockade to reverse catecholamine-induced blood volume contraction and to prevent preoperative orthostatic hypotension and severe hypotension after tumor removal.[131,132,137] Also, volume repletion can support the uteroplacental circulations.[137] In cases of persistent hypertension despite α-adrenergic blockade and no reflex tachycardia, dihydropyridine calcium channel blockers, which are generally considered safe during pregnancy (nifedipine and nicardipine), can be added.[130,137]

In cases of reflex tachycardia that occurs after α-adrenergic receptor blockade, beta-blockers may be used. They should be started only after several days of α-adrenergic receptor blockade because a nonselective β-blockade leads to unopposed α-adrenoreceptor stimulation by catecholamines, resulting in hypertensive crisis.[130] However, beta-blockers have been associated with IUGR, and therefore, it is generally advised to use them only for short periods of time during pregnancy.[137]

Methyldopa is a drug frequently used to treat gestational hypertension. However, it should not be used in the context of PPGL because it can worsen BP.[130,137] Labetalol, a combined α- and β-adrenergic receptor blocker, is also not a recommended option for the treatment of hypertension in the context of PPGL, given that its α-adrenergic blockade is relatively weak, resulting in paroxysmal hypertension in some cases.[137]

25.5.5.2 *Surgical Resection of the Tumor*

After adequate medical preparation, the surgical resection of the PPGL can be done. During pregnancy, the surgery should be done in the second trimester, before 24 weeks' gestation.[131,135] Surgery during the first trimester increases the risk of spontaneous abortion, while after 24 weeks' gestation, uterine growth may preclude the surgery.[131,135] In cases of pheochromocytoma diagnosed before 24 weeks' gestation, laparoscopic adrenalectomy is the treatment of choice when the tumor is < 6–7 cm, given that it is associated with fewer postoperative complications, less postoperative pain, and less perioperative hemodynamic instability than open surgery.[52,130,131,137] In a recent and large series, 16/18 (89%) pheochromocytomas resected before 24 weeks' gestation by laparoscopic adrenalectomy resulted in a healthy mother and baby.[134] In the case of paragangliomas, open surgery is the preferred option, but laparoscopic surgery can be safely done in some instances of small and noninvasive paragangliomas.[130]

When the diagnosis of PPGL is made in early pregnancy and surgery can be performed before 24 weeks of gestation, prolonged medical therapy until term is not recommended. In the series of Biggar et al., 3/8 (38%) of the pregnant patients that had prolonged medical treatment had adverse outcomes: two women experienced intrauterine death and one developed metastatic disease.[134] Therefore, laparoscopic adrenalectomy before 24 weeks' gestation is considered safer and is associated with better outcomes than medical treatment and delayed adrenalectomy.[134]

When laparoscopic adrenalectomy is done before 24 weeks' gestation, the route of delivery can be vaginal delivery or a cesarean section.[131,137] After excision of the tumor, biochemical cure should be confirmed 4–6 weeks after surgery, with plasma-free metanephrines or fractionated urinary metanephrines measured during pregnancy, given that secondary lesions can complicate pregnancy later if they are present.[134,135]

When the diagnosis of PPGL is made after 24 weeks' gestation, medical treatment should be instituted and the adrenalectomy performed when fetal maturity is achieved in the final trimester.[130,137] Laparoscopic adrenalectomy can be done at the same time as the elective cesarean section or a few days or weeks later.[134,137] The advantage of delaying the adrenalectomy by a couple of days or weeks after delivery is that it allows ^{123}I-MIBG and/or ^{18}F-FDG PET/CT scanning to confirm the localization and rule out secondary lesions; it also allows in some cases the improvement of the α-adrenergic blockade.[130,134] Cesarean section is still the suggested route of delivery for cases of PPGL that are not resected before 24 weeks' gestation because vaginal delivery in undiagnosed cases of pheochromocytoma is associated with high maternal and fetal mortality.[130] However, several cases were recently reported of successful vaginal delivery in pregnant patients with PPGL with an adequate medical preparation under epidural analgesia.[137] Also, it is probably safer in multiparous women under epidural anesthesia, who are more likely to have a short and uneventful labor.[130,134]

Overall, cesarean section remains the delivery route of choice in most patients, but vaginal delivery can be considered an adequate way to medically treat multiparous women who are predicted to have an uneventful labor.[130] The timing of surgery depends ultimately on the efficacy of medical treatment to control BP of the mother, as well as fetal well-being.[134] Early delivery should be done with IUGR, decreased fetal movement, deceleration in fetal cardiac monitoring, persistent maternal labile hypertension, or a strong suspicion of malignant PPGL.[134]

25.5.5.3 Medical Treatment of Acute Hypertensive crisis

In cases of acute hypertensive crisis during pregnancy, several drugs can be used. Phentolamine, a competitive α1- and α2-adrenergic receptor antagonist, is a good option, given its fast action.[130,131] Direct vasodilatators, such as hydralazine, nitroglycerine, and sodium nitroprusside, can be effective in treating hypertensive crisis in patients with PPGL. However, the use of sodium nitroprusside is debated because the drug may cause fetal cyanide toxicity if used at an infusion rate ≥ 1 mcg/kg/min.[130,131] Intravenous magnesium sulfate has been reported to be effective in several cases of PPGL hypertensive crisis.[130,145] Magnesium sulfate inhibits catecholamine release, reduces the sensitivity of α-adrenergic receptors to catecholamines, and induces vasodilatation.[131,145] Short-acting calcium channel blockers such as nicardipine also have been used successfully.[130] In cases of significant tachyarrhythmia, esmolol, a short-acting β-blocker that can be given intravenously, can be used, but only after an adequate α-adrenergic blockade.[130,131]

25.5.5.4 Special Considerations in Nursing Mothers

Doxazosin excretion into breast milk is reported in only two cases in the literature. In a mother taking doxazosin 4 mg daily, the relative infant dose was <1%, so doxazosin appears safe under the 10% of the dose considered to be safe for the infant.[146] In another case, there was no doxazosin detected in breast milk in a sample obtained 30 h after the last doxazosin dose in a nursing mother.[144] However, it is impossible to conclude that doxazosin is safe in a mother taking higher doses of doxazosin. No data have been published on the excretion of phenoxybenzamine and prazosin in breast milk, so it is preferable to avoid their use during breastfeeding. Propranolol is the safest beta-blocker to use during breastfeeding because it has an elevated plasma protein binding, very low concentration in breast milk, and no adverse effects reported in breastfed infants.[147,148] Metoprolol is also considered safe, given that the infant relative dose is reported to be 1.4%.[147] But atenolol should be avoided during breastfeeding, given that the relative infant dose is reported to be between 5.7% and 19.2%, and there was a case report of bradycardia and tachypnea in a breastfed infant of a nursing mother taking the drug.[147,148]

25.6 CONGENITAL ADRENAL HYPERPLASIA

Congenital adrenal hyperplasia (CAH) is a group of inherited genetic autosomal recessive disorders involving deficiency in the enzymes that are involved in cortisol synthesis by the zona fasciculata.[15,149] The enzymatic defect results in diminished cortisol synthesis, which in turn results in decreased glucocorticoid receptor-mediated inhibition of the HPA axis and increased secretion of ACTH. The chronically elevated ACTH stimulates adrenal cortex hyperplasia and accumulation of steroid precursors prior to enzymatic defects.[15,149] The clinical presentation depends on the enzymatic defects and the associated elevation in precursors and derived steroid pathways. In this chapter, we will focus on 21-α-hydroxylase (21-OH) deficiency, which accounts for more than 90% of the cases of CAH.[149,150] The 21-OH deficiency results from mutation or deletion in the *CYP21A2* gene, located on chromosome 6p21.[149,151] In cases of 21-OH deficiency, the excess immediate 17-OH-progesterone precursor is diverted to excess adrenal androgen production, resulting in hyperandrogenism in affected females.[150] The diagnosis is made by the demonstration of significantly elevated basal or cosyntropin-stimulated 17-OH-progesterone blood levels.[150]

There are two principal subtypes of 21-OH deficiency that differ in their clinical phenotype: classic 21-OH deficiency CAH and nonclassic CAH.[149,152] Classic CAH affects 1/13,000 to 1/15,000 live births.[149] It is divided into two subtypes of clinical phenotypes, simple virilizing and salt wasting, which differ by the severity of the enzymatic defect and clinical phenotype.[149] Salt-wasting CAH, which accounts for 75% of the cases of classical CAH, is the most severe form; it is associated with severe impairment of the 21-OH enzyme (<2% enzyme activity), which results in insufficient production of aldosterone and cortisol to sustain normal life.[149,150] It usually presents in newborn females with genital ambiguity, and features of salt-wasting/adrenal crisis appear in the first month following delivery in both sexes, including hypovolemia, hyponatremia, hyperkalemia, failure to thrive, seizure, and ultimately death. Male newborns are at high risk of being unrecognized because they do not show the sexual ambiguity that raises suspicion about the diagnosis.[149,151] An activity of 21-OH of 1%–2% over the activity of salt-wasting form results in a simple, virilizing form, representing 25% of classical CAH. In simple, virilizing defects, there is sufficient production of aldosterone, but the cortisol deficiency causes an increase in ACTH secretion and an overproduction of adrenal androgens, resulting in genital ambiguity in females.[149]

In classical CAH, virilization occurs in female fetuses at 7–12 weeks' gestation.[151] Surgical genitoplasty can be done in females with genital ambiguity.[150] Later in childhood and adolescence, if not adequately treated with glucocorticoids, patients with classical CAH will develop signs of androgen excess, such as precocious puberty and accelerated growth, leading to a short adult height.[149,150]

Nonclassic CAH is a mild form of CAH usually associated with variable degrees of postnatal hyperandrogenism, but it also can be asymptomatic. It is usually associated with 20%–50% of 21-OH normal function.[149,150] The incidence of non-classical CAH is about 1/1000.[152] The glucocorticoid or mineralocorticoid deficiency is usually not severe enough to require replacement therapy.[149] However, the glucocorticoid secretion is insufficient to counteract ACTH oversecretion, leading to mild adrenal androgen oversecretion.[149] When symptomatic, nonclassical CAH can present with premature pubarche or adrenarche, accelerated growth, hirsutism, menstrual cycle disorders, acne, and infertility.[149]

The fertility rate is decreased in classic 21-OH CAH, and it is especially diminished in patients with the salt-wasting subtype.[15,153] Various explanations have been proposed to explain that diminished fertility, including frequent irregular menses and anovulation, secondary PCOS, nonsuppressible progesterone levels, endometrial implantation difficulty, a diminished heterosexual relationship, or inadequate introitus in cases of genital ambiguity.[152–154] The development of PCOS may be related to both prenatal and postnatal excess androgen exposure, which can affect the hypothalamic-pituitary-gonadal (HPG) axis.[154] However, with adequate hormonal replacement therapy, a significant proportion of women with classic CAH wishing to conceive were able to become pregnant.[152,153] One major limitation to pregnancy rates appears to be that women with classical CAH are less interested in fertility.[152]

Nonclassical CAH can also be associated with infertility in some women, but the pregnancy and live birth rates appear to be similar to the general population, with appropriate use of glucocorticoid replacement in patients who do not conceive normally without it.[15,154,155]

25.6.1 Treatment of Pregnant Patients with 21-OH Congenital Adrenal Hyperplasia During Pregnancy, Labor, and Postpartum

In the context of classical CAH, there is an AI that necessitates adequate glucocorticoid replacement and, in the salt-wasting subtype, mineralocorticoid (fludrocortisone) replacement. During pregnancy, hydrocortisone is the preferred glucocorticoid, as it is metabolized by the placental 11β-HSD 2.[15] Hydrocortisone and fludrocortisone dosage should be adjusted based on regular clinical evaluation, such as suggested for PAI management during pregnancy.[150,154] Some authors suggest monitoring 17-OH-progesterone, androstenedione, and testosterone levels during pregnancy and adjusting the treatment to target levels in the high-normal range for pregnancy.[152,154] As the levels of these hormones increase during pregnancy in normal women, the replacement therapy dose should be adjusted to pregnancy values to avoid unnecessary excessive treatment. Pregnant women with CAH are at increased risk for developing gestational diabetes and should be monitored with oral glucose tolerance tests frequently throughout pregnancy, but there are no recommendations for the frequency.[29,150,152] Women with classical CAH should receive glucocorticoid stress dosing in the context of labor and delivery to prevent adrenal crisis at dosages similar to those suggested for women with PAI.[15,29,150,154] Elective cesarean is the preferred route for delivery in women with classical CAH who have undergone feminizing genitoplasty.[152,154]

25.6.2 Genetics of 21-OH Congenital Adrenal Hyperplasia and Prenatal Genetic Counseling

Mutations in the CYP21A2 gene cause CAH, but it is the milder of the two affected alleles that usually defines the phenotype.[149] In classical CAH, there is usually a mutation associated with severe loss of function on both alleles.[151] In nonclassical CAH, there can be one severely affected allele and one mildly affected one. Up to 70% of patients with nonclassical CAH are compounds heterozygote carrying one allele with a mutation associated with classic CAH.[149] Therefore, even in nonclassical CAH, there can be a risk of having a newborn with classical CAH if both the mother and the father carry an allele associated with classical CAH.[149] Therefore, preconception genotyping is essential for both parents to determine the risk of classical CAH in their offspring.[149]

25.6.3 Prenatal Treatment to Prevent Virilization in Female Fetuses

The goal of prenatal therapy is to minimize or prevent genital virilization in female fetuses affected with classical CAH in order to limit or eliminate the need for future genitoplasty and gender assignment issues.[149,153] However, prenatal therapy does not eliminate the need for lifelong glucocorticoid/mineralocorticoid replacement therapy for classical CAH.[150] Prenatal treatment remains controversial, and in the most recent clinical guidelines of the Endocrine Society, it is suggested only in the context of research protocols.[150]

One of the main concerns about prenatal treatment is that only 25% of fetuses will be affected by classical CAH, and only 50% of those would be female fetuses. Therefore, of every 8 fetuses, 7 are exposed to unnecessary glucocorticoids, which is associated with potential risk for the fetus, for the 1 female fetus that potentially benefits from being treated.[150] Then, in the context of research protocols, prenatal therapy can be offered for a pregnancy that is at risk of resulting in classical CAH, such as for families with members affected by classical CAH or pregnant women known to carry a severe mutation, and particularly if the partner also carries a severe mutation.[154]

Dexamethasone is used for prenatal therapy because it is not inactivated by placental 11β-HSD 2 and can reach the fetal circulation to suppress fetal pituitary ACTH secretion. The resulting decreased fetal pituitary ACTH secretion minimizes fetal adrenal androgen secretion and limits genital virilization in female fetuses.[149] The treatment should be initiated before 7 weeks of gestation or 9 weeks of amenorrhea to be effective because after that time period, increased fetal androgen secretion initiates genital virilization.[154] The suggested dose for the mother is 20 mg/kg/day based on the maternal prepregnancy body weight, with a maximum dose of 1.5 mg/day divided into three daily doses.[149] However, this dose represents 6 times the dosage of dexamethasone recommended for the mother, and the fetus receives approximately 60 times the usual physiologic glucocorticoid dosage.[151] There were no studies done with lower dosages of dexamethasone, and it is unknown why such high doses would be necessary.[151] When initiated before 9 weeks of amenorrhea and maintained throughout pregnancy, this regimen resulted in normal feminine genitalia in 80%–85% of CAH girls.[151,153] Further, failures are usually due to late initiation therapy, early cessation, or poor compliance with the therapy.[149]

To limit unnecessary exposure of male fetuses, early prenatal sex determination should be done.[153] The identification of the *SRY* gene in fetal deoxyribonucleic acid (DNA) that circulate in maternal plasma can be done as early as 4.5 weeks of gestation (6.5 weeks of amenorrhea), with a reported sensitivity of 96% and no false positives in female fetuses.[156] It avoids prenatal treatment of 68% of male fetuses in one cohort.[156] Sequence analysis comparing the established linkage of SNPs in the CYP21A2 locus of the proband to the fetus allows prenatal diagnosis of 21-OH deficiency CAH by free fetal DNA analysis as early as 6 weeks' gestation[149,153]; this technique can avoid unnecessary treatment in male and female fetuses unaffected by the disease.[149] The other techniques that can be used to identify fetal sex and prenatal CAH diagnosis are chorionic villi sampling, which can be done at 9–11 weeks' gestation, and amniocentesis, which can be done at 15–20 weeks' gestation.[149] Because these procedures cannot be done before 7 weeks' gestation, the fetuses that can be potentially affected by CAH are treated for a few weeks before the treatment can be discontinued for male fetuses or unaffected female fetuses.[151] These techniques are associated with an estimated loss of a fetus of 0.2% for chorionic villi sampling and 0.1% for the amniocentesis.[149] Chorionic villi sampling and amniocentesis also allow prenatal diagnosis of 21-OH deficiency, but a small percentage of patients have undetectable mutations or maternal DNA contamination, which leads to false negative or positive results.[149]

Prenatal therapy is associated with some maternal adverse effects, such as weight gain, edema, mood change, sleep disturbance, acne, and striae.[151,153] However, major side effects, such as gestational hypertension, gestational diabetes, stillbirth, and spontaneous abortion, were not associated with prenatal dexamethasone treatment.[15,153] Thus, prenatal treatment does not represent a major risk for the mother, but if administered, serial monitoring of the weight, BP, and blood glucose should be performed.[150]

Most concerns about prenatal treatment are related to potential adverse effects for the fetus. High-dose glucocorticoids during the first trimester are reported to be anatomically and metabolically teratogenic in animals.[151] Prenatal dexamethasone in rodents is associated with cleft palate; reduced number of kidney cells undergoing mitosis, resulting in postnatal hypertension, albuminuria, and decreased glomerular filtration rate (GFR); impaired thyroid development; reduced birth weight; and susceptibility as adults to develop hypertension, glucose intolerance, and fatty liver.[151]

In nonhuman primates, dexamethasone prenatal exposure is associated with reduced pancreatic beta cell numbers, impaired glucose tolerance, increased systolic and diastolic BP, elevated cortisol levels, and reduced postnatal growth.[151] In animals, high-dose prenatal dexamethasone also exerts negative impacts on brain development.[151] In humans, an increased risk of cleft palate was reported to be associated with high-dose glucocorticoid exposition for multiple reasons in the conception period.[151] However, only one case of cleft palate related to prenatal dexamethasone treatment was recently reported.[157] There were no reported significant differences in head circumference, birth weight or length, and postnatal growth when compared to controls in several cohorts.[153] However, Miller suggested that even if not statistically significant, newborns treated prenatally with dexamethasone have lower birth weight, which can potentially predispose to chronic diseases during adulthood.[151]

There are conflicting results for the potential effect of prenatal treatment for CAH on brain development in humans.[149] New at al. found no adverse long-term effects relating to cognitive function, motor function, or gender identity and behavior in 149 children aged 12 and older, affected and unaffected with CAH, that were exposed in utero to dexamethasone partially or until term.[149] A Polish study reported that prenatal dexamethasone treatment can have a positive effect on the cognition of CAH-affected females, but a negative impact on cognition of females unaffected by CAH.[158] Another study showed no change on working memory globally on individuals exposed to dexamethasone prenatally, but women who were exposed for the long term during pregnancy have lower cognitive processing.[159] Smaller studies from a Swedish group found that in comparison to controls, CAH-unaffected children treated prenatally with dexamethasone for a short period had significantly poorer performance on verbal working memory, lower self-perceived scholastic competence, higher self-perceived social anxiety, and boys had more neutral gender-role behaviors.[160] However, the adult outcomes of those CAH-unaffected patients revealed no significant difference in cognitive abilities or behaviors, such as depression, anxiety, or autistic traits compared to controls.[161]

It should be noted that even if not statistically significant, CAH-unaffected women treated prenatally with dexamethasone scored higher on the anxiety scale and performed worse on verbal intelligence, spatial-working memory, and learning and memory tests.[161] Recent studies have reported that adult women with CAH treated prenatally for the entire gestational period have a poorer performance in tests for all cognitive measures, including self-reported executive functioning and long-term memory.[162] Based on parental ratings, prenatally treated children did not have major behavioral problems or psychopathology, and they were reported to have increased sociability compared to controls.[163] Therefore, concerns remain about the long-term safety of prenatal dexamethasone treatment on cognition and behavior. Long-term observational studies are warranted to assess the potential risks and benefits of this treatment according to the gender and disease status of the exposed patients.

REFERENCES

1. Ganie MA, Bhat RA, Irfan-Ul-Qayoom DMA, Kotwal S, Bhat MA, et al. Unassisted successful pregnancy in a case of Addison's disease with recurrent pregnancy loss. *Indian J Endocrinol Metab* 2012;**16**(3):481–2.
2. Ebeling F, Rahkonen L, Saastamoinen KP, Matikainen N, Laitinen K. Addison's disease presenting as hyperemesis, hyponatremia and pancytopenia in early pregnancy. *Acta Obstet Gynecol Scand* 2011;**90**(1):121–2.
3. George LD, Selvaraju R, Reddy K, Stout TV, Premawardhana LDKE. Vomiting and hyponatraemia in pregnancy. *BJOG An Int J Obstet Gynaecol* 2000;**107**(6):808–9.
4. Hincz P, Lewandowski KC, Cajdler-Luba A, Salata I, Lewinski A. New onset addison's disease presenting as prolonged hyperemesis in early pregnancy. *Endocr Abstr* 2009;**19**(42):P84.
5. Mittal A, Dexter S, Marcus S, Tremble J. First presentation of Addison's disease in the 2nd trimester of pregnancy. *J Obstet Gynaecol (Lahore)* 2011;**31**(4):342.
6. Fux Otta C, Szafryk de Mereshian P, Iraci GS, Ojeda de Pruneda MR. Pregnancies associated with primary adrenal insufficiency. *Fertil Steril* 2008;**90**(4).
7. Gradden C, Lawrence D, Doyle PM, Welch CR. Uses of error: Addison's disease in pregnancy. *Lancet* 2001;**357**:1197.
8. Abu MA, Sinha P, Totoe L. Addison's disease in pregnancy presenting as hyperemesis gravidarum. *J Obstet Gynaecol J Inst Obstet Gynaecol* 1997;**17**(3):278–9.
9. Seaward PGR, Guidozzi F, Sonnendecker EWW. Addisonian crisis in pregnancy: case report. *BJOG An Int J Obstet Gynaecol* 1989;**96**(11):1348–50.
10. Spaniol A, Mulla BM, Daily JG, Ennen CS. Carney complex: a rare cause of Cushing syndrome in pregnancy. *Obstet Gynecol* 2014;**124**(2 Pt 2):426–8.
11. Lindsay JR, Nieman LK. The hypothalamic-pituitary-adrenal axis in pregnancy: challenges in disease detection and treatment. *Endocr Rev* 2005;**26**(6):775–99.
12. Cohade C, Broussaud S, Louiset E, Bennet A, Huyghe E, Caron P. Ectopic Cushing's syndrome due to a pheochromocytoma: a new case in the postpartum and review of literature. *Gynecol Endocrinol* 2009;**25**(9):624–7.
13. Bornstein SR, Allolio B, Arlt W, Barthel A, Don-Wauchope A, Hammer GD, et al. Diagnosis and treatment of primary adrenal insufficiency: an endocrine society clinical practice guideline. *J Clin Endocrinol Metab* 2016;**101**(2):364–89.
14. Anand G, Beuschlein F. Management of endocrine disease: fertility, pregnancy and lactation in women with adrenal insufficiency. *Eur J Endocrinol* 2018;**178**:R45–53.
15. Lekarev O, New MI. Adrenal disease in pregnancy. *Best Pract Res Clin Endocrinol Metab* 2011;**25**(6):959–73.
16. Schneiderman M, Czuzoj-Shulman N, Spence AR, Abenhaim HA. Maternal and neonatal outcomes of pregnancies in women with Addison's disease: a population-based cohort study on 7.7 million births. *BJOG An Int J Obstet Gynaecol* 2017;**124**(11):1772–9.

17. Yuen KCJ, Chong LE, Koch CA. Adrenal insufficiency in pregnancy: challenging issues in diagnosis and management. *Endocrine* 2013;**44**(2):283–92.

18. Björnsdottir S, Cnattingius S, Brandt L, Nordenström A, Ekbom A, Kämpe O, et al. Addison's disease in women is a risk factor for an adverse pregnancy outcome. *J Clin Endocrinol Metab* 2010;**95**(12):5249–57.

19. Langlois F, Lim DST, Fleseriu M. Update on adrenal insufficiency: diagnosis and management in pregnancy. *Curr Opin Endocrinol Diabetes Obes* 2017;**24**(3):184–92.

20. Mweemba DM, Beck I, Tuffnell DJ. Spontaneous maternal adrenal haemorrhage as a cause of intra uterine foetal death. *J Obstet Gynaecol (Lahore)* 2005;**25**(2):194–5.

21. Simon DR, Palese MA. Clinical update on the management of adrenal hemorrhage. *Curr Urol Rep* 2009;**10**(1):78–83.

22. McKenna DS, Wittber GM, Nagaraja HN, Samuels P. The effects of repeat doses of antenatal corticosteroids on maternal adrenal function. *Am J Obstet Gynecol* 2000;**183**(3):669–73.

23. McKenna DS, Fisk AD. The effect of a single course of antenatal corticosteroids on maternal adrenal function at term. *J Matern Neonatal Med* 2004;**16**(1):33–6.

24. Charmandari E, Nicolaides NC, Chrousos GP. Adrenal insufficiency. *Lancet* 2014;**383**(9935):2152–67.

25. Kübler K, Klingmüller D, Gembruch U, Merz WM. High-risk pregnancy management in women with hypopituitarism. *J Perinatol* 2009;**29**(2):89–95.

26. Gei-Guardia O, Soto-Herrera E, Gei-Brealey A, Chen-Ku C. Sheehan syndrome in costa rica: clinical experience with 60 sases. *Endocr Pract* 2011;**17**(3):337–44.

27. Matsuzaki S, Endo M, Ueda Y, Mimura K, Kakigano A, Egawa-Takata T, et al. A case of acute Sheehan's syndrome and literature review: a rare but life-threatening complication of postpartum hemorrhage. *BMC Pregnancy Childbirth* 2017;**17**(1):1–10.

28. Molitch ME, Gillam M. Lymphocytic hypophysitis. *Horm Res* 2007;**68**(Suppl 5):145–50.

29. Kamoun M, Mnif MF, Charfi N, Kacem FH, Naceur BB, Mnif F, et al. Adrenal diseases during pregnancy: pathophysiology, diagnosis and management strategies. *Am J Med Sci* 2014;**347**(1):64–73.

30. Lebbe M, Arlt W. What is the best diagnostic and therapeutic management strategy for an Addison patient during pregnancy? *Clin Endocrinol (Oxf)* 2013;**78**(4):497–502.

31. Fleseriu M, Hashim IA, Karavitaki N, Melmed S, Murad MH, Salvatori R, et al. Hormonal replacement in hypopituitarism in adults: an endocrine society clinical practice guideline. *J Clin Endocrinol Metab* 2016;**101**(11):3888–921.

32. Ambroziak U, Kondracka A, Bartoszewicz Z, Krasnodębska-Kiljańska M, Bednarczuk T. The morning and late-night salivary cortisol ranges for healthy women may be used in pregnancy. *Clin Endocrinol (Oxf)* 2015;**83**(6):774–8.

33. Jung C, Ho JT, Torpy DJ, Rogers A, Doogue M, Lewis JG, et al. A longitudinal study of plasma and urinary cortisol in pregnancy and postpartum. *J Clin Endocrinol Metab* 2011;**96**(5):1533–40.

34. Ospina NS, Al NA, Bancos I, Javed A, Benkhadra K, Kapoor E, et al. ACTH stimulation tests for the diagnosis of adrenal insufficiency: systematic review and meta-analysis. *J Clin Endocrinol Metab* 2016;**101**(2):427–34.

35. Suri D, Moran J, Hibbard JU, Kasza K, Weiss RE. Assessment of adrenal reserve in pregnancy: defining the normal response to the adrenocorticotropin stimulation test. *J Clin Endocrinol Metab* 2006;**91**(10):3866–72.

36. Irani RA, Xia Y. Renin angiotensin signaling in normal pregnancy and preeclampsia. *Semin Nephrol* 2011;**31**(1):47–58.

37. Scrimin F, Panerari F, Guaschino S. Addison's disease and hypothyroidism untreated until twenty-four weeks of pregnancy. *Acta Obstet Gynecol Scand* 2005;**84**(2):198–9.

38. Lindsay JR, Jonklaas J, Oldfield EH, Nieman LK. Cushing's syndrome during pregnancy: personal experience and review of the literature. *J Clin Endocrinol Metab* 2005;**90**(5):3077–83.

39. Chrisoulidou A, Boudina M, Karavitaki N, Bili E, Wass J. Pituitary disorders in pregnancy. *Hormones* 2015;**14**(1):70–80.

40. Remde H, Zopf K, Schwander J. Fertility and pregnancy in primary adrenal insufficiency in Germany. *Horm Metab Res* 2016;**48**(5):306–11.

41. Nieman LK, Biller BMK, Findling JW, Murad MH, Newell-Price J, Savage MO, et al. Treatment of Cushing's syndrome: an endocrine society clinical practice guideline. *J Clin Endocrinol Metab* 2015;**100**(8):2807–31.

42. Lacroix A, Feelders RA, Stratakis CA, Nieman LK. Cushing's syndrome. *Lancet* 2015;**386**(9996):913–27.

43. Caimari F, Valassi E, Garbayo P, Steffensen C, Santos A, Corcoy R, et al. Cushing's syndrome and pregnancy outcomes: a systematic review of published cases. *Endocrine* 2017;**55**(2):555–63.

44. St-Jean M, El Ghorayeb N, Bourdeau I, Lacroix A. Aberrant G-protein coupled hormone receptor in adrenal diseases. *Best Pract Res Clin Endocrinol Metab* 2018;**32**(2):165–87.

45. Andreescu CE, Alwani RA, Hofland J, Looijenga LHJ, De Herder WW, Hofland LJ, et al. Adrenal Cushing's syndrome during pregnancy. *Eur J Endocrinol* 2017 Nov;**177**(5):K13–20.

46. Plockinger U, Chrusciel M, Doroszko M, Saeger W, Blankenstein O, Kroiss M, et al. Functional implications of LH/hCG receptors in pregnancy-induced Cushing syndrome. *J Endocr Soc* 2017;**1**(October 2016):57–71.

47. Lansdown A, Rees DA. Endocrine oncology in pregnancy. *Best Pract Res Clin Endocrinol Metab* 2011;**25**(6):911–26.

48. Jarvis E, Morton A. Adrenal cortical carcinoma mimicking early severe preeclampsia. *Obstet Med* 2014;**7**(1):45–7.

49. Bertherat J, Horvath A, Groussin L, Grabar S, Boikos S, Cazabat L, et al. Mutations in regulatory subunit type 1A of cyclic adenosine 5′-monophosphate-dependent protein kinase (PRKAR1A): phenotype analysis in 353 patients and 80 different genotypes. *J Clin Endocrinol Metab* 2009;**94**(6):2085–91.

50. Caticha O, Barrow R, Lamothe J, Odell D, Wilson DE, Swislocki LM. Estradiol stimulates cortisol production by adrenal cells in estrogen-dependent primary adrenocortical nodular dysplasia. *J Clin Endocrinol Metab* 1993;**77**(2):494–7.

51. Nieman LK, Biller BMK, Findling JW, Newell-Price J, Savage MO, Stewart PM, et al. The diagnosis of Cushing's syndrome: an endocrine society clinical practice guideline. *J Clin Endocrinol Metab* 2008;**93**(5):1526–40.

52. Eschler DC, Kogekar N, Pessah-Pollack R. Management of adrenal tumors in pregnancy. *Endocrinol Metab Clin North Am* 2015;**44**(2):381–97.

53. Caimari F, Corcoy R, Webb SM. Cushing's disease: major difficulties in diagnosis and management during pregnancy. *Minerva Endocrinol* 2018;**43**:1–11.

54. Bronstein MD, Machado MC, Fragoso MCBV. Management of endocrine disease: management of pregnant patients with Cushing's syndrome. *Eur J Endocrinol* 2015;**173**(2):R85–91.

55. Araujo PB, Neto LV, Gadelha MR. Pituitary tumor management in pregnancy. *Endocrinol Metab Clin North Am* 2015;**44**(1):181–97.

56. Manetti L, Rossi G, Grasso L, Raffaelli V, Scattina I, Del Sarto S, et al. Usefulness of salivary cortisol in the diagnosis of hypercortisolism: comparison with serum and urinary cortisol. *Eur J Endocrinol* 2013;**168**(3):315–21.

57. Lopes LML, Francisco RPV, Galletta MAK, Bronstein MD. Determination of nighttime salivary cortisol during pregnancy: comparison with values in non-pregnancy and Cushing's disease. *Pituitary* 2016;**19**(1):30–8.

58. Vilar L, Freitas Mda C, Lima LH, Lyra R, Kater CE. Cushing's syndrome in pregnancy: an overview. *Arq Bras Endocrinol Metab* 2007;**51** (8):1293–302.

59. Schulte HM, Weisner D, Allolio B. The corticotrophin releasing hormone test in late pregnancy: lack of adrenocorticotrophin and cortisol response. *Clin Endocrinol (Oxf)* 1990;**33**(1):99–106.

60. Oh HC, Koh J-M, Kim MS, Park JY, Shong YK, Lee K-U, et al. A case of ACTH-producing pheochromocytoma associated with pregnancy. *Endocr J* 2003;**50**(6):739–44.

61. Jones SE, Carr D, Hoffman J, Macaulay J, Tait P. Cushing's syndrome in pregnancy due to an adrenocorticotropin secreting islet cell tumour. *J Obstet Gynaecol* 1999;**19**(3):303.

62. Asicioglu E, Gonenli G, Kahveci A, Yildizeli B, Deyneli O, Yavuz D, et al. Thymic neuroendocrine carcinoma presenting as Cushing's syndrome: treatment with octreotide combined with surgery and radiotherapy. *Onkologie* 2011;**34**(1–2):46–9.

63. Bombardieri E, Ambrosini V, Aktolun C, et al. 111In-pentetreotide scintigraphy: procedure guidelines for tumour imaging. *Eur J Nucl Med Mol Imaging* 2010;**37**:1441–8.

64. Buescher MA, McClamrock HD, Adashi EY. Cushing syndrome in pregnancy. *Obs Gynecol* 1992;**79**(1):130–7.

65. Karaca Z, Tanriverdi F, Unluhizarci K, Kelestimur F. Pregnancy and pituitary disorders. *Eur J Endocrinol* 2010;**162**:453–75.

66. Abbassy M, Kshettry VR, Hamrahian AH, Johnston PC, Dobri GA, Avitsian R, et al. Surgical management of recurrent Cushing's disease in pregnancy: a case report. *Surg Neurol Int* 2015;**6**(Suppl 25):S640–5.

67. Boronat M, Marrero D, López-Plasencia Y, Barber M, Schamann Y, Nóvoa FJ. Successful outcome of pregnancy in a patient with Cushing's disease under treatment with ketoconazole during the first trimester of gestation. *Gynecol Endocrinol* 2011;**27**(9):675–7.

68. Casson IF, Davis JC, Jeffreys RV, Silas JH, Williams JBP. Successful management of Cushing's disease during pregnancy by transsphenoidal adenectomy. *Clin Endocrinol (Oxf)* 1987;**27**(4):423–8.

69. Coyne TJ, Atkinson RL, Prins J. Adrenocorticotropic hormone-secreting pituitary tumor associated with pregnancy: case report. *Neurosurgery* 1992;**31**(5):953–5.

70. Pickard J, Jochen AL, Sadur CN, Hofeldt FD. Cushing's syndrome in pregnancy. *Obs Gynecol Surv* 1990;**45**(2):87–93.

71. Verdugo SC, Alegría BJ, Grant DC, Briano PE, González GMI, Meza LH, et al. Cirugía transesfenoidal en enfermedad de Cushing durante gestación. *Rev Med Chil* 2004;**132**(1):75–80.

72. Pinette MG, Pan Y, Oppenheim D, Pinette SG, Blackstone J. Bilateral inferior petrosal sinus corticotropin sampling with corticotropin-releasing hormone stimulation in a pregnant patient with Cushing's syndrome. *Am J Obstet Gynecol* 1994;**171**(2):563–4.

73. Ross RJM, Chew SL, Perry L, Erskine K, Medbak S, Afshar F, et al. Diagnosis and selective cure of Cushing's disease during pregnancy by transsphenoidal surgery. *Eur J Endocrinol* 1995;**132**:722–6.

74. Mellor A, Harvey RD, Pobereskin LH, Sneyd JR. Cushing's disease treated by trans-sphenoidal selective adenomectomy in mid-pregnancy. *Br J Anaesth* 1998;**80**(6):850–2.

75. Wang W, Yuan F, Xu D. Cushing's syndrome during pregnancy caused by adrenal cortical adenoma: a case report and literature review. *Front Med* 2015;**9**(3):380–3.

76. Sammour RN, Saiegh L, Matter I, Gonen R, Shechner C, Cohen M, et al. Adrenalectomy for adrenocortical adenoma causing Cushing's syndrome in pregnancy: a case report and review of literature. *Eur J Obstet Gynecol Reprod Biol* 2012;**165**(1):1–7.

77. Aron DC, Schnall AM, Sheeler LR. Cushing's syndrome and pregnancy. *Am J Obstet Gynecol* 1990;**162**(1):244–52.

78. Sun Y, Fang M, Davies H, Hu Z. Mifepristone: a potential clinical agent based on its anti-progesterone and anti-glucocorticoid properties. *Gynecol Endocrinol* 2014;**30**(3):169–73.

79. Lim WH, Torpy DJ, Jeffries WS. The medical management of Cushing's syndrome during pregnancy. *Eur J Obstet Gynecol Reprod Biol* 2013;**168** (1):1–6.

80. Colao A, Petersenn S, Newell-Price J, Findling JW, Gu F, Maldonado M, et al. A 12-month phase 3 study of pasireotide in Cushing's disease. *N Engl J Med* 2012;**366**(10):914–24.

81. Petersenn S, Salgado LR, Schopohl J, Portocarrero-Ortiz L, Arnaldi G, Lacroix A, et al. Long-term treatment of Cushing's disease with pasireotide: 5-year results from an open-label extension study of a phase III trial. *Endocrine* 2017;**57**(1):156–65.

82. Lacroix A, Gu F, Gallardo W, Pivonello R, Yu Y, Witek P, et al. Efficacy and safety of once-monthly pasireotide in Cushing's disease: a 12 month clinical trial. *Lancet Diabetes Endocrinol* 2018;**6**(1):17–26.

83. Abucham J, Bronstein MD, Dias ML. Acromegaly and pregnancy: a contemporary review. *Eur J Endocrinol* 2017;**177**(1):R1–12.

84. Nakhleh A, Saiegh L, Reut M, Ahmad MS, Pearl IW, Shechner C. Cabergoline treatment for recurrent Cushing's disease during pregnancy. *Hormones* 2016;**15**(3):453–8.

85. Berwaerts J, Verhelst J, Mahler C, Abs R. Cushing's syndrome in pregnancy treated by ketoconazole: case report and review of the literature. *Gynecol Endocrinol* 1999;**13**(3):175–82.

86. Woo I, Ehsanipoor RM. Cabergoline therapy for cushing disease throughout pregnancy. *Obstet Gynecol* 2013;**122**(2 Pt 2):485–7.

87. Sek KSY, Deepak DS, Lee KO. Use of cabergoline for the management of persistent Cushing's disease in pregnancy. *BMJ Case Rep* 2017;1–4. table 2.

88. Glezer A, Bronstein MD. Prolactinomas, cabergoline, and pregnancy. *Endocrine* 2014;**47**(1):64–9.

89. Hotham NJ, Ilett KF, Hackett LP, Morton MR, Muller P, Hague WM. Transfer of metyrapone and its metabolite, rac-metyrapol, into breast milk. *J Hum Lact* 2009;**25**(4):451–4.

90. Eglash A. Treatment of maternal hypergalactia. *Breastfeed Med* 2014;**9**(9):423–5.

91. Moretti ME, Ito S, Koren G. Disposition of maternal ketoconazole in breast milk. *Am J Obstet Gynecol* 1995;**173**(5):1625–6.

92. Kurtoğlu S, Sarıcı D, Akın MA, Daar G, Korkmaz L, Memur Ş. Fetal adrenal suppression due to maternal corticosteroid use: case report. *J Clin Res Pediatr Endocrinol* 2011;**3**(3):160–2.

93. Tegethoff M, Pryce C, Meinlschmidt G. Effects of intrauterine exposure to synthetic glucocorticoids on fetal, newborn, and infant hypothalamic-pituitary-adrenal axis function in humans: a systematic review. *Endocr Rev* 2009;**30**(7):753–89.

94. Aydin M, Deveci U, Hakan N. Neonatal hypoglycemia associated with the antenatal corticosteroids may be secondary to fetal adrenal suppression. *J Matern Neonatal Med* 2015;**28**(8):892.

95. Costedoat-Chalumeau N, Amoura Z, Le Thi Hong D, Wechsler B, Vauthier D, Ghillani P, et al. Questions about dexamethasone use for the prevention of anti-SSA related congenital heart block. *Ann Rheum Dis* 2003;**62**(10):1010–2.

96. De Vetten L, Van Stuijvenberg M, Kema IP, Bocca G. Maternal use of prednisolone is unlikely to be associated with neonatal adrenal suppression—a single-center study of 16 cases. *Eur J Pediatr* 2017;**176**(8):1131–6.

97. Saulnier PJ, Piguel X, Perault-Pochat MC, Csizmadia-Bremaud C, Saulnier JP. Hypoglycaemic seizure and neonatal acute adrenal insufficiency after maternal exposure to prednisone during pregnancy: a case report. *Eur J Pediatr* 2010;**169**(6):763–5.

98. Levy RA, De Jesús GR, De Jesús NR, Klumb EM. Critical review of the current recommendations for the treatment of systemic inflammatory rheumatic diseases during pregnancy and lactation. *Autoimmun Rev* 2016;**15**(10):955–63.

99. Lacroix A. Approach to the patient with adrenocortical carcinoma. *J Clin Endocrinol Metab* 2010;**95**(11):4812–22.

100. Homer L, Viatge M, Gayet FX, Laurent Y, Kerlan V. Syndrome de Cushing et grossesse: à propos d'un cas de corticosurrénalome. *Gynecol Obstet Fertil* 2012;**40**(3):e1–4.

101. Klibanski A, Stephen AE, Greene MF, Blake MA, Wu C-L. Case records of the Massachusetts general hospital. case 36-2006. A 35-year-old pregnant woman with new hypertension. *N Engl J Med* 2006;**355**(21):2237–45.

102. Morris LF, Park S, Daskivich T, Churchill BM, Rao CV, Lei Z, et al. Virilization of a female infant by a maternal adrenocortical carcinoma. *Endocr Pract* 2011;**17**(2):e26–31.

103. Jairath A, Aulakh B. Adrenocortical carcinoma in pregnancy: a diagnostic dilemma. *Indian J Urol* 2014;**30**(3):342–4.

104. Kotteas E, Ioachim E, Pavlidis N. A pregnant patient with adrenocortical carcinoma: case report. *Onkologie* 2012;**35**(9):517–9.

105. Anjali A, Nair A, Thomas N, Rajaratnam S, Seshadri MS. Secondary hypertension in pregnancy due to an adrenocortical carcinoma. *Aust New Zeal J Obstet Gynaecol* 2004;**44**(5):466–7.

106. Abiven-Lepage G, Coste J, Tissier F, Groussin L, Billaud L, Dousset B, et al. Adrenocortical carcinoma and pregnancy: clinical and biological features and prognosis. *Eur J Endocrinol* 2010;**163**(5):793–800.

107. Makieva S, Saunders PTK, Norman JE. Androgens in pregnancy: roles in parturition. *Hum Reprod Update* 2014;**20**(4):542–59.

108. Raffin-Sanson ML, Abiven G, Ritzel K, de Corbière P, Cazabat L, Zaharia R, et al. Corticosurrénalome et grossesse. *Ann Endocrinol (Paris)* 2016;**77**(2):139–47.

109. Wy LA, Carlson HE, Kane P, Li X, Lei ZM, Rao CV. Pregnancy-associated Cushing' s syndrome secondary to a luteinizing hormone/human chorionic gonadotropin receptor-positive. *Gynecol Endocrinol* 2002;**16**(November 2017):413–7.

110. Villarroel C, Salinas A, López P, Kohen P, Rencoret G, Devoto L, et al. Pregestational type 2 diabetes and gestational diabetes exhibit different sexual steroid profiles during pregnancy. *Gynecol Endocrinol* 2017;**33**(3):212–7.

111. Leary PO, Boyne P, Flett P, Beilby J, James I. Longitudinal assessment of changes in reproductive hormones during normal pregnancy. *Clin Chem* 1991;**37**(5):667–72.

112. Libé R. Adrenocortical carcinoma (ACC): diagnosis, prognosis, and treatment. *Front Cell Dev Biol* 2015;**3**(July):1–8.

113. Tripto-Shkolnik L, Blumenfeld Z, Bronshtein M, Salmon A, Jaffe A. Pregnancy in a patient with adrenal carcinoma treated with mitotane: a case report and review of literature. *J Clin Endocrinol Metab* 2013;**98**(2):443–7.

114. Landau E, Amar L. Primary aldosteronism and pregnancy. *Ann Endocrinol (Paris)* 2016;**77**(2):148–60.

115. Riester A, Reincke M. Mineralocorticoid receptor antagonists and management of primary aldosteronism in pregnancy. *Eur J Endocrinol* 2015;**172**(1):R23–30.

116. Teo AE, Garg S, Shaikh LH, Zhou J, Karet Frankl FE, Gurnell M, et al. Pregnancy, primary aldosteronism, and adrenal CTNNB1 mutations. *N Engl J Med* 2016;**373**(15):1429–36.

117. Eguchi K, Hoshide S, Nagashima S, Maekawa T, Sasano H, Kario K. An adverse pregnancy-associated outcome due to overlooked primary aldosteronism. *Intern Med* 2014;**53**(21):2499–504.

118. Morton A. Primary aldosteronism and pregnancy. *Pregnancy Hypertens An Int J Women's Cardiovasc Heal* 2015;**5**:259–62.

119. Malha L, August P. Secondary hypertension in pregnancy. *Curr Hypertens Rep* 2015;**17**(7).

120. Campino C, Trejo P, Carvajal CA, Vecchiola A, Valdivia C, Fuentes CA, et al. Pregnancy normalized familial hyperaldosteronism type I: a novel role for progesterone. *J Hum Hypertens* 2015;**29**(2):138–9.

121. Zennaro M-C, Fernandes-Rosa FL, Boulkroun S. Overview of aldosterone-related genetic syndromes and recent advances. *Curr Opin Endocrinol Diabetes Obes* 2018;1.

122. Scholl UI, Stölting G, Schewe J, Thiel A, Tan H, Nelson-Williams C, et al. CLCN2 chloride channel mutations in familial hyperaldosteronism type II. *Nat Genet* 2018;1–6.

123. Albiger NM, Sartorato P, Mariniello B, Iacobone M, Finco I, Fassina A, et al. A case of primary aldosteronism in pregnancy: do LH and GNRH receptors have a potential role in regulating aldosterone secretion? *Eur J Endocrinol* 2011;**164**(3):405–12.

124. Gagnon N, Caceres K, Corbeil G, El Ghoyareb N, Ludwig N, Latour M, et al. Genetic characterization of GnRH/LH-responsive primary aldosteronism. *J Clin Endocrinol Metab* 2018;**103**(8):2926–35.

125. Wyckoff JA, Seely EW, Hurwitz S, Anderson BF, Lifton RP, Dluhy RG. Glucocorticoid-remediable aldosteronism and pregnancy. *Hypertension* 2000;**35**(2):668–72.

126. Mulatero P, Di CSM, Williams TA, Milan A, Mengozzi G, Chiandussi L, et al. Glucocorticoid remediable aldosteronism: low morbidity and mortality in a four-generation Italian pedigree. *J Clin Endocrinol Metab* 2002;**87**(7):3187–91.

127. Funder JW, Carey RM, Mantero F, Murad MH, Reincke M, Shibata H, et al. The management of primary aldosteronism: case detection, diagnosis, and treatment: an endocrine society clinical practice guideline. *J Clin Endocrinol Metab* 2016;**101**(5):1889–916.

128. Magee LA, Pels A, Helewa M, Rey E, Von Dadelszen P. Diagnosis, evaluation, and management of the hypertensive disorders of pregnancy. *Pregnancy Hypertens* 2014;**4**(2):105–45.

129. Pieper PG. Use of medication for cardiovascular disease during pregnancy. *Nat Rev Cardiol* 2015;**12**(12):718–29.

130. Prete A, Paragliola RM, Salvatori R, Corsello SM. Management of catecholamine-secreting tumors in pregnancy: a review. *Endocr Pract* 2016;**22**(3):357–70.

131. Lenders J. Pheochromocytoma and pregnancy: a deceptive connection. *Eur J Endocrinol* 2012;**166**(2):143–50.

132. Lenders JWM, Duh Q-Y, Eisenhofer G, Gimenez-Roqueplo A-P, Grebe SKG, Murad MH, et al. Pheochromocytoma and paraganglioma: an endocrine society clinical practice guideline. *J Clin Endocrinol Metab* 2014;**99**(6):1915–42.

133. Harrington JL, Farley DR, van Heerden JA, Ramin KD. Adrenal tumors and pregnancy. *World J Surg* 1999;**23**(2):182–6.

134. Biggar MA, Lennard TWJ. Systematic review of phaeochromocytoma in pregnancy. *Br J Surg* 2013;**100**(2):182–90.

135. Donatini G, Kraimps JL, Caillard C, Mirallie E, Pierre F, De Calan L, et al. Pheochromocytoma diagnosed during pregnancy: lessons learned from a series of ten patients. *Surg Endosc* 2018;**0**(0):0.

136. Remón-Ruiz P, Aliaga-Verdugo A, Guerrero-Vázquez R. Pheochromocytoma in neurofibromatosis type 1 during pregnancy. *Gynecol Endocrinol* 2017;**33**(2):93–5.

137. Van der Weerd K, Van Noord C, Loeve M, Knapen MFCM, Visser W, De Herder WW, et al. Endocrinology in pregnancy: pheochromocytoma in pregnancy: case series and review of literature. *Eur J Endocrinol* 2017;**177**(2):R49–58.

138. Jóźwik-Plebanek K, Pęczkowska M, Klisiewicz A, Wrzesiński K, Prejbisz A, Niewada M, et al. Pheochromocytoma presenting as takotsubo-like cardiomyopathy following delivery. *Endocr Pract* 2014;**1**:1):1–16.

139. Hamada SI, Hinokio K, Naka O, Higuchi K, Takahashi H, Sumitani H. Myocardial infarction as a complication of pheochromocytoma in a pregnant woman. *Eur J Obstet Gynecol Reprod Biol* 1996;**70**(2):197–200.

140. Mannelli M, Bemporad D. Diagnosis and management of pheochromocytoma during pregnancy. *J Endocrinol Invest* 2002;**25**(6):567–71.

141. Eisenhofer G, Klink B, Richter S, Lenders JWM, Robledo M. Metabologenomics of phaeochromocytoma and paraganglioma: an integrated approach for personalised biochemical and genetic testing. *Clin Biochem Rev* 2017;**38**(2):69–100.

142. Taïeb D, Pacak K. Molecular imaging and theranostic approaches in pheochromocytoma and paraganglioma. *Cell Tissue Res* 2018;1–9.

143. Leide-Svegborn S, Ahlgren L, Johansson L, Mattsson S. Excretion of radionuclides in human breast milk after nuclear medicine examinations. Biokinetic and dosimetric data and recommendations on breastfeeding interruption. *Eur J Nucl Med Mol Imaging* 2016;**43**(5):808–21.

144. Versmissen J, Koch BCP, Roofthooft DWE, ten Bosch-Dijksman W, van den Meiracker AH, Hanff LM, et al. Doxazosin treatment of phaeochromocytoma during pregnancy: placental transfer and disposition in breast milk. *Br J Clin Pharmacol* 2016;568–9.

145. Morton A. Magnesium sulphate for phaeochromocytoma crisis. *Emerg Med Australas* 2007;**19**(5):482.

146. Jensen BP, Dalrymple JM, Begg EJ. Transfer of doxazosin into breast milk. *J Hum Lact* 2013;**29**(2):150–3.

147. Davanzo R, Bua J, Paloni G, Facchina G. Breastfeeding and migraine drugs. *Eur J Clin Pharmacol* 2014;**70**(11):1313–24.

148. Beardmore KS, Morris JM, Gallery EDM. Excretion of antihypertensive medication into human breast milk: a systematic review. *Hypertens Pregnancy* 2002;**21**(1):85.

149. Parsaa AA, New MI. *Steroid 21-hydroxylase deficiency in congenital adrenal hyperplasia.* **165**;2016. p. 2017):2–11.

150. Speiser PW, Azziz R, Baskin LS, Ghizzoni L, Hensle TW, Merke DP, et al. Congenital adrenal hyperplasia due to steroid 21-hydroxylase deficiency: an endocrine society clinical practice guideline. *J Clin Endocrinol Metab* 2010;**95**(9):4133–60.

151. Miller WL. Fetal endocrine therapy for congenital adrenal hyperplasia should not be done. *Best Pract Res Clin Endocrinol Metab* 2015;**29**(3):469–83.

152. Witchel SF. Management of CAH during pregnancy: optimizing outcomes. *Curr Opin Endocrinol Diabetes Obes* 2012;**19**(6):489–96.

153. Bachelot A, Grouthier V, Courtillot C, Dulon J, Touraine P. Management of endocrine disease: congenital adrenal hyperplasia due to 21-hydroxylase deficiency: update on the management of adult patients and prenatal treatment. *Eur J Endocrinol* 2017;**176**(4):R167–81.

154. Nimkarn S, Lin-Su K, New MI. Steroid 21 hydroxylase deficiency congenital adrenal hyperplasia. *Pediatr Clin North Am* 2011;**58**(5):1282–300.

155. Eyal O, Ayalon-Dangur I, Segev-Becker A, Schachter-Davidov A, Israel S, Weintrob N. Pregnancy in women with nonclassic congenital adrenal hyperplasia: time to conceive and outcome. *Clin Endocrinol (Oxf)* 2017;**87**(5):552–6.

156. Tardy-Guidollet V, Menassa R, Costa JM, David M, Bouvattier-Morel C, Baumann C, et al. New management strategy of pregnancies at risk of congenital adrenal hyperplasia using fetal sex determination in maternal serum: French cohort of 258 cases (2002-2011). *J Clin Endocrinol Metab* 2014;**99**(4):1180–8.

157. Rijk Y, van Alfen-van der Velden J, Claahsen-van der Grinten H. Prenatal treatment with dexamethasone in suspected congenital adrenal hyperplasia and orofacial cleft: a case report and review of the literature. *Pediatr Endocrinol Rev* 2017;**15**(1):21–5.

158. Maryniak A, Ginalska-Malinowska M, Bielawska A, Ondruch A. Cognitive and social function in girls with congenital adrenal hyperplasia— influence of prenatally administered dexamethasone. *Child Neuropsychol* 2014;**20**(1):60–70.

159. Meyer-Bahlburg HFL, Dolezal C, Haggerty R, Silverman M, New MI. Cognitive outcome of offspring from dexamethasone-treated pregnancies at risk for congenital adrenal hyperplasia due to 21-hydroxylase deficiency. *Eur J Endocrinol* 2012;**167**(1):103–10.

160. Hirvikoski T, Nordenström A, Wedell A, Ritzén M, Lajic S. Prenatal dexamethasone treatment of children at risk for congenital adrenal hyperplasia: the Swedish experience and standpoint. *J Clin Endocrinol Metab* 2012;**97**(6):1881–3.

161. Karlsson L, Nordenstrom A, Hirvikoski T, Lajic S. Prenatal dexamethasone treatment in the context of at risk CAH pregnancies: long-term behavioral and cognitive outcome. *Psychoneuroendocrinology* 2018;**91**(February):68–74.

162. Karlsson L, Gezelius A, Nordenström A, Hirvikoski T, Lajic S. Cognitive impairment in adolescents and adults with congenital adrenal hyperplasia. *Clin Endocrinol (Oxf)* 2017;**87**(6):651–9.

163. Hirvikoski T, Nordenström A, Lindholm T, Lindblad F, Ritzén EM, Lajic S. Long-term follow-up of prenatally treated children at risk for congenital adrenal hyperplasia: does dexamethasone cause behavioural problems? *Eur J Endocrinol* 2008;**159**(3):309–16.

Chapter 26

Hypertension in Pregnancy

Rosemary Townsend*,† and Asma Khalil*,†

*Department of Fetal Medicine, St George's University of London, London, United Kingdom, †Molecular & Clinical Sciences Research Institute, St. George's University of London, London, United Kingdom

Common Clinical Problems

- Predicting which women will be affected by hypertension in pregnancy is complicated by the variable phenotypes of disease and differing underlying pathologies.
- Most women affected by hypertension in pregnancy are asymptomatic at presentation, so detection must rely on the routine antenatal screening of all women.
- Preeclampsia may present with atypical features, and other conditions may present with features typical of preeclampsia.
- It is easy to say that the "cure" for hypertensive disorders of pregnancy is delivery; however, it is challenging to determine the optimal balance of the competing interests of mother and infant in planning the timing of delivery.
- Women affected by hypertensive disorders of pregnancy are at increased risk of hypertension, diabetes, and cardiovascular and cerebrovascular disease in later life. The postpartum period represents an underutilized opportunity for health education and risk reduction.

26.1 INTRODUCTION

26.1.1 Prevalence and Clinical Significance of Hypertension in Pregnancy

Hypertensive complications of pregnancy are among the top three causes of maternal mortality worldwide, accounting for over 14% of all maternal deaths.[1] Over 99% of maternal deaths are avoidable, including many of those attributable to hypertensive disorders of pregnancy (HDPs). Unlike the other two leading causes of maternal death (hemorrhage and sepsis), hospitalization for hypertension in pregnancy is rising.[2] Although in the United Kingdom, the risk of a mother dying of hypertensive morbidities in pregnancy is now only 1 in 1 million,[3] thanks in large part to increasingly active management of hypertension in pregnancy, HDPs are still associated with significant maternal and perinatal morbidity. In particular, the incidence of iatrogenic preterm delivery continues to rise, and many of these medically indicated deliveries are by cesarean section. HDPs are the indication for between 15% of all premature deliveries and 43% of medically indicated preterm birth,[4] making them the cause of significant neonatal and childhood morbidity associated with prematurity and maternal morbidity associated with both hypertension and surgical delivery.

HDPs include gestational hypertension (GH), preeclampsia, and preexisting hypertension or white coat hypertension syndrome. Preeclampsia is responsible for the most severe instances of maternal and fetal morbidity, including eclampsia, pulmonary edema, HELLP (hemolysis, elevated liver enzymes and low platelets) syndrome, and renal injury. GH and chronic hypertension are more common than preeclampsia, and although considered milder manifestations of the disease, they are still associated with fetal growth restriction, iatrogenic preterm delivery, maternal cardiovascular and hypertensive morbidity, and maternal and perinatal mortality.

Hypertension in pregnancy also has consequences beyond the time of delivery for both mother and offspring. Women who have suffered from hypertension in pregnancy have a 13%–53% risk of recurrence in future pregnancies,[5] and also have an increased risk of hypertension and cardiovascular disease in later life. The risk of recurrence and later morbidity is related to the disease severity in the index pregnancy.[6-9] Children of mothers with HDP are themselves at increased risk of metabolic syndrome, cardiovascular disease, and preeclampsia in adult life.[10]

Maternal-Fetal and Neonatal Endocrinology. https://doi.org/10.1016/B978-0-12-814823-5.00026-X

Preeclampsia is commonly described as arising from failure of the normal maternal adaptation to pregnancy. There is incomplete trophoblast invasion of the maternal spiral arteries, resulting in placental malperfusion. This leads to the release of circulating factors that cause endothelial injury, leading to the maternal features of the disease.[11–13] It has lately been recognized that maternal factors, including prepregnancy cardiovascular function, endothelial health, and impaired lipid and glucose metabolism, play an important role in maldevelopment of the uteroplacental circulation. Moreover, it is very likely that there is more than one pathological pathway that can lead to the syndrome of preeclampsia.

Because the pathophysiology of hypertension in pregnancy involves multiple pathways, it is clear that both in screening for and treatment of HDPs, no single intervention is likely to be appropriate for all cases.

26.2 PHYSIOLOGICAL CHANGES IN NORMAL PREGNANCY

Profound hemodynamic and hormonal changes occur in normal pregnancy in order to support the development of the uteroplacental circulation and growth of the fetus. In general, pregnancy is marked by increased endothelial activity and cardiac work.

The earliest changes can be observed from the luteal phase of the menstrual cycle, when the corpus luteum starts to generate pregnancy-supporting hormones, including relaxin, progesterone, and estrogen. Relaxin plays a key role in inducing renovascular adaptation to pregnancy, as well as reducing myogenic tone in the uterine vessels in order to support the developing pregnancy.[14] It acts to upregulate placental growth factor (PlGF) and vascular endothelial growth factor (VEGF) activity. As the placenta develops, placental hormone production increases, and from 12 weeks onward, this is the principal influence on hemodynamic modulation in pregnancy (Fig. 26.1).

Pregnancies conceived using in vitro fertilization techniques in anovulatory women do not benefit from the hormonal output of the corpus luteum, and despite support from exogenous progesterone, they do not demonstrate the systemic failure of vascular resistance that is typical of normal pregnancy.[15] They are also at increased risk of pregnancy complications, including HDP.

Estrogen is involved in the increase in uterine blood flow via estrogen receptor (ER)-dependent vasodilation of the uterine arteries in early pregnancy, and it also has systemic effects on stroke volume, heart rate, and systemic vascular resistance.[16] Estrogen levels are associated with the expression of endothelial nitric oxide synthase (eNOS), a powerful vasodilator, particularly in uterine vessels, where ER expression is most dense.[17] Flow-mediated dilation (FMD), a marker of endothelial function, steadily increases throughout pregnancy until around 32 weeks' gestation.[18] The levels of prostacyclin, another endothelial dependent relaxation factor, are increased in pregnancy and associated with vascular smooth muscle relaxation, angiogenesis, and inhibition of platelet aggregation.[19]

On its own, progesterone does not increase uterine vasodilation via eNOS activation; however, it may potentiate the effects of estrogen. Progesterone does modulate contractility by increasing alpha-1 adrenergic receptor density in the uterine arterial smooth muscle and sensitizes the uterine vessels to the effect of catecholamines[17] (Fig. 26.2).

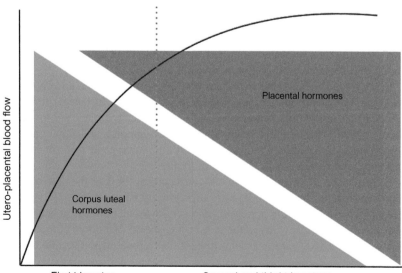

FIG. 26.1 The influence of hormones from the corpus luteum and the placenta on uteroplacental blood flow throughout pregnancy *(Adapted from Conrad KP, Baker VL. Corpus luteal contribution to maternal pregnancy physiology and outcomes in assisted reproductive technologies. Am J Physiol Regul Integr Comp Physiol 2013;304(2):R69–72.)*

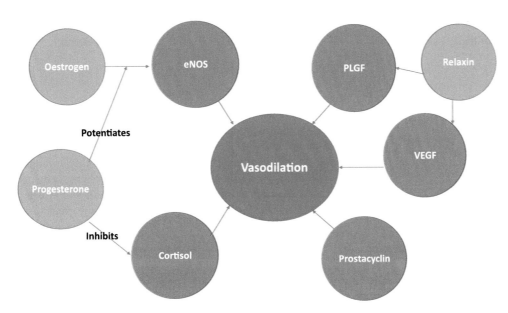

FIG. 26.2 Mechanisms of vasodilation in normal pregnancy.

Maternal cortisol levels double over the course of pregnancy and contribute to maintaining placental perfusion by affecting both systemic and uterine pathways. Maternal adrenal secretion of cortisol and aldosterone increases systemic plasma volume, and cortisol acts locally on the uterine vascular endothelium and smooth muscle. Although in the nonpregnant state, cortisol is associated with the inhibition of eNOS expression and a vasoconstrictive effect on the vascular smooth muscle, this effect is attenuated in pregnancy and posited to be the result of antiglucocorticoid effects of progesterone, which is elevated in pregnancy.[17]

Compared with the nonpregnant state, marked changes in cardiac output (CO) and total peripheral resistance can be seen from very early in gestation.[20] In normal pregnancy, CO increases rapidly, and there is generalized peripheral vasodilation, resulting in a decrease in total peripheral resistance (TPR).[21] Increases in heart rate and stroke volume combine to increase CO from as early as 5 weeks after the last menstrual period, reaching up to 45% above the nonpregnant level by 24 weeks' gestation. Approximately 70% of the increase in CO occurs by the 16th week of gestation, which is well before the marked increase in uterine blood flow. In multiple pregnancy, there is a further increment in CO of around 15%.[22] The increase in CO is linked to an increase in preload, a decrease in afterload, increased compliance of conduit vessels, ventricular remodeling and activation of the renin-angiotensin-aldosterone system.

During an uncomplicated pregnancy, a significant reduction of TPR occurs simultaneously with the increase in CO and a decrease in mean arterial pressure (MAP).[23,24] This reduced TPR represents an important adaptive response that maintains MAP within the normal range despite the greatly increased CO. This occurs in spite of an upregulation of renin and an increase in circulating angiotensin II in pregnancy.[25] This is because pregnancy is typified by a blunting of the pressor response to angiotensin II and other vasopressors[26,27] that facilitate this drop in systemic vascular resistance. Clinically, pregnant women present with a drop in blood pressure during the first trimester, reaching a nadir at 20–22 weeks, after which the increasing plasma volume of pregnancy is associated with steadily increasing MAP until delivery.

Arterial compliance is increased in pregnancy in concert with the generalized fall in TPR. There is a measurable decrease in arterial stiffness from preconception to midpregnancy, as observed in the pulse wave velocity (PWV) and augmentation index (AIx).[18]

Uterine blood flow increases 40 times over the course of pregnancy, initially via vasodilation and later via angiogenesis and remodeling of the uterine vasculature. Despite the overall fall in systemic vascular resistance, uterine perfusion pressure (UPP) and placental perfusion are maintained throughout pregnancy by the increase in uterine blood flow. The key vessels limiting uteroplacental flow have been thought to be the maternal spiral arteries, shed every month with the endometrium during menstruation. Recent evidence suggests that the spiral arteries are actually canalized and allow flow to the intervillous space as early as 7 weeks' gestation, indicating that the key regulators of placental blood flow in the first trimester are actually the proximal radial arteries, which undergo remodeling at a later time than the spiral arteries.[28]

In normal pregnancy, the balance of angiogenic factors is altered to favor placental angiogenesis and uterine vascular remodeling. The levels of the antiangiogenic soluble fms-like tyrosine kinase 1 (sFlt-1) are reduced, while the angiogenic PlGF and VEGF are increased, promoting angiogenesis and vascular remodeling in the uteroplacental circulatory tree, as well as having vasodilatory effects.[19]

Normal pregnancy is also a state of relative insulin resistance and higher-than-normal lipidemia, allowing placental transfer of sufficient nutrition for the developing fetus. This is mediated by human placental lactogen, progesterone, cortisol, and estradiol.[29]

26.2.1 Altered Pregnancy Physiology in HDP

The physiological changes seen in normal pregnancy are altered or absent in pregnancies affected by HDP, with a number of pathways combining to cause the widespread endothelial dysfunction that typifies preeclampsia (Fig. 26.3). Women affected by HDP demonstrate abnormalities of cardiac function on echocardiography that suggest an inability to meet the massive cardiac and metabolic demands of pregnancy. By term, 40% of pregnancies complicated by preeclampsia demonstrate global diastolic dysfunction compared to 14% of controls.[30] The normal inhibition of the pressor response fails in HDP, and preeclamptic women have an increased sensitivity to angiotensin II, particularly in the adrenal cortex and vascular tree.[26] Angiotensin II acts via the regulator of G protein-signaling 5 (RGS5), and expression is reduced in women affected by HDP.[31] The normal decrease in TPR and MAP does not occur in pregnancies complicated by hypertension, and in those affected by preeclampsia with fetal growth restriction, the rise in CO is significantly less than in normal pregnancies.[32]

In pregnancies that will ultimately develop HDP, arterial stiffening and impaired endothelial function can be observed from the first trimester. The degree of impairment correlates with disease severity, with the most severe changes observed in early-onset preeclampsia and milder changes in GH.[33,34]

The angiogenic balance is disturbed in preeclampsia. Levels of sFlt-1, which binds and reduces functional levels of PlGF and VEGF, are increased. Further, sFlt-1 may be released from ischemic placental tissue and also can be induced by platelet-monocyte aggregates.[35] The increase in sFlt-1 observed in HDP is preceded by a fall in PlGF and measurable changes in maternal hemodynamic parameters, suggesting that the release of sFlt-1 by hypoxic placental tissue is not the proximate cause of these changes.[19] The overall effect is to inhibit eNOS and potentiate vascular sensitivity to vasoconstrictors, thereby leading to hypertension.[27]

Although hyperinsulinemia and insulin resistance are features of normal pregnancy, they are exaggerated in HDP. This exaggeration may be greater in GH than in preeclampsia,[29] but it is associated with significant endothelial dysfunction in both conditions via a number of mechanisms. First, hyperinsulinemia increases sodium reabsorption and thereby sympathetic stimulation, which reduces renal perfusion and impairs endothelial function. Second, increased leptin provides increased oxidized lipids that alter the prostacyclin balance and increase thromboxane levels, further impairing endothelial function. Finally, the lipid balance is altered in preeclampsia, with increased levels of triglycerides and low-density lipoprotein/high-density lipoprotein (LDL/HDL) cholesterol ratio.[35] This abnormal lipid profile contributes to inflammation and oxidative stress in HDP.

Preeclampsia is associated with hyperandrogenism, and increased testosterone with reduced sex hormone-binding globulin (SHBG); this situation is also found in polycystic ovarian syndrome (PCOS), which is a predictor of later

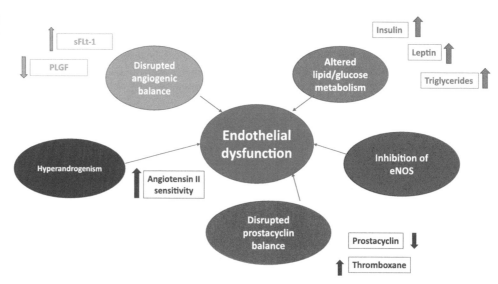

FIG. 26.3 Mechanisms of endothelial dysfunction in preeclamptic pregnancy.

development of preeclampsia. Androgens stimulate the pressor response by increasing angiotensin II receptor sensitivity[36] and further reduce prostacyclin synthesis; therefore, they can be implicated in the vicious cycle of endothelial dysfunction that occurs in preeclampsia.

26.3 SCREENING FOR AND PREVENTION OF PREECLAMPSIA

The finding that early treatment with low-dose aspirin from the first trimester reduces the risk of preeclampsia[37,38] made accurate first-trimester screening tests for preeclampsia a clinical priority. Other plausible potential preventative interventions, including folic acid and vitamin D, have not proved effective in clinical trials.[39,40] Calcium has been shown to reduce the risk of preeclampsia, but primarily in women with low calcium intake, and it is recommended in low-resource settings from 20 weeks of pregnancy.[41] Further study of other agents is warranted; for example, statins have a proven role in the prevention of cardiovascular disease in the nonpregnant population and could potentially affect preeclampsia by modulating inflammation, increasing eNOS activity, inhibiting platelet aggregation, and reducing the LDL/HDL ratio. Pravastatin, the statin least likely to cross the placenta, has been shown to be safe in pregnancy and effective in reducing cholesterol,[42] but further studies are required to establish its efficacy in preventing preeclampsia. Metformin could have a protective effect by improving endothelial function, reducing insulin resistance and sFlt-1 activity,[43] but further research is needed. Peroxisome proliferator-activated receptors (PPARs) regulate RGS5 expression, and in mouse models, the use of PPAR-γ agonists have been shown to abolish GH, but clinical trials are still needed.[31]

Because the benefit of aspirin is greatest when initiated prior to 16 weeks' gestation, the optimal screening test would predict preeclampsia with high sensitivity using data available before then. Because targeted antenatal monitoring could optimize the detection and management of preeclampsia and maximize efficiency in the use of health-care resources, screening models applicable in the second trimester are also of interest to researchers, particularly given that models developed later in pregnancy generally have better predictive performance.

Currently, clinical assessment of the risk of preeclampsia is based mainly on maternal history[44] with limited predictive accuracy.[45–47] Unfortunately, the positive predictive value of this model is low and would lead to nearly half of all women being screen positive.[46] Numerous studies have evaluated the accuracy of various tests, including clinical characteristics, biomarkers, and ultrasound markers, individually or in combination, for predicting early-, late-, and any-onset preeclampsia in the first, second, and third trimesters.[48]

No single test investigated has both sensitivity and specificity above 90%, which would seem to be necessary to make any screening test more cost-effective than a 'treat-all' policy in clinical practice. Body mass index (BMI) > 34 kg/m^2 had a specificity of 93% but a sensitivity of only 18%. Alpha feto protein (AFP) and bilateral uterine artery Doppler (UAD) notching are reported to have a specificity of >90%, but with low sensitivities of 9% and 48%, respectively.[49] Individual markers shown to correlate most strongly with the risk of preeclampsia are UAD indexes and angiogenic biomarkers.[50–52]

A stepwise (sequential) approach, whereby women are identified as high risk in the first trimester and then reevaluated at the time of the midtrimester anomaly scan is promising in terms of picking up most cases of early-onset preeclampsia.[53] The ASPRE trial evaluated the use of a screening model incorporating maternal factors, MAP, uterine artery pulsatility index, pregnancy-associated plasma protein A (PAPP-A), and PlGF applied before 14 weeks of gestaton, then randomized screen-positive women to treatment with 150 mg of aspirin or placebo. There was a significant reduction in preterm (<37 weeks) preeclampsia, but not in term preeclampsia or other secondary maternal and fetal outcomes.[37] The model has not yet been externally validated, and additional factors may be necessary to predict the more common condition of term preeclampsia. Nevertheless, this approach of stepwise screening is likely to form the basis of screening for and prevention of preeclampsia in the future.

26.4 ASSESSMENT OF THE HYPERTENSIVE PREGNANT WOMAN

26.4.1 Diagnostic Criteria for Hypertension in Pregnancy and Considerations Specific to the Measurement of Blood Pressure in Pregnancy

While hypertension is the common feature of all HDPs, criteria for measuring and defining hypertension can vary. Hypertension in pregnancy is generally agreed to be a blood pressure >140 mm Hg (systolic) or 90 mm Hg (diastolic), measured at least twice and separated by a period of rest.[44] Blood pressure should be measured with the woman at rest and with her arm held at the level of the heart with a device validated for use in pregnancy.[54] The measurement of diastolic blood pressure is taken at the fifth Korotkoff (K5) sound because it is more reproducible and better reflects intraarterial pressure.[55] Historically, some preferred to use the fifth Korotkoff sound, on the basis that using the fifth might miss some episodes of hypertension and thereby worsen pregnancy outcomes, but a randomized controlled trial (RCT) published in 1998 demonstrated equivalent outcomes,[56] and the use of K5 is recommended by the National Institute for Health and Care Excellence (NICE).[44]

Manual devices have the advantages of having a low cost and requiring the operator to palpate the pulse herself or himself. Mercury sphygmomanometers have been the gold standard for measurement, but they are being phased out of clinical use because of concerns about the safety of mercury. Aneroid devices are popular, cheap, and portable but easily become inaccurate and require regular calibration. Up to one-third of devices in regular use are inadequately calibrated.[57] Automated devices using oscillometric technology are commonly used in most clinical areas and address systematic errors associated with auscultatory measurements, but most have not been validated for use in pregnancy, and many are also insufficiently calibrated. In preeclampsia in particular, the increased arterial stiffness and marked extravascular edema can compromise the measurement of the intraarterial waveform, leading to the underestimation of blood pressure and the possibility of missed diagnosis.[55] Devices for use in pregnancy, therefore, must be specifically validated in a cohort including patients affected by preeclampsia.

Severe hypertension is defined as a systolic blood pressure of between 160 and 170 mm Hg; the precise cutoff varies among existing guidelines. It is important to understand that because of the increased vascular compliance of pregnancy, neurological complications of hypertension, including cerebral edema and hemorrhage, may be observed at lower levels of hypertension than in the nonpregnant population.[58] Systolic hypertension of >180 mm Hg in a pregnant patient is a medical emergency that requires safe and rapid control.

26.4.2 Diagnostic Criteria for Proteinuria in Pregnancy

Although proteinuria is not necessary to make a diagnosis of preeclampsia, it is a key feature that can be used to discriminate preeclampsia from other forms of pregnancy hypertension. While the basement membrane remains relatively intact in preeclampsia, significant proteinuria usually occurs in conjunction with glomerular endotheliosis. Milder endotheliosis is observed in GH.[59]

Multiple tests for proteinuria are available, but none are ideal. The most accurate is a 24-h urine collection and quantification of protein excretion, but this is cumbersome, time consuming, and susceptible to user error.[60] Simultaneous measurement of creatinine excretion can act as quality control and assist in the interpretation of results, but in practical terms, the delay between suspecting the diagnosis of preeclampsia and obtaining the laboratory results necessarily limits its utility in point-of-care clinical management decisions. It is still the best practice to obtain a 24-h specimen, but other tests may be more appropriate for determining immediate clinical management. A cutoff of 300 mg/day (the 95th percentile for normal women) is accepted as representing significant proteinuria where 24-h urine collection is used and there is no preexisting renal pathology or intercurrent urinary tract infection.

Available tests with a more rapid turnaround time include the urinary dipstick assessment and a spot protein-creatinine ratio (PCR). A dipstick reading >2+ is likely to represent significant proteinuria, but it should always be followed with an additional test, and clinicians must be aware that the negative predictive value of a normal dipstick test is only 0.6, meaning that relying on dipstick testing alone would lead to significant underdiagnosis of preeclampsia.[60] A spot PCR can provide a result within 1 h, and although it is less accurate for quantification of proteinuria than a 24-h collection, it does perform significantly better than dipstick testing to rule out proteinuria.[61] The degree of proteinuria was once incorporated into the classification of severity of preeclampsia, but it is clear that once proteinuria has been established, the degree does not correlate with pregnancy outcomes.[62] When extreme proteinuria in the severe nephrotic range is detected, consideration should be given to the possibility of an alternative or coexisting diagnosis, because preeclampsia is not typically associated with such extreme proteinuria. For this reason, there is little benefit in the more accurate quantification of the 24-h urine collection when the PCR is significantly abnormal, and it is not normally useful to perform serial measurements of proteinuria once it has clearly been established. The degree of proteinuria should not be considered when making the decision to deliver or start antihypertensive therapy or magnesium sulfate.

Hypertension is necessary for a diagnosis of preeclampsia, but a small number of women will initially present with proteinuria without hypertension. These cases should be fully investigated for alternative causes of proteinuria and followed up closely with blood pressure monitoring because up to 51% of these women may go on to develop hypertension and preeclampsia later in pregnancy.[63]

26.4.3 Fetal Assessment

Fetal growth restriction often coexists in hypertensive women and is now considered a diagnostic criterion for preeclampsia.[64] All women presenting with hypertension in pregnancy after 20 weeks should have ultrasound assessment of fetal growth, liquor volume, and umbilical and middle cerebral-artery Dopplers. So long as pregnancy continues, scans should be repeated at fortnightly intervals.[5] Women known to have preexisting hypertension are at increased risk of fetal growth restriction and should routinely be offered serial growth scans throughout pregnancy.

Mothers should be informed of the importance of self-monitoring of fetal movement and where to present if there are subjectively reduced fetal movements. There is no specific evidence related to kick charts or equivalent monitoring tools in preeclampsia, and as these women are high risk for placental insufficiency, it would be reasonable to perform ultrasound assessment at the first presentation with subjectively reduced fetal movement. Where fetal growth restriction has been identified, computerized cardiotocographic (CTG) monitoring and serial assessment of the fetal ductus venosus (DV) Doppler can be used to assess the fetal condition.[65]

26.4.4 Differential Diagnosis of Preeclampsia

Preeclampsia will always be the most common cause of hypertension and organ dysfunction in pregnancy, but many micro-angiopathic disorders can present with similar features. Failure to consider a broad differential diagnosis can lead to unnecessary iatrogenic preterm delivery or missed opportunities to treat deteriorating conditions. Delivery at 28 weeks while in a condition not caused by pregnancy will inevitably risk serious morbidity to the offspring and may well be associated with worsening of the maternal condition by the additional insult of a surgical delivery and the hormonal, fluid, and coagulation shifts that occur at the time of delivery. Table 26.1 describes some of the conditions that may present with some of the typical features of preeclampsia in pregnancy.

For some specific conditions, additional laboratory testing can help to clarify the diagnosis. For example, acute fatty liver of pregnancy (AFLP) is commonly associated with hypoglycemia, hyperammonemia, and jaundice; systemic lupus erythematosus (SLE) will feature antidouble-stranded DNA or antinuclear antibodies.[66] Serum complement levels can indicate the degree of disease activity in SLE and assist in discriminating between a flare of SLE and new preeclampsia. Hemolysis and anemia are common in thrombocytopenic thrombotic purpura (TTP) and hemolytic uremic syndrome (HUS), but von Willebrand factor (vWf) multimers are more commonly elevated than in either AFLP or HELLP. The underlying pathology of TTP relates to a reduced activity of von Willebrand cleaving protease (a disintegrin and metalloproteinase with a thrombospondin type 1 motif, member 13), also called *ADAMTS13*, which is detectable via testing; however, this test may not be available in standard hospital laboratories.

26.4.5 Novel Diagnostic Tests—PLGF/sFlt-1

New tests are clearly necessary to address the diagnostic uncertainty that can arise when a woman presents with suspected preeclampsia. Markers investigated include PLGF, sFlt-1, podocyturia, PAPP-A, placental protein 13 (PP-13), homocysteine, asymmetric dimethylarginine (ADMA), uric acid, and leptin.

Preeclampsia is associated with a disrupted angiogenic balance, and alterations in these circulating factors can be identified several weeks prior to the clinical manifestation of the disease. PlGF is reduced as early as 11–13 weeks' gestation in women destined to develop preeclampsia,[67] while sFlt-1 is elevated up to 5 weeks prior to the onset of clinical signs. PlGF alone and the sFlt-1/PlGF ratio have been evaluated as diagnostic tests and are particularly sensitive for early-onset disease.[68] Neither seems adequate as a diagnostic test by itself, but they perform well as tests to rule out preeclampsia, especially in the context of other diseases causing hypertension.

Where the test gives a low probability of development of preeclampsia within the next 2–4 weeks antenatal monitoring frequency may safely be reduced, improving the mother's experience of care and focusing the use of resources on the highest risk group of patients.[69,70] Observational studies have shown that the use of PlGF in the management of preeclampsia might be associated with earlier delivery, but also with fewer perinatal deaths.[71] RCTs using PlGF to guide clinical management ultimately will determine the clinical utility of these tests, but there is every reason to be optimistic that they will enable more accurate and targeted treatment of preeclampsia in the future.

26.5 CLASSIFICATION OF HYPERTENSIVE DISORDERS OF PREGNANCY

The investigation and management of HDP have been hampered by variable and overlapping definitions in clinical use over time and around the world. International experts are moving toward consensus, although important differences remain between international guideline-issuing bodies, including the American College of Obstetricians and Gynecologists (ACOG), the International Society for the Study of Hypertension in Pregnancy (ISSHP), the National Institute for Clinical Excellence (NICE), the World Health Organization (WHO), and the Society of Obstetricians and Gynecologists of Canada (SOGC).[44,64,72–74]

TABLE 26.1 Differential diagnosis of preeclampsia by organ system

Vascular	Renal	Gastrointestinal	Hematological	Respiratory	Cardiovascular	Neurological
Pheochromocytoma	Lupus nephritis	Acute fatty liver of pregnancy	Gestational thrombocytopenia	Pneumonia	Periaprtum cardiomyopathy	Epilepsy
Hyperaldosteronism	Glomerulonephritis	Obstetric cholestasis	Thrombotic thrombocytopenic purpura	Pulmonary embolus	Myocardial infarction	Brain tumor
Cushing's disease	Interstitial nephritis	Cholecystitis/cholangitis	Hemolytic uremic syndrome			Cerebrovascular accident
Thyrotoxicosis	Pyelonephritis	Viral hepatitis	Idiopathic thrombocytopenic purpura			Hypertensive encephalopathy
Aortic coarctation	Renal artery stenosis	Acute pancreatitis	Antiphospholipid syndrome			
		Gastritis	Folate deficiency			
			Systemic lupus erythematosus (SLE)			

After Steegers EAP, von Dadelszen P, Duvekot JJ, Pijnenborg R. Pre-eclampsia. Lancet 2010;376(9741):631–44.

There are three key hypertensive disorders—essential or chronic hypertension in pregnancy, gestational or pregnancy-induced hypertension, and preeclampsia.[72] Some groups further distinguish preeclampsia superimposed on chronic hypertension and white coat hypertension as separate HDPs.[64] The key differences between international diagnostic criteria chiefly relate to the discrimination between preeclampsia and GH and the classification of preeclampsia as severe or nonsevere. Although each condition increases the risk of maternal and offspring morbidity and mortality, the greatest risks are associated with a diagnosis of preeclampsia, either de novo or superimposed on chronic hypertension.[75,76]

26.5.1 Preexisting Hypertension

Young women of reproductive age may have had little cause to have their blood pressure measured prior to pregnancy, and new diagnosis of hypertension at the time of the first antenatal assessment is not uncommon. The timing of the first visit is important in determining the likely etiology of any hypertension identified for the first time in pregnancy. For the purposes of planning antenatal care and performing screening for aneuploidy, most guidelines recommend that the first antenatal assessment takes place prior to 14 weeks' gestation.[77] At this time, the drop in systemic vascular resistance is not usually great enough to mask preexisting hypertension, but when the first visit takes place between 16 and 20 weeks' gestation, this is a real possibility. If the first blood pressure recorded was in this period and a woman later develops hypertension, it can be unclear whether this represents new-onset or preexisting hypertension. The safest course is to manage the pregnancy as if it were new hypertension and to arrange postnatal follow-up to ensure that the hypertension has resolved.

Young women presenting with hypertension not due to pregnancy should be fully investigated for other underlying pathologies before diagnosing essential hypertension. The prevalence of hypertension in women of reproductive age is between 1% and 10%,[78] and preexisting hypertension complicates 1%–5% of pregnancies.[75] As with all hypertensive patients, the majority are affected by essential hypertension. Key disorders associated with secondary hypertension in women of childbearing age include renovascular stenosis (which is more likely to be secondary to fibromuscular dysplasia than atheromatous disease in this group, and may be present in 5%–10% of hypertensive patients[79]), other renal diseases, primary hyperaldosteronism, Cushing's syndrome, thyroid disease, and pheochromocytoma (affecting only 0.002% of all pregnancies).[80,81] The management of the endocrinological causes of hypertension in pregnancy are dealt with in detail elsewhere. In addition to renal and endocrinological disorders, white coat hypertension is recognized in pregnant women and is not entirely benign. Around 50% of women affected will develop GH, and 8% will develop preeclampsia.[82] Ambulatory blood pressure recording or home blood pressure monitoring programs may be indicated to confirm the diagnosis.

26.5.2 Gestational Hypertension

When hypertension arises de novo in pregnancy, without any features of preeclampsia or other underlying pathology (including primary renal and endocrine disorders), it is classified as GH, also referred to as *pregnancy-induced hypertension (PIH)*. Where hypertension is diagnosed for the first time in pregnancy management is as for GH, but follow-up is required to ensure that hypertension persisting beyond the puerperium can be investigated to identify any other underlying causes of hypertension. Any woman presenting with new hypertension requires assessment of all the possible features of preeclampsia prior to arriving at a diagnosis of GH, and testing for proteinuria and laboratory assessment of the full blood count, creatinine, and liver function should always be performed. In addition, ultrasound assessment of fetal growth should be considered, particularly in women presenting with severe hypertension before 37 weeks' gestation.

The risk of progression to preeclampsia after GH is around 25%,[64] so close monitoring is required throughout pregnancy. GH can be complicated by cerebral hemorrhage, and the absence of proteinuria is not a reason to relax the target blood pressure during antihypertensive treatment.

26.5.3 Preeclampsia

Preeclampsia is classically defined as new-onset hypertension after 20 weeks' gestation in pregnancy with proteinuria. With ongoing study of preeclampsia and advances in diagnostic testing, it is clear that the syndrome of preeclampsia is diverse and that not all cases easily fit into this definition. Preeclampsia may present for the first time postpartum or with eclamptic seizures,[83] may not be associated with proteinuria, and in certain particularly high risk pregnancies (e.g., molar pregnancies), the syndrome may be detected prior to 20 weeks' gestation.

Although all international guidelines require hypertension to make a diagnosis of preeclampsia, the ISSHP recently elected to recognize that preeclampsia may exist in the form of significant hypertension with other evidence of end-organ dysfunction without necessarily presenting with proteinuria.[64] Other international bodies are following suit. This means that a woman presenting with hypertension and severe fetal growth restriction will be recognized as suffering from pre-eclampsia and managed accordingly. In a research setting, it might be appropriate to retain proteinuria as a necessary feature for the diagnosis of preeclampsia to maintain homogeneity in the population under study, but in a clinical setting, recognizing the range of presentations of preeclampsia is pragmatic and minimizes the risk of underdiagnosis and treatment.

Preeclampsia is most commonly diagnosed when hypertension is detected during a routine antenatal visit, and most women are asymptomatic at presentation. The typical symptoms of preeclampsia overlap with common minor complaints of pregnancy such as nausea and vomiting, headache, peripheral edema, and heartburn. More serious symptoms tend to appear later in the disease. Upon examination, patients may be hyperreflexic, and marked clonus is associated with an increased risk of progression to eclampsia. In cases with hepatic involvement, patients may have tenderness in the right upper quadrant, and careful examination must be made to exclude the rare but deadly complication of liver hematoma or capsular rupture. In the most severe cases, women may present with confusion or altered consciousness.

26.5.4 Preeclampsia Superimposed on Preexisting Hypertension

It is particularly difficult to diagnose preeclampsia in women with preexisting hypertension, proteinuria, or both. Hypertension alone is not sufficient to diagnose preeclampsia, and a rise in blood pressure in the third trimester is anticipated in all pregnancies, including those in women affected by preexisting hypertension. Many renal pathologies, including glomerulonephritis and SLE, may worsen or relapse in pregnancy. Increasing antihypertensive requirement, therefore, is also not diagnostic of the development of new preeclampsia. When increasingly refractory hypertension is combined with new-onset proteinuria, fetal growth restriction, or other evidence of new renal or hepatic dysfunction, then the diagnosis of superimposed preeclampsia may be reached. Where hypertension and proteinuria existed prior to pregnancy, no clinical feature can readily discriminate between new-onset preeclampsia and the preexisting disease. This may be problematic because these women are at very high risk of severe preeclampsia, and those who do develop preeclampsia are at risk of long-term deterioration in their renal function, so diagnostic clarity is of key importance.

As described earlier, PlGF is lower in preeclampsia than in normal pregnancies, and the level relates to the severity of the disease. Because placental hypoxia would not be a significant feature in women affected by renal or hypertensive disease alone (i.e., not preeclampsia), sFlt-1 levels should not be increased, nor PlGF suppressed. In the research setting, both PlGF and the sFlt-1-PlGF ratio have demonstrated good diagnostic performance even in women with existing hypertension and proteinuria[84,85] and offer the possibility of discriminating accurately between those with preexisting disease alone and those with superimposed preeclampsia.

26.5.5 Severe Preeclampsia

The majority of patients affected by preeclampsia experience only mild symptoms and minor sequelae, particularly with early identification and active management. Most international guidelines recognize the need to identify those women who experience the more severe manifestations of the disease, but the diagnostic criteria for severe preeclampsia vary (Table 26.2).

26.5.6 Classification of Severity by Gestation at Onset

There is a growing recognition that the most important marker of severity is gestation of onset. ACOG defines early onset as <35 weeks' gestation, while SOGC uses <34 weeks, but both sets of criteria require additional features to classify preeclampsia as severe. Pragmatically, early-onset preeclampsia is usually defined as <34 weeks, reflecting the significantly poorer neonatal prognosis at this time. Early-onset disease is associated with a greater risk of preterm delivery, fetal growth restriction, recurrence in future pregnancies, and later cardiovascular disease and death. Maternal mortality is 20 times higher in preeclampsia diagnosed <32 weeks than when developed at term.[86]

26.5.7 Clinical Features of Severe Preeclampsia

Other features of severe preeclampsia include severe hypertension and the symptoms and development of any of the complications of preeclampsia. Severe hypertension is variously defined as systolic blood pressure >160 mm Hg[74,87] or 170 mm Hg.[44] Severe proteinuria is not a marker of severe disease, but proteinuria in the nephrotic range is an additional risk factor for venous thromboembolism (VTE) over and above the risk of VTE associated with preeclampsia itself.

TABLE 26.2 Classifications of severe preeclampsia

	NICE (2010) (Any of the below features with hypertension and proteinuria)	ACOG (2013) (Any of the below with known preeclampsia)	American Society of Hypertension (2008)
Symptoms	Headache Visual disturbance Vomiting Epigastric pain	Severe persistent right-upper-quadrant or epigastric pain Cerebral or visual disturbance	Headache Visual disturbance Abdominal pain
Signs	Papilledema Clonus Liver tenderness	Pulmonary edema	Oliguria Early-onset disease (<35 weeks) Nonreassuring fetal monitoring
Hypertension	Severe hypertension and proteinuria alone	Systolic BP>160mm Hg Diastolic BP>110mm Hg (on two occasions >4h apart while on bed rest)	Diastolic >110mm Hg
Other maternal disorders	HELLP syndrome Platelets <100×10⁹/L AST or ALT >70	Platelets <100×10⁹/L Liver enzymes > twice normal concentration Progressive renal insufficiency	Elevated creatinine Nephrotic range proteinuria Elevated AST or LDH

BP, blood pressure; *AST*, aspartate transferase; *ALT*, alanine transferase; *LDH*, lactate dehydrogenase; *NICE*, National Institute for Clinical Excellence; *ACOG*, American College of Obstetricians and Gynecologists.

TABLE 26.3 Diagnostic criteria of HELLP syndrome

	Tennessee[89]	Martin[90]	UKOSS[91]
Hemolysis	LDH > 600U/L	Falling HCT, LDH > 164U/L or bleeding diathesis	LDH > 600IU/L or bilirubin >20.5 μmol/L or abnormal peripheral blood smear
Thrombocytopenia	Platelets <100×10³/μL	Platelets <100×10³/μL	Platelets <100×10⁹/L
Hepatocellular injury	AST > 70U/L	AST > 48U/L and ALT >24U/L	GGT, AST or ALT >70U/L

LDH, lactate dehydrogenase; *AST*, aspartame transferase; *ALT*, alananine transferase; *GGT*, gamma glutyl transferase; *HCT*, hematocrit.

Severe disease can develop rapidly in fulminating preeclampsia, and sudden onset of rapidly worsening abdominal pain, nausea and vomiting, or headache should always be taken seriously, particularly in women with a known diagnosis of preeclampsia or GH.

26.6   COMPLICATIONS OF PREECLAMPSIA

Preeclampsia is a multisystem disorder characterized by generalized endothelial damage, which can result in widespread end-organ damage. In current clinical practice, close attention to blood pressure control means that most maternal deaths associated with preeclampsia are attributable to neurological or hepatic complications.[88]

26.6.1   HELLP Syndrome

HELLP syndrome is a serious condition characterized by hemolysis (anemia with blood film appearances of hemolysis), elevated liver enzymes (transaminases greater than twice the upper limit of normal), and low platelets (<150,000/dL). As with preeclampsia, international diagnostic criteria for HELLP syndrome vary (Table 26.3). HELLP syndrome occurs in around 5% of cases of preeclampsia[87] or 10%–20% of severe preeclampsia and is associated with 1.1% maternal mortality and severe morbidity, including disseminated intravascular coagulopathy, liver hematoma, liver failure, and renal failure.[92] The perinatal mortality rate is reported at 6%–17%.[93,94]

Shedding of placental debris into the maternal circulation is thought to provoke a widespread inflammatory response, with a more severe response seen in HELLP syndrome. PP1 is synthesized by syncytiotrophoblast and is detectable at higher levels in the umbilical cord blood in pregnancies affected by HELLP syndrome than in healthy or preeclamptic pregnant patients. This may correlate with the degree of damage to the syncytiotrophoblast membrane, pointing to that damage as a possible causative factor of HELLP syndrome.[95]

As in preeclampsia, endothelial injury results in platelet activation and consumption, vasospasm, release of thromboxane A2 and serotonin, and inhibition of prostacyclin release. The overall effect of the endothelial injury response is to shift the prostacyclin/thromboxane ratio in favor of vasoconstriction. In addition, there are a reduction in endothelium-derived relaxing factor and an increase in fibrin deposition in the endothelium.[96] In HELLP syndrome, a number of other pathological processes create the typical picture of thrombocytopenia, hemolysis, and acute liver injury. Acute activation of the endothelium increases the proportion of active vWf released. Pregnancies affected by preeclampsia and HELLP syndrome have markedly elevated vWf antigen levels,[97] and vWf in the GpIbα-binding conformation (active) can interact spontaneously with platelets without binding to exposed collagen; this is associated with consumptive thrombocytopenia and thrombotic microangiopathy.[98] Although the overall level of vWf antigen is similar in preeclampsia and HELLP syndrome, the proportion of active vWf and the functionality of vWF are greater in patients with HELLP syndrome than in those with preeclampsia.[97] Although high levels of active vWf in TTP are associated with reduced ADAMTS13 activity, in patients with HELLP ADAMTS13 activity is not significantly different from patients with preeclampsia, so it is not a likely cause for the increased vWf activity. It is more plausible that acute endothelial activation leads to release of the large active vWF multimers that then spontaneously interact with platelets, leading to microvascular thrombi and increasing platelet consumption.

Thrombocytopenia is often an early finding in HELLP syndrome, before the hemolysis and liver injury have fully developed. Increasing platelet consumption and formation of microvascular thrombi reduce platelet life span. This, together with increasing adherence to exposed collagen, have the effect of reducing the platelet count. Because the cause of the thrombocytopenia is peripheral, bone marrow aspirate normally demonstrates increased numbers of megakaryocytes, and in fact, megakaryocytes may be detected in the peripheral circulation.

Erythrocytes are damaged by passage through vessels affected by endothelial injury and microvascular thrombi, and the characteristic picture of microangiopathic hemolytic anemia develops, where burr cells, schistocytes, and polychromasia may be detected on peripheral blood film microscopy, and elevated lactate dehydrogenase (LDH), bilirubin, and reticulocyte counts also may be detected.

Fibrin obstruction of the hepatic sinusoids leads to hepatocellular injury. Liver biopsy is nonspecific, but typical features include periportal and focal parenchymal necrosis. Continued swelling of the liver secondary to hepatocellular injury or subcapsular hematoma may lead to the rare but life-threatening complication of rupture of the liver capsule with attendant major hemorrhage; this can occur in 1.8% of HELLP cases. Rupture occurs most frequently in the right lobe and can occur postpartum. This is one of the most serious complications of HELLP syndrome and is associated with an 18%–86% maternal mortality rate and a perinatal mortality rate as high as 80%.[99] Pregnancy and preeclampsia are both prothrombotic states, and where HELLP syndrome occurs in conjunction with antiphospholipid syndrome, there is an increased risk of hepatic infarction.[100]

26.6.2 Renal Dysfunction in Preeclampsia

The kidney is uniquely vulnerable to preeclampsia because of the toxic combination of relative depletion of the intravascular volume and paradoxical renal vasoconstriction mediated by sodium and water retention. In normal pregnancy, the glomerular filtration rate (GFR) is increased and the normal range of creatinine is lower than in the nonpregnant patient, but in preeclampsia, GFR and renal perfusion are reduced.[101] Low or subclinical rises in creatinine can be early signs of severe preeclampsia, and a creatinine >90 mmol/L is a marker of severe disease.[64] In preeclampsia, the typical pathological findings on renal biopsy are glomerular endotheliosis, and milder changes can be observed in GH.[102] The typical glomerular lesion with reduced endothelial fenestration and increased fibrinoid deposits is strongly associated with renal hypofiltration, independent of the renovascular constriction of preeclampsia.[103] Podocyte attachment is damaged in preeclampsia, and podocyturia is detectable prior to the onset of proteinuria.[104]

Renal dysfunction purely secondary to preeclampsia usually resolves after delivery, but it may be worsened in the short term by the practice of fluid restriction in the management of severe preeclampsia. In those who do not recover their renal function, ongoing thrombotic microangiopathy affecting the kidney or thrombosis severely enough to cause renal infarction may be responsible.

26.6.3   Pulmonary Edema

Pulmonary edema is an important cause of death in women with preeclampsia, and yet it is often recognized late. Hypoalbuminemia leads to reduced oncotic pressure and significant interstitial fluid accumulation despite the intravascular depletion of preeclampsia.[105] Fluid accumulation is often exacerbated by the administration of intravenous fluids during labor, whether prior to the use of epidural analgesia or at the time of surgical delivery.

26.6.4   Eclampsia

Eclampsia remains the most feared of all complications of preeclampsia, as indicated by the name of the disease. Eclampsia means lightning, and for centuries, relatives and clinicians have been terrified by the sudden appearance of tonic-clonic seizures in young and apparently healthy pregnant women. Despite all the decades of research that have defined and explored the condition that precedes eclamptic seizures—preeclampsia—the ability to predict the onset of eclampsia remains elusive. Although other pathologies can present with new-onset seizures in pregnancy, eclampsia is the most immediately life-threatening, and treatment should always be initiated in tandem with seeking evidence to support or refute the diagnosis, particularly in a patient not previously known to be hypertensive.

Seizures can arise in a woman who has shown no or minimal preceding symptoms and signs, or who has had stable, mild disease for several weeks. The most common preceding symptoms are severe headache, visual disturbance, and nausea, which are present in 79% of cases who go on to present with eclampsia. Eclampsia is around 10–30 times more common in developing countries, largely because of differences in the quality of antenatal monitoring that lead to missed opportunities to treat preeclampsia and prevent deterioration.[106]

Eclampsia is strongly associated with the finding of posterior reversible encephalopathy syndrome (PRES) on neuroimaging, and it is likely that these changes precede (and in fact may be the mechanism of) eclampsia.[107] It is not clear how many women with preeclampsia might have PRES because neuroimaging is usually reserved for cases with seizures or other neurological features.

The etiology of PRES has not been fully determined, and similar appearances can occur in nonpregnancy-related conditions, including hypertensive encephalopathy, immunosuppressive states, and hepatic failure. It is likely that in preeclampsia, elevated blood pressure that overrides cerebral autoregulation and cerebral hyperperfusion can lead to disruption of the blood-brain barrier and vasogenic edema.[58] Pregnancy enhances the development of edema in response to hypertension, and therefore, the consequences of cerebral edema are observed at lower blood pressure levels than in nonobstetric hypertensive encephalopathy.[13] Mild cognitive impairment is reported by women who have suffered from eclampsia even without focal neurological injury, and this may represent long-term white matter damage as a result of eclamptic seizures.[108]

26.7   ANTENATAL CARE OF WOMEN WITH HYPERTENSIVE DISORDERS IN PREGNANCY

Once hypertension has been identified, subsequent management is determined by the specific diagnosis and gestation at onset. Preexisting hypertension is likely to deteriorate with prolonged pregnancy, and it carries a substantial risk of progression to preeclampsia or GH. GH and preeclampsia are both cured by delivery of the baby, and the only reason to prolong the pregnancy in these conditions is to maximize fetal maturity while avoiding clinical deterioration in the mother.

26.7.1   Periconceptual Care

The antenatal management of women with chronic hypertension should ideally begin preconception. With rising mean maternal age, weight, and medical complexity, it has become increasingly common to meet women with an established diagnosis of essential hypertension in early pregnancy. Ideally, all women with a diagnosis of essential hypertension or previous GH or preeclampsia who are considering pregnancy should be referred to an obstetric medicine service prior to conception. There, they can receive periconceptual advice and then targeted antenatal care and monitoring throughout the pregnancy.

Women with essential hypertension planning a pregnancy should be informed that there is a 20%–25% chance of developing preeclampsia during pregnancy, with the attendant fetal and maternal risks, and that this condition can be mitigated to some extent by the administration of low-dose aspirin from the first trimester. For women who have previously had GH or preeclampsia, the risk of recurrence is related to the gestation at delivery, but all these women are at increased risk compared to normotensive multiparous women. NICE recommends taking 75 mg aspirin once daily until 36 weeks for women at high risk of preeclampsia, although there is emerging evidence that a dose of 150 mg is better at reducing the risk of preeclampsia.[109]

Additionally, when a woman decides to conceive, a review of established antihypertensive therapy and blood pressure control should be undertaken to ensure the suitability of her existing medical therapy for pregnancy. Women on an angiotensin-converting-enzyme inhibitor (ACE-I) or angiotensin receptor blocker (ARB) should be converted to alternative therapies prior to conception. Blood pressure control at conception and in the first trimester is associated with the risk of developing preeclampsia, severe hypertension, and fetal growth restriction later in pregnancy,[110] and ideally, optimal control should be achieved using antihypertensives suitable for use during pregnancy prior to conception.

Optimizing diet and weight prior to pregnancy also may reduce the risk of preeclampsia, along with many other pregnancy and long-term health complications, and folic acid should be taken from preconception until up to 12 weeks' gestation.

26.7.2 Antenatal Treatment of Chronic and Gestational Hypertension

Antihypertensive therapy aims to reduce the risk of severe hypertension and cerebrovascular accidents, cardiovascular strain, and renal injury. The target blood pressure for women with chronic hypertension may differ in pregnancy compared with prepregnancy. Confidential enquiries into maternal mortality in the United Kingdom and United States have stressed repeatedly that failure to control systolic hypertension adequately has been a feature in a number of maternal deaths from aortic dissection and cerebrovascular hemorrhage.[111,112] NICE guidance recommends commencing therapy when blood pressure exceeds 150/100 mm Hg, with the aim of maintaining blood pressure below this level; and the SOGC guidelines are similar.[5,74] The ACOG guidelines are more conservative, citing concerns about the potential effects of antihypertensive therapy in pregnancy on the fetus and the relative rarity of complications at blood pressures of 150/100 mm Hg, and would recommend treatment only for blood pressure over 160/110 mm Hg, or 160/105 in chronic hypertension.

The Control of Hypertension in Pregnancy Study (CHIPS) RCT demonstrated that tight (i.e., target diastolic BP (DBP) < 85 mm Hg) rather than less tight (target DBP < 100 mm Hg) blood pressure control is associated with a lower probability of severe hypertension and no increase in adverse perinatal outcomes in chronic and GH. Bearing in mind the fact that the systemic effects of hypertension may be potentiated in pregnancy by the systemic inflammatory response and altered endothelial function, it is sensible to adopt a tighter approach to blood pressure control for hypertensive pregnant women than for nonpregnant patients.

26.7.3 Choice of Antihypertensive Agents in Pregnancy

The first-line antihypertensive drug in pregnancy is usually labetalol, a mixed beta- and alpha-blocker.[5] Acceptable and commonly used alternatives are methyldopa and nifedipine. There is no good evidence as to the most effective agent, although metaanalysis does suggest that there are differences between drug classes in the effectiveness of preventing severe hypertension.[113] Beta-blockers seem to be associated with good efficacy in the treatment of hypertension, but they also have effects on the fetus, including lower birth weight, neonatal hypoglycemia, and increased neonatal respiratory morbidity. Afro-Caribbean patients often demonstrate relative insensitivity to beta blockers secondary to relatively high renin levels[114] and many argue that calcium channel blockers are the most appropriate first-line agent in these patients. Rapid-release oral nifedipine is as effective at achieving blood pressure control in severe hypertension as intravenous labetalol or hydralazine, but labetalol is associated with fewer adverse perinatal events.[115]

ACE inhibitors, ARBs, and alpha blockers are not appropriate in pregnancy because of the risk of fetal teratogenicity. Polypharmacy might be needed in women with persistent severe hypertension, but as a rule of thumb, the first-line antihypertensive dose should be increased to the maximum before adding a supplementary agent. Table 26.4 outlines commonly used antihypertensive drugs in pregnancy..

26.7.4 Antenatal Monitoring in Gestational and Chronic Hypertension

Because of the ongoing risk of preeclampsia, antenatal care of women with chronic and GH includes regular monitoring for worsening hypertension and new proteinuria. Typically, women are invited to attend the day unit for assessment, with increasing frequency of visits as the estimated due date approaches. Serial ultrasound assessment of fetal growth is recommended.

TABLE 26.4 Commonly used antihypertensives and their application in women of reproductive age

Class of drug	Example	Preconception	Pregnancy	Breastfeeding	Side effects	Contraindications
ACE inhibitor	Enalapril Captopril	Change to alternative antihypertensive	No: associated with severe fetal anomaly, fetal nephropathy and intrauterine death	No known evidence of harm (NICE). May be of particular benefit for women needing cardiac/renal protection	Cough	Peripheral vascular disease, hereditary angiedema, aortic stenosis
Alpha- and beta-blockers	Labetalol	Change to alternative antihypertensive	Yes. Can be given intravenously for rapid control of severe resistant hypertension	Manufacturers recommend avoid. Very small amounts in breast milk. No known evidence of harm (NICE)	Tachycardia	Asthma
Alpha-2 agonists	Clonidine Methyldopa	Methyldopa: can be used in periconceptual period.	Methyldopa: Yes, including first trimester. Longest postmarketing surveillance data. Clonidine: may lower fetal heart rate	No known evidence of harm to infants, but NICE recommends avoiding it because of an association with postpartum depression	Depression Reduced variability on CTG Methyldopa hepatitis	Mental illness Hepatic disease
Angiotensin-receptor blockers	Losartan	Change to alternative antihypertensive	Likely similar risk of teratogenicity as ACE-I. In addition known to cause fetal renal failure and retardation in skull ossification in 2/3rd trimesters	No information available—not recommended.	Dizziness, palpitations, headache, hyperkalemia	Electrolyte imbalance, hepatic or renal impairment
Beta-blockers	Bisprolol Atenolol	Change to alternative antihypertensive.	Avoid in first and second trimesters. Associated with fetal growth restriction and bradycardia, reduces uteroplacental blood flow	No known evidence of harm (NICE). Second line after labetalol	Risk of fetal growth restriction and bradycardia in pregnancy	Asthma
Calcium channel antagonists: Dihydropyridines	Nifedipine Amlodipine	Change to alternative antihypertensive	After 20weeks. Available in short-acting forms for rapid blood pressure control and long-acting forms for maintenance therapy. May be used simultaneously with magnesium sulfate. May inhibit labor	Manufacturers advise avoiding, no known evidence of harm (NICE). Amounts in breast milk too small to be harmful	Headache	Aortic stenosis, acute angina, recent myocardial infarction

Continued

TABLE 26.4 Commonly used antihypertensives and their application in women of reproductive age—cont'd

Class of drug	Example	Preconception	Pregnancy	Breastfeeding	Side effects	Contraindications
Calcium channel antagonists: phenylalkylamines	Verapamil	Change to alternative antihypertensive.	No known teratogenic effect, may relax uterine muscle, may reduce uterine blood flow. Avoid in first trimester.	Excreted in breast milk in very small amounts, unlikely to be significant.	Bradycardia, flushing, peripheral edema	Acute porphyria, accessory conducting pathways, heart failure
Calcium channel antagonists: benzothiazepines	Diltiazem	Change to alternative antihypertensive	Not recommended in pregnancy	Excreted in breast milk in small amounts—avoid breastfeeding if using	Thrombocytopenia, headache, dizziness, AV block, bradycardia	Acute porphyria, LVF, AV block
Mineralocorticoid receptor agonists	Spironolactone Eplerenone	Change to alternative antihypertensive. Spironolactone associated with reduced fertility in mice	Feminization of male fetus in animal studies.	Active metabolite present in milk—avoid	Hyperkalemia, dizziness, leukopenia, hepatic impairment	Renal failure, hyperkalemia, hypercalcemia
Nitroprusside	Nitroprusside	Change to alternative antihypertensive	Although effective for rapid control of hypertension, can lead to accumulation of cyanide in fetus	Caution advised: thiocyanate metabolite	Abdominal pain, phlebitis, thrombotcytopenia, anxiety, and dizziness	Leber's optic atrophy, severe B12 deficiency
Thiazide diuretics	Bendroflumethiazide	Change to alternative antihypertensive	Decrease placental perfusion, stimulation of labor, increase in meconium staining. Can cause neonatal thrombocytopenia, bone marrow suppression, jaundice, and electrolyte disturbance	Amount present in breast milk too small to be harmful, but large doses may inhibit lactation	Hypokalemia, other metabolic and electrolyte disturbance, postural hypotension, gout	Addison's disease, hypokalemia, hypercalcemia, hyponatremia
Vasodilators	Hydralazine	Change to alternative antihypertensive	Avoid before third trimester. May be a risk of neonatal thrombocytopenia	Present in milk, not known to be harmful	Rashes, hepatic dysfunction, anxiety, hemolytic anemia, SLE-like syndrome with long-term therapy	Acute porphyria, cor pulmonale, SLE, severe tachycardia

Although this approach maximizes the early detection of preeclampsia in this high-risk group, women still may develop severe hypertension or new proteinuria between visits. Moreover, the frequency of hospital visits and monitoring unnecessarily add to the anxiety and practical challenges of pregnancy for the majority of the affected women who ultimately will not go on to develop preeclampsia. This is particularly the case for women with chronic hypertension, who will require monitoring throughout pregnancy, compared to women with GH, who may need additional monitoring for only a few weeks in the interval between diagnosis and delivery. In carefully selected women, self-monitoring of blood pressure using approved validated and calibrated devices at home may be an effective way to maintain close monitoring, while reducing the impact of frequent visits on the women and their families. Home monitoring using a clear protocol with triggering of hospital assessment when appropriate can reduce the number of antenatal visits, with no adverse effect on maternal and offspring outcomes.[116]

Although several studies have investigated home monitoring of blood pressure, the problem of testing for proteinuria remains. In fact, most pregnant women have experience with administering home urine tests in the form of beta-human chorionic gonadotropin (bHCG) testing to confirm pregnancy in the first trimester, and it is likely that home testing for proteinuria could further reduce the need for hospital visits. Home testing for proteinuria has been shown to be feasible, accurate, and acceptable to women.[117]

Using home monitoring of blood pressure and proteinuria with appropriate triage protocols can help to individualise antenatal monitoring for women with chronic and gestational hypertension. Incorporating new technologies (including smart phone apps) can facilitate communication of clinical data with the hospital care team and makes home based care, already popular with women, economically viable and more widely accessible.

26.7.5   Timing of Delivery in Chronic and Gestational Hypertension

Blood pressure will continue to rise throughout the third trimester, and ultimately the best way of preventing further progression of hypertension and removing the risk of developing preeclampsia may be to deliver the baby. This would usually be through induction of labor, although in certain cases (very preterm, placenta previa, previous cesarean sections, fetal malposition), this may be contraindicated, and thus a cesarean section would be planned.

The decision to deliver is not as simple as removing the risks of prolonged pregnancy once fetal maturity is achieved. Medically indicated delivery is associated with risks to both mother and baby that need to be weighed against the risks to mother and baby of continuing the pregnancy. Induced labor is associated with increased use of regional analgesia in labor and instrumental delivery; the failure to induce labor and the subsequent need for cesarean section is a possibility, particularly in primigravid women induced remote from term. Although 37 weeks is taken as full term, there is a higher incidence of respiratory morbidity and neonatal unit admission in infants born between 37 and 39 weeks compared to those born between 39 and 41 weeks.[118]

After 37 weeks, any woman with GH or mild-to-moderate disease should have the timing of delivery discussed with her. The HYPITAT trial demonstrated that induction of labor at this gestation time reduces the risk of adverse maternal events and did not carry additional risk for the neonate. In addition, this strategy did not increase the risk of cesarean section, and the women most likely to benefit were those least favorable for induction.[119] This has led many clinicians to recommend the induction of labor from 37 weeks' gestation for women with HDP.

However, clinicians should consider that this trial was conducted in a setting where women are not treated for hypertension <160/100 at term, and may not be directly applicable to the U.K. population, where antihypertensive therapy is offered for lower degrees of hypertension, as one of the primary outcomes was the occurrence of severe hypertension. It also can be reasonable, if the woman wishes, to offer antihypertensive treatment and continue pregnancy under close monitoring, so long as blood pressure is controlled and there are no features of severe disease.[5] A large observational study concluded that, in women with otherwise uncomplicated preexisting hypertension, the optimal balance of fetal and maternal benefit is achieved by planning delivery at 38–39 weeks' gestation.[120]

These considerations should be clearly explained to the mother prior to 37–39 weeks. If she chooses to continue the pregnancy, she should be offered regular monitoring, and a clear plan should be made for when labor will be induced if it has not occurred spontaneously.

26.8   ANTENATAL MANAGEMENT OF PREECLAMPSIA

As in gestational and chronic hypertension, the challenges of management in preeclampsia lie in balancing the maternal and fetal risks of continuing pregnancy (expectant management) against the maternal risks of intervention and the fetal risks of preterm delivery (interventionist management). Women with preeclampsia are at greater risk of sudden deterioration and serious complications, and management protocols for preeclampsia take this into account.

It is important to recognize that, although most guidelines include specific gestational cutoffs for expectant and interventional management, a continuum of risk exists. While opting to continue the pregnancy, the goals of treatment are to maintain a safe blood pressure and monitor the mother for deteriorating disease and the fetus for signs of placental dysfunction and growth restriction.

26.8.1 Inpatient or Outpatient Management?

Most international bodies recommend hospital admission at the point of diagnosis in order to complete a full maternal and fetal assessment, including monitoring of blood pressure over a 24-h period.[64,72,73,121] Many women ultimately will be suitable for home and outpatient management, but blood pressure should be controlled, a full maternal assessment for any complications of preeclampsia completed, and fetal status (as assessed by ultrasound scan of growth and Doppler) determined prior to implementing an outpatient management plan.

Comprehensive maternal assessment should include a thorough clinical examination, including abdominal examination, fundoscopy, and assessment of deep tendon reflexes and clonus. Full blood count, coagulation, creatinine, urea, and liver function should be checked to screen for HELLP syndrome and renal dysfunction. Uric acid testing can be useful to confirm a diagnosis of preeclampsia, but it is not predictive of pregnancy outcome, and a normal result does not rule out preeclampsia.[122]

During admission, blood pressure should be checked at least every 4 h, and a 24-h urine collection for quantification of proteinuria should be performed if not already completed. Antihypertensive therapy should be commenced when the blood pressure consistently exceeds 150/100 mm Hg. While inpatients, women with preeclampsia are at increased risk of VTE and should receive thromboprophylaxis. In most cases, this would be with low-molecular-weight heparin.

There is no evidence to support bed rest in preeclampsia, and hospital admission for this purpose is associated with increased risk of infection, VTE, and psychosocial morbidity.[123] Women with stable blood pressure on treatment, normal laboratory studies, no need for concern about fetal well-being, and a good understanding of their condition are candidates for outpatient management. Outpatient management should be undertaken in the context of a plan for regular monitoring by experienced clinical staff and patient education upon triggers for urgent presentation to hospital services (e.g., headache, abdominal pain, or vaginal bleeding).

Maternal outpatient monitoring should include regular blood pressure measurement in a dedicated day assessment unit, or at home in the context of a clearly structured monitoring protocol. No subsequent quantification of proteinuria is necessary after significant proteinuria has been confirmed. Laboratory tests of biochemical and hematological parameters should be repeated two to three times a week, according to the severity and the progression of the disease.[5]

26.9 TREATMENT OF SEVERE PREECLAMPSIA

26.9.1 Severe Hypertension

Severe hypertension (>160–170/100–110 mm Hg) requires rapid control. The ACOG recommends the initiation of treatment within 1 h[72] and, in the absence of symptoms suggestive of impending eclampsia, it is reasonable to start with oral therapy if it is tolerated by the mother. When severe hypertension is detected in a primary-care or community setting, administration of oral antihypertensives while arranging transfer to secondary care can protect the mother against the risks of severe hypertension in the short term.

Where the systolic blood pressure is >180 mm Hg or refractory to oral therapy, intravenous antihypertensives (usually labetalol or hydralazine) may be required. Because of concerns about potentially compromising uteroplacental circulation by overcorrection of blood pressure (either too rapid or too extreme a drop) using this route, fetal monitoring during therapy is advised, although there is little evidence to support this practice.

Oral, fast-acting nifedipine, intravenous hydralazine and labetalol are equivalent for management of acute severe hypertension in pregnancy.[124] Invasive monitoring via an arterial line may be of benefit in refractory severe hypertension and critical-care medicine and neonatology teams should be involved in management and planning of delivery.

26.9.2 Magnesium Sulfate for Women with Severe Preeclampsia

Women who meet the criteria for the diagnosis of severe preeclampsia (Table 26.2) or have significant signs and symptoms of impending eclampsia (i.e., severe headache, clonus, neurological impairment) should be considered for treatment with magnesium sulfate for eclampsia prophylaxis. Magnesium sulfate reduces cerebral perfusion pressure and the risk of eclampsia in patients with preeclampsia. It is associated with a 50%–67% reduction in the risk of seizures and a reduction in the risk of maternal death, and it may offer a degree of neuroprotection to the baby, which is of particular importance in preterm deliveries.[125] The standard protocol is as described in the Collaborative Eclampsia Trial[126]: a 4-g loading dose with a maintenance infusion of 1 g/h.

Treatment with magnesium sulfate requires at least level 2 care. Monitoring for magnesium toxicity should be continuous, and practitioners should be aware that serum magnesium levels correlate poorly with clinically relevant toxicity. Early signs of magnesium toxicity include respiratory depression and loss of deep tendon reflexes, so respiratory rate and reflexes should be checked at least hourly. Toxicity can occur with therapeutic doses, especially in the context of renal impairment, so urine output also should be monitored closely. Magnesium toxicity is associated with electrocardiogram (ECG) changes and arrhythmias, and where it is suspected or the risk of toxicity is elevated, continuous ECG monitoring may be appropriate.

26.9.3 Plasma Volume Expansion and Fluid Restriction

Because preeclampsia is a state of intravascular depletion despite hypoosmolality and sodium and water retention, fluid management is particularly complex in severe cases. Renal function, if not already compromised, is vulnerable, and there is a significant risk of provoking pulmonary edema. Intensive care and multidisciplinary management incorporating nephrologists, intensivists, and obstetricians is necessary in the complex clinical scenario of coexisting renal injury and pulmonary edema in preeclampsia.

Where a woman is known to have an HDP, the practice of preloading prior to the use of regional anesthesia should be curtailed. In the case of severe preeclampsia, fluid restriction to 1.5 mL/kg/h may be appropriate, with close monitoring of renal function and urine output.

While there has been considerable interest in the possibility of using plasma volume expansion as an intervention to prolong pregnancy at early gestation without worsening extravascular fluid accumulation, it cannot be recommended for routine use.[127] There is evidence that the use of plasma expanders improves measures of maternal and fetal hemodynamics,[128,129] but this does not correlate with improvement in perinatal outcomes.[130]

26.9.4 HELLP Syndrome

In HELLP syndrome, initial minor derangement in transaminases and platelets can deteriorate rapidly, and blood tests should be repeated every 6–12 h if the trend is worsening and the decision has been made to prolong pregnancy to allow administration of corticosteroids for fetal lung maturity. Corticosteroids should not be used to treat HELLP syndrome.[131] HELLP will ultimately be cured by delivery, but clinicians should anticipate an initial worsening in laboratory indexes postdelivery, with recovery typically starting within 24–48 h of delivery.[96]

In severe and refractory HELLP syndrome, therapeutic plasma exchange (TPE) may have the benefit of both removing harmful circulating factors, like ammonia, endotoxins, inflammatory cytokines, vasoactive factors, and antibodies, and of replenishing those coagulation factors and albumin that would normally be produced in the liver.[132] TPE is an established treatment for the phenotypically similar condition of TTP, and also has been used successfully in women with severe HELLP syndrome. TPE is not without risk; complications may include sepsis, anaphylaxis, or plasma-transmitted disease. Patients most likely to benefit from TPE are those with an ongoing deterioration in laboratory parameters postpartum. Because most patients do recover without TPE and there are significant risks associated with this treatment, it should be considered only in exceptional circumstances, such as 48–72 h postpartum in the face of significant and deteriorating thrombocytopenia, anemia, and elevated liver enzymes.

Although liver rupture is rare, it is a surgical emergency and requires multidisciplinary management. A surgical approach should involve both obstetricians and hepatobiliary surgeons, as urgent cesarean section is likely to be necessary before dealing with the liver rupture. Because liver rupture is associated with major hemorrhage in the setting of existing thrombocytopenia and a high risk of disseminated intravascular coagulation, hematology involvement at an early stage is critical, and significant blood product administration is likely to be required. The principle of management is to secure hemostasis, which initially may be achieved by packing the liver, with a planned return to the operating theater 24–48 h later for removal of packs once coagulation has normalized. Alternative strategies include arterial ligation and radiological selective arterial embolization.[133] Resection is likely to provoke massive bleeding. Liver transplantation has been reported as an option of last resort.[134] A subcapsular hematoma should be managed conservatively, and the liver should be handled gently at cesarean section in women with known HELLP syndrome to minimize the risk of additional hepatic trauma.

26.9.5 Acute Management of Eclampsia

Eclampsia is an obstetric emergency, and the first priority is to stabilize the mother through the application of a standard resuscitation principles, first securing the airway and then assessing breathing and circulation (ABC). Most eclamptic seizures are self-terminating and short-lived; however, magnesium sulfate should be commenced as soon as possible, if not already in progress, according to the protocol described previously. If magnesium sulfate has already begun, a further bolus may be given, and the maintenance infusion may be increased to 2 g/h.[126] Hypertension should be controlled as outlined previously; the intravenous route is preferable, as the mother is likely to be in a state of altered consciousness. Recurrent seizures may warrant intubation and paralysis to maintain oxygenation.

Fetal monitoring is not a priority until the mother has been stabilized. Auscultation or CTG will inevitably show fetal bradycardia during and immediately after a seizure, but the primary intervention is controlling seizures and blood pressure, not delivery. As soon as the mother's condition is judged stable, the baby should be delivered by the most expedient route. In certain selected situations, delivery may be achievable vaginally, but it most commonly will occur by cesarean section.

26.10 TIMING AND MODE OF DELIVERY IN PREECLAMPSIA

There is no role for the outpatient management of severe preeclampsia as previously defined. In severe preeclampsia, the clinical scenario is dynamic, and with every advancing day of gestation, the balance of the risks and benefits attending the decision to deliver or continue the pregnancy is altered. Daily review by experienced clinicians is the minimum necessary to ensure that the management plan reflects the current clinical situation. There are general guidelines about the timing of delivery in severe preeclampsia, but the decision must be individualized in every case to the condition of mother and fetus, as well as the ability of local services to meet both of their medical needs.

At any gestation (i.e., even before fetal viability), delivery is indicated for life-threatening maternal disease, which may take the form of severe refractory hypertension, eclampsia, placental abruption, or rapidly deteriorating HELLP syndrome or renal dysfunction. After the age of fetal viability (which may vary depending on the country/setting), delivery also may be indicated for serious fetal compromise with abnormal fetal ductus venosus Doppler or computerized CTG findings. If fetal compromise is the primary indication for delivery at 24–26 weeks, a frank discussion should be held with the parents before proceeding, regarding the poor prognosis for the baby, particularly in the setting of marked intrauterine growth restriction and the potential complications of preterm surgery. Preterm cesarean section is associated with greater maternal blood loss and an increased risk of uterine rupture in subsequent pregnancies, and it may not increase the survival of very-growth-restricted, extremely premature babies.

In all cases, the mother should be stabilized before proceeding to delivery. Performing a Category 1 cesarean section immediately after an eclamptic seizure without full assessment of the condition of mother and baby exposes the mother to severe risks associated with general anesthesia (i.e., failed intubation, severe hypertension, aspiration, or a further cerebral event), bleeding secondary to an undetected coagulopathy, and rushed, potentially complex surgery with a higher risk of intraoperative damage to the bladder and ureters. Once the mother is stable, any blood products ordered, and the appropriate obstetric, anesthetic, and neonatal team assembled, delivery can be accomplished safely if indicated.

In general, at gestations below 34 weeks, the presumption is that expectant management will be preferred in the absence of critical illness in the mother or fetus.[135] Immediate delivery certainly increases neonatal morbidity and may not benefit the mother. A useful clinical tool would be a prediction model that could identify those women likely to develop complications of preeclampsia within the next 7 days. These women then could be offered corticosteroids for fetal lung maturation, transferred to a center with appropriate neonatal care facilities, and receive magnesium sulfate for seizure prophylaxis. Conversely, women identified as being at low risk of disease progression could avoid unnecessary preterm delivery and the attendant neonatal and maternal morbidity. Several such models have been developed and are undergoing investigation in trial settings to inform recommendations for practice.

The fullPIERS model incorporates gestational age, chest pain or dyspnea, SpO_2, platelet count, creatinine, and aspartate transaminase, and it predicts adverse maternal outcomes within 48 h and 7 days, with area under the curve (AUC) of 0.88 and >0.7, respectively.[136] This model has undergone external validation[137] and seems to perform well as a prediction tool, but it has not yet been tested in a clinical context as a decision-making aid. A similar model, miniPIERS, which incorporates physical findings and symptoms rather than the more specialized laboratory tests included in the fullPIERS model, has been developed for use in low-resource clinical settings. The features included are parity, gestational age, systolic blood pressure, degree of proteinuria, vaginal bleeding with abdominal pain, headache and/or visual changes, and chest pain and/or dyspnea; the AUC for this model is 0.768 [95% confidence interval (CI) 0.735–0.801].[138]

The PREP prediction models for the risk of complications in early preeclampsia looked specifically at predicting complications in preeclampsia diagnosed <34 weeks' gestation. The PREP models included maternal age, gestational age at diagnosis, medical history, systolic blood pressure, urine protein-to-creatinine ratio, platelet count, serum urea concentration, oxygen saturation, baseline treatment with antihypertensive drugs, administration of magnesium sulfate, exaggerated tendon reflexes, and serum alanine aminotransaminase and creatinine concentrations.[139] The PREP model has undergone external validation and a trial including the model in the management of patients with early-onset preeclampsia is underway.

Both the PIERS and PREP models are available online. Although no model has yet been proven to be of clinical utility in practice, it is noteworthy that the parameters common to all models, in particular respiratory symptoms (dyspnea and chest pain) and signs (oxygen saturation) present in all three models, are frequently overlooked by obstetric teams fixated on the arm, abdomen, and ankles in examining hypertensive pregnant patients.

After 34 weeks, the threshold for delivery will fall substantially, and any feature of deterioration may prompt consideration of expediting delivery. The HYPITAT II study compared immediate delivery to expectant management between 34 and 37 weeks' gestation. It found a small increase in adverse maternal outcomes with expectant management, offset by a significant increase in neonatal morbidity after immediate delivery. There is insufficient evidence to make prescriptive recommendations in this gestational window; at present, the woman and her medical team must weigh the individual circumstances and review the situation on a daily basis.

In the future, predictive models such as the PIERS and PREP models may assist in making the decision to end a pregnancy. After 37 weeks, a discussion about timing of delivery should take place, even for women with mild and stable preeclampsia. The ideal time of delivery will usually lie between 37 and 39 weeks' gestation, depending on the clinical situation.

Vaginal delivery is preferable to cesarean section because of the lower risk of maternal morbidity, particularly in hypertensive women, who are more vulnerable to the stress of abdominal delivery. Even at preterm gestations, the cervix should be assessed for the possibility of successful induction of labor with cervical-ripening agents. Although half of all inductions before 35 weeks end in cesarean section, and it would be inappropriate to continue an induction for 2–3 days in the presence of severe disease that warrants delivery, sometimes a vaginal delivery is achievable rapidly and may be preferable to operative delivery, with its inherent additional risks of bleeding, thrombosis, infection, and fluid management challenges.

26.11   INTRAPARTUM CARE OF HYPERTENSIVE WOMEN

26.11.1   Normal Intrapartum Hemodynamics and Physiological Changes

The maximum CO in pregnancy occurs during labor and delivery; the expulsion of blood from the uterine vascular bed with each contraction increases circulating volume, and catecholamine release and pain increase heart rate. Preload can be further increased by water retention stimulated by oxytocin release or exogenous administration because oxytocin is an analog of antidiuretic hormone (ADH). CO in labor can increase 40%–60% above the increase already seen in normal pregnancy.[140]

The process of parturition has been described as an inflammatory process and is characterized by proinflammatory cytokines driving an influx of leukocytes into the myometrium and cervix, contributing to uterine contractions and cervical ripening.[141]

26.11.2   Intrapartum Maternal and Fetal Monitoring

The physiological changes of labor can increase the risk of new or worsening hypertension and pulmonary edema by increasing CO and vascular permeability. Women without the cardiac capacity to maintain this increase, particularly those with long-standing hypertension, can be at risk of cardiovascular events in the intrapartum period. Relative underperfusion of the uteroplacental circulation during this time can contribute to fetal hypoxia during labor and increase the risk of neonatal hypoxic ischemic encephalopathy (HIE).

All women with HDP should be offered continuous fetal monitoring in labor. Clinicians interpreting the CTG should take into account the possibility of fetal deterioration occurring more rapidly than would normally be expected because of possible fetal growth restriction, and act accordingly.

Maternal blood pressure should be measured hourly in labor and any antihypertensive medication continued as previously prescribed. Additional antihypertensives are often required. In women with severe preeclampsia, more frequent blood pressure measurement is required, and consideration should be given to invasive monitoring, particularly if intravenous antihypertensive therapy is required. Severe uncontrolled hypertension or neurological symptoms in the second stage of labor may be an indication for assisted vaginal delivery with forceps or vacuum to limit the duration of maternal effort. The use of the forceps is preferable to the use of the ventouse because it is associated with less intracranial bleeding; the ventouse is not appropriate for use at gestations <34 weeks.

26.11.3 Intrapartum Analgesia and Anesthetic Considerations

Early epidural or spinal analgesia reduces the risk of requiring general anesthesia for emergency intervention. It can also assist in blood pressure control by causing vasodilation and removing the noxious stimuli of painful contractions. Pharyngolaryngeal edema in preeclamptic patients increases the chances of failed intubation, and intubation increases the chances of severe hypertension and aspiration. Women with hypertensive disorders should not routinely receive a fluid preload prior to initiating epidural or spinal analgesia.[5]

Although regional anesthesia is preferred, its use may be limited by HDP-associated thrombocytopenia. Epidural hematoma is a feared complication of neuraxial blockade and has been reported in association with pregnancy thrombocytopenia.[142] In the patient with additional risk factors for bleeding such as HELLP syndrome or severe PE, the whole clinical picture should be considered, as regional anesthesia may be contraindicated in the setting of a rapidly falling platelet count and concomitant coagulopathy. Due to a scarcity of cases, definitive guidance on the use of regional anesthesia in pregnancy hypertension-associated thrombocytopenia cannot be determined. Local guidelines recommend a threshold of $75–90 \times 10^9$ g/dL, but ultimately, a clinical risk assessment of the whole clinical picture by an experienced anesthetist is more important than the exact platelet count for determining optimal anesthetic management.[143,144] Options might include platelet transfusion prior to the insertion of spinal for cesarean section in the context of worsening thrombocytopenia, planned general anesthesia, or use of alternative analgesia (e.g., remifentanil) during attempted vaginal delivery.

Consideration should be given to the potential need for blood products based on the hematological and coagulation parameters as measured at the onset of labor, bearing in mind the increased risk of postpartum hemorrhage in preeclampsia. If the platelet count is $<50 \times 10^9$/L, falling rapidly, or there is associated coagulopathy, consideration should be given to ordering platelets and other blood products. Platelet transfusion is required if platelets fall below 20×10^9/L around delivery, whatever the mechanism.

Oxytocin should be used for active management of the third stage of labor to reduce the risk of postpartum hemorrhage. Ergometrine (and therefore Syntometrine) should be avoided for women with known hypertensive disease of any kind, even if blood pressure is normal at the time of delivery. Several maternal deaths have been caused by the hypertension associated with ergometrine use.[111] This does not preclude the use of ergometrine in the event of severe postpartum hemorrhage after the use of alternative drugs and at the discretion of senior clinical staff, but an increase in antihypertensive requirement after the immediate crisis is managed should be anticipated.

26.12 POSTNATAL CARE AND FOLLOW-UP OF WOMEN AFFECTED BY HYPERTENSION IN PREGNANCY

26.12.1 Immediate Postpartum Management of Women Affected by HDP

Although delivery will ultimately cure pregnancy-related hypertension, resolution is not immediate, and hypertension and the abnormalities of HELLP syndrome typically continue to worsen before ultimate improvement. In normal pregnancy, blood pressure falls immediately after delivery due to the blood loss associated with delivery and removal of the sympathetic stimulation associated with labor. As the uterus contracts, around 500–700 mL of blood are returned from the uterine to the systemic circulation. There is further mobilization of extracellular fluid and subsequent expansion of intravascular volume, and most women experience a peak of blood pressure between the third and sixth days postpartum.

In hypertensive women, a similar process will take place, which can lead to the development of severe hypertension a few days after delivery at a time when surveillance may have been relaxed. Other factors that can cause or exacerbate hypertension postpartum are pain, anxiety, the use of certain drugs (e.g., ergometrine), and fluid overload in labor. These factors should be assessed and analgesia and fluid management adjusted as necessary prior to altering antihypertensive management. Women who did not have hypertension during pregnancy may also present with hypertension for the first time during this period, and up to 44% of eclampsia presents postpartum de novo.[78]

After delivery, antihypertensive therapy should be continued and the same targets for control of hypertension apply as during pregnancy—the aim should be to control the blood pressure at <150/100 mm Hg if on medication. If any new features of severe disease develop, mothers should be moved to a higher level of care and consideration given to administering at least 24 h of magnesium sulfate as eclampsia prophylaxis. Any woman with a new-onset severe headache, with or without neurological symptoms, should be assessed to evaluate the possibility of postpartum stroke or venous thrombosis.

Women may be suitable for hospital discharge within 1–2 days of delivery if blood pressure is well controlled and no other complications exist, but arrangements should be made for daily blood pressure assessment in the community by home visits, home monitoring, or an appointment in primary care or the obstetric day assessment unit.

26.12.2   Choice of Antihypertensive in the Puerperium and Lactation

Most women who have required antihypertensive therapy during pregnancy will still require treatment for several days or weeks postpartum. A wider range of effective drugs are available for use in lactating women, so the choice of agent should be reviewed at the earliest opportunity after delivery. An alternative agent might have a more convenient dosing schedule or offer renal protection for women with preexisting hypertensive or renal disease.

No antihypertensive drugs are licensed for use in breastfeeding, so most recommendations are based on observational studies and expert opinion. In addition to the drugs used in pregnancy, ACE-inhibitors (enalapril and captopril) have been shown to be safe and effective in breastfeeding women (Table 26.4). They are particularly appropriate for women needing renal or cardiac protection because of prepregnancy comorbidities. Methyldopa should be avoided because of its side-effect profile, which includes depression and sedation.[5]

26.12.3   Complications of Hypertensive Disease in the Puerperium

GH, proteinuria, and any associated hepatic, renal, or hematological abnormalities should return to baseline by 6 weeks postpartum.[145] Women with persistent hypertension or proteinuria at this time may have had chronic disease revealed by pregnancy and require further investigation in order to establish a diagnosis.

Early-onset preeclampsia is associated with antiphospholipid syndrome, and consideration should be given to screening affected women after the puerperium, particularly if there are other features of the disorder.

Peripartum cardiomyopathy is a rare complication of pregnancy that usually presents within the first few months after delivery. Although only a rare cause, preeclampsia is a risk factor, and symptoms of heart failure (including fatigue, dyspnea, and peripheral edema) may not be recognized immediately in the mother recovering from preeclampsia and managing the demands of a new baby.

26.13   LONG-TERM IMPLICATIONS OF HYPERTENSION IN PREGNANCY

26.13.1   Future Pregnancies

All women affected by HDP should receive postnatal counseling regarding the management of future pregnancies. For women with GH, the risk of recurrence in the next pregnancy is 16%–47% and the risk of preeclampsia is 2%–7%. For women with preeclampsia, the risk of recurrence is 16% if they delivered at term, 25% if they delivered before 34 weeks, and 55% if they delivered before 28 weeks.[78] All women affected by HDP should be considered for administration of low-dose aspirin for preeclampsia prophylaxis in subsequent pregnancies. Most obstetric units will offer more frequent visits or the option of home monitoring for patients at high risk of developing hypertension during pregnancy.

26.13.2   Longer-Term Maternal Health Implications

Hypertension in pregnancy is a risk factor for cardiovascular disease in later life, and postnatal consultation with women affected by preeclampsia represents a pivotal opportunity to inform about and provide advice on risk-reduction strategies.

A year after severe preeclampsia, 42% of women still will have hypertension detectable upon clinical assessment, with around half of them having hypertension uncovered only with a period of ambulatory monitoring.[146] Around 14% of women who had any HDP in their first pregnancy will go on to develop clinically apparent hypertension within the next 10 years, and the risk of developing hypertension within 20 years of pregnancy is doubled in women affected by HDP compared to women normotensive in pregnancy.[147] It is not clear whether the endothelial dysfunction of preeclampsia causes later pathology or whether pregnancy, by increasing the demand on cardiovascular physiology, temporarily unmasks women at risk of dysfunction in later life.

Hypertensive disorders of pregnancy also have been associated with cerebrovascular disease, Type 2 diabetes, hypertension, and VTE.[147–149] The puerperium represents an underutilized opportunity to encourage women to adopt diet and lifestyle changes that may mitigate the increased risk associated with HDP. Women are motivated to improve their health immediately after pregnancy,[78] and clinicians who have been closely involved in detailed counseling and care during pregnancy should not overlook this opportunity to close their therapeutic relationship with the best available advice for their patients' long-term health and quality of life.

26.14 CONCLUSION

- Hypertension in pregnancy is common and extensively investigated, but the precise mechanisms of disease remain unclear.
- Endothelial dysfunction with a background of disrupted maternal hemodynamics, angiogenic balance, lipid and glucose metabolism, and hormonal signaling is typical of hypertension in pregnancy.
- The risk of HDP can be reduced with administration of low-dose aspirin from the first trimester in high-risk women.
- Models combining maternal characteristics, uterine artery Dopplers, and biomarkers can screen effectively for women at high risk of severe and early-onset preeclampsia.
- New technology in validated automated devices for home monitoring of blood pressure, together with digital distance monitoring from the hospital team, can reduce costs and improve women's experience of antenatal monitoring.
- The diagnosis of preeclampsia can be clarified by the use of novel tests including PlGF and the sFlt-1/PlGF ratio.
- Models predicting the development of maternal complications can be used to address the clinical conundrum of timing of delivery in preterm preeclampsia.
- The postnatal period is a critical time for monitoring and prevention of late complications of preeclampsia, as well as health education directed at reducing the risk of cardiovascular disease associated with a history of hypertension in pregnancy.

Directions for future research and investigation include the following:

- Preeclampsia may be the presentation of women with subclinical cardiovascular dysfunction revealed by the stress of pregnancy. Preconception and longitudinal studies of maternal cardiac function could help to clarify this process.
- Models that predict late-onset preeclampsia or perform well as a screening test to rule it out would lead to major changes in antenatal care schedules.
- Additional agents for prevention of preeclampsia beyond aspirin require investigation, and the choice of agent for risk reduction may vary with the maternal phenotype at conception.
- Novel diagnostic tests have been developed for preeclampsia, and trials of management based on these tests now need to be reported to assess clinical effects and cost effectiveness.
- Additional treatments for preeclampsia, including relaxin, PPAR antagonists, nitric oxide donors, and statins, should be evaluated to add to the interventions available to allow prolongation of pregnancy.

REFERENCES

1. Say L, Chou D, Gemmill A, Tunçalp Ö, Moller A-B, Daniels J, et al. Global causes of maternal death: a WHO systematic analysis. *Lancet Glob Health* 2014;**2**(6):e323–33.
2. Kuklina EV, Ayala C, Callaghan WM. Hypertensive disorders and severe obstetric morbidity in the United States. *Obstet Gynecol* 2009; **113**(6):1299–306.
3. Knight M, Nair M, Tuffnell D, Kenyon S, Shakespeare J, Brocklehurst PKJ. *Saving lives, improving mothers' care: surveillance of maternal deaths in the UK 2012–14 and lessons learned to inform maternity care from the UK and Ireland con dential enquiries into maternal deaths and morbidity 2009–14;* 2016.
4. Wong AE, Grobman WA. Medically indicated—Iatrogenic prematurity. *Clin Perinatol* 2011;**38**(3):423–39.
5. NICE. *Hypertension in pregnancy. Guidelines.* NICE; 2010. CG 107.
6. Irgens HU, Reisaeter L, Irgens LM, Lie RT. Long term mortality of mothers and fathers after pre-eclampsia: population based cohort study. *BMJ* 2001;**323**(7323):1213–7.
7. Smith GC, Pell JP, Walsh D. Pregnancy complications and maternal risk of ischaemic heart disease: a retrospective cohort study of 129,290 births. *Lancet* 2001;**357**(9273):2002–6.
8. Ray JG, Vermeulen MJ, Schull MJ, Redelmeier DA. Cardiovascular health after maternal placental syndromes (CHAMPS): population-based retrospective cohort study. *Lancet* 2005;**366**(9499):1797–803.

9. Bellamy L, Casas J-P, Hingorani AD, Williams DJ. Pre-eclampsia and risk of cardiovascular disease and cancer in later life: systematic review and meta-analysis. *BMJ* 2007;**335**(7627):974.

10. Wu CS, Nohr EA, Bech BH, Vestergaard M, Catov JM, Olsen J. Health of children born to mothers who had preeclampsia: a population-based cohort study. *Am J Obstet Gynecol* 2009;**201**(3):269.e1–269.e10.

11. Redman CW. Current topic: pre-eclampsia and the placenta. *Placenta* 1991;**12**(4):301–8.

12. Roberts JM, Redman CW. Pre-eclampsia: more than pregnancy-induced hypertension. *Lancet* 1993;**341**(8858):1447–51.

13. Granger JP, Alexander BT, Llinas MT, Bennett WA, Khalil RA. Pathophysiology of hypertension during preeclampsia linking placental ischemia with endothelial dysfunction. *Hypertension* 2001;**38**(3 Pt 2):718–22.

14. Marshall SA, Senadheera SN, Jelinic M, O'Sullivan K, Parry LJ, Tare M. Relaxin deficiency leads to uterine artery dysfunction during pregnancy in mice. *Front Physiol* 2018;**9**:255.

15. Conrad KP, Baker VL. Corpus luteal contribution to maternal pregnancy physiology and outcomes in assisted reproductive technologies. *Am J Physiol Regul Integr Comp Physiol* 2013;**304**(2):R69–72.

16. Rosenfeld CR, Roy T, Cox BE. Mechanisms modulating estrogen-induced uterine vasodilation. *Vasc Pharmacol* 2002;**38**(2):115–25.

17. Chang K, Lubo ZL. Review article: steroid hormones and uterine vascular adaptation to pregnancy. *Reprod Sci* 2008;**15**(4):336–48.

18. Foo FL, McEniery CM, Lees C, Khalil A, International Working Group on Maternal Hemodynamics. Assessment of arterial function in pregnancy: recommendations of the international working group on maternal hemodynamics. *Ultrasound Obstet Gynecol* 2017;**50**(3):324–31.

19. Possomato-Vieira JS, Khalil RA. Mechanisms of endothelial dysfunction in hypertensive pregnancy and preeclampsia. *Adv Pharmacol* 2016;**77**:361–431.

20. Mahendru AA, Everett TR, Wilkinson IB, Lees CC, McEniery CM. Maternal cardiovascular changes from pre-pregnancy to very early pregnancy. *J Hypertens* 2012;**30**(11):2168–72.

21. Duvekot JJ, Cheriex EC, Pieters FA, Menheere PP, Peeters LH. Early pregnancy changes in hemodynamics and volume homeostasis are consecutive adjustments triggered by a primary fall in systemic vascular tone. *Am J Obstet Gynecol* 1993;**169**(6):1382–92.

22. Valensise H, Vasapollo B, Novelli GP. Maternal cardiovascular haemodynamics in normal and complicated pregnancies. *Fetal Matern Med Rev* 2003;**14**(4):355–85.

23. Tkachenko O, Shchekochikhin D, Schrier RW. Hormones and Hemodynamics in Pregnancy. *Int J Endocrinol Metab* 2014;**12**(2).

24. Valensise H, Novelli GP, Vasapollo B, Borzi M, Arduini D, Galante A, et al. Maternal cardiac systolic and diastolic function: relationship with uteroplacental resistances. A Doppler and echocardiographic longitudinal study. *Ultrasound Obstet Gynecol* 2000;**15**(6):487–97.

25. Irani RA, Xia Y. Renin angiotensin signaling in normal pregnancy and preeclampsia. *Semin Nephrol* 2011;**31**(1):47–58.

26. Gant NF, Daley GL, Chand S, Whalley PJ, PC MD. A study of angiotensin II pressor response throughout primigravid pregnancy. *J Clin Invest* 1973;**52**(11):2682–9.

27. Burke SD, Zsengellér ZK, Khankin EV, Lo AS, Rajakumar A, DuPont JJ, et al. Soluble fms-like tyrosine kinase 1 promotes angiotensin II sensitivity in preeclampsia. *J Clin Invest* 2016;**126**(7):2561–74.

28. Roberts VHJ, Morgan TK, Bednarek P, Morita M, Burton GJ, Lo JO, et al. Early first trimester uteroplacental flow and the progressive disintegration of spiral artery plugs: new insights from contrast-enhanced ultrasound and tissue histopathology. *Hum Reprod* 2017;**32**(12):2382–93.

29. Seely EW, Solomon CG. Insulin resistance and its potential role in pregnancy-induced hypertension. *J Clin Endocrinol Metab* 2003;**88**(6):2393–8.

30. Melchiorre K, Sutherland GR, Baltabaeva A, Liberati M, Thilaganathan B. Maternal cardiac dysfunction and remodeling in women with pre-eclampsia at term. *Hypertension* 2011;**57**(1):85–93.

31. Holobotovskyy V, Chong YS, Burchell J, He B, Phillips M, Leader L, et al. Regulator of G protein signaling 5 is a determinant of gestational hypertension and preeclampsia. *Sci Transl Med* 2015;**7**(290):290ra88.

32. Stott D, Nzelu O, Nicolaides KH, Kametas NA. Maternal haemodynamics in normal pregnancies and in pregnancies affected by pre-eclampsia. *Ultrasound Obstet Gynecol* 2017;.

33. Khalil A, Akolekar R, Syngelaki A, Elkhouli M, Nicolaides KH. Maternal hemodynamics in normal pregnancies at 11-13 weeks' gestation. *Fetal Diagn Ther* 2012;**32**:179–85.

34. Khalil A, Garcia-Mandujano R, Maiz N, Elkhouli M, Nicolaides KH. Longitudinal changes in maternal hemodynamics in a population at risk for pre-eclampsia. *Ultrasound Obstet Gynecol* 2014;**44**(2):197–204.

35. Ganss R. Maternal metabolism and vascular adaptation in pregnancy: the PPAR link. *Trends Endocrinol Metab* 2017;**28**(1):73–84.

36. Chinnathambi V, More AS, Hankins GD, Yallampalli C, Sathishkumar K. Gestational exposure to elevated testosterone levels induces hypertension via heightened vascular angiotensin II type 1 receptor signaling in rats. *Biol Reprod* 2014;**916**(1):1–7.

37. Rolnik DL, Wright D, Poon LC, O'Gorman N, Syngelaki A, de Paco MC, et al. Aspirin versus placebo in pregnancies at high risk for preterm preeclampsia. *N Engl J Med* 2017;**377**(7):613–22.

38. Bujold E, Roberge S, Lacasse Y, Bureau M, Audibert F, Marcoux S, et al. Prevention of preeclampsia and intrauterine growth restriction with aspirin started in early pregnancy: a meta-analysis. *Obstet Gynecol* 2010;**116**(2 Pt 1):402–14.

39. Hyppönen E, Cavadino A, Fraser A. Vitamin D and pre-eclampsia: original data, systematic review, and meta-analysis. *Ann Nutr Metab* 2013;**63**:331–40.

40. Thangaratinam S, Langenveld J, Mol BW, Khan KS. Prediction and primary prevention of pre-eclampsia. *Best Pract Res Clin Obstet Gynaecol* 2011;**25**(4):419–33.

41. Hofmeyr JG, Lawrie TA, Atallah AN, Duley L, Torloni MR. Calcium supplementation during pregnancy for preventing hypertensive disorders and related problems. *Cochrane Database Syst Rev* 2014;**6**.

42. Costantine MM, Cleary K, Hebert MF, Ahmed MS, Brown LM, Ren Z, et al. Safety and pharmacokinetics of pravastatin used for the prevention of preeclampsia in high-risk pregnant women: a pilot randomized controlled trial. *Am J Obstet Gynecol* 2016;**214**(6):720.e1–720.e17.

43. Romero R, Erez O, Hüttemann M, Maymon E, Panaitescu B, Conde-Agudelo A, et al. Metformin, the aspirin of the 21st century: its role in gestational diabetes mellitus, prevention of preeclampsia and cancer, and the promotion of longevity. *Am J Obstet Gynecol* 2017;282–302.

44. Anon. *Hypertension in pregnancy: diagnosis and management, NICE Clinical guideline 107.* NICE; 2010.

45. Poon LCY, Kametas NA, Chelemen T, Leal A, Nicolaides KH. Maternal risk factors for hypertensive disorders in pregnancy: a multivariate approach. *J Hum Hypertens* 2010;**24**(2):104–10.

46. Verghese L, Alam S, Beski S, Thuraisingham R, Barnes I, MacCallum P. Antenatal screening for pre-eclampsia: evaluation of the NICE and pre-eclampsia community guidelines. *J Obstet Gynaecol* 2012;**32**(2):128–31.

47. O'Gorman N, Wright D, Poon LC, Rolnik DL, Syngelaki A, de Alvarado M, et al. Multicenter screening for pre-eclampsia by maternal factors and biomarkers at 11–13 weeks' gestation: comparison with NICE guidelines and ACOG recommendations. *Ultrasound Obstet Gynecol* 2017;**49**(6):756–60.

48. Conde-Agudelo A, Villar J, Lindheimer M. World Health Organization systematic review of screening tests for preeclampsia. *Obstet Gynecol* 2004;**104**(6):1367–91.

49. Meads CA, Cnossen JS, Meher S, Juarez-Garcia A, Ter RGDL, et al. Methods of prediction and prevention of pre-eclampsia. *Heal Technol Assess* 2008;**12**(6):1–270.

50. Kleinrouweler CE, Bossuyt PMM, Thilaganathan B, Vollebregt KC, Arenas Ramírez J, Ohkuchi A, et al. Value of adding second-trimester uterine artery Doppler to patient characteristics in identification of nulliparous women at increased risk for pre-eclampsia: an individual patient data meta-analysis. *Ultrasound Obstet Gynecol* 2013;**42**(3):257–67.

51. Kuc S, Wortelboer EJ, Van Rijn BB, Franx A. First-trimester prediction of preeclampsia: a systematic review. *Obstet Gynecol Surv* 2011;**66**(4):225–39.

52. Cnossen JS, Morris RK, ter Riet G, Mol BWJ, van der Post JAM, Coomarasamy A, et al. Use of uterine artery Doppler ultrasonography to predict pre-eclampsia and intrauterine growth restriction: a systematic review and bivariable meta-analysis. *CMAJ* 2008;**178**(6):701–11.

53. Poon LC, Nicolaides KH. First-trimester maternal factors and biomarker screening for preeclampsia. *Prenat Diagn* 2014;**34**(7):618–27.

54. Petrie JC, O'Brien ET, Littler WA, de Swiet M. Recommendations on blood pressure measurement. *Br Med J (Clin Res Ed)* 1986;**293**(6547):611–5.

55. Nathan HL, Duhig K, Hezelgrave NL, Chappell LC, Shennan AH, Shennan AH. Blood pressure measurement in pregnancy. *Obstet Gynaecol* 2015;**17**:91–8.

56. Brown MA, Buddle ML, Farrell T, Davis G, Jones M. Randomised trial of management of hypertensive pregnancies by Korotkoff phase IV or phase V. *Lancet* 1998;**352**(9130):777–81.

57. de Greeff A, Lorde I, Wilton A, Seed P, Coleman AJ, Shennan AH. Calibration accuracy of hospital-based non-invasive blood pressure measuring devices. *J Hum Hypertens* 2010;**24**(1):58–63.

58. Wagner SJ, Acquah LA, Lindell EP, Craici IM, Wingo MT, Rose CH, et al. Posterior reversible encephalopathy syndrome and eclampsia: pressing the case for more aggressive blood pressure control. *Mayo Clin Proc* 2011;**86**(9):851–6.

59. Hladunewich M, Karumanchi SA, Lafayette R. Pathophysiology of the clinical manifestations of preeclampsia. *Clin J Am Soc Nephrol* 2007;**2**(3):543–9.

60. Chappell LC, Shennan AH. Assessment of proteinuria in pregnancy. *Br Med J* 2008;**336**:968–9.

61. Côté A-M, Brown MA, Lam E, von Dadelszen P, Firoz T, Liston RM, et al. Diagnostic accuracy of urinary spot protein:creatinine ratio for proteinuria in hypertensive pregnant women: systematic review. *BMJ* 2008;**336**(7651):1003–6.

62. Thangaratinam S, Coomarasamy A, O'Mahony F, Sharp S, Zamora J, Khan KS, et al. Estimation of proteinuria as a predictor of complications of pre-eclampsia: a systematic review. *BMC Med* 2009;**7**(10).

63. Morikawa M, Yamada T, Yamada T, Cho K, Yamada H, Sakuragi N, et al. Pregnancy outcome of women who developed proteinuria in the absence of hypertension after mid-gestation. *J Perinat Med* 2008;**36**(5):419–24.

64. Tranquilli AL, Dekker G, Magee L, Roberts J, Sibai BM, Steyn W, et al. The classification, diagnosis and management of the hypertensive disorders of pregnancy: a revised statement from the ISSHP. *Pregnancy Hypertens* 2014;**4**(2):97–104.

65. Lees C, Marlow N, Arabin B, Bilardo CM, Brezinka C, Derks JB, et al. Perinatal morbidity and mortality in early-onset fetal growth restriction: cohort outcomes of the trial of randomized umbilical and fetal flow in Europe (TRUFFLE). *Ultrasound Obstet Gynecol* 2013;**42**(4):400–8.

66. Sibai BM. Imitators of severe pre-eclampsia/eclampsia. *Clin Perinatol* 2004;835–52.

67. Romero R, Nien JK, Espinoza J, Todem D, Fu W, Chung H, et al. A longitudinal study of angiogenic (placental growth factor) and anti-angiogenic (soluble endoglin and soluble vascular endothelial growth factor receptor-1) factors in normal pregnancy and patients destined to develop pre-eclampsia and deliver a small for. *J Matern Fetal Neonatal Med* 2008;**21**(1):9–23.

68. Engels T, Pape J, Schoofs K, Henrich W, Verlohren S. Automated measurement of sFlt1, PlGF and sFlt1/PlGF ratio in differential diagnosis of hypertensive pregnancy disorders. *Hypertens Pregnancy* 2013;**32**(4):459–73.

69. Zeisler H, Llurba E, Chantraine F, Vatish M, Staff AC, Sennström M, et al. Predictive value of the sFlt-1:PlGF ratio in women with suspected pre-eclampsia. *N Engl J Med* 2016;**374**(1):13–22.

70. Chappell LC, Duckworth S, Seed PT, Griffin M, Myers J, Mackillop L, et al. Diagnostic accuracy of placental growth factor in women with suspected preeclampsia: a prospective multicenter study. *Circulation* 2013;**128**(19):2121–31.

71. Sharp A, Chappell LC, Dekker G, Pelletier S, Garnier Y, Zeren O, et al. Placental growth factor informed management of suspected pre-eclampsia or fetal growth restriction: The MAPPLE cohort study. *Pregnancy Hypertens* 2018;.

72. Anon. Hypertension in pregnancy task force. In: *Hypertension in Pregnancy*; 2013.

73. World Health Organisation. *WHO recommendations for prevention and treatment of pre-eclampsia and eclampsia.* Geneva: World Health Organization; 2011.
74. SOGC. Diagnosis, evaluation, and management of the hypertensive disorders of pregnancy: executive summary. *SOGC Clin Pract Guidel* 2014;**307**.
75. Bramham K, Parnell B, Nelson-Piercy C, Seed PT, Poston L, Chappell LC. Chronic hypertension and pregnancy outcomes: systematic review and meta-analysis. *BMJ* 2014;**348**:g2301.
76. Chappell LC, Enye S, Seed P, Briley AL, Poston L, Shennan AH. Adverse perinatal outcomes and risk factors for preeclampsia in women with chronic hypertension: a prospective study. *Hypertension* 2008;**51**:1002–9.
77. NICE (National Institute for Health and Care Excellence). *Antenatal care for uncomplicated pregnancies. Clinical Guideline (CG62).* NICE; 2017.
78. Bramham K, Nelson-Piercy C, Brown MJ, Chappell LC. Postpartum management of hypertension. *BMJ* 2013;**346**. f894.
79. Heyborne KD, Schultz MF, Goodlin RC, Durham JD. Renal artery stenosis during pregnancy: a review. *Obstet Gynecol Surv* 1991;**46**(8):509–14.
80. Gallery ED. Chronic essential and secondary hypertension in pregnancy. *Balliere's Best Pract Res Clin Obstet Gynaecol* 1999;**13**(1):115–30.
81. Lenders JWM. Pheochromocytoma and pregnancy: a deceptive connection. *Eur J Endocrinol* 2012;**166**(2):143–50.
82. Brown MA, Mangos G, Davis G, Homer C. The natural history of white coat hypertension during pregnancy. *BJOG Int J Obstet Gynaecol* 2005;**112**(5):601–6.
83. Knight M. Eclampsia in the United Kingdom 2005. *BJOG Int J Obstet Gynaecol* 2007;**114**:1072–8.
84. Bramham K, Seed PT, Lightstone L, Nelson-Piercy C, Gill C, Webster P, et al. Diagnostic and predictive biomarkers for pre-eclampsia in patients with established hypertension and chronic kidney disease. *Kidney Int* 2016;**89**(4):874–85.
85. Rolfo A, Attini R, Nuzzo AM, Piazzese A, Parisi S, Ferraresi M, et al. Chronic kidney disease may be differentially diagnosed from preeclampsia by serum biomarkers. *Kidney Int* 2013;**83**(1):177–81.
86. von Dadelszen P, Magee LA, Roberts JM. Subclassification of preeclampsia. *Hypertens Pregnancy* 2003;**22**(2):143–8.
87. Lindheimer MD, Taler SJ, Cunningham FG. Hypertension in pregnancy. *J Am Soc Hypertens* 2008;**2**:484–94.
88. Knight M, Nair M, Tuffnell D, Kenyon S, Shakespeare J, Brocklehurst P, et al. *Saving lives, improving mothers' care: Surveillance of maternal deaths in the UK 2012–14 and lessons learned to inform maternity care from the UK and Ireland confidential enquiries into maternal deaths and morbidity 2009–14;* 2016.
89. Sibai BM. The HELLP syndrome (hemolysis, elevated liver enzymes, and low platelets): much ado about nothing? *Am J Obstet Gynecol* 1990;**162**(2):311–6.
90. Martin JN, Blake PG, Perry KG, McCaul JF, Hess LW, Martin RW. The natural history of HELLP syndrome: patterns of disease progression and regression. *Am J Obstet Gynecol* 1991;**164**(6 Pt 1):1500–9 [discussion 1509-13].
91. Fitzpatrick KE, Hinshaw K, Kurinczuk JJ, Knight M. Risk factors, management, and outcomes of hemolysis, elevated liver enzymes, and low platelets syndrome and elevated liver enzymes, low platelets syndrome. *Obstet Gynecol* 2014;**123**(3):618–27.
92. Sibai BM, Ramadan MK, Usta I, Salama M, Mercer BM, Friedman SA. Maternal morbidity and mortality in 442 pregnancies with hemolysis, elevated liver enzymes, and low platelets (HELLP syndrome). *Am J Obstet Gynecol* 1993;**169**(4):1000–6.
93. Malvino E, Muñoz M, Ceccotti C, Janello G, Mc Loughlin D, Pawlak A, et al. Maternal morbidity and perinatal mortality in HELLP syndrome. Multicentric studies in intensive care units in Buenos Aires area. *Medicina (B Aires)* 2005;**65**(1):17–23.
94. Haddad B, Barton JR, Livingston JC, Chahine R, Sibai BM. HELLP (hemolysis, elevated liver enzymes, and low platelet count) syndrome versus severe preeclampsia: onset at < or =28.0 weeks' gestation. *Am J Obstet Gynecol* 2000;**183**(6):1475–9.
95. Abildgaard U, Heimdal K. Pathogenesis of the syndrome of hemolysis, elevated liver enzymes, and low platelet count (HELLP): a review. *Eur J Obstet Gynecol Reprod Biol* 2013;**166**(2):117–23.
96. Baxter JK, Weinstein L. HELLP syndrome: the state of the art. *Obs Gynecol Surv* 2004;**59**:838–45.
97. Hulstein JJJ, van Runnard Heimel PJ, Franx A, Lenting PJ, Bruinse HW, Silence K, et al. Acute activation of the endothelium results in increased levels of active von Willebrand factor in hemolysis, elevated liver enzymes and low platelets (HELLP) syndrome. *J Thromb Haemost* 2006;**4**(12):2569–75.
98. Huizinga EG, Tsuji S, Romijn RAP, Schiphorst ME, de Groot PG, Sixma JJ, et al. Structures of glycoprotein Ibalpha and its complex with von Willebrand factor A1 domain. *Science* 2002;**297**(5584):1176–9.
99. Mihu D, Costin N, Mihu CM, Seicean A, Ciortea R. HELLP syndrome - a multisystemic disorder. *J Gastrointestin Liver Dis* 2007;**16**(4):419–24.
100. Pauzner R, Dulitzky M, Carp H, Mayan H, Kenett R, Farfel Z, et al. Hepatic infarctions during pregnancy are associated with the antiphospholipid syndrome and in addition with complete or incomplete HELLP syndrome. *J Thromb Haemost* 2003;**1**(8):1758–63.
101. Larsson A, Palm M, Hansson L-O, Axelsson O. Reference values for clinical chemistry tests during normal pregnancy. *BJOG Int J Obstet Gynaecol* 2008;**115**(7):874–81.
102. Fisher KA, Luger A, Spargo BH, Lindheimer MD. Hypertension in pregnancy: clinical-pathological correlations and remote prognosis. *Medicine (Baltimore)* 1981;**60**(4):267–76.
103. Lafayette RA, Druzin M, Sibley R, Derby G, Malik T, Huie P, et al. Nature of glomerular dysfunction in pre-eclampsia. 11. See editorial by chapman, p. 1394. *Kidney Int* 1998;**54**(4):1240–9.
104. Craici IM, Wagner SJ, Bailey KR, Fitz-Gibbon PD, Wood-Wentz CM, Turner ST, et al. Podocyturia predates proteinuria and clinical features of preeclampsia: longitudinal prospective study. *Hypertension* 2013;**61**(6):1289–96.
105. Greer IA. *Maternal medicine: medical problems in pregnancy.* Elsevier Health Sciences; 2007. p. 129.
106. Duley L. The global impact of pre-eclampsia and eclampsia. *Semin Perinatol* 2009;130–7.
107. Brewer J, Owens MY, Wallace K, Reeves AA, Morris R, Khan M, et al. Posterior reversible encephalopathy syndrome in 46 of 47 patients with eclampsia. *Am J Obstet Gynecol* 2013;**208**(6):468.e1–6.

108. Aukes AM, Wessel I, Dubois AM, Aarnoudse JG, Zeeman GG. Self-reported cognitive functioning in formerly eclamptic women. *Am J Obstet Gynecol* 2007;**197**(4):365.e1–6.

109. Roberge S, Nicolaides K, Demers S, Hyett J, Chaillet N, Bujold E. The role of aspirin dose on the prevention of preeclampsia and fetal growth restriction: systematic review and meta-analysis. *Am J Obstet Gynecol* 2017;**216**(2):110–120.e6.

110. Nzelu D, Dumitrascu-Biris D, Nicolaides KH, Kametas NA. Chronic hypertension: first-trimester blood pressure control and likelihood of severe hypertension, preeclampsia, and small for gestational age. *Am J Obstet Gynecol* 2018;**218**(3):337.e1–7.

111. Cantwell R, Clutton-Brock T, Cooper G, Dawson A, Drife J, Garrod D, et al. Saving mothers' Lives: reviewing maternal deaths to make motherhood safer: 2006–2008. The Eighth Report of the Confidential Enquiries into Maternal Deaths in the United Kingdom. *BJOG Int J Obstet Gynaecol* 2011;**118**(Suppl):1–203.

112. The joint commission. *Sentinel event alert: preventing maternal death, issue 44;* 2010. p. 45–7.

113. Abalos E, Duley L, Steyn DW. Antihypertensive drug therapy for mild to moderate hypertension during pregnancy. *Cochrane Database Syst Rev* 2014;.

114. Brown MJ. Renin: friend or foe? *Heart* 2007;**93**:1026–33.

115. Magee LA, Cham C, Waterman EJ, Ohlsson A, von Dadelszen P. Hydralazine for treatment of severe hypertension in pregnancy: meta-analysis. *BMJ* 2003;**327**(7421):955–60.

116. Perry H, Sheehan E, Thilaganathan B, Khalil A. Home blood-pressure monitoring in a hypertensive pregnant population. *Ultrasound Obstet Gynecol* 2018;**51**(4):524–30.

117. Tucker KL, Bowen L, Crawford C, Mallon P, Hinton L, Lee M-M, et al. The feasibility and acceptability of self-testing for proteinuria during pregnancy: a mixed methods approach. *Pregnancy Hypertens* 2018;**12**:161–8.

118. Brown HK, Speechley KN, Macnab J, Natale R, Campbell MK. Neonatal morbidity associated with late preterm and early term birth: the roles of gestational age and biological determinants of preterm birth. *Int J Epidemiol* 2014;**43**(3):802–14.

119. Koopmans CM, Bijlenga D, Groen H, Vijgen SMC, Aarnoudse JG, Bekedam DJ, et al. Induction of labour versus expectant monitoring for gestational hypertension or mild pre-eclampsia after 36 weeks' gestation (HYPITAT): a multicentre, open-label randomised controlled trial. *Lancet* 2009;**374**(9694):979–88.

120. Hutcheon J, Lisonkova S, Magee L, Von Dadelszen P, Woo H, Liu S, et al. Optimal timing of delivery in pregnancies with pre-existing hypertension. *BJOG Int J Obstet Gynaecol* 2011;**118**(1):49–54.

121. Milne F, Redman C, Walker J, Baker P, Bradley J, Cooper C, et al. The pre-eclampsia community guideline (PRECOG): how to screen for and detect onset of pre-eclampsia in the community. *BMJ* 2005;**330**(7491):576–80.

122. Thangaratinam S, Ismail KMK, Sharp S, Coomarasamy A, Khan KS. Accuracy of serum uric acid in predicting complications of pre-eclampsia: a systematic review. *BJOG Int J Obstet Gynaecol* 2006;**113**(4):369–78.

123. Meher S, Abalos E, Carroli G. Bed rest with or without hospitalisation for hypertension during pregnancy. John Wiley and Sons, Ltd. for The Cochrane Collaboration. *Cochrane Database Syst Rev* 2010;.

124. Duley L, Meher S, Jones L. Drugs for treatment of very high blood pressure during pregnancy. John Wiley and Sons, Ltd. for The Cochrane Collaboration. *Cochrane Database Syst Rev* 2013;.

125. The Magpie Trial Collaborative Grou. Do women with pre-eclampsia, and their babies, benefit from magnesium sulphate? The magpie trial: a randomised placebo-controlled trial. *Lancet* 2002;**359**(9321):1877–90.

126. The Eclampsia Trial Collaborative Group. Which anticonvulsant for women with eclampsia? Evidence from the collaborative eclampsia trial. *Lancet* 1995;**345**(8963):1455–63.

127. Duley L, Williams J, Henderson-Smart DJ. Plasma volume expansion for treatment of pre-eclampsia. *Cochrane Database Syst Rev* 1999;.

128. Karsdorp VH, van Vugt JM, Dekker GA, van Geijn HP. Reappearance of end-diastolic velocities in the umbilical artery following maternal volume expansion: a preliminary study. *Obstet Gynecol* 1992;**80**(4):679–83.

129. Valensise H, Vasapollo B, Novelli GP, Giorgi G, Verallo P, Galante A, et al. Maternal and fetal hemodynamic effects induced by nitric oxide donors and plasma volume expansion in pregnancies with gestational hypertension complicated by intrauterine growth restriction with absent end-diastolic flow in the umbilical artery. *Ultrasound Obstet Gynecol* 2008;**31**(1):55–64.

130. Ganzevoort W, Rep A, Bonsel GJ, Fetter WPF, Sonderen L, Vries JIP, et al. A randomised controlled trial comparing two temporising management strategies, one with and one without plasma volume expansion, for severe and early onset pre-eclampsia. *BJOG Int J Obstet Gynaecol* 2005;**112** (10):1358–68.

131. Barton JR, Sibai BM. Hepatic imaging in HELLP syndrome (hemolysis, elevated liver enzymes, and low platelet count). *Am J Obstet Gynecol* 1996;**174**(6):1820–5 [discussion 1825-7].

132. Eser B, Guven M, Unal A, Coskun R, Altuntas F, Sungur M, et al. The role of plasma exchange in HELLP syndrome. *Clin Appl Thromb Hemost* 2005;**11**(2):211–7.

133. Rinehart BK, Terrone DA, Magann EF, Martin RW, May WL, Martin JN. Preeclampsia-associated hepatic hemorrhage and rupture: mode of management related to maternal and perinatal outcome. *Obstet Gynecol Surv* 1999;**54**(3):196–202.

134. Wicke C, Pereira PL, Neeser E, Flesch I, Rodegerdts EA, Becker HD. Subcapsular liver hematoma in HELLP syndrome: evaluation of diagnostic and therapeutic options—a unicenter study. *Am J Obstet Gynecol* 2004;**190**(1):106–12.

135. Churchill D, Duley L, Thornton JG, Jones L. Interventionist versus expectant care for severe pre-eclampsia before term. John Wiley and Sons, Ltd. for The Cochrane Collaboration. *Cochrane Database Syst Rev* 2013;.

136. Von Dadelszen P, Payne B, Li J, Ansermino JM, Pipkin FB, Côté AM, et al. Prediction of adverse maternal outcomes in pre-eclampsia: development and validation of the fullPIERS model. *Lancet* 2011;**377**:219–27.

137. Akkermans J, Payne B, von Dadelszen P, Groen H, de Vries J, Magee LA, et al. Predicting complications in pre-eclampsia: external validation of the fullPIERS model using the PETRA trial dataset. *Eur J Obstet Gynecol Reprod Biol* 2014;**179**:58–62.

138. Payne BA, Hutcheon JA, Ansermino JM, Hall DR, Bhutta ZA, Bhutta SZ, et al. A risk prediction model for the assessment and triage of women with hypertensive disorders of pregnancy in low-resourced settings: the miniPIERS (Pre-eclampsia Integrated Estimate of RiSk) multi-country prospective cohort study. Lawn JE, editor. *PLoS Med* 2014;**11**(1):e1001589.

139. Thangaratinam S, Allotey J, Marlin N, Mol BW, Von Dadelszen P, Ganzevoort W, et al. Development and validation of prediction models for risks of complications in early-onset pre-eclampsia (PREP): a prospective cohort study. *Health Technol Assess (Rockv)* 2017;**21**(18):1–100.

140. Sanghavi M, Rutherford JD. Cardiovascular physiology of pregnancy. *Circulation* 2014;**130**(12):1003–8.

141. Norman JE, Bollapragada S, Yuan M, Nelson SM. Inflammatory pathways in the mechanism of parturition. *BMC Pregnancy Childbirth* 2007;**7**(Suppl 1):S7.

142. Douglas JM. *The use of neuraxial anesthesia in parturients with thrombocytopenia: what is an adequate platelet count? Evidence-based obstetric anesthesia*. Oxford, UK: Blackwell Publishing Ltd; 2007. p. 165–77.

143. Douglas MJ. The use of neuraxial anesthesia in parturients with thrombocytopenia: what is an adequate platelet count? In: Halpern SH, Douglas MJ, editors. *Evidence based obstetric anesthesia*. Massachusetts: Blackwell Publishing; 2005. p. 165–177.

144. Obstetric Anaesthetists' Association. *Regional Anaesthesia and Coagulation [Internet]*. [cited July 10], Available from:http://www.oaa-anaes.ac.uk/ui/content/content.aspx?id=188; 2018.

145. Berks D, Steegers EAP, Molas M, Visser W. Resolution of hypertension and proteinuria after preeclampsia. *Obstet Gynecol* 2009;**114**:1307–14.

146. Benschop L, Duvekot JJ, Versmissen J, van Broekhoven V, Steegers EAP, Roeters van Lennep JE. Blood pressure profile 1 year after severe pre-eclampsia. *Hypertension* 2018;**71**(3):491–8.

147. Behrens I, Basit S, Melbye M, Lykke JA, Wohlfahrt J, Bundgaard H, et al. Risk of post-pregnancy hypertension in women with a history of hypertensive disorders of pregnancy: nationwide cohort study. *BMJ* 2017;**358**:j3078.

148. Savitz DA, Danilack VA, Elston B, Lipkind HS. Pregnancy-induced hypertension and diabetes and the risk of cardiovascular disease, stroke, and diabetes hospitalization in the year following delivery. *Am J Epidemiol* 2014;**180**(1):41–4.

149. Lykke JA, Langhoff-Roos J, Sibai BM, Funai EF, Triche EW, Paidas MJ. Hypertensive pregnancy disorders and subsequent cardiovascular morbidity and type 2 diabetes mellitus in the mother. *Hypertension* 2009;**53**(6):944–51.

150. Steegers EAP, von Dadelszen P, Duvekot JJ, Pijnenborg R. Pre-eclampsia. *Lancet* 2010;**376**(9741):631–44.

Chapter 27

Preconception and Pregnancy in Women with Obesity, Postbariatric Surgery, and Polycystic Ovarian Syndrome

Catherine Takacs Witkop

Uniformed Services University of the Health Sciences, Bethesda, MD, United States

---

Common Clinical Problems

- A patient with a history of polycystic ovarian syndrome (PCOS) and body mass index (BMI) of 35 with oligomenorrhea and a 12-month history of trying to conceive presents for infertility workup and treatment.
- A 35-year-old multiparous patient with a prepregnancy BMI of 30 and a history of gestational diabetes (GDM) with her previous pregnancy presents for her first prenatal visit at 8 weeks' gestation. She has many questions about how she can avoid diabetes in this pregnancy, what her risks are, and how she will be screened for congenital anomalies.
- A 32-year-old patient with a prepregnancy BMI of 40 has gained 20 pounds in her current pregnancy. She is now at 40 weeks' gestation, and her physicians suspect that her baby may be large for gestational age (LGA), but they also understand the limitations of estimated fetal weight in this patient. The patient and physician are having a discussion about the risks and benefits of induction.
- A patient recently is 1 week postop from a primary cesarean delivery for failure to progress. Her postpartum course was complicated by wound infection, although she is now discharged from the hospital. She is trying to breastfeed, but she is frustrated and ready to stop. She comes to you for a wound check and tells you that she always wanted three children close in age, but now she is not so sure. Her prepregnancy BMI was 35, and she gained 30 pounds with this pregnancy. She asks how she can avoid some of the problems with future pregnancies.

27.1 OVERALL PERSPECTIVE

Although patients and the general public often assume that obesity is the consequence of a hormonal imbalance or endocrine disorder, this is most often not the case. Nevertheless, a chapter on maternal obesity is relevant in this section on maternal endocrine pathophysiology because obesity plays an important role in the pathogenesis of PCOS (discussed herein) and GDM (discussed in chapter 22).

27.2 EPIDEMIOLOGY OF OVERWEIGHT AND OBESITY AMONG WOMEN DURING PREGNANCY

The prevalence of maternal obesity has increased throughout the world, and it is estimated that over 21% of women globally will be obese by 2025.[1] Populationwide surveillance data are limited in some parts of the world; however, increasing realization of the impact of overweight and obesity on maternal and newborn outcomes, as well as on long-term consequences for mothers and their offspring has led to improved surveillance tools and prevention programs.

The World Health Organization (WHO) classification system is widely used for clinical, surveillance, and research purposes.[2] The WHO classifies obesity as BMI [calculated by the formula weight (kg)/height (m)^2] of 30.0 or above, and overweight as BMI of 25.0–29.9. Obesity is further broken into Class I (30.0–34.9), Class II (35–39.9), and Class III (40 or greater). Extreme obesity is defined as a prepregnancy BMI of 50 or greater. This condition leads to even more complications, with higher odds ratios (ORs) for many complications that will be discussed in this chapter.[3] Because of the significant increase in total body water during pregnancy, BMI is a less useful measure during pregnancy, and prepregnancy BMI is typically used to assess risk and guide recommendations and clinical management during pregnancy. Furthermore, although these classifications are useful for surveillance, research, and counseling about risk, additional risk factors in a given patient may have more of an impact on risk of disease or complication than an isolated BMI at any point in time.

Because obesity during pregnancy is becoming more prevalent each year, efforts to improve surveillance and epidemiologic understanding of the epidemic have increased. In 2003, implementation in the United States of a birth certificate revision in 47 states and the District of Columbia to report prepregnancy height and weight on birth certificates has resulted in the ability to monitor trends in prepregnancy BMI among the majority of the United States, most recently reported for 96% of births in 2014.[4] Although BMI may be slightly underestimated in these self-reported data, the population estimates are well accepted and demonstrate trends, such as the increase in prepregnancy obesity in the vast majority of states that had data between 2011 and 2014. In 2014, 25.6% of women were overweight before pregnancy and 24.8% were obese; prepregnancy obesity increased with increasing parity and was most likely to be seen among non-Hispanic American Indian/Alaska Native women, Hispanic women and non-Hispanic black women.[4] Another commonly used way to estimate prepregnancy obesity in the United States is the National Health and Nutrition Examination Survey (NHANES), which reported that 34% of women between the ages of 20–39 were obese according to measured height and weight.[5]

The issue of overweight and obesity during pregnancy is not confined to the United States. In other high-income countries, trends in rising prevalence reflect what has been seen in the United States, although overweight and obesity rates vary somewhat, with the highest rate in the United Kingdom (25.2%) and the lowest in Poland (7.1%).[6] Historically, low- and middle-income countries (LMIC) have not experienced the same prevalence of conditions related to overeating. However, the nutrition transition in the past 30 years to increased consumption of processed foods and decreased levels of physical activity in the countries designated as LMICs has resulted in a rate of increasing prevalence of overweight and obesity and nutrition deficiencies that has been greater than that seen in developed countries.[6]

27.3 EPIDEMIOLOGY OF EXCESSIVE GESTATIONAL WEIGHT GAIN

A separate but closely related issue is excessive gestational weight gain. In 1990, the Institute of Medicine (IOM), now the National Academy of Science, released recommendations around gestational weight gain. More recently, the IOM released updated recommendations utilizing the WHO BMI categories; one of the significant recommendations was to aim for a lower level of gestational weight gain in obese women, between 5 and 9 kg or 11–20 pounds.[7] Unfortunately, despite the recommendations being adopted by numerous organizations, implementation has been limited at best. A population-based study showed that over half of obese pregnant women in the United States gained more weight than was recommended by the IOM.[8] Efforts to improve counseling of obese women about the increased risks associated with excessive weight gain during pregnancy to help women stay within the IOM-recommended weight range have been ongoing, but it is likely that more systemwide approaches, using evidence-based programs to aid women in lifestyle changes, may be needed.

27.4 OVERVIEW OF MATERNAL COMPLICATIONS RELATED TO OVERWEIGHT/OBESITY

The physiologic changes of pregnancy appear to be different in obese versus lean women, and findings from studies can elucidate why certain complications are more likely in pregnancy. Although both obese and lean women demonstrate a reduction in insulin sensitivity, obese women appear to demonstrate a greater decrease, as well as an increase in certain lipids and amino acids.[9]

Potential maternal complications in obese or overweight women that will be discussed here include increased rates of miscarriage, GDM, hypertensive disorders, stillbirth, abnormal labor patterns, cesarean delivery, operative and postoperative complications, infections, thromboembolism, postpartum hemorrhage, and complications from anesthesia. Longer-term adverse outcomes that could affect subsequent pregnancies, as well as risk of chronic disease later in life, include an increased risk of Type 2 diabetes, hypertension, and heart disease.

Fetal outcomes that may be more prevalent in women with obesity include prematurity, stillbirth, macrosomia, and birth injury. Evidence for each of these conditions and complications will be discussed, followed by recommendations regarding prevention and management, as supported by the literature.

27.5 CARE OF THE OBESE WOMAN BEFORE AND DURING PREGNANCY

27.5.1 Preconception

Obesity alters the hypothalamic-pituitary-ovarian (HPO) axis and is associated with alterations in follicular fluid surrounding the oocyte and ovarian granulosa cells. There is evidence that uterine changes in obese women are also present that affect fertility.[9] Obese women generally have higher levels of circulating insulin, and therefore they are likely to have increased androgen levels, which are then aromatized at increased rates to estrogens (due to excessive adipose tissue). These increased estrogens are thought to impede proper functioning of the HPO axis, affecting gonadotropin production and ovulation.

Although evidence has shown that both PCOS and obesity independently increase the risk of infertility, obesity also increases symptoms and potential complications of PCOS, likely due to an increase in insulin resistance above and beyond that found in women with PCOS. Furthermore, PCOS has been estimated to be present in approximately 30% of obese women, leading to additional impacts on the pathophysiology of pregnancy.[10] Issues specifically related to PCOS for both obese and normal-weight women, including treatments for infertility, will be discussed later in this chapter.

There is a significant amount of evidence that obesity increases the time to successful pregnancy, and this also has been demonstrated in women with normal ovulatory cycles and eumenorrhea.[11, 12] Further evidence that the increased length of time to successful pregnancy outcomes is not simply due to oligoovulation is the impact of obesity on assisted reproductive technologies. Multiple studies have demonstrated an association of obesity with worse live birth rates and other adverse outcomes. High-circulating levels of leptin in obese women may negatively affect assisted reproductive technology and result in less-than-desired outcomes.[13] However, there are no current recommended interventions based only on a woman's BMI. For that reason, it is critical that women who are obese and infertile are counseled on the potential impact that their overweight may have on conceiving, even with current technology.[14] This, in concert with the range of potential complications during pregnancy, may provide incentives for behavioral modification to a woman even before she undergoes a course of treatment for infertility.

Women who are obese are at higher risk for comorbid conditions, some of which require prescription medications. Although many women do not seek preconception counseling, this period before conception is critical for someone who is taking a potentially teratogenic medication. All women of childbearing potential, especially those who are not utilizing effective contraception or who are trying to conceive and who are taking such medication, should be counseled about the risks of continuing treatment, and the risks and benefits of continuing the medication need to be weighed for the individual patient. For example, statins used in the treatment of hyperlipidemia are contraindicated in pregnancy and should be discontinued in someone who is trying to conceive. Similarly, in women with preexisting hypertension, women taking angiotensin-converting enzyme (ACE) inhibitors should be counseled about their risks and benefits. Although the majority of studies have identified risks while taking ACE inhibitors in the second and third trimesters, some evidence has pointed to teratogenic risks in the first trimester as well, so if possible, women should be changed to an alternative treatment prior to conception.

Given the potential negative impact of maternal obesity on pregnancy, the preconception period is also the opportune time to encourage weight loss in overweight or obese individuals. However, a recent systematic review that sought to identify randomized controlled trials (RCTs) of preconception interventions for weight loss in overweight or obese individuals surprisingly turned up no eligible studies.[15] One can speculate about potential reasons for the lack of evidence in this area, including lack of many preconception studies at a time when so many pregnancies are unintended or mistimed, or the difficulty in conducting studies that must begin far in advance of pregnancy and follow women over at least a year from the time of conception to determine any clinically relevant outcomes. Nevertheless, given the fact that studies conducted during pregnancy have not demonstrated effective weight reduction programs, it is absolutely critical that future studies address the preconception period.

Although there are no specific recommendations for addressing overweight and obesity in the prepregnancy population, the U.S. Preventive Services Task Force (USPSTF), which conducts systematic reviews to determine evidence-based recommendations to be applied in the primary-care population, has recommended screening all adults for obesity and states that clinicians should offer or refer patients with BMI of 30 or more to intensive, multicomponent behavioral interventions.[16] Providers caring for obese women can even incorporate some useful techniques for behavior-change counseling into their own practices. For example, social cognitive theory (SCT) has been used to develop a number of behavioral interventions and is based on the theory that the environment, person, and behavior interact, and changes in one affect the other two.[17] The *person* variable includes concepts such as behavioral capability, outcome expectancies, and perceived self-efficacy (e.g., setting realistic goals about exercise and diet early in the process).

Motivational interviewing is another useful technique that providers should consider in caring for their overweight or obese patients, especially those who are considering conception. The goal of motivational interviewing is to use reflective listening and other tools to help the patient move through stages of behavior change.[18] The OARS acronym has been used to describe the key skills of motivational interviewings: *O*pen-ended questions, *A*ffirm, *R*eflect, and *S*ummarize. Motivational interviewing has been effective in helping patients lose weight, as demonstrated in some observational studies.[19] Until clear guidance is available about effective interventions, motivational interviewing appears to be a useful tool; at the very least, it provides the patient an opportunity to think through her ambivalence about weight loss (if present) and feelings about her weight. Furthermore, it serves to likely improve the provider-patient relationship and potentially positively affect behavior change with other issues as well.

At the very least, it is critical that the patient is provided with information about and/or access to resources for healthy diet and physical activity that could lead to weight loss. There is also growing evidence for the benefits of weight loss before pregnancy from the bariatric surgery literature. The pros and cons of bariatric surgery before pregnancy will be discussed later in this chapter under Special Topics.

27.5.2 Early Pregnancy and Antepartum Care

Early pregnancy is a critical time for development of a growing fetus, and obese women experience an increase in risk over their normal-weight peers. Many observational studies have demonstrated an increased risk of miscarriage among those with increasing weight. For example, in a nested case-control study comparing obese primiparous patients with age-matched controls who had normal BMI, the obese women had a significantly higher incidence of early miscarriage, with ORs of 1.2 and 3.5 for early miscarriage and recurrent early miscarriage, respectively.[20] A subsequent meta-analysis demonstrated that the risk of spontaneous miscarriage increases in women who are overweight or obese, with estimated OR of 1.67 [95% confidence interval (CI) 1.25–2.25] in women with BMI of 25 or greater.[21] A more recent prospective observational study demonstrated a greater effect in women with severe obesity; the investigators found an increased rate of late miscarriage in women with Class 2 or 3 obesity when compared with those women with Class 1 obesity or with those who were overweight or of normal weight.[22]

As mentioned earlier, obese women with comorbid conditions ideally should be counseled in the preconception period about discontinuing or changing medications with teratogenic properties. For those women who did not receive preconception counseling, the early pregnancy period may see more women present for care, and their medications need to be addressed. Again, statins for hyperlipidemia should be discontinued, and ACE inhibitors for hypertension need to be discussed and perhaps changed. Discussing potentially teratogenic medications is beyond the scope of this chapter, and new evidence may prompt adding or deleting medications from the list. Providers should refer to current sources, such as the Centers for Disease Control and Prevention (CDC) "Treating for Two" program at https://www.cdc.gov/pregnancy/meds/treatingfortwo/index.html.

Obesity presents a unique issue with regard to congenital anomalies due to the higher risk of occurrence and the concomitant greater difficulty in making a diagnosis. A systematic review and meta-analysis identified several congenital anomalies, including spina bifida, neural tube defects, limb reduction anomalies, cardiovascular anomalies, and cleft lip and palate, that were more likely in obese than in nonobese women.[23] Another meta-analysis focusing specifically on neural tube defects reported an OR of 1.70 (CI 1.34–2.15) and 3.11 (CI 1.75–5.46) for the occurrence of neural tube defects in obese and extremely obese women compared with healthy-weight women.[24] And a 2014 systematic review and meta-analysis of 24 studies demonstrated a pooled OR for all congenital heart disease of 1.12 (1.04–1.20) for moderately obese women and 1.38 (1.20–1.59) for severely obese women.[25]

The epidemiologic data demonstrate associations with congenital anomalies, but strategies for prevention and identification of these anomalies in obese women have proved to be a challenge. The current recommendation for all women of childbearing potential is to take 40 mcg/day of folic acid. Because the pathophysiology of the association between obesity and neural tube defects has not been fully elucidated, it is not clear if increased doses of folic acid would reduce the risk of congenital anomalies. In at least one study, folic acid intake was not associated with a significant attenuation of risk of spina bifida among obese patients.[26] It is critical to ensure that overweight and obese women who are trying to conceive are taking at least the recommended dose of folic acid and beginning at least 1 month before pregnancy.

Some specialty societies have recommendations beyond that dose, based primarily on the observational data of increased risk. The CMACE/RCOG Joint Guideline for Management of Women with Obesity in Pregnancy recommends that women with BMI of 30 or above who are planning to get pregnant should take 5 mg/day folic acid, starting at least 1 month before pregnancy and continuing for at least the first trimester.[27] This recommendation is based on the evidence that obese women are at higher risk for neural tube defects,[24] and women with BMI of 27 or higher in one study had lower serum folate levels even after controlling for folate intake.[28] The CMACE/RCOG guidelines also recommend 10 mcg/day of vitamin D during pregnancy.[27]

A complicating issue is the challenge in identification of congenital anomalies in women who are overweight or obese. In one study using standard or targeted ultrasonography between 18 and 24 weeks' gestation, the detection of anomalies decreased as maternal BMI increased, with only 75% of fetal anomalies detected in women with Class 3 obesity.[29] Although studies are ongoing regarding alternative approaches, there are currently no clearly effective means to improve detection in obese women at this time.

27.5.3 Antepartum Care

As mentioned previously, excessive gestational weight gain can have a compounding effect on the already-increased risks for obese women. In a recent comprehensive systematic review and meta-analysis of over 1.3 million pregnancies in international cohorts, investigators calculated ORs and absolute risk differences (ARDs) for multiple outcomes.[30] The study found that excessive weight gain (i.e., over 2009 IOM-recommended amounts) among obese women was associated with higher risk of having large-for-gestational-age (LGA) infants, defined in most studies as birth weight greater than 90th percentile, with an OR of 1.63 (95% CI 1.56–1.70) and an ARD of 7% (95% CI 5%–8%). Obese women also had increased odds for macrosomia (OR 1.83, 95% CI 1.52–2.22) and cesarean delivery (OR, 1.22, 95% CI 1.05–1.42).[30] Other studies over the years have demonstrated some compelling evidence that excessive gestational weight gain increases the risk for abnormal glucose metabolism during pregnancy, leading to increased risk of GDM, as well as increased risk for hypertensive conditions during pregnancy.[31]

Unfortunately, women with obesity are more likely to gain excessive weight during pregnancy as compared to their normal-weight counterparts; the challenge in counseling obese women about the risks of weight gain is significant, but the importance cannot be overstated. As with any counseling, patients also should be aware of potential risks. In considering the potential risks of weight loss or insufficient weight gain during pregnancy, one study demonstrated that obesity was associated with small-for-gestational-age (SGA) risk, and this risk increased with gestational weight gain below guidelines and with weight loss.[30] However, importantly, weight loss among obese women was also associated with 5% lower risk for LGA and macrosomia, and cesarean delivery risk was 4% lower.[30]

The risk-benefit ratio tends to favor close management of weight gain during pregnancy to remain within the IOM-recommended guidelines. Multiple professional societies have produced guidelines recommending calculation of BMI at the first visit and using it to begin the discussion about benefits of avoiding excessive weight gain. This discussion should include a plan for diet and exercise counseling, as indicated by the woman's current BMI and her current knowledge, skills, and attitudes related to lifestyle modification. Evidence for recommended lifestyle modifications will be cited later in this chapter.

27.5.4 Gestational Diabetes

Multiple studies have demonstrated an increase in diagnosis of GDM in obese women as compared to women with BMI less than 30. The decreased insulin sensitivity among obese women as compared with normal-weight women is partly to blame for this well-established increased risk. Further, GDM and obesity have independent impacts on poor maternal and perinatal outcomes. The Hyperglycemia and Pregnancy Outcome (HAPO) study was an observational experiment examining the outcomes of women diagnosed post hoc with GDM or obesity. Because BMI was measured at the time of the oral glucose tolerance test (OGTT) in this study, the threshold for diagnosis of obesity (for the purpose of comparison groups) was raised to 33. Prenatal care and timing of delivery were determined per standard practice without knowledge of the result of the OGTT. Both obesity and GDM were found to be independently associated with birth weight greater than 90th percentile, increased risk for primary cesarean delivery, and preeclampsia; the negative effects were greater with both obesity and GDM.[32]

Although controversies exist regarding the criteria for diagnosis of GDM, given the significantly increased risk of GDM in obese women, there is no disagreement over the recommendation that women with elevated BMI should be tested. Where variability exists is in the recommended time of initial testing. ACOG recommends early screening for women with BMI over 25 who have one additional risk factor among the following: physical inactivity, first-degree relative with diabetes, high-risk race, history of GDM or previous infant weighing over 4000 g, hypertension, PCOS, impaired glucose tolerance, or other conditions associated with insulin resistance.[33] If BMI is over 40, no other risk factors are needed to justify early screening.

Early screening can be done in a number of ways, and the ideal test has not been established. Options include (1) fasting blood glucose followed by 75-g glucose load and 2-h plasma glucose measurement, as is done to diagnose Type 2 diabetes in nonpregnant patients; (2) 50-g OGTT, as in the two-step process frequently used for GDM screening in the second trimester; and (3) measurement of hemoglobin A1c (HbA1c), although this is not generally recommended because of lower sensitivity.[33] If the screening test is negative in early pregnancy, it should be repeated at 24–28 weeks. If the 50-g OGTT was used and the first step was positive, only the second step is needed. If early testing is not done (e.g., U.K. guidelines), evidence clearly supports testing at 24–28 weeks' gestation. A detailed discussion of screening tests for GDM in general is out of the scope of this chapter, but it is included in Chapter 22.

Management in the patient with GDM is focused on maintaining normoglycemia, which has been shown to reduce the risk of preeclampsia, stillbirth, and LGA infants. Because of the additive effects of obesity on GDM, management of GDM is particularly important.[32, 34–36]

Dietary counseling and nutritional therapy constitute the first-line treatment of GDM. Recommendations generally include a diet controlled in carbohydrates (between 33% and 40%) with the goal of achieving normoglycemia and avoiding ketosis.[33, 37] Exercise is also recommended—namely, approximately 30 min of moderate-intensity aerobic exercise at least five times a week (or minimum of 150 min/week). Exercise is especially important in obese women with GDM, as it has been shown to improve glycemic control.[33]

Surveillance of blood glucose levels is important to monitor glycemic control, although the ideal frequency and whether this changes for obese patients are not clear. ACOG and others generally recommend a goal to keep fasting or preprandial blood glucose values <5.3 mmol/L (95 mg/dL) and postprandial blood glucose values <7.8 mmol/L (140 mg/dL) at 1 h or 6.7 mmol/L (120 mg/dL) at 2 h.

If target glucose levels cannot be accomplished with diet and exercise, pharmacologic treatment is generally begun. A detailed description of ideal medications is outside the scope of this chapter and covered elsewhere. Insulin is generally recommended as the first-line therapy. Multiple studies have investigated the potential benefits of oral agents such as glibenclamide and metformin, and both of them are sometimes used despite not being approved in most countries for treatment of GDM; however, collectively, these studies were of insufficient quality to draw conclusions.[33] A recent systematic review of three RCTs evaluating the use of metformin compared with placebo or no metformin in women who were overweight or obese concluded that metformin seemed to result in a slightly lower gestational weight gain but was not likely to reduce the risk of developing GDM or have an impact on infant birth weight.[38]

Delivery of women with GDM also has been controversial. The current recommendation is that women with GDM who have an estimated fetal weight of 4500 g or more should be counseled regarding the risks and benefits of elective cesarean delivery. While the risks of attempted vaginal delivery are equal or greater in obese women with GDM with a high estimated fetal weight, the ability to estimate fetal weight accurately is less in women who are obese. For that reason, it is critical that shared decision-making play a role in choices about the route of delivery.

Women who are obese are also at increased risk for preeclampsia and gestational hypertension. As for all women, obese women should be screened for prepregnancy hypertension, ensuring appropriate cuff size, and symptoms of obstructive sleep apnea. Women also should be screened for proteinuria. Preeclampsia is twice as likely in obese women as those of normal weight.[39] Multiple studies have been conducted to examine the impact of exercise on reducing the risk of hypertensive disorders of pregnancy, with conflicting results, and it is somewhat difficult to separate any impact on weight as a result of exercise. As with other conditions in obese women, exercise and diet with the goal of avoiding excessive weight gain should be recommended.

Multiple organizations have recommended that women at increased risk of preeclampsia take 75 mg/day of low-dose aspirin for prophylaxis, although how the high-risk pregnancy is defined differs.[40–42] The aspirin should be initiated between 12 and 28 weeks of pregnancy, and ideally before 16 weeks' gestation, and the regimen should be continued until delivery. The recent ACOG guideline, which is also the most specific, makes its recommendation for women who have one or more high-risk factors (i.e., history of preeclampsia, multifetal gestation, renal disease, autoimmune disease, Type 1 or Type 2 diabetes, and chronic hypertension) or who have two or more of the following moderate-risk factors: first pregnancy, maternal age of 35 years or older, a BMI > 30, family history of preeclampsia, sociodemographic characteristics, and personal history factors.[42] The WHO has also issued guidelines for women at increased risk of preeclampsia (i.e., those with previous preeclampsia, obesity, or diabetes) who are thought to have low dietary calcium intake to take calcium supplements during pregnancy.[43] The WHO recommends beginning supplementation at 20 weeks' gestation through delivery; the recommended regimen is 1.5–2.0 g of elemental calcium in 3–4 divided doses per day, taken with food.[43]

Preterm delivery is another complication that is more common in obese women. Given the number of potential conditions for which obese women are at high risk, it is not surprising that obese women may have more indicated preterm deliveries. However, women who are overweight or obese also have been shown to have an increased risk for spontaneous preterm delivery between 22 and 27 weeks' gestation, and this effect increased with each subsequent obesity class.[44]

Unfortunately, 17-alpha hydroxyprogesterone, shown to reduce preterm delivery in numerous studies, did not seem to reduce risk in women who are obese, weigh over 165 pounds, or both.[45] Current research does not support any specific recommendations about dose adjustments, but it is important to keep these data in mind when counseling women with a history of preterm delivery who are obese and making recommendations for their care.

Given the risks for several complications during the prenatal period, one might ask about the potential benefits of life-style modification during pregnancy, with the goal of staying within the recommended gestational weight gain, or perhaps even losing weight. Unfortunately, multiple reviews of lifestyle interventions during pregnancy in overweight or obese patients have demonstrated less-than-optimal outcomes. For example, one systematic review and meta-analysis of 13 RCTs and 6 nonrandomized trials showed that dietary and lifestyle modifications were associated with lower overall gestational weight gain (–2.21 kg; 95% CI, –2.86 to –1.57 kg) and a trend (statistically significant pooled estimate, but OR crossed 1) toward reduction in GDM, but studies were deemed to be poor or medium quality, with small numbers and heterogeneous interventions.[46]

Two more recent large-scale RCTs that were adequately powered to demonstrate differences in maternal and neonatal outcomes demonstrated no clinically significant difference in outcomes such as LGA infants or GDM.[47, 48] These two studies are following the children of participants to early childhood to identify any longer-term outcomes, but results are not yet available. In a recent review focusing on preterm delivery, overweight and obese women who were randomized to aerobic exercise for 30–60 min three to seven times per week were found to have a 37% reduction in preterm delivery as compared to controls, and also had lower risk of GDM. It also did not detect differences in birth weight, gestational age at delivery, cesarean delivery, macrosomia, or stillbirth, similar to some other studies.[49] Lifestyle interventions have been demonstrated to assist women in achieving the recommended gestational weight gain (within the IOM range), and this goal may be sufficient for obese pregnant women.[50]

What also has not been reported in the literature is whether behavioral interventions during pregnancy affect weight loss between pregnancies, outcomes during subsequent pregnancies, and any other long-term outcomes such as diabetes or cardiovascular disease. For the time being, efforts to facilitate implementation of healthy behaviors during pregnancy, such as increasing physical activity and improving diet, should continue.

27.5.5 Intrapartum Care

Several population-based studies have provided evidence about labor abnormalities that could be encountered and should be anticipated for obese women during the intrapartum period. The most common complications, which will be discussed next, include prolonged pregnancy (otherwise known as *postdates*)[51–53], stillbirth, prolonged first stage of labor,[54] failed induction of labor, cesarean delivery,[55–57] and postpartum hemorrhage.[58] Severe maternal morbidity was also more common in obese women compared to their normal-weight counterparts. A recent population-based retrospective cohort study examined the following outcomes as indicators of severe maternal morbidity: sepsis, shock, cardiovascular events, cerebrovascular events, and acute renal failure. Over a 10-year period, the OR for this composite outcome was significantly greater in obese women in each class (Class 1, OR 1.1; Class 2, OR 1.2; and Class 3 OR 1.2), as compared to women with prepregnancy BMIs in the normal range.[59] The only finding that was lower in women with normal BMI in that particular study was risk of transfusion.

Postdates is often defined as a pregnancy extending beyond a certain point (often 290 or 295 days). The challenge with postdates pregnancies is weighing the risks of complications that increase with longer gestation against the potentially difficult induction and risks of failed induction and cesarean delivery. Studies involving labor management, and in particular induction versus expectant management, have been conducted and will be discussed shortly. In one study, 17% of normal-weight women had a pregnancy that extended over 290 days as compared to 30% of obese women, who were more likely to undergo labor induction.[51] In that study, second-degree perineal lacerations and macrosomia were more common in the group of obese women, but other measured outcomes were similar.

The risk for stillbirth has been demonstrated to be higher in obese women than women of normal weight.[60–63] Because of the added risk of prolonged pregnancy, there is a real concern about allowing obese women to progress until they are postdates. Other complications, such as preeclampsia, may lead to an indicated induction of labor, but the concern for stillbirth has led some providers to recommend induction of labor at term, even lacking other complications. Each patient's risk profile should be carefully considered when making this decision.

Understanding the literature around stillbirth can help inform the counseling of obese patients about their options. A recent retrospective cohort study examined the association of BMI with stillbirth and demonstrated an increase in risk with increasing gestational age and increased class of obesity, with the most significant risk among women between 40 and 42 weeks' gestation in women with Class III obesity.[61] Similarly, excessive weight gain (i.e., above IOM-recommended levels) was also associated with increased risk of stillbirth among obese and morbidly obese women, especially after

36 weeks' gestation.[62] A meta-analysis of 38 studies demonstrated a stepwise increase in relative risk for fetal death, still-birth, perinatal, neonatal, and infant death for overweight and obese women as compared with normal-weight women.[63]

Scheduled induction of labor has become common among obese women, primarily due to the manifold other complications of pregnancy. Although the evidence is somewhat contradictory, recent studies have demonstrated that induction of labor increases risks of cesarean delivery, the difficulty of monitoring fetal heart-rate patterns, wound infection, and postpartum hemorrhage—all already risks for obese women.[51, 64] In one recent study, the rate of cesarean delivery was higher in an electively induced group (40.0 versus 25.9%; $P = 0.022$), as was admission to the neonatal intensive care unit (18.3% versus 6.3%; $P = 0.001$) in obese nulliparous women.[64] Multiparity may mitigate the risk of cesarean delivery somewhat.

Whether being induced or in spontaneous labor, obese women tend to have labor patterns that differ from their normal-weight counterparts. These are critical to understand in order to prevent unnecessary interventions. A large study of singleton pregnancies demonstrated a prolonged first stage from lowest-to-highest BMI categories, and this was seen in both induced and spontaneous labor.[56] Theories have included increased fat deposits in the pelvis, decreased uterine contractility, and reduced responsivity to oxytocin, but no definitive etiology is known.[65] The second stage of labor does not appear to be similarly affected.

27.5.6 Prevention of Cesarean Delivery

Rates of cesarean delivery have been on the rise in much of the world over the past several decades. There are many reasons for this trend, but the concomitant increase in prevalence in maternal obesity and the multiple studies demonstrating an increased risk of cesarean delivery in obese women support the notion that obesity may be a significant contributor to the trend of increased cesarean delivery rates. Further, there is a dose-response rate between BMI and risk of cesarean delivery. It can be somewhat difficult to isolate the contributions of obesity to risk of cesarean delivery, given that other risk factors for cesarean delivery occur in greater frequency in women who are obese. For that reason, and because complications such as infection and postpartum hemorrhage are more likely in obese women who undergo cesarean section, it is best to counsel women about this increased risk and ensure that as many preventive measures as possible are put into place to try to prevent the primary cesarean delivery in the first place.

Recently, the American College of Obstetricians and Gynecologists (ACOG) and the Society for Maternal Fetal Medicine (SMFM) jointly developed a consensus document on the "Safe prevention of the primary cesarean delivery."[66] While this document is not necessarily focused on the obese patient, many of its recommendations are particularly applicable to reducing morbidity and mortality in that population. For example, a prolonged latent phase (>20 h in nulliparous women and >14 h in multiparous women) and slow progress through the first stage of labor are not indications for cesarean delivery, and 6-cm cervical dilation should be used as the threshold for active phase of labor.[67] The second stage of labor also should take into account the variability of patients and analgesia, and there is no absolute maximum length of time in the second stage. Operative vaginal delivery should be considered as an alternative if the physicians are experienced and trained in these deliveries.[67]

27.5.7 Prevention of Complications During Cesarean Delivery

The surgical preparations for cesarean delivery in the obese woman are critical, many of which need to be in place long before the obese patient arrives for labor and delivery.[65, 67] The hospital needs appropriately sized chairs, stretchers, and wheelchairs and the physical space (i.e., rooms and hallways) needs to be sufficiently large to accommodate the larger equipment. The operating room itself needs to be equipped with operating tables that have the capacity for morbidly obese patients and, importantly, the surgeon needs to be adequately situated at the bedside to perform the surgery. The operating room staff needs to be able to move around the operating room easily, and there may need to be additional staff support (or specialized equipment) to assist in moving the patient. Visualization within the operative field (especially during closure) may be difficult, so appropriate, specialized retractors and longer instruments need to be on hand.

27.6 VISUALIZATION AND PREVENTING WOUND COMPLICATIONS

Visualization in the surgical field can be extremely difficult in obese women following cesarean delivery of the infant. Furthermore, wound complications are more common with increasing BMI in women undergoing cesarean delivery; wound infections could result in emergency department visits and significantly delayed healing.[68, 69] Given the known risks, multiple studies have examined potential mitigating actions to reduce risks and improve surgical outcomes in overweight and obese women.

Choice of skin incision in women with obesity has been investigated, although studies were of variable quality, with somewhat conflicting results. Options for skin incision include supraumbilical transverse, subumbilical transverse, and vertical. The current evidence suggests that vertical skin incision does not significantly reduce the risk of wound complications compared to horizontal skin incision—indeed, they may actually increase complications.[70] Given the lack of clear evidence, choices should be made based on location of the symphysis pubis, location and size of the pannus, and visualization. Although low transverse incision is most likely to result in decreased morbidity in future deliveries, the decision should be individualized to increase exposure for the obstetrician performing the procedure.[71] Negative pressure dressings have not been shown to reduce the risk of infection or other complications after cesarean delivery compared with standard dressings.[71]

Antibiotics are recommended for all women undergoing cesarean delivery to reduce the risk of endometritis and wound infection.[67] For certain medications, women over a certain BMI may require increased doses. Whether higher doses of antibiotics affect clinical outcomes in obese pregnant women has not been fully elucidated, and recommendations are currently based on evidence from the general surgery literature, which suggests that using a 2-g dose of cefazolin for women who weigh $>80\,kg$ and 3 g for women who weigh $>120\,kg$ may reduce postoperative infection.[67] Canadian clinical practice guidelines recommend doubling the antibiotic dose when maternal BMI is >35.[72] Ideally, providers in a clinical setting will establish protocols for practice based on existing evidence. Local infection rates and other outcomes should guide any modifications to clinical practice.

Suturing of the subcutaneous space when $>2\,cm$ is recommended based on two RCTs that demonstrated reduced risk of wound infection and separation, but the use of drains has not been shown to have similar preventive impact.[73, 74] In fact, drains can actually increase the risk of wound infection and should not be used. Similarly, types of skin preparation, techniques to close the skin, and supplemental oxygen have not been shown to decrease morbidity due to infections after cesarean section.[67]

27.6.1 Postpartum Hemorrhage

Postpartum hemorrhage is responsible for much of the morbidity and mortality of childbirth in many developed countries and seems to be increasing in frequency. Obese women are at an even higher risk than their normal-weight counterparts. In a large, population-based study in New Zealand, nulliparous women with a singleton pregnancy who were obese were twice as likely to be diagnosed with postpartum hemorrhage (defined in that study as loss of 1000 mL or more within 24 h of delivery), independent of confounders or type of delivery (vaginal versus cesarean section) or major perineal trauma.[58] The increase was almost 70% among obese women who underwent cesarean delivery.[58]

The findings of this study support the hypothesis of impaired uterine contractility in obese women, which is also thought to contribute to impaired labor patterns. For overweight and obese women who undergo vaginal delivery, protocols for active management of the third stage of labor have been initiated in many practices to mitigate the risk of postpartum hemorrhage. Such practices are especially important in overweight and obese women, for whom the risk is increased and for whom the consequences can lead to further complications. Postpartum uterotonics also should be considered, including oxytocin and misoprostol (800 mcg per rectum).[65] Labor units should have protocols in place, and all personnel should be aware of the potential increased risk in this population.

27.6.2 Anesthesia

Obese women have increased anesthetic risks, which need to be taken into account. Landmarks for regional anesthesia may be difficult to identify, leading to failed attempts at placement and potentially a need for general anesthesia if cesarean delivery is required. General anesthesia can also be challenging in overweight and obese women, given the potential for edema and a difficult airway. Given that complications are common in obese women, it is prudent to recommend third-trimester consultation with the anesthesiology team for all obese women. Providing the patient with the opportunity to ask questions and understand the risks, benefits, and alternatives of anesthetic options before what could potentially be a traumatic intrapartum experience benefits both her and her family, in addition to providing more information about her to the obstetric and anesthetic teams.

27.6.3 Thromboembolism

Elevated BMI also puts pregnant women at increased risk for thromboembolism. Venous thromboembolism (VTE) is the leading cause of death among pregnant women in North America and the United Kingdom[75] and a significant contributor to maternal morbidity and mortality worldwide. Antenatal thromboprophylactic medications are recommended for specific conditions, including history of previous VTE or the presence of thrombophilia. Several organizations have published guidance on identification, prophylaxis, and treatment of thromboembolic disease in pregnancy, including the Royal College of Obstetricians and Gynaecologists (RCOG),[76] the American College of Chest Physicians,[77] and the ACOG.[78] Of note, one significant difference is that RCOG recommends prophylaxis throughout the whole antenatal period or beginning at 28 weeks' gestation, depending on the number of particular risk factors that may be present, including obesity, even if an individual does not have a personal history of previous VTE or known thrombophilia.[76] Providers caring for obese women need to be apprised of the most up-to-date, evidence-based guidance on the risks of VTE and treatment recommendations, and these are all helpful sources to consult. Because immobility can have a multiplicative effect on the risk of VTE,[79] antenatal bed rest should be avoided if at all possible, and women should be encouraged to ambulate as soon as possible after delivery.

Detailed recommendations about dosing of thromboprophylactic medications for VTE are beyond the scope of this chapter. However, there are a few important notes to consider for an obese woman who requires these prophylactic medications. Low-molecular-weight (LMW) heparin is generally recommended because of convenience of its administration and reliability. Women who are obese, especially with BMI over 40, may benefit from increased doses of LMW heparin. Although few studies have investigated clinical outcomes of LMW heparin, weight-adjusted dosing appears to result in greater thrombin inhibition and can be considered.[80]

After cesarean delivery, pneumatic compression devices should be placed on all women who are not otherwise on thromboprophylaxis and continued through the postpartum period. Furthermore, early mobilization after surgery should be encouraged for all women. For women at very high risk, such as women with a history of VTE, obesity, infection, or immobility, guidelines from the American College of Chest Physicians, RCOG, and ACOG recommend LMW heparin.[76–78] Weight-adjusted dosing was also demonstrated to result in higher anti-Xa concentrations (i.e., in the appropriate range for thromboprophylaxis) in a prospective cohort study among Class III obese women after cesarean delivery.[81] Regardless of the reason for prophylaxis, any woman with antepartum VTE prophylaxis should continue the medication for 6 weeks after either vaginal or cesarean delivery.

27.6.4 Postpartum Care

There are a multitude of benefits of breastfeeding for both the new mother and her infant. However, women with obesity are less likely to initiate and continue breastfeeding than their normal-weight counterparts. Women should be counseled about the benefits of breastfeeding during pregnancy and provided adequate support in the postpartum period. Highlighting the potential positive impact on postpartum weight loss may provide additional motivation for a reluctant obese patient.

The postpartum and interpregnancy periods also should be considered a powerful time to address behaviors contributing to obesity. A large population-based cohort study demonstrated that losing weight between pregnancies was associated with an almost 40% reduction in the risk of having an LGA infant in the next pregnancy, and weight gain between pregnancies increased a woman's risk for an LGA infant by a similar amount.[82] Another study demonstrated that interpregnancy weight loss was associated with a reduced risk of preeclampsia and LGA in future pregnancies.[83]

Fortunately, studies of lifestyle interventions in postpartum women have demonstrated more success than those conducted during pregnancy. A systematic review and meta-analysis of four RCTs showed statistically significant greater postpartum weight loss (–1.22 kg; 95% CI –1.89 to –0.56) in overweight or obese women who received physical activity plus diet intervention than in control women.[84] The most effective interventions were found to be supervised physical activity plus diet intervention, particularly when participants were given a target weight. However, based only on these included studies or the meta-analysis, a specific recommendation cannot be made at this time about the most effective intervention.

None of the studies in this review included an intervention that spanned from the antepartum period through to the postpartum period. Such longitudinal studies could better evaluate the impact of behavioral interventions through the lifespan. However, at least one study demonstrated that while a behavioral intervention did not reduce excessive gestational weight gain in obese women, the intervention during pregnancy did result in 31% of intervention-group participants reaching their preconception weight at 6 months postpartum, as compared to 19% of control participants.[85] Follow-up of these women to 12 months postpartum demonstrated that there was no significant difference in the odds of achieving prepregnancy weight by 12 months postpartum, but 45.3% of women who had been randomly assigned to the intervention group achieved prepregnancy weight and their mean weight retained (above prepregnancy weight) was significantly less (1.4 kg, as compared to 3.0 kg in the control group).[86] Additionally, outcomes of the study included measures of behavior change; women in the intervention group reported higher dietary restraint through 6 months postpartum and had more frequent self-monitoring of body weight.[86] Excess weight retention is associated with long-term obesity, cardiovascular disease, and Type 2 diabetes, so these studies are vital to advancing understanding of how women can prevent long-term chronic disease. Use of technology is also undergoing ongoing study; mobile applications may allow accurate information, monitoring, and feedback for individual women.

27.6.5 Long-Term Outcomes for Offspring

Increasing evidence, both from animal studies and population-based epidemiologic data, supports the premise that maternal obesity can have long-lasting implications for the health of offspring. Animal studies have demonstrated findings of obesity, elevated blood pressure, fatty liver, diabetes, behavior changes, and other metabolic changes in offspring.[87] In humans, both high prepregnancy BMI and excessive gestational weight gain have been associated with increased childhood BMI, and several studies also have demonstrated higher BMI in adolescents and adults.[88] Associations have also been identified with cardiovascular disease, Type 2 diabetes, and stroke for adult offspring of obese mothers.[88] There is also evidence that nonalcoholic fatty liver disease (NAFLD), which affects about 34% of obese children between the ages of 3 and 18, may be related to the in utero environment of an obese mother.[89]

The environmental impact of obesity on the gut microbiome of pregnant women is thought to negatively affect the fetus, potentially leading to increased risk of asthma and other atopic conditions in the offspring.[88] As more is understood about the impact of microbes on the health of an obese adult, there is increasing appreciation that these microbes may cause proinflammatory remodeling in the immune system of the infant, thus affecting long-term health of the offspring.[89] It appears that maternal diet can affect offspring health; for instance, a whole-food, plant-based diet might reduce risk as compared to the typical Western diets. Although a clear recommendation about any particular diet cannot be made, there is increasing evidence that what women eat during pregnancy can directly affect the health of their offspring, even into adulthood. Although not well elucidated at this time, associations with adverse neurocognitive and behavioral outcomes are being investigated as well.

Epigenetics is increasingly being studied as the mechanism for the association between maternal overweight and obesity, and these same conditions in offspring. Of the candidate modifications, deoxyribonucleic acid (DNA) methylation has been studied most extensively, although there remains much to be known about the exact mechanism, as well as the impact of lifestyle modification, weight loss, or both on the process.[88] Whether the impact of the in utero environment on methylation patterns is permanent is an area that requires further study.[89]

27.7 SPECIAL CONSIDERATIONS

27.7.1 Women with History of Bariatric Surgery

A growing number of studies of preconception weight loss have examined the impact of bariatric surgery among women who later become pregnant. Bariatric surgery may be recommended in reproductive-age women when they have a BMI of 40 or greater or a BMI < 35 with comorbidities such as diabetes, severe sleep apnea, or coronary heart disease.[90] Our understanding of the risks and benefits of bariatric surgery before pregnancy have been limited by variability in methodology and inconsistent reporting of prepregnancy BMI, as well as outcomes. However, a few recent studies can help inform the counseling of obese women who are considering bariatric surgery. For example, a recent large cohort study from Sweden found that pregnancies after bariatric surgery, when compared to control pregnancies and matched for prepregnancy and presurgery BMI, had lower risk of GDM and LGA infants, but higher risk of SGA infants and shorter gestation (although not preterm delivery), as well as a borderline significant increase in stillbirth or neonatal death.[91]

There are several important considerations for women who have undergone bariatric surgery who are capable of conceiving or who are pregnant. All women who undergo Roux-en-Y gastric bypass surgery should have a comprehensive evaluation for nutritional deficiencies such as protein, iron, vitamin B12, folate, vitamin D, and calcium, and they also should be provided oral or parenteral supplementation as appropriate.[90] There is no clear evidence that larger doses of folic acid are needed, but it is important to ensure that women are taking at least the recommended 0.4 mg/day to reduce the risk of neural tube defects. Patients should be aware of the possible decreased efficacy of some types of birth control after bariatric surgery. Results from some earlier studies led to recommendations that women wait at least 12 months after bariatric surgery before trying to conceive[90]; however, more recent data do not necessarily support significantly increased adverse events for women who conceive less than 12 months after surgery.[92]

27.7.2 Polycystic Ovarian Syndrome

PCOS, a condition characterized by clinical or biochemical hyperandrogenism, oligomenorrhea related to ovarian dysfunction, and polycystic ovaries on ultrasound, has numerous implications for pregnancy, some of which are related to obesity.[93] The syndrome is heterogeneous, with hirsutism, infertility, amenorrhea, obesity, and irregular bleeding representing the most common symptoms. Endocrine studies have demonstrated elevated luteinizing hormone (LH) levels in the early follicular phase, as well as elevated testosterone levels and insulin resistance.[94]

Although the diagnostic criteria for PCOS remains a favorite controversial topic of discussion, there has been increasing acceptance of the expanded PCOS diagnostic criteria from the European Society of Human Reproduction and Embryology (ESRHE) and the American Society for Reproductive Medicine (ASRM). Women should demonstrate two of the following three symptoms: oligoovulation or anovulation, clinical/biochemical hyperandrogenism, and polycystic ovaries on ultrasound; also, other possible causes should be excluded.

27.7.3 Infertility and Conception

Two of the most important factors that can negatively affect the success of ovulation induction in women with PCOS are insulin resistance and obesity. As a result, most consider lifestyle management a prerequisite to the treatment of obese women with PCOS and anovulatory infertility. Unfortunately, there are few high-quality studies comparing lifestyle and pharmacologic management directly, but the benefits for pregnancy outcomes and the long-term impact on health and wellness make it difficult to argue against providing counseling and support to women with PCOS and infertility prior to undergoing infertility treatment and during the preconception period.[95]

Current first-line pharmacologic treatments for ovulation induction in women with PCOS and anovulatory infertility are letrozole, an aromatase inhibitor, and clomiphene citrate, a selective estrogen receptor modulator.[96] Aromatase inhibitors appear to induce ovulation by reducing inappropriate feedback of weak circulating estrogens, resulting in increased follicle-stimulating hormone (FSH) secretion and follicular development. Prevention of pregnancy complications in women with PCOS in many ways mirrors the prevention of poor outcomes in women with obesity in general. Preconception and inter-pregnancy weight loss, in order to begin pregnancy at a normal or near-normal BMI, are most likely to affect pregnancy outcomes. In particular, given the potential increased risks of complications above and beyond non-PCOS women with obesity, obese women with PCOS need to be counseled about the potential morbidity associated with their BMI, as well as their PCOS status.

Achievement of live birth with letrozole appears to be about 50% more likely than with clomiphene, and initial concerns about teratogenicity seem to have diminished, given that rates are at or below population levels.[93] Rates of multiple gestations also seem to be less than that for clomiphene, and while this finding requires further study, it would have implications for potential reduction in pregnancy complications.

Clomiphene citrate, a selective estrogen receptor modulator (SERM), is the most commonly used and most well studied medication for ovulation induction. Live birth rates range higher for it than for other treatments, such as metformin in women with PCOS, and rates of multiple pregnancies range from 5% to 8%.[93] Recombinant or menopausal gonadotropins are typically second-line treatments, after aromatase inhibitors and/or clomiphene, and have been shown to be effective even at low doses in young women with PCOS (and low doses reduce the risk of multiple gestations).[96]

Metformin, a biguanide, originally held great promise as an ovulation induction agent, especially for women with PCOS because of its impact on circulating androgens and ovulation when compared to placebo. However, the evidence is now clear that pregnancy and live birth rates are lower for metformin as a single agent than for clomiphene.[96] In a large Finnish trial, metformin was found to be effective as an adjuvant therapy, increasing pregnancy rates, especially in an obese subgroup.[97] However, thus far, metformin continued during pregnancy does not appear to lower the rate of miscarriage or reduce adverse outcomes of pregnancy.[98]

Whether weight loss prior to ovulation induction in obese women with PCOS results in higher live birth rates is still a matter of debate,[96] especially after the publication of a study that demonstrated lower live birth rates in women who underwent a 6-month lifestyle management program, as compared to their PCOS counterparts who received immediate pharmacologic treatment.[99] However, women should be counseled about greater success in ovulation induction in women of normal weight compared to their overweight or obese counterparts, as well as improved pregnancy outcomes and the long-term health of both their offspring and themselves.

27.7.4 Complications During Pregnancy

Although the majority of research efforts related to PCOS and pregnancy have focused on conception and achievement of live birth, there is a body of literature that has examined complications that may arise during pregnancy associated with PCOS.[100] It is difficult to clearly delineate complications that can be attributed to PCOS due to the significant heterogeneity of studies and the complicated nature of PCOS itself, including various manifestations of the condition. The majority of studies are retrospective observational studies that make it difficult to attribute causation or even association conclusively. In particular, the individual contributions of BMI and PCOS cannot be distinguished from most of the studies to date. To provide clinical recommendations, we can turn to some systematic reviews and meta-analyses that have included the majority of the higher-quality studies performed.[101–104] As shown in multiple studies, hyperandrogenism, insulin resistance, obesity, dyslipidemia, low-grade inflammation, multiple pregnancy, and placental alteration in gene expression are all believed to contribute to increased complication risks during pregnancy.[105, 106]

Studies addressing miscarriage risk have reported variable outcomes. Although a recent systematic review reports increased risk of miscarriage in women with PCOS, BMI and fertility treatment have been handled in different ways in the studies examining this issue, and the impact of those cannot be reliably accounted for.[104] Multiple pregnancies are more common in women with PCOS, and the complications associated with multiples (e.g., preterm delivery and low birth weight) may account for a substantial portion of the morbidity associated with pregnancy in women with PCOS.[105]

Once pregnant, overweight or obese women with PCOS should be provided with recommendations for avoiding excess weight gain during pregnancy. While no specific dietary or physical interventions have been demonstrated to be most effective for women with PCOS, obese women with PCOS should be provided opportunities for dietary counseling, and attempts to improve system-level interventions may assist these high-risk women in avoiding gestational weight gain above the levels recommended by the WHO.

Women with PCOS and anovulatory infertility should be assessed for other risk factors and, if significant ones are found, such as obesity, being overweight and in a high-risk ethnic group (e.g., Hispanic, Polynesian, South Asian), and family history of Type 2 diabetes, screening with OGTT should be performed.[95] Even if women with PCOS are not undergoing infertility treatment, because of the increased risk of diabetes in such women, pregestational diabetes needs to be considered and women should be tested for Type 2 diabetes at the first prenatal visit, even if they are asymptomatic.[107] If women are found to have pregestational diabetes, management of pregnancy needs to follow recommended guidelines. Some studies have investigated whether monitoring biochemical markers could improve pregnancy outcomes, but no laboratory tests are currently recommended.[105]

In settings where universal screening for GDM is performed, women with PCOS should be screened according to current protocols. In countries or settings that have adopted risk-based screening, a history of PCOS should be considered, along with other risk factors such as ethnicity, high BMI, family history, and previous history of GDM. Many studies have demonstrated that the risk of GDM is higher in women with PCOS; in meta-analyses, the risk is over three times higher.[101–103] In some studies, such as a recent population-based cohort study, women with PCOS and those without had similar prevalence of GDM.[108] In others, it appears that the risk may be somewhat related to obesity, but even when adjusting for BMI, as was done in a large cohort study, women with PCOS had a twofold statistically significant increased risk.[109]

Three separate meta-analyses demonstrated a threefold-to-fourfold increase in the rate of pregnancy-induced hypertension, as well as preeclampsia in women with PCOS.[101–104] Although the confounding effect of obesity is somewhat difficult to tease out, at least one large, population-based cohort study found that the rate of preeclampsia was still higher in women after adjusting for BMI (OR 1.45, 95% CI 1.24–1.69).[110]

Abnormal fetal growth due specifically to PCOS is another complication that is somewhat difficult to isolate, given the association with obesity and GDM in many pregnancies. In one recent study, rates of both LGA and SGA infants were more common in women with PCOS than in those without.[105] Findings from meta-analyses looking at SGA and LGA risks have been somewhat mixed, demonstrating the difficulty in predicting the impact of PCOS alone on this particular outcome.[100]

Results from the most recent meta-analysis demonstrate that women with PCOS are more likely to have cesarean delivery (OR 1.2; 95% CI 1.1–1.7)[104] and three meta-analyses have demonstrated increased risk of admission to the neonatal intensive care unit in infants born to women with PCOS.[101–103]

Given the historical successes of treating PCOS with metformin, pharmacologic treatments have also been suggested for the management of GDM in pregnancy, particularly for women with PCOS. Unfortunately, although an RCT demonstrated reduced maternal weight gain in pregnancy when women with PCOS continued metformin during pregnancy, the rate of GDM was not reduced.[111]

27.7.5 Postpartum

Similar to women with obesity, two important issues to consider postpartum in women with PCOS are follow-up testing for Type 2 diabetes and weight loss. Testing for impaired glucose tolerance and Type 2 diabetes allows not only short-term guidance if another pregnancy is being considered in the near future, but also long-term prevention of Type 2 diabetes and other chronic diseases. As discussed earlier, weight loss between pregnancies can significantly reduce the risk of a number of complications with subsequent pregnancies.

27.8 CONCLUSION

The increasing prevalence of maternal obesity around the world has significant implications for short- and long-term health outcomes of both mother and child. This public health crisis requires a multidisciplinary effort to begin to address its complex and far-reaching impacts. There is a critical need for health-care providers to understand how to care for pregnant patients who are obese in order to optimize outcomes during the pregnancy and positively influence subsequent pregnancies and the future health of offspring. Even more important, everyone—from front-line providers to leaders to researchers to leaders of health-care systems—must be familiar with the evidence concerning preventive interventions that are most effective.

This chapter focused on the role of the clinician in caring for the obese gravida but highlights important gaps that need to be filled by basic and clinical science and health services research. In addition, because many women with PCOS also have elevated BMI, this chapter reviewed the issues unique to PCOS in pregnancy for both obese and normal-weight women.

REFERENCES

1. NCD Risk Factor Collaboration. Worldwide trends in diabetes since 1980: a pooled analysis of 751 population-based studies with 4.4 million participants. *Lancet* 2016;**387**:1513–30.
2. WHO. *Obesity: preventing and managing the global epidemic*. Report of a WHO consultation. WHO Technical Report Series, 894: http://www.who.int/nutrition/publications/obesity/WHO_TRS_894/en/; 2000.
3. Crane JMG, Murphy P, Burrage L, Hutchens D. Maternal and perinatal outcomes of extreme obesity in pregnancy. *JOGC* 2013;**35**:606–11.
4. Branum A, Kirmeyer SE, ECW G. *Prepregnancy body mass index by maternal characteristics and state: data from the birth certificate*. Hyattsville, MD: National Center for Health Statistics; 20142016. National Vital Statistics Reports; 65(6).
5. Ogden CL, Carroll MD, Fryar CD, Flegal KM. *Prevalence of obesity among adults and youth: United States, 2011–2014*. NCHS data brief, no. 219 Hyattsville, MD: National Center for Health Statistics; 2015. Available from: *http://www.cdc.gov/nchs/data/databriefs/db219.pdf*.
6. Poston L, Caleyachetty R, Cnattingius S, Corvalán C, Uauy R, Herring S, Gillman MW. Preconceptional and maternal obesity: epidemiology and health consequences. *Lancet Diabetes Endocrinol* 2016;**4**(12):1025–36.
7. Institute of Medicine and National Research Council. *Weight Gain During Pregnancy: Reexamining the Guidelines*. Washington, DC: National Academies Press; 2009. *https://doi.org/10.17226/12584*.
8. Gavard JA, Artal R. The association of gestational weight gain with birth weight in obese pregnant women by obesity class and diabetic status: a population-based historical cohort study. *Matern Child Health J* 2014;**18**(4):1038–47.
9. Catalano PM, Shankar K. Obesity and pregnancy: mechanisms of short term and long term adverse consequences for mother and child. *BMJ* 2017;**360**.
10. Alvarez-Blasco F, Botella-Carretero JI, San Millan JL, Escobar-Morreale JF. Prevalence and characteristics of the polycystic ovary syndrome in overweight and obese women. *Arch Intern Med* 2006;**166**:2081–6.
11. Law DCG, Maclehose RF, Longnecker MP. Obesity and time to pregnancy. *Hum Reprod* 2007;**22**:414–20.
12. van der Steeg JW, Steures P, Eijkemans MJ, et al. Obesity affects spontaneous pregnancy chances in subfertile ovulatory women. *Hum Reprod* 2008;**23**(2):324-8.f.
13. Broughton DE, Moley KH. Obesity and female infertility: potential mediators of obesity's impact. *Fertil Steril* 2017;**107**(4):840–7.
14. Hanson M, Barker M, Dodd JM, Kumanyika S, Norris S, Steegers E, Stephenson J, Thangaratinam S, Yang H. Interventions to prevent maternal obesity before conception, during pregnancy and postpartum. *Lancet Diabetes Endocrinol* 2017;**5**:65–76.
15. Opray N, Grivell RM, Deussen AR, Dodd JM. Directed preconception health programs and interventions for improving pregnancy outcomes for women who are overweight or obese. *Cochrane Database Syst Rev* 2015;**7**.
16. Moyer VA. Screening for and management of obesity in adults: U.S. Preventive Services Task Force recommendation statement. U.S. Preventive Services Task Force. *Ann Intern Med* 2012;**157**:373–8.
17. Bandura A. Human agency in social cognitive theory. *Am Psychol* 1989;**44**(9):1175–84.
18. Rollnick S, Miller WR. What is motivational interviewing? *Behav Cogn Psychother* 1995;**23**:325–34.
19. Pollak KI, Alexander SC, Coffman CJ, Tulsky JA, Lyna P, Dolor RJ, James IE, Brouwer RJN, Manusov JRE, Ostbye T. Physician communication techniques and weight loss in adults: project CHAT. *Am J Prev Med* 2010;**39**(4):321–8.
20. Lashen H, Fear K, Sturdee DW. Obesity is associated with increased risk of first trimester and recurrent miscarriage: matched case-control study. *Hum Reprod* 2004;**19**(7):1644–6.
21. Metwally M, Ong KJ, Ledger WL, Li TC. Does high body mass index increase the risk of miscarriage after spontaneous and assisted conception? A metaanalysis of the evidence. *Fertil Steril* 2008;**90**:714–26.
22. O'Dwyer V, Monaghan B, Fattah C, Farah N, Kennelly MM. Miscarriage after sonographic confirmation of an ongoing pregnancy in women with moderate and severe obesity. *Obes Facts* 2012;**5**(3):393–8.
23. Stothard KJ, Tennant PW, Bell R, Rankin J. Maternal overweight and obesity and the risk of congenital anomalies: a systematic review and meta-analysis. *JAMA* 2009;**301**:636–50.
24. Rasmussen SA, Chu SY, Kim SY, Schmid CH, Lau J. Maternal obesity and risk of neural tube defects: a metaanalysis. *Am J Obstet Gynecol* 2008;**198**(6):611–9.

25. Cai GJ, Sun XX, Zhang L, Hong Q. Association between maternal body mass index and congenital heart defects in offspring: a systematic review. *Am J Obstet Gynecol* 2014;**211**:91–117.

26. Parker SE, Yazdy MM, Tinker SC, Mitchell AA, Werler MM. The impact of folic acid intake on the association among diabetes mellitus, obesity, and spina bifida. *Am J Obstet Gynecol* 2013;**209**(3):239.e1–8.

27. CMACE/RCOG Joint Guideline: Management of Women With Obesity in Early Pregnancy. Center for Maternal and Child Enquiries and the Royal College of Obstetricians and Gynecologists. March 2010.

28. Mojtabai R. Body mass index and serum folate in childbearing age women. *Eur J Epidemiol* 2004;**19**(11):1029.

29. Dashe JS, McIntire DD, Twickler DM. Effect of maternal obesity on the ultrasound detection of anomalous fetuses. *Obstet Gynecol* 2009;**113**:1001–7.

30. Goldstein RF, Abell SK, Ranasinha S, Misso M, Boyle JA, Black MH, Hu G, Corrado F, Rode L, Kim YJ, Haugen M, Song WO, Kim MH, Bogaerts A, Devlieger R, Chung JH, Teede HJ. Association of gestational weight gain with maternal and infant outcomes: a systematic review and meta-analysis. *JAMA* 2017;**317**(21):2207–25.

31. Ferraro ZM, Contador F, Tawfiq A, Adamo KB, Gaudet L. Gestational weight gain and medical outcomes of pregnancy. *Obstet Med* 2015;**8**(3):133–7.

32. Catalano PM, McIntyre HD, Cruickshank JK, McCance DR, et al. The hyperglycemia and adverse pregnancy outcome study: associations of GDM and obesity with pregnancy outcomes. *Diabetes Care* 2012;**35**:780–6.

33. ACOG Practice Bulletin No 190: gestational diabetes mellitus. Committee on Practice Bulletins—Obstetrics. *Obstet Gynecol* 2018;**131**(2):e49–364.

34. Landon MB, Spong CY, Thom E, et al. A multicenter randomized trial of treatment for mild gestational diabetes. *N Engl J Med* 2009;**361**:1339–48.

35. Crowther CA, Hiller Moss JR, et al. Effect of treatment of gestational diabetes mellitus on pregnancy outcomes. *N Engl J Med* 2005;**352**:2477–86.

36. Landon MB, Mele L, Spong CY, et al. Eunice Kennedy Shriver National Institute of Child Health, and Human Development (NICHD) Maternal–Fetal Medicine Units (MFMU) Network. The relationship between maternal glycemia and perinatal outcome. *Obstet Gynecol* 2011;**117**:218–24.

37. Ma RCW, Schmidt MI, Tam WH, et al. Clinical management of pregnancy in the obese mother: before conception, during pregnancy, and postpartum. *Lancet Diabetes Endocrinol* 2016;**4**(12):1037–49.

38. Dodd JM, Grivell RM, Deussen AR, Hague WM. Metformin for women who are overweight or obese during pregnancy for improving maternal and infant outcomes. *Cochrane Database Syst Rev* 2018;**7**: https://doi.org/10.1002/14651858.CD010564.pub2.

39. Anderson NH, McCowan LM, Em F, et al. The impact of maternal body mass index on the phenotype of pre-eclampsia: a prospective cohort study. *BJOG* 2012;**119**:589–95.

40. WHO. *WHO Recommendations for Prevention and Treatment of Pre-Eclampsia and Eclampsia.* Geneva: World Health Organization; 201138.

41. LeFevre ML, US Preventive Services Task Force. Low-dose aspirin use for the prevention of morbidity and mortality from preeclampsia: U.S. Preventive Services Task Force recommendation statement. *Ann Intern Med* 2014;**161**(11):819–26.

42. American College of Obstetricians and Gynecologists. ACOG Committee Opinion No. 743: low-dose aspirin use during pregnancy. *Obstet Gynecol* 2018;**132**:e44–52.

43. WHO (World Health Organization). *Guideline: Calcium Supplementation in Pregnant Women.* Geneva: World Health Organization; 2013.

44. Cnattingius S, Villamor E, Johansson S, Bonamy AE, Persson M, Wikstrom A, Granath F. Maternal obesity and risk of preterm delivery. *JAMA* 2013;**309**:2362–70.

45. Heyborne KD, Allshouse AA, Carey JC. Does 17-alpha hydroxyprogesterone caproate prevent recurrent preterm delivery in women? *Am J Obstet Gyncol* 2015;**213**(6): https://doi.org/10.1016/j.ajog.2015.08.014. 844.e1–6. Epub 2015 Aug 12.

46. Oteng-Ntim E, Varma R, Croker H, Poston L, Doyle P. Lifestyle interventions for overweight and obese pregnant women to improve pregnancy outcome: systematic review and meta-analysis. *Acta Obstet Gynecol Scand* 2017 Mar;**96**(3):263–73. https://doi.org/10.1111/aogs.13087.

47. Dodd JM, Turnbull D, McPhee AJ, Deussen AR, Grivell RM, Yelland LN, Crowther CA, Wittert G, Owens JA, Robinson JS, LIMIT Randomised Trial Group. Antenatal lifestyle advice for women who are overweight or obese: LIMIT randomised trial. *BMJ* 2014;**10**: 348:g1285.

48. Poston L, Bell R, Corker H, Poston L, Bell R, Croker H, Flynn AC, Godfrey KM, Goff L, Hayes L, Khazaezadeh N, Nelson SM, Oteng-Ntim E, Pasupathy D, Patel N, Robson SC, Sandall J, Sanders TA, Sattar N, Seed PT, Wardle J, Whitworth MK, Briley AL, UPBEAT Trial Consortium. *Effect of a behavioural intervention in obese pregnant women (the UPBEAT study): a multicentre, randomised controlled trial, Lancet Diabetes Endocrinol* 2015;**3**:767–77.

49. Magro-Malosso ER, Saccone G, Di Mascio D, Di Tommaso M, Berghella V. *Exercise during pregnancy and risk of preterm birth in overweight and obese women: a systematic review and meta-analysis of randomized controlled trials. BMC Med* 2012;**10**:47. Published online 2012 May 10. https://doi.org/10.1186/1741-7015-10-47.

50. Thangaratinam S, Rogozinska E, Jolly K, et al. Effects of intervention in pregnancy on maternal weight and obstetric outcomes: meta-analysis of randomized evidence. *BMJ* 2012;**344**.

51. Arrowsmith S, Wray S, Quenby S. Maternal obesity and labour complications following induction of labour in prolonged pregnancy. *BJOG* 2011;**118**:578–88.

52. Denison FC, Price J, Graham C, et al. Maternal obesity, length of gestation, risk of postdates pregnancy and spontaneous onset of labour at term. *BJOG* 2008;**115**:720–5.

53. Olesen AW, Westergaard JG, Olsen J. Prenatal risk indicators of a prolonged pregnancy. The Danish Birth Cohort 1998-2001. *Acta Obstet Gynecol Scand* 2006;**85**(11):1338–41.

54. Kominiarek MA, Zhang J, Vanveldhuisen P, et al. Contemporary labor patterns: the impact of maternal body mass index. *AJOG* 2011;**205**:244. e1–244.e8.

55. Young TK, Woodmansee B. Factors that are associated with cesarean delivery in a large private practice: the importance of prepregnancy body mass index and weight gain. *AJOG* 2002;**187**:312–8.

56. Kominiarek MA, Van Veldhuisen P, Hibbard J, et al. The maternal body mass index: a strong association with delivery route. *AJOG* 2010;**203**: 264. e1–264.e7.

57. Hibbard JU, Gilbert S, Landon MB, et al. Trial of labor or repeat cesarean delivery in women with morbid obesity and previous cesarean delivery. *Obstet Gynecol* 2006;**108**(1):125–33.

58. Fyfe EM, Thompson JM, Anderson NH, Groom KM, McCowan LM. Maternal obesity and postpartum hemorrhage after vaginal and cesarean delivery among nulliparous women at term: a retrospective cohort study. *BMC Pregnancy Childbirth* 2012;**12**:1–8.

59. Lisonkova S, Muraca GM, Potts J, Liauw J, Chan W-S, Skoll A, Lim KI. Association between prepregnancy body mass index and severe maternal mortality. *JAMA* 2017;**318**(18):1777–86.

60. Carmichael SL, Blumenfeld YJ, Mayo J, Wei E, Gould JB, Stevenson DK, Shaw GM. Pre-pregnancy obesity and risks of stillbirth. *PLoS One* 2015;**10**(10).

61. Yao R, Ananth CV, Park BY, Pereira L, Plante LA. Obesity and the risk of stillbirth: a population-based cohort study. Perinatal Research Consortium. *Am J Obstet Gynecol* 2014;**210**: 457.e1–457.e9.

62. Yao R, Park BY, Foster SE, Caughey AB. The association between gestational weight gain and risk of stillbirth: a population-based cohort study. *Ann Epidemiol* 2017;**27**(10): https://doi.org/10.1016/j.annepidem.2017.09.006. 638–644.e1. Epub 2017 Sep 21. Erratum in: Ann Epidemiol 2018;28 (6):420.

63. Aune D, Saugstad OD, Henriksen T, Tonstad S. Maternal body mass index and the risk of fetal death, stillbirth, and infant death: a systematic review and meta-analysis. *JAMA* 2014;**311**:1536–46.

64. Wolfe KB, Rossi RA, Warshak CR. The effect of maternal obesity on the rate of failed induction of labor. *Am J Obstet Gynecol* 2011;**205**:128.

65. Carpenter JR. Intrapartum management of the obese gravida. *Clin Obstet Gynecol* 2016;**59**(1):172–9.

66. American College of Obstetricians and Gynecologists; Society for Maternal-Fetal Medicine, Caughey AB, Ag C, Guise JM, Rouse DJ. Safe prevention of the primary cesarean delivery. *Am J Obstet Gynecol* 2014;**210**(3):179–93.

67. American College of Obstetricians and Gynecologists. Practice Bulletin No. 156: obesity in pregnancy. *Obstet Gynecol* 2015;**126**:e112–26.

68. Tipton AM, Cohen ST, Chelmow D. Wound infection in the obese pregnant woman. *Semin Perinatol* 2011;**35**:345–9.

69. Stamilio DM, Scifres CM. Extreme obesity and postcesarean maternal complications. *Obstet Gynecol* 2014;**124**(2 Pt 1):227–32.

70. Wall PD, Deucy EE, Glantz JC, Pressman EK. Vertical skin incisions and wound complications in the obese parturient. *Obstet Gynecol* 2003;**102**:952–6.

71. Smid MC, Dotters-Katz SK, Grace M, Wright ST, Villers MS, Hardy-Fairbanks A, Stamilio DM. Prophylactic negative pressure wound therapy for obese women after cesarean delivery. *Obstet Gynecol* 2017;**130**(5):969–78.

72. Van Schalkwyk J, Van Eyk N. Antibiotic prophylaxis in obstetric procedures. *J Obstet Gynaecol Can* 2010;**32**:878–92.

73. Allaire AD, Fisch J, McMahon MJ. Subcutaneous drain vs. suture in obese women undergoing cesarean delivery. A prospective, randomized trial. *J Reprod Med* 2000;**45**(4):327–31.

74. Cetin A, Cetin M. Superficial wound disruption after cesarean delivery: effect of the depth and closure of subcutaneous tissue. *Int J Gynaecol Obstet* 1997;**57**(1):17–21.

75. Duhl AJ, Paidas MJ, Ural SH, et al. Antithrombotic therapy and pregnancy:consensus report and recommendations for prevention and treatment of venous thromboembolism and adverse pregnancy outcome. *Am J Obstet Gynecol* 2007;**197**: 457.e1–457.e21.

76. Royal College of Obstetricians and Gynaecologists. *Reducing the risk of venous thromboembolism during pregnancy and the puerperium.* Green Top Guideline No. 37a. London (UK): RCOG: https://www.rcog.org.uk/globalassets/documents/guidelines/gtg-37a.pdf; 2015.

77. Bates SM, Greer IA, Middeldorp S, Veenstra DL, Prabulos AM, Vandvik PO. VTE, thrombophilia, antithrombotic therapy, and pregnancy: antithrombotic therapy and prevention of thrombosis, 9th ed: American College of Chest Physicians Evidence-Based Clinical Practice Guidelines. American College of Chest Physicians. *Chest* 2012;**141**:e691S–736S.

78. American College of Obstetricians and Gynecologists. ACOG Practice Bulletin No. 196: thromboembolism in pregnancy. *Obstet Gynecol* 2018;**132**: e1–17.

79. Jacobsen AF, Skjeldestad FE, Sandset PM. Ante- and postnatal risk factors of venous thrombosis: a hospital-based case-control study. *J Thromb Haemost* 2008;**6**:905–12.

80. Ismail SK, Norris L, O'Shea S, Higgins JR. Weight-adjusted LMWH prophylaxis provides more effective thrombin inhibition in morbidly obese pregnant women. *Thromb Res* 2014;**134**(2):234–9.

81. Overcash RT, Somers AT, La Coursiere DY. Enoxaparin dosing after cesarean delivery in morbidly obese women. *Obstet Gynecol* 2015;**125**:1371–6.

82. Jain AP, Gavard JA, Rice JJ, Cantanzaro RB, Artal R, Hopkins SA. The impact of interpregnancy weight change on birthweight in obese women. *Am J Obstet Gynecol* 2013;**208**:205.

83. Villamor E, Cnattingius S. Interpregnancy weight changes and risk of adverse pregnancy outcomes: a population-based study. *Lancet* 2006;**368**:1164–70.

84. Choi J, Fukuoka Y, Lee JH. The effects of physical activity and physical activity plus diet interventions on body weight in overweight or obese women who are pregnant or postpartum: a systematic review and meta-analysis of randomized controlled trials. *Prev Med* 2013;**56**(6):351–64.

85. Phelan S, Phipps MG, Abrams B, Darroch F, Schaffner F, Wing RR. Randomized trial of a behavioral intervention to prevent gestational weight gain: the Fit for Delivery Study. *Am J Clin Nutr* 2011;**93**:772–9.

86. Phelan S, Phipps MG, Abrams B, Darroch F, Grantham K, Schaffner A, Wing RR. Does behavioral intervention in pregnancy reduce postpartum weight retention? Twelve-month outcomes of the fit for delivery randomized trial. *Am J Clin Nutr* 2014;**99**(2):302–11.

87. Patel N, Pasupathy D, Poston L. Determining the consequences of maternal obesity on offspring health. *Exp Physiol* 2015;**100**:1421–8.
88. Godfrey KM, Reynolds RM, Prescott SL, Nyirenda M, Jaddoe VWV, Eriksson JG, Broekman BFP. Influence of maternal obesity on the long-term health of offspring. *Lancet Diabetes Endocrinol* 2017;**5**:53–64.
89. Dutton H, Borengasser SJ, Gaudet LM, Barbour LA, Keely EJ. Obesity in pregnancy: optimizing outcomes for mom and baby. *Med Clin N Am* 2018;**102**:87–106.
90. American College of Obstetricians and Gynecologists. ACOG Practice Bulletin No. 105: bariatric surgery and pregnancy. *Obstet Gynecol* 2009;**113**:1405–13.
91. Johannson K, Cnattingius S, Naslund I, Roos N, Trolle Lagerros Y, Granath F, Stephansson O, Neovius M. Outcomes of pregnancy after bariatric surgery. *N Engl J Med* 2015;**372**(9):814–24.
92. Dolin C, Welcome AOU, Caughey AB. Management of pregnancy in women who have undergone bariatric surgery. *Obstet Gynecol Survey* 2016;**71**(12):734–40.
93. Legro RS, Arslanian SA, Ehrmann DA, Hoeger KM, Murad MH, Pasquali R, Welt CK. Diagnosis and treatment of polycystic ovary syndrome: an endocrine society clinical practice guideline. *J Clin Endocrinol Metab* 2013;**98**:4565–92.
94. Fauser BCJM, Tarlatzis BC, Rebar RW, et al. Consensus on women's health aspects of polycystic ovary syndrome (PCOS): the Amsterdam ESHRE/ASRM-Sponsored 3rd PCOS ConsensusWorkshop Group. *Fertil Steril* 2012;**97**(1):28–38.
95. Balen AH, Morley LC, Misso M, Franks S, Legro RS, Wijeyaratne CN, Stener-Victorin E, Fauser BCJM, Norman RJ, Teede H. The management of anovulatory infertility in women with polycystic ovary syndrome: an analysis of the evidence to support the development of global WHO guidance. *Hum Reprod Upd* 2016;**22**(6):687–708.
96. Legro RS. Ovulation induction in polycystic ovary syndrome: current options. *Best Pract Res Clin Obstet Gynaecol* 2016;**37**:152–9.
97. Morin-Papunen L, Rantala AS, Unkila-Kallio L, et al. Metformin improves pregnancy and live-birth rates in women with polycystic ovary syndrome (PCOS): a multicenter, double-blind, placebo-controlled randomized trial. *J Clin Endocrinol Metab* 2012;**97**(5):1492–500.
98. Vanky E, Stridskleve S, Heimstad R, et al. Metformin versus placebo from first trimester to delivery in polycystic ovary syndrome: a randomized controlled multicenter study. *J Clin Endocrinol Metab* 2012;**95**:E448–55.
99. Mutsaerts MA, van Oers AM, Groen H, et al. Randomized trial of a lifestyle program in obese infertile women. *NEJM* 2016;**374**:1942–53.
100. Palomba S, de Wilde MA, Falbo A, Koster MPH, LaSala GB, Fauser BCJM. Pregnancy complications in women with polycystic ovary syndrome. *Reprod Upd* 2015;**21**(5):575–92.
101. Boomsma CM, Eijkemans MJ, Hughes EG, Visser GH, Fauser BC, Macklon NS. A meta-analysis of pregnancy outcomes in women with polycystic ovary syndrome. *Hum Reprod Update* 2006;**12**:673–83.
102. Kjerulff LE, Sanchez-Ramos L, Duffy D. Pregnancy outcomes in women with polycystic ovary syndrome: a meta-analysis. *Am J Obstet Gynecol* 2011;**204**: 558.e1–558.e–6.
103. Qin JZ, Pang LH, Li MJ, Fan XJ, Huang RD, Chen HY. Obstetric complications in women with polycystic ovary syndrome: a systematic review and meta-analysis. *Reprod Biol Endocrinol* 2013;**11**:56.
104. Yu HF, Chen HS, Rao DP, Gong J. Association between polycystic ovary syndrome and the risk of pregnancy complications: a PRISMA-compliant systematic review and meta-analysis. *Medicine* 2016;**95**.
105. Palomba S, Chiossi G, Falbo A, Orio F, Tolino A, Colao A, La Sala GB, Zullo F. Low-grade chronic inflammation in pregnant women with polycystic ovary syndrome. *J Clin Endocrinol Metab* 2014;**99**:2942–51.
106. Khomami MB, Boyle JA, Tay CT, Vanky E, Teede HJ, Joham AE, Moran LJ. Polycystic ovary syndrome and adverse pregnancy outcomes: current state of knowledge, challenges and potential implications for practice. *Clin Endocrinol* 2018;**88**:761–9.
107. American Diabetes Association. Standards of medical care in diabetes—2011. *Diabetes Care* 2011;**34**:S11–61.
108. Palm CVB, Glintborg D, Kyhl HB, McIntyre HD, Jensen RC, Jensen TK, Jensen DM, Andersen M. Polycystic ovary syndrome and hyperglycaemia in pregnancy. A narrative review and results from a prospective Danish cohort study. *Diabetes Res Clin Pract* 2018; https://doi.org/10.1016/j.diabres.2018.04.030 pii: S0168-8227(18)30554-0. [Epub ahead of print].
109. Joham AE, Ranasinha S, Zoungas S, Moran L, Teede HJ. Gestational diabetes and type 2 diabetes in reproductive-aged women with polycystic ovary syndrome. *J Clin Endocrinol Metab* 2014;**99**:447–52.
110. Roos N, Kieler H, Sahlin L, Ekman-Ordeberg G, Falconer H, Stephansson O. Risk of adverse pregnancy outcomes in women with polycystic ovary syndrome: population-based cohort study. *Br Med J* 2011;**343**:d6309.
111. Vanky E, Stridsklev S, Heimstad R, Romundstad P, Skogøy K, KleggetveitO HS, von Brandis P, Eikeland T, Flo K, et al. Metformin versus placebo from first trimesterto delivery in polycystic ovary syndrome: a randomized, controlled multicenter study. *J Clin Endocrinol Metab* 2010;**95**:448–55.

Transgendered Issues

Chapter 28

Fertility, Pregnancy, and Chest Feeding in Transgendered Individuals

Alexis Light*, Brett Stark† and Veronica Gomez-Lobo*,‡

*Department of Obstetrics and Gynecology, MedStar Washington Hospital Center, Washington, DC, United States, †Department of OBGYN and Reproductive Science, University of California San Francisco, San Francisco, CA, United States, ‡Children's National Health System and Medstar Washington Hospital Center, Washington, DC, United States

Common Clinical Problems

- Medical providers should be familiar with the social and mental-health risks for the transgender population.
- Terminology related to the transgender experience is evolving, and providers should engage a patient to ensure that they are using terms preferred by that person.
- Fertility desires should be identified and counseling should occur prior to the initiation of gender-affirming hormone therapy.
- While having a transgender identity is not itself a mental disorder, transgender populations are at a higher risk of anxiety and depression, including postpartum depression.
- Chest feeding is possible both before and after gender-affirming surgeries such as breast reduction, and transgender patients should be provided with lactation support as desired.

28.1 INTRODUCTION

Over the last decade and a half, an increasing amount of research has been published about the reproductive health of transgender individuals and the barriers that they experience when trying to access care. In 2011, the American College of Obstetricians and Gynecologists (ACOG) called upon obstetricians and gynecologists to eliminate barriers to the care of transgender patients, including assisting in the reproductive and obstetrical needs of this population.[1] In this chapter, we will briefly summarize the current understanding of fertility, reproduction, and obstetrical care for transgender patients. There is still a significant shortage of research on these topics, and much of what is currently being practiced is extrapolated from other fields.

28.1.1 Terminology and Transgender Identity

While the terms are frequently used interchangeably, there is a distinction between *sex* and *gender* that has significance beyond mere semantics. Historically, *sex* has referred to an individual's sex assigned at birth based on assessment of external genitalia, sex chromosomes, and gonads (i.e., male, female, intersex).[2] *Gender* may refer to the "psychological, social, and cultural aspects of maleness and femaleness".[3] Gender can be analyzed further at the level of identity and expression. *Gender identity* is a person's fundamental, innate sense of being male, female, or somewhere in between.[4] *Gender expression* refers to the outward manner in which an individual expresses or displays their gender.[5] This may include choices in clothing and hairstyle or speech and mannerisms. Gender identity and gender expression may differ; for example, a woman (transgender or nontransgender) may have an androgynous appearance, or a man (transgender or nontransgender) may have a feminine form of self-expression.[6]

When there is a congruence between sex and gender, an individual can be described as being *cisgender*. However, variations in the congruence between sex and gender exist. *Transgender* is an umbrella term used to describe a diverse group of people whose gender identity or expression diverts from societal expectations of gender norms. Historically, gender has

Maternal-Fetal and Neonatal Endocrinology. https://doi.org/10.1016/B978-0-12-814823-5.00028-3

been thought of as dichotomous and bipolar, even with regard to the transgender community. Individuals frequently identify as transgender male (female-to-male) or transgender female (male-to-female). However, identities within the transgender community frequently fall outside this binary categorization. *Genderqueer* and *gender nonconforming* are terms for an individual whose gender identity differs from that which may have been assigned at birth, but the situation also may be more complex, fluid, multifaceted, or otherwise less clearly defined than with a transgender person.[5] *Transmasculine* and *transfeminine* are terms that be used to describe the directionality of gender identity in gender nonconforming or nonbinary persons. A transfeminine person has a feminine-spectrum gender identity, and "Male" is listed as the sex on their original birth certificate.

Note: The authors recognize that terminology related to the transgender experience is evolving. Some terms utilized in this chapter may be offensive to particular individuals but preferable to others. Additionally, there may have been recent shifts in language use that may not be fully reflected in the terms defined in this chapter. This chapter will predominantly utilize *transgender men* and *transgender women* in this discussion. Gender nonconforming or nonbinary individuals are frequently excluded from transgender research; however, this chapter will utilize these terms when possible.

28.1.2 Transgender Statistics

Estimating the prevalence rate of transgender populations is logistically challenging. Recent studies suggest that in the United States, transgender individuals could represent a current population size of 390 adults per 100,000, or almost 1 million adults in total.[7] While transgender individuals constitute a tiny portion of the U.S. population, they frequently experience widespread social and economic marginalization that can negatively affect their health, and this topic is worth exploring. Compared with the general population, a national survey conducted in the United States in 2008 found that transgender individuals were four times more likely to live in extreme poverty, had double the rate of unemployment, and had almost double the rate of being homeless.[8]

The economic and societal exclusion of transgender individuals is associated with higher rates of psychiatric disorders, suicide attempts/ideation, and substance abuse. A U.S. sample of 1093 transgender persons demonstrated a high prevalence of clinical depression (44.1%), anxiety (33.2%), and somatization (27.5%).[9] It is important to note that according to the American Psychiatric Association *Diagnostic and Statistical Manual,* having a transgender identity is not itself a psychiatric disorder. However, the term *gender dysphoria* refers to a potential discomfort or distress that is caused by a discrepancy between a person's gender identity and that person's sex assigned at birth.[10] Only some gender-nonconforming people experience gender dysphoria at some point in their lives.

28.1.3 Heath-Care Discrimination and Barriers to Care

The National Center for Transgender Equality published a report showing that transgender people face multiple barriers to accessing sexual and reproductive health care. One study of 6000 transgender-identifying individuals showed that 28% had postponed care when sick or injured, and 33% had not sought preventive care due to past experiences with transphobia.[11] These barriers include structural and legal factors such as inadequate electronic medical records, challenges with insurance claims, and difficulty obtaining legal gender status.[12] However, discrimination goes beyond structural transphobia, and these individuals frequently experience explicit discrimination. Additionally, transgender treatment is not taught in conventional medical curricula, and too few physicians have the requisite knowledge and comfort level.[9]

Professional heath-care organizations have begun to incorporate transgender antidiscrimination laws into their policy and ethics documents. The American Medical Association explicitly opposes discrimination based on gender identity in health care, physician education and training, and the physician workplace. However, further training in cultural humility is required to reduce these barriers to heath care for transgender individuals.[9]

28.2 REPRODUCTIVE DESIRES

Burgeoning research has begun to explore the reproductive desires and fertility needs of transgender individuals. Some transgender individuals desire to become parents even after following through with gender-affirming therapy.[13] The World Professional Association of Transgender Health (WPATH) and the Endocrine Society recommend that all transgender persons be counseled about the potential impact that gender-affirming therapy could have on their future fertility.[4, 14] Heath-care providers can help assist with reproductive options. While some question the ethics of transgender individuals having and raising children, the American Academy of Child and Adolescent Psychiatry holds that there is no evidence that children are negatively affected by their parents' sexual orientation or gender identity.[15]

As with the general population, a transgender individual may choose to have children for a variety of reasons, including intimacy, nurturance, and desire to have a family. Depending on when a transgender individual "comes out," they may already have children with a partner prior to their transition. Historically, the process of gender affirmation meant the loss of all reproductive potential, not only due to the impact of gender-affirming therapy on reproductive capacity, but also due to exclusion from technology that could help these individuals build their own families. Counter to societal and provider concerns regarding possible risks to the offspring of transgender individuals, data from long-term studies do not support them. Most recently, data from a 12-year follow-up study of 42 French children born into families with a transgender man concluded that the children were healthy, well adjusted, and well attached to their parents, with no evidence of gender-variant behavior.[16]

The fertility desires of transgender populations are as unique and diverse as the individuals within the community itself. One study of 50 transgender men in Belgium showed that half of them stated that they wanted to have children, and if fertility preservation was an option, 38% would use it[17]. As for transgender women, one study found that 77% of 120 trans-women surveyed agreed that cryopreservation of sperm prior to transitioning should be offered.[18] Half of those asked would at least seriously consider preserving their sperm if the option were available. For transgender women who were counseled but chose not to undergo cryopreservation, the option was felt to be limited by time and finances.[19]

Further research is needed to explore the desires of gender nonconforming and nonbinary individuals with regard to their future fertility status. Furthermore, there is little research exploring the desires and needs of transgender adolescents. One pilot study of 25 transgender adolescents showed that many of them wished to parent a child of their own at some point, but few expressed a desire to have their own biological child. However, many of these youths were aware that their feelings about having a biological child might change in the future.[20]

28.3 GENDER-AFFIRMING CARE AND FERTILITY

Transgender individuals may choose to utilize gender-affirming care, including both medical and surgical therapy, as either treatment for the associated gender dysphoria or simply to support their individualized, gender-related needs. Potential elements of gender-affirming care include puberty suppression, gender-affirming hormone therapy (formerly known as *cross-sex hormone therapy*), and surgical interventions such as bilateral mastectomy, hysterectomy with oophorectomy, orchiectomy, vaginoplasty, and phalloplasty. Stages of medical and surgical transitioning are often spread across a treatment spectrum ranging from reversible to irreversible. Current evidence supports beginning reversible hormone blocking on transgender adolescents at Tanner stage 2, and initiating gender-affirming hormones around the age of 16 for the optimization of physical and emotional health.[4, 21] Hormone blockers used in peripubertal children are thought to be reversible, as they can be stopped, and if gender-affirming hormones are not administered, the adolescent will then continue with their natal puberty.[13] Ultimately, surgical interventions may lead to complete sterilization, and further, they are irreversible.[21]

28.3.1 Transgender Men and Fertility

Low levels of testosterone are needed for female fertility. Higher levels of testosterone have been noted in animal studies to be detrimental to ovarian tissue, causing follicular atresia.[22, 23] In cisgender women who experienced excess androgens, secondary to polycystic ovarian syndrome (PCOS) or testosterone-producing tumors, impaired folliculogenesis and anovulation are common.[24, 25] However, fertility can be restored by correcting the underlying disorder. Masculinizing hormones are thought to have a number of effects on the transgender male's natal structures. Studies have shown that androgens alone may have an atrophic effect on the endometrium or cause hyperplasia of the ovarian cortex and stroma.[26] These changes notwithstanding, even if amenorrhea is achieved, the ovarian follicular pool is unaffected.[27] Furthermore, reports demonstrate that transgender-male individuals who have not undergone a hysterectomy are able to conceive, regardless of testosterone utilization.[28]

28.3.2 Transgender Females and Fertility

Analogous to transgender males, low levels of estrogen are necessary in the development of male fertility. However, both animal and human data suggest that higher levels of exogenous estrogen may have a negative impact. Rodent studies suggest that increasing the dose of estrogen can alter sperm counts and the sperm's ability to function.[29] These effects may be reversible.[30] Furthermore, studies of cisgender males suggest that endocrine disruptors with estrogenic properties, such as phthalates, polychlorinated biphenyls (PCBs), and bisphenol A (BPA), may be associated with low semen parameters and increased male factor infertility.[31] The direct effects of exogenous estrogen on fertility, as well as reversibility, need to be demonstrated better in human populations.

28.4 FERTILITY OPTIONS

Infertility in the general population is associated with reduced psychological well-being and quality of life.[32, 33] A range of medical techniques, collectively known as *fertility preservation,* has been developed to preserve reproductive materials for individuals who could become infertile.[15] These fertility-preservation techniques are similarly used by transgender individuals to maintain their options for family-building with biological children. Fertility preservation allows an individual to delay the decision-making process of whether they want to have a child to a later date.

Fertility-preservation options that are considered standard include sperm, oocyte, and, embryo cryopreservation. Ovarian and testicular tissue cryopreservation remains experimental and should be performed only under Institutional Review Board (IRB) approval. These options permit an individual to build a family with their own genetic material, but they also are frequently invasive and cost-prohibitive.[34, 35] Fertility preservation is very different for transgender men and women, requiring varying levels of cost, involvement, invasiveness, and outcomes, as discussed next.

28.4.1 Fertility Preservation and Transgender Men

Transgender men encounter a multitude of issues during the fertility-preservation process, due in particular to the arduous process of harvesting and freezing eggs. Oocyte preservation involves hormonally stimulating the ovaries to produce multiple mature follicles, closely monitoring the development of these oocytes over a 2- to 3-week period, and undergoing an invasive procedure to retrieve the stimulated eggs, often transvaginally.[36] This process is repeated until the desired number of oocytes are accumulated.

It is important to note that gender-affirming hormone therapy is administered during this entire procedure, and natal female hormones are given in order to stimulate oocyte development. The change in hormones may result in a return to menses, which can cause further distress and dysphoria to some transgender males. Furthermore, even in cis-females, the fertility medication regimen may cause mood swings, depression, irritability, anger, tearfulness, and difficulty with decision-making.[27] One mixed-method study of Swedish transgender males showed that many of these individuals experienced gender incongruence and dysphoria due to both the genital examinations necessary during the retrieval process and the physical changes induced by testosterone discontinuation.[27]

28.4.2 Assisted Reproduction and Transgender Men

When a transgender man is ready to have children of their own, one must consider the presence or absence of a uterus. As part of the gender-affirming process, transgender males may choose to undergo a hysterectomy. While these individuals frequently maintain their ovaries as a source of endogenous hormone production, and subsequently may undergo oocyte harvesting, the absence of a uterus precludes them from maintaining a pregnancy without the help of a gestational surrogate. This can be accomplished if the transgender male has a partner who is female at birth with an intact uterus (either cisgender female or another transgender male), or it may be done through third-party surrogacy. Surrogacy may be a preferred option for some transgender men, as the physical process of becoming pregnant and carrying a child may cause dysphoria, presumably due to the association of pregnancy with female identity.[36]

If a transgender man who is ready to have biological children has an intact uterus, hormone therapy must be discontinued in order for the body to return to its natal hormonal and reproductive cycle.[37] Gender-affirming hormones are contraindicated throughout egg maturation, pregnancy, and chest feeding.[37] Sperm may be acquired from a partner, a known donor, or an unknown donor, and the person may be inseminated in many ways (e.g., intercourse, home insemination, or insemination by a medical provider).

For the transgender male without a uterus, or a transgender male who does not wish to carry their own pregnancy, gestational surrogacy is a potential option and can occur in a variety of ways,[38] but it can be costly. It is estimated that the removal, fertilization, and cryopreservation of eggs costs over $10,000—and that does not include annual fees for continued preservation.[37] While fertility preservation and assisted reproduction may be covered by insurance in certain parts of the country, transgender individuals and the lesbian, gay, bisexual, transgender, and questioning (LGBTQ) community as a whole are frequently excluded from this coverage, on the ground that gender identity or sexuality are not true incidences of infertility.[9, 37]

28.4.3 Fertility Preservation and Transgender Women

Transgender women, in comparison to transgender men, experience fewer challenges in preserving fertility. The simplest and most effective method for sperm preservation is through masturbation and subsequent ejaculation, processing of semen in an andrology lab, and storing for later utilization. Other theoretical methods for collection exist, such as testicular aspiration or extraction from a postmasturbation urine sample.[39] Alternative methods may be less necessary, however, as studies show that fertility preservation through ejaculation may not be associated with increasing dysphoria and gender incongruence, as previously thought.[36]

28.4.4 Assisted Reproduction and Transgender Women

When a transgender woman desires to reproduce and has no previously cryopreserved genetic material, feminizing hormone therapy and testosterone blockers are discontinued, and the body returns to its natal hormone levels.[17, 37] These hormone levels must be maintained until the sperm is collected. As transgender women are not yet able to maintain a pregnancy themselves, there is no contraindication for them to continue gender-affirming therapy once viable sperm is collected.

There are multiple sources of egg donors that may be utilized by the transgender woman (e.g., a known donor or an unknown donor),[37] and fertilization may occur through vaginal-penile intercourse or artificial insemination, as previously discussed. However, it is important to note that transgender women, like cisgender men, may experience other types of sperm-related infertility, such as low sperm count or lack of strong motility. If these problems exist, or if the individual has immature sperm, intracytoplastic sperm injection (ICSI) may be beneficial. ICSI is the process by which a single sperm is injected directly into an egg, with the average fertilization rate being over 90%.[40]

Uterus transplant may be a possible option for transgender women in the future. However, the research protocols have excluded transgender individuals from this incipient technology. Interestingly, one study of transgender women showed that they themselves did not wish to become pregnant.[37] The authors of this study extrapolated that this reluctance may be due to the novelty of the technology and an overall lack of knowledge about this future possibility.

28.4.5 Fertility Preservation and Adolescents

As society's understanding of the transgender identity develops, individuals are starting gender-affirming care at younger ages.[41] This phenomenon necessitates the occurrence of fertility counseling earlier than in the past. Adolescents may not always understand the future impact of certain medical interventions.[37, 42] However, we believe that transgender adolescents should always be involved in discussions about their care, in a developmentally appropriate manner.

From the clinical experience of the authors, as well as anecdotal findings at other institutions, it seems that both oocyte and sperm cryopreservation appear to have a low uptake in the adolescent transgender populations in spite of counseling.[43] More research needs to be done to assess why this might be the case, what the long-term implications are, and how to institute fertility-preservation counseling with such people prior to their transition to adolescence.

Gonadal tissue cryopreservation is a potential option for fertility preservation when there are barriers to gamete preservation, such as what is seen in prepubescent adolescents who do not experience natal puberty. To date, over 60 pregnancies have been reported via reimplantation of ovarian tissue, although this approach is still considered experimental. Additionally, adolescents and individuals who have undergone puberty suppression present unique challenges, as they are thought to be too young to undergo permanent surgical elective gonadectomy as they are initiating gender-affirming hormones, but extracting gametes for cryopreservation may not be feasible. It is accepted that the ability to extract sperm requires pubertal development to Tanner stage 3, but it is unknown if ovarian stimulation and egg retrieval can be accomplished in individuals who are Tanner stage 1 in puberty development.[44, 45]

28.5 TRANSGENDER PREGNANCY

28.5.1 Preconception Counseling

For transgender men desiring to become pregnant, preconception counseling should be performed. This process should follow guidelines provided by the ACOG. Providers also should be aware that pregnancy may be an isolating period of time for transgender men.[12] These individuals can be directed to lesbian, gay, bisexual, transgender, questioning, and intersex (LGBTQI) support groups or online community resources, with a growing number of websites, blogs, and social groups. However, many of these sites are not findable through a simple online search.

A discussion regarding gender-affirming hormone therapy should occur, with an emphasis of testosterone cessation throughout the preconception, pregnancy, and chest-feeding periods. Exposure to exogenous testosterone during embryogenesis may lead to virilization, metabolic dysfunction, and future reproductive issues in offspring.[46] Studies also suggest that testosterone exposure may be associated with low birth rate.[47] Anticipatory guidance should be provided to transgender men regarding the potential effects of stopping gender-affirming hormone therapy, such as rapid changes in emotional experiences and a potential increase in gender incongruence and dysphoria.[48]

28.5.2 Obstetrical Care for Transgender Patients

Clinical management of transgender men during pregnancy should follow the same evidence-based guidelines of routine obstetrical care that are practiced with cisgender women.[13] However, there may be a potential difference in the pregnancy of transgender men that is unique. One series found a short interval to pregnancy after stopping testosterone (usually less than 6 months), and even some unplanned pregnancies while on testosterone.[28] This series also revealed significant self-reported rates of hypertension (12%), preterm labor (10%), and placenta abruption (10%).[49] However, more research is needed in this area.

A typical labor process for a vaginal delivery can involve multiple digital vaginal examinations. This possibility should be addressed as part of prenatal care, as multiple studies have linked pelvic examinations in transgender men with increasing dysphoria.[13, 27] In the previously mentioned study, delivery rates were variable[28]: 71% had a vaginal delivery, while 30% had cesarean sections (25% of which were elective). A significant percentage of these study participants choose to deliver at home or in an independent birthing center. In a separate qualitative study of the transgender pregnancy experience, a participant mentioned that they chose to have a home birth out of necessity, due to a lack of culturally competent hospitals in their region.[48] Thus, it is important that the provider elucidates patient expectations early in the pregnancy and that provider and patient work together to develop a birth plan that can maximize the potential for a physically and emotionally safe labor.

28.5.3 Transgender Men and the Labor and Delivery Experience

Multiple qualitative studies have explored the experience of transgender men with pregnancy and the labor-and-delivery process.[27, 48] These experiences included both positive and negative interactions with medical providers and clinic staff. In both studies, positive experiences were associated with the normalization of both the individual and their pregnancy experience through the use of proper gender pronouns, preferred names of private parts, and minimization of examinations perceived to be unnecessary. Negative experiences ranged from aversive features, such as misgendering and exotification, to blatant transphobia and being turned away from medical practices. The study highlighted the need for cultural humility when practicing obstetrics with transgender individuals, and that discomfort relating to gender incongruence and gender dysphoria may be compounded by the general discomfort of labor.

28.6 POSTPARTUM CONSIDERATIONS

28.6.1 Postpartum Contraception

As with cisgender patients, heath-care providers should be prepared to provide appropriate and competent postpartum contraception counseling to transgender patients. This counseling should include a discussion about future desire for children and potential birth control methods to prevent unwanted pregnancy from occurring. Studies assessing the birth control use of transgender men have shown a heavy reliance on condoms for the purpose of pregnancy and prevention of sexually transmitted infection (STI).[28, 50] However, transgender men may be interested in other types of birth control, such as long-acting, reversible contraception or hormonal contraception. Prior studies have showed a utilization rate ranging from 3% to 4% in transgender individuals,[28, 50] compared to 12% in the general cisgender female population.[51]

Importantly, transgender men should be told that testosterone alone is not an appropriate method to prevent pregnancy. Similarly, transgender women should be informed that pregnancy is still possible with penetrative penile sex, regardless of hormone use status, and they also should be counseled regarding condom utilization. Ultimately, a patient should be provided with all contraception options, and the physician should respect their choice about contraception, including the decision not to use contraception at all.

28.6.2 Postpartum Depression

As previously discussed, transgender individuals have a higher rate of depression and suicidal ideation than their cisgender peers—a trend that continues in the postpartum period for transgender men.[13, 28] Studies demonstrate that transgender men who undergo pregnancy experience a high rate of postpartum depression. Given that for a transgender person, pregnancy can pose the unique challenge of losing gender identity, it could be beneficial to openly discuss plans for coping strategies throughout the preconception and prenatal processes, and if desired, to help establish care with a mental health professional prior to pregnancy.[13]

28.7 CHEST FEEDING

Lactation is an important topic to consider when caring for transgender men. Many transgender individuals prefer the term *chest feeding* over the more gendered term *breastfeeding*. However, studies have shown that some individuals use other terms, such as *mammal feeding*.[52] As with their cisgender female counterparts, transgender men should be counseled on the benefits of chest feeding. However, clinicians should maintain open communication with these patients and understand that chest feeding may produce worsening gender incongruence and gender dysphoria in transgender men, and their wishes concerning the option should be supported.

Prior studies show high rates of chest feeding in transgender communities, with as many as 51% of transgender men reporting that they had chest-fed after prior pregnancies. Chest feeding is possible both before and after gender-affirming surgeries such as breast reduction (frequently termed *top surgery*), depending on the technique used during the procedure.[52–54] Optimal counseling and education are key to success. As previously mentioned, the current recommendation is to avoid chest feeding while on testosterone.[37] Providers should be familiar with all chest-feeding options in transgender males and begin the counseling process early in order to build mutual trust with patients and provide culturally sensitive and competent care.

28.8 CONCLUSION

Heath-care providers should offer comprehensive, culturally sensitive, and personally directed care to their transgender patients, just as they should for cisgender patients. Providers should be aware of the many nuances regarding gender-affirming hormones, fertility preservation, and reproductive options for transgender patients. Many of these areas are understudied, and so many exciting areas exist for future research regarding transgender reproductive heath care.

REFERENCES

1. Health care for transgender individuals. Committee Opinion No. 512. *Am Coll Obstet Gynecol: Obstet Gynecol* 2011;**118**:1454–8.
2. Alegria CA. Transgender identity and health care: Implications for psychosocial and physical evaluation. *J Am Assoc Nurse Pract* 2011;**23**(4):175–82.
3. Kessler SJ, McKenna W. *Gender: an ethnomethodological approach.* University of Chicago Press; 1978.
4. Hembree WC, Cohen-Kettenis P, Delemarre-Van De Waal HA, Gooren LJ, Meyer III WJ, Spack NP, Tangpricha V, Montori VM. Endocrine treatment of transsexual persons: an Endocrine Society clinical practice guideline. *J Clin Endocrinol Metab* 2009;**94**(9):3132–54.
5. HJ M. *The Fenway guide to lesbian, gay, bisexual, and transgender health.* ACP Press; 2008.
6. Deutsch MB, editor. *Guidelines for the primary and gender-affirming care of transgender and gender nonbinary people.* San Francisco: University of California; 2016.
7. Meerwijk EL, Sevelius JM. Transgender population size in the United States: a meta-regression of population-based probability samples. *Am J Public Health* 2017;**107**(2):e1–8.
8. Grant JM, Mottet L, Tanis JE, Harrison J, Herman J, Keisling M. *Injustice at every turn: a report of the national transgender discrimination survey.* National Center for Transgender Equality; 2011.
9. Safer JD, Coleman E, Feldman J, Garofalo R, Hembree W, Radix A, Sevelius J. Barriers to health care for transgender individuals. *Curr Opin Endocrinol Diab Obes* 2016;**23**(2):168.
10. Coleman E, Bockting W, Botzer M, Cohen-Kettenis P, DeCuypere G, Feldman J, Fraser L, Green J, Knudson G, Meyer WJ, Monstrey S. Standards of care for the health of transsexual, transgender, and gender-nonconforming people, version 7. *Int J Transgender* 2012;**13**(4):165–232.
11. Grant JM, Mottet LA, Tanis J, Herman JL, Harrison J, Keisling M. *National transgender discrimination survey report on health and health care.* Washington, DC: National Center for Transgender Equality and the National Gay and Lesbian Task Force; 2010.
12. Berger AP, Potter EM, Shutters CM, Imborek KL. Pregnant transmen and barriers to high quality healthcare. *Proc Obstet Gynecol* 2015;**5**(2):1–2.
13. Light AD, Zimbrunes SE, Gomez-Lobo V. Reproductive and obstetrical care for transgender patients. *Curr Obstetr Gynecol Rep* 2017;**6**(2):149–55.
14. Meyer III WJ. World Professional Association for Transgender Health's Standards of Care requirements of hormone therapy for adults with gender identity disorder. *Int J Transgender* 2009;**11**(2):127–32.

15. Ethics Committee of the American Society for Reproductive Medicine. Access to fertility services by transgender persons: an Ethics Committee opinion. *Fertil Steril* 2015;**104**(5):1111–5.

16. Chiland C, Clouet AM, Golse B, Guinot M, Wolf JP. A new type of family: transmen as fathers thanks to donor sperm insemination. A 12-year follow-up exploratory study of their children. *Neuropsychiatr Enfance Adolesc* 2013;**61**(6):365–70.

17. Wierckx K, Stuyver I, Weyers S, Hamada A, Agarwal A, De Sutter P, T'Sjoen G. Sperm freezing in transsexual women. *Arch Sex Behav* 2012;**41**(5):1069–71.

18. Pfäfflin F, Bockting WO, Coleman E, Ekins R, King D, Gray NN, Pellett E. The desire to have children and the preservation of fertility in transsexual women: a survey. *Int J Transgender* 2002;**6**(3) 97–03.

19. De Sutter P. Donor inseminations in partners of female-to-male transsexuals: should the question be asked? *Reprod BioMed Online* 2003;**6**(3):382.

20. Strang JF, Jarin J, Call D, Clark B, Wallace GL, Anthony LG, Kenworthy L, Gomez-Lobo V. Transgender youth fertility attitudes questionnaire: measure development in nonautistic and autistic transgender youth and their parents. *J Adolesc Health* 2018;**62**(2):128–35.

21. Olson J, Forbes C, Belzer M. Management of the transgender adolescent. *Arch Pediatr Adolesc Med* 2011;**165**(2):171–6.

22. Hillier SG, Ross GT. Effects of exogenous testosterone on ovarian weight, follicular morphology and intraovarian progesterone concentration in estrogen-primed hypophysectomized immature female rats. *Biol Reprod* 1979;**20**(2):261–8.

23. Goerlich VC, Dijkstra C, Groothuis TG. Effects of in vivo testosterone manipulation on ovarian morphology, follicular development, and follicle yolk testosterone in the homing pigeon. *J Exp Zool A Ecol Genet Physiol* 2010;**313**(6):328–38.

24. van der Spuy ZM, Dyer SJ. The pathogenesis of infertility and early pregnancy loss in polycystic ovary syndrome. *Best Pract Res Clin Obstet Gynaecol* 2004;**18**(5):755–71.

25. Fong SV, Louwers YV. Causes of anovulation: normogonadotropic normoestrogenic anovulation non-PCOS. In: *Ovulation induction: evidence based guidelines for daily practice*vol. 26. ; 2016. p. 4.

26. Perrone AM, Cerpolini S, Maria Salfi NC, Ceccarelli C, De Giorgi LB, Formelli G, Casadio P, Ghi T, Pelusi G, Pelusi C, Meriggiola MC. Effect of long-term testosterone administration on the endometrium of female-to-male (FtM) transsexuals. *J Sex Med* 2009;**6**(11):3193–200.

27. Armuand G, Dhejne C, Olofsson JI, Rodriguez-Wallberg KA. Transgender men's experiences of fertility preservation: a qualitative study. *Hum Reprod* 2017;**32**(2):383–90.

28. Light AD, Obedin-Maliver J, Sevelius JM, Kerns JL. Transgender men who experienced pregnancy after female-to-male gender transitioning. *Obstet Gynecol* 2014;**124**(6):1120–7.

29. Dumasia K, Kumar A, Kadam L, Balasinor NH. Effect of estrogen receptor-subtype-specific ligands on fertility in adult male rats. *J Endocrinol* 2015;**225**(3):169–80.

30. Robaire B, Duron J, Hales BF. Effect of estradiol-filled polydimethylsiloxane subdermal implants in adult male rats on the reproductive system, fertility, and progeny outcome. *Biol Reprod* 1987;**37**(2):327–34.

31. Skakkebaek NE, et al. Is human fecundity declining? *Int J Androl* 2006;**29**(1):2–11.

32. Canada AL, Schover LR. The psychosocial impact of interrupted childbearing in long-term female cancer survivors. *Psychooncology* 2012;**21**:134–43.

33. Armuand GM, Wettergren L, Rodriguez-Wallberg KA, Lampic C. Desire for children, difficulties achieving a pregnancy, and infertility distress 3 to 7 years after cancer diagnosis. *Support Care Cancer* 2014;**22**:2805–12.

34. De Sutter P. Transgender parenthood: gamete preservation and utilization for transgender people. *Méd Thérap Méd Reprod Gynécol Endocrinol* 2016;**18**(2):109–15.

35. De Sutter P. Gender reassignment and assisted reproduction Present and future reproductive options for transsexual people. *Hum Reprod* 2001;**16**(4):612–4.

36. Mitu K. Transgender reproductive choice and fertility preservation. *AMA J Ethics* 2016;**18**(11):1120.

37. Ducheny KM, Ehrbar RD. Family creation options for transgender and gender nonconforming people. *Psychol Sex Orientat Gend Divers* 2016;**3**(2):173.

38. De Roo C, Tilleman K, T'Sjoen G, De Sutter P. Fertility options in transgender people. *Int Rev Psychiatry* 2016;**28**(1):112–9.

39. Bahadur G, Ling KL, Hart R, Ralph D, Riley V, Wafa R, et al. Semen production in adolescent cancer patients. *Hum Reprod* 2002;**17**:2654–6.

40. Eyler AE, Pang SC, Clark A. LGBT assisted reproduction: Current practice and future possibilities. *LGBT Health* 2014;**1**:151–6.

41. Rosenthal SM. Transgender youth: current concepts. *Ann Pediatr Endocrinol Metab* 2016;**21**(4):185–92.

42. American Psychological Association. Guidelines for psychological practice with transgender and gender nonconforming people. *Am Psychol* 2015;**70**:832–64.

43. Nahata L, Tishelman AC, Caltabellotta NM, Quinn GP. Low fertility preservation utilization among transgender youth. *J Adolesc Health* 2017;.

44. Anderson RA, Mitchell RT, Kelsey TW, Spears N, Telfer EE, Wallace WH. Cancer treatment and gonadal function: experimental and established strategies for fertility preservation in children and young adults. *Lancet Diab Endocrinol* 2015;**3**(7):556–67.

45. Salama M, Isachenko V, Isachenko E, Rahimi G, Mallmann P. Updates in preserving reproductive potential of prepubertal girls with cancer: systematic review. *Crit Rev Oncol Hematol* 2016;**103**:10–21.

46. Connolly F, Rae MT, Bittner L, Hogg K, McNeilly AS, Duncan WC. Excess androgens in utero alters fetal testis development. *Endocrinology* 2013;**154**(5):1921–33.

47. Steckler T, Wang J, Bartol FF, Roy SK, Padmanabhan V. Fetal programming: prenatal testosterone treatment causes intrauterine growth retardation, reduces ovarian reserve and increases ovarian follicular recruitment. *Endocrinology* 2005;**146**(7):3185–93.

48. Hoffkling A, Obedin-Maliver J, Sevelius J. From erasure to opportunity: a qualitative study of the experiences of transgender men around pregnancy and recommendations for providers. *BMC Pregnancy Childbirth* 2017;**17**(2):332.

49. Voegtline K, Costigan K, Kivlighan K, Henderson J, DiPietro J. Sex-specific associations of maternal prenatal testosterone levels with birth weight and weight gain in infancy. *J Dev Orig Health Dis* 2013;**4**(4):280–4.

50. Cipres D, Seidman D, Cloniger C, Nova C, O'Shea A, Obedin-Maliver J. Contraceptive use and pregnancy intentions among transgender men presenting to a clinic for sex workers and their families in San Francisco. *Contraception* 2017;**95**(2):186–9.

51. Daniels K, Daugherty JD, Jones J. *Current contraceptive status among women aged 15–44: United States, 2011–2013*. US Department of Health and Human Services, Centers for Disease Control and Prevention, National Center for Health Statistics; 2014.

52. MacDonald T, Noel-Weiss J, West D, Walks M, Biener M, Kibbe A, Myler E. Transmasculine individuals' experiences with lactation, chestfeeding, and gender identity: a qualitative study. *BMC Pregnancy Childbirth* 2016;**16**(1):106.

53. Farrow A. Lactation support and the LGBTQI community. *J Hum Lact* 2015;**31**(1):26–8.

54. Wolfe-Roubatis E, Spatz DL. Transgender men and lactation: what nurses need to know. *MCN Am J Matern Child Nurs* 2015;**40**(1):32–8.

Section 2

The Child

Facing page: *Nourishing Life*

Christopher Kovacs, 2018. 16 x 10.5 inches, watercolor on 300 lb Arches. *Original painting by Christopher Kovacs based with permission on a reference photo by Melisa Chaulk, Happy Valley – Goose Bay, Labrador. The title was suggested by Lisa Dawe.*

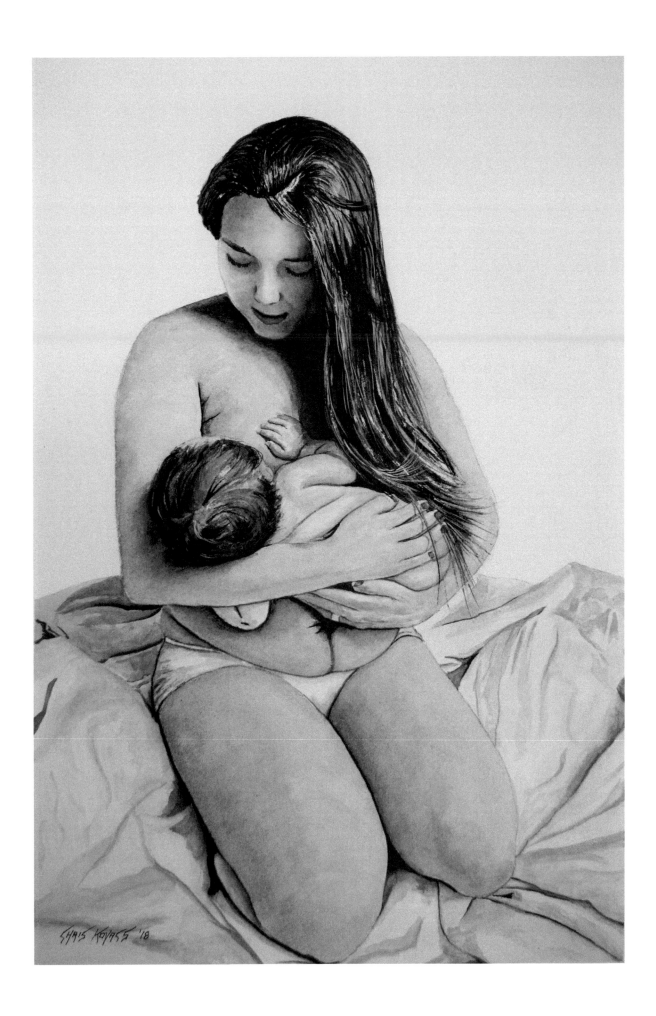

Part D

Normal Endocrine Development and Physiology of the Fetus and Neonate

Chapter 29

Endocrinology of Implantation

Steven L. Young* and Audrey Garneau[†]

*Division of Reproductive Endocrinology and Infertility, Department of Obstetrics and Gynecology and Department of Cell Biology and Physiology, University of North Carolina School of Medicine, Chapel Hill, NC, United States, [†]Department of Obstetrics and Gynecology, University of Kentucky College of Medicine, Lexington, KY, United States

Key Clinical Changes

- Embryo implantation is dependent on the endometrial actions of estradiol and progesterone.
- Estradiol and progesterone induce cellular changes over the menstrual cycle to create a receptive microenvironment that allows apposition, attachment, and invasion of embryo.
- There is an exquisitely complex interplay between the blastocyst and endometrium at implantation, and then a continuingly complex cross-communication as pregnancy progresses.

Normal embryo implantation is the foundation for a successful pregnancy, while abnormalities in implantation appear to underlie infertility, miscarriage, and pregnancy complications, including preeclampsia.[1, 2] The uterine endometrium allows normal implantation during only a few days of the menstrual cycle, which is determined by days of adequate progesterone exposure and response.[2, 3] Blastocyst apposition, attachment, and invasion are optimized further by continued sex steroid action, plus a complex molecular and cellular interchange between the blastocyst and decidualizing endometrium.[4, 5] The factors mediating this interchange include paracrine factors and receptors (e.g., cytokines, chemokines, and growth factors) and extracellular matrix (e.g., collagen and fibronectin), as well the adhesion proteins that bind them (e.g., integrins and selectins). The goal of this chapter is to briefly review the endocrine regulation of embryo implantation, with an emphasis on clinical relevance.

The sequential actions of estradiol (E2) and progesterone (P4) are necessary and sufficient for creating a receptive microenvironment for implantation.[6] Despite the fact that the ovary normally secretes many endocrine factors (aside from E2 and P4, whose cognate receptors are expressed by the endometrium), evidence from oocyte donation cycles in women without ovarian function suggests that excellent endometrial receptivity can be achieved via the provision of only estradiol and progesterone.[7, 8] While the data do not rule out a permissive or minor role for other endocrine factors, the development of endometrial receptivity can be considered simply from the direct and indirect effects of estradiol and progesterone.

The proliferative phase of the menstrual cycle lasts approximately 2 weeks, varying in length from person to person, and is characterized by estrogen secretion from the ovarian follicle. Estrogen (primarily E2) acts on the endometrium to promote the proliferation of both stromal and epithelial cells, expression of both estrogen and progesterone receptors, and endometrial neoangiogenesis. It should be noted that the endometrial basalis responds differently to estrogen and progesterone than does the functionalis layer.[9] However, the basalis is not thought to be an important determinant of embryo implantation, and only the functionalis will considered further in this chapter.

Following ovulation, the corpus luteum secretes both progesterone and estrogen to drive the endometrium's much more temporally constrained secretory phase. Progesterone drives the secretory changes characteristic of this phase, although continued estradiol is likely permissive and very low circulating levels appear completely sufficient.[10, 11] Secretory phase changes include formation and secretion of secretory vacuoles, arrest of epithelial proliferation, immune cell composition changes, increased stroma edema, and coiling of spiral arteries.[12, 13] These changes reflect molecular and cellular alterations that result in a short period of embryo receptivity. Given these essential actions of both estrogen and progesterone, it is important to consider the mechanisms by which these steroidal hormones exert their effects.

Maternal-Fetal and Neonatal Endocrinology. https://doi.org/10.1016/B978-0-12-814823-5.00029-5

Estrogen exerts its effects via highly specific cognate receptors. There are two major types estrogen receptors, ERα and ERβ. Both primarily act as ligand-activated nuclear transcription factors, and each is generated from transcription of a distinct gene (*ESR1* and *ESR2*, respectively). Alternative promoters and splicing allow the generation of multiple mRNA variants that can code for alternate receptor isoforms, although the physiological significance of these alternative isoforms remains unclear. Estrogen can also signal via a G-protein-coupled membrane receptor and a membrane-tethered, palmitoylated ERα. However, physiological actions of estradiol membrane signaling in the endometrium seem largely to augment the canonical nuclear signaling pathway. Overwhelmingly, the most abundant and important receptor for estrogen action on the human endometrium is ERα, and it is likely that nuclear actions of the dominant ERα isoform, by themselves, are sufficient for normal endometrial cyclic development.[14]

The endometrial expression of ERα varies dynamically across the cycle. Epithelial ERα expression increases in response to estrogen in the proliferative phase and then decreases in response to progesterone during the period of receptivity to embryo implantation—not only in humans, but in all placental species studied.[15] In the stromal cells, estrogen induces the production of extracellular matrix proteins and growth factors that act in a paracrine fashion to stimulate epithelial proliferation during the proliferative phase.[16, 17]

Conversely, abnormally increased expression of epithelial ERα during the midsecretory phase in women has been associated with infertility, polycystic ovarian syndrome (PCOS), and endometriosis.[15] Additionally, abnormally increased expression of ERα in the secretory phase has been associated with decreased expression of beta 3 integrin subunit and glycodelin-A, both important, progesterone-regulated markers of endometrial receptivity (*infra vide*),[15] suggesting reciprocal effects of E2 and P4 in the human endometrial epithelium. The cross-species concordance of endometrial epithelial ERα suppression and association between persistent ERα expression and infertility strongly suggests a fundamental role for ERα downregulation in embryo implantation; however, the precise mechanism by which progesterone suppresses epithelial ERα expression remains unknown.

Very low levels of circulating estradiol are sufficient for normal secretory phase function,[7, 8, 10, 11] However, evidence in mice supports an important role for endometrial estradiol production, independent of corpus luteum production as necessary to support endometrial stromal decidualization,[18] which is a necessary step for normal implantation. A role for locally produced estrogens in human endometrial stromal decidualization remains possible, but uncertain.[19] However, an important role for human endometrial estrogen metabolism during decidualization has recently been suggested,[20] indicating that estrogens also may play a role in human endometrial stromal cell function at the time of embryo implantation.

Progesterone, initially produced in large amounts by the corpus luteum after ovulation and later by the placenta, is the critical hormone that allows early pregnancy to survive and thrive. It directs the luminal epithelium to a state that will facilitate trophoblast adhesion and invasion, and the glandular epithelium to produce uterine fluid (histiotroph) that contains factors important for the survival and growth of the early embryo.[21] Furthermore, progesterone acts to halt endometrial epithelial proliferation, suppress expression of epithelial PR and ER, alter blood vessel morphology, expand a specific population of NK cells, and decidualize endometrial stromal cells, all of which are important to implantation.

Progesterone, the key pregnancy hormone, was first isolated by assessing its endometrial effects on the survival of embryos in ovariectomized rabbits, which had very low levels of endogenous estradiol.[22] Furthermore, removal of progesterone by luteectomy,[23] or pharmacological antagonism of progesterone action by mifepristone in early pregnancy, results in pregnancy loss.[24] Given the fundamental and necessary contribution of progesterone to embryo implantation and early pregnancy, it is important to consider the mechanisms of action of progesterone on the endometrium.

Progesterone receptors, like estrogen receptors, are ligand-regulated nuclear transcription factors that alter gene expression by binding directly to specific DNA sequences. There are two isoforms of the progesterone receptor, PRA and PRB, which are encoded by the same gene but utilize different promoters and translation start sites. PRB has an additional 164 amino acids at the amino terminus, which allows it to regulate more transcription factors. The two isoforms may homodimerize or heterodimerize, allowing altered actions in different cells or under different conditions.[25] In the human endometrium, PRB expression predominates in the epithelium, while PRA is more abundant in the stroma. Much like the estrogen receptors, the predominant effects of progesterone receptors occur via binding directly to cognate DNA elements in gene promoters, but progesterone receptors may also act in the cytoplasm by directly modulating cytoplasmic signaling pathways (Fig. 29.1). For example, progesterone receptor can interact directly with the Src tyrosine kinase SH3 domain to activate Ras/mitogen-activated protein kinase (MAPK) signaling.[25]

PR is necessary for embryo implantation and decidualization, as demonstrated by experimental disruption of the progesterone receptor gene in mice.[25] There are many mechanisms by which progesterone induces endometrial receptivity, including direct transcriptional effects of progesterone via its receptors, as well as indirect autocrine and paracrine actions. In humans, direct epithelial actions of progesterone that allow embryo attachment and invasion occur before implantation. Progesterone decreases claudin expression, resulting in reduced tight junctions, which in turn reduce the endometrium's

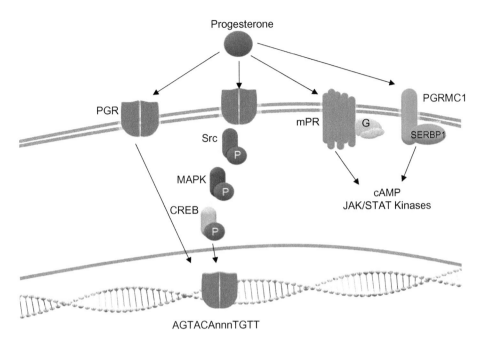

FIG. 29.1 Progesterone signaling complexity. Progesterone can act via rapid nonclassical signaling via various membrane progesterone receptors, or via classical nuclear signaling by the progesterone receptor. Nonclassical signaling may occur through many signaling pathways, including protooncogene tyrosine-protein kinase Src (SRC), cyclic AMP (cAMP), p42/44 MAPK; cAMP response element-binding protein (CREB); Janus-kinase/STAT signaling (JAK/STAT). *PGR*, progesterone receptor (composed of PRA or PRB homodimers or a heterodimer); *mPR*, membrane progesterone receptor; *PGRMC1*, progesterone receptor membrane component 1; *G*, G-protein-signaling complex; *AGTACAnnTGTT*, consensus DNA-binding site for PR; *SERBP1*, plasminogen activator inhibitor 1 RNA-binding protein.

barrier function, promoting invasion.[21] In the stromal compartment, progesterone drives decidualization, a critical mesenchymal-to-epithelial transition, via a number of mechanisms. Progesterone has direct stromal effects, but it also acts via epithelial-to-stromal communication. Direct stromal effects are mediated by the Jun dimerization protein 2 (JPD-2), FOSL1, and activator protein-1 (AP-1).[26] Progesterone acts indirectly on stroma via the induction of epithelial Indian hedgehog protein (IHH), which induces stromal chicken ovalbumin upstream transcription factor II (COUP-TFII), which in turn induces a number of signals that further drive endometrial decidualization.[27]

At the cellular ultrastructural level, progesterone induces the formation of endometrial epithelial pinopodes when the microvilli of surface nonciliated epithelial cells fuse laterally. These unusual structures may aid blastocyst apposition by absorbing uterine fluid, or they may exert direct actions via adhesion proteins. Pinopodes also lack antiadhesive mucins, such as MUC16, which may represent a structural barrier to apposition and adhesion.[28]

As the secretory phase progresses, epithelial progesterone receptor protein abundance is dramatically reduced, especially in the luminal and more superficial glands. Therefore, by the time embryo implantation begins, progesterone effects on the epithelium may occur primarily via paracrine stroma to epithelial actions. The luminal epithelial disappearance of PR itself, promoted by progesterone via poorly understood mechanisms, is critical to murine embryo implantation.[29] The similarities in loss of PR in endometrial luminal epithelium in humans (and other species) suggest a similar importance for PR loss across placental species.

Progesterone-induced cellular changes in the endometrial epithelial cells also seem to be vital, including loss of luminal mucins, increased apical expression of adhesion proteins, such as alphav-beta 3 integrin, and secretion of leukemia inhibiting factor (LIF), all of which play important roles in allowing implantation.[13] LIF promotes the apposition and adhesion of blastocysts, and recurrent pregnancy loss has been associated with decreased secretion of it.[30] Expression of S100P, a calcium-binding protein that is upregulated by progesterone, during the window of implantation is about 100 times higher than in other parts of the menstrual cycle,[31] and it increases 37-fold when cultured with trophoblasts; this suggests its involvement in embryo-uterine communication.[31] Many other progesterone-induced factors likely play a role in early implantation events,[4] but they are too numerous to discuss here, and much of the data are based on mouse models, with human function uncertain.

Optimal receptivity occurs in the midluteal phase at the peak of endometrial secretory activity and cyclic progesterone production. The first phase of implantation, apposition, occurs first as an unstable adhesion of blastocyst to the uterine wall, with increasing communication between the endometrium and the blastocyst enabled by soluble factors, including growth factors and chemokines. Chemokines attract invasive trophoblasts to the decidua.[32] As a complement to endometrial chemokines, the trophectoderm expresses specific chemokine receptors, which likely regulate trophoblast migration and invasion. Interferon-γ induced protein 10 is one such molecule that is secreted by endometrial stromal and glandular cells.[32] It is the ligand for the chemokine receptor CXCR3 expressed on the trophectoderm and IP-10 has been shown to function directly upon blastocyst attraction.[32] It is secreted in gradually increasing levels as the embryo develops to the blastocyst stage, and subsequently promotes blastocyst hatching and trophoblast proliferation.[33] Conversely, trophoblast cells produce CXCL12, which acts on the endometrial cell receptor, CXCR4, to promote trophoblast invasion.[34] Endometrial heparin-binding epidermal growth factor (HB-EGF) expression by luminal epithelial cells is induced at the site of apposition by the blastocyst in mice[35] and induced by progesterone in humans.[36] HB-EGF may function as an adhesion factor for blastocyst attachment and induces complement-protective proteins expressed by the endometrium.[37]

Human chorionic gonadotropin (hCG) plays a critical role in early recognition of pregnancy and deserves mention as an endocrine factor. In human pregnancies, hCG is secreted by blastocysts 7–8 days after fertilization, and mRNA is found as early as 3 days after fertilization.[38] The early production of hCG may act regionally to stimulate the corpus luteum and cause production of higher levels of serum estradiol and progesterone that can be measured prior to measurable amounts of serum hCG. Human syncitiotrophoblasts produce massive amounts of hCG that enter maternal circulation after trophoblast invasion to maintain the corpus luteal production of progesterone until the trophoblasts produce enough progesterone to maintain pregnancy at about 9 weeks. Unless rescued by hCG, the corpus luteum has an average life span of 14.2 days.[38] Removal of the corpus luteum, or lack of corpus luteum in the setting of assisted reproduction, requires progesterone supplementation to prevent abortion.

There is an exquisitely complex interplay between the blastocyst and endometrium at implantation, and then a continuously complex cross-regulation as pregnancy progresses. Given the difficulty of observing human embryo implantation directly, most of our knowledge comes from rodent models, animals whose hormonal cycles (i.e., estrous) differ greatly from those of humans (i.e., menstruation). However, assisted reproduction has given an important window into the larger picture regarding estrogen and progesterone regulation of early pregnancy in women, and technological advances are beginning to bridge the gaps between animal models and humans, which may allow us to identify problems with embryo implantation to improve pregnancy outcomes.

REFERENCES

1. Conrad KP, Rabaglino MB, Post Uiterweer ED. Emerging role for dysregulated decidualization in the genesis of preeclampsia. *Placenta* 2017;**60**:119–29.

2. Garrido-Gomez T, Dominguez F, Quinonero A, Diaz-Gimeno P, Kapidzic M, Gormley M, et al. Defective decidualization during and after severe preeclampsia reveals a possible maternal contribution to the etiology. *Proc Natl Acad Sci U S A* 2017;**114**(40):E8468–77.

3. Prapas Y, Prapas N, Jones EE, Duleba AJ, Olive DL, Chatziparasidou A, et al. The window for embryo transfer in oocyte donation cycles depends on the duration of progesterone therapy. *Hum Reprod* 1998;**13**(3):720–3.

4. Namiki T, Ito J, Kashiwazaki N. Molecular mechanisms of embryonic implantation in mammals: lessons from the gene manipulation of mice. *Reprod Med Biol* 2018;**17**(4):331–42.

5. Paria BC, Song H, Dey SK. Implantation: molecular basis of embryo-uterine dialogue. *Int J Dev Biol* 2001;**45**(3):597–605.

6. Young SL. Oestrogen and progesterone action on endometrium: a translational approach to understanding endometrial receptivity. *Reprod BioMed Online* 2013;**27**(5):497–505.

7. Budak E, Garrido N, Soares SR, Melo MA, Meseguer M, Pellicer A, et al. Improvements achieved in an oocyte donation program over a 10-year period: sequential increase in implantation and pregnancy rates and decrease in high-order multiple pregnancies. *Fertil Steril* 2007;**88**(2):342–9.

8. Younis JS, Simon A, Laufer N. Endometrial preparation: lessons from oocyte donation. *Fertil Steril* 1996;**66**(6):873–84.

9. Slayden OD, Brenner RM. Hormonal regulation and localization of estrogen, progestin and androgen receptors in the endometrium of nonhuman primates: effects of progesterone receptor antagonists. *Arch Histol Cytol* 2004;**67**(5):393–409.

10. Groll JM, Usadi RS, Lessey BA, Lininger R, Young SL, Fritz MA. Effects of variations in serum estradiol concentrations on secretory endometrial development and function in experimentally induced cycles in normal women. *Fertil Steril* 2009;**92**(6):2058–61.

11. Jee BC, Suh CS, Kim SH, Kim YB, Moon SY. Effects of estradiol supplementation during the luteal phase of in vitro fertilization cycles: a meta-analysis. *Fertil Steril* 2010;**93**(2):428–36.

12. Young SL, Loy T. Normal cycling endometrium: molecular, cellular, and histologic perspectives. In: Olive DL, editor. *Endometriosis in clinical practice*; 2004. p. 1–12.

13. Lessey BA, Young SL. The structure, funciton, and evaluation of the female reproductive tract. In: *Yen and Jaffe's reproductive endocrinology: physiology, pathophysiology, and clinical mangement*. Elsevier; 2013.

14. Hewitt SC, Korach KS. Estrogen receptors: new directions in the new millennium. *Endocr Rev* 2018;**39**(5):664–75.

15. Dorostghoal M, Ghaffari HO, Marmazi F, Keikhah N. Overexpression of endometrial estrogen receptor-alpha in the window of implantation in women with unexplained infertility. *Int J Fertil Steril* 2018;**12**(1):37–42.

16. Cooke PS, Uchima FD, Fujii DK, Bern HA, Cunha GR. Restoration of normal morphology and estrogen responsiveness in cultured vaginal and uterine epithelia transplanted with stroma. *Proc Natl Acad Sci U S A* 1986;**83**(7):2109–13.

17. Winuthayanon W, Lierz SL, Delarosa KC, Sampels SR, Donoghue LJ, Hewitt SC, et al. Juxtacrine activity of estrogen receptor alpha in uterine stromal cells is necessary for estrogen-induced epithelial cell proliferation. *Sci Rep* 2017;**7**(1):8377.

18. Das A, Mantena SR, Kannan A, Evans DB, Bagchi MK, Bagchi IC. De novo synthesis of estrogen in pregnant uterus is critical for stromal decidualization and angiogenesis. *Proc Natl Acad Sci U S A* 2009;**106**(30):12542–7.

19. Gibson DA, McInnes KJ, Critchley HO, Saunders PT. Endometrial intracrinology—generation of an estrogen-dominated microenvironment in the secretory phase of women. *J Clin Endocrinol Metab* 2013;**98**(11):E1802–6.

20. Gibson DA, Simitsidellis I, Collins F, Saunders PTK. Endometrial intracrinology: oestrogens, androgens and endometrial disorders. *Int J Mol Sci* 2018;**19**(10).

21. Grund S, Grummer R. Direct cell(−)cell interactions in the endometrium and in endometrial pathophysiology. *Int J Mol Sci* 2018;**19**(8):2227.

22. Allen WM. Recollections of my life with progesterone. *Gynecol Investig* 1974;**5**(3):142–82.

23. Csapo AI, Pulkkinen M. Indispensability of the human corpus luteum in the maintenance of early pregnancy. Luteectomy evidence. *Obstet Gynecol Surv* 1978;**33**(2):69–81.

24. Kahn JG, Becker BJ, MacIsaa L, Amory JK, Neuhaus J, Olkin I, et al. The efficacy of medical abortion: a meta-analysis. *Contraception* 2000;**61**(1):29–40.

25. Wetendorf M, DeMayo FJ. The progesterone receptor regulates implantation, decidualization, and glandular development via a complex paracrine signaling network. *Mol Cell Endocrinol* 2012;**357**(1–2):108–18.

26. Mazur EC, Vasquez YM, Li X, Kommagani R, Jiang L, Chen R, et al. Progesterone receptor transcriptome and cistrome in decidualized human endometrial stromal cells. *Endocrinology* 2015;**156**(6):2239–53.

27. Wang X, Li X, Wang T, Wu SP, Jeong JW, Kim TH, et al. SOX17 regulates uterine epithelial-stromal cross-talk acting via a distal enhancer upstream of Ihh. *Nat Commun* 2018;**9**(1):4421.

28. Gipson IK, Blalock T, Tisdale A, Spurr-Michaud S, Allcorn S, Stavreus-Evers A, et al. MUC16 is lost from the uterodome (pinopode) surface of the receptive human endometrium: in vitro evidence that MUC16 is a barrier to trophoblast adherence. *Biol Reprod* 2008;**78**(1):134–42.

29. Wetendorf M, Wu SP, Wang X, Creighton CJ, Wang T, Lanz RB, et al. Decreased epithelial progesterone receptor A at the window of receptivity is required for preparation of the endometrium for embryo attachment. *Biol Reprod* 2017;**96**(2):313–26.

30. Norwitz ER, Schust DJ, Fisher SJ. Implantation and the survival of early pregnancy. *N Engl J Med* 2001;**345**(19):1400–8.

31. Zhang D, Ma C, Sun X, Xia H, Zhang W. S100P expression in response to sex steroids during the implantation window in human endometrium. *Reprod Biol Endocrinol* 2012;**10**:106.

32. Sela HY, Goldman-Wohl DS, Haimov-Kochman R, Greenfield C, Natanson-Yaron S, Hamani Y, et al. Human trophectoderm apposition is regulated by interferon gamma-induced protein 10 (IP-10) during early implantation. *Placenta* 2013;**34**(3):222–30.

33. Niringiyumukiza JD, Cai H, Xiang W. Prostaglandin E2 involvement in mammalian female fertility: ovulation, fertilization, embryo development and early implantation. *Reprod Biol Endocrinol* 2018;**16**(1):43.

34. Ren L, Liu YQ, Zhou WH, Zhang YZ. Trophoblast-derived chemokine CXCL12 promotes CXCR4 expression and invasion of human first-trimester decidual stromal cells. *Hum Reprod* 2012;**27**(2):366–74.

35. Das SK, Wang XN, Paria BC, Damm D, Abraham JA, Klagsbrun M, et al. Heparin-binding EGF-like growth factor gene is induced in the mouse uterus temporally by the blastocyst solely at the site of its apposition: a possible ligand for interaction with blastocyst EGF-receptor in implantation. *Development* 1994;**120**(5):1071–83.

36. Lessey BA, Gui Y, Apparao KB, Young SL, Mulholland J. Regulated expression of heparin-binding EGF-like growth factor (HB-EGF) in the human endometrium: a potential paracrine role during implantation. *Mol Reprod Dev* 2002;**62**(4):446–55.

37. Young SL, Lessey BA, Fritz MA, Meyer WR, Murray MJ, Speckman PL, et al. In vivo and in vitro evidence suggest that HB-EGF regulates endometrial expression of human decay-accelerating factor. *J Clin Endocrinol Metab* 2002;**87**(3):1368–75.

38. Mesen TB, Young SL. Progesterone and the luteal phase: a requisite to reproduction. *Obstet Gynecol Clin N Am* 2015;**42**(1):135–51.

Chapter 30

Normal Hypothalamic and Pituitary Development and Physiology in the Fetus and Neonate

Harshini Katugampola*,†, Manuela Cerbone*,† and Mehul T. Dattani*,†

*Great Ormond Street Hospital for Children NHS Foundation Trust, London, United Kingdom, †University College London Great Ormond Street Institute of Child Health, London, United Kingdom

Key Clinical Changes

- The hypothalamus, pituitary stalk, and posterior pituitary are mostly developed by 7 weeks' gestation, and at this time, the floor of the sella turcica is evident.
- Hypothalamic neurons containing the somatostatin (SS), growth hormone–releasing hormone (GHRH), thyrotropin-releasing hormone (TRH), and gonadotropin-releasing hormone (GnRH) are present by 10–14 weeks' gestation.
- Maturation of the pituitary portal vascular system continues and becomes functional by 30–35 weeks' gestation when there is portal vascular extension into the hypothalamus.
- Parvocellular hypothalamic neurons secrete hypophysiotrophic hormones that stimulate the release of the seven anterior/intermediate pituitary lobe hormones via the hypophyseal portal system.
- Parvocellular neurons also secrete oxytocin (OT) and arginine-vasopressin (AVP), although at much lower concentrations than the magnocellular neurons.

30.1 INTRODUCTION: THE HYPOTHALAMO-PITUITARY NEUROENDOCRINE AXIS

In postnatal life, the neuroendocrine network between the hypothalamus and the pituitary gland is responsible for the regulation of essential functions such as growth, puberty, reproduction, salt and water balance, stress response, metabolism and homeostasis, behavior, and superior cognitive functions. This network of neurovascular and endocrine structures lies deep within the brain parenchyma. The pituitary gland is located in a bony cavity known as the sella turcica, with the hypothalamus lying superior to this and below the thalamus and formed by a dense conglomeration of nuclei.

The hypothalamus is the master regulatory structure of vital neuroendocrine networks linking the central nervous system (CNS) to the endocrine system via the pituitary gland. To display these functions, the hypothalamus is highly connected to other brain structures (such as the cerebral cortex, brainstem, reticular formation, limbic system, and autonomic nervous system) by numerous axonal projections, and to the pituitary gland by the infundibulum (pituitary stalk), which forms a critical structural connection. The hypothalamus regulates the anterior pituitary gland by secreting stimulatory and inhibitory releasing peptide hormones into the capillary plexus in the median eminence, where they are carried to the pituitary via the hypothalamo-hypophyseal portal vascular system. Magnocellular neurons from the paraventricular and supraoptic nuclei of the hypothalamus have direct axonal projections to the posterior pituitary and are responsible for the synthesis of oxytocin (OT) and arginine-vasopressin (AVP), also known as antidiuretic hormone (ADH). Both the portal system and the axonal projections are carried to the pituitary gland via the infundibulum.

The mature pituitary gland consists of the adenohypophysis (anterior and intermediate lobes) and neurohypophysis (posterior lobe). The adenohypophysis consists of six cell types: somatotrophs [growth hormone (GH)], lactotrophs [prolactin (PRL)], gonadotrophs [luteinizing hormone (LH) and follicle-stimulating hormone (FSH)], corticotrophs [adrenocorticotrophic hormone (ACTH)], thyrotrophs [thyroid-stimulating hormone (TSH)], melanotrophs [α-melanocyte-stimulating hormone (α-MSH) and β-endorphins, both breakdown products of pro-opiomelanocortin (POMC)]. By adulthood,

Maternal-Fetal and Neonatal Endocrinology. https://doi.org/10.1016/B978-0-12-814823-5.00030-1

527

the intermediate lobe, where melanotrophs are largely located, involutes and is avascular.[1] The neurohypophysis contains the termini of hypothalamic axonal projections, which secrete AVP and OT directly into the bloodstream via the surrounding capillary network.

The fetal hypothalamo-pituitary (H-P) neuroendocrine axis develops early in gestation and plays an important modulating role in the various fetal physiological organ systems and prepares the fetus for life after birth. This neuroendocrine system is greatly affected by the placenta, which functions as a unique endocrine system during pregnancy and parturition.

This chapter covers the normal endocrine development of the hypothalamus and the pituitary gland in the fetus and the neonate.

30.2   NORMAL DEVELOPMENT OF THE HYPOTHALAMUS AND PITUITARY (ADENOHYPOPHYSIS AND NEUROHYPOPHYSIS)

The pituitary gland has a dual embryonic origin: the anterior and intermediate lobes derive from oral ectoderm, and the posterior pituitary from neural ectoderm.[2-5] Normal pituitary development is highly reliant on the close apposition and communication between these layers,[5,6] and is linked to the development of the hypothalamus. The formation and function of these organs are dependent upon the sequential temporospatial expression of a cascade of signaling molecules and transcription factors that play a crucial role in organ commitment, cell proliferation, patterning, and terminal differentiation (Fig. 30.1). Although direct evidence for the processes involved in pituitary development in humans is lacking, the process is highly conserved across all vertebrate species, including zebrafish, amphibians, chicks, and rodents,[7-10] and development of the mouse pituitary, in particular, is well characterized.[6]

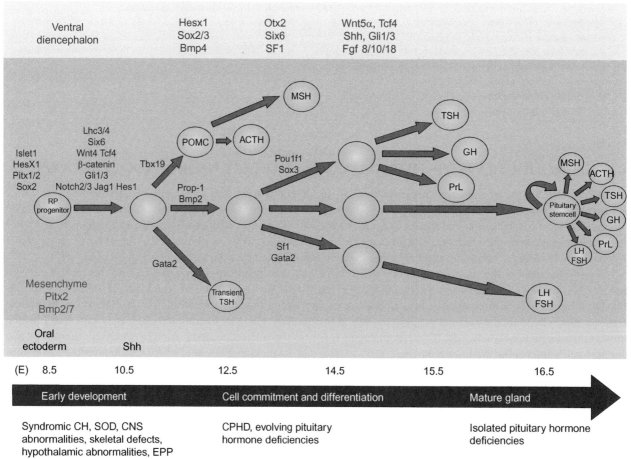

FIG. 30.1   Schematic representation of the developmental cascade of transcription factors and signaling molecules involved in anterior pituitary development. (Taken from Kelberman D, Rizzoti K, Lovell-Badge R, Robinson IC, Dattani M. Genetic regulation of pituitary gland development in human and mouse. Endocr Rev 2009;30(7):790–829.)

The onset of pituitary organogenesis corresponds to 4–6 weeks' gestation in humans. The anterior pituitary is derived from the hypophyseal or pituitary placode, one of six cranial placodes that appear transiently as localized ectodermal thickenings. In the mouse, the pituitary placode appears at embryonic day (E) 7.5. It is located ventrally in the midline of the anterior neural ridge, in continuity with the region located posteriorly in the rostral part of the neural plate that will give rise to the developing hypothalamus and infundibulum. By E8.5, the neural tube bends at the cephalic end, and the pituitary placode is seen as a thickening of the roof of the primitive oral cavity. Invagination of the placode occurs at E9.0 to form the rudimentary Rathke's pouch, and it is from there that the anterior and intermediate lobes of the adenohypophysis develop. By E10.5, Rathke's pouch folds on itself, closing off, and the neural ectoderm located at the base of the developing diencephalon evaginates, giving rise to the posterior pituitary. Proliferation of epithelium occurs between E10.5 and E12.0, and at E12.5, it detaches from the oral cavity, forming the definitive Rathke's pouch. Between E12.5 and E17.5, hormone-secreting progenitor cell types proliferate ventrally from Rathke's pouch to populate the future anterior lobe of the pituitary. The intermediate lobe is formed from the remnants of the dorsal portion of the pouch. The lumen of the pouch persists as the pituitary cleft, separating the two lobes of the adenohypophysis.

In tandem, at E9.5, the hypothalamic primordium becomes morphologically distinct in the neural ectoderm. Hypothalamic neurogenesis is evident at E10, concurrent with the highest expression of genes such as *Arx, Sim1, Sim2,* and *Nr5a1,* which are important for regional patterning of hypothalamic progenitor cells. This process is complete by E16, but the expression of markers of hypothalamic terminal differentiation peaks postnatally.

The posterior lobe comprises axonal projections of neurons, which originate from hypothalamic magnocellular bodies (namely, the supraoptic, suprachiasmatic, and araventricular nuclei). The former two release AVP and the latter releases OT.[11] The neurons traverse the pituitary stalk and median eminence at the base of the hypothalamus.

Differentiation of hormone-producing cells is regulated in a temporospatial manner in the developing pituitary. Transient expression of α-glycoprotein subunit (αGSU, encoded by *Cga*) at E11.5 in a small population of cells located ventrally in Rathke's pouch is one of the earliest markers of anterior pituitary cell differentiation. These cells also express the transcription factor Islet-1 (*Isl1*) and differentiate at E12.5 to prospective thyrotrophs by initiating the expression of TSH subunit-β (*Tshβ*). Definitive thyrotrophs, characterized by *Tshβ* expression, are detected by E14.5. The expression of *Pomc* is the hallmark of corticotroph differentiation, which begins at E12.5, dorsal to the prospective thyrotrophs. By E15.5, the expression of *Gh* in prospective somatotrophs and *Prl* in lactotrophs is seen. Lactotrophs appear anterolaterally in the developing pituitary and proliferate and migrate by E18.5 to the medial zone, adjacent to the ventral surface of the intermediate lobe. Gonadotrophs are the last cell lineage to appear, at E16.5, heralded by expression of the β subunit of LH (*lhβ*) and followed by FSH (*fshb*) a day later.

Birth-dating studies suggest earlier specification of hormone-producing cells, challenging the classical description of sequential differentiation and supporting the concept of plasticity of the pituitary.[12] The structural organization of these cells within the pituitary appears carefully coordinated, with structural and functional homotypic networks forming, which enable synchronized, functional responses to stimuli. For example, the organization of lactotrophs increases their connection and communication, resulting in increased hormone production and also enabling the development of "memory," wherein augmented hormone output is maintained during a second lactation.[13]

The identification of *Sox2*-positive pituitary progenitor (stem) cells in the cleft of the developing and adult pituitary has been seminal in unraveling some of the complexities of pituitary development. These cells form pituispheres *in vitro* and can be induced to differentiate into any pituitary lineage, as demonstrated by the generation of a functional, three-dimensional (3D) anterior pituitary from mouse embryonic stem (ES) cells placed in culture conditions and exposed to various induction factors.[14] Pituitary stem cells generate hormone-producing cells not only during embryonic development, but also adulthood, thereby contributing to pituitary homeostasis. They are implicated in potential regenerative processes of the pituitary and also are able to act in a non-cell-autonomous manner to induce oncogenesis.

30.2.1 Genes Involved in Pituitary Development

Complex genetic interactions dictate normal pituitary development.[6] The development of the anterior pituitary is dependent upon a cascade of extrinsic and intrinsic transcription factors and signaling molecules that are expressed in a temporospatial manner (Fig. 30.1). Extrinsic molecules from the ventral diencephalon [bone morphogenetic protein-4 (BMP4)], fibroblast growth factor-8 (FGF8), fibroblast growth factor-4 (FGF4), NKX2-1, WNT5A, oral ectoderm [sonic hedgehog (SHH)], surrounding mesenchyme [bone morphogenetic protein-2 (BMP2), Indian hedgehog (IHH), chordin], and the pouch itself (BMP2, WNT4) create a network of signaling gradients, which plays a crucial role in organ commitment, cell proliferation, cell patterning, and terminal differentiation. The final product is a culmination of this coordinated process (Fig. 30.1).

Cells within the primordium of the pituitary gland are initially able to differentiate into all cell types. Following expression of the earliest markers of pituitary gland development, such as the homeobox gene expressed in ES cells (*Hesx1*), further signaling pathways direct these cells toward terminal differentiation. Genes expressed early are implicated in organ commitment, but they also are implicated in the repression and activation of downstream target genes that play specific roles in directing the cells toward a particular fate.

30.2.1.1 Morphogenetic Signals (BMPs, FGFs, SHH, Wnt/β-Catenin Pathway)

The induction and maintenance of Rathke's pouch depend on the expression of BMP4 and FGF8. BMP4, detected in the prospective infundibulum from E8.5–E14.5, is the earliest secreted molecule. Following this, FGF8 and other members of the FGF family (e.g., *Fgf1*, *Fgf18*) are expressed in the diencephalon from E9.5.[5,15,16] FGF signaling is important for cell proliferation within the pouch and the activation of LIM homeobox 3 (*Lhx3*) and 4 (*Lhx4*), which is essential for development of the definitive pouch.[3,17]

SHH and its downstream signaling pathway of activators (GLI2) or repressors (GLI3) are also important for the patterning, specification, and expansion of ventral cell types. *Shh* is expressed in the ventral diencephalon until E14.9, as well as the oral ectoderm; its expression is excluded from Rathke's pouch as soon as the pouch appears. A number of Wnt family members (WNT4, WNT5A) and components of the downstream signaling pathway (β-catenin) are expressed within Rathke's pouch, diencephalon, and the surrounding tissues.[18] Members of the Wnt/β-catenin signaling pathway interact with other early transcription factors (SOX2[19] and SOX3[20]), and these interactions are important for numerous developmental processes, including those of the pituitary.

30.2.1.2 Early Transcription Factors

Hesx1, a member of the paired-like class of homeobox genes, is one of the earliest markers of the pituitary primordium. *Hesx1* is a transcriptional repressor and its downregulation is important for downstream activation of *Prop1* and the emergence of the *Pou1f1* cell lineage (somatotrophs, thyrotrophs, and lactotrophs).[3] The simultaneous repression of *Hesx1* and activation of *Pou1f1* is mediated by the direct interaction between β-catenin and PROP1.[21] From E9.0-9.5, *Hesx1* expression is restricted to the ventral diencephalon and Rathke's pouch, and it gradually disappears in a temporospatial sequence that corresponds to progressive pituitary cell differentiation, becoming undetectable by E15.5.[3,22]

The LIM family of homeobox genes includes *Lhx3*, *Lhx4*, and *Lhx2*. *Lhx3* is one of the earliest transcription factors expressed in Rathke's pouch (E9.5), as well as the developing anterior and intermediate pituitary (E16.5), but not in the posterior lobe; its expression persists into adulthood. *Lhx3* is important for the establishment of hormone-producing cell types and the maintenance of at least some cell types in the mature pituitary.[23] *Lhx4* is also expressed in Rathke's pouch and is downregulated by E15.5. In addition, *Lhx4* is expressed in areas of the developing hindbrain, cerebral cortex, and motor neurons of the spinal cord.[23,24] More recently, *Lhx2* was shown to be expressed in the diencephalon and posterior lobe.[25]

The SOX family of transcription factors is characterized by the presence of a 79-amino-acid, high-mobility group (HMG) deoxyribonucleic acid (DNA)-binding domain. *Sox2* and *Sox3* are two of the earliest markers in neuronal determination, and expression of these is seen throughout the developing CNS. During pituitary development, *Sox3* is expressed in the ventral diencephalon and infundibulum, but not in Rathke's pouch. *Sox2* expression in the developing murine CNS is seen in sensory placodes, inner ear, cochlea, lens, retina, and optic nerve. By E11.5, *Sox2* is expressed uniformly in Rathke's pouch and the infundibulum, and expression persists in a small population of cells lining the pituitary cleft of the adult murine pituitary. These cells maintain their potential to proliferate and differentiate into all pituitary cell types, representing a progenitor/stem cell pool.

Members of the T-cell factor/lymphoid enhancer factor (TCF/LEF) family are major targets for interaction with β-catenin. In addition, they have a β-catenin-interacting domain at their N-terminus.[26]

30.2.1.3 Terminal Cell Differentiation

Although corticotrophs are the first cell type to reach terminal differentiation, little is known about the factors that determine their specification and the control of POMC expression. At E12.5, corticotrophs begin differentiation, producing POMC. The transcription factor *Tbx19* (*T-pit*) is expressed in corticotrophs and melanotrophs and, along with *Pitx1*, *Tbx19* activates the *Pomc* promoter.[27,28] More recently, *Pax7* has been described as an important factor in determining the identity of melanotrophs.[29]

Prophet of PIT1 (PROP1) is the earliest expressed pituitary-specific transcription factor, peaking at E12.0 and becoming undetectable by E15.5. *Prop1* expression is required for the emergence of the *Pou1f1* lineage (somatotrophs lactotrophs and thyrotrophs), the activation of NOTCH2 with emergence of the gonadotroph lineage, and the repression of *Hesx1* and *Otx2*.

POU1F1 (previously known as *PIT1*) is a pituitary-specific transcription factor belonging to the POU homeodomain family. It is expressed late during pituitary development (E13.5), and expression persists into adulthood. POU1F1 is important for terminal differentiation and expansion of somatotrophs, lactotrophs, and thyrotrophs. POU1F1 represses gonadotroph cell fate and autoregulates its own transcription.

Several transcription factors govern gonadotroph cell fate (e.g., GATA2, *NR5A1*, EGR1, PITX1, PITX2, and PROP1), and mature cells express terminal cell differentiation markers such as the GnRH receptor (GnRHR) and the hormone-specific β- ubunit of LH (LHβ) and FSH (FSHβ). Centrally, steroidogenic factor-1 (*Nr5a1*) is expressed in gonadotrophs and the ventromedial hypothalamus. Nr5a1 is a zinc-finger nuclear receptor that regulates a number of genes, including *Cga* (producing the protein α-GSU, the common subunit of LH, FSH, and TSH), *lhβ*, *fshb*, and *Gnrhr*. Hypothalamic GnRH regulates the function of gonadotrophs in the anterior pituitary. *Pax6* is required for the generation of GnRH cells, which arise from the olfactory placode and then migrate along the olfactory nerve pathway across the cribiform plate, toward the olfactory bulb and their final position in the hypothalamus. In humans, this migratory process is estimated to begin in the sixth week of gestation. An increasing number of genes are implicated in the migration and maturation of GnRH neurons (including *KAL1, FGFR1, FGF8, PROKR2, KISS1, GPR54, LEP, CHD7, TAC3*, and *TACR3*), and their role is highlighted by mutations found in patients with isolated hypogonadotrophic hypogonadism, with or without other features of Kallmann syndrome.[30–32]

30.2.2 Hypothalamus and Pituitary Stalk Development

The hypothalamus extends from the optic chiasm anteriorly to the mammillary body posteriorly. It is organized into distinct rostral-to-caudal regions (preoptic, anterior, tuberal, and mammillary) and three medial-to-lateral regions (periventricular, medial, and lateral).[33] The preoptic nucleus, anterior hypothalamus, dorsomedial nucleus, ventromedial nucleus, and mammillary nuclei are located within the medial region. The preoptic and hypothalamic areas are found in the lateral zone.[33] As Rathke's pouch invaginates, a portion of the ventral diencephalon evaginates ventrally to form the infundibulum, and subsequently the posterior pituitary lobe and pituitary stalk. The pituitary stalk contains the hypophyseal portal system, as well as the neuronal connections crossing the hypothalamic median eminence. These neurons originate from the supraoptic, suprachiasmatic, and paraventricular nuclei within the periventricular region of the hypothalamus.[33] Hypothalamic development is complex, and perhaps due to its anatomical location and diverse collection of cell groups and neuronal subtypes, there is a paucity of data regarding its regulation at a molecular level.[34,35]

The hypothalamus acting through the pituitary gland is the central mediator of growth, reproduction, and homeostasis.[6] Hypothalamic parvocellular neurons secrete hypophysiotrophic hormones into the capillary bed located within the median eminence. These stimulate the release of the seven anterior/intermediate pituitary-lobe hormones via the hypophyseal portal system. The parvocellular neurons also secrete OT and AVP, although at much lower concentrations than the magnocellular neurons. Parvocellular-derived AVP acts synergistically with corticotrophin-releasing hormone in regulating ACTH release.

30.2.3 Human Hypothalamo-Pituitary Development

The human fetal forebrain is identifiable as early as 3 weeks' gestation, and the diencephalon and telencephalon by 5 weeks. Rathke's pouch, which gives rise to the anterior pituitary, separates from the primitive pharyngeal stomodeum by 5 weeks' gestation.[2,6,36] The definitive Rathke's pouch contains proliferative progenitors that gradually relocate ventrally.[37–39] Specialized anterior pituitary cell types (lactotrophs, somatotrophs, corticotrophs, thyrotrophs, and gonadotrophs) are present at between 7 and 16 weeks.[36] Secretory granules are present in anterior pituitary cells by 10–12 weeks' gestation, and all pituitary hormones can be identified by immunoassay between 10 and 17 weeks.[36,40]

The neural components (hypothalamus, pituitary stalk, and posterior pituitary) are mostly developed by 7 weeks' gestation, and at this time, the floor of the sella turcica is evident, separating the adenohypophysis from the primitive gut. Hypothalamic neurons containing SS, GHRH, TRH, and GnRH are present by 10–14 weeks' gestation. Interconnecting fiber tracts are seen by 15–18 weeks. Maturation of the pituitary portal vascular system continues and becomes functional by 30–35 weeks' gestation, when there is portal vascular extension into the hypothalamus.

Recently, Suga et al. used specific conditions for ES cells to develop into hypothalamic-like neuroepithelium, and developed conditions in which ES cells formed rostral head ectoderm simultaneously.[14] These aggregates expressed markers of neuroepithelium and head ectoderm adjacently. Hedgehog agonist treatment of the cultures increased the

Rathke's pouch marker *Lhx3*. The resulting 3D structures had a central cavity, and the resemblance to Rathke's pouch was striking, as was the topographical location between the neuroepithelium and the rostral headlike ectoderm. The juxtaposition of the two tissues, mimicking the spatial organization in embryonic development, was indeed critical, as Rathke's pouch-like vesicles did not develop when neuroepithelium tissue was not present. ACTH-expressing cells developed from the vesicle-like structures and activation of *Wnt* signaling led to expression of Pit1, GH, and prolactin. LH/FSH/TSH expression was also achieved, albeit after more intense manipulation of the culture conditions. When ES-derived cell aggregates were implanted under the kidney capsule in hypophysectomized mice, corticosterone was produced. This landmark study may mark the first steps toward stem cell treatment for pituitary disorders.

30.3 PHYSIOLOGY OF THE FETAL AND NEONATAL HYPOTHALAMO-PITUITARY HORMONE AXES

30.3.1 GHRH/Somatostatin-GH/PRL

Human GH and PRL are both produced from the somatotroph cells within the anterior pituitary.[41] In postnatal life, GH displays important anabolic functions, including promotion of growth during childhood, while prolactin has a variety of effects during and after pregnancy, including stimulation of lactation and modulation of maternal behavior.

The fetal pituitary gland can synthesize and secrete GH by 8–10 weeks' gestation. Fetal plasma GH concentrations are in the range of 1–4 nmol/L during the first trimester and increase to approximately 6 nmol/L in midgestation.[36] The high plasma GH concentrations at midgestation may reflect unrestrained secretion.[36] Human somatotrophs respond predominantly to GH-releasing hormone (GHRH) at 9–16 weeks, while response to the inhibitory somatostatin develops later in gestation,[42] leading to a progressive fall of plasma GH during the second half of gestation to 1.5 nmoL/L at term.[36] Control of GH secretion matures progressively during the last half of gestation and the early weeks of postnatal life. The responses to somatostatin, GHRH, insulin, and arginine are mature at term in human infants, while mature responses to sleep, glucose, and L-dopa are present by 3 months of age.[36,43]

The ontogenesis of fetal plasma PRL differs significantly from that of GH; concentrations are low until 25–30 weeks' gestation and increase to approximately 11 nmol/L at term.[36] PRL release increases in response to TRH and decreases in response to dopamine. Brain and hypothalamic control of PRL matures late in gestation and during the first months of extrauterine life.[36,43] The marked increase in fetal plasma PRL concentration in the last trimester parallels the increase in fetal plasma estrogen concentrations, although it lags by several weeks.[36,43] During the neonatal period, serum prolactin concentrations fall, but they do not reach normal prepubertal levels until about 6 weeks of age.[44]

The characteristic pulsatile pattern of GH secretion observed in postnatal life is the result of a complex interplay of multiple regulators, with the dual and opposing effects of GHRH and somatostatin being the predominant factors.[45–47] A peak of GH results from a parallel reduction in somatostatin and an increase in GHRH secretion, while a trough of GH secretion results from an increase in somatostatin and a decrease in GHRH secretion.[45] GH secretion is already pulsatile soon after birth in humans, but trough concentrations are still higher than in later life,[48] so that random GH sampling can be used to detect GH deficiency in the neonatal period, which is not possible at a later age. Mean serum GH concentrations remain high during the first week of life (longer in premature infants) and then decline to reach the adult range by the age of 1 month.[49] GHRH stimulates GH secretion through a specialized G-protein-related receptor (GHRHR).[50] Binding of GHRH to the receptor results in the stimulation of adenylate cyclase and transcriptionally mediated increases in intracellular cyclic adenosine monophosphate concentrations that result in increased GH synthesis.[50] Somatostatin inhibits GH secretion through binding to its specific receptor, which then reduces adenylate cyclase activity and concomitantly intracellular calcium concentrations.[47]

The complex pattern of release of these hypothalamic hormones is understood to result from the interaction of multiple neurotransmitters and neuropeptides, including serotonin, histamine, norepinephrine, dopamine, acetylcholine, gamma-aminobutyric acid (GABA), thyroid hormone-releasing hormone (TRH), corticotrophin-releasing hormone (CRH), vasoactive intestinal peptide (VIP), gastrin, neurotensin, substance P, calcitonin, neuropeptide Y, vasopressin, galanin, and the gastric hormone ghrelin.[51,52] The alterations of GH secretion observed in various physiological states (e.g., stress, sleep, hemorrhage, fasting, hypoglycemia, and exercise), are believed to be mediated through these factors.[53] Moreover, the spontaneous and provocative GH secretion is attenuated by increased glucocorticoid and reduced thyroxine concentrations, on the one hand, while on the other, it is amplified by increased sex steroid concentrations.[54] In addition to the complex regulatory processes described previously, the synthesis and secretion of GH are regulated by negative feedback (inhibition) by insulin-like growth factors (IGFs).[55,56]

Human chromosome 17q22-24 contains a growth hormone/placental lactogen (GH/PL) gene cluster containing five related genes: *GH-N* encodes pituitary GH, *GH-V* encodes placental GH, and *PL-A, PL-B,* and *PL-L* encode placental lactogens. GH-V rises sharply after midgestation to a peak at 34–37 weeks and, within 1 h after delivery of the placenta, it disappears from the circulation.[57] Placental GH-V is secreted into the maternal circulation and reduces insulin sensitivity in the mother and so spares glucose and other nutrients for transplacental delivery and fetal growth. Here, PL is structurally homologous to GH but functionally closer to PRL, and it is secreted directly into both fetal and maternal circulations. It is first detected in the mother at 6 weeks' gestation to reach a peak at 32–35 weeks. Lactogens affect insulin production, hypothalamic gene expression, and leptin action in the mother and thus maintain metabolic homeostasis, while providing the substrates for nutrition for the fetus and newborn infant.

Postnatally, GH acts through receptors in liver and other tissues to stimulate production of IGF1 and, to a lesser degree, IGF2. Prenatally, GH receptor messenger ribonucleic acid (mRNA) levels and receptor binding are low in fetal liver, although receptor mRNA is present in other fetal tissues.[36] The growth of anencephalic fetuses and of neonates with congenital GH deficiency is almost normal, suggesting that factors other than GH stimulate fetal IGF production with nutrition probably playing the most important role. Conversely, the birth size may be reduced in infants with a defect in somatomedin generation.[58]

PRL receptors are present in most fetal tissues during the first trimester of gestation, and it is likely that lactogenic hormones play a significant role in organ and tissue development early in gestation,[40,59] and in particular in promoting fetal growth and skeletal/adipose tissue maturation.[60] It has been suggested that prolactin might also stimulate lung surfactant synthesis. Certainly, it appears that cord serum concentrations of prolactin are reduced in infants who develop respiratory distress syndrome.[61]

30.3.2 TRH-TSH

TRH is a hypothalamic neuropeptide pivotal to the regulation of energy metabolism, through both its role in the stimulation of TSH production and its central effects on feeding behavior, thermogenesis, and autonomic regulation.[62] TRH neurons in the hypothalamic paraventricular nucleus (PVN) play a key role in set-point regulation of the hypothalamo-pituitary-thyroid (HPT) axis, adapting thyroid hormone concentrations to environmental factors such as caloric deprivation or infection.[62]

TSH is produced and secreted by the thyrotropic cells of the anterior pituitary. Thyrotropic cells constitute less than 10% of the total number of adenohypophysial cells and are preferentially located in the anteromedial and anterolateral portions of the pituitary. TSH is a heterodimeric glycoprotein consisting of an *a* subunit and a *b* subunit. The *a* subunit is shared with other glycoprotein hormones [i.e., FSH, LH, and chorionic gonadotropin (CG)], whereas the *b* subunit is unique, determining the specificity of TSH. The gene for the human *a* subunit is located on chromosome 6, while the gene for the *b* subunit is located on chromosome 1. TSH plays a critical role in the regulation of the thyroid gland, as it activates the TSH receptor on the thyroid epithelial cell surface, which stimulates the synthesis and secretion of thyroid hormones from the follicular thyrocytes.

In postnatal life, thyroid hormones have pleiotropic effects by acting on virtually every cell of the human body. In childhood, they promote long bone growth (in synergy with GH) and neuronal maturation, but they also play an important role in increasing the basal metabolic rate, regulating protein synthesis, and increasing the body's sensitivity to catecholamines.

In the first trimester of fetal life, extrahypothalamic TRH stimulates pituitary TSH secretion, which mainly increases during the second trimester. Pituitary TSH secretion starts responding to hypothyroxinemia and TRH early in the third trimester.[63] Progressive maturation of hypothalamic-pituitary control and thyroid gland responsiveness to TSH in the late third trimester/early neonatal period leads to increased concentrations of TSH and T4.[64,65]

The maternal and fetal HPT axes operate somewhat independently. The placental deiodinase converts T4 to rT3 and is relatively impermeable to both T4 and T3. The placenta is also impermeable to TRH, TSH, and thyroid-binding globulins. This leads to a gradient of T4 and T3 from maternal to fetal plasma. Early in gestation, placental transfer is the only source of fetal T4 and is essential for normal fetal brain development (between 12 and 20 weeks) before fetal thyroid hormonogenesis begins.[66] With parturition, there is an immediate surge of pituitary TSH release in the neonate, which in turn evokes increased production of thyroid hormones.[67] Serum TSH concentrations reach peaks of approximately 70 μU/mL within 30 min after birth, and then decline over the next few days to the normal range. In response to this phenomenon, mean serum thyroxine concentrations rise to approximately 16 μg/dL at 24–36 h and then fall slowly. Birth also elicits an abrupt increase in peripheral conversion of thyroxine to tri-iodothyronine. Mean serum tri-iodothyronine levels reach 300 ng/dL by 24 h of age and then fall to around 200 ng/dL. In premature infants, similar changes in serum TSH and iodothyronine concentrations occur, but the responses are attenuated.[49]

The regulation of the HPT axis in postnatal life is complex. Thyroid hormone, principally T3, inhibits *TRH* gene expression in hypophysiotropic neurons within the parvocellular subdivision of the hypothalamic PVN. Conversely, *TRH* gene expression increases in response to low serum T4 and T3 concentrations.[62] Hypophysiotropic TRH neurons in the PVN receive monosynaptic input from leptin-responsive neurons in the arcuate nucleus, where the blood–brain barrier is absent. These neurons express either α-MSH and cocaine- and amphetamine-regulated transcript (CART), inhibiting food intake and promoting energy expenditure, or neuropeptide Y (NPY) and agouti-related protein (AGRP), stimulating food intake and decreasing energy expenditure.[68] Various studies in rodents and humans have shown a major downregulation of the HPT axis at the central and peripheral level during fasting, presumably as a homeostatic mechanism to reduce catabolism.[69] Indirect evidence points to similar hypothalamic mechanisms in humans.[70–72] In addition to starvation, the TRH neuron is inhibited during a variety of nonthyroidal illnesses, including infection and inflammation.[73,74] Binding of TRH to the TRH membrane receptor (TRHR) on the thyrotrophs stimulates synthesis and release of TSH. This response is dual, as the rapid release of presynthesized, stored TSH is followed by increased TSH gene expression and TSH production. The TRHR is a member of the seven-transmembrane-spanning, GTP-binding, G-protein-coupled receptor family. TRH binds to the transmembrane helix 3, which results in activation of a G protein and of inositol 1,4,5-triphosphate (IP3). In turn, IP3 stimulates the release of intracellular Ca^{2+}, which is involved in rapid TSH release. Simultaneously, protein kinase C is activated, which is involved in the increase in TSH production. TRH also stimulates the glycosylation of TSH, which is necessary for full biological activity of the hormone.[75] The hypothalamic neuropeptide somatostatin inhibits TSH secretion. Other inhibiting factors include dopamine, which inhibits TSH secretion, and glucocorticoids, which decrease the sensitivity of the pituitary to TRH. In contrast, estrogen increases the sensitivity of the pituitary to TRH. In the context of the HPT axis, TSH secretion is inhibited by circulating thyroid hormones. This so-called negative feedback regulation occurs via binding of T3 to the TRβ2 receptors expressed in the pituitary.

In humans, TSH has a circadian pattern of secretion, with lower plasma TSH concentrations during the daytime and an increase in the early evening and peak values ("nocturnal TSH surge") around the beginning of the sleep period.[76,77] Superimposed upon this diurnal rhythm is a clear ultradian rhythm, as first reported by Parker et al.[78] Later studies showed that the ultradian TSH release follows a high-frequency (approximately 10 pulses/h) and low-amplitude (0.4 mU/L) pulsatile pattern superimposed on the low-frequency, high-amplitude (1.0 mU/L) pattern of the circadian rhythm.[79] In humans, the physiologic meaning of the TSH rhythm is still elusive, and the mechanisms responsible for rhythmic TSH release are incompletely understood. In spite of the clear circadian variation in plasma TSH concentrations, a diurnal rhythm in plasma T4 and T3 concentrations in humans is less obvious,[80] which may be a consequence of the relatively long half-lives of these hormones. There are several physiological[81] and pathological conditions that alter the TSH rhythm.[82] Patients with critical illness show markedly decreased TSH pulsatility, with an absent nocturnal TSH surge and decreased TSH pulse amplitude.[83]

In prolonged critical illness, low circulating thyroid hormone concentrations appear positively correlated with reduced pulsatile TSH secretion.[84] In these conditions, the pituitary is unresponsive to low serum thyroid hormone concentrations, implying that the physiologic negative feedback mechanism of the HPT axis is overruled. Clinical studies in the intensive care setting showed that the continuous intravenous (IV) administration of TRH to patients with prolonged critical illness partially restored the serum concentrations of TSH, T4, and T3.[84,85] Together with the evidence of decreased *TRH* mRNA expression in the PVN of patients with critical illness,[86] these observations support a major role for hypothalamic TRH in the decreased TSH release during critical illness. The nocturnal TSH surge is also diminished in various endocrine pathologies, such as in central hypothyroidism, where a lower absolute and relative nocturnal rise in TSH has been demonstrated.[87] Finally, physiological conditions may affect the TSH rhythm. Examples of physiological modulation include the decreased nocturnal TSH surge during fasting[70] and the increased TSH surge during the first night of sleep deprivation.[88]

30.3.3 GnRH-LH/FSH

The hypothalamic-pituitary-gonadal (HPG) axis is the key regulator of sex development and reproduction. The function of gonadotrophs in the anterior pituitary is under the control of hypothalamic GnRH synthesized by neurons in the preoptic nucleus that project axons to the median eminence where the hormone is secreted. GnRH is released in a pulsatile fashion and binds to its receptors on pituitary gonadotrophs, which in turn respond by synthesizing and releasing the gonadotropins (LH and FSH).

FSH and LH are heterodimeric glycoproteins, consisting of two polypeptide units (α and β). The α subunit is shared between LH, FSH, TSH, and the human chorionic gonadotropin (hCG), while the β subunits vary. However, the LH and hCG β subunits exhibit large homologies and both stimulate the LH receptor. The gene for the shared α subunit is located on chromosome 6q14.3, while the gene for the FSH β subunit is located on chromosome 11p13. The gene for the LH and hCG β subunits is localized in the LHB/CGB gene cluster on chromosome 19q13.32. FSH and LH bind to their cognate receptors in the gonads, where they stimulate the production of sex steroids (androgens or estrogens) and gametogenesis. Similar to other hypothalamic-pituitary-target gland axes, the sex steroids then regulate gonadotropin secretion via negative feedback at the level of the hypothalamus or pituitary.

GnRH neurons migrate from the nasal placode to the hypothalamus during early embryogenesis, and GnRH is detected in the fetal hypothalamus at around 15 weeks' gestation.[89] GnRH is found almost exclusively in the hypothalamus and its content increases with advancing gestation.[49] Factors involved in the regulation of fetal GnRH neuron activity include kisspeptin and KISS1R.[89] LH and FSH are detected in the anterior pituitary and general circulation by 12–14 weeks' gestation.[90] The exact phase when the pituitary gonadotrophin secretion becomes dependent on the control of the hypothalamic GnRH is not fully elucidated; however, a functional connection with respect to GnRH is detected by 16–20 weeks of human gestation. In anencephalic fetuses that lack the hypothalamus but have an intact pituitary, gonadotroph development is normal up to 17–18 weeks' gestation, but thereafter the cells involute,[91] suggesting that hypothalamic input is required for the maintenance of the gonadotrophs from midgestation onward. In sheep fetuses, LH, FSH, and GnRH are present at midgestation or before. Prior to the maturation of the fetal pituitary, hCG from the placenta (the third gonadotrophin) stimulates fetal gonadal growth, differentiation, and secretory activity. Further, hCG concentrations are greater in female fetuses and show pulsatile secretion during the fetal period. This sex difference has been suggested to be due to the negative feedback effects of the fetal testicular hormones. The HPG axis activity peaks at 30%–40% gestation in sheep fetuses, decreasing until birth.[92] The midgestational peak in gonadal steroid hormone secretion stimulates gonadal growth and differentiation. Later in gestation, the placenta also synthesizes estrogens and androgens, controlled by the fetal hypothalamo-pituitary-adrenal (HPA) axis.[93]

At term, presumably because of feedback inhibition by placental estrogens, serum concentrations of FSH and LH are low in both sexes, and the predominant gonadotrophin components found are HCG and free α subunit. After delivery, concentrations of hCG decline rapidly, so that by 72 h, this gonadotrophin is no longer detectable.[49] The restraint mediated by the placental hormones on FSH/LH is removed at birth, leading to reactivation of the axis and an increase in gonadotrophin concentrations. Gonadotrophin concentrations are high during the first 3 months of life but decrease toward the age of 6 months, except for FSH concentrations in girls that remain elevated until 3–4 years of age.[94] The exact role of this transient activity during minipuberty for further reproductive development remains uncertain, although in the context of the perinatal programming theory, this period might be important for further reproductive health and disease.[94]

At birth, gonadotrophin concentrations are higher in premature than in full-term infants.[95] Prematurity appears not to influence the timing of the onset of the postnatal gonadotrophin surge, as the gonadotrophin concentrations begin to increase at the same time after birth as in full-term infants. However, the gonadotrophin surge is augmented in magnitude and also prolonged in premature infants compared to full-term infants, and more clearly in girls than in boys.[96,97]

Postnatal FSH concentrations are also increased in small-for-gestational-age (SGA) infants compared to infants born appropriate for gestational age (AGA).[98] In SGA boys, testosterone concentrations are higher than in full-term, AGA boys.[99] Higher estradiol concentrations have been reported in SGA girls than in AGA girls after a GnRH agonist test, although nonstimulated concentrations have not been significantly different.[100] The reason for the increased HPG axis activity following intrauterine growth restraint is not known.

30.3.4 CRH-ACTH

In humans, corticotroph cells of the anterior pituitary secrete ACTH, and it is derived from posttranslational processing of the precursor molecule proopiomelanocortin in the anterior lobe of the pituitary. This process is modulated by CRH and vasopressin secreted by the PVN of the hypothalamus. ACTH stimulates the biosynthesis of adrenal corticosteroids.

The HPA axis plays a central role in regulating many homeostatic systems in the body, including the metabolic system, cardiovascular system, immune system, reproductive system, and CNS. The HPA axis modulates stress reactions by integrating physical and psychosocial influences to allow the organism to adapt effectively to its environment, use resources, and optimize survival.

Before birth, the HPA axis is an important controller of fetal development and homeostasis.[101] The hypothalamus, pituitary, and adrenal glands are dynamic endocrine organs during fetal development. The adrenal glands, in particular, exhibit remarkable transformation in size, morphology, and function during the prenatal and neonatal periods. It is now recognized that normal development of the HPA axis is essential for the regulation of intrauterine homeostasis, and the timely differentiation and maturation of vital organ systems, including the lungs, liver, and CNS necessary for immediate neonatal survival after birth. In addition, acting together with the placenta, the HPA axis might indirectly control the normal timing of parturition in primates.[102,103]

CRH produced by the fetal hypothalamus is the primary secretagogue controlling POMC and ACTH formation. CRH regulates the growth of pituitary corticotrophs, adrenocortical differentiation, and steroidogenic maturation of the fetal HPA axis. It is also a potent vasodilator of the feto-placental circulation and can potentiate the function of local mediators and hormones, such as prostaglandins and OT, in increasing myometrial contractility during labor.[103] In humans, CRH is expressed in multiple tissues, including the placenta. Similarly, POMC is expressed in multiple tissues, notably in the placenta and fetal lungs. The physiological importance of the extrahypothalamic CRH and the extrapituitary POMC (and POMC-derived peptides) is not yet fully understood. Nevertheless, major roles for these hormones (particularly for placental CRH and ACTH) in fetal physiology have been proposed, including the control of the initiation of parturition and the timing of birth in the sheep and other species.[104] ACTH is the prime trophic hormone controlling fetal adrenocortical growth, differentiation, and steroidogenesis.[103,105]

The fetal development of the HPA axis has been extensively studied in humans, sheep, and rodents. In all these species, pituitary ACTH is observed first during gestation, followed by hypothalamic neuropeptides and the onset of responsiveness to stress or ACTH secretagogues (CRH/AVP).[104] The fetal HPA axis is fully activated progressively throughout latter gestation, leading to increased biosynthesis of hypothalamic CRH, AVP, and POMC in the pituitary, sensitivity of steroidogenic tissue to ACTH, and abundance of steroidogenic enzymes in the adrenal cortex with an increase in its size.[106] ACTH bioactivity is first detected in the 8th week of gestation,[107] although immunoreactive ACTH has been demonstrated later (around 11 weeks' gestation).[108–110] Early studies in the rat suggest that the fetus is competent to respond to stressors a few days after the onset of ACTH synthesis in late embryonic life.[111,112] Placental tissue synthesizes and releases CRH (pCRH) into fetal and maternal blood.[113]

Hypothalamic CRH in the fetus is detected as early as the 12th week of gestation, marking the onset of hypothalamic control of fetal ACTH secretion, although fetal pituitary ACTH can also be stimulated by the earlier pCRH production.[114] The ovine fetus responds to both CRH and AVP[115] with increases in plasma ACTH concentration. The youngest fetal age studied with regard to pituitary responsiveness to CRH is 95 days' gestation.[116] Immunoreactive CRH and AVP peptides have been identified in the ovine fetal hypothalamus as early as day 70 (approximately 50%) of gestation.[117] CRH and AVP regulate the ACTH secretion through the CRHR1 and the V1b receptor, respectively.[118] Recent evidence indicates that the CRHR1 and V1b receptors can heterodimerize, and that this dimerization might form the basis of the interaction between CRH and AVP in the control of ACTH secretion.[119]

The regulation of the fetal HPA axis is extremely complex, and it involves tight interactions with the placenta. The fetal hypothalamus responds to acutely stressful situations, such as arterial hypotension and hemorrhage by releasing CRH. CRH stimulates the production of ACTH from the fetal corticotrophs. ACTH enhances adrenal cortisol secretion, which in turn inhibits excessive CRH and ACTH release from the fetal hypothalamic–pituitary centers. ACTH also promotes dehydroepiandrosterone sulfate (DHEAS) secretion from the adrenocortical fetal zone, which provides substrates for estrogen synthesis. In the later developmental stages, placental estrogens influence the fetal HPA axis by facilitating the conversion of active cortisol into inactive cortisone, thereby reducing the concentration of cortisol in the fetus. This in turn results in decreasing the negative feedback effects of cortisol on the fetal hypothalamic–pituitary centers and causes an increase in fetal POMC, ACTH, and adrenal cortisol production. An increase in fetal ACTH secretion further stimulates DHEAS production.

This positive feedback loop has been proposed to be the mechanism underlying the rapid growth of the fetal adrenal cortex and the efficient production of DHEAS at midgestation.[106,120] Placental CRH, which is identical to hypothalamic CRH in structure, bioactivity, and immunoreactivity, stimulates the expression of fetal pituitary ACTH and effectively establishes another positive feedback circuit, resulting in concomitant increase of CRH, ACTH, and cortisol toward the end of gestation.[103,121] AVP and catecholamines also stimulate fetal ACTH secretion.[106] This self-perpetuating mechanism reaches its peak at the onset of labor, and the positive feedback loop is eventually terminated by delivery of the placenta and the fetus.[103]

Glucocorticoids and estrogens play complex and key roles in the regulation of the HPA axis at the end of gestation and in early neonatal life. In the late-gestation fetus, ACTH secretion is highly sensitive to the negative feedback effects of cortisol.[122] The negative feedback sensitivity of the fetal sheep is high enough that physiological changes in maternal plasma cortisol concentration, which increase fetal plasma cortisol concentration by transplacental transfer, effectively inhibit fetal ACTH.[123] The efficiency of glucocorticoid feedback on HPA activity is critical during development in rodents because abnormally elevated glucocorticoid concentrations have deleterious effects on a number of maturational processes that are still incomplete at birth.[124] In neonates, glucocorticoid feedback efficiency on ACTH secretion is higher than in weaning or adult rats, as shown both *in vivo* and *in vitro*.[125] Estradiol is a potent stimulator of the fetal HPA axis,[108,126] with actions that can be attributed to a site of action within the fetal hypothalamus.[127] Estrogen selectively suppresses fetal zone growth during the second half of pregnancy. At term, human placental estrogen leads to a positive feedback cycle with progressive increase in fetal HPA activity, resulting in an increase in ACTH and cortisol in the last 10 weeks' gestation. This helps in visceral and pulmonary maturity.[104] While the importance of estrogen as a part of the final common pathway to increased myometrial activity and parturition is well known, the importance of estrogens prior to parturition in the fetus has attracted little attention.

The human fetal adrenal gland is characterized by remarkable hyperplasia, the bulk of which is made of the histologically distinct central fetal zone. During the perinatal period, the total mass of adrenal tissue is reduced to less than half by involution of the hyperplastic fetal zone.[49] Despite the dramatic remodeling of the adrenal cortex that occurs immediately after birth, there is no evidence of clinical adrenocortical insufficiency in term infants during this crucial period.[103] The mean cord serum cortisol at term is about 10 µg/dL, in spite of plasma ACTH concentrations in excess of 200 pg/mL. Serum cortisol concentrations remain stable during the neonatal period.[128] Plasma ACTH concentrations fall gradually in the neonate, reaching mean levels of approximately 60 pg/mL at 2 days and 35 pg/mL at 1 week of age.[129,130] Circadian rhythms of ACTH and cortisol secretion become established by about 3 months of age.[131]

In contrast to the physiological neonate, ill and extremely premature infants form a unique group because of their potentially decreased ability to produce stress-induced release of glucocorticoid.[132,133] There is some evidence indicating that the activity of some adrenal steroidogenic enzymes might be reduced as a result of adrenocortical immaturity.[133,134] Additionally, an inability of very low birth weight (VLBW) infants to secrete hypothalamic CRH has also been demonstrated.[135,136] VLBW infants with low or suboptimal serum cortisol concentrations might have a higher risk of developing chronic lung disease.[137] Transient adrenocortical insufficiency has also been described in VLBW infants who present with profound hypotension and shock, which are resistant to volume expansion and inotrope treatment but respond promptly to glucocorticoid replacement.[132]

It is possible that environmental stress might stimulate a precocious rise in fetal hypothalamic and placental CRH production, which triggers the cascade of changes resulting in preterm delivery. This theory is supported by the observation that premature infants have significantly higher concentrations of maternal CRH in the early third trimester than those who deliver at term.[138]

Finally, over the last few years, dysregulation of the HPA axis has been proposed as a key mechanism underlying the link between early-life development and later-life disease (e.g., cardiometabolic disease, mood disorders, and accelerated cognitive decline[139]). Recent epidemiological evidence suggests that stressful events experienced in fetal and early neonatal life can produce enduring changes in the structure and function of the neural pathways, thereby resulting in alteration of the programming process, which predisposes to specific diseases in later life.[140–142] A recent systematic review concluded the presence of a sex difference in early-life programming of the HPA axis in humans, with female offspring exposed to stressors having increased HPA axis reactivity than males. The increased vulnerability of the female's HPA axis to programming suggests a mechanism underlying sex differences in later-life diseases.[143]

30.3.5 POMC and POMC-Derivates

The *POMC* gene is located on chromosome 2p23.3, and it is expressed both in the anterior and intermediate lobes of the pituitary gland. The intermediate lobe of the pituitary gland is prominent in both human and sheep fetuses. Neurointermediate lobe cells mature in late gestation, perhaps in response to cortisol in fetal plasma,[144] and they begin to disappear near term, being virtually absent in the adult human pituitary, although the intermediate lobe in the adult of some lower species is anatomically and functionally distinct.[145]

The intermediate lobe cells synthesize POMC, which after cleavage produces α-MSH, β-endorphin (β-end), ACTH, and β-lipotropin (β-LPH) in the anterior lobe in response to hypoxia.[146] During pregnancy, the placenta produces and secretes ACTH,[147,148] α-MSH, β-LPH, and β-end[149] into embryos and fetuses before the fetal pituitary gland starts to secrete these POMC-derived peptides.

POMC mRNA has been demonstrated in the ovine fetal pituitary as early as 60 days (approximately 40%) of gestation.[150,151] In the human fetus, α-MSH levels decrease with increasing fetal age.[152] Further, α-MSH and corticotropin-like intermediate lobe peptide (CLIP; ACTH18-39) are processed in the hypothalamus, the intermediate lobe of the pituitary, and the skin.[153] Also, α-MSH and CLIP may play roles in fetal adrenal activation, and α-MSH may play a role in fetal growth as well.[154,155]

Melanocortin-2 receptor (MC2R) and melanocortin-5 receptor (MC5R), which are the receptors for ACTH and a-MSH, are expressed in the peripheral tissues in the mouse fetus.[156] Embryonic and fetal melanocortins, through action on their receptors (MCRs), exhibit a variety of functions involving the proliferation and inhibition of ES cell differentiation, HPA axis maturation, induction of lung maturation, and histogenesis of testis and pancreas.[101]

30.3.6 AVP and OT

The posterior pituitary lobe comprises axonal projections of neurons originating from hypothalamic magnocellular bodies termed the *supraoptic, suprachiasmatic,* and *paraventricular* nuclei. The former two release AVP, and the latter releases OT.[11]

The fetal neurohypophysis is well developed by 10–12 weeks' gestation and contains both AVP (also known as ADH) and OT.[157] In addition, arginine vasotocin (AVT), the parent neurohypophyseal hormone in submammalian vertebrates, is present in the fetal pituitary and pineal glands and in adult pineal glands from several mammalian species, including humans.[158] AVT is present in the pituitary during fetal life from 11 to 19 weeks, is secreted by cultured human fetal pineal cells during the second trimester, and disappears in the neonatal period.[157,158] In adult mammals, instillation of AVT into cerebrospinal fluid (CSF) inhibits gonadotropin and corticotropin release, stimulates PRL release by the anterior pituitary, and induces sleep; however, the physiologic importance of these effects remains unclear. The role of AVT in the fetal pineal gland is unknown.[159] Baseline plasma levels of AVT in fetal sheep during the last trimester approximate the values for AVP and OT.[158] Presumably, this AVT is derived from the posterior pituitary, but the stimuli for AVT secretion in the fetus are not defined. By 40 weeks, the concentrations of AVP and OT approximate 20% of those in adults. Fetal pituitary OT concentration, detectable by 11–15 weeks, exceeds AVP concentration by 19 weeks. The AVP-OT ratio falls progressively thereafter.

The AVP and OT genes are located at chromosome 20p13. AVP and OT are both nonapeptides with significant structural analogies. Virtually all vertebrates have an OT-like and a vasopressin-like nonapeptide, with genes usually located close to each other and believed to result from a gene duplication event. Both neurohypophyseal peptides are synthesized as large precursor molecules (neurophysins) and processed to bioactive amidated peptides.[160] Enzymatic processing involves progressive cleavage of carboxyl terminal–extended peptides, sequentially producing OT-glycine-lysine-arginine (OTGKR), OTGK, OTG, and OT (for OT) and AVPG and AVP (for AVP). Enzymatic processing of neurophysins matures progressively in the fetus so that early in gestation, fetal plasma contains relatively large concentrations of the extended peptides.[160] For example, for OT, the ratio of OT-extended peptides to OT in fetal sheep serum is approximately 35:1 early in gestation and 3:1 late in gestation.[160]

In the fetus, AVP has three main biological activities. The vasopressor action on peripheral vessels is mediated by V1a, while V1b and V2 receptors mediate corticotropin-releasing and antidiuretic activity.[101] AVP is an important fetal cardiovascular hormone.[161] Through its vasopressor action, AVP redistributes fetal ventricular output toward the umbilical–placental circulation, maximizing the transfer of gases between maternal and fetal circulations.[101] Despite its main effect being antidiuretic in the postnatal life, AVP appears to function in the fetus as an essential stress-responsive hormone, and to respond to hypoxia, hemorrhage, intrauterine bradycardia, and meconium passage more than to osmolar stimuli.[101] The major potential stress for the fetus is hypoxia, and the response of AVP to hypoxia is increased compared with the maternal and fetal AVP responses to osmolar stimuli.[157,162, 163] Plasma AVP concentrations in human cord blood are elevated in association with intrauterine bradycardia and meconium passage.[162] The vasopressor action of AVP may be important in the maintenance of fetal circulatory homeostasis during hemorrhage and hypoxia.[157] Fetal hypoxia is also a major stimulus for catecholamine release. There is little information on the interactions between AVP and catecholamines during fetal hypoxia, but it is known that both fetal hypoxia and AVP stimulate anterior pituitary function, including ACTH.[164]

During the last trimester, fetal hypothalamic and pituitary responsiveness to both volume and osmolar stimuli for AVP secretion are well developed, and AVP exerts antidiuretic effects on the fetal kidney.[157,165] AVP receptors have been found in renal medullary membranes of newborn sheep.[166,167] Both AVP and AVT evoke antidiuretic actions in the sheep fetus during the last third of gestation, and both hormones act to conserve water for the fetus by inhibiting fluid loss into amniotic fluid through the lungs and kidneys.[157,158] Aquaporin-1, -2, and -3 water channel receptors are present in the human fetal and newborn kidneys, and the ability of the newborn infant to regulate free water clearance in response to volume and osmolar stimuli has been demonstrated.[168,169] Whether AVT exerts its effects through AVP receptors or separate fetal AVT receptors is not clear. The maximal concentrating capacity by the fetal kidney is limited to about 600 mmol/L. This limitation is not related to inadequate AVP stimulation, but rather is inherent to immaturity of the renal tubules.

Finally, a role for AVP as a corticotropin-releasing hormone is established in the adult and the fetal pituitary. ACTH responds separately and synergistically to AVP and CRH early in the third trimester.[170] The role of AVP in controlling fetal corticotropin release seems to decrease with gestational age. It is not known whether AVT functions as a corticotropin-releasing hormone in the fetus.

OT concentrations increase as the fetus matures, and markedly during active labor and delivery; however, there is no evidence that fetal production of OT contributes to the timing or progression of parturition. The placental barrier prevents fetal OT from reaching the myometrium. Given the structural analogies between AVP and OT, it is not surprising that OT also stimulates the release of ACTH via V1b receptor in the fetus.[101] Additionally, recent work shows a role for OT in the development of the neurovascular interface in the posterior pituitary.[159]

30.4 HYPOTHALAMO-PITUITARY REGULATION OF TRANSITION TO EXTRAUTERINE LIFE

The transition to life *ex utero* involves abrupt delivery of the fetus from the protected intrauterine environment into the relatively hostile extrauterine environment. This requires complex physiological adaptations of multiple organ systems, including the hypothalamo-pituitary neuroendocrine system. The neonate must initiate breathing in air, and rapid but careful regulation is required to defend against adverse insults, including hypothermia, hypoglycemia and hypocalcemia.

The placenta supplies continuous IV glucose to meet fetal energy needs, and fetal glucose uptake is directly related to both the maternal blood glucose concentration and the transplacental gradient. There is little endogenous glucose production by the fetus, and fat and glycogen are stored in preparation for birth. During labor, and at delivery following clamping of the cord, maternal supply of glucose ceases. Counterregulatory hormones rapidly become active with a rise in catecholamine, glucagon, GH, and glucocorticoid concentrations, and a fall in insulin, resulting in an increase in fetal blood glucose concentrations.[171,172]

The onset of parturition is likely to involve a complex interplay between maternal, fetal, and placental hormones. The placenta produces vast amounts of estrogens, and biosynthesis relies on a supply of C_{19} androgens (mainly DHEAS, derived principally from the fetal and maternal adrenal cortex).[103,173, 174] ACTH, secreted by the fetal pituitary, is proposed by many to be the primary regulator of fetal adrenocortical development. The fetal pituitary-adrenal axis is postulated to become functional at 50–52 days postconception, with detectable cytoplasmic ACTH, coinciding with the onset of adrenal steroidogenic enzyme expression.[175] Abnormal activation of the fetal H-P adrenal axis and enlargement of the fetal adrenal has been associated with impending preterm birth.[176,177] Hypothalamic CRH stimulates the expression and processing of POMC by pituitary corticotrophs and the secretion of ACTH.

The human placenta, fetal membranes, and decidua also express CRH that is identical to hypothalamic CRH.[178] However, unlike hypothalamic CRH, placental CRH gene expression and production can be stimulated by glucocorticoids.[179] This positive feed-forward system is a unique feature of placental CRH and indicates a distinct role in pregnancy. Therefore, acting together with the placenta, the fetal H-P adrenal axis might indirectly regulate the normal timing of parturition in primates.[180] Delivery results in a reversal of the high fetal cortisone/cortisol ratio and plasma cortisol concentrations are higher in the neonate, despite relatively lower plasma corticotropin concentrations. This increase is presumed to be due to decreased inhibition of the adrenal steroidogenic enzyme, 3β-hydroxysteroid dehydrogenase (3β-HSD) by estrogen, and perhaps removal of a placental CRH action on fetal pituitary corticotropin release. Plasma DHEAS concentrations fall as the fetal adrenal atrophies.

Delivery of the placenta results in decreased fetal blood concentrations of estrogens, progesterone, hCG, and hPL. The reduction in estrogen concentrations is presumed to remove the major stimulus to fetal pituitary PRL release, and PRL concentrations fall over several weeks. This relatively gentle decline may be due to lactotrope hyperplasia in the fetal pituitary or to delayed maturation of hypothalamic dopamine secretion. The gradual fall of GH concentrations during the early weeks of life is due to delayed maturation of H-P feedback regulation of GH release.[36] In the neonatal primate, there are concurrent decreases in plasma GH concentrations and GH responsiveness to exogenous GHRH.[181] The mechanisms are unclear, and changes in secretion or in pituitary sensitivity to GHRH, somatostatin, or both may be involved. IGF-1 and IGF-2 concentrations fall to neonatal values within a few days, presumably because of the removal of placental hPL and placental IGF production.

In male infants, after a transient fall in testosterone concentrations, pituitary LH secretion rebounds as the hCG stimulus subsides, resulting in a secondary surge of plasma testosterone that persists at significant levels for several weeks.[36,182] This surge is mediated by hypothalamic GnRH, and blockade of neonatal activation of the pituitary-testicular axis with a GnRH agonist in neonatal monkeys has been shown to block increments in LH and testosterone.[183] Furthermore, blockade results in low plasma LH and testosterone concentrations and slow testicular enlargement at puberty in these animals, suggesting that neonatal GnRH release with pituitary-testicular activation may be critical for normal sexual maturation of male primates.[183] In females, a brief, secondary surge in FSH may transiently elevate estrogen concentrations.

The thyroid axis matures late in the third trimester, in parallel to the increase in cortisol, with increased TSH, T3, and T4, and decreased rT3 as term approaches.[184] The increase in serum thyrotropin concentrations during the early minutes after birth is due to cooling of the neonate in the extrauterine environment.[63,64] In term infants, the thyrotropin surge peaks at 30 min to reach a concentration of about 70 mU/L, which stimulates increased secretion of T4 and T3 by the thyroid gland. Furthermore, increased conversion of T4–T3 by liver and other tissues maintains the T3 concentration in the extrauterine range of 1.6–3.4 nmol/L (105–220 ng/dL). Serum T3 concentrations and maturation of feedback control of thyrotropin by thyroid hormones during the early weeks of life are thought to subsequently decrease neonatal thyrotropin concentrations.[63,65] Production of rT3 by neonatal tissues ceases by 3–4 weeks of age, at which time serum rT3 reaches adult concentrations.

30.5 CONCLUSIONS

The H-P neuroendocrine axsis starts developing early in fetal life and plays a pivotal role in fetal development and homeostasis, the timing of parturition, and the adaptation of the neonate to the extrauterine environment. These actions are mediated by close interactions with the placental hormones. Perhaps the most unique aspect of fetal endocrine processes is that they operate in the presence of high concentrations of placental estrogens, which are sufficient not only to influence pituitary secretion of hormones such as FSH or prolactin, but also to affect steroidogenesis in the adrenal (and probably the gonad). At birth, fetal endocrine systems, including the H-P neuroendocrine system, must adjust to a new and hostile environment. At the same time, separation from the placenta removes a major source of energy, peptides, and steroid hormones. This initiates a series of adaptive responses, marking the first few days of life as a very unique period for the neuroendocrine activity of the H-P axis.

REFERENCES

1. Saland L. The mammalian pituitary intermediate lobe: an update on innervation and regulation. *Brain Res Bull* 2001;**54**(6):587–93.
2. Cohen LE, Radovick S. Molecular basis of combined pituitary hormone deficiencies. *Endocr Rev* 2002;**23**(4):431–42.
3. Dasen JS, Rosenfeld M. Signaling and transcriptional mechanisms in pituitary development. *Annu Rev Neurosci* 2001;**24**:327–55.
4. Dattani MT, Robinson I. The molecular basis for developmental disorders of the pituitary gland in man. *Clin Genet* 2000;**57**(5):337–46.
5. McCabe MJ, Dattani M. Genetic aspects of hypothalamic and pituitary gland development. *Handb Clin Neurol* 2014;**124**:3–15.
6. Kelberman D, Rizzoti K, Lovell-Badge R, Robinson IC, Dattani M. Genetic regulation of pituitary gland development in human and mouse. *Endocr Rev* 2009;**30**(7):790–829.
7. Kawamura K, Kouki T, Kawahara G, Kikuyama S. Hypophyseal development in vertebrates from amphibians to mammals. *Gen Comp Endocrinol* 2002;**126**:130–5.
8. Rubenstein J, Shimamura K, Martinez S, Puelles L. Regionalization of the prosencephalic neural plate. *Annu Rev Neurosci* 1998;**21**:445–77.
9. Osumi-Yamashita N, Ninomiya Y, Doi H, Eto K. The contribution of both forebrain and midbrain crest cells to the mesenchyme in the frontonasal mass of mouse embryos. *Dev Biol* 1994;**164**:409–19.
10. Pogoda H, Hammerschmidt M. Molecular genetics of pituitary development in zebra fish. *Semin Cell Dev Biol* 2007;**18**:543–58.
11. Pearson C, Placzek M. Development of the medial hypothalamus: forming a functional hypothalamic-neurohypophyseal interface. *Curr Top Dev Biol* 2013;**106**:49–88.
12. Davis SW, Mortensen AH, Camper S. Birthdating studies reshape models for pituitary gland cell specification. *Dev Biol* 2011;**352**(2):215–27.
13. Le Tissier PR, Hodsonm DJ, Martin AO, Romanò N, Mollard P. Plasticity of the prolactin (PRL) axis: mechanisms underlying regulation of output in female mice. *Adv Exp Med Biol* 2015;**846**:139–62.
14. Suga H, Kadoshima T, Minaguchi M, Ohgushi M, Soen M, Nakano T, Takata N, Wataya T, Muguruma K, Miyoshi H, Yonemura S, Oiso Y, Sasai Y. Self-formation of functional adenohypophysis in three-dimensional culture. *Nature* 2011;**480**(7375):57–62.
15. Treier M, O'Connell S, Gleiberman A, Price J, Szeto DP, Burgess R, et al. Hedgehog signaling is required for pituitary gland development. *Development* 2001;**128**(3):377–86.
16. McCabe M, Gaston-Massuet C, Tziaferi V, et al. Novel FGF8 mutations associated with recessive holoprosencephaly, craniofacial defects, and hypothalamo-pituitary dysfunction. *J Clin Endocrinol Metab* 2011;**96**:E1709–18.
17. Zhu X, Gleiberman AS, Rosenfeld M. Molecular physiology of pituitary development: signaling and transcriptional networks. *Physiol Rev* 2007;**87**(3):933–63.
18. Douglas KR, Brinkmeier ML, Kennell JA, Eswara P, Harrison TA, Patrianakos AI, et al. Identification of members of the Wnt signaling pathway in the embryonic pituitary gland. *Mamm Genome* 2001;**12**(11):843–51.
19. Mansukhani A, Ambrosetti D, Holmes G, Cornivelli L, Basilico C. Sox2 induction by FGF and FGFR2 activating mutations inhibits Wnt signaling and osteoblast differentiation. *J Cell Biol* 2005;**168**(7):1065–76.
20. Zorn AM, Barish GD, Williams BO, Lavender P, Klymkowsky MW, Varmus HE. Regulation of Wnt signaling by Sox proteins: XSox17 alpha/beta and XSox3 physically interact with beta-catenin. *Mol Cell* 1999;**4**(4):487–98.
21. Olson D, Skinner K, Challis J. Prostaglandin output in relation to parturition by cells dispersed from human intrauterine tissues. *J Clin Endocrinol Metab* 1983;**57**:694–9.

22. Dattani MT, Martinez-Barbera JP, Thomas PQ, Brickman JM, Gupta R, Mårtensson IL, Toresson H, Fox M, Wales JK, Hindmarsh PC, Krauss S, Beddington RS, Robinson I. Mutations in the homeobox gene HESX1/Hesx1 associated with septo-optic dysplasia in human and mouse. *Nat Genet* 1998;**19**:125–33.

23. Mullen RD, Colvin SC, Hunter CS, Savage JJ, Walvoord EC, Bhangoo AP, et al. Roles of the LHX3 and LHX4 LIM-homeodomain factors in pituitary development. *Mol Cell Endocrinol* 2007;**265–266**:190–5.

24. Raetzman LT, Ward R, Camper S. Lhx4 and Prop1 are required for cell survival and expansion of the pituitary primordia. *Development* 2002;**129**(18):4229–39.

25. Zhao Y, Mailloux CM, Hermesz E, Palkóvits M, Westphal H. A role of the LIM-homeobox gene Lhx2 in the regulation of pituitary development. *Dev Biol* 2010;**337**(2):313–23.

26. Gaston-Massuet C, McCabe MJ, Scagliotti V, Young RM, Carreno G, Gregory LC, et al. Transcription factor 7-like 1 is involved in hypothalamo-pituitary axis development in mice and humans. *Proc Natl Acad Sci U S A* 2016;**113**(5):E548–57.

27. Liu J, Lin C, Gleiberman A, Ohgi KA, Herman T, Huang HP, et al. Tbx19, a tissue-selective regulator of POMC gene expression. *Proc Natl Acad Sci U S A* 2001;**98**(15):8674–9.

28. Pulichino AM, Vallette-Kasic S, Tsai JP, Couture C, Gauthier Y, Drouin J. Tpit determines alternate fates during pituitary cell differentiation. *Genes Dev* 2003;**17**(6):738–47.

29. Budry L, Balsalobre A, Gauthier Y, Khetchoumian K, L'Honore A, Vallette S, et al. The selector gene Pax7 dictates alternate pituitary cell fates through its pioneer action on chromatin remodeling. *Genes Dev* 2012;**26**(20):2299–310.

30. Trarbach EB, Silveira LG, Latronico A. Genetic insights into human isolated gonadotropin deficiency. *Pituitary* 2007;**10**(4):381–91.

31. Hardelin JP, Dodé C. The complex genetics of Kallmann syndrome: KAL1, FGFR1, FGF8, PROKR2, PROK2, et al. *Sex Dev* 2008;**2**(4–5):181–93.

32. Boehm U, Bouloux PM, Dattani MT, de Roux N, Dodé C, Dunkel L, Dwyer AA, Giacobini P, Hardelin JP, Juul A, Maghnie M, Pitteloud N, Prevot V, Raivio T, Tena-Sempere M, Quinton R, Young J. Expert consensus document: European consensus statement on congenital hypogonadotropic hypogonadism—pathogenesis, diagnosis and treatment. *Nat Rev Endocrinol* 2015;**11**(9):547–64.

33. Szarek E, Cheah P, Schwartz J, Thomas P. Molecular genetics of the developing neuroendocrine hypothalamus. *Mol Cell Endocrinol* 2010;**323**:115–23.

34. Tosches M, Arendt D. The bilaterian forebrain: an evolutionary chimaera. *Curr Opin Neurobiol* 2013;**23**:1080–9.

35. Blackshaw S, Scholpp S, Placzek M, Ingraham H, Simerly R, Shimogori T. Molecular pathways controlling development of thalamus and hypothalamus: from neural specification to circuit formation. *J Neurosci* 2010;**30**:14925–30.

36. Grumbach M, Gluckman P. The human fetal hypothalamus and pituitary gland: the maturation of neuroendocrine mechanisms controlling secretion of fetal pituitary growth hormone, prolactin, gonadotropins, adrenocorticotropin-related peptides, and thyrotropin. In: Tulchinsky D, Little A, editors. *Maternal fetal endocrinology*. 2nd ed. Philadelphia, PA: WB Saunders; 1994. p. 193–261.

37. Rizzoti K, Lovell-Badge R. Early development of the pituitary gland: induction and shaping of Rathke's pouch. *Rev Endocr Metab Disord* 2005;**6**:161–72.

38. Fauquier T, Rizzoti K, Dattani M, Lovell-Badge R, Robinson I. SOX2-expressing progenitor cells generate all of the major cell types in the adult mouse pituitary gland. *Proc Natl Acad Sci U S A* 2008;**105**:2907–12.

39. Castinetti F, Davis SW, Brue TCS. Pituitary stem cell update and potential implications for treating hypopituitarism. *Endocr Rev* 2011;**32**:453–71.

40. Gluckman P, Pinal C. Growth hormone and prolactin. In: Polin R, Fox W, Abman S, editors. *Fetal and neonatal physiology*. 3rd ed. Philadelphia, PA: WB Saunders; 2004. p. 1891–5.

41. Masuda N, Watahiki M, Tanaka M, Yamakawa M, Shimizu K, Nagai J, Nakashima K. Molecular cloning of cDNA encoding 20 kda variant human growth hormone and the alternative splicing mechanism. *Biochim Biophys Acta* 1998;**949**:125–31.

42. Anderson LL, Jeftinija S, Scanes C. Growth hormone secretion: molecular and cellular mechanisms and in vivo approaches. *Exp Biol Med* 2004;**229**:291–302.

43. Suganuma N, Seo H, Yamamoto N. The ontogeny of growth hormone in the human fetal pituitary. *Am J Obstet Gynecol* 1989;**160**:729–33.

44. Guyda HJ, Friesen H. Serum prolactin levels in humans from birth to adult life. *Pediatr Res* 1973;**7**(5):534–40.

45. Hartman ML, Faria AC, Vance ML, Johnson ML, Thorner MO, Veldhuis JD. Temporal structure of in vivo growth hormone secretory events in humans. *Am J Phys* 1991;**260**:E101–10.

46. Barinaga M, Yamonoto G, Rivier C, Vale W, Evans R, Rosenfeld MG. Transcriptional regulation of growth hormone gene expression by growth hormone-releasing factor. *Nature* 1983;**306**:84–5.

47. Holl RW, Thorner MO, Leong DA. Intracellular calcium concentration and growth hormone secretion in individual somatotropes: effects of growth hormone-releasing factor and somatostatin. *Endocrinology* 1988;**122**:2927–32.

48. Adcock C, Ogilvy-Stuart A, Robinson I, et al. The use of an automated microsampling system for the characterization of growth hormone pulsatility in newborn babies. *Pediatr Res* 1997;**42**:66–71.

49. Winter J. Hypothalamic—pituitary function in the fetus and infant. *Clin Endocrinol Metab* 1982;**11**(1):41–55.

50. Mayo K. Molecular cloning and expression of a pituitary-specific receptor for growth hormone-releasing hormone. *Mol Endocrinol* 1992;**6**:1734–44.

51. Blanchard MM, Goodyer CG, Charrier J, Barenton B. In vitro regulation of growth hormone (GH) release from ovine pituitary cells during fetal and neonatal development: effects of GH-releasing factor, somatostatin, and insulin-like growth factor I. *Endocrinology* 1988;**122**:2114–20.

52. Hosoda H, Kojima M, Matsuo H, Kangawa K. Purification and characterization of rat des-Gln14-Ghrelin, a second endogenous ligand for the growth hormone secretagogue receptor. *J Biol Chem* 2000;**275**:21995–2000.

53. Giustina A, Veldhuis JD. Pathophysiology of the neuroregulation of growth hormone secretion in experimental animals and the human. *Endocr Rev* 1998;**19**:717–97.

54. Martha PM, Rogol AD, Veldhuis JD, Kerrigan JR, Goodman DW, Blizzard RM. Alterations in the pulsatile properties of circulating growth hormone concentrations during puberty in boys. *J Clin Endocrinol Metab* 1989;**69**:563–70.

55. Berelowitz M, Szabo M, Frohman LA, Firestone S, Chu L, Hintz RL. Somatomedin-C mediates growth hormone negative feedback by effects on both the hypothalamus and the pituitary. *Science (80-)* 1981;**212**:1279–81.

56. Abe H, Molitch ME, Van Wyk JJ, Underwood LE. Human growth hormone and somatomedin C suppress the spontaneous release of growth hormone in unanesthetized rats. *Endocrinology* 1983;**113**:1319–24.

57. Ho Y, Liebhaber S, Cooke N. Activation of the human GH gene cluster: roles for targeted chromatin modification. *Trends Endocrinol Metab* 2004;**15**:40–5.

58. Laron Z, Pertzelan A. Somatotrophin in antenatal and perinatal growth and development. *Lancet* 1969;**1**(7596):680–1.

59. DeLeon D, Cohen P, Katz L. Growth factor regulation of fetal growth. In: Polin R, Fox W, Abman S, editors. *Fetal and neonatal physiology*. 3rd ed. Philadelphia, PA: WB Saunders; 2004. p. 1880–90.

60. Clément-Lacroix P, Ormandy C, Lepescheux L, Ammann P, Damotte D, Goffin V, et al. Osteoblasts are a new target for prolactin: analysis of bone formation in prolactin receptor knockout mice. *Endocrinology* 1999;**140**:96–105.

61. Smith YF, Mullon DK, Hamosh M, Scolon JW, Hamosh P. Serum prolactin and respiratory distress syndrome in the newborn. *Pediatr Res* 1979;**14**:93–5.

62. Fliers E, Boelen A, van Trotsenburg A. Central regulation of the hypothalamo–pituitary–thyroid (HPT) axis: focus on clinical aspects. *Handb Clin Neurol* 2014;**124**:127–38.

63. Brown R, Huang S, Fisher D. The maturation of thyroid function in the perinatal period and during childhood. In: Braverman L, Utiger R, editors. *The thyroid*. Philadelphia, PA: Lippincott; 2005. p. 1013–28.

64. Burrow G, Fisher D, Larsen P. Maternal and fetal thyroid function. *N Engl J Med* 1994;**331**:1072–8.

65. Fisher D, Nelson J, Carlton E. Maturation of human hypothalamic-pituitary-thyroid function and control. *Thyroid* 2000;**10**:229–34.

66. Morreale de Escobar G, Obregon MJ, Escobar del Rey F. Role of thyroid hormone during early brain development. *Eur J Endocrinol* 2004;**151**(3): U25–37.

67. Fisher D, Klein A. Thyroid development and disorders of thyroid function in the newborn. *N Engl J Med* 1981;**304**:702–12.

68. Lechan RM, Fekete C. The TRH neuron: a hypothalamic integrator of energy metabolism. *Prog Brain Res* 2006;**153**:209–35.

69. Boelen A, Wiersinga WM, Fliers E. Fasting-induced changes in the hypothalamus-pituitary-thyroid axis. *Thyroid* 2008;**18**(2):123–9.

70. Romijn JA, Adriaanse R, Brabant G, Prank K, Endert E, Wiersinga W. Pulsatile secretion of thyrotropin during fasting: a decrease of thyrotropin pulse amplitude. *J Clin Endocrinol Metab* 1990;**70**(6):1631–6.

71. Chan JL, Heist K, DePaoli AM, Veldhuis JD, Mantzoros C. The role of falling leptin levels in the neuroendocrine and metabolic adaptation to short-term starvation in healthy men. *J Clin Invest* 2003;**111**(9):1409–21.

72. Snel M, Wijngaarden MA, Bizino MB, van der Grond J, Teeuwisse WM, van Buchem MA, Jazet IM, Pijl H. Food cues do not modulate the neuroendocrine response to a prolonged fast in healthy men. *Neuroendocrinology* 2012;**96**(4):285–93.

73. Boelen A, Kwakkel J, Wiersinga WM, Fliers E. Chronic local inflammation in mice results in decreased TRH and type 3 deiodinase mRNA expression in the hypothalamic paraventricular nucleus independently of diminished food intake. *J Endocrinol* 2006;**191**(3):707–14.

74. Mebis L, van den Berghe G. The hypothalamus-pituitary-thyroid axis in critical illness. *Neth J Med* 2009;**67**(10):332–40.

75. Chiamolera MI, Wondisford F. Minireview: thyrotropin-releasing hormone and the thyroid hormone feedback mechanism. *Endocrinology* 2009;**150**(3):1091–6.

76. Brabant G, Prank K, Ranft U, Schuermeyer T, Wagner TO, Hauser H, Kummer B, Feistner H, Hesch RD, von zur Mühlen A. Physiological regulation of circadian and pulsatile thyrotropin secretion in normal man and woman. *J Clin Endocrinol Metab* 1990;**70**(2):403–9.

77. Allan JS, Czeisler C. Persistence of the circadian thyrotropin rhythm under constant conditions and after light-induced shifts of circadian phase. *J Clin Endocrinol Metab* 1994;**79**(2):508–12.

78. Parker DC, Pekary AE, Hershman J. Effect of normal and reversed sleep-wake cycles upon nyctohemeral rhythmicity of plasma thyrotropin: evidence suggestive of an inhibitory influence in sleep. *J Clin Endocrinol Metab* 1976;**43**(2):318–29.

79. Kalsbeek A, Fliers E. Daily regulation of hormone profiles. *Handb Exp Pharmacol* 2013;**217**:185–226.

80. Greenspan SL, Klibanski A, Schoenfeld D, Ridgway E. Pulsatile secretion of thyrotropin in man. *J Clin Endocrinol Metab* 1986;**63**(3):661–8.

81. Behrends J, Prank K, Dogu E, Brabant G. Central nervous system control of thyrotropin secretion during sleep and wakefulness. *Horm Res* 1998;**49**(3–4):173–7.

82. Roelfsema F, Veldhuis J. Thyrotropin secretion patterns in health and disease. *Endocr Rev* 2013;**34**(5):619–57.

83. Van den Berghe G, de Zegher F, Veldhuis JD, Wouters P, Gouwy S, Stockman W, Weekers F, Schetz M, Lauwers P, Bouillon R, Bowers C. Thyrotrophin and prolactin release in prolonged critical illness: dynamics of spontaneous secretion and effects of growth hormone-secretagogues. *Clin Endocrinol* 1997;**47**(5):599–612.

84. Van den Berghe G, de Zegher F, Baxter RC, Veldhuis JD, Wouters P, Schetz M, Verwaest C, Van der Vorst E, Lauwers P, Bouillon R, Bowers C. Neuroendocrinology of prolonged critical illness: effects of exogenous thyrotropin-releasing hormone and its combination with growth hormone secretagogues. *J Clin Endocrinol Metab* 1998;**83**(2):309–19.

85. Fliers E, Alkemade A, Wiersinga W. The hypothalamic-pituitary-thyroid axis in critical illness. *Best Pract Res Clin Endocrinol Metab* 2001;**15**(4):453–64.

86. Fliers E, Guldenaar SE, Wiersinga WM, Swaab D. Decreased hypothalamic thyrotropin-releasing hormone gene expression in patients with non-thyroidal illness. *J Clin Endocrinol Metab* 1997;**82**(12):4032–6.

87. Adriaanse R, Romijn JA, Endert E, Wiersinga W. The nocturnal thyroid-stimulating hormone surge is absent in overt, present in mild primary and equivocal in central hypothyroidism. *Acta Endocrinol* 1992;**126**(3):206–12.

88. Goichot B, Weibel L, Chapotot F, Gronfier C, Piquard F, Brandenberger G. Effect of the shift of the sleep-wake cycle on three robust endocrine markers of the circadian clock. *Am J Phys* 1998;**275**(2):E243–8.

89. Guimiot F, Chevrier L, Dreux S, Chevenne D, Caraty A, Delezoide AL, de Roux N. Negative fetal FSH/LH regulation in late pregnancy is associated with declined kisspeptin/KISS1R expression in the tuberal hypothalamus. *J Clin Endocrinol Metab* 2012;**97**:E2229.

90. Clements JA, Reyes FI, Winter JS, Faiman C. Studies on human sexual development. III. Fetal pituitary and serum, and amniotic fluid concentrations of LH, CG, and FSH. *J Clin Endocrinol Metab* 1976;**42**:9–19.

91. Pilavdzic D, Kovacs K, Asa S. Pituitary morphology in anencephalic human fetuses. *Neuroendocrinology* 1997;**65**:164–72.

92. Wu Y, He Z, Zhang L, Jiang H, Zhang W. Ontogeny of immunoreactive Lh and Fsh cells in relation to early ovarian differentiation and development in protogynous hermaphroditic ricefield Eel *Monopterus albus*. *Biol Reprod* 2012;**86**:93.

93. Pepe GJ, Albrecht E. Regulation of the primate fetal adrenal cortex. *Endocr Rev* 1990;**11**(1):151–76.

94. Kuiri-Hanninen T. Activation of the hypothalamic-pituitary-gonadal axis in infancy: minipuberty. *Horm Res Paediatr* 2014;**82**:73–80.

95. Shinkawa O, Furuhashi N, Fukaya T, Suzuki M, Kono H, Tachibana Y. Changes of serum gonadotropin levels and sex differences in premature and mature infant during neonatal life. *J Clin Endocrinol Metab* 1983;**56**:1327–31.

96. Kuiri-Hänninen T, Seuri R, Tyrväinen E, Turpeinen U, Hämäläinen E, Stenman UH, Dunkel L, Sankilampi U. Increased activity of the hypothalamic-pituitary-testicular axis in infancy results in increased androgen action in premature boys. *J Clin Endocrinol Metab* 2011;**96**:98–105.

97. Kuiri-Hänninen T, Kallio S, Seuri R, Tyrväinen E, Liakka A, Tapanainen J, Sankilampi U, Dunkel L. Postnatal developmental changes in the pituitary-ovarian axis in preterm and term infant girls. *J Clin Endocrinol Metab* 2011;**96**:3432–9.

98. Ibáñez L, Valls C, Cols M, Ferrer A, Marcos MV, De Zegher F. Hypersecretion of FSH in infant boys and girls born small for gestational age. *J Clin Endocrinol Metab* 2002;**87**:1986–8.

99. Forest MG, de Peretti E, Bertrand J. Testicular and adrenal androgens and their binding to plasma proteins in the perinatal period: developmental patterns of plasma testosterone, 4-androstenedione, dehydroepiandrosterone and its sulfate in premature and small for date infants as compared with that of full-term infants. *J Steroid Biochem* 1980;**12**:25–36.

100. Sir-Petermann T, Hitschfeld C, Codner E, Maliqueo M, Iñiguez G, Echiburú B, Sánchez F, Crisosto N, Cassorla F. Gonadal function in low birth weight infants: a pilot study. *J Pediatr Endocrinol Metab* 2007;**20**:405–14.

101. Kota SK, Gayatri K, Jammula S, Meher LK, Kota SK, Krishna S, Modi K. Fetal endocrinology. *Indian J Endocrinol Metab* 2013;**17**(4):568–79.

102. Winter J, Abman SH. Fetal and neonatal adrenocortical physiology. In: Polin R, Fox W, editors. *Fetal and neonatal physiology*. Philadelphia, PA: WB Saunders; 2004. p. 1915–25.

103. Mesiano S, Jaffe RB. Developmental and functional biology of the primate fetal adrenal cortex. *Endocr Rev* 1997;**18**(3):378–403. https://doi.org/10.1210/edrv.18.3.0304.

104. Wood CE, Walker C-D. Fetal and neonatal HPA axis. *Compr Physiol* 2016;**6**(1):33–62.

105. Snegovskikh V, Park JS, Norwitz E. Endocrinology of parturition. *Endocrinol Metab Clin N Am* 2006;**35AD**:173–91.

106. Rivier C, Vale W. Neuroendocrine interactions between corticotrophin releasing factor and vasopressin on adrenocorticotropic hormone secretion in the rat. In: Schrier W, editor. *Vasopressin*. New York: Raven; 1985. p. 181–8.

107. Pavlova EB, Pronina TS, Skebelskaya Y. Histostructure of adenohypophysis of human fetuses and contents of somatotropic and adrenocorticotropic hormones. *Gen Comp Endocrinol* 1968;**10**:269–76.

108. Saoud CJ, Wood C. Ontogeny and molecular weight of immunoreactive arginine vasopressin and corticotropin-releasing factor in the ovine fetal hypothalamus. *Peptides* 1996;**17**:55–61.

109. Brubaker PL, Baird AC, Bennett HPJ, Browne CA, Solomon E. Corticotropic peptides in the human fetal pituitary. *Endocrinology* 1982;**111**:1150–5.

110. Ackland J, Ratter S, Bourne G, Rees L. Pro-opiomelanocortin peptides in the human fetal pituitary. *Regul Pept* 1983;**6**:51–61.

111. Milkovic S, Milkovic K, Paunovic J. The initiation of fetal adrenocorticotrophic activity in the rat. *Endocrinology* 1973;**92**:380–4.

112. Cohen A, Chatelain A, Dupouy J. Late pregnancy maternal and fetal time-course of plasma ACTH and corticosterone after continuous ether inhalation by pregnant rats. Cytoimmunological study of fetal hypophyseal cells. *Biol Neonate* 1983;**43**:220–8.

113. Power ML, Schulkin J. Functions of corticotropin-releasing hormone in anthropoid primates: from brain to placenta. *Am J Hum Biol* 2006;**18**:431–47.

114. Mastorakos G, Ilias I. Maternal and fetal hypothalamic-pituitary-adrenal axes during pregnancy and postpartum. *Ann N Y Acad Sci* 2003;**997**:136–49.

115. Norman LJ, Challis J. Synergism between systemic corticotropin releasing factor and arginine vasopressin on adrenocorticotropin release in vivo varies as a function of gestational age in the ovine fetus. *Endocrinology* 1987;**120**:1052–8.

116. Hargrave BY, Rose J. By 95 days of gestation CRF increases plasma ACTH and cortisol in ovine fetuses. *Am J Phys* 1986;**250**:e422–7.

117. Currie S, Brooks A. Corticotrophin-releasing factors in the hypothalamus of the developing fetal sheep. *J Dev Physiol* 1992;**17**:241–6.

118. Jard S, Gaillard RC, Guillon G, Marie J, Schoenenberg P, Muller AF, Manning M, Sawyer W. Vasopressin antagonists allow demonstration of a novel type of vasopressin receptor in the rat adenohypophysis. *Mol Pharmacol* 1986;**326**(30):171–7.

119. Young SF, Griffante C, Aguilera G. Dimerization between vasopressin V1b and corticotropin releasing hormone type 1 receptors. *Cell Mol Neurobiol* 2007;**27**:439–61.

120. Pepe G, Albrecht E. Actions of placental and fetal adrenal steroid hormones in primate pregnancy. *Endocr Rev* 1995;**16**:608–48.

121. Wadhwa PD, Sandman CA, Chicz-DeMet A, Porto M. Placental CRH modulates maternal pituitary–adrenal function in human pregnancy. *Ann N Y Acad Sci* 1997;**814**:276–81.

122. Wood CE, Rudolph A. Negative feedback regulation of adrenocorticotropin secretion by cortisol. *Endocrinology* 1983;**112**:1930–6.

123. Wood C. Negative-feedback inhibition of fetal ACTH secretion by maternal cortisol. *Am J Phys* 1987;**252**:R743–8.

124. Moisiadis VG, Matthews S. Glucocorticoids and fetal programming part 1: outcomes. *Nat Rev Endocrinol* 2014;**10**:391–402.

125. Walker CD, Sapolsky RM, Meaney MJ, Vale WW, Rivier C. Increased pituitary sensitivity to glucocorticoid feedback during the stress nonresponsive period in the neonatal rat. *Endocrinology* 1986;**119**:1816–21.

126. Wood C. Estrogen/hypothalamus-pituitary-adrenal axis interactions in the fetus: the interplay between placenta and fetal brain. *J Soc Gynecol Investig* 2005;**12**:67–76.

127. Wood CE, Saoud CJ, Stoner TA, Keller-Wood M. Estrogen and androgen influence hypothalamic AVP and CRF concentrations in fetal and adult sheep. *Regul Pept* 2001;**98**:63–8.

128. Laatikainen T, Pelkonen J, Apter D, Ranta T. Fetal and maternal serum levels of steroid sulfates, unconjugated steroids, and prolactin at term pregnan and in early spontaneous labor. *J Clin Endocrinol Metab* 1980;**50**(3):489–94.

129. Cacciari E, Cicognani A, Pirazzoli P, Dallacasa P, Mazzaracchio MA, Tassoni P, Bernardi F, Salardi S, Zappulla F. Plasma ACTH values during the first seven days of life in infants of diabetic mothers. *J Pediatr* 1975;**87**(6):943–5.

130. Similä S, Kauppila A, Ylikorkala O, Koivisto M, Mäkelä P, Haapalahti J. Adrenocorticotrophic hormone during the first day of life. *Eur J Pediatr* 1977;**124**(3):173–7.

131. Franks R. Diurnal variation of plasma 17-hydroxycorticosteroids in children. *J Clin Endocrinol Metab* 1967;**27**(1):75–8.

132. Helbock HJ, Insoft RM, Conte F. Glucocorticoid-responsive hypotension in extremely low birth weight newborns. *Pediatrics* 1993;**92**:715–7.

133. Hingre RV, Gross SJ, Hingre KS, Mayes DM, Richman R. Adrenal steroidogenesis in very low birth weight preterm infants. *J Clin Endocrinol Metab* 1994;**78**:266–70.

134. Lee MM, Rajagopalan L, Berg GJ, Moshang TJ. Serum adrenal steroid concentrations in premature infants. *J Clin Endocrinol Metab* 1989;**69**:1133–6.

135. Hanna CE, Keith LD, Colasurdo MA, et al. Hypothalamic pituitary adrenal function in the extremely low birth weight infant. *J Clin Endocrinol Metab* 1993;**76**:384–7.

136. Ng PC, Wong GWK, Lam CWK, et al. The pituitary–adrenal responses to exogenous human corticotropin-releasing hormone in preterm, very low birth weight infants. *J Clin Endocrinol Metab* 1997;**82**:797–9.

137. Watterberg KL, Scott S. Evidence of early adrenal insufficiency in babies who develop bronchopulmonary dysplasia. *Pediatrics* 1995;**95**:120–5.

138. Sandman CA, Wadhwa PD, Chicz-DeMet A, Dunkel-Schetter C, Porto M. Maternal stress, HPA activity, and fetal/infant outcome. *Ann N Y Acad Sci* 1997;**814**:266–75.

139. Reynolds R. Glucocorticoid excess and the developmental origins of disease: two decades of testing the hypothesis–2012 Curt Richter award winner. *Psychoneuroendocrinology* 2013;**38**:1–11.

140. Clark P. Programming of the hypothalamo–pituitary–adrenal axis and the fetal origins of adult disease hypothesis. *Eur J Pediatr* 1998;**157**:S7–10.

141. Edward CRW, Benediktsson R, Lindsay RS, Seckl J. Dysfunction of placental glucocorticoid barrier—link between fetal environment and adult hypertension. *Lancet* 1993;**341**:355–7.

142. Hales CN, Barker DJP, Clark PMS, et al. Fetal growth and impaired glucose tolerance at age 64. *BMJ* 1991;**303**:1019–22.

143. Carpenter T, Grecian SM, Reynolds R. Sex differences in early-life programming of the hypothalamic–pituitary–adrenal axis in humans suggest increased vulnerability in females: a systematic review. *J Dev Orig Health Dis* 2017;**8**(2):244–55.

144. Fora MA, Butler TG, Rose JC, Schwartz J. Adrenocorticotropin secretion by fetal sheep anterior and intermediate lobe pituitary cells in vitro: effects of gestation and adrenalectomy. *Endocrinology* 1996;**137**:3394–400.

145. Visser M, Swaab D. Life span changes in the presence of alpha-melanocyte-stimulating-hormone-containing cells in the human pituitary. *J Dev Physiol* 1979;**1**(2):161–78.

146. Perry RA, Mulvogue HM, McMillen IC, Robinson P. Immunohistochemical localization of ACTH in the adult and fetal sheep pituitary. *J Dev Physiol* 1985;**7**(6):397–404.

147. Jailer JW, Knowlton A. Evidence of simulated adrenal cortical activity during pregnancy in an addisonian patient. *J Clin Invest* 1950;**29**(6):825–6.

148. Assali NS, Hamermesz J. Adrenocorticotropic substances from human placenta. *J Clin Endocrinol Metab* 1954;**14**:781–2.

149. Krieger D. Placenta as a source of "brain" and "pituitary" hormones. *Biol Reprod* 1982;**26**:55–71.

150. Keller-Wood M, Powers MJ, Gersting JA, Ali N, Wood C. Genomic analysis of neuroendocrine development of fetal brain-pituitary-adrenal axis in late gestation. *Physiol Genomics* 2006;**24**:218–24.

151. Matthews SG, Han X, Lu F, Challis J. Developmental changes in the distribution of pro-opiomelanocortin and prolactin mRNA in the pituitary of the ovine fetus and lamb. *J Mol Endocrinol* 1994;**13**:175–85.

152. Simamura E, Shimada H, Shoji H, Otani H, Hatta T. Effects of melanocortins on fetal development. *Congenit Anom (Kyoto)* 2011;**51**(2):47–54.

153. Raffin-Sanson ML, de Keyzer Y, Bertagna X. Proopiomelanocortin, a polypeptide precursor with multiple functions: from physiology to pathological conditions. *Eur J Endocrinol* 2003;**149**:79–90.

154. Glickman JA, Carson GD, Challis J. Differential effects of synthetic adrenocorticotropin1-24 and alpha-melanocyte-stimulating hormone on adrenal function in human and sheep fetuses. *Endocrinology* 1979;**104**(1):34–9.

155. Swaab DF, Martin J. Functions of alpha-melanotropin and other opiomelanocortin peptides in labour, intrauterine growth and brain development. *CIBA Found Symp* 1981;**81**:196–217.

156. Nimura M, Udagawa J, Hatta T, Hashimoto R, Otani H. Spatial and temporal patterns of expression of melanocortin type 2 and 5 receptors in the fetal mouse tissues and organs. *Anat Embryol* 2006;**211**(2):109–17.

157. Leake R. The fetal-maternal neurohypophysial system. In: Polin RA, Fox W, editors. *Fetal and neonatal physiology*. 2nd ed. Philadelphia, PA: WB Saunders; 1998.

158. Ervin MG, Leake RD, Ross MG, Calvario GC, Fisher D. Arginine vasotocin in ovine fetal blood, urine, and amniotic fluid. *J Clin Invest* 1985;**75**(5):1696–701.

159. Gutnick A, Blechman J, Kaslin J, Herwig L, Belting HG, Affolter M, Bonkowsky JL, Levkowitz G. The hypothalamic neuropeptide oxytocin is required for formation of the neurovascular interface of the pituitary. *Dev Cell* 2011;**21**:642–54.

160. Morris M, Castro M, Rose J. Alterations in prohormone processing during early development in the fetal sheep. *Am J Phys* 1992;**263**:R738–40.

161. Wood CE, Tong H. Central nervous system regulation of reflex responses to hypotension during fetal life. *Am J Phys* 1999;**277**:R1541–52.

162. DeVane GW, Porter J. An apparent stress-induced release of arginine vasopressin by human neonates. *J Clin Endocrinol Metab* 1980;**51**:1412–6.

163. Matthews SG, Challis J. Regulation of CRH and AVP mRNA in the developing ovine hypothalamus: effects of stress and glucocorticoids. *Am J Phys* 1995;**268**:E1096–107.

164. Brooks AN, White A. Activation of pituitary-adrenal function in fetal sheep by corticotrophin-releasing factor and arginine vasopressin. *J Endocrinol* 1990;**124**(1):27–35.

165. Leake RD, Fisher D. Ontogeny of vasopressin in man. In: Czernichow P, Robinson A, editors. *Diabetes insipidus in man: frontiers in hormone research*. Basel: Karger; 1985.

166. Tribollet E, Charpak S, Schmidt A, Dubois-Dauphin M, Dreifuss J. Appearance and transient expression of oxytocin receptors in fetal, infant and peripubertal rat brain studied by autoradiography and electrophysiology. *J Neurosci* 1989;**9**(5):1764–73.

167. Devuyst O, Burrow CR, Smith BL, Agre P, Knepper MA, Wilson P. Expression of aquaporins-1 and -2 during nephrogenesis and in autosomal dominant polycystic kidney disease. *Am J Phys* 1996;**271**(1):F169–83.

168. Baum MA, Ruddy MK, Hosselet CA, Harris H. The perinatal expression of aquaporin-2 and aquaporin-3 in developing kidney. *Pediatr Res* 1998;**43**(6):783–90.

169. Cryns K, Sivakumaran TA, Van den Ouweland JM, Pennings RJ, Cremers CW, Flothmann K, Young TL, Smith RJ, Lesperance MM, Van Camp G. Mutational spectrum of the WFS1 gene in Wolfram syndrome, nonsyndromic hearing impairment, diabetes mellitus, and psychiatric disease. *Hum Mutat* 2003;**22**(4):275–87.

170. Benedetto MT, De Cicco F, Rossiello F, Nicosia AL, Lupi G, Dell'Acqua S. Oxytocin receptor in human fetal membranes at term and during labor. *J Steroid Biochem* 1990;**35**(2):205–8.

171. Sperling M. Carbohydrate metabolism: insulin and glucagons. In: Tulchinsky D, Little A, editors. *Maternal-fetal endocrinology*. 2nd ed. Philadelphia, PA: WB Saunders; 1994. p. 380–400.

172. Girard J. Control of fetal and neonatal glucose metabolism by pancreatic hormones. *Bailliere Clin Endocrinol Metab* 1989;**3**:817–36.

173. Kaludjerovic J, Ward WE. The interplay between estrogen and fetal adrenal cortex. *J Nutr Metab* 2012;**2012**:837901. https://doi.org/10.1155/2012/837901.

174. Ishimoto H, Jaffe RB. Development and function of the human fetal adrenal cortex: a key component in the feto-placental unit. *Endocr Rev* 2011;**32**(3):317–55. https://doi.org/10.1210/er.2010-0001.

175. Goto M, Piper Hanley K, Marcos J, et al. In humans, early cortisol biosynthesis provides a mechanism to safeguard female sexual development. *J Clin Invest* 2006;**116**(4):953–60. https://doi.org/10.1172/JCI25091.

176. Turan OM, Turan S, Funai EF, et al. Ultrasound measurement of fetal adrenal gland enlargement: an accurate predictor of preterm birth. *Am J Obstet Gynecol* 2011;**204**(4). https://doi.org/10.1016/j.ajog.2010.11.034. 311.e1–10.

177. Lemos A, Feitosa F, Araujo J, et al. Delivery prediction in pregnant women with spontaneous preterm birth using fetal adrenal gland biometry. *J Matern Fetal Neonatal Med* 2016;**29**:3756–61.

178. McLean M, Bisits A, Davies J, Woods R, Lowry P, Smith R. *A placental clock controlling the length of human pregnancy. Nat Med* 1995;**1**(5):460–3. http://www.ncbi.nlm.nih.gov/pubmed/7585095. Accessed 21 March 2014.

179. Robinson BG, Emanuel RL, Frim DM, Majzoub JA. *Glucocorticoid stimulates expression of corticotropin-releasing hormone gene in human placenta. Proc Natl Acad Sci U S A* 1988;**85**(14):5244–8. http://www.pubmedcentral.nih.gov/articlerender.fcgi?artid=281726&tool=pmcentrez&rendertype=abstract. Accessed 23 March 2014.

180. Smith R, Nicholson R. Corticotropin releasing hormone and the timing of birth. *Front Biosci* 2007;**12**:912–8.

181. Wheeler M, Styne D. Longitudinal changes in growth hormone response to growth hormone-releasing hormone in neonatal rhesus monkeys. *Pediatr Res* 1990;**28**:15–8.

182. Penny R, Parlow A, Frasier S. Testosterone and estradiol concentrations in paired maternal and cord sera and their correlation with the concentration of chorionic gonadotropin. *Pediatrics* 1979;**64**:604–8.

183. Mann D, Gould K, Collins D. Blockade of neonatal activation of the pituitary-testicular axis: effect on peripubertal luteinizing hormone and testosterone secretion and on testicular development in male monkeys. *J Clin Endocrinol Metab* 1989;**68**:600–7.

184. Fisher D. Thyroid system immaturities in very low birth weight premature infants. *Semin Perinatol* 2008;**32**(6):387–97.

Chapter 31

The Pineal Gland Development and its Physiology in Fetus and Neonate

Suzana Elena Voiculescu*, Diana Le Duc[†,‡], Adrian Eugen Rosca* and Ana-Maria Zagrean*

*Division of Physiology and Neuroscience, Department of Functional Sciences, "Carol Davila" University of Medicine and Pharmacy, Bucharest, Romania, [†]Institute of Human Genetics, University of Leipzig Hospitals and Clinics, Leipzig, Germany, [‡]Department of Evolutionary Genetics, Max Planck Institute for Evolutionary Anthropology, Leipzig, Germany

Key Clinical Changes

- The pineal gland does not begin secreting melatonin until 3–5 months after birth and coincides with the typical time when sleep patterns are better established in the neonate.
- The fetus is dependent on maternal melatonin crossing the placenta.
- Fetuses display rhythmicity of melatonin and behavior that parallel maternal levels and activity.
- Postnatal production of melatonin is further delayed in premature babies.
- Melatonin has been proposed to affect many aspects of fetal development, but further study is needed to confirm these roles.

31.1 INTRODUCTION

The pineal gland is a nervous system component, a neuroendocrine translator, that in mammals and humans expresses photoperiodicity and a secretory function, all of which are related to and coordinated with the circadian rhythm. Its main hormone and the most studied one is melatonin. The functions of melatonin are a subject of recent research and have been shown to extend to many domains of human physiology. Classically, melatonin is an endogenous synchronizer, and its secretion imprints rhythms in various body functions via the hypothalamus suprachiasmatic nucleus (SCN): body heat, sleep/wake cycle, cortisol secretion, blood pressure, cellular divisions, and immune system function.

Little is known about melatonin's fetal functions and physiology. The passage of maternal melatonin through the placenta exposes the fetus to a daily rhythm of low concentrations during the day and high concentrations at night. Consequently, melatonin is likely involved in inducing a circadian rhythm to fetal physiology and organs (Fig. 31.1).

31.2 PINEAL DEVELOPMENT AND CIRCADIAN RHYTHM ONTOGENESIS

The pineal gland, which is responsible for the circadian endocrine melatonin production, develops from an area of the neuroepithelium that lines the roof of the third ventricle in the prenatal brain. Its maturation continues postnatally with a growth in size until about 2 years of age.[1]

A dynamic and intricate regulatory network of transcription factors is necessary for pineal gland development, among which homeobox transcription factors Pax6, Otx2, and Lhx9 seem to play an essential role.[2, 3] These transcription factors are responsible for regulating pinealocyte specification and prenatal proliferation. In their absence, the pineal gland fails to develop. Hartley and colleagues showed that treating surgically removed neonatal rat pineal glands with norepinephrine, a superior cervical ganglia transmitter, renders their gene expression profile very close to the in vivo state. These findings suggested that, despite the postnatal maturation of the gland, the pineal-defining transcriptome is established prior to birth.[4]

After birth, the newborn no longer receives an infusion of melatonin from the maternal circulation, except through maternal milk, in the case of breastfeeding. Over the following 6 to 8 weeks, the child develops its own circadian rhythm regulated by melatonin secreted by the pineal gland.[5] Detectable circadian variations in melatonin become most apparent

Maternal-Fetal and Neonatal Endocrinology. https://doi.org/10.1016/B978-0-12-814823-5.00031-3

FIG. 31.1 Role of melatonin in the maternal-placental-fetal system. Light detected by the eyes of the mother is transmitted to the circadian pacemaker in the suprachiasmatic nucleus (SCN), which sends a neural signal to the pineal gland to regulate the circadian rhythm of melatonin secretion. Melatonin synthesis is upregulated in pregnant women, possibly via placental signaling to the maternal pineal gland. Melatonin modulates circadian endocrine rhythms and ensures protection via free radical scavenging, indirect antioxidant effects, and immune regulation. Melatonin acts on its MT1/MT2 receptors to promote fetal growth and development. *ROS*, reactive oxygen species; *NO*, nitric oxide.

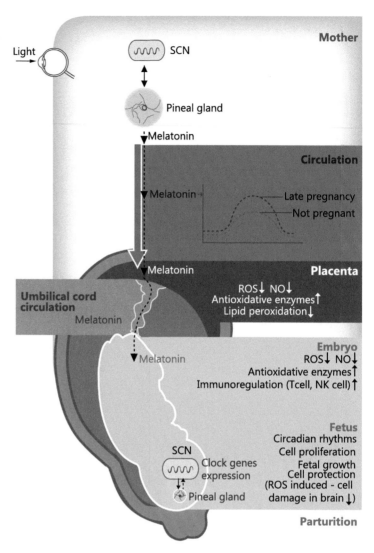

from the 3rd to 6th month of life, which is the period when the newborn develops a normal sleep rhythm. However, the maximal rise in the nocturnal melatonin secretion amplitude occurs between the 4th and 7th year of life.[6]

Circadian rhythm development in humans is a controversial subject with scant human data. We shall instead make some inferences from rodents, which are the most used experimental models. In rats, circadian rhythms per se develop after birth, but in the human fetuses, oscillations have been identified beginning with the 24th intrauterine week, with components of the circadian system appearing well before this. In postnatal rats, basal corticosterone shows 24-h oscillations, beginning at postnatal day 22 (P22).[7] A rhythm in activity period is present starting around day 9 or 10 after birth, and body temperature rhythm begins in the first week after birth.[8, 9]

There are various aspects of fetal physiology, such as body movement, hormonal levels, and heart activity, that exhibit a circadian rhythm, especially during late gestation.[10] It appears that these functions are regulated at least in part by the fetal suprachiasmatic nucleus (SCN) that was first discovered in rodents by Reppert and Schwartz in 1984.[11] It has been shown that fetal tissues contain circadian clock systems that resemble the adult ones, and these rhythms may be regulated by signals coming from the mother across the placenta.[10, 12]

Clock gene expression in fetal and embryonic tissues has been observed mostly in murine models. Mouse embryos express clock genes starting with day 10 of gestation, and this expression increases until day 19, just before birth.[13] The fetal rat SCN exhibits a 24-h rhythm in metabolic activity (specifically use of glucose),[11] and in the expression of various genes, including c-Fos and Avp.[14]

Clock genes are also expressed in the fetal liver, but their expression seems to be arrhythmic.[15] A daily variation of hepatic clock genes develops gradually in the postnatal period, with full rhythmicity apparent by postnatal day 30.[12]

Quite opposite form the fetal SCN and liver, the adrenal clock appears to be functional late during pregnancy.[16]

In rats, the SCN begins to develop around embryonic day (ED) 14 and continues until ED 17. Neurogenesis stops at ED 18, but a progressive maturation in morphology occurs until the 10th day after birth, when synaptic density reaches adult levels. Synaptogenesis happens mostly after birth, but a small number of synapses have been identified, beginning with ED 19.[17] At this time, a rhythm in activity of the internal SCN becomes evident.[11]

Honma et al. found important clues that point to the existence of a maternofetal coordination of circadian rhythms in fetal rats before ED 10, before the SCN is formed. In this experiment, the authors observed that reversal of the light-dark cycle of the pregnant mother at day 10 of pregnancy resulted in an effective reversal of the pup's hormonal rhythm.[18, 19] As to the onset of prenatal entrainment of the circadian oscillation, two possibilities exist. One is that the fetal circadian oscillation entrains to the maternal circadian rhythm before day 10 of gestation and the entrainment continues to the end of pregnancy. If the maternal circadian system is disrupted by the SCN lesion during pregnancy, the fetal circadian oscillation starts to free run, resulting in a negative phase angle difference to the rhythm developed in the control pups. Alternatively, it is possible that the fetal oscillation is unable to entrain to the maternal circadian system until the latter stages of gestation. In this case, we must postulate the phase of oscillation to be preset genetically; this has not been substantiated experimentally yet.

Peripheral circadian systems develop in fetuses before the SCN does and are probably regulated by maternal rhythms. A series of experiments in rats and hamsters showed that fetal circadian systems synchronization is lost after destruction of the maternal SCN.[20]

SCN of the human fetus becomes functional and begins to present periodic 24-h oscillations at midterm (20–25 weeks post conception).[21] This coincides with the first fetal movements felt by the mother. Also, between 24 and 26 weeks of gestation, the eyelids are not fused anymore, and eye movements may be detected by ultrasonography.

In the last trimester, the fetal biological clock develops, and it is sensitive to maternal circadian rhythms, to which it responds by hormonal, behavioral, and sleep fluctuations.[21]

Sladek et al. studied clock genes profile (Per 1, Per2, Cry1, Bmal1, and Clock) at ED 19, and postpartum days 3 and 10 in rats.[12] ED 19 was chosen because at this specific time, neurogenesis of the SCN is complete. All studied genes are present in the SCN, but they either do not have a rhythmic expression, or the amplitude of their expression is too low to be detected. The same study showed a different expression at postnatal day 3, when a high expression of Per1, Per2, Cry1 and Bmal1 is detected, in contrast with the Clock gene. The aim of this study was to discover the development of the clockwork during ontogenesis. Daily profiles of Per1, Per2, Cry1, Bmal1, and Clock mRNA in the SCN of fetuses at the embryonic day 19 and of newborn rats at the postnatal day 3 and 10 were assessed. In addition, daily profiles of PER1, PER2, and CRY1 proteins at ED19 were measured. As early as at ED19, all the studied clock genes were already expressed in the SCN. However, no SCN rhythm in their expression was detected; Per1, Cry1, and Clock mRNA levels were low, whereas Bmal1 mRNA levels were high and Per2 mRNA levels were medium. Moreover, no rhythms of PER1, PER2, and CRY1 were detectable. At P3, rhythms in Per1, Per2, Cry1, and Bmal1, but not in Clock mRNA, were expressed in the SCN. The rhythm matured gradually; at P10, the amplitude of Per1, Per2, and Bmal1 mRNA rhythms were more pronounced than at P3. Altogether, the data show a gradual development of both the positive and negative elements of the molecular clockwork, from no detectable rhythmicity at ED19 to highly developed rhythms at P10.[12]

In conclusion, the animal literature has shown that the constitutive elements of the biological clocks are present during late fetal development, and the molecular elements of these pathways are at least inducible.

The specific maternal signal that induces fetal rhythms is not yet identified, but the main candidate is melatonin. The fetal organism is clearly influenced by many variables in the mother, such as behavior, metabolism, endocrine activity, and cardiovascular function.

31.3 MELATONIN SYNTHESIS

Much of what is known about melatonin and pineal gland function comes from studies of adult humans and animals, and these data are summarized in this section. Melatonin (*N*-acetyl-5 methoxy tryptamine) is a 232 kDa molecular weight indoleamine, synthesized from the essential amino acid tryptophan, via serotonin. Melatonin synthesis primary takes place in the pineal gland. In adults, ectopic melatonin produced by other organs is released in the blood in minimum amounts, having more likely an autocrine or paracrine function than a systemic endocrine function.[2] The pineal gland is a component of the nervous system, being a neuroendocrine translator, by having the capacity to transform a nerve impulse into a neurotransmitter secretion. In invertebrates, it also has a photoreception function, which is lost in mammals and humans.

Melatonin and the synthesis pathway enzymes may be identified at multiple levels in the organism such as retina, nervous organs (cortex, raphe nuclei, striatum), gastrointestinal tract (stomach, intestine), testis, ovary, lymphocytes, lens, cochlea, and skin.[22] Recently, it has been proposed that it is synthesized in mitochondria.[23] High levels of melatonin have been measured in these organelles,[24] which are a major source of free radicals. Pinealocytes secrete melatonin directly into the blood or cerebrospinal fluid. The SCN in the hypothalamus is the major regulator of melatonin release, acting through a multisynaptic pathway. The SCN sends fibers to the superior thoracic spinal cord, and they leave the cord to synapse in the first sympathetic paravertebral ganglion C1. Postganglionic fibers reach the pinealocytes through noradrenergic synapses.[25] In darkness, norepinephrine is released in the synaptic cleft and acts on beta 1 adrenergic receptors, leading to an intracellular cAMP production and subsequently higher melatonin synthesis.[15, 26, 27] cAMP activates N-acetyl transferase enzyme, which catalyzes serotonin to N-acetyl serotonin conversion, the latter being then converted to melatonin with the help of hydroxy-indole-O-methyl transferase (HIOMT).

Although pineal cells are not directly photoreceptive, they do respond to sunlight versus darkness. Optic information reaches the SCN from the retina through the retinal hypothalamic tract, made from axons of a subpopulation of retinal ganglionic cells, melanopsin-positive, that represents 1%–2% of all retinal ganglion cells. In turn, melatonin activates SCN neurons, whose axons project to the adjacent hypothalamic nuclei, synchronizing some of the circadian system components such as body heat, sleep/wake cycle, feeding rhythm, and corticotropin/corticosteroids production.

The SCN receives serotonergic afferent fibers from the raphe nuclei in the midbrain, especially from the median nucleus.[28, 29] It has been shown that serotonin modulates the manner that light influences SCN, by controlling glutamate release from the retinal hypothalamic tract.[30]

Apart from the 24-h circadian rhythm of melatonin secretion (24 ± 4 h in most organisms, 25 h in humans), a variation of secretion with age has also been identified. In humans, melatonin secretion reaches a maximum between 1 and 3 years of age, and then its concentration begins to fall progressively from puberty until 70 years, when it is about 10% of its peak value.[31]

31.3.1 Melatonin Sources for the Fetus

Inferior vertebrates demonstrate secretion of melatonin secretion during embryonic development. Human fetuses and newborns do not produce melatonin. Instead, they are dependent on maternal melatonin, which is transferred via the placenta or maternal milk.

The human pineal gland does not produce melatonin until 3–5 months after birth. In premature babies, this delay is even longer, proportional to the degree of prematurity. The fetal SCN expresses melatonin receptors, and melatonin is one of the few hormones able to cross the placental barrier.[5, 32]

The primary and only source for melatonin in the fetus is the mother via the placenta. Very active melatonin rhythms have been measured in pregnant mammals,[33, 34] which are mirrored and closely paralleled in the fetuses. Melatonin rapidly crosses the placenta, as demonstrated in rodents, sheep, and primates.[35, 36]

31.4 MELATONIN AND OOGENESIS

It has been shown that melatonin has a positive action in human gametogenesis because of a direct action at the level of the ovary. The molecule concentrates at ovary level when injected in the systemic circulation.[33] There are studies that have identified a high concentration of melatonin in the preovulation follicular liquid, higher than in the serum,[33] and that this concentration depends on follicular maturation. It has been stipulated that melatonin has an antioxidative importance in this situation, as follicular maturation is associated with a high production of free radicals. In addition, melatonin can increase glutathione peroxidase activity in the human chorion.[34]

Melatonin has also been studied in the context of assisted reproduction, and it has been shown that it enhances oocyte quality and success rate of in vitro fertilization procedure, when administered before FIV cycle initialization and continued during the entire pregnancy. The fertilization rate was 50% higher in the melatonin-treated group versus controls.[37, 38]

31.5 PINEAL DURING DEVELOPMENT

The outcome of the pregnancy is modified by the environment in which the mother works or lives. Night shifts enhance the risk for prematurity, low birth weight, abortion, and reduced fertility.[39] This may be explained in part by a shorter sleep period. The FSH concentration of women who sleep <8 h per night is reduced by 20%.[40] Plasma concentrations of melatonin and prolactin at 0200 h were significantly lower in nurses working at night than others of the resting group, but plasma concentrations of LH and FSH did not differ between the two groups. These results indicate that night shift suppresses the ovarian function by affecting the circadian rhythm of melatonin and prolactin.

Suppression of maternal melatonin secretion in rats, through continuous light exposure in the second half of the pregnancy, slows intrauterine development and alters mRNA expression of Clock and Clock related genes. It also negatively influences corticosterone secretion by altering its secretion rhythm, lowers ACTH- dependent corticosterone secretion in vitro, and reduces Clock genes expression. All these changes are reversible with melatonin administration.[20]

A study in sheep showed that melatonin administration to pregnant mothers inhibits noradrenalin-induced fetal cerebral artery vasoconstriction, glycerol release from brown adipose tissue, and ACTH-induced cortisol secretion from the fetal adrenal gland. Low corticosterone levels or modified circadian secretion of corticosterone may explain the growth abnormalities mentioned before.[41]

Mice with a Clock Delta 19 mutation were used to determine whether fetal development within a genetically disrupted circadian environment affects pregnancy outcomes and alters the metabolic health of offspring. Circadian abnormality caused hyperleptinemia and excessive adipose tissue development by 3 months after birth. It also leads to altered glucose tolerance and insulin resistance at 1 year.[42]

Multiple animal studies have associated alterations in maternal circadian rhythms during pregnancy with increased risk of different severe pathologies in the fetuses, including metabolic syndrome, obesity, psychiatric conditions (schizophrenia, attention deficit, autistic spectrum disorders).[43]

Melatonin may be essential in the normal development of the placenta; this specific function being in the first place sustained by a high expression of melatonin receptors in the placenta, early during pregnancy.[44] Synthetizing enzymes and melatonin receptors are expressed in the human placenta throughout pregnancy and promote syncytium formation.[45]

Melatonin generating system is expressed throughout pregnancy (from week 7 to term) in placental tissues. AANAT and HIOMT show maximal expression at the third trimester of pregnancy. MT1 receptor expression is maximal at the first trimester compared to the second and third trimesters, while MT2 receptor expression does not change significantly during pregnancy. During primary villous cytotrophoblast syncytialization, MT1 receptor expression increases, while MT2 receptor expression decreases. Treatment of primary villous cytotrophoblast with an increasing concentration of melatonin raises syncytium formation and β-hCG secretion.[45]

31.5.1   Melatonin Levels in the Neonatal Period

Serum samples in the first day of life have been measured in a study that shows a relationship between melatonin concentration and birth weight. If the mean birth weight was <1500 g, melatonin serum level was 63.2 pg/mL, and it has been shown to increase gradually to 79.3 pg/mL at 7 days. If birth weight was >1500 g, melatonin level was 104 pg/mL, and increased at 109.4 at 7 days.[46]

There are studies that have reported different melatonin concentrations in the umbilical artery (UA) and vein (UV), depending on the mode of delivery. The melatonin concentration was not significantly different between UA and UV blood both at daytime and at nighttime. Both in UA and in UV, the melatonin concentration was significantly higher at nighttime than at daytime. Compared with the C-section group, melatonin in the vaginal deliveries group was significantly higher both at night- and daytime. Melatonin both in UA and in UV was found to be not significantly different between patients with and without risk factors for stress including pregnancy complications (e.g., preeclampsia) and intrapartum complications (e.g., emergency section, pathological doppler, and pathological cardiotocography).[47]

31.6   DYNAMICS OF MELATONIN SECRETION DURING NORMAL AND PATHOLOGICAL PREGNANCIES

Serum melatonin concentrations in women exhibit changes in both physiological and pathological pregnancies compared with nonpregnant controls. Although there are no fetal data, these maternal values are in turn expected to determine the fetal concentrations and impact fetal development and behavior. Also, maternal melatonin titers are not constant during the 40 weeks of pregnancy, but they show specific dynamics, which are also presumed to be reflected in what would be present in simultaneous fetal values (see the table with maternal normal levels in Chapter 2).[22] Daytime serum melatonin concentrations were lower in women bearing singletons as compared with women with twins, or pregnancies affected by preeclampsia or intrauterine growth retardation.

Nocturnal serum melatonin in mothers increased after 24 weeks of gestation, with highest levels after 32 weeks. Such values were significantly higher in twin pregnancies after 28 weeks of gestation than in single pregnancies, whereas the patients with severe preeclampsia showed lower serum melatonin levels than in women with mild preeclampsia or normal pregnancies after 32 weeks.[23]

31.7   MELATONIN ANTIOXIDATIVE PROPERTIES DURING FETAL DEVELOPMENT

Melatonin is known for its antioxidative role, being a direct scavenger for hydroxyl groups and peroxynitrite (or other nitrogen reactive species). The mechanism is formation of melatonin groups during its reaction with different radicals, leading to superoxide anions detoxification. More than this, not only melatonin has the capacity of neutralizing free radicals, but also its metabolites that result during the antioxidative fight.[48] Some of them are even more efficient than the melatonin molecule itself.[43]

Melatonin raises the antioxidative potential of the organism by stimulating antioxidative enzyme production and glutathione quantity in the cells.[49]

Melatonin maintains mitochondrial homeostasis; it reduces free radical formation at this level and protects ATP synthesis by direct stimulation of enzymatic complexes I and IV, thus maintaining mitochondrial energy production. Melatonin provides mitochondrial protection, having antiapoptotic effects and keeping mitochondrial integrity. It has the ability to scavenge free oxygen and nitrogen reactive species at mitochondrial level, by this preventing disruption of the membrane and of the electron transport chain (ETC). Melatonin also protects mitochondrial DNA (mtDNA). It inhibits the pathological opening of the mitochondrial permeability transition pore (mPTP). Under normal conditions, this pore allows free exchange of low molecular weight molecules, having an alternating open/close behavior. Under pathological conditions, it gets blocked in a continuous open state and leads to mitochondrial rupture. The inhibition of apoptosis is reached by directly preventing nitro-oxidative damage, and by lowering the expression of the proapoptotic protein BAX. Leakage of cytochrome C is thus prevented, and apoptosis cascade propagation is inhibited (Fig. 31.2).

Melatonin appears to act in a similar way at the level of the placenta: it scavenges free radicals,[29] reduces lipid peroxidation, and enhances antioxidative enzymes production (SOD, glutathione peroxidase and glutathione reductase).[50]

The placenta represents a major source of free radicals. Peroxidation makers, such as lipid hydroxy peroxide and malondialdehyde, are higher in pregnant versus nonpregnant women.[51] Lipid peroxidation begins in the second trimester and progressively increases until delivery.[52] Under normal conditions, these processes that induce oxidative stress are well regulated by placental antioxidative enzymes such as SOD, CAT, GPx, glutathione reductase, glutathione S transferase, and glucose 6 phosphate dehydrogenase. A recent study shows that SOD and CAT levels increase during pregnancy and GPx level lowers in mothers.[53]

Melatonin level is low in pregnant women that associate preeclampsia or intrauterine growth restriction, and this may be explained through a low antioxidative capacity.

Oxidative stress is considered an important cause for intrauterine growth restriction. Some studies show that placental dysfunction leads to a chronic hypoxemic state to which the organism adapts by inhibiting fetal growth.[54] Intrauterine

FIG. 31.2 Melatonin function in the mitochondria. Melatonin reduces free radical formation and protects ATP synthesis by direct stimulation of enzymatic complexes I and IV. Melatonin scavenges free oxygen and nitrogen reactive species at mitochondrial level, by this preventing disruption of the membrane and of the electron transport chain (ETC). It also protects mitochondrial DNA (mtDNA) and inhibits the pathological opening of the mitochondrial permeability transition pore (mPTP). Inhibition of apoptosis is reached by directly preventing nitro-oxidative damage, and by lowering the expression of the proapoptotic protein BAX. Leakage of cytochrome C is thus prevented, and apoptosis cascade propagation is inhibited.

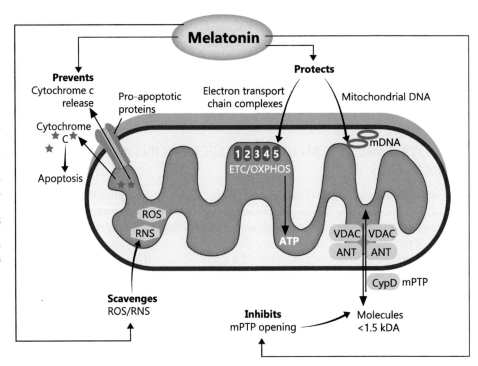

growth restriction is associated with high mortality risk, premature birth, nervous system developmental abnormalities, and potentially severe deficits, such as cerebral palsy.[54,55]

Fetal distress in human infants has been associated with a high level of ROS production and a reduction of melatonin secretion during the first 3 months after birth.[46]

Urinary excretion of 6-sulphatoxy melatonin (6SaMT), a metabolite of melatonin, is reduced in response to infants subjected to life-threatening conditions. Diurnal 6SaMT rhythms in these children exhibit lower 24-h mean values. A follow-up in 6 weeks shows an increased excretion in all groups, which suggests that in these infants there is delayed ontogenesis of melatonin secretion and not a long-term impairment of secretion.[46]

31.8 MELATONIN AND NEURODEVELOPMENT

Melatonin has been shown to have important functions in neurodevelopment, highlighted by the presence of its receptors in the central nervous system of the fetus. The literature describes two types of melatonin receptors: ML1 (high affinity) and ML2 (low affinity). ML1 receptors are further subclassified in Mel1A (MT1), Mel1B (MT2), and Mel1C. The latter are not present in mammals. All of them are classic G-coupled receptors, which inhibit adenylate-cyclase.[49]

There are a lot of available animal studies that determine the presence of MT receptors in the nervous structures in different species.

Melatonin receptors appear to be more highly expressed in developing embryos and neonates than in adults.[56-58] This may suggest a role of melatonin and the pineal gland in fetal and neonatal development. Indeed, melatonin administration in zebrafish has a positive effect on cell proliferation and accelerates embryonic development. Melatonin has a role in extending the safe limit of proliferation rate at night to allow more rapid development when potentially damaging ultraviolet light is absent.[57] In contrast, melatonin receptor antagonists delay neurogenesis in the habenulae, suggesting that melatonin is required for the cell cycle exit of neural progenitors.[59] Moreover, following a metabolic insult in the developing rodent brain, melatonin stimulates the proliferation and differentiation of neuronal stem cells,[60] and increases axonal sprouting and the expression of axonal markers.[61]

In Siberian hamsters, melatonin receptors are first identified during development at gestational day 10, in the primitive pharynx. Until days 12 till 14, these receptors are also present in the nasopharynx, the Rathke pouch, caudal arteries, and the thyroid gland during its migration along the thyroglossal duct. At day 16, the Rathke pouch differentiates into the hypophysis, which continues to express specific receptors until birth. Thyroid receptors are no longer identifiable from day 16 until birth.[62]

In sheep, melatonin receptors were found in the medial cerebral artery, brown adipose tissue, and adrenal gland.[41]

Melatonin receptors are also present in the median eminence. The hypophyseal concentration of ^{125}I-melatonin was highest at ED day 20 in sheep fetuses, progressively lowering after birth until the 29th day, when it reached 10% out of the aforementioned value. In contrast, the median eminence receptor concentration remains the same through the entire developmental period.[41]

Fetal melatonin receptor expression appears to be influenced by the secretion of maternal melatonin. One study compared expression and density of receptors in the fetal brain of rat siblings from mothers with or without pinealectomy. At birth, it appears that in both cases, receptors are expressed by the same nervous organs, but pups born from pinealectomized mothers have a 20% lower receptor density. By day 9 after birth, when pups begin to secrete their own melatonin, these differences disappeared. The conclusion of this study was that melatonin is not essential for the expression of its receptors in fetuses, but it does enhance their density.[63]

Melatonin receptors have been identified in human embryos and fetuses, both in the central nervous system and peripheral organs, such as endocrine glands. One study shows the presence of specific, GTP-sensitive for binding of 2-[(125) I] iodomelatonin in the leptomeninges, cerebellum, thalamus, hypothalamus, and brain stem. In the hypothalamus, one of the specific areas is the SCN itself, but receptors are also present in the arcuate, ventromedial and mamillary nuclei. At the level of the brain stem, there are melatonin receptor-positive areas in the nuclei of cranial nerves, such as oculomotor, trochlear, trigeminal motor and sensory, facial, and cochlear.[64]

31.9 MELATONIN AND PERINATAL NEUROPROTECTION

Melatonin has a neuroprotective function in both adult and fetal brain. In adults, there are many studies that show it has a positive effect in neurodegenerative conditions such as Alzheimer's or Parkinson diseases.[65]

The neuroprotective effect of melatonin in the fetal brain has not been extensively studied as compared with adults. One study shows that melatonin administration at 10 min after a hypoxic and acidemic episode in sheep fetuses lowers the risk of death and the number of activated microglia. It also reduces fetal brain inflammation and cell death.[66] A recent study shows that melatonin treatment before and after temporary fetal asphyxia lowers oxidative stress by reducing free radical formation, lipid peroxidation, and cell death it the fetal brain.[42]

Maternal melatonin administration in an animal model of intrauterine growth restriction in sheep led to reduced oxidative stress and brain damage in newborn lambs.[67] The neuroprotective potential of melatonin is shown also by its positive effect on norepinephrine-induced vasoconstriction in the medial cerebral artery.[68] It also induces vasodilation in the umbilical blood vessels in an ovine model.[69]

Hypothermia represents an efficient therapeutic method used in newborns with neonatal encephalopathy, but even so, 50% suffer long-term consequences. Combined treatment method involving hypothermia associated with melatonin administration had a positive effect on cerebral energetic metabolism and neural apoptosis.[70]

Systemic melatonin administration in newborn rats with intracerebral bleeding leads to a lower degree of cortical atrophy, and better cognitive, sensory, and motor functions in the treated group.[70] Fulia et al. measured malonaldehyde and nitrates before and after melatonin administration in human newborns with perinatal asphyxia. Treatment was applied during the first 6 h after birth, and products of lipid peroxidation were measured at 12 and 24 h. Lipid peroxidation products and nitrites levels went progressively down.[71]

Under pathologic circumstances, melatonin production is greatly influenced, and thus lower and delayed secretion may be found in infants who suffered from preterm delivery, preeclampsia, or growth restriction.[3] However, endogenous melatonin production increases in critically ill children, possibly as a counterresponse to the elevated oxidative stress associated with serious diseases.[72] Indeed, models of neonatal encephalopathy have shown a beneficial neuroprotective effect of melatonin.[66, 69, 70]

At birth, the periventricular white matter is highly susceptible to damage during hypoxic-ischemic episodes, given a blood-vessel density decrease in the region.[34] Hypoxic damage may lead to necrotic lesions of the periventricular white matter, which are described as periventricular leukomalacia. Postasphyxia melatonin treatment (20 mg/kg infusion) attenuated the lipid peroxidation, and reduced the level of oxidative stress and the number of apoptotic cells in the cerebral white matter in midgestational fetal sheep.[66] The protective effects of melatonin on the periventricular white matter of hypoxic neonatal brains were suggested to be due to its antioxidant properties.[73]

Likewise, hypoxic-ischemic brain injury in the neonates results in mitochondrial dysfunction and increased oxidative stress.[74] Hypoxic-ischemic injury induces an increase in deferoxamine (DFO)-chelatable free iron in the rat cerebral cortex, followed by increase in oxidative stress, which may be prevented by melatonin administration.[75] Melatonin treatment before or after hypoxic insults in immature rats was shown to provide a long-lasting benefit, suggesting that melatonin could represent a potentially safe approach to perinatal brain damage in humans.[75]

Human studies have shown melatonin toxicity to be extremely low when including data available from use in children with various neurologically disabling disorders,[76] or even from administration to neonates with sepsis. Hence the neuroprotective outcomes of melatonin on the fetal brain could be assessed in human studies. A randomized controlled pilot study tested the clinical outcomes of melatonin in neonates with hypoxic-ischemic encephalopathy (HIE) including 45 newborns: 30 affected and 15 healthy controls. HIE infants were randomized into a hypothermia group ($N = 15$), which received 72-h whole-body cooling, and a combined melatonin/hypothermia group ($N = 15$), which received hypothermia and five daily enteral doses of melatonin at 10 mg/kg. Serum nitric oxide (NO), plasma superoxide dismutase (SOD), and melatonin levels were measured for the 45 probands on admission and after 5 days. The study concluded that compared with healthy neonates, the HIE groups had increased melatonin, SOD, and NO. However, after 5 days, the melatonin/hypothermia group had a significantly higher level of melatonin and decrease in NO and SOD. This group also had fewer seizures on follow-up electroencephalogram and fewer white matter abnormalities on MRI. Importantly, at 6 months, the melatonin/hypothermia group had significantly better survival rate without developmental or neurological abnormalities.[77]

Melatonin appears thus to be safe and beneficial in HIE treatment. However, larger randomized controlled trials are required before melatonin can be approved for usage in preventing the consequences of HIE.[78] As with the other neuroprotective benefits described earlier in this section, melatonin treatment cannot be recommended for widespread human use due to the lack of data from definitive clinical trials.

31.10 MELATONIN AND BEHAVIOR

Melatonin modulates a sum of physiologic functions such as circadian rhythm, sleep induction, visual, reproductive, neuroendocrine, and immune system functions. It has roles in normal behavior, including learning, stress response,[79–87] memory[88] (especially short-term memory[89]), and pain perception.[90–92]

Changes in melatonin secretion were found in a variety of psychiatric pathologies in humans: seasonal depressive disorder, bipolar disorder, depression, bulimia, anorexia, schizophrenia, panic attack, and obsessive-compulsive disorder.

Memory is a complex process, occurring at an intense rate in the neonatal period and involving distinct phases: acquisition, consolidation, and retrieval. Using an active avoidance conditioning test, it was shown that fish learn better during the day and that melatonin has an adverse effect on mnemonic performance, while pinealectomy improves it.[93] However, under stressful events, melatonin seemed to promote memory formation.[94] Melatonin inhibits the modifications of synaptic strength, the basic cellular mechanism for memory.[95] Yet the mechanism by which melatonin rhythmically influences cognitive processes remains unknown.

Melatonin has broad-spectrum antioxidant properties and potentially modulates inflammation, neurogenesis, and neuroprotection. It seems thus possible that melatonin treatment will be beneficial for a wide range of neonatal conditions. Under these circumstances, the effect of melatonin on mnemonic performance should be better evaluated, given the crucial role of memory formation in the neonatal period.

The pineal gland is a regulator of various functions, among which it influences nervous system function, through a complex interaction with neurotransmitter synthesis and activity, especially monoaminergic system function (serotonin, norepinephrine, and dopamine).

31.10.1 Serotonin

Serotonin is the main coordinator of circadian rhythms. In addition to the known relationship with melatonin on the synthetic pathway, there are other levels at which the two molecules interact. The SCN contains a dense serotonergic terminal plexus.[30] It has been shown that a serotonin agonist administration modifies the SCN rhythm in rats,[96] but the exact pathway through which serotonin influences its function is not known. A few pertinent hypotheses have emerged. One theory shows that serotonin stimulates potassium currents at a postsynaptic level, in a population of SCN neurons,[97] and another shows there is a presynaptic influence of serotonin.[98]

Serotonin is known to influence the synchronization of circadian rhythms, as light does. But serotonin's effect is more evident during day time, because serotonin administration during the night period failed to change Clock genes expression.[99] This effect may be explained by the expression of serotonin receptors in a circadian manner.[100] Serotonin is secreted by the raphe nuclei, while melatonin has an inhibitory effect on its neurons, through an MT1 modulated interaction.[101]

31.10.2 Norepinephrine

Melatonin synthesis at the pineal level depends on the normal function of the key enzyme aryl-alkyl *N*-acetyl transferase (AANAT), which catalyzes serotonin N acetylation and is active during the night.[102] We might say even that AANAT function represents the circadian regulator at the pineal level. Nocturnal release of melatonin is a norepinephrine-dependent process, which induces AANAT synthesis.[103]

31.10.3 Dopamine

Dopamine is the precursor molecule for norepinephrine, being the neurotransmitter of sympathetic nerve endings that leave the pineal gland. The secretory cells present D4 dopamine receptors, and their expression is modulated by the light/dark cycle.[104]

In its turn, melatonin controls dopamine synthesis in specific brain regions such as the hypothalamus, the tubule-infundibular area, and the ventral hippocampus.[105] Some studies show melatonin might have a direct effect on dopamine receptors—for example, it raises D2 expression in the rat striated body.[106] MT1 and MT2 localization overlaps D2 receptors at nervous system: hippocampus, cortex, hypothalamus and brain stem.[107–109] More than this, it has been shown that dopamine receptor expression has a circadian rhythm, with a low concentration during the day.[110]

31.11 MELATONIN ROLE IN IMMUNOMODULATION IN THE FETUS AND NEONATE

While it is generally accepted that the pineal gland has neuroendocrine functions, its involvement in the immune system function has yet to be fully explored. Removal of the pineal gland in neonatal rats results in a reduced number of circulating immune cells, such as lymphocytes and leukocytes, and a worse outcome after an infectious insult.[78] In a small study on septic newborn babies, melatonin was effective in reducing the levels of lipid peroxidation products and improving the survival and overall clinical outcome. This study was conducted to determine the changes in the clinical status and the serum levels of lipid peroxidation products (malondialdehyde [MDA] and 4-hydroxylalkenals [4-HDA]) in 10 septic newborns treated with the antioxidant melatonin, given within the first 12 h after diagnosis. Melatonin improved the clinical outcome of the septic newborns, as judged by measurement of sepsis-related serum parameters after 24 and 48 h. Three of 10 septic children who were not treated with melatonin died within 72 h after diagnosis of sepsis; none of the 10 septic newborns treated with melatonin died.[111]

Also, immune-modulating effects of melatonin have been widely inferred in adult humans who presented higher melatonin metabolites after a viral meningitis infection.[112, 113]

In the cultured rat pineal gland, lipopolysaccharide induced a downregulation of AANAT, the rate-limiting enzyme in melatonin synthesis, implying that infection may itself modulate the endogenous production of melatonin.[114]

These findings are suggestive of an involvement of melatonin in the host immune response. However, exogenous melatonin has shown effects in modulating the host immune response. Melatonin led to an increase in superoxide dismutase antioxidant activity, a reduction in nitric oxide levels, and a decrease in neuronal injury in a rabbit model of *Streptococcus pneumoniae* meningitis.[115]

Furthermore, in a rodent model of *Klebsiella pneumoniae* meningitis, melatonin reversed microglial activation and neuronal apoptosis in a dose-dependent manner.[116] Hypoxia-ischemia at parturition is aggravated by bacterial infection of the immature brain.[117] In a neonatal rat model of lipopolysaccharide (LPS)-sensitized hypoxic-ischemic brain injury, melatonin showed similar beneficial effects as in HIE, with overall reduced oxidative stress and inhibited neuronal apoptosis.[118]

Immunomodulation may also play a role in recovery after surgery. Gitto et al. reported on 10 neonates who received lung or abdominal surgery, and showed lower levels of interleukin-6 and interleukin-8, and a significant clinical improvement after administration of melatonin.[119] Furthermore, melatonin was reported to be as effective as midazolam in achieving sedation and reducing preoperative anxiety in children.[120]

31.12 NORMAL RELATIONSHIP BETWEEN MOTHER AND FETAL CIRCADIAN RHYTHMS

Fetal programming is a newly emerged concept, which connects environmental characteristics present during embryonic and fetal development with an increased risk of different pathologies later in adult life. Beginning with conception and until birth, embryos and fetuses are exposed to a continuous complex flux of chemical signals coming from the maternal organism, with those that are able to cross the placental barrier having potential direct effects on development. Maternal risk factors during development such as gestational diabetes, intrauterine growth restriction, preeclampsia, maternal undernutrition, and maternal stress, may have an important influence on pregnancy outcome.

The pathophysiological basis of this phenomenon could be the existence of high oxidative stress, which in turn may influence fetal development. As previously mentioned, nocturnal melatonin levels in pregnant women with preeclampsia were significantly lower compared with normal pregnancies (48.4 ± 24.7 vs. 85.4 ± 26.9 pg/mL). Blood pressure variations and the melatonin secretion rhythm seem to parallel each other daily during the preeclamptic pregnancy and until 2 months after birth.[121]

Another theory proposes the existence of an epigenetic mechanism, through DNA super structural changes, that come about as an adaptation to potentially harmful external factors exerted during pregnancy. It is believed that melatonin regulates this type of transmission and that it acts through nuclear receptors and not the aforementioned membrane ones. Their activation leads to ultrastructural DNA changes at the oocyte level.[71]

External factors that influence the maternal organism are not necessarily inducing somatic changes in the embryo or fetus, but may also influence the future development of psychiatric issues, behavioral changes, and even diseases.

A study that involves this concept is one developed by Ezra Susser et al., who followed the effects of severe food deprivation in pregnant women during World War II.[122] This study reported, among other things, the association of folate deficiency during pregnancy with neural tube defects. Another discovery was the identification of a high frequency of psychiatric conditions in children resulting from these pregnancies (especially schizophrenia), the risk being higher in those whose mothers were subjected to food deprivation during the second trimester.[122, 123] This result has been confirmed by following studies.[123]

An extensive study on 3099 mother-child pairs that finished in 2014 followed the impact of the maternal state during gestation on adults resulting from these pregnancies. The conclusion was that the offspring of stressed mothers had a high risk of developing behavioral disorders and depression.[124] There are also many available animal studies that point out maternal stress in utero can lead to behavioral abnormalities in the offspring at later ages.

During pregnancy, the maternal organism adapts to support the growth of a full developed fetus, and to maintain maternal metabolic functions. One such adaptation is represented by changes in clock genes expression during pregnancy in the maternal liver and adipose tissue.[15, 125] There are gestational adjustments in the rhythmicity of genes regulating lipogenesis and gluconeogenesis in these tissues.[125] The importance of a normally functioning circadian system in mothers is further highlighted by evidence that disruptions in maternal circadian rhythm (night shifts in pregnant women, or continuous light exposure during pregnancy in animal studies) leads to negative fetal outcomes such as a higher miscarriage risk, preterm labor, low birth weight,[126–128] behavioral alterations,[129, 130] and psychiatric diseases. Whether these disruptions are directly the result of altered pineal function or melatonin release remains to be confirmed.

31.13   CONCLUSION

Melatonin appears to be an important regulator of complex embryo-fetal developmental processes. It induces circadian rhythmicity in the offspring and may have direct developmental effects on nervous and endocrine systems, while also protecting against damage from oxidative stress. Animal models have suggested that melatonin has neuroprotective effects. There is also new evidence of melatonin possibly being an epigenetic transducer. Further studies are required to confirm these postulated roles.

Melatonin is currently an over-the-counter drug. It appears to have no acute adverse effects, based on a few clinical studies of small size that have been done in pregnant women. However, because melatonin's safety or proposed extensive effects on fetal development have not been rigorously confirmed by animal or especially by human studies, it cannot be recommended for use by pregnant women at the present time.

REFERENCES

1. Sumida M, Barkovich A James, Hans Newton T. Development of the pineal gland: measurement with MR. *Am J Neuroradiol* 1996;**17**(2):233–6.
2. Tan DX, Manchester LC, Hardeland R, Lopez-Burillo S, Mayo JC, Sainz RM, et al. Melatonin: a hormone, a tissue factor, an autocoid, a paracoid, and an antioxidant vitamin. *J Pineal Res* 2003;**34**(1):75–8.
3. Kennaway DJ, Goble FC, Stamp GE. Factors influencing the development of melatonin rhythmicity in humans. *J Clin Endocrinol Metab* 1996;**81**(4):1525–32.
4. Hartley SW, Coon SL, Savastano LE, Mullikin JC, Fu C, Klein DC. Neurotranscriptomics: the effects of neonatal stimulus deprivation on the rat pineal transcriptome. *PLoS ONE* 2015;**10**(9):e0137548.
5. Serón-Ferré M, Torres-Farfán C, Forcelledo ML, Valenzuela GJ. The development of circadian rhythms in the fetus and neonate. *Semin Perinatol* 2001;**25**(6):363–70.
6. Arendt J. Melatonin and human rhythms. *Chronobiol Int* 2006;**23**(1–2):21–37.
7. Levin R, Levine S. Development of circadian periodicity in base and stress levels of corticosterone. *Am J Phys* 1975;**229**(5):1397–9.
8. Nuesslein B, Schmidt I. Development of circadian cycle of core temperature in juvenile rats. *Am J Phys* 1990;**259**(2):R270–6.
9. Spiers DE. Nocturnal shifts in thermal and metabolic responses of the immature rat. *J Appl Physiol* 1988;**64**(5):2119–24.
10. Davis FC, Reppert SM. Development of mammalian circadian rhythms, In: Takahashi JS, Turek FW, Moore RY, editors. *Handbook of behavioral neurobiology.* New York: Kluwer; 2001, p. 247–90.
11. Reppert SM, Schwartz WJ. The suprachiasmatic nuclei of the fetal rat: characterization of a functional circadian clock using 14C-labeled deoxyglucose. *J Neurosci* 1984;**4**(7):1677–82.
12. Sládek M, Sumová A, Kováciková Z, Bendová Z, Laurinová K, Illnerová H, et al. Insight into molecular core clock mechanism of embryonic and early postnatal rat suprachiasmatic nucleus. *Proc Natl Acad Sci U S A* 2004;**101**(16):6231–6.
13. Dolatshad H, Cary AJ, Davis FC. Differential expression of the circadian clock in maternal and embryonic tissues of mice. *PLoS ONE* 2010;**5**(3): e9855.
14. Sumova A, Sladek M, Polidarova L, Novakova M, Houdek P. Circadian system from conception till adulthood. *Prog Brain Res* 2012;**5**(3):e9855.
15. Wharfe MD, Mark PJ, Waddell BJ. Circadian variation in placental and hepatic clock genes in rat pregnancy. *Endocrinology* 2011;**152**(9):3552–60.
16. Torres-Farfan C, Mendez N, Abarzua-Catalan L, Vilches N, Valenzuela GJ, Seron-Ferre M. A circadian clock entrained by melatonin is ticking in the rat fetal adrenal. *Endocrinology* 2011;**152**(5):1891–900.
17. Weinert D. Ontogenetic development of the mammalian circadian system. *Chronobiol Int* 2005;**22**(2):179–205.
18. Honma S, Honma KI, Shirakawa T, Hiroshige T. Maternal phase setting of fetal circadian oscillation underlying the plasma corticosterone rhythm in rats. *Endocrinology* 1984;**114**(5):1791–6.
19. Honma S, Honma KI, Shirakawa T, Hiroshige T. Effects of elimination of maternal circadian rhythms during pregnancy on the postnatal development of circadian corticosterone rhythm in blinded infantile rats. *Endocrinology* 1984;**114**(1):44–50.
20. Mendez N, Abarzua-Catalan L, Vilches N, Galdames HA, Spichiger C, Richter HG, et al. Timed maternal melatonin treatment reverses circadian disruption of the fetal adrenal clock imposed by exposure to constant light. *PLoS ONE* 2012;**7**(8):e42713.
21. Rivkees SA, Hao H. Developing circadian rhythmicity. *Semin Perinatol* 2000;**24**(4):232–42.
22. Yonei Y, Hattori A, Tsutsui K, Okawa M, Ishizuka B. Effects of melatonin: basic studies and clinical applications. *Anti Aging Med* 2010;**111**:217–34.
23. Tan DX, Manchester LC, Liu X, Rosales-Corral SA, Acuna-Castroviejo D, Reiter RJ. Mitochondria and chloroplasts as the original sites of melatonin synthesis: a hypothesis related to melatonin's primary function and evolution in eukaryotes. *J Pineal Res* 2013;**54**(2):127–38.

24. Venegas C, García JA, Escames G, Ortiz F, López A, Doerrier C, et al. Extrapineal melatonin: analysis of its subcellular distribution and daily fluctuations. *J Pineal Res* 2012;**52**(2):217–27.

25. Ebadi M, Govitrapong P. Neural pathways and neurotransmitters affecting melatonin synthesis. *J Neural Transm Suppl* 1986;**21**:125–55.

26. Axelrod J. The pineal gland: a neurochemical transducer. *Science* 1974;**184**(4144):1341–8.

27. Reiter RJ. Pineal melatonin: cell biology of its synthesis and of its physiological interactions. *Endocr Rev* 1991;**12**(2):151–80.

28. Hay-Schmidt A, Vrang N, Larsen PJ, Mikkelsen JD. Projections from the raphe nuclei to the suprachiasmatic nucleus of the rat. *J Chem Neuroanat* 2003;**25**(4):293–310.

29. Pontes GN, Cardoso EC, Carneiro-Sampaio MMS, Markus RP. Pineal melatonin and the innate immune response: the TNF-α increase after cesarean section suppresses nocturnal melatonin production. *J Pineal Res* 2007;**43**(4):365–71.

30. Sollars PJ, Pickard GE, Sprouse JS. Serotonin and the regulation of mammalian circadian rhythms. In: *Encyclopedia of neuroscience*, Academic Press; 2010, p. 723–30.

31. Basheer M, Rai S. Melatonin vs. phytomelatonin: therapeutic uses with special reference to polycystic ovarian syndrome (PCOS). *Cogent Biol* 2016;**2**(1):1136257.

32. Torres-Farfan C, Rocco V, Monsó C, Valenzuela FJ, Campino C, Germain A, et al. Maternal melatonin effects on clock gene expression in a non-human primate fetus. *Endocrinology* 2006;**147**(10):4618–26.

33. Brzezinski A, Seibel MM, Lynch HJ, Deng MH, Wurtman RJ. Melatonin in human preovulatory follicular fluid. *J Clin Endocrinol Metab* 1987;**64**(4):865–7.

34. Chen YC, Tain YL, Sheen JM, Huang LT. Melatonin utility in neonates and children. *J Formos Med Assoc* 2012;**111**(2):57–66.

35. Urata Y, Honma S, Goto S, Todoroki S, Iida T, Cho S, et al. Melatonin induces γ-glutamylcysteine synthetase mediated by activator protein-1 in human vascular endothelial cells. *Free Radic Biol Med* 1999;**27**(7–8):838–47.

36. Okatani Y, Wakatsuki A, Reiter RJ, Miyahara Y. Acutely administered melatonin restores hepatic mitochondrial physiology in old mice. *Int J Biochem Cell Biol* 2003;**35**(3):367–75.

37. Tamura H, Nakamura Y, Terron MP, Flores LJ, Manchester LC, Tan DX, et al. Melatonin and pregnancy in the human. *Reprod Toxicol* 2008;**25**(3):291–303.

38. Unfer V, Raffone E, Rizzo P, Buffo S. Effect of a supplementation with myo-inositol plus melatonin on oocyte quality in women who failed to conceive in previous in vitro fertilization cycles for poor oocyte quality: a prospective, longitudinal, cohort study. *Gynecol Endocrinol* 2011;**27**(11):857–61.

39. Chung FF, Yao CCC, Wan GH. The associations between menstrual function and life style/working conditions among nurses in Taiwan. *J Occup Health* 2005;**47**(2):149–56.

40. Davis S, Mirick DK, Chen C, Stanczyk FZ. Night shift work and hormone levels in women. *Cancer Epidemiol Biomarkers Prev* 2012;**21**(4):609–18.

41. Torres-Farfan C, Valenzuela FJ, Mondaca M, Valenzuela GJ, Krause B, Herrera EA, et al. Evidence of a role for melatonin in fetal sheep physiology: direct actions of melatonin on fetal cerebral artery, brown adipose tissue and adrenal gland. *J Physiol* 2008;**586**(16):4017–27.

42. Varcoe TJ, Voultsios A, Gatford KL, Kennaway DJ. The impact of prenatal circadian rhythm disruption on pregnancy outcomes and long-term metabolic health of mice progeny. *Chronobiol Int* 2016;**33**(9):1–11.

43. Hardeland R, Tan DX, Reiter RJ. Kynuramines, metabolites of melatonin and other indoles: the resurrection of an almost forgotten class of biogenic amines. *J Pineal Res* 2009;**47**(2):109–26.

44. Lanoix D, Guérin P, Vaillancourt C. Placental melatonin production and melatonin receptor expression are altered in preeclampsia: new insights into the role of this hormone in pregnancy. *J Pineal Res* 2012;**53**(4):417–25.

45. Soliman A, Lacasse AA, Lanoix D, Sagrillo-Fagundes L, Boulard V, Vaillancourt C. Placental melatonin system is present throughout pregnancy and regulates villous trophoblast differentiation. *J Pineal Res* 2015;**59**(1):38–46.

46. Muñoz-Hoyos A, Bonillo-Perales A, Ávila-Villegas R, González-Ripoll M, Uberos J, Florido-Navío J, et al. Melatonin levels during the first week of life and their relation with the antioxidant response in the perinatal period. *Neonatology* 2007;**92**:209–16.

47. Bagci S, Berner AL, Reinsberg J, Gast AS, Zur B, Welzing L, et al. Melatonin concentration in umbilical cord blood depends on mode of delivery. *Early Hum Dev* 2012;**88**(6):369–73.

48. Tan DX, Manchester LC, Terron MP, Flores LJ, Reiter RJ. One molecule, many derivatives: a never-ending interaction of melatonin with reactive oxygen and nitrogen species? *J Pineal Res* 2007;**42**(1):28–42.

49. Zlotos DP, Jockers R, Cecon E, Rivara S, Witt-Enderby PA. MT1 and MT2 melatonin receptors: ligands, models, oligomers, and therapeutic potential. *J Med Chem* 2014;**57**(8):3161–85.

50. Gupta S, Agarwal A, Sharma RK. The role of placental oxidative stress and lipid peroxidation in preeclampsia. *Obstet Gynecol Surv* 2005;**60**(12):807–16.

51. Morris JM, Gopaul NK, Endresen MJR, Knight M, Linton EA, Dhir S, et al. Circulating markers of oxidative stress are raised in normal pregnancy and pre-eclampsia. *BJOG Int J Obstet Gynaecol* 1998;**105**:1195–9.

52. Little RE, Gladen BC. Levels of lipid peroxides in uncomplicated pregnancy: a review of the literature. *Reprod Toxicol* 1999;**13**(5):347–52.

53. Walsh SW, Wang Y, Jesse R. Peroxide induces vasoconstriction in the human placenta by stimulating thromboxane. *Am J Obstet Gynecol* 1993;**169**(4):1007–12.

54. Gagnon R. Placental insufficiency and its consequences. *Eur J Obstet Gynecol Reprod Biol* 2003;**110**(Suppl 1):S99–S107.

55. Van Wassenaer A. Neurodevelopmental consequences of being born SGA. *Pediatr Endocrinol Rev* 2005;**2**(3):372–7.

56. Bae SE, Wright IK, Wyse C, Samson-Desvignes N, Le Blanc P, Laroche S, et al. Regulation of pituitary MT1 melatonin receptor expression by gonadotrophin-releasing hormone (GnRH) and early growth response factor-1 (Egr-1): in vivo and in vitro studies. *PLoS ONE* 2014;**9**(3):e90056.

57. Danilova N, Krupnik VE, Sugden D, Zhdanova IV. Melatonin stimulates cell proliferation in zebrafish embryo and accelerates its development. *FASEB J* 2004;**18**(6):751–3.
58. Davis FC. Melatonin: role in Development. *J Biol Rhythm* 1997;**12**(6):498–508.
59. de Borsetti NH, Dean BJ, Bain EJ, Clanton JA, Taylor RW, Gamse JT. Light and melatonin schedule neuronal differentiation in the habenular nuclei. *Dev Biol* 2011;**358**(1):251–61.
60. Fu J, Zhao S-D, Liu H-J, Yuan Q-H, Liu S-M, Zhang Y-M, et al. Melatonin promotes proliferation and differentiation of neural stem cells subjected to hypoxia in vitro. *J Pineal Res* 2011;**51**(1):104–12.
61. Husson I, Mespls B, Bac P, Vamecq J, Evrard P, Gressens P. Melatoninergic neuroprotection of the murine periventricular white matter against neonatal excitotoxic challenge. *Ann Neurol* 2002;**51**(1):82–92.
62. Rivkees SA, Reppert SM. Appearance of melatonin receptors during embryonic life in Siberian hamsters (Phodopus sungorous). *Brain Res* 1991;**568** (1–2):345–9.
63. Zitouni M, Masson-Pévet M, Gauer F, Pévet P. Influence of maternal melatonin on melatonin receptors in rat offspring. *J Neural Transm* 1995;**100** (2):111–22.
64. Thomas L, Purvis CC, Drew JE, Abramovich DR, Williams LM. Melatonin receptors in human fetal brain: 2-[125I]iodomelatonin binding and MT1 gene expression. *J Pineal Res* 2002;**33**(4):218–24.
65. Olakowska E, Marcol W, Kotulska K, Lewin-Kowalik J. The role of melatonin in the neurodegenerative diseases. *Bratisl Lek Listy* 2005;**106**(4–5):171–4.
66. Welin AK, Svedin P, Lapatto R, Sultan B, Hagberg H, Gressens P, et al. Melatonin reduces inflammation and cell death in white matter in the midgestation fetal sheep following umbilical cord occlusion. *Pediatr Res* 2007;**61**(2):153–8.
67. Supramaniam VG, Jenkin G, Loose J, Wallace EM, Miller SL. Chronic fetal hypoxia increases activin A concentrations in the late-pregnant sheep. *BJOG Int J Obstet Gynaecol* 2006;**113**(1):102–9.
68. Thakor AS, Herrera EA, Serón-Ferré M, Giussani DA. Melatonin and vitamin C increase umbilical blood flow via nitric oxide-dependent mechanisms. *J Pineal Res* 2010;**49**(4):399–406.
69. Miller SL, Yan EB, Castillo-Meléndez M, Jenkin G, Walker DW. Melatonin provides neuroprotection in the late-gestation fetal sheep brain in response to umbilical cord occlusion. *Dev Neurosci* 2005;**27**(2–4):200–10.
70. Robertson NJ, Faulkner S, Fleiss B, Bainbridge A, Andorka C, Price D, et al. Melatonin augments hypothermic neuroprotection in a perinatal asphyxia model. *Brain* 2013;**136**(1):90–105.
71. Irmak MK, Topal T, Oter S. Melatonin seems to be a mediator that transfers the environmental stimuli to oocytes for inheritance of adaptive changes through epigenetic inheritance system. *Med Hypotheses* 2005;**64**(6):1138–43.
72. Marseglia L, Aversa S, Barberi I, Salpietro CD, Cusumano E, Speciale A, et al. High endogenous melatonin levels in critically ill children: a pilot study. *J Pediatr* 2013;**162**(2):357–60.
73. Kaur C, Sivakumar V, Ling EA. Melatonin protects periventricular white matter from damage due to hypoxia. *J Pineal Res* 2010;**48**(3):185–93.
74. Tataranno ML, Perrone S, Buonocore G. Plasma biomarkers of oxidative stress in neonatal brain injury. *Clin Perinatol* 2015;**42**(3):529–39.
75. Signorini C, Ciccoli L, Leoncini S, Carloni S, Perrone S, Comporti M, et al. Free iron, total F2-isoprostanes and total F4- neuroprostanes in a model of neonatal hypoxic-ischemic encephalopathy: neuroprotective effect of melatonin. *J Pineal Res* 2009;**46**(2):148–54.
76. Gordon N. The therapeutics of melatonin: a paediatric perspective. *Brain Dev* 2000;**22**(4):213–7.
77. Aly H, Elmahdy H, El-Dib M, Rowisha M, Awny M, El-Gohary T, et al. Melatonin use for neuroprotection in perinatal asphyxia: a randomized controlled pilot study. *J Perinatol* 2015;**35**(3):186–91.
78. Beşkonakh E, Palaoğlu S, Renda N, Kulaçoglu S, Turhan T, Taşkm Y. The effect of pinealectomy on immune parameters in different age groups in rats: results of the weekly alteration of the zinc level and the effect of melatonin administration on wound healing. *J Clin Neurosci* 2000;**7**(4):320–4.
79. Arendt J. Melatonin, circadian rhythms, and sleep. *N Engl J Med* 2000;**343**(15):1114–6.
80. Wirz-Justice A. Treatment tools in chronobiology. *Rev Med Interne* 2001;**22**(Suppl 1):37–8.
81. Borjigin J, Li X, Snyder SH. The pineal gland and melatonin: molecular and pharmacologic regulation. *Annu Rev Pharmacol Toxicol* 1999;**39** (1):53–65.
82. Brzezinski A. Melatonin in humans. *N Engl J Med* 1997;**336**(3):186–95.
83. Masana MI, Dubocovich ML. Melatonin receptor signaling: finding the path through the dark. *Sci STKE* 2001;**6**(107):pe36.
84. Vanecek J. Inhibitory effect of melatonin on GnRH-induced LH release. *Rev Reprod* 1999;**4**:67–72.
85. Krause DN, Dubocovich ML. Regulatory sites in the melatonin system of mammals. *Trends Neurosci* 1990;**13**(11):464–70.
86. Millan MJ, Brocco M, Gobert A, Dekeyne A. Anxiolytic properties of agomelatine, an antidepressant with melatoninergic and serotonergic properties: role of 5-HT2Creceptor blockade. *Psychopharmacology* 2005;**177**(4):1–12.
87. Loiseau F, Le Bihan C, Hamon M, Thiébot MH. Effects of melatonin and agomelatine in anxiety-related procedures in rats: interaction with diazepam. *Eur Neuropsychopharmacol* 2006;**16**(6):417–28.
88. Weaver DR, Rivkees SA, Reppert SM. Localization and characterization of melatonin receptors in rodent brain by in vitro autoradiography. *J Neurosci* 1989;**9**(7):2581–90.
89. Argyriou A, Prast H, Philippu A. Melatonin facilitates short-term memory. *Eur J Pharmacol* 1998;**349**(2–3):159–62.
90. Kurtuncu M, Arslan AD, Akhisaroglu M, Manev H, Uz T. Involvement of the pineal gland in diurnal cocaine reward in mice. *Eur J Pharmacol* 2004;**489**(3):203–5.
91. Lakin ML, Miller CH, Stott ML, Winters WD. Involvement of the pineal gland and melatonin in murine analgesia. *Life Sci* 1981;**29**(24):2543–51.

92. Mantovani M, Pértile R, Calixto JB, Santos ARS, Rodrigues ALS. Melatonin exerts an antidepressant-like effect in the tail suspension test in mice: evidence for involvement of N-methyl-D-aspartate receptors and the L-arginine-nitric oxide pathway. *Neurosci Lett* 2003;**343**(1):1–4.

93. Rawashdeh O, De Borsetti NH, Roman G, Cahill GM. Melatonin suppresses nighttime memory formation in zebrafish. *Science* 2007;**318** (5853):1144–6.

94. Rimmele U, Spillmann M, Bärtschi C, Wolf OT, Weber CS, Ehlert U, et al. Melatonin improves memory acquisition under stress independent of stress hormone release. *Psychopharmacology (Berl)* 2009;**202**(4):663–72.

95. Rawashdeh O, Maronde E. The hormonal Zeitgeber melatonin: role as a circadian modulator in memory processing. *Front Mol Neurosci* 2012;**5**:27.

96. Edgar DM, Dean RR, Dement WC, Miller JD, Prosser RA. Serotonin and the mammalian circadian system. II. Phase-shifting rat behavioral rhythms with serotonergic agonists. *J Biol Rhythm* 1993;**8**(1):17–31.

97. Prosser RA, Heller HC, Miller JD. Serotonergic phase advances of the mammalian circadian clock involve protein kinase A and K + channel opening. *Brain Res* 1994;**644**(1):67–73.

98. Esteban S, Garau C, Aparicio S, Moranta D, Barceló P, Fiol MA, et al. Chronic melatonin treatment and its precursor L-tryptophan improve the monoaminergic neurotransmission and related behavior in the aged rat brain. *J Pineal Res* 2010;**48**(2):170–7.

99. Gannon RL, Millan MJ. Evaluation of serotonin, noradrenaline and dopamine reuptake inhibitors on light-induced phase advances in hamster circadian activity rhythms. *Psychopharmacology* 2007;**195**(3):325–32.

100. Cuesta M, Clesse D, Pévet P, Challet E. New light on the serotonergic paradox in the rat circadian system. *J Neurochem* 2009;**110**(1):231–43.

101. Domínguez-López S, Mahar I, Bambico FR, Labonté B, Ochoa-Sánchez R, Leyton M, et al. Short-term effects of melatonin and pinealectomy on serotonergic neuronal activity across the light-dark cycle. *J Psychopharmacol* 2012;**26**(6):830–44.

102. Ackermann K, Dehghani F, Bux R, Kauert G, Stehle JH. Day-night expression patterns of clock genes in the human pineal gland. *J Pineal Res* 2007;**43**(2):185–94.

103. Maronde E, Saade A, Ackermann K, Goubran-Botros H, Pagan C, Bux R, et al. Dynamics in enzymatic protein complexes offer a novel principle for the regulation of melatonin synthesis in the human pineal gland. *J Pineal Res* 2011;**51**(1):145–55.

104. Bailey MJ, Coon SL, Carter DA, Humphries A, Kim JS, Shi Q, et al. Night/day changes in pineal expression of > 600 genes: central role of adrenergic/cAMP signaling. *J Biol Chem* 2009;**284**(12):7606–22.

105. Zisapel N, Egozi Y, Laudon M. Inhibition of dopamine release by melatonin: regional distribution in the rat brain. *Brain Res* 1982;**246**(1):161–3.

106. Hamdi A. Melatonin administration increases the affinity of D2 dopamine receptors in the rat striatum. *Life Sci* 1998;**63**(23):2115–20.

107. Al-Ghoul WM, Herman MD, Dubocovich ML. Melatonin receptor subtype expression in human cerebellum. *Neuroreport* 1998;**9**(18):4063–8.

108. Poirel VJ, Cailotto C, Streicher D, Pévet P, Masson-Pévet M, Gauer F. MT1 melatonin receptor mRNA tissular localization by PCR amplification. *Neuroendocrinol Lett* 2003;**24**(1–2):33–8.

109. Mazzucchelli C, Pannacci M, Nonno R, Lucini V, Fraschini F, Stankov BM. The melatonin receptor in the human brain: cloning experiments and distribution studies. *Mol Brain Res* 1996;**39**(1–2):117–26.

110. Wu YH, Zhou JN, Balesar R, Unmehopa U, Bao A, Jockers R, et al. Distribution of MT1 melatonin receptor immunoreactivity in the human hypothalamus and pituitary gland: colocalization of MT1 with vasopressin, oxytocin, and corticotropin-releasing hormone. *J Comp Neurol* 2006;**499** (6):897–910.

111. Gitto E, Karbownik M, Reiter RJ, Xian Tan D, Cuzzocrea S, Chiurazzi P, et al. Effects of melatonin treatment in septic newborns. *Pediatr Res* 2001;**50**(6):756–60.

112. Carrillo-Vico A, Lardone PJ, Álvarez-Śnchez N, Rodrīguez-Rodríguez A, Guerrero JM. Melatonin: buffering the immune system. *Int J Mol Sci* 2013;**14**(4):8638–83.

113. De Oliveira SS, Ximenes VF, Livramento JA, Catalani LH, Campa A. High concentrations of the melatonin metabolite, N1-acetyl- N2-formyl-5-methoxykynuramine, in cerebrospinal fluid of patients with meningitis: a possible immunomodulatory mechanism. *J Pineal Res* 2005;**39**(3):302–6.

114. Da Silveira C-MS, Carvalho-Sousa CE, Tamura EK, Pinato L, Cecon E, Fernandes PACM, et al. TLR4 and CD14 receptors expressed in rat pineal gland trigger NFKB pathway. *J Pineal Res* 2010;**49**(2):183–92.

115. Gerber J, Lotz M, Ebert S, Kiel S, Huether G, Kuhnt U, et al. Melatonin is neuroprotective in experimental Streptococcus pneumoniae meningitis. *J Infect Dis* 2005;**191**(5):783–90.

116. Wu UI, Mai FD, Sheu JN, Chen LY, Liu YT, Huang HC, et al. Melatonin inhibits microglial activation, reduces pro-inflammatory cytokine levels, and rescues hippocampal neurons of adult rats with acute Klebsiella pneumoniae meningitis. *J Pineal Res* 2011;**50**(2):159–70.

117. Eklind S, Mallard C, Leverin AL, Gilland E, Blomgren K, Mattsby-Baltzer I, et al. Bacterial endotoxin sensitizes the immature brain to hypoxic-ischaemic injury. *Eur J Neurosci* 2001;**13**(6):1101–6.

118. Wang X, Svedin P, Nie C, Lapatto R, Zhu C, Gustavsson M, et al. N-Acetylcysteine reduces lipopolysaccharide-sensitized hypoxic-ischemic brain injury. *Ann Neurol* 2007;**61**(3):263–71.

119. Gitto E, Romeo C, Reiter RJ, Impellizzeri P, Pesce S, Basile M, et al. Melatonin reduces oxidative stress in surgical neonates. *J Pediatr Surg* 2004;**39** (2):184–9.

120. Gitto E, Marseglia L, D'Angelo G, Manti S, Crisafi C, Montalto AS, et al. Melatonin versus midazolam premedication in children undergoing surgery: a pilot study. *J Paediatr Child Health* 2016;**52**(3):291–5.

121. Bouchlariotou S, Liakopoulos V, Giannopoulou M, Arampatzis S, Eleftheriadis T, Mertens PR, et al. Melatonin secretion is impaired in women with preeclampsia and an abnormal circadian blood pressure rhythm. *Ren Fail* 2014;**36**(7):1001–7.

122. Susser E, Neugebauer R, Hoek HW, Brown AS, Lin S, Labovitz D, et al. Schizophrenia after prenatal famine further evidence. *Arch Gen Psychiatry* 1996;**53**(1):25–31.

123. Susser E, Clair DS, He L. Latent effects of prenatal malnutrition on adult health: the example of schizophrenia. *Ann N Y Acad Sci* 2008;**1136**:185–92.

124. Betts KS, Williams GM, Najman JM, Alati R. The relationship between maternal depressive, anxious, and stress symptoms during pregnancy and adult offspring behavioral and emotional problems. *Depress Anxiety* 2015;**32**(2):82–90.

125. Wharfe MD, Wyrwoll CS, Waddell BJ, Mark PJ. Pregnancy-induced changes in the circadian expression of hepatic clock genes: implications for maternal glucose homeostasis. *Am J Physiol-Endocrinol Metab* 2016;**311**(3):E575–86.

126. Knutson KL, von Schantz M. Associations between chronotype, morbidity and mortality in the UK Biobank cohort. *Chronobiol Int* 2018;**35**(8):1045–53.

127. Knutson KL, Wu D, Patel SR, Loredo JS, Redline S, Cai J, et al. Association between sleep timing, obesity, diabetes: the hispanic community health study/study of latinos (hchs/sol) cohort study. *Sleep* 2017;**40**(4).

128. Zhu SH, Valbo A. Depression and smoking during pregnancy. *Addict Behav* 2002;**27**(4):649–58.

129. Voiculescu SE, Le Duc D, Roşca AE, Zeca V, Chiţimuş DM, Arsene AL, et al. Behavioral and molecular effects of prenatal continuous light exposure in the adult rat. *Brain Res* 2016;**1650**:51–9.

130. Voiculescu SE, Rosca AE, Zeca V, Zagrean L, Zagrean AM. Impact of maternal melatonin suppression on forced swim and tail suspension behavioral despair tests in adult offspring. *J Med Life* 2015;**8**(2):202–6.

Chapter 32

Normal Thyroid Development and Function in the Fetus and Neonate

Sarah Elizabeth Lawrence*, Julia Elisabeth von Oettingen[†] and Johnny Deladoëy[‡]

*Children's Hospital of Eastern Ontario, Ottawa, ON, Canada, [†]McGill University Health Centre, Montreal, QC, Canada, [‡]CHU Sainte-Justine, Université de Montréal, Montréal, QC, Canada

---

Key Clinical Changes
- The fetal thyroid reaches the anatomical location at the 7th week of gestation.
- The fetal thyroid gland is capable of iodine concentration at the 11th week (70 days) of gestation.
- Even at term, a substantial amount of fetal thyroid hormone is of maternal origin.

32.1 INTRODUCTION

The thyroid axis is probably the best example of the physiological interactions among the mother, her fetus, and the environment. The discovery of the crucial role of maternal iodine intake for the normal development of the fetus is also a historical tale of the first successful intervention in preventive medicine.[3]

In the early 19th century, some physicians (e.g., Coindet in 1813, Switzerland; Chatin in 1851, France) advocated for the use of iodine to treat endemic goiter, which more frequently plagued women. This idea encountered a lot of resistance from the medical community, as it was believed that iodine was toxic for humans. In 1896, Bauman and Ross demonstrated that 10% of the insoluble fraction of the thyroid was iodine, and they found that this fraction (named thyroiodine) was able to successfully treat myxedema and goiter. The first systematic clinical trial to assess the efficacy of iodized salt for preventing goiter was performed by Marine and Kimball (in Akron, Ohio, in 1916–17), in a cohort of 900 treated girls compared with 1200 untreated girls. It was a success, as the goiter occurrence in the treated group was only 0.2% compared with that of 25% in the control group. Then in 1922, under the impulse of Eggenberger, a Swiss surgeon, one of the first systematic uses of iodized salt at the population level was introduced in the Canton of Appenzel AR, a region of endemic goiter. The results were spectacular: the occurrence of goiter in children decreased sharply, but more stunningly, newborn goiter and cretinism almost disappeared. This was one of the first indirect demonstrations that giving iodine to pregnant women can prevent the development of thyroid disease in the newborn. Indeed, the mother requires double the normal iodine intake to preserve a normal thyroid hormone concentration; therefore mother and newborn were (and still are) very vulnerable in the areas of endemic goiter or iodine deficiency.

In the Western world, endemic goiter and congenital cretinism have all but disappeared thanks the iodination of salt implemented by many countries. Now in these jurisdictions, the most severe cases of congenital hypothyroidism are due to dysgenesis of the pituitary and, more frequently, of the thyroid gland.

32.2 EMBRYOLOGY OF THE HYPOTHALAMIC-PITUITARY-THYROID AXIS

32.2.1 The Pituitary

As for all organs, anatomic development of the hypothalamic-pituitary-thyroid system occurs during the first trimester of gestation. By 3 weeks, a series of homeodomain proteins or transcription factors begin to drive the differentiation of human embryonic forebrain and hypothalamus. Immunoreactive thyrotropin releasing hormone (TRH) becomes detectable in human embryonic hypothalami by 8–9 weeks of postconceptional age and is also produced by the fetal gut and pancreas.[4, 5]

Anatomically, the pituitary gland develops from two ectodermal anlagen: a neural component from the floor of the primitive forebrain, and a Rathke pouch from the primitive oral cavity. The latter is visible by 5 weeks, evolving to a morphologically

Maternal-Fetal and Neonatal Endocrinology. https://doi.org/10.1016/B978-0-12-814823-5.00032-5

mature pituitary gland by 14–15 weeks. The pituitary-portal blood vessels are present by this time and mature further through 30–35 weeks. A wide spectrum of congenital malformations collectively named *midline defects*, including holoprosencephaly and septo-optic dysplasia, may be associated with central hypothyroidism and other anterior pituitary deficiencies.[6] The molecular mechanisms underlying these malformations have been identified in some cases.[7] Within the pituitary itself, PROP-1 and PIT-1 are terminal factors in the differentiation cascade of pituitary cells, and PIT1 or PROP1 deficiency results in profound defects in growth hormone, prolactin and TSH secretion, as well as age-dependent pituitary hypoplasia.[8–10]

32.2.2 The Thyroid

The human thyroid gland develops from a median anlage derived from the primitive pharyngeal floor and from paired lateral anlagen from the fourth pharyngeal pouches. The long-held belief that the lateral anlagen were the only source of calcitonin-producing cells has been challenged by the recent observation that sublingual thyroids that are derived exclusively from the median anlage contain calcitonin mRNA and protein.[11] Conversely, thyroid follicular cells can differentiate within the lateral anlagen, as illustrated by histological observations[12] as well as by patients in whom the only thyroid tissue is a lateral ectopy.[13] Both the median and lateral structures are visible by day 16–17 of gestation; by 50 days, they have fused and the thyroid gland has migrated to its definitive location in the anterior neck. The thyroglossal duct, from the foramen cecum to the final location of the thyroid, may persist and is constituted of degenerated thyroid follicular cells. Within the thyroid gland, iodine concentration, TSH receptors, thyroglobulin, and thyroid peroxidase mRNA and protein can be demonstrated by 70 days.[14]

Thyroid embryogenesis is dependent on the expression of a programmed sequence of homeobox and transcription factors, including thyroid transcription factors-1 and -2 (TTF-1 or TiTF-1, also known as NK2 homeobox 1 (NKX2-1); and TTF-2, also known as Forkhead box E1 (FOXE-1)), and Paired box gene 8 (PAX8).[15] In newborn mice, bi-allelic inactivation of Nkx2.1 results in the absence of both pituitary and thyroid glands, with complete absence of both thyroid follicular cells and of calcitonin-producing C-cells,[16] while that of Pax8 results in a small thyroid gland composed almost exclusively of C cells.[17] FoxE-1 null mouse embryos have either an absent thyroid or an ectopic sublingual gland, but all newborn pups have athyreosis in addition to cleft palate.[18] Mutations in the homologous genes, however, account for at most 2% of cases of thyroid dysgenesis in humans.[18] Therefore, other genes and pathways impacting extrinsic thyroidal factors might be the cause of thyroid dysgenesis.[19, 20]

32.2.3 Possible Role of Embryonic Vasculogenesis on Thyroid Development

A temporal and special connection between vasculogenesis and brain development was already suggested by Vesale, and until recently, angiogenesis was considered to be a passive process occurring secondarily in response to metabolic demands of the growing brain tissue.[21] This view was challenged by works showing that neurons and vessels develop together and follow the same cues.[22]

By analogy, lack of epithelial to mesenchymal translocation (EMT) suggests that the migration of the developing thyroid is not an active process but involves rather movement of the surrounding tissues and vessels.[23] Indeed, growth patterns during thyroid morphogenesis suggest that thyroid inductive signals arise from embryonic vessels.[24] For example, deletion of *Netrin-1* was found in a patient with co-occurring thyroid ectopy and congenital heart disease; phenotypic analysis of *ntn1a* zebrafish morphants indicates that abnormal thyroid morphogenesis resulted from a lack of proper guidance exerted by the dysplastic vasculature of ntn1a-deficient embryos.[25] These data suggest that the thyroid development requires also cues arising from outside the thyroid. These cues can potentially be influenced by maternal factors. Hence, although no seasonality was observed in the occurrence of thyroid dysgenesis, thereby arguing against environmental causes,[26] some data suggest that thyroid dysgenesis occurs more often in newborns borne from mothers with type 1 diabetes,[27] as do other congenital malformations.

32.3 MATERNAL AND PLACENTAL INFLUENCES ON FETAL THYROID HORMONE LEVELS

Iodine is an essential component of thyroid hormones. In this chapter, the term iodine will refer to both iodine itself (I^2) and iodide (I^-). The human placenta expresses the sodium-iodine symporter throughout gestation,[28] which explains why the mother's iodine status is reflected in the fetus. If the mother's iodine intake is suboptimal, the fetal thyroid cannot accrete appropriate stores of iodine and fetal hypothyroidism may ensue. Worldwide, inadequate maternal iodine intake leading to late consequences, known as *endemic cretinism*, remains a major public health problem. Prevention of this condition by supplying the mother with adequate iodine is one of the best and most important examples of considering the fetus as a patient, and of treating this patient through its mother.[29, 30]

In contrast to iodine, thyroxine (T4) was for a long time thought not to cross the placenta in substantial amounts.[31] However, T4 is detectable in human embryonic tissues before the onset of fetal thyroid function and must, therefore, be of maternal origin.[32] Later in gestation, the transfer of T4 from mother to fetus must continue, since the concentration in cord blood from neonates with complete absence of thyroid function is 30%–50% of that of normal neonates.[33] More recently, it was shown that normal neonates born to a mother who has chronically higher T4 concentrations due to a mutation inactivating the thyroid hormone receptor have lower plasma TSH concentrations than those born to normal mothers.[34] Taken together, these data indicate that maternal T4 must cross the placenta in physiologically relevant amounts throughout gestation.

The clinical importance of this transplacental transfer of T4 from mother to fetus was illustrated by the severe developmental delay observed in an infant with central hypothyroidism caused by a maternally inherited heterozygous mutation inactivating PIT1, and whose equally hypothyroid mother had stopped thyroxine treatment at mid-pregnancy.[35] At the population level, children born to mothers who have low T4 concentrations during pregnancy have been reported to have lower IQ than children born to mothers with normal circulating concentrations of thyroid hormones.[36–38] However, in a recent randomized trial, when treatment was begun toward the end of the first trimester, the developmental outcomes were similar in the offspring of T4- and placebo-treated women who had either elevated TSH concentrations (>97.5%ile) or lower circulating T4 concentrations (<2.5%ile).[39] Moreover, in two recent case series of women with severe hypothyroidism diagnosed during pregnancy but corrected by the third trimester, the intellectual outcome of the offspring was normal.[40, 41] Thus universal screening for thyroid dysfunction during pregnancy is not recommended at this time. On the other hand, women with known hypothyroidism require closer monitoring during pregnancy, as 85% of women who are already receiving T4 therapy require a 30%–50% increase in dose during pregnancy, due to the estradiol-induced increase in serum thyroxine-binding globulin.[42]

The transplacental transfer of T4 is not always sufficient to prevent the development of fetal goiter if the fetus has severe thyroid dyshormonogenesis. Fetal goiters may be large enough to interfere with the flow of amniotic fluid into the airways, causing progressive hydramnios and eventual lung hypoplasia. In such occurrences, levothyroxine can be injected into the amniotic fluid, which is then swallowed by the fetus, leading to a decrease in the size of the fetal thyroid and in the degree of hydramnios.[43] The injection of thyroxine into the umbilical vein, which carries an even higher risk of triggering premature labor or fetal loss than amniocentesis, should be restricted to fetuses with a goiter that continues to increase in spite of repeated intra-amniotic injections. Invasive and potentially risky procedures should not be undertaken to protect the brain of affected fetuses: indeed, the fetal brain is, to a large extent, protected from the deleterious effect of hypothyroidism through upregulation of brain type 2 deiodinase, which converts the prohormone T4 into its biologically active derivative, T3.[32] This likely accounts for the observation that even in CH with delayed bone maturation at diagnosis (indicating a prenatal onset), the intellectual outcome is within normal limits if continuous and adequate treatment is instituted shortly after birth.[44] Thus the in utero treatment of fetal hypothyroidism should only be considered in exceptional circumstances, such as for goiter causing progressive hydramnios. Although the identification of a goiter by prenatal ultrasound may be increasing,[45] it remains rare and even direct examination at birth often fails to detect goiters that are obvious on scintigraphy. Goiters can also be observed in fetuses borne by women with Graves disease if they are overtreated with antithyroid drugs, which readily cross the placenta. Reducing the dose of the antithyroid medication given to the mother should decrease the size of the fetal thyroid in such circumstances.[46]

Although a pro-TRH molecule is produced by the placenta, TRH concentrations in the maternal circulation are very low and thus have little effect on fetal thyroid function. However, TRH, with its tripeptide structure (the smallest of the hypothalamic hypophysiotropic peptides), crosses the placenta readily and, when injected to the mother, increases thyroid hormone concentrations in the fetus. Because thyroid hormones stimulate fetal lung maturation, maternal TRH treatment to decrease neonatal respiratory distress syndrome has been attempted, but with negative results.[47]

Because immunoglobulins of the IgG type cross the placenta, transient fetal/neonatal hyperthyroidism from transplacental transfer of TSH-receptor activating antibodies can occur in women with past or present Graves disease. On the other hand, when pregnant women are overtreated with antithyroid drugs, which also cross the placenta readily, their fetuses may develop goitrous hypothyroidism, as noted previously; however, only one case of CH out of 30,000 births is attributable to this in the Québec database (unpublished observations). Lastly, transient neonatal hypothyroidism from maternofetal transfer of TSH-receptor blocking antibodies can also occur but only accounts for 2% of cases of neonatal hypothyroidism identified by screening,[48] and a specific screening strategy is not required for babies born to women with Hashimoto thyroiditis.

Thyroid function tests are often ordered clinically in newborns whose mother has a history of thyroid disease and, if abnormal, require special consideration of optimal approach to therapy. For example, hypothyroidism at birth caused by treatment of maternal Graves disease with antithyroid medication may only require observation, in the expectation that the effects of the drugs will dissipate over a few days; hyperthyroidism may follow, albeit exceptionally. For hypothyroidism or hyperthyroidism resulting respectively from maternal blocking or stimulating antibodies, treatment will be required, as these effects may last several months.[49]

32.4   MATURATION OF THYROID HORMONE SYNTHESIS AND SECRETION

Maturation of thyroid function in the fetus reflects changes at the level of the hypothalamus, pituitary, and thyroid. Serum TRH concentrations are relatively high in the human fetus, because it is produced at both hypothalamic and extrahypothalamic sites and because the TRH-degrading activity of fetal blood is low.[50] Fetal serum TSH increases from a low level at 18 to 20 weeks to a peak value of approximately 7 to 10 mU/L at term. After delivery, in response to exposure to the cold extrauterine environment, there is an acute release of TSH with mean serum levels peaking at 30 min at concentrations of approximately 70 mU/L. The increase in serum T4 levels immediately after birth is TSH-dependent.

Only free thyroid hormones enter cells, and hormones bound to serum TBG and other transport proteins are not available to tissues. In addition, T4 is a prohormone, and it is T3 that is biologically active to exert intracellular effects, so that deiodination of T4 is essential for tissue euthyroidism. Both serum transport proteins and intracellular deiodination change during development. As previously mentioned, the fetal thyroid gland is capable of iodine concentration and iodothyronine synthesis as early as 70 days of gestation, a reflection of a sharp increase in the expression of the sodium-iodine symporter and of the appearance of a follicular architecture.[51] Starting at 18–20 weeks, TBG and total T4 concentrations in fetal serum increase steadily until the final weeks of pregnancy.

The study of free T4 concentrations in fetal/neonatal blood has been hampered by the relative inadequacy of the commercially available immunoassay systems for measurements in these samples.[52] The fetal serum T3 concentration remains low until 30 weeks due to two factors: first, the low activities of type I iodothyronine monodeiodinase result in relatively low rates of T4 to T3 conversion in fetal tissues; second, active type III monodeiodinase in placenta and selected fetal tissues degrades T3 to T2. After 30 weeks, serum T3 increases slowly until birth. This prenatal increase in serum T3 is due to progressive maturation of liver type I deiodinase activity increasing hepatic conversion of T4 to T3, and to decreased placental T3 degradation. Postnatally, T3 and T4 serum concentrations increase two- to sixfold within the first few hours, peaking on the 2nd day of life. These levels then gradually decline to levels characteristic of infancy over the first 4–5 weeks of life.

In the human, the fetal thyroid gland grows and its production increases under the influence of the increasing serum TSH level during the second half of gestation, as evidenced by the severely atrophic and hypofunctional glands observed in newborns with mutations that inactivate either the beta-subunit of TSH[53] or the TSH receptor.[54] On the other hand, the maturation of the negative feedback control system appears to occur earlier than previously thought, since an elevated TSH in serum obtained at cordocentesis can be seen in fetuses with primary hypothyroidism as early as 18 weeks.[55]

Thyroid function in the premature infant (before 30–32 weeks) is characterized by low circulating concentrations of T4 and free T4, a normal or low concentration of TSH, and a normal or prolonged TSH response to TRH, suggesting a degree of relative hypothalamic (tertiary) hypothyroidism.

In summary, fetal thyroid hormone secretion results from increasing hypothalamic TRH secretion and increasing thyroid follicular cell sensitivity to TSH, and is regulated by increasing pituitary sensitivity to thyroid hormone inhibition of TSH release. The marked cold-stimulated TRH-TSH surge at birth is associated with a marked increase in T4 secretion and free T4 concentration with a new equilibrium reached by 1–2 months. During infancy and childhood, there is a progressive decrease in T4 secretion rate (based on a μg/kg/day) correlating with a decreasing metabolic rate (Table 32.1).

32.5   MATURATION OF THYROID HORMONE METABOLISM AND TRANSPORT

The thyroid gland is the sole source of T4. Most of the circulating T3 after birth is derived from conversion of T4 to T3 via monodeiodination in peripheral tissues. Deiodination of the iodothyronines is the major route of metabolism, and monodeiodination may occur either at the outer (phenolic) ring or the inner (tyrosyl) ring of the iodothyronine molecule. Outer ring monodeiodination of T4 produces T3, the form of thyroid hormone with greatest affinity for the thyroid nuclear receptor. Inner ring monodeiodination of T4 produces reverse T3 (rT3), an inactive metabolite. In adults, between 70% and 90% of circulating T3 is derived from peripheral conversion of T4 and 10% to 30% from direct glandular secretion. Nearly all circulating rT3 derives from peripheral conversion, with only 2% to 3% coming directly from the thyroid gland. T3 and rT3 are progressively metabolized to diiodo, monoiodo, and noniodinated forms of thyroxine, none of which possess biologic activity.

TABLE 32.1 Normal values for fetal thyroid volume, cord TSH and total thyroxine levels according to gestation age

Gestational age (weeks)	Mean FTP in cm³ (SD)	Mean fetal cord TSH in mU/L (SD)	Mean fetal cord total T4 in nmol/L (SD)
20–23	0.08 (0.05)	NA	NA
24–27	0.15 (0.09)	6.8 (2.93)	69.6 (25.5)
28–31	0.24 (0.10)	7.0 (3.73)	81.2 (26.4)
32–35	0.42 (0.21)	8.0 (5.15)	97.0 (29.0)
>36	0.62 (0.22)	6.4 (4.85)	116.5 (20.6)

Mean fetal thyroid volume (FTP),[1] cord TSH and total thyroxine.[2]
(Adapted from Hume R, Simpson J, Delahunty C, van Toor H, Wu SY, Williams FL, et al. Human fetal and cord serum thyroid hormones: developmental trends and interrelationships. *J Clin Endocrinol Metab* 2004;**89(8)**:4097–103.)

Two types of outer ring iodothyronine monodeiodinases have been described.[56] Type I deiodinase (predominantly expressed in liver, kidney, and thyroid) is a high-Km enzyme inhibited by propylthiouracil and stimulated by thyroid hormone. Type II deiodinase (predominantly located in brain, pituitary, placenta, skeletal muscle, heart, thyroid, and brown adipose tissue) is a low-Km enzyme insensitive to propylthiouracil and inhibited by thyroid hormone. Types I and II deiodinases contribute to circulating T3 production, whereas type II acts to increase local tissue levels of T3 as well. An inner ring deiodinase (type III deiodinase) has been characterized in most fetal tissues, including placenta. This enzyme system catalyzes the conversion of T4 to rT3 and T3 to diiodothyronine. All three deiodinase enzymes are selenoproteins.

Deiodination is developmentally and thyroid-state regulated. In the human fetal brain, type II deiodinase activity in the cortex increases between 13 and 20 weeks' gestation and by about 50% over the last third of gestation. There is a general inverse correlation of type II and type III activities. Both of these deiodinase species are thyroid hormone responsive.

Fetal thyroid hormone metabolism is characterized by a predominance of type III enzyme activity (particularly in liver, kidney, and placenta), accounting for the increased circulating concentrations of rT3 observed in the fetus. However, the persistence of high circulating rT3 concentrations for several weeks in the newborn indicate that type III deiodinase activity expressed in nonplacental tissues is important. The mixture of type II and type III deiodinase activities in the placenta provides for the conversion of T4 to T3 and of T4 and T3 to rT3 and T2, respectively.

Sulfated iodothyronines are the major thyroid hormone metabolites circulating in the fetus.[57] Sulfokinase enzymes are present early in fetal life, and sulfation of the phenolic hydroxyl group of the iodothyronine molecule may be a normal prerequisite step for monodeiodination. The sulfated iodothyronines are preferred substrates for the type I deiodinase, and concentrations are high in fetal serum in part because of low type I deiodinase activity. However, increased production of sulfated metabolites is also involved. There is evidence that T3S has biologic activity (i.e., suppresses TSH in vivo), suggesting that it can be de-sulfated by one or more tissue sulfatase enzymes. The low production rates and low levels of T3 metabolites and the high ratio of inactive to active metabolites suggest that fetal thyroid hormone metabolism is largely oriented to inactivating T4, presumably to avoid tissue thermogenesis and to potentiate the anabolic state of the rapidly growing fetus. This is mediated by early activation of type III monodeiodinase, inactivation of type I monodeiodinase, and augmented iodothyronine sulfation.

The developmental expression of type II deiodinase in brain and other tissues provides for local T3 supply to specific tissues (particularly in the event of T4 deficiency) and helps guarantee provision of T3 during gestation, when brain development is thyroid hormone-dependent.[32]

32.6 EXTRAUTERINE THYROID ADAPTATION

At the time of parturition, the neonate must rapidly convert from the fetal state of predominant thyroid hormone inactivation to a state of relative thyroidal hyperactivity. During the first hours after birth, there is an abrupt increase in circulating T4 and T3 levels. This is due to the abrupt increase in hypothalamic TRH and pituitary TSH secretion stimulating increased thyroid hormone secretion. The cold-stimulated TRH-TSH surge is short-lived, and mean TSH concentrations decrease progressively to normal infant levels by 3–5 days, but the serum free T4 level remains elevated for several weeks.[58]

Serum T3 levels increase in response to the TSH surge, because of stimulation of thyroidal T3 secretion and of a combined cortisol- and T4-stimulated increase in hepatic type I deiodinase activity. Placental separation decreases T3 deiodination (to inactive T2), contributing to the early postnatal increase in serum T3 concentration. The type II deiodinase activity in brown adipose tissue increases during the last weeks of gestation to potentiate catecholamine-stimulated brown adipose tissue thermogenesis, thereby contributing to the maintenance of the body temperature of the neonate.[56]

32.7 THYROID HORMONE ACTIONS

Recent evidence suggests that all thyroid-sensitive cell populations express iodothyronine membrane transporters. These belong to several families of integrin, organic anion, amino acid, and monocarboxylate solute carriers. The importance of these transporters is highlighted by the role of mutations inactivating human monocarboxylate transporter 8 (MCT8) in an X-linked syndrome of severe psychomotor retardation (previously called the Allan-Herndon-Dudley syndrome), combined with mild abnormalities of thyroid function, characterized by high T3, low T4 and normal or high TSH.[59, 60] MCT8 is thought to play a role in the entry of T3 into neurons, after deiodination of T4 to T3 in neighboring astrocytes. In addition, MCT8 is involved in the transfer of T3 across the blood-brain barrier. Lastly, the abnormalities in thyroid hormone levels and TSH are also due to the effect of MCT8 on deiodination.[61]

Thyroid hormone effects are mediated predominantly via nuclear thyroid hormone protein receptors (TR), which act as DNA-binding transcription factors regulating gene transcription. Two mammalian genes code for TR, TRα, and TRβ, and alternative mRNA splicing lead to the production of four major thyroid hormone-binding transcripts: TRα1, TRα2, TRβ1, and TRβ2. The TRs exist as monomers, homodimers, and heterodimers with other nuclear receptor family members, such as the retinoid X receptors. TRα1 is the predominant subtype in bone, gastrointestinal tract, heart, and brain. TRβ1 is expressed in liver, kidney, heart, lung, brain, cochlea, and pituitary. TRβ2 is expressed in the pituitary gland, retina, and cochlea. The receptors function redundantly, as indicated by knockout studies in mice, but predominant effects of one or another TR have been described.

In humans, the specific roles of TRα and TRβ are illustrated by the phenotypes observed in patients with inactivating mutations in the corresponding genes. The syndrome of thyroid hormone resistance initially described in 1967 was later found to be due to mutations inactivating TRβ that either occur de novo or are inherited in an autosomal dominant fashion; however, in some patients with thyroid hormone resistance, TRβ is normal and the molecular defect remains elusive.[62] Recently, mutations in TRα have been described, occurring de novo in one patient[63] and transmitted from father to daughter in one pedigree.[64]

Thyroid hormone-programmed development of fetal tissues requires the interaction of local tissue monodeiodinase I and II, TRs, thyroid receptor coactivators, and thyroid-responsive genes. In most responsive tissues, the timing of maturation events is controlled by the TRs acting as a molecular switch. In the absence of T3, the unliganded receptor recruits corepressors, thereby repressing gene transcription. Local tissue maturation events are stimulated by the coincident availability of T3, liganded T3 receptor, T3-mediated receptor exchange of corepressors with coactivators, and activation of responsive gene transcription.[65]

In the human fetus, low levels of TR binding have been detected in brain tissue at 10 weeks gestational age, and liver, heart, and lung TR binding is observed at 16–18 weeks. TR levels in human fetal cerebral cortex and cerebellum increase markedly during the second and third trimesters. Information is limited regarding the timing of appearance of thyroid hormone tissue effects in the human fetus.

The birth length of the athyroid human neonate is within normal limits: the linear growth of the human fetus is programmed independently of thyroid hormones by a complex interplay of genetic, nutritional, and hormonal factors, as well as by the mechanical uterine constraint.[66] However, 50%–60% of athyroid newborns manifest delayed epiphyseal maturation and have large fontanelles.[67] Neonates with severe CH may have large fontanelles, macroglossia, and umbilical hernia, and develop prolonged jaundice and feeding difficulties.[68] However, the classic clinical manifestations of CH appear progressively during the early months of life. These include soft-tissue myxedema, a slow linear growth, metabolic derangements, and retarded central nervous system (CNS) development.[66] The normal IQ in most early treated athyroid infants thanks to newborn screening[69] seems attributable to the low but significant levels of maternal thyroxine derived from placental transfer, as shown in humans,[33] and the upregulation of type II monodeiodinase in fetal brain tissue in the face of low fetal serum thyroxine concentrations, as shown in rats.[32]

Postnatal thermogenesis is mediated via the brown adipose tissue prominent in subscapular and perirenal areas in the mammalian fetus and neonate. Heat production in brown adipose tissue is stimulated by catecholamines via β-adrenergic receptors and is thyroid hormone dependent. The uncoupling protein thermogenin unique to brown adipose tissue is located on the inner mitochondrial membrane and uncouples phosphorylation by dissipating the proton gradient created by the mitochondrial respiratory chain. The type II monodeiodinase in brown adipose tissue mediates local T4 to T3 conversion. Full thermogenin expression in brown adipose tissue requires both catecholamine and T3 stimulation.[70] Brown adipose tissue matures progressively in the fetus but remains thermoneutral until stimulated by catecholamines in the perinatal period. Brown adipose tissue thermogenesis is immature in small premature infants, and brown adipose tissue mass decreases in the neonatal period in full-term infants as the capacity for nonshivering thermogenesis develops in other tissues.[70] Uncoupling protein-2 is found in many tissues but does not appear to be regulated by β-adrenergic agonists or thyroid hormone. Uncoupling protein-3 is expressed in muscle and white adipose tissue as well as brown adipose tissue. Muscle uncoupling protein-3 is regulated by β3-adrenergic stimulation and thyroid hormone, and presumably contributes to nonshivering thermogenesis in humans. mRNA levels for uncoupling protein-3 are also regulated by dexamethasone, leptin, and starvation, but the regulation differs in brown adipose tissue and muscle. Starvation increases muscle and decreases brown adipose tissue uncoupling protein-3, suggesting that muscle serves a larger role in thermoregulation during starvation.[71]

The critical role of thyroid hormones in CNS maturation has long been recognized. Nervous system development involves neurogenesis, gliogenesis, neural cell migration, neuronal differentiation, dendritic and axonal growth, synaptogenesis, myelination, and neurotransmitter synthesis. Thyroid hormones have been shown to stimulate a number of developmentally regulated nervous tissue genes, but the role of these factors in the CNS developmental program remains undefined. Available evidence suggests that the deficiency or excess of thyroid hormones alters the timing or synchronization of the CNS developmental program, presumably by initiating critical gene actions or other genetic CNS maturation events.[72]

There is increasing evidence for a critical period for thyroid-dependent brain maturation in utero. Early maternal hypothyroxinemia in the rat alters histogenesis and cerebral cortical architecture of the progeny.[73] As noted previously, maternal hypothyroxinemia in humans has been reported to be associated with IQ reduction in offspring,[36–38] but association does not mean causation, as shown by the negative results of the RCT of T4 treatment.[39] In contrast, the impact of iodine supplementation in pregnant women in geographic areas of severe iodine deficiency has suggested a critical period of hormone action on CNS maturation during a narrow interval of time at the beginning of the third trimester of gestation.[29] The reasons for the discrepancy between the effect of iodine in this situation and the lack of effect of T4 in mildly hypothyroid women are unknown. Recent studies of the dose and timing of thyroid hormone therapy in infants with CH suggest a second critical period of thyroid hormone action during the very early neonatal period,[74] but the period of CNS thyroid hormone dependency extends further, to at least 2 years of age.[75]

REFERENCES

1. Ho SS, Metreweli C. Normal fetal thyroid volume. *Ultrasound Obstet Gynecol* 1998;**11**(2):118–22.
2. Hume R, Simpson J, Delahunty C, van Toor H, Wu SY, Williams FL, et al. Human fetal and cord serum thyroid hormones: developmental trends and interrelationships. *J Clin Endocrinol Metab* 2004;**89**(8):4097–103.
3. Zimmermann MB. Research on iodine deficiency and goiter in the 19th and early 20th centuries. *J Nutr* 2008;**138**(11):2060–3.
4. Winters AJ, Eskay RL, Porter JC. Concentration and distribution of TRH and LRH in the human fetal brain. *J Clin Endocrinol Metab* 1974;**39**(5):960–3.
5. Morley JE. Extrahypothalamic thyrotropin releasing hormone (TRH)—its distribution and its functions. *Life Sci* 1979;**25**(18):1539–50.
6. Nebesio TD, McKenna MP, Nabhan ZM, Eugster EA. Newborn screening results in children with central hypothyroidism. *J Pediatr* 2010;**156**(6):990–3.
7. McCabe MJ, Alatzoglou KS, Dattani MT. Septo-optic dysplasia and other midline defects: the role of transcription factors: HESX1 and beyond. *Best Pract Res Clin Endocrinol Metab* 2011;**25**(1):115–24.
8. Ward L, Chavez M, Huot C, Lecocq P, Collu R, Decarie JC, et al. Severe congenital hypopituitarism with low prolactin levels and age-dependent anterior pituitary hypoplasia: a clue to a PIT-1 mutation. *J Pediatr* 1998;**132**(6):1036–8.
9. Deladoey J, Fluck C, Buyukgebiz A, Kuhlmann BV, Eble A, Hindmarsh PC, et al. "Hot spot" in the PROP1 gene responsible for combined pituitary hormone deficiency. *J Clin Endocrinol Metab* 1999;**84**(5):1645–50.
10. Pfaffle R, Klammt J. Pituitary transcription factors in the aetiology of combined pituitary hormone deficiency. *Best Pract Res Clin Endocrinol Metab* 2011;**25**(1):43–60.
11. Vandernoot I, Sartelet H, Abu-Khudir R, Chanoine JP, Deladoey J. Evidence for calcitonin-producing cells in human lingual thyroids. *J Clin Endocrinol Metab* 2012;**97**(3):951–6.
12. Williams ED, Toyn CE, Harach HR. The ultimobranchial gland and congenital thyroid abnormalities in man. *J Pathol* 1989;**159**(2):135–41.
13. Kumar R, Gupta R, Bal CS, Khullar S, Malhotra A. Thyrotoxicosis in a patient with submandibular thyroid. *Thyroid* 2000;**10**(4):363–5.
14. De Felice M, Di Lauro R. Thyroid development and its disorders: genetics and molecular mechanisms. *Endocr Rev* 2004;**25**(5):722–46.
15. De Felice M, Di Lauro R. Minireview: intrinsic and extrinsic factors in thyroid gland development: an update. *Endocrinology* 2011;**152**(8):2948–56.
16. Kimura S, Hara Y, Pineau T, Fernandez-Salguero P, Fox CH, Ward JM, et al. The T/EBP null mouse: thyroid-specific enhancer-binding protein is essential for the organogenesis of the thyroid, lung, ventral forebrain, and pituitary. *Genes Dev* 1996;**10**(1):60–9.
17. Mansouri A, Chowdhury K, Gruss P. Follicular cells of the thyroid gland require Pax8 gene function. *Nat Genet* 1998;**19**(1):87–90.

18. De Felice M, Ovitt C, Biffali E, Rodriguez-Mallon A, Arra C, Anastassiadis K, et al. A mouse model for hereditary thyroid dysgenesis and cleft palate. *Nat Genet* 1998;**19**(4):395–8.

19. Vassart G, Dumont JE. Thyroid dysgenesis: multigenic or epigenetic... or both? *Endocrinology* 2005;**146**(12):5035–7.

20. Deladoey J, Vassart G, Van Vliet G. Possible non-Mendelian mechanisms of thyroid dysgenesis. *Endocr Dev* 2007;**10**:29–42.

21. Risau W. Mechanisms of angiogenesis. *Nature* 1997;**386**(6626):671–4.

22. Vasudevan A, Bhide PG. Angiogenesis in the embryonic CNS: a new twist on an old tale. *Cell Adhes Migr* 2008;**2**(3):167–9.

23. Fagman H, Grande M, Edsbagge J, Semb H, Nilsson M. Expression of classical cadherins in thyroid development: maintenance of an epithelial phenotype throughout organogenesis. *Endocrinology* 2003;**144**(8):3618–24.

24. Fagman H, Andersson L, Nilsson M. The developing mouse thyroid: embryonic vessel contacts and parenchymal growth pattern during specification, budding, migration, and lobulation. *Dev Dyn* 2006;**235**(2):444–55.

25. Opitz R, Hitz MP, Vandernoot I, Trubiroha A, Abu-Khudir R, Samuels M, et al. Functional zebrafish studies based on human genotyping point to netrin-1 as a link between aberrant cardiovascular development and thyroid dysgenesis. *Endocrinology* 2015;**156**(1):377–88.

26. Deladoey J, Belanger N, Van Vliet G. Random variability in congenital hypothyroidism from thyroid dysgenesis over 16 years in Quebec. *J Clin Endocrinol Metab* 2007;**92**(8):3158–61.

27. Medda E, Olivieri A, Stazi MA, Grandolfo ME, Fazzini C, Baserga M, et al. Risk factors for congenital hypothyroidism: results of a population case-control study (1997–2003). *Eur J Endocrinol* 2005;**153**(6):765–73.

28. Di Cosmo C, Fanelli G, Tonacchera M, Ferrarini E, Dimida A, Agretti P, et al. The sodium-iodide symporter expression in placental tissue at different gestational age: an immunohistochemical study. *Clin Endocrinol* 2006;**65**(4):544–8.

29. Cao XY, Jiang XM, Dou ZH, Rakeman MA, Zhang ML, O'Donnell K, et al. Timing of vulnerability of the brain to iodine deficiency in endemic cretinism. *N Engl J Med* 1994;**331**(26):1739–44.

30. Glinoer D. The importance of iodine nutrition during pregnancy. *Public Health Nutr* 2007;**10**(12A):1542–6.

31. Fisher DA, Lehman H, Lackey C. Placental transport of thyroxine. *J Clin Endocrinol Metab* 1964;**24**:393–400.

32. Calvo RM, Jauniaux E, Gulbis B, Asuncion M, Gervy C, Contempre B, et al. Fetal tissues are exposed to biologically relevant free thyroxine concentrations during early phases of development. *J Clin Endocrinol Metab* 2002;**87**(4):1768–77.

33. Vulsma T, Gons MH, de Vijlder JJ. Maternal-fetal transfer of thyroxine in congenital hypothyroidism due to a total organification defect or thyroid agenesis. *N Engl J Med* 1989;**321**(1):13–6.

34. Anselmo J, Cao D, Karrison T, Weiss RE, Refetoff S. Fetal loss associated with excess thyroid hormone exposure. *JAMA* 2004;**292**(6):691–5.

35. de Zegher F, Pernasetti F, Vanhole C, Devlieger H, Van den Berghe G, Martial JA. The prenatal role of thyroid hormone evidenced by fetomaternal Pit-1 deficiency. *J Clin Endocrinol Metab* 1995;**80**(11):3127–30.

36. Man EB, Brown JF, Serunian SA. Maternal hypothyroxinemia: psychoneurological deficits of progeny. *Ann Clin Lab Sci* 1991;**21**(4):227–39.

37. Haddow JE, Palomaki GE, Allan WC, Williams JR, Knight GJ, Gagnon J, et al. Maternal thyroid deficiency during pregnancy and subsequent neuropsychological development of the child. *N Engl J Med* 1999;**341**(8):549–55.

38. Pop VJ, Kuijpens JL, van Baar AL, Verkerk G, van Son MM, de Vijlder JJ, et al. Low maternal free thyroxine concentrations during early pregnancy are associated with impaired psychomotor development in infancy. *Clin Endocrinol* 1999;**50**(2):149–55.

39. Lazarus JH, Bestwick JP, Channon S, Paradice R, Maina A, Rees R, et al. Antenatal thyroid screening and childhood cognitive function. *N Engl J Med* 2012;**366**(6):493–501.

40. Momotani N, Iwama S, Momotani K. Neurodevelopment in children born to hypothyroid mothers restored to normal thyroxine (T(4)) concentration by late pregnancy in Japan: no apparent influence of maternal T(4) deficiency. *J Clin Endocrinol Metab* 2012;**97**(4):1104–8.

41. Downing S, Halpern L, Carswell J, Brown RS. Severe maternal hypothyroidism corrected prior to the third trimester is associated with normal cognitive outcome in the offspring. *Thyroid* 2012;**22**(6):625–30.

42. Alexander EK, Marqusee E, Lawrence J, Jarolim P, Fischer GA, Larsen PR. Timing and magnitude of increases in levothyroxine requirements during pregnancy in women with hypothyroidism. *N Engl J Med* 2004;**351**(3):241–9.

43. Stoppa-Vaucher S, Francoeur D, Grignon A, Alos N, Pohlenz J, Hermanns P, et al. Non-immune goiter and hypothyroidism in a 19-week fetus: a plea for conservative treatment. *J Pediatr* 2010;**156**(6):1026–9.

44. Simoneau-Roy J, Marti S, Deal C, Huot C, Robaey P, Van Vliet G. Cognition and behavior at school entry in children with congenital hypothyroidism treated early with high-dose levothyroxine. *J Pediatr* 2004;**144**(6):747–52.

45. Stewart CJ, Constantatos S, Joolay Y, Muller L. In utero treatment of fetal goitrous hypothyroidism in a euthyroid mother: a case report. *J Clin Ultrasound* 2012;**40**(9):603–6.

46. Stoppa-Vaucher S, Van Vliet G, Deladoey J. Discovery of a fetal goiter on prenatal ultrasound in women treated for Graves' disease: first, do no harm. *Thyroid* 2011;**21**(8):931 [author reply 932–3].

47. Ballard RA, Ballard PL, Cnaan A, Pinto-Martin J, Davis DJ, Padbury JF, et al. Antenatal thyrotropin-releasing hormone to prevent lung disease in preterm infants. North American Thyrotropin-Releasing Hormone Study Group. *N Engl J Med* 1998;**338**(8):493–8.

48. Brown RS, Bellisario RL, Botero D, Fournier L, Abrams CA, Cowger ML, et al. Incidence of transient congenital hypothyroidism due to maternal thyrotropin receptor-blocking antibodies in over one million babies. *J Clin Endocrinol Metab* 1996;**81**(3):1147–51.

49. Zakarija M, McKenzie JM, Hoffman WH. Prediction and therapy of intrauterine and late-onset neonatal hyperthyroidism. *J Clin Endocrinol Metab* 1986;**62**(2):368–71.

50. Aratan-Spire S, Czernichow P. Thyrotropin-releasing hormone-degrading activity of neonatal human plasma. *J Clin Endocrinol Metab* 1980;**50**(1):88–92.

51. Szinnai G, Lacroix L, Carre A, Guimiot F, Talbot M, Martinovic J, et al. Sodium/iodide symporter (NIS) gene expression is the limiting step for the onset of thyroid function in the human fetus. *J Clin Endocrinol Metab* 2007;**92**(1):70–6.

52. Deming DD, Rabin CW, Hopper AO, Peverini RL, Vyhmeister NR, Nelson JC. Direct equilibrium dialysis compared with two non-dialysis free T4 methods in premature infants. *J Pediatr* 2007;**151**(4):404–8.

53. Heinrichs C, Parma J, Scherberg NH, Delange F, Van Vliet G, Duprez L, et al. Congenital central isolated hypothyroidism caused by a homozygous mutation in the TSH-beta subunit gene. *Thyroid* 2000;**10**(5):387–91.

54. Gagne N, Parma J, Deal C, Vassart G, Van Vliet G. Apparent congenital athyreosis contrasting with normal plasma thyroglobulin levels and associated with inactivating mutations in the thyrotropin receptor gene: are athyreosis and ectopic thyroid distinct entities? *J Clin Endocrinol Metab* 1998;**83**(5):1771–5.

55. Ribault V, Castanet M, Bertrand AM, Guibourdenche J, Vuillard E, Luton D, et al. Experience with intraamniotic thyroxine treatment in nonimmune fetal goitrous hypothyroidism in 12 cases. *J Clin Endocrinol Metab* 2009;**94**(10):3731–9.

56. Bianco AC. Minireview: cracking the metabolic code for thyroid hormone signaling. *Endocrinology* 2011;**152**(9):3306–11.

57. Stanley EL, Hume R, Visser TJ, Coughtrie MW. Differential expression of sulfotransferase enzymes involved in thyroid hormone metabolism during human placental development. *J Clin Endocrinol Metab* 2001;**86**(12):5944–55.

58. Djemli A, Van Vliet G, Belgoudi J, Lambert M, Delvin EE. Reference intervals for free thyroxine, total triiodothyronine, thyrotropin and thyroglobulin for Quebec newborns, children and teenagers. *Clin Biochem* 2004;**37**(4):328–30.

59. Dumitrescu AM, Liao XH, Best TB, Brockmann K, Refetoff S. A novel syndrome combining thyroid and neurological abnormalities is associated with mutations in a monocarboxylate transporter gene. *Am J Hum Genet* 2004;**74**(1):168–75.

60. Friesema EC, Grueters A, Biebermann H, Krude H, von Moers A, Reeser M, et al. Association between mutations in a thyroid hormone transporter and severe X-linked psychomotor retardation. *Lancet* 2004;**364**(9443):1435–7.

61. Visser WE, Friesema EC, Visser TJ. Minireview: thyroid hormone transporters: the knowns and the unknowns. *Mol Endocrinol* 2011;**25**(1):1–14.

62. Refetoff S, Weiss RE, Usala SJ. The syndromes of resistance to thyroid hormone. *Endocr Rev* 1993;**14**(3):348–99.

63. Bochukova E, Schoenmakers N, Agostini M, Schoenmakers E, Rajanayagam O, Keogh JM, et al. A mutation in the thyroid hormone receptor alpha gene. *N Engl J Med* 2012;**366**(3):243–9.

64. van Mullem A, van Heerebeek R, Chrysis D, Visser E, Medici M, Andrikoula M, et al. Clinical phenotype and mutant TRalpha1. *N Engl J Med* 2012;**366**(15):1451–3.

65. Flamant F, Gauthier K. Thyroid hormone receptors: the challenge of elucidating isotype-specific functions and cell-specific response. *Biochim Biophys Acta* 2013;**1830**(7):3900–7.

66. Andersen HJ. Studies of hypothyroidism in children. *Acta Paediatr Suppl* 1961;**50**(Suppl 125):1–150.

67. Smith DW, Popich G. Large fontanels in congenital hypothyroidism: a potential clue toward earlier recognition. *J Pediatr* 1972;**80**(5):753–6.

68. Lenz AM, Root AW. Congenital hypothyroidism: a forgotten clinical diagnosis? *J Pediatr Endocrinol Metab* 2008;**21**(7):623–4.

69. Grosse SD, Van Vliet G. Prevention of intellectual disability through screening for congenital hypothyroidism: how much and at what level? *Arch Dis Child* 2011;**96**(4):374–9.

70. Silva JE. Physiological importance and control of non-shivering facultative thermogenesis. *Front Biosci (Schol Ed)* 2011;**3**:352–71.

71. Sluse FE. Uncoupling proteins: molecular, functional, regulatory, physiological and pathological aspects. *Adv Exp Med Biol* 2012;**942**:137–56.

72. Morreale de Escobar G, Obregon MJ, Escobar del Rey F. Role of thyroid hormone during early brain development. *Eur J Endocrinol* 2004;**151**(Suppl. 3):U25–37.

73. Lavado-Autric R, Auso E, Garcia-Velasco JV, Arufe Mdel C, Escobar del Rey F, Berbel P, et al. Early maternal hypothyroxinemia alters histogenesis and cerebral cortex cytoarchitecture of the progeny. *J Clin Invest* 2003;**111**(7):1073–82.

74. Bongers-Schokking JJ, de Muinck Keizer-Schrama SM. Influence of timing and dose of thyroid hormone replacement on mental, psychomotor, and behavioral development in children with congenital hypothyroidism. *J Pediatr* 2005;**147**(6):768–74.

75. Joergensen JV, Oerbeck B, Jebsen P, Heyerdahl S, Kase BF. Severe hypothyroidism due to atrophic thyroiditis from second year of life influenced developmental outcome. *Acta Paediatr* 2005;**94**(8):1049–54.

Chapter 33

Physiology of Calcium, Phosphorus, and Bone Metabolism During Fetal and Neonatal Development

Christopher S. Kovacs* and Leanne M. Ward[†,‡]

*Faculty of Medicine, Endocrinology, Memorial University of Newfoundland, St. John's, NL, Canada, [†]Department of Pediatrics, Faculty of Medicine, University of Ottawa, Ottawa, ON, Canada, [‡]Division of Endocrinology, Children's Hospital of Eastern Ontario, Ottawa, ON, Canada

Key Clinical Changes

- Serum calcium and phosphorus are maintained at high levels in the fetal circulation to facilitate skeletal mineralization.
- Parathyroid hormone (PTH) and calcitriol both circulate at low levels, while PTH-related protein (PTHrP) is present at high concentrations in plasma.
- PTHrP stimulates placental calcium transport, while PTH and PTHrP together regulate skeletal development and serum mineral concentrations.
- Calcitriol may not be required for fetal mineral homeostasis and skeletal development, but becomes important after birth to regulate intestinal calcium and phosphorus absorption.
- Fibroblast growth factor-23 is not required by the fetus, but begins to regulate phosphorus metabolism within hours after birth.

33.1 INTRODUCTION

Parathyroid hormone (PTH), calcitriol, fibroblast growth factor-23 (FGF23), calcitonin, and the sex steroids (largely estradiol and testosterone) each play important roles in regulating mineral and bone homeostasis in the child and adult. Loss of any one of these can have significant consequences. But each hormone's roles differ during fetal development, such that absence of calcitriol or FGF23 cause minimal to no disturbances. Another hormone, PTH-related protein (PTHrP), has key roles to regulate fetal bone and mineral metabolism.

The average human baby has 30 g of calcium at term, of which 80% is accreted during the third trimester.[1] The kidneys and intestines are not important sources of mineral; instead, the placenta actively transports calcium, phosphorus, and magnesium from the maternal circulation (Fig. 33.1). Calcium transport increases from a rate of 60 mg/day at week 24 to between 300 and 350 mg/day during the last 6 weeks.[1] Serum minerals are maintained at higher concentrations as compared with the mother, which facilitates mineralization of the fetal skeleton.

After birth, the placental pump is lost, the intestines become the main source of mineral, the kidneys reabsorb calcium and excrete phosphorus, and bone turnover contributes minerals to the circulation. Over hours to days, mineral metabolism changes to resemble that of the adult.

Human data pertinent to fetal development consist mainly of cord blood samples, and pathological examination of embryos and fetuses that died due to congenital abnormalities or obstetrical accidents. Consequently, this chapter will also make reference to studies in fetal animal models. Owing to restrictions on the reference list, a comprehensive review will be principally cited that contains more than 700 citations of the relevant primary literature.[1]

33.2 OVERVIEW OF FETAL MINERAL METABOLISM

The normal circulating concentrations of minerals and calciotropic and phosphotropic hormones are schematically depicted in Fig. 33.2.

Maternal-Fetal and Neonatal Endocrinology. https://doi.org/10.1016/B978-0-12-814823-5.00033-7

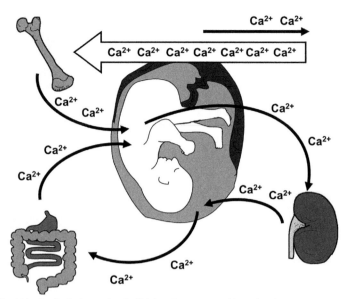

FIG. 33.1 Circulation of mineral within the fetal-placental unit. Calcium is represented here, but these statements also apply to phosphorus and magnesium. At the *top right*, the main flux of mineral is across the placenta and through the fetal circulation into bone; however, some mineral returns to the maternal circulation (backflux). On the *bottom right*, the fetal kidneys filter the blood and excrete mineral into urine, which in turn makes up much of the amniotic fluid. On the *bottom left*, amniotic fluid is swallowed and its mineral content can be absorbed, thereby restoring it to the circulation. The renal-amniotic-intestinal loop is likely a minor component for fetal mineral homeostasis. On the *top left*, although the net flux of mineral is into bone, some mineral is resorbed from the developing skeleton to reenter the fetal circulation. If placental delivery of mineral is deficient, fetal secondary hyperparathyroidism ensues, which resorbs mineral from the fetal skeleton, reduces skeletal mineral content, and may cause fractures in utero or during delivery. *(Reproduced with permission from Kovacs CS. Fetal control of calcium and phosphate homeostasis. In: Thakker RV, Whyte MP, Eisman JA, Igarashi T, editors.* Genetics of bone biology and skeletal disease. *2nd ed. San Diego: Academic Press/Elsevier; 2017. p. 329–47 ©2017 Elsevier.)*

33.2.1 Serum Mineral Concentrations

From at least 15 weeks of gestation onward, human fetuses maintain serum calcium and ionized calcium about 0.30–0.50 mmol/L above the maternal level.[1] Serum phosphorus and magnesium are respectively about 0.5 and 0.05 mmol/L higher than in the mother.[1] Consequently, fetal blood has a high calcium × phosphorus product (Ca × P). In adults, a Ca × P value greater than 5.6 $mmol^2/L^2$ or 70 mg^2/dL^2 causes spontaneous calcium-phosphate crystals to form, which lead to soft tissue calcifications, calciphylaxis, coronary artery calcifications, and increased mortality. But the high Ca × P product is nonhazardous in utero, likely due to rapid uptake into bone and the relatively short duration of gestation. Studies in rodents have shown that if serum calcium is reduced to the maternal level, then the fetal skeleton is undermineralized.[1] Therefore, physiological hypercalcemia in the fetus facilitates skeletal mineralization; it may also reduce the likelihood of hypocalcemia after birth (discussed later).

Animal studies have shown that the high fetal serum calcium is not set by the calcium-sensing receptor (CaSR) on the fetal parathyroids; instead, the elevated fetal ionized calcium acts through the CaSR to suppress PTH (Fig. 33.3).[1] Fetuses set their ionized calcium independent of the maternal calcium concentration, and can maintain that level despite maternal hypocalcemia due to a calcium-restricted diet, vitamin D deficiency, genetic disorders of vitamin D metabolism (loss of calcitriol or vitamin D receptor), and absence of PTH or parathyroids.[1]

33.2.2 Calciotropic and Phosphotropic Hormone Concentrations

33.2.2.1 Parathyroid Hormone

PTH is produced starting at 10 weeks of gestation, but low concentrations are present in cord blood as compared with adult values.[1] As noted previously, the CaSR keeps PTH synthesis and release suppressed.[2] However, PTH release can be stimulated by chronic maternal hypocalcemia (such as from hypoparathyroidism) or acute hypocalcemia (after EDTA or calcitonin).[1] Maternal PTH does not cross the placenta.[1]

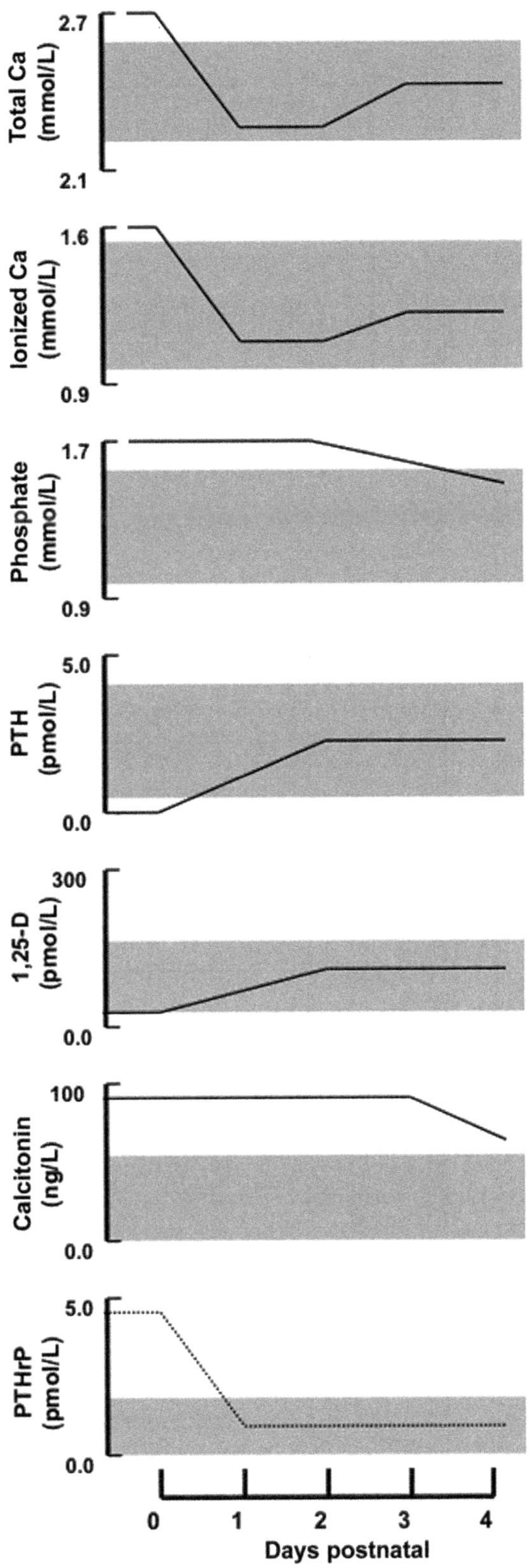

FIG. 33.2 Schematic illustration of the longitudinal changes in calcium, phosphate, and calciotropic hormone levels that occur during the fetal and neonatal period in humans. Normal adult ranges are indicated by the *shaded areas*. The progression in PTHrP has been depicted by a *dashed line* to reflect that it is speculative. *(Reproduced with permission from Kovacs CS, Kronenberg HM. Maternal-fetal calcium and bone metabolism during pregnancy, puerperium, and lactation. Endocr Rev 1997;18(6):832–72 ©1997 The Endocrine Society.)*

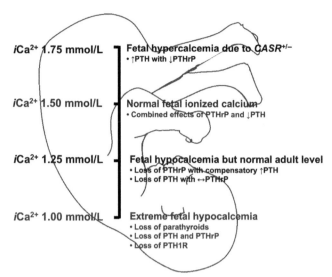

FIG. 33.3 Regulation of fetal ionized calcium. This schematic illustrates changes in ionized calcium as observed in murine fetuses and extrapolated to humans; the levels shown are meant as a relative guide only. The normal ionized calcium level is higher in fetuses than in the normal adult, and is maintained by the combined effects of high concentrations of PTHrP and low levels of PTH in the circulation. CaSR likely suppresses PTH in response to the normal high level of calcium in fetal blood. The high fetal blood calcium may be set by a novel calcium-sensing receptor (other than the known CaSR), which regulates PTHrP release from the placenta and possibly other fetal tissues. In the absence of PTHrP, serum calcium falls but is then maintained at the normal adult level through the normal actions of CaSR to regulate PTH. Loss of PTH leads to a similar blood calcium value, approximately equal to the maternal calcium concentration, without a compensatory increase in circulating PTHrP. Combined loss of PTH and PTHrP, loss of parathyroids, or loss of PTH1R, each result in the lowest fetal ionized calcium values. Conversely, inactivating mutations of *CASR* cause PTH and the blood calcium to increase above normal, in turn causing a decrease in PTHrP. *(Reproduced with permission from Kovacs CS. Fetal control of calcium and phosphate homeostasis. In: Thakker RV, Whyte MP, Eisman JA, Igarashi T, editors. Genetics of bone biology and skeletal disease. 2nd ed. San Diego: Academic Press/Elsevier; 2017. p. 329–47 ©2017 Elsevier.)*

33.2.2.2 Calcitriol

25-Hydroxyvitamin D (25OHD) readily crosses the placenta, resulting in cord blood levels that are 75%–100% of the maternal value at term.[1] In contrast, cord blood calcitriol is typically less than 50% of the maternal value.[1] The fetal kidneys are the main source of calcitriol, not the placenta, because the concentration of calcitriol is greater in the umbilical artery than in the umbilical vein.[3] Animal studies have confirmed that fetal nephrectomy causes a substantial fall in serum calcitriol.[1] Recent studies in *Cy27b1* null mice, which cannot make calcitriol, have confirmed that maternal calcitriol does cross the placenta.[4]

The placenta expresses 1α-hydroxylase (Cyp27b1), which converts 25OHD to calcitriol, and the 24-hydroxylase (Cyp24a1), which catabolizes 25OHD and calcitriol into inactive forms.[5–7] It has generally been assumed that the placenta is the source of a two- to threefold increase calcitriol within the maternal circulation during pregnancy. However, the placenta does not contribute substantial calcitriol to the mother. This has been shown by animal studies,[1,4] and by an anephric woman on dialysis who had low serum calcitriol before, during, and after her pregnancy.[8]

Calcitriol is maintained at low levels in part due to suppression of its synthesis by the ambient high serum calcium, high phosphorus, and low PTH.[1] Furthermore, there is increased 24-hydroxylation of 25OHD and calcitriol by the placenta, resulting in up to 40-fold higher concentrations of 24-hydroxylated forms as compared with calcitriol in cord blood.[9,10] The fetal kidneys are capable of upregulating calcitriol's synthesis, as shown by high calcitriol concentrations in *Vdr* null fetal mice that lacked the vitamin D receptor (VDR)[11] and *Casr* null fetuses that have increased PTH.[12]

FGF23 may contribute to keeping calcitriol low in fetal blood by inhibiting 1α-hydroxylase and stimulating 24-hydroxylase. Animal data indicate that FGF23's effect may be largely through 24-hydroxylase, but only in the extremes of absence or excess of FGF23. *Fgf23* null fetal mice had a modest reduction in renal expression of *Cyp24a1* but no change in *Cyp27b1* or serum calcitriol. Conversely, in a mouse model of X-linked hypophosphatemic rickets (XLH), affected fetuses have very high FGF23, significantly increased expression of *Cyp24a1*, no change in *Cyp27b1*, and only a small decrease in serum calcitriol.[13]

33.2.2.3 Parathyroid Hormone-Related Protein

Cord blood contains low immunoreactive levels (0.2–0.5 pmol/L) of PTH, while simultaneously displaying high PTH-like bioactivity.[1] This discrepancy is due PTHrP, which typically circulates at 2–4 pmol/L, or up to 15-fold higher than PTH.[1]

Animal studies have similarly shown high immunoreactive PTHrP concentrations in fetal plasma, which explains why PTH-like bioactivity is increased while PTH immunoreactivity is low.[1] PTHrP is subject to rapid degradation in serum, and even when rigorously collected in chilled tubes containing protease inhibitors, it begins to degrade within 15 min of collection. Additional problems with PTHrP assays contribute to failure to detect PTHrP, and these are discussed elsewhere.[1]

Diverse fetal tissues express PTHrP, but the placenta and fetal parathyroids are the likeliest sources of it in the fetal circulation.[1] Maternally derived PTHrP does not cross the placenta.[1]

33.2.2.4 FGF23

FGF23 is produced mainly by osteoblasts and osteocytes in fetal bone. Intact FGF23 concentrations in human cord blood have ranged from low to identical to the maternal values.[14–18] Three studies also used a C-terminal assay for FGF23 (which detects both intact FGF23 and biologically inactive C-terminal fragments), and found that the FGF23 concentration in cord blood was up to twice that of expected adult values.[14,16,17] Collectively, these results suggest that FGF23 is abundantly produced but rapidly cleaved in utero, thereby resulting in elevated levels of the nonfunctional fragments.

FGF23 does not cross the placenta in rodents.[13] Animal models have similarly shown that fetal FGF23 concentrations range from low to equal to maternal values.[13,19]

33.2.2.5 Calcitonin

C-cells of the thyroid differentiate in the human embryo around the 12th week, and calcitonin becomes detectable within those cells by the 15th week.[1] Placental trophoblasts also express calcitonin, but how much is contributed to the circulation is unknown. Cord blood calcitonin is as high as twice the maternal level, and it does not cross the placenta.[1]

33.2.2.6 Sex Steroids

The sex steroids, largely estradiol and testosterone, are considered here because they are calciotropic hormones postnatally. Embryonic and fetal production of the gonadotropins and sex steroids are discussed in greater detail in other chapters. In brief, luteinizing hormone and follicle stimulating hormone are produced by the embryonic pituitary as early as 5 weeks.[1] These gonadotropins and chorionic gonadotropin (originating in the placenta) drive the Leydig cells of testes to produce testosterone, whereas the ovaries and the adrenals of both sexes produce only negligible amounts. Very little estradiol is produced by the ovaries, testes, and adrenals until late gestation.

Male fetuses show a surge in testosterone between 11 and 17 weeks before the level declines and remains there.[1] In cord blood, there may be no difference in testosterone or estradiol levels between male and female fetuses. In most studies, estradiol and testosterone are present at low levels in cord blood. However, in a few studies, fetal values were not low, which may be dependent on whether the umbilical vein, artery, or mixed cord blood were sampled. By the third trimester, the placenta produces nearly all of the estrogens (estradiol, estrone, and estriol) in the maternal circulation, synthesizing them by aromatizing androgens from fetal and maternal adrenals. Consequently, sampling the umbilical vein or mixed cord blood will result in high concentrations of sex steroids due to placental production, whereas the lower values in the umbilical artery are likely a better reflection of fetal systemic concentrations.[1]

33.2.3 Fetal Parathyroids

One pair of parathyroids and the thymus develop together within the third pharyngeal pouch, whereas the second pair of parathyroids derives from the fourth pouch. The parathyroids migrate during embryonic development to their final positions adjacent to the thyroid, but their friable nature can result in parathyroid tissue ending up in thymic or other ectopic sites.

PTH has been detected in fetal parathyroids by as early as 10 weeks of gestation.[20] Although PTHrP has been found in adult parathyroids,[1] no studies have assessed its expression in human fetal parathyroids. There are contradictory reports from animal models as to whether the fetal parathyroids express PTHrP,[1] while two different models of aparathyroid fetal mice showed no alteration in plasma PTHrP.[21,22]

Although PTH is present at low levels in the fetal circulation, studies in fetal animal models have consistently shown that the fetal parathyroids and PTH are required to maintain the high concentration of calcium in blood. Loss of parathyroids from surgical removal in lambs or rats, and genetic ablation in mice, results in hypocalcemia and hyperphosphatemia. Whether this results from the combined actions of PTH and PTHrP originating from the parathyroids, or PTH alone, remains to be clarified. However, it is clear that PTH and PTHrP both regulate fetal serum calcium and phosphorus. Loss of either hormone leads to hypocalcemia and hyperphosphatemia, while loss of both results in more marked hypocalcemia.[21–24]

The fetal parathyroids are capable of secreting more PTH, such as in response to maternal hypocalcemia. This may lead to hyperplasia of the fetal parathyroids with cord blood findings of increased PTH and normal calcium, skeletal resorption and demineralization, and fractures.[1] Conversely, maternal hypercalcemia causes increased flow of calcium across the placenta, which leads to suppression of the fetal parathyroids. After birth, this suppression can result in hypocalcemia due to neonatal hypoparathyroidism that may be prolonged or permanent.[1]

33.2.4 Renal Mineral Reabsorption and Excretion, and the Amniotic Fluid

There are no measurements of serum mineral or calciotropic hormones from anephric babies to confirm what role the fetal kidneys might play in regulating fetal mineral and bone metabolism. Anephric human fetuses have exhibited skeletal anomalies (scoliosis, rib anomalies, and absent toes, radii, or thumbs), but whether these result from the underlying genetic disturbances or absent kidney function is unknown. Bilateral renal agenesis causes oligohydramnios or anhydramnios, due to the lack of fetal urine.

Studies in animal models suggest that the fetal kidneys are of far lesser importance for mineral homeostasis than they are postnatally. The placenta fulfills the functions that the postnatal kidneys have, including import and export of fluid and minerals, and synthesis of calcitriol. Mineral that is excreted into the urine becomes part of the amniotic fluid that is swallowed (autourophagia), absorbed, and thereby recycled (Fig. 33.1). Renal blood flow and glomerular filtration rate are low until after birth.

There is contradictory evidence from animal models as to whether loss of kidney function disturbs fetal mineral metabolism. Bilateral nephrectomy in fetal lambs caused hypocalcemia and hyperphosphatemia in some studies but not others, while in fetal rats the procedure did not alter serum calcium or phosphorus.[1]

Fetal kidneys respond to the parathyroids, since thyroparathyroidectomy in fetal lambs caused increased renal fractional excretion of calcium, and reduced phosphorus excretion.[1] In turn, pharmacological treatment with N-terminal PTH or PTHrP reduced renal calcium excretion, but had no effect on urine phosphorus excretion.[1] In contrast, loss of parathyroids, PTH, or the PTH receptor caused reduced renal calcium excretion in fetal mice.[1] It appears that hypocalcemia in murine fetuses leads to a reduced renal filtered load of calcium and hypocalciuria, in contrast to the postnatal finding of hypercalciuria. Conversely, high blood calcium in murine fetuses leads to increased urine calcium excretion, likely from an increased filtered load.[2] The CaSR is minimally expressed within fetal kidneys, which contributes to why filtered renal calcium is handled differently in utero.[1]

The fetal kidneys likely produce much of the calcitriol in the fetal circulation.[25] However, calcitriol may have little importance for fetal mineral and bone homeostasis. As discussed in Chapter 44, severe vitamin D deficiency, or genetic loss of calcitriol or the vitamin D receptor, do not alter fetal serum calcium, phosphorus, PTH, urine or amniotic fluid concentrations of calcium and phosphorus, and skeletal morphology or mineralization.[1,4]

Fetal kidneys show abundant expression of FGF23's co-receptor Klotho and receptor Fgfr1c, and its downstream targets, the sodium-phosphate co-transporters NaPi2a and NaPi2c. However, in murine fetuses, loss of FGF23 or Klotho and high circulating levels of FGF23 each failed to alter serum phosphorus, amniotic fluid phosphorus excretion, or renal expression of NaPi2a and NaPi2c.[13,26] These results suggest that the fetal kidneys are not important for renal phosphorus handling, and that FGF23 plays no role in phosphorus handling in utero.

33.2.5 Intestinal Mineral Absorption

The placenta is the organ of mineral delivery during fetal development, and so the fetal intestines are relatively unimportant for fetal mineral homeostasis. However, fetal urine (which is the main content of the amniotic fluid) can be swallowed and reabsorbed, thereby enabling recycling of minerals. Gastrointestinal atresias cause increased amniotic fluid (polyhydramnios), but whether this disturbs fetal mineral homeostasis is unknown.

Although intestinal mineral absorption cannot be studied in human fetuses, intestinal function in preterm babies is likely indicative of what should be present in utero at that gestational age. In preterm babies, calcium absorption is proportional to intake and nonsaturable, consistent with passive absorption.[27–29] It is also unresponsive to vitamin D or calcitriol at this stage of development.[30] The fetal skeleton is normally accreting about 300 mg of calcium per day at this gestational age,[31] which exceeds what the preterm intestines are capable of absorbing. Consequently, parenteral administration of calcium is needed to avoid rickets of prematurity.[32]

33.2.6 Placental Mineral Transport

As noted earlier, the human skeleton accretes at least 80% of its mineral during the third trimester, with a high rate of flow that requires active transport across the placenta. Human placentas have been perfused in vitro, from which it has been estimated that active transport explains at least one-third of the forward flow of calcium from mother to fetus.[1] Trophoblasts express many of the genes and proteins that are involved in intestinal calcium absorption (transient receptor potential cation channel, subfamily V, member 6 [TRPV6], calbindin-D_{9k}, and Ca^{2+}-ATPase [isoforms 1 through 4]) and phosphorus absorption (NaPi2b), and so placental absorption is thought to occur through similar mechanisms. Trophoblasts also express PTHrP, the PTH receptor, VDR, 1α-hydroxylase, calcitonin, and the calcitonin receptor.

It is not possible to study placental mineral transport in human fetuses. However, it may be inferred that substantial maternal hypocalcemia (such as from hypoparathyroidism) reduces placental calcium transport because it can cause intrauterine fetal hyperparathyroidism, skeletal demineralization, intrauterine fractures, and bowing of the long bones.[1] Conversely, maternal hypercalcemia likely increases placental calcium transport because it causes suppression of the fetal parathyroid glands.[1] These conditions are discussed in more detail in Chapter 44.

The bulk of the mechanistic studies come from animal models, which have confirmed that diffusional or passive flow is insufficient to account for the rapidity of mineral exchanges, the transport of calcium and phosphorus occurs against substantial electrochemical and concentration gradients, and that placental transport is dependent on Mg^{2+} and ATP.[1] Active transport has been estimated to explain about two-thirds of the forward flow from mother to fetus.

Calcium transport begins with opening of gated calcium channels (TRPV6) on maternal-facing basement membranes that brings calcium into trophoblasts. Calcium is carried by proteins (such as calbindin-D_{9k}) intracellularly to the fetal-facing basement membrane, from where the Ca^{2+}-ATPase actively pumps calcium into the fetal circulation.[1] Within rodents, trophoblasts and cells of the intraplacental yolk sac (IPYS) transport minerals, with the IPYS cells showing the most intense expression of calcium-transporting genes and proteins.[1] Human placentas lack the IPYS, and so calcium transport likely occurs solely across trophoblasts.

Calbindin-D_{9k}, Ca^{2+}-ATPase, and TRPV6 all show marked upregulation of expression during the last 5 days of gestation in rodents, corresponding with the interval of active transport of calcium.[1] There is evidence to support that each is required for placental calcium transport.[1]

Midmolecular regions of PTHrP, which may act on a unique receptor, have been shown to stimulate placental calcium transport in fetal lambs, rats, and sheep.[1] Loss of PTHrP leads to a reduced rate of placental calcium transport, which can be increased by treating with midmolecular PTHrP. This midmolecular region has no similarity to PTH and cannot activate the PTH receptor. There is inconsistent evidence that PTH may have a lesser role in regulating placental calcium transport.

Calcitriol and VDR do not appear to be required, since placental expression of calciotropic factors, and the rate of placental calcium transport, are not reduced by absence of vitamin D, calcitriol, or VDR. These issues are discussed in more detail in Chapter 44.

Placental phosphorus transport increases in rodents during late gestation, accompanied by increased expression of NaPi2b, Klotho, and Fgfr1c.[1] There is also a very low level of expression of FGF23 within murine placentas.[13] The factors that regulate placental phosphorus transport are unknown, with PTH, PTHrP, calcitriol, VDR, and FGF23 failing to show effects in animals.

Active placental transport of magnesium transport has been demonstrated in fetal lambs, and to be dependent upon PTHrP,[1] but the mechanisms by which it is transported are unknown.

33.2.7 Endochondral Bone Formation, Mineralization, and Remodeling

In developing humans, a cartilaginous scaffold for the endochondral skeleton forms by the 8th gestational week.[1] Primary ossification centers then begin to form in vertebrae and long bones between the 8th and 12th weeks, but substantial mineralization of these structures doesn't occur until the third trimester. Secondary ossification centers form in the femurs by the 34th week. Although the flow of mineral is into the skeleton, skeletal turnover likely contributes to maintaining normal mineral concentrations within the fetal circulation. This becomes more exaggerated with marked skeletal resorption and demineralization resulting when substantial maternal hypocalcemia is present.

Early embryonic development of the skeleton is beyond the scope of this chapter, but will be summarized briefly here. Detailed studies in mouse models have revealed that Hox genes, Wnts, Hedgehogs, bone morphogenetic proteins, fibroblast growth factors, and Notch/Delta are among the important genes and signaling pathways.[33] Mesenchymal cells are first laid down to pattern the skeleton. Where the flat bones of the skull and a few other bones are destined to form, these mesenchymal cells differentiate directly into osteoblasts (intramembranous bone formation). But in the bulk of the skeleton, these mesenchymal progenitors differentiate into chondroblasts and chondrocytes, which form a cartilaginous scaffold for the vertebrae and most of the appendicular skeleton. Proliferating and early differentiating cells respond to growth factors and hormonal signals such as PTHrP, which prevents chondrocytes from terminally differentiating. Older chondrocytes are further away from the source of PTHrP, and the loss of its suppressive signal causes them to undergo terminal differentiation into hypertrophic chondrocytes, after which they undergo apoptosis. Chondroclasts remove these cells and the surrounding matrix, new blood vessels invade, and osteoblasts differentiate to lay down the primary spongiosa of bone where the cartilaginous scaffold has been torn down. Primary ossification centers form in the mouse before term, while most secondary ossification centers develop after birth. Concurrent with formation of primary ossification centers, the placenta ramps up its expression of calciotropic genes and its rate of mineral delivery, and the skeleton in turn accretes much of its mineral content. In contrast to humans, the fetal rat skeleton accretes 95% of its mineral content during the last 5 days of gestation.[34]

Murine models have confirmed that some degree of bone turnover likely contributes to maintenance of normal serum mineral concentrations. Osteoclasts are active within fetal bones, releasing products of bone resorption into fetal serum and amniotic fluid.[2] Loss of the PTH receptor within bone reduces blood calcium, while a constitutively active PTH receptor causes increased serum calcium.[1] Furthermore, fetal skeletal resorption can be exaggerated by significant maternal hypocalcemia[1] or by inactivating mutations of CaSR.[2]

PTHrP's role to regulate the terminal fate of chondrocytes is exemplified by the *Pthrp* null mouse, which displays a short-limb chondrodysplasia, in addition to some normally cartilaginous structures (such as the medial ribs) being transformed into rigid bone.[35] PTHrP also supports skeletal development by stimulating calcium delivery across the placenta and maintaining the serum at a high level. Conversely, PTH's main role is to support mineralization of the skeleton, since absence of PTH results in reduced mineral content in an otherwise morphologically normal structure.[1] Calcitriol and calcitonin do not appear to be required at all, since endochondral bone development and skeletal mineralization are normal despite absence of these hormones. The data pertaining to these models are discussed in greater detail in Chapter 44.

The relative contributions of PTH and PTHrP to endochondral bone formation and mineralization are summarized in Fig. 33.4.

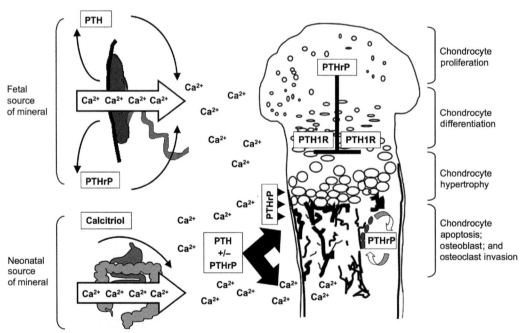

FIG. 33.4 Relative roles of PTH, PTHrP, calcitriol, and FGF23 during fetal and neonatal life. The placenta is the main source of mineral during fetal life. PTH and PTHrP are expressed within the placenta but may also act on it from systemic sources to stimulate calcium transfer. The intestines are a trivial source of mineral in the fetus but are the main source for the neonate. Intestinal calcium absorption is initially passive but later becomes active, saturable, and calcitriol-dependent in the infant. Within the endochondral skeleton, PTHrP is produced by proliferating chondrocytes and perichondral cells *(arrowheads)* and delays terminal differentiation of prehypertrophic chondrocytes. PTHrP is also produced within preosteoblasts and osteoblasts and stimulates bone formation *(semicircular arrows)*. During fetal life PTHrP and PTH act together to maintain high blood calcium and phosphorus levels in order to facilitate mineralization; loss of either PTHrP or PTH causes hypocalcemia and hyperphosphatemia. Calcitriol and FGF23 are not required to regulate serum minerals, endochondral bone formation, or skeletal mineralization in the fetus. *(Reproduced with permission from Kovacs CS. Fetal control of calcium and phosphate homeostasis. In: Thakker RV, Whyte MP, Eisman JA, Igarashi T, editors.* Genetics of bone biology and skeletal disease, *2nd ed. San Diego: Academic Press/Elsevier; 2017. p. 329–47 ©2017 Elsevier.)*

33.3 OVERVIEW OF NEONATAL MINERAL HOMEOSTASIS

The normal changes in circulating minerals and hormones that occur during neonatal development are also depicted in Fig. 33.2.

33.3.1 Serum Mineral Concentrations

With loss of the placenta and the first breaths, serum calcium falls and initiates substantial changes in the regulation of mineral homeostasis.

Serum and ionized calcium typically decline 20%–30% over the first 12–24 h,[1] with the ionized calcium dropping from 1.45 mmol/L in cord blood to a mean of 1.20 mmol/L by 24 h.[36] The initial high level in fetal blood may reduce the likelihood that this obligatory fall in calcium causes symptomatic hypocalcemia. After the trough level is reached, serum and ionized calcium progressively increase over several days to reach adult normal values. Newborns fed formula will experience a greater drop in serum calcium compared to breastfed babies, because the high phosphorus content of formula causes hyperphosphatemia and complexes calcium.[1]

Phosphorus is high at birth and continues to increase over the 24–48 h.[1] The value subsequently declines toward expected pediatric levels.

The evolution of serum calcium and phosphorus are consistent with transient hypoparathyroidism in the newborn, and a triggered awakening of the parathyroids from their suppressed state in utero.

33.3.2 Calciotropic and Phosphotropic Hormone Concentrations

The fall in calcium after birth sparks the neonatal parathyroids to upregulate PTH. This was first delineated using older C-terminal PTH assays, which found that PTH remained low over the first 12–24 h, and reached its highest levels after 48 h.[1] Modern intact PTH assays have shown simply that PTH increases between measurements at birth and 24 h, without delineating the time course.[37–43] In newborn rats, PTH surges to high levels by 6–12 h after birth, with the highest level corresponding to the low point in the time course of serum calcium.[1] After that, PTH slowly falls to adult values over 2 weeks.

The rise in PTH upregulates renal 1α-hydroxylase, which causes an increase in serum calcitriol over the succeeding 2 days.[44,45] In neonatal rodents and lambs, the rise in calcitriol is more delayed until 2–3 weeks after birth (the time of weaning in rodents); before that time, a high level of 24-hydroxylase continues to metabolize 25OHD and contribute to low levels of calcitriol, even despite pharmacological treatment with PTH.[46–48] These studies suggest a developmental preference to suppress calcitriol formation and maintain increased catabolism until the intestines are developmentally ready to respond to calcitriol.

PTHrP eventually becomes undetectable in normal adults, but whether the neonatal parathyroids synthesize it, or how soon it disappears from the circulation of neonates, are unknown. A single study found that the plasma PTHrP declined 50% over the first 24 h, but returned to the cord blood value a day later.[49] Human milk contains very high concentrations of PTHrP that conceivably may be absorbed into the circulation; conversely, infant formulas have low PTHrP content. Clinical studies have not examined neonatal PTHrP blood levels timed with breastfeeding to determine if PTHrP is absorbed into the circulation.

Limited data have shown a marked increase in intact FGF23 over the first few days in humans,[14,15] while C-terminal FGF23 remained unchanged.[14]

Calcitonin increases as much as 10-fold during the first 48 h after birth, after which it declines slowly to expected pediatric and adult values.[1]

Estradiol persists at very low concentrations in male and female newborns until puberty. Testosterone remains very low in females, but in male newborns, it briefly spikes within the first 24 h.[50] A second spike occurs during the 2nd week, and this is maintained until about 4 months of age, after which testosterone returns to very low levels until puberty.[51,52]

33.3.3 Neonatal Parathyroid Function

The fall in ionized calcium and rise in phosphorus after birth trigger increased PTH synthesis and release. In turn, the rise in PTH precedes a subsequent rise in ionized calcium and calcitriol, and a fall in phosphorus. This is a transient, physiological hypoparathyroidism. The parathyroids are initially sluggish in their response to acute hypocalcemia,[53–56] but as the postnatal days pass, responsiveness becomes normal.[55,56]

Studies in neonatal rodents have shown a similar pattern of increasing parathyroid responsiveness. However, neonatal parathyroidectomy did not alter the length, morphology, trabecular content, and calcium or phosphorus content of the developing skeleton as compared with sham controls.[57] This suggests that PTH is not required for neonatal mineral homeostasis and skeletal development. It may imply a role for PTHrP during the neonatal transition, and that intestinal calcium absorption is still passive and not dependent upon PTH or calcitriol.

33.3.4 Renal Mineral Reabsorption and Excretion

During the neonatal period, the kidneys begin to actively reabsorb and excrete minerals. Although cord blood calcium is high and PTH is low at birth, which would predict increased urine calcium excretion, the neonatal kidneys output a low amount of calcium over the first 5–7 days. After this, urine calcium excretion increases over the subsequent weeks, despite serum calcium being lower and PTH higher than early neonatal values.[40,58] The pattern of changes in renal calcium excretion are likely the result of multiple factors, including a developmental increase in renal blood flow and glomerular filtration rate,[58–60] possible effects of PTHrP to stimulate reabsorption of calcium, a developmental increase in renal expression of the CaSR, and increased renal responsiveness to calcitriol.

Similar to calcium, phosphorus excretion is also low at birth but shows a significant increase as the days pass.[61,62] This likely reflects the increasing concentration of PTH, and increased renal responsiveness to PTH, which have been demonstrated in term and preterm infants.[62,63]

As noted previously, calcitriol increases after birth in response to the rising concentration of PTH, and it largely originates from the neonatal kidneys.

Studies in neonatal rodents have confirmed that there is reduced renal responsiveness to PTH during the first days after birth.[64] There is low expression of VDR and responsiveness to calcitriol until the 3rd week,[65] while TRPV6 and calbindin-D_{9k} show a similar time course of rising from low levels to maximum expression by 3 weeks.[66] CaSR is also expressed at very low levels in newborn kidneys, but begins to increase after the first postnatal day in mice.[67]

33.3.5 Intestinal Mineral Absorption

In the fetal section, it was noted that preterm human infants, which are developmentally equivalent to fetus, display passive, nonvitamin D-dependent absorption of calcium. An interventional study has shown that preterm infants are not responsive to supraphysiological doses of calcitriol (0.1–3.0 μg/kg), which suggests that the preterm intestines are refractory to calcitriol (for comparison, adults with hypoparathyroidism require only 0.25–1.0 μg total).[68] Another interventional study used 4.0 μg/kg for 3 consecutive days and found a significant increase in serum calcium; however, there were indications, from bone markers and renal calcium excretion, that the increased serum calcium may have been due to increased bone resorption rather than intestinal calcium absorption.[69]

Additional studies in preterm neonates support that vitamin D or calcitriol are not effective at stimulating intestinal calcium absorption at this early developmental stage, but calcitriol becomes more effective by 4 weeks of age.[70,71]

The lactose content of milk facilitates calcium absorption,[72,73] which contributes to the lack of dependence on calcitriol-regulated mechanisms during early postnatal life. As postnatal and gestational age increases, intestinal calcium absorption and retention of calcium both increase, consistent with the intestines maturing toward an active, calcitriol-dependent, saturable mechanism of calcium absorption.[27,71,74–77]

As noted earlier, the preterm infant requires a very high rate of daily calcium delivery that is beyond the capability of the preterm intestines to absorb from breast milk or formula; a high intake of phosphate is also required. Consequently, parenteral nutrition must be provided during the first week or more after birth to provide the needed calcium and phosphorus.[32] After this, special oral formulas can be administered that are high in calcium in order to meet the ongoing needs. In very low birth weight preterm neonates, the recommended calcium intake is 120–200 mg/kg daily, with most of that given parenterally.[32] As the postnatal days pass, the skeletal demand for mineral declines, while the efficiency of intestinal calcium and phosphate absorption increases. Consequently, the preterm neonate's demand for calcium and phosphorus can eventually be met with normal volumes of breast milk or formula.

Absorption of calcium is more efficient from breast milk than from infant formula, regardless of vitamin D supplementation.[71,78, 79] More than 90% of phosphate in breast milk and formula is absorbed.[71] The higher phosphate content of formula leads to a doubling of serum phosphorus, a lowering of serum calcium, and an increase in the risk of neonatal hypocalcemia, as compared with breastfed babies.[56,71,79,80]

More extensive studies in neonatal rodents have confirmed that intestinal calcium absorption is mainly passive, nonsaturable, and not dependent on calcitriol,[81–83] facilitated by the effect of lactose to increase paracellular calcium absorption.[84–86] The neonatal intestines show developmental changes from low to high levels of relevant genes and proteins over the first several weeks, including VDR,[87] calbindin-D$_{9k}$,[66,88] and TRPV6.[66] By the time of weaning at 3 weeks of age, the intestines display reduced passive absorption, and increased active, calcitriol-dependent absorption of calcium.[81–83]

33.3.6 Skeletal Metabolism

Whereas skeletal mineral accretion is over 300 mg/day or about 150 mg/kg/day near term, it drops to 30–40 mg/kg/day in normal neonates.[1] The skeleton requires efficient intestinal delivery of mineral in order to undergo an ongoing increase in mineral content. Failing to provide that mineral will result in secondary hyperparathyroidism and a lack of growth plate and skeletal mineralization, as seen in rickets and osteomalacia of prematurity.

A similar effect has been demonstrated in children who lack functional VDRs, in which lack of responsiveness to calcitriol causes impaired intestinal calcium absorption and, in turn, reduced skeletal mineral accrual and rachitic deformities. Special oral calcium formulas or parenteral calcium will correct the skeletal abnormalities and allow normal growth. These findings point to calcitriol's postnatal role as being indirect with respect to the skeleton (Fig. 33.4). It acts mainly to stimulate intestinal calcium delivery rather than directly stimulating osteoblasts, and it can be completely bypassed by use of high calcium diets or parenteral calcium. The same has been demonstrated in animal models. Data relevant to this are discussed in more detail in Chapter 44.

33.4 CONCLUSIONS

Fetuses and neonates must maintain adequate mineral delivery to sustain normal circulating concentrations for diverse physiological functions, and to support ongoing growth and mineralization of the skeleton normally (Fig. 33.4). Active transport of minerals across the placenta requires PTHrP and possibly PTH, but not calcitriol, calcitonin, or FGF23. PTH and PTHrP are both required to maintain serum calcium and phosphorus and optimal endochondral bone development and mineralization, whereas calcitriol, calcitonin, FGF23, and the sex steroids are not required (Fig. 33.4). During the neonatal period, intestinal calcium absorption is initially passive, facilitated by lactose, and not dependent upon calcitriol; it later becomes calcitriol-dependent. This means that skeletal development and mineralization are initially independent of calcitriol but later become dependent on it. However, calcitriol isn't absolutely required because calcitriol's role can be bypassed by increasing the calcium content of the diet or by administering parenteral calcium (Fig. 33.4).

REFERENCES

1. Kovacs CS. Bone development and mineral homeostasis in the fetus and neonate: roles of the calciotropic and phosphotropic hormones. *Physiol Rev* 2014;**94**(4):1143–218.
2. Kovacs CS, Ho-Pao CL, Hunzelman JL, Lanske B, Fox J, Seidman JG, et al. Regulation of murine fetal-placental calcium metabolism by the calcium-sensing receptor. *J Clin Invest* 1998;**101**:2812–20.
3. Wieland P, Fischer JA, Trechsel U, Roth HR, Vetter K, Schneider H, et al. Perinatal parathyroid hormone, vitamin D metabolites, and calcitonin in man. *Am J Phys* 1980;**239**:E385–90.
4. Ryan BA, Alhani K, Sellars KB, Kirby BJ, St-Arnaud R, Kaufmann M, et al. Mineral homeostasis in murine fetuses is sensitive to maternal calcitriol, but not to absence of fetal calcitriol. *J Bone Miner Res* 2019;**34**:669–80.
5. Weisman Y, Harell A, Edelstein S, David M, Spirer Z, Golander A. 1 alpha, 25-Dihydroxyvitamin D3 and 24,25-dihydroxyvitamin D3 in vitro synthesis by human decidua and placenta. *Nature* 1979;**281**(5729):317–9.
6. Danan JL, Delorme AC, Mathieu H. Presence of 25-hydroxyvitamin D3 and 1,25-dihydroxyvitamin D3 24-hydroxylase in vitamin D target cells of rat yolk sac. *J Biol Chem* 1982;**257**(18):10715–21.
7. Avila E, Diaz L, Halhali A, Larrea F. Regulation of 25-hydroxyvitamin D3 1alpha-hydroxylase, 1,25-dihydroxyvitamin D3 24-hydroxylase and vitamin D receptor gene expression by 8-bromo cyclic AMP in cultured human syncytiotrophoblast cells. *J Steroid Biochem Mol Biol* 2004;**89–90**(1–5):115–9.
8. Turner M, Barre PE, Benjamin A, Goltzman D, Gascon-Barre M. Does the maternal kidney contribute to the increased circulating 1,25-dihydroxyvitamin D concentrations during pregnancy? *Miner Electrolyte Metab* 1988;**14**:246–52.
9. Delvin EE, Glorieux FH, Salle BL, David L, Varenne JP. Control of vitamin D metabolism in preterm infants: feto-maternal relationships. *Arch Dis Child* 1982;**57**:754–7.
10. Higashi T, Mitamura K, Ohmi H, Yamada N, Shimada K, Tanaka K, et al. Levels of 24,25-dihydroxyvitamin D3, 25-hydroxyvitamin D3 and 25-hydroxyvitamin D3 3-sulphate in human plasma. *Ann Clin Biochem* 1999;**36**(Pt 1):43–7.
11. Fudge NJ, Kovacs CS. Pregnancy up-regulates intestinal calcium absorption and skeletal mineralization independently of the vitamin D receptor. *Endocrinology* 2010;**151**(3):886–95.

12. Kovacs CS, Woodland ML, Fudge NJ, Friel JK. The vitamin D receptor is not required for fetal mineral homeostasis or for the regulation of placental calcium transfer. *Am J Physiol Endocrinol Metab* 2005;**289**(1):E133–44.

13. Ma Y, Samaraweera M, Cooke-Hubley S, Kirby BJ, Karaplis AC, Lanske B, et al. Neither absence nor excess of FGF23 disturbs murine fetal-placental phosphorus homeostasis or prenatal skeletal development and mineralization. *Endocrinology* 2014;**155**(5):1596–605.

14. Takaiwa M, Aya K, Miyai T, Hasegawa K, Yokoyama M, Kondo Y, et al. Fibroblast growth factor 23 concentrations in healthy term infants during the early postpartum period. *Bone* 2010;**47**(2):256–62.

15. Ohata Y, Arahori H, Namba N, Kitaoka T, Hirai H, Wada K, et al. Circulating levels of soluble alpha-Klotho are markedly elevated in human umbilical cord blood. *J Clin Endocrinol Metab* 2011;**96**(6):E943–7.

16. Holmlund-Suila E, Viljakainen H, Ljunggren O, Hytinantti T, Andersson S, Makitie O. Fibroblast growth factor 23 concentrations reflect sex differences in mineral metabolism and growth in early infancy. *Horm Res Paediatr* 2016;**85**(4):232–41.

17. Ali FN, Josefson J, Mendez AJ, Mestan K, Wolf M. Cord blood ferritin and fibroblast growth factor-23 levels in neonates. *J Clin Endocrinol Metab* 2016;**101**(4):1673–9.

18. Godang K, Froslie KF, Henriksen T, Isaksen GA, Voldner N, Lekva T, et al. Umbilical cord levels of sclerostin, placental weight, and birth weight are predictors of total bone mineral content in neonates. *Eur J Endocrinol* 2013;**168**(3):371–8.

19. Fukumoto S. Phosphate metabolism and vitamin D. *Bonekey Rep* 2014;**3**:497.

20. Leroyer-Alizon E, David L, Anast CS, Dubois PM. Immunocytological evidence for parathyroid hormone in human fetal parathyroid glands. *J Clin Endocrinol Metab* 1981;**52**:513–6.

21. Kovacs CS, Manley NR, Moseley JM, Martin TJ, Kronenberg HM. Fetal parathyroids are not required to maintain placental calcium transport. *J Clin Invest* 2001;**107**(8):1007–15.

22. Simmonds CS, Karsenty G, Karaplis AC, Kovacs CS. Parathyroid hormone regulates fetal-placental mineral homeostasis. *J Bone Miner Res* 2010;**25**(3):594–605.

23. Kovacs CS, Lanske B, Hunzelman JL, Guo J, Karaplis AC, Kronenberg HM. Parathyroid hormone-related peptide (PTHrP) regulates fetal-placental calcium transport through a receptor distinct from the PTH/PTHrP receptor. *Proc Natl Acad Sci U S A* 1996;**93**:15233–8.

24. Kovacs CS, Chafe LL, Fudge NJ, Friel JK, Manley NR. PTH regulates fetal blood calcium and skeletal mineralization independently of PTHrP. *Endocrinology* 2001;**142**(11):4983–93.

25. Moore ES, Langman CB, Favus MJ, Coe FL. Role of fetal 1,25-dihydroxyvitamin D production in intrauterine phosphorus and calcium homeostasis. *Pediatr Res* 1985;**19**:566–9.

26. Ma Y, Kirby BJ, Fairbridge NA, Karaplis AC, Lanske B, Kovacs CS. FGF23 is not required to regulate fetal phosphorus metabolism but exerts effects within 12 hours after birth. *Endocrinology* 2017;**158**(2):252–63.

27. Giles MM, Fenton MH, Shaw B, Elton RA, Clarke M, Lang M, et al. Sequential calcium and phosphorus balance studies in preterm infants. *J Pediatr* 1987;**110**:591–8.

28. Barltrop D, Mole RH, Sutton A. Absorption and endogenous faecal excretion of calcium by low birthweight infants on feeds with varying contents of calcium and phosphate. *Arch Dis Child* 1977;**52**:41–9.

29. Salle B, Senterre J, Putet G, Rigo J. Effects of calcium and phosphorus supplementation on calcium retention and fat absorption in preterm infants fed pooled human milk. *J Pediatr Gastroenterol Nutr* 1986;**5**(4):638–42.

30. Bronner F, Salle BL, Putet G, Rigo J, Senterre J. Net calcium absorption in premature infants: results of 103 metabolic balance studies. *Am J Clin Nutr* 1992;**56**(6):1037–44.

31. Ziegler EE, O'Donnell AM, Nelson SE, Fomon SJ. Body composition of the reference fetus. *Growth* 1976;**40**:329–41.

32. Mimouni FB, Mandel D, Lubetzky R, Senterre T. Calcium, phosphorus, magnesium and vitamin D requirements of the preterm infant. *World Rev Nutr Diet* 2014;**110**:140–51.

33. Yang Y. Skeletal morphogenesis during embryonic development. *Crit Rev Eukaryot Gene Expr* 2009;**19**(3):197–218.

34. Comar CL. Radiocalcium studies in pregnancy. *Ann N Y Acad Sci* 1956;**64**:281–98.

35. Karaplis AC, Luz A, Glowacki J, Bronson RT, Tybulewicz VL, Kronenberg HM, et al. Lethal skeletal dysplasia from targeted disruption of the parathyroid hormone-related peptide gene. *Genes Dev* 1994;**8**:277–89.

36. Loughead JL, Mimouni F, Tsang RC. Serum ionized calcium concentrations in normal neonates. *Am J Dis Child* 1988;**142**:516–8.

37. Saggese G, Baroncelli GI, Bertelloni S, Cipolloni C. Intact parathyroid hormone levels during pregnancy, in healthy term neonates and in hypocalcemic preterm infants. *Acta Paediatr Scand* 1991;**80**:36–41.

38. Bagnoli F, Bruchi S, Garosi G, Pecciarini L, Bracci R. Relationship between mode of delivery and neonatal calcium homeostasis. *Eur J Pediatr* 1990;**149**:800–3.

39. Martinez ME, Catalan P, Lisbona A, Sanchez-Cabezudo MJ, Pallardo F, Jans I, et al. Serum osteocalcin concentrations in diabetic pregnant women and their newborns. *Horm Metab Res* 1994;**26**:338–42.

40. Nishioka T, Yasuda T, Niimi H. A discordant movement in urine calcium excretion in relation to serum calcium and parathyroid function occurring immediately after birth. *Acta Paediatr Scand* 1991;**80**:590–5.

41. Loughead JL, Mimouni F, Tsang RC, Khoury JC. A role for magnesium in neonatal parathyroid gland function? *J Am Coll Nutr* 1991;**10**:123–6.

42. Mimouni F, Loughead JL, Tsang RC, Khoury J. Postnatal surge in serum calcitonin concentrations: no contribution to neonatal hypocalcemia in infants of diabetic mothers. *Pediatr Res* 1990;**28**:493–5.

43. Loughead JL, Mimouni F, Ross R, Tsang RC. Postnatal changes in serum osteocalcin and parathyroid hormone concentrations. *J Am Coll Nutr* 1990;**9**:358–62.

44. Davis OK, Hawkins DS, Rubin LP, Posillico JT, Brown EM, Schiff I. Serum parathyroid hormone (PTH) in pregnant women determined by an immunoradiometric assay for intact PTH. *J Clin Endocrinol Metab* 1988;**67**:850–2.

45. Steichen JJ, Tsang RC, Gratton TL, Hamstra A, DeLuca HF. Vitamin D homeostasis in the perinatal period: 1,25-dihydroxyvitamin D in maternal, cord, and neonatal blood. *N Engl J Med* 1980;**302**:315–9.

46. Garel JM, Barlet JP. Calcium metabolism in newborn animals: the interrelationship of calcium, magnesium, and inorganic phosphorus in newborn rats, foals, lambs, and calves. *Pediatr Res* 1976;**10**:749–54.

47. Weisman Y, Sapir R, Harell A, Edelstein S. Maternal-perinatal interrelationships of vitamin D metabolism in rats. *Biochim Biophys Acta* 1976;**428**:388–95.

48. Kooh SW, Vieth R. 25-hydroxyvitamin D metabolism in the sheep fetus and lamb. *Pediatr Res* 1980;**14**(4 Pt 1):360–3.

49. Briana DD, Boutsikou M, Baka S, Hassiakos D, Gourgiotis D, Marmarinos A, et al. N-terminal parathyroid hormone-related protein levels in human intrauterine growth restricted pregnancies. *Acta Obstet Gynecol Scand* 2007;**86**(8):945–9.

50. Corbier P, Edwards DA, Roffi J. The neonatal testosterone surge: a comparative study. *Arch Int Physiol Biochim Biophys* 1992;**100**(2):127–31.

51. Winter JS, Hughes IA, Reyes FI, Faiman C. Pituitary-gonadal relations in infancy: 2. Patterns of serum gonadal steroid concentrations in man from birth to two years of age. *J Clin Endocrinol Metab* 1976;**42**(4):679–86.

52. Cuttler L, Palmert MR. Luteinizing hormone and follicle-stimulating hormone secretion in the fetus and newborn infant. In: Polin RA, Fox WW, Abman SH, editors. *Fetal and neonatal physiology.* 3rd ed. Philadelphia, PA: Saunders; 2004. p. 1896–906.

53. David L, Anast CS. Calcium metabolism in newborn infants. The interrelationship of parathyroid function and calcium, magnesium, and phosphorus metabolism in normal, sick, and hypocalcemic newborns. *J Clin Invest* 1974;**54**:287–96.

54. Schedewie HK, Odell WD, Fisher DA, Krutzik SR, Dodge M, Cousins L, et al. Parathormone and perinatal calcium homeostasis. *Pediatr Res* 1979;**13**:1–6.

55. Tsang RC, Chen IW, Friedman MA, Chen I. Neonatal parathyroid function: role of gestational age and postnatal age. *J Pediatr* 1973;**83**:728–38.

56. Tsang RC, Light IJ, Sutherland JM, Kleinman LI. Possible pathogenetic factors in neonatal hypocalcemia of prematurity. The role of gestation, hyperphosphatemia, hypomagnesemia, urinary calcium loss, and parathormone responsiveness. *J Pediatr* 1973;**82**:423–9.

57. Krukowski M, Kahn AJ. The role of parathyroid hormone in mineral homeostasis and bone modeling in suckling rat pups. *Metab Bone Dis Relat Res* 1980;**2**:257–60.

58. Karlén J, Aperia A, Zetterström R. Renal excretion of calcium and phosphate in preterm and term infants. *J Pediatr* 1985;**106**:814–9.

59. Edelmann Jr CM, Spitzer A. The maturing kidney. A modern view of well-balanced infants with imbalanced nephrons. *J Pediatr* 1969;**75**(3):509–19.

60. Guignard JP, Torrado A, Da Cunha O, Gautier E. Glomerular filtration rate in the first three weeks of life. *J Pediatr* 1975;**87**:268–72.

61. Senterre J, Salle B. Renal aspects of calcium and phosphorus metabolism in preterm infants. *Biol Neonate* 1988;**53**:220–9.

62. Linarelli LG. Newborn urinary cyclic AMP and developmental renal responsiveness to parathyroid hormone. *Pediatrics* 1972;**50**:14–23.

63. Mallet E, Basuyau JP, Brunelle P, Devaux AM, Fessard C. Neonatal parathyroid secretion and renal receptor maturation in premature infants. *Biol Neonate* 1978;**33**:304–8.

64. Thomas ML, Anast CS, Forte LR. Regulation of calcium homeostasis in the fetal and neonatal rat. *Am J Phys* 1981;**240**:E367–72.

65. Somjen D, Weisman Y, Berger E, Earon Y, Kaye AM, Binderman I. Developmental changes in the responsiveness of rat kidney to vitamin D metabolites. *Endocrinology* 1986;**118**(1):354–9.

66. Song Y, Peng X, Porta A, Takanaga H, Peng JB, Hediger MA, et al. Calcium transporter 1 and epithelial calcium channel messenger ribonucleic acid are differentially regulated by 1,25 dihydroxyvitamin D3 in the intestine and kidney of mice. *Endocrinology* 2003;**144**(9):3885–94.

67. Chattopadhyay N, Baum N, Bai M, Riccardi D, Hebert SC, Harris EW, et al. Ontogeny of the extracellular calcium-sensing receptor in rat kidney. *Am J Phys* 1996;**271**:F736–43.

68. Venkataraman PS, Tsang RC, Steichen JJ, Grey I, Neylan M, Fleischman AR. Early neonatal hypocalcemia in extremely preterm infants. High incidence, early onset, and refractoriness to supraphysiologic doses of calcitriol. *Am J Dis Child* 1986;**140**(10):1004–8.

69. Koo WW, Tsang RC, Poser JW, Laskarzewski P, Buckley D, Johnson R, et al. Elevated serum calcium and osteocalcin levels from calcitriol in preterm infants. A prospective randomized study. *Am J Dis Child* 1986;**140**(11):1152–8.

70. Senterre J, Putet G, Salle B, Rigo J. Effects of vitamin D and phosphorus supplementation on calcium retention in preterm infants fed banked human milk. *J Pediatr* 1983;**103**(2):305–7.

71. Senterre J, Salle B. Calcium and phosphorus economy of the preterm infant and its interaction with vitamin D and its metabolites. *Acta Paediatr Scand Suppl* 1982;**296**:85–92.

72. Kobayashi A, Kawai S, Obe Y, Nagashima Y. Effects of dietary lactose and lactase preparation on the intestinal absorption of calcium and magnesium in normal infants. *Am J Clin Nutr* 1975;**28**:681–3.

73. Kocian J, Skala I, Bakos K. Calcium absorption from milk and lactose-free milk in healthy subjects and patients with lactose intolerance. *Digestion* 1973;**9**:317–24.

74. Barltrop D, Oppe TE. Absorption of fat and calcium by low birthweight infants from milks containing butterfat and olive oil. *Arch Dis Child* 1973;**48**(7):496–501.

75. Shaw JC. Evidence for defective skeletal mineralization in low-birthweight infants: the absorption of calcium and fat. *Pediatrics* 1976;**57**:16–25.

76. Okamoto E, Muttart CR, Zucker CL, Heird WC. Use of medium-chain triglycerides in feeding the low-birth-weight infant. *Am J Dis Child* 1982;**136**(5):428–31.

77. Hillman LS, Tack E, Covell DG, Vieira NE, Yergey AL. Measurement of true calcium absorption in premature infants using intravenous 46Ca and oral 44Ca. *Pediatr Res* 1988;**23**(6):589–94.

78. Widdowson EM. Absorption and excretion of fat, nitrogen, and minerals from "filled" milks by babies one week old. *Lancet* 1965;**2**(7422):1099–105.

79. Gittleman IF, Pincus JB. Influence of diet on the occurrence of hyperphosphatemia and hypocalcemia in the newborn infant. *Pediatrics* 1951;**8**(6):778–87.

80. Bagnoli F, Bruchi S, Sardelli S, Buonocore G, Vispi L, Franchi F, et al. Calcium homeostasis in the first days of life in relation to feeding. *Eur J Pediatr* 1985;**144**:41–4.

81. Ghishan FK, Jenkins JT, Younoszai MK. Maturation of calcium transport in the rat small and large intestine. *J Nutr* 1980;**110**:1622–8.

82. Ghishan FK, Parker P, Nichols S, Hoyumpa A. Kinetics of intestinal calcium transport during maturation in rats. *Pediatr Res* 1984;**18**:235–9.

83. Halloran BP, DeLuca HF. Calcium transport in small intestine during early development: role of vitamin D. *Am J Phys* 1980;**239**:G473–9.

84. Buchowski MS, Miller DD. Lactose, calcium source and age affect calcium bioavailability in rats. *J Nutr* 1991;**121**:1746–54.

85. Pansu D, Chapuy MC, Milani M, Bellaton C. Transepithelial calcium transport enhanced by xylose and glucose in the rat jejunal ligated loop. *Calcif Tissue Res* 1976;**21**(Suppl):45–52.

86. Leichter J, Tolensky AF. Effect of dietary lactose on the absorption of protein, fat and calcium in the postweaning rat. *Am J Clin Nutr* 1975;**28**:238–41.

87. Halloran BP, DeLuca HF. Appearance of the intestinal cytosolic receptor for 1,25-dihydroxyvitamin D_3 during neonatal development in the rat. *J Biol Chem* 1981;**256**:7338–42.

88. Bruns ME, Bruns DE, Avioli L. Vitamin D-dependent calcium-binding protein of rat intestine: changes during postnatal development and sensitivity to 1,25-dihydroxycholecalciferol. *Endocrinology* 1979;**105**:934–8.

89. Kovacs CS. Fetal control of calcium and phosphate homeostasis. In: Thakker RV, Whyte MP, Eisman JA, Igarashi T, editors. *Genetics of bone biology and skeletal disease*. 2nd ed. San Diego: Academic Press/Elsevier; 2017. p. 329–47.

90. Kovacs CS, Kronenberg HM. Maternal-fetal calcium and bone metabolism during pregnancy, puerperium, and lactation. *Endocr Rev* 1997;**18**(6):832–72.

Chapter 34

Developmental Physiology of Carbohydrate Metabolism and the Pancreas

Kathryn Beardsall[*,†] and Amanda L. Ogilvy-Stuart[†]

*Department of Paediatrics, University of Cambridge, Cambridge, United Kingdom, †Neonatal Unit, Rosie Hospital, Cambridge University Hospitals NHS Foundation Trust, Cambridge, United Kingdom

Key Clinical Changes

- 80% of the fetal energy requirement is met by glucose, with most coming from transplacental passage.
- Fetal glucose production is usually negligible, unless placental insufficiency drives the need for gluconeogenesis.
- The placenta helps buffer the fetus against maternal hyperglycemia and hypoglycemia.
- The fetal liver does not normally produce glucose, but is focused on the anabolic processes of glycogen storage.
- Immediately after birth, there is a catabolic phase, and upregulation of gluconeogenic enzymes is required to prevent hypoglycemia.
- With feeding insulin, secretion and incretins are linked to the intermittent delivery of milk.
- At this time of physiological adaptation, infants are at risk of both hyperglycemia and hypoglycemia.

34.1 INTRODUCTION

The growing fetus has a high energy requirement to satisfy the needs of metabolism and growth, 80% of which is met by glucose.[1] In healthy pregnancies, the majority of this glucose requirement is maintained by a continuous and well-regulated placental transfer from mother to fetus.[2] The role of the fetal pancreas and insulin secretion at this time is to promote fetal growth and to ensure there are adequate fat and glycogen stores to maintain glucose homeostasis in the transition to independent life. After delivery and clamping of the umbilical cord, there is a transitional period of catabolism before the primary energy source becomes milk, which is high in fat but low in carbohydrate. During this transition period, it is vital that there is upregulation of the enzymes involved in gluconeogenesis if glucose homeostasis is to be maintained.[3–5] Then insulin secretion and incretins become linked to enteral milk supply to allow physiological adaptation to the challenges of preserving homeostasis during fasting and feeding.[6] These changes are under the control of a cascade of hormones, including catecholamines, cortisol, glucagon, and insulin.[6] During this critical period of physiological adaptation, infants are at risk of both hyperglycemia and hypoglycemia if the appropriate regulation of these processes and the availability of the necessary substrates for glucose metabolism are not available.[7]

34.2 PRENATAL

In utero, the high energy requirements of the growing and developing fetus are predominantly met by glucose oxidation.[1] Glucose also provides the precursor for other carbon-containing compounds, including protein and glycogen, and is a precursor for fat synthesis.[8] Fetal glucose utilization rates average 5 mg/kg/min, which are nearly double the adult requirement of 2–3 mg/kg/min. The placenta and fetal liver are the principal organs that maintain nutrient supply and production to meet the high fetal requirements.[8, 9] In healthy pregnancies, the majority of this is achieved by transplacental glucose transport from mother to fetus and is dependent on maternal glycemia, as there is a direct relationship between maternal and fetal glucose levels.[10] Fetal glycemia also influences the levels of fetal insulin and growth factor production.[11] Fetal carbohydrate metabolism is therefore influenced by the relationship between placental function, which is affected by uterine blood flow and maternal health, and the fetal endocrine system.

Maternal-Fetal and Neonatal Endocrinology. https://doi.org/10.1016/B978-0-12-814823-5.00034-9

34.2.1 Placental Function and Glucose Transport

Transplacental transfer of glucose, from mother to fetus, through facilitated transport meets the majority of fetal carbohydrate requirements.[12-16] There is a family of glucose transporters with various isoforms found in the syncytiotrophoblast, including GLUT 1, 3, 4, and 12, of which 4 and 12 are insulin sensitive.[12-16] GLUT1 is the most abundant transporter and is expressed in almost every fetal tissue.[12] Increases in GLUT1 levels on the maternal facing placental membrane in early pregnancy increases the transport of glucose from mother into the placenta, the placenta itself using 30%–40%, and the rest is transferred to the growing fetus. In later pregnancy, the GLUT1 receptors on the fetal facing basal membrane increase in number, and activity to support the increased glucose transfer required in later gestation by the growing fetus. The expression of the placental glucose transporters is also affected by maternal diabetes mellitus, placental hypoxia, and exogenous glucocorticoid administration.[10, 15]

Normal fetal glucose uptake in humans is estimated to range from 4 to 6 mg/kg/min, but placental glucose transport does not become saturated until >360 mg/dL (>20 mmol/L). There are limited animal studies in the lamb and rat of the effect of uterine blood flow on fetal glucose levels, but an acute compromise to placental blood flow leads to a reactive increase in blood glucose and lactate and increased glucose delivery and uptake.[17-20] However, chronic placental insufficiency is associated with a reduced glucose delivery and fetal hypoglycemia. The placenta also has a large capacity for storage, and therefore this blunts the transfer of glucose in the case of maternal hyperglycemia.[21]

34.2.2 Maternal Effects

The fetal glucose level is about 70% of maternal levels, and the gravid mother increases glucose production by 15%–30% in late gestation to provide for the increasing needs of the growing fetus.[22] During the first trimester, maternal insulin sensitivity is increased, which increases fat deposition, and this is reversed in later pregnancy when increasing insulin resistance allows mobilization of these stores.[23, 24] A global perspective shows that relative maternal malnutrition is a significant cause of fetal growth restriction and women carrying growth retarded fetuses have lower rates of lipolysis in the third trimester.[25, 26] However, it is increasingly being appreciated that the differences in maternal physiology, which have not previously been considered pathological, can also play a significant role in fetal health. This is highlighted in the results of the HAPO study, where fetal outcomes were related to levels of maternal glucose control that were below those previously considered pathological, in the setting of diabetes.[27]

34.2.3 Fetal Role

34.2.3.1 Fetal Metabolism

In healthy pregnancies, fetal glucose uptake from the placenta is equivalent to fetal glucose utilization. Fetal liver and kidneys do not produce glucose, but are focused on the anabolic processes of glycogen and lipid storage.[2] However, in the setting of placental insufficiency or maternal starvation, the fetus is then able to adapt with upregulation of enzymes for gluconeogenesis (GNG) and by using alternative fuels such as ketones (Fig. 34.1).[28] The fetus is required to maintain oxidative phosphorylation in the face of low oxygen tension, and although energy is produced predominantly by aerobic metabolism, the fetus has the potential for a significant level of anaerobic metabolism and can use lactate efficiently.[29] Ketone bodies can be used as an alternative source of fuel by the fetus as well as a precursor for glucose (Fig. 34.1).[23, 28, 30]

34.2.3.2 Fetal Glycogen Metabolism

In addition to providing the predominant source of energy to the fetus, 40% of the glucose taken up by the fetus is converted into glycogen or to lipid for storage. In humans, glycogen is synthesized from the 9th week of gestation from glucose and lactate and is stored in the liver lung, heart, and skeletal muscle, and to a lesser extent, kidney, intestine, and brain (Fig. 34.1).[8] The fetus can also synthesize glycogen from pyruvate, acetate, and alanine. Liver glycogen storage increases throughout gestation but mostly occurs in the third trimester, and is dependent on both substrate availability and hormonal regulation by the activity of the enzyme glycogen synthetase.[31] By term in healthy pregnancies, glycogen stores are two to three times adult levels.[32] Corticosteroids induce glycogen synthetase, which is activated by insulin. Fetal cells have an increased number and receptor affinity for insulin (and delayed hepatic glycogen receptor activation), which favors the storage of glucose as glycogen and fat (and inhibits catabolism).[33, 34]

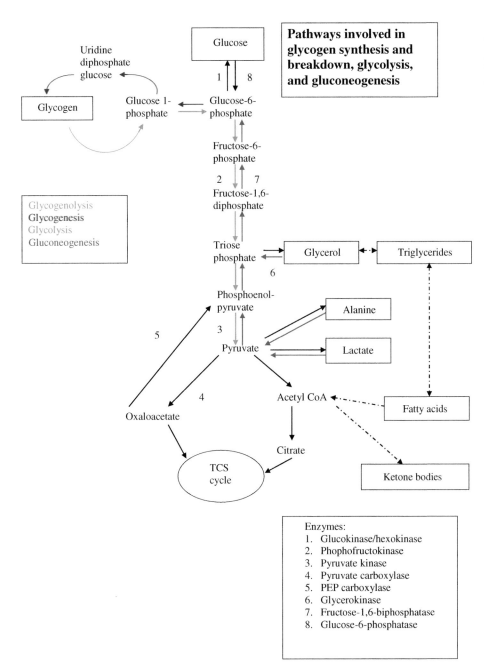

Pathways involved in glycogen synthesis and breakdown, glycolysis, and gluconeogenesis

FIG. 34.1 Pathways in glycogen synthesis and breakdown, glycolysis, and gluconeogenesis. *(With permission from Cambridge University Press (Practical Neonatal Endocrinology).)*

Enzymes:
1. Glucokinase/hexokinase
2. Phophofructokinase
3. Pyruvate kinase
4. Pyruvate carboxylase
5. PEP carboxylase
6. Glycerokinase
7. Fructose-1,6-biphosphatase
8. Glucose-6-phosphatase

Other growth factors such as epidermal growth factor (EGF) and insulin-like growth factors I and II (IGF-I and IGF-II) have also been shown to stimulate glycogen synthesis in the fetal rat.[35] In keeping with this, knockout IGF-II mice have low glycogen stores and low glycogen synthetase activity at birth.[36] Glucose conversion to fat occurs predominantly in the third trimester, with the fat mass at term in the human fetus reaching 16% of body mass.[37] The human transfer of free fatty acids is not sufficient to account for the amount of adipose tissue that is accumulated, and therefore triglycerides must be synthesized from glucose. Therefore, if glucose supplies are limited, there is a reduction in both adipose tissue and glycogen stores.

34.2.3.3 Fetal Glucose Production

Although some of the enzymes required for GNG are present from the 3rd month of gestation, fetal glucose production is usually negligible until the last few days of gestation.[38, 39] In many species, the activities of the key gluconeogenic enzymes glucose 6 phosphatase (G6P), and phosphoenolpyruvate carboxykinase (PEPCK) are dependent on the prepartum cortisol surge for activation.[40, 41] In animal studies, this can be inhibited by adrenalectomy and stimulated by exogenous infusion of cortisol.[42] With adequate maternal nutrition, GNG and ketogenesis are not seen in the fetus, and the fetus cannot acutely induce these enzymes in response to hypoglycemia. However, if there is impaired placental glucose supply, the fetus can use alternative fuels, and with chronic deprivation, glucose can be produced by glycogenolysis and GNG, but this is following the upregulation of the enzyme pathways secondary to increased cortisol levels.[42]

34.2.3.4 Fetal Pancreatic Development

The pancreas is formed from two separate embryonic rudiments, which come together to form one organ. The principle endocrine function of the pancreas is the regulation of blood glucose, through the release of hormones from the islets of Langerhans. The islets are scattered throughout the pancreas and contain three types of cells: 60%–80% beta cells that secrete insulin to increase glucose cellular uptake and utilization, 15%–20% alpha cells that secrete glucagon to increase GNG, 5%–10% delta cells that release somatostatin, and a small number of cells that release incretins (peptides which act on the gut). Numerous transcription factors control differentiation and development of the islets in organogenesis (HIX, PDX1, CDX1, NKx2.3, PAX4) and insulin gene expression (e.g., HNF1 alpha, HNF4 alpha, PDX1). PDX1 seems to be essential for normal islet development and function.[43, 44] Beta cells are detected from 14 weeks' gestation and insulin secretion by 18 weeks. The main phase of islet differentiation and development occurs in the second trimester with further remodeling in late gestation.[45] Fetal pancreatic development appears to be regulated by the in utero environment with glucose and amino acid availability, as well as growth factors including insulin and insulin-like growth factors impacting on longer-term structure and function.[45–48]

Insulin secretion by the beta cell is stimulated by increases in blood glucose (Fig. 34.2). At rest the potassium ATP (KATP) channels on beta cells are open. When blood glucose rises it enters the cell through the cell membrane-bound GLUT2 glucose transporter. Glucose inside the beta cell is then phosphorylated by glucokinase, which leads to an increase in ATP/ADP ratio. As the ATP rises, the KATP channel closes causing depolarization of the cell, which in turn opens voltage-dependent calcium channels, resulting in an influx of calcium. High calcium in the cytosol stimulates exocytosis of insulin from secretory granules (Fig. 34.2). Fetal insulin secretion increases during the last trimester of pregnancy and is critical for normal fetal growth, with increased insulin concentrations leading to increased rates of protein synthesis and increased glucose uptake. The high insulin/glucagon ratio also appears to be important in maintaining glycogen synthesis whilst suppressing GNG during fetal life. There are also maturational changes toward term indicating that the pancreatic beta cell's response to glucose-stimulated insulin secretion may be influenced by the rise in cortisol levels in late gestation.[49]

Glucose is the primary regulator of fetal insulin secretion (although in the fetus amino acids also play a role), with insulin levels having a positive correlation with plasma glucose particularly after 20 weeks gestation. In healthy pregnancies, the continuous delivery of glucose to the fetus is well regulated by the placenta to meet requirements for metabolism and growth. Insulin and glucagon do not cross the placenta, and the levels detected in fetal plasma are dependent on fetal pancreatic secretion. Fetal insulin secretion acts to promote fetal growth and to ensure there are adequate fetal fat and glycogen stores in late gestation to maintain glucose homeostasis immediately after birth.

FIG. 34.2 The beta cell. *(With permission from Cambridge University Press (Practical Neonatal Endocrinology).)*

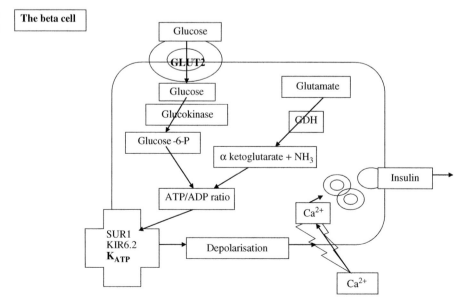

34.2.3.5 The Insulin/IGF-I Axis

The fetus is not generally exposed to large fluctuations in glucose levels, and acute changes in glucose (leading to hypoglycemia or hyperglycemia) do not lead to significant changes in either insulin or glucagon, as would be seen in adults. However, chronic changes such as the hyperglycemia present in a diabetic mother leads to increased fetal insulin secretion and beta-cell hyperplasia. This then leads to increased fetal glycogen and fat deposition and neonatal macrosomia. Insulin also has indirect actions on growth through its positive regulation of IGF-I and increasing the cellular availability of glucose. IGF-I and IGF-II are also primary endocrine regulators of fetal growth, and levels increase gradually toward about 33 weeks of gestation and then increase two- to threefold until term.[50] Cord blood levels correlate with birth weight, and low levels of IGF-I are found following fetal growth restriction.[51, 52] IGFs have roles in cell proliferation, differentiation, and metabolism, and are found in the circulation by 15 weeks gestation, but activity is regulated by a family of binding proteins, which are developmentally and nutritionally regulated. Glucose transfer across the placenta stimulates insulin secretion, and this stimulates IGF production. This then increases fetal anabolism, which further increases placental uptake of glucose and other nutrients to support fetal growth.[50]

In contrast, in pregnancies complicated by placental insufficiency where there is reduced glucose delivery to the fetus, there are low insulin levels and reduced growth and fat deposition. Insulin deficiency leads to reduced plasma IGF-I and IGF-II, which play key roles in the regulation of fetoplacental growth, with cord blood insulin and C-peptide as well as IGF-I correlating with size at birth. The fetal insulin/glucose ratio is lower in small for gestational age fetuses compared with those where growth is appropriate for gestational age.[53] Glucagon can also be detected in fetal plasma by 15 weeks gestation and peaks at 24–26 weeks gestation. At this time, the relatively low levels of hepatic glucagon receptors compared with adulthood help decrease glucagon-mediated catabolism. The actions of insulin and other hormones of the insulin-IGF-I axis are shown in Table 34.1.

34.3 TRANSITION

Increasing gestational age and birth itself have maturational effects on enzyme systems, glucose transporter levels, and hormone and hormone receptor levels. These effects, combined with substrate availability, clinical morbidities, and clinical interventions, all impact on glucose levels during the transition to independent life for the newborn. During the first 4–6 h after birth, glucose values fall and stabilize at about 50–60 mg/dL (2.8–3.3 mmol/L). This decrease can be influenced by maternal glucose infusion during labor, and is earlier and lower in preterm and small for gestational age infants.[54] However, by 2–3 days of age, plasma glucose levels average 70–80 mg/dL (3.9–4.4 mmol/L) in healthy term neonates (Fig. 34.3).[55]

The stresses of birth, including transient hypoxia, cold exposure, and cutting of the cord, lead to increases in catecholamines, which in turn leads to a fall in insulin and a rise in glucagon and growth hormone. The elevated glucagon and noradrenaline activate adenylate cyclase, which causes an increase in intracellular cyclic AMP and promotes glycogenolysis, lipolysis, and GNG. Glucocorticoids also promote lipolysis and protein breakdown, increasing the availability of gluconeogenic substrate. Healthy term infants are therefore able to mobilize free fatty acids and oxidize ketones to maintain their blood glucose levels. In keeping with this rapid change to a "catabolic state," there is a decrease in glycogen

TABLE 34.1 Primary metabolic actions of insulin (and the IGF axis)

Glucagon	Insulin	GLP1	IGF-I/IGF-II
Stimulates glycogenolysis	Promotes cellular glucose uptake and utilization in muscle and adipose cells	Enhances glucose dependent insulin secretion	Stimulates protein synthesis
Promotes hepatic gluconeogenesis production of glucose from alanine	Suppresses postprandial glucagon secretion	Slows gastric emptying	Stimulates free fatty acid utilization
Promotes hepatic ketogenesis and lipolysis	Promotes protein and fat synthesis (glyconeogenesis) and glycogen synthesis from carbohydrate (glycogenesis)	Reduces food intake and body weight	Increased insulin sensitivity and glucose utilization
Decreases glycogen synthesis	Reduces gluconeogenesis and lipolysis—formation of glucose from fats		

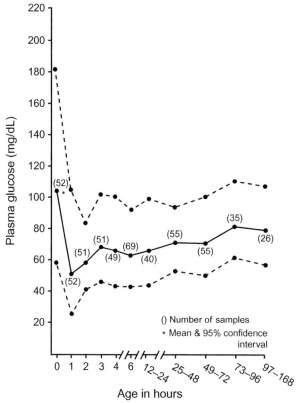

FIG. 34.3 Plasma glucose levels in healthy term neonates postdelivery. *(With permission from Srinivasan G, Pildes RS, Cattamanchi G, et al. Plasma glucose values in normal neonates: a new look.* J Pediatr *1986;**109(1)**:114–7.)*

synthetase activity and an increase in glycogen phosphorylase activity, which is mediated by enzyme phosphorylation, activated by cAMP. Immediately after delivery glycogenolysis is critical in maintaining glucose levels, however, liver stores are rapidly diminished within 2–3 h of birth, are almost entirely depleted by 12 h, and then remain low for several days.[4]

During this time, GNG is required if glucose levels are to be maintained, and this is dependent on the availability of gluconeogenic precursors, as well as activation of the enzymes for GNG. There is upregulation of hepatic glucagon receptors, which become linked to the cyclic 3,5 adenosine monophosphate protein kinase and induction of the key enzymes for GNG, PEPCK, and G6P. The low blood glucose levels and increased cortisol levels at birth stimulate hepatic G6P activity, which in term infants is low before birth and rises rapidly after birth, reaching adult levels within 3 days of age.[5] Also, reversal of the insulin:glucagon ratio through a reduction in insulin levels induces PEPCK, which is the rate-limiting enzyme in GNG. The concentration of PEPCK continues to increase during the first of after birth, regardless of gestation. Together these adaptations lead to increase hepatic glucose release from GNG to maintain glucose supplies to vital organs in the newborn infant.[5]

The mobilization of muscle stores of glycogen is a much longer process, and due to a lack of muscle G6P, these stores can only be used by the muscles themselves. Lactate, however, that has been formed by glycolysis can leave the muscle and be converted into glucose in the liver, or oxidized by other tissues. Animal studies have also demonstrated that stimulation of the vagus nerve increases activation of hepatic glycogen synthetase, whereas stimulation of the splanchnic nerve induces glycogen phosphorylase and increases glycogenolysis.

34.4 NEWBORN

After birth, the newborn baby has to maintain independent carbohydrate homeostasis during the fed and fasting state. Newborn glucose requirements are high due to the relatively large brain to body weight ratio (13% in the newborn and 2% in the adult), as the brain is primarily dependent on glucose as its energy source. Steady-state glucose utilization in the term newborn is two- to threefold higher than in the adult (relative to body weight) at 4–6 mg/kg/min. In the preterm and growth-restricted newborn, it is even higher at 6–8 mg/kg/min. Glucose utilization is also increased with hypoxia, hyperinsulinism, and respiratory or cold stress.[56, 57]

Low blood sugar levels are the norm in healthy term newborns during adaptation to postnatal life, and low levels may play a role in the induction of enzymes involved in GNG.[58] However, the levels of exposure to low glucose levels that are physiological versus pathological remain controversial,[59] with the clinical signs of hypoglycemia and consequences being nonspecific and difficult to identify. On the basis of historical neurophysiological and neurodevelopmental outcome studies, hypoglycemia in the newborn has been defined as <46 mg/dL (<2.6 mmol/L), although this threshold remains controversial.[60, 61] The neonatal brain is thought to be able to use alternative fuels, such as ketones and lactate, and therefore to be resistant to relatively low glucose levels that would not be tolerated later in life.[62] Ketones are provided by increased hepatic ketogenesis, which occurs in the 24 h after delivery, leading to a high ketone body concentration and turnover rate (12–22 μmol/min). This, however, is not the case in preterm infants, and those of low birthweight, where there is limited availability of substrates for alternative fuel production.

There is also controversy over the definition of hyperglycemia in the newborn.[63] In utero, and in healthy term infants, blood glucose levels are rarely >126 mg/dL (>7 mmol/L). Traditionally, hyperglycemia has been viewed as a physiological response to stress,[64] and most neonatologists would not intervene to treat blood glucose levels until they rose to 180–216 mg/dL (>10–12 mmol/L). However, there is evidence linking early hyperglycemia with both mortality and morbidity, but intervention studies are required to determine if this relationship is merely an association, or is causal.[65, 66]

34.4.1 Postprandial State: Glycogen Storage and Fat Metabolism

The gradual rise in cortisol levels in the fetus in the last trimester not only cause maturation of enzymes for GNG but also lead to increased pancreatic sensitivity to insulin.[49] These changes are thought to prepare the fetus to be able to regulate glucose control after delivery. Animal studies have also shown that the newborn liver is resistant to the suppressive effect of insulin on hepatic glucose production. Glucose production rates have been found to persist until glucose infusion rates reached 21.7 mg/kg/min, whereas in adults, glucose production is suppressed with glucose infusion rates of 5.7 mg/kg/min.[67]

34.4.2 Intestinal Transport

Lactase, which is present in the brush border of the intestinal villi, hydrolyzes the disaccharide lactose in milk, to the monosaccharides glucose and galactose.[68] Intestinal lactase activity is detectable as early as 8 weeks of gestation in the fetal gut, but activity rises gradually from 8 to 34 weeks, and then rises rapidly from that time until term.[69] With oral feeding in the postnatal period, lactase activity increases in both preterm and term infants.[70, 71] Increasing intestinal lactase activity after birth is critical in maintaining normoglycemia for infants on milk feeds. Breastfed babies have lower blood glucose levels than bottle-fed babies, but these levels have been associated with higher ketone levels, which are thought to provide an alternative fuel during the transition period when breastfeeding is being established.[58, 72] This is thought to be particularly important for the neonatal brain, which may use ketones and lactate as an alternative energy source to glucose.[62]

34.4.2.1 Glucose Uptake

Glucose uptake is dependent on a family of eight developmentally regulated glucose transporters, each of which has a specific tissue distribution. GLUT 1 has a high affinity for glucose and is insulin independent, being responsible for basal glucose uptake.[73–75] It is found in most tissues, but particularly in the brain, and maintains glucose transport across the blood-brain barrier. GLUT 1 appears to be downregulated by high glucose concentrations and upregulated by low glucose concentrations.[76] After birth, GLUT 1 levels decrease, and the other isoforms increase: GLUT 2 in the liver, GLUT 3 in the brain, and GLUT 4 in the muscle.[74, 76] Insulin's actions on glucose uptake are predominantly mediated by GLUT 4, which is found in muscle, fat, and heart, where glucose uptake is insulin-mediated. GLUT 4 is usually found in intracellular vesicles, but in adults, insulin stimulates the migration of GLUT 4 transporters to the plasma membrane.[77] However, in the newborn, upregulation of GLUT 4 transporters in muscle only respond modestly to insulin.[78]

34.4.2.2 Glucose Utilization

Glucose utilization rates in the newborn can far exceed the levels found in adults, as demonstrated by the effect of increasing dextrose or insulin infusion. The mean glucose oxidation rate in the term newborn has been estimated to be 6 mg/kg/min (3.8–9.7 mg/kg/min) compared with an adult rate of 3 mg/kg/min.[79–81] In preterm infants, glucose oxidation rates have also been reported to be high, ranging from 2.9 to 7.9 mg/kg/min[82] or 4.3 to 8.5 mg/kg/min.[81] In addition, there is a switch during the 1st week of life from the percentage of total energy expenditure utilized for oxidative versus nonoxidative glucose metabolism, with an increase in nonoxidative disposal marking the change from a catabolic to an anabolic state.[75] Insulin stimulates nonoxidative glucose disposal through lipogenesis, glycogenesis, and protein synthesis, impacting on growth both directly and indirectly through the regulation of IGF-I and IGF binding protein one (IGFBP-1).[83–85]

34.4.2.3 Insulin Secretion

Insulin is the primary hormonal regulator of glucose uptake, and utilization in the newborn and its secretion is under the influence of neural and enteroendocrine mechanisms. Glucoreceptor neurons are present in the ventromedial hypothalamic nucleus and the portal vein, causing an increase in insulin secretion in response to hyperglycemia.[86] Insulin secretion is coupled to the enteric supply of milk and release of incretins.[87–89] However, in the newborn, there is initially reduced insulin secretion in response to glucose with maturation in the weeks after birth.[90, 91] Also, animal models have demonstrated remodeling of the pancreas after birth and associated weaning with increased levels of apoptosis and neogenesis that can be influenced by nutritional intake.[92–95]

There is similar postmortem evidence of beta cell apoptosis in humans with a new population of beta cells compensating for the perinatal loss.[96] This may be important in responding to the change from continuous placental glucose delivery to the intermittent enteral supply of nutrients. The secretion of incretins may be necessary for the remodeling of a new population of beta cells that are better suited to metabolic control in postnatal life. Any interference with this process of remodeling may have a critical impact on the ability of the pancreas to meet requirements for insulin secretion later in life.[97] In rats, this period of apoptosis occurs at the same time as a significant fall in levels of IGF-II expression, and overexpression of IGF-II leads to a reduction in the level of apoptosis, suggesting a protective role for IGF-II.[98]

34.4.3 Preprandial State and Gluconeogenesis

After birth, as the glycogen reserves are rapidly diminished, the newborn quickly becomes dependent on GNG. There are four gluconeogenic enzymes in the liver (pyruvate carboxylase [PC]), PEPCK, fructose 1,6-bisphosphatase, and glucose-6-phosphate dehydrogenase (G6PD). Of these, PC and PEPCK are only present in negligible amounts in the fetal liver and require upregulation after birth to allow GNG.[56]

34.4.3.1 Enzyme Induction

As described previously, the increase in glucagon and catecholamines and fall in insulin levels at birth increase PEPCK and PC expression. The hepatic enzyme G6P, which catalyzes the last step of both GNG and glycogenolysis, has only 10% of adult activity by term, but in the 1st week after birth activity rises rapidly to adult levels. This is thought to be dependent on the postnatal drop in plasma glucose levels and the high glucagon:insulin ratio.[59]

34.4.3.2 Substrate Availability

Glucose obtained by hydrolysis of lactose from milk provides approximately 6.1 g/kg/day of glucose, 20% to 40% of the newborn's energy requirements. Of the remaining gluconeogenic substrates, galactose provides the most significant amount, with smaller amounts available from lactate, amino acids, and glycerol. Galactose from milk is mainly converted to glucose by G6PD. Uptake is independent of insulin concentrations, and clearance is very rapid compared with that of glucose (6.9%/min disappearance compared with 1.4%/min). Glycerol accounts for approximately 10%–20% of glucose production. The first step of GNG from glycerol is not influenced by glucagon, insulin, or glucocorticoids, which regulate the rate of GNG from nonglycerol precursors, but is related to changes in blood glycerol concentration.

In healthy full-term newborns, GNG via pyruvate contributes significantly to glucose appearance rates (31%), similar rates to those seen in normal healthy adults after an overnight fast. GNG from lactate occurs soon after birth, and it contributes approximately 30% of the total glucose production in the healthy term newborn. The rate of lactate turnover is almost twofold higher than the rate of glucose turnover. This is in contrast to the situation in adults when lactate turnover is much lower than the rate of glucose turnover. Only one study has measured the contribution of alanine to glucose production in the human newborn and found that at 8 h of age, 9.3 ± 2.3% of blood glucose was derived from alanine.[75]

34.5 CLINICAL IMPLICATIONS

The transition from fetal to independent life requires a rapid and complex orchestration of enzyme induction and change in resource utilization to ensure adequate energy supplies to the baby and for glucose homeostasis to be maintained. It is not surprising therefore that the newborn period is one when physiological glucose levels are more varied and less well controlled than later in life. However, it is also a time when there is a risk of clinically significant derangements in metabolic processes, and some metabolic disorders of carbohydrate metabolism may present. It is therefore essential that a clinical assessment is made to determine the likely etiology and potential consequences of any "derangements" in glucose control at this time. Avoiding overtreatment while knowing when clinically intervention may be beneficial can be challenging when there is limited evidence regarding "optimal" glucose control at this time.

REFERENCES

1. Kalhan SC. Metabolism of glucose and methods of investigation in the fetus and newborn. In: Fox WW, Polin RA, Abman SH, editors. *Fetal and neonatal physiology*. 3rd ed. Philadelphia, PA: Saunders; 2003. p. 449–64.
2. Kalhan SC, D'Angelo LJ, Savin SM, et al. Glucose production in pregnant women at term gestation. Sources of glucose for human fetus. *J Clin Investig* 1979;**63**(3):388–94.
3. Sperling MA, DeLamater PV, Phelps D, et al. Spontaneous and amino acid-stimulated glucagon secretion in the immediate postnatal period. Relation to glucose and insulin. *J Clin Invest* 1974;**53**(4):1159–66.
4. Ward Platt M, Deshpande S. Metabolic adaptation at birth. *Semin Fetal Neonatal Med* 2005;**10**(4):341–50. https://doi.org/10.1016/j.siny.2005.04.001.
5. Hillman NH, Kallapur SG, Jobe AH. Physiology of transition from intrauterine to extrauterine life. *Clin Perinatol* 2012;**39**(4):769–83. https://doi.org/10.1016/j.clp.2012.09.009.
6. Aynsley-Green A, Lucas A, Bloom SR. The effect of feeds of differing composition on entero-insular hormone secretion in the first hours of life in human neonates. *Acta Paediatr Scand* 1979;**68**(2):265–70.
7. Stomnaroska O, Petkovska E, Ivanovska S, et al. Hypoglycaemia in the newborn. *Pril (Makedon Akad Nauk Umet Odd Med Nauki)* 2017;**38**(2):79–84. https://doi.org/10.1515/prilozi-2017-0025.
8. Hay Jr WW, Sparks JW. Placental, fetal, and neonatal carbohydrate metabolism. *Clin Obstet Gynecol* 1985;**28**(3):473–85.
9. Homko CJ, Sivan E, Reece EA, et al. Fuel metabolism during pregnancy. *Semin Reprod Endocrinol* 1999;**17**(2):119–25. https://doi.org/10.1055/s-2007-1016219.
10. Baumann MU, Deborde S, Illsley NP. Placental glucose transfer and fetal growth. *Endocr J* 2002;**19**(1):13–22.
11. Higgins M, Mc Auliffe F. A review of maternal and fetal growth factors in diabetic pregnancy. *Curr Diabetes Rev* 2010;**6**(2):116–25.
12. Illsley NP. Glucose transporters in the human placenta. *Placenta* 2000;**21**(1):14–22.
13. Arnott G, Coghill G, McArdle HJ, et al. Immunolocalization of GLUT1 and GLUT3 glucose transporters in human placenta. *Biochem Soc Trans* 1994;**22**(3):272S.
14. Jansson T, Wennergren M, Illsley NP. Glucose transporter protein expression in human placenta throughout gestation and in intrauterine growth retardation. *J Clin Endocrinol Metab* 1993;**77**(6):1554–62. https://doi.org/10.1210/jcem.77.6.8263141.
15. Jansson T, Ekstrand Y, Wennergren M, et al. Placental glucose transport in gestational diabetes mellitus. *Am J Obstet Gynecol* 2001;**184**(2):111–6. https://doi.org/10.1067/mob.2001.108075.
16. Takata K, Kasahara T, Kasahara M, et al. Localization of erythrocyte/HepG2-type glucose transporter (GLUT1) in human placental villi. *Cell Tissue Res* 1992;**267**(3):407–12.
17. Lasuncion MA, Lorenzo J, Palacin M, et al. Maternal factors modulating nutrient transfer to fetus. *Biol Neonate* 1987;**51**(2):86–93.
18. Wesolowski SR, Hay Jr WW. Role of placental insufficiency and intrauterine growth restriction on the activation of fetal hepatic glucose production. *Mol Cell Endocrinol* 2016;**435**:61–8. https://doi.org/10.1016/j.mce.2015.12.016.
19. Limesand SW, Rozance PJ, Smith D, et al. Increased insulin sensitivity and maintenance of glucose utilization rates in fetal sheep with placental insufficiency and intrauterine growth restriction. *Am J Physiol Endocrinol Metab* 2007;**293**(6):E1716–25. https://doi.org/10.1152/ajpendo.00459.2007.
20. Hay Jr WW. Placental-fetal glucose exchange and fetal glucose metabolism. *Trans Am Clin Climatol Assoc* 2006;**117**:321–39 [discussion 39–40].
21. Illsley NP. Placental glucose transport in diabetic pregnancy. *Clin Obstet Gynecol* 2000;**43**(1):116–26.
22. Bozzetti P, Ferrari MM, Marconi AM, et al. The relationship of maternal and fetal glucose concentrations in the human from midgestation until term. *Metabolism* 1988;**37**(4):358–63.
23. Herrera E. Lipid metabolism in pregnancy and its consequences in the fetus and newborn. *Endocrine* 2002;**19**(1):43–55.
24. Schaefer-Graf UM, Graf K, Kulbacka I, et al. Maternal lipids as strong determinants of fetal environment and growth in pregnancies with gestational diabetes mellitus. *Diabetes Care* 2008;**31**(9):1858–63.
25. Diderholm B, Stridsberg M, Ewald U, et al. Increased lipolysis in non-obese pregnant women studied in the third trimester. *BJOG* 2005;**112**(6):713–8.
26. Diderholm B, Beardsall K, Murgatroyd P, et al. Maternal rates of lipolysis and glucose production in late pregnancy are independently related to foetal weight. *Clin Endocrinol* 2017;**87**(3):272–8. https://doi.org/10.1111/cen.13359.
27. Catalano PM, McIntyre HD, Cruickshank JK, et al. The hyperglycemia and adverse pregnancy outcome study: associations of GDM and obesity with pregnancy outcomes. *Diabetes Care* 2012;**35**(4):780–6.

28. Ogata ES. Carbohydrate metabolism in the fetus and neonate and altered neonatal glucoregulation. *Pediatr Clin N Am* 1986;**33**(1):25–45.

29. Sparks JW, Hay Jr WW, Bonds D, et al. Simultaneous measurements of lactate turnover rate and umbilical lactate uptake in the fetal lamb. *J Clin Invest* 1982;**70**(1):179–92.

30. Bougneres PF, Lemmel C, Ferre P, et al. Ketone body transport in the human neonate and infant. *J Clin Invest* 1986;**77**(1):42–8. https://doi.org/10.1172/JCI112299.

31. Devi BG, Habeebullah CM, Gupta PD. Glycogen metabolism during human liver development. *Biochem Int* 1992;**28**(2):229–37.

32. Shelley HJ. Carbohydrate reserves in the newborn infant. *Br Med J* 1964;**1**(5378):273–5.

33. Plas C, Nunez J. Role of cortisol on the glycogenolytic effect of glucagon and on the glycogenic response to insulin in fetal hepatocyte culture. *J Biol Chem* 1976;**251**(5):1431–7.

34. Gruppuso PA, Brautigan DL. Induction of hepatic glycogenesis in the fetal rat. *Am J Phys* 1989;**256**(1 Pt 1):E49–54. https://doi.org/10.1152/ajpendo.1989.256.1.E49.

35. Menuelle P, Binoux M, Plas C. Regulation by insulin-like growth factor (IGF) binding proteins of IGF-II-stimulated glycogenesis in cultured fetal rat hepatocytes. *Endocrinology* 1995;**136**(12):5305–10. https://doi.org/10.1210/endo.136.12.7588275.

36. Lopez MF, Dikkes P, Zurakowski D, et al. Regulation of hepatic glycogen in the insulin-like growth factor II-deficient mouse. *Endocrinology* 1999;**140**(3):1442–8. https://doi.org/10.1210/endo.140.3.6602.

37. Catalano PM, Thomas AJ, Huston LP, et al. Effect of maternal metabolism on fetal growth and body composition. *Diabetes Care* 1998;**21**(Suppl. 2): B85–90.

38. Teng C, Battaglia FC, Meschia G, et al. Fetal hepatic and umbilical uptakes of glucogenic substrates during a glucagon-somatostatin infusion. *Am J Physiol Endocrinol Metab* 2002;**282**(3):E542–50. https://doi.org/10.1152/ajpendo.00248.2001.

39. Gleason CA, Rudolph AM. Gluconeogenesis by the fetal sheep liver in vivo. *J Dev Physiol* 1985;**7**(3):185–94.

40. Fowden AL, Mijovic J, Silver M. The effects of cortisol on hepatic and renal gluconeogenic enzyme activities in the sheep fetus during late gestation. *J Endocrinol* 1993;**137**(2):213–22.

41. Fowden AL, Mundy L, Silver M. Developmental regulation of glucogenesis in the sheep fetus during late gestation. *J Physiol* 1998;**508**(Pt 3):937–47.

42. Fowden AL, Forhead AJ. Adrenal glands are essential for activation of glucogenesis during undernutrition in fetal sheep near term. *Am J Physiol Endocrinol Metab* 2011;**300**(1):E94–102. https://doi.org/10.1152/ajpendo.00205.2010.

43. Piper K, Brickwood S, Turnpenny LW, et al. Beta cell differentiation during early human pancreas development. *J Endocrinol* 2004;**181**(1):11–23.

44. Wilson ME, Scheel D, German MS. Gene expression cascades in pancreatic development. *Mech Dev* 2003;**120**(1):65–80.

45. Fowden AL, Hill DJ. Intra-uterine programming of the endocrine pancreas. *Br Med Bull* 2001;**60**:123–42.

46. Garofano A, Czernichow P, Breant B. In utero undernutrition impairs rat beta-cell development. *Diabetologia* 1997;**40**(10):1231–4.

47. Garofano A, Czernichow P, Breant B. Beta-cell mass and proliferation following late fetal and early postnatal malnutrition in the rat. *Diabetologia* 1998;**41**(9):1114–20.

48. Limesand SW, Hay Jr WW. Adaptation of ovine fetal pancreatic insulin secretion to chronic hypoglycaemia and euglycaemic correction. *J Physiol* 2003;**547**(Pt 1):95–105.

49. Fowden AL, Gardner DS, Ousey JC, et al. Maturation of pancreatic beta-cell function in the fetal horse during late gestation. *J Endocrinol* 2005;**186**(3):467–73.

50. Hellstrom A, Ley D, Hansen-Pupp I, et al. Insulin-like growth factor 1 has multisystem effects on foetal and preterm infant development. *Acta Paediatr* 2016;**105**(6):576–86. https://doi.org/10.1111/apa.13350.

51. Bhatia S, Faessen GH, Carland G, et al. A longitudinal analysis of maternal serum insulin-like growth factor I (IGF-I) and total and nonphosphorylated IGF-binding protein-1 in human pregnancies complicated by intrauterine growth restriction. *J Clin Endocrinol Metab* 2002;**87**(4):1864–70.

52. Ozkan H, Aydin A, Demir N, et al. Associations of IGF-I, IGFBP-1 and IGFBP-3 on intrauterine growth and early catch-up growth. *Biol Neonate* 1999;**76**(5):274–82.

53. Bazaes RA, Salazar TE, Pittaluga E, et al. Glucose and lipid metabolism in small for gestational age infants at 48 hours of age. *Pediatrics* 2003;**111**(4 Pt 1):804–9.

54. Kaiser JR, Bai S, Rozance PJ. Newborn plasma glucose concentration nadirs by gestational-age group. *Neonatology* 2018;**113**(4):353–9. https://doi.org/10.1159/000487222.

55. Srinivasan G, Pildes RS, Cattamanchi G, et al. Plasma glucose values in normal neonates: a new look. *J Pediatr* 1986;**109**(1):114–7.

56. Thureen P. *Neonatal nutrition and metabolism*. 2nd ed. Cambridge University Press; 2006.

57. Boardman JP, Hawdon JM. Hypoglycaemia and hypoxic-ischaemic encephalopathy. *Dev Med Child Neurol* 2015;**57**(Suppl. 3):29–33. https://doi.org/10.1111/dmcn.12729.

58. Hawdon JM, Ward Platt MP, Aynsley-Green A. Patterns of metabolic adaptation for preterm and term infants in the first neonatal week. *Arch Dis Child* 1992;**67**(4 Spec):357–65.

59. Hay Jr WW, Raju TN, Higgins RD, et al. Knowledge gaps and research needs for understanding and treating neonatal hypoglycemia: workshop report from Eunice Kennedy Shriver National Institute of Child Health and Human Development. *J Pediatr* 2009;**155**(5):612–7.

60. Lucas A, Morley R, Cole TJ. Adverse neurodevelopmental outcome of moderate neonatal hypoglycaemia. *BMJ* 1988;**297**(6659):1304–8.

61. Koh TH, Aynsley-Green A, Tarbit M, et al. Neural dysfunction during hypoglycaemia. *Arch Dis Child* 1988;**63**(11):1353–8.

62. Harris DL, Weston PJ, Harding JE. Lactate, rather than ketones, may provide alternative cerebral fuel in hypoglycaemic newborns. *Arch Dis Child Fetal Neonatal Ed* 2015;**100**(2):F161–4. https://doi.org/10.1136/archdischild-2014-306435.

63. Alsweiler JM, Kuschel CA, Bloomfield FH. Survey of the management of neonatal hyperglycaemia in Australasia. *J Paediatr Child Health* 2007;**43**(9):632–5.

64. Szymonska I, Jagla M, Starzec K, et al. The incidence of hyperglycaemia in very low birth weight preterm newborns. Results of a continuous glucose monitoring study–preliminary report. *Dev Period Med* 2015;**19**(3 Pt 1):305–12.

65. Ogilvy-Stuart AL, Beardsall K. Management of hyperglycaemia in the preterm infant. *Arch Dis Child Fetal Neonatal Ed* 2010;**95**(2):F126–31.

66. Beardsall K, Vanhaesebrouck S, Ogilvy-Stuart AL, et al. *Prevalence and determinants of hyperglycemia in very low birth weight infants: cohort analyses of the NIRTURE study. J Pediatr* 2010;**157**(5):715–9. e1–3, https://doi.org/10.1016/j.jpeds.2010.04.032.

67. Cowett RM, Susa JB, Oh W, et al. Endogenous glucose production during constant glucose infusion in the newborn lamb. *Pediatr Res* 1978;**12**(8):853–7.

68. Antonowicz I, Lebenthal E. Developmental pattern of small intestinal enterokinase and disaccharidase activities in the human fetus. *Gastroenterology* 1977;**72**(6):1299–303.

69. Lacroix B, Kedinger M, Simon-Assmann P, et al. Developmental pattern of brush border enzymes in the human fetal colon. Correlation with some morphogenetic events. *Early Hum Dev* 1984;**9**(2):95–103.

70. Mayne A, Hughes CA, Sule D, et al. Development of intestinal disaccharidases in preterm infants. *Lancet* 1983;**2**(8350):622–3.

71. Boellner SW, Beard AG, Panos TC. Impairment of intestinal hydrolysis of lactose in newborn infants. *Pediatrics* 1965;**36**(4):542–50.

72. Hawdon JM, Weddell A, Aynsley-Green A, et al. Hormonal and metabolic response to hypoglycaemia in small for gestational age infants. *Arch Dis Child* 1993;**68**(3 Spec):269–73.

73. Mitanchez D. Glucose regulation in preterm newborn infants. *Horm Res* 2007;**68**(6):265–71.

74. Santalucia T, Camps M, Castello A, et al. Developmental regulation of GLUT-1 (erythroid/Hep G2) and GLUT-4 (muscle/fat) glucose transporter expression in rat heart, skeletal muscle, and brown adipose tissue. *Endocrinology* 1992;**130**(2):837–46.

75. Cowett RM, Farrag HM. Selected principles of perinatal-neonatal glucose metabolism. *Semin Neonatol* 2004;**9**(1):37–47.

76. Sadiq HF, Das UG, Tracy TF, et al. Intra-uterine growth restriction differentially regulates perinatal brain and skeletal muscle glucose transporters. *Brain Res* 1999;**823**(1–2):96–103.

77. Slot JW, Geuze HJ, Gigengack S, et al. Translocation of the glucose transporter GLUT4 in cardiac myocytes of the rat. *Proc Natl Acad Sci U S A* 1991;**88**(17):7815–9.

78. He J, Thamotharan M, Devaskar SU. Insulin-induced translocation of facilitative glucose transporters in fetal/neonatal rat skeletal muscle. *Am J Phys Regul Integr Comp Phys* 2003;**284**(4):R1138–46.

79. Bier DM, Leake RD, Haymond MW, et al. Measurement of "true" glucose production rates in infancy and childhood with 6,6-dideuteroglucose. *Diabetes* 1977;**26**(11):1016–23.

80. Sunehag AL, Haymond MW, Schanler RJ, et al. Gluconeogenesis in very low birth weight infants receiving total parenteral nutrition. *Diabetes* 1999;**48**(4):791–800.

81. Sauer PJ, Van Aerde JE, Pencharz PB, et al. Glucose oxidation rates in newborn infants measured with indirect calorimetry and [U-13C]glucose. *Clin Sci (Lond)* 1986;**70**(6):587–93.

82. Farrag H, Cowett RM. Glucose homeostasis in the micropremie. *Clin Perinatol* 2000;**27**:1–22.

83. Iniguez G, Ong K, Bazaes R, et al. Longitudinal changes in insulin-like growth factor-I, insulin sensitivity, and secretion from birth to age three years in small-for-gestational-age children. *J Clin Endocrinol Metab* 2006;**91**(11):4645–9.

84. Fant ME, Weisoly D. Insulin and insulin-like growth factors in human development: implications for the perinatal period. *Semin Perinatol* 2001;**25**(6):426–35.

85. Woods KA, Camacho-Hubner C, Savage MO, et al. Intrauterine growth retardation and postnatal growth failure associated with deletion of the insulin-like growth factor I gene. *N Engl J Med* 1996;**335**(18):1363–7.

86. Heijboer AC, Pijl H, Van den Hoek AM, et al. Gut-brain axis: regulation of glucose metabolism. *J Neuroendocrinol* 2006;**18**(12):883–94.

87. Amin H, Holst JJ, Hartmann B, et al. Functional ontogeny of the proglucagon-derived peptide axis in the premature human neonate. *Pediatrics* 2008;**121**(1):e180–6.

88. Padidela R, Patterson M, Sharief N, et al. Elevated basal and post feed glucagon like peptide 1 (GLP-1) concentrations in the neonatal period. *Eur J Endocrinol* 2009;**160**(1):53–8. https://doi.org/10.1530/EJE-08-0807.

89. Aynsley-Green A. The endocrinology of feeding in the newborn. *Bailliere Clin Endocrinol Metab* 1989;**3**(3):837–68.

90. Philipps AF, Dubin JW, Raye JR. Maturation of early-phase insulin release in the neonatal lamb. *Biol Neonate* 1981;**39**(5–6):225–31.

91. King RA, Smith RM, Dahlenburg GW. Long term postnatal development of insulin secretion in early premature infants. *Early Hum Dev* 1986;**13**:285–94.

92. Reusens B, Remacle C. Programming of the endocrine pancreas by the early nutritional environment. *Int J Biochem Cell Biol* 2006;**38**(5–6):913–22.

93. Scaglia L, Cahill CJ, Finegood DT, et al. Apoptosis participates in the remodeling of the endocrine pancreas in the neonatal rat. *Endocrinology* 1997;**138**(4):1736–41.

94. Hill DJ, Strutt B, Arany E, et al. Increased and persistent circulating insulin-like growth factor II in neonatal transgenic mice suppresses developmental apoptosis in the pancreatic islets. *Endocrinology* 2000;**141**(3):1151–7.

95. Kaung HL. Growth dynamics of pancreatic islet cell populations during fetal and neonatal development of the rat. *Dev Dyn* 1994;**200**(2):163–75.

96. Kassem SA, Ariel I, Thornton PS, et al. Beta-cell proliferation and apoptosis in the developing normal human pancreas and in hyperinsulinism of infancy. *Diabetes* 2000;**49**(8):1325–33.

97. Hill DJ, Duvillie B. Pancreatic development and adult diabetes. *Pediatr Res* 2000;**48**(3):269–74.

98. Agudo J, Ayuso E, Jimenez V, et al. IGF-I mediates regeneration of endocrine pancreas by increasing beta cell replication through cell cycle protein modulation in mice. *Diabetologia* 2008;**51**(10):1862–72.

Chapter 35

Developmental Origins and Roles of Intestinal Enteroendocrine Hormones

Venkata S. Jonnakuti, Diana E. Stanescu and Diva D. De Leon

The Children's Hospital of Philadelphia, Perelman School of Medicine at the University of Pennsylvania, Philadelphia, PA, United States

Key Clinical Changes

- Enteroendocrine cells differentiate from multipotent endodermal precursors during intestinal villus formation.
- Enteroendocrine cells (EECs) secrete more than 30 peptide hormones and biogenic amines and collectively represents the largest endocrine organ in the body.
- The upper gastrointestinal tract secretes secretin, gastric inhibitory peptide (GIP), xenin, cholecystokinin, motilin, neurotensin, peptide YY, glucagon-like peptide 1 (GLP-1), glucagon-like peptide 2 (GLP-2), glicentin, and oxyntomodulin.
- The lower gastrointestinal tract secretes serotonin and somatostatin.
- GLP-1 plays important roles in adult glucose homeostasis, but its role in fetal and neonatal physiology is overall poorly understood.

35.1 DEVELOPMENTAL ORIGINS OF ENTEROENDOCRINE CELLS

In light of the many pathologies affecting the gut and their potential multisystemic effects, the scientific community has become increasingly interested in the developmental origins of these conditions and the possibility of applying this knowledge to develop new pharmacologic or transplant-based therapies.

35.1.1 Gastrulation and Endoderm Specification

The development of gastrointestinal (GI) lineages begins with gastrulation, which gives rise to the three primary germ layers: ectoderm, mesoderm, and endoderm. The process of gastrulation starts in the epiblast of the blastocyst and results in the formation of the primitive streak.[1] In mice, the first cells to migrate through and emerge from the primitive streak define the anterior definitive endoderm, with the mid and posterior definitive endoderm forming afterward.[2–4] Throughout this process, the newly specified definitive endoderm intercalates with the underlying visceral endoderm.[5]

As gastrulation continues, mesendoderm progenitor cells contribute to either the mesoderm or endoderm.[6,7] Exposure to Nodal, a TGF-β superfamily member, is necessary for this process, as mesendoderm progenitors exposed to low levels of Nodal specify the mesoderm while higher levels of Nodal specify the endoderm.[8–11] Activin, another TGF-β superfamily member, mimics Nodal activity and specification patterns.[12] Together, Nodal/Activin signaling separates the mesoderm and endoderm lineages.

35.1.2 Gut Tube Formation and Patterning

Upon establishment of the primary germ layers, the endodermal sheet undergoes complex morphogenetic movements to give rise to the gut tube. Invaginations of the anterior and posterior ends of the endoderm initiate gut tube closure. The anterior endodermal invagination contributes to the anterior intestinal portal (AIP), while the posterior endodermal invagination contributes to the caudal intestinal portal (CIP).[5,13] At embryonic day (e)9.0 in mouse development, the lateral endoderm of the midgut folds ventrally, allowing opposing ends of both the AIP and CIP to fuse together.[14]

Upon the conclusion of gastrulation and formation of the gut tube, anterior-posterior (A-P) domains pattern the endoderm with distinct anterior expression of Hhex, FoxA2, and Sox2 markers and posterior Cdx expression.[7,15–17] Nodal, fibroblast growth factor (FGF), Wnt, bone morphogenetic protein (BMP), and retinoic acid (RA) signaling pathways play crucial roles in the A-P patterning of the endoderm.[6,18–21] For instance, Nodal signaling establishes anterior identity while FGF4 and RA work synergistically to induce Cdx2 expression and specify posterior identity.[22] Hox factors also play important roles in gut tube patterning, with Cdx2, a ParaHox gene cluster member, driving hindgut and intestinal specification and patterning.[23,24] In fact, studies in mice have shown that conditional loss of Cdx2 in the endoderm at embryonic day (e)9.5 results in loss of intestinal identity while preserving other facets of A-P patterning.[24] As expected, the aforementioned signaling pathways regulate Cdx2 in a complex temporal, spatial, and context-specific manner.[25–28]

Throughout gut tubulogenesis and patterning, extensive cross-talk and inductive cues exist between the mesoderm and endoderm, setting the stage for organ-specific molecular domains.[17,29–31] Notably, however, cell labeling experiments show that mesodermal movements are not directly tethered to endodermal movements, allowing previously adjacent mesoderm and endoderm to localize differently.[32] Ultimately, the anterior gut tube gives rise to the esophagus, lungs, thyroid, liver, pancreas, and biliary system, while the midgut gives rise to the stomach and small intestine. The hindgut gives rise to the large intestines and the lining of the genitourinary system.[6,7, 33, 34]

35.1.3 Early Intestinal Development

Following formation of the hindgut epithelium, the intestine increases in circumference and length in accordance with the growing embryo.[35,36] Wnt and FGF signaling are critically involved in this stage of early intestinal development. For instance, Wnt5a controls gut elongation and epithelial architecture via a noncanonical Wnt signaling schema, as Wnt5a null mice exhibit greatly reduced intestinal length and disrupted apical-basal polarity of the intestinal epithelium.[36]

The pseudostratified intestinal epithelium undergoes extensive reorganization to ultimately give rise to simple columnar epithelium and nascent villi. This process begins when the endoderm transitions from a pseudostratified arrangement, in which the nuclei in a single layer of cells exist in different levels, to a stratified columnar positioning, in which cells are arranged in multiple layers.[37] Subsequently, rostral-to-caudal intestinal epithelial reorganization initiates formation of intraepithelial cavities and nascent junctional complexes within the basal layers of the stratified epithelium. Fusion of the junctional complexes with the intraepithelial cavities expands the secondary lumina, which coalesces with the primary intestinal epithelium in a simple columnar arrangement. Simultaneously, the intestinal mesenchyme invaginates into the developing columnar epithelium to form nascent villi in a rostral-to-caudal fashion.[38,39] Cellular proliferation then increases at the epithelium near the bases of these villi and becomes restricted to the intervillous epithelium and eventually only to the crypts of Lieberkuhn.

At present, the molecular mechanisms behind the morphological changes leading to intestinal epithelial reorganization and villus emergence are incompletely understood. Some known factors important for this stage of development are listed and described in Table 35.1.

35.1.4 Development of Enteroendocrine Cells

During villus emergence, most daughter cells of pluripotent stem cells migrate from the crypt base to the surface epithelial cuff, while others migrate downwards. Morphological and molecular markers begin to mark distinct epithelial cell types, such as enterocytes/colonocytes, goblet cells, tuft cells, and enteroendocrine cells. After villus and crypt development, Paneth cells begin to appear in the crypt base of the small intestine.

Enteroendocrine, goblet, tuft, and Paneth cells contain secretory granules and are collectively called *secretory cells*. Enterocytes/colonocytes, commonly referred to as *absorptive cells*, are columnar cells bearing microvilli to absorb nutrients and electrolytes. The adult intestinal epithelium is essentially composed of these secretory and absorptive cellular subtypes.

Though enteroendocrine cells (EECs) constitute less than 1% of the intestinal epithelium, this population secretes more than 30 peptide hormones and biogenic amines and collectively represents the largest endocrine organ in the body.[60,61] EECs that reach the lumen with their microvilli and can dynamically secrete hormones in response to lumen content are classified as open-type, while those that are separated by tight junctions and do not reach the lumen are classified as closed-type.[62] EECs are further subclassified by their localization to gastrointestinal tract region and specific hormone expression. The upper GI tract contains the secretin-secreting S cells; gastric inhibitory peptide (GIP) and xenin-secreting K cells; cholecystokinin-secreting I cells; motilin-secreting M cells; neurotensin-secreting N cells; and peptide YY (PYY), glucagon-like peptide 1 (GLP-1), glucagon-like peptide 2 (GLP-2), glicentin, and oxyntomodulin (OXM)-secreting L cells. The lower GI tract contains the serotonin-secreting EC cells, somatostatin-secreting D cells, and L cells.[63,64] Recent studies have shown that, regardless of subtype, individual EECs can cross-secrete variable mixtures of these hormones.[65] Therefore, an alternative EEC classification schema based on primary secretion hormone and anatomic location has been proposed.[66] Drucker suggested a classification system composed of region of the GI tract (G, gastric; J, jejunum; I, ileum; C, colon), species (M, mouse; H, human), then presence or absence of specific hormone gene expression.[66]

TABLE 35.1 Important factors for early intestinal development

Important factors	Role of the factor	Mouse phenotype of loss of function	Human phenotype
Ezrin	Apical membrane organizing protein Defines normal parameters for epithelial polarization	Gross disorganization of intestinal mucosa Aberrant villus fusion[40]	Not described
Shh and Ihh	Mediate hedgehog signaling regulating underlying mesenchyme	Shh exhibit villus overgrowth Ihh mutant mice exhibit villus undergrowth, suggesting opposing functions of these proteins.[41]	Not described
Gli/Fox transcription factors (Gli2, Gli3, FoxF1, FoxF2)	Mediate epithelial-mesenchymal crosstalk by regulating other morphogenic pathways such as Wnt and BMP signaling Facilitate villus emergence and mesenchymal expansion[42, 43]	Defective intestinal mesenchymal development Disrupted crypt-villus axis formation[44, 45]	Not described
BMPR1a receptor	Mediates BMP signaling occurring within the mesenchyme underlying nascent villi	Ectopic crypt formation on villi[46–48] Aberrant activity of Wnt, PDGF, and Hedgehog pathways[49]	Not described
PDGF-A/ PDGFR-α receptor	Mediates PDGF signaling	Abnormal folding of small intestinal villi[50]	Not described
EGF receptor	Mediates EGF signaling	Delays in intestinal epithelial reorganization Blunted villus formation[51, 52]	Not described
Epimorphin	Targets secretory vesicles to the plasma membrane of mesenchymal cells	Defects in epithelial morphogenesis and proliferation[53]	Not described
HNF4α	Maintains crypt-villus axis, mesenchymal maturation, and epithelial proliferation during early embryonic endoderm development[54]	HNF4α-null colons fail to form normal crypts. Globet-cell maturation is also perturbed.	Maturity onset diabetes of the young type 1. Gastrointestinal phenotype not described.
Elf3/Crif1	Regulates intestinal epithelial differentiation[55, 56]	Fewer, abnormal villi with defective epithelial cells and disorganized mesenchyme[57]	Not described
Nkx2.3	Regulates mesenchymal cell differentiation, villus formation, and epithelial proliferation	Significant defects in intestinal architecture[58]	Not described
Dnmt1	DNA methyltransferase Maintains genomic integrity during intestinal development and establishes crypts during perinatal intestinal development	Loss of Dnmt1 in intervillous progenitors results in DNA damage, premature differentiation, and loss of villi[59]	Not described

The other secretory and absorptive intestinal epithelial subtypes are crucial for mucus production, immune response, and nutrient absorption.[67,68] However, further discussion of the development of these cells is beyond the scope of this chapter.

Sequential binary fate decisions determine the terminal differentiation status of a pluripotent intestinal crypt stem cell. Notch signaling plays a crucial role in this process, as it separates absorptive and secretory lineages. For instance, Notch ligands Dll1 and Dll4 drive differentiation toward intestinal secretory progenitors. This signaling pathway promotes the expression of transcription factors like Neurogenin3, which marks early enteroendocrine progenitors, and BETA2/NeuroD, HES-1, and Atoh1, which mark committed endocrine precursors.[69,70] Subsequent differentiation of these progenitors into specific enteroendocrine lineages involves a complex network of transcription factors such as Nkx2.2, Insm1, Arx, Pax4, Pdx, and Pax6.[71–73]

176   Cell 161, March 26, 2015 ©2015 Elsevier Inc.   DOI http://dx.doi.org/10.1016/j.cell.2015.03.014   See online version for legend and references.

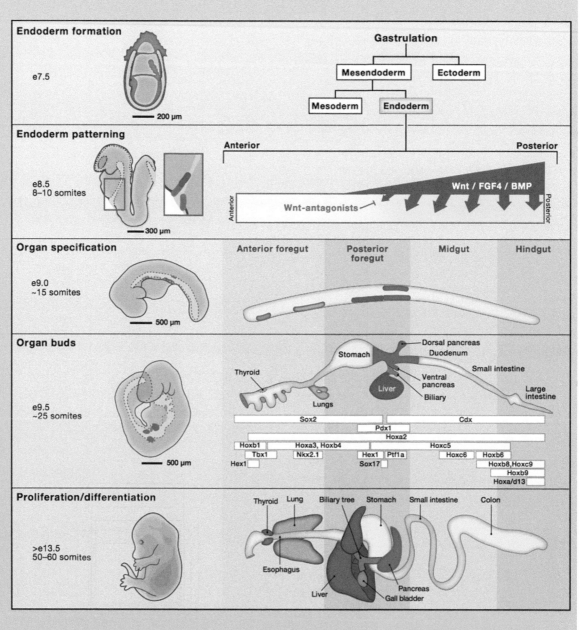

(Figure reproduced with permission from McGrath PS, Wells JM. SnapShot: GI tract development. Cell 2015;16(1):176–176.)

35.2 ROLE OF ENTEROENDOCRINE HORMONES IN FETAL AND NEONATAL HOMEOSTASIS

Unlike other endocrine glands, the enteroendocrine system is heterogenous and diffuse, allowing vigilant surveillance of luminal contents (e.g., nutrients or bacterial components) throughout the gastrointestinal tract. Many EECs possess basal cytoplasmic processes, which contain hormone vesicles and extend beneath the absorptive intestinal epithelium.[74] Presumably, these appendages function to monitor absorbed nutrients, relay electrochemical information to nerves and intestinal subepithelial myofibroblasts, and secrete hormones, the chemical messengers of the body.

In recent years, the enteroendocrine hormones have been investigated due to their pharmacologic potential in modulating metabolism and appetite. Most notably, GLP-1 agonists have become one of the main treatments for adults with type 2 diabetes and/or obesity. Other enteroendocrine hormones are under intense investigations for wide range of gastrointestinal conditions such as short bowel syndrome and inflammatory bowel disease.[66,75] Although these treatments are yet not approved for use in pediatric patients, the hope is that they will become more widely available in the years to come.

Enteroendocrine hormones, short peptides that relay information between cells of the gastrointestinal tract, are synthesized, stored, and secreted by highly specialized EECs. These hormones are implicated in several physiological functions such as food intake, postprandial digestion, gut motility, exocrine and endocrine pancreatic secretion, as well as cellular growth. This section will discuss the specific role(s) that these hormones play in the regulation of homeostasis.

35.2.1 Cholecystokinin

Meals consisting of fats and proteins stimulate small intestinal I cell-mediated secretion of cholecystokinin (CCK).[76] This hormone binds to the CCK-1 receptor found on pancreatic acinar cells, gastric smooth muscle, peripheral nerves, and the gallbladder. Primary functions include potent stimulation of pancreatic secretion and gallbladder contraction, as well as regulation of gastric and intestinal motility. CCK also plays a role in inducing satiety.

35.2.2 Glucose-Dependent Insulinotropic Peptide

In the presence of nutrients, namely glucose and fat, within the lumen of the GI tract, small intestinal K cells secrete glucose-dependent insulinotropic peptide or gastric inhibitory polypeptide (GIP). This 42-amino acid hormone functions to inhibit gastric acid secretion while also enhancing insulin secretion.[77] The GIP receptor is expressed in adipocytes and in pancreatic beta cells. In adipocytes, GIP functions to increase triglyceride storage, leading to fat accumulation.

35.2.3 Glicentin

Intestinal enteroendocrine hormones belonging to the proglucagon family include GLP-1, GLP-2, OXM, and glicentin. While other members have been well studied, glicentin, mainly produced by L cells, has not yet been fully characterized. Food intake and loading of glucose, lipids, and proteins into the duodenum stimulates glicentin secretion.[78,79] Glicentin primarily functions to stimulate intestinal mucosal enterocyte proliferation as well as inhibit gastric emptying, the phenomenon by which the contents of the stomach enter the small intestine.[80] In addition, a recent study has suggested that this hormone protects the mucosa by preventing *bacterial* translocation.[81]

35.2.4 Glucagon-Like Peptide-1

Meals containing carbohydrates, fat, and protein result in GABA-mediated activation of L cells, which release GLP-1.[82–84] The incretin effect is defined as enhanced insulin secretion after ingestion of glucose compared with insulin secretion after an intravenous glucose load.[85] Both GLP-1 and GIP (described previously) are incretin hormones. GLP-1 has a complex role in glucose homeostasis and metabolism in general by acting on GLP-1 receptors found in multiple organs.[85] It delays gastric emptying and inhibits gastric acid and pancreatic exocrine secretions presumably via neural circuitry.[86,87] Studies have also suggested that GLP-1 negatively regulates energy intake by inducing postprandial satiety by acting on the hypothalamus and brain stem.[88,89] In preclinical and clinical studies, GLP-1 agonists were shown to increase lipolysis and glucose uptake by adipocytes and to increase glycogen synthesis and glucose oxidation in the muscle.[90] Lastly, GLP-1 has a crucial impact on pancreatic islet function: it stimulates insulin secretion from pancreatic beta cells and inhibits glucagon secretion from pancreatic alpha cells.[91] It also stimulates beta cell mass expansion by increasing beta cell proliferation and promoting beta cell survival.[92] However, at least in mice, loss of GLP-1 receptors (GLP-1R) on pancreatic beta cells did not affect normal oral glucose tolerance in lean mice.[93]

The role of GLP-1 secretion in fetal and neonatal physiology is overall poorly understood. Padidela et al. showed that both preterm and term neonates show very high elevated circulating amidated GLP-1 ([7–36] amide and [9–36] amide) in response to feeding. They postulated that this significant elevation in GLP-1 in neonatal period may have a role in EEC maturation or in ensuring the well-described pancreatic beta cell mass expansion characteristic of this age.[94] In parallel, Salis et al. showed that very preterm infants (less than 32 weeks gestation) were more insulin resistant and fed neonates had higher GLP-1 levels compared with never fed babies, confirming that onset of enteral feeding is important in modulating insulin secretion partially through a GLP-1 dependent mechanism.[95]

As pharmacologic agents, GLP-1 agonists are widely used for treatment of type 2 diabetes and obesity in adults. Recent studies have proposed the use of the GLP-1 receptor antagonist exendin-(9–39) in the treatment of hyperinsulinemic hypoglycemia.[96,97]

A more intriguing GLP-1 role in neonatal metabolism comes from studies in mice. Rozo et al. found that administration of a GLP-1 agonist to mice in the first week of life reduced adult body weight and fat mass, increased energy expenditure, and protected female mice from diet-induced obesity.[98] These effects were due to durable GLP-1-induced changes both in adipose tissue and in hypothalamic architecture.[98] Their findings suggest that a short-term intervention in neonatal period could have a long-lasting impact on risk of diabetes and obesity in adulthood.

35.2.5 Glucagon-Like Peptide-2

The same conditions for GLP-1 release apply for GLP-2, as these hormones are often co-secreted by L cells. However, unlike GLP-1, GLP-2 does not affect plasma glucose homeostasis; rather, this hormone stimulates mucosal epithelial growth and proliferation, especially within the small intestine.[80,99,100] Similar to GLP-1, GLP-2 concentrations increase after feeding. GLP-2 is present during fetal and neonatal gut development in rat and pig, and it is thought to play a role in the maturation of the intestine.[101,102]

In line with this proposed role, neonatal piglets with distal intestinal resection treated with intravenous GLP-2 showed improved intestinal adaptation and supported a potential clinical use for GLP-2 in neonatal-pediatric short bowel syndrome.[103] Furthermore, GLP-2 treatment was shown to have a beneficial role in a neonatal piglet model of parental nutrition associated liver disease, by regulating bile acid synthesis and increasing bile acid export.[104]

35.2.6 Motilin

A time-dependent cyclical pattern rather than bolus ingestion triggers motilin secretion by M cells embedded in the duodenal epithelium. This hormone binds to specific GPCRs on smooth muscle and other receptors found throughout the GI tract. Its key role is to regulate GI motility by stimulating smooth muscle contraction and propulsion in the third trimester of fetal life.[105] Motilin levels were significantly higher in full term neonates that had passed meconium antenatally, compared with those neonates that had not.[106]

35.2.7 Neurotensin

Ingested fat potently stimulates neurotensin (NT) release by N cells, which are scattered throughout the jejuno-ileum epithelium.[107] Gastric acid facilitates protein digestion; iron, calcium, vitamin B12, and thyroxin absorption; as well as prevention of bacterial overgrowth and infection. Neurotensin is a brain-gut peptide, acting as a neurotransmitter in the CNS and a hormone in the GI tract. In the intestine, neurotensin acts in concert with other enteroendocrine hormones, such as GIP, GLP-1, and secretin, to negatively regulate gastric acid secretion, as uninhibited levels of gastric acid can lead to maldigestion and ulcers.[108] In addition, NT inhibits gastric and duodenal motor activity and coordinates blood flow to optimize digestion and postprandial distribution of absorbed fat.[109,110] Several studies have also implicated NT in mediating intestinal inflammatory responses by activating mast cells, neutrophils, T cells, and macrophages.[111–115]

35.2.8 Oxyntomodulin

Ingestion of nutrients triggers the release of oxyntomodulin (OXM) from intestinal L-cells. Acting as an anorectic peptide, OXM inhibits calorie intake by suppressing plasma ghrelin levels and signaling satiety.[116,117] OXM can further enhance weight loss by augmenting energy expenditure, as studies have reported increases in voluntary activity in humans and increases in heart rate in rodents following OXM infusions.[118,119] In addition, this hormone mediates the incretin effect and inhibits gastric emptying.[120,121] Studies suggest that these effects are typically exerted through the GLP-1 receptor, but similar dosage effects of both OXM and GLP-1, despite the significantly lower binding affinity of OXM to GLP-1 receptor compared with GLP-1, indicate that another receptor for OXM may have yet to be identified.[122]

35.2.9 Peptide YY

Meals containing fat stimulate the secretion of peptide YY (PYY), especially by intestinal L-cells situated in the ileum and colon. Acting as an "ileal brake," this hormone inhibits GI motility as well as chloride, gastric, and pancreatic exocrine secretions.[123] Notably, PYY has also been implicated in decreasing appetite and food intake by producing postprandial satiety.[124-126] Studies have also suggested that PYY stimulates colonic epithelial cell growth and proliferation to maintain mucosal integrity.[127]

PYY levels surge after birth in neonates and is thought to be part of the postnatal adaptation to enteral nutrition.[128] Similar to GLP-1, PYY levels are higher in preterm than in full-term infants, and levels had a negative correlation with anthropometric measurements at birth.[129]

35.2.10 Secretin

In response to acidification of the duodenum, small intestinal S cells secrete secretin, which bind and activate receptors on pancreatic acinar cells, stimulating pancreatic exocrine secretions.[130] This hormone is most notably known to increase levels of pancreatic fluid and bicarbonate to neutralize the otherwise acidic chime.[131] Other effects of secretin include inhibition of gastric acid secretion and regulation of GI motility. Secretin has been found in cord blood, and levels increased after birth.[132]

35.2.11 Serotonin

Though commonly thought of as only a neurotransmitter of the central nervous system, serotonin (5-hydroxytryptamine, 5-HT) is predominantly secreted by enterochromaffin (EC) cells embedded in the intestinal mucosa.[133] At present, the secretory conditions for this hormone are incompletely understood, though studies have implicated chemical stimulants such as short-chain fatty acids, neural reflexes, and mechanical activation of EC cells caused by distention of the GI tract.[134-136] Within the GI tract, 5-HT binds to receptors that activate neural circuitry, interstitial cells, and myocytes to ultimately stimulate gut motility and secretion, visceral sensation, appetite, as well as cellular growth and proliferation.[137] Based on studies in neonatal guinea pigs, Bian et al. postulated that the postnatal maturation of the 5HT signaling may contribute to the development of intestinal motor reflexes.[138]

35.2.12 Somatostatin

Somatostatin is secreted by neural cells in the hypothalamus, delta cells in the pancreas, and D cells in the GI tract.[139] Meals consisting of fats and glucose, low gastric pH, and neural input stimulate somatostatin release within the GI tract. Somatostatin reduces the release of all other known GI hormones and primarily works to inhibit the actions of these compounds via endocrine, paracrine, or neuroendocrine mechanisms. A recent study shows that somatostatin results in EEC contraction, whereby hormone-carrying secretory vesicles translocate from the cell periphery to the perinuclear region.[140] Within the GI tract, somatostatin decreases acid secretion, pancreatic endocrine/exocrine function, splanchnic blood flow, GI motility, as well as cell growth and proliferation. In addition to its inhibitory effects, somatostatin also facilitates activity of the migrating myoelectric complex (MMC), patterns of GI smooth muscle contractions between meals to clear residual undigested material through the digestive tract.[141] The somatostatin analogue octreotide has been used off-label to treat a variety of neonatal conditions, such as chylothorax, congenital hyperinsulinism, GI bleeding, and pleural effusion; however, significant side effects limit its use.[142,143]

35.2.13 Xenin

Xenin, a NT-related hormone with poorly understood physiological functions, is secreted by K cells in the duodenal mucosa.[144] It is known, though, that xenin increases the rate of duodenal ion secretion. In fact, studies have shown that postprandial, peripherally released xenin augments HCO_3^- and Cl^- secretion through the activation of afferent nerves.[145] Xenin also augments the release of calcium and acetylcholine from myenteric neurons.[146]

35.3 CONCLUSION

Remarkable progress has been made in identifying the pathways and molecular mechanisms responsible for the development of endocrine and neuroendocrine hormone-producing intestinal cells. Despite these efforts, understanding the fetal and neonatal physiology of enteric hormones remains limited. However, therapies aimed at modulating their action have proven to benefit a variety of conditions in the neonatal and pediatric age group. One of the directions of investigation remains in vitro differentiation of stem cells to recapitulate all intestinal cellular fates. Unfortunately, differentiation protocols do not completely recapitulate embryonic development, and cells made via these techniques often fail to attain their mature form and function, highlighting gaps in our understanding of GI development and cytodifferentiation of the intestinal epithelium. Additional work is required to ultimately develop robust pharmacologic and transplantation-based therapies for use in the pediatric age group.

REFERENCES

1. Lawson KA, Pedersen RA. Cell fate, morphogenetic movement and population kinetics of embryonic endoderm at the time of germ layer formation in the mouse. *Development* 1987;**101**(3):627–52.
2. Lawson KA, Meneses JJ, Pedersen RA. Cell fate and cell lineage in the endoderm of the presomite mouse embryo, studied with an intracellular tracer. *Dev Biol* 1986;**115**(2):325–39.
3. Kimura W, Yasugi S, Stern CD, Fukuda K. Fate and plasticity of the endoderm in the early chick embryo. *Dev Biol* 2006;**289**(2):283–95.
4. Tam PP, Loebel DA. Gene function in mouse embryogenesis: get set for gastrulation. *Nat Rev Genet* 2007;**8**(5):368–81.
5. Franklin V, Khoo PL, Bildsoe H, Wong N, Lewis S, Tam PP. Regionalisation of the endoderm progenitors and morphogenesis of the gut portals of the mouse embryo. *Mech Dev* 2008;**125**(7):587–600.
6. Zorn AM, Wells JM. Molecular basis of vertebrate endoderm development. *Int Rev Cytol* 2007;**259**:49–111.
7. Zorn AM, Wells JM. Vertebrate endoderm development and organ formation. *Annu Rev Cell Dev Biol* 2009;**25**:221–51.
8. Ben-Haim N, Lu C, Guzman-Ayala M, Pescatore L, Mesnard D, Bischofberger M, Naef F, Robertson EJ, Constam DB. The nodal precursor acting via activin receptors induces mesoderm by maintaining a source of its convertases and BMP4. *Dev Cell* 2006;**11**(3):313–23.
9. Hagos EG, Dougan ST. Time-dependent patterning of the mesoderm and endoderm by nodal signals in zebrafish. *BMC Dev Biol* 2007;**7**:22.
10. Tada S, Era T, Furusawa C, Sakurai H, Nishikawa S, Kinoshita M, Nakao K, Chiba T, Nishikawa S. Characterization of mesendoderm: a diverging point of the definitive endoderm and mesoderm in embryonic stem cell differentiation culture. *Development* 2005;**132**(19):4363–74.
11. Shen MM. Nodal signaling: developmental roles and regulation. *Development* 2007;**134**(6):1023–34.
12. Gray PC, Harrison CA, Vale W. Cripto forms a complex with activin and type II activin receptors and can block activin signaling. *Proc Natl Acad Sci U S A* 2003;**100**(9):5193–8.
13. Tam PP, Khoo PL, Wong N, Tsang TE, Behringer RR. Regionalization of cell fates and cell movement in the endoderm of the mouse gastrula and the impact of loss of Lhx1(Lim1) function. *Dev Biol* 2004;**274**(1):171–87.
14. Lewis SL, Tam PP. Definitive endoderm of the mouse embryo: formation, cell fates, and morphogenetic function. *Dev Dyn* 2006;**235**(9):2315–29.
15. Chawengsaksophak K, de Graaff W, Rossant J, Deschamps J, Beck F. Cdx2 is essential for axial elongation in mouse development. *Proc Natl Acad Sci U S A* 2004;**101**(20):7641–5.
16. Kinkel MD, Eames SC, Alonzo MR, Prince VE. Cdx4 is required in the endoderm to localize the pancreas and limit beta-cell number. *Development* 2008;**135**(5):919–29.
17. Sherwood RI, Chen TY, Melton DA. Transcriptional dynamics of endodermal organ formation. *Dev Dyn* 2009;**238**(1):29–42.
18. Vincent SD, Dunn NR, Hayashi S, Norris DP, Robertson EJ. Cell fate decisions within the mouse organizer are governed by graded nodal signals. *Genes Dev* 2003;**17**(13):1646–62.
19. Duboc V, Rottinger E, Besnardeau L, Lepage T. Nodal and BMP2/4 signaling organizes the oral-aboral axis of the sea urchin embryo. *Dev Cell* 2004;**6**(3):397–410.
20. Lu CC, Robertson EJ. Multiple roles for nodal in the epiblast of the mouse embryo in the establishment of anterior-posterior patterning. *Dev Biol* 2004;**273**(1):149–59.
21. Pan FC, Chen Y, Bayha E, Pieler T. Retinoic acid-mediated patterning of the pre-pancreatic endoderm in Xenopus operates via direct and indirect mechanisms. *Mech Dev* 2007;**124**(7–8):518–31.
22. Johannesson M, Stahlberg A, Ameri J, Sand FW, Norrman K, Semb H. FGF4 and retinoic acid direct differentiation of hESCs into PDX1-expressing foregut endoderm in a time- and concentration-dependent manner. *PLoS ONE* 2009;**4**(3).
23. Gao N, White P, Kaestner KH. Establishment of intestinal identity and epithelial-mesenchymal signaling by Cdx2. *Dev Cell* 2009;**16**(4):588–99.
24. Grainger S, Savory JG, Lohnes D. Cdx2 regulates patterning of the intestinal epithelium. *Dev Biol* 2010;**339**(1):155–65.
25. Beland M, Lohnes D. Chicken ovalbumin upstream promoter-transcription factor members repress retinoic acid-induced Cdx1 expression. *J Biol Chem* 2005;**280**(14):13858–62.
26. Keenan ID, Sharrard RM, Isaacs HV. FGF signal transduction and the regulation of Cdx gene expression. *Dev Biol* 2006;**299**(2):478–88.
27. Pilon N, Oh K, Sylvestre JR, Bouchard N, Savory J, Lohnes D. Cdx4 is a direct target of the canonical Wnt pathway. *Dev Biol* 2006;**289**(1):55–63.
28. Joo JH, Taxter TJ, Munguba GC, Kim YH, Dhaduvai K, Dunn NW, Degan WJ, Oh SP, Sugrue SP. Pinin modulates expression of an intestinal homeobox gene, Cdx2, and plays an essential role for small intestinal morphogenesis. *Dev Biol* 2010;**345**(2):191–203.

29. Sugi Y, Markwald RR. Endodermal growth factors promote endocardial precursor cell formation from precardiac mesoderm. *Dev Biol* 2003;**263**(1):35–49.

30. Serls AE, Doherty S, Parvatiyar P, Wells JM, Deutsch GH. Different thresholds of fibroblast growth factors pattern the ventral foregut into liver and lung. *Development* 2005;**132**(1):35–47.

31. Wandzioch E, Zaret KS. Dynamic signaling network for the specification of embryonic pancreas and liver progenitors. *Science* 2009;**324**(5935):1707–10.

32. Tremblay KD, Zaret KS. Distinct populations of endoderm cells converge to generate the embryonic liver bud and ventral foregut tissues. *Dev Biol* 2005;**280**(1):87–99.

33. Seifert AW, Harfe BD, Cohn MJ. Cell lineage analysis demonstrates an endodermal origin of the distal urethra and perineum. *Dev Biol* 2008;**318**(1):143–52.

34. McLin VA, Henning SJ, Jamrich M. The role of the visceral mesoderm in the development of the gastrointestinal tract. *Gastroenterology* 2009;**136**(7):2074–91.

35. Lepourcelet M, Tou L, Cai L, Sawada J, Lazar AJ, Glickman JN, Williamson JA, Everett AD, Redston M, Fox EA, et al. Insights into developmental mechanisms and cancers in the mammalian intestine derived from serial analysis of gene expression and study of the hepatoma-derived growth factor (HDGF). *Development* 2005;**132**(2):415–27.

36. Cervantes S, Yamaguchi TP, Hebrok M. Wnt5a is essential for intestinal elongation in mice. *Dev Biol* 2009;**326**(2):285–94.

37. Trier JS, Moxey PC. Morphogenesis of the small intestine during fetal development. *CIBA Found Symp* 1979;(70):3–29.

38. Matsumoto A, Hashimoto K, Yoshioka T, Otani H. Occlusion and subsequent re-canalization in early duodenal development of human embryos: integrated organogenesis and histogenesis through a possible epithelial-mesenchymal interaction. *Anat Embryol* 2002;**205**(1):53–65.

39. Toyota T, Yamamoto M, Kataoka K. Light and electron microscope study on developing intestinal mucosa in rat fetuses with special reference to the obliteration of the intestinal lumen. *Arch Histol Cytol* 1989;**52**(1):51–60.

40. Saotome I, Curto M, McClatchey AI. Ezrin is essential for epithelial organization and villus morphogenesis in the developing intestine. *Dev Cell* 2004;**6**(6):855–64.

41. Ramalho-Santos M, Melton DA, McMahon AP. Hedgehog signals regulate multiple aspects of gastrointestinal development. *Development* 2000;**127**(12):2763–72.

42. Kaestner KH, Silberg DG, Traber PG, Schutz G. The mesenchymal winged helix transcription factor Fkh6 is required for the control of gastrointestinal proliferation and differentiation. *Genes Dev* 1997;**11**(12):1583–95.

43. Ormestad M, Astorga J, Landgren H, Wang T, Johansson BR, Miura N, Carlsson P. Foxf1 and Foxf2 control murine gut development by limiting mesenchymal Wnt signaling and promoting extracellular matrix production. *Development* 2006;**133**(5):833–43.

44. Mao J, Kim BM, Rajurkar M, Shivdasani RA, McMahon AP. Hedgehog signaling controls mesenchymal growth in the developing mammalian digestive tract. *Development* 2010;**137**(10):1721–9.

45. Madison BB, Braunstein K, Kuizon E, Portman K, Qiao XT, Gumucio DL. Epithelial hedgehog signals pattern the intestinal crypt-villus axis. *Development* 2005;**132**(2):279–89.

46. Batts LE, Polk DB, Dubois RN, Kulessa H. Bmp signaling is required for intestinal growth and morphogenesis. *Dev Dyn* 2006;**235**(6):1563–70.

47. Howe JR, Bair JL, Sayed MG, Anderson ME, Mitros FA, Petersen GM, Velculescu VE, Traverso G, Vogelstein B. Germline mutations of the gene encoding bone morphogenetic protein receptor 1A in juvenile polyposis. *Nat Genet* 2001;**28**(2):184–7.

48. He XC, Zhang J, Tong WG, Tawfik O, Ross J, Scoville DH, Tian Q, Zeng X, He X, Wiedemann LM, et al. BMP signaling inhibits intestinal stem cell self-renewal through suppression of Wnt-beta-catenin signaling. *Nat Genet* 2004;**36**(10):1117–21.

49. Haramis AP, Begthel H, van den Born M, van Es J, Jonkheer S, Offerhaus GJ, Clevers H. De novo crypt formation and juvenile polyposis on BMP inhibition in mouse intestine. *Science* 2004;**303**(5664):1684–6.

50. Karlsson L, Lindahl P, Heath JK, Betsholtz C. Abnormal gastrointestinal development in PDGF-A and PDGFR-(alpha) deficient mice implicates a novel mesenchymal structure with putative instructive properties in villus morphogenesis. *Development* 2000;**127**(16):3457–66.

51. Miettinen PJ, Berger JE, Meneses J, Phung Y, Pedersen RA, Werb Z, Derynck R. Epithelial immaturity and multiorgan failure in mice lacking epidermal growth factor receptor. *Nature* 1995;**376**(6538):337–41.

52. Duh G, Mouri N, Warburton D, Thomas DW. EGF regulates early embryonic mouse gut development in chemically defined organ culture. *Pediatr Res* 2000;**48**(6):794–802.

53. Hirai Y, Takebe K, Takashina M, Kobayashi S, Takeichi M. Epimorphin: a mesenchymal protein essential for epithelial morphogenesis. *Cell* 1992;**69**(3):471–81.

54. Garrison WD, Battle MA, Yang C, Kaestner KH, Sladek FM, Duncan SA. Hepatocyte nuclear factor 4alpha is essential for embryonic development of the mouse colon. *Gastroenterology* 2006;**130**(4):1207–20.

55. Ng AY, Waring P, Ristevski S, Wang C, Wilson T, Pritchard M, Hertzog P, Kola I. Inactivation of the transcription factor Elf3 in mice results in dysmorphogenesis and altered differentiation of intestinal epithelium. *Gastroenterology* 2002;**122**(5):1455–66.

56. Kwon MC, Koo BK, Kim YY, Lee SH, Kim NS, Kim JH, Kong YY. Essential role of CR6-interacting factor 1 (Crif1) in E74-like factor 3 (ELF3)-mediated intestinal development. *J Biol Chem* 2009;**284**(48):33634–41.

57. Flentjar N, Chu PY, Ng AY, Johnstone CN, Heath JK, Ernst M, Hertzog PJ, Pritchard MA. TGF-betaRII rescues development of small intestinal epithelial cells in Elf3-deficient mice. *Gastroenterology* 2007;**132**(4):1410–9.

58. Pabst O, Zweigerdt R, Arnold HH. Targeted disruption of the homeobox transcription factor Nkx2-3 in mice results in postnatal lethality and abnormal development of small intestine and spleen. *Development* 1999;**126**(10):2215–25.

59. Elliott EN, Sheaffer KL, Schug J, Stappenbeck TS, Kaestner KH. Dnmt1 is essential to maintain progenitors in the perinatal intestinal epithelium. *Development* 2015;**142**(12):2163–72.

60. Gunawardene AR, Corfe BM, Staton CA. Classification and functions of enteroendocrine cells of the lower gastrointestinal tract. *Int J Exp Pathol* 2011;**92**(4):219–31.

61. Rehfeld JF. A centenary of gastrointestinal endocrinology. *Horm Metab Res* 2004;**36**(11–12):735–41.

62. Tolhurst G, Reimann F, Gribble FM. Intestinal sensing of nutrients. *Handb Exp Pharmacol* 2012;**209**:309–35.

63. Coate KC, Kliewer SA, Mangelsdorf DJ. SnapShot: hormones of the gastrointestinal tract. *Cell* 2014;**159**(6):1478 [e1471].

64. Posovszky C, Wabitsch M. Regulation of appetite, satiation, and body weight by enteroendocrine cells. Part 1: characteristics of enteroendocrine cells and their capability of weight regulation. *Horm Res Paediatr* 2015;**83**(1):1–10.

65. Grun D, Lyubimova A, Kester L, Wiebrands K, Basak O, Sasaki N, Clevers H, van Oudenaarden A. Single-cell messenger RNA sequencing reveals rare intestinal cell types. *Nature* 2015;**525**(7568):251–5.

66. Drucker DJ. Evolving concepts and translational relevance of enteroendocrine cell biology. *J Clin Endocrinol Metab* 2016;**101**(3):778–86.

67. Grencis RK, Worthington JJ. Tuft cells: a new flavor in innate epithelial immunity. *Trends Parasitol* 2016;**32**(8):583–5.

68. Clevers HC, Bevins CL. Paneth cells: maestros of the small intestinal crypts. *Annu Rev Physiol* 2013;**75**:289–311.

69. Li HJ, Ray SK, Singh NK, Johnston B, Leiter AB. Basic helix-loop-helix transcription factors and enteroendocrine cell differentiation. *Diabetes Obes Metab* 2011;**13**(Suppl. 1):5–12.

70. Jenny M, Uhl C, Roche C, Duluc I, Guillermin V, Guillemot F, Jensen J, Kedinger M, Gradwohl G. Neurogenin3 is differentially required for endocrine cell fate specification in the intestinal and gastric epithelium. *EMBO J* 2002;**21**(23):6338–47.

71. Beucher A, Gjernes E, Collin C, Courtney M, Meunier A, Collombat P, Gradwohl G. The homeodomain-containing transcription factors Arx and Pax4 control enteroendocrine subtype specification in mice. *PLoS ONE* 2012;**7**(5).

72. Du A, McCracken KW, Walp ER, Terry NA, Klein TJ, Han A, Wells JM, May CL. Arx is required for normal enteroendocrine cell development in mice and humans. *Dev Biol* 2012;**365**(1):175–88.

73. Engelstoft MS, Egerod KL, Lund ML, Schwartz TW. Enteroendocrine cell types revisited. *Curr Opin Pharmacol* 2013;**13**(6):912–21.

74. Bohorquez DV, Liddle RA. Axon-like basal processes in enteroendocrine cells: characteristics and potential targets. *Clin Transl Sci* 2011;**4**(5):387–91.

75. Mace OJ, Tehan B, Marshall F. Pharmacology and physiology of gastrointestinal enteroendocrine cells. *Pharmacol Res Perspect* 2015;**3**(4).

76. Iwai K, Fukuoka S, Fushiki T, Tsujikawa M, Hirose M, Tsunasawa S, Sakiyama F. Purification and sequencing of a trypsin-sensitive cholecystokinin-releasing peptide from rat pancreatic juice. Its homology with pancreatic secretory trypsin inhibitor. *J Biol Chem* 1987;**262**(19):8956–9.

77. Usdin TB, Mezey E, Button DC, Brownstein MJ, Bonner TI. Gastric inhibitory polypeptide receptor, a member of the secretin-vasoactive intestinal peptide receptor family, is widely distributed in peripheral organs and the brain. *Endocrinology* 1993;**133**(6):2861–70.

78. Ohneda A, Takahashi H, Maruyama Y. Response of plasma glicentin to fat ingestion in piglets. *Diabetes Res Clin Pract* 1987;**3**(2):103–9.

79. Ohneda A, Kobayashi T, Nihei J, Takahashi H. Effect of intraluminal administration of amino acids upon plasma glicentin. *Diabetes Res Clin Pract* 1988;**5**(4):265–70.

80. Drucker DJ. Biological actions and therapeutic potential of the glucagon-like peptides. *Gastroenterology* 2002;**122**(2):531–44.

81. Chiba M, Sanada Y, Kawano S, Murofushi M, Okada I, Yoshizawa Y, Gomi A, Yatsuzuka M, Toki A, Hirai Y. Glicentin inhibits internalization of enteric bacteria by cultured INT-407 enterocytes. *Pediatr Surg Int* 2007;**23**(6):551–4.

82. Gameiro A, Reimann F, Habib AM, O'Malley D, Williams L, Simpson AK, Gribble FM. The neurotransmitters glycine and GABA stimulate glucagon-like peptide-1 release from the GLUTag cell line. *J Physiol* 2005;**569**(3Pt. 3):761–72.

83. Tian L, Jin T. The incretin hormone GLP-1 and mechanisms underlying its secretion. *J Diabetes* 2016;**8**(6):753–65.

84. Elliott RM, Morgan LM, Tredger JA, Deacon S, Wright J, Marks V. Glucagon-like peptide-1 (7-36)amide and glucose-dependent insulinotropic polypeptide secretion in response to nutrient ingestion in man: acute post-prandial and 24-h secretion patterns. *J Endocrinol* 1993;**138**(1):159–66.

85. Andersen A, Lund A, Knop FK, Vilsboll T. Glucagon-like peptide 1 in health and disease. *Nat Rev Endocrinol* 2018;**14**(7):390–403.

86. Wettergren A, Schjoldager B, Mortensen PE, Myhre J, Christiansen J, Holst JJ. Truncated GLP-1 (proglucagon 78-107-amide) inhibits gastric and pancreatic functions in man. *Dig Dis Sci* 1993;**38**(4):665–73.

87. Holst JJ. The physiology of glucagon-like peptide 1. *Physiol Rev* 2007;**87**(4):1409–39.

88. Verdich C, Flint A, Gutzwiller JP, Naslund E, Beglinger C, Hellstrom PM, Long SJ, Morgan LM, Holst JJ, Astrup A. A meta-analysis of the effect of glucagon-like peptide-1 (7-36) amide on ad libitum energy intake in humans. *J Clin Endocrinol Metab* 2001;**86**(9):4382–9.

89. Tang-Christensen M, Vrang N, Larsen PJ. Glucagon-like peptide 1(7-36) amide's central inhibition of feeding and peripheral inhibition of drinking are abolished by neonatal monosodium glutamate treatment. *Diabetes* 1998;**47**(4):530–7.

90. Villanueva-Penacarrillo ML, Marquez L, Gonzalez N, Diaz-Miguel M, Valverde I. Effect of GLP-1 on lipid metabolism in human adipocytes. *Horm Metab Res* 2001;**33**(2):73–7.

91. Mari A, Schmitz O, Gastaldelli A, Oestergaard T, Nyholm B, Ferrannini E. Meal and oral glucose tests for assessment of beta -cell function: modeling analysis in normal subjects. *Am J Physiol Endocrinol Metab* 2002;**283**(6):E1159–66.

92. Buteau J. GLP-1 receptor signaling: effects on pancreatic beta-cell proliferation and survival. *Diabetes Metab* 2008;**34**(Suppl. 2):S73–7.

93. Smith EP, An Z, Wagner C, Lewis AG, Cohen EB, Li B, Mahbod P, Sandoval D, Perez-Tilve D, Tamarina N, et al. The role of beta cell glucagon-like peptide-1 signaling in glucose regulation and response to diabetes drugs. *Cell Metab* 2014;**19**(6):1050–7.

94. Padidela R, Patterson M, Sharief N, Ghatei M, Hussain K. Elevated basal and post-feed glucagon-like peptide 1 (GLP-1) concentrations in the neonatal period. *Eur J Endocrinol* 2009;**160**(1):53–8.

95. Salis ER, Reith DM, Wheeler BJ, Broadbent RS, Medlicott NJ. Insulin resistance, glucagon-like peptide-1 and factors influencing glucose homeostasis in neonates. *Arch Dis Child Fetal Neonatal Ed* 2017;**102**(2):F162–6.

96. Calabria AC, Charles L, Givler S, De Leon DD. Postprandial hypoglycemia in children after gastric surgery: clinical characterization and pathophysiology. *Horm Res Paediatr* 2016;**85**(2):140–6.

97. Calabria AC, Li C, Gallagher PR, Stanley CA, De Leon DD. GLP-1 receptor antagonist exendin-(9-39) elevates fasting blood glucose levels in congenital hyperinsulinism owing to inactivating mutations in the ATP-sensitive K+ channel. *Diabetes* 2012;**61**(10):2585–91.

98. Rozo AV, Babu DA, Suen PA, Groff DN, Seeley RJ, Simmons RA, Seale P, Ahima RS, Stoffers DA. Neonatal GLP1R activation limits adult adiposity by durably altering hypothalamic architecture. *Mol Metab* 2017;**6**(7):748–59.

99. Tsai CH, Hill M, Asa SL, Brubaker PL, Drucker DJ. Intestinal growth-promoting properties of glucagon-like peptide-2 in mice. *Am J Phys* 1997;**273**(1 Pt 1):E77–84.

100. Ghatei MA, Goodlad RA, Taheri S, Mandir N, Brynes AE, Jordinson M, Bloom SR. Proglucagon-derived peptides in intestinal epithelial proliferation: glucagon-like peptide-2 is a major mediator of intestinal epithelial proliferation in rats. *Dig Dis Sci* 2001;**46**(6):1255–63.

101. Lovshin J, Yusta B, Iliopoulos I, Migirdicyan A, Dableh L, Brubaker PL, Drucker DJ. Ontogeny of the glucagon-like peptide-2 receptor axis in the developing rat intestine. *Endocrinology* 2000;**141**(11):4194–201.

102. Burrin DG, Stoll B, Guan X, Cui L, Chang X, Holst JJ. Glucagon-like peptide 2 dose-dependently activates intestinal cell survival and proliferation in neonatal piglets. *Endocrinology* 2005;**146**(1):22–32.

103. Suri M, Turner JM, Sigalet DL, Wizzard PR, Nation PN, Ball RO, Pencharz PB, Brubaker PL, Wales PW. Exogenous glucagon-like peptide-2 improves outcomes of intestinal adaptation in a distal-intestinal resection neonatal piglet model of short bowel syndrome. *Pediatr Res* 2014;**76**(4):370–7.

104. Lim DW, Wales PW, Mi S, Yap JY, Curtis JM, Mager DR, Mazurak VC, Wizzard PR, Sigalet DL, Turner JM. Glucagon-like peptide-2 alters bile acid metabolism in parenteral nutrition—associated liver disease. *JPEN J Parenter Enteral Nutr* 2016;**40**(1):22–35.

105. Peeters TL, Depoortere I. Motilin receptor: a model for development of prokinetics. *Dig Dis Sci* 1994;**39**(12 Suppl):76S–78S.

106. Mahmoud EL, Benirschke K, Vaucher YE, Poitras P. Motilin levels in term neonates who have passed meconium prior to birth. *J Pediatr Gastroenterol Nutr* 1988;**7**(1):95–9.

107. Zhao D, Pothoulakis C. Effects of NT on gastrointestinal motility and secretion, and role in intestinal inflammation. *Peptides* 2006;**27**(10):2434–44.

108. Schubert ML. Hormonal regulation of gastric acid secretion. *Curr Gastroenterol Rep* 2008;**10**(6):523–7.

109. Kihl B, Rokaeus A, Rosell S, Olbe L. Fat inhibition of gastric acid secretion in man and plasma concentrations of neurotensin-like immunoreactivity. *Scand J Gastroenterol* 1981;**16**(4):513–26.

110. Thor K, Rokaeus A, Kager L, Rosell S. (Gln4)-neurotensin and gastrointestinal motility in man. *Acta Physiol Scand* 1980;**110**(3):327–8.

111. Goldman R, Bar-Shavit Z. On the mechanism of the augmentation of the phagocytic capability of phagocytic cells by Tuftsin, substance P, neurotensin, and kentsin and the interrelationship between their receptors. *Ann N Y Acad Sci* 1983;**419**:143–55.

112. Lazarus LH, Perrin MH, Brown MR. Mast cell binding of neurotensin. I. Iodination of neurotensin and characterization of the interaction of neurotensin with mast cell receptor sites. *J Biol Chem* 1977;**252**(20):7174–9.

113. Lazarus LH, Perrin MH, Brown MR, Rivier JE. Mast cell binding of neurotensin. II. Molecular conformation of neurotensin involved in the stereospecific binding to mast cell receptor sites. *J Biol Chem* 1977;**252**(20):7180–3.

114. Robbins RA, Nelson KJ, Gossman GL, Rubinstein I. Neurotensin stimulates neutrophil adherence to bronchial epithelial cells in vitro. *Life Sci* 1995;**56**(16):1353–9.

115. Evers BM, Bold RJ, Ehrenfried JA, Li J, Townsend Jr CM, Klimpel GR. Characterization of functional neurotensin receptors on human lymphocytes. *Surgery* 1994;**116**(2):134–9 [discussion 139–140].

116. Dakin CL, Gunn I, Small CJ, Edwards CM, Hay DL, Smith DM, Ghatei MA, Bloom SR. Oxyntomodulin inhibits food intake in the rat. *Endocrinology* 2001;**142**(10):4244–50.

117. Cohen MA, Ellis SM, Le Roux CW, Batterham RL, Park A, Patterson M, Frost GS, Ghatei MA, Bloom SR. Oxyntomodulin suppresses appetite and reduces food intake in humans. *J Clin Endocrinol Metab* 2003;**88**(10):4696–701.

118. Dakin CL, Small CJ, Batterham RL, Neary NM, Cohen MA, Patterson M, Ghatei MA, Bloom SR. Peripheral oxyntomodulin reduces food intake and body weight gain in rats. *Endocrinology* 2004;**145**(6):2687–95.

119. Wynne K, Park AJ, Small CJ, Meeran K, Ghatei MA, Frost GS, Bloom SR. Oxyntomodulin increases energy expenditure in addition to decreasing energy intake in overweight and obese humans: a randomised controlled trial. *Int J Obes* 2006;**30**(12):1729–36.

120. Schjoldager B, Mortensen PE, Myhre J, Christiansen J, Holst JJ. Oxyntomodulin from distal gut. Role in regulation of gastric and pancreatic functions. *Dig Dis Sci* 1989;**34**(9):1411–9.

121. Dakin CL, Small CJ, Park AJ, Seth A, Ghatei MA, Bloom SR. Repeated ICV administration of oxyntomodulin causes a greater reduction in body weight gain than in pair-fed rats. *Am J Physiol Endocrinol Metab* 2002;**283**(6):E1173–7.

122. Baggio LL, Huang Q, Brown TJ, Drucker DJ. Oxyntomodulin and glucagon-like peptide-1 differentially regulate murine food intake and energy expenditure. *Gastroenterology* 2004;**127**(2):546–58.

123. Ballantyne GH. Peptide YY(1-36) and peptide YY(3-36): part I. Distribution, release and actions. *Obes Surg* 2006;**16**(5):651–8.

124. Suzuki K, Simpson KA, Minnion JS, Shillito JC, Bloom SR. The role of gut hormones and the hypothalamus in appetite regulation. *Endocr J* 2010;**57**(5):359–72.

125. Batterham RL, Cohen MA, Ellis SM, Le Roux CW, Withers DJ, Frost GS, Ghatei MA, Bloom SR. Inhibition of food intake in obese subjects by peptide YY3-36. *N Engl J Med* 2003;**349**(10):941–8.

126. Dietrich MO, Horvath TL. Feeding signals and brain circuitry. *Eur J Neurosci* 2009;**30**(9):1688–96.

127. Mannon PJ. Peptide YY as a growth factor for intestinal epithelium. *Peptides* 2002;**23**(2):383–8.

128. Adrian TE, Smith HA, Calvert SA, Aynsley-Green A, Bloom SR. Elevated plasma peptide YY in human neonates and infants. *Pediatr Res* 1986; **20**(12):1225–7.

129. Siahanidou T, Mandyla H, Vounatsou M, Anagnostakis D, Papassotiriou I, Chrousos GP. Circulating peptide YY concentrations are higher in preterm than full-term infants and correlate negatively with body weight and positively with serum ghrelin concentrations. *Clin Chem* 2005; **51**(11):2131–7.

130. Bayliss WM, Starling EH. The mechanism of pancreatic secretion. *J Physiol* 1902;**28**(5):325–53.

131. Li P, Lee KY, Chang TM, Chey WY. Mechanism of acid-induced release of secretin in rats. Presence of a secretin-releasing peptide. *J Clin Invest* 1990;**86**(5):1474–9.

132. Rogers IM, Davidson DC, Lawrence J, Buchanan KD. Neonatal secretion of secretin. *Arch Dis Child* 1975;**50**(2):120–2.

133. Hasler WL. Serotonin and the GI tract. *Curr Gastroenterol Rep* 2009;**11**(5):383–91.

134. Fukumoto S, Tatewaki M, Yamada T, Fujimiya M, Mantyh C, Voss M, Eubanks S, Harris M, Pappas TN, Takahashi T. Short-chain fatty acids stimulate colonic transit via intraluminal 5-HT release in rats. *Am J Phys Regul Integr Comp Phys* 2003;**284**(5):R1269–76.

135. Modlin IM, Kidd M, Pfragner R, Eick GN, Champaneria MC. The functional characterization of normal and neoplastic human enterochromaffin cells. *J Clin Endocrinol Metab* 2006;**91**(6):2340–8.

136. Spiller R. Serotonin and GI clinical disorders. *Neuropharmacology* 2008;**55**(6):1072–80.

137. Costedio MM, Hyman N, Mawe GM. Serotonin and its role in colonic function and in gastrointestinal disorders. *Dis Colon Rectum* 2007; **50**(3):376–88.

138. Bian X, Patel B, Dai X, Galligan JJ, Swain G. High mucosal serotonin availability in neonatal Guinea pig ileum is associated with low serotonin transporter expression. *Gastroenterology* 2007;**132**(7):2438–47.

139. Low MJ. Clinical endocrinology and metabolism. The somatostatin neuroendocrine system: physiology and clinical relevance in gastrointestinal and pancreatic disorders. *Best Pract Res Clin Endocrinol Metab* 2004;**18**(4):607–22.

140. Saras J, Gronberg M, Stridsberg M, Oberg KE, Janson ET. Somatostatin induces rapid contraction of neuroendocrine cells. *FEBS Lett* 2007; **581**(10):1957–62.

141. Peeters TL, Janssens J, Vantrappen GR. Somatostatin and the interdigestive migrating motor complex in man. *Regul Pept* 1983;**5**(3):209–17.

142. McMahon AW, Wharton GT, Thornton P, De Leon DD. Octreotide use and safety in infants with hyperinsulinism. *Pharmacoepidemiol Drug Saf* 2017;**26**(1):26–31.

143. Testoni D, Hornik CP, Neely ML, Yang Q, McMahon AW, Clark RH, Smith PB. Best pharmaceuticals for children act—pediatric trials network administrative core C: safety of octreotide in hospitalized infants. *Early Hum Dev* 2015;**91**(7):387–92.

144. Cho YM, Kieffer TJ. K-cells and glucose-dependent insulinotropic polypeptide in health and disease. *Vitam Horm* 2010;**84**:111–50.

145. Kaji I, Akiba Y, Kato I, Maruta K, Kuwahara A, Kaunitz JD. Xenin augments duodenal anion secretion via activation of afferent neural pathways. *J Pharmacol Exp Ther* 2017;**361**(1):151–61.

146. Zhang S, Hyrc K, Wang S, Wice BM. Xenin-25 increases cytosolic free calcium levels and acetylcholine release from a subset of myenteric neurons. *Am J Physiol Gastrointest Liver Physiol* 2012;**303**(12):G1347–55.

Chapter 36

Development and Function of the Adrenal Cortex and Medulla in the Fetus and Neonate

Sonir R. Antonini, Monica F. Stecchini and Fernando S. Ramalho
Ribeirao Preto Medical School, University of Sao Paulo, Sao Paulo, Brazil

Key Clinical Changes

- A common embryonic origin explains the co-occurrence of adrenal cortex and gonadal defects in some patients.
- The adrenal cortex and adrenal medulla have different origins, functions, and regulations. Therefore, defects affecting these two components are extremely rare.
- Neonatal levels of dehydroepiandrosterone/dehydroepiandrosterone sulfate (DHEA/DHEAS) are very high due to the presence of the fetal zone in the adrenal cortex. However, in the weeks and months after birth, DHEA/DHEAS levels decline rapidly due to the involution of this zone.
- A normal diurnal cortisol circadian rhythm is established early (between birth and 3 months of life).

36.1 INTRODUCTION

The adrenal glands are bilateral structures located above the kidneys. They consist of two parts, the cortex and the medulla, which differ in origin, composition, and function. The adrenal cortex, the outer part, derives from the mesoderm, is composed of steroidogenic cells, and synthetizes steroid hormones. The adrenal medulla, the inner part, derives from the neuroectoderm, is composed of chromaffin cells, and synthetizes catecholamines. Cortical and medullary cells have intimate contact during both the prenatal and postnatal periods.[1]

These glands are an important element for fetal development and maturation, and, hence, for the transition from fetal to neonatal life. Their appropriate function during the prenatal period involves maternal, placental, and fetal interactions, and is crucial for several processes that can affect the fetus itself, the neonate, and even the future adult. After birth, they play an essential role in survival, adaptive responses to stress, fluid homeostasis, and development of secondary sexual characteristics.[2, 3]

This chapter reviews the embryology, physiology, and endocrinology of the adrenals. Although there has been considerable advance in the knowledge about these glands, some aspects of their development and function during the fetal and the neonatal periods have not been fully described or understood.

36.2 ADRENAL DEVELOPMENT

The development of the human adrenals begins early in embryogenesis and continues into adult life. Although the most important milestones of this process are known, the exact timing in which they occur varies among the studies in this area.[2, 4–11] Figs. 36.1 and 36.2 illustrate the stages of adrenal prenatal and postnatal development.

36.2.1 Prenatal Period

The two components of the adrenals have different embryologic origins. While the cortex is derived from cells of the intermediate mesoderm,[2, 5] the medulla is derived from cells of the neuroectoderm.[8] The urogenital ridge is the common embryologic precursor of the adrenal cortex, gonad, and kidney.[2, 5]

Maternal-Fetal and Neonatal Endocrinology. https://doi.org/10.1016/B978-0-12-814823-5.00036-2

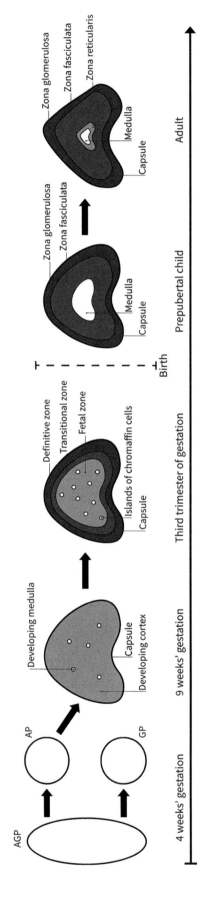

FIG. 36.1 Development of the adrenal cortex and medulla. At 4 weeks' gestation, cells from the intermediate mesoderm start to form the AGP, which will later originate both the adrenal and the gonadal primordium (AP and GP, respectively). At 7 weeks, sympathogonia cells from the neuroectoderm start to migrate into the AP, forming islands of cells, which will later differentiate into neuroblasts and pheochromoblasts to form the adrenal medulla after birth. The adrenal continues to develop during the postnatal period, until it is fully differentiated in adulthood. The major postnatal changes are the involution of the fetal zone right after birth and the development of the zona reticularis during childhood.

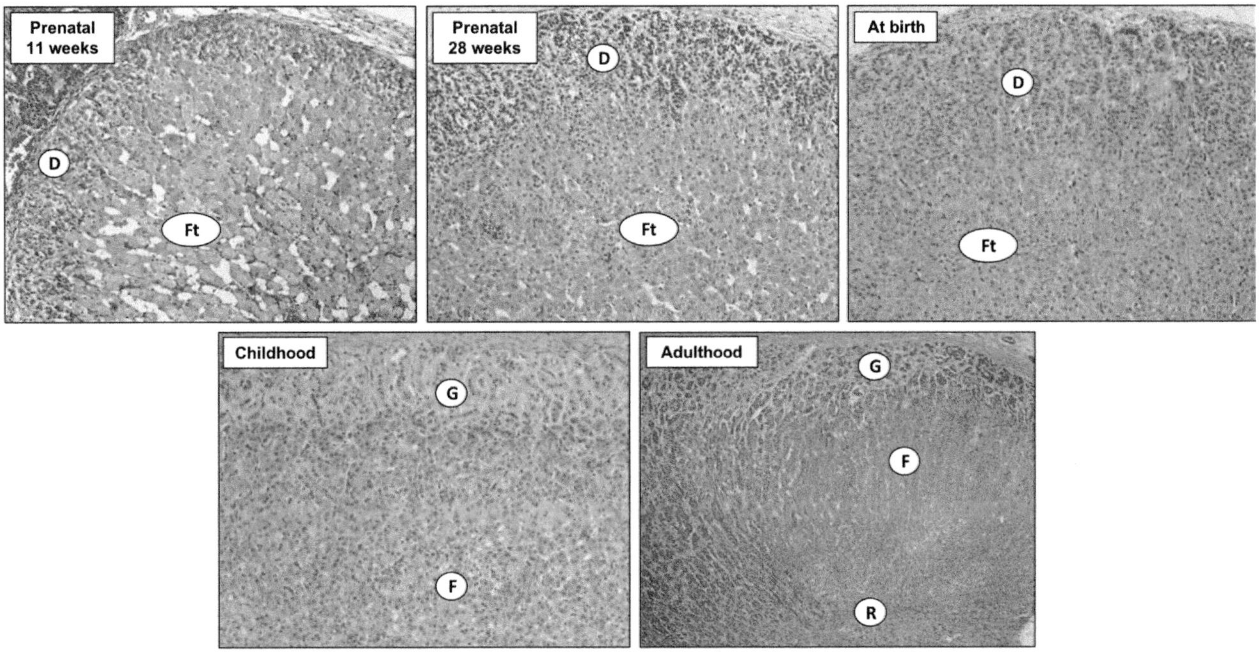

FIG. 36.2 Photomicrographs of the adrenal cortex, showing the spectrum of morphological changes during the development of the gland. In the fetus, the fetal zone (Ft) corresponds to 80%–90% of the adrenal cortex (*Prenatal 11 and 28 weeks—HE 100 × magnification*). At birth, the fetal zone begins its regression, concomitant with the modification of the definitive (D) and transitional zones (*HE 100 × magnification*). The prepubertal adrenal cortex consists only of the zona glomerulosa (G) and fasciculata (F). In the adult cortex, the innermost layer is the zona reticularis (R—*Childhood and adulthood—HE 100 × and 40 × magnification, respectively*).

At about 4 weeks' gestation, a group of cells arises from the coelomic epithelium (intermediate mesoderm), to form the bilateral **adrenogonadal primordium** (AGP). Each AGP contains a mixed population of adrenocortical and gonadal progenitor cells. A subset of cells from the cephalic part of the AGP migrates dorsomedially to form the **adrenal primordium** (AP), which settles ventrolateral to the dorsal aorta.[2, 5]

At about 7 weeks' gestation, cells from the primitive sympathetic nervous system—which are derived from the neural crest and located dorsally to the aorta—migrate to the AP area. These cells, called *sympathogonia*, enter the AP and form small islands, which remain scattered throughout the developing cortex until birth. They differentiate into two types of cells, neuroblasts and pheochromoblasts, to form the future adrenal medulla.[8]

Concomitantly, mesenchymal cells from the area of the Bowman's capsule migrate to form a fibrous **capsule** around the developing adrenal. This process is usually complete at about 9 weeks.[2, 5] At 8 weeks, the rudimentary adrenal cortex consists of an inner layer, the **fetal zone**, and a newly emerging outer layer, the **definitive zone**. After midgestation, a third layer, the **transitional zone,** which is derived from the definitive zone, appears between these two zones.[2, 5, 10]

The prenatal adrenals are very large in proportion to other structures; at midgestation, their size is similar to that of the kidneys, and they continue to grow until the third trimester of gestation. This intrauterine growth depends mostly on the enlargement of the fetal zone and involves a complex interplay of cell proliferation, hypertrophy, migration, and apoptosis. The mass of the fetal zone increases exponentially in late gestation, especially in the last 6 weeks, and reaches more than 80% of the adrenal gland.[2, 5]

36.2.2 Postnatal Period

During the neonatal period, the adrenals continue to undergo significant remodeling. At birth, their weight is 8–10 g, which is twice the weight of adult adrenals, but it decreases to about 2 g during the first 2 weeks of postnatal life. The involution of the fetal zone by apoptosis is responsible for this reduction. This process can be divided into two distinct phases: the rapid one—from birth until the end of the second week—and the subsequent slower one, which is usually complete by 3–6 months. However, there are marked individual variations in the rate of involution, and elements of the fetal zone may persist until the end of the second year.[7, 12, 13] As the fetal zone regresses, chromaffin cells coalesce to form a rudimentary medulla; the medulla only becomes mature at the age of 12–18 months.[8]

Meanwhile, the definitive and transitional zones form the adult adrenal cortex. The zona glomerulosa and the zona fasciculata, which may begin to differentiate during the late prenatal period or even after birth, proliferate and become mature by the age of 2–3 years. The zona reticularis appears only at the age of 6–8 years in girls and 7–9 years in boys, during a process named *adrenarche*. Until then, only focal islands of reticularis cells can be identified after the age of 3–4 years. The development of this zone, however, may not be complete until the age of 10–20 years.[10, 14–16]

36.3 ADRENAL CORTEX

36.3.1 Structure and Function

The adrenal cortex is composed of morphologically and functionally distinct zones during both the prenatal and the postnatal periods. Its main function is to synthetize a variety of steroid hormones. The specific characteristics and steroidogenic enzymes present in each zone define their function and, hence, their hormone synthesis. Based on these features, it has been proposed that the prenatal zones are analogous to the adult ones. Therefore, the definitive, the transitional, and the fetal zones correspond to the zona glomerulosa, the zona fasciculata, and the zona reticularis, respectively.[2, 5]

The origin and maintenance of the distinct adrenocortical zones are not fully understood, but numerous studies suggest the involvement of stem or progenitor cells. According to the most accepted hypothesis, these cells, located in the periphery of the adrenals, proliferate and migrate centripetally to populate the zones. As the cells move toward the center, they become functionally differentiated in the appropriate environment. Conversely, most of the cell deaths occur in the central area of the adrenals, between the cortex and the medulla. There is evidence to support this theory in both the prenatal and the postnatal periods.[2, 15–17]

36.3.1.1 Prenatal Adrenal Cortex

By the third trimester of gestation, three adrenocortical zones are morphologically and functionally distinguishable.[2, 7, 10] The definitive zone—the outermost layer—is composed of small and densely packed cells with basophilic cytoplasm. These cells exhibit typical ultrastructural characteristics of cells in the proliferative state: free ribosomes, small and dense mitochondria with lamelliform cristae, and scant lipids. As gestation advances, some of these cells also accumulate cytoplasmic lipids and begin to resemble cells with steroidogenic activity. During late gestation, they acquire the capacity to synthetize mineralocorticoids (aldosterone), which only seem to be required postnatally.[1, 2, 7, 10, 18]

The transitional zone—the middle layer—has cells that are arranged as cords, with intermediate characteristics from the two other zones. During the third trimester, this zone begins to synthetize glucocorticoids (cortisol). The increased cortisol levels in this period induce the differentiation of fetal tissues and the maturation necessary for postnatal life.[2, 7, 10, 18, 19]

The fetal zone—the innermost and largest layer—is composed of large cells with abundant eosinophilic cytoplasm and round nucleus (high cytoplasmic/nuclear ratio). During most of gestation, this zone has the highest steroidogenic activity and synthetizes large quantities of DHEA and DHEAS. DHEA and DHEAS, the main steroids produced during fetal life, are used by the placenta as estrogen precursors. Mitotic figures are scant in the fetal zone, as opposed to the definitive zone.[2, 5, 7, 19]

The extent of the contribution of the fetal adrenal steroids in the maintenance of pregnancy, in the maturation of fetal organs, and in the initiation of parturition, is still unclear and a matter of debate.[1]

36.3.1.2 Neonatal Adrenal Cortex

The neonatal period is a transition phase, critical to the adaptation to extrauterine life. The significant morphological and functional changes that begin in the late prenatal period and continue in the neonatal period prepare the adrenal cortex for its essential postnatal roles and ensure its autonomy once the placenta is separated. It is not clear, however, whether some of these changes are determined by gestational age or by birth itself.[2, 20–23]

The histologic regression of the fetal zone is accompanied by a rapid decrease in DHEA and DHEAS levels. Nevertheless, they may still be abundant in the neonate, especially in the first few days of postnatal life. The development of the zona glomerulosa and the zona fasciculata is accompanied by increased aldosterone secretion and a surge—followed by a gradual decline—of cortisol levels. While aldosterone secretion is essential to avoid salt loss, cortisol is required to prevent adrenal insufficiency in the neonatal period. After this period of adaptation, in contrast to DHEA and DHEAS, the synthesis and secretion of both aldosterone and cortisol remain somewhat constant postnatally.[1, 2, 19]

36.3.1.3 Adult Adrenal Cortex

The adult adrenal cortex represents 80%–90% of the size of the adrenal. In comparison to the correspondent prenatal zones, there is a significant change in the proportion that the zona glomerulosa, the zona fasciculata, and the zona reticularis occupy in the adult adrenal cortex.[1, 9, 10]

The zona glomerulosa, located under the capsule, comprises about 15% of the cortex and is composed of ovoid cells that synthetize mineralocorticoids (mainly aldosterone). Although this zone presents as a full zone in children with low salt diets, in adults with high salt consumption, its cells are scattered in clusters beneath the capsule, called *aldosterone-producing cell clusters (APCCs)*. Aldosterone is involved in the maintenance of intravascular volume and electrolyte balance.[1, 9, 10]

The zona fasciculata, in the middle, becomes the largest layer—it comprises about 75% of the cortex. It is composed of large cells, organized into radial cords or bundles (known as *fascicles*), which synthetize glucocorticoids (mainly cortisol). Cortisol is involved in glucose homeostasis and in the mobilization of energy stores.[1, 9, 10]

The zona reticularis, in contact with the medulla, comprises about 10% of the cortex. It is composed of cords of cells, projected in different directions, similar to a net (*reticulum* means "net"), which synthetize androgen precursors (mainly DHEA, which is mostly sulfated to DHEAS, and androstenedione) after adrenarche. DHEA and androstenedione serve as substrates for sex steroid (testosterone and estradiol) synthesis in peripheral tissues and, therefore, contribute to secondary sexual characteristics.[1, 9, 10, 14]

36.3.2 Physiology

36.3.2.1 Prenatal Period

36.3.2.1.1 Fetal Hypothalamic-Pituitary-Adrenal Axis

The fetal hypothalamic-pituitary-adrenal (HPA) axis (Fig. 36.3) begins to function early in the prenatal period: its hormone activity can be detected at 8–12 weeks' gestation. However, fine-tuning among the elements of this axis is not reached until late gestation. This axis is stimulated by stress and mediates the physiological responses to it, in coordination with the sympathetic nervous system. The magnitude of these responses matures with gestational age.[3, 24–26]

In the fetal hypothalamus, the parvocellular neurons of the paraventricular nucleus (PVN) synthetize corticotropin-releasing hormone (CRH), which stimulates the pituitary corticotrophs through CRH receptor 1. Consequently, the fetal anterior pituitary synthetizes pro-opiomelanocortin (POMC), which is subsequently cleaved to the adrenocorticotrophic hormone (ACTH). ACTH binds to the transmembrane melanocortin-receptor 2 (MC2R) in adrenocortical cells and enhances cortisol and DHEAS synthesis. In turn, cortisol inhibits excessive further CRH and ACTH release by negative feedback.[1, 3]

ACTH from the fetal pituitary is considered the main regulator of adrenocortical development and function. However, placental factors, as well as locally produced factors, also contribute significantly to the regulation of these processes by acting independent of, or in concert with, this hormone.[2, 3, 27]

ACTH effects on growth are partially mediated by locally produced growth factors, such as insulin-like growth factor 2 (IGF2), basic fibroblast growth factor (bFGF), and epidermal growth factor (EGF), which stimulate cellular hyperplasia and hypertrophy. In addition, ACTH promotes the transcription of genes that encode various steroidogenic enzymes and other factors involved in hormone synthesis.[2, 5, 27]

Disorders in which ACTH signaling is impaired—such as congenital malformations with absence of the pituitary gland—result in adrenal hypoplasia. Anencephalic fetuses, for example, develop significantly smaller adrenals due to

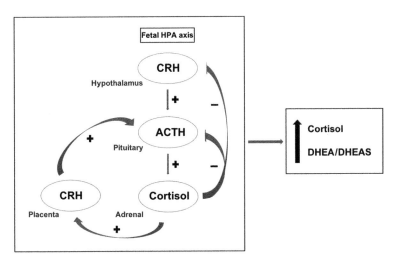

FIG. 36.3 The fetal HPA axis. The fetal hypothalamus synthetizes CRH, which stimulates the pituitary corticotrophs to synthetize and release ACTH. ACTH enhances the synthesis of cortisol and DHEA, as well as its sulfate (DHEAS), in adrenocortical cells. In turn, cortisol inhibits excessive further CRH and ACTH release by negative feedback. Placental CRH stimulates the fetal HPA axis. However, unlike pituitary CRH, placental CRH is stimulated by cortisol. The consequent feed-forward loop increases the synthesis of cortisol and DHEA/DHEAS.

reduced size of the fetal zone and the medulla. However, normal adrenal development is observed until 10–15 weeks' gestation, the size of the definitive zone is preserved, and the overall steroidogenic capacity is retained. These observations suggest that the trophic effects of this hormone may be zone-specific, and that adrenal growth and steroidogenesis may be indeed regulated by both ACTH-dependent and independent mechanisms. Besides the evidence that structural development of the definitive zone is not completely dependent on ACTH, the rapid postnatal involution of the fetal zone in normal newborns also reinforces that ACTH is not the only factor that regulates the growth and maintains the structure and function of this zone.[2, 5, 7]

36.3.2.1.2 Placental Factors

The placenta is also an important source of CRH, which is released into fetal and maternal circulation. Placental CRH is identical to hypothalamic CRH in structure and bioactivity. Nevertheless, in contrast to hypothalamic CRH, which is inhibited by elevated cortisol levels, placental CRH is stimulated by cortisol. In the fetus, placental CRH stimulates the synthesis and secretion of pituitary ACTH, as well as enhances the adrenal response to ACTH. This positive feedback loop (known as a *feed-forward loop*) leads to increased cortisol and DHEA/DHEAS synthesis. Because the concentration of placental CRH increases as gestation advances toward term and reaches its peak at the onset of labor, it is thought to play a role in the parturition process.[2, 5, 19, 28]

Another crucial placental factor is 11β-HSD2 (11β-hydroxysteroid dehydrogenase type 2), which inactivates cortisol to cortisone. This enzyme is an essential regulator of fetal exposure to maternal cortisol. It inactivates 80%–90% of cortisol, thus avoiding the possible detrimental effects of excessive maternal cortisol in fetal circulation. During the first half of gestation, its activity is low, allowing passive transmission of maternal cortisol to the fetus. During the last trimester, however, its activity increases markedly, converting both maternal and fetal cortisol to cortisone. Hence, it decreases cortisol negative feedback on the fetal HPA, stimulating the synthesis of fetal ACTH, cortisol, and DHEA/DHEAS and contributing to further development of the adrenals. Placental estrogen, synthetized from fetal DHEAS, stimulates 11β-HSD2, and this feed-forward loop continues until parturition.[2, 5, 19, 28, 29]

36.3.2.1.3 Prenatal Exposure to Glucocorticoids

As a consequence of fetal-placental-maternal interactions, cortisol levels in the fetal circulation are usually very low until the third trimester of gestation. However, perturbation of any of these three elements may result in fetal exposure to elevated cortisol levels. The fetus may be passively exposed to excess maternal cortisol, either from maternal production (due to increased maternal stress or under nutrition, for example) or from decreased activity of placental 11β-HSD2. Conversely, the fetus may actively secrete increased amounts of cortisol in response to stimulatory factors, such as in the event of inflammation (chorioamnionitis).[19, 29–31]

Increased fetal exposure to glucocorticoids in late gestation may influence the responses of fetal and neonatal HPA axis.[3, 19] While passive exposure to glucocorticoids suppresses the HPA axis, stimulus of this axis enhances its responses to stress. Transient suppression of the HPA axis may follow the use of exogenous prenatal glucocorticoids for the advancement of lung maturation, but this practice is considered safe because recovery of the axis is achieved by most newborns at the end of the first week of life.[24, 32] Because the HPA axis is highly susceptible to programming by early environmental changes, different forms of prenatal stress may permanently affect neuroendocrine and cognitive/behavioral responses. This condition has been associated with the development of diseases in adulthood, such as cardiovascular disease and type 2 diabetes mellitus.[33–35]

36.3.2.2 Neonatal Period

At birth, placental supply of CRH, estrogen, and progesterone to the fetus is suddenly discontinued, and 11β-HSD2 activity is suddenly collapsed.[2, 3, 31]

The HPA axis is upregulated toward the time of delivery, leading to a surge in cortisol levels at birth, followed by a gradual decline. As in the late prenatal period, cortisol is synthetized by the developing zona fasciculata at a basal level, but it can be stimulated by CRH (and, hence, ACTH) under stress. As part of the feedback control of the HPA axis, cortisol then inhibits CRH and ACTH.[2, 3]

The transition from the intrauterine "aquatic" environment to the extrauterine "terrestrial" life leads to hyperactivation of the renin-angiotensin-aldosterone system, and, consequently, to increased aldosterone secretion by the developing zona glomerulosa. In this system, renin (from the juxtaglomerular cells of the kidney) converts angiotensinogen (synthetized in the liver) to angiotensinogen I, which is converted to angiotensin II by angiotensin-converting enzyme (ACE) in the lung. Despite the hyperactivation of this system, neonates have transient and partial aldosterone resistance, associated with undetectable renal mineralocorticoid receptor expression. This is an adaptive mechanism to prevent excessive water and salt reabsorption and to remove extracellular volume excess.[36, 37]

36.3.2.3 Adulthood

In the adult adrenal, the HPA axis regulates cortisol synthesis in the zona fasciculata and androgen synthesis in the zona reticularis, while the renin-angiotensin-aldosterone system regulates aldosterone synthesis in the zona glomerulosa. The mechanisms that regulate the development and function of the zona reticularis, however, have not been fully elucidated. Although ACTH secretion is constant throughout the postnatal period, androgen secretion resumes only after adrenarche.[1, 10, 14]

36.3.3   Adrenal Steroidogenesis

To understand the peculiarities of prenatal and neonatal steroidogenesis, it is important to review the adrenal steroidogenic process in the adult adrenal (Fig. 36.4). The hormones produced in the adult adrenal cortex—aldosterone, cortisol, and DHEA/DHEAS—have a common precursor: cholesterol. The steroidogenic acute regulatory protein (**StAR**) transfers cholesterol from the outer to the inner mitochondrial membrane. It, therefore, provides the substrate for the initial, rate-limiting, and hormonally regulated step of steroidogenesis: the conversion of cholesterol to pregnenolone by **P450scc** (the cholesterol side-chain cleavage enzyme—the *CYP11A1* gene). Subsequently, the specific enzymes expressed in each zone determine the fate of pregnenolone metabolism.[1]

In the zona glomerulosa, the coexpression of **3βHSD2** (3β-hydroxysteroid dehydrogenase—the *HSD3B2* gene), **P450c21** (21-hydroxylase—the *CYP21A2* gene) and **P450c11AS** (aldosterone synthase—the *CYP11B2* gene) leads aldosterone synthesis.[1] In the zona fasciculata, the coexpression of **P450c17** (with its 17α-hydroxylase activity—the *CY17A1* gene), **3βHSD2**, **P450c21**, and **P450c11β** (11β-hydroxylase—the *CYP11B1* gene) results in cortisol synthesis.[1]

In the zona reticularis, the coexpression of **P450c17** and **cytochrome *b*5** (the *CYB5A* gene) selectively activates the 17,20-lyase activity of P450c17, resulting in the synthesis of DHEA, much of which is sulfated to DHEAS, by **SULT2A1** (DHEA-sulfotransferase—the *SULT2A1* gene). In this zone, small amounts of accumulated DHEA may be converted by **3βHSD2** to androstenedione, little of which is then converted by **17βHSD5** (17β-hydroxysteroid dehydrogenase type 5—the *ARK1C3* gene) to testosterone. However, unlike in the other zones, there is little expression of **3βHSD2** in zona reticularis. Importantly, after the first year of life, DHEA, DHEAS, and androstenedione synthesis is very low and increases only after adrenarche.[1, 14]

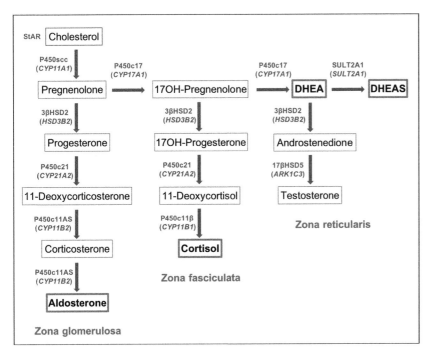

FIG. 36.4 Adrenal steroidogenesis. The main hormones produced in the adult adrenal cortex are aldosterone, cortisol and DHEA, as well as its sulfate (DHEAS). Initially, StAR transfers cholesterol to the inner mitochondrial membrane, providing the substrate for the initial step of steroidogenesis: the conversion of cholesterol to pregnenolone by the cholesterol side-chain cleavage enzyme (P450scc). Subsequently, the specific enzymes expressed in each zone—glomerulosa, fasciculata, or reticularis—determine the fate of pregnenolone metabolism.

36.3.3.1 Prenatal Period

The fetal adrenal cortex and the placenta are responsible for most aspects of prenatal steroidogenesis, with participation of the fetal liver and the testes (in male fetuses). Close interaction between the fetal adrenal cortex and the placenta is required because both of them have incomplete steroidogenic pathways. This cooperation, which enables adequate hormone synthesis and intrauterine homeostasis, has been named "the fetoplacental unit."[1–3, 7]

The adrenal cortex acquires the ability to synthetize and to secrete steroid hormones as early as 6–8 weeks' gestation, but it lacks certain enzymes required for complete steroidogenesis until late gestation. The time course of expression of steroidogenic enzymes determines the zonal differential steroidogenic activity and its onset. Basically, the prenatal steroidogenic activity is characterized by early transient cortisol synthesis, followed by its suppressed synthesis until late gestation, and extensive DHEA/DHEAS synthesis during most of the gestation period.[1–3, 7]

Among the three zones, the fetal zone has the highest steroidogenic activity. Its expression of **P450c17, cytochrome** $b5$, and **SULT2A1** enables the synthesis of large quantities of DHEA and DHEAS. The placenta uses these androgen precursors for estrogen synthesis because it lacks the enzyme P450c17 and cannot synthesize estrogen de novo. While most of DHEAS undergoes modifications in the fetal liver and then in the placenta to produce estriol, small amounts of it bypass the liver and are directly converted to estrone and estradiol in the placenta. The fetoplacental unit is responsible for 50% of the estrone and estradiol, and for 90% of the estriol in the maternal circulation.[1–3, 7]

An important characteristic of the fetal zone is that it does not express 3βHSD2, which is necessary for de novo cortisol and aldosterone synthesis. However, transient expression of this enzyme at about 7–12 weeks enables cortisol synthesis, with a peak at 8–9 weeks. Although the physiological significance of cortisol synthesis in the first trimester remains unclear, the concomitance with the period of sexual differentiation of the external genitalia (7–10 weeks) provides a clue. It is presumed that the transient early adrenal cortisol synthesis causes suppression of the HPA axis to inhibit adrenal androgen secretion and, therefore, to prevent virilization of the female fetus. After this period, the expression of this enzyme decreases, and the cortisol de novo synthesis is suppressed.[1–3, 7, 38]

After 23–24 weeks, the transitional zone expresses **3βHSD2**. However, de novo cortisol synthesis only begins in this zone in late gestation (after 30 weeks).[1–3, 7]

The definitive zone does not express the enzymes required for aldosterone synthesis until after midgestation. It only acquires the ability to synthesize mineralocorticoids in late gestation.[1–3, 7]

36.3.3.2 Neonatal Period

There is a pronounced change in the pattern of adrenal steroidogenesis during early adaptation to extrauterine life. The rapid clearance of placental steroids, such as progesterone and estrogens, from the neonatal circulation removes the inhibiting effect on adrenal 3βHSD2 activity, which is essential for the synthesis of cortisol and aldosterone. Concomitantly, involution of the fetal zone leads to a significant decrease in the synthesis and secretion of DHEA and DHEAS.[1–3, 7]

36.3.4 Circadian Rhythm

The HPA axis has a well-documented endogenous circadian rhythm, with consequent daily variations in plasma cortisol. Peak concentrations of this hormone occur prior to or at the time of activity in the morning, with a decline over the remaining 24 h. This rhythm is regulated by a complex brain-adrenal neurohumoral circuit. It involves the endogenous cycles of clock genes and is partially synchronized by environmental elements, such as periodic factors (light-dark, rest-activity, and sleep-wake cycles), food ingestion, and social cues.[39]

The circadian system is functional in fetal life. Maternal circadian inputs provide the main entrainment factors to the programming of the fetal circadian cycles. At birth, however, there is no circadian rhythm of sleep, body temperature, melatonin production, or cortisol secretion. Although the period of light-dark cycle is a dominant environmental synchronizer, mother-infant interactions and a household's social routine are important nonphotic-synchronizer factors.[39, 40]

The age of appearance of cortisol rhythm is still a matter of debate: comprehensive studies have shown that both term and preterm infants present a normal circadian rhythm in a variable period—soon after birth until the age of 3 months.[40–47] Different definitions of circadian rhythm, sampling times, and methods of data analysis may account for these variations among the studies.

36.3.5 Molecular Aspects

Adrenocortical development, growth, and maintenance depend on the interaction of sequential gene expression, local paracrine signaling molecules, and endocrine regulators.[48] The role of some essential transcription factors and signaling pathways in these processes is discussed next.[2, 9, 10, 27, 48–51]

36.3.5.1 SF1 (NR5A1)

Steroidogenic factor 1 (SF1) is a transcription factor that regulates several genes involved in the HPA and gonadal axis.[2, 9, 10, 52, 53] It is also called *NR5A1* (nuclear receptor subfamily 5, group A, member 1). Although it belongs to the superfamily of nuclear receptors, SF1 is considered an orphan receptor because it has no known ligand.[54–56]

SF1 is essential for adrenocortical development (for both initiation and maturation) and steroidogenesis. The AGP is characterized by the expression of SF1, and the specification of the AP requires higher expression of this transcription factor.[57, 58] As adrenal differentiation progresses, SF1 is expressed in the definitive, the transitional, and the fetal zones during the prenatal period, and in the zona glomerulosa, the zona fasciculata, and the zona reticularis after birth. Its role in steroidogenesis is based on the regulation of the promoter of cytochrome P450 and other enzymes involved in hormone synthesis. In addition, SF1 expression seems to be essential to the proliferation of progenitor cells.[2, 9, 10]

36.3.5.2 DAX1 (NR0B1)

DAX1 [dosage-sensitive sex reversal (DSS), adrenal hypoplasia critical (AHC) region, on chromosome X, gene 1], also called NR0B1 (nuclear receptor subfamily 0, group B, member 1), is another orphan nuclear receptor, which acts as a key transcription factor for adrenocortical development and function.[59]

DAX1 is a target gene for SF1. In turn, DAX1 negatively regulates the transcriptional activity of SF1, and therefore plays an essential role in the inhibition of SF1-mediated adrenocortical steroidogenesis. In addition, DAX1, which is mostly expressed in the subcapsular region of the adrenals, seems to play a role in the maintenance of the pluripotency of stem/progenitor cells.[2, 9, 10]

36.3.5.3 IGF2

The IGF-signaling pathway is involved in the differentiation and growth of the adrenal cortex. Both IGF1 and IGF2 are expressed in the adrenals.[2, 9, 10, 60–62] IGF2 is highly expressed in human fetal adrenal glands and is considered the most important controller of fetal zone growth. It is thought to act as a mediator, in concert with bFGF and EGF, of the trophic actions of ACTH. At birth, IGF2 expression decreases dramatically, coincident with fetal zone regression. It appears to be expressed postnatally only in the adrenal capsule and in the periphery of the cortex. This location coincides with the stem/progenitor cell niche.[2, 9, 10, 60–62]

Although IGF1 is also expressed during adrenal development, it is dominant in the adult adrenal gland. IGF1 functions as a regulator of postnatal growth maintenance.[2, 9, 10, 60–62]

36.3.5.4 WNT/β-Catenin-Signaling Pathway

The Wnt/β-catenin-signaling pathway plays an important role in adrenal development. β-catenin can be a coactivator for multiple nuclear receptors, such as SF1. In the absence of Wnt signaling, β-catenin is in a complex with axin, APC, and GSK3-β. Within this complex, β-catenin is phosphorylated and targeted for degradation. When Wnt signaling is activated, β-catenin is uncoupled from the degradation complex and translocates to the nucleus, where it activates target genes.[9, 10, 63]

In the adrenal, there is an activation of the Wnt/β-catenin-signaling pathway in the subcapsular region. β-catenin plays a role in the maintenance of stem/progenitor cells and may be considered a major regulator of adrenocortical cell proliferation. It is essential for the development and maintenance of the definitive cortex.[9, 10, 63] There is also some initial evidence that this signaling pathway also has a role in adrenal steroidogenesis.[64]

36.3.5.5 Sonic Hedgehog-Signaling Pathway

The sonic hedgehog (SHH)-signaling pathway is central to adrenocortical development. It contains three ligands: SHH, desert hedgehog (DHH), and Indian hedgehog (IHH). The activation of this signaling pathway prevents the cleavage of GLI Kruppel family member 3 (GLI3), which acts as a transcriptional activator.[9, 10, 65]

The sonic hedgehog (SHH)-signaling pathway is important for adrenal cortex development and maintenance. Components of this pathway are expressed during both prenatal and postnatal periods. Their localization in the subcapsular region of the adrenals suggests that they serve as progenitor cells for the adrenal cortex.[9, 10, 65]

36.4 ADRENAL MEDULLA

36.4.1 Structure and Function

Due to its origin and function, the adrenal medulla may be considered a modified sympathetic ganglion. It synthetizes and secretes catecholamines (adrenaline or epinephrine—predominantly—and also noradrenaline or norepinephrine), as part of the sympathetic nervous system. The adrenal medulla is the body's most abundant source of adrenaline.[66]

36.4.1.1 Prenatal Adrenal Medulla

During most of gestation, the adrenal medulla is not recognized as a distinct structure, as there are only clusters of primitive medullary cells and a plexus of nerves scattered throughout the developing cortex. Two types of cells are derived from the sympathogonia: neuroblasts and pheochromoblasts. While neuroblasts have scarce cytoplasm and darkly staining nucleus, pheochromoblasts are larger cells, with basophilic cytoplasm and vesicular nucleus. The latter differentiate into pheochromocytes, also called *chromaffin cells,* which are neuroendocrine cells.[8]

At 7–12 weeks' gestation, synthesis and storage of catecholamines and opioids begin. Noradrenaline synthesis begins at 11–16 weeks, while adrenalin synthesis begins at 17–23 weeks. At this stage, chromaffin cells attain their maximal proliferation and develop the adrenergic phenotype (predominant synthesis and secretion of adrenaline over noradrenaline), which remains in the postnatal period.[8] Catecholamines synthetized during the prenatal period are important to regulate fetal heart rate.[67]

36.4.1.2 Neonatal Adrenal Medulla

After birth, as the fetal zone regresses, the clusters of medullary cells coalesce to form a rudimentary medulla in the center of the adrenal. The effects of catecholamines are particularly important to regulate thermogenesis and cardiovascular response to stress during delivery and further adaptation to extrauterine life.[8, 68]

36.4.1.3 Adult Adrenal Medulla

The adrenal medulla is considered mature only after 12–18 months of postnatal life. In the adult, it represents 10%–20% of the size of the gland and rarely measures more than 2 mm in thickness. The junction between the zona reticularis of the cortex and the medulla has minimal intervening connective tissue, leaving cortical and medullary cells in direct contact. One of the main roles of catecholamines is to ensure adequate blood flow and energy supply to vital organs during stressful situations.[8, 66]

36.4.2 Physiology

Under basal conditions, small amounts of catecholamines are released into the circulatory system. During a stress response, however, their plasma concentration increases up to 60 times, with a predominance of adrenaline (70%) over noradrenaline (30%) in most situations. The secretion of catecholamines is part of the fight-or-flight reaction, which is triggered by activation of the sympathetic nervous system. Catecholamine release may be triggered by splanchnic nerve activity (in fear, anxiety, or organic stress) or by endogenous compounds (histamine, bradykinin, or angiotensin II) that reach the adrenal medulla through the bloodstream—in allergic reactions or hypotension.[8, 66]

Glucocorticoids play an essential role in chromaffin-cell catecholamine synthesis by regulating the expression of the **phenylethanolamine *N*-methyltransferase enzyme (PNMT)**. They selectively stimulate adrenaline synthesis, and therefore are considered critical for the development and maintenance of the adrenergic phenotype.[8, 10, 66, 69]

36.4.3 Catecholamine Synthesis

The enzyme **tyrosine hydroxylase (TH)** catalyzes the initial and rate-limiting step of catecholamine synthesis: the conversion of tyrosine to L-dihydroxyphenylalanine (L-DOPA). The **aromatic amino acid decarboxylase** subsequently converts L-DOPA to dopamine. The expression of the **dopamine β-hydroxylase enzyme (DBH)** from 11 to 16 weeks' gestation onward enables the conversion of dopamine to noradrenaline. Finally, the expression of PNMT from 17 to 23 weeks' gestation onward enables the conversion of noradrenaline to adrenaline. After synthesis, catecholamines are stored by the chromaffin cells in vesicles, along with other peptides, such as enkephalins, chromogranin A (CgA), and neuropeptide Y (NPY).[8, 66]

36.5   CONCLUSION

The development of the adrenal glands begins early during the prenatal period and continues during the first postnatal years until reaching the adult morphology and function. Although the adrenal cortex and the adrenal medulla have different origins, regulations, and functions, glucocorticoids from the cortex are crucial for the synthesis of catecholamines in the medulla.

The formation of the adrenal cortex is regulated by several well-known transcription factors. Before birth, the adrenal cortex is regulated not only by the fetal HPA axis, but also by placental CRH. In this context, fetal cortisol levels are regulated by fetal-placental-maternal interactions. The main steroids produced by the fetal adrenal cortex, however, are DHEA and DHEAS, which are converted by the placenta to estrogens. Right after birth, one of the most important changes is the involution of the fetal zone, resulting in dramatically decreased DHEA/DHEAS. Only a few years later, during childhood, the zona reticularis develops and the synthesis of significant amounts of DHEA/DHEAS returns. In addition, to adapt in a terrestrial environment after birth, there is increased secretion of aldosterone, which becomes essential in the postnatal period.

Knowledge about the embryogenesis of the adrenal gland, as well as the regulation of its main parts, cortex and medulla, both prenatally and postnatally, is essential to understand not only the physiology of these glands, but also the pathophysiology of diseases that affect them.

REFERENCES

1. Miller WL, Auchus RJ. The molecular biology, biochemistry, and physiology of human steroidogenesis and its disorders. *Endocr Rev* 2011;**32**(1):81–151.
2. Ishimoto H, Jaffe RB. Development and function of the human fetal adrenal cortex: a key component in the feto-placental unit. *Endocr Rev* 2011;**32**(3):317–55.
3. Wood CE, Walker C-D. Fetal and neonatal HPA axis. *Compr Physiol* 2016;**6**:33–62.
4. Sucheston M, Cannon M. Development of zonular patterns in the human adrenal gland. *J Morphol* 1968;**126**(4):477–91.
5. Mesiano S, Jaffe RB. Developmental and functional biology of the primate fetal adrenal cortex. *Endocr Rev* 1997;**18**(3):378–403.
6. Kempna P, Fluck CE. Adrenal gland development and defects. *Best Pract Res Clin Endocrinol Metab* 2008;**22**(1):77–93.
7. Malendowicz LK. 100th anniversary of the discovery of the human adrenal fetal zone by Stella Starkel and Leslaw Wegrzynowski: how far have we come? *Folia Histochem Cytobiol* 2010;**48**(4):491–506.
8. Pérez-Alvarez A, Hernández-Vivanco A, Albillos A. Past, present and future of human chromaffin cells: role in physiology and therapeutics. *Cell Mol Neurobiol* 2010;**30**:1407–15.
9. Lefrevre L, Bertherat J, Ragazzon B. Adrenocortical growth and cancer. *Compr Physiol* 2015;**5**:293–326.
10. Xing Y, Lerario A, Rainey W, Hammer GD. Development of adrenal cortex zonation. *Endocrinol Metab Clin N Am* 2015;**44**(2):243–74.
11. Lodish M. Genetics of adrenocortical development and tumors. *Endocrinol Metab Clin N Am* 2017;**46**:419–33.
12. Bocian-Sobkowska J, Wozniak W, Malendowicz L. Postnatal involution of the human adrenal fetal zone: stereologic description and apoptosis. *Endocr Res* 1998;**24**(3–4):969–73.
13. Spencer SJ, Mesiano S, Lee JY, Jaffe RB. Proliferation and apoptosis in the human adrenal cortex during the fetal and perinatal periods: implications for growth and remodeling. *J Clin Endocrinol Metab* 1999;**84**(3):1110–5.
14. Belgorosky A, Sonia M, Gabriela B, Marco G. Adrenarche: postnatal adrenal zonation and hormonal and metabolic regulation. *Horm Res* 2008;**70**:257–67.
15. Vinson GP. Functional zonation of the adult mammalian adrenal cortex. *Front Neurosci* 2016;**10**:1–23.
16. Baquedano MS, Belgorosky A. Human adrenal cortex: epigenetics and postnatal functional zonation. *Horm Res Paediatr* 2018;**89**(5):331–40.
17. Wood MA, Hammer GD. Adrenocortical stem and progenitor cells: unifying model of two proposed origins. *Mol Cell Endocrinol* 2011;**336**:206–12. https://doi.org/10.1016/j.mce.2010.11.012.
18. Johnston ZC, Bellingham M, Filis P, Soffientini U, Hough D, Bhattacharya S, et al. The human fetal adrenal produces cortisol but no detectable aldosterone throughout the second trimester. *BMC Med* 2018;**16**:1–16.
19. Watterberg KL. Adrenocortical function and dysfunction in the fetus and neonate. *Semin Perinatol* 2004;**9**:13–21.
20. Heckmann M, Hartmann M, Kampschulte B, Gack H, Bödeker R, Gortner L, et al. Persistent high activity of the fetal adrenal cortex in preterm infants: is there a clinical significance? *J Pediatr Endocrinol Metab* 2006;**19**(11):1303–12.
21. Honour J, Wickramaratne K, Valman H. Adrenal function in preterm infants. *Biol Neonate* 1992;**61**(4):214–21.
22. Midgley P, Russell K, Oates N, Shaw J, Honour J. Activity of the adrenal fetal zone in preterm infants continues to term. *Endocr Res* 1996;**22**(4):729–33.
23. Midgley P, Russell K, Oates N, Holownia P, Shaw J, Honour J. Adrenal function in preterm infants: ACTH may not be the sole regulator of the fetal zone. *Pediatr Res* 1998;**44**(6):887–93.
24. Ng PC. The fetal and neonatal hypothalamic -pituitary-adrenal axis. *Arch Dis Child Fetal Neonatal Ed* 2000;**82**:250–4.
25. Brosnan PG. The hypothalamic pituitary axis in the fetus and newborn. *Semin Perinatol* 2001;**25**(6):371–84.

26. Bagnoli F, Mori A, Fommei C, Coriolani G, Badii S, Tomasini B. ACTH and cortisol cord plasma concentrations in preterm and term infants. *J Perinatol* 2013;**33**:520–4. https://doi.org/10.1038/jp.2012.165.

27. Jaffe R, Mesiano S, Smith R, Coulter C, Spencer S, Chakravorty A. The regulation and role of fetal adrenal development in human pregnancy. *Endocr Res* 1998;**24**(3–4):919–26.

28. Gilles M, Otto H, Wolf IAC, Scharnholz B, Peus V, Schredl M, et al. Maternal hypothalamus-pituitary-adrenal (HPA) system activity and stress during pregnancy: effects on gestational age and infant's anthropometric measures at birth. *Psychoneuroendocrinology* 2018;**94**:152–61. https://doi.org/10.1016/j.psyneuen.2018.04.022.

29. Duthie L, Reynolds RM. Changes in the maternal hypothalamic-pituitary-adrenal axis in pregnancy and postpartum: influences on maternal and fetal outcomes. *Neuroendocrinology* 2013;**98**:106–15.

30. Stirrat LI, Reynolds RM. The effect of fetal growth and nutrient stresses on steroid pathways. *J Steroid Biochem Mol Biol* 2016;**160**:214–20. https://doi.org/10.1016/j.jsbmb.2015.07.003.

31. Alcántara-Alonso V, Panetta P, de Gortari P, Grammatopoulos DK. Corticotropin-releasing hormone as the homeostatic rheostat of feto-maternal symbiosis and developmental programming in utero and neonatal life. *Front Endocrinol (Lausanne)* 2017;**8**:1–10.

32. Manabe M, Nishida T, Imai T, Kusaka T, Kawada K, Okada H, et al. Cortisol levels in umbilical vein and umbilical artery with or without antenatal corticosteroids. *Pediatr Int* 2005;**47**:60–3.

33. Heckmann M, Hartmann MF, Kampschulte B, Gack H, Bodeker R, Gortner L, et al. Cortisol production rates in preterm infants in relation to growth and illness: a noninvasive prospective study using gas chromatography-mass spectrometry. *J Clin Endocrinol Metab* 2005;**90**(10):5737–42.

34. Matthews SG. Early programming of the hypothalamo-pituitary-adrenal axis. *Trends Endocrinol Metab* 2002;**13**(9):373–80.

35. Cheung P. Effect of stress on the hypothalamic-pituitary-adrenal axis in the fetus and newborn. *J Pediatr* 2011;**158**:e41–3. https://doi.org/10.1016/j.jpeds.2010.11.012.

36. Martinerie L, Pussard E, L LF, Petit F, Cosson C, Boileau P. Physiological partial aldosterone resistance in human newborns. *Pediatr Res* 2009;**66**(3):323–8.

37. Martinerie L, Viengchareun S, Delezoide A, Jaubert F, Sinico M, Prevot S, et al. Low renal mineralocorticoid receptor expression at birth contributes to partial aldosterone resistance in neonates. *Endocrinology* 2009;**150**(9):4414–24.

38. Goto M, Hanley KP, Marcos J, Wood PJ, Wright S, Postle AD, et al. In humans, early cortisol biosynthesis provides a mechanism to safeguard female sexual development. *J Clin Invest* 2006;**116**(4):953–60.

39. Moreira AC, Antonini SR, Castro MA. Sense of time of the glucocorticoid circadian clock: from the ontogeny to the diagnosis of Cushing's syndrome. *Eur J Endocrinol* 2018;**179**:R1–18.

40. Custodio RJ, Eduardo C, Junior M, Lopes S, Milani S, Simões AL, et al. The emergence of the cortisol circadian rhythm in monozygotic and dizygotic twin infants: the twin-pair synchrony. *Clin Cancer Res* 2007;**66**:192–7.

41. Vermes I, Dohanics J, Tóth G, Pongrácz J. Maturation of the circadian rhythm of the adrenocortical functions in human neonates and infants. *Horm Res* 1980;**12**(5):237–44.

42. Price D, Close G, Fielding B. Age of appearance of circadian rhythm in salivary cortisol values in infancy. *Arch Dis Child* 1983;**58**:454–6.

43. Spangler G. The emergence of adrenocortical circadian function in newborns and infants and its relationship to sleep, feeding and maternal adreno-cortical activity. *Early Hum Dev* 1991;**25**(3):197–208.

44. Antonini S, Jorge S, Moreira A. The emergence of salivary cortisol circadian rhythm and its relationship to sleep activity in preterm. *Clin Endocrinol* 2000;**52**(4):423–6.

45. Serón-Ferré M, Riffo R, Valenzuela G, Germain A. Twenty-four-hour pattern of cortisol in the human fetus at term. *Am J Obstet Gynecol* 2001;**184**(6):1278–83.

46. Iwata O, Okamura H, Saitsu H, Saikusa M, Kanda H, Eshima N. Diurnal cortisol changes in newborn infants suggesting entrainment of peripheral circadian clock in utero and at birth. *J Clin Endocrinol Metab* 2013;**98**(1):e25–32.

47. Kinoshita M, Iwata S, Okamura H, Saikusa M, Hara N, Urata C, et al. Paradoxical diurnal cortisol changes in neonates suggesting preservation of foetal adrenal rhythms. *Nat Sci Rep* 2016;**6**:1–7. https://doi.org/10.1038/srep35553.

48. Else T, Hammer GD. Genetic analysis of adrenal absence: agenesis and aplasia. *Trends Endocrinol Metab* 2005;**16**(10):458–68.

49. Keegan CE, Hammer GD. Recent insights into organogenesis of the adrenal cortex. *Trends Endocrinol Metab* 2002;**13**(5):200–8.

50. Hammer GD, Parker KL, Schimmer BP. Minireview: transcriptional regulation of adrenocortical development. *Endocrinology* 2005;**146**(3):1018–24.

51. Morohashi K, Zubair M. Molecular and cellular endocrinology the fetal and adult adrenal cortex. *Mol Cell Endocrinol* 2011;**336**:193–7. https://doi.org/10.1016/j.mce.2010.11.026.

52. Ozisik G, Achermann C, Meeks JJ, Larry J. SF1 in the development of the adrenal gland and gonads. *Horm Res* 2003;**59**(suppl 1):94–8.

53. Hammer GD, Ingraham HA. Steroidogenic Factor-1: its role in endocrine organ development and differentiation. *Front Neuroendocrinol* 1999;**20**:199–223.

54. Lala DS, Rice DA, Parker KL. Steroidogenic factor I, a key regulator of steroidogenic enzyme expression, is the mouse homolog of fushi tarazu-factor. *Mol Endocrinol* 1992;**6**(8):1249–58.

55. Morohashi K, Honda S, Inomata Y, Handa H, Omura T. A common trans-acting factor, Ad4-binding protein, to the promoters of steroidogenic P-450s. *J Biol Chem* 1992;**267**(25):17913–9.

56. Honda S, Morohashi K, Nomura M, Takeya H, Kitajimaf M. Ad4BP regulating steroidogenic P-450 gene is a member of steroid hormone receptor superfamily. *J Biol Chem* 1993;**268**(10):7494–502.

57. Luo X, Ikeda Y, Parker KLA. Cell-specific nuclear receptor is essential for adrenal and gonadal development and sexual differentiation. *Cell* 1994;**77** (May):481–90.

58. Hatano O, Takakusu A, Nomura M, Morohashi K. Identical origin of adrenal cortex and gonad revealed by expression profiles of Ad4BP/SF. *Genes Cells* 1996;**1**:663–71.

59. Suntharalingham JP, Buonocore F, Duncan AJ, Achermann JC. DAX-1 (NR0B1) and steroidogenic factor-1 (SF-1, NR5A1) in human disease. *Best Pract Res Clin Endocrinol Metab* 2015;**29**(4):607–19.

60. Mesiano S, Mellon S, Jaffe R. Mitogenic action, regulation, and localization of insulin-like growth factors in the human fetal adrenal. *J Clin Endocrinol Metab* 1993;**76**(4):968–76.

61. Mesiano S, Jaffe RB. Role of growth factors in the developmental regulation of the human fetal adrenal cortex. *Steroids* 1997;**62**:62–72.

62. Ilvesmaki V, Blum W, Voutilainen R. Insulin-like growth factor-II in human fetal adrenals: regulation by ACTH, protein kinase C and growth factors. *J Endocrinol* 1993;**137**(3):533–42.

63. Kim AC, Reuter AL, Zubair M, Else T, Serecky K, Bingham NC, et al. Targeted disruption of β-catenin in Sf1-expressing cells impairs development and maintenance of the adrenal cortex. *Development* 2008;**135**:2593–602.

64. Leal LF, Mermejo LM, Ramalho LZ, Martinelli CE, Yunes A, Seidinger AL, et al. Wnt/beta-catenin pathway deregulation in childhood adrenocortical tumors. *J Clin Endocrinol Metab* 2011;**96**:3106–14.

65. Gomes DC, Leal LF, Mermejo LM, Scrideli CA, Martinelli Jr CE, Fragoso MC, et al. Sonic hedgehog signaling is active in human adrenal. *J Clin Endocrinol Metab* 2014;**99**:1209–16.

66. Wong DL. Why is the adrenal adrenergic? *Endocr Pathol* 2003;**14**(1):25–36.

67. Artal R. Fetal adrenal medulla. *Clin Obstet Gynecol* 1980;**23**(3):825–36.

68. Lagercrantz H, Bistoletti P. Catecholamine release in the newborn infant at birth. *Pediatr Res* 1973;**11**:889–93.

69. Chung K, Qin N, Androutsellis-Theotokis A, Bornstein S. Effects of dehydroepiandrosterone on proliferation and differentiation of chromaffin progenitor cells. *Mol Cell Endocrinol* 2011;**336**(1–2):141–8.

Chapter 37

Development and Function of the Ovaries and Testes in the Fetus and Neonate

Analía V. Freire*, María Gabriela Ropelato* and Rodolfo A. Rey*,†

*Centro de Investigaciones Endocrinológicas "Dr. César Bergadá" (CEDIE), CONICET-FEI-División de Endocrinología, Hospital de Niños Ricardo Gutiérrez, Buenos Aires, Argentina, †Departamento de Histología, Biología Celular, Embriología y Genética, Facultad de Medicina, Universidad de Buenos Aires, Buenos Aires, Argentina

Key Clinical Changes

- The chromosomal sex of the embryo is established at fertilization; however, XX and XY embryos develop undifferentiated bipotential primordia of the gonads, urogenital sinus and external genitalia, as well as unipotential Wolffian and Müllerian ducts during the first 6 weeks of gestation.
- Sex determination, i.e., the commitment of the gonadal ridges into testes or ovaries, depends on the presence or absence of SRY expression and occurs independently of gonadotropins during the 7th week.
- Testes secrete anti-Müllerian hormone (AMH), responsible for the regression of Müllerian ducts, and androgens, which drive the virilization of Wolffian ducts, the urogenital sinus, and external genitalia.
- Ovaries do not have any influence on fetal differentiation of the genitalia: in the absence of AMH, Müllerian ducts form the fallopian tubes, the uterus, and the upper vagina, whereas lack of androgens results in the feminization of the urogenital sinus and external genitalia.
- Fetal gonadotropins regulate testicular and ovarian hormone production during the second and third trimesters of fetal life.
- After birth, the hypothalamic-pituitary-gonadal axis is active for 3–6 months in boys and up to 2 years in girls, showing a sexual dimorphism: FSH is higher than LH in girls, while the opposite occurs in boys, and AMH, inhibin B, and testosterone are clearly higher in boys.

37.1 SEX DIFFERENTIATION OF THE REPRODUCTIVE SYSTEM

Developmental sex biology may be approached at different levels: chromosomal, genetic, gonadal, and genital. These characteristics usually show a marked sexual dimorphism. In this chapter, we will address the various aspects of differentiation of the gonads and the genitalia, which set the basis for the comprehension of the pathogenesis, diagnosis, and management of disorders of sex development (DSD). The focus will be set on the pathways having clinical relevance in humans, although the largest part of the available information originates in observations made in experimental mammalian species, especially the mouse.

The initial mechanisms governing sex determination vary across species: in reptiles, for instance, environmental factors like temperature are determinant for early differentiation of the gonads, whereas in birds and mammals heteromorphic sex chromosomes rule gonadal fate.[1] The chromosomal sex of the embryo is established at the very moment of fertilization (Fig. 37.1), but no evident difference exists between XX and XY embryos in the gonads or the genital tracts until the 6th week. Embryonic and fetal development consists of three sequential periods: (i) sexually undifferentiated, characterized by the organogenesis of the gonadal and genital primordia; (ii) differentiation of the gonads (or sex determination); and (iii) sexual differentiation of the internal and external genitalia.

Sex differentiation is largely independent of fetal pituitary gonadotropins. Thus, we will only make a brief description of the hypothalamic-pituitary development, and the major focus will be set on the gonads and the reproductive tracts.

37.2 THE HYPOTHALAMIC-PITUITARY-GONADAL AXIS

GnRH neurons derive from neuroepithelial cells present in the olfactory placode in the 5th–6th weeks after conception. They migrate in close association with the terminal olfactory nerve and enter the forebrain by week 6.5, reaching the

Maternal-Fetal and Neonatal Endocrinology. https://doi.org/10.1016/B978-0-12-814823-5.00037-4

FIG. 37.1 Chromosomal, gonadal, and genital sex. Chromosomal sex is defined at fertilization by the sex chromosome of the spermatozoon. Gonadal sex differentiation from the undifferentiated gonadal ridge takes place during the 7th week; the testes produce androgens and anti-Müllerian hormone (AMH), which drive genital sex differentiation in the first trimester of fetal life. The ovaries do not secrete androgens and AMH in the first trimester. Genital differentiation is dependent on testicular hormones: AMH, secreted by Sertoli cells, acts on the AMH receptor (AMHR) inducing Müllerian duct regression; in the absence of AMH action, Müllerian ducts form the fallopian tubes, the uterus, and the upper vagina. Androgens, acting on the androgen receptor (AR), induce the differentiation of the Wolffian ducts into the epididymides, the vasa deferentia, and the seminal vesicles, and the virilization of the urogenital sinus and the external genitalia. In the absence of androgen action, the Wolffian ducts regress, and the urogenital sinus and the external genitalia feminize. *(Reproduced with modifications from Rey RA, Racine C, Josso N. Sexual Differentiation. In: De Groot LJ, Beck-Peccoz P, Chrousos G, Dungan K, Grossman A, Hershman JM, Koch C, McLachlan R, New M, Rebar R, Singer F, Vinik A, Weickert MO, editors. Endotext [Internet]. South Dartmouth (MA): MDText.com, Inc.; 2000–2016 June 1. http://www. endotext.org/chapter/sexual-differenti ation/ Copyright © 2000–2018, MDText. com, Inc. This electronic version has been made freely available under a Creative Commons (CC-BY-NC-ND) license. A copy of the license can be viewed at http://creativecommons.org/licenses/by-nc-nd/2.0/.)*

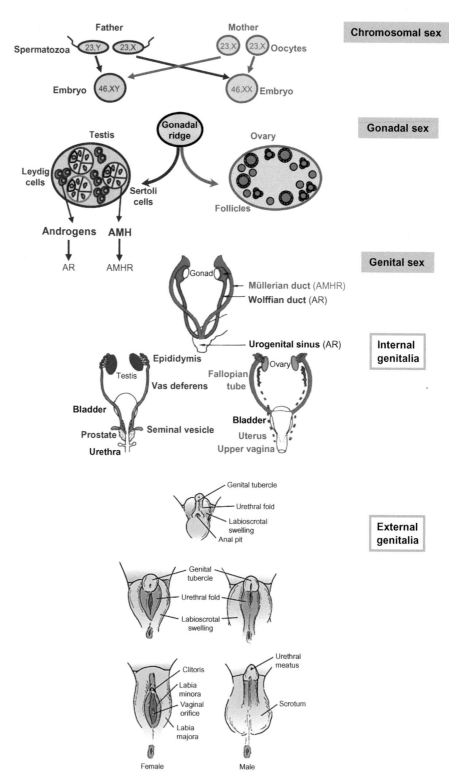

hypothalamus by week 9. GnRH neuron migration is considered complete between the 13th and 16th weeks of gestation.[2] An increasing number of molecules are involved in differentiation, proliferation/apoptosis, and migration of the GnRH neurons. Their mutations result in congenital central hypogonadism usually associated with hyposmia, a condition known as Kallmann syndrome.[3]

The pituitary gland has two embryonic origins: the adenohypophysis or anterior pituitary derives from the Rathke's pouch, an invagination of the oral ectoderm, whereas the neurohypophysis or posterior pituitary originates from the diencephalon. The development of the anterior pituitary involves a coordinated temporal and spatial sequence that ultimately gives rise to five distinct pituitary cell populations: somatotroph, thyrotroph, lactotroph, gonadotroph, and corticotroph.[4]

The gonadotroph is capable of responding to GnRH from week 11, when the portal system for the transport of hypothalamic releasing hormones is established.[5] The pituitary content of LH and FSH reaches maximum levels between 25 and 29 weeks of fetal life. Subsequently the pituitary activity decreases, so that near birth the gonadotropin levels are lower than in the second trimester. Fetal pituitary gonadotropins have a role in regulating gonadal function during the second and third trimesters of gestation; in the first trimester placental hCG is the main regulator of gonadal function.

After birth, the hypothalamic-gonadotroph function is active for 3–6 months in the boy and 1–2 years in the girl. Thereafter, a quiescent period exists until the onset of puberty. A detailed description of the development of the hypothalamic pituitary axes is available in Chapter 30.

37.3 EARLY ORGANOGENESIS OF THE REPRODUCTIVE ORGANS

The genital and urinary systems have a common origin: the urogenital ridges and derivatives of the cloaca. The anlagen of the gonads and reproductive ducts stem from the intermediate and the lateral mesoderm between the 4th and the 6th weeks of embryonic development, i.e., the 6th and 8th weeks from the last menstrual cycle. The cloaca, the dilated distal part of the hindgut formed essentially by endoderm surrounded by mesoderm, also contributes to the urinary and genital excretory tracts. Finally, the cloacal membrane, formed by endoderm and ectoderm, and the surrounding ectodermic structures give rise to the anlagen of the external genitalia.

A thickening of the intermediate mesoderm protrudes into the coelomic cavity—the future abdominal cavity—and gives rise to the urogenital ridges, covered by the coelomic epithelium, a derivative of lateral mesoderm. Subsequently, two distinct portions differentiate in each urogenital ridge: the urinary ridge laterally and the adreno-gonadal ridge medially. The caudal end of the urinary ridge, called metanephros, gives rise to most of the kidney. The mesonephros lying between them provides mesenchymal components to the adreno-gonadal ridge and gives rise as well to the mesonephric (Wolffian) ducts. The normal organogenesis and development of the Wolffian ducts is essential for most of male internal reproductive ducts but also for the urinary system in both sexes. Laterally to the Wolffian ducts, the paramesonephric (Müllerian) ducts arise as a cleft covered by coelomic epithelium and surrounded by mesodermal mesenchyme. Müllerian ducts are the main component of the female internal reproductive tract.

These processes taking place during early embryonic development are induced by regulatory pathways that involve secreted or intracellular factors ubiquitously expressed. Their deficiency may be lethal or result in multiple malformations. Examples of these are the transcription factors EMX2, LHX1, PAX3, SIX1, and WT1 involved in early intermediate mesoderm stabilization (reviewed in ref.[6]).

37.4 THE BIPOTENTIAL GONAD

37.4.1 The Gonadal Ridge

The adreno-gonadal ridge, the common precursor of the gonads and adrenal cortex, forms in the medial portion of each urogenital ridge under the control of transcription factors SF1, DAX1, CBX2, LHX9, GATA4, and SIX1/4.[7] Cells originate from the coelomic epithelium and the mesonephric mesoderm. By the beginning of the 5th embryonic week, distinct cell populations progressively separate to form the adrenal primordium and the gonadal ridge. However, cells of a common origin may remain in adrenals and gonads, which may explain the finding of adrenal rests in the testes of male patients with congenital adrenal hyperplasia.[8]

The gonadal ridge is bipotential and can develop into an ovary or a testis, irrespective of its chromosomal constitution. XX and XY gonads are indistinguishable until the end of the 5th embryonic week. Furthermore, identical expression profiles are seen for purportedly ovarian factors like WNT4, RSPO1, and DAX1 or male factors like SOX9 and FGF9. Somatic cell proliferation is an essential process at this stage. LHX9 regulates cell proliferation of the gonadal ridge by interacting with WT1 and modulating SF1 expression, which are both highly expressed irrespective of chromosomal sex. Other factors involved in somatic cell proliferation in the bipotential gonad are TCF21 and members of the insulin family, like INSR, IGF1R, and INSRR. Cell proliferation seems to be more critical in the male than in the female in early gonadal development, which may explain the finding of gonadal dysgenesis leading to undervirilization in 46,XY patients with no male-specific gene mutations. An insufficient number of SRY-expressing cells would result in a failure of the testicular differentiation triggering process (reviewed in ref.[6]).

WT1 and SF1 play major roles in the process of urogenital organogenesis. WT1, named after Wilms tumor (nephroblastoma), is a transcriptional and/or posttranscriptional regulator.[9,10] WT1 is expressed early in the urogenital ridge and is essential for the development of the kidneys and gonads. SF1, also called Ad4BP or FTZF1 and encoded by the *NR5A1* gene, is an orphan nuclear receptor, initially described as a regulator of steroid hydroxylases in the adrenal cortex, and subsequently found in the hypothalamus, the pituitary, and the gonads.[11] In early embryogenesis, SF1 plays a role in the stabilization of the intermediate mesoderm and the formation of the adreno-gonadal primordium. Later, SF1 also plays an important role in testicular spermatogenesis and ovarian follicle development and ovulation.[12]

37.4.2 The Germ Cells

Until the beginning of the 6th embryonic week, the undifferentiated gonads are only formed by the coelomic epithelium and the mesenchyme of the intermediate mesoderm. At approximately day 37, primordial germ cells, of extragonadal origin, reach the gonadal anlagen.

Primordial germ cells differentiate from pluripotent cells of the proximal epiblast in the 3rd week; factors involved in early germ cell specification vary between species, and include BLIMP1, BMP2, BMP4, BMP8B, NANOG, OCT3/4 (encoded by *POU5F1*), PRDM1, PMRD14, SOX2, and SOX17.[13] Primordial germ cell precursors migrate through the primitive streak into the extraembryonic region at the base of the allantois and can be seen in the yolk sac during the 4th embryonic week, where they express BLIMP1, alkaline phosphatase, OCT3/4, and the tyrosine kinase receptor C-KIT.[14] Later, primordial germ cells migrate along the wall of the hind gut and through the dorsal mesentery to reach the gonadal ridges during the 6th week. Several factors drive the differentiation, migration, proliferation, and apoptosis of primordial germ cells.[15]

Chromatin modifications are observed at this stage: genome-wide demethylation leads to erasure of epigenetic marks imprinted during parental gametogenesis. Methylation of the genome of germ cells is recovered later during fetal life. Like somatic cells of the gonadal ridges, germ cells are bipotential. Chromosomal constitution does not influence sex differentiation of germ cells.[16] However, germ cells whose karyotype is discordant with the somatic lineages fail to progress through gametogenesis and enter apoptosis later in life. The influence of germ cells on the developing gonad is sexually dimorphic: germ cell progression through meiosis is essential for the maintenance of the fetal ovary; otherwise prospective follicular cells degenerate and streak gonads result. In contrast, the development of the somatic component of the testis is not hindered by the lack of germ cells.

37.5 THE TESTES

37.5.1 Fetal Sex Determination and Differentiation

The central dogma of fetal sexual determination and differentiation in mammals states that: (i) the existence of a Y chromosome leads the gonadal ridges, though the expression of the *SRY* gene, to differentiate into testes (testis determination), and (ii) fetal testes secrete two distinct hormones, namely anti-Müllerian hormone (AMH) and androgens, responsible for the differentiation of the internal and external genitalia along the male pathway (sex differentiation). The pioneering experiments performed by Alfred Jost in the mid-20th century showed that when testes are present internal and external genitalia virilize, whereas when testes are absent internal and external genitalia differentiate along the female pathway.[17] The presence or absence of ovaries has no influence whatsoever on genital differentiation during fetal life (Fig. 37.1).

37.5.1.1 Seminiferous Cord Formation. Differentiation of Sertoli and Leydig Cells

Testis differentiation is initiated in the XY fetus by the beginning of the 7th embryonic week. Cells derived from the coelomic epithelium and mesonephric mesenchyme and primordial germ cells become segregated in two compartments: testicular cords and interstitial tissue. These changes are preceded by the formation of the coelomic vessel below the coelomic epithelium.[7,18] Endothelial cells migrating from the mesonephros to the coelomic zone of the gonad are essential for cord formation. Coelomic cells differentiate to form Sertoli cells, which aggregate and enclose the primordial germ cells. Sertoli cells also interact with differentiating peritubular myoid cells, probably derived from the mesonephric mesenchyme, resulting in the formation of basement membrane of the testicular cords. Testicular cords are seen by day 43, beginning in the central part of the gonad.[19] The differentiating Sertoli cells are characterized by a polarized, large and clear cytoplasm and the expression of SOX9, AMH, and DHH. Sertoli and germ cell numbers increase exponentially in the human fetal testis during the second trimester,[20] reflecting a direct FSH action on Sertoli cells and an indirect androgen action through the peritubular myoid cells.[21] This explains the finding of small testes and low AMH levels in newborns with congenital hypogonadotropic hypogonadism.[22] Sertoli cells do not reach a mature state, and meiosis is not initiated in the human testis until pubertal age, when all Sertoli cells reach a high expression level of the androgen receptor.[23–27]

Mesenchymal cells and matrix and blood vessels fill the interstitial space. The interstitial tissue of the fetal testis is characterized by the differentiation of Leydig cells by the 8th week, after testicular cords have completely formed. Leydig cells produce androgens, which drive the stabilization of Wolffian ducts and the masculinization of external genitalia, and insulin-like growth factor 3 (INSL3), responsible for the transabdominal phase of testicular descent. The origin of fetal Leydig cells is controversial: they might have the same origin as Sertoli cells in the coelomic epithelium,[28] but other origins, including pericytes of the coelomic vessel and neural crest, cannot be ruled out.[29]

The basement membrane layer that surrounds the developing gonad beneath the coelomic epithelium thickens to form the tunica albuginea.

37.5.1.2   Molecular Pathways

The currently prevailing theory on the molecular mechanisms driving the undifferentiated bipotential gonadal ridge to enter the testicular or the ovarian pathway, i.e. sex determination, is that the balance between "pro-testis/anti-ovary" and "pro-ovary/anti-testis" factors is disrupted in the XY gonad by SRY, favoring the testicular pathway.[1] Conversely, in the XX gonad, the lack of SRY leans the scale towards the ovarian pathway (Fig. 37.2).

Until the end of the 6th embryonic week, purported "pro-testis" (e.g. SOX9, FGF9) and "pro-ovary" (e.g. RSPO1, FOXL2) genes are expressed at similar levels in the XY and the XX gonadal ridges.[30] In the XY embryo, at the beginning

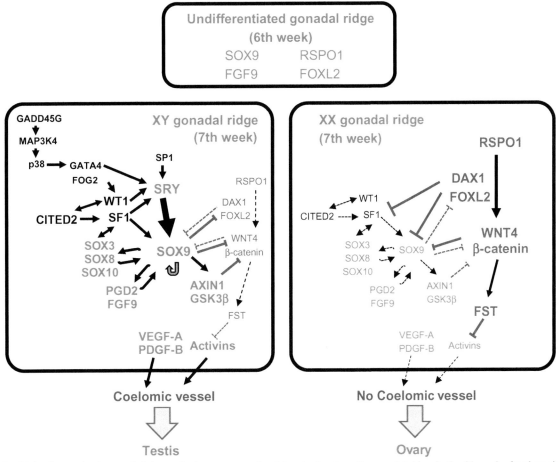

FIG. 37.2   Molecular mechanisms underlying testicular versus ovarian determination from the gonadal ridge. In the 6th week of embryonic life, the gonadal ridge is sexually undifferentiated, and various factors are expressed at the same levels in the XX and the XY gonads. During the 7th week, in the XY gonad, SRY expression is triggered, and the male pathway prevails driving to the formation of the coelomic vessel. In the XX gonad, the female pathway prevails, and there is no formation of the coelomic vessel.

of the 7th week, SF1, SP1, and WT1 initiate *SRY* expression. CITED2 cooperation with SF1 and WT1 and interaction between GATA4 and its cofactor FOG2 are involved in further *SRY* upregulation, following GADD45G- and MAP3K4-mediated phosphorylation reactions.[9] *SRY* expression initiates between days 41 and 44 postconception in pre-Sertoli cells of the middle of the gonad and expands towards the poles. Peak levels of SRY are attained at day 44,[30] reaching the critical threshold that triggers testicular differentiation.[6] SRY expression levels and timing seem critical for normal Sertoli cells differentiation, and decreased or delayed expression levels may lead to testicular dysgenesis or the formation of ovotestes.[31]

SOX9 is the earliest SRY-upregulated gene in differentiating Sertoli cells, followed by *SOX3, SOX8, SOX10* and many other genes that are critical for testicular differentiation.[7] SOX9 seems to be the master regulator of testis differentiation since it is able to mimic SRY in its absence.[32] Unlike SRY, SOX9 is not testis-specific: it is also expressed in chondrocytes, bile duct, central nervous system, hair follicles, heart, lung, pancreas, and retina. SOX9 is able to maintain its own expression via two different mechanisms: (1) SOX9 itself or other SOX factors upregulate *SOX9* promoter,[33,34] and (2) SOX9 triggers a feed-forward pathway involving FGF9 and PGD2. FGF9 and SOX9 also upregulate AXIN1 and GSK3β, which block ovarian development by destabilizing β-catenin (Fig. 37.2).[35] The signaling cascade initiated by SRY and SOX9 counteracts the WNT4/β-catenin/FST pathway[36] (see following, "The ovaries"). In the XY fetus, the prevalence of SRY/SOX9 results in the activation of activin B, VEGF, PDGF, and other unidentified factors that facilitate endothelial migration and formation of the testis-specific vasculature, including the coelomic vessel.[18]

Sertoli cells are essential for the maintenance of testicular differentiation, including the development of the germ and Leydig cell populations. Initially, Sertoli cell-secreted PDGFs, FGF9, and DHH promote the differentiation of fetal Leydig cells,[37] but further functional differentiation depends on placental hCG in the first and second trimesters of fetal life and on fetal pituitary LH thereafter, both acting on the same LH/CG receptor.

37.5.1.3 Spermatogenic Development

As already stated, primordial germ cells are bipotential, i.e., they can commit to spermatogenesis or oogenesis independently of their own XX or XY constitution. Indeed, the functional characteristics of the surrounding somatic cells of the gonads regulate germ cell sexual differentiation.[38] In the fetal testis, primordial germ cells differentiate to gonocytes, which proliferate by mitosis but do not enter meiosis as in the fetal ovary. Meiosis onset and progression is dependent upon retinoic acid availability.[39] Germ cells embedded in the seminiferous cords are not exposed to retinoic acid, which is catabolized by the enzyme of the cytochrome P450 family CYP26B1. Fetal Sertoli cells also prevent germ cells from entering meiosis by repressing STRA8 expression in germ cells via FGF9 and NANOS2.[39] Germ cells are the most sensitive testicular cell population to testicular dysgenesis, with decreased numbers observed as the first sign of mild dysgenesis. Nonetheless, germ cell loss does not hinder Sertoli and Leydig cell development during fetal life.

37.5.1.4 Hormone Synthesis and Secretion

AMH. Sertoli cells begin producing AMH as soon as they differentiate, i.e., at the beginning of the 7th embryonic week.[40] AMH is responsible for the regression of Müllerian ducts in the male fetus. Initially, AMH expression is triggered by SOX9, independently of gonadotropins, and SF1, GATA4, and WT1 synergize to increase SOX9-activated AMH transcription. Subsequently, during the second and third trimesters of fetal life and after birth, testicular AMH production is further increased by FSH, which induces Sertoli cell proliferation and upregulates AMH transcription. Although Müllerian duct regression takes place in the 8th and 9th weeks of fetal life, Sertoli cells continue to produce high amounts of AMH until puberty (reviewed in ref.[6]).

Androgens. Leydig cells secrete androgens from the beginning of the 9th week. In the first half of fetal life, Leydig cell function is mainly regulated by placental hCG, whereas fetal pituitary LH progressively takes over during the second half. Both hCG and LH act on the same LH/CG receptor. Androgen levels peak between 11 and 14 weeks in the male fetus,[41] and are responsible for the differentiation of the Wolffian ducts, the virilization of the urogenital sinus and the external genitalia, and the descent of the testes into the scrotum.

Steroidogenesis involves a series of enzymatic reactions, most of which also take place in the adrenal cortex (Fig. 37.3).[42] The initial step is the transfer of cholesterol from the cytosol into the mitochondria mediated by the steroidogenic acute regulatory protein (StAR) and TSPO. Then, cholesterol is converted to pregnenolone by the P450 side-chain cleavage enzyme (P450scc) in the inner mitochondrial membrane. The Δ5 steroid pregnenolone is subsequently metabolized by the cytochrome P450c17, which has two activities: 17α-hydroxylase is responsible for pregnenolone hydroxylation to 17α-hydroxypregnenolone and 17–20 lyase accounts for its conversion to dehydroepiandrosterone (DHEA). The flavoprotein P450 oxidoreductase (POR) and the cytochrome *b*5 are required for optimal 17,20 lyase activity. P450c17, together

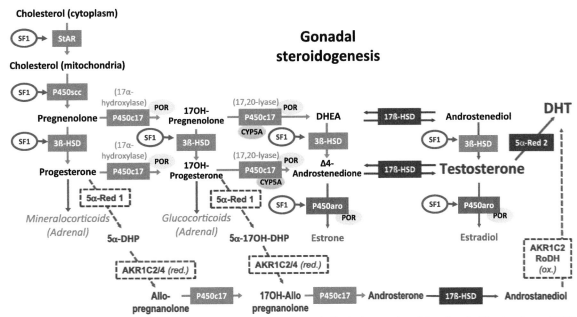

FIG. 37.3   Steroidogenesis in the gonads. The first steps of steroidogenesis are similar in the gonads and the adrenals. The steps beyond P450c17 are specific to the gonads. DHT can be synthesized via the classical pathway involving 5α-reductase type 2 conversion of testosterone, or through the alternative "backdoor" pathway *(dotted lines)* not involving testosterone. *(Reproduced with permission from Rey RA, Grinspon RP. Normal male sexual differentiation and etiology of disorders of sex development. Best Pract Res Clin Endocrinol Metab. 2011;25:221–238. Copyright 2010 Elsevier Ltd.)*

with POR and cytochrome *b*5, also transform the Δ4 compound progesterone into 17α-hydroxyprogesterone and Δ4-androstenedione. The next step in testicular testosterone synthesis is mediated by 17ß-hydroxysteroid dehydrogenase type 3 (17β-HSD-3), responsible for the conversion of Δ4-androstenedione to testosterone and the Δ5 steroid DHEA to androstenediol. Several 17β-HSD isoforms have been identified, but only the type 3 is expressed in the testis. Another hydroxysteroid dehydrogenase, 3ß-HSD type 2, is responsible for the conversion of Δ5 to Δ4 steroids. Androgens can be transformed to estrogens by the P450 enzyme aromatase.

Dihydrotestosterone (DHT) is a more potent androgen, which cannot be aromatized. At least two pathways are involved in DHT biosynthesis. In the classic pathway, testosterone is converted to DHT in target tissues by the enzyme 5α-reductase type 2. The alternative, also known as the "backdoor" pathway, does not involve testosterone as a precursor [43] (Fig. 37.3). Instead, progesterone and 17-hydroxyprogesterone are respectively converted to dihydroprogesterone and 17-hydroxydihydroprogesterone by 5α-reductase type 1, and to allopregnanolone and 17-hydroxyallopregnanolone by 3αHSD. P450c17 converts them to androsterone, which is finally metabolized to DHT via androstanediol or androstenedione by 17β-HSD types 3 or 5, and 17β-HSD type 6 together with 3αHSD.

INSL3. Leydig cells also synthesize insulin-like factor 3 (INSL3), a protein hormone that is involved in the first phase of testicular descent by binding to the seven transmembrane domain receptor RXFP2.[44]

37.5.2   Postnatal Changes

37.5.2.1   Anatomical Aspects and Histological Changes

At birth, the testes are formed by solid seminiferous cords with no lumen; their mean diameter is approximately 50 μm. Sertoli cells are the most abundant cell type and divide by mitosis in response to FSH. Some large gonocytes are still lying in the center of the cords while others have differentiated to spermatogonia, which are placed against the basement membrane. Mitotic, but not meiotic, divisions occur at this stage. In the interstitial tissue, typical Leydig cells are present and respond to LH.

37.5.2.2   The Physiology of the Postnatal Activation

The activity of the hypothalamic-pituitary-testicular axis declines over the 3rd trimester of fetal life.[45] A further dramatic decline is observed in gonadotropins and testosterone on the first day after birth. FSH and LH levels do not differ between boys and girls, but AMH, inhibin B, and testosterone are clearly higher in the male (Table 37.1).[45–48] Serum levels of

TABLE 37.1 Hormone levels in the newborn period

Hormone	Day 2	Day 7	Day 10	Day 14	Day 20	Day 30
FSH (IU/L)						
Boys	ND–1.2	ND–4.4	0.9–3.6	0.3–6.9	0.5–2.3	0.6–2.5
Girls	0.1–0.6					0.6–21.5
LH (IU/L)						
Boys	ND–1.1	0.1–8.1	1.7–9.6	1.2–5.8	0.5–5.9	1.1–5.2
Girls	ND–0.45					ND–1.9
T (ng/dL)						
Boys	105–450	90–216	102–209	70–223	95–168	100–210
Girls	14–42					25–48
AMH (pmol/L)						
Boys	140–819	114–856	254–703	374–892	324–858	438–1197
Girls	ND–25					ND–64
Inhibin B (ng/L)						
Boys	18–192	18–147	21–117	17–325	43–322	98–508
Girls	ND–ND					65–215

Data correspond to the 3rd and 97th centiles. FSH and LH measured by time-resolved immunofluorometric assays (DELFIA), testosterone by RIA after ethyl ether extraction, and AMH and Inhibin B by enzyme-linked immunosorbent assays (ELISA).
(Data obtained from Bergadá I, Milani C, Bedecarrás P, Andreone L, Ropelato MG, Gottlieb S, et al. Time course of the serum gonadotropin surge, inhibins, and anti-Mullerian hormone in normal newborn males during the first month of life. J Clin Endocrinol Metab 2006;91(10):4092–8.)

reproductive hormones should be interpreted with caution, strictly compared to age-specific normal ranges, during the first week. From the second week of life there is a progressive surge in all reproductive hormones. Gonadotropins increase more rapidly, and are high by the 8th day of life, whereas testosterone remains relatively low until the 3rd–4th weeks.[45,46] Gonadotropins and testosterone peak during the 2nd month of life, with a clear predominance of LH over FSH levels in the male, and then start declining after the 3rd month.[45,49] This timing differs in preterm newborns and infants: a slight delay is observed in the reactivation of gonadotropin and testosterone secretion, but peak levels are higher and the rate of decrease is slower.[45,49,50]

AMH and inhibin B show fewer variations than gonadotropins and androgens: although somewhat lower in the first days of life, they show a slight but constant increase during the first year of postnatal life,[45,46] probably reflecting the effect of FSH on Sertoli cell proliferation and secretory activity (Table 37.1). The germ cell population shows an increased mitotic activity, but meiosis is not initiated.

This period of postnatal activation of the reproductive axis is usually called "mini-puberty." However, notorious differences are observed when compared with true pubertal development occurring later in life.[26] Indeed, in spite of the high levels of intratesticular androgen concentrations seminiferous cords are exposed to during fetal life and "mini-puberty," no maturation occurs. Sertoli cells go on proliferating by mitosis, do not develop the cell-cell junctions typical of the blood-testis barrier, continue to produce high amounts of AMH, and are incapable of triggering meiosis and adult spermatogenesis. This physiological androgen insensitivity of the seminiferous cords is due to the lack of androgen receptor expression in Sertoli cells during fetal and early postnatal life.[27]

37.5.2.3 Childhood and Puberty: Brief Description

After the 4th–6th months of life, gonadotropins and testosterone are very low: the decline is more evident in LH and testosterone, which usually are nondetectable in serum during childhood. Only Sertoli cell activity remains clinically detectable, by means of the assessment of AMH and inhibin B levels, in this period of life.

Between 9 and 14 years of age, there is a progressive increase in gonadotropin pulse amplitude and frequency that triggers testicular pubertal maturation. Once again, LH induces Leydig cells to secrete androgen, which results in an increase in intratesticular testosterone concentration. Since Sertoli cells now express the androgen receptor, they acquire a mature phenotype characterized by the development of the blood-testis barrier and a downregulation of AMH production. Germ cells enter meiosis and go through the complete spermatogenic process giving rise to spermatozoa. The rise in serum testosterone is a somewhat late event in male pubertal development.[26]

37.6 THE OVARIES

37.6.1 Fetal Differentiation

The ovaries have no physiologic role in fetal differentiation of the genitalia,[17] which probably explains why less was known on ovarian than on testicular development until recent years.

37.6.1.1 Oogenesis and Folliculogenesis

Ovarian development begins with differentiation and proliferation of Gonadal Ridge Epithelial-Like (GREL) cells from mesonephric epithelial cells. When the underlying basal lamina breaks down, it allows stromal cells, vasculature and pluripotential primordial germ cells to migrate into the future ovary interspersed between the GREL cells (Fig. 37.4).[51] GREL cells present an initial differentiation as pregranulosa cells, only in XX gonads. Primordial germ cells proliferate and differentiate to oogonia for an extended period, from arrival at the developing XX genital ridges until the 7th month of gestation. Ovarian maturation proceeds from the center to the periphery. Beginning on week 11, oogonia in the deepest layers of the ovary enter meiotic prophase by a process that requires retinoic acid.[39,52] The stroma penetrates further towards the ovarian surface and then spreads laterally. GREL cells undergo continuous proliferation, expansion, and invagination towards the interior of the gonads and enclose oogonia forming ovigerous cords. The cords are arranged in the ovarian cortex surrounded by a basal lamina and stromal areas that contain capillaries, radially orientated towards and open to the surface of the ovary. The medulla is characterized by stromal cells, vasculature, and tubules originating from the mesonephros (rete ovarii).

Ovigerous cords are partitioned into smaller cords and eventually into follicles. GREL cells from ovigerous cords become pregranulosa cells. The oogonia enter meiosis and form oocytes, which become closely associated with pregranulosa. Primordial follicles arise, composed of one oocyte surrounded by a layer of flattened granulosa cells (Fig. 37.4). As follicles grow, the granulosa cells become cuboidal (primary follicle) and proliferate into multilayers (secondary follicle). At this stage the steroidogenic cell population called theca cells appears and surrounds the granulosa cell layers outside of the basal lamina. The progenitors of steroidogenic theca cells derive from two sources: the coelomic epithelium and the mesonephros. The first primary follicles appear during weeks 15 to 16, while the earliest antral follicles can be seen by weeks 23 to 24.[53,54] The first wave of granulosa cells contribute to ovarian follicles localized in the medullar part of the ovary.[55] There is a second population of granulosa cells that derive from the surface epithelium and give rise to cortical follicles. The latter seem to be the main contributor to continuous ovulation throughout reproductive life, and their gradual but steady loss leads to reproductive aging. By the 8th month of fetal life, there is no more mitosis of the oogonia and almost all germ cells have entered meiosis. Oocytes become arrested at the diplotene stage, where they remain until meiosis is completed with each cycle during puberty and adulthood. Noteworthy is the fact that only a minor proportion of oocytes undergo the full process: from 6 to 7 million ovarian follicles at 25 weeks, only 300,000 to 1 million persist at term.[54] Most oocytes undergo apoptosis and follicles become atretic. Primary and secondary follicles synthesize AMH in low amounts after the 23rd week of development.[56,57] Germ cells are critical in the ovaries in order to maintain the somatic component, i.e., granulosa and theca cells. If germ cells are lost, follicles rapidly degenerate.[53,58] Estrogen secretion by the ovaries is negligible compared to high placental estrogen production.

Finally, the ovarian surface undergoes further changes: surface cells no longer move into the ovary. GREL cells begin to differentiate into typical ovarian single-layered surface epithelium and are lined by a basal laminal that is thickened by the stroma underlying the surface forming the tunica albuginea.[59]

37.6.1.2 Molecular Pathways

The "default pathway" theory, suggesting that in the absence of *SRY* ovarian differentiation occurs, may apply to specific experimental conditions in rodents but not to humans, where mutations or deletions of the *SRY* gene result in gonadal dysgenesis, but not in ovarian differentiation with follicle development.[53] Recent findings indicate that the coordinated action of several factors is needed for the differentiation and stabilization of the ovaries. Two pathways are crucial in ovarian determination: one involving RSPO1/WNT4/CTNNB1 (β-catenin) and the other with FOXL2 as the major player. Both

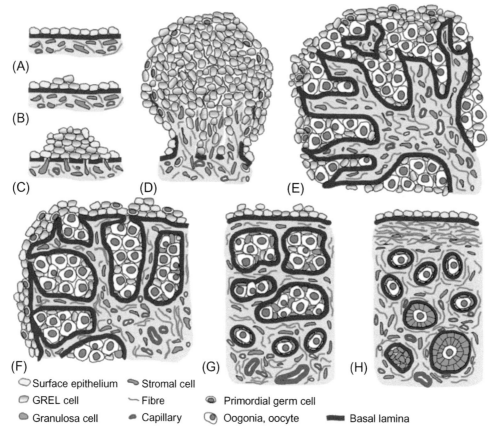

FIG. 37.4 Schematic diagram of ovarian development. (A) The development of the ovary commences at the mesonephric surface epithelium (*yellow* cells) in the location of the future gonadal ridge. (B) Some mesonephric surface epithelial cells change phenotype into GREL cells (*yellow-blue* cells). (C) The GREL cells proliferate and the basal lamina underlying the mesonephric surface epithelium breaks down, allowing stromal cells *(green)* to penetrate into the gonadal ridge. (D) GREL cells continue to proliferate and PGCs *(gray)* migrate into the ridge between the GREL cells. Mesonephric stroma including vasculature *(red)* continues to penetrate and expand in the ovary. (E) Oogonia proliferate and stroma penetrates further towards the ovarian surface enclosing oogonia and GREL cells into ovigerous cords. The cords are surrounded by a basal lamina at their interface with stroma but are open to the ovarian surface. Stromal areas, including those between the ovigerous cords, contain capillaries. (F) A compartmentalization into cortex and medulla becomes obvious. The cortex is characterized by alternating areas of ovigerous cords and stroma, whereas the medulla is formed by stromal cells, vasculature, and tubules originating from the mesonephros (rete ovarii). Once stroma penetrates below the cells on the surface it spreads laterally. The GREL cells at the surface are then aligned by a basal lamina at their interface with the stroma and begin to differentiate into typical ovarian surface epithelium (*yellow* cells). Some germ cells at the surface are also compartmentalized to the surface as stroma expands below it. (G) Ovigerous cords are partitioned into smaller cords and eventually into follicles. These contain GREL cells that form granulosa cells (*blue* cells) and oogonia that form oocytes. The first primordial follicles appear in the inner cortex-medulla region, surrounded by a basal lamina. A now fully intact basal lamina underlies multiple layers of surface epithelial cells. (H) At the final stage the surface epithelium becomes mostly single-layered and a tunica albuginea, densely packed with fibers, develops from the stroma below the surface epithelial basal lamina. Some primordial follicles become activated and commence development into primary and preantral follicles. *(Reproduced from Hummitzsch K, Irving-Rodgers HF, Hatzirodos N, Bonner W, Sabatier L, Reinhardt DP, Sado Y, Ninomiya Y, Wilhelm D, Rodgers RJ. A new model of development of the mammalian ovary and follicles. PloS One 2013;8(2):e55578.)*

are involved in activating the ovarian-specific genetic cascade and antagonizing testicular differentiation.[7,60] While they are two separate routes, β-catenin is the main candidate to promote the upregulation of FOXL2 that would be partially dependent on it.

WNT4, expressed at similar levels in the XY and XX undifferentiated gonads, is silenced by the SOX9-FGF9 pathway in the XY gonad (Fig. 37.2) but increases in the XX gonad and stabilizes β-catenin.[61] In the nucleus, β-catenin activates ovary-specific genes, resulting in granulosa cell differentiation.[60,62] WNT4 and β-catenin compete against FGF9 and SOX9.[35] β-catenin also stimulates follistatin (FST), which antagonizes the masculinizing factors Activin A and B, thus repressing endothelial cell migration and the coelomic vessel formation.[18] WNT4 also upregulates DAX1, which antagonizes SF1 and thereby inhibits steroidogenic enzymes involved in androgen biosynthesis.[63] WNT4 also acts as a germ cell survival factor in females.[64] Meiosis is triggered in response to upregulation of STRA8 induced by the high levels of retinoic acid synthesized by retinaldehyde dehydrogenases (ALDHs, also known as RALDHs).[9,15]

RSPO1 expression is present in the undifferentiated XX and XY gonads, but increases in the XX gonad before week 9, where it facilitates WNT signaling.[65]

FOXL2 is activated by β-catenin in the XX gonad from the 8th fetal week and is involved in granulosa cell differentiation. The high levels of WNT4, β-catenin and FOXL2 counteract FGF9 and SOX9, thus stabilizing the ovarian pathway.[7,66] FOXL2 is required to continuously suppress SOX9, thus preventing ovarian cells from transdifferentiating into "testis-like" cells, at least in the mouse.[67]

Finally, an increasing number of factors are essential for folliculogenesis.[14] Neurotrophins and their receptors facilitate follicle assembly and early follicular development. FIGα plays a crucial role in primordial follicle formation. NOBOX, SOHLH1, and SOHLH2 are involved in the transition to primary follicles, and GDF9 and BMP15 are essential in later stages of folliculogenesis.

37.6.2 Postnatal Changes

37.6.2.1 Anatomical Aspects and Histological Changes

In the newborn, the ovaries are a mass of elongated tissue lying in the abdominal cavity, not descending to the pelvis until the age of approximately 6 years. They are grayish in color, with an uneven surface covered by a modified peritoneum. The size of the ovaries varies with age: 0.3–3 cm^3 at birth and, during the first year of life, the volume decreases from the 2nd year to approximately 0.15–1.5 cm^3.[68–70] Thereafter, ovarian volume is below 1 cm^3 until 8–9 years when pubertal changes start.[69] In the outer cortex follicles (approximately 300 thousand to 1 million) are found at various stages of development, from primordial to small antral (<9 mm) and degeneration. The stroma of the cortex is a connective tissue composed of theca cells that respond to LH stimulation. The medulla contains the ovarian vasculature. Primary (noncyclic) follicle recruitment, i.e. the transition from a nongrowing primordial stage to a small growing stage, happens without interruption from the time of follicle assembly until the last one is recruited soon after menopause.

37.6.2.2 The Physiology of the Postnatal Activation

The transient postnatal pituitary-gonadal activation, or "mini-puberty," is longer in girls than in boys. There is a significant gonadotropin and steroid hormone secretion but, in contrast with the true puberty, ovulation does not happen. As in boys, all hormones are low at birth (Table 37.1). Gonadotropins increase and peak between the first and third month, with a predominance of FSH in the female newborn and infant.[45,46,49] LH levels decrease by the 6th month, but FSH remains high for 1 or 2 years. Estradiol increases, in association with follicular development, and is clearly higher than in infant boys; levels fluctuate, probably reflecting cyclic follicular maturation and atrophy, and decrease after the second year.[49] AMH and inhibin B are undetectable or very low at birth and increase during the first month and then stabilize but remain significantly lower than in boys.[45,46] The gonadotropin surge is bigger and prolonged in premature girls.[49] Testosterone levels are usually low; to avoid cross-reactions leading to falsely elevated androgen levels, measurements should be done after submitting serum samples to extractive procedures that eliminate other steroids.[46]

In preterm newborns and infants, gonadotropins are higher during the first 2 to 3 months of postnatal life; then they normalize in coincidence with the elevation of estradiol levels.[50]

37.6.2.3 Childhood and Puberty: Brief Description

During childhood the ovary is rather quiescent, with little follicular activity. Gonadotropin levels are low, especially LH. Estrogens are usually undetectable or very low, whereas AMH[71] and inhibin B[72] are low and stable.

The reactivation of the GnRH pulse leads to an increase in gonadotropin release and to ovarian stimulation. LH and FSH secretion take place initially at night and then, as puberty advances, throughout the day. Serum LH concentrations rise at puberty to levels 10–50 times higher than prepubertal levels, while FSH concentrations increase 2–3 times during female puberty.[73] Secondary or "cyclic" follicular recruitment begins. Oocytes arrested in diplotene resume the first meiotic division. One dominant follicle containing a secondary oocyte is ovulated every 21 to 35 days. However, the cycles may be irregular and anovulatory for 2–5 years.[74] Ovarian volume increases (>1 mL) owing largely to follicular development. The clinical onset of puberty or gonadarche is marked by breast development or thelarche, which reflects estradiol production. Gonadotropins, estrogens, progesterone, and inhibins A and B show typical cyclic changes, whereas AMH is stable.

37.7 THE REPRODUCTIVE TRACT AND EXTERNAL GENITALIA

37.7.1 The Sexually Undifferentiated Embryo

Like the gonadal ridges, the reproductive duct system and the external genitalia are sexually undifferentiated during early embryonic life. Up to the 8th week, the internal reproductive tract consists of a set of two unipotential ducts, the Wolffian (mesonephric) and Müllerian (paramesonephric) ducts, which run into the urogenital sinus (Fig. 37.1). The opening of the urogenital sinus, the ostium, is surrounded by labioscrotal swellings, which develop on each side of the urogenital folds. The genital tubercle emerges as a ventral medial outgrowth just cranial to the opening of the ostium. All these structures are sexually bipotential, i.e., they can differentiate following the male or the female pathway depending on the hormonal context.

37.7.1.1 Morphogenesis of the Anlagen

Wolffian ducts originate in the mesonephros in embryos 25 to 32 days old. They participate in the formation of the male internal ducts and of the urinary system, which explains the existence of associated malformations of the Wolffian ducts and the kidneys or ureters.

Müllerian ducts arise approximately 1 week later as a cleft lined by the coelomic epithelium, laterally to the Wolffian ducts in the urogenital ridge.[75] By the 8th week, the growing Müllerian ducts, now in the pelvis, cross the Wolffian duct ventrally. The two Müllerian ducts fuse in the midline, giving rise to the uterovaginal canal, which contacts the posterior wall of the urogenital sinus.

The cloaca, the distal portion of the hindgut, is covered by endoderm surrounded by mesoderm. Distally, it is closed by the cloacal membrane, formed by ectoderm and endoderm, with no mesoderm in between. During the 5th week, mesodermal cells spread along the cloacal membrane and give rise to the cloacal folds. The cloaca and the cloacal membrane are divided by the urorectal septum, giving rise ventrally to the urogenital sinus and the urogenital folds, and dorsally to the rectal sinus and the anal folds. The urogenital folds fuse ventrally in the midline to form the genital tubercle, which consists of mesoderm and surface ectoderm.[76] Endodermal cells from the urogenital sinus invade the genital tubercle to form the urethral plate, in the roof of the urethral groove.[77,78] The corpora cavernosa and glans differentiate from the mesoderm and are localized laterally to the urethral groove. Laterally to the urogenital folds are the labioscrotal folds (Fig. 37.1). The external genitalia remain undifferentiated up to approximately 9 weeks and are represented by the genital tubercle, the urogenital folds, and the labioscrotal folds.[79]

37.7.1.2 Molecular Pathways

The development of the Wolffian ducts depends on several factors (for review see ref.[6]). PAX2, PAX8, and GATA3 induce the initial formation, while LIM1 promotes the extension. EMX2 and FGF8 signaling through FGFR1 and FGFR2 play a role in the development and maintenance of the Wolffian ducts. RET signaling is involved in several steps of early development.

Three phases are described in the development of the Müllerian ducts.[75] During the first phase, coelomic epithelium specification is dependent on DACH1 and DACH2, which regulate the expression of LHX1 and WNT7A. This phase is characterized by the expression of LHX1 and AMH receptor type 2 (AMHR2). In the second phase, WNT4 expression is essential in the mesonephros for the Müllerian duct invagination. Finally, the elongation phase needs an integrity of protein kinase pathways. Because close contact with the Wolffian duct is necessary, Müllerian growth is also dependent on factors required for Wolffian development, such as LIM1 or PAX2, and on WNT9B, secreted by the Wolffian epithelial cells.[80]

Many growth factors involved in the initial formation of internal ducts, such as EMX2, HOXA13, LIM1, PAX2, and VANGL2, are ubiquitously expressed and necessary also for the development of other organs. For instance, the cystic fibrosis transmembrane conductance regulator (CFTR) is involved in the formation of Wolffian ducts as well as ducts of the respiratory system and the pancreas.[81] Others, like WNT4A and WNT7A, are restricted to the formation of Müllerian ducts.[75]

SOX9[82] and FGF10[83] play a role in early prostate bud differentiation from the urogenital sinus. The secreted frizzled-related proteins (SFRP1 and 2) are required for correct gubernaculum development and testicular descent.[84]

The formation of the anlagen of the external genitalia is regulated by a cascade of signaling molecules that shows similarities with that involved in distal limb development, e.g., BMPs,[76,85] FGF8, FGF10, and HOX factors.[86] β-catenin regulates FGF8 in genital tubercle outgrowth.[87] Ephrins mediate cell adhesion and patterning events occurring at the midline, including urethral closure, scrotal fusion, and palate fusion.[76,88] Diacylglycerol kinase K (DGKK) seems important for urethral plate development.[89]

37.7.2 Male Differentiation

The pioneering experiments performed by Jost in the 1940s[17] led to the currently valid paradigm of fetal differentiation of internal and external genitalia: the existence of two functional testicular hormones, testosterone and AMH, are necessary and sufficient to drive male differentiation. In their absence, female differentiation proceeds (Fig. 37.1).

37.7.2.1 Anatomic Aspects and Hormonal Regulation

The Müllerian ducts begin to regress under the effect of AMH during the 8th week and has completely disappeared by week 10. AMH signals through two membrane receptors with serine/threonine kinase activity. AMHR2 is specific for AMH, expressed in the mesenchymal cells surrounding the Müllerian duct epithelium. AMH binding to AMHR2 requires proteolytic cleavage of the AMH precursor.[90] Subsequently, AMHR2 assembles with type 1 receptor ALK3.[91] Intracellular signaling is mediated by Smad-1/5/8 phosphorylation and association with Smad4, and shuttling to the nucleus where they regulate transcription of target genes.

Wolffian ducts differentiate exclusively along the male pathway, in response to androgens, to form the epididymides, the vasa deferentia, and the seminal vesicles during the 9th to 12th weeks of fetal life. Testosterone, the main androgen produced by the fetal testis, acts locally on the Wolffian ducts through its nuclear receptor. Because the androgen receptor is not expressed in the epithelium but in the stroma of the Wolffian ducts, the process seems to be dependent on androgen-mediated signaling from the stroma to the epithelium.[92]

The urogenital sinus gives rise to the bladder in both sexes. Male differentiation of the urogenital sinus is characterized by prostatic development and by the repression of vaginal development. Prostatic buds grow into solid branching cords during the 10th week. Additionally, two sino-utricular bulbs develop close to the opening of the Wolffian ducts and grow inwards, fusing with the medial Müllerian tubercle, to form the prostatic utricle, the male equivalent of the vagina, at 18 weeks.[93]

Male differentiation of the external genitalia, beginning in the 9th week, is characterized by the lengthening of the anogenital distance and the fusion of the labioscrotal and urogenital folds, in a dorsal to ventral fashion.[79,94] Fusion of the labioscrotal folds gives rise to the scrotum by week 12. Penile development is a controversial issue: some authors propose that the proximal urethra forms by fusion of the urogenital folds and the distal urethra arises from an invagination of the apical ectoderm, while others suggest that the entire urethra is of endodermal origin, formed by the urethral plate dorsally and the fused urethral folds ventrally.[95] Urethral formation is complete by the 14th week, although a physiological ventral curvature can persist up to the 6th month. Differential penile growth, as compared to the clitoris, does not occur until 14 weeks.[96] Maximal phallic growth occurs during the third trimester of fetal life, even though testosterone levels are declining.

The masculinization of the urogenital sinus and external genitalia occurs mainly in response to DHT, which has 5 to 10 times higher activity than testosterone[97,98] because it binds to the androgen receptor with greater affinity. Furthermore, DHT cannot be aromatized to estrogen; thus it has a purely androgenic effect.

37.7.2.2 Testicular Descent

The testes, initially formed in the abdominal cavity near the kidneys, normally descend to their final location in the scrotum by term in >97% of the cases. Preterm birth is associated with higher incidence of cryptorchidism, and testicular descent can occur during the first year of postnatal life.[99] The testes are attached to the cranial abdominal wall by the suspensory ligament and to the scrotum by the gubernaculum testis and descend to the scrotum in a two-phase process. The first or transabdominal phase is controlled by INSL3,[44] which acts on the gubernaculum testis. The second or inguino-scrotal phase is mainly dependent on androgens, which mediate the disappearance of the cranial suspensory ligament and the shrinkage of the gubernaculum.

37.7.2.3 Postnatal Changes

At birth, the penis measures >2.5 cm, with the urethral meatus at the tip, and the testes are in the scrotum; their volume is usually clinically estimated at 1–2 mL when measured by comparison with Prader's orchidometer and approximately 0.25 mL when measured by ultrasonography.[70] The penis enlarges during the first 3–6 months, due to androgen action. Concomitantly, there is a slight increase in testicular volume, which may not be noticeable by palpation but can be measured by ultrasonography[100] and reflects FSH action on Sertoli cells.

During the rest of infancy and childhood, the changes in penile size and testicular volume are negligible. Pubertal onset is clinically defined by a testicular volume of 4 mL or more, which is associated with reddening of the scrotal skin, and corresponds to stage 2 as defined by Marshall and Tanner.[101] Spermatogenic development is mainly responsible for the remarkable increase of testis volume during puberty. FSH and germ cells induce an increase in inhibin B. Serum levels of inhibin B increase concomitantly with testicular volume and attain adult levels as early as pubertal stage 2.[72]

37.7.3 Female Differentiation

37.7.3.1 Anatomic Aspects and Hormonal Regulation

If there is no AMH action by the end of the 9th week, Müllerian ducts differentiate into the fallopian tubes, uterus, and upper vagina. The two Müllerian ducts are initially separated by an intermediate septum, which decreases in a caudal-rostral sense, leading to the formation of a unicavitary uterus and vagina. In the absence of androgen action, the lower portion of the vagina and the vestibulum vaginae are formed from the urogenital sinus. The lower end of the vagina slides down along the urethra until the vaginal rudiment opens directly on the surface of the perineum at 22 weeks. The hymen marks the separation between the vagina and the diminutive urogenital sinus, which becomes the vestibule. Lack of androgen action also leads to Wolffian duct regression, which starts on the 10th week, and to the feminization of the external genitalia. The urogenital folds give rise to the labia minora and the labioscrotal folds to the labia majora (Fig. 37.1). Fetal estrogens are not necessary for feminization of the internal and external genitalia, as shown by Jost's experiments.[17]

37.7.3.2 Postnatal Changes

In the postnatal period, girls do not show significant changes in the external genital appearance. An edema of the labia majora may occur and usually resolves in the first days of life; this condition is more usual in fetuses that present pelvic position at birth. A sparse genital bleeding may occur between 3 and 5 days of life secondary to endometrial proliferation due to the passage of placental estrogens and their descent after birth. Likewise, a transient mammary gland development can occur during the postnatal period of pituitary-gonadal activation ("mini-puberty"). During childhood there are no evident changes. Pubertal onset is clinically defined by breast bud development, corresponding to stage 2 as described by Marshall and Tanner,[102] due to estrogen activity.

37.8 THE ROLE OF EPIGENETICS

Epigenetic mechanisms are involved in the regulation of gene expression without changing the DNA sequence. These mechanisms result from the effect of environmental factors and produce changes in chromatin structure. Histone acetylation, methylation, and demethylation, DNA methylation, and ATP-dependent chromatin remodeling are the best-characterized mechanisms underlying epigenetic regulation.[103]

Under normal conditions, epigenetic regulation guarantees the expected spatial and temporal expression of developmentally regulated genes. In reptiles, temperature is an environmental stimulus that affects sex determination by changing DNA methylation patterns in the promoter of the aromatase gene, which seems essential in the commitment to the female pathway. On the other hand, environmental toxicants, like polychlorinated biphenyls, may lead to epigenetic changes, resulting in altered expression profiles of genes responsible for gonadal differentiation turtles. (Reviewed in ref.[1]).

The involvement of histone methylation and demethylation in sex differentiation has been clearly demonstrated in the mouse. While methylation of histone H3 lysine 4 (H3K4) is seen in the promoter regions of actively transcribed genes, methylation of H3K9 is enriched in transcriptionally silenced gene promoters.[103] The activation of *Sry* transcription in the fetal male gonad requires demethylation of H3K9. In XY mice deficient for the H3K9-demethylating enzyme JMJD1A, there is a decrease in *Sry* expression leading to sex reversal.[104] The importance of histone acetylation in gonadal determination is illustrated by the experimental mouse model in which loss of p300 and CBP disrupts histone acetylation at the mouse *Sry* promoter, causing XY sex reversal.[105] ATP-dependent chromatin remodeling complexes include four different families: switch/sucrose nonfermentable (SWI/SNF), ISWI, CHD, and INO80 families. While our understanding of the role of epigenetics in the human is not as advanced as in the murine model, it is likely a key player in ovarian and testicular development. For example, mutations in the *ATRX* gene, which encodes the SWI/SNF-like chromatin remodeling protein, are responsible for a congenital disorder in humans characterized by alpha-thalassemia, mental retardation, and sex reversal due to gonadal dysgenesis in XY individuals.[106] Future insights into normal gonadal development will likely come from the identification of additional disorders of the epigenome.

REFERENCES

1. Capel B. Vertebrate sex determination: evolutionary plasticity of a fundamental switch. *Nat Rev Genet* 2017;**18**(11):675–89.
2. Quinton R, Hasan W, Grant W, Thrasivoulou C, Quiney RE, Besser GM, et al. Gonadotropin-releasing hormone immunoreactivity in the nasal epithelia of adults with Kallmann's syndrome and isolated hypogonadotropic hypogonadism and in the early midtrimester human fetus. *J Clin Endocrinol Metab* 1997;**82**(1):309–14.
3. Valdes-Socin H, Rubio Almanza M, Tomé Fernández-Ladreda M, Debray FG, Bours V, Beckers A. Reproduction, smell, and neurodevelopmental disorders: genetic defects in different hypogonadotropic hypogonadal syndromes. *Front Endocrinol* 2014;**5**:109; 1–8.
4. Romero CJ, Pine-Twaddell E, Radovick S. Novel mutations associated with combined pituitary hormone deficiency. *J Mol Endocrinol* 2011;**46**(3): R93–R102.
5. Thliveris JA, Currie RW. Observations on the hypothalamo-hypophyseal portal vasculature in the developing human fetus. *Am J Anat* 1980;**157**(4):441–4.
6. Rey R, Josso N, Racine C. *Sexual differentiation*. In: De Groot LJ, Chrousos G, Dungan K, Feingold KR, Grossman A, Hershman JM, et al. *Endotext*. South Dartmouth, MA: MDText.com, Inc.; 2016 http://www.endotext.org/chapter/sexual-differentiation/ [Accessed 1 June 2017].
7. Lin YT, Capel B. Cell fate commitment during mammalian sex determination. *Curr Opin Genet Dev* 2015;**32**:144–52.
8. Martinez-Aguayo A, Rocha A, Rojas N, García C, Parra R, Lagos M, et al. Testicular adrenal rest tumors and Leydig and Sertoli cell function in boys with classical congenital adrenal hyperplasia. *J Clin Endocrinol Metab* 2007;**92**(12):4583–9.
9. Sekido R, Lovell-Badge R. Genetic control of testis development. *Sex Dev* 2013;**7**(1–3):21–32.
10. Hastie ND. Wilms' tumour 1 (WT1) in development, homeostasis and disease. *Development* 2017;**144**(16):2862–72.
11. Suntharalingham JP, Buonocore F, Duncan AJ, Achermann JC. DAX-1 (NR0B1) and steroidogenic factor-1 (SF-1, NR5A1) in human disease. *Best Pract Res Clin Endocrinol Metab* 2015;**29**(4):607–19.
12. Jeyasuria P, Ikeda Y, Jamin SP, Zhao L, De Rooij DG, Themmen AP, et al. Cell-specific knockout of steroidogenic factor 1 reveals its essential roles in gonadal function. *Mol Endocrinol* 2004;**18**(7):1610–9.
13. Surani MA. Human germline: a new research frontier. *Stem Cell Rep* 2015;**4**(6):955–60.
14. Edson MA, Nagaraja AK, Matzuk MM. The mammalian ovary from genesis to revelation. *Endocr Rev* 2009;**30**(6):624–712.
15. Bowles J, Koopman P. Precious cargo: regulation of sex-specific germ cell development in mice. *Sex Dev* 2013;**7**(1–3):46–60.
16. McLaren A. Germ and somatic cell lineages in the developing gonad. *Mol Cell Endocrinol* 2000;**163**(1–2):3–9.
17. Jost A. Problems of fetal endocrinology: the gonadal and hypophyseal hormones. *Recent Prog Horm Res* 1953;**8**:379–418.
18. Ungewitter EK, Yao HH. How to make a gonad: cellular mechanisms governing formation of the testes and ovaries. *Sex Dev* 2013;**7**(1–3):7–20.
19. Bendsen E, Byskov AG, Laursen SB, Larsen HP, Andersen CY, Westergaard LG. Number of germ cells and somatic cells in human fetal testes during the first weeks after sex differentiation. *Hum Reprod* 2003;**18**(1):13–8.
20. O'Shaughnessy PJ, Baker PJ, Monteiro A, Cassie S, Bhattacharya S, Fowler PA. Developmental changes in human fetal testicular cell numbers and messenger ribonucleic acid levels during the second trimester. *J Clin Endocrinol Metab* 2007;**92**(12):4792–801.
21. O'Shaughnessy PJ, Morris ID, Huhtaniemi I, Baker PJ, Abel MH. Role of androgen and gonadotrophins in the development and function of the Sertoli cells and Leydig cells: data from mutant and genetically modified mice. *Mol Cell Endocrinol* 2009;**306**:2–8.
22. Braslavsky D, Grinspon RP, Ballerini MG, Bedecarrás P, Loreti N, Bastida G, et al. Hypogonadotropic hypogonadism in infants with congenital hypopituitarism: a challenge to diagnose at an early stage. *Hormone Research in Paediatrics* 2015;**84**(5):289–97.
23. Berensztein EB, Baquedano MS, Gonzalez CR, Saraco NI, Rodriguez J, Ponzio R, et al. Expression of aromatase, estrogen receptor alpha and beta, androgen receptor, and cytochrome P-450scc in the human early prepubertal testis. *Pediatr Res* 2006;**60**(6):740–4.
24. Chemes HE, Rey RA, Nistal M, Regadera J, Musse M, Gonzalez-Peramato P, et al. Physiological androgen insensitivity of the fetal, neonatal, and early infantile testis is explained by the ontogeny of the androgen receptor expression in Sertoli cells. *J Clin Endocrinol Metab* 2008;**93**(11):4408–12.
25. Boukari K, Meduri G, Brailly-Tabard S, Guibourdenche J, Ciampi ML, Massin N, et al. Lack of androgen receptor expression in Sertoli cells accounts for the absence of anti-Mullerian hormone repression during early human testis development. *J Clin Endocrinol Metab* 2009;**94**(5):1818–25.
26. Rey RA. Mini-puberty and true puberty: differences in testicular function. *Ann Endocrinol* 2014;**75**(2):58–63.
27. Rey RA, Musse M, Venara M, Chemes HE. Ontogeny of the androgen receptor expression in the fetal and postnatal testis: its relevance on Sertoli cell maturation and the onset of adult spermatogenesis. *Microsc Res Tech* 2009;**72**(11):787–95.
28. Stevant I, Neirijnck Y, Borel C, Escoffier J, Smith LB, Antonarakis SE, et al. Deciphering cell lineage specification during male sex determination with single-cell RNA sequencing. *Cell Rep* 2018;**22**(6):1589–99.
29. Wen Q, Cheng CY, Liu YX. Development, function and fate of fetal Leydig cells. *Semin Cell Dev Biol* 2016;**59**:89–98.
30. Mamsen LS, Ernst EH, Borup R, Larsen A, Olesen RH, Ernst E, et al. Temporal expression pattern of genes during the period of sex differentiation in human embryonic gonads. *Sci Rep* 2017;**7**(1).
31. Bullejos M, Koopman P. Delayed Sry and Sox9 expression in developing mouse gonads underlies B6-YDOM sex reversal. *Dev Biol* 2005;**278**(2):473–81.
32. Huang B, Wang SB, Ning Y, Lamb AN, Bartley J. Autosomal XX sex reversal caused by duplication of SOX9. *Am J Med Genet* 1999;**87**(4):349–53.
33. Sutton E, Hughes J, White S, Sekido R, Tan J, Arboleda V, et al. Identification of SOX3 as an XX male sex reversal gene in mice and humans. *J Clin Investig* 2011;**121**(1):328–41.
34. Georg I, Barrionuevo F, Wiech T, Scherer G. Sox9 and Sox8 are required for basal lamina integrity of testis cords and for suppression of FOXL2 during embryonic testis development in mice. *Biol Reprod* 2012;**87**(4):99 1–11.

35. Kim Y, Kobayashi A, Sekido R, DiNapoli L, Brennan J, Chaboissier M-C, et al. Fgf9 and Wnt4 act as antagonistic signals to regulate mammalian sex determination. *PLoS Biol* 2006;**4**(6):e187.

36. Eggers S, Ohnesorg T, Sinclair A. Genetic regulation of mammalian gonad development. *Nat Rev Endocrinol* 2014;**10**:673–83.

37. Shima Y, Morohashi KI. Leydig progenitor cells in fetal testis. *Mol Cell Endocrinol* 2017;**445**:55–64.

38. Adams IR, McLaren A. Sexually dimorphic development of mouse primordial germ cells: switching from oogenesis to spermatogenesis. *Development* 2002;**129**(5):1155–64.

39. Feng CW, Bowles J, Koopman P. Control of mammalian germ cell entry into meiosis. *Mol Cell Endocrinol* 2014;**382**(1):488–97.

40. Josso N, Lamarre I, Picard JY, Berta P, Davies N, Morichon N, et al. Anti-Müllerian hormone in early human development. *Early Hum Dev* 1993;**33**(2):91–9.

41. Scott HM, Mason JI, Sharpe RM. Steroidogenesis in the fetal testis and its susceptibility to disruption by exogenous compounds. *Endocr Rev* 2009;**30**(7):883–925.

42. Auchus RJ, Miller WL. Defects in androgen biosynthesis causing 46,XY disorders of sexual development. *Semin Reprod Med* 2012;**30**(5):417–26.

43. Flück CE, Pandey AV. Steroidogenesis of the testis – new genes and pathways. *Ann Endocrinol* 2014;**75**(2):40–7.

44. Ivell R, Anand-Ivell R. Biological role and clinical significance of insulin-like peptide 3. *Curr Opin Endocrinol Diabetes Obes* 2011;**18**(3):210–6.

45. Kuijper EA, Ket JC, Caanen MR, Lambalk CB. Reproductive hormone concentrations in pregnancy and neonates: a systematic review. *ReprodBiomedOnline* 2013;**27**(1):33–63.

46. Bergadá I, Milani C, Bedecarrás P, Andreone L, Ropelato MG, Gottlieb S, et al. Time course of the serum gonadotropin surge, inhibins, and anti-Mullerian hormone in normal newborn males during the first month of life. *J Clin Endocrinol Metab* 2006;**91**(10):4092–8.

47. Bergadá I, Ballerini MG, Ayuso S, Groome NP, Bergadá C, Campo S. High serum concentrations of dimeric inhibins A and B in normal newborn girls. *Fertil Steril* 2002;**77**(2):363–5.

48. Garagorri JM, Rodriguez G, Lario-Elboj AJ, Olivares JL, Lario-Munoz A, Orden I. Reference levels for 17-hydroxyprogesterone, 11-desoxycortisol, cortisol, testosterone, dehydroepiandrosterone sulfate and androstenedione in infants from birth to six months of age. *Eur J Pediatr* 2008;**167**(6):647–53.

49. Kuiri-Hänninen T, Sankilampi U, Dunkel L. Activation of the hypothalamic-pituitary-gonadal axis in infancy, minipuberty. *Hormone Res Paediatr* 2014;**82**:73–80.

50. Kuiri-Hänninen T, Dunkel L, Sankilampi U. Sexual dimorphism in postnatal gonadotrophin levels in infancy reflects diverse maturation of the ovarian and testicular hormone synthesis. *Clin Endocrinol* 2018;**89**:85–92.

51. Hummitzsch K, Irving-Rodgers HF, Hatzirodos N, Bonner W, Sabatier L, Reinhardt DP, et al. A new model of development of the mammalian ovary and follicles. *PLoS One* 2013;**8**(2).

52. Le Bouffant R, Guerquin MJ, Duquenne C, Frydman N, Coffigny H, Rouiller-Fabre V, et al. Meiosis initiation in the human ovary requires intrinsic retinoic acid synthesis. *Hum Reprod* 2010;**25**(10):2579–90.

53. Reynaud K, Cortvrindt R, Verlinde F, De Schepper J, Bourgain C, Smitz J. Number of ovarian follicles in human fetuses with the 45,X karyotype. *Fertil Steril* 2004;**81**(4):1112–9.

54. Kerr JB, Myers M, Anderson RA. The dynamics of the primordial follicle reserve. *Reproduction* 2013;**146**(6):R205–15.

55. Zheng W, Zhang H, Gorre N, Risal S, Shen Y, Liu K. Two classes of ovarian primordial follicles exhibit distinct developmental dynamics and physiological functions. *Hum Mol Genet* 2014;**23**(4):920–8.

56. Kuiri-Hänninen T, Kallio S, Seuri R, Tyrvainen E, Liakka A, Tapanainen J, et al. Postnatal developmental changes in the pituitary-ovarian axis in preterm and term infant girls. *J Clin Endocrinol Metab* 2011;**96**(11):3432–9.

57. Rey R, Sabourin JC, Venara M, Long WQ, Jaubert F, Zeller WP, et al. Anti-Mullerian hormone is a specific marker of sertoli- and granulosa-cell origin in gonadal tumors. *Hum Pathol* 2000;**31**(10):1202–8.

58. Singh RP, Carr DH. The anatomy and histology of XO human embryos and fetuses. *Anat Rec* 1966;**155**(3):369–83.

59. Smith P, Wilhelm D, Rodgers RJ. Development of mammalian ovary. *J Endocrinol* 2014;**221**(3):R145–61.

60. Pannetier M, Chassot AA, Chaboissier MC, Pailhoux E. Involvement of FOXL2 and RSPO1 in ovarian determination, development, and maintenance in mammals. *Sex Dev* 2016;**10**(4):167–84.

61. Biason-Lauber A. WNT4, RSPO1, and FOXL2 in sex development. *Semin Reprod Med* 2012;**30**(5):387–95.

62. Chassot AA, Gillot I, Chaboissier MC. R-spondin1, WNT4, and the CTNNB1 signaling pathway: strict control over ovarian differentiation. *Reproduction* 2014;**148**(6):R97–110.

63. Heikkila M, Prunskaite R, Naillat F, Itaranta P, Vuoristo J, Leppaluoto J, et al. The partial female to male sex reversal in Wnt-4-deficient females involves induced expression of testosterone biosynthetic genes and testosterone production, and depends on androgen action. *Endocrinology* 2005;**146**(9):4016–23.

64. Rastetter RH, Bernard P, Palmer JS, Chassot AA, Chen H, Western PS, et al. Marker genes identify three somatic cell types in the fetal mouse ovary. *Dev Biol* 2014;**394**(2):242–52.

65. Tomaselli S, Megiorni F, Lin L, Mazzilli MC, Gerrelli D, Majore S, et al. Human RSPO1/R-spondin1 is expressed during early ovary development and augments beta-catenin signaling. *PLoS One* 2011;**6**(1).

66. Biason-Lauber A, Chaboissier MC. Ovarian development and disease: the known and the unexpected. *Semin Cell Dev Biol* 2015;**45**:59–67.

67. Uhlenhaut NH, Jakob S, Anlag K, Eisenberger T, Sekido R, Kress J, et al. Somatic sex reprogramming of adult ovaries to testes by FOXL2 ablation. *Cell* 2009;**139**(6):1130–42.

68. Cohen HL, Shapiro MA, Mandel FS, Shapiro ML. Normal ovaries in neonates and infants: a sonographic study of 77 patients 1 day to 24 months old. *AJR Am J Roentgenol* 1993;**160**(3):583–6.

69. Khadilkar VV, Khadilkar AV, Kinare AS, Tapasvi HS, Deshpande SS, Maskati GB. Ovarian and uterine ultrasonography in healthy girls between birth to 18 years. *Indian Pediatr* 2006;**43**(7):625–30.

70. Kaplan SL, Edgar JC, Ford EG, Adgent MA, Schall JI, Kelly A, et al. Size of testes, ovaries, uterus and breast buds by ultrasound in healthy full-term neonates ages 0-3 days. *Pediatr Radiol* 2016;**46**(13):1837–47.

71. Hagen CP, Aksglæde L, Sorensen K, Main KM, Boas M, Cleemann L, et al. Serum levels of anti-Mullerian hormone as a marker of ovarian function in 926 healthy females from birth to adulthood and in 172 turner syndrome patients. *J Clin Endocrinol Metab* 2010;**95**(11):5003–10.

72. Bergadá I, Bergadá C, Campo SM. Role of inhibins in childhood and puberty. *J Pediatr Endocrinol Metab* 2001;**14**(4):343–53.

73. Oerter KE, Uriarte MM, Rose SR, Barnes KM, Cutler Jr GB. Gonadotropin secretory dynamics during puberty in normal girls and boys. *J Clin Endocrinol Metab* 1990;**71**(5):1251–8.

74. Rosenfield RL. Clinical review: adolescent anovulation: maturational mechanisms and implications. *J Clin Endocrinol Metab* 2013;**98**(9):3572–83.

75. Mullen RD, Behringer RR. Molecular genetics of Mullerian duct formation, regression and differentiation. *Sex Dev* 2014;**8**(5):281–96.

76. Bouty A, Ayers KL, Pask A, Heloury Y, Sinclair AH. The genetic and environmental factors underlying hypospadias. *Sex Dev* 2015;**9**(5):239–59.

77. Penington EC, Hutson JM. The urethral plate: does it grow into the genital tubercle or within it? *Br J Urol* 2002;**89**:733–9.

78. Blaschko SD, Cunha GR, Baskin LS. Molecular mechanisms of external genitalia development. *Differentiation* 2012;**84**(3):261–8.

79. Jirásek JE. Morphogenesis of the genital system in the human. *Birth Defects Orig Artic Ser* 1977;**13**(2):13–39.

80. Carroll TJ, Park JS, Hayashi S, Majumdar A, McMahon AP. Wnt9b plays a central role in the regulation of mesenchymal to epithelial transitions underlying organogenesis of the mammalian urogenital system. *Dev Cell* 2005;**9**(2):283–92.

81. Chen H, Ruan YC, Xu WM, Chen J, Chan HC. Regulation of male fertility by CFTR and implications in male infertility. *Hum Reprod Update* 2012;**18**(6):703–13.

82. Thomsen MK, Butler CM, Shen MM, Swain A. Sox9 is required for prostate development. *Dev Biol* 2008;**316**(2):302–11.

83. Donjacour AA, Thomson A, Cunha G. FGF-10 plays an essential role in the growth of the fetal prostate. *Dev Biol* 2003;**261**(1):39–54.

84. Warr N, Siggers P, Bogani D, Brixey R, Pastorelli L, Yates L, et al. Sfrp1 and Sfrp2 are required for normal male sexual development in mice. *Dev Biol* 2009;**326**(2):273–84.

85. Suzuki K, Bachiller D, Chen YP, Kamikawa M, Ogi H, Haraguchi R, et al. Regulation of outgrowth and apoptosis for the terminal appendage: external genitalia: development by concerted actions of BMP signaling. *Development* 2003;**130**(25):6209–20.

86. Klonisch T, Fowler PA, Hombach-Klonisch S. Molecular and genetic regulation of testis descent and external genitalia development. *Dev Biol* 2004;**270**(1):1–18.

87. Lin C, Yin Y, Long F, Ma L. Tissue-specific requirements of beta-catenin in external genitalia development. *Development* 2008;**135**(16):2815–25.

88. Yucel S, Dravis C, García N, Henkemeyer M, Baker LA. Hypospadias and anorectal malformations mediated by Eph/ephrin signaling. *J Pediatr Urol* 2007;**3**(5):354–63.

89. Shen J, Liu B, Sinclair A, Cunha G, Baskin LS, Choudhry S. Expression analysis of DGKK during external genitalia formation. *J Urol* 2015;**194**(6):1728–36.

90. di Clemente N, Jamin SP, Lugovskoy A, Carmillo P, Ehrenfels C, Picard J-Y, et al. Processing of anti-Mullerian hormone regulates receptor activation by a mechanism Distinct from TGF-β. *Mol Endocrinol* 2010;**24**(11):2193–206.

91. Jamin SP, Arango NA, Mishina Y, Hanks MC, Behringer RR. Requirement of Bmpr1a for Mullerian duct regression during male sexual development. *Nat Genet* 2002;**32**(3):408–10.

92. Welsh M, Saunders PT, Sharpe RM. The critical time window for androgen-dependent development of the Wolffian duct in the rat. *Endocrinology* 2007;**148**(7):3185–95.

93. Glenister TW. The development of the utricle and of the so-called "middle" or "median" lobe of the human prostate. *J Anat* 1962;**96**:443–55.

94. Baskin LS, Erol A, Jegatheesan P, Li Y, Liu W, Cunha GR. Urethral seam formation and hypospadias. *Cell Tissue Res* 2001;**305**(3):379–87.

95. Cunha GR, Sinclair A, Risbridger G, Hutson J, Baskin LS. Current understanding of hypospadias: relevance of animal models. *Nat Rev Urol* 2015;**12**(5):271–80.

96. Zalel Y, Pinhas-Hamiel O, Lipitz S, Mashiach S, Achiron R. The development of the fetal penis – an in utero sonographic evaluation. *Ultrasound Obstet Gynecol* 2001;**17**(2):129–31.

97. Pihlajamaa P, Sahu B, Jänne OA. Determinants of receptor- and tissue-specific actions in androgen signaling. *Endocr Rev* 2015;**36**(4):357–84.

98. Liao S, Liang T, Fang S, Castaneda E, Shao TC. Steroid structure and androgenic activity. Specificities involved in the receptor binding and nuclear retention of various androgens. *J Biol Chem* 1973;**248**(17):6154–62.

99. Virtanen HE, Toppari J. Epidemiology and pathogenesis of cryptorchidism. *Hum Reprod Update* 2008;**14**(1):49–58.

100. Joustra SD, van der Plas EM, Goede J, Oostdijk W, Delemarre-van de Waal HA, Hack WW, et al. New reference charts for testicular volume in Dutch children and adolescents allow the calculation of standard deviation scores. *Acta Paediatr* 2015;**104**(6):e271–8.

101. Marshall WA, Tanner JM. Variations in the pattern of pubertal changes in boys. *Arch Dis Child* 1970;**45**(239):13–23.

102. Marshall WA, Tanner JM. Variations in pattern of pubertal changes in girls. *Arch Dis Child* 1969;**44**(235):291–303.

103. Miyawaki S, Tachibana M. Role of epigenetic regulation in mammalian sex determination. *Curr Top Dev Biol* 2019;**134**:195–221.

104. Kuroki S, Matoba S, Akiyoshi M, Matsumura Y, Miyachi H, Mise N, et al. Epigenetic regulation of mouse sex determination by the histone demethylase Jmjd1a. *Science* 2013;**341**(6150):1106–9.

105. Carré GA, Siggers P, Xipolita M, Brindle P, Lutz B, Wells S, et al. Loss of p300 and CBP disrupts histone acetylation at the mouse Sry promoter and causes XY gonadal sex reversal. *Hum Mol Genet* 2018;**27**(1):190–8.

106. Gibbons R. Alpha thalassaemia-mental retardation, X linked. *Orphanet J Rare Dis* 2006;**1**:15.

Chapter 38

Development of Renin-Angiotensin-Aldosterone and Nitric Oxide System in the Fetus and Neonate

Jiaqi Tang*, Bailin Liu*, Na Li*, Mengshu Zhang*, Xiang Li*, Qinqin Gao*, Xiuwen Zhou*, Miao Sun*, Zhice Xu*,[†] and Xiyuan Lu*

*Institute for Fetology, First Hospital of Soochow University, Suzhou, China, [†]Center for Perinatal Biology, Loma Linda University, Loma Linda, CA, United States

> **Key Clinical Changes**
> - RAAS and NO are involved in placental development and function.
> - RAAS and NO play roles in fetal cardiovascular system, brain, and kidney.
> - RAAS and NO regulate vascular tone.
> - RAAS is important for regulation of body fluid homeostasis in the fetus.

38.1 INTRODUCTION OF RENIN-ANGIOTENSIN-ALDOSTERONE SYSTEM AND NITRIC OXIDE

38.1.1 Renin-Angiotensin-Aldosterone System

The renin-angiotensin-aldosterone system (RAAS) is a peptidergic system with endocrine characteristics. It has been studied over a century, since the first identification of renin by Tigerstedt and Bergman in 1898. Traditionally, the liver synthesizes and releases angiotensinogen (AGT), a glycoprotein, which serves as the substrate of the systemic RAAS.[1] It is cleaved in the circulation by renin produced by the juxtaglomerular apparatus in the kidney,[1] to generate decapeptide angiotensin (Ang) I. Ang I is then converted to the octapeptide Ang II by angiotensin converting enzyme (ACE), a membrane-bound metalloproteinase, which is in high density on the surface of endothelial cells in the pulmonary circulation.[1] Ang II stimulates the adrenal cortex to secrete aldosterone, which acts on renal mineralocorticoid receptors (MR) to maintain sodium-potassium homeostasis by increasing sodium reabsorption in renal proximal tubules and excreting potassium.

Apart from the well-known systemic RAAS pathway, additional RAAS pathways exist. Angiotensin converting enzyme 2 (ACE2), a homologue of ACE, cleaves one amino acid from Ang I to convert Ang I to Ang-(1–9).[2] Ang-(1–9) is subsequently converted to Ang-(1–7) by ACE. Ang-(1–7) is known to act on Mas receptors to antagonize the Ang II/AT1R pathway. In addition, aminopeptidase A can metabolize Ang II into Ang III.[3]

Traditionally, the physiological effects of RAAS are well known in the regulation of the arterial blood pressure, renal functions, and the homeostasis of body fluids. In addition to those "classic" roles, the RAAS is found to mediate a number of physiological processes, including proliferation, apoptosis, angiogenesis, neuroendocrinology, and secretion of placental hormones, thereby playing essential roles in development of fetuses and neonates. This chapter summarizes the ontogenesis of RAAS (especially in the placenta, cardiovascular systems, brain, and kidney of fetuses and neonates) and its functions during development.

38.1.2 Nitric Oxide

Nitric oxide (NO) is one of the simplest gaseous molecules, and it exerts significant signaling functions in nearly every organ and system in the body. NO is responsible to modulate a diverse range of physiological and cellular processes,

Maternal-Fetal and Neonatal Endocrinology. https://doi.org/10.1016/B978-0-12-814823-5.00038-6

including endothelial cell proliferation, migration, angiogenesis, and extracellular matrix degradation. Moreover, as a signaling molecule in endothelium-dependent regulation of vascular tension, angiogenesis, mitogenesis, and platelet functions, NO is critical regulator in cardiovascular physiology.

NO plays an important role in regulating the physiological adaptations and pathophysiology of adapting to pregnancy. This chapter reviews our current understanding of the physiological functions of NO during gestation and fetal development.

38.2 ENDOCRINE PHYSIOLOGY OF RAAS IN PLACENTA, FETUS, AND NEONATE

38.2.1 Placental RAAS

38.2.1.1 Components of RAAS in the Placenta

The placenta is derived from cells of the extraembryonic conceptus and maternal decidua. It is responsible for maternal-fetal exchange of nutrients and wastes. All the components of the RAAS have been shown to be present locally in the placenta (Table 38.1).

38.2.1.1.1 Renin

In human placental tissue, a placental renin-angiotensin-system (RAS) was found and a renin-like substance identified as early as 1967.[9] Renin mRNA expression in cultured chorionic cells was first reported in 1968.[10] Prorenin, the biosynthetic precursor of active renin in renin-producing cells, is the predominant form of renin in the human placenta.[11] In human placenta, prorenin mRNA level is the highest level of expression between 6 and 16 weeks of gestation,[4] and a high ratio of prorenin to renin receptor expression is detected. In contrast, in animals such as pigs and cows, placental prorenin concentrations are relatively lower, and the major form is active renin.[11]

38.2.1.1.2 ACE and ACE2

Human placenta contains high levels of ACE, and it is specifically present in the fetal vascular endothelium of the placental villi during early gestation. ACE2 is abundant in the syncytiotrophoblast layer and villous stroma, but not in the fetal vascular endothelium. Low ACE2 immunoreactivity is also detected in cytotrophoblasts.[4] ACE activity in the human placenta increases during the course of pregnancy, whereas the ACE mRNA expression initially increases and then decreases near term.[12] ACE2 mRNA expression in human placenta reached the highest levels in early gestation. And there was a negative correlation between ACE and ACE2 mRNA expression.[4]

TABLE 38.1 Component of local RAAS in human placenta

	mRNA expression	Protein localization
Prorenin	Predominant form, highest in early gestation (6–9 weeks)[4]	Early STB, CTB, EVT[4] Term STB, vascular endothelium
Renin	Highest in early gestation (8–14 weeks)[4] Decreased near term[4]	STB, CTB, villous stroma[5]
ACE	Higher at term than in early gestation[4]	Fetal vascular endothelium[4]
ACE2	Highest in early gestation placentae (6–16 weeks)[4]	STB, CTB, villous stroma[4]
AGT	Start at 6 weeks, relatively low but higher in early gestation (6–16 weeks) than at term[4]	STB, CTB, villous stroma[4]
AT1	Predominant and present from first trimester to term[5]	STB, CTB, EVT, chorionic villi, fetal endothelium[6, 7]
AT2	Typically low but highest in early gestation[5]	CTB, EVT[5]
MR	Throughout gestation (5–40 weeks)[8]	STB, CTB[8]

CTB, cytotrophoblasts; *EVT*, extravillous trophoblasts; *STB*, syncytiotrophoblasts.

38.2.1.1.3 Angiotensinogen

AGT mRNA is present in the entire human placenta, starting at 6 weeks of gestation[13] and higher in early gestation than at term.[4] Most of AGT is the high-molecular-weight species, and the proportion of it in placenta is much higher than that in plasma.[14]

38.2.1.1.4 Angiotensin Receptors

A majority of Ang II receptors in human placenta are AT1 receptors, localized in the syncytiotrophoblast and cytotrophoblast of the placental villi, extravillous trophoblast, and blood vessels of the placental villi.[6, 7] In addition, low expression of Ang II receptors is present in fetal membranes, and the proportion of AT1 and AT2 receptors is similar.[15] In human placenta, mRNA and protein of AT1 receptors are increased from the first trimester and reach the highest levels at term.[16] Ang II concentrations have a positive relationship to AT1 receptor levels in human placenta, suggesting that Ang II plays a role in regulating AT1 receptor expression in this organ.[17]

38.2.1.1.5 Aldosterone

Aldosterone regulates blood pressure (BP) and homeostasis of body fluids via binding with mineralocorticoid receptors (MR). As with "classical" mineralocorticoid target tissues (kidney and colon), MR is also expressed in the placenta. MR mRNA expression in human placenta tissues and MR immunoreactivity in syncytiotrophoblasts, cytotrophoblasts, and interstitial cells of the villous core are moderately detected throughout all gestational stages.[8]

38.2.1.2 Functions of RAAS in the Placenta

38.2.1.2.1 Placentation

The development of the placenta is a complex process, including trophoblast invasion, proliferation, differentiation, and placental angiogenesis. At early developmental stages, trophoblast cells invade the uterus and remodel spiral arteries for adequate maternal blood supply to the placenta and fetus, which is an important adaptation mechanism in human pregnancy.[18]

The RAAS, highly expressed in the placenta at early gestation,[4] plays a critical role in placental development. Angiotensin II via AT1 receptors can regulate cytotrophoblast differentiation in vitro, promote cellular outgrowth of human villous explant cultures,[19] and contribute to placental angiogenesis through increasing the production of vascular endothelial growth factor (VEGF).[20] Furthermore, uterine RAAS in primates and rodents assumes an important role in decidualization of the endometrium and implantation of the blastocyst.[21] Aldosterone is also important for placental growth because plasma aldosterone is positively related to placental size in human pregnancy. Studies have revealed that activating MR by aldosterone directly stimulates trophoblast growth.[22]

38.2.1.2.2 Placental Hormone Secretion

The placenta produces and releases various hormones and biofactors in expressing its functions to maintain normal pregnancy and trigger natural delivery. The RAAS plays a critical role in regulating secretion of placental hormones. Renin has been shown to promote prostaglandin E2 (PGE2) biosynthesis in human amnion cells in vitro.[23] However, locally generated hormones in trophoblastic tissues, including estrogens, progesterone, prostaglandins (PGE2, PGI2), and endothelins, may control secretion of renin. The biosynthesis of these hormones is in turn modulated by Ang II.[24] Furthermore, in the human placenta, Ang II stimulates the secretion of human placental lactogen and pregnancy-specific β_1 glycoprotein from the villous tissue and trophoblastic cells by interacting with Ang II receptors.[15]

38.2.1.2.3 Placental Vascular Function

The placenta is very rich in blood vessels, which supply oxygen and nutrients to the fetus, and remove waste products in utero. Human placental villous blood vessels contain almost exclusively AT1-R.[6, 7, 13] Ang II acts as a typical vasoconstrictor to cause dose-dependent vasoconstrictions not only in nonplacental vessels (human umbilical cord vein and artery) but also in human placenta vessels.[25] However, the placental vascular responses to Ang II are significantly more sensitive than those of the nonplacental vessels[25] (Fig. 38.1). In general, catecholamines are dominant in the control and maintain baseline vascular tone in the peripheral vascular systems (nonplacental vessels). However, recent progress has demonstrated that Ang II-mediated vasoconstriction in placental vessels is stronger than that induced by catecholamines, indicating that Ang II is critical in maintaining vascular baseline vascular tension for the placenta (Fig. 38.1).

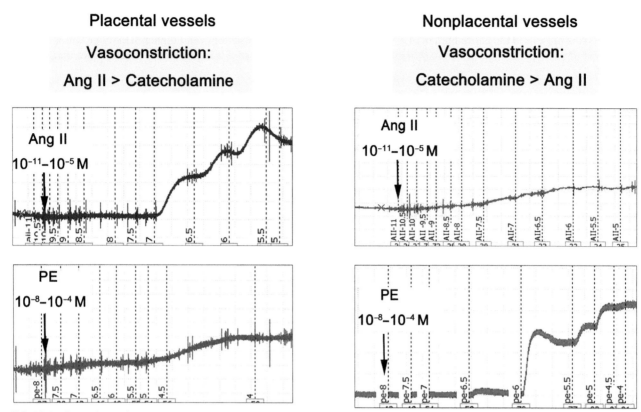

FIG. 38.1 Comparisons of vasoconstriction induced by Ang II and PE between placental and nonplacental vessels. The placental vascular responses to Ang II are significantly more sensitive than those of the nonplacental vessels. Ang II induces more vasoconstriction than catecholamines in placental vessels, whereas the reverse is true in nonplacental vessels. *PE*, Phenylephrine; *Ang II*, angiotensin II.

In the placenta, the regulation of the vascular tone and blood flow is complex. During human pregnancies, the level of Ang II in both maternal and fetal circulations is high and temporally associated with dramatically increased placental blood flow.[26] Angiotensin II stimulates the synthesis of prostanoids (PGE and PGI) that oppose the vasoconstrictory effect of Ang II in the uteroplacental unit.[27] In addition, changes in vascular responsiveness or sensitivity to Ang II are demonstrated in pregnant women developing attenuated pressor responses to infused Ang II.[28] The low doses of Ang II increase uteroplacental blood flow partly due to an elevation of the systemic blood pressure induced by Ang II. However, Ang II in high doses decreases uteroplacental blood flow,[29] which is the result of the increased uteroplacental vascular resistance. It has also been demonstrated that functional aldosterone deficiency could result in reduced fetal umbilical blood flow in pregnant mice, suggesting that aldosterone also plays an important role in regulating uteroplacental blood flow.[22]

38.2.2 Fetal and Neonate RAAS

38.2.2.1 Components of RAAS in Fetus and Neonate

38.2.2.1.1 Systemic RAAS in Fetus and Neonate

In human embryos, all components of the RAS are expressed as early as 5 weeks of gestation, when most tissues undergo organogenesis.[30] Fetal renin of renal origin is first detected in human fetuses at 5 weeks of gestation, and rises to much higher levels by 16 weeks.[31] The level of AGT mRNA expression is very high in hepatocytes as soon as they differentiate and migrate to form the liver (23–27 days of gestation). Thus, at a very early developmental stage, the human embryo is capable of producing AGT.[30] Since metabolic clearance rate of Ang II in fetuses is about 10-fold higher than that in adults,[26] more ACE activity is required to maintain the early functioning of the RAAS during the fetal period. In humans, fetal lung ACE activity is increased with gestational age and at the end of the second trimester was already 70% of that present in the adult human lung.[32] The plasma ACE activity in premature infants is higher than that in term infants.[33] The circulating levels of Ang II in normal pregnant women are increased progressively and about 2.7 times higher than non-pregnant women at late pregnancy.[34] More impressively, Ang II production in human fetuses is even higher than that in mothers.[35] Aldosterone is synthesized by human fetal adrenal glands from 15 weeks of gestation,[36] and its plasma levels increase with gestational age.[37] Aldosterone has been shown to cross the human placenta during cesarean sections, and plasma aldosterone levels in the fetus[38] are 2–12 times higher than in the mother, suggesting that aldosterone is secreted and released in human fetus at the time of birth.

38.2.2.1.2 Local RAAS in the Fetus and Neonate

In humans and other mammals, in addition to systemic RAAS, production of multiple RAAS components has been found in a variety of organs. During development, almost all components of RAAS are widely distributed and localized throughout embryonic tissues and organs (such as kidneys, adrenal glands, cardiovascular tissues, and brain) in fetuses and neonates (Table 38.2).

Kidney The development of the fetal kidneys begins as early as the 3rd week of gestation. The nephrotome develops from the intermediate mesoderm and undergoes three probably overlapped stages: the pronephros (the rudimentary kidney), mesonephros (the nonfunctional kidney), and the metanephros (the permanent kidney).

The mesonephros is present in the human fetus from 23 days of gestation. Although the AGT, renin, ACE, AT1-receptors, and AT2-receptors can be simultaneously observed in the mesonephros at 30–35 days of gestation, all of them have particular expression and distribution patterns. AT2-receptor is the component that is expressed first (23–24 days of gestation) in the undifferentiated mesenchyme of the mesonephros. AT1-receptor mRNA is found in glomeruli beginning at 25 days of gestation. AGT is present in the proximal portion of the primitive tubules at 25–30 days of gestation. Renin is highly expressed in capillaries within glomeruli and arteries in the interstitium from 28 days of gestation. ACE is observed in the apical membrane of the mesonephric tubule cells from 30 days of gestation.[30]

In the human metanephros, ATG mRNA and protein are expressed in proximal tubules beginning at 8 weeks and then throughout gestation. Renin mRNA and protein are confined to the juxtaglomerular apparatus at the vascular pool of glomeruli, as well as to dispersed cells of arteries adjacent to glomeruli, which is slightly different from that in the mesonephros. An increase of ACE protein can be detected in proximal convoluted tubules and collecting ducts from 8 weeks of gestation until birth.[30] AT1 receptor mRNA is observed in glomeruli, proximal tubular epithelium, and juxtaglomerular cells during metanephric kidney development. AT2 receptor mRNA, detected in undifferentiated mesenchyme surrounding tubules and immature glomeruli, reaches its peak level in the human metanephros at 8–9 weeks of gestation and declines after 20 weeks but remains detectable until birth. MR is transiently expressed in human distal tubule cells between 15 and 24 weeks of gestation,[39] but then is downregulated in the prenatal period and especially at birth.

TABLE 38.2 Components of local RAAS in fetus and neonate

Organs	Renin	ACE	AGT	AT1	AT2	MR
Kidney *Mesonephros* *Metanephros*	+++, h, 28 GD +++, h, 8 GW	++, h, 30 GD +++, h, 8 GW	++, h, 25–30 GD +, h, 8 GW	++, h, 25 GD ++, h, 8 GW	++, h, 23–24 GD +++, h, 8–9 GW ++, h, 20 GW +, h, birth	– ++, h, 15–24 GW Down at birth
Adrenal gland	++, m, 13–14 GD	–	–	++, h, 8 GW	++, h, 5–6 GW[a]	–
Heart	++, h, 25 GD	++, h, 30 GD +, o, 80 GD	++, r, 10.5 GD	++, h, 35–37 GD	++, h, 23–27 GD	++, m, 13.5 GD +, m, 18.5 GD
Vasculature	–	–	–	++, o, 120 GD ++, r, 14 GD +++, r, 16 GD	++, o, 120 GD ++, r, 16 GD +++, r, 19 GD	–
Brain	++, r, 19 GD	++, r, 19 GD	++, r, 18 GD	++, r, 18 GD	++, r, 13 GD	++, h, 24 GW

[a]*Expressed in condensed cells in the adrenal zone in the fetal kidney.*
(+) low levels; (++) moderate levels; (+++) high levels. GD, gestation days; GW, gestation weeks; h, human; m, mouse; o, ovine; r, rat.

Adrenal glands The adrenal glands, composed of a cortex and medulla, are important for the RAAS, because aldosterone secretion from the zona glomerulosa classically follows stimulation by Ang II. In human fetuses, it is still unclear whether renin is expressed in the adrenal glands. However, in mouse fetuses, renin is detected in the cortex at embryonic day (E) 13–14. AT1 receptor mRNA is expressed in the neocortex of the human fetal adrenal glands at 8 weeks and throughout gestation. The AT2 receptor mRNA expression can be detected at 5–6 weeks of gestation in a mass of condensed cells (named the future adrenal fetal zone) within the developing kidneys.[30] However, no expression of AT2 receptor mRNA has been found so far in adrenal medulla of human kidneys.[30] Studies have shown that the human fetal adrenal glands are capable of secreting aldosterone as early as 15 weeks of gestation.[36]

Heart Whether ATG is expressed in the human fetal heart is unclear. However, in rats, ATG mRNA is detected as early as E10.5 in the embryonic heart,[40] and it is also detected in both left and right ventricles in ovine fetuses.[41] Those studies on animal fetuses strongly suggest ATG should be present in the human fetal heart.

Renin mRNA begins to be expressed gestational day 25 in human embryonic heart, mainly located in the inner parts of the myocardium, and becomes abundant during the course of gestation. ACE is detected from gestational day 30, within the inner layers of the human embryonic heart, and slightly later than when renin first appears.[30]

In ovine fetuses, ACE and ACE2 mRNA are found in the left and right ventricles, and the ACE/ACE2 ratio at term is about 15-fold than that at gestational day.[41] In rat fetuses, ACE mRNA is expressed in the cardiac vasculature and heart valves at E19. ACE expression could also be detected in the myocardium during the fetal and neonatal stage and is increased during development. The expression and localization of cardiac ACE2 in rodent fetuses has not been determined, but evidence indicates that ACE2 might be important in heart development.[42]

The cardiac AT1 receptor transcript is diffusely expressed over the human embryonic myocardium around stage 15, whereas AT2 receptor mRNA is expressed in the innermost layers of the myocardium earlier and higher than that of AT1 receptors (about stage 11–12).[30] The mRNA expression of both AT1 and AT2 receptors are detected in the left and right ventricles of ovine fetuses[41] and in the embryonic heart of rats.[40] AT1 receptors are relatively unchanged in the heart during late fetal and early neonatal periods in sheep,[43] while only the AT1a mRNA but not AT1b mRNA in myocardium of the developing rodent shows sustained expression.[44] However, AT2 receptor levels are highly expressed during the late fetal and immediate neonatal periods, and decrease rapidly thereafter to adult levels within 2 days after birth in valvular tissues of rats.[45] MR mRNA expression is presented in the mouse fetal heart starts from E13.5, decreases by E18.5, and reappears postnatally.[46] In the hearts of sheep fetuses, MR expression also can be detected from 80 days of gestation and significantly decreases in the left rather than in the right ventricle to the postnatal stage.[41]

Vasculature Except for angiotensin receptors, knowledge regarding dynamical expression and distribution patterns of other key elements of RAAS (including ATG, renin, and ACE) in human embryonic/fetal vasculature is limited. Both AT1 and AT2 receptors are detected in the vasculature of ovine fetuses around 120 gestational days. Notably, the AT1 receptor is predominantly expressed in VSMC(vascular smooth muscle cell) of umbilical cord vessels, while the AT2 receptor seems to be preferentially distributed in VSMC of systemic blood vessels.[47] In fetal aorta of rats, expression of the AT1 receptor is detected at E14, increases until E16, and then remains at similar levels throughout postnatal development. Compared with AT1, the expression of AT2 receptors appears later (about E16) and reaches maximal levels between E19 and neonatal day 1, followed by a rapid decline in rats.[48] High levels of AT2 receptor mRNA are detected in the aortic arch and pulmonary arteries from 15 days of gestation to 15 days postpartum, while it is transiently expressed in the coronary arteries before and after birth.[49]

Brain Although the expression and distribution of components of RAAS are still relatively unclear in the human fetal brain, it has been widely studied in other species. In the brain of rat fetuses, mRNA and protein of ATG has been detected at E18 in the choroid plexus and ependymal cells lining the third ventricle, and increases until birth.[50] During early postnatal development, a rapid progression of ATG expression is detected in the astrocytes of the paraventricular nucleus, medial preoptic area, and ventromedial and arcuate hypothalamic nuclei.[50] Renin activity could also be detected in the fetal brain of rodents. Immunostaining for ACE can be observed in the fetal nervous system and dermomyotome. In the rodent brain, ACE is detected in the choroid plexus, subfornical organ (SFO), and posterior pituitary at E19.[51]

Expression of AT1 and AT2 receptors in the fetal brain is detected in rodents at E18.[52] Using radiolabeled cRNA probes for in situ hybridization, expression of AT1a mRNA is found in many regions of the fetal brain at E19, and that of AT2 mRNA is located in the differentiating lateral hypothalamus at E13.[53] Notably, unlike that of adults, the AT2 receptor is more abundant than AT1 receptor in the fetal brain. In the developing brain of rat fetuses, the AT1 receptor is mainly located to the paraventricular nucleus (PVN), subfornical organ, nucleus of the solitary tract (NTS), anterior pituitary, and choroid plexus. Expression of AT2 receptor transiently appears earlier than that of AT1 receptor. AT2 receptor mRNA is presented in the lateral hypothalamic neuroepithelium at E13. Later, at E15, it can be detected in hypoglossus and subthalamic nuclei; at E17, in the pedunculopontine nucleus, motor facial nucleus, cerebellum, and the inferior olivary complex; at E19, in the thalamus, locus coeruleus, supragenual nucleus, nuclei of the lateral lemniscus, interstitial nucleus of Cajal, and bed nucleus of the supraoptic decussation; and at E21, in the medial geniculate body, lateral septal and medial amygdaloid nuclei, and the superior colliculus.[54] In the developing brain of ovine fetuses at 70% of gestational age, both AT1 and AT2 receptors are detected and associated with central pathways in cardiovascular and body fluid regulation.[55] MR is expressed in the human hippocampus at 24 weeks of gestation, and is maintained at a constant level until the 34th week of gestation.[56] In contrast, in mouse fetuses, hippocampal expression of MR is presented between E14 and E15.5, and MR decreases until postnatal day 10.[56]

38.2.2.2 Functions of RAAS in Fetus and Neonate

38.2.2.2.1 The RAAS in the Kidney

Numerous studies using animal models have demonstrated the important role of RAAS in renal organogenesis. In humans, nephrogenesis is completed before gestational week 36, whereas in rodents nephrogenesis can last for about 2 weeks after birth.[57] Thus neonatal rats and mice born with immature kidneys are extensively used as a model for nephrogenesis. The deletion of renin, ATG, ACE, AT1, or AT2 receptor by genetic manipulations in mice can result in pathological phenotypes in the kidney both prenatally and postnatally, including papillary atrophy, hydronephrosis, impaired medulla, renal fibrosis, hyperplasia of vascular smooth muscle cells, and thickening of renal vessels.[58] The pharmacological experiments further demonstrated the critical role of RAAS in normal renal development.[59] Administration of ACE inhibition or Ang II antagonism to neonatal rodents could result in the delay of nephrogenesis, papillary atrophy, and a decrease in number and size of glomeruli. In human, the use of these drugs for maternal antihypertensive therapy in pregnancy can cause renal lesions in the newborns.[60]

A balance between cellular proliferation and apoptosis is extremely important for nephrogenesis. During prenatal nephrogenesis, signaling of Ang II via AT2 receptors promotes proliferation and differentiation, as well as apoptosis of tubular cells through upregulating the paired homeobox 2 gene (Pax-2), which mediates the mesenchymal to epithelial transformation and the clearance of unnecessary cells.[61] However, Ang II inhibits growth of cultured embryonic renomedullary interstitial cells via AT2 receptors, while promoting its growth via AT1 receptors, suggesting the dual effects of Ang II on the proliferation of embryonic renomedullary interstitial cells.[62]

In the fetus, body fluid and electrolyte homeostasis is regulated primarily by signals from the placenta, and the role of the fetal kidney in homeostasis is not well defined. The fetal kidney produces urine, which is the main source of amniotic fluid in the third trimester. The RAAS plays an important role in renal regulation of body fluid homeostasis. The Ang II acting as the main effector of RAAS is important for increasing blood pressure, maintaining a high urine flow and adequate volume of fetal fluids.[63] Angiotensin II modulates renal vasoconstriction to regulate the renal blood flow and glomerular filtration rate via directly acting on Ang II receptors in glomerular and proximal tubular cells.[64] Angiotensin converting enzyme inhibitors reduce the availability of Ang II and can decrease glomerular filtration rate and renal vascular resistance, leading to restricted or no urine flow in the fetus at late gestation.[63] Although studies show that absence of aldosterone biosynthesis does not alter fetal development, renal aldosterone has a critical role in neonatal adaptation to a new environment. For example, MR knockout mice exhibit no gross developmental defects, but develop serious hyponatremia, hyperkalemia, dehydration, and high renal salt wasting that threaten life after both (postnatal day 8 in mice).[65] Inactivating mutations of the MR gene in humans also result in a very similar phenotype.[66]

38.2.2.2.2 The RAAS in the Cardiovascular System

Heart development begins from induction of primary cardiac field formation at the trilaminar embryonic disc stage. Although there is limited information on the role of RAS in very early cardiac development, accumulated evidence indicates that Ang II via AT1 receptors could increase cardiac loop inversion in rats at early embryonic stage.[40] The RAAS also may mediate cardiovascular remolding and growth during development since atrophy of myocardium, and reduction of heart/body weight ratio, can be caused by the deficiency of AT1 receptors.[67] Other findings in experimental models show that Ang II influences cellular differentiation or proliferation during development. For example, in immature ovine cardiomyocytes in vitro, Ang II acts probably via AT1 receptors to stimulate cellular proliferation via ERK and PI3K/Akt pathways.[68] Moreover, in the pressure-overloaded fetal heart in vivo, Ang II is able to elicit hypertrophy of myocardium, particularly in the left ventricle.[69] Furthermore, it is well known that activation of RAAS, especially Ang II/AT2 receptor signaling, plays critical roles in apoptosis during the fetal heart development.

The RAAS is also involved in the development of vasculature. In general, Ang II promotes proliferation and hypertrophy on VSMC via AT1 receptors, while eliciting antiproliferative effects via AT2 receptors. During fetal vasculogenesis, Ang II may contribute to VSMC differentiation and vasculogenesis by stimulating AT1 and AT2 receptors, suggesting the synergistical regulatory roles of the two receptors in the development of vasculature during the perinatal period.[70] Nevertheless, overexpression of AT2 receptors may attenuate neointimal formation and DNA synthesis during vascular development in the aorta.[71] It remains to be determined in detail how AT1 and AT2 receptors regulate vasculogenesis during early development.

Increasing evidence has demonstrated that the abnormal activation of RAS during the fetal period significantly contributes to the development of hypertension in adult offspring. It is clear now that fetal AT1 receptors are important for the regulation of vascular tone and blood pressure.[72] In many instances, AT2 receptors could mediate the counteracting effects to AT1 receptors.[71, 72] In spite of the increasing evidence shows the important roles of AT2 in cardiovascular regulations, fetal data remain limited.

38.2.2.2.3 The RAAS in the Central Nervous System

The RAAS components are expressed and detected very early in the fetal brain, suggesting important roles of RAAS in the development of nervous systems. Using antisense deoxyoligonucleotides to ATG mRNA in vitro inhibits the growth of neuroblastoma cells.[73] Angiotensin II, acting via AT1 receptors, has neurotropic roles in regulating neuritogenesis processes. Ang II could stimulate AT2 receptors to induce neuronal differentiation and neurite outgrowth in cell lines of neural origin (NG108-15 cells).[74] AT2 receptors are highly expressed in the neonate brain and contribute to apoptosis in cultured neurons from newborn rat.[75] Genetic deletion of AT2 receptors results in increased neural cell numbers in different brain regions of mice,[76] demonstrating that AT2 receptors may contribute to cellular apoptosis during the development of the fetal brain. MR can act as a neuroprotective factor during neurogenesis and exerts a protective effect against neuron apoptosis.

Fetal RAAS in the brain also plays an important role in the control of fetal blood pressure. Intracerebroventricular (icv) application of either Ang I or Ang II can increase fetal blood pressure, associated with a significant decrease in heart rate in both near-term and preterm ovine fetuses. The central Ang-induced elevation of fetal blood pressure depends partially on AVP that is released from the fetal hypothalamus, since the pressor effects can be inhibited by V1 receptor, an AVP blocker.[77] Thus local RAS in the fetal brain can regulate fetal blood pressure, and its regulating roles are associated with central neuroendocrine pathways.

Local RAS in the fetal brain is also important in regulating body fluid balance, including intake of water and salt, renal excretion and reabsorption, and vascular volumes.[78] In ovine fetuses, intensive AT1 receptors have been detected in the brain, especially in the paraventricular nucleus (PVN) and supraoptic nuclei (SON).[54] These two central regions are closely associated with neuroendocrine releases that are critical in renal excretions and salt appetite. AVP and oxytocin (OT) are two major neuropeptides synthesized and released by magnocellular neuroendocrine cells of the hypothalamus in response to the signals, including changes of osmotic pressure and application of central Ang II.[78] Angiotensin II or its precursor Ang I increase both AVP and OT levels in the fetal circulation, suggesting that the developed central RAAS plays critical roles in the control of the neuroendocrine responses that contribute to body fluid regulation.[79] Furthermore, losartan (a specific inhibitor of AT1R), but not PD123319 (a specific inhibitor of AT2R), inhibits the elevation of plasma AVP levels in response to icv Ang II,[80] thereby demonstrating that AT1 receptors in the developing fetal brain are important for the central Ang II-mediated neuroendocrine responses.

Fetal swallowing activity also plays a role in regulating fetal body fluid homeostasis. Multiple factors, including amniotic fluid availability, dipsogenic stimulation, and behavioral status, influence fetal swallowing activity. Swallowing activity in utero is controlled by hypovolemic, hyperosmotic, and chemical stimuli such as Ang II in late gestation.[81] Application of icv hypertonic saline, icv Ang II, and dehydration stimulate the fetal swallowing or dipsogenic responses.[81] Icv Ang II-induced fetal swallowing responses can be blocked by AT1 receptor antagonists, suggesting that Ang II via AT1 receptors mediates the fetal swallowing activity.[82]

Although there still is missing information regarding the presence and time of appearance for all components of the RAAS in all major organs in fetuses and neonates, it is clear that both systemic RAAS and local RAS exist during fetal stages, and in the placenta. Notably, there are three endocrine systems for RAAS during pregnancy. These include systemic RAAS and local RAS and/or RAAS in the maternal body, local RAS and RAAS in the placenta, and systemic RAAS and local RAS in the fetus, while the placental barrier should prevent large molecules entering the fetus in utero under normal

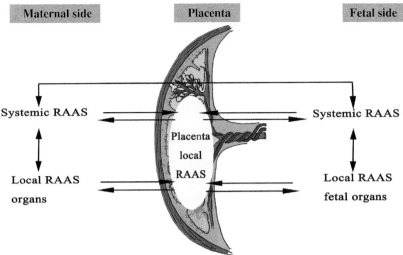

FIG. 38.2 Interactions of systemic and local RAAS among mother, placenta, and fetus.

physiological conditions. Rationally, there should be interactions among the three endocrine systems in the mother, placenta, and fetus (Fig. 38.2). Those interactions play important roles in fetal growth, as well as in development of diseases during pregnancy, for both mother and fetus. However, studies on those endocrine interactions among mother, placenta, and fetus are still limited, and further investigations are needed.

38.3 PHYSIOLOGICAL FUNCTIONS OF NO IN PREGNANCY AND FETUSES

38.3.1 Signaling Pathway in Regulation of NO Generation

38.3.1.1 Synthesis of NO

Nitric oxide, a gaseous messenger molecule, is generated from L-arginine by the catalytic action of the NO synthases (NOS; Fig. 38.3). There are three different isoforms of NOS. Neuronal (nNOS), endothelial (eNOS), and inducible (iNOS) have been identified, cloned, and characterized. While the nNOS and eNOS isoforms are constitutively expressed in a variety of tissues, expression of iNOS can be induced by cytokines and other agents.[83] The powerful vasodilatory effect of NO in resistance vessels throughout the body is mediated by locally produced NO and by the subsequently produced guanosine 3–5 cyclic monophosphate (cGMP).

38.3.1.2 Regulation of NO Synthesis

Endothelial NO production is largely dependent on eNOS activity, which is regulated by canonical Ca^{2+}/calmodulin-dependent and Ca^{2+}-independent mechanisms. The Ca^{2+}/calmodulin-dependent pathway mediates actions by acetylcholine, ATP, thrombin, and bradykinin B2 receptor agonists, to increase eNOS activity.[84] Those agonists bind to G-protein-dependent receptors and activate phospholipase C, then catalyze the cell membrane component phosphatidylinositol 4,5-triphosphate into diacylglycerol and inositol 1,4,5-triphosphate (IP_3), which acts on endoplasmic IP_3 receptors, thereby increasing intracellular Ca^{2+} levels. Then Ca^{2+} binds to calmodulin-dependent protein kinase II (CaM kinase II) to

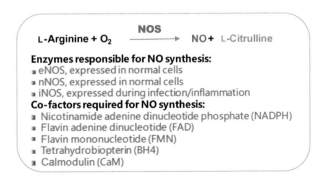

FIG. 38.3 Nitric oxide syntheses. Enzymes and cofactors for L-arginine pathway for synthesis of nitric oxide (NO).

enhance eNOS activity. Although eNOS activity is related to changes in intracellular Ca^{2+}, it is not the only factor required for the modulation of the enzyme activity. The binding of calmodulin (CaM) and the electrons transferring from the reductase to the oxygenase domain of eNOS are also dependent on its phosphorylation states.[85] For example, phosphorylation of Ser617, 635, and 1179 promotes an increase in eNOS activity, while phosphorylation of Ser 116, Thr497, and Tyr659 inhibits eNOS function.[86] There are numerous protein kinases that could phosphorylate Ser 1179 of eNOS, including CaM kinase II kinase (CaMKII), Akt (protein kinase B), AMP-activated protein kinase (AMPK), cyclic AMP dependent protein kinase (PKA), and cyclic GMP dependent protein kinase (PKG). Among them, except for CaMKII, the others are involved in Ca^{2+}-independent regulation of eNOS activity. A number of lines of evidence have supported that Ca^{2+}-independent mechanisms contribute to substantial NO generation in endothelial cells.[87] In addition, other associated regulatory proteins like Caveolin-1, a major caveolae-localized protein through caveolae internalization, Hsp90 and gp60, also play an important role in Ca^{2+}-independent activation of eNOS and NO generation.[86]

38.3.2 Nitric Oxide and Pregnancy

38.3.2.1 Circulating NO Concentration During Pregnancy

Pregnancy is associated with significant changes in maternal cardiovascular systems that regulate oxygen and nutrient supply to the growing fetus. Nitric oxide, a physiologic vascular smooth muscle relaxant, regulates blood flow and therefore plays a role in the cardiovascular changes in pregnancy. NO is unstable and is determined by its stable metabolites, including nitrite (NO_2) and nitrate (NO_3). As a gaseous signaling molecule, NO plays roles in a variety of biological processes. Endothelial NO produces vascular smooth muscle relaxation through a cGMP-dependent pathway. NO is one of the downstream factors of relaxin, a key hormone in pregnancy.

The relationship between serum NO levels and gestational periods is not certain due to inconsistent data. Some researchers showed that serum NO levels were the same between nonpregnant and normal pregnant women.[88] Others suggested that, in normal pregnancy, there was a negative correlation between NO production and gestational weeks.[88] In addition, there are reports demonstrating that in normal pregnant women, the serum NO level and cGMP levels gradually increase from 28 to 36 gestational weeks. The highest level of serum NO and cGMP is in 33–34 gestational weeks.[89] During the puerperium, serum NO products are decreased when compared with pregnancy.[88]

L-Arginine is the substrate for NOS. Maternal arginine concentrations decrease significantly during the first trimester, and then rise toward term, to almost similar levels in nonpregnant women.[90] NO production is also downregulated by asymmetric dimethylarginine (ADMA). The level of ADMA in the maternal circulation declines during the first half of pregnancy, reaching its nadir at 24 weeks' gestation, and then increases again to the prepregnancy levels toward term.[91] The arginine/ADMA ratio, a determinant of NO production by NOS, remains unchanged throughout pregnancy.[90] Following 3 days of postpartum, there is an increase in plasma ADMA, leading to a decline of NO, in normotensive women.[92]

38.3.2.2 NO and Maternal Cardiovascular Systems

Significant cardiovascular changes occur to meet the metabolic demands of the placenta, fetus, and pregnant woman. Plasma volume expands about 30% above the nonpregnant value during the third trimester. Despite plasma volume expansion, a decrease of maternal blood pressure is a consequence of reduced peripheral vascular tone, which results from an increased production of vasodilators, including NO and prostaglandins.[93]

The vasculature is in a constant state of active dilation mediated by nitric oxide. Endothelial cells continuously release small amounts of nitric oxide, producing a basal level of vascular smooth muscle relaxation. NO dilates blood vessels by directly acting on underlying vascular smooth muscle cells. Since NO is a small and highly diffusible molecule, it can adjust blood flow in response to changes in local regions of the vasculature.

Nitric oxide plays a vital role in vascular dilation during pregnancy. Its production is implicated in the maternal hemodynamic changes, by inducing vasodilatory responses in the maternal vasculature. In pregnancy, vascular NO production is increased due to an increase in expression/activity of NOS in maternal systemic vasculature.[94] The pregnancy-related increases of NOS are likely due to the increased levels of sex hormones and corticotrophin releasing hormone.[95] Meanwhile, during pregnancy, an elevation of cytosolic calcium stimulates the production of NO and prostacyclin in endothelial cells.[96]

38.3.2.3 NO and Uterine Arteries

Despite dramatic changes in cardiovascular function, little is known about how pregnancy affects the uterine and intrauterine vasculature. A vessel of particular interest is the myometrial artery, because it is a principal site of uterine vascular resistance, and hence may contribute to the regulation of maternal uteroplacental blood flow. Uterine arteries from non-pregnant women respond to NO with relaxation, and endothelial NO release is affected by the phase of the menstrual cycle. The release of NO enhances at the follicular phase when the estrogen is at a high level. Evidence has shown that NO is a potent vasodilator in human uterine arteries, and there is normally a physiological increase in uterine blood flow during pregnancy. The increased uterine blood flow during pregnancy is associated with NO liberated from the endothelium.[97] The bioavailability of NO in the uteroplacental circulatory system gradually increases during gestation.

Nitric oxide synthesis and its downstream signaling are also increased in pregnancy. Expression of eNOS and nNOS, but not iNOS, are demonstrated in human uterine arteries.[98] eNOS is located in the endothelium, and nNOS is distributed in the adventitia of human uterine arteries. During pregnancy, NOS is enhanced in human myometrial and uterine arteries.[98] The increase in NOS contributes to the enhanced production of NO in human uterine vasculature, supporting maximal perfusion of the uterus during pregnancy. Nitric oxide diffuses to the vascular smooth muscle layer, where it activates soluble guanylyl cyclase, producing cGMP, and induces vasorelaxation. Pregnancy augments NO-dependent vasodilatation in response to acetylcholine in the human uterine artery.[99] Nitric oxide-mediated vasodilatation effects and myogenic responses are increased in human myometrial vasculature during pregnancy.[100]

In addition to inducing vasodilatation, NO is also a key player in maternal uterine vascular remodeling, a process that is essential for normal fetal growth and pregnancy outcome. In pregnancy, NO is necessary for the formation of healthy endothelium and induces endovascular invasion by the cytotrophoblast. As interstitial trophoblasts invade maternal spiral arteries in the uterine, NO production creates a low-resistance and high-caliber uteroplacental unit.

38.3.2.4 NO and Ovulation, Implantation, Uterine Contractility, and Cervical Ripening

Nitric oxide is a major paracrine mediator and plays an important role in various reproductive processes, such as ovulation, implantation, uterine contractility, and cervical ripening (Fig. 38.4).

38.3.2.4.1 Follicular Development and Ovulation

Ovulation is a complicated process that is regulated by various factors or mechanisms. In animal models, circulating NO products (NO_2/NO_3) increase with the follicular development and decline after ovulation.[101] Inhibition of iNOS results in a 50% reduction of ovulation in rats, an effect completely reversed by NO donor.[102] There is a positive correlation between NO synthesis and estrogen levels, and estrogen regulates NO synthesis during follicular development and ovulation.[103] Similar changes in circulating NO concentrations with follicular development have been seen in women undergoing in vitro fertilization, and some related hormones (human chorionic gonadotrophin, follicle stimulating hormone, luteinizing hormone, and progesterone) play roles in the regulation of NO synthesis and folliculogenesis.[103]

38.3.2.4.2 Implantation

Implantation is subject to the interaction between trophoblast cells and the decidua. NO also regulates endometrial functions such as endometrial receptivity, implantation, and decidualization.[101] NO donors may be useful for promoting fertility, while NO inhibitors could be considered for contraception. All three NOS isoforms were present within the mouse implantation site, with iNOS and eNOS being the most prominent.[104] There is an elevation of iNOS and eNOS expression in implantation sites versus intervening tissue sites on days 6–8 in mice pregnancy.

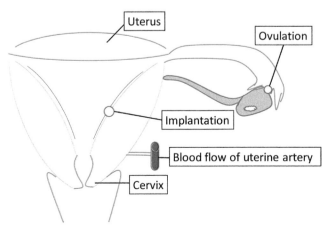

FIG. 38.4 Sites and major roles of nitric oxide prior to and during pregnancy.

38.3.2.4.3 Uterine Contractility

The uterus undergoes important structural alterations during pregnancy. NO is present in the human uterus and is a potent relaxant of the myometrium. The relaxation responsiveness to NO is elevated to maintain uterine quiescence during pregnancy, and reduced to induce uterine contraction at the end of pregnancy and during labor.[105, 106]

All three NOS isoforms (eNOS, iNOS, and nNOS) are present in human uterus, and eNOS is the predominant isoform in the nonpregnant human uterus. There is growing evidence indicating that iNOS turns into a dominant NOS isoform during early pregnancy.[107] Some investigators reported that NOS expression in the human uterus is increased during pregnancy,[108] while others found NOS was either downregulated or even unchanged during pregnancy. Besides inducing dilation, NO regulates spontaneous contractions and distension of the uterus. NO is also generated in trophoblasts and placenta, where it may play a role in maintaining uterine quiescence.[109] Clinical trials have demonstrated that NO donors are effective tocolytics.[110] With the onset of labor, some showed the expression of myometrial NOS mRNA was not changed, while others reported a decline in myometrial NOS expression associated with labor and delivery.

There have been various and contradictory research results regarding systemic and local NO concentrations, and effects of NO on the uterine vascular systems during pregnancy. There are two main possible causes for this: First, the study of human samples requires large sample sizes due to variability from genetic, dieting, and many other factors, but many previous studies had only small sample sizes. Second, well-controlled experimental models should be helpful for removing such variability. Unfortunately, very limited animal studies have been done thus far.

38.3.2.4.4 Cervical Ripening

As in the myometrium, all three NOS isoforms are observed in the human cervix, suggesting an important role of NO production. In contrast to the myometrium, NO production in the cervix is lower during gestation and becomes upregulated when pregnancy advances to term.[111] The expression of iNOS isoforms in the human cervix is highest at the end of pregnancy, suggesting that NO may be involved in cervical ripening. Cervical NOS activity is progesterone dependent.[112] Animal studies and clinical trials demonstrate that NO donors are effective and safe cervical ripening agents.[113, 114]

38.3.3 Nitric Oxide and Placenta

38.3.3.1 *Nitric Oxide and Fetoplacental Circulation and Placenta*

In human placentas, NOS is mainly expressed in the syncytiotrophoblast, macrophages, and villous endothelium, the major isoform being eNOS. eNOS expression has been identified in trophoblasts of early-trimester placentas. It is present in the cell columns of anchoring villi and extravillous trophoblasts at the implantation site, and in villous syncytiotrophoblasts of the first-trimester placenta, indicating that in situ generated NO by trophoblasts may participate in the dilation of vascular tone at the implantation site. iNOS expression is not detectable in the syncytiotrophoblast cell layer.[115] The multinucleated syncytiotrophoblast layer lining the chorionic villi is the interface between the maternal and fetal vascular systems, which could contribute to NO circulation.[116]

eNOS is the only isoform of NOS family expressed in the endothelium of the ovine fetoplacental vascular bed.[117] In ovine placentas, the concentration of NO and its second messenger cyclic guanosine monophosphate (cGMP) are substantially increased during normal pregnancy,[118, 119] especially in the fetoplacental units.[120] Furthermore, eNOS protein expression in fetoplacental artery endothelium and NO generation in ovine placenta are elevated gradually during the third trimester, specifically from days 110 to 130.[120]

38.3.3.2 *Nitric Oxide and Vasoreactivity of Fetoplacental Vessels*

The placental vasculature lacks adrenergic and cholinergic innervation, and NO is its most important fetoplacental vasodilator. Several early studies showed that the placental endothelium releases NO. In normal pregnancy, NO is the major vasodilator in the placenta. Similar to nonplacental vascular beds, the placental vasculature expresses the signal mediators of the classical NO-dependent vessel relaxation pathway, such as soluble guanylate cyclase (sGC), cyclic guanosine monophosphate (cGMP)-dependent protein kinase, and cGMP-specific phosphodiesterases. NO induces dilation in placental vessels through activation of the sGC and modulates larger conductance-, calcium-, and voltage-gated potassium (BK) channel activity.[121] NO synthesis at this level can be induced by shear stress, which is an important activator of eNOS by its phosphorylation at serine 1177, via ERK1/2 and Akt in placental endothelium, ATP, adenosine, calcitonin gene-related peptide (CGRP), and histamine.

O_2 level is an important factor regulating the vasoreactivity of fetoplacental vessels; whether in vivo or ex vivo, hypoxia increases placental vascular resistance. In low oxygen levels, the maximal response to vasodilator agents is impaired in isolated placental vessels. For instance, NO plays a key role maintaining sheep placental blood flow under conditions of normoxia and acute hypoxia.[122] A reduction in basal NO release causes hypoxic fetoplacental vasoconstriction in the perfused human placental cotyledon in vitro,[123] suggesting that the effect of hypoxia-mediated vasoconstriction is in part via weaker NOS activity. However, vasodilatation in response to the NO donor sodium nitroprusside (SNP) was increased in reduced oxygenation in placental veins but not in arteries.[124] SNP could dilate the human placental chorionic plate veins greater than those in nonplacental vessels,[125] even under basal conditions. The same finding has also been found in the $PGF_{2\alpha}$-preconstricted placental vessels.[126] L-NAME (an inhibitor of NOS) had no effect on Ang-II-induced contraction in placental vessels. Furthermore, the concentrations of L-arginine, NOS, and NO in placental tissue were significantly higher than those in placental vasculature, indicating that, unlike nonplacental vessels, dilated effects caused by endothelial NO systems of placental vessels are very weak, and NO-mediated placental vasodilatation was mainly induced by NO from other site, and not from placental vessels.[127]

A recent study has provided solid evidence to demonstrate that acetylcholine (ACh) showed no classic NO-mediated relaxation in human placental vasculature, whereas exogenous NO donor SNP could reliably decrease the basal vascular tension in human and sheep (Fig. 38.5).[127] These and other related data allow the conclusion that (1) placental vascular endothelial eNOS has limited roles in mediating the classic vasodilatation, and (2) exogenous NO is a strong stimulator for vasorelaxation in placental vessels.[128]

38.3.3.3 Nitric Oxide and Placental Vascular Development

38.3.3.3.1 Vasculogenesis

Placental vasculogenesis, the de novo formation of blood vessels, occurs very early in pregnancy (e.g., in humans about 6 weeks' gestation and in rhesus monkeys approximately 19 days postfertilization),[129] resulting in the formation of tertiary villi.

Human placental vessels

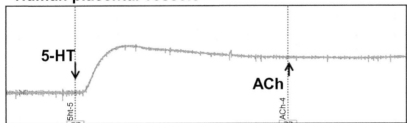

Human placental vessels

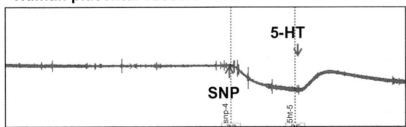

Sheep placental vessels

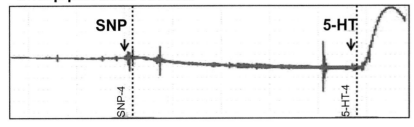

FIG. 38.5 Effects of acetylcholine (ACh) and sodium nitroprusside (SNP) on placenta vessels. In contrast to what occurs in most blood vessels, endogenous NO plays little role in regulating placental vessels, but exogenous NO showed a major role in regulating placental tone.

Nitric oxide is crucial for placental vasculogenesis. The spatiotemporal expression patterns of eNOS and iNOS are related to vasculogenesis in the yolk sac. In the first stage, iNOS-derived NO induces the mesodermal cells differentiation of adjacent extra-embryonic to form a primary capillary plexus at 7 days of embryonic development (E7.0) in rodents. Subsequently, a decrease in iNOS expression in the endoderm is accompanied by increasing eNOS expression in the yolk sac mesodermal cells.[130] At E6.5, pharmacologic inhibition of NOS activity completely retards the development of the primary capillary plexus.[130] In addition, more and more evidence has demonstrated that a crucial role of the yolk sac in embryo and placental vascular development.[131] Moreover, vasculogenesis at mice yolk sac is initiated by NO.[130] eNOS activity in embryonic vascular development represents a late hallmark of differentiation during vasculogenesis, which could be related to the formation of cardiac muscle contractions.[132]

38.3.3.3.2 Angiogenesis

Angiogenesis is the growth of new blood vessels from preexisting vessels through sprouting, migration, and proliferation of endothelial cells (ECs), which is critical in keeping the growth and consolidation of the placental vascular tree. Two types of angiogenesis pathway are involved in increasing placental vascular surface areas: (1) branching angiogenesis, as multiple short capillary loops are formed; and (2) nonbranching angiogenesis, with an increase in the length of the villous vessels.

It is known that eNOS produced NO is critical for placental angiogenesis. For example, vascularization is dramatically reduced in the placenta of *eNOS*-null pregnant mice. During normal gestation in sheep, placental NO production is increased in association with enhanced local expression of FGF2 and VEGF, vascular density, and blood flow to the placenta,[133] suggesting that eNOS-derived NO is important in placental angiogenesis. Nitric oxide is not only an effector of angiogenic pathways, but a stimulator and positive feedback signal for VEGF- and angiotensin-induced placental angiogenesis. For instance, NO donors stimulate ovine placental endothelial cell proliferation via activation of mitogen-activated protein kinase (MEK1/2) pathway. Akt[134] and eNOS[132] knockout mice showed reduced placental vascularization.

38.3.3.4 Nitric Oxide and Trophoblast Invasion

Trophoblasts are cells that form the outer layer of a blastocyst, which provides nutrients to the embryo, and then develop into a large part of the placenta. Trophoblast invasion is a critical process in the establishment of a successful pregnancy. But abnormal trophoblast invasion is associated with pathological conditions such as IUGR, stillbirth, spontaneous abortion, and preeclampsia. Trophoblasts constitutively express two isoforms of NOS (eNOS and iNOS), which produce NO in cells. Previous studies have identified positive staining of eNOS expression on cytotrophoblast columns and interstitial cytotrophoblasts. Taken together with the evidence of sGC expression in extravillous cytotrophoblasts, these findings indicate a role for NO in the process of trophoblast invasion.[135] NO might be instrumental to endovascular invasion and vascular remodeling in the developing placenta because (i) NO production mediates vascular endothelial-growth-factor-induced and hepatocyte growth-factor-induced human trophoblast invasion; (ii) NO is required for human trophoblast cell invasion during embryo implantation by upregulating the expression and activity of MMP-2 and MMP-9; and (iii) NO induces relaxation of the uteroplacental arteries, which is another prerequisite for trophoblast invasion. These findings indicate that low levels of NO might lead to the impaired cytotrophoblast invasion observed in preeclampsia.

38.3.3.5 Nitric Oxide and Placental Glucocorticoid Metabolism

Evidence obtained from cultured human trophoblasts indicates a role of NO in placental glucocorticoid metabolism. For example, NO regulates placental trophoblast steroidogenic capacity by attenuating, partially through a sGC-cGMP dependent mechanism, the 11β-hydroxysteroid dehydrogenase type 2 (11β-HSD2) oxidase activity and its mRNA expression. 11β-HSD2 is responsible for the conversion of cortisol into cortisone in the placenta.[136] The high affinity of placental 11β-HSD2 for its substrates might enable it to modulate the level of maternal glucocorticoids that flow into fetal circulation. Thus downregulation of NOS activity would lead to increasing the levels of bioactive cortisol in the placenta, the effect of which is likely to be physiologically important. The cortisol level in the fetal circulation is crucial for fetal organ maturation, while excessive cortisol could cause fetal growth retardation.

38.3.4 Nitric Oxide and the Fetus

Nitric oxide plays a vital role in the fetus, including cardiovascular systems and organ development.

38.3.4.1 Brain

Functional NOS is present in the fetal brain. Neuronal NOS and eNOS are constitutively expressed and their proteins are present in fetal brain. Moreover, during fetal brain development, the isoforms of NOS are regulated differentially. Among them, the expression of eNOS is consistent with maturation of the cerebral vasculature. Fetal brain nNOS is differentially regulated according to brain regions,[137] indicating a restricted role in the maturation of specific neuronal populations in the developing brain.[138] Nitric oxide is involved in regulating fetal cerebral blood flow. Endothelial NOS, instead of nNOS, may contribute to the maintenance of cerebral blood flow in response to hypoxia in the fetal brain in rats.[139]

38.3.4.2 Pulmonary System

In the fetal lung development, NO plays roles in regulating several biological processes, including pulmonary vascularization, airway branching morphogenesis, lung liquid production, and pulmonary vascular tone. All three NOS isoforms are primarily expressed in the respiratory epithelium in the fetus, and their abundance and NO production increase in accordance with maturation in the primate.[140, 141]

Expression of eNOS is increased toward term gestation in fetal lungs to prepare for successful transition at birth. When exposed to high oxygen tension, fetal pulmonary vascular resistance declines, mainly through increased eNOS. Nitric oxide synthesis increases and induces dilation in neonatal pulmonary arteries. Endothelial NOS can target mitochondria and decrease endothelial oxidative stress, and ultimately mediate pulmonary vasodilatation at birth. The increase in airway NO production is associated with a decrease in expiratory resistance.[141]

38.3.4.3 Ductus Arteriosus

The fetal ductus arteriosus (DA) is in an environment with a low oxygen tension, and NO is involved in the regulation of the fetal DA patency. NOS isoforms are expressed and functional in the mouse DA endothelium in the third trimester. eNOS is the dominant isoform. After birth, eNOS expression is maintained at a stable state throughout the postnatal period,[142] indicating NO plays a major role in regulating DA during the earlier developmental periods.

38.3.4.4 Heart

Nitric oxide has also been shown to play an important role in the regulation of blood pressure, peripheral resistance, and maintenance of cardiac functions in the fetus. It also regulates coronary artery tone in the heart. Among all NOS isoforms, eNOS and nNOS are the most important ones constitutively expressed in cardiomyocytes of fetal lambs.[143]

38.3.4.5 Adrenal Glands

Nitric oxide regulates the blood flow of adrenal gland and adrenal corticomedullary functions during the late gestation of the llama fetus.[144]

REFERENCES

1. Hall JE. Historical perspective of the renin-angiotensin system. *Mol Biotechnol* 2003;**24**(1):27–39 [Epub 2003/05/02].
2. Tipnis SR, Hooper NM, Hyde R, Karran E, Christie G, Turner AJ. A human homolog of angiotensin-converting enzyme. Cloning and functional expression as a captopril-insensitive carboxypeptidase. *J Biol Chem* 2000;**275**(43):33238–43 [Epub 2000/08/05].
3. Wolf G, Mentzel S, Assmann KJ. Aminopeptidase A: a key enzyme in the intrarenal degradation of angiotensin II. *Exp Nephrol* 1997;**5**(5):364–9 [Epub 1997/12/05].
4. Pringle KG, Tadros MA, Callister RJ, Lumbers ER. The expression and localization of the human placental prorenin/renin-angiotensin system throughout pregnancy: roles in trophoblast invasion and angiogenesis? *Placenta* 2011;**32**(12):956–62.
5. Marques FZ, Pringle KG, Conquest A, Hirst JJ, Markus MA, Sarris M, et al. Molecular characterization of renin-angiotensin system components in human intrauterine tissues and fetal membranes from vaginal delivery and cesarean section. *Placenta* 2011;**32**(3):214–21 [Epub 2011/01/11].
6. Li X, Shams M, Zhu J, Khalig A, Wilkes M, Whittle M, et al. Cellular localization of AT1 receptor mRNA and protein in normal placenta and its reduced expression in intrauterine growth restriction. Angiotensin II stimulates the release of vasorelaxants. *J Clin Invest* 1998;**101**(2):442–54.
7. Knock GA, Sullivan MH, McCarthy A, Elder MG, Polak JM, Wharton J. Angiotensin II (AT1) vascular binding sites in human placentae from normal-term, preeclamptic and growth retarded pregnancies. *J Pharmacol Exp Ther* 1994;**271**(2):1007–15.
8. Hirasawa G, Takeyama J, Sasano H, Fukushima K, Suzuki T, Muramatu Y, et al. 11Beta-hydroxysteroid dehydrogenase type II and mineralocorticoid receptor in human placenta. *J Clin Endocrinol Metab* 2000;**85**(3):1306–9 [Epub 2000/03/17].
9. Hodari AA, Smeby R, Bumpus FM. A renin-like substance in the human placenta. *Obstet Gynecol* 1967;**29**(3):313–7 [Epub 1967/03/01].

10. Symonds EM, Stanley MA, Skinner SL. Production of renin by in vitro cultures of human chorion and uterine muscle. *Nature* 1968;**217**(5134):1152–3 [Epub 1968/03/23].

11. Kalenga MK, Thomas K, de Gasparo M, De Hertogh R. Determination of renin, angiotensin converting enzyme and angiotensin II levels in human placenta, chorion and amnion from women with pregnancy induced hypertension. *Clin Endocrinol* 1996;**44**(4):429–33 [Epub 1996/04/01].

12. Yagami H, Kurauchi O, Murata Y, Okamoto T, Mizutani S, Tomoda Y. Expression of angiotensin-converting enzyme in human placenta and its physiologic role in the fetal circulation. *Obstet Gynecol* 1994;**84**(3):453–7 [Epub 1994/09/01].

13. Cooper AC, Robinson G, Vinson GP, Cheung WT, Broughton PF. The localization and expression of the renin-angiotensin system in the human placenta throughout pregnancy. *Placenta* 1999;**20**(5–6):467–74 [Epub 1999/07/27].

14. Lenz T, Sealey JE, Tewksbury DA. Regional distribution of the angiotensinogens in human placentae. *Placenta* 1993;**14**(6):695–9 [Epub 1993/11/01].

15. Kalenga MK, de Gasparo M, de Hertogh R, Whitebread S, Vankrieken L, Thomas K. Angiotensin II receptors in the human placenta are type AT1 [Les recepteurs de l'angiotensine II dans le placenta humain sont de type AT1]. *Reprod Nutr Dev* 1991;**31**(3):257–67 [Epub 1991/01/01].

16. Petit A, Geoffroy P, Belisle S. Expression of angiotensin II type-I receptor and phospholipase C-linked G alpha q/11 protein in the human placenta. *J Soc Gynecol Investig* 1996;**3**(6):316–21 [Epub 1996/11/01].

17. Kalenga MK, De Hertogh R, Whitebread S, Vankrieken L, Thomas K, De Gasparo M. Distribution of the concentrations of angiotensin II (A II), A II receptors, hPL, prolactin, and steroids in human fetal membranes [Distribution des concentrations de l'angiotensine II (A II), des recepteurs A II, de l'hPL, de la prolactine et des steroides dans les annexes foetales humaines]. *Rev Fr Gynecol Obstet* 1991;**86**(10):585–91.

18. Hering L, Herse F, Geusens N, Verlohren S, Wenzel K, Staff AC, et al. Effects of circulating and local uteroplacental angiotensin II in rat pregnancy. *Hypertension* 2010;**56**(2):311–8 [Epub 2010/06/10].

19. Araki-Taguchi M, Nomura S, Ino K, Sumigama S, Yamamoto E, Kotani-Ito T, et al. Angiotensin II mimics the hypoxic effect on regulating trophoblast proliferation and differentiation in human placental explant cultures. *Life Sci* 2008;**82**(1–2):59–67 [Epub 2007/12/01].

20. Zhao Q, Ishibashi M, Hiasa K, Tan C, Takeshita A, Egashira K. Essential role of vascular endothelial growth factor in angiotensin II-induced vascular inflammation and remodeling. *Hypertension* 2004;**44**(3):264–70 [Epub 2004/07/21].

21. Squires PM, Kennedy TG. Evidence for a role for a uterine renin-angiotensin system in decidualization in rats. *J Reprod Fertil* 1992;**95**(3):791–802 [Epub 1992/08/01].

22. Gennari-Moser C, Khankin EV, Schuller S, Escher G, Frey BM, Portmann CB, et al. Regulation of placental growth by aldosterone and cortisol. *Endocrinology* 2011;**152**(1):263–71.

23. Lundin-Schiller S, Mitchell MD. Renin increases human amnion cell prostaglandin E2 biosynthesis. *J Clin Endocrinol Metab* 1991;**73**(2):436–40 [Epub 1991/08/01].

24. Hackenthal E, Paul M, Ganten D, Taugner R. Morphology, physiology, and molecular biology of renin secretion. *Physiol Rev* 1990;**70**(4):1067–116.

25. Gao Q, Tang J, Li N, Zhou X, Li Y, Liu Y, et al. A novel mechanism of angiotensin II-regulated placental vascular tone in the development of hypertension in preeclampsia. *Oncotarget* 2017;**8**(19):30734–41 [Epub 2017/04/22].

26. Rosenfeld CR, Gresores A, Roy TA, Magness RR. Comparison of ANG II in fetal and pregnant sheep: metabolic clearance and vascular sensitivity. *Am J Phys* 1995;**268**(2 Pt 1):E237–47 [Epub 1995/02/01].

27. Speroff L, Haning Jr. RV, Levin RM. The effect of angiotensin II and indomethacin on uterine artery blood flow in pregnant monkeys. *Obstet Gynecol* 1977;**50**(5):611–4 [Epub 1977/11/01].

28. Gant NF, Daley GL, Chand S, Whalley PJ, MacDonald PC. A study of angiotensin II pressor response throughout primigravid pregnancy. *J Clin Invest* 1973;**52**(11):2682–9 [Epub 1973/11/01].

29. Naden RP, Rosenfeld CR. Effect of angiotensin II on uterine and systemic vasculature in pregnant sheep. *J Clin Invest* 1981;**68**(2):468–74 [Epub 1981/08/01].

30. Schutz S, Le Moullec JM, Corvol P, Gasc JM. Early expression of all the components of the renin-angiotensin-system in human development. *Am J Pathol* 1996;**149**(6):2067–79 [Epub 1996/12/01].

31. Symonds EM, Craven DJ, Rodeck CH. Fetal plasma renin and renin substrate in mid-trimester pregnancy. *Br J Obstet Gynaecol* 1985;**92**(6):618–21 [Epub 1985/06/01].

32. Sim MK, Seng KM. Development of angiotensin converting enzyme in fetal lung and placenta of the rat and human. *Clin Exp Pharmacol Physiol* 1984;**11**(5):497–501 [Epub 1984/09/01].

33. Bender JW, Davitt MK, Jose P. Angiotensin-I-converting enzyme activity in term and premature infants. *Biol Neonate* 1978;**34**(1–2):19–23 [Epub 1978/01/01].

34. Magness RR, Cox K, Rosenfeld CR, Gant NF. Angiotensin II metabolic clearance rate and pressor responses in nonpregnant and pregnant women. *Am J Obstet Gynecol* 1994;**171**(3):668–79 [Epub 1994/09/01].

35. Oparil S, Koerner TJ, Lindheimer MD. Plasma angiotensin converting enzyme activity in mother and fetus. *J Clin Endocrinol Metab* 1978;**46**(3):434–9 [Epub 1978/03/01].

36. Beitins IZ, Bayard F, Levitsky L, Ances IG, Kowarski A, Migeon CJ. Plasma aldosterone concentration at delivery and during the newborn period. *J Clin Invest* 1972;**51**(2):386–94 [Epub 1972/02/01].

37. Procianoy RS, de Oliveira-Filho EA. Aldosterone cord levels in preterm newborn infants. *Acta Paediatr* 1996;**85**(5):611–3 [Epub 1996/05/01].

38. Bayard F, Ances IG, Tapper AJ, Weldon VV, Kowarski A, Migeon CJ. Transplacental passage and fetal secretion of aldosterone. *J Clin Invest* 1970;**49**(7):1389–93 [Epub 1970/07/01].

39. Baxter JD, James MN, Chu WN, Duncan K, Haidar MA, Carilli CT, et al. The molecular biology of human renin and its gene. *Yale J Biol Med* 1989;**62**(5):493–501 [Epub 1989/09/01].

40. Price RL, Carver W, Simpson DG, Fu L, Zhao J, Borg TK, et al. The effects of angiotensin II and specific angiotensin receptor blockers on embryonic cardiac development and looping patterns. *Dev Biol* 1997;**192**(2):572–84 [Epub 1998/01/27].

41. Reini SA, Wood CE, Keller-Wood M. The ontogeny of genes related to ovine fetal cardiac growth. *Gene Expr Patterns* 2009;**9**(2):122–8 [Epub 2008/10/07].

42. Crackower MA, Sarao R, Oudit GY, Yagil C, Kozieradzki I, Scanga SE, et al. Angiotensin-converting enzyme 2 is an essential regulator of heart function. *Nature* 2002;**417**(6891):822–8 [Epub 2002/06/21].

43. Cox BE, Liu XT, Fluharty SJ, Rosenfeld CR. Vessel-specific regulation of angiotensin II receptor subtypes during ovine development. *Pediatr Res* 2005;**57**(1):124–32 [Epub 2004/11/24].

44. Gasc JM, Shanmugam S, Sibony M, Corvol P. Tissue-specific expression of type 1 angiotensin II receptor subtypes. An in situ hybridization study. *Hypertension* 1994;**24**(5):531–7 [Epub 1994/11/01].

45. Saavedra JM, Viswanathan M, Shigematsu K. Localization of angiotensin AT1 receptors in the rat heart conduction system. *Eur J Pharmacol* 1993;**235**(2–3):301–3 [Epub 1993/04/28].

46. Brown RW, Diaz R, Robson AC, Kotelevtsev YV, Mullins JJ, Kaufman MH, et al. The ontogeny of 11 beta-hydroxysteroid dehydrogenase type 2 and mineralocorticoid receptor gene expression reveal intricate control of glucocorticoid action in development. *Endocrinology* 1996;**137**(2):794–7 [Epub 1996/02/01].

47. Rosenfeld CR, Cox BE, Magness RR, Shaul PW. Ontogeny of angiotensin II vascular smooth muscle receptors in ovine fetal aorta and placental and uterine arteries. *Am J Obstet Gynecol* 1993;**168**(5):1562–9.

48. Hutchinson HG, Hein L, Fujinaga M, Pratt RE. Modulation of vascular development and injury by angiotensin II. *Cardiovasc Res* 1999;**41**(3):689–700 [Epub 1999/08/06].

49. Shanmugam S, Corvol P, Gasc JM. Angiotensin II type 2 receptor mRNA expression in the developing cardiopulmonary system of the rat. *Hypertension* 1996;**28**(1):91–7 [Epub 1996/07/01].

50. Mungall BA, Shinkel TA, Sernia C. Immunocytochemical localization of angiotensinogen in the fetal and neonatal rat brain. *Neuroscience* 1995;**67**(2):505–24 [Epub 1995/07/01].

51. Tsutsumi K, Seltzer A, Saavedra JM. Angiotensin II receptor subtypes and angiotensin-converting enzyme in the fetal rat brain. *Brain Res* 1993;**631**(2):212–20 [Epub 1993/12/24].

52. Tsutsumi K, Viswanathan M, Stromberg C, Saavedra JM. Type-1 and type-2 angiotensin II receptors in fetal rat brain. *Eur J Pharmacol* 1991;**198**(1):89–92 [Epub 1991/05/30].

53. Nuyt AM, Lenkei Z, Palkovits M, Corvol P, Llorens-Cortes C. Ontogeny of angiotensin II type 2 receptor mRNA expression in fetal and neonatal rat brain. *J Comp Neurol* 1999;**407**(2):193–206 [Epub 1999/04/23].

54. Mao C, Shi L, Xu F, Zhang L, Xu Z. Development of fetal brain renin-angiotensin system and hypertension programmed in fetal origins. *Prog Neurobiol* 2009;**87**(4):252–63 [Epub 2009/05/12].

55. Hu F, Morrissey P, Yao J, Xu Z. Development of AT(1) and AT(2) receptors in the ovine fetal brain. *Brain Res Dev Brain Res* 2004;**150**(1):51–61 [Epub 2004/05/06].

56. Noorlander CW, De Graan PN, Middeldorp J, Van Beers JJ, Visser GH. Ontogeny of hippocampal corticosteroid receptors: effects of antenatal glucocorticoids in human and mouse. *J Comp Neurol* 2006;**499**(6):924–32 [Epub 2006/10/31].

57. Lumbers ER. Development of renal function in the fetus: a review. *Reprod Fertil Dev* 1995;**7**(3):415–26 [Epub 1995/01/01].

58. Mao C, Shi L, Li N, Xu F, Xu Z. Development of local RAS in cardiovascular/body fluid regulatory systems and hypertension in fetal origins. In: De Luca Jr. LA, Menani JV, Johnson AK, editors. *Neurobiology of body fluid homeostasis: transduction and integration*. Boca Raton, FL: CRC Press, Taylor & Francis Group; 2014.

59. Miyazaki Y, Tsuchida S, Fogo A, Ichikawa I. The renal lesions that develop in neonatal mice during angiotensin inhibition mimic obstructive nephropathy. *Kidney Int* 1999;**55**(5):1683–95 [Epub 1999/05/07].

60. Scott AA, Purohit DM. Neonatal renal failure: a complication of maternal antihypertensive therapy. *Am J Obstet Gynecol* 1989;**160**(5 Pt 1):1223–4 [Epub 1989/05/01].

61. Zhang SL, Moini B, Ingelfinger JR. Angiotensin II increases Pax-2 expression in fetal kidney cells via the AT2 receptor. *J Am Soc Nephrol* 2004;**15**(6):1452–65 [Epub 2004/05/22].

62. Maric C, Aldred GP, Harris PJ, Alcorn D. Angiotensin II inhibits growth of cultured embryonic renomedullary interstitial cells through the AT2 receptor. *Kidney Int* 1998;**53**(1):92–9 [Epub 1998/02/07].

63. Lumbers ER, Burrell JH, Menzies RI, Stevens AD. The effects of a converting enzyme inhibitor (captopril) and angiotensin II on fetal renal function. *Br J Pharmacol* 1993;**110**(2):821–7 [Epub 1993/10/01].

64. Lumbers ER. Functions of the renin-angiotensin system during development. *Clin Exp Pharmacol Physiol* 1995;**22**(8):499–505 [Epub 1995/08/01].

65. Berger S, Bleich M, Schmid W, Greger R, Schutz G. Mineralocorticoid receptor knockout mice: lessons on Na+ metabolism. *Kidney Int* 2000;**57**(4):1295–8 [Epub 2000/04/12].

66. Fernandes-Rosa FL, Hubert EL, Fagart J, Tchitchek N, Gomes D, Jouanno E, et al. Mineralocorticoid receptor mutations differentially affect individual gene expression profiles in pseudohypoaldosteronism type 1. *J Clin Endocrinol Metab* 2011;**96**(3):E519–27 [Epub 2010/12/17].

67. Gembardt F, Heringer-Walther S, van Esch JH, Sterner-Kock A, van Veghel R, Le TH, et al. Cardiovascular phenotype of mice lacking all three subtypes of angiotensin II receptors. *FASEB J* 2008;**22**(8):3068–77 [Epub 2008/05/24].

68. Sundgren NC, Giraud GD, Stork PJ, Maylie JG, Thornburg KL. Angiotensin II stimulates hyperplasia but not hypertrophy in immature ovine cardiomyocytes. *J Physiol* 2003;**548**(Pt 3):881–91 [Epub 2003/03/11].

69. Segar JL, Dalshaug GB, Bedell KA, Smith OM, Scholz TD. Angiotensin II in cardiac pressure-overload hypertrophy in fetal sheep. *Am J Physiol Regul Integr Comp Physiol* 2001;**281**(6):R2037–47 [Epub 2001/11/14].

70. Yamada H, Akishita M, Ito M, Tamura K, Daviet L, Lehtonen JY, et al. AT2 receptor and vascular smooth muscle cell differentiation in vascular development. *Hypertension* 1999;**33**(6):1414–9 [Epub 1999/06/18].

71. Nakajima M, Hutchinson HG, Fujinaga M, Hayashida W, Morishita R, Zhang L, et al. The angiotensin II type 2 (AT2) receptor antagonizes the growth effects of the AT1 receptor: gain-of-function study using gene transfer. *Proc Natl Acad Sci U S A* 1995;**92**(23):10663–7 [Epub 1995/11/07].

72. Reaves PY, Beck CR, Wang HW, Raizada MK, Katovich MJ. Endothelial-independent prevention of high blood pressure in L-NAME-treated rats by angiotensin II type I receptor antisense gene therapy. *Exp Physiol* 2003;**88**(4):467–73 [Epub 2003/07/16].

73. Sernia C, Zeng T, Kerr D, Wyse B. Novel perspectives on pituitary and brain angiotensinogen. *Front Neuroendocrinol* 1997;**18**(2):174–208 [Epub 1997/04/01].

74. Laflamme L, Gasparo M, Gallo JM, Payet MD, Gallo-Payet N. Angiotensin II induction of neurite outgrowth by AT2 receptors in NG108-15 cells. Effect counteracted by the AT1 receptors. *J Biol Chem* 1996;**271**(37):22729–35 [Epub 1996/09/13].

75. Shenoy UV, Richards EM, Huang XC, Sumners C. Angiotensin II type 2 receptor-mediated apoptosis of cultured neurons from newborn rat brain. *Endocrinology* 1999;**140**(1):500–9 [Epub 1999/01/14].

76. von Bohlen und Halbach O, Walther T, Bader M, Albrecht D. Genetic deletion of angiotensin AT2 receptor leads to increased cell numbers in different brain structures of mice. *Regul Pept* 2001;**99**(2–3):209–16 [Epub 2001/06/01].

77. Xu Z, Shi L, Hu F, White R, Stewart L, Yao J. In utero development of central ANG-stimulated pressor response and hypothalamic fos expression. *Brain Res Dev Brain Res* 2003;**145**(2):169–76 [Epub 2003/11/08].

78. Fitzsimons JT. Angiotensin, thirst, and sodium appetite. *Physiol Rev* 1998;**78**(3):583–686 [Epub 1998/07/23].

79. Shi L, Mao C, Zeng F, Hou J, Zhang H, Xu Z. Central angiotensin I increases fetal AVP neuron activity and pressor responses. *Am J Physiol Endocrinol Metab* 2010;**298**(6):E1274–82 [Epub 2010/04/08].

80. Shi L, Mao C, Wu J, Morrissey P, Lee J, Xu Z. Effects of i.c.v. losartan on the angiotensin II-mediated vasopressin release and hypothalamic fos expression in near-term ovine fetuses. *Peptides* 2006;**27**(9):2230–8 [Epub 2006/05/09].

81. Ross MG, Kullama LK, Ogundipe A, Chan K, Ervin MG. Ovine fetal swallowing response to intracerebroventricular hypertonic saline. *J Appl Physiol (1985)* 1995;**78**(6):2267–71 [Epub 1995/06/01].

82. El-Haddad MA, Ismail Y, Gayle D, Ross MG. Central angiotensin II AT1 receptors mediate fetal swallowing and pressor responses in the near-term ovine fetus. *Am J Physiol Regul Integr Comp Physiol* 2005;**288**(4):R1014–20 [Epub 2004/11/20].

83. Ignarro LJ. Signal transduction mechanisms involving nitric oxide. *Biochem Pharmacol* 1991;**41**(4):485–90 [Epub 1991/02/15].

84. Mombouli JV, Vanhoutte PM. Kinins and endothelial control of vascular smooth muscle. *Annu Rev Pharmacol Toxicol* 1995;**35**:679–705 [Epub 1995/01/01].

85. Fleming I, Busse R. Molecular mechanisms involved in the regulation of the endothelial nitric oxide synthase. *Am J Physiol Regul Integr Comp Physiol* 2003;**284**(1):R1–12 [Epub 2002/12/17].

86. Schell W. Patient information [Patientenaufklarung]. *Kinderkrankenschwester* 1991;**10**(4):159–61 [Epub 1991/04/01].

87. Fleming I, Bauersachs J, Busse R. Calcium-dependent and calcium-independent activation of the endothelial NO synthase. *J Vasc Res* 1997;**34**(3):165–74 [Epub 1997/05/01].

88. Garmendia JV, Gutierrez Y, Blanca I, Bianco NE, De Sanctis JB. Nitric oxide in different types of hypertension during pregnancy. *Clin Sci (Lond)* 1997;**93**(5):413–21 [Epub 1998/03/05].

89. Zhou R, Xlong Q, You Y, Qiu D, Zhang K, Liu S. The use of serum nitric oxide level and cyclic guanosine monophosphate level as predictors of preterm delivery. *Sichuan Da Xue Xue Bao Yi Xue Ban* 2003;**34**(1):115–6 [Epub 2004/12/17].

90. Valtonen P, Laitinen T, Lyyra-Laitinen T, Raitakari OT, Juonala M, Viikari JS, et al. Serum L-homoarginine concentration is elevated during normal pregnancy and is related to flow-mediated vasodilatation. *Circ J* 2008;**72**(11):1879–84 [Epub 2008/09/20].

91. Holden DP, Fickling SA, Whitley GS, Nussey SS. Plasma concentrations of asymmetric dimethylarginine, a natural inhibitor of nitric oxide synthase, in normal pregnancy and preeclampsia. *Am J Obstet Gynecol* 1998;**178**(3):551–6 [Epub 1998/04/16].

92. Pettersson A, Hedner T, Milsom I. Increased circulating concentrations of asymmetric dimethyl arginine (ADMA), an endogenous inhibitor of nitric oxide synthesis, in preeclampsia. *Acta Obstet Gynecol Scand* 1998;**77**(8):808–13 [Epub 1998/10/17].

93. West CA, Sasser JM, Baylis C. The enigma of continual plasma volume expansion in pregnancy: critical role of the renin-angiotensin-aldosterone system. *Am J Physiol Ren Physiol* 2016;**311**(6):F1125–34 [Epub 2016/10/22].

94. Sladek SM, Magness RR, Conrad KP. Nitric oxide and pregnancy. *Am J Phys* 1997;**272**(2 Pt 2):R441–63 [Epub 1997/02/01].

95. Hillhouse EW, Grammatopoulos DK. Role of stress peptides during human pregnancy and labour. *Reproduction* 2002;**124**(3):323–9 [Epub 2002/08/31].

96. Adamova Z, Ozkan S, Khalil RA. Vascular and cellular calcium in normal and hypertensive pregnancy. *Curr Clin Pharmacol* 2009;**4**(3):172–90 [Epub 2009/06/09].

97. Toda N, Toda H, Okamura T. Regulation of myometrial circulation and uterine vascular tone by constitutive nitric oxide. *Eur J Pharmacol* 2013;**714**(1–3):414–23 [Epub 2013/07/23].

98. Nelson SH, Steinsland OS, Wang Y, Yallampalli C, Dong YL, Sanchez JM. Increased nitric oxide synthase activity and expression in the human uterine artery during pregnancy. *Circ Res* 2000;**87**(5):406–11 [Epub 2000/09/02].

99. Nelson SH, Steinsland OS, Suresh MS, Lee NM. Pregnancy augments nitric oxide-dependent dilator response to acetylcholine in the human uterine artery. *Hum Reprod* 1998;**13**(5):1361–7 [Epub 1998/07/01].

100. Kublickiene KR, Cockell AP, Nisell H, Poston L. Role of nitric oxide in the regulation of vascular tone in pressurized and perfused resistance myometrial arteries from term pregnant women. *Am J Obstet Gynecol* 1997;**177**(5):1263–9 [Epub 1997/12/16].

101. Maul H, Longo M, Saade GR, Garfield RE. Nitric oxide and its role during pregnancy: from ovulation to delivery. *Curr Pharm Des* 2003;**9**(5):359–80 [Epub 2003/02/07].

102. Shukovski L, Tsafriri A. The involvement of nitric oxide in the ovulatory process in the rat. *Endocrinology* 1994;**135**(5):2287–90 [Epub 1994/11/01].

103. Rosselli M, Imthurn B, Macas E, Keller PJ, Dubey RK. Circulating nitrite/nitrate levels increase with follicular development: indirect evidence for estradiol mediated NO release. *Biochem Biophys Res Commun* 1994;**202**(3):1543–52 [Epub 1994/08/15].

104. Purcell TL, Given R, Chwalisz K, Garfield RE. Nitric oxide synthase distribution during implantation in the mouse. *Mol Hum Reprod* 1999;**5**(5):467–75 [Epub 1999/05/25].

105. Norman JE, Thompson AJ, Telfer JF, Young A, Greer IA, Cameron IT. Myometrial constitutive nitric oxide synthase expression is increased during human pregnancy. *Mol Hum Reprod* 1999;**5**(2):175–81 [Epub 1999/03/05].

106. Buhimschi I, Yallampalli C, Dong YL, Garfield RE. Involvement of a nitric oxide-cyclic guanosine monophosphate pathway in control of human uterine contractility during pregnancy. *Am J Obstet Gynecol* 1995;**172**(5):1577–84 [Epub 1995/05/01].

107. Telfer JF, Irvine GA, Kohnen G, Campbell S, Cameron IT. Expression of endothelial and inducible nitric oxide synthase in non-pregnant and decidualized human endometrium. *Mol Hum Reprod* 1997;**3**(1):69–75 [Epub 1997/01/01].

108. Kakui K, Itoh H, Sagawa N, Yura S, Korita D, Takemura M, et al. Augmented endothelial nitric oxide synthase (eNOS) protein expression in human pregnant myometrium: possible involvement of eNOS promoter activation by estrogen via both estrogen receptor (ER)alpha and ERbeta. *Mol Hum Reprod* 2004;**10**(2):115–22 [Epub 2004/01/27].

109. Ramsay B, Sooranna SR, Johnson MR. Nitric oxide synthase activities in human myometrium and villous trophoblast throughout pregnancy. *Obstet Gynecol* 1996;**87**(2):249–53 [Epub 1996/02/01].

110. Leszczynska-Gorzelak B, Laskowska M, Marciniak B, Oleszczuk J. Nitric oxide for treatment of threatened preterm labor. *Int J Gynaecol Obstet* 2001;**73**(3):201–6 [Epub 2001/05/30].

111. Buhimschi I, Ali M, Jain V, Chwalisz K, Garfield RE. Differential regulation of nitric oxide in the rat uterus and cervix during pregnancy and labour. *Hum Reprod* 1996;**11**(8):1755–66 [Epub 1996/08/01].

112. Rosselli M, Keller PJ, Dubey RK. Role of nitric oxide in the biology, physiology and pathophysiology of reproduction. *Hum Reprod Update* 1998;**4**(1):3–24 [Epub 1998/06/11].

113. Promsonthi P, Preechapornprasert A, Chanrachakul B. Nitric oxide donors for cervical ripening in first-trimester surgical abortion. *Cochrane Database Syst Rev* 2015;**2**: [Epub 2015/05/01].

114. Vaisanen-Tommiska MR. Nitric oxide in the human uterine cervix: endogenous ripening factor. *Ann Med* 2008;**40**(1):45–55 [Epub 2008/02/05].

115. Motta-Mejia C, Kandzija N, Zhang W, Mhlomi V, Cerdeira AS, Burdujan A, et al. Placental vesicles carry active endothelial nitric oxide synthase and their activity is reduced in preeclampsia. *Hypertension* 2017;**70**(2):372–81 [Epub 2017/06/14].

116. Redman CW. Current topic: pre-eclampsia and the placenta. *Placenta* 1991;**12**(4):301–8 [Epub 1991/07/01].

117. Zheng J, Li Y, Weiss AR, Bird IM, Magness RR. Expression of endothelial and inducible nitric oxide synthases and nitric oxide production in ovine placental and uterine tissues during late pregnancy. *Placenta* 2000;**21**(5–6):516–24 [Epub 2000/08/15].

118. Rosenfeld CR, Cox BE, Roy T, Magness RR. Nitric oxide contributes to estrogen-induced vasodilation of the ovine uterine circulation. *J Clin Invest* 1996;**98**(9):2158–66 [Epub 1996/11/01].

119. Magness RR, Rosenfeld CR, Hassan A, Shaul PW. Endothelial vasodilator production by uterine and systemic arteries. I. Effects of ANG II on PGI2 and NO in pregnancy. *Am J Phys* 1996;**270**(6 Pt 2):H1914–23 [Epub 1996/06/01].

120. Sheppard C, Shaw CE, Li Y, Bird IM, Magness RR. Endothelium-derived nitric oxide synthase protein expression in ovine placental arteries. *Biol Reprod* 2001;**64**(5):1494–9 [Epub 2001/04/25].

121. Sand A, Andersson E, Fried G. Nitric oxide donors mediate vasodilation in human placental arteries partly through a direct effect on potassium channels. *Placenta* 2006;**27**(2–3):181–90 [Epub 2005/12/13].

122. Coumans AB, Garnier Y, Supcun S, Jensen A, Hasaart TH, Berger R. The role of nitric oxide on fetal cardiovascular control during normoxia and acute hypoxia in 0.75 gestation sheep. *J Soc Gynecol Investig* 2003;**10**(5):275–82 [Epub 2003/07/11].

123. Byrne BM, Howard RB, Morrow RJ, Whiteley KJ, Adamson SL. Role of the L-arginine nitric oxide pathway in hypoxic fetoplacental vasoconstriction. *Placenta* 1997;**18**(8):627–34 [Epub 1997/11/19].

124. Wareing M, Greenwood SL, Baker PN. Reactivity of human placental chorionic plate vessels is modified by level of oxygenation: differences between arteries and veins. *Placenta* 2006;**27**(1):42–8 [Epub 2005/11/29].

125. Sprague B, Chesler NC, Magness RR. Shear stress regulation of nitric oxide production in uterine and placental artery endothelial cells: experimental studies and hemodynamic models of shear stresses on endothelial cells. *Int J Dev Biol* 2010;**54**(2–3):331–9 [Epub 2009/10/31].

126. Read MA, Giles WB, Leitch IM, Boura AL, Walters WA. Vascular responses to sodium nitroprusside in the human fetal-placental circulation. *Reprod Fertil Dev* 1995;**7**(6):1557–61 [Epub 1995/01/01].

127. Gao Q, Tang J, Li N, Zhou X, Zhu X, Li W, et al. New conception for the development of hypertension in preeclampsia. *Oncotarget* 2016;**7**(48):78387–95 [Epub 2016/11/20].

128. Gao Q, Tang J, Li N, Liu B, Zhang M, Sun M, et al. What is precise pathophysiology in development of hypertension in pregnancy? Precision medicine requires precise physiology and pathophysiology. *Drug Discov Today* 2018;**23**(2):286–99 [Epub 2017/11/05].

129. Kaufmann P, Mayhew TM, Charnock-Jones DS. Aspects of human fetoplacental vasculogenesis and angiogenesis. II. Changes during normal pregnancy. *Placenta* 2004;**25**(2–3):114–26 [Epub 2004/02/20].

130. Nath AK, Enciso J, Kuniyasu M, Hao XY, Madri JA, Pinter E. Nitric oxide modulates murine yolk sac vasculogenesis and rescues glucose induced vasculopathy. *Development* 2004;**131**(10):2485–96 [Epub 2004/05/07].

131. Freyer C, Renfree MB. The mammalian yolk sac placenta. *J Exp Zool B Mol Dev Evol* 2009;**312**(6):545–54 [Epub 2008/11/06].

132. Teichert AM, Scott JA, Robb GB, Zhou YQ, Zhu SN, Lem M, et al. Endothelial nitric oxide synthase gene expression during murine embryogenesis: commencement of expression in the embryo occurs with the establishment of a unidirectional circulatory system. *Circ Res* 2008;**103**(1):24–33 [Epub 2008/06/17].

133. Zheng J, Vagnoni KE, Bird IM, Magness RR. Expression of basic fibroblast growth factor, endothelial mitogenic activity, and angiotensin II type-1 receptors in the ovine placenta during the third trimester of pregnancy. *Biol Reprod* 1997;**56**(5):1189–97.

134. Yang ZZ, Tschopp O, Hemmings-Mieszczak M, Feng J, Brodbeck D, Perentes E, et al. Protein kinase B alpha/Akt1 regulates placental development and fetal growth. *J Biol Chem* 2003;**278**(34):32124–31 [Epub 2003/06/05].

135. Martin D, Conrad KP. Expression of endothelial nitric oxide synthase by extravillous trophoblast cells in the human placenta. *Placenta* 2000;**21**(1):23–31 [Epub 2000/02/29].

136. Sun K, Yang K, Challis JR. Differential regulation of 11 beta-hydroxysteroid dehydrogenase type 1 and 2 by nitric oxide in cultured human placental trophoblast and chorionic cell preparation. *Endocrinology* 1997;**138**(11):4912–20 [Epub 1997/11/05].

137. Massmann GA, Zhang J, Sallah J, Figueroa JP. Developmental and regional expression patterns of Type I Nitric Oxide Synthase mRNA and protein in fetal sheep brain during the last third of gestation. *Brain Res Dev Brain Res* 2000;**124**(1–2):141–52 [Epub 2000/12/13].

138. Northington FJ, Koehler RC, Traystman RJ, Martin LJ. Nitric oxide synthase 1 and nitric oxide synthase 3 protein expression is regionally and temporally regulated in fetal brain. *Brain Res Dev Brain Res* 1996;**95**(1):1–14 [Epub 1996/08/20].

139. Nakata M, Anno K, Sugino N, Matsumori LT, Nakamura Y, Kato H. Effect of intrauterine ischemia-hypoxia on endothelial nitric oxide synthase in fetal brain in rats. *Biol Neonate* 2002;**82**(2):117–21 [Epub 2002/08/10].

140. McCurnin DC, Pierce RA, Willis BC, Chang LY, Yoder BA, Yuhanna IS, et al. Postnatal estradiol up-regulates lung nitric oxide synthases and improves lung function in bronchopulmonary dysplasia. *Am J Respir Crit Care Med* 2009;**179**(6):492–500 [Epub 2009/01/20].

141. Shaul PW, Afshar S, Gibson LL, Sherman TS, Kerecman JD, Grubb PH, et al. Developmental changes in nitric oxide synthase isoform expression and nitric oxide production in fetal baboon lung. *Am J Physiol Lung Cell Mol Physiol* 2002;**283**(6):L1192–9 [Epub 2002/10/22].

142. Richard C, Gao J, LaFleur B, Christman BW, Anderson J, Brown N, et al. Patency of the preterm fetal ductus arteriosus is regulated by endothelial nitric oxide synthase and is independent of vasa vasorum in the mouse. *Am J Physiol Regul Integr Comp Physiol* 2004;**287**(3):R652–60 [Epub 2004/05/15].

143. Kameny RJ, He Y, Morris C, Sun C, Johengen M, Gong W, et al. Right ventricular nitric oxide signaling in an ovine model of congenital heart disease: a preserved fetal phenotype. *Am J Physiol Heart Circ Physiol* 2015;**309**(1):H157–65 [Epub 2015 May 1].

144. Riquelme RA, Sánchez G, Liberona L, Sanhueza EM, Giussani DA, Blanco CE, et al. Nitric oxide plays a role in the regulation of adrenal blood flow and adrenocorticomedullary functions in the llama fetus. *J Physiol* 2002;**544**(Pt 1):267–76.

Chapter 39

Origins of Adipose Tissue and Adipose Regulating Hormones

Declan Wayne*, T'ng Chang Kwok*, Shalini Ojha†, Helen Budge* and Michael E. Symonds*,‡

*Division of Child Health, Obstetrics and Gynaecology, University of Nottingham, Nottingham, United Kingdom, †Division of Medical Sciences and Graduate Entry Medicine, School of Medicine, University of Nottingham, Derby, United Kingdom, ‡Nottingham Digestive Disease Centre and Biomedical Research Centre, The School of Medicine, University of Nottingham, Nottingham, United Kingdom

Key Clinical Changes

- Increasing evidence supports the hypothesis that there may be a developmental origin of health and disease beginning within the pre- and perinatal period.
- Dysregulation of prenatal adipose tissue development and regulating hormones may lead to a predisposition of adulthood obesity.
- Adulthood obesity has been linked to a range of acute and chronic diseases, including cardiovascular disease, cancer, and diabetes.
- Our understanding of these hormones in utero, specifically in the human population, are still lacking.

39.1 ADIPOSE TISSUE

Adipose tissue plays a major role in a range of physiological processes throughout the life course. This ranges from providing a source of heat by thermoregulation, to maintaining and orchestrating metabolic control, to the release of a range of hormones responsible for regulating reproduction and satiety. All forms of adipose tissue provide an intricate and crucial role in the maintenance of homeostasis, originating in the earliest stages of neonatal development and continuing throughout life.[1]

39.1.1 Evolutionary Origins of Adipose Tissue Storage and Regulation

The primary role for adipose tissue is that of a lipid store utilized as an energy source in times of nutritional scarcity. The evolutionary benefit of being able to retain excess calorific intake during times of hardship is seen throughout nature. Both vertebrates and invertebrates therefore possess the ability to utilize energy consumed through feeding as a source of both immediate and prolonged energy. However, the complex nature and role of deposited adipose tissue extends beyond energy storage. Adipose tissue is the body's largest endocrine organ. It is responsible for a range of metabolic functions, including the control and release of lipid, adipokines, and cytokines. It also includes the regulation of a range of physiological actions, including satiety, insulin sensitivity, glucose homeostasis, and thermoregulation.[2]

Adipocytes originate within the mesoderm which are formed during embryogenesis.[3] Each form of adipose tissue (WAT and BAT) demonstrates a unique cell lineage, but the timing of initial deposition varies between adipose subtypes. In humans, for example, BAT emerges first, followed later in midgestation by WAT.[4] With a basic composition of adipocytes (the fat storing cell), adipose stem cells (the adipocyte precursor), alongside neuronal, mural, and endothelial cells, each aid in the endocrine and energy storing function of the cell type.[5] Adipose tissues are located throughout the body, including depots within the interscapular, inguinal, perigonadal, mesenteric, and retroperitoneal depots.

39.1.2 White and Brown Adipose Tissue: Physiological Role and Developmental Origins

Mammals possess two physiologically distinct forms of adipose tissue WAT and BAT that are histologically different. Each are deposited in different depots in the body that reflect their physiological and metabolic demand.[6] WAT provides a long-term energy storage and endocrine function[7], while BAT plays a crucial role during the early stages of development and early postnatal period, where it acts as a source of nonshivering thermogenesis (NST) but remains active into adulthood.[8]

39.1.3 Adipose Tissue Cell Lineage

Adipose tissue has a mesodermal origin alongside bone and muscle.[9] The mesoderm is formed by the migration of a layer of cells between the primitive endo and ectoderm. It then spreads along the dorsoventral and anteroposterior axes, forming the paraxial, intermediate, and axial mesoderm of the developing embryo.[10] These regions then go on to form the axial skeleton and musculature of the trunk through segmentation of the paraxial mesoderm and the lateral plate, which forms the musculature and skeleton responsible for the limbs.[10] The progenitor cell for the adipocyte is the mesenchymal or mesodermal stem cell (MSC). MSCs can give rise to a range of cell types, including osteoblasts, chondrocytes, and adipocytes.[11] Both brown and white adipocytes are thought to share a similar cell lineage in the form of the "preadipocyte." However, since these cells show no defining white or brown cellular characteristics at this stage, it is not yet fully established whether preadipocytes exist for the differing adipocyte subtypes or whether they share the same progenitor.[1] Preadipocytes then follow four stages of differentiation from preadipocyte to distinct brown or white adipocyte that includes cessation of cell growth, clonal expansion, primary differentiation, and final stage differentiation[12] (Fig. 39.1).

39.2 BROWN ADIPOSE TISSUE

39.2.1 Structure and Physiology

Brown adipocytes share a similar stem cell origin with myocytes, both carrying the myogenic factor 5 (Myf5) marker.[13] They are regulated by the Zn-finger transcriptional regulator PRD1-BF1-RIZ1 homologous domain, which contains the 16 (PRDM16) transcription coregulator, and enforces the cell fate, switching between myoblast and BAT cell lines.[14] Once mature, both cell types demonstrate similarities in the form of a large core sympathetic innervation, abundant mitochondria, and an ability to facilitate thermogenesis.[13]

Brown adipocytes are specially adapted for thermogenesis, a crucial physiological process in many large mammals around the time of birth, following cold exposure to the extrauterine environment.[15] BAT cells are unique in their composition, containing mitochondria with a unique thermogenic protein, called uncoupling protein 1 (UCP1). It is a 32 kDa protein located within the inner mitochondrial membrane that allows the cell to utilize stored fatty acids to generate heat by a process of energy uncoupling within the mitochondria. This is achieved by modifying the proton conductance pathway, rather than converting adenosine diphosphate (ADP) to adenosine triphosphate (ATP). When maximally stimulated, heat is produced at a rate of 300 W/kg compared with 1 W/kg in all other tissues.[16] The heat-generating capacity of BAT plays a role in thermogenesis and the maintenance and control of the core body temperature.

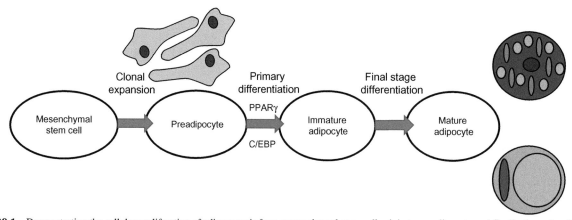

FIG. 39.1 Demonstrating the cellular proliferation of adipogenesis from mesenchymal stem cell origin to preadipocyte and finally through a differentiation process resulting in the production of brown or white adipose tissue, instigated by transcription factors C/EBP and PPARγ.

Brown adipocytes can be found in a number of anatomical locations, which include (at birth) perirenal, cervical, axillary, and periadrenal regions, with discrete depots surrounding the jugular vein and carotid artery.[17] These can be directly impacted by endocrine and environmental changes in utero.[18] Unlike WAT, BAT is highly abundant during early life and is usually reduced during early postnatal development, as the body becomes more adapted to controlling temperature through means such as shivering thermogenesis.[16] While BAT was not considered to be found in significant amounts in adults, recent imaging studies utilizing positron emission tomography (PET-CT)[19] and thermal imaging[20] have demonstrated active BAT within the supraclavicular region of adults, which may impact metabolism and energy expenditure.

39.3 WHITE ADIPOSE TISSUE

39.3.1 Structure and Physiology

WAT provides a range of metabolic functions, both as an energy source and an endocrine organ.[21] Histologically, WAT is subdivided into two forms based on gross anatomical location, subcutaneous (found beneath the skin) and visceral (found close to and surrounding many internal organs). These WAT subtypes can be distinguished by specific features, including their developmental timing, histology, and function.[22]

Subcutaneous WAT can be distinguished by its heterogeneous mix of both mature unilocular adipocytes, interspersed with smaller multilocular adipocytes. While visceral adipose tissue has a much more uniform histological appearance of mainly larger unilocular adipocytes[6], the lipid contained within each cell consists of triglycerides that can be stored and utilized as an energy source when required. Due to the large lipid component of each adipocyte, the mitochondria contained within each cell are elongated and can vary in number.[23] It has been noted that both visceral and subcutaneous WAT depots are able to respond differently to a range of external factors based on the stimulus itself and the depot's location. For example, in mice and humans, estrogen has been shown to enlarge the size of subcutaneous depots, whereas visceral depots are more responsive to glucocorticoids.[24]

Gene expression profiling of both visceral and subcutaneous adipose tissues have demonstrated each has distinct molecular phenotypes[2] and overall adipocyte size.[25] Endocrine function also differs between WAT subtypes. For example, visceral WAT found in the omentum express greater amounts of the insulin receptor 11β hydroxysteroid dehydrogenase (11β HSD) and interleukin 6 (IL6), whereas subcutaneous fat has more leptin and glycogen synthase.[2] These variations in gene expression between depots and tissue type are particularly important during early development of the tissue[26] (Table 39.1).

TABLE 39.1 Histological changes seen in white adipocytes and brown adipocytes, based on their physiological function and depot location

	White	Brown
Anatomical location	Found dispersed throughout body, with major visceral depots within the perirenal areas, omentum, and intestines, and subcutaneously surrounding the abdomen and thighs as well as interspersed within a range of other areas	(At birth): perirenal, cervical, axillary and periadrenal regions, with discrete depots surrounding the jugular vein and carotid artery
Lipid component	Uniocular	Multiocular
Mitochondrial concentration	Low levels of mitochondria	High levels of mitochondria
Vascularization	Low levels of vascularization	High levels of vascularization
Thermogenic capacity	Nonthermogenic	Thermogenic
Characterizing protein	Leptin	UCP1
Functional role	Energy storage, insulation, and endocrine functionality	Able to produce heat via UCP1 for nonshivering thermogenesis

39.4 NEONATAL AND FETAL ADIPOSE TISSUE DEVELOPMENT

Developmentally, adipose tissue usually contributes to a small proportion of total fetal body weight in most mammalian species. Fat deposition is determined in part by the overall glucose environment, with higher maternal glucose availability resulting in an increase in adipose tissue deposition.[15] In human development, the longer gestation period results in larger amounts of WAT deposition during midgestation and of subcutaneous BAT deposition during the late gestation period.[15] Adipose tissue deposition within the human fetus begins around 14 weeks' gestation within the head and neck, followed by the trunk and limbs.[27] Within the hypoxic and hypoglycemic uterine environment, fetal temperature is reliant on maternal regulation and usually remains at a steady state. It is therefore unsurprising that due to the higher metabolic demands of lipid deposition, when compared to carbohydrate or protein, the amount of fat deposited is low during fetal development. Fat deposition increases postnatally, as available oxygen and glucose is much higher and lipid supply increases.[28]

During fetal development in humans and sheep, adipose tissue is present from midgestation. It continues to develop throughout the remainder of pregnancy, with the highest rates of deposition occurring toward term. This coincides with the increased demand for heat generation following exposure to the extrauterine environment.[29] The longer gestation of precocial mammals, such as humans and sheep, allows for the complete maturation of the hypothalamic pituitary axis prior to birth. The development of this system prior to birth allows for the autonomic control of nonshivering thermogenesis under extrauterine conditions.[29] In humans, subcutaneous adipose tissue depots represent the primary stage of adipose tissue development, predating the deposition of visceral depots, and account for the highest proportion of adipose tissue in humans at birth. This is also true throughout the life course, as adipose tissue is continually developed and deposited based on metabolic and physiological demands.[30]

Adipose tissues are in a continual state of growth and development based on nutritional availability.[3] Based on early anatomical investigation,[27] prenatal adipose tissue development can be divided into morphological developmental phases:

- Phase one can be seen prior to 14 weeks' gestation, wherein adipocyte precursor cells consist of loose connective tissue.
- Phase two demonstrates the earliest signs of adipogenesis. During this phase, mesenchymal cells begin to aggregate into a dense mass. This stage also coincides with the proliferation of early stage vessels and ends the undifferentiated cell phase.[27]
- Development of adipocyte vasculature begins with a network of capillaries stemming from these vessels forming a rich network of capillaries, which the mesenchymal cells differentiate into preadipocytes. These mesenchymal cells organized within a glomerulus represent phase 3 of the developmental process and at this stage do not contain the lipid droplet characteristic of the adipocyte.
- As the vascular network continues to proliferate and increase in density, development of early adipocytes occurs within the mesenchymal lobules, as lipid vacuoles form within the cytoplasm concluding phase 4.
- During the final stage of adipocyte development, fat lobules are surrounded by perilobular mesenchyme, which condenses at a high rate and eventually thickens to form interlobular septa[27] (Fig. 39.2).

Fetal adipose tissue development is highly reliant on a well-established vascularization of the surrounding cells. This allows for the secretion and mobilization of a range of endocrine factors, including a range of cytokines.[31] With the expansion of fat mass toward the end of the gestation period, there is a marked increase in the number of hormone receptors. This,

Developmental stage of fetus	Primary adipose tissue characteristic	Fetal adipose tissue adaptation
Mid-to late gestation	Early growth shows signs of WAT deposition	Increase in fat mass promotes energy storage
Final stage of gestation prior to birth	Build up to birth shows increase in BAT deposition, increase in UCP1 in preparation for birth	Represents the highest levels of human BAT and UCP1 presence
Postpartum	Slow decline in BAT mass and increase in WAT over time	An increase in glucose and oxygen availability and decrease in requirement for NST. Initiates a phase of WAT development and BAT loss.

FIG. 39.2 Summarizes the changes in adipose tissue deposition characteristics in humans over the course of the pregnancy and following birth. White adipose tissue growth and development is increased at midgestation to supplement energy demands, whereas brown adipose tissue deposition is increased toward the final stages of gestation to coincide with the increased UCP1 requirement following birth into the extrauterine environment.

alongside the development of the sympathetic nervous system, results in increased abundance of UCP1 at the time of birth, ensuring thermoregulation in the extrauterine environment.[32]

39.4.1   The Endocrine System and Adipose Tissue Regulating Hormones

Adipose tissue is a highly adapted and specialized tissue. Renowned for its role as an energy store and thermal insulator, adipose tissue is now regarded as the body's largest endocrine organ. It is highly innervated and composed of a range of cell types, including adipocytes, macrophages, and endothelial cells.[33] Adipose tissue regulates and secretes a range of hormones, including cytokines and growth factors.[34]

39.4.2   Adipose Tissue Regulating Hormones

The process of adipogenesis is tightly controlled during fetal development. The hormones governing adipose tissue growth and differentiation are able to act in a paracrine or endocrine manner, utilizing adipose tissue vascularization to affect both their surrounding tissues and those within the vicinity.[30] Adipose regulating hormones are often classified as adipokines (cytokines secreted from adipocytes), hormones, and growth factors, with each class of secretion having a distinct role in the overall maintenance of fetal health and development.[34]

39.5   CYTOKINES

39.5.1   Insulin

Insulin is a form of an anorexigenic hormone. Insulin is seen in the fetus as early as 8 weeks of gestation.[32] The main source of insulin in the fetus is the β-cells in the islets of Langerhans in the fetal pancreas, as the transfer of maternal insulin by the placenta is not possible.

Insulin plays an important role in energy homeostasis through its action on the hypothalamus. Insulin diffuses directly around the Arc nucleus and binds to the insulin receptor (InsR) on POMC/CART as well as NPY/AgRP neurons.[35] This induces receptor tyrosine autophosphorylation and activation of a signaling pathway involving the phosphatidylinositol (3,4,5)-triphosphate (PIP 3).[36, 37] As a result, there is increased expression of α-MSH from POMC/CART neurons and reduced expression of NPY and AgRP from NPY/AgRP neurons. Anorexigenic second-order neurons are subsequently activated, which send signals to the nucleus of solitary tract to induce satiety.[32]

Insulin may also have a neurotrophic role in the hypothalamus, whereby it activates the differentiation of hypothalamic neural progenitor cells.[38] This is seen especially in the PVN in animal models like rodents. In adipocytes, insulin directly activates adipogenesis and lipogenesis while inhibiting lipolysis.[36] Insulin also has an important role in energy generation through oxidation of acetyl-CoA and converting glucose into pyruvate in the tricarboxylic acid (TCA) cycle.[39]

39.5.2   Ghrelin

Ghrelin was first discovered in 1999 as a 28 amino acid residue peptide hormone. It is an endogenous ligand for growth hormone secretagogue receptor (GHS-R).[40] In adults, ghrelin is mainly secreted by the gastric body and fundus.[32] Other organs that secrete ghrelin in smaller quantities include the Arc nucleus in the hypothalamus, pituitary gland, gut, pancreas, immune system, lungs, and placenta.[32] Ghrelin is also found in the fetal circulation throughout gestation, irrespective of the gender of the fetus. The larger concentration of ghrelin-secreting cells in the fetus (108 cells/mm^2) compared with a healthy adult (60 cells/mm^2) suggests the importance of ghrelin during the prenatal period in fetal development.[41] Ghrelin in the fetus is thought to be secreted from the fetal pancreas or stomach from 11 weeks of gestation. From rodent studies, it is postulated that fetal ghrelin may be mainly secreted from the fetal pancreas and has a close relationship with the development of the fetal pancreas in utero. Fetal ghrelin concentration are six to seven times higher in the fetal pancreas than that in the fetal stomach.[42] Fetal pituitary gland somatotroph is also found to secrete ghrelin from 18 to 36 weeks of gestation, suggesting that fetal ghrelin may regulate the secretion of fetal growth hormone from the pituitary gland.[32]

Ghrelin has an orexigenic action on the hypothalamus. Animal studies, especially in rodents, found ghrelin receptor afferent neurons around the vagus nerve. This suggests that ghrelin's action on the hypothalamus is through the vagus nerve rather than a direct transfer of peripheral ghrelin in the circulation.[32] In a human study,[43] patients who underwent subdiaphragmatic vagotomy showed the elimination of hunger induced by ghrelin post vagotomy. The administration of peripheral ghrelin postvagotomy did not increase the food-seeking behavior. However, it is still possible that there may be another compensatory mechanism for peripheral ghrelin to communicate with hypothalamic arc nucleus postvagotomy. Indeed, some studies found that not all of ghrelin's actions are mediated by the vagus nerve.[32]

Ghrelin receptor afferent neurons send signals from the stomach to the nucleus of solitary tract via the vagus nerve. The vagus nerve also stimulates ghrelin production in the hypothalamus. It then binds to the receptor around the POMC/CART, as well as NPY/AgRP neurons in the hypothalamus. This results in an increased expression for NPY and AgRP while reducing expression of α-MSH. Anorexigenic neurons in the PVN are inhibited, while orexigenic neurons in the LHN are stimulated, sending signals to the nucleus of solitary tract, leading to hunger and food-seeking behavior.[32]

Ghrelin is also a potent stimulator of growth hormone and regulates the secretion of growth hormone directly by the GHS-R 1a receptor. When bound to the GHS-R 1a receptor, a cascade of signaling pathways involving the phospholipase C and protein kinase C are activated. This releases calcium from the endoplasmic reticulum and stimulates the secretion of growth hormone.[42] Ghrelin also regulates the secretion of growth hormone indirectly by modulating the expression of the Pit-1 transcription factor in the anterior pituitary gland. This leads to increased expression of the growth hormone gene in somatotrophs.[42] The regulation of growth hormones is independent of ghrelin's orexigenic role in the hypothalamus.

39.5.3 Glucocorticoids

Glucocorticoids are steroid hormones secreted by the adrenal gland under the regulation of the hypothalamus-pituitary-adrenal axis. They play an important role in regulating appetite and energy homeostasis.[44] At the hypothalamus, glucocorticoids bind to and activate the intracellular glucocorticoid receptor (GR) in the arc nucleus.[37] This triggers a cascade of events, resulting in the activated GR functioning as a transcription factor, binding to glucocorticoid response elements (GREs).[44] GREs are present in the promoter regions of AgRP, NPY, and POMC genes in animal studies.[37] Hence this modulates the gene expression of orexigenic and anorexigenic neuropeptides in Arc. In animals, AgRP gene is positively regulated by glucocorticoids. The effect is less clear in NPY and POMC genes in animal studies. Dexamethasone, a synthetic glucocorticoid is found to stimulate NPY expression, while corticosterone, an endogenous corticosteroid, is found to have no effect on NPY expression.[37] Although POMC is thought to be positively regulated by glucocorticoids, there are studies showing negative regulation as well.[37]

Obesity in humans is associated with greater ability for WAT to bind to glucocorticoids due to higher expression of GR in WAT. Glucocorticoids stimulate adipogenesis by increasing key adipogenic transcription factors[45] and differentiation of preadipocytes. They also inhibit lipolysis on mature adipocytes.[45] Hence it is postulated that high glucocorticoid levels in adipose tissues result in adiposity.[46] Obesity is often seen as a chronic inflammatory response. Chronic hypercorticosteronemia also induces expression of proinflammatory genes leading to macrophage infiltration and inflammation.[47] In some rodent studies, changes in the perinatal maternal nutrition are associated with elevated perinatal circulatory glucocorticoid levels.[48] This could permanently change the hypothalamus-pituitary-adrenal axis with permanent hypercorticosteronemia. In turn, this may modulate the postnatal leptin surge, contributing to leptin resistant state and increasing the susceptibility to obesity in adulthood.[47]

UCP1 has been demonstrated (in sheep) to be maximally abundant at birth and shows a subsequent decline over the course of the first month following birth.[49] During this period, a range of steroid hormones, including glucocorticoids (cortisol) and thyroid hormones (triiodothyronine (T_3)), has been shown to be upregulated in accordance with this increase in UCP1 at birth.[26]

The changes required for adipose tissue maturation to start during gestation rely on an increase in plasma glucocorticoid concentration within the fetus leading up to term.[50] This surge in cortisol levels has been shown to affect a range of proteins during this late stage of development in preparation for birth including a range of receptors, enzymes, and hormones.[51] An increase in fetal cortisol levels toward term leads to an upregulation of prolactin receptors (PRLRs), coinciding with an increase in hepatic 5′-monodeiodinase.[51] This upregulation then leads to an increase in deiodination of the thyroid hormone thyroxine (T_4) to T_3, increasing circulating T_3 toward term.[51] This increase in thyroid hormone and glucocorticoid closely increases at the same time that we see an increase in UCP1 abundance, ensuring the fetus is adapted to thermoregulation in the extrauterine environment.[29]

The thyroid hormones, T_3 and T_4, are present within the fetal circulation from the early phase of fetal development and provide an important developmental and metabolic function.[52] The availability of thyroid hormones in fetal tissues is tightly regulated and can be affected by the gestational age of the fetus, nutrition, and oxygen availability.[53] The impact of dysfunctional availability of thyroid hormones have been demonstrated to impact fetal growth in utero and impact adaptation to survive the extrauterine environment[52], while thyroid hormone treatment of cells (including adipocytes) has been shown to promote cell differentiation.[54]

39.5.4 Leptin

Leptin is a form of anorexigenic adipocytokine, which comprises 167 amino acid residues and is commonly referred to as the "fullness hormone," and is a product of the ob gene, which is made almost exclusively by the WAT.[32] The amount of leptin circulating in the body is in direct proportion to the adipose tissue amount. It is also secreted in small quantities by the placenta, gonads, stomach, pituitary gland, vascular endothelium, BAT, and skeletal muscle.[55] Leptin displays pleiotropic roles, as the leptin receptor (Ob-R) has multiple isoforms that are present in various organs in the body, including the hypothalamus.[56] One of its main actions is the regulation of energy homeostasis through its effect on the hypothalamus.[32, 39] Leptin reaches the hypothalamus through the circulation and binds to the Ob-R receptor of the POMC/CART and NPY/AgRP neurons around the Arc nucleus.[35] This activates a cascade of intracellular signaling pathways involving the janus activating kinase-signal transducer and activator of transcription 3 (JAK-STAT3).[56] The resulting activated STAT 3 then dimerizes and translocates into the nucleus to modulate the expression of target genes such as increasing the expression α-MSH from POMC/CART neurons and suppressing the expression of NPY and AgRP from NPY/AgRP neurons.[36, 37] α-MSH then binds to the MC4R receptor, especially around the PVN, activating anorexigenic secondary neurons to send a signal along the nucleus of solitary tract to suppress appetite and reduce lipogenesis, thereby controlling body weight.[32, 39] Besides that, the previously described activated STAT3 also modulates the expression of suppressors of cytokine signaling 3 (SOCS3). SOCS3 inhibits the leptin-induced tyrosine phosphorylation of the JAK-STAT3 pathway.[37] This is postulated to be a potential mechanism for neuronal leptin resistance, which is associated with obese adults.

Leptin also shares a common pathway with insulin in the hypothalamus at the level of PIP3, allowing cross-interaction between insulin and leptin.[36, 37] Both hormones ultimately lead to a reduced expression of orexigenic neuropeptide with an increased expression of anorexigenic neuropeptides. It plays a neurotrophic role in the hypothalamus as well. This is crucial in the plasticity or programming of the appetite regulatory pathway in the hypothalamus. It has a trophic effect on the hypothalamic neural progenitor cells[38] and promotes neuronal outgrowth from Arc to PVN during the early postnatal period.[57] Leptin also affects growth by its interaction with the somatotroph, which is also known as the growth hormone-producing cell. It inhibits the secretion of somatostatin in the hypothalamus, besides having a direct effect on the somatotroph cells in the pituitary gland.[35] It may play a role in fetal adipose tissue formation. Leptin is noted in the fetus between 6 and 10 weeks of gestation, coinciding with the beginning of lipogenesis,[32] and promotes the differentiation of preadipocytes and hence directly activating adipogenesis.

39.5.5 Others

Nutrients such as glucose also interact with the arc nucleus in the hypothalamus in regulating energy homeostasis. Glucose is taken up by the POMC/CART neurons through glucose transporter GLUT 2. Glucose is then phosphorylated and metabolized to generate ATP, which binds to and blocks the K_{ATP} channel. As a result, the POMC neuron is depolarized, activating the anorexigenic secondary order neurons.[37]

39.5.6 Adiponectin

Adiponectin is an adipocyte secreted protein that controls lipid and glucose metabolism within insulin sensitive tissues and is negatively correlated with adult body weight.[33] It is a 30 kDa protein that circulates in relatively high concentrations, compared to leptin, with a primary structure composed of a collagen-like tail, N-terminal signal sequence, a variable domain region, and C-terminal globular head, which resembles that of TNF-α.[33] Adiponectin receptors mediate the phosphorylation of AMPK (AMP-activated protein kinase) and are composed of seven transmembrane domains and found in two forms, ApidoR1 and AdipoR2.[58] AdipoR1 receptors show a high affinity for binding the globular form of adiponectin, with low affinity for full length adiponectin. AdipoR2 receptors are found in high abundance within the liver and demonstrate a high affinity for binding both forms of adiponectin (full length and globular).[59]

Adiponectin bound receptors mediate the oxidation of fatty acids and suppress gluconeogenesis through activation of AMPK, insulin receptor phosphorylation, and the modulation of nuclear factor κB (NF-κB).[59]

Due to the importance of maternal gluconeogenesis and the concentrations of insulin and glucose affecting fetal growth and development, circulating levels of maternal adiponectin impact fetal development.[60] Adiponectin within the fetus is produced through endocrine tissues, including adipocytes as well as a range of fetal vascular tissues. It has been demonstrated to be highly abundant within fetal plasma and closely related to lower insulin concentration and increased insulin sensitivity.[61] Adiponectin therefore demonstrates a clear role in multiple areas of neonatal development and could contribute to insulin sensitivity.[62]

39.5.7 Resistin

Resistin is an adipocyte and mononuclear cell secreted hormone, believed to play a key functional role in the regulation of energy homeostasis through a functional action which slows glucose metabolism and drives insulin resistance.[63] While leptin is seen in lower concentrations within those who are obese or over weight, resistin has been found at higher concentrations and may play a key role in linking insulin resistance.[33] With a relative mass of 12 kDa, resistin belongs to a family of proteins known as RELMs (resistin-like molecules) and has a composition cysteine rich at the C terminal domain.[64] Resistin proliferates within murine white adipocytes, while in humans it is secreted from activated macrophages and monocular cells, and localized to the bone marrow.[65]

Resistin circulates in a hexamer or trimer structure due the proteins ability to associate with itself. Composed of an N-terminal α-helical tail section, among a C-terminal disulphide-rich β-sandwich head. The N-terminal α-helical tail is able to bind itself forming an interchain disulphide link composed of three stranded coils.[64] Circulating resistin is known to impact the action of insulin on peripheral tissues, including muscle tissues where overexpression of the resistin gene leads to impaired functionality of insulin.[64] It is expressed within the placenta, elucidating an important endocrine function in maintenance of energy homeostasis within the developing fetus and deposition of adipose tissue.[66] High levels of circulating resistin at term may aid in the prevention of hyperglycemia through a mechanism involving the liver and hepatic production of glucose.[67] While adipogenesis may also be impacted through a negative feedback mechanism on resistin, which may play a crucial role in the prevention of an overabundance of adipocyte proliferation and fat deposition.[67] The high impact on glucose metabolism and insulin sensitivity point to a key role for resistin in the maintenance of fetal energy homeostasis and utilization that may impact CNS functionality of the newborn and glucose availability.

39.6 PERSPECTIVES

Continued research has demonstrated that the adipose organ has a much more profound impact on growth and development than being a mere energy store. It is evident that the development and deposition of adipose tissue in utero and following birth is an intricate and finely balanced process, reliant on a range of maternal, nutritional, and hormonal factors. The newly established resurgence of interest and research into BAT as a thermogenic tissue with potential antiobesity implications highlights the importance of adipose tissue regulation and genesis throughout the life cycle.

The sheer presence of a range of adipocytokines within the cord blood and fetal tissues implies a role in fetal growth and development. Our understanding of these hormones in utero, specifically in the human population, is still lacking. However, as new evidence emerges linking deficiencies in fetal adipose tissue development and the hormones that regulate these tissues with a predisposition to a range of adulthood metabolic disease, our increased understanding may lead us to new therapeutic approaches in the midst of a worldwide epidemic of obesity and type 2 diabetes.

REFERENCES

1. Ali AT, Hochfeld WE, Myburgh R, Pepper MS. Adipocyte and adipogenesis. *Eur J Cell Biol* 2013;**92**(6–7):229–36.
2. Gesta S, Tseng Y, Kahn CR. Developmental origin of fat: tracking obesity to its source. *Cell* 2007;**131**:242 Cell 2008;**135**(2):366.
3. Arner P, Bernard S, Salehpour M, Possnert G, Liebl J, Steier P, et al. Dynamics of human adipose lipid turnover in health and metabolic disease. *Nature* 2011;**478**(7367):110.
4. Symonds ME, Pope M, Budge H. Adipose tissue development during early life: novel insights into energy balance from small and large mammals. *Proc Nutr Soc* 2012;**71**(3):363–70.
5. Smorlesi A, Frontini A, Giordano A, Cinti S. The adipose organ: white-brown adipocyte plasticity and metabolic inflammation. *Obes Rev* 2012;**13**:83–96.
6. Tchkonia T, Lenburg M, Thomou T, Giorgadze N, Frampton G, Pirtskhalava T, et al. Identification of depot-specific human fat cell progenitors through distinct expression profiles and developmental gene patterns. *Am J Physiol Endocrinol Metab* 2007;**292**(1):E298.
7. Badoud F, Perreault M, Zulyniak MA, Mutch DM. Molecular insights into the role of white adipose tissue in metabolically unhealthy normal weight and metabolically healthy obese individuals. *FASEB J* 2015;**29**:748–58.
8. Nedergaard J, Bengtsson T, Cannon B. Unexpected evidence for active brown adipose tissue in adult humans. *Am J Physiol Endocrinol Metab* 2007;**293**(2):E444.
9. Nnodim JO. Development of adipose tissues. *Anat Rec* 1987;**219**(4):331.
10. Bronnerfraser M. Neural crest cell-formation and migration in the developing embryo. *FASEB J* 1994;**8**:699–706.
11. Bunnell BA, Flaat M, Gagliardi C, Patel B, Ripoll C. Adipose- derived stem cells: isolation, expansion and differentiation. *Methods* 2008;**45**(2):115–20.
12. Evan DR, Ormond AM. Adipocyte differentiation from the inside out. *Nat Rev Mol Cell Biol* 2006;**7**(12):885.
13. Ravussin E, Galgani JE. The implication of brown adipose tissue for humans. *Annu Rev Nutr* 2011;**31**(1):33–47.

14. Seale P, Kajimura S, Yang W, Chin S, Rohas L, Uldry M, et al. Transcriptional control of brown fat determination by PRDM16. *Cell Metab* 2007;**6**(1):38–54.

15. Symonds M, Pope M, Sharkey D, Budge H. Adipose tissue and fetal programming. *Diabetologia* 2012;**55**(6):1597–606.

16. Symonds ME. Brown adipose tissue growth and development. *Scientifica (Cairo)* 2013;**2013**:305763.

17. Carter BW, Schucany WG. Brown adipose tissue in a newborn. *Proc (Baylor Univ Med Cent)* 2008;**21**(3):328.

18. Cannon B, Nedergaard J. Brown adipose tissue: function and physiological significance. *Physiol Rev* 2004;**84**:277–359.

19. Lee P, Zhao JT, Swarbrick MM, Gracie G, Bova R, Greenfield JR, et al. High prevalence of brown adipose tissue in adult humans. *J Clin Endocrinol Metab* 2011;**96**(8):2450.

20. Law J, Morris DE, Izzi Engbeaya C, Salem V, Coello C, Robinson LJ, et al. Thermal imaging is a non-invasive alternative to PET-CT for measurement of brown adipose tissue activity in humans. *J Nucl Med* 2018;**59**(3):516–22.

21. Berry DC, Stenesen D, Zeve D, Graff J. The developmental origins of adipose tissue. *Development* 2013;**140**:3939–49.

22. Saely C, Geiger K, Drexel H. Brown versus white adipose tissue: a mini-review. *Gerontology* 2012;**58**:15–23.

23. Cinti S. Adipocyte differentiation and transdifferentiation: plasticity of the adipose organ. *J Endocrinol Investig* 2002;**25**(10):823.

24. Shi H, Clegg DJ. Sex differences in the regulation of body weight. *Physiol Behav* 2009;**97**(2):199–204.

25. Jernås M, Palming J, Sjöholm K, Jennische E, Svensson P-A, Gabrielsson BG, et al. Separation of human adipocytes by size: hypertrophic fat cells display distinct gene expression. *FASEB J* 2006;**20**(9):1540.

26. Budge H, Gnanalingham MG, Gardner DS, Mostyn A, Stephenson T, Symonds ME. Maternal nutritional programming of fetal adipose tissue development: long-term consequences for later obesity. *Birth Defects Res C Embryo Today* 2005;**75**:193–9.

27. Poissonnet CM, Burdi AR, Bookstein FL. Growth and development of human adipose tissue during early gestation. *Early Hum Dev* 1983;**8**(1):1–11.

28. Symonds ME, Mostyn A, Pearce S, Budge H, Stephenson T. Endocrine and nutritional regulation of fetal adipose tissue development. *J Endocrinol* 2003;**179**:293–9.

29. Clarke L, Buss D, Juniper D, Lomax M, Symonds M. Adipose tissue development during early postnatal life in ewe-reared lambs. *Exp Physiol* 1997;**82**(6):1015–27.

30. Kiess W, Petzold S, Töpfer M, Garten A, Blüher S, Kapellen T, et al. Adipocytes and adipose tissue. *Best Pract Res Clin Endocrinol Metab* 2008;**22**(1):135.

31. Stephenson T, Budge H, Mostyn A, Pearce S, Webb R, Symonds ME. Fetal and neonatal adipose maturation: a primary site of cytokine and cytokine-receptor action. *Biochem Soc Trans* 2001;**29**:80–5.

32. Warchol M, Krauss H, Wojciechowska M, Opala T, Pieta B, Zukiewicz-Sobczak W, et al. The role of ghrelin, leptin and insulin in foetal development. *Ann Agric Environ Med* 2014;**21**:349–52.

33. Poulos SP, Hausman DB, Hausman GJ. The development and endocrine functions of adipose tissue. *Mol Cell Endocrinol* 2010;**323**(1):20–34.

34. Ronti T, Lupattelli G, Mannarino E. The endocrine function of adipose tissue: an update. *Clin Endocrinol* 2006;**64**:355–65.

35. Horvath TL. The hardship of obesity: a soft-wired hypothalamus. *Nat Neurosci* 2005;**8**(5):561–5.

36. Breton C. The hypothalamus-adipose axis is a key target of developmental programming by maternal nutritional manipulation. *J Endocrinol* 2013;**216**(2):R19–31.

37. Wattez JS, Delahaye F, Lukaszewski MA, Risold PY, Eberle D, Vieau D, et al. Perinatal nutrition programs the hypothalamic melanocortin system in off spring. *Horm Metab Res* 2013;**45**(13):980–90.

38. Desai M, Li T, Ross MG. Hypothalamic neurosphere progenitor cells in low birth-weight rat newborns: neurotrophic effects of leptin and insulin. *Brain Res* 2011;**1378**:29–42.

39. Dessi A, Puddu M, Ottonello G, Fanos V. Metabolomics and fetal-neonatal nutrition: between "not enough" and "too much". *Molecules* 2013;**18**(10):11724–32.

40. Gillman MW. Early infancy—a critical period for development of obesity. *J Dev Orig Health Dis* 2010;**1**(5):292–9.

41. Cortelazzi D, Cappiello V, Morpurgo PS, Ronzoni S, De Santis MSN, Cetin I, et al. Circulating levels of ghrelin in human fetuses. *Eur J Endocrinol* 2003;**149**(2):111–6.

42. Kedzia A, Obara-Moszynska M, Chmielnicka-Kopaczyk M. Assessment of ghrelin, GHS-R, GH, and neurohormones in human fetal pituitary glands and central nervous system: an immunohistochemical study. *Folia Histochem Cytobiol* 2009;**47**(3):505–10.

43. le Roux CW, Neary NM, Halsey TJ, Small CJ, Martinez-Isla AM, Ghatei MA, et al. Ghrelin does not stimulate food intake in patients with surgical procedures involving vagotomy. *J Clin Endocrinol Metab* 2005;**90**(8):4521–4.

44. Ramamoorthy TG, Begum G, Harno E, White A. Developmental programming of hypothalamic neuronal circuits: impact on energy balance control. *Front Neurosci* 2015;**9**:16.

45. Campbell JE, Peckett AJ, D'Souza AM, Hawke TJ, Riddell MC. Adipogenic and lipolytic effects of chronic glucocorticoid exposure. *Am J Phys Cell Phys* 2011;**300**(1):C198–209.

46. Lukaszewski MA, Mayeur S, Fajardy I, Delahaye F, Dutriez-Casteloot I, Montel V, et al. Maternal prenatal undernutrition programs adipose tissue gene expression in adult male rat offspring under high-fat diet. *Am J Physiol Endocrinol Metab* 2011;**301**(3):E548–59.

47. Lukaszewski MA, Eberle D, Vieau D, Breton C. Nutritional manipulations in the perinatal period program adipose tissue in offspring. *Am J Physiol Endocrinol Metab* 2013;**305**(10):E1195–207.

48. Lesage J, Sebaai N, Leonhardt M, Dutriez-Casteloot I, Breton C, Deloof S, et al. Perinatal maternal undernutrition programs the offspring hypothalamo-pituitary-adrenal (HPA) axis. *Stress* 2006;**9**(4):183–98.

49. Mostyn A, Pearce S, Budge H, Elmes M, Forhead AJ, Fowden AL, et al. Influence of cortisol on adipose tissue development in the fetal sheep during late gestation. *J Endocrinol* 2003;**176**(1):23.

50. Chida D, Miyoshi K, Sato T, Yoda T, Kikusui T, Iwakura Y. The role of glucocorticoids in pregnancy, parturition, lactation, and nurturing in melanocortin receptor 2-deficient mice. *Endocrinology* 2011;**152**(4):1652.

51. Liggins GC. The role of cortisol in preparing the fetus for birth. *Reprod Fertil Dev* 1994;**6**(2):141–50.

52. Forhead A, Fowden AL. Thyroid hormones in fetal growth and prepartum maturation. *J Endocrinol* 2014;**221**:R87–R103.

53. Fowden AL, Mapstone J, Forhead AJ. Regulation of glucogenesis by thyroid hormones in fetal sheep during late gestation. *J Endocrinol* 2001;**170**(2):461–9.

54. Fowden AL, Li J, Forhead AJ. Glucocorticoids and the preparation for life after birth: are there long-term consequences of the life insurance? *Proc Nutr Soc* 1998;**57**(1):113–22.

55. Zhang Y, Scarpace PJ. The role of leptin in leptin resistance and obesity. *Physiol Behav* 2006;**88**(3):249–56.

56. Bjorbaek C, Kahn BB. Leptin signaling in the central nervous system and the periphery. *Recent Prog Horm Res* 2004;**59**:305–31.

57. Bouret SG, Draper SJ, Simerly RB. Trophic action of leptin on hypothalamic neurons that regulate feeding. *Science* 2004;**304**(5667):108–10.

58. Wagner de Jesus P. The endocrine function of adipose tissue. *Rev Facul Ciênc Méd Soroc* 2014;**16**(3):111–20.

59. Fasshauer M, Blüher M. Adipokines in health and disease. *Trends Pharmacol Sci* 2015;**36**(7):461–70.

60. Luo ZC, Nuyt AM, Delvin E, Fraser WD, Julien P, Audibert F, et al. Maternal and fetal leptin, adiponectin levels and associations with fetal insulin sensitivity. *Obesity* 2013;**21**(1):210–6.

61. Pinar H, Basu S, Hotmire K, Laffineuse L, Presley L, Carpenter M, et al. High molecular mass multimer complexes and vascular expression contribute to high adiponectin in the fetus. *J Clin Endocrinol Metab* 2008;**93**(7):2885.

62. Hansen-Pupp I, Hellgren G, Hård A-L, Smith L, Hellström A, Löfqvist C. Early surge in circulatory adiponectin is associated with improved growth at near term in very preterm infants. *J Clin Endocrinol Metab* 2015;**100**(6):2380–7.

63. Angelidis G, Dafopoulos K, Messini CI, Valotassiou V, Tsikouras P, Vrachnis N, et al. The emerging roles of adiponectin in female reproductive system-associated disorders and pregnancy. *Reprod Sci* 2013;**20**(8):872–81.

64. Jackson MB, Ahima R. Neuroendocrine and metabolic effects of adipocyte-derived hormones. *Clin Sci (Lond)* 2006;**110**:143–52.

65. Guerre-Millo M. Adipose tissue hormones. *J Endocrinol Investig* 2002;**25**(10):855–61.

66. Wang J, Shang LX, Dong X, Wang X, Wu N, Wang SH, et al. Relationship of adiponectin and resistin levels in umbilical serum, maternal serum and placenta with neonatal birth weight. *Aust N Z J Obstet Gynaecol* 2010;**50**(5):432–8.

67. Pak-Cheng N, Cheuk HL, Christopher WKL, Iris HSC, Eric W, Tai FF. Resistin in preterm and term newborns: relation to anthropometry, leptin, and insulin. *Pediatr Res* 2005;**58**(4):725.

Chapter 40

Fetal and Placental Growth Physiology and Pathophysiology

Victor Han[*,†,‡], Bethany Radford[†,‡] and Zain Awamleh[†,‡]

[*]Division of Neonatal-Perinatal Medicine Department of Paediatrics, Schulich School of Medicine & Dentistry, Western University, London, Canada, [†]Department of Biochemistry, Schulich School of Medicine & Dentistry, Western University, London, Canada, [‡]Children's Health Research Institute, Lawson Health Research Institute and Western University, London, Canada

Key Clinical Changes

- Fetal genome that orchestrates the normal physiological growth and development is greatly impacted by the microenvironment within which it develops.
- Placental development precedes fetal development, and its growth/development determines the successful outcome of each pregnancy.
- Maternal physical and chemical environment and microbiome influence fetal development through epigenetic mechanisms.
- Autocrine/paracrine mechanisms are of greater importance than endocrine mechanisms in fetal and placental development.
- Pregnancy-associated diseases are both genomic and epigenomic in origin.
- Normal and abnormal fetal growth has lifelong health implications.

40.1 NORMAL PHYSIOLOGICAL GROWTH OF THE FETUS AND PLACENTA

Normal growth and development of the fetus, including fetal organs and tissues, occur in a series of coordinated cellular processes tightly orchestrated by the fetal genome (contributed by both maternal and paternal genomes) and modulated by the cellular microenvironment (gene-environment interaction). The latter is determined by the fetal environment, which in turn is determined by the maternal and external environments. Growth and development of both the fetus and placenta occur within the maternal uterine environment, but the processes are distinctive as well as interdependent. The development of a lung was elegantly described recently, as to how the organ is constructed on a cell-by-cell basis.[1] Normal placental growth and development occur in a similar series of processes with some unique features, including: (1) placental development precedes embryonic development, (2) it interacts and crosstalks with the maternal environment as it is in direct contact with the mother's uterine environment, (3) it is critical to the pregnancy outcome and any disruption of the process leads to failure of the pregnancy (miscarriage or prematurity) or pregnancy-associated diseases (fetal growth restriction and preeclampsia).

40.1.1 Normal Growth—Cell-Based

40.1.1.1 Cell Replication in Development

Cells replicate in an orderly manner through the resting phase (G_0), an activation or gap phase (G_1) during which protein synthesis is initiated, DNA synthesis (S), a second gap phase (G_2), and finally mitosis (M). The cell cycle is regulated at two checkpoints during the G_1/S and G_2/M phases. Cyclins and cyclin-dependent protein kinases (cdks) regulate progression through the cell cycle. Cyclins function as regulatory subunits of the cdks, which in turn phosphorylate and regulate key cell cycle protein substrates such as retinoblastoma protein (Rb). Growth and differentiation factors (GDFs), such as platelet-derived growth factor (PDGF), insulin-like growth factors (IGFs), fibroblast growth factor (FGF), epidermal growth factor (EGF), colony stimulating factor-1 (CSF-1) and transforming growth factors (TGFs), modulate (stimulate or impede) cells to progress through the checkpoints of the cell cycle. Growth factors originate as autocrine, paracrine, or endocrine factors.

Maternal-Fetal and Neonatal Endocrinology. https://doi.org/10.1016/B978-0-12-814823-5.00040-4

Mostly, they bind to cognate receptors on the cell surfaces and transduce their signals to the nucleus via a variety of signaling molecules. In some cases, growth factors may be transported into the nucleus by specific transport mechanisms and have direct actions on the regulatory regions of the genes. Gene targeting studies using a variety of animal models (*Drosophila*, zebrafish, and mouse) have clearly demonstrated the vital importance of local autocrine/paracrine factors, compared to endocrine factors, in fetal and organ/tissue development.[2]

Differentiation factors like WNT and hedgehog are involved not only in growth and cell survival, but also in the critical phases of embryonic development of specific tissues and organs, such as migration and tissue polarity. There are at least 15 different WNT genes and they act through members of the frizzled family of proteins. WNT proteins are involved in regulating stem cell differentiation,[3] limb patterning, midbrain development, and some aspects of somite and urogenital differentiation. In mammals, there are three hedgehog genes (Desert, Indian, and sonic). Sonic hedgehog is involved in limb patterning, neural tube induction and patterning, somite differentiation, and gut regionalization. The receptor for hedgehog is Patched, which binds to another protein called Smoothened. The Smoothened protein transduces the hedgehog signal, but it is inhibited by Patched until the hedgehog protein binds to this receptor.[4]

40.1.2 Totipotency, Pluripotency, and Differentiation

Embryonic cells, within the first few cell divisions up to the morula stage, consist of cells that are totipotent (can form all the cell types of the body including extraembryonic or placental cells). The first differentiation event that occurs in an early embryo is the formation of an inner cell mass that gives rise to the embryo proper, and an outer cell mass, which forms the trophoblast and later contributes to the placenta. Cells of the inner cell mass are pluripotent (can give rise to all cells of three germ layers) and provide a source for the generation of embryonic stem cells.[5, 6] At around 6 days postfertilization, the embryo reaches the blastocyst stage in the uterine cavity, and the trophoblast cells in the outside of the embryo begin to express L-selectin and the uterine epithelial cells express carbohydrate receptors called pinopodia.[7] Following capture by selectins, the embryo invades further into the endometrium, which involves expression of integrins by the trophoblasts and laminin (for attachment) and fibronectin (for invasion).[8]

Somatic or fully differentiated cells can be artificially induced to become pluripotent and the cells derived are called induced pluripotent cells (iPSCs).[9] This requires a process of forced expression of certain genes and transcription factors, initially including Oct4, Sox2, Klf4 and c-Myc (reprogramming). Subsequently, it was demonstrated that iPSCs can be derived using less than all four of the transcription factors. In addition, the original methods used virus-mediated procedures and were deemed not suitable for regenerative therapies in humans due to their oncogenic potential. More recently, reprogramming methods have focused on using RNA, proteins, and small molecules, which improved the safety and efficiency.

40.1.3 Regulation of Cell Replication and Differentiation

In mammals, cell replication and differentiation are regulated by the human genome via an intrinsic mechanism of coordinated expression of a series of transcription factors orchestrated by the epigenome.[1] The latter is in turn modulated by the environment, which has been termed the epigenetic cascade.

One mechanism by which prenatal and postnatal environmental factors influence normal development and the predisposition to develop chronic diseases in the offspring as children or adults is the alteration of epigenetic marks, which have a central role in determining gene expression. The term epigenetics ("above genetics") refers to changes in gene expression without alteration in DNA sequence.[10–13] The mechanisms of molecular modifications to DNA and chromatin include (1) DNA methylation at the 5-carbon position of cytosine in CpG dinucleotides[14]; (2) modifications of histones involving acetylation, phosphorylation, ubiquitinylation, and sumoylation that result in changes in chromatin packaging of DNA allowing or inhibiting transcriptional machinery to have access to the DNA[15]; and (3) regulation by noncoding RNAs such as microRNAs and lnRNAs.[16–18] The classic phenomena in mammals are X-chromosome inactivation and genomic imprinting.[19]

During development, epigenetic regulation is involved in tissue-specific expression and in the silencing of transposable elements and preventing insertional mutagenesis. One important consequence of epigenetics is the mitotic inheritance in somatic cells that leads to long-term effects on gene expression. Epigenetics also play a significant role in preimplantation development to ensure correct progression of development. During this phase, the control of development passes from the gametes to the embryo, a process called maternal-to-zygotic transition (MZT). MZT involves the depletion of maternal RNAs and proteins and the transcriptional activation of the zygotic genome. The latter, called the zygotic genome activation (ZGA), is a highly coordinated process following which the first cell-fate decisions are made. In mice and humans, ZGA occurs in two transcription bursts, termed the minor and major waves.[20] In humans, low transcription rates are detected from the zygote to four-cell embryo and the major wave occurs at the eight-cell stage. In addition to protein-coding transcripts, transcription waves of noncoding RNAs include small noncoding RNAs (sncRNAs),[21] long noncoding RNAs (lncRNAs), and endogenous repeats or transposons. During this time, early embryos undergo extensive global DNA demethylation from the zygote through to blastocyst before methylation levels are reestablished during gastrulation. Demethylation occurs either passively or actively through DNA repair pathways; methylation occurs actively by DNA methyltransferase 3A (DNMT3A) and DNMT3B and is maintained through mitosis by DNMT1. Considering the global loss of DNA methylation during preimplantation development, maternal mutations in components of the DNA methylation machinery cause defects in the imprinting maintenance. The paternal genome undergoes rapid and active demethylation, possibly driven by TET3, whereas the maternal genome is protected from demethylation through the binding of STELLA.[22]

All cells in the body have essentially the same DNA, yet different organs and tissues serve vastly different functions and retain their identity as the cells divide. This cellular identity is epigenetic information, or information that is added to the genes themselves.[23, 24] Waddington described the process by which a pluripotent cell acquires differentiated properties as the "epigenetic landscape",[25] recognizing that the environment has a profound effect on developmental plasticity; modifications of DNA or associated factors are maintained during DNA replication, which allows stable changes in gene expression.

Human epidemiologic studies have indicated that diet/nutrition is one of the most important environmental factors that impact gene expression over multiple generations[26, 27] via alteration of the epigenome. For example, folate deficiency impairs biosynthesis of S-adenosylmethionine, which is the active precursor of DNA methylation. Epigenetic epidemiology, a new field of study, incorporates genetic variation with environmental exposure to explain disease susceptibility (e.g., diabetes, metabolic diseases) mediated by the epigenome. The principal tool for epigenetic epidemiology is the epigenome-wide association study, which currently is based on DNA methylation only.

40.1.4 Cell Type-Specific Adaptation During Development

Cell division coupled with proliferation is required for growth and renewal of many cell types during embryonic development. The DNA replication program must change during embryonic development, when undifferentiated cells are proliferating at a high rate, while some of the cells are transitioning to primordial cells and then into differentiation. Undifferentiated cells are proliferating at a high rate, which requires a high DNA synthesis rate, whereas differentiated cells have a reduced DNA synthesis rate. DNA synthesis occurs during the S phase of the cell cycle by a molecular machinery made up of many proteins acting in a coordinated manner to synthesize DNA at many genomic locations.[28]

Recent studies have demonstrated that regulation of DNA replication is influenced by the fate of a given cell. In eukaryotes, replication origins are licensed through a chronological order that requires binding of the origin recognition complex (ORC), Cdc6, and Cdt1 into chromatin. MCM2-7 helicase complexes are then loaded in an inactive state prior to the S phase, whereby Cdt1 and MCM2-7 form a complex before being recruited into replication origins by ORC and Cdc6. Most replication origins being activated are associated with unmethylated CpG islands. G-rich elements, transcription start sites, and histone modifications are related to open chromatin marks.[29]

The placenta is the critical gatekeeper of the fetal environment and, under normal conditions, it functions to promote development. However, under conditions of limited availability, it may compete with the fetus for its own metabolism.[30] As a target of both maternal (hypertension, renal, coagulopathies) and pregnancy diseases (preeclampsia), it may be poorly developed or damaged, leading to poor function (placental insufficiency). The cellular processes of growth and differentiation are regulated by complex cell-cell and cell matrix interactions, which are mediated by locally expressed soluble or structural peptide factors (growth factors, cytokines, and matrix). The regulation of the expression of genes that control these intricate processes in various tissues of the embryo/fetus can be categorized into intrinsic (genomic and epigenomic) and extrinsic (environment). The genome of the developing embryo consists of all the information needed to develop from a single cell zygote to a complex multicellular and multiorgan/tissue structure of the fetus/newborn and placenta. The epigenetic or epigenomic influence of gene expression is defined as the molecular changes to DNA and its organization into chromatin, independent of genomic sequence. Once established, it is erased and reestablished during gametogenesis. This includes DNA methylation, histone modifications, and noncoding RNAs. This epigenetic or epigenomic influence is also the major mechanism by which the environment (nutrition, chemicals) regulates gene expression that may be long lasting and sometimes deleterious to the individual's health and may be responsible for developmental programming.[31]

One of the critical processes in the development of a hemochorial placenta in humans and primates is the remodeling of the spiral arteries by the extravillous trophoblast cells, which originate from the developing early placenta through the anchoring villi attached to the maternal endometrium.[32] Adequate and/or complete invasion and spiral artery remodeling allow the adequate perfusion of the maternal venous sinuses and good exchange of nutrients and substrates between the maternal and fetal circulations (Fig. 40.1). Shallow invasion and/or incomplete remodeling lead to hypoxia and the resultant

FIG. 40.1 Timeline of normal placental development with highlight on spiral artery remodeling. *(Adapted from Redman CW, Sargent IL. Latest advances in understanding preeclampsia. Science 2005;308(5728):1592–4.)*

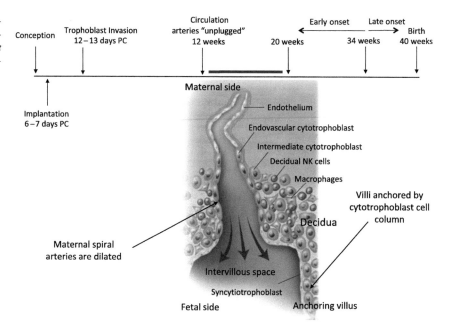

release of syncytiotrophoblastic factors, micromolecules (DNA and RNAs), and debris into the maternal circulation, which have been suggested as the basis for the development of pregnancy-associated diseases such as preeclampsia and/or fetal growth restriction.

40.1.5 Regulation of Growth

40.1.5.1 Mechanistic Target of Rapamycin

Recent studies have brought prominence to the roles of the mechanistic target of rapamycin (mTOR) complexes in both normal and abnormal development of the embryo and placenta; mTOR is a serine/threonine protein kinase in the PI3K-related kinase (PIKK) family that coordinates cell growth with environmental conditions, and plays a fundamental role in the cell and organismal physiology and pathology.[33] It forms the catalytic subunit of two distinct protein complexes known as mTOR Complex 1 (mTORC1) and 2 (mTORC2). Note that mTORC1 consists of three core components: mTOR, Raptor (regulatory protein associated with mTOR), and mLST8 (mammalian lethal with Sec13 protein 8). Raptor facilitates substrate recruitment to mTORC1 through binding to the TOR signaling motif, which is required for the cellular localization of mTORC1. It also contains two inhibitory subunits: PRAS40 (proline-rich Akt substrate of 40 kDa) and DEPTOR (DEP domain containing mTOR interacting protein). Note that mTORC2 contains mTOR and MLST8, but instead of Raptor, it contains Rictor (rapamycin insensitive companion of mTOR), and DEPTOR and regulatory subunits mSin1 and Protor1/2.

In addition to playing a central role in regulating the cellular processes that are required for cell growth, such as increased production of proteins, lipids, and nucleotides, while suppressing catabolic pathways such as autophagy,[34, 35] mTORC1 controls the balance between anabolism and catabolism in response to environmental conditions, of which nutrition is a critical part of cellular metabolism. It promotes protein synthesis through the phosphorylation of two key effectors, S6K1 and 4EBP. It promotes de novo lipid synthesis through the sterol responsive element binding protein (SREBP) transcription, which controls the expression of metabolic genes involved in fatty acid and cholesterol biosynthesis, the processes important for cellular growth. Also, mTORC1 promotes the synthesis of nucleotides required for DNA replication and ribosome biogenesis in proliferating and differentiating cells. It promotes a shift in glucose metabolism from oxidative phosphorylation to glycolysis, increasing the translation of HIF1α, which drives the expression of several glycolytic enzymes such as phosphor-fructo kinase (PFK); it regulates autophagy by activation of ULK1 and TFEB, which drives genes for lysosomal biogenesis. As for mTORC2, it controls cellular proliferation and survival by phosphorylating several members of the AGC (PKA/PKG/PKC) family of protein kinases.

Because of the ability to integrate environmental cues and coordinate metabolic changes in a cell, mTOR signaling is critical for many cellular processes and cell survival, and mTOR function is important in various physiologic and pathologic processes in many tissues, including the nervous system, immune system, and skeletal muscle, and in glucose and lipid homeostasis. During fetal development, mTOR function has been closely linked to placental function and disorders associated with intrauterine growth restriction, and its impaired function has been suggested to be an underlying pathophysiology of placental insufficiency. The placenta senses and responds to changes in the maternal environment by altering its structure and function, which can lead to changes in blood flow, fetal nutrient supply, and secretion of hormones and other signaling molecules.[36] Changes in transplacental nutrient transport may influence fetal nutrient availability, which determines fetal growth and body composition. Two nutrient-sensing proteins involved in placental development and glucose and amino acid transport are mTOR and O-linked N-acetylglucosamine transferase (OGT), which in turn are regulated by availability of oxygen. Impairment in either of these pathways is associated with fetal growth restriction and is accompanied by cellular stress in the forms of hypoxia, oxidative and endoplasmic reticulum (ER) stress, metabolic dysfunction, and nutrient starvation of the placenta. This disturbance in the nutrient-sensing pathways is believed to be the underlying pathophysiology leading to placental insufficiency and fetal growth restriction.

40.2 DEVELOPMENTAL ORIGINS OF HEALTH AND DISEASE

Since Barker and colleagues first described in 1989 that low birth weight and weight at 1 year (proxies for fetal growth restriction) are associated with an individual's risk for developing hypertension and cardiovascular disease,[37, 38] many reports from around the world have not only supported the concept but expanded it to the risk for many adult onset diseases (diabetes, metabolic syndrome) and chronic disorders (neuroendocrine disorders, reproductive disorders, obesity).[39]

One of the most intriguing observations was a series of epidemiological studies associated with the tragic Dutch Winter Hunger of 1944–45.[26] Early undernutrition due to famine during pregnancy has a negative effect on an individual's health and wellness over their life course. This unfortunate tragedy provided a rare proof in humans that maternal undernutrition and stress are linked to adult onset diseases by altering the developmental trajectory of the fetus newborn and infant, which has been demonstrated in many animal models. Epigenetic modifications in response to in utero stresses have been suggested as the underlying pathophysiological mechanism.[31] The adaptive response of restricting an energy-dependent growth may confer immediate advantage and, perhaps more importantly, fetal survival; however, the resulting smaller body size (proxy measure) may incur a cost later in life by increasing susceptibility to chronic diseases. The relationship between birth size and disease outcome is not linear, but more U-shaped, with birthweights in either extremes being vulnerable to adult onset diseases, in particular diabetes and metabolic syndrome.[40]

40.3 PLACENTAL GROWTH AND DEVELOPMENT

Fetal growth is closely intertwined with the growth and development of the placenta. The placenta is a unique organ that conducts the functional activities of most fetal organs, to substitute for the maturing embryonic and fetal organs. Its control of the traffic of substrates and nutrients between the mother and the fetus is an important rate-limiting factor for fetal growth.[41–43] Equally important is its function as an endocrine organ that provides many of the peptide and steroid hormones essential for a successful pregnancy, and the preparation of maternal reproductive organs and breast for the immediate postnatal life of the newborn.[36] In addition, the placenta is a metabolically active organ that competes with the fetus for nutrients and substrates.[44, 45]

Placental growth is not just a uniform progression of cellular replication from early trophectoderm to a complex multicellular organ, but is also a series of fundamentally different anabolic processes that include proliferation, differentiation, migration, aggregation, and apoptosis. The latter has been increasingly recognized as an important process in the development of the placenta.[46] A successful implantation and receptivity by the maternal endometrium require important communication between the developing early embryo and the maternal tissues. The important molecular and cellular events that are critically required for the development of a well-developed and functioning hemochorial placenta are well described.[7] These molecular and cellular events are orchestrated by the placental genome via autocrine/paracrine factors, including growth factors, which are synthesized by the developing placenta and the receiving endometrium and uterus in a precisely integrated manner. Of the multitude of growth factors (GFs) described to date, IGFs and their binding proteins (IGFBPs) are the most important and best studied. Several other growth factors, namely EGF, TGF-α, TGF-β, FGF, and VEGF, also play important roles in placental development. Recent evidence from null mutants of EGFR and *flt1* and *flk1* (VEGF receptors), in which embryonically lethal phenotypes are observed, indicates their importance. However, only some of the GFs are not expressed locally within the developing placenta (e.g., EGF), and therefore their potential role as a local autocrine/paracrine factor is questioned. Null mutants of some GF genes that are expressed in the developing placenta fail to show any placental phenotype (e.g., TGF-α, TGF-β, FGF). Biological redundancy, as a result of multiple growth factors responsible for the same function, is a possible explanation. It is also possible that some GF biological effects may be due to interactions among them. Evidence of abundant expression of IGF, its receptors and the binding proteins, in a specific spatial and temporal manner; of null mutants of *Igf2* and *Igf2r* showing placental phenotype; and of IGF system genes expressed in the placentae of all species studied indicates that the IGF system is the most important GF family in placental development.[47]

Cellular sites of expression of the genes of the IGF system in the placenta will also determine the phenotype observed. Our studies of the expression of IGF system genes in the mouse placenta demonstrate that IGF-II mRNA is abundantly expressed in the labyrinthine- and spongio-trophoblasts, glycogen cells, yolk sac, and vasculogenic mesenchyme, and IGFBPs in the decidua, endometrial stroma, and myometrium early in gestation, and in the endothelium of the maternal blood vessels in the junctional zone. These findings provide the reason for impaired placental development in *Igf2* null mutant mice. Placental phenotypes in the *Igfbp* targeted animals have not been studied in detail, and our data of specific cell types in the decidua, myometrium, placenta, and endothelium of maternal blood vessels suggest the possibility of abnormalities in these animals. It is more likely that altered phenotypic and pathophysiologic responses will be seen when these null mutant animals are subjected to conditions such as hypoxia or undernutrition.

Our previous in situ hybridization studies in the human placenta[47] have shown a clear demarcation of expression of IGF-II mRNA in fetal trophoblasts and IGFBP mRNAs (IGFBP-1 being the most abundant) in the maternal decidual cells. This observation forms the basis of many studies in the human placenta to delineate the functional significance of the IGF system at the fetomaternal interface. IGF-II promotes trophoblast invasion and has no effect on proliferation.

40.3.1 Evidence from Gene Targeting Studies

Gene targeting is a powerful tool to determine the biological significance of different genes, including those of the IGF system, during development.[48, 49] Since most placental cells are derived from the primitive trophectoderm of fetal origin, targeting also affects these cells.[50] However, placental development involves interaction between fetal and maternal cells, and therefore the final placental phenotype is dependent on the maternal genome as well. However, evidence to date suggests that the presence or absence of maternal expression does not influence the placental phenotype. The different placental phenotypes described in the various targeted and transgenic mouse models are summarized in Table 40.1. Biological redundancy among different IGFBP genes could be a factor in the lack of phenotype for the *Igfbp2*(-/-), and the structural and functional changes may become apparent only when all the IGFBP genes are collectively disrupted.

TABLE 40.1 Birth size and placental phenotypes resulting from the IGF system and insulin knockout and transgenic mice

Genotype	Birth size	Placental phenotype
Igf1(−/−)	60% of WT	Normal size
Igf2(−/−)	60% of WT	Size smaller (51% of WT at E15, 80% of WT at E18); smaller total number of cells; smaller proportion of glycogen cells
Placental *Igf2*(+/−)	78% of WT	76% of WT; all cell types proportionately smaller; diffusion capacity 40%
Igf1r(−/−)	30% of WT	Normal size
Igf2r(m−/p+)	Larger than WT	Larger; continues to grow until term (WT completes growth at E17)
Igfbp2(−/−)	Normal	Normal size
Igfbp4(−/−)	Normal	Placental phenotype not described
Igfbp5(−/−)		Placental phenotype not described
Igfbp6(−/−)	Normal	Placental phenotype not described
Paternal *Igf2* disomy	Larger	Larger
Igfbp1 overexpression	85% of WT	Placental phenotype not described
Ins1/Ins2(−/−)	78% of WT	Not described
Insr(−/−)	Normal	Not described

WT = wild type

40.4 FETAL GROWTH AND DEVELOPMENT

40.4.1 Optimal Fetal Growth

With the recognition that appropriateness of an individual's intrauterine growth is the determinant of both short- and long-term outcomes, many epidemiological studies have used birth weight as a proxy measure for the quality of fetal development, as it is a commonly recorded parameter at birth in most countries. However, it is a problematic measure because different prenatal environmental exposures, patterns of fetal growth, and durations of pregnancy can lead to similar birth weights. It was suggested that, instead of using one's birth weight relative to the population, we should determine the appropriateness of one's birth weight to one's own estimated "optimal fetal growth".[51] Appropriateness of growth can be inferred from the ratio of the value of the observed dimension to that of the optimal dimension. Nonpathological determinants of fetal size—gestational duration, fetal gender, and maternal height, age, and parity—were used to predict birth weight, birth length, and head circumference. Optimal birth weight is defined as that achieved when no factors are present that can exert a pathological effect on growth. However, this concept was questioned recently as the trajectory of fetal growth, especially in the second half of gestation, is more important in determining the susceptibility of an individual to chronic morbidities.[52] Historically, the median birth weight has been regarded as normal or even supernormal in some more refined clinical studies.

40.4.2 Normal Growth—Population-Based

Normal growth of the fetus is estimated clinically by the estimated fetal weight (EFW), which is a synthesis of biometric parameters measured using a 2-D ultrasound.[53] Many formulae exist for computing EFW with varying accuracy.[54–56] The Hadlock third formula with three parameters (abdominal circumference, head circumference, and femur length) is one of the most widely used[57, 58] because of its good performance in unselected populations as well as among high-risk fetuses. This formula was developed based on a study of 392 white healthy women from a single center in Texas, where each fetus contributed a single ultrasound. Until recently, longitudinal ultrasound-based references were based on relatively small studies. Three intrauterine fetal growth charts have been developed recently, using three longitudinal cohort studies: one in the United States by the Eunice Kennedy Shriver National Institutes of Child Health and Human Development (NICHD) Fetal Growth Studies[59]; second by the INTERGROWTH-21st (INTERGROWTH)[60, 61]; and third by the World Health Organization Multicentre Growth Reference Study (WHO Fetal).[62] However, each has slightly different research aims that have impact on the interpretation and utility of the findings (Table 40.2).[57, 58]

One of the two most commonly used growth curves was updated to complement the WHO postnatal growth curves.[63] Two recent studies, one from France and another from United States, compared Hadlock EFW with INTERGROWTH-21st and NICHD FGS, respectively, and found that the Hadlock standard is superior to both for preterm fetuses delivered between 22–34 weeks gestation and for the prediction of both neonatal morbidity and small for gestational age. It has also been suggested that estimation of fetal weight using MRI, which is done by measuring the fetal body volume and converting to EFW using a formula, may be better.[64] However, a large-scale longitudinal population-based study has yet to be completed. Similarly, placental weight or volume has been studied longitudinally using MRI in limited population-based studies, although ultrasound is still the imaging modality of practical choice.[65]

40.4.3 Parturition

Preterm births (<37 weeks gestation) occur in 5%–15% of pregnancies worldwide and are associated with 70% of neonatal deaths, and there is a strong inverse association between perinatal mortality and the duration of gestation. Human parturition is now recognized as a distinctly human event, with animal models revealing only limited, however valuable, insights. Endocrine and paracrine factors play significant roles in all species. Parturition in sheep is initiated by the fetal hypothalamo-pituitary-adrenal axis, whereas in goats it is dependent on the dissolution of the maternal corpus luteum. In humans, the timing of birth is associated with the development of the placenta, in particular with the expression of the gene encoding corticotrophin-releasing hormone. In addition, the placenta also produces a circulating CRH binding protein, the production of which falls just prior to parturition, allowing an increase in free CRH. Glucocorticoids stimulate the expression of the placental CRH gene, which in turn stimulates the pituitary to produce corticotropin, which then stimulates the adrenal to produce cortisol. Placental CRH production is inhibited by estrogen, progesterone, and nitric oxide. During pregnancy, CRH receptors (CRHR1α) in the myometrium when activated by CRH cause the dissociation of the α subunit of the G-protein, leading to the relaxation of the myometrium. However, at term, CRH receptors activate the Gaq pathway,

TABLE 40.2 Cohort profiles of the three longitudinal growth studies

Study	Location	Race & Ethnic	Inclusion/ Exclusion	Analytical Approaches	Estimated Fetal Weight
NICHD	**12 US sites:** New York (2), New Jersey, Delaware, Rhode Island, Massachusetts, South Carolina, Alabama, Illinois, California (3)	Highly significant difference in fetal growth by race/ethnicity; Racial/ethnic-specific derived standards	**Exclusion:** Pregnancy-associated complications Preterm delivery Stillbirth Fetal factors, including structural and karyotype abnormalities	**Data information:** log **Model assumptions:** linear mixed models, assuming a normal distribution of the fetal growth trajectories **Smoothing technique over gestational age:** cubic splines	Calculated EFW from HC, AC, and FL using the Hadlock 1985 formula
INTERGROWTH	**8 countries:** Brazil, China, India, Italy, Kenya, Oman, UK, and US	One overall growth chart; No statistical testing for differences among countries	**Exclusion:** Pregnancy complications; Fetal factors, including congenital anomalies and stillbirth	**Data transformation:** none **Model assumptions:** linear mixed models with location and scale assumptions, assuming a normal distribution of the fetal growth trajectories **Smoothing technique over gestational age:** second-degree fractional polynomials	Created a new formula for EFW based on only HC and AC, making the comparison of EFW less meaningful
WHO	**10 countries:** Argentina, Brazil, Democratic Republic of Congo, Denmark, Egypt, France, Germany, India, Norway and Thailand	One overall growth chart; Fetal growth standard showed natural variation, differing significantly between countries which largely followed ethnic distribution	Inclusion: Only optimal health No complications excluded	**Data transformation:** log **Model assumptions:** quantile regression without distributional assumptions **Smoothing technique over gestational age:** polynomial functions	Calculated EFW from HC, AC, and FL using the Hadlock 1985 formula

Bold is used to highlight the differences among the three studies.
Adapted from Grantz KL, Sungkuk K, Grobman WA, et al. Fetal growth velocity: the NICHD fetal growth studies. *Am J Obstetr Gynecol* 2018;**219**:285e1–e36. Grantz KL, Hediger ML, Liu D, Buck Louis GM. Fetal growth standards: the NICHD fetal growth study approach in context with INTERGROWTH-21st and the World Health Organization multicenter growth reference study. *Am J Obstetr Gynecol* 2018:S641–55.

which activates protein kinase-C and the contractile pathway. CRH potentiates the contractile effects of several uterotonins, such as oxytocin and prostaglandin $F_{2\alpha}$, that promote uterine contraction.[66]

Preterm birth in humans is caused by multiple etiological factors such as chorioaminionitis, maternal infections (e.g., urinary tract infection), vascular disorders, decidual senescence, decline in progesterone action, uterine over distension, cervical incompetence, or maternal stress. A short cervix is a significant risk factor for spontaneous preterm birth. Vaginal progesterone therapy has been shown to be able to decrease the risk of preterm birth in single gestations with short cervix.[67] The shortened cervix may be due to the increased activity of 20α-hydroxysteroid dehydrogenase (20αHSD) in the cervix, which inactivates placental progesterone, leading to a localized progestin deficiency. Vaginal progesterone therapy acts by correcting the local progestin deficiency and reverses shortened cervix.[68]

40.4.4 Antenatal Corticosteroid Therapy

Antenatal corticosteroid therapy is one of the most important endocrine interventions that has improved neonatal mortality and morbidity in early preterm newborns (<34 weeks) and reduced respiratory morbidity in late preterm newborns (34–36 weeks). Antenatal corticosteroids were initially discovered to rapidly mature lungs (surfactant system as well as lung elasticity) and reduce the incidence and severity of respiratory distress syndrome in mid- to high-income countries.[69] However, it was also found to decrease intraventricular hemorrhage, necrotizing enterocolitis, and early onset neonatal sepsis. The impact of antenatal corticosteroids is not as apparent in low-income countries; however, WHO still recommends cautious use in these countries. Betamethasone or dexamethasone are the corticosteroids of choice and are most effective when a pregnant mother receives a complete course (2 doses 24 hours apart). Unlike the natural corticosteroid, cortisol, the synthetic corticosteroids are not inactivated by the 11β-hydroxysteroid dehydrogenase enzyme in the syncytiotrophoblast of the placenta, and are transported across the placental barrier to the fetus, where they act on lungs and many organs and tissues.[70]

40.5 NEONATAL, INFANTILE, AND EARLY CHILDHOOD GROWTH AND DEVELOPMENT

40.5.1 Normal Neonatal, Infantile, and Early Childhood Growth

Recently developed postnatal growth curves provide guidance for the goals of holistic care for all newborns and infants in conditions as physiologic as possible to optimum survival and long-term outcomes. Identification of growth patterns within the normal range requires comparison with prescriptive standards based on growth of healthy infants. Standards are critically important to monitor and assess the effectiveness of interventions and avoid negative effects, such as overnutrition.[60, 61] WHO and INTERGROWTH 21st complement each other in providing guidelines towards achievement of newborns at 26 weeks to term. These growth curves for both boys and girls were derived from adequately grown newborns from accurately dated, uncomplicated pregnancies. The cohorts were normally breast fed without morbidity and were assumed to be as healthy as possible.

40.6 REGULATION OF NORMAL NEONATAL, INFANTILE, AND EARLY CHILDHOOD GROWTH

Early postnatal growth is influenced by both genetic and environmental factors. In early infancy, growth is rapid but rapidly decelerating, followed by a steady growth in childhood and a growth spurt in puberty.[71] Growth in infancy is regulated by nutrition and less by growth hormone and thyroid hormone, in childhood by nutrition and growth hormone, and in puberty by sex hormones and growth hormone. Although there is no difference in average adult height among early, normal, and late maturing children, the timing of puberty influences the peak height velocity. Organ and tissue growth generally parallel skeletal growth with some notable exceptions. Brain and eyes are highly developed at birth and attain adult size within the first few years. Reproductive tissues are relatively underdeveloped until puberty.

There is significant difference in size, body proportions, and timing of puberty among different races. Sexual differences are apparent at birth—males have slightly higher birth weights than females, but the growth during childhood is similar between males and females. There is also a genetic determinant of an offspring's overall height from parents, with a correlation coefficient between parents and child of 0.33 and midparent height and child of 0.65. However, the most important environmental factor that influences infant and child growth is nutrition. Malnutrition, which is often observed in developing countries, especially in areas of conflict, not only leads to growth failure but also poor brain development. Nutritional status interacts with endocrine regulation of growth via the growth hormone and IGF axis. In contrast, in developed countries, obesity has become a significant problem in children with the development of type-2 diabetes and metabolic disorders in youth. In small for gestational age children, an early catch-up growth is associated with the development of metabolic syndrome in young adults.

40.7 SUMMARY AND CLINICAL IMPLICATIONS

The delineation of the human genome and the recognition that the attainment of the fetal size within normal parameters is not based in large part on the genetic sequence of the fetus or the placenta but on the environment that regulates gene expression via epigenetic mechanisms has provided clinicians with improved understanding of the physiology of normal growth as well as the pathophysiology of abnormal growth. However, attempts at improving growth of growth-restricted fetuses have not yielded positive outcomes, mainly because interventions have been initiated only after the FGR has been diagnosed. This is because the placenta has been damaged by pathological processes that have occurred early in pregnancy (early second trimester). Healthcare providers have a reasonably good idea of factors that may influence normal fetal growth such as adequate nutrition pre- and intrapregnancy; avoidance of environmental toxins, especially smoking and substance abuse; adequate management of maternal medical conditions; etc. New noninvasive imaging technologies to assess fetal and placental growth, such as MRI,[65, 72, 73] 3-D ultrasound and functional spectrophotometric technologies, single-cell genomic analysis,[74–76] and identification of small nucleic acids within the maternal circulation such as microRNAs and noncoding RNAs using next-generation sequencing early in pregnancy, will allow identification of mothers at high risk for pregnancy-associated disorders and allow clinicians to develop new intervention strategies to prevent poor fetal growth or minimize the impact of FGR in the fetus and newborns. The ultimate outcome will be to reduce the development of chronic diseases in children and adults.

REFERENCES

1. Whitsett JA, Kalin TV, Xu Y, Kalinichenko VV. Building and regenerating the lung cell by cell. *Physiol Rev* 2019;**99**:513–54.
2. Yakar S, Liu JL, Stannard B, Butler A, Accili D, Sauer B, LeRoith D. Normal growth and development in the absence of hepatic insulin-like growth factor I. *Proc Natl Acad Sci U S A* 1999;**96**:7324–9.
3. Steinhart Z, Angers S. Wnt signaling in development and tissue homeostasis. *Development* 2018;**145**(11). https://doi.org/10.1242/dev.146589. pii: dev146589.
4. Fernandes-Silva H, Correria-Pinto J, Moura RS. Canonical sonic hedgehog signaling in early lung development. *J Dev Biol* 2017;**5**(3):1–14.
5. Liu N, Lu M, Tian X, Han Z. Molecular mechanisms involved in self-renewal and pluripotency of embryonic stem cells. *J Cell Physiol* 2007;**211**:279–86.
6. Martello G, Smith A. The nature of embryonic stem cells. *Ann Rev Cell Dev* 2014. https://doi.org/10.1146/annurev-cellbio-100913-013116.
7. Norwitz ER, Schust DJ, Fisher SJ. Implantation and survival of early pregnancy. *New Engl J Med* 2001;**345**:19.
8. Cha J, Sun X, Dey SK. Mechanisms of implantation: strategies for successful pregnancy. *Nat Med Rev* 2012;**18**(12):1754–67.
9. Karagiannis P, Takahashi K, Saito M, Yoshida Y, Okita K, Watanabe A, Inoue H, Yamashita JK, Todani M, Nakagawa M, Osawa M, Yashiro Y, Yamanaka S, Osafune K. Induced pluripotent stem cells and their use in human models of disease and development. *Physiol Rev* 2019;**99**(1):79–114.
10. Feinberg AP. The key role of epigenetics in human disease prevention and mitigation. *New Engl J Med* 2018;**378**(14):1323–33.
11. Jirtle RL, Skinner MK. Environmental epigenomics and disease susceptibility. *Nat Rev* 2007;**8**:253–62.
12. Kaelin WG, McKnight SL. Influence of metabolism on epigenetics and disease. *Cell* 2013;**153**:56–69.
13. Rodenhiser D, Mann M. Epigenetics and human disease: translating basic biology into clinical applications. *Can Med Assoc J* 2006;**174**:341–7.
14. Roost MS, Slieker RC, Bialecka M, et al. DNA methylation and transcriptional trajectories during human development and reprogramming of isogenic pluripotent stem cells. *Nature* 2018;**8**:908.
15. Skvortsova K, Iovino N, Bogdanovic O. Functions and mechanisms of epigenetic inheritance in animals. *Nat Rev* 2018;**19**. https://doi.org/10.1038/s41580-0180-0074-2.
16. Esteller M. Non-coding RNAs in human disease. *Nat Rev* 2011;**12**:861–73.
17. Ransohof JD, Wei Y, Khavari PA. The functions and unique features of long intergenic non-coding RNA. *Nat Rev* 2018;**19**:143–57.
18. Yang Q, Vijayakumar A, Kahn BB. Metabolites as regulators of insulin sensitivity and metabolism. *Nat Rev* 2018;**19**. s41580-018-0044-8.
19. Cassidy FC, Charalambous M. Genomic imprinting, growth and maternal-fetal interactions. *J Exp Biol* 2018;**221**.
20. Eckelsley-Maslin MA, Alda-Catalinas C, Reik W. Dynamics of the epigenetic landscape during the maternal-to-zygotic transition. *Nat Rev* 2018;**19**:436–50.
21. Treiber T, Treiber N, Meister G. Regulation of microRNA biogenesis and its crosstalk with other cellular pathways. *Nat Rev* 2019;**20**:5–19.
22. Berdasco M, Esteller M. Clinical epigenetics: seizing opportunities for translation. *Nat Rev* 2019;**20**.
23. Moore-Morris T, van Vliet PP, Andelfinger G, Puceat M. Role of epigenetics in cardiac development and congenital diseases. *Physiol Rev* 2018;**98**:2453–75.
24. Morrisey EE, Hogan BLM. Preparing for the first breath: genetic and cellular mechanisms in lung development. *Dev Cell Rev* 2010;**18**:8–22.
25. Slack JM. Conrad Hal Waddington: the last Renaissance biologist? *Nat Rev Genet* 2002;**3**(11):889–95.
26. Roseboom TJ. Epidemiological evidence for the developmental origins of health and disease: effects of prenatal undernutrition in humans. *J Encrinol* 2019;**242**(1):T135–44. https://doi.org/10.1530/JOE-18-0683.
27. Vagero D, Pinger PR, Aronsson V, van den Berg GJ. Paternal grandfather's access to food predicts all-cause and cancer mortality in grandsons. *Nat Commun* 2018;**9**(1):5124. https://doi.org/10.1038/s41467-018-07617-9.
28. Aze A, Maiorano D. *Recent advances in understanding DNA replication: cell type-specific adaptation of the DNA replication program. F1000 Res 7:1351; 2018. p.* 1–10.
29. Crews D, Gillette R, Miller-Crews I, Gore AC, Skinner MK. Nature, nurture and epigenetics. *Mol Cell Endocrinol* 2014;**398**:42–52.
30. Bloomfield FH, Spiroski AM, Harding JE. Fetal growth factors and fetal nutrition. *Sem Fetal Neonatal Med* 2013;**18**:118–23.
31. Gluckman PD, Hanson MA, Low FM. The role of developmental plasticity and epigenetics in human health. *Birth Defects Res* 2011;**93**:12–8.
32. Redman CW, Sargent IL. Latest advances in understanding preeclampsia. *Science* 2005;**308**(5728):1592–4.
33. Saxton R, Sabatini DM. mTOR signaling in growth, metabolism and disease. *Cell Rev* 2017;**169**(2):361–71.

34. Hart B, Morgan E, Alejandro EU. Nutrient sensor signaling pathways and cellular stress in fetal growth restriction. *J Mol Endocrinol* 2019;**62**(2): R155–65.
35. Hiani YE, Egom EEA, Dong X-P. mTOR signaling: jack-of-all-trades. *Biochem Cell Biol* 2019;**97**:58–67.
36. Dimasuay KG, Boeuf P, Powell TL, Jansson T. Placental responses to changes in the maternal environment determine feta growth. *Front Physiol* 2016;**7**:12.
37. Barker DJ, Winter PD, Osmond C, Margetts B, Simmonds SJ. Weight in infancy and death from ischaemic heart disease. *Lancet* 1989; **2**(8663):577–80.
38. Calkins K, Devaskar SU. Fetal origins of adult diseases. *Curr Probl Pediatr Adolesc Health Care* 2011;**41**:158–76.
39. Limesand SW, Thornburg KL, Harding JE. 30th anniversary for the developmental origins of endocrinology. *J Endocrinol* 2019. 19-0227.R1.
40. Godfrey KM, Gluckman PD, Hanson MA. Developmental origins of metabolic disease: life course and intergenerational perspectives. *Trends Endocrinol Metabol* 2010;**21**:199–205.
41. Gaccioli F, Lager S. Placental nutrient transport and intra uterine growth restriction. *Front Physiol* 2016;**7**:40.
42. Jones HN, Powell T, Jansson T. Regulation of placental nutrient transport—a review. *Placenta* 2007;**28**:763–74.
43. Lager S, Powell T. Regulation of nutrient transport across the placenta. *J Pregnancy* 2012;.
44. Baker BC, Hayes DJL, Jones RL. Effects of micronutrients on placental function: evidence from clinical studies to animal models. *Reproduction* 2018;**136**:R69–82.
45. Burton GJ, Jauniaux E. Pathophysiology of placental-derived fetal growth restriction. *Am J Obstetr Gynecol* 2018;S745–61.
46. Desforges M, Sibley C. Placental nutrient supply and fetal growth. *Int J Dev Biol* 2010;**54**:377–90.
47. Han VK, Bassett N, Walton J, Challis JR. The expression of insulin-like growth factor (IGF) and IGF-binding protein (IGFBP) genes in the human placenta and membranes: evidence for IGF-IGFBP interactions at the feto-maternal interface. *J Clin Endocrinol Metab* 1996;**81**(7):2680–93.
48. LeRoith D, Scavo L, Butler A. What is the role of circulating IGF-1? *Trends Endocrinol Metabol* 2001;**12**(2):48–52.
49. Woods L, Perez-Garcia V, Hemberger M. Regulation of placental development and its impact on fetal growth—new insights from mouse models. *Front Endocrinol* 2018;**9**:570. https://doi.org/10.3389/fendo.2018.00570.
50. Namiki T, Iton J, Kashiwazaki N. Molecular mechanisms of embryonic implantation in mammals: lessons from gene manipulation of mice. *Reprod Med Biol* 2018;**17**:331–42.
51. Blair EM, Liu Y, de Klerk NH, Lawrence DM. Optimal fetal growth for the Caucasian singleton and assessment of appropriateness of fetal growth: an analysis of a total population perinatal database. *BMC Pediatr* 2005;**5**(13):1–12.
52. Hanson M, Kiserud T, Visser GHA, Brockehurst P, Schneider EB. Optimal fetal growth: a misconception? *Am J Obstetr Gynecol* 2015;332–4.
53. Hiersch L, Melamed N. Fetal growth velocity and body proportion in the assessment of growth. *Am J Obstetr Gynecol* 2018;S700–11.
54. Gardosi J, Francis A, Turner S, Williams M. Customized growth charts: rationale, validation and clinical benefits. *Am J Obstetr Gynecol* 2018; S609–18 (Hadlock).
55. Ohuma EO, Njim T, Sharps MC. Current issues in the development of foetal growth references and standards. *Curr Epidemiol Rep* 2018;**5**:388–98.
56. Pugh SJ, Ortega-Villa AM, Grobman W, Newman RB, Owen J, Wing DA, Albert PS, Grantz KL. Estimating gestational age at birth from fundal height and additional anthropormetrics: a prospective cohort study. *Br J Obstetr Gynaecol* 2013;https://doi.org/10.1111/1471-0528.15179.
57. Grantz KL, Sungkuk K, Grobman WA, et al. Fetal growth velocity: the NICHD fetal growth studies. *Am J Obstetr Gynecol* 2018;**219**:285e1–285e36.
58. Grantz KL, Hediger ML, Liu D, Buck Louis GM. Fetal growth standards: the NICHD fetal growth study approach in context with INTERGROWTH-21st and the World Health Organization multicenter growth reference study. *Am J Obstetr Gynecol* 2018;S641–55.
59. Grewal J, Grantz KL, Zhang C, et al. *Cohort profile: NICHD fetal growth studies—singletons and twins.* .
60. Villar J, Papageorghiou AT, Pang R, et al. Monitoring human growth and development: a continuum from the womb to the classroom. *Am J Obstetr Gynecol* 2015;**213**(4):494–9.
61. Villar J, Giuliani F, Bhutta ZA, et al. Postnatal growth standards for preterm infants: the Preterm Postnatal Follow-up Study of the INTERGROWTH-21st project. *Lancet* 2015;**3**:e681–91.
62. Kiserud T, Benachi A, Hecher K, Gonzalez P, Carvalho J, Piaggio G, Platt LD. The World Health Organization fetal growth charts: concept, findings, interpretation, and application. *Am J Obstetr Gynecol* 2017;S619–29.
63. Fenton TR, Kim JH. A systemic review and meta-analysis to revise the Fenton growth chart for preterm infants. *BMC Pediatr* 2013;**13**(59):1–13.
64. Blue NR, Beddow ME, Savabi M, Katukuri VR, Chao CR. Comparing the Hadlock fetal growth standard to the Eunice Kennedy Shriver National Institute of Child Health and Human Development racial/ethnic standard for the prediction of neonatal morbidity and small for gestational age. *Am J Obstetr Gynecol* 2018;**474**:e1–e12.
65. Kadji CC, Cannie MM, Resta S, Guez D, Abi-Khalil F, De Angelis R, Jani JC. Magnetic resonance imaging for prenatal estimation of birthweight in pregnancy: review of available data, techniques, and future perspectives. *Am J Obstetr Gynecol* 2019;1–12.
66. Smith R. Parturition. *New Engl J Med* 2007;**356**(3):271–83.
67. Romero R, Conde-Agudelo A, Da Fonseca E, O'Brien JM, Cetingoz E, Creasy GW, Hassan S, Nicolaides K. Vaginal progesterone for preventing preterm birth and adverse perinatal outcomes in singleton gestations with a short cervix: a meta-analysis of individual patient data. *Am J Obstetr Gynecol* 2018;161–80.
68. Weatherborn M, Mesiano S. Rationale for current and future progestin-based therapies to prevent preterm birth. *Best Pract Res Clin Obstetr Gynecol* 2018;**52**:114–25.
69. Smith LJ, McKay KO, van Asperen PP, Selvadurai H, Fitzgerald DC. Normal development of the lung and premature birth. *Pediatr Resp Rev* 2010;**11**:135–42.

70. Zhu P, Wang W, Zuo R, Sun K. Mechanisms for establishment of the placental glucocorticoid barrier, a guard for life. *Cell Mol Life Sci* 2019;**76**:13–26.

71. Wilbaux M, Kasser S, Wellmann S, Lapaire O, van den Anker JN, Pfister M. Characterizing and forecasting individual weight changes in term neonates. *J Pediatr* 2016;**173**:101–7.

72. Dahdouh S, Andescavage N, Yewale S, Yarish A, Lanham D, Bulas D, du Plessis AJ, Limperopoulos C. In vivo placental MRI shape and textural features predict fetal growth restriction and postnatal outcome. *J Magn Reson Imaging* 2018;**47**:449–58.

73. Leon R, Li KT, Brown BP. A retrospective segmentation analysis of placental volume by magnetic resonance imaging from first trimester to term gestation. *Pediatr Radiol* 2018;**48**:1936–44.

74. Chen HH, Jin Y, Huang Y, Chen Y. Detection of high variability in gene expression from single-cell RNA-seq profiling. *BMC Genomics* 2016;**17**:508.

75. Risso D, Perraudeau F, Gribkova S, Dudoit S, Vert JP. A general and flexible method for signal extraction from single-cell RNA seq data. *Nat Commun* 2018;**9**:284.

76. Schwartzman O, Tanay A. Single cell epigenomics: techniques and emerging applications. *Nat Rev* 2015;**16**:716–26.

Chapter 41

Placental Production of Peptide, Steroid, and Lipid Hormones

Jerome F. Strauss, III* and Sam A. Mesiano[†,‡]

*Department of Obstetrics and Gynecology, Division of Reproductive Biology and Research, Virginia Commonwealth University, Richmond, VA, United States, [†]Department of Reproductive Biology, Case Western Reserve University, Cleveland, OH, United States, [‡]Department of Obstetrics and Gynecology, University Hospitals Cleveland Medical Center, Cleveland, OH, United States

Key Clinical Changes
- The placenta is the principle source of hormones that control the physiology of pregnancy.
- Trophoblast cells within the placenta are the main site of hormone production.
- Placental hormonal products include proteins, glycoproteins, steroids and bioactive lipids that are either identical to or homologous to hormones produced by the hypothalamus, anterior pituitary gland, and ovary.
- The biosynthesis of estrogens requires the contribution of precursors from the fetal adrenal glands, such that estrogens are formed by the "fetoplacental unit."
- The amounts of placental hormones produced are largely determined by the mass of trophoblast tissue, although there is evidence for local control of hormone production within the placenta.
- Placental hormones are secreted mainly into the maternal circulation.
- The placenta serves as a barrier to some maternal hormones; in other cases, the placenta metabolizes the hormones into active or inactive metabolites.
- Placental progesterone maintains uterine quiescence, and withdrawal of its activity triggers parturition and the onset of lactation.

41.1 INTRODUCTION: THE PLACENTA-MATERNAL ENDOCRINE INTERFACE

The hormonal milieu of pregnancy is dominated by a wide variety factors synthesized by the placenta and secreted mainly into the maternal compartment. Most hormones produced by the placenta are identical, or close structural and functional homologues, of maternal hormones, and as such they interact with cognate receptors on maternal cells. Consequently, placental hormones that are secreted in relatively large amounts to achieve high levels (compared with levels in nonpregnant women) in the maternal circulation override maternal counterparts and have profound effects on maternal physiology. In this way, placental hormones can be considered as allocrine factors: hormones produced by one organism, the fetus, that affect the function of another organism, the mother.

The human placenta develops early in embryogenesis. The main cells of the placenta, the trophoblasts, arise shortly after formation of the blastocyst, and are morphologically distinct from other cells of the early embryo. Cytotrophoblasts are proliferative mononuclear epithelial cells that give rise to the various cells of the developed placenta. Important among these is the syncytiotrophoblast, a large multinucleated cell formed by the fusion of underlying trophectodermal/cytotrophoblast cells. The syncytiotrophoblast lines the maternal surface of the placental villi and is in direct contact with maternal blood (Fig. 41.1). Most placental hormones are synthesized by the syncytiotrophoblast. This vascular arrangement of the human placenta is referred to as hemochorial: direct contact of maternal blood with placental cells. The syncytiotrophoblast is anatomically positioned to perform gas exchange and transfer of nutrients from the maternal blood to the fetus. It also metabolizes maternal hormones (e.g., glucocorticoid and insulin) to prevent fetal exposure and thus separates components of the maternal and fetal endocrine systems. Importantly, the hemochorial arrangement allows hormones produced by the syncytiotrophoblast to directly access the maternal circulation. In contrast, the syncytiotrophoblast prevents most maternal hormones from entering the fetal compartment.

Maternal-Fetal and Neonatal Endocrinology. https://doi.org/10.1016/B978-0-12-814823-5.00041-6

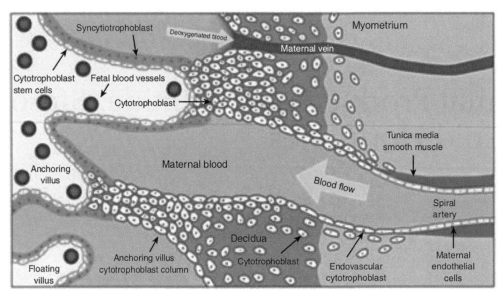

FIG. 41.1 Anatomic arrangement of the human hemochorial placenta. Maternal blood bathes the placental villi that are lined with the syncytiotrophoblast. Cytotrophoblasts invade the spiral arteries to increase their diameter and therefore placental perfusion. *(Upper panel only from Fig. 11.2,* Yen and Jaffe's Reproductive endocrinology. *8th ed., [chapter 11].)*

Animals have been used to study placental physiology in vivo and in vitro, but it is important to keep in mind that there are anatomical and structural differences from the human placenta, which in turn imply functional differences. The vascular arrangement of placentas from sheep, goats, and pigs is epitheliochorial, which means that a full thickness of maternal tissues prevents maternal blood from directly contacting placental cells of fetal origin. In contrast, rodents (mice, rats) and monkeys have a hemochorial structure similar to human placentas, in which maternal blood directly contacts placental cells of fetal origin. There are differences in macrostructure as well, with ovine placentas arranged into cotyledons, and rodent and monkey placentas arranged in a single discoid structure, whereas human placentas have a villous structure. Rodent placentas also contain the intraplacental yolk sac, which produces hormones and appears to be a route of maternal-fetal exchange separate from trophoblasts, but this structure is absent in placentas of humans and other primates. This chapter focuses on the human placenta.

The hormones known to be produced by the human placenta are listed in Table 41.1. The generally accepted reason for such variety of hormones is that it reflects the importance of modifying maternal physiology to satisfy the nutritional needs of the developing conceptus. Given the profound evolutionary importance of ensuring appropriate maternal adaptations to pregnancy, it is plausible that considerable redundancy exists and that some hormones and the pattern of their production are evolutionary holdovers that no longer have a specific function. Nonetheless, a case can be made that the fetus via placental hormones exerts fine control of maternal physiology to favor fetal well-being and pregnancy success while also protecting maternal health. Some of the key hormones produced by the human placenta and how they may affect pregnancy are discussed as follows.

41.2 HYPOTHALAMIC-PITUITARY HORMONE ANALOGUES

41.2.1 Gonadotropin-Releasing Hormone/Gonadotropin

Placental hormone production begins during the early stages of blastocyst formation and before implantation when trophoblast cells secreted chorionic gonadotropin (CG; designated hCG in humans) into the maternal blood. The production of CG is essential for the establishment of pregnancy. In a nonconception cycle, the corpus luteum (CL) usually regresses at about the 2nd week after ovulation, and the subsequent decline in progesterone leads to menstruation. For pregnancy to be established, CL regression and the associated decrease in systemic progesterone must be prevented. The principal function of CG is to prevent regression of the ovarian corpus luteum, leading to sustained generation of CL progesterone during the first several weeks of pregnancy. CG is structurally similar to LH, a heterodimeric glycoprotein that is composed of an α-subunit, common to LH and CG, and a separate but very similar β-subunit. The CG β-subunit has a C-terminal extension

TABLE 41.1 Major hormones and bioactive lipids produced by the human placenta

Neuropeptides	Pituitary-like hormones	Adipokines	Growth factors	Steroid hormones	Monoamines and adrenal-like peptides	Bioactive lipids
CRH	ACTH	Adiponectin	IGF-I/-II	Progesterone	Epinephrine	$PGF_{2\alpha}$
TRH	TSH	Leptin	VEGF	Estradiol	Norepinephrine	PGE_2
GnRH	PGH	Resistin	EGF	Estrone	Dopamine	PGI
Melatonin	PL	Visfatin	Activins	Estriol	Serotonin	PGI_2
Cholecystokinin	CG	Ghrelin	Inhibins	Estetrol	Adrenomedullin	TX_{A2}
Met-enkephalin	LH	FGF21	Follistatin	2-Methoxyestradiol		
Dynorphin	FSH			Allopregnanolone		
Neurotensin	β-Endorphin			Pregnenolone		
VIP	Prolactin			5α-Dihydroprogesterone		
Galanin	Oxytocin					
Somatostatin						
CGRP						
Neuropeptide Y						
Substance P						
Endothelin						
ANP						
Renin						
Angiotensin						
Urocortin						
Kisspeptin						

(Adapted from Reis FM, Petraglia F. The placenta as a neuroendocrine organ. *Front Horm Res* 2001;**27**:216; Costa MA. The endocrine function of the human placenta: an overview. *Reprod BioMed Online* 2016;**32**:14–43.)

and a glycosylation profile that increases its half-life in the circulation. Like LH, it predominantly functions through the LH/CG receptor. The affinity of CG for the LH/CG receptor is greater than that of LH.

Immunoassays detecting the distinct CG β-subunit are used for the clinical evaluation of CG in maternal blood and urine. The levels of CG in the maternal blood and urine are clinically used to diagnose pregnancy. It is the earliest clinically recognized hormone secreted by the conceptus. The capacity of the conceptus to produce CG may provide a test of endocrine competence for natural selection because pregnancy will not occur if the embryo cannot gain control of the maternal CL and prevent its regression. Thus one of the first endocrine interactions between the conceptus and the mother involves signaling by the early embryo to promote intrauterine conditions that will allow implantation and the establishment of pregnancy. This is referred to as the maternal recognition of pregnancy and involves extending the functional lifespan of the CL to ensure the presence of progesterone, which is essential for the establishment and maintenance of pregnancy.

CG produced by the peri-implantation blastocyst may affect the implantation process via paracrine effects on the endometrium, particularly endometrial stromal cells. CG produced by the blastocyst is thought to extend the time of implantation receptivity by inhibiting insulin-like growth factor (IGF) binding protein-1 (IGFBP-1) production by endometrial cells, thereby increasing the bioactivity of IGF-1 in the endometrium. CG also may increase angiogenesis by increasing vascular endothelial growth factor (VEGF) and local cytokine and chemokine expression, and local protease activity to augment invasive potential.[1, 2]

FIG. 41.2 Schematic representation of concentrations of human chorionic gonadotropin (hCG) and placental lactogen (hPL) throughout gestation. Note differences in the magnitude of the concentrations of the two
hormones in early and late gestation. *LMP*, last menstrual period.
(Fig. 11.3 from Yen and Jaffe's Reproductive endocrinology. *8th ed.,
[chapter 11].)*

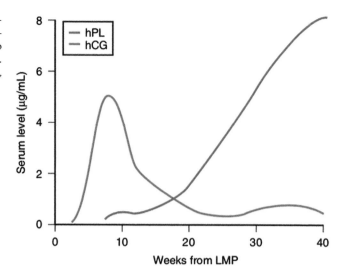

If conception occurs, CG is detectable in the maternal blood around 10 days after the midcycle LH surge and ovulation.
Thus existence of a conceptus can be detected before the first missed menstrual period. During early pregnancy, the level of
CG in the maternal blood doubles every 2–3 days and reaches a peak at around the end of the first trimester. Thereafter, CG
levels decrease to a plateau that is maintained during the remainder of the pregnancy (Fig. 41.2).

Maternal CG levels are used clinically to establish the existence of pregnancy and assist in assessing viability of the
early conceptus and the possibility ectopic implantation. In addition, the maternal blood CG level has been included in some
first and second trimester screening paradigms to predict genetic abnormalities such as trisomy 13, 18, and 21. Maternal CG
levels are also used to determine the existence of choriocarcinomas and molar pregnancy, and can be used to monitor
treatment and recurrence of such conditions.

CG levels in maternal blood are determined by trophoblast mass and trophoblast viability in early pregnancy, but they
also appear to be influenced over time by a placental hypothalamic-pituitary-like axis, as demonstrated by in vitro studies.
The production of CG by the human placenta is stimulated by gonadotropin-releasing hormone (GnRH) that is also produced by placental cells.[3] Levels of GnRH in the circulation of pregnant women are highest in the first trimester and correlate closely with CG levels.[4] Other factors that regulate pituitary gonadotropin secretion also affect placental CG
production. These include inhibin, activin, and progesterone. Thus, there appears to be autoregulation of CG production
by that placenta that is analogous to the hypothalamic-pituitary-gonadal axis.

41.2.2 Corticotrophin-Releasing Hormone/Pro-Opiomelanocortin Derivatives

The human placenta expresses the gene encoding corticotropin-releasing hormone (CRH) beginning at around the 6th to 8th
week of gestation,[5] and placental CRH can be detected in the maternal blood as early as the 15th week of gestation, and then
levels increase exponentially as pregnancy advances.[6, 7] The level of placental CRH in the maternal blood at midgestation
and the trajectory of its increase for the remainder of pregnancy are directly predictive of the risk for preterm or postterm
birth.[8] For most of pregnancy, CRH circulates in association with a binding protein that is thought sequester CRH and
prevent it from exerting biological activity. At the end of pregnancy (4–5 weeks before parturition), levels of the CRH
binding protein in the maternal blood decrease, and this is associated with an exponential increase in placental CRH production,[9] which is thought to result in increased CRH biological activity.

Placental CRH production (based on in vitro studies of placental explants) is increased by prostaglandins (PGs) E_2 and
$F_{2\alpha}$, norepinephrine, acetylcholine, vasopressin, angiotensin-II, oxytocin, interleukin-I, and neuropeptide-Y,[10] and
decreased by progesterone and nitric oxide donors.[10, 11] Although glucocorticoids inhibit expression and secretion of
CRH by the hypothalamus, they increase CRH expression and secretion by the human placenta, especially during the third
trimester.[12–14] This effect of glucocorticoids may have implications for the activity of the fetal pituitary-adrenal axis in the
context of parturition and fetal maturation. Placental CRH may stimulate adrenocorticotropin (ACTH) production by the
fetal pituitary, which would increase cortisol and dehydroepiandrosterone (DHEA)-sulfate (DHEA-S) secretion by the fetal
adrenals (discussed later). The increase in cortisol may prepare the fetus for parturition because cortisol promotes the

maturation of organ systems, especially the lungs, needed for its survival as a neonate. A parallel increase in fetal adrenal DHEA-S would increase placental estrogen synthesis by providing substrate (mainly DHEA) for placental aromatization. CRH also may directly and preferentially increase DHEA-S production by the fetal adrenal glands.[15–17] Interestingly, placental CRH and fetal adrenal DHEA-S increase concordantly during the third trimester, suggesting that production of these two hormones is physiologically linked.

The syncytiotrophoblast and extravillous trophoblasts also produce, albeit to a lesser extent relative to CRH, a group of structurally and functionally related neuropeptides known as *urocortins*.[18] Consistent with the hypothalamic-pituitary analogy within placental tissue, CRH and urocortins stimulate ACTH production by trophoblast cells. Interestingly, CRH and urocortins cause vasodilation of the uteroplacental vasculature.[19–21] Women with preeclampsia have reduced placental vasculature responsiveness to urocortin, suggesting that a principal role of urocortin is to facilitate vasodilation in the fetoplacental circulation.[22]

The gene encoding pro-opiomelanocortin (POMC), a 31-kDa glycoprotein that can be enzymatically cleaved to produce ACTH, β-lipotrophic hormone (β-LPH), α-melanocyte-stimulating hormone (α-MSH), and β-endorphin (β-EP), is expressed by the syncytiotrophoblast in a transcriptional pattern resembling extra-pituitary tumors.[23, 24] Each of the POMC-derived peptides, including full-length POMC, has been detected in the human placenta.[24] The physiological role of placental POMC derivatives is unclear. Although the placenta produces ACTH in response to placental CRH, it is not sufficient to prevent fetal adrenal hypoplasia in fetal hypopituitarism, suggesting a negligible role in the fetal compartment. Placental ACTH may affect glucocorticoid production by the maternal adrenals and disrupt the negative feedback between the adrenals and the hypothalamus-pituitary in the mother. The roles of placental α-MSH, β-LPH, and β-EP are also not known. The placenta also produces enkephalins and dynorphins.[25, 26] In vitro studies suggest that dynorphin acts in a paracrine manner to stimulate the production of placental lactogen.[27]

41.2.3 Somatotropins

The human placenta expresses genes encoding members of the growth hormone (GH)-placental lactogen (PL) family.[28] The genes are derived from duplications of a common ancestral gene *GH1* gene that encodes pituitary GH. The placental GH (*PGH*) genes encode 2 variants of pituitary GH and are expressed exclusively by the syncytiotrophoblast.[29] PL has 96% homology with pituitary GH and can be detected in the placenta from around day 18 of pregnancy, and in the maternal circulation by the 3rd week of pregnancy. At term, the syncytiotrophoblast produces 1–4 g of PL per day, which represents a major biosynthetic commitment.[30]

PL is preferentially secreted into the maternal compartment, and maternal blood levels increase exponentially during gestation[31] (Fig. 41.2). The rise in PL production is thought to be due to the increase in placental mass, as the extent of PL gene expression by the syncytiotrophoblast does not change during the course of pregnancy, and maternal PL levels rise concordantly with the amount of syncytiotrophoblast tissue with advancing gestation.[32] PGH production is significantly less than that of PL. PGH is not secreted into the fetal compartment and is exclusively a maternal hormone.[33] During the third trimester, maternal PGH levels increase exponentially, in concert with PL. During the same period, pituitary GH production decreases progressively, and by 30 weeks cannot be detected.

In cytotrophoblast cells, PGH and PL production are stimulated by insulin and growth hormone-releasing factor (GRF) and inhibited by somatostatin (SS). SS and GRF are expressed by the syncytiotrophoblast, and the level of GRF correlates closely with PL,[34] suggesting that PL and PGH are controlled by a paracrine autoregulatory loop analogous to the hypothalamic-pituitary axis. Although maternal PL levels do not change in association with normal metabolic fluctuations,[35] prolonged fasting at midgestation[36] and insulin-induced hypoglycemia raise maternal PL concentrations,[37] suggesting the role of PL in metabolic homeostasis.

The physiologic actions of PGH and PL are not clearly understood. Pregnancy, fetal development, and parturition are normal in cases of complete PL deficiency.[38] Thus, despite remarkably high levels of PL, it is not essential for normal pregnancy. However, mutations in the GH/PL gene cluster that cause co-deficiency in PL and PGH are associated with severe fetal growth restriction in an otherwise normal pregnancy. Pregnancies in which only PGH is deficient have not been identified, suggesting that it plays an essential role in normal fetal development. Taken together, these observations indicate that PL and PGH influence fetal growth through effects on the mother. This is consistent with the thesis that PL and PGH modulate maternal metabolism to meet fetal energy requirements. In the second half of pregnancy, maternal physiology is in a mildly a diabetogenic state (i.e., cells become increasingly resistant to insulin) that is thought to be promoted by the combined GH-like and contra-insulin activity of PGH and PL. The consequent decrease in glucose uptake and increase in free fatty acid release increases the availability of free fatty acids, glucose, and amino acids for fetal consumption. Thus, during the second half of pregnancy, PGH and PL direct maternal metabolism toward mobilization of maternal energy resources to furnish the needs of the developing fetus.[39]

41.3 GROWTH FACTORS

The human placenta secretes multiple growth factors and cytokines,[40, 41] whose exact functions are not clearly defined. Growth of the placenta involves trophoblast proliferation, migration, differentiation, and fusion, and as such, growth factors are likely to be involved in these processes. Development of the placenta also involves extensive angiogenesis and vascularization at the implantation site, and modulation of the maternal immune system to prevent rejection of the allogeneic fetal tissue. These processes likely involve a complex autocrine/paracrine communication that involves a plethora of growth factors, angiogenic factors, and cytokines. Some of these factors are discussed as below.

41.3.1 Insulin-Like Growth Factors

Cytotrophoblasts, syncytiotrophoblast, and extravillous trophoblasts in the human placenta produce IGF-I and IGF-II from as early as the 8th week of pregnancy.[42] Studies in mice show that placental IGF-I and IGF-II are key regulators of placental and fetal growth. In mice lacking IGF-I, fetal growth is normal, but pups have poor postnatal growth and die before adulthood. In mice lacking IGF-II, fetal growth is restricted but postnatal growth is normal.[43] Mice lacking only placental IGF-II expression have placental and fetal growth restriction.[44, 45] Thus IGF-II appears to play a key role in fetal and placental growth, whereas IGF-I is important for postnatal growth. Interestingly, IGF-II is an imprinted gene, expressed only by the paternal allele.[46] In Beckwith-Wiedemann syndrome, abnormal methylation of the imprinting centers on chromosome 11 leads to additional expression of IGF-II from the maternal allele, which is normally suppressed. The extra IGF-II produced in this condition causes fetal macrosomia.[47] Loss of IGF-II imprinting is associated with fetal growth restriction that is thought to be secondary to placental dysfunction.[48]

41.3.2 Vascular Endothelial Growth Factor Family

Uterine vascular remodeling and continued angiogenesis through pregnancy is necessary to match blood flow to the placenta with placental growth and fetal requirements. These events are affected by the VEGF family of peptides expressed by cytotrophoblasts, the syncytiotrophoblast, and villous stromal cells in the placenta.[49] Placental growth factor (PGF) is a member of this family that shares about 50% homology with VEGF-A. It is expressed by villous and extravillous trophoblast cells. The role of these peptides is especially evident in the etiology of preeclampsia. In this disease, restricted invasion of trophoblasts into the uterine spiral arteries early in pregnancy is thought to compromise placental perfusion later in gestation.[50, 51] The resultant hypoxia increases cytotrophoblast expression of VEGF peptides, which in turn increases production of a soluble splice variant of VEGF receptor-1, sFLT-1, that binds to VEGF peptides and PGF in the maternal circulation and neutralizes their angiogenic activity.[52] Excess sFLT1 in the maternal circulation may disrupt maternal endothelium function, leading to the symptoms of preeclampsia, especially hypertension and proteinuria.[53] Circulating sFLT1 levels in the maternal blood are increased compared with normal pregnancies in women with preeclampsia,[54–56] and consequently, sFLT1 levels and the FLT1/PGF ratio have biomarker potential to assess risk for preeclampsia.[57, 58] Variants in the fetal genome near FLT1 gene are associated with the risk of preeclampsia.[59]

41.3.3 Fibroblast Growth Factor Family

Members of the fibroblast growth factor (FGF) family are expressed by villous trophoblasts and connective tissue stroma of mesenchymal villi in the human placenta,[60] and FGF receptors are expressed by placental mononuclear phagocytes (also known as Hofbauer cells).[61] FGF induces Hofbauer cells to produce multiple growth factors and cytokine involved in tissue repair. Activation of Hofbauer cells by FGF may promote placental growth by facilitating the outgrowth of syncytiotrophoblast buds.

41.3.4 Transforming Growth Factor β Family

Transforming growth factor β (TGF-β) influences both the proliferation and differentiation of trophoblast cells acting through receptors that include endoglin (ENG), a co-receptor for TGF-β1 and TGF-β3, which is expressed by the syncytiotrophoblasts and by endothelial cells. Trophoblast cells produce a soluble truncated ENG (sENG) consisting of the extracellular domain. sENG expression is upregulated in preeclampsia and may act as a decoy to sequester and block TGF-β1 binding to its endothelial cell receptor, preventing vasodilation. sENG appears to augment the endothelial dysfunction caused by elevated sFLT1.[62]

41.3.5 Activins and Inhibins

Activins and inhibins are disulfide-linked homo- and heterodimeric members of the TGF-β family that derive their names from their ability to activate or inhibit, respectively, pituitary follicle stimulating hormone (FSH) secretion. An inhibin is a heterodimer composed of an α-subunit and one of two β-subunits, βA or βB (αβA and αβB). Activins are composed of βA or βB homodimers (βAβA and βBβB). Both hormones affect target cell function via specific cell surface receptors. The capacity for activin to stimulate FSH secretion is restricted by follistatin, which binds activin and limits its bioavailability to interact with receptors on target cells. Each of the activin/inhibin subunits and follistatin are expressed in the syncytiotrophoblast, and the levels of expression do not change with advancing gestation.[63–65] Activin-A is also produced by the CL, decidua, and fetal membranes during human pregnancy. These factors are secreted into the maternal and fetal circulations and amniotic fluid, and their production varies with stage of gestation.[66]

Activins and inhibins may affect placental CG production. In cultured trophoblast cells, inhibin suppresses GnRH-induced CG expression, whereas activin augments the GnRH-induced release of CG.[67] Thus, at least in vitro, activin and inhibin via paracrine effects on placental GnRH production may contribute to the regulation of CG secretion in a manner similar to their effect on hypothalamic-pituitary gonadotropin secretion.[68] Interestingly, levels of inhibin-A and activin-A in the maternal circulation have been reported to have predictive value for pathologies such as placental tumors, hypertensive disorders of pregnancy, intrauterine growth restriction, fetal hypoxia, Down syndrome, fetal demise, preterm delivery, and intrauterine growth restriction.[69–72]

41.3.6 Epidermal Growth Factor Family

Cytotrophoblasts and the syncytiotrophoblast in the human placenta express epidermal growth factors (EGF) early in pregnancy, and the level of expression decreases with advancing gestation.[73] EGF is thought to promote trophoblast invasion during implantation, and deficiency in EGF expression and/or signaling is associated with preeclampsia and fetal growth restriction.[74, 75]

41.4 ADIPOKINES

The adipokines, leptin, adiponectin, resistin, ghrelin, and visfatin (nicotinamide phosphoribosyltransferase), are expressed by the human placenta and secreted into the maternal circulation. They are thought to regulate maternal metabolic adaptation to pregnancy, especially increased insulin resistance.[76]

Leptin levels during pregnancy are relatively high, due mainly to placental production.[77] Leptin acts in a similar manner to PL on maternal metabolism. It promotes fatty acid mobilization from adipose tissue and acts in the liver, pancreas, and muscle to decrease insulin sensitivity and mobilize glucose, thus increasing the availability nutrients for fetal use. Pregnancy is considered to be a state of hyperleptinemia and selective leptin resistance. During pregnancy, leptin effects on eating behavior, satiety, and certain metabolic activities, typically observed in the nonpregnancy sate, are lost, whereas effects on metabolism appear to be maintained.[78] Placental leptin production is abnormally high in maternal diabetes mellitus and hypertension, and umbilical leptin levels correlate with fetal adiposity.[79] As with most hormone-receptor systems in the placenta, leptin and its receptors are expressed by trophoblast cells, suggesting that it acts in a paracrine manner to modulate placental function. Consistent with this, leptin induces CG production in trophoblast cells and is also thought to increase placental growth by augmenting mitogenesis, amino acid uptake, and extracellular matrix synthesis.[80, 81]

41.5 STEROID HORMONES

For the majority of pregnancy, and especially during the second and third trimesters, the human placenta produces large amounts of progesterone and estrogens that are secreted mainly into the maternal compartment. Steroid hormone production occurs in cytotrophoblasts and the syncytiotrophoblast, and is dependent on precursors provided by the fetus and mother to form an integrated fetal-placental-maternal steroidogenic unit (Fig. 41.3).

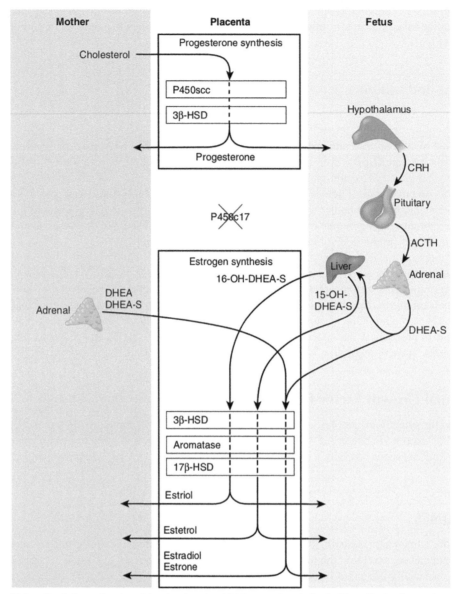

FIG. 41.3 Functional interaction between the placental and maternal and fetal compartments for the biosynthesis of progesterone and estrogens by the human placenta. Progesterone is produced mainly from maternal cholesterol. P450c17 is not expressed in the human placenta and, therefore, progesterone cannot be converted to C19 androgens. Instead, estrogens are biosynthesized from C19-androgen precursors (mainly DHEA-S) provided by the maternal and fetal adrenals. *(Fig. 11.8 from* Yen and Jaffe's Reproductive endocrinology. *8th ed., [chapter 11].)*

41.5.1 Progesterone

Progesterone is aptly referred to as the "hormone of pregnancy." In all viviparous species examined so far, it is essential for the establishment and maintenance of pregnancy. Among its critical progestational actions, progesterone prepares the endometrium for successful implantation, modulates the maternal immune system, especially at the implantation site, to accept the allogenic embryo, and for the duration of pregnancy promotes myometrial relaxation and quiescence, cervical closure, and prevents weakening of the fetal membranes. The importance of progesterone for pregnancy maintenance is demonstrated by clinical studies showing that inhibition of its activity by treatment with progesterone receptor (PR) antagonists (e.g., mifepristone) increases uterine contractility, and in most cases induces the full parturition cascade.

Before pregnancy is established and during most of the first trimester, progesterone is produced by the maternal CL. During this time, ovariectomy induces abortion. However, during weeks 6–10 of pregnancy, cytotrophoblasts and the syncytiotrophoblast begin synthesizing progesterone from maternal low-density lipoprotein cholesterol. At around the same time, progesterone production by the CL decreases. The transfer of progesterone synthesis from the CL to the placenta is referred to as the luteal-placental shift. Removal of the maternal ovaries after the luteal-placental shift does not affect the continuation of pregnancy, and for the remainder of pregnancy, the placenta is the principal source of progesterone.

The amount of progesterone secreted by the placenta increases through most of human pregnancy and appears to be a function of syncytiotrophoblast mass and synthetic capacity, and the availability of low-density lipoprotein cholesterol in the maternal circulation. Placental cells contain the cholesterol side-chain cleavage enzyme (CYP11A1), efficiently converting cholesterol into pregnenolone, which is then converted by 3β-hydroxysteroid dehydrogenase/$\Delta^{5 \to 4}$-isomerase type I (HSD3B1) into progesterone. Unlike gonadal and adrenal cortical tissue, the human placenta does not express the steroidogenic acute regulatory protein (StAR), encoded by the STARD1 gene, which controls the access of cholesterol to the inner mitochondrial membrane, where CYP11A1 and its electron transport chain reside. This is the rate-limiting step in gonadotropin- and ACTH-stimulated steroidogenesis. The fact that the human placenta does not express StAR is consistent with the absence of a rapid action trophic regulator of placental progesterone synthesis. Instead the placenta expresses a related StAR-like protein encoded by STARD3, known as metastatic lymph node 64 protein (MLN64), that acts tonically to promote cholesterol access to the inner mitochondrial membrane. Further metabolism of progesterone into 17α-hydroxyprogesterone or deoxycorticosterone in the human placenta is highly inefficient due to low to negligible expression of 17α-hydroxtlase-17/20 desmolase (CYP17A1). During the third trimester, the placenta produced 250–300 mg of progesterone per day, and maternal circulating levels of progesterone are 100–200 ng/mL (318–636 nM)[82–84] (Fig. 41.4). This is remarkably high, considering that the dissociation constant for the nuclear progesterone receptors is approximately 1 nM. Interestingly, fetal mutations in the CYP11A1 gene which markedly impair enzyme activity are still compatible with term pregnancy despite diminished placental capacity for progesterone production. In these rare cases, placental estrogen production would also be diminished due to reduced fetal adrenal DHEA synthesis, suggesting that either the CL compensates for reduced placental progesterone elaboration, or that the ratio of placental progesterone to estrogen production is critical for maintenance of gestation. It is also possible that the levels of progesterone and estrogen produced by the placenta during pregnancy far exceed the amounts needed for normal pregnancy.

The main function of placental progesterone is to maintain pregnancy by promoting uterine quiescence. In the myometrium, progesterone suppresses contractility by inhibiting the responsiveness of myometrial cells to uterotonic hormones such as oxytocin and PGF$_{2\alpha}$ (see below) and increasing the resting membrane potential. It also decreases the expression of

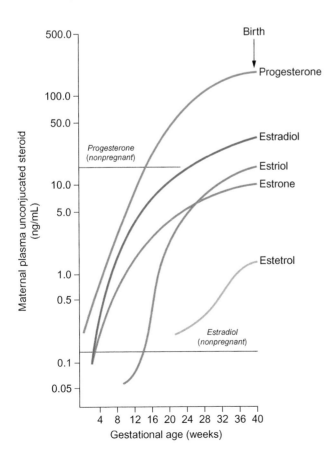

FIG. 41.4 Maternal progesterone and estrogen (estrone, estradiol, estriol, and estetrol) concentrations during human pregnancy compared with average levels in normal cycling women. *(Fig. 11.9 from* Yen and Jaffe's Reproductive endocrinology. *8th ed., [chapter 11].)*

genes encoding other contraction associated proteins such as gap junction proteins that connect myometrial cells and allow for action potential propagation and synchronous contractions.[85–87] In the uterine cervix, progesterone promotes extracellular matrix rigidity by preventing water absorption and collage dissolution in the cervical extracellular matrix.[88–91] In the decidua, progesterone exerts antiinflammatory and immunosuppressive actions to prevent maternal rejection of the adjacent fetal tissue and to prevent inflammation-induced weakening of the amnion membrane.[92, 93] Antiinflammatory actions of progesterone also occur in the myometrium and cervix.[94–98] Pro-gestation effects of progesterone are mediated by its genomic mode of action, whereby it interacts with the nuclear progesterone receptor (PR) isoforms, PR-A and PR-B, that then affect expression of specific cohorts of genes in myometrial, cervical, and decidual cells. The importance of progesterone/PR signaling for the maintenance of human pregnancy is reflected by the fact that disruption of PR signaling (e.g., by treatment with mifepristone, a PR antagonist) increases myometrial contractility and excitability, promotes cervical softening, and increases inflammatory activity in the decidua.[99–102]

Placental progesterone also may serve as substrate for the production of metabolites with specific bioactivity in the physiology of pregnancy.[103] In particular, 5β-reduced progesterone (5β-dihydroprogesterone) promotes relaxation in myometrial strips and decreases basal and oxytocin-induced contractile activity.[104–107] Circulating levels of 5β-dihydroprogesterone and expression of the 5β-reductase enzyme in the placenta and myometrium decrease in association with the onset of labor.[108] This suggests that metabolites of placental progesterone may contribute to promoting myometrial relaxation. Interestingly, some studies suggest that 5β-dihydroprogesterone (and other reduce progesterone metabolites) do not act via the nuclear PRs but instead promote myometrial quiescence by binding to other cells surface receptors such as the gamma-aminobutyric acid-A (GABA$_A$) receptor.[109, 110] Interaction of progesterone metabolites with the GABA$_A$ receptor is thought to be the main mechanism for neuroactivity of progesterone metabolites and especially their anesthetic effects.[111]

The rapid fall in progesterone with delivery serves as a key trigger for milk production, as discussed in Chapter 14.

41.5.2 Estrogens

Estrogens favor pregnancy by stimulating uterine growth and increasing uteroplacental blood flow. Estrogens also promote breast development in preparation for lactation. The human placenta produces large amounts of estrogens in the form of estrone, estradiol, estriol, and estetrol, especially during the second and third trimesters (Figs. 41.3 and 41.4). The syncytiotrophoblast synthesizes estrogens from C19 steroids, primarily dehydroepiandrosterone (DHEA), derived mainly from the fetal compartments, a symbiotic interaction referred to as the *fetoplacental steroidogenic unit* (Fig. 41.3). The syncytiotrophoblast has a remarkably high capacity to convert DHEA to estrogens due to high levels of expression of aromatase (CYP19A1), but lacks the capacity to synthesize estrogens de novo from cholesterol. Thus placental estrogen synthesis is directly affected by the availability of DHEA. Throughout pregnancy, maternal DHEA is also used for placental estrogen synthesis. However, at 12–15 weeks of pregnancy, the fetal adrenal glands begin to produce sulfated DHEA (DHEA-S) in response to fetal pituitary ACTH. The syncytiotrophoblast removes the sulfate and converts DHEA to estradiol and estrone. The DHEA-S synthetic activity of the fetal hypothalamic-pituitary-adrenal axis increases significantly with advancing gestation and surpasses maternal DHEA levels such that in the latter half of pregnancy ~90% of estrogens in the maternal blood are derived from placental aromatization of fetal adrenal DHEA-S.[112] Thus the exponential increase in maternal estrogens during human pregnancy is attributable directly to the steroidogenic activity of the fetal hypothalamic-pituitary adrenal axis.

The fetal liver expresses the 16α-hydroxylase enzyme that converts DHEA-S to 16α-hydroxy-DHEA-S (16αOH-DHEA-S). Hepatic 16α-hydroxylase activity decreases soon after birth and is minimal during postnatal life. 16αOH-DHEA-S production increases with advancing gestation, mainly due to increased DHEA-S substrate from the fetal adrenal glands. 16αOH-DHEA-S is metabolized by the syncytiotrophoblast to estriol. Estriol production by the placenta increases with advancing gestation, and ranges from approximately 2 mg/day at 26 weeks to 35–45 mg/day at term. In contrast, ovarian production of estriol in nonpregnant women is barely detectable. Consequently, the level of estriol in the maternal circulation reflects the activity of fetal hypothalamic-pituitary adrenal axis.[113]

The fetal liver can also 15-hydroxylate C19 steroids, resulting in placental production of estetrol from 15-hydroxy-DHEA. Estetrol levels increase as pregnancy progresses, particularly after 30 weeks of gestation, and the increases occur more rapidly than estriol in both blood and urine. Interestingly, estetrol levels are higher in the fetus than in the maternal compartment.[114]

The role of placental estrogens in the physiology of human pregnancy is unclear. In most biological systems, estriol is a weak estrogen with approximately 1% the potency of estradiol. However, estriol is as effective as estradiol and estrone in promoting uteroplacental blood flow,[115] suggesting a specialized role during pregnancy. Estetrol has been proposed to be a selective estrogen receptor modulator; it may protect fetal tissues from the action of other more potent estrogens.

Conditions of placental estrogen deficiency or excess show that placental estrogens are not necessary for normal pregnancy outcome. Pregnancy and parturition are normal in pregnancies bearing a fetus that produces excessive DHEA-S due to congenital adrenal hyperplasia arising from 21-hydroxylase deficiency.[116–119] Similarly, pregnancy and parturition timing are not affected by abnormalities that decrease placental estrogen production, such as anencephaly or placental aromatase deficiency.[120–124] Thus high levels of placental estrogens are not essential for normal pregnancy and parturition. It is important to note that maternal estrogen level in all cases of placental estrogen deficiency were low but not absent. Levels in most cases were in a physiologically relevant range (1–1.6 nmol/L)[122, 125] and comparable to levels reached in the midcycle and luteal phase of the menstrual cycle (0.6–2 nmol/L). It is also noteworthy that no conditions are known in which pregnancy occurs in the complete absence of estrogens. This suggests that a minimal level of estrogen is necessary for human pregnancy and that the excessive levels produced by the placenta are redundant.

Estrogen metabolites, other than the major metabolites produced by the fetal placental-unit, and found in maternal blood during pregnancy, may have important pro- and antiangiogenic activities. These metabolites include 2-methoxyestradiol and 2-methoxyestrone, which have antiangiogenic activity, and 16-keto-estradiol and 4-hydroxyestrone, which have proangiogenic activity in vitro.[126–129] The catechol estrogens, particularly 2-methoxyestradiol, are produced from catechol estrogens, generated mainly by the action of cytochrome P4501A1, with the catechol estrogens subsequently being methylated by catechol-*O*-methyltransferase. The biological activity of 2-methoxyestradiol includes its ability to antagonize hypoxia-inducible factor-1α (HIF-1α), a major transcription factor driving expression of VEGF. 2-Methoxyestradiol downregulates HIF-1α expression and prevents HIF-1α translocation into the nucleus. In human pregnancies complicated by preeclampsia, 2-methoxyestradiol levels are reduced in maternal blood, suggesting that a state of accentuated response to reduced perfusion and hypoxia may contribute to preeclampsia. 16-Ketoestradiol, 16α-hydroxyestrone, and 4-hydroxyestrone have proangiogenic activity in vitro, and in the case of the 16-oxo molecules correlated with systolic blood pressure in nonpregnant women. However, these metabolites have not been well studied in pregnancy. 4-Hydroxyestrone was found to be elevated in severe preeclampsia, while 16α-hydroxyestrone was higher in mild preeclampsia, and 16-keto-estradiol-17β levels were significantly higher in severe preeclampsia. The molecular mechanisms underlying the proangiogenic effects of these estrogen metabolites are not known.

41.5.3 Glucocorticoid Metabolism

The syncytiotrophoblast plays an important role in regulating the passage of maternal steroid hormones into the fetal compartment. For most of pregnancy the placenta expresses the 11β-hydroxysteroid dehydrogenase type 2 (11β-HSD-2) enzyme, which converts cortisol to cortisone, thereby inactivating its glucocorticoid activity.[130, 131] This biochemical barrier serves to prevent exposure of the fetus to maternal cortisol that could interfere with the fetal HPA activity.[132–134] To circumvent the placental barrier to maternal cortisol, synthetic glucocorticoids such as betamethasone and dexamethasone, which are not metabolized by 11β-HSD2, are used clinically in cases of threatened preterm birth to promote maturation of fetal organ systems, especially the lungs. On the other hand, as noted in Chapter 25, very high endogenous levels of cortisol from Cushing syndrome, or from use of high pharmacological doses of hydrocortisone, may overwhelm the capacity of placental 11β-HSD2 and lead to exposure of the fetus to high cortisol.

41.6 LIPID MEDIATORS

The placenta influences the maternal plasma lipidome through (1) uptake of free fatty acids and lipoproteins for transfer of their lipid components to the fetus; (2) metabolism of circulating maternal lipids into bioactive compounds (e.g., lipoprotein-carried cholesterol is metabolized into progesterone by the syncytiotrophoblast); and (3) release or secretion of lipids in the form of microvesicles (e.g., exosomes) limited by a lipid membrane derived either from the plasma membrane or endosomal vesicles, or secretion of lipid products produced in the placenta and fetal membranes (e.g., prostanoids) derived from enzyme-catalyzed reactions (e.g., cyclooxygenases [COXs] and lipoxygenases [LOXs]), as well as nonenzymatic processes like lipid peroxidation (e.g., formation of isoprostanes). Pathological states such as gestational diabetes and preeclampsia alter the maternal lipidome, impacting maternal physiology. The development of untargeted mass spectrometry-based methods to assess the plasma lipidome promises to yield new biomarkers for pregnancy-related conditions and longitudinal assessment of placental function.

41.6.1 Prostanoids

Prostanoids are COX-derived products that have been the most studied bioactive lipids produced by the placenta and fetal membranes (Fig. 41.5). Although they mainly act locally (e.g., fetal membrane prostanoids acting on the myometrium),

H.N. peiris et aL /Placenta 54 (2017) 95–103 97

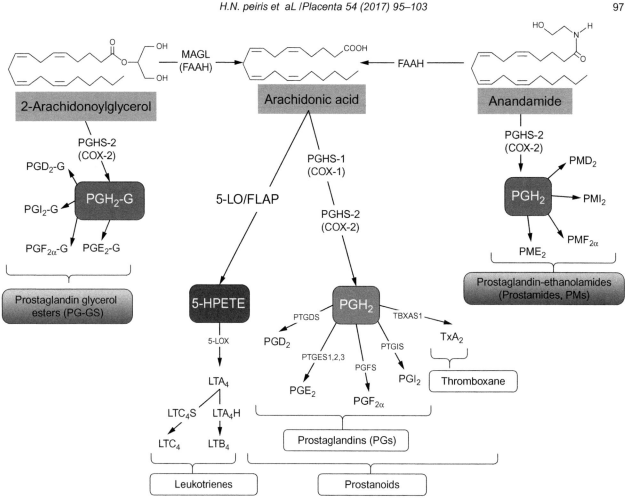

FIG. 41.5 The metabolism of arachidonic acid into prostanoids, leukotrienes, prostaglandin glycerol esters, and prostamides. *(From Peiris, et al.* Placenta *2017;54:95–103 with permission.)*

they are released into the maternal circulation and can affect the function of maternal vascular tissue and formed blood elements. Prostanoids also play an important role in the fetus, for example by promoting closure of the ductus arteriosus.

Prostanoids are synthesized de novo when cells are activated by hormonal or mechanical stimuli. The first and often rate-limiting step in eicosanoid (20-carbon lipid compounds) biosynthesis is the release of arachidonic acid from phospholipids.[135, 136] This process is regulated by a number of enzymes, particularly several types of phospholipase A2 (PLA2).[137] There at least three types of PLA2: the Ca^{2+}-independent PLA2 involved in the liberation of arachidonic acid and other polyunsaturated fatty acids from membrane phospholipids, the Ca^{2+}-dependent cytosolic PLA2 activated by receptor-ligand interactions, and secreted PLA2 family members.

After release from membrane phospholipids, arachidonic acid is transformed enzymatically through multiple pathways. One pathway is initiated by the enzyme PGH synthase (PGHS, also known as COX)[138] and results in the production of PGs, thromboxane (TX), and prostacyclin (PGI_2). The initial cyclized fatty acid derivative formed in this reaction is PG G_2 (PGG_2). The peroxide moiety at the 15-carbon position of PGG_2 is subsequently reduced to an alcohol group to form PGH_2 as a result of the inherent peroxidase activity of PGHS. Both PGG_2 and PGH_2 are unstable intermediates with very short half-lives. The production of specific PGs depends on the local expression of specific PG-synthesizing enzymes.[138, 139] Two COX enzymes, COX-1 and COX-2, that initiate the formation of PGs are encoded by separate genes.[138, 140] COX-1 is largely constitutively expressed, whereas the COX-2 is more often inducible by cytokines, growth factors, and hormones. This categorization as constitutive COX-1 and inducible COX-2 is useful, but is not always accurate. The subsequent conversion of PGH_2 to individual prostanoids is relatively tissue-specific and is catalyzed by the corresponding isomerases and synthases.[140] Anandamide, another lipid molecule, is converted by COX-2 and PGH2 into prostaglandin-ethanolamines (prostamides), which have not been well-studied with respect to pregnancy.

The second major pathway of arachidonic acid metabolism is initiated by LOX. Like COXs, LOXs are dioxygenases that catalyze the insertion of molecular oxygen into arachidonic acid to form a hydroperoxyl derivative.[141]

Arachidonic acid can also be metabolized through the activity of cytochrome P450 enzymes.[142] Unlike the COX or LOX enzymes, cytochrome P450 enzymes catalyze the mono-oxygenation (insertion of one atom of oxygen from O_2) of arachidonic acid, with hydroxy- or epoxy-derivatives of arachidonic acid as their major products.[142] Some cytochrome P450-derived epoxy metabolites of arachidonic acid are elevated in women with pregnancy-induced hypertension,[143] and others may have antiinflammatory activities.[144]

Peroxidation of arachidonic acid and cyclization to PG-like compounds called *isoprostanes* can also occur nonenzymatically by free radical-catalyzed reactions. The F_2-isoprostane, 8-epi-PGF$_{2\alpha}$, is an example of one of these molecules that is elevated in the plasma of women with severe preeclampsia. Urine and plasma isoprostane levels have proven to be reliable markers of lipid peroxidation and oxidant stress in vivo.[145, 146]

There are at least two types of glutathione-dependent PGE$_2$ synthases.[147–150] One is PGE$_2$ synthase, cPGES, a constitutively expressed cytosolic enzyme functionally coupled to COX-1; the other is a microsomal and inducible enzyme, mPGES-1, which appears to be coupled to COX-2.[147–150] Another enzyme, mPGES-2, is less well characterized, and its role in PGE2 synthesis is unclear.[151]

Although eicosanoids are lipid compounds, they do not permeate the cell membrane freely. A PG transporter (PGT), belonging to the organic anion transporter polypeptide family, has been identified and is found in a limited range of cells, where it is subject to humoral and physical stimuli.[152] PGT mediates the cellular uptake of most prostanoids, but not PGI$_2$.[152] On the other hand, multidrug-resistance protein 4 (MRP4) functions as a PG efflux transporter.[153]

A hallmark of prostanoids is their short lifespan. PGI$_2$ and TX$_{A2}$ are chemically unstable and are degraded spontaneously through hydrolysis in aqueous solutions. TX$_{A2}$ rapidly undergoes hydrolysis to form the inactive product TX$_{B2}$. Plasma or urinary TX$_{B2}$ metabolites have served as useful indices of TX$_{A2}$ formation in vivo.

The most important catabolic step for PGs is the conversion of the 15-hydroxy group to a 15-keto group by a NAD(+)-dependent 15-hydroxyprostaglandin dehydrogenase (15-OH-PGDH).[154] 15-OH-PGDH is a cytosolic protein with highest concentrations in the placenta. PGE$_2$ and PGF$_{2\alpha}$ are excellent substrates for 15-OH-PGDH.[154] The second notable step in the degradation of PGs is reduction of the double bond at position 13 by $\Delta^{13,14}$-PG reductase. This enzyme has a tissue distribution similar to that of 15-OH-PGDH.

There are 13 distinct eicosanoid receptors cloned and characterized: 9 for COX-derived prostanoids and 4 for LTs.[155–157] All eicosanoid receptors characterized so far are rhodopsin-like, seven transmembrane domain-containing, G-protein-coupled receptors.[156, 157] The nine G-protein-coupled prostanoid receptors, conserved in mammals from mouse to human, are the TX receptor (TP), the prostacyclin receptor (IP), the PGF$_{2\alpha}$ receptor (FP), two PGD receptors (DP1 and DP2), and four PGE2 receptors (EP1, EP2, EP3, and EP4). These receptors are encoded by separate genes. In addition, there are several splice variants for the EP3, FP, and TP receptors, which differ only in their C-terminal tails.[157–161]

Although there is high ligand selectivity for each of the prostanoid receptors, cross-activation by prostanoids other than the cognate ligand may occur; coupling to alternative downstream signaling pathways at different concentrations of the same ligand may also take place.[156, 161] The multiplicity in prostanoid receptor subtypes and signaling pathways, coupled with their differential tissue expression, explains why the same PG at different concentrations or in different tissues can sometimes produce opposing effects.

41.6.2 Prostanoids and Parturition

There is an abrupt increase in amniotic fluid prostanoid concentrations (particularly PGF$_{2\alpha}$, which increases 25-fold) before the onset of spontaneous labor at term.[162] Prostacyclin is the predominant prostanoid in nonlaboring and laboring myometrium, with PGD$_2$ and PGF$_{2\alpha}$ being the second most abundant, suggesting that PGF$_{2\alpha}$ plays an important role in parturition, while the increase in PGE$_2$ probably facilitates relaxation of the lower uterine segment myometrium and cervical dilation.[163]

Aspirin-like drugs, which inhibit COX enzymes, were shown to delay parturition in humans >30 years ago,[164] and nonsteroidal antiinflammatory drugs (NSAIDs) are also well known to be effective agents in attenuating the progression of term and preterm labor in various species.[165, 166] PGE$_2$ and PGF$_{2\alpha}$, stimulate uterine contractions in vitro and in vivo; they also promote the coordinated inflammatory response that results in dilation and thinning of the cervix.[167]

Although COX-1 is involved in term labor, COX-2 induction is likely to be primarily responsible for PG-mediated preterm labor. COX-2, but not COX-1, is induced during inflammation-mediated preterm labor elicited by lipopolysaccharide (LPS) administration.[168] Indomethacin, an inhibitor of both COX-1 and COX-2, has been used successfully in treating human preterm labor, both when given systemically and when delivered locally through the vaginal route.[169, 170] The clinical utility of indomethacin as a tocolytic agent, however, is tempered by concerns over fetal and neonatal complications, such as constriction of the ductus arteriosus.[169, 170] The adverse effects associated with indomethacin use in preterm labor have been mainly linked to inhibition of COX-2 based on mouse studies using selective COX-1 and COX-2 inhibitors.[171, 172]

41.6.3 Prostanoids and Pregnancy-Induced Hypertension/Preeclampsia

The possible involvement of placenta PGs in pregnancy-induced hypertension (PIH) and preeclampsia, and the potential therapeutic efficacy of low-dose aspirin in their prophylactic treatment, have received considerable attention. Although the exact cause of the disease is unknown, dysregulated production of PGI_2 and TX_{A2} has been postulated as one of many potential etiologic factors.[173] Decreased urinary PGI_2 metabolites are found to precede the development of PIH,[174] and increased TX_{A2} metabolite excretion occurs in patients with severe preeclampsia.[175, 176] Such changes may predispose to vasoconstriction of small arteries, activation of platelets, and uteroplacental insufficiency—clinical outcomes that are associated with PIH and preeclampsia. Clinical trials have been conducted to evaluate the use of aspirin in the prevention of preeclampsia. A metaanalysis revealed that aspirin reduces the risk of preterm preeclampsia, but not term preeclampsia, when it is initiated at ≤16 weeks of gestation at a daily dose of ≥100 mg.[177, 178] Moreover, in pregnancies at high risk of preeclampsia, aspirin treatment reduced the length of stay in the neonatal intensive care unit by approximately 70%, due to the reduction in the births at <32 weeks' gestation.[179] Aspirin also appears to reduce the risk of placental abruption and antepartum hemorrhage.[178] Based on the existing literature, the US Preventive Services Task Force recommends low-dose aspirin for prevention of preeclampsia among women at high risk.

41.6.4 Other Lipid Mediators

Other lipid mediators have been implicated in reproductive function, including the lysophospholipids, lysophosphatidic acid (LPA), and sphingosine-1-phosphate (S1P).[180, 181] These lipids may, in part, originate from the placenta and are postulated to have significant roles in pregnancy, but their roles in normal and pregnancy and pregnancy complications are less well studied than roles and actions of the prostanoids.

41.7 EXTRAVILLOUS TROPHOBLASTS, SYNCYTIAL FRAGMENTS, MICROVESICLES, EXOSOMES, AND CELL FREE NUCLEIC ACIDS

Extravillous trophoblasts, placental cell fragments, including apoptotic bodies, and vesicles containing placental cell nuclear and cytoplasmic material enter into the maternal blood stream and are distributed throughout the maternal circulation. Once thought to be merely debris, there is now consensus that these placental products perform important regulatory functions in the maternal compartment (Fig. 41.6).[182] The best characterized placental "deported" products are placental exosomes and cell-free nucleic acids.

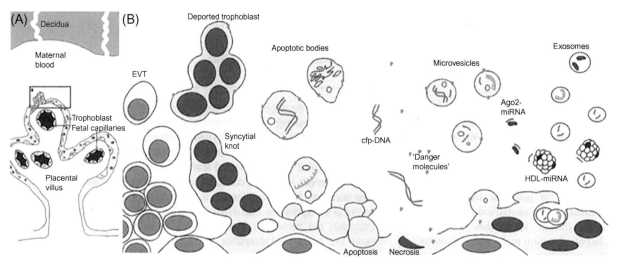

FIG. 41.6 Placental material released into the maternal circulation. (A) Placental villous. (B) Cytotrophoblast and syncytiotrophoblast and their deported products. *Arg2*, argonaute-2 protein; *cfpDNA*, cell free placental DNA; *EVT*, extravillous trophoblast; *HDL*, high density lipoprotein; *miRNA*, microRNA. *(From Manokhina I, Wilson SL, Robinson WP. Noninvasive nucleic acid-based approaches to monitor placental health and predict pregnancy-related complications.* Am J Obstet Gynecol *2015;**213(4 Suppl.)**:S197–206.)*

41.7.1 Exosomes

Exosomes are 30–100 nm extracellular spherical or cup-shaped vesicles, enriched with certain proteins, including CD9, CD63, and CD81, that contain biologically active signaling factors in the form of nucleic acids (messenger RNA, microRNA, and noncoding RNA), proteins and lipids. Exosomes exert biological effects by fusing with the target cell plasma membrane and depositing their cargo of bioactive factors into the cytoplasm.[183] Villous trophoblasts and the syncytiotrophoblast produce exosomes that are shed via endosomal trafficking primarily into the maternal compartment.[184] Placental exosomes can been detected in the maternal circulation from the 6th week of gestation, and their levels increase gradually with advancing gestation in proportion to the increased size of the placenta[184] (Fig. 41.7). In this context, placental exosomes may be critical vectors for communication from the fetus/placenta to the mother via the packaging of a specific cargo of signaling molecules. MicroRNAs in placental exosomes affect the function of local immune cells to boost resistance to viral infection.[185–188] Levels of exosomes (placental and nonplacental) in the maternal circulation and the composition of their cargo has been associated with pregnancy complications such as preeclampsia, preterm birth, intrauterine growth restriction, and gestational diabetes.[189] This suggests that the content of placental exosomes can be used as biomarkers to predict specific pregnancy complications.

41.7.2 Cell-Free Fetal Nucleic Acids

Cell-free DNA (cfDNA) originates in trophoblast cells and can be assayed in the maternal blood as biomarkers of placental health and function.[190, 191] cfDNA is detectable in the maternal circulation from around the 7th week of gestation, and the amount increases with advancing gestation such that late in pregnancy it represents ~4% of the cfDNA in maternal blood.[192] After delivery of the placenta, the amount of cfDNA in maternal blood rapidly decreases. The physiologic role of cfDNA and why it is shed from trophoblast cells into the maternal compartment is not known. The amount of cfDNA in maternal blood has been used as a biomarker of placental health, with increases in cfDNA noted in nonviable pregnancies, preeclampsia, and intrauterine growth restriction associated with placental insufficiency. It is hyothesized that declining telomere length of cfDNA derived from the placenta represents a signal of placental senescence and that lacenta-derived reduced telomere length of cfDNA is a trigger for parturition through its ability to stimulate the innate immune system via toll-like receptor 9 (TLR9).[193] This model supports the notion of a placental "biological clock" that links placental age/senescence with the timing of birth via activation of local inflammatory pathways.

Because it can be isolated and sequenced, cfDNA is used for noninvasive prenatal diagnosis, and testing for conditions such as X-linked genetic disorders and aneuploidies, as well as fetal sex determination.[194]

Cell-free mRNA derived from the placenta has been detected in maternal blood by 8 weeks of gestation.[195] The cell-free mRNA has been evaluated quantitatively for specific transcripts, particularly those encoding proteins expressed uniquely by the placenta (e.g., CG β-subunit, PL, PLAC4). It has been found that some of these transcript levels in maternal blood are

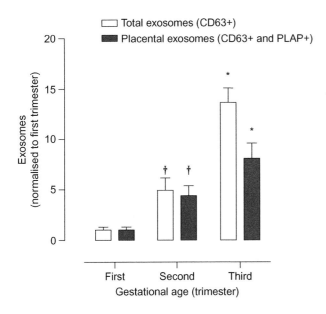

FIG. 41.7 Exosomes in maternal blood by trimester. Total exosomes (CD63+) and placental exosomes (CD63+ and containing placental alkaline phosphatase (PLAP) are shown. *(From Mitchell MD, Peiris HN, Kobayashi M, Koh YQ, Duncombe G, Illanes SE, et al. Placental exosomes in normal and complicated pregnancy. Am J Obstet Gynecol 2015;213(4 Suppl.):S173–81 with permission.)*

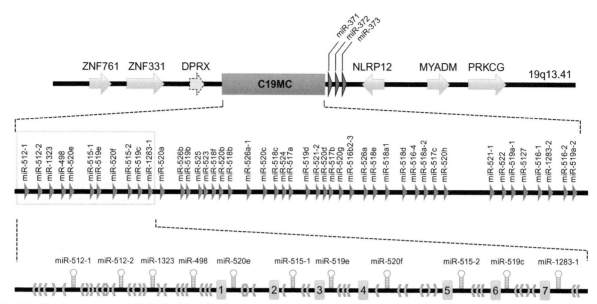

FIG. 41.8 The human genomic C19MC microRNA cluster and the position of microRNA genes (middle section). The bottom panel shows an enlargement of the 5′ end of the region, showing genes *(green)*, the microRNA cluster *(orange)*, and individual microRNAs. The light blue chevrons denote Alu sequences in an antisense orientation and the dark blue chevrons in a sense orientation. The seven first-expressed exons are indicated by green rectangles. *(From Mouillet JF, Ouyang Y, Coyne CB, Sadovsky Y. MicroRNAs in placental health and disease. Am J Obstet Gynecol 2015;213(4 Suppl): S163–72, with permission).*

elevated in preeclampsia and intrauterine growth restriction. These analyses are confounded by the relative instability of mRNA.

MicroRNAs, short noncoding single strand RNA molecules, are known to be epigenetic factors regulating gene expression by targeting specific sequences in mRNAs and destabilizing the transcripts and/or inhibiting or reducing translation. The microRNAs released from the placenta may be incorporated into microvesicles, including exosomes, in apoptotic bodies, or protein-bound. The placenta-derived microRNAs are thought to influence maternal gene expression, particularly in vascular endothelial cells. The placental-specific microRNAs include those encoded in clusters on chromosomes 14 and 19, with the best studied being the microRNAs from the chromosome 19 cluster (C19MC)[196] (Fig. 41.8). Alterations in levels of specific microRNAs in maternal blood have been reported on nonviable pregnancies and preeclampsia.[182]

REFERENCES

1. Licht P, Fluhr H, Neuwinger J, Wallwiener D, Wildt L. Is human chorionic gonadotropin directly involved in the regulation of human implantation? *Mol Cell Endocrinol* 2007;**269**(1–2):85–92.
2. Banerjee P, Fazleabas AT. Extragonadal actions of chorionic gonadotropin. *Rev Endocr Metab Disord* 2011;**12**(4):323–32.
3. Gibbons JM, Mitnick M, Chieffo V. In vitro biosynthesis of TSH- and LH-releasing factors by the human placenta. *Am J Obstet Gynecol* 1975;**121**(1):127–31.
4. Siler-Khodr TM, Khodr GS, Valenzuela G. Immunoreactive gonadotropin-releasing hormone level in maternal circulation throughout pregnancy. *Am J Obstet Gynecol* 1984;**150**(4):376–9.
5. McLean M, Smith R. Corticotropin-releasing hormone in human pregnancy and parturition. *Trends Endocrinol Metab* 1999;**10**(5):174–8.
6. Goland RS, Wardlaw SL, Stark RI, Brown LSJ, Frantz AG. High levels of corticotropin-releasing hormone immunoactivity in maternal and fetal plasma during pregnancy. *J Clin Endocrinol Metab* 1986;**63**:1199–203.
7. Frim DM, Emanuel RL, Robinson BG, Smas CM, Adler GK, Majzoub JA. Characterization and gestational regulation of corticotropin-releasing hormone messenger RNA in human placenta. *J Clin Invest* 1988;**82**:287–92.
8. McLean M, Bisits A, Davies J, Walters W, Hackshaw A, De Voss K, et al. Predicting risk of preterm delivery by second-trimester measurement of maternal plasma corticotropin-releasing hormone and alpha-fetoprotein concentrations. *Am J Obstet Gynecol* 1999;**181**:207–15.
9. McLean M, Bisits A, Davies J, Woods R, Lowry P, Smith R. A placental clock controlling the length of human pregnancy. *Nat Med* 1995;**1**:460–3.
10. Petraglia F, Sutton S, Vale W. Neurotransmitters and peptides modulate the release of immunoreactive corticotropin-releasing factor from cultured human placental cells. *Am J Obstet Gynecol* 1989;**160**(1):247–51.

11. Ni X, Chan EC, Fitter JT, Smith R. Nitric oxide inhibits corticotropin-releasing hormone exocytosis but not synthesis by cultured human trophoblasts. *J Clin Endocrinol Metab* 1997;**82**(12):4171–5.

12. Robinson BG, Emanuel RL, Frim DM, Majzoub JA. Glucocorticoid stimulates expression of corticotropin-releasing hormone gene in human placenta. *Proc Natl Acad Sci U S A* 1988;**85**(14):5244–8.

13. Korebrits C, Yu DH, Ramirez MM, Marinoni E, Bocking AD, Challis JR. Antenatal glucocorticoid administration increases corticotrophin-releasing hormone in maternal plasma. *Br J Obstet Gynaecol* 1998;**105**(5):556–61.

14. Marinoni E, Korebrits C, Di Iorio R, Cosmi EV, Challis JR. Effect of betamethasone in vivo on placental corticotropin-releasing hormone in human pregnancy. *Am J Obstet Gynecol* 1998;**178**(4):770–8.

15. Smith R, Mesiano S, Chan EC, Brown S, Jaffe RB. Corticotropin-releasing hormone directly and preferentially stimulates dehydroepiandrosterone sulfate secretion by human fetal adrenal cortical cells. *J Clin Endocrinol Metab* 1998;**83**(8):2916–20.

16. Chakravorty A, Mesiano S, Jaffe RB. Corticotropin-releasing hormone stimulates P450 17alpha-hydroxylase/17,20-lyase in human fetal adrenal cells via protein kinase C. *J Clin Endocrinol Metab* 1999;**84**(10):3732–8.

17. Ibanez L, Potau N, Marcos MV, de Zegher F. Corticotropin-releasing hormone as adrenal androgen secretagogue. *Pediatr Res* 1999;**46**(3):351–3.

18. Glynn BP, Wolton A, Rodriguez-Linares B, Phaneuf S, Linton EA. Urocortin in pregnancy. *Am J Obstet Gynecol* 1998;**179**(2):533–9.

19. Clifton VL, Read MA, Leitch IM, Giles WB, Boura AL, Robinson PJ, et al. Corticotropin-releasing hormone-induced vasodilatation in the human fetal-placental circulation: involvement of the nitric oxide-cyclic guanosine 3′,5′-monophosphate-mediated pathway. *J Clin Endocrinol Metab* 1995;**80**(10):2888–93.

20. Leitch IM, Boura AL, Botti C, Read MA, Walters WA, Smith R. Vasodilator actions of urocortin and related peptides in the human perfused placenta in vitro. *J Clin Endocrinol Metab* 1998;**83**(12):4510–3.

21. Petraglia F, Florio P, Benedetto C, Marozio L, Di_Blasio AM, Ticconi C, et al. Urocortin stimulates placental adrenocorticotropin and prostaglandin release and myometrial contractility in vitro. *J Clin Endocrinol Metab* 1999;**84**(4):1420–3.

22. Karteris E, Vatish M, Hillhouse EW, Grammatopoulos DK. Preeclampsia is associated with impaired regulation of the placental nitric oxide-cyclic guanosine monophosphate pathway by corticotropin-releasing hormone (CRH) and CRH-related peptides. *J Clin Endocrinol Metab* 2005;**90**(6):3680–7.

23. Chen CL, Chang CC, Krieger DT, Bardin CW. Expression and regulation of proopiomelanocortin-like gene in the ovary and placenta: comparison with the testis. *Endocrinology* 1986;**118**(6):2382–9.

24. Grigorakis SI, Anastasiou E, Dai K, Souvatzoglou A, Alevizaki M. Three mRNA transcripts of the proopiomelanocortin gene in human placenta at term. *Eur J Endocrinol* 2000;**142**(5):533–6.

25. Sastry BV, Barnwell SL, Tayeb OS, Janson VE, Owens LK. Occurrence of methionine enkephalin in human placental villus. *Biochem Pharmacol* 1980;**29**(3):475–8.

26. Valette A, Desprat R, Cros J, Pontonnier G, Belisle S, Lemaire S. Immunoreactive dynorphine in maternal blood, umbilical vein and amniotic fluid. *Neuropeptides* 1986;**7**(2):145–51.

27. Ahmed MS, Horst MA. Opioid receptors of human placental villi modulate acetylcholine release. *Life Sci* 1986;**39**(6):535–40.

28. Anthony RV, Limesand SW, Fanning MD, Liang R. Placental lactogen and growth hormone. In: Bazer FW, editor. *The endocrinology of pregnancy*. Totowa: Humana Press Inc; 1998. p. 461–90.

29. Liebhaber SA, Urbanek M, Ray J, Tuan RS, Cooke NE. Characterization and histologic localization of human growth hormone-variant gene expression in the placenta. *J Clin Invest* 1989;**83**(6):1985–91.

30. Kaplan SL, Gurpide E, Sciarra JJ, Grumbach MM. Metabolic clearance rate and production rate of chorionic growth hormone-prolactin in late pregnancy. *J Clin Endocrinol Metab* 1968;**28**(10):1450–60.

31. Crosignani PG, Nencioni T, Brambati B. Concentration of chorionic gonadotrophin and chorionic somatomammotrophin in maternal serum, amniotic fluid and cord blood serum at term. *J Obstet Gynaecol Br Commonw* 1972;**79**(2):122–6.

32. Hoshina M, Boothby M, Boime I. Cytological localization of chorionic gonadotropin alpha and placental lactogen mRNAs during development of the human placenta. *J Cell Biol* 1982;**93**(1):190–8.

33. Frankenne F, Closset J, Gomez F, Scippo ML, Smal J, Hennen G. The physiology of growth hormones (GHs) in pregnant women and partial characterization of the placental GH variant. *J Clin Endocrinol Metab* 1988;**66**(6):1171–80.

34. Jeske W, Soszynski P, Rogozinski W, Lukaszewicz E, Latoszewska W, Snochowska H. Plasma GHRH, CRH, ACTH, beta-endorphin, human placental lactogen, GH and cortisol concentrations at the third trimester of pregnancy. *Acta Endocrinol* 1989;**120**(6):785–9.

35. Gillmer MD, Oakley NW, Beard RW, Brooke FM, Brudenell M, Chard T. Plasma human placental lactogen profiles over 24 hours in normal and diabetic pregnancy. *Br J Obstet Gynaecol* 1977;**84**(3):197–204.

36. Tyson JE, Austin K, Farinholt J, Fiedler J. Endocrine-metabolic response to acute starvation in human gestation. *Am J Obstet Gynecol* 1976;**125**(8):1073–84.

37. Hochberg Z, Perlman R, Brandes JM, Benderli A. Insulin regulates placental lactogen and estradiol secretion by cultured human term trophoblast. *J Clin Endocrinol Metab* 1983;**57**(6):1311–3.

38. Rygaard K, Revol A, Esquivel-Escobedo D, Beck BL, Barrera-Saldana HA. Absence of human placental lactogen and placental growth hormone (HGH-V) during pregnancy: PCR analysis of the deletion. *Hum Genet* 1998;**102**(1):87–92.

39. Samaan N, Yen SC, Gonzalez D, Pearson OH. Metabolic effects of placental lactogen (HPL) in man. *J Clin Endocrinol Metab* 1968;**28**(4):485–91.

40. Deal CL, Guyda HJ, Lai WH, Posner BI. Ontogeny of growth factor receptors in the human placenta. *Pediatr Res* 1982;**16**(10):820–6.

41. Bowen JM, Chamley L, Keelan JA, Mitchell MD. Cytokines of the placenta and extra-placental membranes: roles and regulation during human pregnancy and parturition. *Placenta* 2002;**23**(4):257–73.

42. Demendi C, Borzsonyi B, Nagy ZB, Rigo Jr J, Pajor A, Joo JG. Gene expression patterns of insulin-like growth factor 1, 2 (IGF-1, IGF-2) and insulin-like growth factor binding protein 3 (IGFBP-3) in human placenta from preterm deliveries: influence of additional factors. *Eur J Obstet Gynecol Reprod Biol* 2012;**160**(1):40–4.

43. Sferruzzi-Perri AN, Vaughan OR, Forhead AJ, Fowden AL. Hormonal and nutritional drivers of intrauterine growth. *Curr Opin Clin Nutr Metab Care* 2013;**16**(3):298–309.

44. Constancia M, Hemberger M, Hughes J, Dean W, Ferguson_Smith A, Fundele R, et al. Placental-specific IGF-II is a major modulator of placental and fetal growth. *Nature* 2002;**417**:945–8.

45. Crossey PA, Pillai CC, Miell JP. Altered placental development and intrauterine growth restriction in IGF binding protein-1 transgenic mice. *J Clin Invest* 2002;**110**(3):411–8.

46. Wu HK, Squire JA, Song Q, Weksberg R. Promoter-dependent tissue-specific expressive nature of imprinting gene, insulin-like growth factor II, in human tissues. *Biochem Biophys Res Commun* 1997;**233**(1):221–6.

47. Eggenschwiler J, Ludwig T, Fisher P, Leighton PA, Tilghman SM, Efstratiadis A. Mouse mutant embryos overexpressing IGF-II exhibit phenotypic features of the Beckwith-Wiedemann and Simpson-Golabi-Behmel syndromes. *Genes Dev* 1997;**11**(23):3128–42.

48. Koukoura O, Sifakis S, Soufla G, Zaravinos A, Apostolidou S, Jones A, et al. Loss of imprinting and aberrant methylation of IGF2 in placentas from pregnancies complicated with fetal growth restriction. *Int J Mol Med* 2011;**28**(4):481–7.

49. Clark DE, Smith SK, Sharkey AM, Charnock_Jones DS. Localization of VEGF and expression of its receptors flt and KDR in human placenta throughout pregnancy. *Hum Reprod* 1996;**11**(5):1090–8.

50. Zhou Y, Damsky CH, Chiu K, Roberts JM, Fisher SJ. Preeclampsia is associated with abnormal expression of adhesion molecules by invasive cytotrophoblasts. *J Clin Invest* 1993;**91**(3):950–60.

51. Meekins JW, Pijnenborg R, Hanssens M, McFadyen IR, van Asshe A. A study of placental bed spiral arteries and trophoblast invasion in normal and severe pre-eclamptic pregnancies. *Br J Obstet Gynaecol* 1994;**101**(8):669–74.

52. Kendall RL, Thomas KA. Inhibition of vascular endothelial cell growth factor activity by an endogenously encoded soluble receptor. *Proc Natl Acad Sci U S A* 1993;**90**(22):10705–9.

53. Zhou Y, McMaster M, Woo K, Janatpour M, Perry J, Karpanen T, et al. Vascular endothelial growth factor ligands and receptors that regulate human cytotrophoblast survival are dysregulated in severe preeclampsia and hemolysis, elevated liver enzymes, and low platelets syndrome. *Am J Pathol* 2002;**160**(4):1405–23.

54. Torry DS, Wang HS, Wang TH, Caudle MR, Torry RJ. Preeclampsia is associated with reduced serum levels of placenta growth factor. *Am J Obstet Gynecol* 1998;**179**(6 Pt 1):1539–44.

55. Maynard SE, Min JY, Merchan J, Lim KH, Li J, Mondal S, et al. Excess placental soluble fms-like tyrosine kinase 1 (sFlt1) may contribute to endothelial dysfunction, hypertension, and proteinuria in preeclampsia. *J Clin Invest* 2003;**111**(5):649–58.

56. Tripathi R, Rath G, Jain A, Salhan S. Soluble and membranous vascular endothelial growth factor receptor-1 in pregnancies complicated by preeclampsia. *Ann Anat* 2008;**190**(5):477–89.

57. Levine RJ, Maynard SE, Qian C, Lim KH, England LJ, Yu KF, et al. Circulating angiogenic factors and the risk of preeclampsia. *N Engl J Med* 2004;**350**(7):672–83.

58. Smith GC, Crossley JA, Aitken DA, Jenkins N, Lyall F, Cameron AD, et al. Circulating angiogenic factors in early pregnancy and the risk of preeclampsia, intrauterine growth restriction, spontaneous preterm birth, and stillbirth. *Obstet Gynecol* 2007;**109**(6):1316–24.

59. McGinnis R, Steinthorsdottir V, Williams NO, Thorleifsson G, Shooter S, Hjartardottir S, et al. Variants in the fetal genome near FLT1 are associated with risk of preeclampsia. *Nat Genet* 2017;**49**(8):1255–60.

60. Di Blasio AM, Carniti C, Vigano P, Florio P, Petraglia F, Vignali M. Basic fibroblast growth factor messenger ribonucleic acid levels in human placentas from normal and pathological pregnancies. *Mol Hum Reprod* 1997;**3**(12):1119–23.

61. Arany E, Hill DJ. Fibroblast growth factor-2 and fibroblast growth factor receptor-1 mRNA expression and peptide localization in placentae from normal and diabetic pregnancies. *Placenta* 1998;**19**(2–3):133–42.

62. Gregory AL, Xu G, Sotov V, Letarte M. Review: the enigmatic role of endoglin in the placenta. *Placenta* 2014;**35**(Suppl):S93–9.

63. Petraglia F, Sawchenko P, Lim AT, Rivier J, Vale W. Localization, secretion, and action of inhibin in human placenta. *Science* 1987;**237**(4811):187–9.

64. Rabinovici J, Goldsmith PC, Librach CL, Jaffe RB. Localization and regulation of the activin-A dimer in human placental cells. *J Clin Endocrinol Metab* 1992;**75**(2):571–6.

65. Yokoyama Y, Nakamura T, Nakamura R, Irahara M, Aono T, Sugino H. Identification of activins and follistatin proteins in human follicular fluid and placenta. *J Clin Endocrinol Metab* 1995;**80**(3):915–21.

66. Florio P, Cobellis L, Luisi S, Ciarmela P, Severi FM, Bocchi C, et al. Changes in inhibins and activin secretion in healthy and pathological pregnancies. *Mol Cell Endocrinol* 2001;**180**(1–2):123–30.

67. Petraglia F, Vaughan J, Vale W. Inhibin and activin modulate the release of gonadotropin-releasing hormone, human chorionic gonadotropin, and progesterone from cultured human placental cells. *Proc Natl Acad Sci U S A* 1989;**86**(13):5114–7.

68. De Bonis M, Torricelli M, Severi FM, Luisi S, De Leo V, Petraglia F. Neuroendocrine aspects of placenta and pregnancy. *Gynecol Endocrinol* 2012;**28**(Suppl. 1):22–6.

69. Muttukrishna S, Knight PG, Groome NP, Redman CW, Ledger WL. Activin A and inhibin A as possible endocrine markers for pre-eclampsia. *Lancet* 1997;**349**(9061):1285–8.

70. Petraglia F, Di_Blasio AM, Florio P, Gallo R, Genazzani AR, Woodruff TK, et al. High levels of fetal membrane activin beta A and activin receptor IIB mRNAs and augmented concentration of amniotic fluid activin A in women in term or preterm labor. *J Endocrinol* 1997;**154**(1):95–101.

71. Reddy A, Suri S, Sargent IL, Redman CW, Muttukrishna S. Maternal circulating levels of activin A, inhibin A, sFlt-1 and endoglin at parturition in normal pregnancy and pre-eclampsia. *PLoS ONE* 2009;**4**(2).

72. Rosenberg VA, Buhimschi IA, Dulay AT, Abdel-Razeq SS, Oliver EA, Duzyj CM, et al. Modulation of amniotic fluid activin-a and inhibin-a in women with preterm premature rupture of the membranes and infection-induced preterm birth. *Am J Reprod Immunol* 2012;**67**(2):122–31.

73. Jessmon P, Leach RE, Armant DR. Diverse functions of HBEGF during pregnancy. *Mol Reprod Dev* 2009;**76**(12):1116–27.

74. Leach RE, Romero R, Kim YM, Chaiworapongsa T, Kilburn B, Das SK, et al. Pre-eclampsia and expression of heparin-binding EGF-like growth factor. *Lancet* 2002;**360**(9341):1215–9.

75. Moll SJ, Jones CJ, Crocker IP, Baker PN, Heazell AE. Epidermal growth factor rescues trophoblast apoptosis induced by reactive oxygen species. *Apoptosis* 2007;**12**(9):1611–22.

76. Briana DD, Malamitsi-Puchner A. Reviews: adipocytokines in normal and complicated pregnancies. *Reprod Sci* 2009;**16**(10):921–37.

77. Beck S, Wojdyla D, Say L, Betran AP, Merialdi M, Requejo JH, et al. The worldwide incidence of preterm birth: a systematic review of maternal mortality and morbidity. *Bull World Health Organ* 2010;**88**(1):31–8.

78. Mukherjea R, Castonguay TW, Douglass LW, Moser-Veillon P. Elevated leptin concentrations in pregnancy and lactation: possible role as a modulator of substrate utilization. *Life Sci* 1999;**65**(11):1183–93.

79. Hauguel-de Mouzon S, Lepercq J, Catalano P. The known and unknown of leptin in pregnancy. *Am J Obstet Gynecol* 2006;**194**(6):1537–45.

80. Chardonnens D, Cameo P, Aubert ML, Pralong FP, Islami D, Campana A, et al. Modulation of human cytotrophoblastic leptin secretion by interleukin-1alpha and 17beta-oestradiol and its effect on HCG secretion. *Mol Hum Reprod* 1999;**5**(11):1077–82.

81. Jansson N, Greenwood SL, Johansson BR, Powell TL, Jansson T. Leptin stimulates the activity of the system A amino acid transporter in human placental villous fragments. *J Clin Endocrinol Metab* 2003;**88**(3):1205–11.

82. Tulchinsky D, Hobel CJ, Yeager E, Marshall JR. Plasma estrone, estradiol, estriol, progesterone, and 17-hydroxyprogesterone in human pregnancy. I. Normal pregnancy. *Am J Obstet Gynecol* 1972;**112**(8):1095–100.

83. Johansson E. Plasma levels of progesterone in pregnancy measured by a rapid competitive protein binding technique. *Acta Endocrinol* 1979;**61**:607.

84. Strauss JF, Martinez F, Kiriakidou M. Placental steroid hormone synthesis: unique features and unanswered questions. *Biol Reprod* 1996;**54**(2):303–11.

85. Sakai N, Tabb T, Garfield RE. Studies of connexin 43 and cell-to-cell coupling in cultured human uterine smooth muscle. *Am J Obstet Gynecol* 1992;**167**(5):1267–77.

86. Petrocelli T, Lye SJ. Regulation of transcripts encoding the myometrial gap junction protein, connexin-43, by estrogen and progesterone. *Endocrinology* 1993;**133**(1):284–90.

87. Goodenough DA, Goliger JA, Paul DL. Connexins, connexons, and intercellular communication. *Annu Rev Biochem* 1996;**65**:475–502.

88. Sato T, Ito A, Mori Y, Yamashita K, Hayakawa T, Nagase H. Hormonal regulation of collagenolysis in uterine cervical fibroblasts. Modulation of synthesis of procollagenase, prostromelysin and tissue inhibitor of metalloproteinases (TIMP) by progesterone and oestradiol-17 beta. *Biochem J* 1991;**275**(Pt 3):645–50.

89. Ito A, Imada K, Sato T, Kubo T, Matsushima K, Mori Y. Suppression of interleukin 8 production by progesterone in rabbit uterine cervix. *Biochem J* 1994;**301**(Pt 1):183–6.

90. Tanaka K, Nakamura T, Ikeya H, Higuchi T, Tanaka A, Morikawa A, et al. Hyaluronate depolymerization activity induced by progesterone in cultured fibroblasts derived from human uterine cervix. *FEBS Lett* 1994;**347**(1):95–8.

91. Imada K, Ito A, Sato T, Namiki M, Nagase H, Mori Y. Hormonal regulation of matrix metalloproteinase 9/gelatinase B gene expression in rabbit uterine cervical fibroblasts. *Biol Reprod* 1997;**56**(3):575–80.

92. Cakmak H, Schatz F, Huang ST, Buchwalder L, Rahman M, Arici A, et al. Progestin suppresses thrombin- and interleukin-1beta-induced interleukin-11 production in term decidual cells: implications for preterm delivery. *J Clin Endocrinol Metab* 2005;**90**(9):5279–86.

93. Kumar D, Springel E, Moore RM, Mercer BM, Philipson E, Mansour JM, et al. Progesterone inhibits in vitro fetal membrane weakening. *Am J Obstet Gynecol* 2015;**213**(4):520.e1–9.

94. Hardy DB, Janowski BA, Corey DR, Mendelson CR. Progesterone receptor plays a major antiinflammatory role in human myometrial cells by antagonism of nuclear factor-kappaB activation of cyclooxygenase 2 expression. *Mol Endocrinol* 2006;**20**(11):2724–33.

95. Yellon SM, Burns AE, See JL, Lechuga TJ, Kirby MA. Progesterone withdrawal promotes remodeling processes in the nonpregnant mouse cervix. *Biol Reprod* 2009;**81**(1):1–6.

96. Tan H, Yi L, Rote NS, Hurd WW, Mesiano S. Progesterone receptor-A and -B have opposite effects on proinflammatory gene expression in human myometrial cells: implications for progesterone actions in human pregnancy and parturition. *J Clin Endocrinol Metab* 2012;**97**(5):E719–30.

97. Amini P, Michniuk D, Kuo K, Yi L, Skomorovska-Prokvolit Y, Peters GA, et al. Human parturition involves progesterone receptor-A phosphorylation at serine-345 in myometrial cells. *Endocrinology* 2016;**157**(11):4434–45.

98. Kirby MA, Heuerman AC, Custer M, Dobyns AE, Strilaeff R, Stutz KN, et al. Progesterone receptor-mediated actions regulate remodeling of the cervix in preparation for preterm parturition. *Reprod Sci* 2016;**23**(11):1473–83.

99. Avrech OM, Golan A, Weinraub Z, Bukovsky I, Caspi E. Mifepristone (RU486) alone or in combination with a prostaglandin analogue for termination of early pregnancy: a review. *Fertil Steril* 1991;**56**(3):385–93.

100. Ikuta Y, Matsuura K, Okamura H, Oyamada I, Usuku G. Effects of RU486 on the interstitial collagenase in the process of cervical ripening in the pregnant rat. *Endocrinol Jpn* 1991;**38**(5):491–6.

101. Carbonne B, Brennand JE, Maria B, Cabrol D, Calder AA. Effects of gemeprost and mifepristone on the mechanical properties of the cervix prior to first trimester termination of pregnancy. *Br J Obstet Gynaecol* 1995;**102**(7):553–8.

102. Cadepond F, Ulmann A, Baulieu EE. RU486 (mifepristone): mechanisms of action and clinical uses. *Annu Rev Med* 1997;**48**:129–56.

103. Hill M, Parizek A, Kancheva R, Jirasek JE. Reduced progesterone metabolites in human late pregnancy. *Physiol Res* 2011;**60**(2):225–41.

104. Kubli-Garfias C, Hoyo-Vadillo C, Lopez-Nieto E, Ponce-Monter H. Inhibition of spontaneous contractions of the rat pregnant uterus by progesterone metabolites. *Proc West Pharmacol Soc* 1983;**26**:115–8.

105. Kubli-Garfias C, Medrano-Conde L, Beyer C, Bondani A. In vitro inhibition of rat uterine contractility induced by 5 alpha and 5 beta progestins. *Steroids* 1979;**34**(**6 Spec no**):609–17.

106. Perusquia M, Jasso-Kamel J. Influence of 5alpha- and 5beta-reduced progestins on the contractility of isolated human myometrium at term. *Life Sci* 2001;**68**(26):2933–44.

107. Thornton S, Terzidou V, Clark A, Blanks A. Progesterone metabolite and spontaneous myometrial contractions in vitro. *Lancet* 1999; **353**(9161):1327–9.

108. Sheehan PM, Rice GE, Moses EK, Brennecke SP. 5 Beta-dihydroprogesterone and steroid 5 beta-reductase decrease in association with human parturition at term. *Mol Hum Reprod* 2005;**11**(7):495–501.

109. Sergeev PV, Sizov PI, Dukhanin AS, Mineeva EN. Study of the GABA-benzodiazepine receptor system of the human myometrium. *Biull Eksp Biol Med* 1990;**110**(10):382–4.

110. Putnam CD, Brann DW, Kolbeck RC, Mahesh VB. Inhibition of uterine contractility by progesterone and progesterone metabolites: mediation by progesterone and gamma amino butyric acidA receptor systems. *Biol Reprod* 1991;**45**(2):266–72.

111. Mellon SH, Griffin LD. Neurosteroids: biochemistry and clinical significance. *Trends Endocrinol Metab* 2002;**13**(1):35–43.

112. Mesiano S, Jaffe RB. Developmental and functional biology of the primate fetal adrenal cortex. *Endocr Rev* 1997;**18**(3):378–403.

113. Tulchinsky D. Placental secretion of unconjugated estrone, estradiol and estriol into the maternal and the fetal circulation. *J Clin Endocrinol Metab* 1973;**36**(6):1079–87.

114. Holinka CF, Diczfalusy E, Coelingh Bennink HJ. Estetrol: a unique steroid in human pregnancy. *J Steroid Biochem Mol Biol* 2008;**110**(1–2):138–43.

115. Resnik R, Killam AP, Battaglia FC, Makowski EL, Meschia G. The stimulation of uterine blood flow by various estrogens. *Endocrinology* 1974; **94**(4):1192–6.

116. Price HV, Cone BR, Keogh M. Length of gestation in congenital adrenal hyperplasia. *J Obstet Gynaecol Br Commonw* 1971;**78**:430–4.

117. Miller W, Levine L. Molecular and clinical advances in congenital adrenal hyperplasia. *J Pediatr* 1987;**111**:1–71.

118. Morel Y, Miller W. Clinical and molecular genetics of congenital adrenal hyperplasia due to 21-hydroxylase deficiency. *Adv Hum Genet* 1991;**20**:1–68.

119. New MI. Diagnosis and management of congenital adrenal hyperplasia. *Annu Rev Med* 1998;**49**:311–28.

120. Milic AB, Adamsons K. The relationship between anencephaly and prolonged pregnancy. *J Obstet Gynaecol Br Commonw* 1969;**76**(2):102–11.

121. Honnebier WJ, Swaab DF. The influence of anencephaly upon intrauterine growth of fetus and placenta and upon gestation length. *J Obstet Gynaecol Br Commonw* 1973;**80**:577–88.

122. Shozu M, Akasofu K, Harada T, Kubota Y. A new cause of female pseudohermaphroditism: placental aromatase deficiency. *J Clin Endocrinol Metab* 1991;**72**(3):560–6.

123. Harada N, Ogawa H, Shozu M, Yamada K. Genetic studies to characterize the origin of the mutation in placental aromatase deficiency. *Am J Hum Genet* 1992;**51**(3):666–72.

124. Mullis PE, Yoshimura N, Kuhlmann B, Lippuner K, Jaeger P, Harada H. Aromatase deficiency in a female who is compound heterozygote for two new point mutations in the P450arom gene: impact of estrogens on hypergonadotropic hypogonadism, multicystic ovaries, and bone densitometry in childhood. *J Clin Endocrinol Metab* 1997;**82**(6):1739–45.

125. Harada N, Ogawa H, Shozu M, Yamada K, Suhara K, Nishida E, et al. Biochemical and molecular genetic analyses on placental aromatase (P-450AROM) deficiency. *J Biol Chem* 1992;**267**(7):4781–5.

126. Kanasaki K, Palmsten K, Sugimoto H, Ahmad S, Hamano Y, Xie L, et al. Deficiency in catechol-O-methyltransferase and 2-methoxyoestradiol is associated with pre-eclampsia. *Nature* 2008;**453**(7198):1117–21.

127. Zhang Y, Wang T, Shen Y, Wang X, Baker PN, Zhao A. 2-Methoxyestradiol deficiency is strongly related to hypertension in early onset severe pre-eclampsia. *Pregnancy Hypertens* 2014;**4**(3):215–9.

128. Devoto L, Henriquez S, Kohen P, Strauss 3rd JF. The significance of estradiol metabolites in human corpus luteum physiology. *Steroids* 2017;**123**:50–4.

129. Wantania J, Attamimi A, Siswishanto R. A comparison of 2-methoxyestradiol value in women with severe preeclampsia versus normotensive pregnancy. *J Clin Diagn Res* 2017;**11**(3):QC35–8.

130. Mitchell BF, Seron-Ferre M, Jaffe RB. Cortisol-cortisone interrelationship in the late gestation rhesus monkey fetus in utero. *Endocrinology* 1982;**111**:1837–42.

131. Yang K. Placental 11ß hydroxysteroid dehydrogenase: barrier to maternal glucocorticoids. *Rev Reprod* 1997;**2**:129–32.

132. Seckl R. Glucocorticoids and small babies. *Q J Med* 1994;**87**:259–62.

133. Seckl JR, Benediktsson R, Lindsay RS, Brown RW. Placental 11ß-hydroxysteroid dehydrogenase and the programming of hypertension. *J Steroid Biochem Mol Biol* 1995;**55**:447–55.

134. Burton PJ, Waddell BJ. Dual function of 11ß-hydroxysteroid dehydrogenase in placenta: modulating placenta glucocorticoid passage and local steroid action. *Biol Reprod* 1999;**60**:234–40.

135. Brash AR. Arachidonic acid as a bioactive molecule. *J Clin Invest* 2001;**107**(11):1339–45.

136. Fitzpatrick FA, Soberman R. Regulated formation of eicosanoids. *J Clin Invest* 2001;**107**(11):1347–51.

137. Burke JE, Dennis EA. Phospholipase A2 structure/function, mechanism, and signaling. *J Lipid Res* 2009;**50**(Suppl):S237–42.

138. Smith WL, DeWitt DL, Garavito RM. Cyclooxygenases: structural, cellular, and molecular biology. *Annu Rev Biochem* 2000;**69**:145–82.

139. Smith W. Molecular biology of prostanoid biosynthetic enzymes and receptors. *Adv Exp Med Biol* 1997;**400B**:989–1011.

140. Smith WL, Urade Y, Jakobsson PJ. Enzymes of the cyclooxygenase pathways of prostanoid biosynthesis. *Chem Rev* 2011;**111**(10):5821–65.

141. Brash AR. Lipoxygenases: occurrence, functions, catalysis, and acquisition of substrate. *J Biol Chem* 1999;**274**(34):23679–82.

142. Spector AA. Arachidonic acid cytochrome P450 epoxygenase pathway. *J Lipid Res* 2009;**50**(Suppl):S52–6.

143. Catella F, Lawson JA, Fitzgerald DJ, FitzGerald GA. Endogenous biosynthesis of arachidonic acid epoxides in humans: increased formation in pregnancy-induced hypertension. *Proc Natl Acad Sci U S A* 1990;**87**(15):5893–7.

144. Node K, Huo Y, Ruan X, Yang B, Spiecker M, Ley K, et al. Anti-inflammatory properties of cytochrome P450 epoxygenase-derived eicosanoids. *Science* 1999;**285**(5431):1276–9.

145. Roberts 2nd LJ, Morrow JD. Isoprostanes. Novel markers of endogenous lipid peroxidation and potential mediators of oxidant injury. *Ann N Y Acad Sci* 1994;**744**:237–42.

146. Milne GL, Yin H, Hardy KD, Davies SS, Roberts 2nd LJ. Isoprostane generation and function. *Chem Rev* 2011;**111**(10):5973–96.

147. Murakami M, Kambe T, Shimbara S, Kudo I. Functional coupling between various phospholipase A2s and cyclooxygenases in immediate and delayed prostanoid biosynthetic pathways. *J Biol Chem* 1999;**274**(5):3103–15.

148. Murakami M, Naraba H, Tanioka T, Semmyo N, Nakatani Y, Kojima F, et al. Regulation of prostaglandin E2 biosynthesis by inducible membrane-associated prostaglandin E2 synthase that acts in concert with cyclooxygenase-2. *J Biol Chem* 2000;**275**(42):32783–92.

149. Tanioka T, Nakatani Y, Semmyo N, Murakami M, Kudo I. Molecular identification of cytosolic prostaglandin E2 synthase that is functionally coupled with cyclooxygenase-1 in immediate prostaglandin E2 biosynthesis. *J Biol Chem* 2000;**275**(42):32775–82.

150. Samuelsson B, Morgenstern R, Jakobsson PJ. Membrane prostaglandin E synthase-1: a novel therapeutic target. *Pharmacol Rev* 2007;**59**(3):207–24.

151. Parent J, Fortier MA. Expression and contribution of three different isoforms of prostaglandin E synthase in the bovine endometrium. *Biol Reprod* 2005;**73**(1):36–44.

152. Schuster VL. Molecular mechanisms of prostaglandin transport. *Annu Rev Physiol* 1998;**60**:221–42.

153. Reid G, Wielinga P, Zelcer N, van der Heijden I, Kuil A, de Haas M, et al. The human multidrug resistance protein MRP4 functions as a prostaglandin efflux transporter and is inhibited by nonsteroidal antiinflammatory drugs. *Proc Natl Acad Sci U S A* 2003;**100**(16):9244–9.

154. Ensor CM, Yang JY, Okita RT, Tai HH. Cloning and sequence analysis of the cDNA for human placental NAD(+)-dependent 15-hydroxyprostaglandin dehydrogenase. *J Biol Chem* 1990;**265**(25):14888–91.

155. Funk CD. Prostaglandins and leukotrienes: advances in eicosanoid biology. *Science* 2001;**294**(5548):1871–5.

156. Narumiya S, Furuyashiki T. Fever, inflammation, pain and beyond: prostanoid receptor research during these 25 years. *FASEB J* 2011;**25**(3):813–8.

157. Woodward DF, Jones RL, Narumiya S. International Union of Basic and Clinical Pharmacology. LXXXIII: classification of prostanoid receptors, updating 15 years of progress. *Pharmacol Rev* 2011;**63**(3):471–538.

158. Raychowdhury MK, Yukawa M, Collins LJ, McGrail SH, Kent KC, Ware JA. Alternative splicing produces a divergent cytoplasmic tail in the human endothelial thromboxane A2 receptor. *J Biol Chem* 1994;**269**(30):19256–61.

159. Narumiya S. Molecular diversity of prostanoid receptors; subtypes and isoforms of prostaglandin E receptor. *Adv Exp Med Biol* 1997;**400A**:207–13.

160. Pierce KL, Bailey TJ, Hoyer PB, Gil DW, Woodward DF, Regan JW. Cloning of a carboxyl-terminal isoform of the prostanoid FP receptor. *J Biol Chem* 1997;**272**(2):883–7.

161. Sugimoto Y, Inazumi T, Tsuchiya S. Roles of prostaglandin receptors in female reproduction. *J Biochem* 2015;**157**(2):73–80.

162. Lee SE, Romero R, Park IS, Seong HS, Park CW, Yoon BH. Amniotic fluid prostaglandin concentrations increase before the onset of spontaneous labor at term. *J Matern Fetal Neonatal Med* 2008;**21**(2):89–94.

163. Durn JH, Marshall KM, Farrar D, O'Donovan P, Scally AJ, Woodward DF, et al. Lipidomic analysis reveals prostanoid profiles in human term pregnant myometrium. *Prostaglandins Leukot Essent Fat Acids* 2010;**82**(1):21–6.

164. Lewis RB, Schulman JD. Influence of acetylsalicylic acid, an inhibitor of prostaglandin synthesis, on the duration of human gestation and labour. *Lancet* 1973;**2**(7839):1159–61.

165. Skarnes RC, Harper MJ. Relationship between endotoxin-induced abortion and the synthesis of prostaglandin F. *Prostaglandins* 1972;**1**(3):191–203.

166. Fidel Jr PL, Romero R, Wolf N, Cutright J, Ramirez M, Araneda H, et al. Systemic and local cytokine profiles in endotoxin-induced preterm parturition in mice. *Am J Obstet Gynecol* 1994;**170**(5 Pt 1):1467–75.

167. Olson DM, Ammann C. Role of the prostaglandins in labour and prostaglandin receptor inhibitors in the prevention of preterm labour. *Front Biosci* 2007;**12**:1329–43.

168. Gross G, Imamura T, Vogt SK, Wozniak DF, Nelson DM, Sadovsky Y, et al. Inhibition of cyclooxygenase-2 prevents inflammation-mediated preterm labor in the mouse. *Am J Phys Regul Integr Comp Phys* 2000;**278**(6):R1415–23.

169. Vermillion ST, Landen CN. Prostaglandin inhibitors as tocolytic agents. *Semin Perinatol* 2001;**25**(4):256–62.

170. Stika CS, Gross GA, Leguizamon G, Gerber S, Levy R, Mathur A, et al. A prospective randomized safety trial of celecoxib for treatment of preterm labor. *Am J Obstet Gynecol* 2002;**187**(3):653–60.

171. Takahashi Y, Roman C, Chemtob S, Tse MM, Lin E, Heymann MA, et al. Cyclooxygenase-2 inhibitors constrict the fetal lamb ductus arteriosus both in vitro and in vivo. *Am J Phys Regul Integr Comp Phys* 2000;**278**(6):R1496–505.

172. Loftin CD, Trivedi DB, Langenbach R. Cyclooxygenase-1-selective inhibition prolongs gestation in mice without adverse effects on the ductus arteriosus. *J Clin Invest* 2002;**110**(4):549–57.

173. Friedman SA. Preeclampsia: a review of the role of prostaglandins. *Obstet Gynecol* 1988;**71**(1):122–37.

174. Fitzgerald DJ, Entman SS, Mulloy K, FitzGerald GA. Decreased prostacyclin biosynthesis preceding the clinical manifestation of pregnancy-induced hypertension. *Circulation* 1987;**75**(5):956–63.

175. Fitzgerald DJ, Mayo G, Catella F, Entman SS, FitzGerald GA. Increased thromboxane biosynthesis in normal pregnancy is mainly derived from platelets. *Am J Obstet Gynecol* 1987;**157**(2):325–30.

176. Fitzgerald DJ, Rocki W, Murray R, Mayo G, FitzGerald GA. Thromboxane A2 synthesis in pregnancy-induced hypertension. *Lancet* 1990; **335**(8692):751–4.

177. Roberge S, Bujold E, Nicolaides KH. Aspirin for the prevention of preterm and term preeclampsia: systematic review and metaanalysis. *Am J Obstet Gynecol* 2018;**218**(3):287–93. e1.

178. Roberge S, Bujold E, Nicolaides KH. Meta-analysis on the effect of aspirin use for prevention of preeclampsia on placental abruption and antepartum hemorrhage. *Am J Obstet Gynecol* 2018;**218**(5):483–9.

179. Wright D, Rolnik DL, Syngelaki A, de Paco Matallana C, Machuca M, de Alvarado M, et al. Aspirin for evidence-based preeclampsia prevention trial: effect of aspirin on length of stay in the neonatal intensive care unit. *Am J Obstet Gynecol* 2018;.

180. Ye X. Lysophospholipid signaling in the function and pathology of the reproductive system. *Hum Reprod Update* 2008;**14**(5):519–36.

181. Guo L, Ou X, Li H, Han Z. Roles of sphingosine-1-phosphate in reproduction. *Reprod Sci* 2014;**21**(5):550–4.

182. Manokhina I, Wilson SL, Robinson WP. Noninvasive nucleic acid-based approaches to monitor placental health and predict pregnancy-related complications. *Am J Obstet Gynecol* 2015;**213**(4 Suppl):S197–206.

183. Raposo G, Stoorvogel W. Extracellular vesicles: exosomes, microvesicles, and friends. *J Cell Biol* 2013;**200**(4):373–83.

184. Mitchell MD, Peiris HN, Kobayashi M, Koh YQ, Duncombe G, Illanes SE, et al. Placental exosomes in normal and complicated pregnancy. *Am J Obstet Gynecol* 2015;**213**(4 Suppl):S173–81.

185. Southcombe J, Tannetta D, Redman C, Sargent I. The immunomodulatory role of syncytiotrophoblast microvesicles. *PLoS ONE* 2011;**6**(5).

186. Abumaree MH, Chamley LW, Badri M, El-Muzaini MF. Trophoblast debris modulates the expression of immune proteins in macrophages: a key to maternal tolerance of the fetal allograft? *J Reprod Immunol* 2012;**94**(2):131–41.

187. Delorme-Axford E, Donker RB, Mouillet JF, Chu T, Bayer A, Ouyang Y, et al. Human placental trophoblasts confer viral resistance to recipient cells. *Proc Natl Acad Sci U S A* 2013;**110**(29):12048–53.

188. Mincheva-Nilsson L, Baranov V. Placenta-derived exosomes and syncytiotrophoblast microparticles and their role in human reproduction: immune modulation for pregnancy success. *Am J Reprod Immunol* 2014;**72**(5):440–57.

189. Ezrin AM, Brohman B, Willmot J, Baxter S, Moore K, Luther M, et al. Circulating serum-derived microparticles provide novel proteomic biomarkers of spontaneous preterm birth. *Am J Perinatol* 2015;**32**(6):605–14.

190. Gupta AK, Holzgreve W, Huppertz B, Malek A, Schneider H, Hahn S. Detection of fetal DNA and RNA in placenta-derived syncytiotrophoblast microparticles generated in vitro. *Clin Chem* 2004;**50**(11):2187–90.

191. Alberry M, Maddocks D, Jones M, Abdel Hadi M, Abdel-Fattah S, Avent N, et al. Free fetal DNA in maternal plasma in anembryonic pregnancies: confirmation that the origin is the trophoblast. *Prenat Diagn* 2007;**27**(5):415–8.

192. Lo YM, Tein MS, Lau TK, Haines CJ, Leung TN, Poon PM, et al. Quantitative analysis of fetal DNA in maternal plasma and serum: implications for noninvasive prenatal diagnosis. *Am J Hum Genet* 1998;**62**(4):768–75.

193. Phillippe M. Cell-free fetal DNA, telomeres, and the spontaneous onset of parturition. *Reprod Sci* 2015;**22**(10):1186–201.

194. Mackie FL, Hemming K, Allen S, Morris RK, Kilby MD. The accuracy of cell-free fetal DNA-based non-invasive prenatal testing in singleton pregnancies: a systematic review and bivariate meta-analysis. *BJOG* 2016;.

195. Heung MM, Jin S, Tsui NB, Ding C, Leung TY, Lau TK, et al. Placenta-derived fetal specific mRNA is more readily detectable in maternal plasma than in whole blood. *PLoS ONE* 2009;**4**(6).

196. Mouillet JF, Ouyang Y, Coyne CB, Sadovsky Y. MicroRNAs in placental health and disease. *Am J Obstet Gynecol* 2015;**213**(4 Suppl):S163–72.

Part E

Endocrine Disorders Affecting the Fetus or Neonate

Chapter 42

Hypothalamic and Pituitary Disorders Affecting the Fetus and Neonate

Manuela Cerbone*,†, Harshini Katugampola*,† and Mehul T. Dattani*,†

*University College London Great Ormond Street Institute of Child Health, London, United Kingdom, †Great Ormond Street Hospital for Children NHS Foundation Trust, London, United Kingdom

---

Common Clinical Problems

- In the presence of a neonate with hypoglycemia (with or without jaundice, micropenis, or cryptorchidism), it is important to diagnose and treat potential pituitary hormone deficits, to avoid adverse cognitive outcomes.
- Congenital hypopituitarism may arise from mutations in any of the genes involved in pituitary development, although it is more commonly associated with pituitary stalk interruption syndrome where the genetic/epigenetic cause(s) remain illusive.
- The finding of other brain anomalies and/or syndromic features merits a more thorough genetic work-up, particularly in the context of consanguinity.
- Anterior and posterior pituitary hormone deficiencies can occur as single hormone deficiencies, but depending on the etiology of these defects, it may be necessary to consider potentially evolving phenotypes.

42.1 INTRODUCTION: CONGENITAL DISORDERS OF HYPOTHALAMO-PITUITARY (H-P) DEVELOPMENT

The most common neonatal disorders of the hypothalamo-pituitary axis (HPA) are represented by congenital defects of the H-P development leading to pituitary hormone deficiencies, while acquired forms of hypopituitarism are much rarer, and pituitary diseases leading to hormonal excess are virtually absent in the neonatal period.

Congenital hypopituitarism (CH) is characterized by the deficiency of one or more pituitary hormones. The prevalence of hypopituitarism in the general population is estimated to be between 290 and 455 per million.[1] The annual incidence has been reported to be between 42.1 cases per million in one study[1] and 1 in 3000–4000 births in another study.[2]

CH is a life-long disorder causing significant morbidity and mortality.[3] It is a highly heterogeneous disorder that may manifest either as an isolated hormone deficiency, the commonest being isolated GH deficiency (IGHD), or as combined pituitary hormone deficiency (CPHD) when two or more pituitary hormones are affected. The clinical features vary in severity and time of presentation (from neonatal period to adulthood). CH may also be part of a syndrome where abnormalities in extra-pituitary structures which share a common embryologic origin with the pituitary gland (such as eye, midline, and forebrain abnormalities) are also present.

CH may arise from mutations in any of the genes involved in pituitary development. As a general rule, mutations in genes implicated in the early stages of H-P development tend to result in syndromic forms of hypopituitarism in association with extra-pituitary deficits and midline abnormalities, while mutations in genes required for the specification of particular cell types or encoding specific hormone subunits give rise to isolated pituitary hormone deficiencies.[4] However, the etiology remains unknown in the majority of patients with hypopituitarism with causative mutations being identified only in a small proportion (<10%) of cases, thus suggesting that other genes and/or environmental or epigenetic factors may play a key role.

42.2 COMBINED PITUITARY HORMONE DEFICIENCIES (TABLE 42.1)

CPHD is characterized classically by GH deficiency and deficiency of at least one other pituitary hormone. The prevalence of CPHD is estimated to be 1 in 8000 individuals worldwide (Genetics Home Reference at NIH, https://www.ghr.nlm.nih.gov).

TABLE 42.1 Clinical syndromes associated with pituitary deficiencies in the neonatal period and early infancy/childhood

Syndrome/ Phenotype	MIM number Gene/ Locus[a] Phenotype[b]	Gene	Inheritance	Clinical features in the neonatal period and infancy/childhood	MRI findings	Pituitary deficiencies
CPHD1	601538[a] 262600[b]	PROP1	AR	Early onset GH deficiency—growth failure, neonatal hypoglycemia, prominent forehead, mid-facial hypoplasia, deep-set eyes, depressed nasal bridge with anteverted nostrils; developmental delay; hypogonadism—microphallus, undescended testes	APH, normal or enlarged; AP that may change over time, normal PP and stalk	GH, TSH, PRL, LH, FSH and evolving ACTH deficiencies with variable time of onset and severity
CPHD2	173110[a] 613038[b]	POUF1[c] (PIT1)	AD, AR	Early onset GH deficiency—growth failure, neonatal hypoglycemia, prominent forehead, mid-facial hypoplasia, deep-set eyes, depressed nasal bridge with anteverted nostrils; developmental delay; CCH	APH or normal AP, normal PP and infundibulum, no extra-pituitary abnormalities	GH, PRL and TSH (TSH deficiency may present early or develop later)
CPHD3	600577[a] 221750[b]	LHX3	AR	GH deficiency—Growth failure, neonatal hypoglycemia, mid-facial hypoplasia; variable sensorineural deafness; short cervical spine with limited rotation; loose skin; developmental delay; vertebral abnormalities Neck rotation and hearing are normal	APH, enlarged/cystic AP, normal PP and stalk	GH, TSH, PRL, LH, FSH deficiencies; reported ACTH deficiency
CPHD4	602146[a] 262700[b]	LHX4 Patients with LHX4 mutations may have a partial loss of LHX3 function	AD	SGA; GH deficiency—growth failure, mid-facial hypoplasia; hypogonadism—small phallus, undescended testes; severe respiratory distress after birth reported	APH, normal PP or EPP, Chiari malformation, cerebellar abnormalities	GH with variable TSH, ACTH, LH and FSH deficiencies
			AR	Lethality in the first weeks of life with severe sepsis, poor tone, lung atelectasis, mid-facial hypoplasia, low-set ears	APH, EPP	ACTH, TSH, PRL and probable GH deficiencies

Disorder	OMIM	Gene	Inheritance	Clinical features	Radiological features	Phenotype
CPHD5 SOD (de Morsier syndrome)	601802[a] 182230[b]	HESX1		Mutation in HESX1 can cause SOD, CPHD without associated optic nerve hypoplasia or defects of midline brain structures, and growth hormone deficiency with pituitary anomalies Visual impairment; developmental delay; supernumerary digits, hypoplastic digits; early onset GH deficiency—neonatal hypoglycemia, prolonged jaundice, growth failure	Radiological features of SOD include ONH, APH, and midline abnormalities of the brain, including ACC and absent septum pellucidum	Variably penetrant phenotypes, ranging from IGHD, evolving hypopituitarism without midline and eye defects, to SOD and pituitary aplasia with undetectable concentrations of all AP hormones
			AD		APH, EPP, ONH, ACC; normal AP with EPP and ONH	Pan-hypopituitarism; GH deficiency with evolving ACTH and TSH deficiencies
			AR		APH, EPP, ONH, ACC; normal ON with EPP and APH; pituitary aplasia with normal PP and ON; pituitary aplasia with normal PP and ON coloboma	Pan-hypopituitarism; GH, LH, FSH, evolving ACTH and TSH deficiencies
CPHD6 SOD Microphthalmia, syndromic 5, MCOPS5	600037[a] 613986[b] 610125[b]	OTX2	AD	Mutation in OTX2 can cause CPHD, microphthalmia with associated features, including pituitary dysfunction, coloboma, cataract, retinal dystrophy, hypoplasia or agenesis of the optic nerves, ACC, developmental delay; joint laxity, hypotonia, and seizures GH deficiency—Growth failure, mid-face hypoplasia; hypogonadism—microphallus, undescended testes. Variable ocular malformations (anophthalmia, microphthalmia, bilateral/ unilateral retinal dystrophy; normal eye phenotype) Manifestation of craniofacial defects, in particular those that affect the lower jaw such as otocephaly and dysgnathia, may be exacerbated in patients with biallelic OTX2 mutations	Normal pituitary; APH, EPP, Chiari malformation	Highly variable phenotypes including IGHD or partial GH deficiency; GH, TSH, ACTH, LH and FSH deficiencies
SOD	604652[a]	TCF7L1	AD	Nystagmus; GH deficiency—Growth failure	APH, absent PP, ONH, thin optic tracts, partial ACC, absent septum pellucidum, thin anterior commissure	Isolated GH deficiency or low IGF1, mildly elevated TSH with normal ft_4

Continued

TABLE 42.1 Clinical syndromes associated with pituitary deficiencies in the neonatal period and early infancy/childhood—cont'd

Syndrome/Phenotype	MIM number Gene/Locus[a] Phenotype[b]	Gene	Inheritance	Clinical features in the neonatal period and infancy/childhood	MRI findings	Pituitary deficiencies
SOD/CPHD/KS	300836[a]	KAL1[c]	XL	GH deficiency—Growth failure; females affected	APH, ONH	GH, ACTH and TSH deficiencies
SOD/CPHD/KS	136350[a]	FGFR1[c]	AD	Cleft lip/palate; brachydactyly; single central incisor	APH, ACC, ONH, ectopic PP; thin or normal pituitary stalk	GH, TSH, LH/FSH DI
SOD Micropthalmia, syndromic 3 MCOPS 3 (anophthalmia-esophageal-genital syndrome, AEG syndrome)	184429[a] 206900[b]	SOX2	AD	Bilateral/unilateral anophthalmia; trachea-oesophageal atresia/fistula; hypospadias, undescended testis, small phallus; sensorineural deafness; spastic diplegia, developmental delay, learning difficulties	APH, midline or forebrain defects Absent septum pellucidum, dysgenesis or partial ACC; hippocampal abnormalities; hypothalamic hamartoma; slow-progressing hypothalamo-pituitary tumor	LH and FSH deficiencies, rarely GH deficiency
SOD/CPHD/KS	607123[a]	PROKR2[c]	AD	Facial asymmetry; hypoplastic optic discs	APH or normal AP, EPP, absent pituitary stalk, CC dysgenesis, Schizencephaly, Cerebellar hypoplasia	GH, ACTH, TSH, LH and FSH deficiencies; isolated GH deficiency
X-linked panhypopituitarism	313430[a] 312000[b] 300123[b]	SOX3[c]	XL	CPHD and IGHD, with and without learning difficulties. GH deficiency—neonatal hypoglycemia	APH, EPP; persistent craniopharyngeal canal	GH, TSH, ACTH, LH and FSH deficiencies; isolated GH deficiency
CPHD	6000288[a]	FOXA2[d]		CPHD and variable accompanying variants. Rare. One case had CH and congenital hyperinsulinism (HI) with craniofacial dysmorphic features, choroidal coloboma and endoderm-derived organ malformations in the liver, lung, and gastrointestinal tract. Another had CH with childhood-onset diabetes, cardiac malformation and anal atresia; previous report of a pedigree with CH, situs inversus, polysplenia, dysmorphic features, and cardiovascular and gastrointestinal defects with biliary atresia	APH, absent PP, thin pituitary stalk, and corpus callosum	TSH, ACTH, and GH deficiencies

Disorder	OMIM	Gene	Inheritance	Clinical features	Imaging	Hormone deficiencies
Congenital hypopituitarism	607542[a]	KCNQ1		Rare. Growth failure. Heart defects such as cardiac arrhythmia syndromes; maternally inherited gingival fibromatosis, and accompanying mild craniofacial dysmorphic features	Normal pituitary; APH, thin stalk	GH. Reported ACTH, FSH LH TSH
Pituitary Stalk Interruption syndrome	608707[a] 614226[b]	CDON	AD	Neonatal hypoglycemia and cholestatic jaundice	Thin or discontinuous pituitary stalk, a hypoplastic anterior pituitary gland, EPP	GH, TSH, and ACTH deficiencies
Pituitary Stalk Interruption syndrome	602430[a]	ROBO1		Growth failure; ocular anomalies including hypermetropia with strabismus, and ptosis	Thin or discontinuous pituitary stalk, APH EPP	GH
MEHMO syndrome	300161[a] 300148[b]	EIF2S3	XL	Mental retardation, epileptic seizures, hypogonadism with hypogenitalism, microcephaly and obesity; severe intellectual disability, GHD and microcephaly, with a few reports of hypoglycemia. Reported unique form of glucose dysregulation that fluctuates between hyperinsulinemic hypoglycemia and postprandial hyperglycemia, with only mild learning difficulties	APH	GH, LH, FSH, TSH
Holoprosencephaly	600483[a]	FGF8[c]	AR	Mid-line facial defects include cyclopia, anophthalmia, hypotelorism, mid-face hypoplasia, cleft lip/palate, single central incisor	ACC	Central DI; anterior pituitary hormone deficiencies have also been described
Holoprosencephaly	165230[a] 610829[b]	GLI2	AD	Mid-line facial defects including cleft lip/palate, single central incisor; postaxial polydactyly	APH, normal PP or EPP, hypoplastic PP, ONH, holoprosencephaly, cavum septum pellucidum	GH, TSH, ACTH, LH and FSH deficiencies; IGHD DI
Holoprosencephaly	601881[a]	RAX		Variable clinical features; most severe phenotype to date corresponds to a homozygous truncating mutation in a patient with anophthalmia, CH, DI, bilateral cleft lip and palate, microphallus	Absent anterior and posterior pituitary gland on MRI	GH, TSH and ACTH deficiencies, probable LH, FSH deficiency, DI
Hartsfield syndrome	136350[a] 615465[b]	FGFR1	AD	Holoprosencephaly; ectrodactyly; cleft/lip palate; severe developmental delay; growth failure; small phallus, undescended testes	Mid-line brain defects, Diminished cortical thickening, ACC	GH, Central DI, LH and FSH deficiencies

Continued

TABLE 42.1 Clinical syndromes associated with pituitary deficiencies in the neonatal period and early infancy/childhood—cont'd

Syndrome/Phenotype	MIM number Gene/Locus[a] Gene/Phenotype[b]	Gene	Inheritance	Clinical features in the neonatal period and infancy/childhood	MRI findings	Pituitary deficiencies
Ectrodactyly—ectodermal dysplasia—cleft Syndrome 1 (EEC1)	129900[b]	Unknown	AD	Ectodermal dysplasia (subjective hypohidrosis, nail dysplasia, sparse hair, tooth abnormalities); cleft lip/palate; split-hand/foot malformation/syndactyly; mid-face hypoplasia; hypertelorism; lacrimal duct obstruction; hypopigmentation; microphallus, undescended testes; growth failure	APH, Absent septum pellucidum	GH, Central DI
Oliver-McFarlane syndrome Laurence-Moon syndrome	603197[a] 275400[b] 245800[b]	PNPLA6	AR	Oliver-McFarlane syndrome—Thyroid and GH abnormalities may be present at birth and, if untreated, result in intellectual impairment and profound short stature; trichomegaly; progressive cerebellar ataxia or atrophy; chorioretinal dystrophy Laurence-Moon syndrome—chorioretinopathy and pituitary dysfunction, but with childhood onset of ataxia, peripheral neuropathy, and spastic paraplegia and without trichomegaly	APH, cerebellar hypoplasia	GH, TSH, LH and FSH deficiencies; isolated hypogonadotrophic hypogonadism
Axenfeld-Rieger syndrome	601542[a] 180500[b]	PITX2	AD	Anomalies of anterior chamber of the eye, hypoplasia of iris; dental hypoplasia; protuberant umbilicus; learning difficulties; pituitary abnormalities	May have an abnormal sella turcica without endocrine dysfunction	Reduced GH concentration
Webb-Dattani syndrome (WEDAS)	606036[a] 615926[b]	ARNT2	AR	Abnormal pattern of growth, with either growth failure or maintenance of linear growth in conjunction with obesity; congenital hypothyroidism; postnatal microcephaly, seizures, severe visual impairment, developmental delay, abnormalities of the kidneys and urinary tract. Prominent forehead, deep-set eyes, well-grooved philtrum, retrognathia	APH, absent PP, thin CC; frontal and temporal lobe hypoplasia; large Sylvian fissure	Central DI, GH, ACTH, TSH deficiencies

Disorder	OMIM	Gene	Inheritance	Clinical features	Imaging	Hormone deficiencies
Hallermann-Streiff syndrome		Unknown		Typical skull shape (brachycephaly with frontal bossing), hypotrichosis, microphthalmia, cataracts, beaked nose, micrognathia, skin atrophy, dental anomalies; obstruction of the upper airway, apnoea, feeding, swallowing, and/or breathing difficulties; severe early respiratory infections; respiratory insufficiency resulting in cor pulmonale and heart failure; GH deficiency—growth failure, short stature. Hypogonadism—microphallus	ACC, APH, ONH	GH, LH/FSH deficiencies, TSH, ACTH rare
Pallister-Hall syndrome	165240[a] 146510[b]	GLI3	AD	Polydactyly; imperforate anus; potential neonatal death due to untreated adrenal insufficiency	APH, absent pituitary, hypothalamic hamartoma	GH, ACTH, TSH, LH/FSH deficiencies
Isolated GH deficiency (IGHD) Type 1A	139250[a] 262400[b]	GH1	Type 1A AR	Type 1A—Early severe growth failure; mid-face hypoplasia; neonatal hypoglycemia; micro-phallus	Normal pituitary, APH	Undetectable GH within 6 months postnatally; anti-GH antibodies on rhGH treatment
Type 1B	612781[b]		Type 1B AR	Type 1B—Early severe growth failure; Mid-face hypoplasia; neonatal hypoglycemia; micro-phallus	Normal pituitary, APH	Low, detectable GH; no antibodies on rhGH treatment
Type 2	173100[b]		Type 2 AD	Type 2—Variable short stature (severe to normal height without treatment); reversibility of GHD has also been observed; most common genetic form of IGDH	Normal pituitary, APH	Low but detectable GH. May develop additional pituitary hormone deficits including ACTH, TSH, PRL, and gonadotrophin deficiencies; requires life-long follow-up
Isolated GH deficiency (IGHD) Type 3	300300[a] 307200[b]	BTK	XLR	Short stature; agammaglobulinemia	APH	GH
Isolated GH deficiency Type 4 (Sindh Dwarfism)	139191[a]	GHRHR	AR	Severe growth failure; phenotypically distinct from the classical GHD phenotype, minimal mid-facial hypoplasia; neonatal hypoglycemia and microphallus are uncommon	APH	Undetectable GH concentrations, a blunted GH response to provocation, low IGF-1 and IGF-BP3 good response to treatment with GH
	618157[b]		AR	Severe postnatal growth failure, delayed bone age without bone dysplasia, mild microcephaly	APH	Undetectable GH response to provocation

Continued

TABLE 42.1 Clinical syndromes associated with pituitary deficiencies in the neonatal period and early infancy/childhood—cont'd

Syndrome/Phenotype	MIM number Gene/Locus[a] Phenotype[b]	Gene	Inheritance	Clinical features in the neonatal period and infancy/childhood	MRI findings	Pituitary deficiencies
Isolated GH deficiency Type 5	618016[a] 618160[b]	RNPC3	AR	Growth failure—50% have GH deficiency; progressive cone-rod dystrophy leading to blindness, sensorineural hearing loss, childhood obesity associated with hyperinsulinemia, and Type 2 diabetes mellitus; dilated cardiomyopathy occurs in ~70% during infancy or adolescence. Renal failure, pulmonary, hepatic, and urologic dysfunction	Normal pituitary; partial empty sella	GH
Alström syndrome	606884[a] 203800[b]	ALMS1	AR	Early growth retardation, retinopathy, and hypertension with renal failure. The phenotype was consistent with a ciliopathy	APH, EPP	GH
Ciliopathy	607386[a]	IFT172	AD, AR	Short stature	APH	GH
Isolated partial GH deficiency	601898[a] 615925[b]	GHSR	AR	Severe isolated CCH of neonatal onset with high α-GSU	Normal pituitary, APH	TSH concentrations are highly variable, occasionally being undetectable
CCH	188540[a] 275100[b]	TSHβ	Unknown	Isolated CCH; apparently uneventful infantile development, delayed diagnosis from childhood (growth failure) to adulthood	Normal pituitary	TSH deficiency with absent TSH and PRL responses to exogenous TRH
CCH	188545[a,b]	TRHR	XLR	Males with CCH, either in isolation, or associated with hypoprolactinemia; later growth failure in childhood and macroorchidism in adolescence with one report of hypothyroidism and macroorchidism in early childhood	Normal pituitary	TSH, PRL; reported reduced TSH biopotency and increased FSH secretion in neonatal minipuberty Female carriers have also been described with low FT4 concentrations, necessitating treatment; Transient/partial GH deficiency in childhood

Disorder	Gene/locus (MIM)	Gene	Inheritance	Clinical features	Imaging	Hormone
IGSF1 deficiency syndrome CCH	300137[a] 300888[b]	IGSF1				
ACTH deficiency	176830[a] 609734[b]	POMC	AR	Nonspecific symptoms (poor feeding, failure to thrive, hypoglycemia) or more acute neonatal presentation with signs of adrenal insufficiency (vascular collapse, shock). Red hair due to lack of MSH production. Early-onset obesity	Normal pituitary, APH	ACTH
ACTH deficiency	604614[a] 201400[b]	TBX19 (TPIT)	AR	Mutations in TBX19 have been identified in >60% of neonatal early-onset isolated ACTH deficiency; profound hypoglycemia associated with seizures and prolonged cholestatic jaundice; unexplained recurrent infections; acute neonatal presentation with signs of adrenal insufficiency (vascular collapse, shock). Risk of neonatal death reported in 25% of cases	Normal pituitary, APH	ACTH. Low basal plasma concentrations of ACTH and cortisol with no significant ACTH response to CRH
Proprotein convertase 1/3 deficiency ACTH deficiency	162150[a] 600955[b]	PCSK1	AR	Hypoadrenalism, reactive hypoglycemia, Red hair; severe enteropathy, malabsorptive severe refractory neonatal diarrhoea, extreme early-onset obesity; defective processing of other pro-hormones such as GH and vasopressin, and glucose dysregulation insulin-dependent diabetes mellitus	Normal pituitary	ACTH LH/FSH elevated circulating prohormones

ACC, absent corpus callosum; ACTH, adrenocorticotrophic hormone; AD, autosomal dominant; AP, anterior pituitary; APH, anterior pituitary hypoplasia; AR, autosomal recessive; CC, corpus callosum; CCH, central congenital hypothyroidism; CPHD, combined pituitary hormone deficiency; DI, diabetes insipidus ; EPP, ectopic posterior pituitary; FSH, follicle stimulating hormone; GH, growth hormone; IGF1, insulin-like growth factor 1; LH, luteinizing hormone; ON, optic nerves; ONH, optic nerve hypoplasia; PP, posterior pituitary; PRL, prolactin; rhGH, recombinant human growth hormone; SGA, small for gestational age; fT$_4$, free T$_4$ thyroxine; TSH, thyroid-stimulating hormone; TRH-R, thyroid releasing hormone receptor; XL, X-linked; XLR, X-linked recessive.

[a]Gene/locus.

[b]Phenotype those are specified in the heading on the second column and then in the MIM number for each syndrome/phenotype.

[c]These genes are also known to cause isolated pituitary hormone deficiencies.

[d]Fang Q, George AS, Brinkmeier ML, Mortensen AH, Gergics P, Cheung LY, et al. genetics of combined pituitary hormone deficiency: roadmap into the genome era. Endocr Rev 2016;37(6):636–75.

The risk of progression to CPHD in children varies depending on the etiology, and the highest risks are displayed by children with abnormalities of the H-P region (in particular pituitary stalk abnormalities, empty sella, and ectopic posterior pituitary), midline brain (corpus callosum) anomalies, abnormalities of the optic nerves, and genetic defects.[5] Significant insight has been gleaned from spontaneous and artificially induced mutations in the mouse, and the identification of mutations associated with human pituitary disease. Furthermore, the explosion in new technologies such as whole genome sequencing has helped to define the genetic cascade of pituitary development and factors involved in disease. To date, over 30 genes implicated in the pathogenesis of CPHD have been reported.[2, 5–7] However the majority of patients have no genetic diagnosis, and the phenotypic spectrum is broad.

42.2.1 Nonsyndromic CPHD

42.2.1.1 PROP1 Mutations

PROP1 (prophet of PIT1) mutations are the most common cause of CPHD and account for approximately 50% of familial cases.[8] PROP1-related CPHD is associated with deficiencies of GH, TSH, LH/FSH, PRL, and occasionally ACTH, but the time of onset and severity of hormone deficiencies varies, suggesting that as yet unidentified genetic/epigenetic modifying factors may play a role in the pathogenesis.[9] Most patients present with early onset GH deficiency and growth retardation. Hypogonadism can present in the neonatal period with microphallus and undescended testes. TSH and ACTH deficiencies present later in childhood.[10, 11] The evolving nature of hormone deficiencies suggests a gradual decline in the function of the anterior pituitary, indicating a need for regular follow-up with clinical and biochemical monitoring. Pituitary morphology in these patients is variable. Most have a small or normal anterior pituitary with a normal posterior lobe and pituitary stalk, but a large anterior pituitary that waxes and wanes in size and later involutes has also been reported.[12–15]

42.2.1.2 POU1F1 Mutations

Mutations in *POU1F1* (previously known as *PIT1*, OMIM 173110) are associated with GH, TSH, and PRL deficiencies.[16] The incidence of *POU1F1* mutations is low in cases of sporadic CPHD (3-6%) and higher in familial cases (25%).[17] Patients with *POU1F1* mutations present early in life with GH and PRL deficiencies. TSH deficiency can be highly variable with the majority of patients presenting early, but hypothyroidism also has been reported later in childhood and early adulthood.[14] Patients with *POU1F1* mutations have a small or normal sized anterior pituitary gland with a normal posterior pituitary and infundibulum and no extra-pituitary abnormalities.

42.2.2 Syndromic CPHD

42.2.2.1 Septo-Optic Dysplasia (SOD) and its Variants

SOD is a rare, heterogeneous congenital disorder comprising forebrain, eye, and pituitary abnormalities. The prevalence of SOD varies between 6.3 and 10.9 per 100,000. It is defined by at least 2 of optic nerve hypoplasia (ONH), midline forebrain defects (for example, agenesis of the corpus callosum, absent septum pellucidum), and pituitary hypoplasia with variable hypopituitarism.[18] Approximately 30% of patients are reported to have the full triad of features; 60% have an absent septum pellucidum, and 62% have variable hypopituitarism.[19] Associated features include cavum septum pellucidum, cerebellar hypoplasia, schizencephaly, and aplasia of the fornix. Neurological manifestations are common (75%–80%) and range from focal deficits to global developmental delay.[18] ONH may be unilateral (12%) or bilateral (88%) and may be the first presenting feature, antenatally or postnatally, with development of pituitary hormone deficiencies later in life. More severe ocular abnormalities include bilateral anophthalmia or severe microphthalmia. Approximately 75%–80% of patients with ONH have evidence of abnormal neuroimaging. Anterior pituitary hypoplasia, an undescended (ectopic) posterior pituitary, and an absent pituitary stalk predispose to hypopituitarism (ranging from IGHD to CPHD). The most common endocrinopathy is GH deficiency followed by TSH and ACTH deficiencies, while gonadotrophin secretion may be retained. It is important to appreciate that endocrinopathies can evolve over time.

The etiology of SOD is probably multifactorial with both genetic and environmental factors (viral infections, vascular or degenerative changes, exposure to alcohol or drugs) playing a role. SOD is seen more commonly in children born to younger mothers and as clusters in geographical areas with a high frequency of teenage pregnancies.[20, 21] Prenatal ethanol exposure in mouse embryos with mutations in the Sonic hedgehog (Shh) pathway have been associated with an increased risk of ONH, supporting the hypothesis of a multifactorial etiology in SOD.[22]

Early development of the forebrain and pituitary are intricately linked, occurring at 3-6 weeks of gestation. During these stages, signaling molecules and transcription factors have extensive and overlapping patterns of expression in the developing forebrain, pituitary, and sensory placodes. There is now increasing evidence of overlap in the etiology of conditions that were previously considered to be discrete, such as SOD, CPHD, and Kallmann syndrome, likely due to mutations in the same array of genes (e.g., *KAL1, PROKR2, FGF8, FGFR1*) implicated in their etiologies.[23–26] A number of mutations have now been described in association with SOD and SOD variants, including *HESX1, TCF7L1, KAL1, FGFR1, SOX2, and OTX2*.

HESX1 mutations are an uncommon cause of hypopituitarism and SOD, accounting for <1% of cases.[27] Both homozygous and heterozygous *HESX1* mutations have been described in patients with highly variable phenotypes and with no obvious genotype-phenotype correlation.[7, 9, 28, 29] The posterior pituitary may be undescended/ectopic whereas the anterior pituitary is usually hypoplastic, although it may be absent in rare cases. To date, diabetes insipidus has not been described in patients with *HESX1* mutations, whereas deficiencies in all of the anterior pituitary hormones have been described. Additionally, both midline forebrain defects and eye defects have been variably described.

Two variants of *TCF7L1* associated with variable forms of SOD in humans have recently been reported.[30] TCF7LI is a target of the Wnt signaling pathway and is implicated in forebrain and pituitary development. The two variants identified were both associated with impaired function, but partially penetrant. This data paralleled those in the mouse, where a conditional loss of function allele was associated with variable pituitary deficits. These findings therefore suggest a role for further genetic and/or environmental modifiers.

Two loss-of-function variants in *KAL1* in females with hypopituitarism/SOD reflect the overlap between Kallman syndrome and SOD that has also been observed with *FGF8, FGFR1,* and *PROKR2* variants. Affected females presented with GH, ACTH, and TSH deficiencies with anterior pituitary hypoplasia and ONH seen on neuroimaging.[31]

Patients with SOD/CPHD have also been reported to harbor mutations in *FGFR1* with GH, TSH, and gonadotrophin deficiencies and DI.[25] Anterior pituitary hypoplasia, agenesis of the corpus callosum, ONH, and an ectopic posterior pituitary/thin or normal pituitary stalk are seen on MRI. Associated features include cleft lip/palate, brachydactyly, and a single central incisor.[32]

Association of the loss of *SOX2* with hypopituitarism was first reported in a cohort of patients with severe eye abnormalities (anophthalmia, bilateral microphthalmia) ± other developmental defects. All patients had isolated gonadotrophin deficiency with variable anterior pituitary hypoplasia and midline or forebrain defects, suggesting a clinical phenotype within the SOD spectrum.[33, 34] In addition to anterior pituitary hypoplasia, other abnormalities include generalized defects in white matter, hippocampal hypoplasia, rotated mesial temporal structures, hydrocephalus or cystic dilatation of single ventricle, hypothalamic hamartoma (or slowly progressing hypothalamo-pituitary tumors), absent septum pellucidum and hypoplasia, dysgenesis, or partial agenesis of the corpus callosum. Hypogonadotrophic hypogonadism is a recurrent finding in these patients, and GH insufficiency may be seen in some cases.[35]

Orthodenticle homeobox 2 (*OTX2*) is a transcription factor implicated in 2%–3% of anophthalmia or microphthalmia cases in humans. Heterozygous *OTX2* mutations have been described in patients with variable ocular malformations (anophthalmia, microphthalmia, retinal degeneration) and rarely in patients with no eye abnormality. The pituitary phenotype ranges from partial to complete GH deficiency or hypopituitarism ± an ectopic posterior pituitary on MRI. There is no clear genotype-phenotype correlation, even among patients with the same mutation.[36–39] GH deficiency is the most frequently observed pituitary hormone abnormality, although the development of other pituitary hormone deficiencies over time cannot be excluded due to the relative short-term follow-up of these patients.

42.2.2.2 *Hypopituitarism with Associated Learning Difficulties*

SOX3 has been implicated in the etiology of X-linked hypopituitarism with a highly variable phenotype. In patients with over- and under-dosage of *SOX3*, CPHD, and IGHD are seen with and without learning difficulties.[40] Most patients have anterior pituitary hypoplasia and an ectopic posterior pituitary, but a eutopic posterior pituitary or additional abnormalities, including a persistent craniopharyngeal canal, have also been reported.[41] Large or submicroscopic duplications encompassing *SOX3* have also been associated with hypopituitarism. In addition, polyalanine tract expansions and deletions have been reported in association with a variable phenotype (IGHD or CPHD).[42, 43] Recently, a complete SOX3 deletion in male with Hemophilia due to factor IX deficiency also has been described in association with CPHD. MRI revealed a eutopic posterior pituitary with anterior pituitary hypoplasia and a persistent craniopharyngeal canal.[41]

42.2.2.3 *Holoprosencephaly*

Holoprosencephaly (HPE) is a structural malformation of the forebrain with an incidence of 1 in 10,000–20,000 live births. It is defined by complete or incomplete separation of the cerebral hemispheres and ventricles, and failure of posterior division of the frontal and parietal lobes resulting in an absent corpus callosum. Midline facial defects associated with

HPE include cyclopia, anophthalmia, hypotelorism, midfacial hypoplasia, cleft lip/palate, and a single central incisor. DI is the most common pituitary hormone deficiency, although anterior pituitary hormone deficiencies have also been described. Mutations in *FGF8* have been identified as the first genetic cause of autosomal recessive HPE in association with pituitary dysfunction.[24] Additionally, an increasing number of genes are implicated in the etiology of HPE, including members of the Shh signaling pathway. Heterozygous, variably penetrant mutations in *GLI2*, for example, have been reported in patients with variable craniofacial abnormalities, IGHD or panhypopituitarism, and an absent or hypoplastic anterior pituitary.[44–46] Polydactyly may be seen in some of these patients.

42.2.2.4 Congenital Hypopituitarism with Neck or Cerebellar Abnormalities

Mutations in *LHX3* are reported to present as congenital hypopituitarism in the neonatal period with a short neck, loose skin, vertebral abnormalities, and variable sensorineural hearing loss.[47–50] The limited rotation associated with a short neck is variably present. The anterior pituitary may be normal, hypoplastic, or enlarged on neuroimaging. Patients with homozygous or compound heterozygous *LHX3* mutations present with GH deficiency associated with TSH, gonadotrophin or PRL deficiency, ± ACTH deficiency. Early-onset ACTH deficiency has been reported in one patient who presented with severe hypopituitarism, neonatal hypoglycemia, and low random cortisol concentrations with an impaired cortisol response to stimulation. Variably penetrant heterozygous *LHX4* mutations have been reported in patients with GH deficiency and short stature in association with other pituitary deficits (ACTH, TSH, gonadotrophin deficiency) or panhypopituitarism.[51, 52] Significant variability in the phenotype is seen, even within the same family. Radiological abnormalities include a hypoplastic, normal or enlarged anterior pituitary, ectopic posterior pituitary (in almost a third of cases), hypoplastic corpus callosum, and Chiari malformation. Neck rotation and hearing are normal. The first homozygous missense *LHX4* mutation was reported in two male infants of Pakistani origin, who died within the first week of life. Both had severe panhypopituitarism, anterior pituitary aplasia, and an ectopic posterior pituitary and were born small for gestational age with a small phallus, undescended testes, and mid-facial hypoplasia. They developed severe respiratory distress after birth, mirroring the mouse model, in which null mutants die within the first week of life from immature lungs that fail to inflate.[53] Despite rapid commencement of hydrocortisone and thyroxine replacement, both died within the first week of life.

Loss-of-function *PNPLA6* mutations have been reported in patients with progressive cerebellar ataxia or atrophy, chorioretinal dystrophy, and variable pituitary dysfunction, including GH and TSH deficiencies and normosmic hypogonadotrophic hypogonadism (manifesting as pubertal failure).[54] *PNPLA6* encodes a lysophospholipase that is expressed in neurons throughout the brain, including the cortex and Purkinje cells of the cerebellum. These findings suggest a genetic overlap between the previously unexplained Oliver-McFarlane and Laurence-Moon syndromes.[55]

42.2.2.5 Other Syndromic Forms

Mutations within *PITX2* are associated with Axenfeld-Rieger syndrome. Axenfeld-Rieger syndrome is a heterogeneous autosomal dominant condition with variable manifestations including anomalies of the anterior chamber of the eye, dental hypoplasia, a protuberant umbilicus, learning difficulties, and pituitary abnormalities. All mutations identified within *PITX2* to date are heterozygous, affecting the homeodomain of the gene. Some patients have reduced GH concentration and anterior pituitary hypoplasia, while others may have an abnormal sella turcica without endocrine dysfunction.[56, 57] Although these observations suggest a role for *PITX2* in pituitary development, its importance and role remain to be elucidated.

Homozygous mutations in *ARNT2* (c.1373_1374dupTC), a gene implicated in hypothalamic development, have been reported in six affected children of a highly consanguineous family. All patients presented in the first month of life with hypernatremia secondary to DI and cortisol insufficiency. Some children presented with, or subsequently developed, central hypothyroidism (CeH) and/or demonstrated an abnormal pattern of growth with either growth failure or maintenance of linear growth in conjunction with obesity. In this cohort, MPHD was associated with postnatal microcephaly, frontotemporal lobe hypoplasia, seizures, severe visual impairment, and abnormalities of the kidneys and urinary tract. An absent posterior pituitary with a thin pituitary stalk and anterior pituitary hypoplasia, as well as a thin corpus callosum and a global delay in brain myelination, were seen on neuroimaging.[58]

Recently, mutations have been reported in *MAGEL2* and *L1CAM* in four unrelated pedigrees with variable hypopituitarism (GHD, DI and GHD, GH and ACTH deficiency) and arthrogryposis.[59] This novel finding suggests that patients with syndromic arthrogryposis, for example, Schaaf-Yang syndrome (which has phenotypic overlap with Prader-Willi syndrome), and L1 syndrome, a group of X-linked disorders including hydrocephalus and spasticity of the lower limbs, should be screened for pituitary dysfunction.[60]

42.3 ISOLATED PITUITARY HORMONE DEFICIENCIES (TABLE 42.1)

42.3.1 Isolated GH Deficiency

Congenital IGHD is the most common pituitary hormone deficiency with an incidence of 1 in 4000–10,000 live births.[61]

The last two decades have witnessed an explosion of our understanding of the phenotype of patients with IGHD. It has now become clear that the phenotype of these children is highly heterogeneous and that these so called "isolated" GHD conditions can instead evolve and include multiple additional pituitary deficits, thus suggesting that lifelong follow-up is needed in these patients.

The diagnosis of IGHD is rarely suspected in the neonatal period and in early infancy, unless there is a known family history of genetic forms of GH deficiency or there is a history of hypoglycemia. Indeed, it is very well documented that fetal growth is not affected in children with congenital forms of GH Deficiency, and they are generally born with a normal weight, length, and head circumference, although the mean birth weight SDS has been reported to be −0.4 SDS in patients with IGHD, significantly lower than patients with CPHD associated with midline defects (+0.1 SDS).[62] Growth restriction can become evident in the first few weeks/months of life, but the variable degrees of height deficit can make a clinical diagnosis difficult. In some cases, the presence of clinical signs/symptoms of GH deficiency (such as frontal bossing, mid-facial hypoplasia, micropenis, and hypoglycemia) can aid the diagnosis.

Although most cases are sporadic, 3%–30% are familial.[63] IGHD has been classically categorized into four genetic types depending on the pattern of inheritance: autosomal recessive (types IA and IB), autosomal dominant (type II), and X-linked recessive (type III).[61] However, the expanding knowledge on the molecular defects leading to IGHD and the emerging patterns of phenotype/genotype correlations may challenge this classification in the future.[63]

The most common genes implicated are those encoding GH (*GH1*) and the receptor for GHRH (*GHRHR*). IGHD also can result from heterozygous mutations in early developmental transcription factors of development of the anterior pituitary and somatotrophs (*HESX1, SOX3, SOX2, OTX2*). IGHD may be the initial presentation before the development of multiple pituitary hormone deficiencies, as is the case with mutations in transcription factors involved in the later stages of pituitary cell differentiation, such as *PROP1* or *POU1F1*.

42.3.1.1 IGHD Caused by GH1 Mutations

The *GH1* gene is located on the long arm of chromosome 17 (17q22-24) within a cluster of five homologous genes. It consists of five exons, and its full-length product is a 191 amino acid (22 kDa) peptide representing about 75% of the circulating GH. Alternative splicing may result in complete skipping of exon 3 and the generation of a 17.5 kDa variant, which lacks amino acids 32–71, representing 1%–5% of circulating GH. Another product of aberrant splicing is the 20 kDa molecule, which represents 5%–10% of circulating GH.

Homozygous *GH1* deletions of various size (*autosomal recessive IGHD type IA*) were first described in families with early severe growth failure (height <−4.5 SDS), undetectable GH concentration, and poor response to GH treatment because of the development of antibodies.[64] Similar phenotypes can result from homozygous or compound heterozygous mutations that result in a severely truncated or absent GH molecule. On the other hand, patients with *type IB IGHD* due to *GH1* mutations also have marked short stature with low but detectable GH concentrations and a good response to GH treatment.[63]

The most common genetic form of IGHD is inherited in an autosomal dominant manner (*type II IGHD*), accounting for 73% of genetic changes in *GH1*.[65] In contrast to the previous two forms, patients with *type II IGHD* vary in the age of presentation and the degree of growth failure from severe short stature to even normal height. They tend to have low but detectable GH with or without anterior pituitary hypoplasia on MRI (35%–80%).[65] There is substantial variation in the severity of GH deficiency and patients of the same pedigree having the same mutation (e.g., p.R183H) can vary considerably in height (≤−4 SDS to normal) and even attain normal adult height without treatment.[65–68] These patients also may develop additional pituitary hormone deficits including ACTH, TSH, PRL and gonadotrophin deficiencies; hence they require life-long follow-up.[66, 69] The evolving phenotype can be explained by the mechanism by which heterozygous *GH1* mutations cause IGHD since the 17.5 kDa isoform exerts a dominant effect on the production of the 22 kDa molecule with a dose-dependent deleterious effect demonstrated in in vitro and in vivo studies.[69] In particular, the 17.5 kDa molecule is retained in the endoplasmic reticulum and triggers a misfolded protein response and the accumulation of macrophages resulting in the disruption of the Golgi apparatus. The tracking and secretory pathway of GH and other hormones such as ACTH, TSH, and LH is thereby impaired.

Another heterozygous *GH1* mutation (p.R77C) has been reported in a patient with growth retardation and delayed puberty who showed normal catch-up growth with GH replacement therapy, but there is no clear phenotype-genotype correlation as the same mutation also has been identified in family members of normal height.[67] Patients with this mutation may have normal or slightly increased GH secretion and low IGF-1 and GH-binding protein (GHBP) concentrations. Functional studies do not show a difference between the mutant and wild-type GH molecule in terms of binding to the GH receptor and activation of the downstream JAK2/STAT5 pathway, but it is possible that the mutation results in reduced capability to induce *GHR/GHBP* gene transcription compared to the wild-type molecule.

42.3.1.2 IGHD Caused by GHRHR Mutations

The gene encoding GHRHR maps to chromosome 7p15 and consists of 13 exons spanning approximately 15 kb. It encodes a 423-amino acid G-protein-coupled receptor comprising seven transmembrane domains. The expression of *GHRHR* is up-regulated by *POU1F1* and required for the proliferation of somatotrophs.

GHRHR mutations were first reported in two patients of a consanguineous Indian pedigree who had severe IGHD resulting from the homozygous p.E72X *GHRHR* mutation that caused premature termination and a truncated protein missing all transmembrane domains of the receptor.[70] A number of homozygous or compound heterozygous mutations have since been reported (missense, nonsense splice site, deletions, or regulatory mutations) leading to autosomal recessive *type IB IGHD*. Patients are usually of consanguineous pedigrees and from specific ethnic backgrounds, including the Indian subcontinent, Pakistan, Sri Lanka, Somalia, and Brazil.[63]

Children usually have severe growth failure with heights up to −7.4 SDS, undetectable GH concentrations, a blunted GH response to various stimuli, low IGF-1 and IGF-BP3, and a good response to treatment with GH.[63] Compared to patients with recessive *GH1* mutations, mid-facial hypoplasia, neonatal hypoglycemia, and microphallus are uncommon. However, recently, a 2-year-old child from a consanguineous pedigree with severe short stature (−5 SDS) was reported to present with hypoglycemia leading to convulsions. GH deficiency was subsequently diagnosed, and the child was found to be homozygous for the p.C64G mutation in exon 3.[71]

Due to the role of GHRH in the proliferation of somatotrophs, the finding of anterior pituitary hypoplasia on MRI has been considered to be almost invariable in these patients.[63] A number of reports suggest variability of anterior pituitary size, even among family members having the same *GHRHR* mutation. This finding may be explained by the fact that patients were of different ages and by the lack of well-defined age-matched reference standards for the normal pituitary size.[63]

With regard to the mechanism of action, mutations in *GHRHR* may impair ligand binding and signal transduction or affect the trafficking and localization of the receptor to the cell membrane.[63]

A heterozygous change in *GHRH* has been reported in patients with sporadic IGHD.[72] Although a digenic effect cannot be excluded in these patients, it has been proposed that this may represent a novel form of IGHD caused by dominant mutations in *GHRHR* with variable penetrance.[63]

42.3.1.3 Other Genetic Factors and IGHD

The GH secretagogue receptor (*GHSR*) is expressed in the H-P area and its endogenous ligand, ghrelin, is known to have a role in the regulation of the release of GH. Recessive and dominant *GHSR* mutations (p.W2X, p.R237W, p.A204E) have been reported to result in phenotypes that range from normal to partial IGHD[73, 74] with a mechanism of action that is not fully elucidated but may be associated with loss of the constitutive activity of the receptor.

Severe IGHD and anterior pituitary hypoplasia also has been reported in patients with biallelic *RNPC3* mutations.[75] The gene codes for a minor spliceosome protein. Three sisters with *RNPC3* mutation from a nonconsanguineous pedigree were born with normal length and weight and showed severe postnatal proportionate growth retardation (height −5 to −6.6 SDS), typical physical features of GH deficiency, delayed bone maturation without bone dysplasia, and mild microcephaly. They had undetectable GH after stimulation, undetectable IGF-1 and IGF-BP3, and low-normal PRL concentrations. Pituitary MRI confirmed anterior pituitary hypoplasia.

X-linked GHD in association with agammaglobulinemia has long been recognized as a distinct entity. Although the *Btk* (Bruton tyrosine kinase) gene, a key regulator of β cell development, has been associated with this condition, its genetic etiology remains unknown.[76]

Finally, mutations in early and later transcription factors responsible for CPHD (such as SOX3, HESX1, OTX2, LHX4, POU1F1) can also more rarely be responsible for isolated forms of GH deficiency.[63]

42.3.2 Isolated TSH Deficiency

CeH is a rare condition. However, its prevalence is probably higher than that previously suggested ranging between 1 in 50,000 and 1 in 20,000.[77] Analysis of the Dutch neonatal CeH screening program revealed the prevalence of permanent congenital CeH to be approximately 1 in 18,000.[78–80] If the prevalence of acquired CeH equals this number, the combined prevalence of permanent congenital and acquired CeH may be as high as 1 in 8000–10,000.[77] However, variable prevalences have been reported in the literature ranging between 1:16,000 and 1:100,000. Such heterogeneity probably depends upon several factors, including ethnicity, but also differences in sensitivity of the diagnostic strategies.[81]

CeH can be defined as reduced thyroid hormone secretion resulting from insufficient thyroid stimulation due to disturbed pituitary and/or hypothalamic functioning.[81] It is usually caused by a functional or anatomic disorder of the hypothalamus, the pituitary gland, or both.[82] TSH secretion may be insufficient not only in quantitative terms, but also in qualitative terms, resulting from decreased biological activity.[82]

Worldwide, most national neonatal screening programs for congenital hypothyroidism are TSH-based and effectively detect neonates with congenital hypothyroidism of thyroidal origin. However, only screening programs that combine measurement of thyroxine (T4) or free T4 (FT4) with the measurement of TSH are able to detect congenital CeH. Therefore, congenital hypothyroidism represents a major false-negative result of the "reflex TSH strategy," which is a worldwide diffuse method to screen thyroid function by the first-line TSH measurement.[83]

Inheritable conditions are the major cause of CeH in newborns and infants, while expansive lesions of the H-P region constitute the major cause of acquired CeH,[81] mostly occurring beyond the neonatal period.

CeH is generally clinically milder than primary hypothyroidism, and neonates may present with nonspecific symptoms such as lethargy, poor feeding, failure to thrive, prolonged hyperbilirubinemia, and cold intolerance. Hence, this condition can be easily clinically missed. If congenital CeH is part of multiple pituitary hormone deficiencies, there may be signs and symptoms of cortisol, GH, and testosterone deficiency as well, such as hypoglycemia, sepsis-like illness, conjugated hyperbilirubinemia, and micropenis. In addition, in syndromic forms, there may be other associated abnormalities such as midline or optic nerve defects that can aid the diagnosis. Indeed, the majority of neonates with permanent congenital CeH (approximately 75%) will have hypothyroidism within the framework of MPHD,[79, 84, 85] while only the remaining 25% will present with isolated forms.

When the diagnosis of congenital CeH is suspected in the neonatal period based on an abnormal neonatal screening result or on clinical grounds, the diagnosis should be confirmed by measurement of plasma or serum FT4 [or total T4 + thyroid binding globulin (TBG)] and TSH concentrations. FT4 concentrations below the age-specific reference interval in the presence of a TSH concentration within, below, or just above the reference interval support the diagnosis.

However, the biochemical diagnosis of CeH in the neonatal period has several caveats and a number of other thyroidal and nonthyroidal conditions should be considered in the differential diagnosis.

First, it is important to remember that neonates with a normal hypothalamo-pituitary-thyroid (HPT) axis may have low FT3 and FT4 concentrations because of nonthyroidal illness (NTI). If the medical history reveals severe birth asphyxia, (proven) bacterial sepsis, or major surgery in the first days of life, NTI is a more likely diagnosis than CeH. In this situation, FT4 measurement should be repeated once or twice weekly until a normal concentration is established. If not, the diagnosis of congenital CeH should be reconsidered.[77]

When the medical history does not point to NTI, a second alternative diagnosis to consider is transient congenital CeH related to maternal Graves' disease.[86, 87] The mother's medical history followed by an immediate TSH measurement in the mother will provide the diagnosis in most cases.

Rarer causes of a low plasma or serum FT4 concentration in the presence of a normal or mildly elevated TSH concentration are a defective monocarboxylate transporter 8 (MCT8) and resistance to thyroid hormone caused by a mutation in the thyroid hormone receptor α (TRα) gene.[88, 89] Finding a high serum or plasma T3 concentration is suggestive of a MCT8 defect, while clinical signs suggestive of severe congenital hypothyroidism in the presence of only slightly lowered FT4 concentrations may be a clue to a TRα mutation.

Once NTI and transient CeH related to maternal Graves' disease have been ruled out or unlikely, the further diagnostic workup should focus on the question of whether the neonate has MPHD or isolated congenital CeH. Considering the high mortality and morbidity associated with congenital MPHD,[90] this workup should be immediate and carried out by an experienced pediatric endocrinologist.

Finally, the clinical scenario of serum or plasma FT4 concentrations just below or fluctuating around the lower end of the age-specific reference interval in an asymptomatic neonate represents a diagnostic challenge. Although, by definition, 2.5% of a group of individuals has a FT4 concentration below the reference interval, the possible serious sequelae of a missed diagnosis of MPHD in a neonate warrant a very low threshold for the above-mentioned diagnostic workup and, if necessary, treatment. Additionally, low FT4 concentrations may be associated with neurodevelopmental deficit if left untreated.

Among pedigrees with confirmed permanent isolated congenital CeH, familial cases have been reported, although the condition may also be sporadic. Recent European Thyroid Association (ETA) consensus guidelines recommend genetic analyses in congenital cases and in cases of CeH onset during childhood or at any age when CeH remains unexplained or to support the diagnosis of idiopathic mild forms of CeH (borderline low FT4).[81]

Congenital isolated TSH deficiency may result from homozygous or compound heterozygous mutations of the TSHβ-subunit gene[91] or in the TRH receptor gene.[4] Patients classically present with absence of TSH and PRL responses to TRH and with clinically severe hypothyroidism in the latter.

Mutations in the immunoglobulin superfamily member 1 (*IGSF1*) are the most recently identified cause of CeH with an estimated incidence of up to 1 in 100,000. *IGSF1* is located on the X-chromosome and encodes a membrane glycoprotein expressed in Rathke's pouch, in the adult pituitary gland, and in testis. IGSF1 protein is detected in thyrotrophs, somatotrophs, and lactotrophs but not gonadotrophs. The function of the gene remains unclear, but it may be involved in TRH signaling.[92, 93] Loss of function mutations in *IGSF1* have been reported in males with CeH, either in isolation, or associated with hypoprolactinemia. A minority of patients require treatment for transient/partial GH deficiency in childhood. There is a variably delayed pubertal growth spurt, but all affected individuals develop macroorchidism in adulthood. Males may present with early severe CeH. Female carriers have also been described with low FT4 concentrations, often necessitating treatment.[94]

42.3.3 Isolated ACTH Deficiency

Congenital isolated ACTH deficiency is rare, although the exact prevalence is unknown. As for TSH deficiency, ACTH deficiency is more commonly associated with other pituitary hormone deficiencies than present in isolation.

The clinical features are poorly defined, and patients usually present in the neonatal period with nonspecific symptoms (poor feeding, failure to thrive, hypoglycemia) or more acutely with signs of adrenal insufficiency (vascular collapse, shock). Abnormalities in salt excretion are unusual because aldosterone secretion is largely controlled by the renin-angiotensin system.

A few cases of isolated ACTH deficiency have been reported due to mutations in *POMC* and *TBX19* (*T-PIT*).

Patients with homozygous or compound heterozygous mutations in *POMC* present with early-onset isolated ACTH deficiency, obesity, and red hair due to a lack of MSH production.

Recessive *TBX19/T-PIT* mutations are the main molecular cause of congenital neonatal isolated ACTH deficiency,[95] which tends to be severe and results in profound hypoglycemia associated with seizures and prolonged cholestatic jaundice. Neonatal deaths have been reported in up to 25% of families with these mutations, suggesting that isolated ACTH deficiency may be an underestimated cause of neonatal death. Patients present with very low basal plasma concentrations of ACTH and cortisol with no significant ACTH response to CRH.

Recently, a heterozygous nonsense mutation in NFKB2 also has been reported in a patient presenting with isolated ACTH Deficiency associated with common variable immunodeficiency.[96] De novo NFKB2 mutations also have been identified in patients with DAVID syndrome, a rare condition combining various anterior pituitary hormone deficiencies and anatomical pituitary abnormalities with common variable immunodeficiency. This finding expands the potential phenotype of NFKB2 mutations to include additional pituitary deficits and anatomical pituitary abnormalities, although a direct role of NFKB pathways on pituitary development in mice has not been demonstrated.[97]

PC1 mutations are rare and lead to ACTH deficiency in association with hypogonadotrophic hypogonadism and a complex phenotype including red hair and severe enteropathy.[98, 99] A compound heterozygous *PC1* mutation also has been described in a female patient with extreme early-onset obesity and ACTH deficiency, hypogonadotrophic hypogonadism, defective processing of other pro-hormones such as GH and vasopressin, and insulin-dependent diabetes mellitus.[100]

42.3.4 Isolated Hypogonadotrophic Hypogonadism

Hypogonadotrophic hypogonadism is a disorder caused by insufficient GnRH stimulation of an otherwise intact pituitary-gonadal axis.

Isolated hypogonadotrophic hypogonadism (IHH) is rare with a reported incidence of 1–10 cases per 100,000 births[101] and of 1:8000 males and 1:40,000 females.[102] The major underlying cause of IHH is failure to activate pulsatile secretion of gonadotropin-releasing hormone (GnRH) during puberty, a developmental stage characterized by a substantial increase in the frequency and amplitude of pulses of this hormone.

IHH is a clinically and genetically heterogeneous condition.[103] Congenital disorders of gonadotropin secretion can be divided in two groups: (1) normosomic isolated gonadotropin-releasing hormone deficiency causing hypogonadotropic hypogonadism (40% of cases) and (2) Kallmann syndrome (KS) (60% of cases), a disorder characterized by a variable combination of hypogonadotropic hypogonadism, anosmia/hyposmia, cleft lip/palate, sensorineural hearing loss, dental anomalies, synkinesia, cerebellar ataxia, mental retardation, and unilateral renal agenesis.

Patients with IHH may present in the neonatal period with micropenis and cryptorchidism (in males, while the condition is silent in females), but they more commonly manifest in adolescence and adulthood with delayed or arrested puberty and subfertility. Other features associated with specific mutations also may be present, including synkinesis and renal agenesis (*ANOS1*), coloboma, heart defects, choanal atresia, retardation of growth, genitourinary defects and ear abnormalities (the CHARGE association, *CHD7*), or marked obesity (*LEP, LEPR, PROK2*). Anosmia/hyposmia is the most frequent associated feature, which is explained by the common embryonic origins and developmental pathways of GnRH and olfactory neurons.[101] In some cases, the severity of hypogonadism and the presence of associated phenotypes in a pedigree present in a dimorphic distribution with incomplete penetrance. This pattern suggests that changes may occur in more than one gene and/or that sex-associated modifying factors may contribute to the phenotype.[104, 105] Evidence for the contribution of sex-associated factors in IHH is reinforced by the 5:1 male predominance of the disorder. In addition, male patients often present with a more severe phenotype than affected female individuals within a given family.

Mutations in genes encoding proteins that regulate GnRH neuronal development, migration from the nasal placode to the hypothalamus, GnRH secretion, or GnRH action have been identified in patients with IHH ± anosmia.

A number of genes have been reported to date in Kallmann syndrome, namely: *KAL1, CCDC141, FEZF1, IL17RD, SEMA3A*, SEMA3E, and *SOX10*.[106–109] Pathogenic variants in *CHD7, FGF8, FGF17, FGFR1, DUSP6, SPRY4, FLRT3, HS6ST1, NSMF (NELF), PROK2, PROKR2*, and *WDR11* cause both KS and normosmic hypogonadotropic hypogonadism.[109, 110] Variants in *PROKR2* and *PROK2*, encoding prokineticin receptor-2 and prokineticin-2, respectively, have been identified in approximately 9% of patients with KS.[111] Prokineticins are secreted cysteine-rich proteins that possess diverse biologic activities including effects on neuronal survival, gastrointestinal smooth muscle contraction, circadian locomotor rhythm, and appetite regulation.[111] Variations in *PROKR2 also* have been associated with hypo-pituitarism, pituitary stalk interruption syndrome, and SOD but are unlikely to be causative in isolation and more likely contribute to the phenotype in combination with other genetic mutations or environmental factors. Heterozygous pathogenic variants or microdeletions in *CHD7* can cause CHARGE syndrome, characterized by *c*oloboma, *h*eart abnormalities, choanal *a*tresia, *r*etardation of growth and development, *g*enital hypoplasia, and *e*ar abnormalities.[112] The genital abnormalities in CHARGE syndrome are caused by hypogonadotropic hypogonadism and are frequently accompanied by olfactory defects and cleft lip/palate.[113]

Mutations in a number of genes have been identified in association with normosmic hypogonadotropic hypogonadism, and these mutations include genes encoding for GnRH1 and its receptor GnRHR, kisspeptin *(KISS1)* and its receptor KISS1R, and neurokinin B (encoded by tachykinin 3, TAC3), and its receptor TACR3.[109, 114–117]

More recently, mutations in genes such as *RNF216, OTUD4, STUB1,* and *PNPLA6* have been found in syndromic forms of GnRH deficiency that have associated features such as ataxia and dementia, as part of Gordon Holmes syndrome *(RNF216, OTUD4, STUB1)*[118, 119] and Boucher-Neuhäuser syndrome *(PNPLA6)*.[120] *RNF216, OTUD4,* and *STUB1* are involved in protein ubiquitination; *PNPLA6* encodes an enzyme involved in the production of the neurotransmitter acetylcholine.

Advances in our understanding of the molecular basis of CHH have helped explain the genetic cause in 50% of cases and uncovered a complex model of genetics (oligogenicity) that might apply to a large proportion of patients.[103] Despite these recent advances, much room remains for further discovery.

42.3.5 Isolated Central Diabetes Insipidus (ICDI)

Central diabetes insipidus (CDI) is a disease in which large volumes of dilute urine are excreted due to partial or complete vasopressin (AVP) deficiency.

Congenital CDI is rare and may be found in association with other anterior pituitary deficits in the context of syndromic forms with midline disorders (such as SOD and HPE) or, more rarely (<10% of the cases), may be present in isolation and be due to mutations in genes involved in the secretion of AVP.[121]

The classic clinical signs/symptoms of CDI are polyuria, polydipsia, and weight loss, although overt clinical features might not be present until late childhood/adolescence (even in congenital/genetic forms). Nephrogenic DI is more likely to present in the neonatal period than CDI. The diagnosis is made by documentation of inability to concentrate the urine (inappropriately low urine osmolality) in the presence of plasma hyperosmolality and hypernatremia. The biochemical diagnosis can be difficult, and the interpretation of the water deprivation test requires considerable expertise.

At present, more than 70 different mutations resulting in defective prohormone and a deficiency of AVP have been identified in familial forms of CDI with all except a few showing an autosomal dominant pattern of inheritance.[121]

A number of mutations have been described in the gene that encodes the AVP preprohormone, AVP-neurophysin II (*AVP-NPII*), resulting in autosomal dominant CDI.[122] The gene is located on chromosome 20 and consists of three exons. Exon 1 encodes the signal peptide of the preprohormone and AVP; exon 3 encodes the glycoprotein copeptin, while the carrier protein NPII is encoded by all three exons. In this rare familial disorder of AVP secretion, patients usually present in the first 10 years of life, but neonatal manifestations are uncommon, which suggests that the pathophysiology of familial CDI involves progressive postnatal degeneration of AVP-producing magnocellular neurons. The proposed mechanism is that the mutant allele exerts a dominant negative effect; the misfolded mutant hormone precursor accumulates in the endoplasmic reticulum, resulting in progressive damage to the AVP neurons and the eventual clinical manifestation of DI.

Autosomal recessive mutations in the AVP gene also have been reported, but they are much more rare than the autosomal dominant forms.[122] Only one family pedigree consistent with X-linked inheritance of neurohypophyseal DI has been described to date.[123] The phenotype has been linked to chromosome Xq28, a region that also harbors the renal AVP receptor; however, the AVPR2 gene is unaltered in affected individuals, as is the AVP gene. The genetic background of this form of DI has not been elucidated.

Finally, CDI is a feature of Wolfram syndrome, a rare recessive disorder characterized additionally by insulin dependent juvenile-onset diabetes mellitus, optic atrophy, sensorineural deafness, and progressive neurodegeneration (DIDMOAD syndrome). The gene, *WFS1*, is located on 4p16.1 and encodes wolframin. The protein is localized in the endoplasmic reticulum and is a component of the misfolded protein/stress response mechanism. *WFS1* expression has been detected in selected neurons in the hippocampus, amygdala, and olfactory tubercle. CDI occurs in 70% of these patients, but it usually manifests during the second or third decade of life after diabetes mellitus and optic atrophy.[122]

42.4 ACQUIRED FORMS OF NEONATAL HYPOPITUITARISM

Acquired forms of hypopituitarism rarely occur in the neonatal period.

Hypopituitarism has been occasionally reported following neonatal/infantile sepsis from Group B streptococcus[124, 125] and Salmonella enteritidis.[126] Neonatal hypopituitarism also has been reported in association with head trauma following traumatic delivery.[127, 128] However, the direct causality between brain infections/trauma and the occurrence of hypopituitarism has not been clearly ascertained in these cases. It is also unclear whether these forms of hypopituitarism persist later in life or whether they are transient. Finally, patients with congenital forms of hypopituitarism are also known to have a high incidence of abnormal deliveries (breech, instrumental) and perinatal asphyxia, making the interpretation of the relationship between traumatic neonatal events possibly affecting the HPA and the onset of hypopituitarism even more difficult.

Other inflammatory/autoimmune and oncological causes of acquired hypopituitarism, which account for a significant proportion of the cases occurring in childhood and adolescence, are virtually absent in the neonatal period. Craniopharyngioma is a rare embryonic tumor of low-grade histological malignancy with a peak incidence of childhood-onset forms at 5–14 years of age.[129] However, nine cases presenting in the neonatal period have been reported to date.[130]

42.5 APPROACH TO THE NEONATE WITH SUSPECTED CONGENITAL HYPOPITUITARISM

Congenital hypopituitarism may present nonspecifically in the neonatal period with a spectrum of symptoms that vary in severity, depending on the hormone deficiencies that exist (see Table 42.2). Pituitary problems may be part of a syndrome, and abnormalities in other structures, such as eye and forebrain, also may be evident. Associated congenital abnormalities include HPE/anencephaly, agenesis of the corpus callosum, cleft lip/palate, and features of SOD. There may be a family history of hypopituitarism or consanguinity, and genetic counseling is important for inherited causes.

Infants with MPHD commonly present with hypoglycemia, most likely due to ACTH deficiency. Neonatal hypoglycemia also has been reported in cases of isolated growth hormone deficiency.[62] A capillary blood glucose is checked routinely in sick infants, and if this is <3.0 mmol/L, a hypoglycemia screen should be taken to include insulin, C-peptide, GH, cortisol, nonesterified fatty acids, and ketones. Low concentrations of serum GH and/or cortisol in the face of hypoglycemia suggest a diagnosis of hypopituitarism and warrant further investigation.

Polyuria and polydipsia indicative of CDI are uncommon presentations in a neonate, apart from patients with associated midline defects. Cortisol is necessary for free water excretion, and therefore, the diagnosis of CDI may be masked if the infant also has ACTH deficiency. Hypernatremia may be indicative of CDI.

Management includes replacement therapy with the appropriate hormone(s) once any deficiencies are confirmed. Pituitary deficiencies can evolve over time, and pituitary function should be reassessed at regular intervals. Patients with a *PROP1* mutation, for example, rarely present in the neonatal period, and cortisol secretion may be normal initially; later,

TABLE 42.2 Clinical presentation of hypopituitarism in a neonate

Symptom/sign	Pituitary hormone deficiency
Poor feeding	GH, ACTH
Poor weight gain	GH, ACTH, DI
Jitteriness	GH, ACTH
Lethargy	GH, ACTH
Seizures	ACTH
Recurrent sepsis	ACTH
Apnoea	ACTH
Conjugated jaundice	ACTH
Prolonged unconjugated jaundice	TSH
Temperature instability	TSH
Respiratory difficulties	TSH
Polyuria	ADH, diabetes insipidus
Polydipsia	ADH, diabetes insipidus
Undescended testes	Gonadotropin
Micropenis	Gonadotropin, GH

GH, growth hormone; ACTH, adrenocorticotrophic hormone; TSH, thyroid-stimulating hormone; ADH, antidiuretic hormone.

however, these patients can develop ACTH deficiency. Cranial ultrasound is useful in the immediate postnatal period to assess for structural anomalies of the brain; however, the pituitary gland will not be visible. Magnetic resonance imaging (MRI) with pituitary views are important to assess the size/location of the pituitary in the neonate. If a pituitary mass is present, serial scans are indicated to monitor size, as the mass will often then involute. Infants with visual abnormalities require ophthalmological review to assess for ONH. Patients with SOD may additionally require a neurodevelopmental assessment, as well as social, psychological, and educational support.

42.6 MANAGEMENT OF CONGENITAL HYPOPITUITARISM PRESENTING IN THE NEONATAL PERIOD

Neonates diagnosed with CH require lifelong follow-up by a multidisciplinary team. The mainstay of treatment is replacement of the lacking pituitary hormones. However, it is crucial to recognize the potential for evolution of endocrine deficits over time,[5] and all patients with documented endocrine dysfunction require careful lifelong monitoring and appropriate transition into adulthood. Additionally, genetic counseling should be offered in the cases where a genetic defect is detected. Finally, patients with syndromic forms of hypopituitarism (such as SOD) will also need visual assessment and neurodevelopmental support to address their complex needs.

42.6.1 GH Treatment

Growth and puberty should be monitored in these patients, and GH deficiency should be treated with recombinant human GH (rhGH) until linear growth ceases, although there is increasing evidence for the use of continued GH treatment into adulthood due to its possible metabolic effects on body composition and bone mineral density.

Regardless of the age when starting GH treatment, the recommended initial GH dose is 0.16–0.24 mg/kg/week (22–35 µg/kg/day) with individualization of subsequent dosing.[131] We advocate minimum effective doses for GH replacement, aiming for normal IGF-1 concentrations and an age-appropriate height velocity. GH treatment is uncommonly initiated in the early phases of life (particularly before the first year of life), but it can be considered in congenital cases with documented early-onset growth restriction and/or in those presenting with associated hypoglycemia.

42.6.2 Treatment of Micropenis and Cryptorchidism

Disorders of the hypothalamo-pituitary-gonadal (HPG) axis are not usually diagnosed, managed, and treated in the neonatal period as they manifest more frequently in adolescence (at the expected times of onset of puberty). In these cases, oestrogen/testosterone replacement therapy is recommended in cases presenting with delayed puberty/pubertal arrest, while GnRH analogues can be offered to patients developing precocious onset of puberty.

Male neonates presenting with micropenis and/or cryptorchidism possibly suggestive of hypogonadotrophic hypogonadism represent an exception.

Testosterone treatment can be offered to the families of male neonates presenting with micropenis for the following reasons: (1) cosmetic, to provide a future body image that will not cause embarrassment for the patient when seen by others, (2) to try and preserve the patient's future sexual function, and (3) to enable the patient to urinate standing up.[132] Testosterone can be administered intramuscularly or topically. In the first case, a short trial of 25 mg of testosterone cypionate or enanthate every 4 weeks for 3 months is usually sufficient to achieve a good response in terms of penile length. Topical applications of 5-α dihydrotestosterone (DHT) gel have also been shown to be effective in increasing the penile length at various dosage regimens (between 3 applications/day for 4 weeks to 1 application/day for 3–4 months).[132]

In males born with cryptorchidism, early referral (by 6 months of age) to the surgical team is the key aspect of the management, with recent guidelines advocating orchidopexy by 18 months of age to maximize potential for fertility and perhaps reduce the risk for testicular carcinoma in the future.[133, 134] These surgical guidelines additionally do not recommend performing imaging prior to referral and recommend against hormonal treatment, although the latter still remains a very controversial topic.[135]

Gonadotropins (LH and FSH) have been used to treat patients with micropenis and evidence of absent minipuberty.[136, 137] Such an approach might be beneficial for the additional stimulatory effect on gonadal development. Although initial studies involving neonatal administration of gonadotropins have been promising, these studies are limited, both in number of studies and number of participants, and further studies are needed to examine the effectiveness of gonadotropin treatment and its effect on long-term outcomes such as fertility.[103]

42.6.3 Levo-Thyroxine (L-T4) Treatment

CeH is an indisputable indication for thyroxine treatment. TSH deficiency is easily replaced with L-T4, which is effectively converted into triiodothyronine, the active hormone, by the type 1 and 2 deiodinases in the target tissues.

Consensus guidelines on the management of congenital hypothyroidism recommend a starting dose of 10–15 µg/kg/day shortly after birth with subsequent dose titrations being based entirely on FT4 concentrations (and not TSH) every 2–4 weeks until the concentrations settle.[138, 139] Consensus guidelines focusing on patients with CeH recommend a different treatment strategy in severe versus milder forms. Initiation of treatment with L-T4 doses similar to the ones used in primary congenital hypothyroidism are recommended in severe cases (e.g., *TSHβ* mutations), in order to rapidly restore serum FT4 concentrations to the normal range and secure optimal treatment as quickly as possible. Lower L-T4 doses (5–10 µg/kg/day) are recommended in milder forms of congenital CeH to avoid the risk of over-treatment.[81] The same guidelines recommend checking adequacy of replacement therapy 6–8 weeks after the start of L-T4 replacement with concomitant FT4 and TSH measurements, provided that blood is withdrawn before the morning replacement dose or at least 4 h after L-T4 administration, and to maintain FT4 above the median value of the normal range with the aim of optimizing the intellectual outcome.[81] In CeH, this could also be particularly beneficial in terms of limiting weight gain, given the risk of hypothalamic obesity in many forms of hypopituitarism. However, in CeH patients, replacement treatment with L-T4 should be initiated only after evidence of preserved cortisol secretion. If coexistent central adrenal insufficiency is not ruled out, thyroid replacement must be commenced after glucocorticoid therapy in order to prevent the possible induction of an adrenal crisis.[81]

In neonates and infants, most centers use initial intervals of 2–3 weeks for thyroid function monitoring, followed by 1–3 monthly assessments.

42.6.4 Hydrocortisone Treatment

In neonates with ACTH deficiency, replacement doses of Hydrocortisone (8–10 mg/m^2/day) should be given orally at least three times daily and titrated in the growing infant against trough concentrations. Doses should be doubled or even trebled in the face of illness, with patient education on how to administer emergency intramuscular hydrocortisone (doses < 1 year 25 mg, 1–5 years 25–50 mg, > 5 years 100 mg) and correct hypoglycemia during crises. Intravenous Hydrocortisone at a dose of 1–2 mg/kg 4–6 hourly should be administered to patients unable to tolerate oral Hydrocortisone (for example, severe gastrointestinal illnesses, patients undergoing surgery, or general anesthesia for investigations/procedures), followed by double/triple oral Hydrocortisone dose in the recovery phase and then titration down to the standard oral dose. When a neonate is commenced on hydrocortisone treatment, it is important to monitor for DI, as glucocorticoid therapy will unmask this in patients with multiple pituitary hormone deficiencies.

42.6.5 Desmopressin (DDAVP) Treatment

Management of CDI, particularly in patients with coexisting ACTH deficiency, is complex and needs specialist care. CDI in a neonate is best managed with fluid therapy alone. Untreated patients with an intact thirst axis and free access to fluid are able to maintain euvolemia and eunatremia by adjusting their oral intake appropriately. In neonates, given their limited ability to express a sense of thirst and given that their fluid intake is mandated by parents/care givers, this condition is even more difficult to manage.

If an infant with CDI cannot concentrate urine sufficiently to reach an osmolality greater than the renal solute concentration of the feed, this results in polyuria and hypernatremia. A balance needs to be struck between adding large volumes of water and the need to provide adequate calories for growth. In infants who are able to partially concentrate their urine between 70 and 100 mOsm/L, the use of a low-solute formula or breast milk will reduce the obligate urine output and hence the volume of free-water supplementation. In severe CDI where the concentration of urine is less than 70 mOsm/L, the use of a thiazide diuretic may be helpful. DDAVP should only be used sparingly with close titration of plasma sodium concentrations. DDAVP treatment generally aims to provide the patient with a relatively normal quality of life by reducing the burden of polyuria and polydipsia, and to allow the infant to thrive. Doses should be titrated against trough paired plasma and urine osmolalities and against the patient's symptoms, and treatment should ideally be started as an inpatient. Treatment should generally err on the side of under-dosing, since overdosing DDAVP can result in hyponatremia and rapid fluid shifts, which are difficult to correct safely, with the attendant risk of cerebral edema, or even death. Patients with hypothalamic adipsia require a strict fluid intake regimen to maintain euvolemia, and the DDAVP dose is then adjusted around this.

Oral, intranasal, and subcutaneous DDAVP preparations are commercially available.

The recommended starting dose oral dose is 1–4 µg 2–3 times/day in neonates and 10 µg 2–3 times/day in infants, to be adjusted according to response.

However, DDAVP doses are particularly difficult to titrate in neonates and infants, in whom smaller dose adjustments are required. In this age-group, buccal DDAVP formulation has recently been proposed as a practical and safe treatment alternative for CDI.[140]

Another management option in infantile DI is the use of low-renal solute load formula and thiazide diuretics. Low-renal solute load formula reduces obligatory urinary water losses, and thiazide diuretics concentrate the urine to levels seen in normal formula-fed infants. This approach has been reported to be effective in achieving consistent eunatremia and reducing the risk of hyponatremia.[141, 142]

42.7 CONCLUSIONS

In the neonatal period, the hypothalamo-pituitary neuroendocrine network is more often disrupted by congenital than by acquired etiologies. Many genetic causes have been discovered in association with congenital forms of hypopituitarism, with several single gene mutations identified. However, the vast majority of cases remain idiopathic, and the etiology of this condition is likely to involve the contribution of multiple genes and environmental factors. Regardless of the cause, the mainstay of treatment is replacement of the lacking pituitary hormones. Lifelong follow-up of such patients is required as pituitary deficits can potentially evolve over time.

REFERENCES

1. Regal M, Paramo C, Sierra SM, Garcia-Mayor RV. Prevalence and incidence of hypopituitarism in an adult Caucasian population in northwestern Spain. *Clin Endocrinol* 2001;**55**(6):735–40.
2. Castinetti F, Reynaud R, Saveanu A, Quentien MH, Albarel F, Barlier A, et al. Clinical and genetic aspects of combined pituitary hormone deficiencies. *Ann Endocrinol* 2008;**69**(1):7–17.
3. Tomlinson JW, Holden N, Hills RK, Wheatley K, Clayton RN, Bates AS, et al. Association between premature mortality and hypopituitarism. West Midlands Prospective Hypopituitary Study Group. *Lancet* 2001;**357**(9254):425–31.

4. Alatzoglou KS, Dattani MT. Genetic forms of hypopituitarism and their manifestation in the neonatal period. *Early Hum Dev* 2009;**85**(11):705–12.

5. Cerbone M, Dattani MT. Progression from isolated growth hormone deficiency to combined pituitary hormone deficiency. *Growth Hormone IGF Res* 2017;**37**:19–25.

6. Kelberman D, Dattani MT. Hypothalamic and pituitary development: novel insights into the aetiology. *Eur J Endocrinol/Eur Feder Endocr Soc* 2007;**157**(Suppl 1):S3–14.

7. Fang Q, George AS, Brinkmeier ML, Mortensen AH, Gergics P, Cheung LY, et al. Genetics of combined pituitary hormone deficiency: roadmap into the genome Era. *Endocr Rev* 2016;**37**(6):636–75.

8. Wu W, Cogan JD, Pfaffle RW, Dasen JS, Frisch H, O'Connell SM, et al. Mutations in PROP1 cause familial combined pituitary hormone deficiency. *Nat Genet* 1998;**18**(2):147–9.

9. Kelberman D, Rizzoti K, Lovell-Badge R, Robinson IC, Dattani MT. Genetic regulation of pituitary gland development in human and mouse. *Endocr Rev* 2009;**30**(7):790–829.

10. Vallette-Kasic S, Barlier A, Teinturier C, Diaz A, Manavela M, Berthezene F, et al. PROP1 gene screening in patients with multiple pituitary hormone deficiency reveals two sites of hypermutability and a high incidence of corticotroph deficiency. *J Clin Endocrinol Metab* 2001;**86**(9): 4529–35.

11. Ohta K, Nobukuni Y, Mitsubuchi H, Fujimoto S, Matsuo N, Inagaki H, et al. Mutations in the Pit-1 gene in children with combined pituitary hormone deficiency. *Biochem Biophys Res Commun* 1992;**189**(2):851–5.

12. Bas F, Uyguner ZO, Darendeliler F, Aycan Z, Cetinkaya E, Berberoglu M, et al. Molecular analysis of PROP1, POU1F1, LHX3, and HESX1 in Turkish patients with combined pituitary hormone deficiency: a multicenter study. *Endocrine* 2015;**49**(2):479–91.

13. Fluck C, Deladoey J, Rutishauser K, Eble A, Marti U, Wu W, et al. Phenotypic variability in familial combined pituitary hormone deficiency caused by a PROP1 gene mutation resulting in the substitution of Arg→Cys at codon 120 (R120C). *J Clin Endocrinol Metab* 1998;**83**(10):3727–34.

14. Turton JP, Mehta A, Raza J, Woods KS, Tiulpakov A, Cassar J, et al. Mutations within the transcription factor PROP1 are rare in a cohort of patients with sporadic combined pituitary hormone deficiency (CPHD). *Clin Endocrinol* 2005;**63**(1):10–8.

15. Voutetakis A, Argyropoulou M, Sertedaki A, Livadas S, Xekouki P, Maniati-Christidi M, et al. Pituitary magnetic resonance imaging in 15 patients with Prop1 gene mutations: pituitary enlargement may originate from the intermediate lobe. *J Clin Endocrinol Metab* 2004;**89**(5):2200–6.

16. Pfaffle RW, Blankenstein O, Wuller S, Kentrup H. Combined pituitary hormone deficiency: role of Pit-1 and Prop-1. *Acta Paediatr (Oslo, Norway: 1992) Suppl* 1999;**88**(433):33–41.

17. Rainbow LA, Rees SA, Shaikh MG, Shaw NJ, Cole T, Barrett TG, et al. Mutation analysis of POUF-1, PROP-1 and HESX-1 show low frequency of mutations in children with sporadic forms of combined pituitary hormone deficiency and septo-optic dysplasia. *Clin Endocrinol* 2005;**62**(2):163–8.

18. Webb EA, Dattani MT. Septo-optic dysplasia. *Eur J Hum Genet: EJHG* 2010;**18**(4):393–7.

19. Morishima A, Aranoff GS. Syndrome of septo-optic-pituitary dysplasia: the clinical spectrum. *Brain Dev* 1986;**8**(3):233–9.

20. Kelberman D, Dattani MT. Genetics of septo-optic dysplasia. *Pituitary* 2007;**10**(4):393–407.

21. McCabe MJ, Alatzoglou KS, Dattani MT. Septo-optic dysplasia and other midline defects: the role of transcription factors: HESX1 and beyond. *Best Pract Res Clin Endocrinol Metab* 2011;**25**(1):115–24.

22. Kahn BM, Corman TS, Lovelace K, Hong M, Krauss RS, Epstein DJ. Prenatal ethanol exposure in mice phenocopies Cdon mutation by impeding Shh function in the etiology of optic nerve hypoplasia. *Dis Model Mech* 2017;**10**(1):29–37.

23. McCabe MJ, Gaston-Massuet C, Gregory LC, Alatzoglou KS, Tziaferi V, Sbai O, et al. Variations in PROKR2, but not PROK2, are associated with hypopituitarism and septo-optic dysplasia. *J Clin Endocrinol Metab* 2013;**98**(3):E547–57.

24. McCabe MJ, Gaston-Massuet C, Tziaferi V, Gregory LC, Alatzoglou KS, Signore M, et al. Novel FGF8 mutations associated with recessive holo-prosencephaly, craniofacial defects, and hypothalamo-pituitary dysfunction. *J Clin Endocrinol Metab* 2011;**96**(10):E1709–18.

25. Raivio T, Avbelj M, McCabe MJ, Romero CJ, Dwyer AA, Tommiska J, et al. Genetic overlap in Kallmann syndrome, combined pituitary hormone deficiency, and septo-optic dysplasia. *J Clin Endocrinol Metab* 2012;**97**(4):E694–9.

26. Falardeau J, Chung WC, Beenken A, Raivio T, Plummer L, Sidis Y, et al. Decreased FGF8 signaling causes deficiency of gonadotropin-releasing hormone in humans and mice. *J Clin Invest* 2008;**118**(8):2822–31.

27. McNay DE, Turton JP, Kelberman D, Woods KS, Brauner R, Papadimitriou A, et al. HESX1 mutations are an uncommon cause of septooptic dysplasia and hypopituitarism. *J Clin Endocrinol Metab* 2007;**92**(2):691–7.

28. Thomas PQ, Dattani MT, Brickman JM, McNay D, Warne G, Zacharin M, et al. Heterozygous HESX1 mutations associated with isolated congenital pituitary hypoplasia and septo-optic dysplasia. *Hum Mol Genet* 2001;**10**(1):39–45.

29. Sobrier ML, Maghnie M, Vie-Luton MP, Secco A, di Iorgi N, Lorini R, et al. Novel HESX1 mutations associated with a life-threatening neonatal phenotype, pituitary aplasia, but normally located posterior pituitary and no optic nerve abnormalities. *J Clin Endocrinol Metab* 2006;**91**(11): 4528–36.

30. Gaston-Massuet C, McCabe MJ, Scagliotti V, Young RM, Carreno G, Gregory LC, et al. Transcription factor 7-like 1 is involved in hypothalamo-pituitary axis development in mice and humans. *Proc Natl Acad Sci U S A* 2016;**113**(5):E548–57.

31. McCabe MJ, Hu Y, Gregory LC, Gaston-Massuet C, Alatzoglou KS, Saldanha JW, et al. Novel application of luciferase assay for the in vitro functional assessment of KAL1 variants in three females with septo-optic dysplasia (SOD). *Mol Cell Endocrinol* 2015;**417**:63–72.

32. Correa FA, Trarbach EB, Tusset C, Latronico AC, Montenegro LR, Carvalho LR, et al. FGFR1 and PROKR2 rare variants found in patients with combined pituitary hormone deficiencies. *Endocr Connect* 2015;**4**(2):100–7.

33. Kelberman D, de Castro SC, Huang S, Crolla JA, Palmer R, Gregory JW, et al. SOX2 plays a critical role in the pituitary, forebrain, and eye during human embryonic development. *J Clin Endocrinol Metab* 2008;**93**(5):1865–73.

34. Kelberman D, Rizzoti K, Avilion A, Bitner-Glindzicz M, Cianfarani S, Collins J, et al. Mutations within Sox2/SOX2 are associated with abnormalities in the hypothalamo-pituitary-gonadal axis in mice and humans. *J Clin Invest* 2006;**116**(9):2442–55.

35. Schneider A, Bardakjian T, Reis LM, Tyler RC, Semina EV. Novel SOX2 mutations and genotype-phenotype correlation in anophthalmia and microphthalmia. *Am J Med Genet A* 2009;**149a**(12):2706–15.

36. Ashkenazi-Hoffnung L, Lebenthal Y, Wyatt AW, Ragge NK, Dateki S, Fukami M, et al. A novel loss-of-function mutation in OTX2 in a patient with anophthalmia and isolated growth hormone deficiency. *Hum Genet* 2010;**127**(6):721–9.

37. Dateki S, Kosaka K, Hasegawa K, Tanaka H, Azuma N, Yokoya S, et al. Heterozygous orthodenticle homeobox 2 mutations are associated with variable pituitary phenotype. *J Clin Endocrinol Metab* 2010;**95**(2):756–64.

38. Diaczok D, Romero C, Zunich J, Marshall I, Radovick S. A novel dominant negative mutation of OTX2 associated with combined pituitary hormone deficiency. *J Clin Endocrinol Metab* 2008;**93**(11):4351–9.

39. Tajima T, Ohtake A, Hoshino M, Amemiya S, Sasaki N, Ishizu K, et al. OTX2 loss of function mutation causes anophthalmia and combined pituitary hormone deficiency with a small anterior and ectopic posterior pituitary. *J Clin Endocrinol Metab* 2009;**94**(1):314–9.

40. Laumonnier F, Ronce N, Hamel BC, Thomas P, Lespinasse J, Raynaud M, et al. Transcription factor SOX3 is involved in X-linked mental retardation with growth hormone deficiency. *Am J Hum Genet* 2002;**71**(6):1450–5.

41. Alatzoglou KS, Azriyanti A, Rogers N, Ryan F, Curry N, Noakes C, et al. SOX3 deletion in mouse and human is associated with persistence of the craniopharyngeal canal. *J Clin Endocrinol Metab* 2014;**99**(12):E2702–8.

42. Alatzoglou KS, Kelberman D, Cowell CT, Palmer R, Arnhold IJ, Melo ME, et al. Increased transactivation associated with SOX3 polyalanine tract deletion in a patient with hypopituitarism. *J Clin Endocrinol Metab* 2011;**96**(4):E685–90.

43. Burkitt Wright EM, Perveen R, Clayton PE, Hall CM, Costa T, Procter AM, et al. X-linked isolated growth hormone deficiency: expanding the phenotypic spectrum of SOX3 polyalanine tract expansions. *Clin Dysmorphol* 2009;**18**(4):218–21.

44. Franca MM, Jorge AA, Carvalho LR, Costalonga EF, Vasques GA, Leite CC, et al. Novel heterozygous nonsense GLI2 mutations in patients with hypopituitarism and ectopic posterior pituitary lobe without holoprosencephaly. *J Clin Endocrinol Metab* 2010;**95**(11):E384–91.

45. Gregory LC, Gaston-Massuet C, Andoniadou CL, Carreno G, Webb EA, Kelberman D, et al. The role of the sonic hedgehog signalling pathway in patients with midline defects and congenital hypopituitarism. *Clin Endocrinol* 2015;**82**(5):728–38.

46. Roessler E, Du YZ, Mullor JL, Casas E, Allen WP, Gillessen-Kaesbach G, et al. Loss-of-function mutations in the human GLI2 gene are associated with pituitary anomalies and holoprosencephaly-like features. *Proc Natl Acad Sci U S A* 2003;**100**(23):13424–9.

47. Bhangoo AP, Hunter CS, Savage JJ, Anhalt H, Pavlakis S, Walvoord EC, et al. Clinical case seminar: a novel LHX3 mutation presenting as combined pituitary hormonal deficiency. *J Clin Endocrinol Metab* 2006;**91**(3):747–53.

48. Netchine I, Sobrier ML, Krude H, Schnabel D, Maghnie M, Marcos E, et al. Mutations in LHX3 result in a new syndrome revealed by combined pituitary hormone deficiency. *Nat Genet* 2000;**25**(2):182–6.

49. Pfaeffle RW, Savage JJ, Hunter CS, Palme C, Ahlmann M, Kumar P, et al. Four novel mutations of the LHX3 gene cause combined pituitary hormone deficiencies with or without limited neck rotation. *J Clin Endocrinol Metab* 2007;**92**(5):1909–19.

50. Rajab A, Kelberman D, de Castro SC, Biebermann H, Shaikh H, Pearce K, et al. Novel mutations in LHX3 are associated with hypopituitarism and sensorineural hearing loss. *Hum Mol Genet* 2008;**17**(14):2150–9.

51. Pfaeffle RW, Hunter CS, Savage JJ, Duran-Prado M, Mullen RD, Neeb ZP, et al. Three novel missense mutations within the LHX4 gene are associated with variable pituitary hormone deficiencies. *J Clin Endocrinol Metab* 2008;**93**(3):1062–71.

52. Tajima T, Hattori T, Nakajima T, Okuhara K, Tsubaki J, Fujieda K. A novel missense mutation (P366T) of the LHX4 gene causes severe combined pituitary hormone deficiency with pituitary hypoplasia, ectopic posterior lobe and a poorly developed sella turcica. *Endocr J* 2007;**54**(4):637–41.

53. Gregory LC, Humayun KN, Turton JP, McCabe MJ, Rhodes SJ, Dattani MT. Novel lethal form of congenital hypopituitarism associated with the first recessive LHX4 mutation. *J Clin Endocrinol Metab* 2015;**100**(6):2158–64.

54. Topaloglu AK, Lomniczi A, Kretzschmar D, Dissen GA, Kotan LD, McArdle CA, et al. Loss-of-function mutations in PNPLA6 encoding neuropathy target esterase underlie pubertal failure and neurologic deficits in Gordon Holmes syndrome. *J Clin Endocrinol Metab* 2014;**99**(10):E2067–75.

55. Hufnagel RB, Arno G, Hein ND, Hersheson J, Prasad M, Anderson Y, et al. Neuropathy target esterase impairments cause Oliver-McFarlane and Laurence-Moon syndromes. *J Med Genet* 2015;**52**(2):85–94.

56. Tumer Z, Bach-Holm D. Axenfeld-Rieger syndrome and spectrum of PITX2 and FOXC1 mutations. *Eur J Hum Genet: EJHG* 2009;**17**(12):1527–39.

57. Wang Y, Zhao H, Zhang X, Feng H. Novel identification of a four-base-pair deletion mutation in PITX2 in a Rieger syndrome family. *J Dent Res* 2003;**82**(12):1008–12.

58. Webb EA, AlMutair A, Kelberman D, Bacchelli C, Chanudet E, Lescai F, et al. ARNT2 mutation causes hypopituitarism, post-natal microcephaly, visual and renal anomalies. *Brain J Neurol* 2013;**136**(Pt 10):3096–105.

59. Gregory LC, Pratik S, JRF S, Arancibia M, Hurst J, Jones WD, Spoudeas H, Le Quesne Stabej P, Ocaka L, Loureiro C, Martinez-Aguayo A, Williams H, Dattani MT. Mutations in MAGEL2 and L1CAM are associated with congenital hypopituitarism and arthrogryposis. *ESPE Abstr* 2018;**89**:FC93.

60. Jobling R, Stavropoulos DJ, Marshall CR, Cytrynbaum C, Axford MM, Londero V, et al. Chitayat-Hall and Schaaf-Yang syndromes:a common aetiology: expanding the phenotype of MAGEL2-related disorders. *J Med Genet* 2018;**55**(5):316–21.

61. Mullis PE. Genetics of growth hormone deficiency. *Endocrinol Metab Clin N Am* 2007;**36**(1):17–36.

62. Mehta A, Hindmarsh PC, Stanhope RG, Turton JP, Cole TJ, Preece MA, et al. The role of growth hormone in determining birth size and early postnatal growth, using congenital growth hormone deficiency (GHD) as a model. *Clin Endocrinol* 2005;**63**(2):223–31.

63. Alatzoglou KS, Webb EA, Le Tissier P, Dattani MT. Isolated growth hormone deficiency (GHD) in childhood and adolescence: recent advances. *Endocr Rev* 2014;**35**(3):376–432.

64. Laron Z, Kelijman M, Pertzelan A, Keret R, Shoffner JM, Parks JS. Human growth hormone gene deletion without antibody formation or growth arrest during treatment—a new disease entity? *Isr J Med Sci* 1985;**21**(12):999–1006.

65. Alatzoglou KS, Turton JP, Kelberman D, Clayton PE, Mehta A, Buchanan C, et al. Expanding the spectrum of mutations in GH1 and GHRHR: genetic screening in a large cohort of patients with congenital isolated growth hormone deficiency. *J Clin Endocrinol Metab* 2009;**94**(9):3191–9.

66. Turton JP, Buchanan CR, Robinson IC, Aylwin SJ, Dattani MT. Evolution of gonadotropin deficiency in a patient with type II autosomal dominant GH deficiency. *Eur J Endocrinol/Eur Feder Endocr Soc* 2006;**155**(6):793–9.

67. Petkovic V, Lochmatter D, Turton J, Clayton PE, Trainer PJ, Dattani MT, et al. Exon splice enhancer mutation (GH-E32A) causes autosomal dominant growth hormone deficiency. *J Clin Endocrinol Metab* 2007;**92**(11):4427–35.

68. Hess O, Hujeirat Y, Wajnrajch MP, Allon-Shalev S, Zadik Z, Lavi I, et al. Variable phenotypes in familial isolated growth hormone deficiency caused by a G6664A mutation in the GH-1 gene. *J Clin Endocrinol Metab* 2007;**92**(11):4387–93.

69. Mullis PE, Robinson IC, Salemi S, Eble A, Besson A, Vuissoz JM, et al. Isolated autosomal dominant growth hormone deficiency: an evolving pituitary deficit? A multicenter follow-up study. *J Clin Endocrinol Metab* 2005;**90**(4):2089–96.

70. Wajnrajch MP, Gertner JM, Harbison MD, Chua Jr SC, Leibel RL. Nonsense mutation in the human growth hormone-releasing hormone receptor causes growth failure analogous to the little (lit) mouse. *Nat Genet* 1996;**12**(1):88–90.

71. Demirbilek H, Tahir S, Baran RT, Sherif M, Shah P, Ozbek MN, et al. Familial isolated growth hormone deficiency due to a novel homozygous missense mutation in the growth hormone releasing hormone receptor gene: clinical presentation with hypoglycemia. *J Clin Endocrinol Metab* 2014;**99**(12):E2730–4.

72. Godi M, Mellone S, Petri A, Arrigo T, Bardelli C, Corrado L, et al. A recurrent signal peptide mutation in the growth hormone releasing hormone receptor with defective translocation to the cell surface and isolated growth hormone deficiency. *J Clin Endocrinol Metab* 2009;**94**(10):3939–47.

73. Pantel J, Legendre M, Cabrol S, Hilal L, Hajaji Y, Morisset S, et al. Loss of constitutive activity of the growth hormone secretagogue receptor in familial short stature. *J Clin Invest* 2006;**116**(3):760–8.

74. Pantel J, Legendre M, Nivot S, Morisset S, Vie-Luton MP, le Bouc Y, et al. Recessive isolated growth hormone deficiency and mutations in the ghrelin receptor. *J Clin Endocrinol Metab* 2009;**94**(11):4334–41.

75. Argente J, Flores R, Gutierrez-Arumi A, Verma B, Martos-Moreno GA, Cusco I, et al. Defective minor spliceosome mRNA processing results in isolated familial growth hormone deficiency. *EMBO Mol Med* 2014;**6**(3):299–306.

76. Stewart DM, Tian L, Notarangelo LD, Nelson DL. X-linked hypogammaglobulinemia and isolated growth hormone deficiency: an update. *Immunol Res* 2008;**40**(3):262–70.

77. Fliers E, Boelen A, van Trotsenburg AS. Central regulation of the hypothalamo-pituitary-thyroid (HPT) axis: focus on clinical aspects. *Handb Clin Neurol* 2014;**124**:127–38.

78. Lanting CI, van Tijn DA, Loeber JG, Vulsma T, de Vijlder JJ, Verkerk PH. Clinical effectiveness and cost-effectiveness of the use of the thyroxine/thyroxine-binding globulin ratio to detect congenital hypothyroidism of thyroidal and central origin in a neonatal screening program. *Pediatrics* 2005;**116**(1):168–73.

79. van Tijn DA, de Vijlder JJ, Verbeeten Jr B, Verkerk PH, Vulsma T. Neonatal detection of congenital hypothyroidism of central origin. *J Clin Endocrinol Metab* 2005;**90**(6):3350–9.

80. Kempers MJ, Lanting CI, van Heijst AF, van Trotsenburg AS, Wiedijk BM, de Vijlder JJ, et al. Neonatal screening for congenital hypothyroidism based on thyroxine, thyrotropin, and thyroxine-binding globulin measurement: potentials and pitfalls. *J Clin Endocrinol Metab* 2006;**91**(9):3370–6.

81. Persani L, Brabant G, Dattani M, Bonomi M, Feldt-Rasmussen U, Fliers E, Gruters A, Maiter D, Schoenmakers N, van Trotsenburg ASP. European Thyroid Association (ETA) guidelines on the diagnosis and management of central hypothyroidism. *Eur Thyroid J* 2018;**7**(5):225–37.

82. Persani L. Clinical review: Central hypothyroidism: pathogenic, diagnostic, and therapeutic challenges. *J Clin Endocrinol Metab* 2012;**97**(9):3068–78.

83. Price A, Weetman AP. Screening for central hypothyroidism is unjustified. *BMJ (Clin Res Ed)* 2001;**322**(7289):798.

84. Hanna CE, Krainz PL, Skeels MR, Miyahira RS, Sesser DE, LaFranchi SH. Detection of congenital hypopituitary hypothyroidism: ten-year experience in the Northwest Regional Screening Program. *J Pediatr* 1986;**109**(6):959–64.

85. Adachi M, Soneda A, Asakura Y, Muroya K, Yamagami Y, Hirahara F. Mass screening of newborns for congenital hypothyroidism of central origin by free thyroxine measurement of blood samples on filter paper. *Eur J Endocrinol/Eur Feder Endocr Soc* 2012;**166**(5):829–38.

86. Kempers MJ, van Tijn DA, van Trotsenburg AS, de Vijlder JJ, Wiedijk BM, Vulsma T. Central congenital hypothyroidism due to gestational hyperthyroidism: detection where prevention failed. *J Clin Endocrinol Metab* 2003;**88**(12):5851–7.

87. Matsuura N, Konishi J. Transient hypothyroidism in infants born to mothers with chronic thyroiditis—a nationwide study of twenty-three cases. The Transient Hypothyroidism Study Group. *Endocrinol Japonica* 1990;**37**(3):369–79.

88. Friesema EC, Grueters A, Biebermann H, Krude H, von Moers A, Reeser M, et al. Association between mutations in a thyroid hormone transporter and severe X-linked psychomotor retardation. *Lancet* 2004;**364**(9443):1435–7.

89. Bochukova E, Schoenmakers N, Agostini M, Schoenmakers E, Rajanayagam O, Keogh JM, et al. A mutation in the thyroid hormone receptor alpha gene. *N Engl J Med* 2012;**366**(3):243–9.

90. Nebesio TD, McKenna MP, Nabhan ZM, Eugster EA. Newborn screening results in children with central hypothyroidism. *J Pediatr* 2010;**156**(6):990–3.

91. Ramos HE, Labedan I, Carre A, Castanet M, Guemas I, Tron E, et al. New cases of isolated congenital central hypothyroidism due to homozygous thyrotropin beta gene mutations: a pitfall to neonatal screening. *Thyroid* 2010;**20**(6):639–45.

92. Sun Y, Bak B, Schoenmakers N, van Trotsenburg AS, Oostdijk W, Voshol P, et al. Loss-of-function mutations in IGSF1 cause an X-linked syndrome of central hypothyroidism and testicular enlargement. *Nat Genet* 2012;**44**(12):1375–81.

93. Joustra SD, van Trotsenburg AS, Sun Y, Losekoot M, Bernard DJ, Biermasz NR, et al. IGSF1 deficiency syndrome: a newly uncovered endocrinopathy. *Rare Dis (Austin, TX)* 2013;**1**:e24883.

94. Joustra SD, Schoenmakers N, Persani L, Campi I, Bonomi M, Radetti G, et al. The IGSF1 deficiency syndrome: characteristics of male and female patients. *J Clin Endocrinol Metab* 2013;**98**(12):4942–52.

95. Pulichino AM, Vallette-Kasic S, Couture C, Gauthier Y, Brue T, David M, et al. Human and mouse TPIT gene mutations cause early onset pituitary ACTH deficiency. *Genes Dev* 2003;**17**(6):711–6.

96. Shi C, Wang F, Tong A, Zhang XQ, Song HM, Liu ZY, et al. NFKB2 mutation in common variable immunodeficiency and isolated adrenocorticotropic hormone deficiency: a case report and review of literature. *Medicine* 2016;**95**(40).

97. Brue T, Quentien MH, Khetchoumian K, Bensa M, Capo-Chichi JM, Delemer B, et al. Mutations in NFKB2 and potential genetic heterogeneity in patients with DAVID syndrome, having variable endocrine and immune deficiencies. *BMC Med Genet* 2014;**15**:139.

98. Farooqi IS, Volders K, Stanhope R, Heuschkel R, White A, Lank E, et al. Hyperphagia and early-onset obesity due to a novel homozygous missense mutation in prohormone convertase 1/3. *J Clin Endocrinol Metab* 2007;**92**(9):3369–73.

99. Jackson RS, Creemers JW, Farooqi IS, Raffin-Sanson ML, Varro A, Dockray GJ, et al. Small-intestinal dysfunction accompanies the complex endocrinopathy of human proprotein convertase 1 deficiency. *J Clin Invest* 2003;**112**(10):1550–60.

100. O'Rahilly S, Gray H, Humphreys PJ, Krook A, Polonsky KS, White A, et al. Brief report: impaired processing of prohormones associated with abnormalities of glucose homeostasis and adrenal function. *N Engl J Med* 1995;**333**(21):1386–90.

101. Bianco SD, Kaiser UB. The genetic and molecular basis of idiopathic hypogonadotropic hypogonadism. *Nat Rev Endocrinol* 2009;**5**(10):569–76.

102. Network for Central Hypogonadism (Network Ipogonadismo Centrale, NICe) of Italian Societies of Endocrinology (SIE), of Andrology and Sexual Medicine (SIAMS) and of Peadiatric Endocrinology and Diabetes (SIEDP). Kallmann's syndrome and normosmic isolated hypogonadotropic hypogonadism: two largely overlapping manifestations of one rare disorder. *J Endocrinol Investig* 2014;**37**(5):499–500.

103. Boehm U, Bouloux PM, Dattani MT, de Roux N, Dode C, Dunkel L, et al. Expert consensus document: European Consensus Statement on congenital hypogonadotropic hypogonadism—pathogenesis, diagnosis and treatment. *Nat Rev Endocrinol* 2015;**11**(9):547–64.

104. Pitteloud N, Meysing A, Quinton R, Acierno Jr JS, Dwyer AA, Plummer L, et al. Mutations in fibroblast growth factor receptor 1 cause Kallmann syndrome with a wide spectrum of reproductive phenotypes. *Mol Cell Endocrinol* 2006;**254–255**:60–9.

105. Pitteloud N, Quinton R, Pearce S, Raivio T, Acierno J, Dwyer A, et al. Digenic mutations account for variable phenotypes in idiopathic hypogonadotropic hypogonadism. *J Clin Invest* 2007;**117**(2):457–63.

106. Valdes-Socin H, Rubio Almanza M, Tome Fernandez-Ladreda M, Debray FG, Bours V, Beckers A. Reproduction, smell, and neurodevelopmental disorders: genetic defects in different hypogonadotropic hypogonadal syndromes. *Front Endocrinol* 2014;**5**:109.

107. Pingault V, Bodereau V, Baral V, Marcos S, Watanabe Y, Chaoui A, et al. Loss-of-function mutations in SOX10 cause Kallmann syndrome with deafness. *Am J Hum Genet* 2013;**92**(5):707–24.

108. Hutchins BI, Kotan LD, Taylor-Burds C, Ozkan Y, Cheng PJ, Gurbuz F, et al. CCDC141 mutation identified in anosmic hypogonadotropic hypogonadism (Kallmann syndrome) alters GnRH neuronal migration. *Endocrinology* 2016;**157**(5):1956–66.

109. Balasubramanian R, Crowley Jr WF. Reproductive endocrine phenotypes relating to CHD7 mutations in humans. *Am J Med Genet C Semin Med Genet* 2017;**175**(4):507–15.

110. Miraoui H, Dwyer AA, Sykiotis GP, Plummer L, Chung W, Feng B, et al. Mutations in FGF17, IL17RD, DUSP6, SPRY4, and FLRT3 are identified in individuals with congenital hypogonadotropic hypogonadism. *Am J Hum Genet* 2013;**92**(5):725–43.

111. Sarfati J, Fouveaut C, Leroy C, Jeanpierre M, Hardelin JP, Dode C. Greater prevalence of PROKR2 mutations in Kallmann syndrome patients from the Maghreb than in European patients. *Eur J Endocrinol/Eur Feder Endocr Soc* 2013;**169**(6):805–9.

112. Vissers LE, van Ravenswaaij CM, Admiraal R, Hurst JA, de Vries BB, Janssen IM, et al. Mutations in a new member of the chromodomain gene family cause CHARGE syndrome. *Nat Genet* 2004;**36**(9):955–7.

113. Pinto G, Abadie V, Mesnage R, Blustajn J, Cabrol S, Amiel J, et al. CHARGE syndrome includes hypogonadotropic hypogonadism and abnormal olfactory bulb development. *J Clin Endocrinol Metab* 2005;**90**(10):5621–6.

114. Bouligand J, Ghervan C, Tello JA, Brailly-Tabard S, Salenave S, Chanson P, et al. Isolated familial hypogonadotropic hypogonadism and a GNRH1 mutation. *N Engl J Med* 2009;**360**(26):2742–8.

115. de Roux N, Young J, Misrahi M, Genet R, Chanson P, Schaison G, et al. A family with hypogonadotropic hypogonadism and mutations in the gonadotropin-releasing hormone receptor. *N Engl J Med* 1997;**337**(22):1597–602.

116. Topaloglu AK, Reimann F, Guclu M, Yalin AS, Kotan LD, Porter KM, et al. TAC3 and TACR3 mutations in familial hypogonadotropic hypogonadism reveal a key role for Neurokinin B in the central control of reproduction. *Nat Genet* 2009;**41**(3):354–8.

117. Topaloglu AK, Tello JA, Kotan LD, Ozbek MN, Yilmaz MB, Erdogan S, et al. Inactivating KISS1 mutation and hypogonadotropic hypogonadism. *N Engl J Med* 2012;**366**(7):629–35.

118. Shi CH, Schisler JC, Rubel CE, Tan S, Song B, McDonough H, et al. Ataxia and hypogonadism caused by the loss of ubiquitin ligase activity of the U box protein CHIP. *Hum Mol Genet* 2014;**23**(4):1013–24.

119. Seminara SB, Acierno Jr JS, Abdulwahid NA, Crowley Jr WF, Margolin DH. Hypogonadotropic hypogonadism and cerebellar ataxia: detailed phenotypic characterization of a large, extended kindred. *J Clin Endocrinol Metab* 2002;**87**(4):1607–12.

120. Synofzik M, Hufnagel RB, Zuchner S. PNPLA6-related disorders. In: Adam MP, Ardinger HH, Pagon RA, Wallace SE, LJH B, Stephens K, et al., editors, *GeneReviews((R))*. Seattle (WA): University of Washington, Seattle; 1993. GeneReviews is a registered trademark of the University of Washington, Seattle. All rights reserved.

121. Di Iorgi N, Napoli F, Allegri AE, Olivieri I, Bertelli E, Gallizia A, et al. Diabetes insipidus—diagnosis and management. *Hormone Res Paediatr* 2012;**77**(2):69–84.

122. Rutishauser J, Spiess M, Kopp P. Genetic forms of neurohypophyseal diabetes insipidus. *Best Pract Res Clin Endocrinol Metab* 2016;**30**(2):249–62.

123. Habiby RLRG, Kaplowitz PB, Rittig S. A novel X-linked form of familial neurohypophyseal diabetes insipidus [abst]. *J Investig Med* 1996;**44** (341A).

124. Ferreira AS, Fernandes AL, Guaragna-Filho G. Hypopituitarism as consequence of late neonatal infection by Group B streptococcus: a case report. *Pan Afr Med J* 2015;**20**:308.

125. Pai KG, Rubin HM, Wedemeyer PP, Linarelli LG. Hypothalamic-pituitary dysfunction following group B beta hemolytic streptococcal meningitis in a neonate. *J Pediatr* 1976;**88**(2):289–91.

126. Saranac L, Bjelakovic B, Djordjevic D, Novak M, Stankovic T. Hypopituitarism occurring in neonatal sepsis. *J Pediatr Endocrinol Metab: JPEM* 2012;**25**(9-10):847–8.

127. Minutti CZ, Zimmerman D. Traumatic hypopituitarism due to maternal uterine leiomyomas. *J Endocrinol Investig* 2002;**25**(2):158–62.

128. Gacs G. Perinatal factors in the aetiology of hypopituitarism. *Helv Paediatr Acta* 1987;**42**(2-3):137–44.

129. Olsson DS, Andersson E, Bryngelsson IL, Nilsson AG, Johannsson G. Excess mortality and morbidity in patients with craniopharyngioma, especially in patients with childhood onset: a population-based study in Sweden. *J Clin Endocrinol Metab* 2015;**100**(2):467–74.

130. do Prado Aguiar U, Araujo JL, Veiga JC, Toita MH, de Aguiar GB. Congenital giant craniopharyngioma. *Child's Nervous Syst: ChNS* 2013;**29**(1): 153–7.

131. Grimberg A, DiVall SA, Polychronakos C, Allen DB, Cohen LE, Quintos JB, et al. Guidelines for growth hormone and insulin-like growth factor-I treatment in children and adolescents: growth hormone deficiency, idiopathic short stature, and primary insulin-like growth factor-I deficiency. *Hormone Res Paediatr* 2016;**86**(6):361–97.

132. Hatipoglu N, Kurtoglu S. Micropenis: etiology, diagnosis and treatment approaches. *J Clin Res Pediatr Endocrinol* 2013;**5**(4):217–23.

133. Kolon TF, Herndon CD, Baker LA, Baskin LS, Baxter CG, Cheng EY, et al. Evaluation and treatment of cryptorchidism: AUA guideline. *J Urol* 2014;**192**(2):337–45.

134. Elder JS. Surgical management of the undescended testis: recent advances and controversies. *Eur J Pediatr Surg* 2016;**26**(5):418–26.

135. Ludwikowski B, Gonzalez R. The controversy regarding the need for hormonal treatment in boys with unilateral cryptorchidism goes on: a review of the literature. *Eur J Pediatr* 2013;**172**(1):5–8.

136. Main KM, Schmidt IM, Toppari J, Skakkebaek NE. Early postnatal treatment of hypogonadotropic hypogonadism with recombinant human FSH and LH. *Eur J Endocrinol/Eur Feder Endocr Soc* 2002;**146**(1):75–9.

137. Bouvattier C, Maione L, Bouligand J, Dode C, Guiochon-Mantel A, Young J. Neonatal gonadotropin therapy in male congenital hypogonadotropic hypogonadism. *Nat Rev Endocrinol* 2011;**8**(3):172–82.

138. Leger J, Olivieri A, Donaldson M, Torresani T, Krude H, van Vliet G, et al. European Society for Paediatric Endocrinology consensus guidelines on screening, diagnosis, and management of congenital hypothyroidism. *J Clin Endocrinol Metab* 2014;**99**(2):363–84.

139. Rose SR, Brown RS, Foley T, Kaplowitz PB, Kaye CI, Sundararajan S, et al. Update of newborn screening and therapy for congenital hypothyroidism. *Pediatrics* 2006;**117**(6):2290–303.

140. Smego AR, Backeljauw P, Gutmark-Little I. Buccally administered intranasal desmopressin acetate for the treatment of neurogenic diabetes insipidus in infancy. *J Clin Endocrinol Metab* 2016;**101**(5):2084–8.

141. Pogacar PR, Mahnke S, Rivkees SA. Management of central diabetes insipidus in infancy with low renal solute load formula and chlorothiazide. *Curr Opin Pediatr* 2000;**12**(4):405–11.

142. Rivkees SA, Dunbar N, Wilson TA. The management of central diabetes insipidus in infancy: desmopressin, low renal solute load formula, thiazide diuretics. *J Pediatr Endocrinol Metab: JPEM* 2007;**20**(4):459–69.

Chapter 43

Fetal and Postnatal Disorders of Thyroid Function

Sarah Elizabeth Lawrence*, Julia Elisabeth von Oettingen[†] and Johnny Deladoëy[‡]

*Children's Hospital of Eastern Ontario, Ottawa, ON, Canada, [†]McGill University Health Centre, Montreal, QC, Canada, [‡]CHU Sainte-Justine, Université de Montréal, Montréal, QC, Canada

---

Common Clinical Problems

- A 6-day-old infant has had a positive newborn screening test for congenital hypothyroidism.
  - Is this a true positive screen? If so, what is the etiology? Is this due to transient or permanent congenital hypothyroidism (CH)?
  - How would you manage a child with CH?
- A child is born to a mother with a history of Graves' disease. How would you monitor and manage this infant?
- A neonate has suspected hypopituitarism. How does central hypothyroidism present, and how is it diagnosed and managed?

43.1 CONGENITAL HYPOTHYROIDISM

43.1.1 Newborn Screening

CH is the most common preventable cause of neurodevelopmental delay and affects 1 in 2500 newborns.[1, 2] Newborn screening for CH has been widely adopted since its first introduction in Quebec in 1975[3] due to its public health success and breakthrough achievement to eliminate preventable mental retardation. The screening classically consists of the following: (1) a newborn heel-prick blood specimen obtained onto filter paper at 36–72 h of life (Fig. 43.1), (2) transport to a central laboratory for analysis, (3) communication with the infant's treating physician if results are positive, and (4) immediate treatment initiation with once-daily levothyroxine[4] if diagnostic testing is consistent with a diagnosis of CH. Alternatively, cord blood can be used, although the physiologic thyroid-stimulating hormone (TSH) rise after birth must be taken into account for interpretation of the results.[5] The infrastructure, logistics, and coordination of clinical follow-up required challenging implementation of newborn screening in many low- and middle-income countries. As a result, 70% of newborns globally do not have access to this essential public health measure.[6] In some settings, point-of-care testing may be more appropriate to overcome some of the logistical challenge with specimen transport and feedback loop, although adequate technological devices are not yet readily available.

Screening is most effective when it is universal, and when a centralized approach is used whereby a central laboratory oversees specimen collection; manages reception, analysis, interpretation, and results communication; and provides quality assurance. Possible screening approaches include primary T4 screening,[3] primary TSH screening,[7] or a combination of the two. Primary hypothyroidism being by far the most common etiology of CH, a primary TSH approach has emerged as the preferred screening approach worldwide,[6] especially after 1990, when precise, reliable TSH assays emerged. While a primary TSH-screening strategy will not detect central hypothyroidism,[8] its incidence is low, and it is often also missed on primary T4 screening due to normal T4 values in over 80% of newborns with central hypothyroidism.[9] Two examples of a TSH-based screening algorithm in Quebec and a primary T4 algorithm used in the Netherlands are shown in Fig. 43.2.

Due to the neonatal TSH surge after birth, the timing of screening for CH should be *after* a minimum of 24 h of life to avoid a high number of false positives. Values above 15 mU/L are seen in 9% versus 0.2%–0.3% of neonates when TSH is measured within the first 24 h versus at 2–5 days of life.[10] Further, TSH values obtained before 24 h do not correlate well with measurements obtained at 2–3 days of life.[11] This necessity to wait until 24 h after birth to obtain the newborn screening specimen can be logistically challenging, especially in settings where otherwise healthy babies are discharged

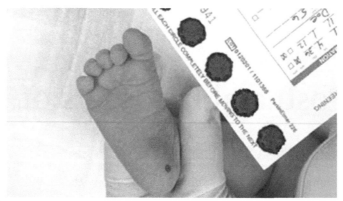

FIG. 43.1 Newborn screening dried blood spot.

Quebec NBS algorithm

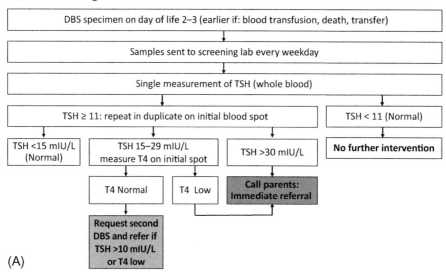

(A)

The Netherlands NBS algorithm

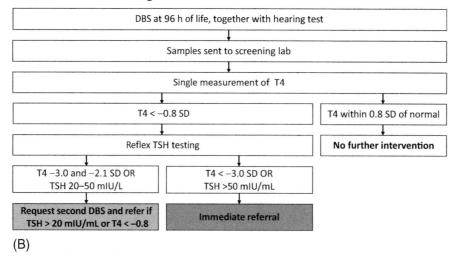

(B)

FIG. 43.2 Examples of congenital hypothyroidism screening logic. (A) Quebec NBS Algorithm, (B) The Netherlands NBS Algorithm.

from the hospital within hours after birth. In these situations, postnatal or vaccine visits within the first week of life could potentially be used as alternative platforms for newborn screening.

Over the past two decades, controversy about the optimal TSH cutoff to use in screening algorithms has been ongoing.[12] The historically used values of 20–50 mU/L to determine a positive screen have been lowered in most programs to 6–20 mU/L. The main benefit has been an improved sensitivity, although at the expense of higher false positive rates. Most additional cases detected are mild and often transient,[13, 14] and whether treatment of these infants who mostly have eutopic, normally formed thyroid glands[2, 14] affects developmental outcomes has been subject to debate.[12] On the other hand, false negative results are rare and are most commonly due to problems in specimen collection, handling, processing, analysis, or results reporting. Premature, low-birth-weight infants may represent an exception, in that their TSH rise can be delayed and as a result missed on the newborn screening specimen obtained at 2–5 days of life.[15–17] While this has led to the introduction of a second specimen collection for these infants in some screening programs, data suggest the TSH rise is often transient and may not warrant treatment.[18, 19] A special situation where initial screening can be falsely negative, warranting repeat sampling, is fetal blood mixing in monozygotic twins who are discordant for CH.[20]

From an epidemiological standpoint, the increased detection rate has led to an apparent increase in the prevalence of CH from 1:4000 at first introduction of newborn screening to estimates closer to 1:2000 using today's screening algorithms,[6] with some countries reporting a prevalence lower than 1:1000.[21, 22] Similarly, most of the geographic variability in reported prevalence is likely due to the difference in screening algorithms in the respective jurisdictions.[23] In fact, rates of permanent CH from thyroid dysgenesis (TD) confirmed by radionuclide scanning remain stable despite changes in screening approaches and across populations. However, some epidemiologic differences based on geography and ethnicity are independent of screening algorithms, including higher prevalence rates of autosomal recessively inherited forms of dyshormonogenesis in populations with high rates of consanguinity[24, 25] and a somewhat lower prevalence of CH in Hispanic and Black infants than in Caucasian infants.[26]

43.1.2 Thyroid Dysgenesis

43.1.2.1 General Features

TD describes an abnormal organogenesis of the thyroid and includes thyroid ectopy, agenesis, hypoplasia, and hemiagenesis. It is to be distinguished from dyshormonogenesis (reviewed later in this chapter), which consists of a defect in thyroid hormone synthesis by an otherwise normally developed, eutopic gland. Traditionally, TD is estimated to underly 80%–85% and dyshormonogenesis about 10%–15% of CH, although recent studies suggest that in non-Western populations, the proportion of CH due to dyshormonogenesis may account for up to 50%.[27–29]

These data need to be interpreted with caution, as lower TSH-screening cutoffs will pick up on milder and transient cases of CH, which are more frequently seen in patients with DUOX2 mutations (discussed later in this chapter). TD occurs most often in isolation, but it may be associated with extrathyroidal organ manifestations such as congenital heart malformations (2%–5% of cases) and, more rarely, lung, kidney, or pancreas.[30]

43.1.2.2 Thyroid Ectopy

Thyroid ectopy is the most common form of TD and underlies about half of CH cases.[2] It results from a defect in thyroid migration during embryonic development from the sublingual location downward to the anterior neck, and leads to a small, round, often dumbbell-shaped dystopic thyroid gland that is located along its migratory pathway but most commonly remains in the sublingual space (for details, see Chapter 32). The molecular mechanism that regulates this active migration of thyroid is not fully understood. While the location and size are aberrant, ectopic thyroids are fully differentiated and have a normal follicular architecture. A reduced number of cells and smaller size due to absent lateral lobes and limited TSH-induced cell growth result in CH severities ranging from severe to transient.[31]

43.1.2.3 Athyreosis, Hypoplasia, and Hemiagenesis

Athyreosis describes the absence of orthotopic or ectopic thyroid follicular cells that results from an absent formation or differentiation and proliferation of the thyroid anlage. Given that almost one in two infants have measurable thyroglobulin levels despite undetectable thyroid tissue on radionucleide imaging,[32] it has also been suggested to be called "apparent athyreosis."[33] A heterogeneous entity, athyreosis can range from permanent severe CH in the case of completely inactivating TSH receptor mutations and associated severely hypofunctional, hypoplastic, or aplastic thyroid glands,[34] to transient, mild CH due to maternal TSH receptor-blocking antibodies that are passed through the placenta.[33]

Hypoplastic thyroids are orthotopic but smaller than normal glands. They represent approximately 5% of CH cases[35] and likely represent a genetic, heterogeneous form of dysgenesis.[36]

Thyroid hemiagenesis describes another form of TD, whereby one of the two thyroid lobes (most commonly the left lobe) does not develop. Segregation in families suggests contribution of genetic factors, and although recently emerging data implicate alterations in proteasome-associated genes,[37] the exact molecular mechanisms are unknown. Most patients are clinically and biochemically euthyroid and are picked up incidentally.[36, 38] Some have asymptomatic compensatory hypertrophy of the normally developed lobe, and average TSH levels may be higher than in bilobed controls.[39] In a recent review, both thyroidal and exrathyroidal pathologies associated with hemiagenesis were described, including a potentially increased risk for thyroid pathologies such as autoimmune thyroid disease and thyroid cancer.[38]

43.1.2.4 Genetics and Inheritance

A common underlying molecular mechanism likely underlies TD, representing a continuum of disease from athyreosis, ectopy, hypoplasia, and hemiagenesis to a normal thyroid.[40] However, the full picture of the genetic background remains to be elucidated, and inheritance patterns of TD have been subject to debate. Almost all modes of inheritance have been suggested, including sporadic, monogenic, polygenic, epigenetic, and multifactorial inheritance.

Sporadic mutations are thought to account for most cases, a hypothesis that is supported by the finding that the majority of monozygotic twins are discordant for TD.[20] On the other hand, prevalence in first-degree relatives is up to 15 times higher than would be expected by chance alone,[41] and extrathyroidal congenital malformations (particularly heart septation defects) are more common than in healthy controls.[42, 43] However, a twofold higher prevalence of TD in females compared to males[44] implies a non-Mendelian inheritance pattern, and the higher prevalence in Caucasian populations compared to Black populations supports an oligogenic inheritance of susceptibility to TD.[26]

An identifiably genetic cause of TD is found in about 5% of cases, mainly in the genes implicated in thyroid morphogenesis (i.e., thyroid transcription factors and the TSH receptor gene).[35] While these mutations have been shown to cause athyreosis and hypoplasia, they do not seem to account for thyroid ectopy. Further, in linkage analyses of TD, an association between the phenotypes and the transcription factors or TSHR gene could not be established, suggesting genetic heterogeneity and the involvement of other, potentially novel genes.[45]

Reconciliation of these seemingly contradictory findings may be provided by a two-hit hypothesis, whereby an underlying first-hit, germline susceptibility predisposes to an effect from a second-hit, early postzygotic mutation.[46] However, in at least one case report of thyroid ectopy that included information on the genetics of the removed ectopic thyroid, none of three thyroid transcription factors contained mutations in their respective genes; this finding suggests that they may not be implicated in the pathogenesis of thyroid ectopy.[31] Extrathyroidal genes that are involved in thyroid migration, including those encoding for adhesion molecules and vascular factors, have been postulated as possible somatic targets. A similar effect may be attributable to epigenetic changes in the regulation of promotors of thyroid transcription factors.[47]

Although a number of genes have been associated with syndromic thyroid hypoplasia, monogenic forms of TD, including true ectopy and athyreosis, stem from germline mutations in the TSH receptor and in the abovementioned transcription factors. The following section, therefore, focuses on these genes.

43.1.2.5 TSH Receptor Mutations

TSH receptor (TSHR)-inactivating mutations occur in an estimated 3%–6% of CH[48] and represent the most common cause of monogenic TD and isolated, nonsyndromic CH (OMIM#275200). There may be a founder effect with loss of genetic variation in Asian populations that carry a specific missense mutation (R450H) with higher frequencies of up to 16.5%.[49–51] Since its first description in 1968,[52] over 30 mutations have been reported.[53] Molecular characterization of the G-protein-coupled TSH receptor in1995[54] led to the discovery of both homozygote and heterozygote loss-of-function mutations.[34, 55, 56]

Depending on the severity of TSH resistance, the phenotype of CH varies from apparent athyreosis in homozygous-complete inactivating mutations[55] to milder presentations, often biallelic or only present on one allele, leading to compensatory hyperthyrotropinemia and normally developed thyroid glands.[57–60] Mutations affecting the receptor's Gs subunit are likewise typically mild, and although they may be picked up on newborn screening,[60] the presentation is that of subclinical hypothyroidism with typically normal thyroid hormone concentrations.

43.1.2.6 Thyroid Transcription Factor Mutations

The thyroid transcription factors, and more specifically their combined presence in thyroid tissue, lead to the correct formation of the thyroid anlage and morphogenesis.[61] Given the expression of transcription factors in many other extrathyroidal tissues, mutations mostly lead to syndromic phenotypes.[62–65] A recent systematic review summarizes mutations in the transcription factor-encoding genes.[31] Of note, most of the cases presenting with mutations are syndromic, and mutations in transcription factors account for only a small fraction of the patients.

43.1.2.7 NKX2-1

NK2 homeobox-1 (*NKX2-1*, formerly thyroid transcription factor 1, *TTF1*), as one of the essential transcription factors for thyroid development and maintenance, is involved in activating the thyroglobulin (TG), thyroid peroxidase (TPO), TSH receptor (TSHR), and Pendred syndrome (PDS) genes. Extrathyroidal effects include the lung and brain, and de novo or autosomal-dominantly inherited deleterious mutations lead to the brain-lung-thyroid (BLT) syndrome. The associated CH phenotype ranges from a normal thyroid gland with mild hypothyroidism[66, 67] to apparent athyreosis.[62]

43.1.2.8 FOXE1

Forkhead box E1 (*FOXE1*, formerly thyroid transcription factor 2, *TTF-2*) recognizes and binds to TG and TPO promoters and interacts with regulatory regions of genes implicated in hormonogenesis, including dual oxidase 2 (*DUOX2*) and sodium/iodide symporter (*NIS*). It is one of the least common causes of athyreosis, with only three homozygous mutations described[68, 69] that lead to Bamforth-Lazarus syndrome (OMIM#241850), with a variable phenotype of athyreosis, cleft palate, and spiky hair, with or without bifid epiglottis and choanal atresia. A more important role of *FOXE1* may be its modulation of TD risk, especially ectopy, through its alanine-containing stretch.[70]

43.1.2.9 PAX8

Paired box transcription factor 8 (*PAX8*) is relevant for both thyroid and kidney development. The phenotypic spectrum of de novo or autosomal-dominantly inherited mutations varies widely, both among individuals and within families carrying the same mutations, and ranges from normal thyroid morphology to TD, including hypoplasia, ectopy and athyreosis, with or without renal manifestations.[63, 71]

43.1.2.10 GLIS3

GLI-similar3 (GLIS3) is a zinc finger protein that plays a role in both activating and repressing transcription during development of most organ tissues.[65] In the thyroid, it is essential for TSH/TSHR-mediated proliferation of thyroid follicular cells and hormone biosynthesis.[72] Mutations in humans are exceedingly rare, and while CH is present in most (but not all) cases of neonatal diabetes seems to be ubiquitous. Other features include congenital glaucoma, sensorineural deafness, craniosynostosis, cardiac, liver, kidney, and exocrine pancreatic manifestations.[65]

43.1.2.11 HHEX

Hematopoietically expressed homeobox protein (HHEX) plays a role in thyroid follicular precursor cell survival by maintaining the expression of thyroid transcription factors Nkx2-1, Pax8, and Foxe1.[35] Only one potential monoallelic mutation was detected during genetic screening of 110 Chinese patients with CH,[27] although a genetic variant in intron 2 was observed in another series of 234 Chinese patients, and no causative mutations were detected.[73]

43.1.2.12 NKX2.5

NK2 homeobox-5 (*NKX2.5*), a gene primarily known for its role in heart development, was initially described for its role in thyroid organogenesis and its causing TD in mice. In humans, heterozygous mutations have been described that cause a dominant negative effect on wild-type *Nkx2.5*, resulting in TD,[74] potentially due to reduced TG and TPO promoter transactivation.[75] Nonetheless, the role of this *NKX2.5* mutation in the pathogenesis of TD has perhaps been overestimated because it was also carried by a healthy parent, sibling, and grandmother. Given these observations, it is now generally accepted that *NKX2.5* mutations are not a major contributor to the pathogenesis of TD, although their role as a genetic modifier cannot be excluded.[76]

43.1.3 Thyroid Dyshormonogenesis

43.1.3.1 General Features

The thyroid gland is likened to a factory that uses an intake pump and a series of biochemical steps to organify nutritionally uptaken iodide to manufacture and secrete thyroid hormone into the bloodstream.[77] Iodine, as an essential trace element for thyroid hormone production, can be rate limiting for thyroid hormone synthesis, and thus a recycling mechanism exists to conserve it maximally. TSH is the main regulator of hormone biosynthesis: Binding of the TSH receptor on the follicular cell surface triggers cyclic adenosine monophosphate (cAMP) activation, which in turn stimulates iodine transport across the cell membrane and initiates the synthesis cascade.[78] First, iodine is trapped in the follicular cell, diffuses to the apex, and is transported into the colloid. Next, oxidation and incorporation into tyroxine residues within the thyroglobulin molecules

FIG. 43.3 Thyroid hormone biosynthesis.

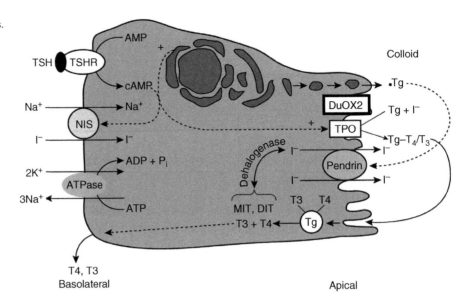

take place. Thyroglobulin is then endocytosed and fuses with intracellular phagolysosome. Proteolysis leads to the release of iodotyrosines [monoiodotyrosine (MIT) and diiodotyrosine (DIT)] and iodothyronine (T4 and T3) residue. Lastly, deiodination of MIT and DIT by a dehalogenase leads to intracellular iodine recycling and release of T4 and T3 into the circulation.[79] Thyroglobulin that escapes from the gland via the lymphatic system can be detected in blood and can be used as a marker for the presence of thyroid tissue. A schematic representation of thyroid hormone biosynthesis is shown in Fig. 43.3.

Dyshormonogenesis is thought to contribute to 10%–15% of CH, with higher percentages observed in populations with high rates of consanguinity. With a few exceptions,[80] and in contrast to the multiple inheritance modes in TD, thyroid dyshormonogenesis follows a classically Mendelian, autosomal-recessive pattern.[79] Even further distinct from TD, the molecular mechanisms for most of dyshormonogenesis are well described and mostly can be derived from the steps in hormone biosynthesis: Decreased iodine trapping, defective organification of trapped iodine, abnormalities of thyroglobulin structure, and deficiency of iodotyrosine deiodination and recycling have all been described. TPO mutations are reported as the most common cause of dyshormonogenesis in Caucasians,[81] while recent reports from Asia suggest that *DUOX2* may be the most frequent underlying etiology in Asian populations.[27, 28]

Other than a higher frequency of familial occurrence of CH and the possible presence of a goiter, individuals with CH due to dyshormonogenesis present a similar clinical picture as individuals affected by CH due to TD. Goitrous enlargement of the thyroid can be seen as early as in utero or at birth, but in many infants, thyroid enlargement goes unnoticed or onset of goiter occurs later. Of note, on an individual level, diagnosis of the specific underlying genetic disorder may not be necessary, as management is usually unchanged: Treatment is initiated as for CH, and a 25% recurrence risk for siblings of affected subjects can be given empirically.

43.1.3.2 Sodium-Iodine Symporter Defects

Mutations in the *SLC5A5* gene encoding the sodium-iodine symporter impair the first step of thyroid hormone biosynthesis, whereby iodine is transported across the plasma membrane into the follicular cell cytosol. The symporter pump is stimulated by TSH and by TSH-receptor antibodies, such as those for Graves' disease, and generates a gradient between the thyroid cells and serum of >1:20–30 that can increase up to hundredfold when the thyroid is deprived of iodine.

NIS is present in several other tissues as well, including the salivary glands, gastric mucosa, mammary glands, ciliary body, choroid plexus, and placenta. While these tissues can concentrate iodine (and thus can be visible on iodine scintigraphy), the capacity to organify inorganic iodine is limited to the thyroid gland. Since its first description in 1997,[80] several deleterious mutations in *SLC5A5* have been reported.[82] Based on the degree of residual NIS activity, patients may present as neonates, infants, or during childhood. Diagnosis is based on detection of a goiter (on exam or by ultrasound) in the context of absent or reduced iodine uptake on scintigraphy. Infants may present after normal newborn screening, risking neurodevelopmental sequelae.[82]

43.1.3.3 Pendred Syndrome

Biallelic loss-of-function mutations in the *SLC26A4* gene encoding for the anion exchanger protein pendrin are the underlying cause for PDS.[83] A wealth of pathogenic mutations have been described to date.[84] In the thyroid, the defect leads to a partial iodide organification defect due to impaired iodide efflux. Pendrin is also expressed in the inner ear, where it is implicated in normal anion transport and maintenance of the endocochlear potential, and in the kidney, where it functions as a chloride/bicarbonate exchanger. Clinical features of PDS include congenital bilateral neurosensory deafness and goiter, but no renal abnormalities. The thyroid phenotype is usually mild: Development of goiter and mild hypothyroidism depend on nutritional iodine intake, often only develop over time, and show variable onset within the same families. PDS is seldom identified by elevated TSH on newborn screening.[84, 85]

43.1.3.4 Thyroperoxidase Defects

Mutations in the *TPO* gene cause a dysfunction in one of the main enzymes involved in thyroid hormone biosynthesis. The heme protein TPO is membrane-bound at the apex of follicular cells, where it catalyzes the iodination of thyroglobulin-bound tyrosyl residues to form the iodotyrosines MIT and DIT, and the coupling of these in association with thyroid [nicotinamide adenine dinucleotide phosphate (NADPH)] oxidases. Defective TPO constitutes one of the most common causes of dyshormonogenesis. Over 100 mutations, including homozygous, compound heterozygous, missense, frame-shift, base pair duplications, and single nucleotide substitutions, have been described.[86, 87] One report suggests that up to 17% of patients have a phenotype of TPO deficiency but carry monoallelic mutations that lead to mutant TPO in the thyroid.[88] Overall, no clear genotype-phenotype correlations have been established, and phenotypes may vary even within the same families.[89, 90]

Clinically, TPO deficiency manifests as goitrous CH with elevated levels of thyroglobulin (if measured) and high iodine uptake on scintigraphy. The historically used perchlorate discharge test characteristically shows a rapid discharge of trapped iodine after administration of perchlorate.[79] Of note, this test is also usually positive in other causes of dyshormonogenesis, such as *PDS* and *DUOX2* deficiency, and thus lacks specificity. A diagnosis made by TPO sequencing may be important in cases of uniparental disomy[91] or when an inheritance pattern other than autosomal-recessive may be suspected.[80]

43.1.3.5 DUOX2 Defects

DUOX2, like *TPO*, is located at the apical membrane of thyroid follicular cells, and its H_2O_2 generation is the rate-limiting factor for thyroglobulin iodination during thyroid hormone biosynthesis. Only biallelic inactivating *DUOX2* mutations cause thyroid dyshormonogenesis and goitrous or nongoitrous CH,[79, 92] while both biallelic and monoallelic mutations can lead to transient CH.[93] The phenotype seems to be variable even within the same family, possibly at least in part due to disease modifiers such as iodine intake[94] and genetic variants in DuOX1, the other thyroidal H2O2-generating enzyme.[93] Mutation of the *DUOX2* maturation factor, *DUOXA2*, which translocates *DUOX2* to the plasma,[95] can mimic a *DUOX2*-deficiency phenotype,[96] although generally, the two DUOX enzymes and their maturation factors are thought to be redundant.[79]

43.1.3.6 Thyroglobulin (TG) Defects

Mutations in the *TG* gene affect the organification step of thyroid hormone biosynthesis. To date, 117 homozygous or compound heterozygous splice site mutations, premature stop codons, deletions, and nucleide insertions have been described,[87] which variably cause structural changes in the thyroglobulin glycoprotein affecting normal folding, assembly, and biosynthesis of thyroid hormones; defective transport; deficient tyrosine residues; those that are unable to be iodized; or defective iodotyrosine coupling. Clinically, the result is goitrous CH as early as in utero or at birth, with undetectable serum TG levels.[97]

43.1.3.7 Iodotyrosine Deiodinase (IYD) Mutations

The *IYD* gene (also referred to as *DEHAL1*) encodes iodotyrosine deiodinase, the enzyme responsible for iodine recycling in the follicular cell, to avoid leaking of iodine and loss of the precious mineral in urine. Mutations in a handful of pedigrees have been described to date. The thyroid phenotype is variable and, as in *PDS* and *DUOX2* deficiency, seems dependent on iodine intake and likely other not-yet-identified modifier genes.[98–100] The onset of hypothyroidism may be congenital or occur during infancy or childhood, and in the latter cases, it may be missed and lead to neurodevelopmental sequelae.[98] Upon scintigraphy, iodine uptake is early, rapid, and with rapid spontaneous discharge. Urinary MIT and DIT concentrations are elevated.

43.1.4 Transient Neonatal Hyperthyrotropinemia and Hypothyroidism

Transient congenital hypothyroidism (TCH) is a temporary deficiency of the thyroid hormone that occurs postnatally, with eventual restoration of normal thyroid function over time—typically within weeks to months. This may be primary hypothyroidism (elevated TSH, low T4) or isolated hyperthyrotropinemia (elevated TSH, normal T4). Identification and treatment of TCH are likely the reasons for the apparent increase in prevalence of CH since the onset of screening.[2, 101, 102] The reported proportion of those diagnosed with CH who have transient CH is widely disparate, ranging from 17%–40% depending on the study,[102–107] and approaching 50% when including only those with in situ glands.[104, 108] The variability between studies largely reflects the various TSH thresholds in screening, as well as the lack of a standardized definition and evaluation strategy for transient CH.

43.1.4.1 Iodine Deficiency

Worldwide, iodine deficiency is the most common cause of transient CH. The addition of iodine to salt has significantly reduced the risk of iodine deficiency, and yet maternal diets continue to be deficient in developed countries, including European countries and the United States. National Health and Nutrition Examination Surveys (NHANES) demonstrated a decline in iodine nutrition from NHANES I to III, with an apparent stabilization thereafter, but evidence of persistent mild deficiency exists.[85, 105, 109] The American Thyroid Association recommends that women take a dietary supplement containing 150 μg of iodine daily during preconception, pregnancy, and lactation, but uptake has been poor.[110] Premature newborns are at higher risk of iodine deficiency due to inadequate time for accumulation of iodine within the gland. With iodine deficiency, the duration of the effect on thyroid function varies. Radionuclide and ultrasound imaging are typically normal.[102]

43.1.4.2 Iodine Excess

Excessive iodine exposure can also cause hypothyroidism due to the Wolff-Chaikoff effect. Prenatal exposure may occur through maternal use of amiodarone, iodine antiseptics, and exposure to iodinated contrast agents or amniofetography. A systematic review found that neonates exposed postnatally to iodinated contrast media are at risk of abnormal thyroid function and development of hypothyroidism, and that the risk might be higher in premature infants.[111]

Exposure can occur through the use of iodinated skin preparations, as well as contrast media for cardiac catheterization, urinary and gut imaging, or treatment with amiodarone. This has led to many nurseries discontinuing the use of iodine containing antiseptics. Hypothyroidism may not be detected on newborn screening, as low T4 and high TSH levels generally appear 2–3 days after exposure. Some nurseries have recommendations for thyroid function testing after exposure to iodine. The duration of the effect of iodine excess on thyroid function is variable, ranging between 1 and 3 months.[112] Based on systematic review, Ahmet et al. recommend, following neonatal exposure to iodinated contrast media, doing thyroid function (TSH, FreeT4) tests at baseline, day 5, and weekly for 3–4 weeks unless abnormalities of thyroid function persist.[111] Upon imaging following excess iodine, radionuclide uptake is blocked, but an ultrasound will show a normal thyroid location.[102]

43.1.4.3 Maternal Factors

Maternal use of antithyroid drugs (ATDs) at the time of delivery can result in transient hypothyroidism in the neonate, with return of normal thyroid hormone metabolism typically within 2–5 days.[113] Radionuclide and ultrasound imaging are typically normal.

Thyrotropin receptor-blocking antibodies (TRABs) block TSH receptors in the thyroid gland of the newborn, resulting in transient hypothyroidism. This resolves within 3–6 months as the antibody levels decline. This should be a diagnostic consideration in babies born to women with known autoimmune thyroid disease (Graves' disease or autoimmune thyroiditis) and families with a previous sibling detected with CH. Radionucide uptake might be blocked partially or completely, but ultrasound will show a normal thyroid location and thyroglobulin levels will be normal.[102]

43.1.4.4 Other Causes of Persistent Neonatal hyperthyrotropinemia

Neonatal factors causing to transient CH may also include prematurity, low birth weight and intrauterine growth restriction (IUGR), critical illness, and the use of dopamine or steroids. Autosomal recessive loss of function mutations in *DUOX2* (*THOX2*) and *DUOXA2* can also cause transient hyperthyrotropinemia. Children with Down syndrome have mildly elevated TSH levels and decreased T4 concentration, with left-shifted normal distribution. This points to a mild hypothyroid state and a Down syndrome-specific thyroid regulation disorder in newborns with Down syndrome. The question remains whether this contributes to brain maldevelopment.[114]

43.1.4.5 Diagnosis and Management of TCH

At birth, one cannot reliably distinguish transient from permanent CH as, by definition, this only becomes evident with time. Some programs define TCH as a return to normal TSH within weeks, while others say it takes place by 3 years. Some include FT4 levels in the definition. Imaging is helpful, but not absolute. For instance, those with agenesis will have permanent CH, but TRAb can cause apparent thyroid agenesis on a thyroid scan. An in situ gland is suggestive of either transient CH or permanent dyshormonogenesis. Most with an ectopic thyroid would be expected to have permanent CH, but transient CH has been reported in this group.[115]

Screening and diagnostic thyroid functions have been inconsistent predictors of transient versus permanent CH. Baseline TSH levels alone may not be helpful, as even mild CH is permanent in 75%–89% of cases,[2] and transient CH has been described in patients with extremely elevated TSH levels of >500 mL U/L.[104] Other studies have found initial TSH cut points for distinguishing TSH and PCH of 30.5 IU/L,[116] 31 mL U/L,[108] and 34 IU/L.[117] An initial above-average level of free T4 may also be predictive of TCH in neonates with mild elevation of TSH.[108]

A summary of initial TSH and free T4 levels in studies evaluating predictors of TCH versus PCH is shown in Table 43.1. Practice guidelines recommend treating all those with presumptive CH on diagnostic testing for a period of 3 years during

TABLE 43.1 Summary of studies evaluating the role of thyroxine dose requirements and initial TSH and free T4 levels to distinguish TCH from PCH

Author	Number	Dose of thyroxine (mg/kg/day)	Initial TSH (mL U/L)	Initial freeT4 (pmol/L)

Cho[117]	56 eutopic thyroid (25 TCH, 31 PCH)	Optimum cutoff <3.3 at 1 and 2 years for TCH
		Highest sensitivity (100%)
		  at 1 year was 1.9
		  at 2 years was 2.8
		Highest specificity (100%)
		  at 1 year was 5.55
		  at 2 years was 5.0
			Cutpoint of 34 mL U/L suggestive of TCH
			TCH 60.5 ± 78.3
			PCH 89.4 ± 67.1
			(P = 0.038)
				TCH 9.8 ± 4.8
				PCH 10.0 ± 4.8
				NS

Messina[118]	64 eutopic thyroid (46 TCH, 18 PCH)	Highly suggestive of PCH if
		  >4.9 at 12 months or
		  >4.27 at 24 months
		Highly suggestive of TCH if
		  <1.7 at 12 months or
		  <1.45 at 24 months
			TCH median 29 (IQR 100–400)
			PCH 64.8 (IQR 29.6–137.5)
			NS
				Not reported

Kang[72]	79 (37 TCH, 42 PCH)	Predictive of PCH if
		  >4.1 at 2 years of age and maximal thyroxine dose >50 µg/day
		  3.6 (TCH) versus 4.6 (PCH) at 1 year, P < 0.001
		  3.1 (TCH) versus 4.3 (PCH) at 2 years, P < 0.001
		  2.8 (TCH) versus 4.1 (PCH) at 3 years, P < 0.001
			Cut point of 31 mL U/L suggestive of TCH
			TCH 22 (16.5–25.6)
			PCH 49.1 (27.5–150)
			(P < 0.01)
				Above-average free T4 with TSH < 27.2 mL U/L, predictive of TCH
				TCH 7.2 (5.5–12.0)
				PCH 6.4 (2.4–11.8)
				NS

Zdraveska[116]	76 (34 TCH, 42 PCOH)	Optimal cutoff of <2.6 at 3 years predictive of TCH (sensitivity 100%, specificity 76%)
		  2.4 (TCH) versus 3.7 (PCH) at 1 year, P < 0.001
		  1.9 (TCH) versus 3.3 (PCH) at 2 years, P < 0.001
		  1.7 (TCH) versus 3.2 (PCH) at 3 years, P < 0.001
			Cutpoint of 30.5 mL U/L suggestive of TCH
			TCH 22.7 ± 10.9
			PCH 81.9 ± 56.8
			(P < 0.001)
				TCH 8.6 ± 3.0
				PCH 6.2 ± 5.0

Oron[119]	84 eutopic (17 TCH, 67 PCH)	Optimal cutoff of <2.2 after 6 months predictive of TCH (sensitivity 90%, specificity 57%)
		  2.7 (TCH) versus 4.1 (PCH) at 1 year, P = 0.004
		  2.1 (TCH) versus 3.4 (PCH) at 2 years, P = 0.003
		  1.9 (TCH) versus 3.0 (PCH) at 3 years, P = 0.027
			Eutopic only
			TCH 42.5 ± 29.1
			PCH 49.1 ± 27.9
			NS
				Eutopic only
				TCH 11.4 ± 6.4
				PCH 12.5 ± 5.1
				NS

Saba[120]	92 eutopic (49 TCH, 43 PCH)	Cutoff of 3.2 µg/kg/day at 6 months predictive of TCH with sensitivity of 71% and specificity of 79%	TCH TSH 49 (23–89) PCH 142 (57–366) (P < 0.001)	TCH 12.8 (10.3–15.2) PCH 11.8 (4.9–16.0) NS

TCH, transient congenital hypothyroidism; *PCH*, permanent congenital hypothyroidism; *NS*, not significant.
Data shown preferentially include only those with eutopic glands when data allows this distinction.

the critical period of neurocognitive development, followed by a controlled withdrawal. This is prudent, but it also can result in unnecessary treatment, monitoring, and cost to families and the healthcare system for many of these children who were not the intended targets of newborn screening. No controlled trials exist to determine if there is a neurocognitive benefit to treating those with mild CH or TCH. An evidence-based algorithm is needed to guide monitoring, treatment, and safe timing for a trial of treatment to distinguish permanent from transient CH. The 2014 European Society for Pediatric Endocrinology (ESPE) consensus guidelines recommend starting treatment if venous FT4 is below norms for age or if venous TSH is >20 mL U/L, even if the FT4 concentration is normal.[121]

For those who are started on treatment, some potential predictors have been reported that may support an earlier ree-valuation off treatment. Several studies have shown lower thyroxine requirements at 1–3 years of age in the TCH group compared to PCH,[104, 116–120] but there is considerable overlap, as shown in Table 43.1. A larger study is needed to identify a clearer threshold to distinguish TCH from PCH, but these studies suggest that consideration of an earlier trial off treatment is feasible for children on relatively low-dose thyroxine who do not have increasing dose requirements over time. Further studies are required to systematically evaluate these potential predictors of transient CH.

43.1.5 Thyroid Function and Prematurity

Maturation of the hypothalamic-pituitary-thyroid (HPT) axis starts at around 20 weeks and completes close to term. At birth, premature neonates are unable to generate sufficient levels of bioactive thyroid hormones, resulting in a relative deficiency and a dip in hormone levels at about 1 week of age. Preterm infants are at risk of iodine deficiency secondary to lower iodine stores, and standard formulas provide less than the recommended 30 μg/kg/day of iodine.[122] They are also more vulnerable to iodine excess, as the Wolff-Chiakoff effect does not mature until 36 weeks. They may be critically ill, with low T3 and T4 levels from nonthyroidal illness. As a result, several patterns of thyroid dysfunction are seen in preterm infants.

The most common pattern is transient hypothyroxinemia of prematurity (THOP), low T4 with normal TSH, which is observed in up to 50% of infants born before 28 weeks.[123] The question arises whether we should be supplementing with thyroxine to bring thyroxine levels to postnatal levels. While several observational studies showed a correlation between THOP, low IQ, and neurologic sequelae, they did not establish causality,[105] and a recent study showed no association.[124] A Cochrane review does not support the use of prophylactic thyroid hormone,[125] and two more recent randomized controlled trials showed no benefit[126, 127] and indeed, that thyroxine may increase the risk of circulatory collapse or necrotizing enterocolitis.

Another pattern seen in premature neonates is that of primary hypothyroidism (low T4 and elevated TSH), which is 14 times more common in VLBW babies than normal-weight babies[15] and nearly two-thirds of them demonstrated a delayed TSH rise (normal TSH at birth, and elevated later).[15] Based on this finding, routine rescreening for VLBW/premature infants has been implemented in some programs. A 2011 study found that CH with a delayed TSH elevation occurred in 1 in 58 extremely low birth weight (ELBW) infants, 1 in 95 VLBW infants, and 1 in 30,329 infants weighing ≥1500 g (P < 0.0001) and was transient in all, lasting a mean of 51 days. Neurodevelopmental outcomes in follow-up to 18 months were equivalent to matched controls.[18] This brings in question whether rescreening is indicated.

43.1.6 Consumptive Hypothyroidism

Congenital large hepatic hemangiomas produce large amounts of enzyme-type 3-iodothyronine deiodinase, resulting in high levels of reverse T3 and low levels of T4. Hypothyroidism is usually not present at birth, but it develops with the rapid growth of the hemangioma in the first weeks or months of life, and it may be the presenting feature for the hemangioma. High doses of thyroxine are required to maintain physiologic levels of T4. Hypothyroidism resolves with spontaneous involution, medical or surgical treatment of the hemangioma.

43.1.7 Central Congenital Hypothyroidism

Central congenital hypothyroidism (CCH) is an uncommon condition resulting from inadequate stimulation of the thyroid by TSH. The previously reported prevalence varied from 1 in 25,000 to 1 in 100,000 live births, but a systematic screening program in the Netherlands using T4, TSH, and TBG testing identified a prevalence of up to 1 in 16,000 neonates.[128] The majority of patients will have hypothalamic and/or pituitary pathology with multiple pituitary hormone deficiencies, with or without structural anomalies of the pituitary and additional syndromic features. Magnetic resonance imaging (MRI) may show elements of the classic triad of ectopic posterior pituitary, absent pituitary stalk, and small or absent anterior pituitary. A minority of these individuals will have mutations in known transcription factors, such as POU1F1, PROP1, HESX1, LHX3, LHX4, SOX3, or ORX3. Genetic causes of isolated central hypothyroidism have an estimated incidence of 1 in 65,000, caused by mutations in genes controlling the TSH biosynthetic pathway, including *TSHB, TRHR,* and *IGSF1*.

Primary TSH screening is most commonly used as the most sensitive test for identifying primary CH, but it will not identify CCH. Primary T4 screening or a combination of primary T4 and TSH screening has the potential to identify CCH, but the sensitivity is low, as one can only measure total T4, not free T4 on blood spots. The Netherlands program reported that the addition of TBG raised the sensitivity for identifying CCH from 22%–92%, with only a small incremental cost. Although definitive studies are lacking, early identification of CCH through newborn screening has the potential to positively affect IQ and psychomotor development, as it does for primary CH. It also allows the early detection and treatment of complications of other hormone deficiencies, such as life-threatening hypoglycemia.

43.2   EVALUATION OF INFANTS WITH A POSITIVE NEWBORN SCREENING TEST

Any positive CH newborn screening test should be acted on immediately to confirm the diagnosis and promptly initiate treatment. Beyond acting on the screening result, it is important for the individual and for public health purposes to establish the etiology of CH and document outcomes.

43.2.1   History and Physical Examination

Perinatal history should include exposure to maternal thyroid disease during pregnancy, including maternal thyroid auto-immune antibody status, adherence to iodine-supplemented prenatal vitamins (particularly in iodine-deficient regions), and consumption of additional iodine supplements or an iodine-rich diet. Birth weight and length should be documented, as well as history of jaundice, hypotonia, poor feeding, and sleepiness. A family history of consanguinity and/or familial cases of CH should be elicited, as they can point to an increased risk of dyshormonogenesis. A thorough physical examination, including anthropometric measurements and vital signs, should be documented. Jaundice, hypotonia, dry skin, large fontanelles (including an open posterior fontanelle), coarse facial features, macroglossia, and umbilical hernia are all classic features of CH and may help assess CH severity. Evaluation for dysmorphisms may elicit syndromic CH and a careful cardiac exam can suggest the more commonly associated heart septation defects. Thyroid examination and evaluation for presence of a goiter should be performed by propping up the prone infant's shoulders to hyperextend the neck (Fig. 43.4).

43.2.2   Laboratory Investigations

Confirmatory thyroid function tests, including serum TSH and free T4, should be obtained on any newborn with a positive screening test. However, treatment initiation should never be delayed while awaiting test results, especially if TSH on the screening sample is >40 mU/L.[129] TSH correlates with CH severity, but only pretreatment free T4 predicts neurocognitive sequelae, with lower values implying greater risk.[130, 131] If radionuclide imaging (outlined next) does not unequivocally show ectopy or goiter, thyroglobulin may be helpful to distinguish apparent from true athyreosis. In the former case, thyroid autoantibodies may be added to differentiate antibody blockage from TSH receptor resistance-mediated, apparent athyreosis (Fig. 43.5).

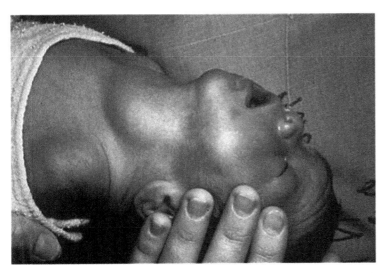

FIG. 43.4   Neonatel goiter.

43.2.3 Imaging

Radionuclide scanning is the gold standard of imaging modality to visualize thyroid tissue in situ, and the only technique that can unequivocally detect ectopic glands. The use of sodium pertechnate may be preferable over iodine, as imaging is faster (20 min versus several hours) and the tracer is more readily available. Babies should be fed after the injection of the tracer to keep it from accumulating in their salivary glands.[132] Advantages of performing the scan at diagnosis include easier administration of the test in newborns who usually fall asleep following an oral feeding (as opposed to an older child, who may not cooperate with the test), immediate etiologic diagnosis and assessment of recurrence risk, and likelihood of CH permanence (Fig. 43.5). Ideally, testing should be performed before therapy is begun, although it should never delay the initiation of hormone replacement.[129] After starting treatment, the time window to perform imaging depends on CH severity, but it usually can be performed for a few days, so long as TSH remains >30 mU/L.[133]

Neck ultrasound can be considered as an alternative when nuclear technology is not available, although its lower sensitivity and specificity may yield equivocal, false positive, and false negative results. Anteroposterior X-ray and ultrasound of the knee may help to assess the severity and duration of prenatal hypothyroidism and predict hormone replacement needs[134] and neurocognitive outcomes.[135, 136]

Some clinicians opt to forgo any imaging altogether, as it may be perceived as cumbersome to organize and does not alter immediate management. However, this should be weighed against the parental and public health benefits from a confirmed diagnosis; planning of long-term management, including risk assessment of trial off therapy at age 3 years to distinguish transient from permanent CH; and quality assurance of laboratory testing.

43.3 TREATMENT OF AFFECTED INFANTS WITH CONGENITAL HYPOTHYROIDISM

43.3.1 Initial Therapy

Thyroid hormone replacement in the form of levothyroxine should be commenced promptly after diagnosis, and by 2 weeks of life at the latest,[129] as later treatment initiation correlates with lower IQ.[137] The goal of treatment is to restore normal thyroid function as quickly as possible and maintain normal thyroid function thereafter. While the optimal dose of levothyroxine was long subject to debate, results of the only randomized controlled trial to date (performed in 2002, with follow-up data in 2005) provided convincing evidence that in term newborns, a starting dose of 50 μg/day (about 15 μg/kg/day) was more effective than a dose of 37.5 μg/day (about 10 μg/kg/day) at normalizing TSH earlier and optimizing neurodevelopment at 5–6 years of age.[138, 139]

Subsequent studies have confirmed that optimal neurodevelopmental outcomes with similar IQs as healthy controls are achieved at higher doses.[140] Most professional society guidelines have endorsed this approach, although tiered dosing recommendations based on estimated severity using thyroid function test results, imaging, and clinical presentation may be considered.[129, 141] Local T4-to-T3 conversion is the major source of thyroid hormone in the brain, and thus thyroxine is the hormone replacement of choice, with the addition of T3 unlikely to convey further benefits.[142]

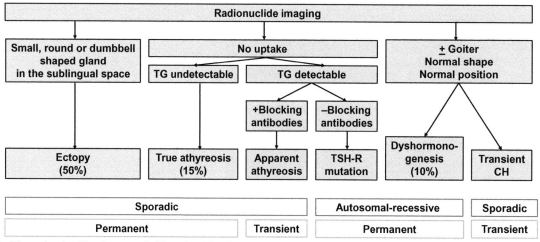

FIG. 43.5 Diagnositc algorithm for congenital hypothyroidism based on radionuclide imaging.

43.3.2 Follow-Up

As clinical signs and symptoms are not sufficiently reliable to assess thyroid hormone status, thyroid function needs to be monitored frequently following the initiation of therapy, with progressively decreasing follow-up intervals over time. The first clinical and biochemical follow-up is recommended within 1–2 weeks of initiating therapy, and every 2 weeks thereafter until TSH has normalized. Generally, subsequent visits are at least every 3 months for the first year of life, and every 6 months thereafter, until growth is completed.

As both overtreatment and undertreatment are associated with adverse school outcomes,[143, 144] the goal is to maintain TSH within the age-appropriate reference range and free T4 within the upper half of the normal range. At a starting dose of 15 µg/kg/day, mean serum free T4 concentrations increase to slightly above average for age, but T3 is generally normal. Likewise, a higher T4 suppression threshold for TSH exists early on, which only resets later in infancy.[145] Especially early on, TSH is the main treatment target, and so long as it is not persistently suppressed, or if the child is not clinically hyperthyroid, the dose does not need to be reduced.

Clinical monitoring during follow-up visits should focus on growth and cognitive, motor, and behavior development. If treated adequately, length and weight curves fall within genetic potential and complete catch-up, including normalization of the bone age, is expected by age 3 years. In severe CH, head circumference tends to be slightly above average, likely reflecting an immaturity of the skeleton rather than true pathology.[146] With appropriate treatment, children with CH usually have normal neurocognitive development, although some may have language delays or other learning difficulties, including deficits in psychomotricity, reaction time, memory, and attention.[147] Socioeconomic status implications on development may interact with the biologic effects of CH, causing a more significant decline in IQ with decreasing social status.[131] Thus, CH severity, treatment adequacy, and social determinants should be considered for inclusion in the management plan and decisions for support interventions.

43.4 NEONATAL HYPERTHYROIDISM

The incidence of neonatal Graves' disease (NGD) in the offspring of women with a history of Graves' disease is 1%–5%,[113] even if previously ablated with ^{131}I or athyreotic following surgery. Fetal and neonatal morbidity and mortality are significant. Untreated or poorly controlled maternal disease can result in poor fetal growth, oligohydramnios, goiter, prematurity, and fetal death.[148] The predominant prenatal manifestations of fetal Graves' disease are fetal tachycardia, poor fetal growth, and goiter. Postnatal morbidity is primarily related to high-output cardiac failure and craniosynostosis. Prenatal manifestations are also discussed in Chapter 19. Symptoms after birth include tachycardia; hyperexcitability; poor weight gain despite high food intake; staring, lid retraction, and/or exophthalmos; small anterior fontanel; microcephaly; and hepatomegaly and/or splenomegaly.[149] This underscores the importance of early detection and treatment.

Concentrations of circulating TRAb should be assessed at initial thyroid function testing in early pregnancy, and if TRAb is positive, again at weeks 18–22.[113] Management of the pregnant woman with Graves' disease is detailed in the *ATA Guidelines,*[113] and this includes careful monitoring guided by TRAb levels, consideration of ATDs with preference for PTU in the first 16 weeks, and then conversion to methimazole (MMI) due to teratogenic risks.

NGD typically shows up at the end of the first week of life, after the effects of ATDs have waned but TRAb remains high. As such, a normal newborn screen does not rule out NGD and monitoring with TSH, and free T4 between days 3 and 7 are recommended. A recent study on the prediction of neonatal hyperthyroidism found that a TSH level < 0.90 mL U/L between days 3 and 7 of life predicted neonatal hyperthyroidism, with a sensitivity of 78%, a specificity of 99%, a positive predictive value of 90%, and a negative predictive value of 98%.[150] TRAb levels of ≥6.8 mL U/L between days 0 and 5 is an independent predictor of NGD risk.[151]

Bescanon et al. found that no infants of third-trimester TRAb-negative mothers developed NGD, but in 33 TRAb-positive pregnancies, 24 had positive cord blood TRAb, and 7 went on to develop NG. FT4 elevation between days 3 and 7, but not at birth, was predictive of the development of hyperthyroidism. They recommend FT4 measurement at birth and then repeated between days 3 and 5 (and by day 7 at the latest).[152] Putting this together, at a minimum, TSH and free T4 levels should be measured in at-risk neonates at birth and repeated at 3–7 days of life, with TRAb levels providing further information if available. Some will repeat TSH and FT4 levels in the second week of life.[149]

If NGD is confirmed, treatment is recommended with MMI/carbimazole therapy (0.5–1 mg/day, divided into three doses). Propranolol (2 mg/kg, divided into two doses) may be added if the hyperthyroidism is severe. Dose titration is based on thyroid function tests and TRAb levels until stimulating antibodies disappear (usually 1–3 months).[113]

According to the *ATA Thyroid and Pregnancy Guidelines,* when antithyroid medication is indicated for women who are lactating, both MMI (up to a maximal dose of 20 mg/d) and propylthiouracil (PTU; up to a maximal dose of 450 mg/day) can be administered. Given a small but detectable amount of both PTU and MMI transferred into breast milk, the lowest effective doses of MMI/carbimazole or PTU should always be administered. Breastfed children of women who are treated with ATDs should be monitored for appropriate growth and development during routine pediatric health and wellness evaluations. Routine assessment of serum thyroid function in the child is not recommended.[113]

Nonimmune causes of neonatal hyperthyroidism are rare and should be considered when a family history of Graves' disease is absent. They include activating mutations of the *GNAS* gene in McCune-Albright syndrome, or of the TSH receptor. Presentation and management are similar to NGD, but hyperthyroidism may be permanent.

43.5 IMPAIRED SENSITIVITY TO THYROID HORMONE

In addition to defects in thyroid hormone production, there can be defects in downstream thyroid hormone action. These disorders were initially referred to as thyroid hormone resistance (THR) due to mutations in the thyroid hormone receptor (TR). The more current resistance to thyroid hormone (RTH) nomenclature describes impairment based on whether the molecular defect is in the alpha or beta TR genes (i.e., *RTH-α* and *RTH-β*). Other mechanisms of impaired sensitivity to thyroid hormone have been identified, including impaired conversion of T4 to T3 and defective transport of T4 and T3 into the cell. While these are congenital defects, most are not identified through newborn screening, as TSH levels are variable and often normal.

43.5.1 Thyroid Hormone Metabolism Defects

T4 is converted to biologically active T3 in the cell cytoplasm through deiodination by the selenoenzymes, DI01 and DI02, mainly in the liver and the thyroid itself. No disease has been reported in humans from mutations in DI01 or DI02, presumably because, through compensation, both DIOs would need to be affected for symptoms to develop.[153] SBP2 mutations affect the larger group of selenoenzymes, including deiodinases. Patients have been reported to have high-normal T4 and low-normal T3 levels with normal TSH. Growth retardation is common, and other common features include hearing impairment, vertigo, muscle weakness, infertility, and mild developmental delay.[153, 154] Limited reports of treatment with T3 resulted in only minimal improvement in growth and neurodevelopment.

43.5.2 Thyroid Hormone Cell Membrane Transport Defects

T4 and T3 are actively transported into the cells, where they bind to the intracellular thyroid hormone receptor. The expression of these transporters is tissue dependent. Monocarboxylate transporter 8 (MTC8) plays an important role in the transport of thyroid hormone into the brain. Individuals with an MTC8 defect have thyroid hormone deprivation in the brain during embryonic and early postnatal life, resulting in varying degrees of psychomotor delay, but typically severe, presenting during infancy or early childhood. They have characteristically high serum T3 and low rT3 concentrations, low T4 levels, and normal or slightly elevated TSH levels.

The high T3 may cause hyperthyroidism symptoms in peripheral tissues that are not dependent on MTC8, resulting in tachycardia, increased metabolic rate, and sleep disturbances. Treatment with levothyroxine is not effective due to poor uptake. Thyroid hormone analogs to bypass the defect have been tried. A small trial of a thyroid hormone analog, diiodothyropropionic acid (DITPA) treatment, almost completely normalized thyroid tests and reduced the hypermetabolism and the tendency for weight loss, but did not improve neurocognitive function.[155] Other treatment strategies are being tested.

43.5.3 Thyroid Hormone Action Defects

The active hormone T3 binds with equal affinity to both TR-α and TR-β receptors with variable expression ratios in various tissues and individuals. For example, the pituitary thyrotrophs express primarily TR-β, while other brain areas express only TR-α and the heart expresses both. As a result, the clinical phenotype of THADs varies between TR-α and TR-β mutations. Even family members with the same mutations will have variable phenotypes.[153]

The most common resistance to thyroid hormone (RTH) defect is an autosomal, dominantly inherited defect in the *TR-β* gene (RTH-β), with >3000 cases reported and an estimated incidence of 1 in 40,000 patients, as identified through a primary T4 screening program.[156] Pituitary resistance to thyroid hormone results in elevated TSH, with high T4 and T3 levels. Supraphysiologic doses of levothyroxine are required to normalize the TSH concentration. Symptoms depend on the relative expression of TR-α and TR-β in a given tissue. Because the increased thyroid hormone levels are secondary to hormone resistance, many with RTH will be clinically euthyroid, but goiter is common. Hyperthyroid symptoms may occur in tissues expressing predominantly TR-α, such as the heart (tachycardia) and some brain regions (hyperactivity), and increased metabolic rate. Hypothyroid symptoms predominate in TR-β-expressing tissues and may include growth failure, delayed bone maturation, learning disabilities, and sensorineural deafness.[153, 154] Treatment is usually not required, but it may be indicated in those with significant hypothyroid or hyperthyroid symptoms.

RTH-α mutations have been identified only recently, with the increasing use of exome sequencing. They are characterized by tissue-specific thyroid hormone resistance with a phenotype much like untreated true CH, but near-normal thyroid function levels. Because the thyrotophs respond to TH-β, TSH levels are typically normal. T4 is low/low normal, with a high/high normal T3.[157] An overview of inheritable forms of thyroid hormone resistance is provided in Table 43.1.[154]

43.6 DISORDERS OF THYROID HORMONE TRANSPORT

Newborn screening programs that measure total T4 may detect infants with abnormalities of the serum proteins that bind thyroid hormone—namely, thyroid-binding globulin (TBG), transthyretin (TTR, also called *prealbumin*), and albumin. Genetic mutations causing excess, deficiency, or abnormal affinity or binding to thyroid hormone exist and are all benign. Higher total T4 is seen in TBG excess, and when albumin or TTR have lower affinity but higher capacity for T4 (i.e., familial dysalbuminemic hyperthyroxinemia and abnormal TTR binding). The level of total T4 is lower in TBG deficiency. Importantly, because the hypothalamic-pituitary (H-P) axis responds to the free T4 fraction, TSH and free T4 are normal, and patients are therefore euthyroid.

Thus, in institutions where total T4 is still routinely measured, in order to avoid erroneous diagnoses, clinicians should be aware of protein-binding abnormalities, interpret T4 conjointly with TSH, and obtain a free T4 level if possible.

References

1. Deladoey J, Belanger N, Van Vliet G. Random variability in congenital hypothyroidism from thyroid dysgenesis over 16 years in quebec. *J Clin Endocrinol Metab* 2007;**92**(8):3158–61.
2. Deladoey J, Ruel J, Giguere Y, Van Vliet G. Is the incidence of congenital hypothyroidism really increasing? A 20-year retrospective population-based study in quebec. *J Clin Endocrinol Metab* 2011;**96**(8):2422–9.
3. Dussault JH, Coulombe P, Laberge C, Letarte J, Guyda H, Khoury K. Preliminary report on a mass screening program for neonatal hypothyroidism. *J Pediatr* 1975;**86**(5):670–4.
4. Van Vliet G, Czernichow P. Screening for neonatal endocrinopathies: rationale, methods and results. *Semin Neonatol* 2004;**9**(1):75–85.
5. Virtanen M, Maenpaa J, Pikkarainen J, Pimnen L, Perheentupa J. Aetiology of congenital hypothyroidism in finland. *Acta Paediatr Scand* 1989;**78**:67–73.
6. Ford G, Lafranchi SH. Screening for congenital hypothyroidism: a worldwide view of strategies. *Best Pract Res Clin Endocrinol Metab* 2014;**28** (2):175–87.
7. Delange F, Camus M, Winkler M, Dodion J, Ermans AM. Serum thyrotrophin determination on day 5 of life as screening procedure for congenital hypothyroidism. In: *Arch Disease Child* **52**:; 1977. p. 89–96.
8. LaFranchi SH. Newborn screening strategies for congenital hypothyroidism: an update. *J Inherit Metab Dis* 2010;**33**(Suppl. 2):S225–33.
9. Nebesio T, McKenna M, Nabhan ZM, Eugster EA. Newborn screening results in children with central hypothyroidism. *J Pediatr* 2010;**156**(6):990–3.
10. Dussault JH, Grenier A, Morissette J, Mitchell M. Preliminary report on filter paper TSH levels in the first 24h of life and the following days in a program screening for congenital hypothyroidism. In: Pass KA, Levy HL, editors. *Early hospital discharge: impact on newborn screening*. Atlanta, GA: Council of Regional Networks for Genetics Services, Emory University School of Medicine; 1995. p. 267–9.
11. Fagela-Domingo C, Padilla CD. Newborn screening for congenital hypothyroidism in early discharged infants. *Southeast Asian J Trop Med Public Health* 2003;**34**(Suppl. 3):165–9.
12. Lain S, Trumpff C, Grosse SD, Olivieri A, Van Vliet G. Are lower tsh cutoffs in neonatal screening for congenital hypothyroidism warranted? *Eur J Endocrinol* 2017;**177**(5):D1–D12.
13. Zung A, Tenenbaum-Rakover Y, Barkan S. Neonatal hyperthyrotropinemia: population characteristics, diagnosis, management and outcome after cessation of therapy. *Clin Endocrinol (Oxf)* 2010;**72**:264–71.
14. Corbetta C, Webert G, Fea C. A 7-year experience with low blood tsh cutoff levels for neonatal screening reveals an unsuspected frequency of congenital hypothyroidism (ch). *Clin Endocrinol (Oxf)* 2009;**71**:739–45.
15. Larson C, Hermos R, Delaney A, Daley D, Mitchell M. Risk factors associated with delayed thyrotropin elevations in congenital hypothyroidism. *J Pediatr* 2003;**143**(5):587–91.
16. Bijarnia S, Wilcken B, Wiley VC. Newborn screening for congenital hypothyroidism in very-low-birth-weight babies: the need for a second test. *J Inherit Metab Dis* 2011;**34**(3):827–33.

17. Hyman SJ, Greig F, Holzman I, Patel A, Wallach E, Rapaport R. Late rise of thyroid stimulating hormone in ill newborns. *J Pediatr Endocrinol Metab* 2007;**20**(4):501–10.

18. Woo HC, Lizarda A, Tucker R, Mitchell ML, Vohr B, Oh W, et al. Congenital hypothyroidism with a delayed thyroid-stimulating hormone elevation in very premature infants: incidence and growth and developmental outcomes. *J Pediatr* 2011;**158**(4):538–42.

19. Vincent MA, Rodd C, Dussault JH, Van Vliet G. Very low birth weight newborns do not need repeat screening for congenital hypothyroidism. *J Pediatr* 2002;**140**(3):311–4.

20. Perry R, Heinrichs C, Bourdoux P, Khoury K, Fo S, Dussault JH, et al. Discordance of monozygotic twins for thyroid dysgenesis: Implications for screening and for molecular pathophysiology. *J Clin Endocrinol Metabol* 2002;**87**(9):4072–7.

21. Hashemipour M, Hovsepian S, Kelishadi R, Iranpour R, Hadian R, Haghighi S, et al. Permanent and transient congenital hypothyroidism in isfahan–iran. *J Med Screen* 2009;**16**(1):11–6.

22. Erdenechimeg S. National neonatal hypothyroid screening program in mongolia. *Southeast Asian J Trop Med Public Health* 2003;**34**(Suppl. 3):85–6.

23. Olney RS, Grosse SD, Vogt RF. *Prevalence of congenital hypothyroidism—current trends and future directions: workshop summary. Pediatrics* 2010;**125**(Suppl. 2)https://doi.org/10.1542/peds.2009-1975Cwww.pediatrics.org/cgi/doi/10.1542/peds.2009-1975C.

24. Majeed-Saidan MA, Joyce B, Khan M, Hmam HD. Congenital hypothyroidism: the Riyadh Military Hospital experience. *Clin Endocrinol (Oxf)* 1993;**38**:191–5.

25. Albert BB, Cutfield WS, Webster D, Carll J, Derraik JGB, Jefferies C, et al. Etiology of increasing incidence of congenital hypothyroidism in new zealand from 1993–2010. *J Clin Endocrinol Metabol* 2012;**97**(9):3155–60.

26. Stoppa-Vaucher S, Van Vliet G, Deladoëy J. Variation by ethnicity in the prevalence of congenital hypothyroidism due to thyroid dysgenesis. *Thyroid* 2011;**21**(1):13–8.

27. Sun F, Zhang JX, Yang CY, Gao GQ, Zhu WB, Han B, et al. The genetic characteristics of congenital hypothyroidism in china by comprehensive screening of 21 candidate genes. *Eur J Endocrinol* 2018;**178**(6):623–33.

28. Matsuo K, Tanahashi Y, Mukai T, Suzuki S, Tajima T, Azuma H, et al. High prevalence of duox2 mutations in japanese patients with permanent congenital hypothyroidism or transient hypothyroidism. *J Pediatr Endocrinol Metab* 2016;**29**(7):807–12.

29. Zou M, Alzahrani AS, Al-Odaib A, Alqahtani MA, Babiker O, Al-Rijjal RA, et al. Molecular analysis of congenital hypothyroidism in saudi arabia: Slc26a7 mutation is a novel defect in thyroid dyshormonogenesis. *J Clin Endocrinol Metab* 2018;**103**(5):1889–98.

30. Reddy PA, Rajagopal G, Harinarayan CV, Vanaja V, Rajasekhar D, Suresh V, et al. High prevalence of associated birth defects in congenital hypothyroidism. *Int J Pediatr Endocrinol* 2010;**2010**:940980.

31. Stoppa-Vaucher S, Lapointe A, Turpin S, Rydlewski C, Vassart G, Deladoëy J. Ectopic thyroid gland causing dysphonia: imaging and molecular studies. *J Clin Endocrinol Metabol* 2010;**95**(10):4509–10.

32. Djemli A, Fillion M, Belgoudi J, Lambert R, Delvin EE, Schneider W, et al. Twenty years later: a reevaluation of the contribution of plasma thyroglobulin to the diagnosis of thyroid dysgenesis in infants with congenital hypothyroidism. *Clin Biochem* 2004;**37**(9):818–22.

33. Van Vliet G, Deladoey J. Disorders of the thyroid in the newborn and infant. In: Sperling M, editor. *Pediatric endocrinology*. 4th ed. Elsevier; 2014.

34. Gagné N, Parma J, Deal C, Vassart G, Van Vliet G. Apparent congenital athyreosis contrasting with normal plasma thyroglobulin levels and associated with inactivating mutations in the thyrotropin receptor gene: are athyreosis and ectopic thyroid distinct entities? *J Clin Endocrinol Metabol* 1998;**83**(5):1771–5.

35. Nettore IC, Cacace V, De Fusco C, Colao A, Macchia PE. The molecular causes of thyroid dysgenesis: a systematic review. *J Endocrinol Invest* 2013;**36**(8):654–64.

36. De Felice M, Di Lauro R. Thyroid development and its disorders: genetics and molecular mechanisms. *Endocr Rev* 2004;**25**(5):722–46.

37. Budny B, Szczepanek-Parulska E, Zemojtel T, Szaflarski W, Rydzanicz M, Wesoly J, et al. Mutations in proteasome-related genes are associated with thyroid hemiagenesis. *Endocrine* 2017;**56**(2):279–85.

38. Szczepanek-Parulska E, Zybek-Kocik A, Wartofsky L, Ruchala M. Thyroid hemiagenesis: incidence, clinical significance, and genetic background. *J Clin Endocrinol Metab* 2017;**102**(9):3124–37.

39. Maiorana R, Carta A, Floriddia G, Leonardi D, Buscema M, Sava L, et al. Thyroid hemiagenesis: prevalence in normal children and effect on thyroid function. *J Clin Endocrinol Metab* 2003;**88**(4):1534–6.

40. Stoupa A, Kariyawasam D, Carré A, Polak M. Update of thyroid developmental genes. *Endocrinol Metab Clin North Am* 2016;**45**(2):243–54.

41. Leger J, Marinovic D, Garel C, Bonaiti-Pellie C, Polak M, Czernichow P. Thyroid developmental anomalies in first degree relatives of children with congenital hypothyroidism. *J Clin Endocrinol Metab* 2002;**87**(2):575–80.

42. Castanet M, Polak M, Bonaiti-Pellie C, Lyonnet S, Czernichow P, Leger J. Nineteen years of national screening for congenital hypothyroidism: familial cases with thyroid dysgenesis suggest the involvement of genetic factors. *J Clin Endocrinol Metab* 2001;**86**(5):2009–14.

43. Olivieri A, Stazi MA, Mastroiacovo P, Fazzini C, Medda E, Spagnolo A, et al. A population-based study on the frequency of additional congenital malformations in infants with congenital hypothyroidism: data from the italian registry for congenital hypothyroidism (1991–1998). *J Clin Endocrinol Metab* 2002;**87**(2):557–62.

44. Devos H, Rodd C, Gagné N, Laframboise R, Van Vliet G. A search for the possible molecular mechanisms of thyroid dysgenesis: sex ratios and associated malformations. *J Clin Endocrinol Metabol* 1999;**84**(7):2502–6.

45. Castanet M, Sura-Trueba S, Chauty A, Carre A, de Roux N, Heath S, et al. Linkage and mutational analysis of familial thyroid dysgenesis demonstrate genetic heterogeneity implicating novel genes. *Eur J Hum Genet* 2005;**13**(2):232–9.

46. Deladoëy J, Vassart G, Van Vliet G. Possible non-mendelian mechanisms of thyroid dysgenesis. In: Van Vliet G, Polak M, editors. *Thyroid gland development and function*. vol. 10. Karger Publishers; 2007. p. 29–42.

47. Abu-Khudir R, Magne F, Chanoine J-P, Deal C, Van Vliet G, Deladoëy J. Role for tissue-dependent methylation differences in the expression of foxe1 in nontumoral thyroid glands. *J Clin Endocrinol Metab* 2014;**99**(6):E1120–9.
48. Szinnai G. Genetics of normal and abnormal thyroid development in humans. *Best Pract Res Clin Endocrinol Metab* 2014;**28**(2):133–50.
49. Chang W-C, Liao C-Y, Chen W-C, Fan Y-C, Chiu S-J, Kuo H-C, et al. R450h tsh receptor mutation in congenital hypothyroidism in taiwanese children. *Clin Chim Acta* 2012;**413**(11):1004–7.
50. Lee S-T, Lee DH, Kim J-Y, Kwon M-J, Kim J-W, Hong Y-H, et al. Molecular screening of the tsh receptor (tshr) and thyroid peroxidase (tpo) genes in korean patients with nonsyndromic congenital hypothyroidism. *Clin Endocrinol (Oxf)* 2011;**75**(5):715–21.
51. Narumi S, Muroya K, Asakura Y, Adachi M, Hasegawa T. Transcription factor mutations and congenital hypothyroidism: systematic genetic screening of a population-based cohort of japanese patients. *J Clin Endocrinol Metabol* 2010;**95**(4):1981–5.
52. Stanbury JB, Rocmans P, Buhler UK, Ochi Y. Congenital hypothyroidism with impaired thyroid response to thyrotropin. *N Engl J Med* 1968;**279** (21):1132–6.
53. Stenson PD, Mort M, Ball EV, Shaw K, Phillips AD, Cooper DN. The human gene mutation database: building a comprehensive mutation repository for clinical and molecular genetics, diagnostic testing and personalized genomic medicine. *Hum Genet* 2014;**133**(1):1–9.
54. Parmentier M, Libert F, Maenhaut C, Lefort A, Gerard C, Perret J, et al. Molecular cloning of the thyrotropin receptor. *Science (New York, NY)* 1989;**246**(4937):1620–2.
55. Abramowicz MJ, Duprez L, Parma J, Vassart G, Heinrichs C. Familial congenital hypothyroidism due to inactivating mutation of the thyrotropin receptor causing profound hypoplasia of the thyroid gland. *J Clin Invest* 1997;**99**(12):3018–24.
56. Biebermann H, Schöneberg T, Krude H, G S, Gudermann T, Grüters A. Mutations of the human thyrotropin receptor gene causing thyroid hypoplasia and persistent congenital hypothyroidism. *J Clin Endocrinol Metabol* 1997;**82**(10):3471–80.
57. Calebiro D, Gelmini G, Cordella D, Bonomi M, Winkler F, Biebermann H, et al. Frequent tsh receptor genetic alterations with variable signaling impairment in a large series of children with nonautoimmune isolated hyperthyrotropinemia. *J Clin Endocrinol Metabol* 2012;**97**(1):E156–60.
58. Sunthornthepvarakul T, Gottschalk ME, Hayashi Y, Refetoff S. Resistance to thyrotropin caused by mutations in the thyrotropin-receptor gene. *N Engl J Med* 1995;**332**(3):155–60.
59. de Roux N, Misrahi M, Brauner R, Houang M, Carel JC, Granier M, et al. Four families with loss of function mutations of the thyrotropin receptor. *J Clin Endocrinol Metabol* 1996;**81**(12):4229–35.
60. Yokoro S, Matsuo M, Ohtsuka T, Ohzeki T. Hyperthyrotropinemia in a neonate with normal thyroid hormone levels: the earliest diagnostic clue for pseudohypoparathyroidism. *Neonatology* 1990;**58**(2):69–72.
61. Parlato R, Rosica A, Rodriguez-Mallon A, Affuso A, Postiglione MP, Arra C, et al. An integrated regulatory network controlling survival and migration in thyroid organogenesis. *Dev Biol* 2004;**276**(2):464–75.
62. Krude H, Schutz B, Biebermann H, von Moers A, Schnabel D, Neitzel H, et al. Choreoathetosis, hypothyroidism, and pulmonary alterations due to human nkx2-1 haploinsufficiency. *J Clin Invest* 2002;**109**(4):475–80.
63. Macchia PE, Lapi P, Krude H, Pirro MT, Missero C, Chiovato L, et al. Pax8 mutations associated with congenital hypothyroidism caused by thyroid dysgenesis. *Nat Genet* 1998;**19**(1):83–6.
64. Clifton-Bligh RJ, Wentworth JM, Heinz P, Crisp MS, John R, Lazarus JH, et al. Mutation of the gene encoding human ttf-2 associated with thyroid agenesis, cleft palate and choanal atresia. *Nat Genet* 1998;**19**(4):399–401.
65. Dimitri P, Habeb AM, Garbuz F, Millward A, Wallis S, Moussa K, et al. Expanding the clinical spectrum associated with glis3 mutations. *J Clin Endocrinol Metab* 2015;**100**(10):E1362–9.
66. Carré A, Szinnai G, Castanet M, Sura-Trueba S, Tron E, Broutin-L'Hermite I, et al. Five new ttf1/nkx2.1 mutations in brain–lung–thyroid syndrome: Rescue by pax8 synergism in one case. *Hum Mol Genet* 2009;**18**(12):2266–76.
67. Maquet E, Costagliola S, Parma J, Christophe-Hobertus C, Oligny LL, Fournet J-C, et al. Lethal respiratory failure and mild primary hypothyroidism in a term girl with a de novo heterozygous mutation in the titf1/nkx2.1 gene. *J Clin Endocrinol Metabol* 2009;**94**(1):197–203.
68. Castanet M, Polak M. Spectrum of human foxe1/ttf2 mutations. *Horm Res Paediatr* 2010;**73**(6):423–9.
69. Bamforth JS, Hughes IA, Lazarus JH, Weaver CM, Harper PS. Congenital hypothyroidism, spiky hair, and cleft palate. *J Med Genet* 1989;**26** (1):49–51.
70. Carré A, Castanet M, Sura-Trueba S, Szinnai G, Van Vliet G, Trochet D, et al. Polymorphic length of foxe1 alanine stretch: evidence for genetic susceptibility to thyroid dysgenesis | springerlink. *Hum Genet* 2007;**122**(5):467–76.
71. Ramos HE, Carré A, Chevrier L, Szinnai G, Tron E, Cerqueira TLO, et al. Extreme phenotypic variability of thyroid dysgenesis in six new cases of congenital hypothyroidism due to pax8 gene loss-of-function mutations. *Eur J Endocrinol* 2014;**171**(4):499.
72. Kang HS, Kumar D, Liao G, Lichti-Kaiser K, Gerrish K, Liao X-H, et al. Glis3 is indispensable for tsh/tshr-dependent thyroid hormone biosynthesis and follicular cell proliferation. *J Clin Invest* 2017;**127**(12):4326–37.
73. Liu S, Chai J, Zheng G, Li H, Lu D, Ge Y. Screening of hhex mutations in chinese children with thyroid dysgenesis. *J Clin Res Pediatr Endocrinol* 2016;**8**(1):21–5.
74. Dentice M, Cordeddu V, Rosica A, Ferrara AM, Santarpia L, Salvatore D, et al. Missense mutation in the transcription factor nkx2–5: a novel molecular event in the pathogenesis of thyroid dysgenesis. *J Clin Endocrinol Metabol* 2006;**91**(4):1428–33.
75. Hermanns P, Grasberger H, Refetoff S, Pohlenz J. Mutations in the nkx2.5 gene and the pax8 promoter in a girl with thyroid dysgenesis. *J Clin Endocrinol Metab* 2011;**96**(6):E977–81.
76. van Engelen K, Mommersteeg MT, Baars MJ, Lam J, Ilgun A, van Trotsenburg AS, et al. The ambiguous role of nkx2-5 mutations in thyroid dysgenesis. *PLoS One* 2012;**7**(12).

77. Polak M, Van Vliet G. Disorders of the thyroid gland. In: Sarafoglou K, Hoffmann GF, Roth KS, editors. *Pediatric endocrinology and inborn errors of metabolism*. New York: McGraw-Hill; 2008. p. 355–82.

78. Vassart G, Dumont JE. The thyrotropin receptor and the regulation of thyrocyte function and growth. *Endocr Rev* 1992;**13**(3):596–611.

79. Grasberger H, Refetoff S. Genetic causes of congenital hypothyroidism due to dyshormonogenesis. *Curr Opin Pediatr* 2011;**23**(4):421–8.

80. Deladoëy J, Pfarr N, Vuissoz J-M, Parma J, Vassart G, Biesterfeld S, et al. Pseudodominant inheritance of goitrous congenital hypothyroidism caused by tpo mutations: molecular and in silico studies. *J Clin Endocrinol Metab* 2008;**93**(2):627–33.

81. Avbelj M, Tahirovic H, Debeljak M, Kusekova M, Toromanovic A, Krzisnik C, et al. High prevalence of thyroid peroxidase gene mutations in patients with thyroid dyshormonogenesis. *Eur J Endocrinol* 2007;**156**(5):511.

82. Szinnai G, Kosugi S, Cl D, Lucidarme N, Vr D, Czernichow P, et al. Extending the clinical heterogeneity of iodide transport defect (itd): a novel mutation r124h of the sodium/iodide symporter gene and review of genotype-phenotype correlations in itd. *J Clin Endocrinol Metabol* 2006;**91**(4):1199–204.

83. Everett LA, Glaser B, Beck JC, Idol JR, Buchs A, Heyman M, et al. Pendred syndrome is caused by mutations in a putative sulphate transporter gene (pds). *Nat Genet* 1997;**17**(4):411–22.

84. Bizhanova A, Kopp P. Genetics and phenomics of pendred syndrome. *Mol Cell Endocrinol* 2010;**322**(1):83–90.

85. Gaudino R, Garel C, Czernichow P, Léger J. Proportion of various types of thyroid disorders among newborns with congenital hypothyroidism and normally located gland: a regional cohort study. *Clin Endocrinol (Oxf)* 2005;**62**(4):444–8.

86. Belforte FS, Miras MB, Olcese MC, Sobrero G, Testa G, Muñoz L, et al. Congenital goitrous hypothyroidism: mutation analysis in the thyroid peroxidase gene. *Clin Endocrinol (Oxf)* 2012;**76**(4):568–76.

87. Targovnik HM, Citterio CE, Rivolta CM. Iodide handling disorders (nis, tpo, tg, iyd). *Best Pract Res Clin Endocrinol Metab* 2017;**31**(2):195–212.

88. Fugazzola L, Cerutti N, Mannavola D, Vannucchi G, Fallini C, Persani L, et al. Monoallelic expression of mutant thyroid peroxidase allele causing total iodide organification defect. *J Clin Endocrinol Metab* 2003;**88**(7):3264–71.

89. Stoupa A, Chaabane R, Gueriouz M, Raynaud-Ravni C, Nitschke P, Bole-Feysot C, et al. Thyroid hypoplasia in congenital hypothyroidism associated with thyroid peroxidase mutations. *Thyroid* 2018;**28**(7):941–4.

90. Lee CC, Harun F, Jalaludin MY, Heh CH, Othman R, Kang IN, et al. Variable clinical phenotypes in a family with homozygous c.1159g > a mutation in the thyroid peroxidase gene. *Horm Res Paediatr* 2014;**81**(5):356–60.

91. Bakker B, Bikker H, Hennekam RCM, Lommen EJP, Schipper MGJ, Vulsma T, et al. Maternal isodisomy for chromosome 2p causing severe congenital hypothyroidism. *J Clin Endocrinol Metab* 2001;**86**(3):1164–8.

92. Moreno JC, Bikker H, Kempers MJE, van Trotsenburg ASP, Baas F, de Vijlder JJM, et al. Inactivating mutations in the gene for thyroid oxidase 2 (thox2) and congenital hypothyroidism. *N Engl J Med* 2002;**347**(2):95–102.

93. Hoste C, Rigutto S, Van Vliet G, Miot F, De Deken X. Compound heterozygosity for a novel hemizygous missense mutation and a partial deletion affecting the catalytic core of the H_2O_2-generating enzyme duox2 associated with transient congenital hypothyroidism. *Hum Mutat* 2010;**31**(4):E1304–19.

94. Vigone MC, Fugazzola L, Zamproni I, Passoni A, Di Candia S, Chiumello G, et al. Persistent mild hypothyroidism associated with novel sequence variants of the duox2 gene in two siblings. *Hum Mutat* 2005;**26**(4):395.

95. Grasberger H, Refetoff S. Identification of the maturation factor for dual oxidase. Evolution of an eukaryotic operon equivalent. *J Biol Chem* 2006;**281**(27):18269–72.

96. Zamproni I, Grasberger H, Cortinovis F, Vigone MC, Chiumello G, Mora S, et al. Biallelic inactivation of the dual oxidase maturation factor 2 (duoxa2) gene as a novel cause of congenital hypothyroidism. *J Clin Endocrinol Metab* 2008;**93**(2):605–10.

97. Targovnik HM, Citterio CE, Rivolta CM. Thyroglobulin gene mutations in congenital hypothyroidism. *Horm Res Paediatr* 2011;**75**(5):311–21.

98. Moreno JC, Klootwijk W, van Toor H, Pinto G, D'Alessandro M, Lèger A, et al. Mutations in the iodotyrosine deiodinase gene and hypothyroidism. *N Engl J Med* 2008;**358**(17):1811–8.

99. Afink G, Kulik W, Overmars H, de Randamie J, Veenboer T, van Cruchten A, et al. Molecular characterization of iodotyrosine dehalogenase deficiency in patients with hypothyroidism. *J Clin Endocrinol Metab* 2008;**93**(12):4894–901.

100. Burniat A, Pirson I, Vilain C, Kulik W, Afink G, Moreno-Reyes R, et al. Iodotyrosine deiodinase defect identified via genome-wide approach. *J Clin Endocrinol Metab* 2012;**97**(7):E1276–83.

101. Krude H, Blankenstein O. Treating patients not numbers: the benefit and burden of lowering tsh newborn screening cut-offs. *Arch Dis Child* 2011;**96**(2):121–2.

102. Parks JS, Lin M, Grosse SD, Hinton CF, Drummond-Borg M, Borgfeld L, et al. The impact of transient hypothyroidism on the increasing rate of congenital hypothyroidism in the United States. *Pediatrics* 2010;**125**(Suppl. 2):S54–63.

103. Gaudino R, Garel C, Czernichow P, Leger J. Proportion of various types of thyroid disorders among newborns with congenital hypothyroidism and normally located gland: a regional cohort study. *Clin Endocrinol (Oxf)* 2005;**62**(4):444–8.

104. Eugster EA, LeMay D, Michael Zerin J, Pescovitz OH. Definitive diagnosis in children with congenital hypothyroidism. *J Pediatr* 2004;**144**(5):643–7.

105. Kanike N, Davis A, Shekhawat PS. Transient hypothyroidism in the newborn: to treat or not to treat. *Transl Pediatr* 2017;**6**(4):349–58.

106. Bekhit OE, Yousef RM. Permanent and transient congenital hypothyroidism in fayoum, egypt: a descriptive retrospective study. *PLoS One* 2013;**8**(6).

107. Korzeniewski SJ, Grigorescu V, Kleyn M, Young WI, Birbeck G, Todem D, et al. Transient hypothyroidism at 3-year follow-up among cases of congenital hypothyroidism detected by newborn screening. *J Pediatr* 2013;**162**(1):177–82.

108. Kang MJ, Chung HR, Oh YJ, Shim YS, Yang S, Hwang IT. Three-year follow-up of children with abnormal newborn screening results for congenital hypothyroidism. *Pediatr Neonatol* 2017;**58**(5):442–8.

109. Caldwell KL, Makhmudov A, Ely E, Jones RL, Wang RY. Iodine status of the U.S. Population, national health and nutrition examination survey, 2005–2006 and 2007–2008. *Thyroid* 2011;**21**(4):419–27.

110. Gupta PM, Gahche JJ, Herrick KA, Ershow AG, Potischman N, Perrine CG. Use of iodine-containing dietary supplements remains low among women of reproductive age in the United States: Nhanes 2011–2014. *Nutrients* 2018;**10**(4). pii: E422.

111. Ahmet A, Lawson ML, Babyn P, Tricco AC. Hypothyroidism in neonates post-iodinated contrast media: a systematic review. *Acta Paediatr* 2009;**98**(10):1568–74.

112. Aitken J, Williams FL. A systematic review of thyroid dysfunction in preterm neonates exposed to topical iodine. *Arch Dis Child Fetal Neonatal Ed* 2014;**99**(1):F21–8.

113. Alexander EK, Pearce EN, Brent GA, Brown RS, Chen H, Dosiou C, et al. 2017 Guidelines of the american thyroid association for the diagnosis and management of thyroid disease during pregnancy and the postpartum. *Thyroid* 2017;**27**(3):315–89.

114. van Trotsenburg AS, Vulsma T, van Santen HM, Cheung W, de Vijlder JJ. Lower neonatal screening thyroxine concentrations in down syndrome newborns. *J Clin Endocrinol Metab* 2003;**88**(4):1512–5.

115. Schoen EJ, Clapp W, To TT, Fireman BH. The key role of newborn thyroid scintigraphy with isotopic iodide (123i) in defining and managing congenital hypothyroidism. *Pediatrics* 2004;**114**(6):e683–8.

116. Zdraveska N, Zdravkovska M, Anastasovska V, Sukarova-Angelovska E, Kocova M. Diagnostic re-evaluation of congenital hypothyroidism in macedonia: predictors for transient or permanent hypothyroidism. *Endocr Connect* 2018;**7**(2):278–85.

117. Cho MS, Cho GS, Park SH, Jung MH, Suh BK, Koh DG. Earlier re-evaluation may be possible in pediatric patients with eutopic congenital hypothyroidism requiring lower l-thyroxine doses. *Ann Pediatr Endocrinol Metab* 2014;**19**(3):141–5.

118. Messina MF, Aversa T, Salzano G, Zirilli G, Sferlazzas C, De Luca F, et al. Early discrimination between transient and permanent congenital hypothyroidism in children with eutopic gland. *Horm Res Paediatr* 2015;**84**(3):159–64.

119. Oron T, Lazar L, Ben-Yishai S, Tenenbaum A, Yackobovitch-Gavan M, Meyerovitch J, et al. Permanent vs transient congenital hypothyroidism: assessment of predictive variables. *J Clin Endocrinol Metab* 2018;**103**(12):4428–36.

120. Saba C, Guilmin-Crepon S, Zenaty D, Martinerie L, Paulsen A, Simon D, et al. Early determinants of thyroid function outcomes in children with congenital hypothyroidism and a normally located thyroid gland: a regional cohort study. *Thyroid* 2018;**28**(8):959–67.

121. Leger J, Olivieri A, Donaldson M, Torresani T, Krude H, van Vliet G, et al. European society for paediatric endocrinology consensus guidelines on screening, diagnosis, and management of congenital hypothyroidism. *Horm Res Paediatr* 2014;**81**(2):80–103.

122. Belfort MB, Pearce EN, Braverman LE, He X, Brown RS. Low iodine content in the diets of hospitalized preterm infants. *J Clin Endocrinol Metab* 2012;**97**(4):E632–6.

123. Wassner AJ, Brown RS. Hypothyroidism in the newborn period. *Curr Opin Endocrinol Diabetes Obes* 2013;**20**(5):449–54.

124. Hollanders JJ, van der Pal SM, Verkerk PH, Rotteveel J, Finken MJ. Transient hypothyroxinemia of prematurity and problem behavior in young adulthood. *Psychoneuroendocrinology* 2016;**72**:40–6.

125. Osborn DA, Hunt RW. Prophylactic postnatal thyroid hormones for prevention of morbidity and mortality in preterm infants. *Cochrane Database Syst Rev* 2007;(1).

126. Uchiyama A, Kushima R, Watanabe T, Kusuda S. Effect of l-thyroxine supplementation on very low birth weight infants with transient hypothyroxinemia of prematurity at 3 years of age. *J Perinatol: official journal of the California Perinatal Association* 2017;**37**(5):602–5.

127. Ng SM, Turner MA, Gamble C, Didi M, Victor S, Manning D, et al. An explanatory randomised placebo controlled trial of levothyroxine supplementation for babies born <28 weeks' gestation: results of the tipit trial. *Trials* 2013;**14**:211.

128. van Tijn DA, de Vijlder JJM, Verbeeten JB, Verkerk PH, Vulsma T. Neonatal detection of congenital hypothyroidism of central origin. *J Clin Endocrinol Metab* 2005;**90**(6):3350–9.

129. Leger J, Olivieri A, Donaldson MDC, Torresani T, Krude H, van Vliet G, et al. European society for paediatric endocrinology consensus guidelines on screening, diagnosis, and management of congenital hypothyroidism. *J Clin Endocrinol Metab* 2014;**99**:363–84.

130. Kempers MJE, van der Sluijs VL, der Sanden RWG N-v, Lanting CI, Kooistra L, Wiedijk BM, et al. Neonatal screening for congenital hypothyroidism in the netherlands: cognitive and motor outcome at 10 years of age. *J Clin Endocrinol Metab* 2007;**92**(3):919–24.

131. Dimitropoulos A, Molinari L, Etter K, Torresani T, Lang-Muritano M, Jenni OG, et al. Children with congenital hypothyroidism: long-term intellectual outcome after early high-dose treatment. *Pediatr Res* 2009;**65**:242.

132. Verelst J, Chanoine JP, Delange F. Radionuclide imaging in primary permanent congenital hypothyroidism. *Clin Nucl Med* 1991;**16**(9):652–5.

133. Delange F. Neonatal screening for congenital hypothyroidism: results and perspectives. *Hormones* 1997;**48**(2):51–61.

134. Ogawa E, Kojima-Ishii K, Fujiwara I. Ultrasound appearance of thyroid tissue in hypothyroid infants. *J Pediatr* 2008;**153**(1):101–4.

135. Glorieux J, Desjardins M, Letarte J, Morissette J, Dussault JH. Useful parameters to predict the eventual mental outcome of hypothyroid children. *Pediatr Res* 1988;**24**:6.

136. Wasniewska M, De Luca F, Cassio A, Oggiaro N, Gianino P, Delvecchio M, et al. In congenital hypothyroidism bone maturation at birth may be a predictive factor of psychomotor development during the first year of life irrespective of other variables related to treatment. *Eur J Endocrinol* 2003;**149**(1):1–6.

137. Najmi SB, Hashemipour M, Maracy MR, Hovsepian S, Ghasemi M. Intelligence quotient in children with congenital hypothyroidism: the effect of diagnostic and treatment variables. *J Res Med Sci* 2013;**18**(5):395–9.

138. Selva KA, Harper A, Downs A, Blasco PA, LaFranchi SH. Neurodevelopmental outcomes in congenital hypothyroidism: comparison of initial t_4 dose and time to reach target t_4 and tsh. *J Pediatr* 2005;**147**(6):775–80.

139. Selva KA, Mandel SH, Rien L, Sesser D, Miyahira R, Skeels M, et al. Initial treatment dose of l-thyroxine in congenital hypothyroidism. *J Pediatr* 2002;**141**(6):786–92.

140. Aleksander PE, Bruckner-Spieler M, Stoehr AM, Lankes E, Kuhnen P, Schnabel D, et al. Mean high-dose l-thyroxine treatment is efficient and safe to achieve a normal iq in young adult patients with congenital hypothyroidism. *J Clin Endocrinol Metab* 2018;**103**(4):1459–69.

141. Nagasaki K, Minamitani K, Anzo M, Adachi M, Ishii T, Onigata K, et al. Guidelines for mass screening of congenital hypothyroidism (2014 revision). *Clin Pediatr Endocrinol* 2015;**24**(3):107–33.

142. Cassio A, Cacciari E, Cicognani A, Damiani G, Missiroli G, Corbelli E, et al. Treatment for congenital hypothyroidism: thyroxine alone or thyroxine plus triiodothyronine? *Pediatrics* 2003;**111**:1055–60.

143. Álvarez M, Iglesias Fernández C, Rodríguez Sánchez A, Dulín Íñiguez E, Rodríguez Arnao MD. Episodes of overtreatment during the first six months in children with congenital hypothyroidism and their relationships with sustained attention and inhibitory control at school age. *Horm Res Paediatr* 2010;**74**(2):114–20.

144. Leger J, Larroque B, Norton J. Influence of severity of congenital hypothyroidism and adequacy of treatment on school achievement in young adolescents: a population-based cohort study. *Acta Paediatr* 2001;**90**(11):1249–56.

145. Fisher DA, Schoen EJ, Franchi SL, Mandel SH, Nelson JC, Carlton EI, et al. The hypothalamic-pituitary-thyroid negative feedback control axis in children with treated congenital hypothyroidism. *J Clin Endocrinol Metab* 2000;**85**(8):2722–7.

146. Bucher H, Prader A, Illig R. Head circumference, height, bone age and weight in 103 children with congenital hypothyroidism before and during thyroid hormone replacement. *Helv Paediatr Acta* 1985;**40**(4):305–16.

147. Leger J. Congenital hypothyroidism: a clinical update of long-term outcome in young adults. *Eur J Endocrinol* 2015;**172**(2):R67–77.

148. Cooper DS, Laurberg P. Hyperthyroidism in pregnancy. *Lancet Diabetes Endocrinol* 2013;**1**(3):238–49.

149. Leger J. Management of fetal and neonatal graves' disease. *Horm Res Paediatr* 2017;**87**(1):1–6.

150. Banige M, Polak M, Luton D. Prediction of neonatal hyperthyroidism. *J Pediatr* 2018;**197**:249–254.e1.

151. Banige M, Estellat C, Biran V, Desfrere L, Champion V, Benachi A, et al. Study of the factors leading to fetal and neonatal dysthyroidism in children of patients with graves disease. *J Endocr Soc* 2017;**1**(6):751–61.

152. Besancon A, Beltrand J, Le Gac I, Luton D, Polak M. Management of neonates born to women with graves' disease: a cohort study. *Eur J Endocrinol* 2014;**170**(6):855–62.

153. Krude H, Kühnen P, Biebermann H. Treatment of congenital thyroid dysfunction: achievements and challenges. *Best Pract Res Clin Endocrinol Metab* 2015;**29**(3):399–413.

154. Refetoff S, Bassett JH, Beck-Peccoz P, Bernal J, Brent G, Chatterjee K, et al. Classification and proposed nomenclature for inherited defects of thyroid hormone action, cell transport, and metabolism. *J Clin Endocrinol Metab* 2014;**99**(3):768–70.

155. Verge CF, Konrad D, Cohen M, Di Cosmo C, Dumitrescu AM, Marcinkowski T, et al. Diiodothyropropionic acid (ditpa) in the treatment of mct8 deficiency. *J Clin Endocrinol Metab* 2012;**97**(12):4515–23.

156. Lafranchi SH, Snyder DB, Sesser DE, Skeels MR, Singh N, Brent GA, et al. Follow-up of newborns with elevated screening t4 concentrations. *J Pediatr* 2003;**143**(3):296–301.

157. Moran C, Chatterjee K. Resistance to thyroid hormone due to defective thyroid receptor alpha. *Best Pract Res Clin Endocrinol Metab* 2015;**29**(4):647–57.

Chapter 44

Disorders of Calcium, Phosphorus, and Bone Metabolism During Fetal and Neonatal Development

Christopher S. Kovacs* and Leanne M. Ward[†,‡]

*Faculty of Medicine, Endocrinology, Memorial University of Newfoundland, St. John's, NL, Canada, [†]Department of Pediatrics, Faculty of Medicine, University of Ottawa, Ottawa, ON, Canada, [‡]Division of Endocrinology, Children's Hospital of Eastern Ontario, Ottawa, ON, Canada,

Common Clinical Problems

- Maternal hypercalcemia can suppress the fetal parathyroids, leading to neonatal hypocalcemia that may be prolonged and, sometimes, permanent.
- Maternal hypocalcemia provokes secondary hyperparathyroidism in the fetus, which can lead to substantial resorption of the fetal skeleton, and fractures occurring in utero or during delivery.
- Hypocalcemia develops in utero with congenital causes of hypoparathyroidism, but may be asymptomatic.
- Vitamin D deficiency, and genetic disorders of vitamin D physiology, may not affect the fetus, but instead will lead to hypocalcemia and rickets postnatally.
- Disorders due to excess or absence of FGF23 do not disturb phosphorus metabolism in utero, but lead to altered serum phosphorus and renal phosphorus excretion within weeks after birth.

44.1 INTRODUCTION

An earlier chapter (33) on normal physiology of fetal and neonatal bone and mineral metabolism explained how the main calciotropic and phosphotropic hormones play somewhat different roles than in the adult. Parathyroid hormone (PTH) and calcitriol normally circulate at very low levels, whereas calcium and phosphorus are maintained at high concentrations in the fetal circulation. The placenta actively pumps minerals against concentration and electrochemical gradients, while the fetal intestines and kidneys do not play critical roles in providing minerals. The human skeleton typically accretes 30 g of calcium by term, with 80% of that obtained in the third trimester.[1] This corresponds to 100–150 mg/kg/day of calcium being transported across the placenta during the third trimester, or more than 300 mg per day between weeks 35 and 38.[1] PTH and PTH-related protein (PTHrP) play key roles in fetal bone and mineral homeostasis, while vitamin D/calcitriol, fibroblast growth factor-23 (FGF23), calcitonin, and the sex steroids may not be required.

The placental pump is lost at birth. The intestines immediately become the main source of mineral delivery, while the kidneys begin to reabsorb mineral, and bone turnover contributes additional mineral to the circulation. PTH surges in the circulation, followed by a rise in calcitriol. Calcium is initially absorbed largely through passive mechanisms facilitated by lactose, but this later becomes an active and calcitriol-dependent process.

This chapter reviews the pathophysiology of disorders of bone and mineral metabolism that are caused by the absence or excess of the main calciotropic or phosphotropic hormones. In addition, the effects of maternal bone and mineral metabolism disorders on the fetus and neonate are also described.

There are only limited human fetal data, which at times consist of cord blood samples, and pathological examination of embryos and fetuses that died due to congenital abnormalities or obstetrical accidents. The main exception is with respect to vitamin D deficiency and insufficiency, for which there have been many randomized interventional trials, cohort studies, and associational studies.

This chapter will rely in part on discussion of data from animal models, which have included surgical, genetic, and pharmacological approaches to mimic the human conditions. In order to avoid any confusion between sources of data, within each subsection of this chapter, animal data will be followed by any human data.

Due to limits on the number of references, a longer review with over 750 citations of the primary literature will be mainly cited.[1] Only selected and recent papers can be cited within this chapter.

44.2 ABSENCE OF PTH (HYPOPARATHYROIDISM, APARATHYROIDISM, PTH RECEPTOR)

44.2.1 Fetal Animal Data

Although PTH typically circulates at low levels in all fetal models that have been studied, it remains critically important in regulating fetal mineral and bone metabolism. Fetal hypocalcemia and hyperphosphatemia have resulted when genes encoding PTH or the parathyroids have been ablated in mice, when PTH antiserum is infused in rats, or after parathyroid-ectomy in fetal lambs and rats.[1] Loss of parathyroids leads to more marked hypocalcemia than loss of PTH, which suggests that the fetal parathyroids produce factors in addition to PTH, such as PTHrP.

The PTH/PTHrP receptor (PTH1R) is expressed by murine trophoblasts and cells of the intraplacental yolk sac. This implies that N-terminal PTH (or PTHrP) has some placental role, but most studies have found no effect of PTH on placental mineral transport.[1] The main evidence that PTH may have a role comes from study of *Pth* null fetuses, which have reduced placental expression of several genes involved in mineral transport.[2] Furthermore, although placental calcium transport was normal in *Pth* null fetuses, treatment with full-length PTH resulted in a 30% increase in calcium transport.[2]

The ash weight, calcium, and phosphorus content of the skeleton has been consistently reduced by loss of PTH, as observed in thyroparathyroidectomized (i.e., both glands removed, but thyroid hormone replacement given) fetal lambs, aparathyroid fetal mice (Fig. 44.1), and *Pth* null fetuses.[1] However, the development of the skeleton may be otherwise normal. *Pth* null fetuses were initially reported (within an inbred mouse strain) to have slightly shorter tibial metaphyses, shortened metacarpals and metatarsals, smaller vertebrae, reduced trabecular bone volumes, fewer osteoclasts and osteo-blasts, and reduced expression of some osteoblast-specific genes.[3] But when back-crossed into an outbred mouse strain, *Pth* null fetuses had normal lengths of the long bones, normal cellular morphology of the tibial growth plate and trabecular compartment, and normal expression of chondrocyte and osteoblast-specific genes.[4, 5] The only consistent finding across both background strains was the reduction in skeletal mineral content.

Overall, the animal models confirm that hypoparathyroidism and aparathyroidism result in hypocalcemia, hyperpho-sphatemia, and reduced skeletal mineral content. Since placental calcium transport is normal in the absence of PTH or parathyroids, the reduced skeletal mineral content may indicate that low serum calcium impairs mineral accretion by the developing skeleton. The underlying structure of the hypoparathyroid skeleton may be completely normal, or it may display evidence of modest osteoblast-specific deficits, depending on the genetic background.

44.2.2 Neonatal Animal Data

PTH normally becomes a key regulator of mineral and bone homeostasis in the hours after birth. The parathyroids upre-gulate the synthesis and secretion of PTH, which in turn has its effects to increase blood calcium, reduce serum phosphorus, stimulate calcitriol synthesis and reduce its catabolism, reabsorb calcium in the kidney tubules, excrete phosphorus, and increase bone turnover.

Aparathyroid and *Pth* null fetuses are hypocalcemic and hyperphosphatemic at birth, and 2 weeks later they are slightly smaller than their wild-type (WT) siblings, due to reduced osteoblast function that leads to slower bone lengthening.[1] It is not until weaning at 3 weeks of age that sporadic deaths begin to occur from presumed hypocalcemia.[1] This timing is con-sistent with intestinal calcium absorption undergoing a developmental change from passive to active, calcitriol-dependent absorption. Prior to 3 weeks of age, lactose in milk facilitates calcium absorption and calcitriol is not required. It is after weaning that calcitriol becomes important, but in the absence of PTH, calcitriol synthesis is markedly reduced and its catab-olism is increased. Sudden deaths in *Pth* null fetuses are prevented by providing a calcium-phosphate-lactose-enriched "rescue diet" that increases passive absorption of mineral, thereby bypassing the need for calcitriol.[1]

Hypocalcemia in *Pth* nulls contributes to their increased mortality and reduced skeletal mineralization independent of PTH or calcitriol. This has been shown by double mutant mice that lack PTH and calcitriol. They are hypocalcemic, hyper-phosphatemic, and hypercalciuric, have shortened skeletal lengths and reduced trabecular bone volumes, and die before weaning at 3 weeks of age.[6] In the first study, when either PTH or PTHrP were injected daily starting at 4 days after birth,

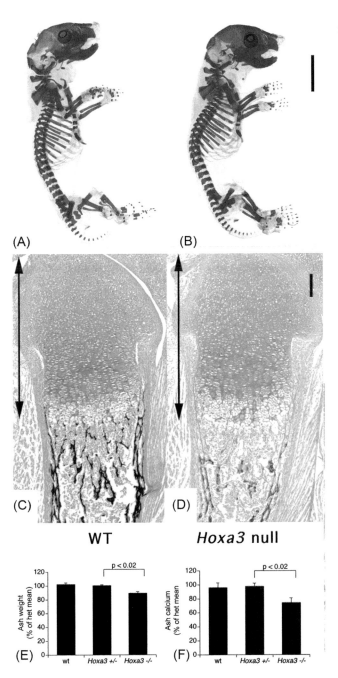

WT   *Hoxa3* null

(E)   (F)

FIG. 44.1 Skeletal morphology and mineral content in aparathyroid fetuses. Panels (A) and (B) show images of fetal skeletons (ED 18.5) stained with alizarin *red* (for mineral) and alcian *blue* (for cartilage). Skeletal morphology of the aparathyroid *Hoxa3* null was consistently normal, as shown by the normal crown-rump length, lengths of long bones, and mineralization pattern of the *Hoxa3* null (B) and its WT sibling (A). Subtle changes in the hyoid bone and other derivatives of the third and fourth pharyngeal arches in the *Hoxa3* null are not evident in these views. Panels (C) and (D) are von Kossa preparations (counterstained with *methyl green*) of the upper halves of fetal tibias (ED 18.5), which include the growth plates and part of the tibial shafts. The overall morphology of the tibias, the lengths of the growth plates, and periosteal thickness were normal in *Hoxa3* null (D) as compared with WT (C), but a marked reduction in the amount of mineral *(black)* was evident in the shaft of the *Hoxa3* null tibia. Panel (E) shows the skeletal ash weight, and panel (F) shows the ash skeletal ash calcium content, both of which were significant reduced in aparathyroid *Hoxa3* null fetuses as compared with the heterozygous (*Hoxa3$^{+/-}$* or het) littermate values. Scale bars indicate 0.5 cm in ABCD, and 100 μm in EF. As discussed within the text, loss of PTH alone (in *Pth* null fetal mice) also leads to reduced skeletal mineral content. *(Adapted with permission from Kovacs CS, Chafe LL, Fudge NJ, Friel JK, Manley NR. PTH regulates fetal blood calcium and skeletal mineralization independently of PTHrP. Endocrinology 2001;**142(11)**:4983–93; copyright © The Endocrine Society.)*

survival improved significantly.[7] Serum calcium increased, hyperphosphatemia persisted, urine calcium excretion decreased, while skeletal lengths, trabecular bone volumes, and mineral content were all increased.[7] The double-mutants lacked the ability to stimulate calcitriol synthesis, and so the observed improvements were not due to calcitriol.[7] In the second study, the double mutants were treated with exogenous calcitriol. They too demonstrated improved survival, increased serum calcium, lowered serum phosphorus, reduced urine calcium excretion, and improved skeletal lengths, trabecular bone volumes, and mineral content.[8] These effects were not due to PTH, since the double-mutants lacked it. Because identical outcomes occurred when serum calcium of double mutants was increased, regardless of whether it was by treatment with PTH, PTHrP, or calcitriol, these results confirm the importance of normal serum calcium to prevent deaths due to hypocalcemia, support osteoblast function, and improve skeletal mineralization. Calcium is itself a growth factor that stimulates the function of osteoblasts; it is not simply a mineral to be accreted by bone tissue.

44.2.3 Human Data

Human trophoblasts express PTH1R, while several in vitro studies have suggested that PTH can stimulate calcium transport, although less potently than PTH.[1] Whether placental calcium transport is reduced by absence of PTH remains unknown.

Congenital hypoparathyroidism occurs from multiple different gene deletions that lead to the absence of parathyroids (DiGeorge and other 22q11.2 deletion syndromes, ablation of *GCM2*, etc.) and from activating mutations of the calcium sensing receptor.[9] The animal data uniformly indicate that hypoparathyroid babies should have hypocalcemia, hyperphosphatemia, and impaired skeletal mineralization at birth. However, congenital hypoparathyroidism occurs sporadically and is often asymptomatic at birth; consequently, no cord blood data, skeletal radiographs, or bone density measurements have been reported for isolated hypoparathyroidism. A newborn with multiple congenital anomalies, including DiGeorge syndrome with hypoparathyroidism, was noted to have hypocalcemia, hyperphosphatemia, and low PTH upon admission to the neonatal intensive care unit.[10]

Symptomatic hypocalcemia isn't inevitable with congenital absence of parathyroids, as confirmed by a large series of 22q11.2 deletions in which only 60% of affected individuals displayed hypocalcemia at some point.[11] Many presented as neonates, but presentations later in childhood and as teenagers were noted.[11] In a series of 12 cases with confirmed hypocalcemia, only 4 were symptomatic, 10 were diagnosed before 1 month of age, one at 2 months, and another at 12 years of age.[12] Serum phosphorus was not consistently increased at diagnosis. In another series of 10 cases of congenital hypoparathyroidism, the diagnosis was made between 9 days and 13 years of age.[13] The animal studies indicate that hypocalcemia begins in utero with congenital hypoparathyroidism. This appears to result in adaptation to the neurological effects of low calcium, thereby making it less likely to be symptomatic after birth. This is in marked contrast to the symptoms that occur after surgically induced hypoparathyroidism in children or adults.

Hypoparathyroidism may be recognized because of associated congenital anomalies in 22q11.2 deletion syndromes, but if hypoparathyroidism is isolated, it may not be recognized until hypocalcemia provokes neonatal jitteriness, tetany, or seizures. The case series indicate that the presentation is most often in the neonatal period, but it could be delayed into the second decade or later. The animal data suggest that the skeleton will be undermineralized at birth, whereas with time, the skeleton will develop the low turnover and high mineralization state that is characteristic of longstanding hypoparathyroidism.

44.2.4 Clinical Management

Symptomatic hypocalcemia is treated aggressively with parenteral calcium to stop tetany and seizures, and to prevent or interrupt cardiac dysrhythmias.

For chronic management, PTH analogs are the ideal treatment, but their cost is prohibitive, and the need for daily subcutaneous injections is a substantial deterrent. Furthermore, there is a black box warning against the use of PTH in children due to observations of osteosarcoma when used at high doses in growing rats.[14, 15] Other modes of PTH delivery (such as sublingual, buccal, and oral) have been reportedly under investigation,[16] which could prove to be more affordable and acceptable. In the present day, hypoparathyroidism is treated with oral calcium supplementation and either calcitriol or 1α-cholecalciferol D (alfacalcidol) to stimulate intestinal calcium absorption. Hypercalciuria is inevitable in the absence of PTH, followed by eventual development of nephrocalcinosis and renal insufficiency if prolonged and severe. This may be delayed by targeting an ionized calcium or albumin-corrected serum calcium at the lower end of the normal range or just below it (i.e., an ionized calcium of 1.00 mmol/L), and by using a thiazide diuretic to reduce urine calcium excretion.

44.3 PSEUDOHYPOPARATHYROIDISM

44.3.1 Animal Data

A mouse model of pseudohypoparathyroidism has not been studied during fetal or neonatal development, while the homozygous condition is genetically lethal.[1] Affected heterozygotes display normal serum calcium and phosphorus, and have no skeletal abnormalities. They do display renal resistance to PTH upon provocative testing.

44.3.2 Human Data

A few case series have shown that the manifestations of pseudohypoparathyroidism begin later in childhood.[1] Hyperphosphatemia and elevated PTH begin first, followed eventually by hypocalcemia. Pseudohypoparathyroidism may occur in conjunction with the skeletal abnormalities of Albright hereditary osteodystrophy. The documented childhood onset indicates that affected newborns should have normal cord blood calcium and are unlikely to be hypocalcemic as neonates. Hypocalcemia is typically unveiled at puberty when bone mineral accrual ramps up. Therefore, when a family history of pseudohypoparathyroidism is present, monitoring is increased around expected puberty. There are different genetic subtypes of pseudohypoparathyroidism, but that is beyond the scope of this chapter.

Vitamin D deficiency (discussed in Section 44.8) provokes secondary hyperparathyroidism and skeletal resistance to PTH, which can mimic the features of pseudohypoparathyroidism.[17] The clue to vitamin D deficiency-induced PTH resistance is the ability to wean from active forms of vitamin D following replacement of 25-hydroxyvitamin D (25OHD) stores.

44.3.3 Clinical Management

The clinical management of pseudohypoparathyroidism is similar to that of hypoparathyroidism, with use of oral calcium and calcitriol, and possibly the use of a thiazide diuretic to reduce renal calcium excretion.

44.4 PRIMARY HYPERPARATHYROIDISM

Multiple cases of primary hyperparathyroidism diagnosed during the early neonatal period have been described[1]; in retrospect, these likely represent neonatal severe primary hyperparathyroidism due to homozygous or compound heterozygous inactivating mutations of the calcium sensing receptor. This condition is discussed in Section 44.6.

The earliest that primary hyperparathyroidism due to single adenomas or four-gland hyperplasia has been reported is 4 years of age.[18] The younger that the patient, the more likely a genetic predisposition may be present, such as multiple endocrine neoplasia types 1 or 2, or familial primary hyperparathyroidism.

Fetal secondary hyperparathyroidism can result in neonatal hypercalcemia that persists for days or weeks and be mistaken for primary hyperparathyroidism until the hypercalcemia and elevated PTH resolve; this is discussed in Section 44.9.3.

44.5 ABSENCE OF PTHRP

Fetal blood contains high PTH-like bioactivity but low immunoreactive levels of PTH.[1] This is explained by the presence of high circulating concentrations of PTHrP, which mimics many of the biological activities of PTH. PTHrP acts as both a hormone and a paracrine factor during fetal life, and its role has been elucidated by studying the effect of its absence in the *Pthrp* null mouse fetus.

44.5.1 Fetal Animal Data

Loss of PTHrP has diverse effects on fetal development, contributing to early mortality in the first minutes to hours after birth. *Pthrp* null fetuses have a hypoparathyroid-like phenotype characterized by modest hypocalcemia and hyperphosphatemia.[19] PTH is increased threefold, a result of the low serum calcium leading to less activation of the calcium-sensing receptor (CaSR), and release of its inhibition of PTH synthesis and release.[1] PTH raises the blood calcium of *Pthrp* nulls to the maternal level, which is the value normally set by the CaSR.

Pthrp null fetuses have a 25% reduction in placental calcium transport compared with their WT littermates.[19] Placental magnesium and phosphorus have not be assessed, but studies in ovine placentas suggest that loss of PTHrP causes reduced placental magnesium transport but has no effect on phosphorus transport.[1]

PTHrP has a paracrine role to regulate the development of the endochondral skeleton. It is produced by perichondrial cells and proliferating chondrocytes, and it acts on the PTH1R expressed by prehypertrophic chondrocytes, preosteoblasts, and osteoblasts. PTHrP delays the terminal differentiation and hypertrophy of chondrocytes.[1] In the absence of PTHrP, hypertrophy and apoptosis of chondrocytes occur prematurely, followed by initiation of primary bone formation. The result is a short-limbed chondrodysplasia that also features a shortened mandible.[20] Bones that normally mineralize after birth become mineralized in utero, while the cartilaginous portions of ribs turn abnormally into bone. (In contrast, overexpression of PTHrP or PTH1R has the opposite effect of delayed chondrocyte hypertrophy, which leads to a wholly cartilaginous skeleton at birth that undergoes a slow, postnatal conversion into bone.[21])

Although the reduced serum calcium and placental calcium transport might be expected to cause reduced skeletal ash weight and mineral content, this is not the case. The ash weight and mineral content of the *Pthrp* null skeleton has been reported by independent investigators as normal or even modestly increased.[1] This is explained by the early, accelerated, and abnormal mineralization that occurs within the *Pthrp* null. Bones become prematurely mineralized in utero, while normally cartilaginous structures (such as the medial ribs and the sternum) are transformed into bone.[20] The *Pthrp* null skeleton undergoes a more rapid development with faster accretion of mineral in normal and abnormal locations, thereby leading to a seemingly normal or increased mineral content.

PTHrP has nonskeletal actions, including to regulate the development of alveolar type II cells in the lungs and the production of surfactant.[1] The *Pthrp* null fetus displays stiff lungs with reduced alveolar type II cells and surfactant, which are the characteristics that can lead to respiratory distress syndrome in the newborn. The short mandible and protruding tongue may contribute to difficulty suckling and breathing.

44.5.2 Neonatal Animal Data

Most *Pthrp* null pups die within a few minutes of birth. A few have lived for a maximum of 5 days, during which they became progressively smaller than their littermates. The cause of early death may be multifactorial, including hypocalcemia with tetany or cardiac arrhythmias, a rigid rib cage that restricts ventilation, and stiff lungs due to abnormal development of alveolar type II cells and low surfactant.[1] Since the *Pthrp* null fetus starts with a lower serum calcium than normal, the obligatory fall in calcium at birth may lead to a severely low calcium that triggers cardiac and neurological events.

44.5.3 Human Data

Inactivating, recessive mutations in the human PTHrP gene (*PTHLH*) have not yet been identified. Based on the experience with murine fetuses, it is expected that homozygous loss of PTHrP will result in multiple congenital abnormalities and intrauterine death. Surprisingly, an autosomal dominant microdeletion in *PTHLH* has been linked to brachydactyly type E, which displays shortened stature, metacarpals, and metatarsals. These findings have some similarity to the *Pthrp* null fetuses and confirm that PTHrP plays a role in regulating the formation of the endochondral skeleton in humans. However, why the microdeletion has autosomal dominant effects, rather than being recessive, remains unclear. Furthermore, there are in vitro data from cultured human trophoblasts that show PTHrP stimulates calcium uptake, which suggests that in the absence of PTHrP, placental calcium transport will be reduced.[1]

44.5.4 Clinical Management

The expected recessive PTHrP-devoid condition has not yet been identified in humans and is likely to be prenatally lethal, and thus no clinical management can be proposed at present.

44.6 ABSENCE OF THE PTH1R OR BOTH PTH AND PTHRP

PTHrP and PTH are both present in the fetal circulation, have similar actions on the PTH1R, and seemingly overlap in the regulation of fetal bone and mineral metabolism. Loss of PTHrP and PTH, PTHrP and the parathyroids, or PTH1R causes more severe abnormalities than loss of PTH or PTHrP alone.

44.6.1 Fetal Animal Data

Loss of *Pthrp* and the parathyroids, or the PTH1R, results in more marked hypocalcemia than in fetuses lacking PTHrP, PTH, or the parathyroids alone.[1] Taken together, these data confirm that the fetal ionized calcium is determined by the combined actions of both PTHrP and PTH, since loss of the PTH1R led to the same reduction in blood calcium as loss of PTHrP and parathyroids combined.[4] Although *Pthrp/Pth* double mutants have been created, fetal blood calcium has not been measured, and so it is unknown if that level is similar to what is observed in *Pth1r* null fetuses.

Pth1r null fetuses have 11-fold increased plasma PTHrP and 10-fold increased PTH, which is a compensatory response to loss of their common N-terminal receptor.[4, 5] Placental calcium transport is significantly increased in *Pth1r* null fetuses,[19] which may result from the high circulating levels of midmolecular PTHrP being able to act on a mid-molecular receptor (independent of PTH1R) to stimulate placental calcium transport. These results are consistent with studies in fetal lambs and *Pthrp* null fetuses, which showed that mid-molecular PTHrP stimulated placental calcium transport while N-terminal PTHrP and PTH did not.[1]

The skeletal phenotype of fetuses that lack PTHrP and parathyroids, or PTHrP and PTH, combine the *Pthrp* null chondrodysplasia with the undermineralized skeleton of fetuses lacking PTH; they are also globally smaller.[4] *Pth1r* nulls have a more severe phenotype with accelerated endochondral ossification, dysplasia, ossification of the cartilaginous portions of ribs, and small size.[22] Their skeletal mineral content is markedly reduced, despite the elevated rate of placental calcium transport.[4, 19] The very low ionized calcium concentration in these fetuses likely contributes to their reduced skeletal mineral content, in addition to loss of the actions of PTH and PTHrP to stimulate osteoblast activity.

The opposite skeletal phenotype has been created through an activating mutation of the PTH1R, which exaggerates PTHrP's N-terminal actions to delay chondrocyte hypertrophy, and resulted in a largely cartilaginous skeleton at term.[23] This was similar to the effect of overexpression of PTHrP on the developing skeleton.[21]

44.6.2 Fetal Neonatal Data

The *Pth1r* null fetuses, *Pthrp/Pth* double mutants, and *Pthrp*/aparathyroid double mutants all die within minutes after birth. Consequently, there are no neonatal data. The cause of death may be multifactorial, similar to the early mortality of *Pthrp* null mice. In addition, some *Pth1r* null fetuses die at midgestation due to widespread cardiomyocyte apoptosis.

44.6.3 Human Data

The human equivalent of homozygous inactivating mutations of PTH1R is Blomstrand chondrodysplasia, which is characterized by a chondrodysplasia quite similar to what has been found in *Pth1r* null fetal mice.[1] It is embryonically lethal; therefore, there are no cord blood measurements of calcium, phosphorus, and so on. The existence of this condition reaffirms that the *Pthrp* null state is likely also likely to be embryonically lethal in humans.

44.6.4 Clinical Management

Blomstrand chondrodysplasia is an embryonically lethal, autosomal recessive condition. Genetic counseling is available for parents who are known carriers.

44.7 DISORDERS OF THE CASR

Calcium functions like a calciotropic hormone by binding to the CaSR in the parathyroids, C-cells of the thyroid, kidney tubules, osteoblasts, chondrocytes, and placenta. Calcium appears to have direct actions that influence the function of osteoblasts and chondrocytes.

44.7.1 Fetal Animal Data

The high concentration of calcium in the fetal circulation is not set by the CaSR; instead, PTH is suppressed to low levels by increased binding of calcium to the CaSR.[1]

Inactivating mutations of the CaSR have an autosomal dominant effect to cause hypercalcemia and hypocalciuria in the adult, a condition known as *familial hypocalciuric hypercalcemia*. As shown in the murine knockout model, this hypercalcemia begins in utero.[24] But ablation of one ($Casr^{+/-}$) or both alleles ($Casr$ null) alleles results in the same elevation in fetal blood calcium above that of the WT littermates, despite a dose-dependent increase in circulating PTH and calcitriol. The intrauterine environment may constrain $Casr$ null fetuses from achieving the much higher blood calcium level that they reach after birth. PTH mediates the hypercalcemia caused by ablation of $Casr$, because simultaneous ablation of PTH1R results in hypocalcemia regardless of CaSR ablation.[24]

Although inactivating mutations of CaSR cause a dose-dependent decrease in renal calcium clearance,[25] $Casr^{+/-}$ and $Casr$ null fetuses have hypercalciuria or increased amniotic fluid calcium.[24] The opposing fetal phenotype is due in part to the fetal kidneys having very low expression of CaSR until after birth, such that ablating the CaSR will have no effect on the fetal kidneys. Instead, fetal hypercalcemia increases the renal filtered load of calcium, and without modulation by CaSR, this leads to increased renal excretion of calcium into the amniotic fluid.

Bone resorption is increased in $Casr$-null fetuses, and this contributes to reduced ash weight and mineral content.[24, 26] In turn, this likely compromises bone strength at a time when skeletal mineralization and strength are normally increasing rapidly. The underlying structure and cellular morphology of the endochondral skeleton is normal at birth in $Casr$ null mice, apart from the reduced mineral content.[24, 26]

Placental calcium transport is dose-dependently reduced in $Casr^{+/-}$ and $Casr$ null fetuses, accompanied by a dose-dependent decrease in PTHrP.[24] CaSR is normally expressed in the placenta, specifically within trophoblasts and intraplacental yolk sac. Together these data may indicate CaSR senses calcium flow within the placenta, or that it regulates placental expression of PTHrP. Alternatively, the hypercalcemia and elevated PTH in $Casr^{+/-}$ and $Casr$ null fetuses may cause a compensatory downregulation of placental calcium transport.

Activating mutations of CaSR leads to hypoparathyroidism, hypocalcemia, and hypercalciuria. Nuf mice have such an activating mutation of $Casr$, but no fetal data have been reported.[1] The phenotype should be similar to Pth null fetuses, with hypocalcemia, low PTH, increased phosphorus, and reduced skeletal mineralization.

44.7.2 Neonatal Animal Data

$Casr^{+/-}$ neonates accurately model the human condition of FHH by displaying hypercalcemia, hypocalciuria, normal to elevated PTH, and normal life-spans and fertility.[25]

$Casr$ nulls model the human condition of neonatal severe primary hyperparathyroidism from homozygous inactivating mutations of CaSR. They develop marked hypercalcemia, very high PTH, grossly enlarged parathyroids, fluid depletion, and growth failure.[25] They generally die before the normal end of weaning, but surgical or genetic ablation of the parathyroids allows them to survive.[1]

The early neonatal phenotype of Nuf mice has not been reported. By 4 weeks of age they show hypocalcemia, hyperphosphatemia, low PTH, and ectopic calcifications in multiple tissues; they are also prone to sudden death.[1]

44.7.3 Human Data

Cord blood calcium and PTH values have not been reported for fetuses or newborns with heterozygous inactivating mutations of $CASR$, owing to the fact that the mother is often not known to be affected, and serum calcium is not routinely measured. The murine data indicate that hypercalcemia should begin in utero and that the cord blood calcium will be higher than expected. Early developmental onset of hypercalcemia likely explains why children and adults with FHH are adapted to a high-ionized calcium, and develop symptoms of hypocalcemia if their blood calcium is lowered toward the usual adult normal values.

Hypercalcemia is not inevitable in a baby with FHH immediately following birth when the disorder is inherited from the mother. In one published case, the baby had transient hypoparathyroidism and hypocalcemia before later developing hypercalcemia.[27] This is consistent with maternal hypercalcemia suppressing the fetal parathyroids despite the baby having an inactivating mutation in $CASR$.

Neonatal severe primary hyperparathyroidism is due to homozygous or compound heterozygous inactivating mutations of $CASR$, although single heterozygous mutations have been identified that presumably had a dominant-negative effect.[1] Again, there are no cord blood data owing to its sporadic nature, but data from $Casr$ null fetal mice predict that hypercalcemia onsets in utero. Affected neonates can develop severe and life-threatening hypercalcemia, dehydration, failure to thrive, neurological disturbances, nephrocalcinosis, and skeletal demineralization with fractures. The presentation can be delayed as much as a month after birth because the mother will have FHH with hypercalcemia, which can suppress the fetal parathyroids and lead to a slower emergence of hyperparathyroidism after birth.[28] Affected neonates will have very high calcium and PTH, and gross enlargement of the parathyroids.

Activating $CASR$ mutations cause autosomal dominant hypocalcemia with hyperphosphatemia and normal (inappropriately low) PTH.[1] However, hypocalcemia and hypercalciuria are only variably present, and hypocalcemia will not necessarily be symptomatic, as noted in several published cases.[1] The best example of how variable the postnatal presentation can be is shown by a baby that developed hypocalcemic seizures at postnatal day 7.[29] Genetic testing later confirmed that his sister (age 3), mother (age 31), and grandfather (age 63) all shared the activating mutation that caused hypocalcemia, low PTH, hypercalciuria, nephrolithiasis, and nephrocalcinosis. But none of the affected relatives were symptomatic. Another survey of 25 patients with activating $CASR$ mutations found that only two developed hypocalcemia within 30 days after birth.[30] The mean age of confirmed hypocalcemia was 28 years, with only 50% ever being symptomatic.[30]

44.7.4 Clinical Management

FHH requires no intervention apart from confirming that it is not primary hyperparathyroidism. The diagnosis may be confirmed biochemically (documenting hypocalciuria) or through genetic testing. It should be kept in mind that a neonate who presents with hypocalcemia can still prove to have FHH.

Neonatal severe primary hyperparathyroidism is almost invariably fatal unless parathyroidectomy is urgently performed, although some rare cases have appeared to spontaneously resolve into milder hypercalcemia that did not require surgery.[1] Surgery carries substantial risks of mortality when performed in newborns. Bisphosphonates and the calcimimetic drug Cinacalcet have been used to lower the serum calcium temporarily in order to enable the newborn to have surgery at an older age.[31] A three-and-a-half gland parathyroidectomy is typically carried out, with the remnant parathyroid tagged and left in place.

Autosomal dominant hypocalcemia is biochemically indistinguishable from hypoparathyroidism. Genetic testing is needed to confirm the presence of an activating mutation, or a calcilytic drug could conceivably be used to stimulate release of PTH. Since the parathyroids are normal except for being suppressed by an overly sensitive CASR, their function may be normalized by calcilytic medications that are currently under development.[32] In the absence of such medications, the treatment is identical to that of hypoparathyroidism, described previously.

44.8 VITAMIN D DEFICIENCY, GENETIC VITAMIN D RESISTANCE, AND 24-HYDROXYLASE DEFICIENCY

44.8.1 Preamble About Rickets And Osteomalacia

Rickets is often thought to be synonymous with vitamin D deficiency, but this is erroneous. Rickets is defined by the histological presence of an undermineralized growth plate. Its bone tissue corollary, osteomalacia, is characterized by an increase in unmineralized osteoid associated with prolongation of the mineralization lag time. Both rickets and osteomalacia result from inadequate available calcium, phosphorus, or both. Undermineralized growth plates and bone tissue deform easily with weight bearing, and cause clinically apparent widening of the growth plates and deformity of the long bones. In addition to clinical features, rickets and osteomalacia can be diagnosed radiologically. Rickets appears on X-rays as widening of the growth plate with growth plate cupping, fraying, and metaphyseal splaying (Fig. 44.2A). Osteomalacia is characterized by Looser zones, which appear as incomplete cracks in the bone cortex (commonly referred to as *pseudofractures*; Fig. 44.2B). Looser zones occur most often along the medial shafts of long bones, pubic rami, ribs, and scapulae. Any condition that impairs calcium or phosphate delivery to the bone surface can lead to rickets or osteomalacia; vitamin D deficiency is only one of many causes.

44.8.2 Fetal Animal Data: Vitamin D Deficiency and Genetic Vitamin D Resistance

Studies in multiple different animal models have confirmed that vitamin D, calcitriol, and the vitamin D receptor are not required for the fetus to maintain normal serum mineral concentrations. The models have included severely vitamin D deficient rats, 1α-hydroxylase-null pigs, *Vdr* null fetuses, and *Cyp27b1* null fetuses, in which serum calcium, ionized calcium, phosphorus, and PTH were all normal in utero.[1, 33]

Placental calcium transport was normal in severely vitamin D deficient rats,[34] increased in *Vdr* null fetal mice,[35, 36] and normal in *Cyp27b1* null fetuses.[33] Placentas of severely vitamin D deficient rats, and *Vdr* null and *Cyp27b1* null fetal mice, displayed normal expression of calbindinD-$_{9k}$ and Ca^{2+}-ATPase, while PTHrP and TRPV6 were upregulated in *Vdr* null placentas.[1, 33, 35, 36] These findings indicate that placental calcium transport does not require calcitriol. The increased rate of placental calcium transport seen in *Vdr* null fetuses may indicate that calcitriol can act on a receptor other than VDR, such that its high concentrations in the *Vdr* null stimulate placental calcium transport. This would explain why placental calcium transport is not increased in vitamin D deficient and *Cyp27b1* null fetuses, both of which lack calcitriol.[33, 34]

Calcitriol is similarly not required for the formation and mineralization of the endochondral skeleton during fetal development. Severely vitamin D deficient rats, *Vdr* null fetuses, and *Cyp7b1* null fetuses have normal skeletal lengths, morphology, histology, ash weight, and mineral content at term when compared with their normal counterparts (Fig. 44.3).[1, 33] However, maternal *Vdr* null status does influence the fetal phenotype independent of the fetal genotype. WT, *Vdr*$^{+/-}$, and *Vdr* null fetuses born of *Vdr*$^{+/-}$ mothers were indistinguishable from each other, but had a slightly larger size, weight, and skeletal mineral content than their *Vdr*$^{+/-}$ and *Vdr* null counterparts born of *Vdr* null mothers.[35] When adjusted for their smaller size or weight, the ash weight and mineral content of the *Vdr* null mothers' offspring were no different from that of *Vdr*$^{+/-}$ mothers.[35] However, this difference in size was not seen with the offspring of *Cyp27b1* null mothers compared with the offspring of WT mothers.[33] The influence of maternal VDR on fetal size is discussed further in Section 44.12.5.

There are additional studies in the older literature, including some that examined guinea pigs, the pharmacological effects of calcitriol or 1α-calcidiol administered to the mother, or the effects of fetal nephrectomy as a model of calcitriol deficiency. These relevance of these studies and problems with the data are discussed elsewhere.[1]

FIG. 44.2 Radiographic features of rickets versus osteomalacia. In panel (A), an 8-year-old boy with XLH displays the undermineralized and widened growth plates characteristic of rickets *(white arrows)*. In (B), a 10-month-old girl has osteomalacia resulting from feeding challenges. In addition to undermineralized growth plates, she shows a pseudofracture or "Looser zone" in the ulnar diaphysis *(white arrow)*.

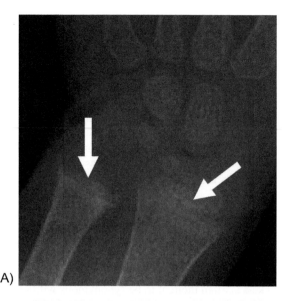

(A)

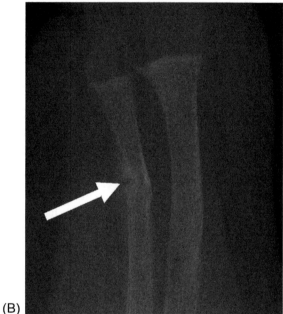

(B)

Overall, vitamin D deficient rat fetuses, *Vdr* null fetal mice, and *Cyp27b1* null fetal mice all show normal serum calcium, phosphorus, PTH, endochondral bone development, and skeletal mineralization at term. Placental calcium transport is normal to increased, with normal to increased expression of some factors involved in calcium transport. Collectively, this is convincing evidence that calcitriol is not required during fetal development to regulate these processes. The placenta provides calcium and phosphorus without requiring calcitriol to regulate the process; the intestines and kidneys, which are regulated by calcitriol postnatally, have an inconsequential role in fetal mineral physiology.

44.8.3 Fetal Animal Data: 24-Hydroxylase Deficiency

A mouse model of 24-hydroxylase deficiency has not been studied during fetal development.[37]

44.8.4 Neonatal Animal Data: Vitamin D Deficiency and Genetic Vitamin D Resistance

Severely vitamin D deficient rats, four different *Vdr* null mouse models, and two different *Cyp27b1* null mouse models have been studied during early postnatal development.[1] All appear normal at birth, as noted previously in the discussion of fetal

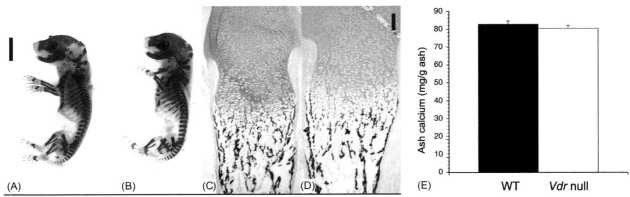

FIG. 44.3 Skeletal morphology and mineral content in *Vdr* null fetal mice. Panels (A) and (B) show images of fetal skeletons (ED 18.5) stained with alizarin *red* (for mineral) and alcian *blue* (for cartilage). Skeletal morphology of the *Vdr* null was consistently normal, as shown by the normal crown-rump length, lengths of long bones, and mineralization pattern of the *Vdr* null (B) and its WT sibling (A). Panels (C) and (D) are von Kossa preparations (counterstained with *methyl green*) of the upper halves of fetal tibias (ED 18.5), which include the growth plates and part of the tibial shafts. The overall morphology of the tibias, the lengths of the growth plates, and periosteal thickness were normal in *Vdr* null (D) as compared with WT (C), and a normal amount of mineral *(black)* was present in the shafts of the tibias. Panel (E) shows the skeletal ash calcium content, which was also no different between WT and *Vdr* null. Scale bars indicate 0.5 cm in AB, and 100 μm in CD. As discussed in the text, vitamin D deficiency and genetic inability to make calcitriol similarly have no effect on fetal skeletal development in animal models. *(Adapted with permission from Kovacs CS, Woodland ML, Fudge NJ, Friel JK. The vitamin D receptor is not required for fetal mineral homeostasis or for the regulation of placental calcium transfer. Am J Physiol Endocrinol Metab 2005;289(1): E133–E44.)*

data. The neonates of each model remain phenotypically and biochemically normal through 3 weeks of lactation. Near the time of weaning, which coincides with the intestines becoming dependent on active, calcitriol-dependent intestinal calcium absorption, all of these models begin to display hypocalcemia, hypophosphatemia, secondary hyperparathyroidism, and histological evidence of rickets.[1] Provision of a calcium, phosphate, and lactose-enriched "rescue diet" increases passive absorption of calcium, and enables each of these models to maintain normal serum chemistries, skeletal morphology, and skeletal mineral content.[1] The rescue diet effectively bypasses the need for vitamin D/calcitriol or its receptor.

These animal data clearly show that it is at the time of weaning, when the intestines are the route of mineral delivery and dependent upon calcitriol, that the effects of vitamin D deficiency or disrupted vitamin D physiology will begin to be seen. Furthermore, since the skeletal manifestations of vitamin D-related rickets are prevented by the rescue diet, the main role of calcitriol with respect to the skeleton must be indirect through upregulation of intestinal mineral delivery to provide the calcium and phosphorus that chondrocytes and osteoblasts require. This has been reaffirmed by the following series of studies. Selective expression of *Vdr* in intestinal cells rescues the skeletal phenotype of *Vdr* null mice, whereas selective ablation of *Vdr* from intestinal cells recreates the rachitic phenotype, and a similar phenotype will also develop simply from dietary calcium restriction.[1]

44.8.5 Neonatal Animal Data: 24-Hydroxylase Deficiency

24-Hydroxylase deficiency causes perinatal lethality in about 50% of affected pups prior to weaning, with severe hypercalcemia (twice the WT value), marked elevation in calcitriol, and undetectable PTH.[37] This is similar to infantile hypercalcemia in humans. The survivors have mild hypercalcemia that is exacerbated by vitamin D supplementation and pregnancy.

44.8.6 Human Data: Vitamin D Deficiency and Genetic Vitamin D Resistance

The potential role of vitamin D/calcitriol during fetal and neonatal development has not only been extensively studied, but it is a subject of ongoing controversy. Consequently, this topic will be dealt with in greater detail. It is not possible to cite all of the relevant primary literature, and so the reader is again referred to a comprehensive review.[1]

In the following discussion, fetal and prenatal are used synonymously to indicate findings that onset during fetal development and would be present before or at the time of birth. Conversely, early postnatal and neonatal indicates the first 30 days after birth, while late postnatal or infant means more than 30 days after birth.

44.8.6.1 Observational Studies and Case Reports

The most rigorous possible assessment for prenatal rickets would compare severely vitamin D deficient to vitamin D replete fetuses, carry out detailed radiological assessment of the skeleton, and determine the ash weight and mineral content of bone. Such a study was done on babies that had died of obstetrical accidents: seven from mothers with clinically diagnosed osteomalacia and vitamin D deficiency, and eight from otherwise healthy mothers.[38] Plain radiographs were obtained of the long bones, while the femurs were reduced to ash and skeletal mineral content was assayed by atomic absorption spectroscopy. One fetus from an osteomalacic mother was born prematurely at 7.5 months, and had the expected finding of an ash weight less than half that of the remaining 14 near-term or term fetuses (more than 80% of the mineral content of the fetal skeleton is accreted during the third trimester).[1] That single fetus's low ash weight gave the investigators the early impression that babies born of osteomalacic mothers had softer bone and lower ash weight compared with normal babies. However, analysis of the raw data displayed in that publication reveals that the calcium content (mean $\pm$ SE) was 374.2 ± 3.0 per thousand in "osteomalacic parent" babies versus 371.8 ± 13.9 per thousand in normal babies, while phosphorus content was respectively 189.0 ± 1.1 versus 189.6 ± 1.6 per thousand.[38] Rickets could not be present because unmineralized osteoid is pathognomonic for the condition, yet skeletal mineral content was normal. The skeletal radiographs revealed no signs of rickets and normal centers of ossification in the long bones.[38] The authors noted "a curious cupping" at the ulnar ends in two babies born to osteomalacic mothers and speculated that it might be evidence of rickets,[38] but that is now recognized to be a normal variant.[39] Overall, the authors concluded "there is no evidence of pre-natal rickets." Oddly, this 1925 report has been cited at times as confirming the existence of prenatal rickets, despite what the data revealed.

Epidemiological surveys have found that hypocalcemia and rickets from vitamin D deficiency are not usually diagnosed until weeks to months after birth, with the highest incidence between 6 and 18 months, even where vitamin D deficiency is endemic.[1, 40] For example, clinical suspicion runs high in India, but in Teotia's series of 165 babies born of women with severe osteomalacia from vitamin D deficiency, no babies had fetal abnormalities, and only 6 had postnatal abnormalities that included hypocalcemia or the later development of rachitic changes.[41] Teotia concluded that congenital rickets is "uncommon and develops only when maternal mineral and vitamin D stores have been completely exhausted."[42]

The clinical data described thus far are in agreement with the animal models, that the fetal skeleton should be normal at birth (because the placenta supplies the needed mineral) with rickets developing postnatally (when the intestines become the route of mineral delivery), and rarely during the early postnatal period. Intestinal calcium absorption is largely passive at birth but becomes calcitriol-dependent as the baby matures, and that is when the presence of vitamin D deficiency is likely to lead to hypocalcemia or the more gradual emergence of an undermineralized, rachitic skeleton. (As an aside, vitamin D-deficiency rickets is not the same as rickets of prematurity, which results from the preterm skeleton having a much higher demand for calcium and phosphorus than what the intestines can absorb from milk or formula at that gestational age. Key risk factors with rickets of prematurity are prolonged use of total parenteral nutrition and low phosphorus intake.)

Despite these assertions, a few isolated reports from the past 100 years (all cited in a comprehensive review[1]) have suggested that physical, radiographic, or histological changes consistent with rickets may rarely be present at birth, so-called congenital rickets.[1] Such cases would suggest that vitamin D deficiency does affect fetal bone and mineral homeostasis; consequently, these cases will now be scrutinized in some detail. In almost all, no measurements of 25OHD were done (or were possible at the time) to confirm vitamin D deficiency as the cause. This is a critical point because, as noted in the preamble to this section, rickets is not synonymous with vitamin D deficiency, but refers instead to lack of mineralization of the growth plate and bone tissue due to deficiency of calcium and/or phosphorus. Vitamin D deficiency and genetic forms of vitamin D resistance cause rickets due to the lack of available calcium and/or phosphorus. On the other hand, there are more than 50 different conditions that can lead to an abnormal radiographic appearance of the fetal growth plate and/or bone that is consistent with rickets.[43] These include fetal hypoparathyroidism (which, unlike in the adult, causes reduced skeletal mineralization), hyperparathyroidism, skeletal dysplasias,[44] metaphyseal chondrodysplasias,[43] hypophosphatasias,[45, 46] types V and VI osteogenesis imperfecta,[47, 48] and scurvy.[49] Some of the purported cases of congenital rickets were clearly not due to vitamin D deficiency, such as many that had normal cord blood calcium, and a half-dozen that hemorrhaged from multiple orifices before dying. The horrific end for those cases is more consistent with scurvy, vitamin K deficiency, or multiple nutritional deficiencies as the cause of the growth plate and bone abnormalities, rather than deficiency of vitamin D somehow causing rickets despite normal cord blood calcium and phosphorus.[1]

In other reports claiming recognition of rickets at birth caused by vitamin D deficiency, the diagnosis was not made until the first or second week after birth, which is consistent with early postnatal rickets.[1] In such cases, the term "neonatal rickets" is more appropriate than "congenital rickets," since the latter term implies that the condition is present at birth. The pathogenesis for early postnatal rickets is quite clear. The neonate normally accretes about 100 mg of calcium per day into the skeleton while simultaneously maintaining normal calcium and phosphorus levels in the circulation.[1] Reduced intestinal absorption of calcium can quickly lead to hypocalcemia, followed by secondary hyperparathyroidism, hypophosphatemia, and progressive undermineralization of the skeleton. This has been documented in one neonate who had unremarkable radiographs at day 2, but radiographic evidence of rickets by day 16.[50]

In additional cases of rickets diagnosed at or soon after birth, the mothers had significant concurrent medical problems such as severe anorexia, malnutrition, malabsorption from celiac disease or pancreatic insufficiency, lactose intolerance, extreme avoidance of calcium and dairy food sources, use of drugs that interfere with vitamin D metabolism, or very low intakes of both calcium and vitamin D.[1] Many of the mothers were in an extreme state with serum calcium at half normal values, globally poor nutrition, carpopedal spasms, positive Chvostek signs, hypotonia, severe osteomalacia, severe back pain, and a waddling gait.[1] The confounding presence of other nutritional deficiencies makes it unlikely that vitamin D deficiency alone can explain these rare cases.

In such cases, it was not isolated vitamin D deficiency but instead multiple nutritional deficiencies that likely contributed to skeletal abnormalities at birth.

Finally, some case reports and series have used the isolated finding of craniotabes (the subjective determination that the skull is softer than normal), distal ulnar cupping, or a widened fontanelle as evidence of vitamin D-deficiency rickets in the newborn. However, public health data from several countries have shown craniotabes to be present in 30%–50% of healthy infants, and to have no correlation with maternal or neonatal 25OHD levels or radiographic evidence of rickets.[1] Distal ulnar cupping is a normal variant that should not be used in isolation to diagnose rickets.[39] A widened anterior fontanelle can be seen with rickets, but it is a nonspecific change shared among more than 25 metabolic, genetic, and skeletal disorders.[51, 52] It is clear that these isolated criteria are not sufficient to diagnose rickets of any etiology. Despite this, large case series have purported to diagnose congenital rickets in 9%–24% of otherwise healthy neonates who have nonspecific findings of distal ulnar cupping,[53, 54] or craniotabes,[55] despite normal values of serum calcium, ionized calcium, phosphorus, and alkaline phosphatase.[1, 53, 54]

Overall, out of 100 years of rare cases suggesting that vitamin D deficiency rickets can be diagnosed prenatally or at the time of birth, most do not satisfy that diagnosis. Instead, many used invalid criteria, substantial nutritional deficiencies were present in the mother that would adversely affect the fetal skeleton, and other disorders were likely the cause of the rachitic skeleton. Furthermore, when vitamin D deficiency was likely the cause, the diagnosis was not made at birth but in the early postnatal period.

If hypocalcemia or rickets from vitamin D deficiency can be present at birth, such are exceptional cases and do not reflect the degree of vitamin D deficiency commonly seen today. Although severe maternal hypocalcemia of any cause can lead to an undermineralized fetal skeleton, this is uncommon in vitamin D deficiency because secondary hyperparathyroidism in the mother minimizes the fall in calcium, thereby maintaining the supply of mineral to the fetus.

Additional cohort studies have examined bone mineral content in newborns stratified by cord blood 25OHD levels. Congdon studied infants born of 45 untreated Asian women, 19 Asian women who received 1000 IU of vitamin D daily during the third trimester, and 12 unsupplemented Caucasian women.[56] Mean cord blood 25OHD levels were 5.9, 15.2, and 33.4 nmol/L, respectively. Serum calcium, phosphorus, alkaline phosphatase, and bone mineral content of the forearm (measured within 5 days of birth) did not differ among groups.[56] Weiler measured bone mineral content of the lumbar spine, femur, and whole body by DXA within 15 days after birth in 50 healthy term infants.[57] Cord blood 25OHD was 73 and 36 nmol/L in sufficient and insufficient Caucasians, 44 nmol/L in Asians, and 27 nmol/L in First Nations infants. Ethnicity contributed to differences in bone mineral content but not the mean 25OHD levels.[57]

Viljakainen used DXA soon after birth and at 14 months in a cohort of 87 children.[58] When divided into two groups, above and below the median cord blood 25OHD, there were no differences in anthropometric parameters or tibial bone mineral density at either time point. Cross-sectional area and mineral content of the tibia were slightly lower at baseline in the cohort below the median 25OHD; the difference in mineral content was gone at 14 months while a difference in cross-sectional area persisted. The investigators acknowledged that there were disparities in sex and size of the newborns above and below the median 25OHD, which may account for some of the differences in baseline readings.

If vitamin D deficiency could cause fetal rickets, then this should be more prominent in inherited forms of vitamin D resistance. This includes the inability to synthesize calcitriol because of 1α-hydroxylase deficiency (pseudovitamin D deficiency rickets or vitamin D dependent rickets type I; VDDR-I), and the lack of functional vitamin D receptors (hereditary vitamin D-resistant rickets; vitamin D dependent rickets type II; VDDR-II). But apart from alopecia in VDDR-II, these babies are phenotypically normal at birth and have normal cord blood calcium levels.[1] In both conditions, hypocalcemia, hypophosphatemia, and rickets will inevitably develop if left untreated. VDDR-I presents within the first 3–12 months after birth; VDDR-II can present in infancy but has more often been diagnosed during the second year or even later.[1] Severe hypocalcemia can lead to infantile or childhood mortality.[1] Bowing of the long bones and metaphyseal widening can occur, with pseudofractures and true fractures being much less common.[1] VDDR-II is often recognizable for total alopecia, which VDDR-I does not cause.

Data from older children with VDDR-II children confirm that, as in the animal model, calcitriol's role to regulate intestinal calcium absorption can be bypassed. Repeated intravenous or intracaval calcium infusions, or high oral dose calcium, will normalize calcium, phosphorus, PTH, alkaline phosphatase; rickets was prevented or healed.[1] Rickets heals more rapidly with parenteral instead of high dose oral calcium; less severely affected patients can be successfully treated with high dose oral calcium alone. For VDDR-I, high-dose parenteral or oral calcium is not needed because physiological doses of calcitriol or 1α-cholecalciferol should normalize intestinal calcium absorption.

It is after weight bearing begins that untreated vitamin D deficiency, VDDR-I, or VDDR-II will lead to progressive deformities of the long bones (enlargement of the wrist, bowing of the distal radius and ulna, lateral bowing of the femur and tibia), abnormal growth plates, and short stature.[1] The unmineralized osteoid in these conditions makes the bone soft, such that it bends in response to weight bearing. Fractures of the long bones do not occur any more commonly in untreated vitamin D deficiency compared with normal children.[59]

In summary, case series data from vitamin D deficiency, VDDR-I, and VDDR-II are consistent with the animal models. Hypocalcemia and rickets are not likely to be present at birth in these conditions, but instead will develop in the early to late postnatal period with a peak incidence between 6 and 18 months when left untreated. Furthermore, calcitriol's role is not a direct one to stimulate skeletal development, but instead an indirect one through stimulating the intestinal absorption of calcium. This role can be completely bypassed through the use of a high-dose calcium diet or parenteral calcium treatment.

44.8.6.2 Randomized Interventional Studies

Large randomized interventional studies have the potential to provide the highest level and quality of clinical evidence. There have been many randomized studies of vitamin D supplementation during pregnancy that have examined fetal and neonatal outcomes. Unfortunately, many of them were very small, randomization methods and not clearly specified, and the risk of bias appears high. Still others measured only cord blood 25OHD and anthropometrics in the newborn, which are inadequate to determine if vitamin D supplementation had any beneficial impact on fetal mineral homeostasis or skeletal development and mineralization. Ideally, a definitive trial would compare babies of mothers with severe vitamin D deficiency (mean 25OHD <20 nmol/L) to those who are indisputably vitamin D replete (mean 25OHD >50 or perhaps >75 nmol/L).[60] However, most studies did not compare those extremes, or used too modest a dose of vitamin D to create a substantial difference between groups. It is not possible to review and cite all studies in this section; instead, the reader is referred to two recent comprehensive reviews[1, 61] and a metaanalysis.[62] This section will focus on the few studies that included severely vitamin D deficient mothers and babies, in addition to others that were more recent or were well publicized.

One of the earliest randomized trials is still perhaps the most definitive because it compared severe vitamin D deficiency with an unarguably replete state.[63] Brooke studied 126 Asian women living in England, 59 who were treated with 1000 IU of vitamin D daily versus 67 controls. The dose administered may have been closer to 10,000 IU daily because maternal 25OHD rose from 20 nmol/L at baseline to 168 nmol/L at term in the treated group. Mean cord blood 25OHD was 10 nmol/L in control babies and 138 nmol/L in babies born of vitamin D-supplemented mothers; this extreme difference was ideal to determine if correction of vitamin D deficiency conferred any benefit on fetal mineral or bone metabolism. There were no differences at birth in cord blood calcium and phosphorus, in radiological assessment for evidence of rickets, or in standard anthropometrics.[63] Alkaline phosphatase was higher in control babies, but this was due to the placental fraction and not the bone-specific fraction. Anterior fontanelle diameter was slightly smaller in babies born of vitamin D-supplemented mothers.

Most interestingly, control infants had lower blood calcium at day 3 and 6 after birth, with five developing symptomatic hypocalcemia (none in offspring of the vitamin D-supplemented mothers).[63] These results corroborate the previously discussed animal studies, in which serum calcium and phosphorus are normal at birth, but decline postnatally with severe vitamin D deficiency or genetic absence of calcitriol or VDR.

Delvin randomized 40 women to receive 1000 IU vitamin D$_3$ daily or placebo starting at 6 months of pregnancy. Cord blood 25OHD increased from 17.5 to 45 nmol/L, but there were no differences between groups in skeletal parameters, cord blood calcium, phosphorus, and PTH.[64] Similar to Brooke's study, babies born of vitamin D-supplemented mothers had significantly higher total and ionized calcium at 5 days of age.[64]

Roth studied 160 women who were randomized to 35,000 IU per week of vitamin D$_3$ or placebo beginning at 26–29 weeks until delivery.[65] Cord blood 25OHD was 103 nmol/L in the offspring of supplemented mothers versus 30 nmol/L in babies of placebo-treated mothers. There was no effect on anthropometric parameters at birth, including length, weight, head circumference, and femur length.[66] In a follow-up report, there was also no effect on albumin-corrected cord blood calcium, but the fall in serum calcium by 3 days after birth was blunted in babies from the vitamin D group.[67]

Hashemipour randomized 160 women to receive 50,000 IU vitamin D per week or 400 IU daily beginning at 26–28 weeks for 8 weeks total.[68] Cord blood 25OHD was 69 nmol/L in babies of supplemented mothers versus 27 nmol/L in babies of placebo-treated mothers. Cord blood calcium (not corrected for albumin) was significantly increased by vitamin D supplementation (2.48 vs 2.28 mmol/L), but there was no difference in the incidence of hypocalcemia. There were also small but statistically significant increases in newborn weight, length, and head circumference of babies born of vitamin D-treated mothers.

Grant randomized 260 women to placebo, 1000 IU vitamin D daily, or 2000 IU vitamin D daily, which resulted in cord blood 25OHD values of 33, 60, and 65 nmol/L, respectively.[69] There was no difference in serum calcium among the three groups at 2.58, 2.62, and 2.60 mmol/L, respectively.[69]

Hollis and Wagner completed two larger trials. The first had 350 women complete the study after randomization at 12–16 weeks to receive 400, 2000, or 4000 IU of vitamin D₃ per day.[70] The primary outcome was a combination of the 25OHD concentrations and bone mineral density of both mother and infant; however, the infant BMD values have not been published. Achieved cord blood 25OHD was 46, 57, and 66 nmol/L, respectively. The second study had 160 women randomized to receive 2000 or 4000 IU of vitamin D₃ per day starting at 12–16 weeks of gestation.[71] Achieved cord blood 25OHD was 55 and 68 nmol/L, respectively. The cord blood calcium values for both studies, and the bone density results for the first study, have not been published, but have been described by the authors in public presentations as showing no significant differences between groups.[72] In the first study, 4000 IU of vitamin D had no effect on gestational age at delivery, birth weight, mode of delivery, need for level II or III neonatal care, cord blood calcium, preterm birth, preterm labor, preeclampsia, infection, or BMD.[70, 72, 73] Post hoc analyses of combined data from both studies have suggested that some combinations of nonskeletal obstetric or neonatal outcomes appear improved by high 25OHD values, but only after arbitrary exclusion of certain races from the analyses and without adjustments for multiple comparisons.[70, 72–74]

MAVIDOS is a well-publicized UK-based study that involved 900 women who received either 1000 IU of vitamin D or placebo beginning at 14 weeks of pregnancy.[75] Baseline 25OHD was close to sufficient at 45 nmol/L (18 ng/mL), did not change in placebo-treated women, and rose to 68 nmol/L (27 ng/mL) in vitamin D-supplemented women. Cord blood 25OHD, calcium, phosphorus, and PTH have not been reported. The study proved negative in both its primary (neonatal bone area, bone mineral content, and bone mineral density within the first 14 days after birth) and secondary outcomes (anthropometric and body composition parameters within 48 h of birth). A post hoc associational analysis, which was not prespecified in the clinical trial registrations (ISRCTN 82927713 and EUDRACT 2007-001716-23), regrouped the neonates by season of birth. A possible benefit of vitamin D supplementation was seen in BMC and BMD in winter-born babies, but a similar magnitude of negative effect of vitamin D supplementation was seen in autumn-born babies. The apparent differences in these subgroup analyses may be chance findings, especially given that the negative trends in the autumn-born babies do not make obvious physiological sense.[76] But a possible benefit in winter-born babies could have developed during the early postnatal period, rather than during fetal development. As noted earlier, the neonatal skeleton accrues about 100 mg of calcium daily.[1] In this study, the DXA measurements were obtained up to 14 days after birth.[75] This is sufficient time for vitamin D sufficiency to have improved intestinal calcium absorption and, thereby, skeletal mineral accrual in autumn-born neonates whose mothers received vitamin D supplementation.

Vaziri treated 127 women with either 2000 IU of vitamin D or placebo. Maternal 25OHD was 45 nmol/L in the treated group versus 30 nmol/L in the placebo group; cord blood 25OHD was not measured. There was no effect on anthropometric parameters at birth, or whole body BMC and BMD measured within 5 weeks after birth.[77]

Sahoo randomized pregnant women to receive 60,000 IU monthly, 60,000 IU every 2 months, or 400 IU daily.[78] Mean cord blood 25OHD was 47.8, 31.0, and 17.8 in the respective groups. Anthropometric parameters did not differ among the groups at birth. Whole body BMC and BMD were measured in 52 infants at 12–18 months, and were unexpectedly lower in the groups with higher 25OHD. However, the small group sizes and disparities in the postnatal ages at which the measurements were done (2 months older in the lowest-dose group) may have contributed to the apparent differences in BMC and BMD.

Most recently, Roth randomized 1298 women in Bangladesh to one of five interventions beginning at 17–24 weeks of gestation: placebo, three arms receiving weekly dosing of vitamin D₃ (4200 IU, 16,800 IU, and 28,000 IU), and one arm in which 28,000 IU vitamin D₃ per week was continued until 26 weeks postpartum.[79] The study compared clear-cut vitamin D deficiency with sufficiency, as confirmed by maternal 25OHD values at term that ranged from 23.8 ± 13.9 nmol/L in the placebo group to 113.6 ± 25.7 nmol/L in the high dose group.[79] The study was powered to reveal differences in infant length at birth, but none were seen—nor did vitamin D supplementation alter any other clinical or anthropometric outcome in the mothers or their babies.[79] This study, like the earlier one of Brooke but with 10 times the number of participants, provides convincing evidence that vitamin D or calcitriol are not required during fetal development for regulation of mineral homeostasis or skeletal development.

Overall these trials, and others cited in reviews[1, 61] and a metaanalysis,[62] have not shown compelling evidence that prenatal vitamin D supplementation achieves any benefit related to calcium and bone metabolism in the babies prior to birth. On the other hand, some of the studies have confirmed that vitamin D supplementation does reduce the risk of hypocalcemia developing in the infants 48 h or more after birth, where the control group had a mean 25OHD below 20 nmol/L. Most of the studies have compared neonates with cord blood 25OHD levels that were well above that value and found no differences between groups. This is consistent with no added benefit from vitamin D supplementation if the 25OHD level already supports a normal rate of intestinal calcium absorption.

The focus in this chapter is on calcium and bone physiology. Vitamin D supplementation has been theorized to confer nonskeletal benefits to the fetus or neonate, but a recent metaanalysis found that the data from these trials are inconsistent and not compelling.[62]

44.8.6.3 Associational Studies

Associational studies can involve many more subjects than are seen in clinical trials, and therefore have more power to detect associations between measurements of vitamin D sufficiency and an outcome of interest. Several have drawn attention for conclusions that higher intakes of vitamin D may be needed during pregnancy to optimize bone health in the fetus, infant, and child. What these studies have examined are associations between single measurements of maternal 25OHD during pregnancy (less commonly, cord blood 25OHD or estimates of maternal vitamin D intake) and several skeletal outcomes in the offspring. In agreement with the previously described observational studies and randomized trials, these studies have generally found no significant associations of maternal vitamin D status with newborn weight, skeletal lengths, or bone mineral density.[1]

Morley concluded that maternal 25OHD below 28 nmol/L predicted a slightly shorter knee-heel length in newborns.[80] However, the association was not statistically significant after correcting for gestational age.

A pair of studies by Mahon and Viljakainen found seemingly opposing results in which increased metaphyseal area of the offspring femur or tibia was associated with lower[81] or higher[82] maternal 25OHD. Mahon considered greater cross-sectional area of the femoral metaphysis in 242 babies to be evidence of prenatal rickets,[81] while Viljakainen considered greater cross-sectional area of the tibial metaphysis in 125 babies to indicate stronger bones.[82] Ioannou, together with Mahon and colleagues, adapted their ultrasound technique to calculate femoral volumes in 357 mother-baby pairs, and found that maternal 25OHD below 75 nmol/L was associated with slightly smaller femur length, width, and volume, which is in the opposite direction from Mahon's original analysis.[83] Although maternal 25OHD predicted fetal femoral volume in a univariate analysis, there was no association after adjustments for maternal height and skinfold thickness.[84] These studies by Mahon, Viljakainen, and Ioannou have provided seemingly contradictory results. This may mean that there is no causal link between maternal 25OHD during pregnancy and the areas or volumes of long bones in the fetus or newborn.

Javaid examined 198 mother-child pairs and reported no significant associations between maternal 25OHD during pregnancy and birth weight, length, placental weight, abdominal circumference, head circumference, or cord blood calcium.[85] At 9 months of age, there were still no associations between maternal 25OHD during pregnancy and infant skeletal and anthropometric parameters. But at *9 years of age*, there was slightly but significantly lower whole body BMC by DXA in children whose mothers had a 25OHD level below 27.5 nmol/L during pregnancy as compared with children of women whose 25OHD had been ≥50 nmol/L (1.04 ± 0.16 vs 1.16 ± 0.17 kg, $P < .002$).[85] There was no difference when the values were adjusted to estimate volumetric BMD or bone mineral apparent density.[85] These data have been touted to prove that fetal exposure to vitamin D programs the bone mass that will be reached later in childhood.[86] However, Lawlor analyzed 20 times the number of mother-child pairs (3960 vs 198), and found no association between maternal 25OHD during pregnancy and offspring bone mass at age 9 years, as assessed by DXA.[87] Lawlor had eight times the number of women with 25OHD below 27.5 nmol/L (220 vs 28 mothers); therefore, the study had greater power to detect any association of low maternal 25OHD with childhood bone mass.[87] More recently, Garcia examined 5294 mother-child pairs and found the opposite results to Javaid's original report, in that lower maternal and cord blood 25OHD were associated with *increased* BMC at 6 years of age.[88] This association disappeared after adjusting for childhood 25OHD, and the authors concluded that childhood 25OHD level was more relevant for childhood bone outcomes than the fetal 25OHD level.

Considering the studies by Javaid, Lawlor, and Garcia together, it seems likely that there is no real causative association between 25OHD measures during pregnancy (or at birth) and childhood bone mass. Instead, the 25OHD level and general nutrition during childhood are more likely to be significant factors in determining childhood bone mass.

All of the aforementioned associational studies are confounded by factors that will cause a low maternal 25OHD. These include maternal obesity, lower socioeconomic status, poorer nutrition, and lack of exercise, prenatal care, vitamin supplementation, and so on. In this context, a lower 25OHD may simply predict a less healthy pregnant woman, rather than revealing any direct effects that maternal 25OHD might have on fetal bone health. Furthermore, if maternal 25OHD is low during pregnancy, it may remain low in both mother and child because of shared factors that may not change over years (lower socioeconomic status, poorer nutrition, obesity, etc.), thereby influencing childhood growth and bone mass without implicating an effect of 25OHD exposure prior to birth.

The larger sample sizes of association studies, as compared with clinical trials, provide power to detecting real differences that the trials cannot detect. But associational studies may also be reporting "noise" caused by residual confounding, which in turn could explain why results from one study to the next appear contradictory. Associational studies cannot prove causation, but instead may generate hypotheses that warrant testing through careful clinical trials.

44.8.6.4 Overall Conclusions From Observational, Clinical Trial, and Associational Studies

The bulk of available data are consistent with the animal data, in which vitamin D or calcitriol are not required to regulate fetal calcium homeostasis or skeletal development and mineralization. Instead, calcitriol becomes important after birth, when the intestines become the route of mineral delivery and their efficiency at absorbing calcium is increased by calcitriol. Several comprehensive reviews and metaanalyses have concluded that the available data are insufficient to conclude that there are any skeletal or nonskeletal benefits achieved by higher levels of vitamin D sufficiency during pregnancy and, thereby, in the fetus.[60, 62, 89, 90]

The preceding is not meant to infer that vitamin D deficiency does not require treatment during pregnancy. Instead, the available data should reassure that if a woman is not recognized to have severe vitamin D deficiency, VDDR-I, or VDDR-II, and the condition remains untreated during pregnancy, the fetus will likely have normal calcium and bone metabolism. It is after birth that the neonate can be adversely impacted by vitamin D deficiency or inheritance of VDDR-I or VDDR-II. Nevertheless, vitamin D sufficiency should be maintained during pregnancy whenever possible, since calcitriol become important soon after birth to regulate intestinal mineral delivery.

44.8.7 Human Data: 24-Hydroxylase Deficiency

It is unknown whether 24-hydroxylase deficiency alters fetal mineral metabolism because no cord blood data are available from these sporadic cases. Instead, 24-hydroxylase deficiency due to mutations in *CYP24A1* is now recognized as a cause of idiopathic infantile hypercalcemia. Affected neonates have hypercalcemia, suppressed PTH, elevated calcitriol, reduced 24-hydroxylase activity detected in fibroblasts, and reduced 24-hydroxylated metabolites in the circulation.[91] Homozygous or compound heterozygous inactivating mutations in *CYP24A1* can present with severe hypercalcemia in infancy, whereas some have been asymptomatic, detected as older children or adults with milder hypercalcemia, hypercalciuria, nephrocalcinosis, and nephrolithiasis. The heterozygous state causes hypercalcemia in some patients as well.

44.8.8 Clinical Management

44.8.8.1 Vitamin D Deficiency

The Institute of Medicine recommends that neonates and infants receive an intake of 400 IU of vitamin D daily, which has been shown to raise the 25OHD level above 50 nmol/L in most normal infants in the first year of life.[60] If a neonate is recognized to have asymptomatic vitamin D deficiency, this dose may be all that is needed to quickly achieve vitamin D sufficiency. In a preterm infant, the use of calcitriol may be needed to simulate intestinal calcium absorption. Doses higher than 400 IU/day are given to rescue infants from severe symptomatic vitamin D deficiency (i.e., hypocalcemia seizures) and rickets; intravenous calcium infusions and calcitriol may be needed in severe symptomatic vitamin D deficiency associated with neurological or cardiac instability, such as infants and toddlers with seizures.[92] Furthermore, calcium intake must be assessed and optimized, since deficient calcium intake is often present with vitamin D deficiency.[92]

44.8.8.2 VDDR-I and II

VDDR-I results in the inability to make calcitriol. As soon as it is recognized, then treatment with calcitriol or 1α-cholecalciferol should be instituted in combination with optimization of oral calcium intake. In contrast, VDDR-II is characterized by lack of functional VDRs. In some patients, the VDRs are subfunctional, and consequently high-dose calcitriol (or high-dose vitamin D) may be effective at normalizing serum calcium. But in most subjects, high-dose calcitriol is ineffective, and instead the oral intake of calcium must be increased significantly to maximize passive intestinal absorption of calcium. Periodic parenteral administration of calcium may be required, especially during times of rapid growth, or if high dose oral calcium is not tolerated.

44.8.8.3   24-Hydroxylase Deficiency

Infants presenting with hypercalcemia should be treated with adequate hydrations and a low-calcium and vitamin D-restricted diet. The use of vitamin D supplements should be avoided. If the hypercalcemia is refractory to these measures, additional options to consider include blocking bone resorption (intravenous bisphosphonate), suppressing intestinal calcium absorption (glucocorticoids), or reducing calcitriol synthesis (ketoconazole or fluconazole).

44.9   CALCITONIN DEFICIENCY

The gene *CALCA* encodes both calcitonin and calcitonin gene-related peptide-α, while *CALCR* encodes the calcitonin receptor. Calcitonin is expressed in the endometrium during implantation, and blocking its expression results in reduced implantations of early embryos.[1] The *Calcr* or *Ctr* null condition in mice is embryonically lethal at midgestation,[93, 94] whereas *Calca* or *Ctcgrp* null mice are born in expected Mendelian ratios and are fully viable. Pregnancies in *Ctcgrp* null mice result in a small but significant reduction in the numbers of viable pups.[95] Considering all of these data, it appears that calcitonin plays a critical role during implantation and until midgestation, as seen by the embryonic demise of *Ctr* nulls. Maternal calcitonin may enable *Ctcgrp* null embryos to implant and develop until placentation, whereas the lack of receptor in *Ctr* nulls would prevent rescue by maternal calcitonin.

44.9.1   Fetal Animal Data

Loss of calcitonin from thyroidectomy or ablation of the gene has had no effect on fetal serum calcium, phosphorus, or PTH.[1, 95] However, serum magnesium was significantly reduced in *Ctgrp* null fetuses. Placental transport of calcium was unaltered in *Ctcgrp* nulls.[95] Endochondral bone development is normal in *Ctcgrp* null fetuses, as was the ash weight and mineral content, with the exception of a small decrease in skeletal magnesium content.[95] Collectively the findings suggest that calcitonin and CGRP-α play some role in regulating serum magnesium and skeletal magnesium accretion, but otherwise these hormones are not required for fetal mineral and bone homeostasis.

44.9.2   Neonatal Animal Data

No disturbances in mineral metabolism have been reported in *Ctcgrp* null neonates.

44.9.3   Human Data

A *CALCA* or *CALCR* null state has not been described in humans. Therefore it is unknown whether these conditions are embryonic lethal, or not recognized because there is obvious phenotype.

44.10   FGF23: DEFICIENCY OR EXCESS

FGF23 plays a key role in regulating phosphorus metabolism in postnatal mice and humans. It complexes with its coreceptor Klotho and the FGF23 receptor (specifically FGFR1c), and downregulates expression of sodium-phosphate cotransporters within the proximal renal tubules to promote renal phosphorus excretion.[96] FGF23 also inhibits the renal 1α-hydroxylase (CYP27B1), increases expression of 24-hydroxylase (CYP24A1), and may inhibit PTH.[96] FGF23's principal actions serve to lower serum phosphorus.

Genetic disorders leading to loss of FGF23 or Klotho cause impaired renal phosphorus excretion, hyperphosphatemia, increased calcitriol, increased intestinal phosphorus absorption, skeletal abnormalities, extraskeletal calcifications, and early mortality. In contrast, genetic disorders leading to inappropriately high levels of FGF23, such as from X-linked hypophosphatemic rickets (XLH), cause hyperphosphaturia, hypophosphatemia, low calcitriol, reduced intestinal phosphorus absorption, and rickets and/or osteomalacia.

44.10.1   Fetal Animal Data

Fgf23 null and *Klotho* null fetuses have normal serum phosphorus and calcium, amniotic fluid phosphorus and calcium, calcitriol, and PTH.[97, 98] *Phex* or *Hyp* null male fetuses, which have 8–1000-fold increased circulating FGF23, have normal serum phosphorus and calcium, amniotic fluid phosphorus and calcium, and PTH.[97, 99] Serum calcitriol was reduced 50% in *Phex* null male fetuses.[97, 99]

Although fetal kidneys abundantly express the downstream targets of FGF23, the only abnormality in *Fgf23* null and *Klotho* fetal kidneys was downregulation of *Cyp24a1* expression.[97, 98] Conversely *Phex* null male fetal kidneys displayed significantly increased expression of *Cyp24a1*.[97, 99]

Placental transport of phosphorus was also normal in all three models, as was endochondral bone development, ash weight, and skeletal content of phosphorus and calcium.[97, 98]

These results show that loss of FGF23, loss of Klotho, or excess FGF23 each fail to alter fetal phosphorus homeostasis or skeletal development. The only abnormalities seen were that excess FGF23 led to a reduced serum calcitriol with normal phosphorus parameters, while renal Cyp24a1 expression was altered by excess or deficiency of FGF23 action. These modest changes contrast markedly with the postnatal phenotypes caused by these same disorders.

44.10.2 Neonatal Animal Data

Fgf23 nulls and *Klotho* nulls are normal at birth, but develop hyperphosphatemia, increased renal expression of phosphate transporters, and reduced renal phosphorus excretion between 5 and 7 days after birth.[98] They are smaller than their littermates by 2 weeks of age.[100] By 3 weeks, progressive limb deformities and undermineralization of the skeleton have developed, but whole body mineral content is increased because of excessive mineralization of soft tissues, including the heart, lungs, and kidneys.[100–103] The mice begin dying by 5 weeks, and mortality is 100% by 10–12 weeks.[100–103]

In contrast, high levels of FGF23 in *Phex* null males cause abnormal phosphorus metabolism within 12 h after birth, with the onset of hypophosphatemia, reduced renal expression of phosphate transporters, and increased renal phosphorus excretion.[98] By 72 h after birth, the tibias are slightly shortened, with histomorphometric analysis showing fewer osteoblasts and osteoclasts.[104]

The neonatal findings reveal that absence or excess FGF23 exerts substantial effects in the neonate, in striking contrast to a lack of effect of these conditions in the fetus.

44.10.3 Human Data

Familial hyperphosphatemic tumor calcinosis is caused by genetic loss of FGF23 action. It typically presents during the first two decades with calcific tumor masses, hyperphosphatemia, elevated calcitriol, and normal or elevated serum calcium.[1] The masses typically occur around large joints such as elbows, hips, and knees, and can be exacerbated by trauma. The earliest documented presentation is 18 days after birth with a calcific mass and hyperphosphatemia.[105, 106] Tumor calcinosis may be caused missense mutations in *FGF23*, inactivating mutations in *GALNT3*, and inactivating mutations in *KLOTHO* (Fig. 44.4).

Excessive FGF23 action can be caused by such hereditary disorders as XLH, autosomal dominant hypophosphatemic rickets, autosomal recessive hypophosphatemic rickets, and McCune-Albright syndrome with fibrous dysplasia of bone.[107] These conditions are characterized by hypophosphatemia, inappropriately normal to high FGF23, inappropriately normal to low calcitriol, normal to low PTH, normal calcium, myopathy, and rickets (in children) or osteomalacia (in children or adults).

XLH is the best characterized disorder of excess FGF23 action. It most often presents at 2 or 3 years of age with bowed limb or growth failure, or at later ages with short stature. However, it has been diagnosed during the first year when family history and early onset of hypophosphatemia led to clinical suspicion of its presence. In four newborns that were examined carefully because of affected parents, serum phosphorus was low between 2 and 6 weeks of age, tubular reabsorption of phosphorus became low between 9 days and 6 months of age, but rachitic changes were not seen on radiographs until 3–6 months of age.[108]

The most dramatic clinical example of FGF23 overproduction in humans is a condition called *tumor-induced osteomalacia (TIO)*. It is typically produced by otherwise benign mucinous tumors that may be very difficult to locate, and leads to acquired renal phosphate wasting, hypophosphatemia, osteomalacia, and profound myopathy.[109]

44.10.4 Clinical Management

Hereditary hyperphosphatemic tumor calcinosis does not require any management until the serum phosphorus begins to rise weeks to months postnatally. Phosphate binders and dietary phosphorus restriction are potential options, as well as avoidance of vitamin D supplementation. Acetazolamide (ACTZ) can also be used to promote renal phosphorus excretion; in addition, the mild acidosis resulting from ACTZ reduces calcium-phosphate precipitation, and can lead to a reduction in tumor burden when administered in combination with a phosphate binder such as sevelamer carbonate.[110]

FIG. 44.4 Radiographic features of familial tumoral calcinosis. A 13-year-old boy with a homozygous loss of function in the *GALNT3* gene displays tumoral calcinosis of the left elbow.

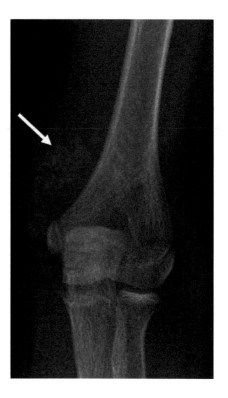

Topical thiosulfate has recently been shown to have benefit on calcinotic tumors.[111] Calcific masses may need to be excised when they become troublesome; however, the trauma caused by surgery can perpetuate the calcinotic tumors and, overall, surgery is to be avoided if possible.

XLH and other disorders related to excess FGF23 action have typically been managed with increased oral phosphorus and calcitriol, which has some benefit to raise serum phosphorus, improve bone mineralization, and reduce myopathy. However, its use provokes secondary hyperparathyroidism. Nephrocalcinosis is a common side effect of combined oral phosphorus and calcitriol therapy, and tertiary hyperparathyroidism has been reported, necessitating 3.5 gland parathyroidectomy. A new treatment strategy is burosumab, an antiFGF23 antibody, which has shown benefit in restoring phosphorus homeostasis to near-normal in adults[112]; similar trials are presently underway in children.[113]

When the tumor causing TIO can be localized, it is preferentially managed with surgical removal; burosumab is an option for unresectable or nonlocalizable tumors.

44.11 SEX STEROID DEFICIENCY

44.11.1 Animal Data

Mice lacking estrogen receptor alpha or beta, or the aromatase, have not been studied during fetal development. At birth, they have normal skeletal lengths and morphology, and do not develop altered skeletal metabolism until several weeks later.[1] It is likely that mineral metabolism is undisturbed until after weaning, but this has not been studied either.

Estradiol acts on osteoblasts to downregulate the expression of receptor activator of nuclear factor kappa-B ligand (RANKL) and upregulate expression of its decoy receptor osteoprotegerin (OPG). The RANKL-OPG-RANK system regulates the formation, recruitment, and function of osteoclasts within the adult. However, this system may be relatively unimportant for development of the fetal skeleton and regulation of mineral homeostasis, and in turn explains why loss of the estrogen receptor causes no obvious fetal development. Deletion of RANKL, RANK, and OPG result in unremarkable pups at birth that develop the expected phenotypes over days to weeks after birth.[1]

44.11.2 Human Data

There are no fetal data and only scant data from early childhood. A man with an inactivating mutation of the estrogen receptor presented with severe osteoporosis. His pediatric record showed normal birth weight, length, and early development.[114]

44.12 FETAL AND NEONATAL RESPONSES TO MATERNAL MINERAL DISTURBANCES

44.12.1 Primary Hyperparathyroidism in the Mother

44.12.1.1 Animal data

Acute infusions of calcium into the mother will increase fetal serum calcium and suppress PTH, consistent with suppression of the fetal parathyroids.[1] Furthermore, maternal hypercalcemia from an inactivating mutation in CaSR causes suppression of PTH in normal fetuses.[24]

44.12.1.2 Human Data

Consistent with the animal studies, maternal hypercalcemia is expected to increase the flow of calcium across the placenta, raise the fetal blood calcium, and suppress the fetal parathyroids. The consequences of fetal hypoparathyroidism have included miscarriage, stillbirth, and neonatal hypocalcemia with tetany, but these outcomes appear less likely to occur with milder maternal hypercalcemia that is commonly seen today. However, neonatal hypocalcemia and tetany have occurred with seemingly mild primary hyperparathyroidism.[115] Furthermore, a modern survey reported fetal death during the second or third trimester in 30 of 62 medically managed cases, which was a 3.5-fold increase in fetal mortality as compared with surgically treated cases.[116]

The suppression of fetal parathyroids leads to delayed upregulation of parathyroid function in the neonate, which in turn can provoke hypocalcemia and tetany. The condition is quite serious. Among case series, up to 50% of neonates had tetany or other complications of maternal hypercalcemia, with 25%–30% mortality.[117–120] Hypoparathyroidism can be delayed in onset, typically resolves after several weeks, but can be permanent. The variability of the condition is exemplified by a twin pregnancy complicated by maternal hypercalcemia: one neonate was normocalcemic while the other had hypocalcemic seizures.[121]

44.12.1.3 Clinical Management

Whenever a woman has been hypercalcemic during pregnancy, increased monitoring of the newborn is required to detect biochemical and clinical evidence of hypocalcemia. The hypocalcemia typically onsets within 48 h, but delayed presentations have occurred. Calcium infusions or oral calcium are used to support the blood calcium until such time as the neonatal parathyroids are able to regulate the blood calcium.

44.12.2 Familial Hypocalciuric Hypercalcemia in the Mother

44.12.2.1 Animal Data

As noted previously, in the mouse model of FHH, maternal hypercalcemia leads to reduced fetal PTH, indicating suppression of the fetal parathyroids.[24]

44.12.2.2 Human Data

Although FHH is generally considered benign and asymptomatic, the often milder hypercalcemia that occurs in this condition has been sufficient during pregnancy to suppress the fetal parathyroids, and leads to neonatal hypocalcemia and tetany.[1] Even a heterozygous neonate—destined to be hypercalcemic because of the inherited mutation—has presented with hypocalcemia and tetany.[27]

44.12.2.3 Clinical Management

Expectant observation of newborns from women with FHH should be carried out similar to that of women who had primary hyperparathyroidism during pregnancy.

44.12.3 Hypoparathyroidism and Activating Mutations of the Calcium-Sensing Receptor in the Mother

44.12.3.1 Animal Data

Maternal hypocalcemia, especially of the degree that can be caused by hypoparathyroidism, will compromise the mineral supply available to the fetus. This has been assessed in both surgical and genetic models of maternal hypoparathyroidism.[1]

Fetuses of rats, lambs, and mice have shown resiliency in being able to maintain normal serum calcium and phosphorus, and skeletal mineral content, despite hypocalcemia and hyperphosphatemia in their mothers.[1] These findings imply that placental calcium transport upregulates to compensate for the low maternal blood calcium. But in other studies, placental delivery of calcium must have been insufficient, because despite normal serum calcium, the fetuses displayed parathyroid hyperplasia, and lower skeletal ash weight and mineral content.[1] In such cases, the fetal skeletal resorption is evidently contributing to the normal serum calcium.

44.12.3.2 Human Data

It is quite clear that prolonged and severe maternal hypocalcemia during pregnancy has serious adverse consequences on fetal development, including spontaneous abortion, stillbirth, and neonatal death. Morbidity has included fetal hyperparathyroidism, severe resorption of the developing skeleton, and fractures occurring in utero or during birth. Similar to the animal studies, cord blood calcium may be normal, low, or even increased, whereas the fetal parathyroids may be enlarged and hyperplastic. Normal cord blood calcium does not reassure that the fetus will be normal, because it may have been maintained by fetal skeletal resorption rather than inflow of calcium across the placenta.

The parathyroid hyperplasia that occurs represents secondary hyperparathyroidism, but it can remain autonomous for a time after birth, leading to hypercalcemia and progressive skeletal resorption before parathyroid function subsides to normal.

Activating mutations of the CaSR have led to similar complications, with low-normal cord blood calcium and elevated PTH at birth,[122] whereas other newborns have appeared normal.[123]

44.12.3.3 Clinical Management

If the maternal serum calcium is maintained in the midnormal range during pregnancy, that should prevent fetal secondary hyperparathyroidism and other complications. Babies born of poorly controlled hypoparathyroid mothers should have cord blood calcium and PTH measured and observed for fractures and the emergence of hypercalcemia.

44.12.4 Pseudohypoparathyroidism in the Mother

44.12.4.1 Animal Data

The relevant animal models have not been studied during pregnancy.

44.12.4.2 Human Data

When women with pseudohypoparathyroidism have been hypocalcemic during pregnancy, this has led to the same fetal outcomes observed with maternal hypoparathyroidism, including parathyroid hyperplasia, skeletal demineralization, and fractures.[124, 125] Postnatally, neonatal hypercalcemia can develop before the autonomous parathyroid function subsides.

44.12.4.3 Clinical Management

As with hypoparathyroidism, maintaining normocalcemia in the mother during pregnancy should prevent these complications. Babies should have their cord blood calcium and PTH measured, examined for fractures, and monitored for emergence of hypercalcemia.

44.12.5 Vitamin D-Related Disorders in the Mother

44.12.5.1 Animal Data

Severe maternal vitamin D deficiency and genetic absence of VDR or calcitriol all cause maternal hypocalcemia and hypophosphatemia. As discussed previously, the fetuses in these models have shown normal serum minerals, PTH, skeletal lengths, and mineral content.[1] This differs from the fetal hyperparathyroidism that can develop in response to more marked maternal hypocalcemia, such as from maternal hypoparathyroidism. Maternal hypocalcemia is generally more modest with disorders of vitamin D physiology because secondary hyperparathyroidism offsets the fall in maternal serum calcium. In this setting, the fetus seems able to upregulate placental calcium transport to maintain an adequate delivery of mineral content.

Female mice that are homozygous for 24-hydroxylase deficiency are hypercalcemic, and their null fetuses show abnormal mineralization of intramembranous bone, a finding that is not seen in null fetuses born of mothers that are heterozygous for the mutation.[37] It is possible that the very high calcitriol levels in the null mothers cross the placenta in increased amounts to adversely affect their null fetuses, which are incapable of catabolizing calcitriol normally.

44.12.5.2 Human Data

The potential effects of maternal vitamin D deficiency, VDDR-I, or VDDR-II during pregnancy have already been addressed in the earlier section. At the time of birth, the baby can be expected to have normal serum calcium, phosphorus, and PTH, and likely a normal skeletal and mineral content. It is in the days to months after birth that hypocalcemia and hypophosphatemia may develop in vitamin D deficient neonates and any neonates who inherited the genetic disorder. This will be accompanied by secondary hyperparathyroidism, and eventually the development of rachitic changes in the neonatal skeleton.

If maternal hypocalcemia was more marked during pregnancy, especially if confounded by low calcium intake or other nutritional deficits, then the newborn could show early evidence of secondary hyperparathyroidism and a rachitic skeleton.

Maternal hypercalcemia can occur from excess consumption of calcitriol, 1α-cholecalciferol, or vitamin D (hypervitaminosis D). It can also occur from 24-hydroxylase deficiency, which leads to a marked increase in maternal calcitriol and, thereby, intestinal calcium absorption during pregnancy. Each of these conditions in turn can lead to fetal parathyroid suppression, neonatal hypocalcemia, and prolonged to permanent hypoparathyroidism. It is the maternal calcium concentration, and not the vitamin D metabolite levels, that are most relevant. If women consume moderate to high doses of vitamin D during pregnancy but remain normocalcemic, the neonate should be normal. Furthermore, high 24-hydroxylase activity in the fetus and placenta help protect against hypervitaminosis D and hypercalcemia in the newborn.[1]

44.12.5.3 Clinical Management

Babies born of mothers with overt vitamin D deficiency should receive prompt treatment with vitamin D to replenish body stores, and be urgently managed with calcium and calcitriol treatment if presenting with symptomatic hypocalcemia.

Offspring of mothers with VDDR-I or VDDR-II are most likely to be heterozygous and, therefore, clinically normal with no need for intervention. However, consanguinity has been increased in some reports of VDDR-I and VDDR-II, and so clinical assessment or genetic testing may be warranted to determine if the baby is unaffected or not.

Neonates born of mothers with hypercalcemia due to hypervitaminosis D or 24-hydroxylase deficiency should be observed for evidence of hypocalcemia due to transient to prolonged hypoparathyroidism, a consequence of maternal hypercalcemia causing fetal parathyroid suppression.

44.12.6 Maternal Magnesium Infusions (Tocolytic Therapy)

Intravenous magnesium inhibits uterine contractions from premature labor and also helps prevent seizures from eclampsia. Magnesium readily crosses the placenta and causes fetal hypermagnesemia, parathyroid suppression, and variable effects on the total and ionized calcium of neonates.[1] Prolonged exposure can lead to defective ossification of bone and enamel in the teeth, and abnormal mineralization of long bones. Severe hypermagnesemia ($>7\,mg/dL$) may also cause hypotonia and respiratory depression in the newborn.

The general principle is that the more prolonged the use of tocolytic therapy, the more alert the neonatologist should be to adverse effects of that treatment on the newborn.

44.12.7 Hypercalcemia of Malignancy in the Mother

Hypercalcemia of malignancy can cause more marked maternal hypercalcemia and, thereby, more marked suppression of the fetal parathyroids. This in turn can lead to severe neonatal hypocalcemia, tetany, and even permanent hypoparathyroidism. The initial cord blood calcium may be high because of the maternal hypercalcemia leading to increased transplacental delivery of calcium to the fetus, but the calcium will fall and may reach severely low values that cause respiratory distress, tetany, and seizures.[1] In published case reports, one of four babies died, but in other cases the outcome wasn't reported.

44.12.8 Pseudohyperparathyroidism in the Mother

Pseudohyperparathyroidism is excess production of PTHrP from breasts or placenta, which leads to maternal hypercalcemia. In turn, this can cause the same effects on the fetus and neonate as maternal hypercalcemia does from primary hyperparathyroidism during pregnancy. Hypercalcemia may be present in cord blood, but this may be followed by symptomatic hypocalcemia, and the parathyroid suppression becomes evident. Clinical management should be similar to that for observation and management of babies born of mothers with primary hyperparathyroidism.

44.12.9 Maternal Diabetes Causing Fetal and Neonatal Hypoparathyroidism

Poorly controlled maternal diabetes during pregnancy is known to increase the risk of neonatal hypocalcemia, seizures, and tetany within the first 24–72 h after birth. Hyperphosphatemia may be present, which suggests that some degree of neonatal hypoparathyroidism is present. However, the mechanism by which maternal diabetes leads to fetal and neonatal hypoparathyroidism is unknown. In one case series, the cord blood ionized and total serum calcium levels were increased in infants of diabetic mothers,[126] which could explain suppression of the fetal parathyroids. But it is unclear how maternal diabetes would in turn cause fetal hypercalcemia. The glucosuria of uncontrolled diabetes may cause renal wasting of magnesium, and if maternal stores are sufficiently depleted, this could conceivably lead to fetal hypomagnesemia and parathyroid suppression. However, magnesium supplementation had no effect on preventing neonatal hypocalcemia in infants of diabetic mothers.[127] Additional risks for hypocalcemia in neonates born of diabetic mothers include preterm birth, lung immaturity, and asphyxia.

Clinical management should consist of increased awareness and monitoring for hypocalcemia in neonates born of diabetic mothers, especially those with poorly controlled diabetes.

44.13 CONCLUSIONS

Fetal mineral homeostasis and skeletal development are dependent on adequate delivery of mineral by the placenta. Placental calcium transfer requires PTHrP and possibly PTH, but not calcitriol, calcitonin, or FGF23. In turn, PTH and PTHrP each contribute to regulating endochondral bone development, bone mineralization, and serum calcium and phosphorus in utero, whereas calcitriol, calcitonin, FGF23, and the sex steroids are not required. These aspects of fetal physiology explain why the clinical presentation of a newborn with deficiency in one of these hormones will differ from how such deficiency will present in the child or adult. After birth, the intestines become the route of mineral delivery, and calcitriol is of critical importance in regulating that process. This explains why hormonal deficiency or excess will affect the fetus differently than the adult. Fetal and neonatal bone and mineral metabolism can also be affected by maternal disorders that, for example, lead to fetal parathyroid suppression or hyperplasia.

REFERENCES

1. Kovacs CS. Bone development and mineral homeostasis in the fetus and neonate: roles of the calciotropic and phosphotropic hormones. *Physiol Rev* 2014;**94**(4):1143–218.
2. Simmonds CS, Karsenty G, Karaplis AC, Kovacs CS. Parathyroid hormone regulates fetal-placental mineral homeostasis. *J Bone Miner Res* 2010;**25**(3):594–605.
3. Miao D, He B, Karaplis AC, Goltzman D. Parathyroid hormone is essential for normal fetal bone formation. *J Clin Invest* 2002;**109**(9):1173–82.
4. Kovacs CS, Chafe LL, Fudge NJ, Friel JK, Manley NR. PTH regulates fetal blood calcium and skeletal mineralization independently of PTHrP. *Endocrinology* 2001;**142**(11):4983–93.
5. Kovacs CS, Manley NR, Moseley JM, Martin TJ, Kronenberg HM. Fetal parathyroids are not required to maintain placental calcium transport. *J Clin Invest* 2001;**107**(8):1007–15.
6. Xue Y, Karaplis AC, Hendy GN, Goltzman D, Miao D. Genetic models show that parathyroid hormone and 1,25-dihydroxyvitamin D3 play distinct and synergistic roles in postnatal mineral ion homeostasis and skeletal development. *Hum Mol Genet* 2005;**14**(11):1515–28.
7. Xue Y, Zhang Z, Karaplis AC, Hendy GN, Goltzman D, Miao D. Exogenous PTH-related protein and PTH improve mineral and skeletal status in 25-hydroxyvitamin D-1alpha-hydroxylase and PTH double knockout mice. *J Bone Miner Res* 2005;**20**(10):1766–77.
8. Xue Y, Karaplis AC, Hendy GN, Goltzman D, Miao D. Exogenous 1,25-dihydroxyvitamin D3 exerts a skeletal anabolic effect and improves mineral ion homeostasis in mice that are homozygous for both the 1alpha-hydroxylase and parathyroid hormone null alleles. *Endocrinology* 2006;**147**(10):4801–10.
9. Brandi ML. Genetics of hypoparathyroidism and pseudohypoparathyroidism. *J Endocrinol Investig* 2011;**34**(7 Suppl):27–34.
10. Inoue H, Takada H, Kusuda T, Goto T, Ochiai M, Kinjo T, et al. Successful cord blood transplantation for a CHARGE syndrome with CHD7 mutation showing DiGeorge sequence including hypoparathyroidism. *Eur J Pediatr* 2010;**169**(7):839–44.
11. Ryan AK, Goodship JA, Wilson DI, Philip N, Levy A, Seidel H, et al. Spectrum of clinical features associated with interstitial chromosome 22q11 deletions: a European collaborative study. *J Med Genet* 1997;**34**(10):798–804.
12. Brauner R, Le Harivel de Gonneville A, Kindermans C, Le Bidois J, Prieur M, Lyonnet S, et al. Parathyroid function and growth in 22q11.2 deletion syndrome. *J Pediatr* 2003;**142**(5):504–8.

13. Adachi M, Tachibana K, Masuno M, Makita Y, Maesaka H, Okada T, et al. Clinical characteristics of children with hypoparathyroidism due to 22q11.2 microdeletion. *Eur J Pediatr* 1998;**157**(1):34–8.

14. Vahle JL, Sato M, Long GG, Young JK, Francis PC, Engelhardt JA, et al. Skeletal changes in rats given daily subcutaneous injections of recombinant human parathyroid hormone (1–34) for 2 years and relevance to human safety. *Toxicol Pathol* 2002;**30**(3):312–21.

15. Vahle JL, Long GG, Sandusky G, Westmore M, Ma YL, Sato M. Bone neoplasms in F344 rats given teriparatide [rhPTH(1–34)] are dependent on duration of treatment and dose. *Toxicol Pathol* 2004;**32**(4):426–38.

16. Morley P. Delivery of parathyroid hormone for the treatment of osteoporosis. *Expert Opin Drug Deliv* 2005;**2**(6):993–1002.

17. Akin L, Kurtoglu S, Yildiz A, Akin MA, Kendirici M. Vitamin D deficiency rickets mimicking pseudohypoparathyroidism. *J Clin Res Pediatr Endocrinol* 2010;**2**(4):173–5.

18. Kollars J, Zarroug AE, van Heerden J, Lteif A, Stavlo P, Suarez L, et al. Primary hyperparathyroidism in pediatric patients. *Pediatrics* 2005;**115**(4):974–80.

19. Kovacs CS, Lanske B, Hunzelman JL, Guo J, Karaplis AC, Kronenberg HM. Parathyroid hormone-related peptide (PTHrP) regulates fetal-placental calcium transport through a receptor distinct from the PTH/PTHrP receptor. *Proc Natl Acad Sci U S A* 1996;**93**:15233–8.

20. Karaplis AC, Luz A, Glowacki J, Bronson RT, Tybulewicz VL, Kronenberg HM, et al. Lethal skeletal dysplasia from targeted disruption of the parathyroid hormone-related peptide gene. *Genes Dev* 1994;**8**:277–89.

21. Weir EC, Philbrick WM, Amling M, Neff LA, Baron R, Broadus AE. Targeted overexpression of parathyroid hormone-related peptide in chondrocytes causes chondrodysplasia and delayed endochondral bone formation. *Proc Natl Acad Sci U S A* 1996;**93**(19):10240–5.

22. Lanske B, Karaplis AC, Lee K, Luz A, Vortkamp A, Pirro A, et al. PTH/PTHrP receptor in early development and Indian hedgehog-regulated bone growth. *Science* 1996;**273**:663–6.

23. Schipani E, Lanske B, Hunzelman J, Luz A, Kovacs CS, Lee K, et al. Targeted expression of constitutively active PTH/PTHrP receptors delays endochondral bone formation and rescues PTHrP-less mice. *Proc Natl Acad Sci U S A* 1997;**94**(25):13689–94.

24. Kovacs CS, Ho-Pao CL, Hunzelman JL, Lanske B, Fox J, Seidman JG, et al. Regulation of murine fetal-placental calcium metabolism by the calcium-sensing receptor. *J Clin Invest* 1998;**101**:2812–20.

25. Ho C, Conner DA, Pollak MR, Ladd DJ, Kifor O, Warren HB, et al. A mouse model of human familial hypocalciuric hypercalcemia and neonatal severe hyperparathyroidism. *Nat Genet* 1995;**11**:389–94.

26. Kovacs CS. Fetal mineral homeostasis. In: Glorieux FH, Pettifor JM, Jüppner H, editors. *Pediatric bone: biology and diseases.* San Diego: Academic Press; 2003. p. 271–302.

27. Thomas AK, McVie R, Levine SN. Disorders of maternal calcium metabolism implicated by abnormal calcium metabolism in the neonate. *Am J Perinatol* 1999;**16**(10):515–20.

28. Rodrigues LS, Cau AC, Bussmann LZ, Bastida G, Brunetto OH, Correa PH, et al. New mutation in the CASR gene in a family with familial hypocalciuric hypercalcemia (FHH) and neonatal severe hyperparathyroidism (NSHPT). *Arq Bras Endocrinol Metabol* 2011;**55**(1):67–71.

29. Chikatsu N, Watanabe S, Takeuchi Y, Muraosa Y, Sasaki S, Oka Y, et al. A family of autosomal dominant hypocalcemia with an activating mutation of calcium-sensing receptor gene. *Endocr J* 2003;**50**(1):91–6.

30. Raue F, Pichl J, Dorr HG, Schnabel D, Heidemann P, Hammersen G, et al. Activating mutations in the calcium-sensing receptor: genetic and clinical spectrum in 25 patients with autosomal dominant hypocalcaemia-a German survey. *Clin Endocrinol* 2011;**75**(6):760–5.

31. Wilhelm-Bals A, Parvex P, Magdelaine C, Girardin E. Successful use of bisphosphonate and calcimimetic in neonatal severe primary hyperparathyroidism. *Pediatrics* 2012;**129**(3):e812–6.

32. Nemeth EF, Van Wagenen BC, Balandrin MF. Discovery and development of calcimimetic and calcilytic compounds. *Prog Med Chem* 2018;**57**(1):1–86.

33. Ryan BA, Alhani K, Sellars KB, Kirby BJ, St-Arnaud R, Jones G, et al. Mineral homeostasis in murine fetuses is sensitive to maternal calcitriol but not to absence of fetal calcitriol. *J Bone Miner Res* 2019;**34**:669–80.

34. Glazier JD, Mawer EB, Sibley CP. Calbindin-D$_{9K}$ gene expression in rat chorioallantoic placenta is not regulated by 1,25-dihydroxyvitamin D$_3$. *Pediatr Res* 1995;**37**:720–5.

35. Kovacs CS, Woodland ML, Fudge NJ, Friel JK. The vitamin D receptor is not required for fetal mineral homeostasis or for the regulation of placental calcium transfer. *Am J Physiol Endocrinol Metab* 2005;**289**(1):E133–44.

36. Lieben L, Stockmans I, Moermans K, Carmeliet G. Maternal hypervitaminosis D reduces fetal bone mass and mineral acquisition and leads to neonatal lethality. *Bone* 2013;**57**(1):123–31.

37. St-Arnaud R, Arabian A, Travers R, Barletta F, Raval-Pandya M, Chapin K, et al. Deficient mineralization of intramembranous bone in vitamin D-24-hydroxylase-ablated mice is due to elevated 1,25-dihydroxyvitamin D and not to the absence of 24,25-dihydroxyvitamin D. *Endocrinology* 2000;**141**(7):2658–66.

38. Maxwell JP, Miles LM. Osteomalacia in China. *J Obstet Gynaecol Br Emp* 1925;**32**(3):433–73.

39. Glaser K. Double contour, cupping and spurring in roentgenograms of long bones in infants. *Am J Roentgenol Radium Ther* 1949;**61**(4):482–92.

40. Ward LM, Gaboury I, Ladhani M, Zlotkin S. Vitamin D-deficiency rickets among children in Canada. *CMAJ* 2007;**177**(2):161–6.

41. Teotia M, Teotia SP, Nath M. Metabolic studies in congenital vitamin D deficiency rickets. *Indian J Pediatr* 1995;**62**(1):55–61.

42. Teotia M, Teotia SPS, Singh RK. Metabolism of fluoride in pregnant women residing in endemic fluorosis areas. *Fluoride* 1979;**12**(2):58–64.

43. Pitt MJ. Rickets and osteomalacia are still around. *Radiol Clin N Am* 1991;**29**(1):97–118.

44. Heo JS, Choi KY, Sohn SH, Kim C, Kim YJ, Shin SH, et al. A case of mucolipidosis II presenting with prenatal skeletal dysplasia and severe secondary hyperparathyroidism at birth. *Korean J Pediatr* 2012;**55**(11):438–44.

45. Rockman-Greenberg C. Hypophosphatasia. *Pediatr Endocrinol Rev* 2013;**10**(Suppl. 2):380–8.

46. Samson GR. Skeletal dysplasias with osteopenia in the newborn: the value of alkaline phosphatase. *J Matern Fetal Neonatal Med* 2005;**17**(3):229–31.

47. Arundel P, Offiah A, Bishop NJ. Evolution of the radiographic appearance of the metaphyses over the first year of life in type V osteogenesis imperfecta: clues to pathogenesis. *J Bone Miner Res* 2011;**26**(4):894–8.

48. Glorieux FH, Ward LM, Rauch F, Lalic L, Roughley PJ, Travers R. Osteogenesis imperfecta type VI: a form of brittle bone disease with a mineralization defect. *J Bone Miner Res* 2002;**17**(1):30–8.

49. Brickley M, Ives R. Skeletal manifestations of infantile scurvy. *Am J Phys Anthropol* 2006;**129**(2):163–72.

50. Sann L, David L, Frederich A, Bovier-Lapierre M, Bourgeois J, Romand-Monier M, et al. Congenital rickets. Study of the evolution of secondary hyperparathyroidism. *Acta Paediatr Scand* 1977;**66**(3):323–7.

51. Kiesler J, Ricer R. The abnormal fontanel. *Am Fam Physician* 2003;**67**(12):2547–52.

52. Rothman SM, Lee BC. What bulges under a bulging fontanel? *Arch Pediatr Adolesc Med* 1998;**152**(1):100–1.

53. Owada C. Are there New-born Rickets? *Tohoku J Exp Med* 1956;**64**(Suppl):37–43.

54. Ramavat LG. Vitamin D deficiency rickets at birth in Kuwait. *Indian J Pediatr* 1999;**66**(1):37–43.

55. Yorifuji J, Yorifuji T, Tachibana K, Nagai S, Kawai M, Momoi T, et al. Craniotabes in normal newborns: the earliest sign of subclinical vitamin D deficiency. *J Clin Endocrinol Metab* 2008;**93**(5):1784–8.

56. Congdon P, Horsman A, Kirby PA, Dibble J, Bashir T. Mineral content of the forearms of babies born to Asian and white mothers. *Br Med J (Clin Res Ed)* 1983;**286**(6373):1233–5.

57. Weiler HA, Fitzpatrick-Wong SC, Schellenberg JM. Bone mass in first nations, Asian and white newborn infants. *Growth Dev Aging* 2008;**71**(1):35–43.

58. Viljakainen HT, Korhonen T, Hytinantti T, Laitinen EK, Andersson S, Makitie O, et al. Maternal vitamin D status affects bone growth in early childhood—a prospective cohort study. *Osteoporos Int* 2011;**22**(3):883–91.

59. Thacher TD, Fischer PR, Pettifor JM. The usefulness of clinical features to identify active rickets. *Ann Trop Paediatr* 2002;**22**(3):229–37.

60. Ross AC, Abrams SA, Aloia JF, Brannon PM, Clinton SK, Durazo-Arvizu RA, et al. Ross AC, Taylor CL, YA L, Del Valle HB, editors. *Dietary reference intakes for calcium and vitamin D*. Washington, DC: Institute of Medicine; 2011.

61. Kovacs CS. Maternal mineral and bone metabolism during pregnancy, lactation, and post-weaning recovery. *Physiol Rev* 2016;**96**(2):449–547.

62. Roth DE, Leung M, Mesfin E, Qamar H, Watterworth J, Papp E. Vitamin D supplementation during pregnancy: state of the evidence from a systematic review of randomised trials. *BMJ* 2017;**359**.

63. Brooke OG, Brown IR, Bone CD, Carter ND, Cleeve HJ, Maxwell JD, et al. Vitamin D supplements in pregnant Asian women: effects on calcium status and fetal growth. *Br Med J* 1980;**280**:751–4.

64. Delvin EE, Salle BL, Glorieux FH, Adeleine P, David LS. Vitamin D supplementation during pregnancy: effect on neonatal calcium homeostasis. *J Pediatr* 1986;**109**:328–34.

65. Roth DE, Al Mahmud A, Raqib R, Akhtar E, Perumal N, Pezzack B, et al. Randomized placebo-controlled trial of high-dose prenatal third-trimester vitamin D3 supplementation in Bangladesh: the AViDD trial. *Nutr J* 2013;**12**(1):47.

66. Roth DE, Perumal N, Al Mahmud A, Baqui AH. Maternal vitamin D3 supplementation during the third trimester of pregnancy: effects on infant growth in a longitudinal follow-up study in Bangladesh. *J Pediatr* 2013;**163**(6):1605–11 e3.

67. Harrington J, Perumal N, Al Mahmud A, Baqui A, Roth DE. Vitamin D and fetal-neonatal calcium homeostasis: findings from a randomized controlled trial of high-dose antenatal vitamin D supplementation. *Pediatr Res* 2014;**76**(3):302–9.

68. Hashemipour S, Lalooha F, Zahir Mirdamadi S, Ziaee A, Dabaghi Ghaleh T. Effect of vitamin D administration in vitamin D-deficient pregnant women on maternal and neonatal serum calcium and vitamin D concentrations: a randomised clinical trial. *Br J Nutr* 2013;**110**(9):1611–6.

69. Grant CC, Stewart AW, Scragg R, Milne T, Rowden J, Ekeroma A, et al. Vitamin D during pregnancy and infancy and infant serum 25-hydroxyvitamin D concentration. *Pediatrics* 2014;**133**(1):e143–53.

70. Hollis BW, Johnson D, Hulsey TC, Ebeling M, Wagner CL. Vitamin D supplementation during pregnancy: double-blind, randomized clinical trial of safety and effectiveness. *J Bone Miner Res* 2011;**26**(10):2341–57.

71. Wagner CL, McNeil R, Hamilton SA, Winkler J, Rodriguez Cook C, Warner G, et al. A randomized trial of vitamin D supplementation in 2 community health center networks in South Carolina. *Am J Obstet Gynecol* 2013;**208**(2):137. e1–13.

72. Wagner CL, editor. *Vitamin D supplementation during pregnancy: impact on maternal outcomes. Centers for disease control and prevention conference on vitamin D physiology in pregnancy: implications for preterm birth and preeclampsia, Atlanta, April 26–27*, Georgia: Centers for Disease Control and Prevention; 2011.

73. Hollis BW. *Vitamin D supplementation in pregnancy & breastfeeding-effectiveness and safety/the vitamin D requirement during pregnancy and lactation*. Available from: http://www.youtube.com/watch?v=O0elnh4D08g; 2011. Accessed 12 October 2011.

74. Hollis BW, Wagner CL. Vitamin D and pregnancy: skeletal effects, nonskeletal effects, and birth outcomes. *Calcif Tissue Int* 2013;**92**(2):128–39.

75. Cooper C, Harvey NC, Bishop NJ, Kennedy S, Papageorghiou AT, Schoenmakers I, et al. Maternal gestational vitamin D supplementation and offspring bone health (MAVIDOS): a multicentre, double-blind, randomised placebo-controlled trial. *Lancet Diabetes Endocrinol* 2016;**4**(5):393–402.

76. Kovacs CS. Does fetal exposure to vitamin D programme childhood bone mass? *Lancet Diabetes Endocrinol* 2017;**5**(5):317–9.

77. Vaziri F, Dabbaghmanesh MH, Samsami A, Nasiri S, Shirazi PT. Vitamin D supplementation during pregnancy on infant anthropometric measurements and bone mass of mother-infant pairs: a randomized placebo clinical trial. *Early Hum Dev* 2016;**103**:61–8.

78. Sahoo SK, Katam KK, Das V, Agarwal A, Bhatia V. Maternal vitamin D supplementation in pregnancy and offspring outcomes: a double-blind randomized placebo-controlled trial. *J Bone Miner Metab* 2017;**35**(4):464–71.

79. Roth DE, Morris SK, Zlotkin S, Gernand AD, Ahmed T, Shanta SS, et al. Vitamin D supplementation in pregnancy and lactation and infant growth. *N Engl J Med* 2018;**379**(6):535–46.

80. Morley R, Carlin JB, Pasco JA, Wark JD. Maternal 25-hydroxyvitamin D and parathyroid hormone concentrations and offspring birth size. *J Clin Endocrinol Metab* 2006;**91**(3):906–12.

81. Mahon P, Harvey N, Crozier S, Inskip H, Robinson S, Arden N, et al. Low maternal vitamin D status and fetal bone development: cohort study. *J Bone Miner Res* 2010;**25**(1):14–9.

82. Viljakainen HT, Saarnio E, Hytinantti T, Miettinen M, Surcel H, Makitie O, et al. Maternal vitamin D status determines bone variables in the newborn. *J Clin Endocrinol Metab* 2010;**95**(4):1749–57.

83. Ioannou C, Javaid MK, Mahon P, Yaqub MK, Harvey NC, Godfrey KM, et al. The effect of maternal vitamin D concentration on fetal bone. *J Clin Endocrinol Metab* 2012;**97**(11):E2070–7.

84. Ioannidis G, Papaioannou A, Hopman WM, Akhtar-Danesh N, Anastassiades T, Pickard L, et al. Relation between fractures and mortality: results from the Canadian Multicentre Osteoporosis Study. *CMAJ* 2009;**181**(5):265–71.

85. Javaid MK, Crozier SR, Harvey NC, Gale CR, Dennison EM, Boucher BJ, et al. Maternal vitamin D status during pregnancy and childhood bone mass at age 9 years: a longitudinal study. *Lancet* 2006;**367**(9504):36–43.

86. Cooper C, Westlake S, Harvey N, Javaid K, Dennison E, Hanson M. Review: developmental origins of osteoporotic fracture. *Osteoporos Int* 2006; **17**(3):337–47.

87. Lawlor DA, Wills AK, Fraser A, Sayers A, Fraser WD, Tobias JH. Association of maternal vitamin D status during pregnancy with bone-mineral content in offspring: a prospective cohort study. *Lancet* 2013;**381**(9884):2176–83.

88. Garcia AH, Erler NS, Jaddoe VWV, Tiemeier H, van den Hooven EH, Franco OH, et al. 25-hydroxyvitamin D concentrations during fetal life and bone health in children aged 6 years: a population-based prospective cohort study. *Lancet Diabetes Endocrinol* 2017;**5**(5):367–76.

89. Rosen CJ, Adams JS, Bikle D, Black DM, Demay MB, Manson JE, et al. The nonskeletal effects of vitamin D: an endocrine society scientific statement. *Endocr Rev* 2012;**33**(3):456–92.

90. Harvey NC, Holroyd C, Ntani G, Javaid K, Cooper P, Moon R, et al. Vitamin D supplementation in pregnancy: a systematic review. *Health Technol Assess* 2014;**18**(45):1–190.

91. Carpenter TO. CYP24A1 loss of function: clinical phenotype of monoallelic and biallelic mutations. *J Steroid Biochem Mol Biol* 2017;**173**:337–40.

92. Munns CF, Shaw N, Kiely M, Specker BL, Thacher TD, Ozono K, et al. Global consensus recommendations on prevention and management of nutritional rickets. *J Clin Endocrinol Metab* 2016;**101**(2):394–415.

93. Dacquin R, Davey RA, Laplace C, Levasseur R, Morris HA, Goldring SR, et al. Amylin inhibits bone resorption while the calcitonin receptor controls bone formation in vivo. *J Cell Biol* 2004;**164**(4):509–14.

94. Laplace C, Li X, Goldring SR, Galson DL. Homozygous deletion of the murine calcitonin receptor gene is an embryonic lethal [abstract]. *J Bone Miner Res* 2002;**17**(Suppl):S166.

95. McDonald KR, Fudge NJ, Woodrow JP, Friel JK, Hoff AO, Gagel RF, et al. Ablation of calcitonin/calcitonin gene related peptide-α impairs fetal magnesium but not calcium homeostasis. *Am J Physiol Endocrinol Metab* 2004;**287**(2):E218–26.

96. Kovesdy CP, Quarles LD. FGF23 from bench to bedside. *Am J Phys Renal Phys* 2016;**310**(11):F1168–74.

97. Ma Y, Samaraweera M, Cooke-Hubley S, Kirby BJ, Karaplis AC, Lanske B, et al. Neither absence nor excess of FGF23 disturbs murine fetal-placental phosphorus homeostasis or prenatal skeletal development and mineralization. *Endocrinology* 2014;**155**(5):1596–605.

98. Ma Y, Kirby BJ, Fairbridge NA, Karaplis AC, Lanske B, Kovacs CS. FGF23 is not required to regulate fetal phosphorus metabolism but exerts effects within 12 hours after birth. *Endocrinology* 2017;**158**(2):252–63.

99. Ohata Y, Yamazaki M, Kawai M, Tsugawa N, Tachikawa K, Koinuma T, et al. Elevated fibroblast growth factor 23 exerts its effects on placenta and regulates vitamin d metabolism in pregnancy of hyp mice. *J Bone Miner Res* 2014;**29**(7):1627–38.

100. Shimada T, Kakitani M, Yamazaki Y, Hasegawa H, Takeuchi Y, Fujita T, et al. Targeted ablation of Fgf23 demonstrates an essential physiological role of FGF23 in phosphate and vitamin D metabolism. *J Clin Invest* 2004;**113**(4):561–8.

101. Sitara D, Kim S, Razzaque MS, Bergwitz C, Taguchi T, Schuler C, et al. Genetic evidence of serum phosphate-independent functions of FGF-23 on bone. *PLoS Genet* 2008;**4**(8).

102. Sitara D, Razzaque MS, Hesse M, Yoganathan S, Taguchi T, Erben RG, et al. Homozygous ablation of fibroblast growth factor-23 results in hyper-phosphatemia and impaired skeletogenesis, and reverses hypophosphatemia in Phex-deficient mice. *Matrix Biol* 2004;**23**(7):421–32.

103. Nakatani T, Sarraj B, Ohnishi M, Densmore MJ, Taguchi T, Goetz R, et al. In vivo genetic evidence for klotho-dependent, fibroblast growth factor 23 (Fgf23) -mediated regulation of systemic phosphate homeostasis. *FASEB J* 2009;**23**(2):433–41.

104. Bai X, Miao D, Goltzman D, Karaplis AC. Early lethality in Hyp mice with targeted deletion of Pth gene. *Endocrinology* 2007;**148**(10):4974–83.

105. Slavin RE, Wen J, Barmada A. Tumoral calcinosis—a pathogenetic overview: a histological and ultrastructural study with a report of two new cases, one in infancy. *Int J Surg Pathol* 2012;**20**(5):462–73.

106. Polykandriotis EP, Beutel FK, Horch RE, Grunert J. A case of familial tumoral calcinosis in a neonate and review of the literature. *Arch Orthop Trauma Surg* 2004;**124**(8):563–7.

107. Hori M, Shimizu Y, Fukumoto S. Minireview: fibroblast growth factor 23 in phosphate homeostasis and bone metabolism. *Endocrinology* 2011; **152**(1):4–10.

108. Moncrieff MW. Early biochemical findings in familial hypophosphataemic, hyperphosphaturic rickets and response to treatment. *Arch Dis Child* 1982;**57**(1):70–2.

109. Carpenter TO. The expanding family of hypophosphatemic syndromes. *J Bone Miner Metab* 2012;**30**(1):1–9.

110. Finer G, Price HE, Shore RM, White KE, Langman CB. Hyperphosphatemic familial tumoral calcinosis: response to acetazolamide and postulated mechanisms. *Am J Med Genet A* 2014;**164a**(6):1545–9.

111. Jost J, Bahans C, Courbebaisse M, Tran TA, Linglart A, Benistan K, et al. Topical sodium thiosulfate: a treatment for calcifications in hyperphosphatemic familial tumoral calcinosis? *J Clin Endocrinol Metab* 2016;**101**(7):2810–5.

112. Imel EA, Zhang X, Ruppe MD, Weber TJ, Klausner MA, Ito T, et al. Prolonged correction of serum phosphorus in adults with X-linked hypophosphatemia using monthly doses of KRN23. *J Clin Endocrinol Metab* 2015;**100**(7):2565–73.

113. Linglart A, Carpenter T, Imel E, Boot A, Högler W, Padidela R, et al. Effect of KRN23, a fully human anti-FGF23 monoclonal antibody, on rickets in children with X-linked hypophosphatemia (XLH): 40-week interim results from a randomized, open-label phase 2 study. *Ann Endocrinol (Paris)* 2016;**77**(4):440.

114. Smith EP, Boyd J, Frank GR, Takahashi H, Cohen RM, Specker B, et al. Estrogen resistance caused by a mutation in the estrogen-receptor gene in a man. *N Engl J Med* 1994;**331**(16):1056–61.

115. Pieringer H, Hatzl-Griesenhofer M, Shebl O, Wiesinger-Eidenberger G, Maschek W, Biesenbach G. Hypocalcemic tetany in the newborn as a manifestation of unrecognized maternal primary hyperparathyroidism. *Wien Klin Wochenschr* 2007;**119**(3–4):129–31.

116. Norman J, Politz D, Politz L. Hyperparathyroidism during pregnancy and the effect of rising calcium on pregnancy loss: a call for earlier intervention. *Clin Endocrinol* 2009;**71**(1):104–9.

117. Kelly TR. Primary hyperparathyroidism during pregnancy. *Surgery* 1991;**110**(6):1028–33. discussion 33–34.

118. Wagner G, Transhol L, Melchior JC. Hyperparathyroidism and pregnancy. *Acta Endocrinol* 1964;**47**:549–64.

119. Ludwig GD. Hyperparathyroidism in relation to pregnancy. *N Engl J Med* 1962;**267**:637–42.

120. Delmonico FL, Neer RM, Cosimi AB, Barnes AB, Russell PS. Hyperparathyroidism during pregnancy. *Am J Surg* 1976;**131**:328–37.

121. McDonnell CM, Zacharin MR. Maternal primary hyperparathyroidism: discordant outcomes in a twin pregnancy. *J Paediatr Child Health* 2006;**42**(1–2):70–1.

122. Pagan YL, Hirschhorn J, Yang B, D'Souza-Li L, Majzoub JA, Hendy GN. Maternal activating mutation of the calcium-sensing receptor: implications for calcium metabolism in the neonate. *J Pediatr Endocrinol Metab* 2004;**17**(4):673–7.

123. Adeniyi JO, Esen U, Parr J. Pregnancy outcome in women with autosomal dominant hypocalcaemic hypercalciuric nephrocalcinosis. *J Matern Fetal Neonatal Med* 2014;**27**:1826–8.

124. Glass EJ, Barr DG. Transient neonatal hyperparathyroidism secondary to maternal pseudohypoparathyroidism. *Arch Dis Child* 1981;**56**:565–8.

125. Vidailhet M, Monin P, Andre M, Suty Y, Marchal C, Vert P. Neonatal hyperparathyroidism secondary to maternal hypoparathyroidism. *Arch Fr Pediatr* 1980;**37**:305–12.

126. Tsang RC, Chen I, Friedman MA, Gigger M, Steichen J, Koffler H, et al. Parathyroid function in infants of diabetic mothers. *J Pediatr* 1975;**86**:399–404.

127. Mehta KC, Kalkwarf HJ, Mimouni F, Khoury J, Tsang RC. Randomized trial of magnesium administration to prevent hypocalcemia in infants of diabetic mothers. *J Perinatol* 1998;**18**(5):352–6.

Chapter 45

Pathophysiology and Management of Disorders of Carbohydrate Metabolism and Neonatal Diabetes

Amanda L. Ogilvy-Stuart* and Kathryn Beardsall*,†

*Neonatal Unit, Rosie Hospital, Cambridge University Hospitals NHS Foundation Trust, Cambridge, United Kingdom, †Department of Paediatrics, University of Cambridge, Cambridge, United Kingdom

Common Clinical Problems

- When the fetus is exposed to chronically high or low glucose levels because of maternal or placental abnormal glucose delivery, this leads to physiological changes in the fetus and potentially abnormal glucose regulation in the newborn.
- Neonatal hypoglycemia can be caused by defective counterregulatory hormone secretion (GH, cortisol, glucagon, catecholamines) or excess insulin; additional metabolic disorders are rare but must be considered.
- Neonatal hypoglycemia must be rapidly treated in order to avoid neurocognitive impairment.
- Hyperglycemia is not commonly seen in infants born at term but occurs frequently in extremely preterm infants, and in rare cases of neonatal diabetes.
- In utero exposure to a deranged metabolic environment leads to fetal programming, predisposing offspring to adverse cardiometabolic outcomes in later life.

45.1 INTRODUCTION

In utero, the mother, placenta, and fetus all play a role in regulating glucose control for the growing fetus. The supply of glucose at this time is critical for the increasing demands for fetal metabolism and growth. The placenta plays a central role in delivery and buffering of acute fluctuations in glucose supply to the fetus, but chronic exposure to high or low glucose levels leads to physiological changes in the fetus. These changes may be beneficial in the short term, but can have consequences both immediately after birth for the newborn, and for future adult health. With the fundamental physiological changes required at birth, to ensure upregulation of enzymes required for gluconeogenesis, and the fact that insulin secretion becomes linked to intermittent feeding, it is not surprising that in the perinatal period glucose levels are more varied than later in life. An adverse in utero environment, prematurity, or stress during delivery make infants more at risk from these transient derangements in glucose control.

Hypoglycemia is the most common metabolic disorder found in the neonatal period but is variably defined. It is usually the consequence of impaired counterregulation but, if severe, persistent, or in the setting of hyperinsulinism, it can cause significant long-term neurocognitive impairment. A range of metabolic disorders can also present immediately after birth and early identification and intervention is critical to avoid long-term harm. Hyperglycemia is not commonly seen at term but occurs frequently in extremely preterm infants and in rare cases of neonatal diabetes. There is increased awareness that in utero exposure to a deranged metabolic environment leads to fetal programming, predisposing offspring to adverse cardiometabolic outcomes in later life.[1,2]

45.2 IN UTERO PATHOPHYSIOLOGICAL EFFECTS ON FETAL GLUCOSE

In a healthy, nonstressed pregnancy, fetal blood glucose levels are predominantly determined by the placenta, the levels reflecting maternal levels with no endogenous glucose production. Placental glucose transfer occurs by carrier-mediated facilitated diffusion involving several glucose transporters that are not insulin regulated.[3] Placental function, however, can be impaired in conditions such as preeclampsia, in mothers who smoke, or in starvation. Chronic impaired glucose transport and lower maternal and fetal glucose levels result in suppressed insulin and greater glucagon secretion. In contrast, chronic hyperglycemia will result in increased insulin secretion and suppression of glucagon such as in diabetes in pregnancy.[4]

45.2.1 Placental Dysfunction and Intrauterine Growth Restriction

Placental insufficiency leading to intrauterine growth restriction (IUGR) affects approximately 8% of all pregnancies and is associated with short- and long-term disturbances in metabolism. In this setting reduced glucose transfer and hypoxia result in limited fetal glycogen stores as well as reduced fat free mass. Cord blood shows elevated free fatty acid and lactate levels with low levels of glucose and insulin. Experimental models of placental insufficiency show low fetal blood oxygen and increased plasma catecholamine concentrations, which lower fetal insulin concentrations. These observations in animal models are consistent with findings in humans. Sustained high catecholamine concentrations observed in the IUGR fetus produce developmental adaptations in pancreatic β cells that impair fetal insulin secretion. The elevated catecholamines allow for maintenance of a normal fetal basal metabolic rate, despite low fetal insulin and glucose concentrations, while suppressing fetal growth. However, a compensatory increase in insulin secretion occurs following delivery when there is inhibition or cessation of catecholamine signaling in IUGR fetuses. This finding has been replicated in normally grown sheep in utero following a 7-day noradrenaline (norepinephrine) infusion. Together, these programmed effects will potentially create an imbalance between insulin secretion and insulin-stimulated glucose utilization in the neonate, which probably explains the transient hyperinsulinism and hypoglycemia in some IUGR infants.

45.2.2 Maternal Diabetes

Acute hypoglycemia in the mother with diabetes mellitus will result in hypoglycemia in the fetus. While acute hypoglycemia or hyperglycemia do not cause significant change to fetal insulin and glucagon levels, chronic maternal hyperglycemia will result in increased glucose delivery to the fetus and increased fetal insulin secretion and suppression of glucagon.[4] It was Pedersen in 1952 who first hypothesized this and the association with the various aspects of diabetic fetopathy including increased fat deposition and characteristic macrosomic appearance. Fetal hyperinsulinemia, in the absence of maternal diabetes, also causes macrosomia in animal models, and in clinical cases of congenital hyperinsulinism. The increased fetal weight is in part attributable to increased fat accretion, with body fat being more affected by the in utero environment than lean body mass, which is determined more by genetic aspects of growth.[5] Further studies have demonstrated a continuous positive relationship between maternal glucose levels below those diagnostic of diabetes and fetal hyperinsulinemia, although the association with neonatal hypoglycemia is weaker.[6]

45.2.3 Maternal Obesity

In the landmark Hyperglycemia and Adverse Pregnancy Outcomes (HAPO) study, obesity (OR ∼ 1.7) was nearly equivalent to gestational diabetes mellitus (GDM) (OR ∼ 2.2) as a risk factor for large for gestational age (LGA), and these infants are at increased risk of obesity in later life.[7] In addition to glucose, obese mothers have higher triglycerides (TGs) and free fatty acids (FFAs), and greater insulin resistance, lipolysis, and inflammatory cytokines than normal-weight women. The increased insulin resistance may act to increase shunting of glucose, FFAs, and amino acids to the fetoplacental unit. If excess maternal calorie consumption occurs, fetal glucose exposure becomes excessive and results in fetal hyperinsulinemia and excess fat accretion linked to an increased risk for childhood obesity and metabolic disease, particularly with further exposure to an unhealthy postnatal environment (Fig. 45.1).[8]

45.2.4 Fetal Genotype

Polymorphic variation in the fetal genome, in particular in fetal growth genes, can lead to alterations in maternal metabolism in pregnancy and can alter a mother's risk of developing GDM.[9] Many well-characterized fetal growth genes are imprinted, meaning that their expression is dependent on the parent that contributed them. Haig's kinship, or conflict hypothesis, suggests that paternally expressed fetal imprinted genes will tend to increase fetal growth, whereas maternally expressed genes will tend to restrain it.[10] This is thought to be achieved through modifying fetal and placental nutritional demand and supply, such as altering maternal glucose concentrations. Animal studies have shown that alterations in the imprinted H19 gene and insulin-like growth factor 2 (IGF-II) control element lead to pups born 30% heavier than unaffected

Altered fetal growth:
More than mother's glucose

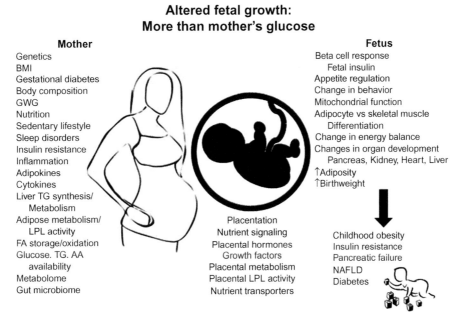

Mother
Genetics
BMI
Gestational diabetes
Body composition
GWG
Nutrition
Sedentary lifestyle
Sleep disorders
Insulin resistance
Inflammation
Adipokines
Cytokines
Liver TG synthesis/
    Metabolism
Adipose metabolism/
    LPL activity
FA storage/oxidation
Glucose. TG. AA
    availability
Metabolome
Gut microbiome

Placentation
Nutrient signaling
Placental hormones
Growth factors
Placental metabolism
Placental LPL activity
Nutrient transporters

Fetus
Beta cell response
Fetal insulin
Appetite regulation
Change in behavior
Mitochondrial function
Adipocyte vs skeletal muscle
    Differentiation
Change in energy balance
Changes in organ development
    Pancreas, Kidney, Heart, Liver
↑Adiposity
↑Birthweight

Childhood obesity
Insulin resistance
Pancreatic failure
NAFLD
Diabetes

FIG. 45.1 Factors impacting on fetal growth: maternal, placental, and fetal effects.

litter mates.[11] In addition, intraperitoneal glucose tolerance tests indicated that mice carrying knockout offspring have increased circulating glucose concentrations in late pregnancy in comparison with those of genetically matched controls.[12] Similarly, associations have been shown in humans between SNP alleles from 15 fetal imprinted genes and maternal glucose concentrations in late pregnancy. This suggests that polymorphic variation in fetal imprinted genes, particularly in the IGF2-INS region, can contribute a small but significant part to the risk of raised late pregnancy maternal glucose concentrations.[13]

45.2.5 Drugs

Drugs that alter maternal carbohydrate metabolism have the potential to impact on fetal and then neonatal metabolism, placing a baby at risk of either hypoglycemia or hyperglycemia. Drugs causing maternal hyperglycemia may result in elevated glucose levels in the fetus, which in turn stimulate the β cells of the fetal pancreas to produce excessive insulin. Once the umbilical cord is clamped, the glucose supply from the mother is interrupted, and the inappropriately high insulin levels in the baby may result in hypoglycemia. Drugs that cause hypoglycemia when used in pregnant women may theoretically result in lower blood glucose levels in the fetus, in whom there is no significant endogenous glucose production. Such side effects (neonatal hypoglycemia), are most commonly reported following the use in late pregnancy of both β-blockers (which are often used to manage preeclampsia) and thiazide diuretics.[14] The use of antidepressants during pregnancy also significantly increases the risk of hypoglycemia in the newborn.[15,16] These babies are at risk of hypoglycemia but whether they need to be routinely monitored after birth is debated.[17]

Corticosteroids may be used in pregnancy to treat maternal disease or to treat the fetus.[18,19] Steroids can be metabolized by the placental enzyme 11 beta-hydroxy steroid dehydrogenase type 2. Prednisolone and methylprednisolone are highly sensitive to this enzyme, and therefore use in pregnancy has little effect on the fetus, and they are the steroids of choice to treat maternal diseases such as adrenal insufficiency or autoimmune disorders. However, in long-term use or in high doses, placental enzyme saturation occurs and fetal adrenal suppression may result.[20] In contrast, dexamethasone and betamethasone are less well metabolized by the placenta, and are therefore used to treat a fetus at risk from congenital adrenal hyperplasia or in anticipation of preterm birth, where they are used to enhance lung maturation and reduce the risks associated with preterm birth.[19] However, their use in later preterm birth has been associated with a 1.6 times increased risk of hypoglycemia.[21,22] This may be multifactorial, related to the increase in maternal hyperglycemia, which leads to fetal pancreatic β-cell hyperplasia/hyperinsulinemia and subsequent neonatal hypoglycemia[21]; or may be secondary to fetal adrenal suppression leading to hyponatremia, hypoglycemia, and hypotension, which become prominent on postnatal day three.[23]

45.3 POSTNATAL GLUCOSE METABOLISM

The dramatic changes that are required for adaptation for independent life after birth mean that derangements in glucose control are not uncommon but can also be a result of underlying pathophysiology. Hypoglycemia is the most common metabolic disorder in the neonatal period but is variably defined, with hyperglycemia much less commonly seen. There remains significant controversy regarding the definitions and clinical significance of glucose levels in the newborn. Some of this relates historically to the limited accuracy of different methods to measure glucose levels, combined with the overlap in what may be physiologically normal glucose levels for one infant but that may place another at risk, and also the challenges in assessing either acute signs and symptoms or long-term outcomes.

45.3.1 Measurement of Glucose in the Newborn

Accurate measurement of blood glucose levels across the range of levels that are considered physiological in the newborn is challenging. Glucose levels in whole blood are lower than in plasma and it is important that clinicians are aware of what level is being reported. Biological variables that are common in the newborn, such as high hematocrit and hyperbilirubinemia, can lead to inaccuracies in the measurement of glucose levels.[24] In addition, the thresholds that are considered of clinical significance are relatively extreme and at the limits of many analytical methodologies.[25] Point of care technology has progressed greatly, but not all devices correct for hematocrit and many are subject to interference. In contrast, laboratory analysis is limited by long turn-around times for results, making it unhelpful in acute management, and it has to be remembered that glucose levels will fall by up to 25% in the first hour while being delivered to the laboratory. Blood gas analyzers are often used to balance these different challenges. All these methods are limited by the intermittent nature of the measurement. The use of continuous glucose monitoring has revealed that glucose levels in the newborn can fluctuate widely and current standard blood glucose measurements fail to identify potentially clinically significant (but silent) episodes of glucose dysregulation.[26] There have been developments in continuous glucose monitoring techniques, but further studies are required, particularly for validation at low glucose levels, before they can replace current methods of monitoring. In the future they may provide an opportunity for improved glucose monitoring in neonatal intensive care; exposure to these clinically silent periods of hypoglycemia has been associated with adverse outcomes in infants at risk.[27–29]

45.3.2 Defining Euglycemia in the Newborn

Much controversy remains regarding what should be considered euglycemia for the newborn, and at what glucose level clinical intervention is required. In relation to hypoglycemia, Koh et al. used a physiological approach to evaluate functional effects, using auditory evoked response waveforms in children including neonates, and reporting changes at a cut off of <2.6 mmol/L (<42 mg/dL).[30] Data based on neurodevelopmental outcomes are limited. The landmark paper by Lucas et al. showed that in a cohort of preterm infants, worse Bayley motor and mental developmental scores at 18 months of age were associated with persistent hypoglycemia <2.6 mmol/L (<42 mg/dL).[31] However, there was a very high prevalence of hypoglycemia lasting for a period of 3–30 days, and others undertaking longer follow up, to 15 years of age, of a cohort of infants <32-week gestation were not able to replicate this finding.[32] Duvanel reported that recurrent hypoglycemia was a more predictable factor for long-term effects than the severity of a single hypoglycemic episode.[33] These findings are not surprising as the clinical significance of any one glucose level is dependent on many other clinical variables, and the critical level below which brain injury may occur depends on the baby's energy demands and the balance of available fuels.

The clinical definition of hyperglycemia also remains controversial but is often defined as plasma glucose >8.3 mmol/L (150 mg/dL). Most neonatologists become concerned when plasma glucose concentration exceeds 10 mmol/L (180 mg/dL) or is associated with an osmotic diuresis, as this has been independently associated with worse outcomes.[34–36] Such levels are frequently observed in extremely preterm infants or more rarely may be a sign of neonatal diabetes.[37]

45.3.3 Timing and Transition

Hypoglycemia most commonly occurs in the first 24 h after birth and the majority of these episodes will be transient. The most common cause of transient hypoglycemia is failure of metabolic adaptation in the "at-risk" infant during the period of establishment of feeding. If hypoglycemia occurs after 48 h of life, it may be considered persistent and is likely to be due to more significant underlying pathology. Similarly, hyperglycemia is not uncommon in the setting of infection or "stress" when inflammatory mediators lead to a catabolic state with increased catecholamines and cortisol, suppression of insulin secretion, and increase in glucose levels. This transient response is a normal physiological response but if high glucose levels persist, they can be harmful.

45.4 HYPOGLYCEMIA IN THE NEWBORN

45.4.1 Clinical Approach to Hypoglycemia

Clinical manifestations of hypoglycemia are notoriously nonspecific in the newborn and infants can have extremely low blood glucose (BG) levels while being reported to be "asymptomatic." However, what is a normal BG for one baby may make another at risk from long-term neurological sequelae, due to coexistent pathology and increased metabolic vulnerability.[38–41] Symptoms such as change in neurological behavior, exaggerated Moro reflex, irritability, jitteriness, tremors, high-pitched cry, seizures, lethargy, or poor feeding should arouse suspicions of hypoglycemia. Other symptoms include cyanosis, hypothermia, apnea, and floppiness. A detailed history related to pregnancy (diabetes/diet/insulin), delivery (asphyxia), gestational age (SGA, LGA), and birth weight (low birth weight/macrosomia) is important in elucidating potential pathophysiology. Similarly, a family history of in utero demise may increase the likelihood of an inborn error of metabolism. Physical examination of the infant is valuable in identifying growth restriction or features such as macrosomia, macroglossia, ear pits, hemi-hypertrophy, and omphalocele that suggest Beckwith-Wiedemann syndrome. Midline defects, micropenis, and hypoglycemia point to congenital hypopituitarism. Hypoglycemia, dehydration, and shock in the presence of genital anomalies point to a diagnosis of congenital adrenal hyperplasia. Sudden cardiorespiratory collapse, acidosis, and hypoglycemia following feeds in an otherwise healthy neonate indicate a metabolic disorder.

45.4.2 Clinical Intervention and Investigation

Cornblath et al. suggested that immediate intervention should be taken for any infant with a BG <2.5 mmol/L and who shows neurological signs suggestive of hypoglycemia. In "at risk" (due to potential impaired counterregulation) but asymptomatic (or rather those without overt signs) patients, urgent interventions should be considered only after two consecutive BG levels <2.0 mmol/L, or with a single BG level <1.0 mmol/L. These thresholds have been reiterated by the recent British Association of Perinatal Medicine framework for practice. It is also highlighted that blood glucose levels <2.2 mmol/L, or >6.9 mmol/L after 48 h of life, are abnormal.[40,42] Further assessment and investigations must be undertaken to exclude endocrine or metabolic disease. It is imperative that alongside these investigations glucose levels are optimized to reduce the risk of neurological impairment. Detailed clinical assessment and screening investigations need to be performed urgently at the time of hypoglycemia if results such as insulin levels are to be interpretable.

45.5 TRANSIENT HYPOGLYCEMIA IN INFANTS AT RISK

Newborns exposed to an abnormal metabolic environment in utero can be at risk from transient hypoglycemia due to pancreatic hyperplasia and hyperinsulinism or limited alternative fuels such as ketones and lactate. Transient forms can follow preterm birth or appear in babies born SGA, growth restricted, or following perinatal stress/asphyxia or sepsis, or can be due to transient hyperinsulinism in infants of diabetic mothers (IDM).

45.5.1 Preterm

These infants have limited fat and protein stores related to prematurity and many of these babies are also growth restricted and have increased metabolic demands because of the relatively large head. A poor ketogenic response can also be related to immaturity of the normal homeostatic mechanisms, which may therefore result in hypoglycemia in these babies with a lack of alternative metabolic fuels.

45.5.2 Small for Gestational Age and Growth Restriction

The SGA baby's risk of hypoglycemia is multifactorial. If these babies are growth restricted, they will have limited fat and protein stores as well as increased demands because of the relatively large head and a poor ketogenic response related to low substrate levels. Studies of the endocrine status of SGA infants in the perinatal period have been inconsistent. This is likely to reflect the range of underlying pathologies encompassing the diagnosis of SGA. One study showed that SGA infants have lower blood glucose and insulin levels than appropriate for gestational age (AGA) infants, and higher glucose/insulin ratios.

SGA infants also had higher levels of insulin-like binding protein-1 (IGFBP-1), free fatty acids, and beta-hydroxy butyrate.[43] This demonstrates that these infants display increased insulin sensitivity with respect to glucose disposal but not with respect to suppression of lipolysis, ketogenesis, and hepatic production of IGFBP-1. This can be seen as advantageous in serving to ensure alternative energy sources are available for these neonates who have limited glucose reserves.[44] Normal insulin-glucose relationships have been reported by others in the setting of intrauterine growth restriction.[45,46]

Others have shown that both full-term and preterm SGA neonates had higher insulin concentrations, insulin-to-glucose ratios, triglycerides, total cholesterol, and low-density lipoprotein cholesterol concentrations than AGA neonates.[47] This is suggestive of lower insulin sensitivity and less favorable lipid metabolism in the early postnatal period. Hyperinsulinism and increased sensitivity to insulin and gluconeogenesis are limited by low cytosolic phosphoenolpyruvate carboxykinase (PEPCK) activity[48] reflected in higher concentration of gluconeogenic precursors, and limited mobilization and oxidation of fatty acids.

Hypoglycemia secondary to hyperinsulinism is usually transient, but some extremely growth-restricted infants occasionally require prolonged treatment (up to 9 months) with diazoxide and chlorothiazide.[49] The etiology of prolonged hypoglycemic hyperinsulinism in these growth-restricted babies appears to be a combination of lack of exogenous substrate supply, depletion of hepatic glycogen stores, defective gluconeogenesis, hyperinsulinism and increased sensitivity to insulin, and adrenocortical insufficiency. It has been shown that insulin sensitivity is reduced in the liver but increased in the periphery in these growth-restricted infants. Growth restriction may be secondary to congenital abnormalities such as Silver Russell syndrome, which may be caused by maternal uniparental disomy (mUPD) of chromosome 7 (5%–10%) or hypomethylation of the imprinting control region (ICR) 1 on chromosome 11p15 (60%).[50] However, the possible genetic etiology of prolonged hyperinsulinemic hypoglycemia due to growth restriction is still unclear. In contrast, babies born SGA who are constitutionally or genetically small or have not been growth restricted are not at the same risk of hypoglycemia. The causes of SGA births are described more in depth in Chapter 51.

45.5.3 Hypoxic-Ischemic Encephalopathy

Both hypoglycemia and hyperglycemia occur frequently in babies with hypoxic ischemic encephalopathy, with both being associated with an unfavorable outcome.[36] The etiology is likely to be multifactorial and secondary to severe metabolic and hormonal disruption.[51] In perinatal asphyxia, increasing metabolic and energy demands are achieved transiently by increasing glucose production through glycogenolysis.[52] Due to hypoxia, the infant switches to anaerobic metabolism, resulting in rapid exhaustion of glycogen stores, hypoglycemia, and lactic academia. The mechanism for hyperglycemia is likely to include an impaired insulin response, excessive hepatic glucose production with stress-induced increase in counterregulatory hormones. Animal models suggest that hypoglycemia worsens the effects of hypoxia by reducing brain glucose reserves, which attenuates anaerobic glycolysis, resulting in a reduction in high-energy phosphates.

45.5.4 Infants of Diabetic Mothers

If antenatal control of maternal diabetes has been poor, high maternal blood glucose levels may have induced fetal hyperinsulinism, which will persist after delivery and may result in an exaggerated and/or prolonged postnatal fall in glucose concentration. After delivery, the infant of a diabetic mother will no longer be receiving the maternal glucose supply and high insulin levels may also impair hormonal counterregulation with a blunted glucagon response.[53]

45.5.5 Large for Gestational Age Babies

There is debate as to whether babies who are LGA and not infants of diabetic mothers are at risk of hypoglycemia.[54] It is suggested that these babies may have hyperinsulinism secondary to undiagnosed maternal diabetes or prediabetes, or that there may be other insulin-like growth factors that lead to hypoglycemia.[55,56] While there are studies to support this, other studies have shown no difference in the incidence of hypoglycemia compared with healthy term AGA infants. When blood glucose levels are monitored "routinely" in these babies, the incidence of hypoglycemia has been reported to be 12%–16%, with the majority of babies being hypoglycemic in the first 4 h, when the blood glucose would be anticipated to be low even in AGA babies.[57] The causes of LGA newborns is discussed in Chapter 51.

45.5.6 Other Risk Factors

Other causes of transient hyperinsulinism immediately after delivery include the administration of intravenous glucose to mothers in labor and the use of drugs that may cause maternal (and hence fetal) hyperglycemia in pregnancy, such as maternal steroids or betamimetics (see previous). Transient dysregulation of other counterregulatory hormones are uncommon (glucagon, adrenaline, cortisol, and growth hormone). Rhesus hemolytic disease has been associated with fetal and neonatal hyperinsulinism, which may be the result of islet cell hyperplasia secondary to the release of metabolic by-products from lysed red blood cells, but the precise mechanism is unknown.[58] Cold stress is also associated with hypoglycemia, and should be avoided by encouraging skin-to-skin contact in a warm environment.

45.6 PERSISTENT OR SEVERE HYPOGLYCEMIA

The most common cause of persistent hypoglycemia is hyperinsulinemia (HH) caused by dysregulation of insulin secretion from pancreatic β cells. Other rarer disorders include hormonal dysregulation, such as hypopituitarism and adrenal insufficiency, leading to deficiencies in growth hormone and cortisol. Inborn errors of metabolism such as disorders of glycogen storage, fatty acid oxidation, and gluconeogenesis also require consideration and investigation. Sometimes there may be diagnostic clues such as hyperpigmentation of the skin, suggesting the diagnosis of familial glucocorticoid deficiency (FGD), or genital anomalies, but typically no other signs are present and extensive laboratory evaluation is required, guided by specialist advice.

45.6.1 Congenital Hyperinsulinism

Congenital hyperinsulinism (CHI) usually presents in the first few days after birth with symptomatic hypoglycemia. Symptoms of hypoglycemia are nonspecific, including hypotonia, cyanosis, hypothermia, and abnormal movements before evolving into increased irritability, poor feeding, and lethargy, and may progress to seizures or coma. Due to in utero exposure to high insulin levels, babies may be macrosomic or have facial dysmorphism, but lack of these features does not exclude the diagnosis. Diagnosis should be suspected if there is a glucose requirement of >8 mg/kg/min and is confirmed if in the presence of hypoglycemia (BG < 2.6 mmol/L (<42 mg/dL)), and there is still detectable plasma insulin and/or C-peptide. In this setting there are low plasma levels of ketone bodies, FFAs, and branched chain amino acids, making these infants at increased risk from hypoglycemia. Initial intervention should be to support glucose levels with intravenous dextrose and this often requires central access to allow the use of high concentrations of dextrose solutions, to provide adequately for demands while avoiding fluid overload. The first choice of medication is diazoxide (which should always be given with chlorothiazide to counteract the fluid retention caused by diazoxide), with octreotide and nifedipine as second line if the former is ineffective.

In about 50% of cases of CHI a genetic basis can be determined, with 9 different genes (*ABCC8, KCNJ11, GLD1, GCK, HADH, SLC16A1, HNF4A, HNF1A* and *UCP2*) having been identified in which abnormalities can lead to unregulated insulin secretion. These mutations either have a direct effect on the β-cell adenosine triphosphate (ATP)-sensitive potassium channel, or impact on increased ATP generation in the β cell with indirect effects. Most cases of the diffuse form of CHI are inherited in an autosomal recessive pattern, although less frequently it may involve an autosomal dominant pattern. In contrast, the inheritance of the focal form of CHI is more complex. In these cases, two independent events are required: first a paternally inherited mutation in *ABCC8* or *KCNJ11* gene and then a somatic loss of function mutation in the maternal allele within the affected cells, thus leading to a focal pattern of pathology.

The most common mutations identified involve genes located on Chr 11p15.1, where the SUR (β-cell sulphonylurea receptor *ABCC8*) gene (50% of genetic cases), and KIR6.2 (β-cell K+ inward rectifier channel *KCNJ11*) gene (10% of genetic cases) are situated. Mutations in these genes *ABCC8* and *KCNJ11*, which encode the two subunits of the β-cell ATP-sensitive potassium channel, have a variable effect on channel activity. Mutations inactivating the K_{ATP} channels leave the voltage-dependent calcium channels open continuously, resulting in continuous insulin release.

There are also a collection of genetic mutations that impact on insulin secretion by affecting the glucose-sensing mechanisms that control insulin secretion. These include activating mutations in the gene encoding glucokinase (*GCK*) as glucokinase is a key regulator of glucose stimulated insulin secretion by the pancreas. Glucokinase phosphorylates glucose and increases ATP with the increase in the ATP: adenosine triphosphate (ADP) ratio leading to closure of the K_{ATP} channel and unregulated secretion of insulin. In these cases, there is a reduced threshold for insulin secretion to be switched off, i.e., the blood glucose has to fall to a lower level than normal before insulin secretion is switched off. Hypoglycemia is usually milder and inheritance is autosomal dominant. Uncoupling proteins regulate ATP production by uncoupling oxidative phosphorylation and lowering ATP production. Therefore loss of function mutations will increase ATP synthesis and glucose-sensitive insulin secretion. The *HNF4A* gene encodes for a nuclear transcription factor that controls the expression of several genes, including hepatocyte nuclear factor 1 alpha, a transcription factor that regulates the expression of several hepatic genes and also impacts on glucose-stimulated insulin secretion. There are other rarer mutations such as *GLUD1* mutations that impact on glutamate dehydrogenase expression and are classically associated with postprandial hypoglycemia and hyperammonia, *HADH* (gene for Hydroxyacyl-CoA Dehydrogenase) mutations that have been associated with protein (leucine) induced hyperinsulinemic hypoglycemia, and activating mutations in the *SLC16A1* gene, which codes for a monocarboxylic acid transporter that can lead to increased insulin secretion in response to exercise.

Differentiation between diffuse and focal forms of CHI is not possible on clinical presentation alone but is important, as focal lesions can be excised discretely, avoiding the long-term complications of subtotal (95%) pancreatectomy. There is also no easy diagnostic test that can distinguish between the two forms. Routine imaging (USS, CT, MRI) is not helpful. Pancreatic venous sampling can be performed to map the site of the lesions using the concentrations of insulin in the head, body, and tail of the pancreas, but has been superseded by [18]Fluoro-dopa PET (positron emission tomography) scanning and pancreatic biopsy. PET scanning can delineate a focus/foci and is sometimes performed with simultaneous CT or MRI to enhance anatomical localization. PET scanning can also identify an ectopic pancreatic focus. There are currently about 10 centers worldwide performing PET scanning. Laparoscopic biopsy of the tail of the pancreas provides histological information but can be difficult to interpret, particularly in diffuse disease. If focal disease is identified, then the focus is removed surgically. With diffuse disease conservative management may be tried, on the basis that diffuse disease may burn itself out over time (although this may take 5 years or longer). Even children who have not had a pancreatic resection occasionally go on to develop diabetes, suggesting either an excessive apoptotic process in the β cells, and/or that the β cells remain "blind" to glucose.

Most infants with HH have no other abnormal clinical signs, but the condition is associated with several recognizable syndromes including Beckwith-Wiedemann syndrome, Turner's syndrome, Costello syndrome, Prader-Willi syndrome, and Sotos syndrome. Other features of Beckwith-Wiedemann syndrome include macrosomia, visceromegaly, macroglossia, exomphalos or umbilical hernia, hemihypertrophy, ear creases; these infants also need to be monitored for a later risk of Wilms' tumor and hepatoblastoma. The hypoglycemia secondary to the hyperinsulinism is usually apparent in the early neonatal period and resolves within a few weeks.[59] Careful clinical examination and involvement of a clinical geneticist and genetic testing can be helpful in evaluating longer term prognosis.

45.6.2 Disorders of Carbohydrate Metabolism/Inborn Errors of Metabolism

Unexpected hypoglycemia in the newborn may be one of the presenting features of an inborn error of metabolism, including defects in gluconeogenesis but also fatty acid oxidation defects, mitochondrial disorders, disorders of amino acid metabolism, and some organic acidurias. Assessment of the constellation of other symptoms and signs related to deficiency or excess of intermediate metabolites helps to guide the diagnosis. Following we highlight some rare but more common inborn errors of metabolism. However, obtaining early specialist advice about recent developments in investigations and management is important to optimize the care of babies with a suspected inborn error of metabolism.

45.6.2.1 Galactosemia

Symptoms appear in the second half of the first week and include refusal to feed, vomiting, jaundice, and lethargy and it is important that milk feeds are stopped until the diagnosis is excluded. Hepatomegaly, edema, and ascites may follow but on withholding milk, galactosuria ceases, but excess amino acids continue to be excreted for a few days. Galactosemia is an autosomal recessive inborn error of carbohydrate metabolism caused by a defect in one of the enzymes in galactose metabolism galactokinase (GALK), galactose-1-phosphate uridylyltransferase (GALT), and UDP-galactose 4-epimerase (GALE). Classical galactosemia, caused by GALT, is the most frequent and most severe of the three enzyme deficiencies and is life-threatening in the newborn period. It presents in the first week of life once milk feeds have commenced with vomiting and feed intolerance, hypoglycemia, and jaundice. Neurological symptoms (hypotonia) and cataracts may be present and *Escherichia coli* sepsis occurs in up to 40%, often starting as a urinary tract infection, and there may be renal tubular dysfunction. The gold standard for diagnosis of classical galactosemia is measurement of GALT activity in erythrocytes. Gas-chromatographic determination of urinary sugars and sugar alcohols demonstrates elevated concentrations of galactose and galactitol. Treatment is dietary restriction of lactose as soon as the diagnosis is suspected and replacement with a soya-based formula. Although this results in recovery of liver dysfunction and regression of cataracts, neurodevelopmental outcome is poor with learning difficulties and motor symptoms, most commonly tremor and dystonia, as well as cerebellar signs.[60,61]

45.6.2.2 Fructose-1,6-Diphosphatase (or Biphosphatase) Deficiency

Fructose-1,6-biphosphatase deficiency is a rare autosomal recessive disorder with an incidence between 1/350,000 and 1/900,000.[62] Symptoms usually present early in postnatal life and include hyperventilation, hypoglycemia, severe lactic acidosis, hepatomegaly, and hypotonia, and these infants can deteriorate rapidly with apnea, coma, and death. In later infancy, hypoglycemic episodes are triggered by fasting or intercurrent infections. As gluconeogenesis is severely impaired, in addition to hypoglycemia, there is accumulation of gluconeogenic precursors (lactate, amino acids, and ketones) and there is increased urinary glycerol excretion (picked up on urinary organic acid analysis). Patients do not vomit after ingesting fructose or develop an aversion to sweets (unlike hereditary fructose intolerance). The diagnosis is made on enzyme activity measurement on mononuclear white blood cells and mutation analysis.[62] Treatment is avoidance of fasting and avoiding fructose-containing food and glycerol. Acute crises usually respond to intravenous glucose.

45.6.2.3 Glycogen Storage Diseases

Glycogen storage disease (GSD) type 0 is an autosomal recessive disease caused by deficiency of the hepatic isoform of glycogen sythase. Mutations in (*GYS2*) cause fasting hypoglycemia, high levels of ketones and free fatty acids, and low levels of alanine and lactate, usually presenting in infancy or early childhood. In contrast to the classic glycogen storage diseases, the liver is not enlarged and hypoglycemia is typically milder than other types of GSD. Muscle symptoms are not prominent. Most children are cognitively and developmentally normal. The inability to synthesize hepatic glycogen results in postprandial hyperglycemia, hyperlactatemia, and hyperlipidemia as glucose shifts from glycogenesis to the glycolytic pathway. Molecular analysis of the affected gene (*GYS2*) has replaced the need of measuring glycogen synthase activity in a liver biopsy to make the diagnosis.[63] Management includes preventing hypoglycemia by the use of frequent feeds and uncooked cornstarch may be used to reduce overnight hypoglycemia.

All variants of GSD type I can present in the neonatal period with profound hypoglycemia. The two main subtypes are GSD-Ia, caused by a deficiency of glucose-6-phosphatase (G6Pase), and GSD-Ib, which together maintain glucose homeostasis. In addition to hypoglycemia, there is lactic acidosis, hyperuricemia and hyperlipidemia as well as hepatomegaly and nephromegaly. Diagnosis is by mutation analysis (which has replaced liver biopsy). Hypoglycemia is managed by frequent daytime feeds and continuous overnight nasogastric support. Patients with GSD-Ib also have chronic neutropenia and functional deficiencies of neutrophils and monocytes, which is treated with granulocyte colony stimulating factor to restore myeloid function.[64]

45.6.2.4 Maple Syrup Urine Disease

This is a rare autosomal recessive disorder caused by a pathogenic variation in genes encoding the E1alpha, E1beta, and E2 subunits of the branched-chain alpha-ketoacid dehydrogenase enzyme complex, resulting in elevated levels of the branch-chain amino acids (valine, leucine, and isoleucine) in blood and urine as well as their corresponding alpha-ketoacids. The pathognomonic disease marker is the production of alloisoleucine. Although the clinical spectrum is broad, the classical presentation is with vomiting and encephalopathy (feeding difficulties, lethargy, seizures, apnea, dystonia, coma) in the neonatal period.[65] In addition to ketosis, these babies are often hypoglycemic with mildly elevated ammonia levels. Treatment is by restriction of branched-chain amino acids in the diet.[65]

45.6.3 Deficiencies of Counterregulatory Hormones

Hypothalamic pituitary dysfunction in the neonate can present with hypoglycemia, which may be associated with prolonged jaundice, and micropenis. It is the deficiency in adrenocorticotropic hormone (ACTH) leading to adrenal insufficiency, with a lack of production of glucocorticoids such as cortisol by the adrenal gland, that is the cause of hypoglycemia. Congenital hypopituitarism may be the result of complications around delivery, or holoprosencephaly, or it may be the result of hypoplasia of the gland, sometimes in the context of specific genetic abnormalities. Mutations may cause either insufficient development of the gland or decreased function. Hormone deficiencies may be isolated, involving the somatotrophes (*GH1*, *GHRHR*) and the corticotrophes (*TPIT*) or multiple and may be the result of mutations in any of the genes involved in pituitary development. Forms of combined pituitary hormone deficiency ("CPHD") include septic optic dysplasia (CPHD5, due to a mutation in the *HESX1* gene), which is associated with midline defects but may be caused by mutations in a number of other genes, including *POU1F1, PROP1, LHX3, and LHX4*.[66] A discussion of the clinical presentation and genetics of these disorders can be found in Chapter 42.

Severe primary adrenal disease, caused by congenital adrenal hyperplasia (a defect in an enzyme involved in cortisol synthesis), aplasia or hypoplasia of the adrenal gland, or adrenal hemorrhage, which lead to primary cortisol deficiency, may also cause hypoglycemia.[67] Cortisol deficiency leads to diminished liver glycogen reserves as well as impaired release of amino acids from skeletal muscle for hepatic gluconeogenesis. Congenital adrenal hyperplasia may be associated with genital anomalies (virilization of females and undervirilization of males) as well as electrolyte disturbance (hyperkalemia and hyponatremia) depending on the site of the enzyme block. (See also Chapter 47 for a complete discussion of causes of hypocortisolemia in the neonate.)

Primary hypothyroidism may cause hypoglycemia in the neonatal period. In the newborn, the growth hormone-insulin-like growth factor I axis is closely related to feeding.[68] Glucagon deficiency resulting in neonatal hypoglycemia has been described but is very rare.[69] Decreased adrenomedullary function may also be a feature of maternal or neonatal β-blocker use and should be considered if there is a family history of dysautonomia.

45.7 HYPERGLYCEMIA IN THE NEWBORN

45.7.1 Prematurity

The frequency of hyperglycemia in preterm infants has been reported to vary between 20%–86%[70–72] and can be considered the result of the inadequate insulin response to the insulin resistance found at this time; the potential role of insulin in management in the early neonatal period has been reviewed.[73]

45.7.1.1 Pathology

45.7.1.1.1 Central Insulin Resistance: Hepatic Glucose Production

Although glucose infusions of 6 mg/kg/min completely suppress endogenous glucose production in the adult, they fail to suppress glucose production in the preterm newborn.[74] Farrag reported that complete suppression of glucose production in the preterm infant was not present until glucose levels were > 13.9 mmol/L (250 mg/dL), and at a glucose infusion rate of 16 mg/kg/min.[75] It has been suggested that suppression of endogenous glucose production may be incomplete if glucose is the sole substrate infused, without the addition of either amino acids or lipid augmenting insulin secretion and the suppression of endogenous glucose production.[76,77] In the mature hepatocyte, the GLUT 2 glucose transporters tightly regulate glucose release in response to increases in glucose and insulin.[78] However, GLUT 2 levels only increase after birth,[79] and the low levels of GLUT2 may result in the lack of sensitivity of the preterm infant to hyperglycemia, resulting in insulin resistance and continued hepatic glucose production.

45.7.1.1.2 Peripheral Insulin Resistance

GLUT4 expression in muscle is lower in the newborn than in the adult and this may result in reduced insulin mediated glucose uptake by muscle and adipocytes.[80] In contrast to the marked insulin responsiveness in adults, with upregulation of GLUT 4 transporters, normal fetal rat muscle GLUT 4 transporters only respond modestly to insulin.[81] Additionally, insulin sensitive tissues such as adipose tissue and skeletal muscle are less abundant in preterm infants than in term infants.[82]

45.7.1.1.3 Relative Insulin Deficiency

There are a number of different reasons why insulin secretion may be impaired in the preterm infant and result in an inability to compensate for any insulin resistance, leading to hyperglycemia. In utero studies suggest that there is a steady increase in insulin levels towards term[83] and immaturity of the β cells may result in insufficient insulin secretion. Comparisons of the insulin response to a 30-min glucose infusion in term and preterm infants demonstrated that the preterm infant's insulin response was reduced compared with the term infant.[84] The response increased postnatally, but some preterm infants were only fully responsive 18 weeks postnatally.[84] In preterm infants the pancreas responds to increasing glucose levels by secretion of both insulin and proinsulin.[85] Proinsulin is 10-fold less active than mature insulin and is not able to control blood glucose levels.[86] Some assays do not adequately distinguish insulin from proinsulin and this may explain the very variable insulin levels and poor relationship between glucose and insulin levels often reported in the newborn.[85]

Feeding and Incretins In the preterm infant there is often a delay in the normal establishment of enteral feeds, and the provision of glucose via the intravenous route means that the normal postnatal association of nutritional delivery with stimulation of incretins does not occur.[87] The role for incretins in the newborn has not been well studied, but in adults it is clear that incretins play an important role in augmenting insulin secretion postprandially.[88,89] Studies in the newborn lamb have shown increased insulin release in response to an oral glucose load compared to one given intravenously.[90] In the preterm infant, glucose control often improves once enteral feeds have been established, and the lack of enteral stimulation may add to the relative insulin deficiency.[91] Even when enteral feeds are given, preterm infants do not demonstrate an equivalent incretin response to that seen in term infants.[92] Regular boluses of milk result in cyclical hormonal responses to feeding that may be important in adaptation to glucose control in postnatal life.[87]

Growth Restriction Some infants born preterm will also be growth restricted and animal studies have shown growth restriction to be associated with reduced β-cell mass.[93,94] However, these changes seem dependent on the model and timing of growth restriction[95] and data from human studies has not confirmed these findings compared with appropriately grown infants.[96]

Pancreatic Glucose Sensitivity GLUT 2 is involved in glucose transport in the liver and in glucose-stimulated insulin secretion from the pancreas.[97] Hepatic GLUT 2 transporters increase dramatically shortly after birth and at the time of weaning.[98] In rats GLUT 2 content of the fetal pancreas is about half that of adults.[99] Human fetal pancreatic β cells do not express GLUT 2 until 7 months.[100] In the pancreatic β cell, GLUT2 acts as a glucose sensor that detects small changes in glucose levels leading to increased insulin secretion. The lack of GLUT2 transporters in the immature pancreas is likely to impact on the β cell's response to hyperglycemia, and it has been demonstrated that the insulin secretory response to glucose is age related[74] (Fig. 45.2).

45.7.1.2 Clinical Consequences

Transient hyperglycemia may be beneficial in the acute stress response but prolonged hyperglycemia in critical illness has been associated with a poor prognosis.[101–103] It has been suggested that by causing a significant osmotic diuresis and hence electrolyte imbalance, hyperglycemia may lead to an increased risk of intraventricular hemorrhage (IVH).[101,104,105] Additionally, morbidities such as retinopathy of prematurity (ROP), necrotizing enterocolitis (NEC),[34] and neonatal sepsis[106] have been associated with neonatal hyperglycemia,[103,107,108] and have been linked to longer hospital admission.[34,101–103]

Hays et al. (2006) performed a retrospective study ($n = 82$) and examined the outcome of death or severe IVH before 10 days. They found an association, after adjusting for oxygen requirement and CRIB score, between death or IVH and hyperglycemia. Kao et al. (2006) in a cohort of 201 extremely low birthweight (ELBW) infants found that, after adjustment for gestational age, early hyperglycemia increased the risk of death or sepsis, OR 5.07 (95% CI 1.06 to 24.3). Persistent hyperglycemia was also associated with NEC, OR 9.49 (95% CI 1.52 to 59.3). The relationship with IVH was not examined.[102] Blanco et al. (2006) investigated the data from a cohort of 169 ELBW infants and found 88% of the infants to have hyperglycemia (>10 mmol/L) during the first 2 weeks of life.[103] However, no association between death or IVH and hyperglycemia was found after adjusting for age, birth weight, and postnatal steroids although there was an association with ROP OR 4.6 (95% CI 1.12 to 18.9).

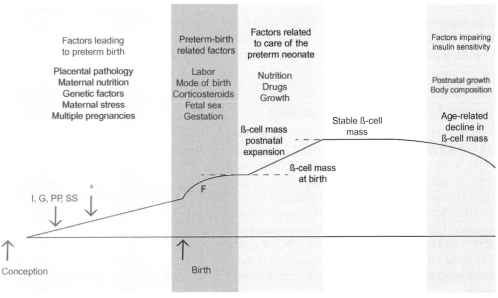

FIG. 45.2 Factors related to preterm birth that may affect β-cell mass and glucose control.

The mechanisms underlying the relationship between hyperglycemia and mortality and morbidity remain to be established. Hyperglycemia itself can be harmful to cells but is also a marker of relative insulin deficiency, and insulin has a number of independent actions that may impact on clinical outcomes.

45.7.1.2.1 Primary Role of Hyperglycemia

Hyperglycemia is harmful to cells and can lead to an overexpression of insulin independent glucose transporters (GLUT-1, GLUT-2, and GLUT 3), which leads to an increase in glucose uptake by endothelial, hepatic, immune, and nerve cells.[109] This glucose overload can cause an increased generation of oxygen free radicals, which can cause mitochondrial dysfunction and increased apoptosis.[110] Ellger et al. independently manipulated blood glucose and insulin levels in a burn injured parenterally fed rabbit model to determine the importance of glucose control, versus insulin independent actions of insulin, and demonstrated survival to be better in the normoglycemic groups.[111] Hyperglycemia also impairs leukocyte phagocytic function,[112] increases a number of proinflammatory cytokines,[113] and impairs neutrophil chemotaxis.[114]

45.7.1.2.2 Relative Insulin Deficiency

In both animal and human models insulin has been shown to improve innate immunity and suppress proinflammatory products while increasing antiinflammatory cytokines.[115–119] One mechanism of insulin action may be through increased expression of nitric oxide synthase (iNOS), and therefore increased nitric oxide.[114,120] In adult studies it has been found that there was suppression of iNOS by intensive insulin intervention,[121] suggesting a protective effect of insulin by prevention of excess nitric oxide release. In an animal burns model, insulin improved cardiac function[111] and in patients postmyocardial infarction and in sepsis the combination of glucose and insulin infusions improve cardiac function.[122] Insulin infusions can reduce proteolysis and in burns have a positive impact on protein synthesis and wound healing.[123–125]

45.7.1.2.3 Association with Impaired IGF-I Generation

Hyperglycemia may also be related to low insulin-like growth factor (IGF) levels, which are important mediators of growth in utero and in the neonatal period. IGF-I synthesis by the liver requires normal portal insulin levels.[126] In adults and children, starvation and critical illness[127] lead to suppression of IGF-I levels, and IGF-I administration has been shown to increase nitrogen balance in catabolic states such as starvation[128] and in patients with acquired immune deficiency.[129] This is likely to be important in preterm infants.

45.7.2 Neonatal Diabetes Mellitus

Neonatal diabetes mellitus (NDM), defined as persistent hyperglycemia in the first 6 months of life, is a rare disease that occurs in approximately 1 in 300,000–400,000 live births and is associated with a clinical picture of growth restriction and polyuria. It can be classified as either transient (TNDM) (50%–60% of cases), which disappears in the first 6 months but may reappear later in life, or permanent (PNDM), which persists throughout infancy into childhood. Although TNDM and PNDM cannot be distinguished on clinical features alone, certain features are more prominent in cases with TNDM (Table 45.1).[37]

45.7.2.1 Transient Neonatal Diabetes Mellitus

Transient neonatal diabetes mellitus typically presents within the first few days to weeks of life (earlier than PNDM) with features of IUGR (which are less prominent in PNDM). The insulin requirements of TNDM infants are often lower than in PNDM and resolve at an average age of 12 weeks. Relapses occur in 50% of cases (usually during childhood or young adulthood at a median age of 14 years) and coincide with a period of increased insulin demand such as puberty or pregnancy. The majority of cases (70%) of TNDM are caused by defects in imprinted genes in chromosome 6q24 and lead to overexpression of the chromosomal regions 6q24. Three mechanisms have been identified to cause 6q24-related TNDM: uniparental isodisomy (UPD), an inherited duplication of 6q24 and maternal DNA methylation. In addition, a small number of cases of TNDM can be caused by KCNJ11 or ABCC8 mutations that encode the K_{ATP} channel. Other rarer causes include mutations in the HNF-1B and recessive mutations in the INS gene encoding insulin that leads to decreased insulin biosynthesis. Although called "transient" it is likely to be a permanent β-cell defect with variable expression during development and growth.

TABLE 45.1 All known monogenic causes of neonatal diabetes with associated features, from more common to less common (top to bottom)

Gene	Transient vs. permanent	Inheritance	Features	Treatment
KCNJ11	Either	Spontaneous (80%), AD (20%)	Low birthweight, developmental delay, seizures (DEND syndrome), may have other neurologic features	Insulin SU
ABCC8	Either	Spontaneous, AD	Low birthweight	Insulin SU
6q24	Transient	Spontaneous, AD for paternal duplications	Low birthweight, possible IUGR, diagnosed earlier than channel mutations (closer to birth), relapsed cases may respond to SU	Insulin
INS	Either	Spontaneous (80%), AD (20%) AR (rare: T or P)	Low birthweight	Insulin
GATA6	Permanent	Spontaneous, AD	Pancreatic hypoplasia or agenesis, exocrine insufficiency, cardiac defect	Insulin
EIF2AK3[a]	Permanent	Spontaneous, AR	Wolcott-Rallison syndrome, skeletal dysplasia (1–2 year old) Episodic acute liver failure, exocrine pancreatic insufficiency	Insulin
GCK[a]	Permanent	Spontaneous, AR (neonatal diabetes), AD (GCK-MODY)	Low birthweight	Insulin
PTF1A	Permanent	Spontaneous, AR	Neurologic abnormalities, exocrine insufficiency, kidney involvement	Insulin
FOXP3	Permanent	X-linked	Autoimmune thyroid disease, exfoliative dermatitis, enteropathy (IPEX syndrome)	Insulin
ZFP57	Transient	Spontaneous, maternal Hypomethylation Imprinting	Variable phenotype Low birthweight, macroglossia, developmental delay	Insulin
GLIS3[a]	Permanent	Spontaneous, AR	Hypothyroidism, kidney cysts, glaucoma, hepatic fibrosis	Insulin
PDX1	Permanent	Spontaneous, AR (neonatal diabetes), AD (PDX1-MODY)	Pancreatic hypoplasia or agenesis, exocrine insufficiency	Insulin
SLC2A2	Either	Spontaneous, AR	Fanconi-Bickel syndrome (hepatomegaly, RTA)	Insulin
SLC19A2	Permanent	Spontaneous, AR	Neurologic deficit (stroke, seizure) Visual disturbance; cardiac abnormality	Insulin Thiamine (rarely)
GATA4	Permanent	Spontaneous, AR	Pancreatic hypoplasia or agenesis, exocrine insufficiency, cardiac defect	Insulin
NEUROD1	Permanent	Spontaneous, AR	Neurologic abnormalities (later), learning difficulties, sensorineural deafness	Insulin
NEUROG3	Permanent	Spontaneous, AR	Diarrhea (due to lack of enteroendocrine cells)	Insulin
NKX2-2	Permanent		Neurologic abnormalities (later), very low birthweight	Insulin
RFX6[a]	Permanent	Spontaneous, AR	Low birthweight, intestinal atresia, gallbladder hypoplasia, diarrhea	Insulin
IER3IP1[a]	Permanent	Spontaneous, AR	Microcephaly, infantile epileptic encephalopathy	Insulin
MNX1[a]	Permanent	Spontaneous, AR	Neurologic abnormalities (later)	Insulin
HNF1B	Transient	Spontaneous, AD	Pancreatic atrophy, abnormal kidney, and genitalia development	Insulin

Abbreviations: *AD*, autosomal dominant; *AR*, autosomal recessive; *DEND*, developmental delay, epilepsy, and neonatal diabetes; *DM*, diabetes mellitus; *IUGR*, intrauterine growth restriction; *MODY*, maturity onset diabetes of the young; *RTA*, renal tubular acidosis; *SGA*, small for gestational age.
[a]*Autosomal recessive forms may be more likely in populations or families with known consanguinity.*

45.7.2.2 Permanent Neonatal Diabetes Mellitus

Approximately 50% of permanent neonatal diabetes mellitus are associated with β-cell potassium channel defects caused by mutations in KCNJ11 and ABCC8. KCNJ11 encodes Kir6.2 (a protein coding gene in the potassium channel) and ABCC8 encodes the gene SUR1 (the type 1 subunit of the sulfonylurea receptor), the two components of the K_{ATP} channel. This channel links glucose metabolism to insulin secretion by closing in response to increased ATP levels. Increased blood glucose levels and transport into the β cell leads to increased glycolysis and increased ATP generation. The elevated ATP/ADP ratio causes closure of the K_{ATP} channel and inhibits potassium efflux, which leads to depolarization of the βcell membrane. Calcium flows into the cell where there is exocytosis of insulin-containing granules.

Mutations of the KCNJ11 or ABCC8 genes make the K_{ATP} channel less sensitive and result in more channels being in an open state, therefore preventing cell depolarization and insulin secretion, despite high levels of glucose (Fig. 45.3). Identification of these mutations as causative is critical, as it means that patients will be sensitive to treatment with sulfonylureas as they bind to the SUR1 subunits of the KATP channel and close the channel in an ATP-dependent manner. This causes cell membrane depolarization and insulin secretion and patients can be weaned off insulin. Studies have shown that, despite tolerance developing in patients with type 2 diabetes mellitus, sulphonylureas can be used long term with good effect in the majority of patients with PNDM who are responsive.[130] Other causes of PNDM include genes encoding GCK, insulin promoter factor 1, and pancreas transcription factor 1 alpha.

45.7.2.3 Treatment and Prognosis

Although primary management requires the use of insulin, this can be challenging due to the small doses required and variable insulin sensitivity. Treatment of hyperglycemia with insulin can easily result in hypoglycemia. Continuous insulin pump therapy has been found to be a solution to some of these challenges.[132] Once a genetic diagnosis has been made it may be possible (if the defect is due to a mutation in a gene for the KATP channel) for infants to be transitioned onto oral

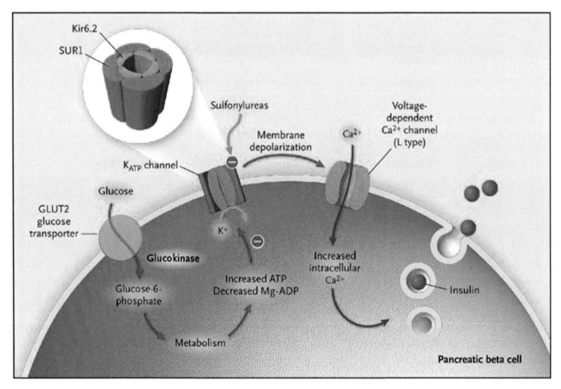

FIG. 45.3 Schematic representation of the pancreatic β cell, illustrating the role of the ATP-sensitive potassium (K_{ATP}) channel in insulin secretion. Glucose enters the β cell by way of the GLUT2 glucose transporter. Once inside the cell, glucose is metabolized, leading to changes in the intracellular concentration of adenine nucleotides that inhibit the K_{ATP} channel and thus cause channel closure. The K_{ATP} channel consists of four sulphonylurea-receptor (SUR1) subunits and four Kir6.2 subunits in an octomeric structure. Channel closure leads to membrane depolarization, which subsequently activates voltage-dependent calcium (Ca^{2+}) channels, leading in turn to an increase in intracellular Ca^{2+}, which triggers insulin exocytosis. Sulphonylureas initiate secretion by directly binding to the SUR1 subunits of K_{ATP} channels and causing channel closure. Mg-ADP denotes magnesium ADP.[131]

sulphonylureas such as Glibenclamide. Long-term follow-up of all cases is important to prevent acute and long-term complications. The course and severity is dependent on the genetic cause; some patients with PNDM secondary to KATP channel mutations have associated neurological features, developmental delay, and epilepsy believed to be related to the effect of the mutation in the brain.

45.8 LONG-TERM CONSEQUENCES: PROGRAMMING OF GLUCOSE METABOLISM

The work of Barker and colleagues in the 1980s showed that early life had a significant impact on long-term health and chronic diseases. Recent studies have tried to elucidate the underlying mechanisms that lead to this finding and the evolving concept of fetal origins of adult disease. It has been shown that physiological adaptation to the in utero and postnatal environment, related to reduced or excess nutrient delivery, can alter organ development and endocrine function. The adaptation may be optimal for the current physiological environment but with different environmental pressures later in life these adaptations may not be beneficial and can lead to altered glucose, insulin, and lipid metabolism. These effects may not be immediately apparent but have been associated with early programming and increased adiposity and insulin resistance, high blood pressure, and type 2 diabetes in later life (Fig. 45.4).

Animal models have demonstrated remodeling of the pancreas after birth and at the time of weaning, with increased levels of apoptosis and βcell neogenesis associated with hypoinsulinemia.[133–136] IGF-I has been associated with increased proliferation of precursor β cells,[137] and the period of apoptosis occurs at the same time as a significant fall in the levels of IGF-II expression.[138] Overexpression of IGF-II and IGF-I can lead to a reduction in the level of apoptosis, suggesting a protective role.[139,140] Postmortem studies in humans have shown similar increases in apoptosis in the perinatal period.[141] In addition it has been suggested that the secretion of incretins in response to enteral feeds may influence βcell neogenesis with the establishment of a population of cells that is nonproliferative and better suited to metabolic control in postnatal life.[142] Adaptive changes in insulin secretion have been shown with alteration in the neonatal diet.[143] The perinatal period may therefore be a critical time for programming of the endocrine pancreas. Interference with this process of remodeling may have a significant impact on the ability of the pancreas to meet requirements for insulin secretion both perinatally and in later life (Fig. 45.5).[144]

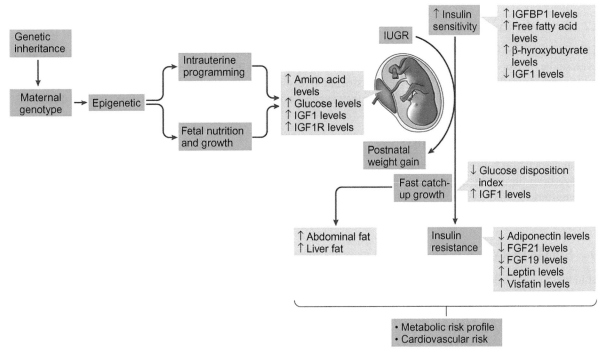

FIG. 45.4 Risk of diabetes in later life: relationship between size at birth and later lifestyle. *(Reproduced with permission from Wells JCK. The Metabolic Ghetto. An evolutionary perspective on nutrition, power relations and chronic disease. UK: Cambridge University Press; 2016.)*

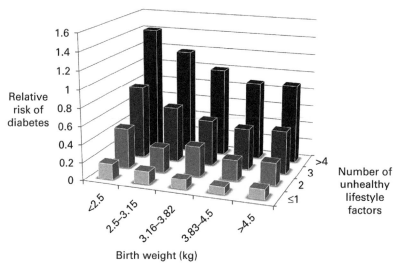

FIG. 45.5   The fetal insulin hypothesis and risk of metabolic disease. *(Reproduced with permission from Mericq V, Martinez-Aguayo A, Uauy R, Iñiguez G, Van der Steen M, Hokken-Koelega A. Long-term metabolic risk among children born premature or small for gestational age.* Nat Rev Endocrinol *2017;**13**(1):50–62. https://doi.org/10.1038/nrendo.2016.127.)*

45.8.1   Small for Gestational Age

SGA individuals' increased risk of metabolic disease in later life most likely reflects the association with growth restriction; those with greatest weight gains having the highest incidences of cardiovascular disease, hypertension, and type 2 diabetes mellitus. Critical to the risk of developing glucose intolerance is the relationship between insulin sensitivity and compensatory insulin secretion. The reduced disposition index (the product of insulin secretion and sensitivity) in SGA children at 3 years of age may indicate early deficiency in their first phase insulin response. In the ALSPAC cohort the compensatory increased insulin secretion for the degree of insulin resistance was related to height gain and IGF-I levels and it is possible that the insulin secretion response in relation to growth hormone mediated insulin resistance could be a factor in promoting early catch-up growth, particularly growth in length.

45.8.2   Prematurity

Population studies in the UK and Australia have shown 17%–43% increased risk of type I diabetes following preterm birth.[145,146] However, studies in Norway[147] and Europe[148] did not show this association, although these studies were smaller and did not go beyond 15 years of age. There is also evidence of an association between preterm birth and type 2 diabetes. Although studies are small and do not show consistent findings, together they suggest a 50% increased risk of developing type I diabetes.[149–155]

45.8.3   Infants of Diabetic Mothers

There is an association between maternal gestational diabetes and offspring's insulin resistance in later childhood. Most studies have been limited by a retrospective study design and lack of controlling for multiple confounders. However, a prospective study of children exposed to maternal GDM, in utero hyperinsulinemia predicted children's abnormal glucose tolerance at 8 and 15 years of age.[156–158]

45.9   SUMMARY

Whilst in utero glucose delivery to the growing fetus is normally well controlled, chronic exposure to either hypoglycemia or hyperglycemia can lead to metabolic adaptation. This can lead to impaired metabolic counterregulation immediately after birth, with infants at risk from hypoglycemia, the commonest metabolic abnormality in the newborn. Although hypoglycemia is usually transient, there are a range of metabolic disorders that can present immediately after birth and early identification and intervention is critical to avoid long-term harm. Hyperglycemia occurs frequently in extremely preterm infants but is rare in term babies and may indicate neonatal diabetes. There is also increasing evidence that the perinatal metabolic environment is important in programming risk of adverse cardiometabolic outcomes in later life.

REFERENCES

1. Armitage JA, Poston L, Taylor PD. Developmental origins of obesity and the metabolic syndrome: the role of maternal obesity. *Front Horm Res* 2008;**36**:73–84. https://doi.org/10.1159/0000115355.

2. Heerwagen MJ, Miller MR, Barbour LA, et al. Maternal obesity and fetal metabolic programming: a fertile epigenetic soil. *Am J Physiol Regul Integr Comp Physiol* 2010;**299**(3):R711–22. https://doi.org/10.1152/ajpregu.00310.2010.

3. Illsley NP. Glucose transporters in the human placenta. *Placenta* 2000;**21**(1):14–22.

4. Artal R, Doug N, Wu P, et al. Circulating catecholamines and glucagon in infants of strictly controlled diabetic mothers. *Biol Neonate* 1988;**53**(3):121–5.

5. Friedman JE. Obesity and gestational diabetes mellitus pathways for programming in mouse, monkey, and man-where do we go next? The 2014 Norbert Freinkel award lecture. *Diabetes Care* 2015;**38**(8):1402–11. https://doi.org/10.2337/dc15-0628.

6. International Association of Diabetes & Pregnancy Study Groups (IADPSG) Consensus Panel Writing Group and the Hyperglycemia & Adverse Pregnancy Outcome (HAPO) Study Steering Committee, et al. The diagnosis of gestational diabetes mellitus: New paradigms or status quo? *J Matern Fetal Neonatal Med* 2012;**25**(12):2564–9. https://doi.org/10.3109/14767058.2012.718002.

7. Catalano PM, McIntyre HD, Cruickshank JK, et al. The hyperglycemia and adverse pregnancy outcome study: associations of GDM and obesity with pregnancy outcomes. *Diabetes Care* 2012;**35**(4):780–6. https://doi.org/10.2337/dc11-1790.

8. Barbour LA, Hernandez TL. Maternal non-glycemic contributors to fetal growth in obesity and gestational diabetes: spotlight on lipids. *Curr Diab Rep* 2018;**18**(6):37. https://doi.org/10.1007/s11892-018-1008-2.

9. Petry CJ, Mooslehner K, Prentice P, et al. Associations between a fetal imprinted gene allele score and late pregnancy maternal glucose concentrations. *Diabetes Metab* 2017;**43**(4):323–31. https://doi.org/10.1016/j.diabet.2017.03.002.

10. Haig D. Genomic imprinting and kinship: how good is the evidence? *Annu Rev Genet* 2004;**38**:553–85. https://doi.org/10.1146/annurev.genet.37.110801.142741.

11. Angiolini E, Coan PM, Sandovici I, et al. Developmental adaptations to increased fetal nutrient demand in mouse genetic models of Igf2-mediated overgrowth. *FASEB J* 2011;**25**(5):1737–45. https://doi.org/10.1096/fj.10-175273.

12. Petry CJ, Evans ML, Wingate DL, et al. Raised late pregnancy glucose concentrations in mice carrying pups with targeted disruption of H19delta13. *Diabetes* 2010;**59**(1):282–6. https://doi.org/10.2337/db09-0757.

13. Petry CJ, Ong KK, Dunger DB. Does the fetal genotype affect maternal physiology during pregnancy? *Trends Mol Med* 2007;**13**(10):414–21. https://doi.org/10.1016/j.molmed.2007.07.007.

14. Senior B, Slone D, Shapiro S, et al. Letter: benzothiadiazides and neonatal hypoglycaemia. *Lancet* 1976;**2**(7981):377.

15. Davis RL, Rubanowice D, McPhillips H, et al. Risks of congenital malformations and perinatal events among infants exposed to antidepressant medications during pregnancy. *Pharmacoepidemiol Drug Saf* 2007;**16**(10):1086–94. https://doi.org/10.1002/pds.1462.

16. Forsberg L, Naver L, Gustafsson LL, et al. Neonatal adaptation in infants prenatally exposed to antidepressants – clinical monitoring using neonatal abstinence score. *PLoS One* 2014;**9**(11)https://doi.org/10.1371/journal.pone.0111327.

17. Daskas N, Crowne E, Shield JP. Is labetalol really a culprit in neonatal hypoglycaemia? *Arch Dis Child Fetal Neonatal Ed* 2013;**98**(2):F185. https://doi.org/10.1136/archdischild-2012-303057.

18. Kemp MW, Schmidt AF, Jobe AH. Optimizing antenatal corticosteroid therapy. *Semin Fetal Neonatal Med* 2019. https://doi.org/10.1016/j.siny.2019.05.003.

19. Briceno-Perez C, Reyna-Villasmil E, Vigil-De-Gracia P. Antenatal corticosteroid therapy: Historical and scientific basis to improve preterm birth management. *Eur J Obstet Gynecol Reprod Biol* 2019;**234**:32–7. https://doi.org/10.1016/j.ejogrb.2018.12.025.

20. Saulnier PJ, Piguel X, Perault-Pochat MC, et al. Hypoglycaemic seizure and neonatal acute adrenal insufficiency after maternal exposure to prednisone during pregnancy: a case report. *Eur J Pediatr* 2010;**169**(6):763–5. https://doi.org/10.1007/s00431-009-1095-9.

21. Pettit KE, Tran SH, Lee E, et al. The association of antenatal corticosteroids with neonatal hypoglycemia and hyperbilirubinemia. *J Matern Fetal Neonatal Med* 2014;**27**(7):683–6. https://doi.org/10.3109/14767058.2013.832750.

22. Gyamfi-Bannerman C, Thom EA. Antenatal betamethasone for women at risk for late preterm delivery. *N Engl J Med* 2016;**375**(5):486–7. https://doi.org/10.1056/NEJMc1605902.

23. Aydin M, Deveci U, Hakan N. Neonatal hypoglycemia associated with the antenatal corticosteroids may be secondary to fetal adrenal suppression. *J Matern Fetal Neonatal Med* 2015;**28**(8):892. https://doi.org/10.3109/14767058.2014.936002.

24. Beardsall K. Measurement of glucose levels in the newborn. *Early Hum Dev* 2010;**86**(5):263–7.

25. Ghosh A, Banerjee I, Morris AA. Recognition, assessment and management of hypoglycaemia in childhood. *Arch Dis Child* 2016;**101**(6):575–80. https://doi.org/10.1136/archdischild-2015-308337.

26. Beardsall K, Dunger D. Insulin therapy in preterm newborns. *Early Hum Dev* 2008;.

27. Saha P, Beardsall K. Perioperative continuous glucose monitoring in a preterm infant. *BMJ Case Rep* 2018;**2018**:https://doi.org/10.1136/bcr-2018-224728.

28. Thomson L, Elleri D, Bond S, et al. Targeting glucose control in preterm infants: pilot studies of continuous glucose monitoring. *Arch Dis Child Fetal Neonatal Ed* 2018;https://doi.org/10.1136/archdischild-2018-314814.

29. Burakevych N, McKinlay CJ, Alsweiler JM, et al. Bayley-III motor scale and neurological examination at 2 years do not predict motor skills at 4.5 years. *Dev Med Child Neurol* 2017;**59**(2):216–23. https://doi.org/10.1111/dmcn.13232.

30. Koh TH, Aynsley-Green A, Tarbit M, et al. Neural dysfunction during hypoglycaemia. *Arch Dis Child* 1988;**63**(11):1353–8.

31. Lucas A, Morley R, Cole TJ. Adverse neurodevelopmental outcome of moderate neonatal hypoglycaemia. *BMJ* 1988;**297**(6659):1304–8.

32. Tin W, Brunskill G, Kelly T, et al. 15-year follow-up of recurrent "hypoglycemia" in preterm infants. *Pediatrics* 2012;**130**(6):e1497–503. https://doi.org/10.1542/peds.2012-0776.

33. Duvanel CB, Fawer CL, Cotting J, et al. Long-term effects of neonatal hypoglycemia on brain growth and psychomotor development in small-for-gestational-age preterm infants. *J Pediatr* 1999;**134**(4):492–8.

34. Hall NJ, Peters M, Eaton S, et al. Hyperglycemia is associated with increased morbidity and mortality rates in neonates with necrotizing enterocolitis. *J Pediatr Surg* 2004;**39**(6):898–901 [discussion 898-901].

35. Banik SK, Baki MA, Sarker S, et al. Hyperglycemia is a predictor of mortality and morbidity in low birth weight newborn. *Mymensingh Med J* 2014;**23**(3):480–4.

36. Basu SK, Kaiser JR, Guffey D, et al. Hypoglycaemia and hyperglycaemia are associated with unfavourable outcome in infants with hypoxic ischaemic encephalopathy: a post hoc analysis of the CoolCap study. *Arch Dis Child Fetal Neonatal Ed* 2016;**101**(2):F149–55. https://doi.org/10.1136/archdischild-2015-308733.

37. Lemelman MB, Letourneau L, Greeley SAW. Neonatal diabetes mellitus: an update on diagnosis and management. *Clin Perinatol* 2018;**45**(1):41–59. https://doi.org/10.1016/j.clp.2017.10.006.

38. Adamkin DH. Neonatal hypoglycemia. *Semin Fetal Neonatal Med* 2017;**22**(1):36–41. https://doi.org/10.1016/j.siny.2016.08.007.

39. Committee on Fetus and Newborn, Adamkin DH. Postnatal glucose homeostasis in late-preterm and term infants. *Pediatrics* 2011;**127**(3):575–9. https://doi.org/10.1542/peds.2010-3851.

40. Cornblath M, Hawdon JM, Williams AF, et al. Controversies regarding definition of neonatal hypoglycemia: suggested operational thresholds. *Pediatrics* 2000;**105**(5):1141–5.

41. Diwakar KK, Sasidhar MV. Plasma glucose levels in term infants who are appropriate size for gestation and exclusively breast fed. *Arch Dis Child Fetal Neonatal Ed* 2002;**87**(1):F46–8.

42. Hay Jr. WW, Raju TN, Higgins RD, et al. Knowledge gaps and research needs for understanding and treating neonatal hypoglycemia: workshop report from Eunice Kennedy Shriver National Institute of Child Health and Human Development. *J Pediatr* 2009;**155**(5):612–7.

43. Iniguez G, Ong K, Bazaes R, et al. Longitudinal changes in insulin-like growth factor-I, insulin sensitivity, and secretion from birth to age three years in small-for-gestational-age children. *J Clin Endocrinol Metab* 2006;**91**(11):4645–9.

44. Bazaes RA, Salazar TE, Pittaluga E, et al. Glucose and lipid metabolism in small for gestational age infants at 48 hours of age. *Pediatrics* 2003;**111**(4):804–9. Pt 1.

45. Hawdon J, Aynsley-Green A, Bartlett K, et al. The role of pancreatic insulin secretion in neonatal glucoregulation. II. Infants with disordered blood glucose homeostasis. *Arch Dis Child* 1993;**68**:280–5.

46. Collins JE, Leonard JV, Teale D, et al. Hyperinsulinaemic hypoglycaemia in small for dates babies. *Arch Dis Child* 1990;**65**(10):1118–20.

47. Wang HS, Lim J, English J, et al. The concentration of insulin-like growth factor-I and insulin-like growth factor-binding protein-1 in human umbilical cord serum at delivery: relation to fetal weight. *J Endocrinol* 1991;**129**(3):459–64.

48. Girard J. Gluconeogenesis in late fetal and early neonatal life. *Biol Neonate* 1986;**50**(5):237–58. https://doi.org/10.1159/000242605.

49. Fafoula O, Alkhayyat H, Hussain K. Prolonged hyperinsulinaemic hypoglycaemia in newborns with intrauterine growth retardation. *Arch Dis Child Fetal Neonatal Ed* 2006;**91**(6):F467. https://doi.org/10.1136/adc.2006.095919.

50. Wakeling EL. Silver-Russell syndrome. *Arch Dis Child* 2011;**96**(12):1156–61. https://doi.org/10.1136/adc.2010.190165.

51. Basu P, Som S, Choudhuri N, et al. Contribution of the blood glucose level in perinatal asphyxia. *Eur J Pediatr* 2009;**168**(7):833–8. https://doi.org/10.1007/s00431-008-0844-5.

52. Boardman JP, Hawdon JM. Hypoglycaemia and hypoxic-ischaemic encephalopathy. *Dev Med Child Neurol* 2015;**57**(Suppl 3):29–33. https://doi.org/10.1111/dmcn.12729.

53. Bloom SR, Johnston DI. Failure of glucagon release in infants of diabetic mothers. *Br Med J* 1972;**4**(5838):453–4.

54. Ward Platt MP. Big fat babies. *Arch Dis Child Fetal Neonatal Ed* 2014;**99**(5):F348. https://doi.org/10.1136/archdischild-2013-305894.

55. Elhddad AS, Lashen H. Fetal growth in relation to maternal and fetal IGF-axes: a systematic review and meta-analysis. *Acta Obstet Gynecol Scand* 2013;**92**(9):997–1006. https://doi.org/10.1111/aogs.12192.

56. Elhddad AS, Fairlie F, Lashen H. Impact of gestational weight gain on fetal growth in obese normoglycemic mothers: a comparative study. *Acta Obstet Gynecol Scand* 2014;**93**(8):771–7. https://doi.org/10.1111/aogs.12427.

57. Schaefer-Graf UM, Rossi R, Buhrer C, et al. Rate and risk factors of hypoglycemia in large-for-gestational-age newborn infants of nondiabetic mothers. *Am J Obstet Gynecol* 2002;**187**(4):913–7.

58. Bennardello F, Coluzzi S, Curciarello G, et al. Recommendations for the prevention and treatment of haemolytic disease of the foetus and newborn. *Blood Transfus* 2015;**13**(1):109–34. https://doi.org/10.2450/2014.0119-14.

59. Vajravelu ME, De Leon DD. Genetic characteristics of patients with congenital hyperinsulinism. *Curr Opin Pediatr* 2018;**30**(4):568–75. https://doi.org/10.1097/MOP.0000000000000645.

60. Rubio-Agusti I, Carecchio M, Bhatia KP, et al. Movement disorders in adult patients with classical galactosemia. *Mov Disord* 2013;**28**(6):804–10. https://doi.org/10.1002/mds.25348.

61. Demirbas D, Coelho AI, Rubio-Gozalbo ME, et al. Hereditary galactosemia. *Metabolism* 2018;**83**:188–96. https://doi.org/10.1016/j.metabol.2018.01.025.

62. Lebigot E, Brassier A, Zater M, et al. Fructose 1,6-bisphosphatase deficiency: clinical, biochemical and genetic features in French patients. *J Inherit Metab Dis* 2015;**38**(5):881–7. https://doi.org/10.1007/s10545-014-9804-6.

63. Weinstein DA, Correia CE, Saunders AC, et al. Hepatic glycogen synthase deficiency: an infrequently recognized cause of ketotic hypoglycemia. *Mol Genet Metab* 2006;**87**(4):284–8. https://doi.org/10.1016/j.ymgme.2005.10.006.

64. Rake JP, Visser G, Labrune P, et al. Guidelines for management of glycogen storage disease type I – European study on glycogen storage disease type I (ESGSD I). *Eur J Pediatr* 2002;**161**(Suppl 1):S112–9. https://doi.org/10.1007/s00431-002-1016-7.

65. Blackburn PR, Gass JM, Vairo FPE, et al. Maple syrup urine disease: mechanisms and management. *Appl Clin Genet* 2017;**10**:57–66. https://doi.org/10.2147/TACG.S125962.

66. Alatzoglou KS, Dattani MT. Genetic forms of hypopituitarism and their manifestation in the neonatal period. *Early Hum Dev* 2009;**85**(11):705–12. https://doi.org/10.1016/j.earlhumdev.2009.08.057.

67. Kim MS, Ryabets-Lienhard A, Bali B, et al. Decreased adrenomedullary function in infants with classical congenital adrenal hyperplasia. *J Clin Endocrinol Metab* 2014;**99**(8):E1597–601. https://doi.org/10.1210/jc.2014-1274.

68. Ogilvy-Stuart AL, Hands SJ, Adcock CJ, et al. Insulin, insulin-like growth factor I (IGF-I), IGF-binding protein-1, growth hormone, and feeding in the newborn. *J Clin Endocrinol Metab* 1998;**83**(10):3550–7. https://doi.org/10.1210/jcem.83.10.5162.

69. Kollee LA, Monnens LA, Cecjka V, et al. Persistent neonatal hypoglycaemia due to glucagon deficiency. *Arch Dis Child* 1978;**53**(5):422–4.

70. Ng SM, May JE, Emmerson AJ. Continuous insulin infusion in hyperglycaemic extremely-low-birth-weight neonates. *Biol Neonate* 2005;**87**(4):269–72.

71. Hey E. Hyperglycaemia and the very preterm baby. *Semin Fetal Neonatal Med* 2005;**10**(4):377–87.

72. Louik C, Mitchell AA, Epstein MF, et al. Risk factors for neonatal hypeglycaemia associated with 10% dextrose infusion. *AJDC* 1985;**139**:783–6.

73. Sinclair JC, Bottino M, Cowett RM. Interventions for prevention of neonatal hyperglycemia in very low birth weight infants. *Cochrane Database Syst Rev* 2009;**10**. https://doi.org/10.1002/14651858.CD007615.pub3.

74. Cowett RM, Oh W, Schwartz R. Persistent glucose production during glucose infusion in the neonate. *J Clin Invest* 1983;**71**(3):467–75.

75. Farrag H, Nawrath L, Healey J, et al. Persistent glucose production and greater peripheral sensitivity to insulin in the neoante vs the adult. *Am J Physiol* 1997;**272**(Endocrinol Metab 35):E86–93.

76. Anderson TL, Muttart CR, Bieber MA, et al. A controlled trial of glucose versus glucose and amino acids in premature infants. *J Pediatr* 1979;**94**(6):947–51.

77. Yunis KA, Oh W, Kalhan S, et al. Glucose kinetics following administration of an intravenous fat emulsion to low-birth-weight neonates. *Am J Physiol* 1992;**263**(5 Pt 1):E844–9.

78. Scheepers A, Joost HG, Schurmann A. The glucose transporter families SGLT and GLUT: molecular basis of normal and aberrant function. *JPEN J Parenter Enteral Nutr* 2004;**28**(5):364–71.

79. Lane RH, Crawford SE, Flozak AS, et al. Localization and quantification of glucose transporters in liver of growth-retarded fetal and neonatal rats. *Am J Physiol* 1999;**276**(1 Pt 1):E135–42.

80. Santalucia T, Camps M, Castello A, et al. Developmental regulation of GLUT-1 (erythroid/Hep G2) and GLUT-4 (muscle/fat) glucose transporter expression in rat heart, skeletal muscle, and brown adipose tissue. *Endocrinology* 1992;**130**(2):837–46.

81. He J, Thamotharan M, Devaskar SU. Insulin-induced translocation of facilitative glucose transporters in fetal/neonatal rat skeletal muscle. *Am J Physiol Regul Integr Comp Physiol* 2003;**284**(4):R1138–46.

82. Ogata ES. Carbohydrate homeostasis. In: Avery GB, Fletcher MA, MacDonald MG, editors. *Neonatology pathophysiology and management of the newborn*. 5th ed. Philadelphia: Lippincott Williams&Wilkins; 1999. p. 699–714.

83. Economides DL, Proudler A, Nicolaides KH. Plasma insulin in appropriate and small for gestational age fetuses. *Am J Obstet Gynecol* 1989;**160**:1091–4.

84. King RA, Smith RM, Dahlenburg GW. Long term postnatal development of insulin secretion in early premature infants. *Early Human Development* 1986;**13**:285–94.

85. Mitanchez-Mokhtari D, Lahlou N, Kieffer F, et al. Both relative insulin resistance and defective islet beta-cell processing of proinsulin are responsible for transient hyperglycemia in extremely preterm infants. *Pediatrics* 2004;**113**(3):537–41. Pt 1.

86. Revers RR, Henry R, Schmeiser L, et al. The effects of biosynthetic human proinsulin on carbohydrate metabolism. *Diabetes* 1984;**33**(8):762–70.

87. Aynsley-Green A. The endocrinology of feeding in the newborn. *Baillieres Clin Endocrinol Metab* 1989;**3**(3):837–68.

88. Holst JJ, Gromada J. Role of incretin hormones in the regulation of insulin secretion in diabetic and nondiabetic humans. *Am J Physiol Endocrinol Metab* 2004;**287**(2):E199–206.

89. Baggio LL, Drucker DJ. Biology of incretins: GLP-1 and GIP. *Gastroenterology* 2007;**132**(6):2131–57.

90. Oliven A, King KC, Kalhan SC. Gastrointestinal enhanced insulin release in response to glucose in newborn infants. *J Pediatr Gastroenterol Nutr* 1986;**5**(2):220–5.

91. Ekblad H, Kero P, Takala J. Stable glucose balance in premature infants with fluid restriction and early enteral feeding. *Acta Paediatr Scand* 1987;**76**(3):438–43.

92. Lucas A, Bloom SR, Aynsley-Green A. Metabolic and endocrine events at the time of the first feed of human milk in preterm and term infants. *Arch Dis Child* 1978;**53**(9):731–6.

93. Garofano A, Czernichow P, Breant B. In utero undernutrition impairs rat beta-cell development. *Diabetologia* 1997;**40**(10):1231–4.

94. Limesand SW, Rozance PJ, Zerbe GO, et al. Attenuated insulin release and storage in fetal sheep pancreatic islets with intrauterine growth restriction. *Endocrinology* 2006;**147**(3):1488–97.

95. Alvarez C, Martin MA, Goya L, et al. Contrasted impact of maternal rat food restriction on the fetal endocrine pancreas. *Endocrinology* 1997;**138**(6):2267–73.

96. Beringue F, Blondeau B, Castellotti MC, et al. Endocrine pancreas development in growth-retarded human fetuses. *Diabetes* 2002;**51**:385–91.

97. Permutt MA, Koranyi L, Keller K, et al. Cloning and functional expression of a human pancreatic islet glucose-transporter cDNA. *Proc Natl Acad Sci U S A* 1989;**86**(22):8688–92.

98. Postic C, Leturque A, Printz RL, et al. Development and regulation of glucose transporter and hexokinase expression in rat. *Am J Physiol* 1994;**266** (4 Pt 1):E548–59.

99. Navarro-Tableros V, Fiordelisio T, Hernandez-Cruz A, et al. Physiological development of insulin secretion, calcium channels, and GLUT2 expression of pancreatic rat beta-cells. *Am J Physiol Endocrinol Metab* 2007;**292**(4):E1018–29.

100. Richardson CC, Hussain K, Jones PM, et al. Low levels of glucose transporters and K + ATP channels in human pancreatic beta cells early in development. *Diabetologia* 2007;**50**(5):1000–5.

101. Hays SP, Smith EO, Sunehag AL. Hyperglycemia is a risk factor for early death and morbidity in extremely low birth-weight infants. *Pediatrics* 2006;**118**(5):1811–8.

102. Kao LS, Morris BH, Lally KP, et al. Hyperglycemia and morbidity and mortality in extremely low birth weight infants. *J Perinatol* 2006;.

103. Blanco CL, Baillargeon JG, Morrison RL, et al. Hyperglycemia in extremely low birth weight infants in a predominantly Hispanic population and related morbidities. *J Perinatol* 2006.

104. Finberg L. Dangers to infants caused by changes in osmolal concentration. *Pediatrics* 1967;**40**(6):1031–4.

105. Dweck HS, Cassady G. Glucose intolerance in infants of very low birth weight. I. Incidence of hyperglycemia in infants of birth weights 1,100 grams or less. *Pediatrics* 1974;**53**(2):189–95.

106. Fanaroff AA, Korones SB, Wright LL, et al. Incidence, presenting features, risk factors and significance of late onset septicemia in very low birth weight infants. The National Institute of Child Health and Human Development Neonatal Research Network. *Pediatr Infect Dis J* 1998;**17**(7):593–8.

107. Garg R, Agthe AG, Donohue PK, et al. Hyperglycemia and retinopathy of prematurity in very low birth weight infants. *J Perinatol* 2003;**23** (3):186–94.

108. Ertl T, Gyarmati J, Gaal V, et al. Relationship between hyperglycemia and retinopathy of prematurity in very low birth weight infants. *Biol Neonate* 2006;**89**(1):56–9.

109. Van den Berghe G. How does blood glucose control with insulin save lives in intensive care? *J Clin Invest* 2004;**114**(9):1187–95.

110. Vanhorebeek I, De Vos R, Mesotten D, et al. Protection of hepatocyte mitochondrial ultrastructure and function by strict blood glucose control with insulin in critically ill patients. *Lancet* 2005;**365**(9453):53–9.

111. Ellger B, Debaveye Y, Vanhorebeek I, et al. Survival benefits of intensive insulin therapy in critical illness: impact of maintaining normoglycemia versus glycemia-independent actions of insulin. *Diabetes* 2006;**55**(4):1096–105.

112. Nielson CP, Hindson DA. Inhibition of polymorphonuclear leukocyte respiratory burst by elevated glucose concentrations in vitro. *Diabetes* 1989;**38** (8):1031–5.

113. Turina M, Fry DE, Polk Jr. HC. Acute hyperglycemia and the innate immune system: clinical, cellular, and molecular aspects. *Crit Care Med* 2005;**33** (7):1624–33.

114. Marik PE, Raghavan M. Stress-hyperglycemia, insulin and immunomodulation in sepsis. *Intensive Care Med* 2004;**30**(5):748–56.

115. Jeschke MG, Klein D, Thasler WE, et al. Insulin decreases inflammatory signal transcription factor expression in primary human liver cells after LPS challenge. *Mol Med* 2008;**14**(1–2):11–9.

116. Leffler M, Hrach T, Stuerzl M, et al. Insulin attenuates apoptosis and exerts anti-inflammatory effects in endotoxemic human macrophages. *J Surg Res* 2007;**143**(2):398–406.

117. Klein D, Schubert T, Horch RE, et al. Insulin treatment improves hepatic morphology and function through modulation of hepatic signals after severe trauma. *Ann Surg* 2004;**240**(2):340–9.

118. Jeschke MG, Klein D, Bolder U, et al. Insulin attenuates the systemic inflammatory response in endotoxemic rats. *Endocrinology* 2004;**145** (9):4084–93.

119. Krogh-Madsen R, Moller K, Dela F, et al. Effect of hyperglycemia and hyperinsulinemia on the response of IL-6, TNF-alpha, and FFAs to low-dose endotoxemia in humans. *Am J Physiol Endocrinol Metab* 2004;**286**(5):E766–72.

120. Aljada A, Saadeh R, Assian E, et al. Insulin inhibits the expression of intercellular adhesion molecule-1 by human aortic endothelial cells through stimulation of nitric oxide. *J Clin Endocrinol Metab* 2000;**85**(7):2572–5.

121. Langouche L, Vanhorebeek I, Vlasselaers D, et al. Intensive insulin therapy protects the endothelium of critically ill patients. *J Clin Invest* 2005;**115** (8):2277–86.

122. Hinshaw LB, Archer LT, Benjamin B, et al. Effects of glucose or insulin on myocardial performance in endotoxin shock. *Proc Soc Exp Biol Med* 1976;**152**(4):529–34.

123. Sakurai Y, Aarsland A, Herndon DN, et al. Stimulation of muscle protein synthesis by long-term insulin infusion in severely burned patients. *Ann Surg* 1995;**222**(3):283–94; 94-7.

124. Shiozaki T, Tasaki O, Ohnishi M, et al. Paradoxical positive nitrogen balance in burn patients receiving high-dose administration of insulin for nutritional care. *Surgery* 1997;**122**(3):527–33.

125. Ferrando AA, Chinkes DL, Wolf SE, et al. A submaximal dose of insulin promotes net skeletal muscle protein synthesis in patients with severe burns. *Ann Surg* 1999;**229**(1):11–8.

126. Pao CI, Farmer PK, Begovic S, et al. Expression of hepatic insulin-like growth factor-I and insulin-like growth factor-binding protein-1 genes is transcriptionally regulated in streptozotocin-diabetic rats. *Mol Endocrinol* 1992;**6**(6):969–77.

127. Gardelis JG, Hatzis TD, Stamogiannou LN, et al. Activity of the growth hormone/insulin-like growth factor-I axis in critically ill children. *J Pediatr Endocrinol Metab* 2005;**18**(4):363–72.

128. Clemmons DR, Smith-Banks A, Underwood LE. Reversal of diet-induced catabolism by infusion of recombinant insulin-like growth factor-I in humans. *J Clin Endocrinol Metab* 1992;**75**(1):234–8.

129. Lieberman SA, Butterfield GE, Harrison D, et al. Anabolic effects of recombinant insulin-like growth factor-I in cachectic patients with the acquired immunodeficiency syndrome. *J Clin Endocrinol Metab* 1994;**78**(2):404–10.

130. Bowman P, Sulen A, Barbetti F, et al. Effectiveness and safety of long-term treatment with sulfonylureas in patients with neonatal diabetes due to KCNJ11 mutations: an international cohort study. *Lancet Diabetes Endocrinol* 2018;**6**(8):637–46. https://doi.org/10.1016/S2213-8587(18)30106-2.

131. Gloyn AL, Pearson ER, Antcliff JF, et al. Activating mutations in the gene encoding the ATP-sensitive potassium-channel subunit Kir6.2 and permanent neonatal diabetes. *N Engl J Med* 2004;**350**(18):1838–49. https://doi.org/10.1056/NEJMoa032922.

132. Beardsall K, Pesterfield CL, Acerini CL. Neonatal diabetes and insulin pump therapy. *Arch Dis Child Fetal Neonatal Ed* 2011;**96**(3):F223–4. https://doi.org/10.1136/adc.2010.196709.

133. Reusens B, Remacle C. Programming of the endocrine pancreas by the early nutritional environment. *Int J Biochem Cell Biol* 2006;**38**(5–6):913–22.

134. Scaglia L, Cahill CJ, Finegood DT, et al. Apoptosis participates in the remodeling of the endocrine pancreas in the neonatal rat. *Endocrinology* 1997;**138**(4):1736–41.

135. Hill DJ, Strutt B, Arany E, et al. Increased and persistent circulating insulin-like growth factor II in neonatal transgenic mice suppresses developmental apoptosis in the pancreatic islets. *Endocrinology* 2000;**141**(3):1151–7.

136. Kaung HL. Growth dynamics of pancreatic islet cell populations during fetal and neonatal development of the rat. *Dev Dyn* 1994;**200**(2):163–75.

137. Lingohr MK, Buettner R, Rhodes CJ. Pancreatic beta-cell growth and survival–a role in obesity-linked type 2 diabetes? *Trends Mol Med* 2002;**8**(8):375–84.

138. Petrik J, Arany E, McDonald TJ, et al. Apoptosis in the pancreatic islet cells of the neonatal rat is associated with a reduced expression of insulin-like growth factor II that may act as a survival factor. *Endocrinology* 1998;**139**(6):2994–3004.

139. George M, Ayuso E, Casellas A, et al. Beta cell expression of IGF-I leads to recovery from type 1 diabetes. *J Clin Invest* 2002;**109**(9):1153–63.

140. Petrik J, Reusens B, Arany E, et al. A low protein diet alters the balance of islet cell replication and apoptosis in the fetal and neonatal rat and is associated with a reduced pancreatic expression of insulin-like growth factor-II. *Endocrinology* 1999;**140**(10):4861–73.

141. Kassem SA, Ariel I, Thornton PS, et al. Beta-cell proliferation and apoptosis in the developing normal human pancreas and in hyperinsulinism of infancy. *Diabetes* 2000;**49**(8):1325–33.

142. Xu G, Stoffers DA, Habener JF, et al. Exendin-4 stimulates both beta-cell replication and neogenesis, resulting in increased beta-cell mass and improved glucose tolerance in diabetic rats. *Diabetes* 1999;**48**(12):2270–6.

143. Srinivasan M, Aalinkeel R, Song F, et al. Adaptive changes in insulin secretion by islets from neonatal rats raised on a high-carbohydrate formula. *Am J Physiol Endocrinol Metab* 2000;**279**(6):E1347–57.

144. Bonner-Weir S. Perspective: Postnatal pancreatic beta cell growth. *Endocrinology* 2000;**141**(6):1926–9.

145. Goldacre RR. Associations between birthweight, gestational age at birth and subsequent type 1 diabetes in children under 12: a retrospective cohort study in England, 1998-2012. *Diabetologia* 2018;**61**(3):616–25. https://doi.org/10.1007/s00125-017-4493-y.

146. Haynes A, Bower C, Bulsara MK, et al. Perinatal risk factors for childhood type 1 diabetes in Western Australia – a population-based study (1980-2002). *Diabet Med* 2007;**24**(5):564–70. https://doi.org/10.1111/j.1464-5491.2007.02149.x.

147. Stene LC, Magnus P, Lie RT, et al. Birth weight and childhood onset type 1 diabetes: population based cohort study. *BMJ* 2001;**322**(7291):889–92.

148. Dahlquist GG, Patterson C, Soltesz G. Perinatal risk factors for childhood type 1 diabetes in Europe. The EURODIAB substudy 2 study group. *Diabetes Care* 1999;**22**(10):1698–702.

149. Li S, Zhang M, Tian H, et al. Preterm birth and risk of type 1 and type 2 diabetes: systematic review and meta-analysis. *Obes Rev* 2014;**15**(10):804–11. https://doi.org/10.1111/obr.12214.

150. Kajantie E, Hovi P. Is very preterm birth a risk factor for adult cardiometabolic disease? *Semin Fetal Neonatal Med* 2014;**19**(2):112–7. https://doi.org/10.1016/j.siny.2013.11.006.

151. Sipola-Leppanen M, Vaarasmaki M, Tikanmaki M, et al. Cardiometabolic risk factors in young adults who were born preterm. *Am J Epidemiol* 2015;**181**(11):861–73. https://doi.org/10.1093/aje/kwu443.

152. Tinnion R, Gillone J, Cheetham T, et al. Preterm birth and subsequent insulin sensitivity: a systematic review. *Arch Dis Child* 2014;**99**(4):362–8. https://doi.org/10.1136/archdischild-2013-304615.

153. Hovi P, Andersson S, Eriksson JG, et al. Glucose regulation in young adults with very low birth weight. *N Engl J Med* 2007;**356**(20):2053–63.

154. Willemsen RH, de Kort SW, van der Kaay DC, et al. Independent effects of prematurity on metabolic and cardiovascular risk factors in short small-for-gestational-age children. *J Clin Endocrinol Metab* 2008;**93**(2):452–8. https://doi.org/10.1210/jc.2007-1913.

155. Hofman PL, Regan F, Jackson WE, et al. Premature birth and later insulin resistance. *N Engl J Med* 2004;**351**(21):2179–86.

156. Tam WH, Ma RC, Yang X, et al. Glucose intolerance and cardiometabolic risk in children exposed to maternal gestational diabetes mellitus in utero. *Pediatrics* 2008;**122**(6):1229–34. https://doi.org/10.1542/peds.2008-0158.

157. Tam WH, Ma RC, Yang X, et al. Glucose intolerance and cardiometabolic risk in adolescents exposed to maternal gestational diabetes: a 15-year follow-up study. *Diabetes Care* 2010;**33**(6):1382–4. https://doi.org/10.2337/dc09-2343.

158. Silverman BL, Metzger BE, Cho NH, et al. Impaired glucose tolerance in adolescent offspring of diabetic mothers. Relationship to fetal hyperinsulinism. *Diabetes Care* 1995;**18**(5):611–7.

Chapter 46

Intestinal Enteroendocrine Disorders in the Fetus and Neonate

Jessica S. Yang, Venkata S. Jonnakuti, Diana E. Stanescu and Diva D. De Leon

The Children's Hospital of Philadelphia, Perelman School of Medicine at the University of Pennsylvania, Philadelphia, PA, United States

> **Common Clinical Problems**
>
> - Congenital malabsorptive diarrhea can result from loss-of-function mutations in determinants of neuroendocrine cell function or differentiation.
> - These conditions have neonatal onset and are inapparent in fetuses.
> - Loss-of-function mutations in *NEUROG3* cause severe congenital malabsorptive diarrhea and diabetes.
> - Mutations in genes such as *PCSK1*, *RFX6*, *NEUROD1*, *FOXP3*, *ARX*, and *AIRE* also cause severe congenital malabsorptive diarrhea.
> - Dumping syndrome, a complication of gastric fundoplication, causes hypoglycemia due to rapidgastric emptying and absorption of nutrients.

Congenital malabsorptive diarrhea is most commonly due to loss-of-function mutations in endodermal factors important for the differentiation or function of enteroendocrine cells. Although these are rare conditions, the limited available therapeutic interventions severely affect the quality of life and life expectancy of these children.

The fetal intestine has a limited role in fetal physiology as nutrients are delivered via the placenta. Fetal gastrointestinal blockage usually results in polyhydramnios due to decreased swallowing of amniotic fluid. As such, there is no other overt fetal phenotype of the enteroendocrine intestinal disorders. Upon birth and transition to extrauterine life, the intestine becomes the main route of fluid and nutrient delivery for the developing neonate. Hence, the intestinal enteroendocrine disorders become clinically apparent only during or after the neonatal period and not during the fetal life.

Developmental modeling in mice has provided a wealth of information, and many of the factors implicated in enteroendocrine cell differentiation have been found to cause chronic diarrhea and malabsorption in newborns or in young children. Loss of other factors found to impair differentiation in mice have as yet no known human phenotype. In this chapter, we will describe known genetic disorders causing congenital malabsorptive diarrhea in humans. We will also summarize data from animal studies that could expand the list of genes to be tested in clinical situations where defects in enteroendocrine cell differentiation is strongly suspected.

46.1 PART 1. DISORDERS RESULTING FROM DEFECTS IN ENTEROENDOCRINE CELLS

46.1.1 NEUROG3

Neurogenin-3 (NEUROG3) is a key transcription factor that is crucial for the fate of both pancreatic and intestinal endocrine cells.[1,2] Loss-of-function mutations in *NEUROG3* in humans have been associated with a phenotype characterized by severe congenital malabsorptive diarrhea and diabetes resulting from abnormal enteroendocrine and pancreatic endocrine cell differentiation, respectively.[3,4] The severe malabsorption has an early onset, often in the first few days of life after introduction of enteral feeds, and is present in all described cases. The osmotic diarrhea affects all nutrients, and it usually improves by cessation of enteral feeds. Water can be absorbed when administered alone.[5] Hyperchloremic acidosis is a common initial finding.[6] Pancreatic exocrine insufficiency with low fecal elastase and trypsin levels has been described in some of the cases and contributes to malabsorption. It has been suggested that the pancreatic exocrine insufficiency is due to an indirect role of NEUROG3 in exocrine cell development, or that the absence of enteroendocrine secreted cholecystokinin and secretin fails to

Maternal-Fetal and Neonatal Endocrinology. https://doi.org/10.1016/B978-0-12-814823-5.00047-7

stimulate pancreatic exocrine secretion.[7] Clinical evidence shows that pancreatic enzyme replacement leads to only minor clinical improvement, suggesting that the primary mechanism of malabsorption is intestinal.[6]

Intestinal biopsies show a complete loss of enteroendocrine cells (enteric anendocrinosis) in the small intestine and colon by chromogranin staining, while goblet and Paneth cells are not affected[4,6] and gastric endocrine cells have a normal distribution. There is also an arrest of enteroendocrine cell development in the small intestine and colon.[8] Enteroendocrine cell dysgenesis has no inflammatory and autoimmunity component.

Unlike the congenital malabsorptive diarrhea, diabetes mellitus has an incomplete penetrance and variable presentation, even among members of the same family. Both permanent and relapsing transient diabetes requiring insulin have been described in neonates and in older children.[4,5,9] The development of diabetes may be multifactorial, the phenotype may be explained by both abnormal differentiation of insulin producing pancreatic beta cells and lack of incretin hormones (glucagon-like peptide-1 [GLP1] and glucose-dependent insulinotropic peptide [GIP]) secretion from affected enteroendocrine cells.

It is important to note that there are significant differences in the phenotype of human and mouse models of NEUROG3 deficiency. Mice deficient in NEUROG3 exhibit impaired lipid absorption, reduced weight, and altered intestinal architecture,[10] similar to clinical features in humans. The mouse phenotype includes lack of gastric antral endocrine cells, while this does not occur in humans. Homozygous loss of *NEUROG3* in the pancreas of mice leads to complete loss of all endocrine lines and death from diabetes in the first 3 days of life.[1] By comparison, homozygous mutations in humans lead to diabetes in only some cases, with variable age of onset from the neonatal period to later childhood years.[6,9] The differences between the two models may be ascribed to the severity of the genetic defect, since the mouse models are created by completely deleting the coding sequence, whereas reported cases have been due to point mutations. It is possible that point mutations in *NEUROG3* lead to the formation of a NEUROG3 protein with decreased function, which results in some endocrine cells developing and ultimately leading to apparent normal cells numbers in the antrum.[11] This is supported by the finding that as little as 10% NEUROG3 in human embryonic stem cell lines is sufficient for the formation of pancreatic endocrine cells.[12]

The only treatment available for these children is parenteral nutrition, which has been used in the management of all published cases. However, it seems that some children are completely dependent on parenteral nutrition, while others can obtain part of caloric needs from a regular diet.[9] Unfortunately, severe cholestatic liver disease and recurrent central line sepsis episodes are common complications associated with long-term use of parental nutrition and contribute to increased mortality in early childhood.[3,6] Intestine-liver transplantation is often the only hope for these children.[3]

46.1.2 PCSK1

Proprotein convertase 1/3 (PC1/3) deficiency, an autosomal-recessive disorder, results from homozygous mutations in the proprotein convertase subtilisin kexin type 1 (*PCSK1*) gene. PC1/3 is a calcium-dependent serine endoprotease that is responsible for endocrine and neuronal prohormone processing including pro-opiomelanocortin, proinsulin, proglucagon, and progonadotropin releasing hormone.[13–17] PC1/3 is composed of three common domain structures—a prodomain involved in proper folding, a catalytic domain with a highly conserved catalytic triad of three amino acids, and a P domain with roles in protein stability—and a unique C-terminal region.[18] Most patients have mutations in the catalytic domain or P domain of the gene.[18] PC1/3 is expressed abundantly in the enteroendocrine cells, arcuate and paraventricular hypothalamic cells, pituitary cells, and pancreatic beta cells.[19]

Affected newborns usually have a normal birth weight and present with severe malabsorptive diarrhea in the first weeks of life.[20] The severe diarrhea has clinical characteristics similar to those seen in patients with *NEUROG3* mutations: early onset osmotic diarrhea, improved with cessation of feeds, causing metabolic acidosis and requiring complete or partial parenteral nutrition.[20,21] The diarrhea does not improve with selective elimination of nutrients including carbohydrates, amino acids, and lipids.[20] Unlike the cases of *NEUROG3* mutations, intestinal biopsies in children with *PCSK1* mutations are normal or show mild villus atrophy without overt inflammation,[20] suggesting the function and not the number of enteroendocrine cells is affected.

Similar to cases with *NEUROG3* mutations, PC1/3 deficiency cases have early poor weight gain, which requires the initiation of parenteral nutrition. Interestingly, the dependency on parenteral nutrition decreases over time, despite the persistence of diarrhea.[20] By early childhood, these children are often obese.[20] Obesity is often present in adults, and most exhibit severe hyperphagia.[18]

In addition to these clinical findings, children carrying homozygous mutations in *PCSK1* can develop several other endocrine abnormalities. As the disease progresses, pituitary hormone deficiencies, such as diabetes insipidus, growth hormone deficiency, primary hypogonadism, adrenal insufficiency, and central hypothyroidism, occur. In general, these endocrine abnormalities can develop at any time, after the first month of life.[20] Testing the pituitary function is likely necessary as soon as the genetic diagnosis is made in the neonatal period, in order to limit long-term complications due to hormone deficiencies.

Interestingly, a *PCSK1* mutation has been recentlyassociated with the Blue Diaper Syndrome (BDS). BDS is a clinical syndrome with no prior known genetic cause, characterized by neonatal malabsorptive diarrhea, poor weight gain, hypercalcemia, and nephrocalcinosis associated with characteristic blue-tinged urine spots on diapers. Whole exome sequencing identified a homozygous *PCSK1* frameshift mutation in a child with neonatal diarrhea, metabolic acidosis, recurrent hypoglycemia, and blue urine spots. Distelmaier et al. postulated that the blue urine spots might be caused by a direct impact of PC1/3 on tryptophan uptake or metabolism.[22]

46.1.3 RFX6

A downstream transcription factor of NEUROG3, Regulatory Factor 6 (RFX6), directs islet cell differentiation. Mutations in RFX6 can cause neonatal diabetes as well as other digestive system defects. RFX6 mutations present clinically as the Mitchell-Riley syndrome, which includes hypoplastic or annular pancreas, intestinal atresia or stenosis, intestinal malrotation, gallbladder hypoplasia or agenesis, cholestatic disease, and/or abnormal biliary tract.[23,24] There has been a report of a patient whose symptoms started within 24 h of birth and had chronic diarrhea feeding intolerance and cholestatic jaundice, which led to liver failure, eventually leading to death at 4 months.[25] Mice lackingRFX6 fail to generate any normal islet cell types, except for pancreatic polypeptide producing cells.[23]

46.1.4 NEUROD1

NEUROD1 (also known as BETA2) is a basic helix-loop-helix transcription factor that is important in endocrine cell lineage, downstream of NEUROG3, important for the specification of the endocrine lineage in both pancreas and intestine.[26] Mice lacking NEUROD1 die shortly after birth from severe diabetic ketoacidosis.[27] Furthermore, loss of NEUROD1 in the mouse intestine impairs the differentiation of secretin and cholecystokinin enteroendocrine cells, while the other EEC lineages appeared unaffected.[27] A lack of the two pancreatic secretagogues, secretin and cholecystokinin, leads to abnormalities in pancreatic acinar cell polarity and inability to secrete zymogen.[27] *NEUROD1* mutations in humans have been implicated as a very rare cause of maturity-onset diabetes of the young (MODY),[28] permanent neonatal diabetes (PNDM),[29] and late-onset diabetes.[30] In two patients with *NEUROD1* mutations with PNDM, there was also developmental delay, cerebella hypoplasia, and hearing as well as visual impairment. Although no intestinal phenotype was described in human mutations, data from mice suggest that alterations in EEC lineages could occur in these cases.[27]

46.1.5 FOXP3

FOXP3 is a transcription factor on the X chromosome, involved in thymus-derived regulatory T-cell development and homeostasis.[31] Mutations in *FOXP3* mutations can result in immune dysfunction, polyendocrinopathy, enteropathy, and X-linked inheritance (termed IPEX) and result in immune dysregulation secondary to a deficiency of regulatory T cells.[32] IPEX may be a subtype of autoimmune enteropathy and causes severe inflammation with ulceration and villus atrophy.[11] The disease, which affects males, typically causes death in the first year of life, though bone marrow transplants and immunosuppression can be done with variable success early in diagnosis.[33] Although similar to enteroendocrine dysgenesis, as they share enteropathy and diabetes mellitus, IPEX also causes eczema, thyroiditis and hypothyroidism, hemolytic anemia, and diabetes in the first year of life. The enteropathy of IPEX syndrome is characterized by abundant mucosal inflammation with ulcerations and changes in villus architecture, sometimes with loss of enteroendocrine, goblet, and Paneth cells.[11] Interesting to note is that the syndrome can present differently in patients, despite identical mutations, and has a continuum of clinical manifestations.[31]

46.1.6 ARX

Aristaless-related homeobox (ARX) is a paired-domain transcription factor on the X-chromosome. It is associated with neurologic disease, loss of pancreatic alpha cells, and early onset, severe diarrhea.[34-36] Fifty percent of patients with missense or nonsense ARX mutations present with congenital diarrhea that leads to early death. The ARX-deficient mouse model supports this finding.[37] ARX polyalanine insertion leads to loss of CCK and GLP-1 cells but an increase in SST-expressing populations, results of which are also supported by a mouse model.[38]

46.1.7 AIRE

Mutations in the autoimmune regulator gene (AIRE) leading to loss of function[39] can result in autoimmune-polyendocrinopathy-candidiasis-endodermal-dystrophy (APECED), a monogenetic disorder characterized by chronic mucocutaneous candidiasis, hypoparathyroidism, adrenal failure, hypergonadotropic hypogonadism, type 1 diabetes, autoimmune thyroid diseases, and pituitary defects.[40] Intestinal biopsies of patients with APECED and chronic diarrhea show an almost complete loss of enteroendocrine and enterochromaffin cells in the stomach, duodenum, and colon.[41] Although the typical age of onset of symptoms is in early childhood, gastrointestinal symptoms can precede the onset of the typical diagnostic features of APECED.[41]

46.1.8 Gene Mutations that Could Affect Enteroendocrine Cell Populations

Several genes have been implicated in neuroendocrine and/or enteroendocrine cell differentiation in mice. Loss of these genes has been shown to impact enteroendocrine cell differentiation in mice and could potentially have similar effects in humans.

MATH1/ATOH1: Similar to NEUROG3, MATH1 is a basic loop helix protein, with roles in enteroendocrine cell development. Loss of MATH1 in mice causes impairment of all three secretory cell types in the intestine (goblet, Paneth, and enteroendocrine cells).[42] These findings are consistent with a role of MATH1 in the specification of these three lineages. No loss-of-function mutations have been yet found in humans.

PAX6: Paired box-6 (PAX6) is a transcription factor that is an important determinant of islet cell development, proglucagon gene expression in pancreatic islet alpha cells and proglucagon gene transcription in the small and large intestine. In mice with homozygous dominant negative Pax6 allele, SEY^{Neu} mutation, there are significantly reduced levels of proglucagon mRNA transcripts in both the small and large intestine, as well as a lack of GLP-1 and GLP-2 immunopositive enteroendocrine cells in the intestinal mucosa.[43]

ISL1: ISLET1 (ISL1), a LIM homeodomain transcription factor, is upstream of ARX.[44,45] ISL1 plays an important role in promoting expression of somatostatin and preproglucagon in endocrine cell lines and functions in the heart, brain, hindlimb, and pancreas formation.[45–50] It also is expressed in many intestinal endocrine cells, such as incretin-expressing cells. An intestinal epithelial-specific ablation of *Isl1* mouse model was found to have loss of GLP-1, GIP, cholecystokinin (CCK), and somatostatin expressing cells, as well as an increase in serotonin-producing cells. Chromogranin A population was unchanged. Animals were also found to have lipid malabsorption. Oral glucose tolerance in the mouse demonstrated impaired glucose tolerance.[51]

46.2 PART 2. DISORDERS RESULTING FROM EXCESS ENTEROENDOCRINE HORMONE SECRETION

46.2.1 Dumping Syndrome

Dumping syndrome is an often unrecognized complication of gastric fundoplication, a surgery performed for managing severe gastroesophageal reflux disease in neonates and children. Dumping syndrome is characterized by an early phase (early dumping) manifesting with gastrointestinal symptoms—bloating, diarrhea, and a late phase (late dumping or postprandial hypoglycemia). The postprandial hypoglycemia typically occurs 1–3 h after a meal and can be severe, resulting in seizures. The pathophysiology of postprandial hypoglycemia after fundoplication involves rapid gastric emptying and rapid absorption of nutrients, triggering early hyperglycemia and an exaggerated GLP-1 response, followed by an exaggerated insulin surge and subsequent hypoglycemia.[52]

The reported prevalence of postprandial hypoglycemia after fundoplication varies widely and is mostly dependent on the screening practices.[53,54] In our experience at the Children's Hospital of Philadelphia, postsurgical surveillance of NICU patients showed a high incidence of postprandial hypoglycemia of 25% following fundoplication, while the incidence in non-NICU patients was slightly lower at 23%.[55] Our standard protocol involves postprandial glucose measurements on a bedside glucose meter at 60, 90 and 120 min after goal bolus feedings, for at least 72 h. Critical hypoglycemia is diagnosed when plasma glucose reaches a level below 60 mg/dL (3.3 mmol/L), confirmed via a laboratory venous sample.

Several factors may worsen this phenomenon in neonates and young infants. These children are fed an exclusively liquid diet, which increases the rate of gastric emptying and leads to faster nutrient absorption, thus contributing to the exaggerated GLP-1 secretion. GLP-1 actions on nonbeta cell targets, including effects on appetite and glucagon secretion, may also play a role in the pathophysiology.[56]

Several therapies have been used to limit hypoglycemia, most aimed at decreasing the speed of nutrient absorption. Pectin, cornstarch, and dietary manipulations have had limited success. Acarbose, an α-glucosidase inhibitor that slows the digestion of complex carbohydrates, is effective but is of limited use at very young ages, and can cause significant gastrointestinal side effects. Continuous enteral feeding is commonly used in the NICU setting, but also poses significant limitations and does not prevent hypoglycemia when the feeding is inadvertently stopped. The use of GLP-1 antagonists (exendin 9–39) has been proposed as a potential therapy aimed at decreasing GLP-1 mediated effects.[57] Although not yet in clinical use, this type of therapy has greater promise, since it addresses the role of GLP-1 in inducing the excessive insulin response to a glucose load.

REFERENCES

1. Gradwohl G, Dierich A, LeMeur M, Guillemot F. neurogenin3 is required for the development of the four endocrine cell lineages of the pancreas. *Proc Natl Acad Sci* 2000;**97**(4):1607–11.
2. Jenny M, Uhl C, Roche C, Duluc I, Guillermin V, Guillemot F, Jensen J, Kedinger M, Gradwohl G. Neurogenin3 is differentially required for endocrine cell fate specification in the intestinal and gastric epithelium. *EMBO J* 2002;**21**(23):6338–47.
3. Wang J, Cortina G, Wu SV, Tran R, Cho J-H, Tsai M-J, Bailey TJ, Jamrich M, Ament ME, Treem WR, et al. Mutant neurogenin-3 in congenital malabsorptive diarrhea. *N Engl J Med* 2006;**355**(3):270–80.
4. Hancili S, Bonnefond A, Philippe J, Vaillant E, De Graeve F, Sand O, Busiah K, Robert J-J, Polak M, Froguel P, et al. A novel NEUROG3 mutation in neonatal diabetes associated with a neuro-intestinal syndrome. *Pediatr Diabetes* 2018;**19**(3):381–7.
5. Rubio-Cabezas O, Codner E, Flanagan SE, Gómez JL, Ellard S, Hattersley AT. Neurogenin 3 is important but not essential for pancreatic islet development in humans. *Diabetologia* 2014;**57**(11):2421–4.
6. Pinney SE, Oliver-Krasinski J, Ernst L, Hughes N, Patel P, Stoffers DA, Russo P, De León DD. Neonatal diabetes and congenital malabsorptive diarrhea attributable to a novel mutation in the human neurogenin-3 gene coding sequence. *J Clin Endocrinol Metab* 2011;**96**:1960–5.
7. Sayar E, Islek A, Yilmaz A, Akcam M, Flanagan SE, Artan R. Extremely rare cause of congenital diarrhea: enteric anendocrinosis. *Pediatr Int* 2013;**55** (5):661–3.
8. Ohsie S, Gerney G, Gui D, Kahana D, Martin MG, Cortina G. A paucity of colonic enteroendocrine and/or enterochromaffin cells characterizes a subset of patients with chronic unexplained diarrhea/malabsorption. *Hum Pathol* 2009;**40**(7):1006–14.
9. Rubio-Cabezas O, Jensen JN, Hodgson MI, Codner E, Ellard S, Serup P, Hattersley AT. Permanent neonatal diabetes and enteric anendocrinosis associated with biallelic mutations in NEUROG3. *Diabetes* 2011;**60**(4):1349–53.
10. Mellitzer G. Loss of enteroendocrine cells in mice alters lipid absorption and glucose homeostatsis and impairs postnatal survival. *J Clin Investig* 2010;**120**(5):1708–21.
11. Cortina G, Smart CN, Farmer DG, Bhuta S, Treem WR, Hill ID, Martín MG. Enteroendocrine cell dysgenesis and malabsorption, a histopathologic and immunohistochemical characterization. *Hum Pathol* 2007;**38**(4):570–80.
12. McGrath PS, Watson CL, Ingram C, Helmrath MA, Wells JM. The basic helix-loop-helix transcription factor NEUROG3 is required for development of the human endocrine pancreas. *Diabetes* 2015;**64**(7):2497–505.
13. Smeekens SP, Montag AG, Thomas G, Albiges-Rizo C, Carroll R, Benig M, Phillips LA, Martin S, Ohagi S, Gardner P, et al. Proinsulin processing by the subtilisin-related proprotein convertases furin, PC2, and PC3. *Proc Natl Acad Sci U S A* 1992;**89**(18):8822–6.
14. Rouille Y, Martin S, Steiner DF. Differential processing of proglucagon by the subtilisin-like prohormone convertases PC2 and PC3 to generate either glucagon or glucagon-like peptide. *J Biol Chem* 1995;**270**(44):26488–96.
15. Dong W, Seidel B, Marcinkiewicz M, Chrétien M, Seidah NG, Day R. Cellular localization of the prohormone convertases in the hypothalamic paraventricular and supraoptic nuclei: selective regulation of PC1 in corticotrophin-releasing hormone parvocellular neurons mediated by glucocorticoids. *J Neurosci Off J Soc Neurosci* 1997;**17**(2):563–75.
16. Benjannet S, Rondeau N, Day R, Chrétien M, Seidah NG. PC1 and PC2 are proprotein convertases capable of cleaving proopiomelanocortin at distinct pairs of basic residues. *Proc Natl Acad Sci U S A* 1991;**88**(9):3564–8.
17. Schaner P, Todd RB, Seidah NG, Nillni EA. Processing of prothyrotropin-releasing hormone by the family of prohormone convertases. *J Biol Chem* 1997;**272**(32):19958–68.
18. Stijnen P, Ramos-Molina B, O'Rahilly S, Creemers JWM. PCSK1 mutations and human endocrinopathies: from obesity to gastrointestinal disorders. *Endocr Rev* 2016;**37**:347–71.
19. Hoshino A, Lindberg I. Peptide biosynthesis: prohormone convertases 1/3 and 2. *Coll Ser Neuropept* 2012;**1**(1):1–112.
20. Martín MG, Lindberg I, Solorzano-Vargas RS, Wang J, Avitzur Y, Bandsma R, Sokollik C, Lawrence S, Pickett LA, Chen Z, et al. Congenital proprotein convertase 1/3 deficiency causes malabsorptive diarrhea and other endocrinopathies in a pediatric cohort. *Gastroenterology* 2013;**145** (1):138–48.
21. Härter B, Fuchs I, Müller T, Akbulut UE, Cakir M, Janecke AR. Early clinical diagnosis of PC1/3 deficiency in a patient with a novel homozygous PCSK1 splice-site mutation. *J Pediatr Gastroenterol Nutr* 2016;**62**(4):577–80.
22. Distelmaier F, Herebian D, Atasever C, Beck-Woedl S, Mayatepek E, Strom TM, Haack TB. Blue diaper syndrome and PCSK1 mutations. *Pediatrics* 2018;**141**:S501–5.
23. Smith SB, Qu HQ, Taleb N, Kishimoto NY, Scheel DW, Lu Y, Patch AM, Grabs R, Wang J, Lynn FC, et al. Rfx6 directs islet formation and insulin production in mice and humans. *Nature* 2010;**463**(7282):775–80.

24. Spiegel R, Dobbie A, Hartman C, de Vries L, Ellard S, Shalev SA. Clinical characterization of a newly described neonatal diabetes syndrome caused by RFX6 mutations. *Am J Med Genet A* 2011;**155**(11):2821–5.

25. Concepcion JP, Reh CS, Daniels M, Liu X, Paz VP, Ye H, Highland HM, Hanis CL, Greeley SAW. Neonatal diabetes, gallbladder agenesis, duodenal atresia, and intestinal malrotation caused by a novel homozygous mutation in RFX6. *Pediatr Diabetes* 2014;**15**(1):67–72.

26. Bernardo AS, Hay CW, Docherty K. Pancreatic transcription factors and their role in the birth, life and survival of the pancreatic beta cell. *Mol Cell Endocrinol* 2008;**294**(1–2):1–9.

27. Naya FJ, Huang HP, Qiu Y, Mutoh H, DeMayo FJ, Leiter AB, Tsai MJ. Diabetes, defective pancreatic morphogenesis, and abnormal enteroendocrine differentiation in BETA2/NeuroD-deficient mice. *Genes Dev* 1997;**11**(18):2323–34.

28. Kristinsson SY, Thorolfsdottir ET, Talseth B, Steingrimsson E, Thorsson AV, Helgason T, Hreidarsson AB, Arngrimsson R. MODY in Iceland is associated with mutations in HNF-1alpha and a novel mutation in NeuroD1. *Diabetologia* 2001;**44**(11):2098–103.

29. Rubio-Cabezas O, Minton JAL, Kantor I, Williams D, Ellard S, Hattersley AT. Homozygous mutations in NEUROD1 are responsible for a novel syndrome of permanent neonatal diabetes and neurological abnormalities. *Diabetes* 2010;**59**(9):2326–31.

30. Malecki MT, Jhala US, Antonellis A, Fields L, Doria A, Orban T, Saad M, Warram JH, Montminy M, Krolewski AS. Mutations in NEUROD1 are associated with the development of type 2 diabetes mellitus. *Nat Genet* 1999;**23**(3):323–8.

31. Bacchetta R, Barzaghi F, Roncarolo M-G. From IPEX syndrome to FOXP3 mutation: a lesson on immune dysregulation. *Ann N Y Acad Sci* 2018;**1417**(1):5–22.

32. Gambineri E, Torgerson TR, Ochs HD. Immune dysregulation, polyendocrinopathy, enteropathy, and X-linked inheritance (IPEX), a syndrome of systemic autoimmunity caused by mutations of FOXP3, a critical regulator of T-cell homeostasis. *Curr Opin Rheumatol* 2003;**15**:430–5.

33. Baud O, Goulet O, Canioni D, Le Deist F, Radford I, Rieu D, Dupuis-Girod S, Cerf-Bensussan N, Cavazzana-Calvo M, Brousse N, et al. Treatment of the immune dysregulation, polyendocrinopathy, enteropathy, X-linked syndrome (IPEX) by allogeneic bone marrow transplantation. *N Engl J Med* 2001;**344**(23):1758–62.

34. Marsh ED, Golden JA. Developing models of Aristaless-related homeobox mutations. In: Noebels JL, Avoli M, Rogawski MA, Olsen RW, Delgado-Escueta AV, editors. *Jasper's basic mechanisms of the epilepsies [Internet]*. 4th ed. Bethesda (MD): National Center for Biotechnology Information (US); 2012. p. 1–16.

35. Jackson RS, Creemers JWM, Farooqi IS, Raffin-Sanson ML, Varro A, Dockray GJ, Holst JJ, Brubaker PL, Corvol P, Polonsky KS, et al. Small-intestinal dysfunction accompanies the complex endocrinopathy of human proprotein convertase 1 deficiency. *J Clin Investig* 2003;**112**(10):1550–60.

36. Collombat P, Mansouri A, Hecksher-Sørensen J, Serup P, Krull J, Gradwohl G, Gruss P. Opposing actions of Arx and Pax4 in endocrine pancreas development. *Genes Dev* 2003;**17**(20):2591–603.

37. Du A, McCracken KW, Walp ER, Terry NA, Klein TJ, Han A, Wells JM, May CL. Arx is required for normal enteroendocrine cell development in mice and humans. *Dev Biol* 2012;**365**(1):175–88.

38. Terry NA, Lee RA, Walp ER, Kaestner KH, Lee May C. Dysgenesis of enteroendocrine cells in aristaless-related homeobox polyalanine expansion mutations. *J Pediatr Gastroenterol Nutr* 2015;**60**(2):192–9.

39. Kisand K, Peterson P. Autoimmune polyendocrinopathy candidiasis ectodermal dystrophy. *J Clin Immunol* 2015;**35**:463–78.

40. Perheentupa J. Extensive clinical experience—autoimmune polyendocrinopathy-candidiasis-ectodermal dystrophy. *J Clin Endocrinol Metab* 2006;**91**:2843–50.

41. Posovszky C, Lahr G, Von Schnurbein J, Buderus S, Findeisen A, Schröder C, Schütz C, Schulz A, Debatin KM, Wabitsch M, et al. Loss of enteroendocrine cells in autoimmune-polyendocrine-candidiasis- ectodermal-dystrophy (APECED) syndrome with gastrointestinal dysfunction. *J Clin Endocrinol Metab* 2012;**97**(2):292–300.

42. Yang Q, Bermingham NA, Finegold MJ, Zoghbi HY. Requirement of Math1 for secretory cell lineage commitment in the mouse intestine. *Science* 2001;**294**(5549):2155–8.

43. Hill ME, Asa SL, Drucker DJ. Essential requirement for Pax 6 in control of enteroendocrine proglucagon gene transcription. *Mol Endocrinol* 1999;**13**(9):1474–86.

44. Hunter CS, Rhodes SJ. LIM-homeodomain genes in mammalian development and human disease. *Mol Biol Rep* 2005;**32**(2):67–77.

45. Lu KM, Evans SM, Hirano S, Liu FC. Dual role for Islet-1 in promoting striatonigral and repressing striatopallidal genetic programs to specify striatonigral cell identity. *Proc Natl Acad Sci* 2014;**111**(1):E168–77.

46. Leonard J, Serup P, Gonzalez G, Edlund T, Montminy M. The LIM family transcription factor Isl-1 requires cAMP response element binding protein to promote somatostatin expression in pancreatic islet cells. *Proc Natl Acad Sci U S A* 1992;**89**(14):6247–51.

47. Ehrman LA, Mu X, Waclaw RR, Yoshida Y, Vorhees CV, Klein WH, Campbell K. The LIM homeobox gene Isl1 is required for the correct development of the striatonigral pathway in the mouse. *Proc Natl Acad Sci* 2013;**110**(42):E4026–35.

48. Kawakami Y, Marti M, Kawakami H, Itou J, Quach T, Johnson A, Sahara S, O'Leary DDM, Nakagawa Y, Lewandoski M, et al. Islet1-mediated activation of the -catenin pathway is necessary for hindlimb initiation in mice. *Development* 2011;**138**(20):4465–73.

49. Wang M, Drucker DJ. The LIM domain homeobox gene isl-1 is a positive regulator of islet cell-specific proglucagon gene transcription. *J Biol Chem* 1995;**270**(21):12646–52.

50. Du A, Hunter CS, Murray J, Noble D, Cai CL, Evans SM, Stein R, May CL. Islet-1 is required for the maturation, proliferation, and survival of the endocrine pancreas. *Diabetes* 2009;**58**(9):2059–69.

51. Terry NA, Walp ER, Lee RA, Kaestner KH, May CL. Impaired enteroendocrine development in intestinal-specific Islet1 mouse mutants causes impaired glucose homeostasis. *Am J Physiol Gastrointest Liver Physiol* 2014;**307**(10):G979–91.
52. Palladino AA, Sayed S, Levitt Katz LE, Gallagher PR, De Leon DD. Increased glucagon-like peptide-1 secretion and postprandial hypoglycemia in children after Nissen fundoplication. *J Clin Endocrinol Metab* 2009;**94**(1):39–44.
53. Samuk I, Afriat R, Horne T, Bistritzer T, Barr J, Vinograd I. Dumping syndrome following Nissen fundoplication, diagnosis, and treatment. *J Pediatr Gastroenterol Nutr* 1996;**23**(3):235–40.
54. Gilger MA, Yeh C, Chiang J, Dietrich C, Brandt ML, El-Serag HB. Outcomes of surgical fundoplication in children. *Clin Gastroenterol Hepatol* 2004;**2**(11):978–84.
55. Calabria AC, Gallagher PR, Simmons R, Blinman T, De Leon DD. Postoperative surveillance and detection of postprandial hypoglycemia after fundoplasty in children. *J Pediatr* 2011;**159**(4):597–601 [e591].
56. van Bloemendaal L, RG IJ, Ten Kulve JS, Barkhof F, Konrad RJ, Drent ML, Veltman DJ, Diamant M. GLP-1 receptor activation modulates appetite- and reward-related brain areas in humans. *Diabetes* 2014;**63**(12):4186–96.
57. Calabria AC, Charles L, Givler S, De Leon DD. Postprandial hypoglycemia in children after gastric surgery: clinical characterization and pathophysiology. *Horm Res Paediatr* 2016;**85**(2):140–6.

Chapter 47

Disorders of the Adrenal Cortex in the Fetus and Neonate

Ahmed Khattab[†], Mithra L. Narasimhan[*], Anne Macdonald[*], Gertrude Costin[*] and Maria New[*]

[*]Department of Pediatrics, Icahn School of Medicine at Mount Sinai, New York, NY, United States, [†]Division of Pediatric Endocrinology, Rutgers-Robert Wood Johnson Medical School, Child Health Institute of New Jersey, New Brunswick, NJ, United States

---

Common Clinical Problems

- The implementation of newborn screening programs permits early treatment and reduces neonatal morbidity and mortality. Worldwide expansion of newborn screening programs is needed.
- Prenatal diagnosis, including noninvasive prenatal diagnosis, is available for a few adrenal disorders, with CAH being one of the few where prenatal treatment may be beneficial.
- The debate over prenatal treatment of CAH with dexamethasone to prevent genital ambiguity continues. To date, prenatal dexamethasone therapy is considered experimental.
- Prenatal estriol levels are markers of fetal adrenal well-being and low prenatal estriol levels and, although not specific to them, have been associated with pregnancies carrying fetuses with adrenal insufficiency.
- The treatment for adrenal disorders has not been perfected to mimic adrenal physiology.
- In many parts of the world where molecular diagnostic resources are not readily available, physicians are then dependent on clinical and biochemical values that may be misleading in the diagnosis of adrenal steroid disorders.

47.1 ANCIENT HISTORY OF ADRENAL STEROID DISORDERS

The history of steroid disorders, particularly congenital adrenal hyperplasia (CAH), goes back centuries. The first published report of a cadaver with ambiguous genitalia was by Luigi de Crecchio in 1865. The male cadaver was found to have ovaries, a uterus, fallopian tubes, and massively enlarged adrenal glands. De Creccio's publication is the first report of a virilized female with the clinical constellation of CAH who was reared as a male. Further, one of the earliest accounts of consanguinity, frequently associated with autosomal recessive disorders and in particular adrenal disorders, is found in the Old Testament of the Bible in a description of the ancient pedigree of Abraham that delineates how his wife Sarah was the daughter of his dead brother Haran and therefore his niece (Fig. 47.1).[1]

More recently, developments after 1930 furthered our modern scientific understanding of CAH and the field of adrenal steroid disorders (Fig. 47.2). Following advances in the field of molecular genetics, extensive research has contributed to our understanding of the various genetic mutations that result in adrenal steroid disorders.

47.2 ADRENAL DEVELOPMENT AND FUNCTION

The adrenal cortex is of mesodermal origin. The adrenocortical primordial cells appear at around the 4th week of gestation from proliferation of the coelomic epithelium (mesothelium) forming small buds that differentiate from the epithelium, after which the adrenal primordium migrates retroperitoneally. These progenitor cells give rise to the steroidogenic cells of the adrenals and gonads. At 6 weeks of gestation, the mesenchymal cells surrounding the developing medulla cells differentiate from the fetal adrenal cortex, which is later replaced by the adult cortex. By the 8th to 9th week of gestation the fetal adrenal cortex develops a small **definitive zone**, which is the site of glucocorticoid and mineralocorticoid production, and a larger **fetal zone** that produces the androgenic precursors required for the production of estriol by the placenta. The fetal adrenal cortex is responsive to adrenocorticotropic hormone (ACTH) by the 8th to 9th week of gestation; early stages

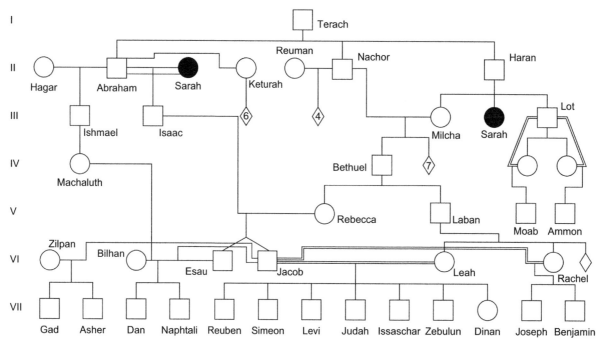

FIG. 47.1 Pedigree of Abraham and Sarah. *(Reproduced with permission from Fig. 1.1 – Chapter 1* Genetic Steroid Disorders *(Copyright Elsevier 2014). Source: Old Testament of Bible. New MI, et al.* Genetic steroid disorders. *Amsterdam; Boston; Heidelberg; London; New York; Oxford; Paris; San Diego; Singapore; Sydney; Tokyo: Elsevier; 2014. xiii, 392 pages.)*

of adrenal differentiation and development involve numerous signaling pathways. Subsequent fetal adrenal growth is dependent on ACTH, its receptor, and its downstream signaling pathways as well as growth factor signaling pathways (insulin like growth factor II (IGF-II), basic fibroblast growth factor (bFGF), and epidermal growth factor (EGF)). The fetal adrenals are huge compared to other structures and continue to grow until the end of the third trimester. Although at birth the fetal adrenals represent 0.4% of the total body weight, by 6–12 months postnatally the weight of the adrenal gland regresses to about 0.01% of the total body weight owing to the disappearance of the fetal zone postnatally.

The adrenal gland itself is divided into three zones: the zona glomerulosa, zona fasciculata, and zona reticularis. The zona glomerulosa and zona fasciculata are histologically distinct and behave hormonally and histologically as two separate sections.[2,3]

Steroidogenesis in the zona fasciculata is regulated by ACTH, which stimulates the secretion of corticosteroids and androgens as well as desoxycorticosterone, and corticosterone. Mutations or deletions in the various enzymes involved in adrenal steroidogenesis result in abnormalities of the adrenal cortex production. Steroidogenesis in the zona glomerulosa is regulated by angiotensin II and potassium.[4]

47.3 SIGNS AND SYMPTOMS OF ADRENAL DISEASE IN THE NEWBORN PERIOD

The clinical presentation of monogenic adrenal disorders is variable even within the same disorder and within the same family. Since many of these disorders are autosomal recessive conditions, there may be a history of consanguinity. The most frequently occurring genetic disorder of the adrenal gland that manifests in the newborn period is by far CAH, with an overall incidence of 1:15,000.

Before the implementation of newborn screening for CAH, and in countries where newborn screening is not yet available, physicians relied solely on the clinical presentation of the newborn for initial diagnosis. Newborn girls with salt wasting 21-hydroxylase deficiency CAH present with different degrees of virilization of the external genitalia, whereas boys may present with hyperpigmentation or a potentially fatal adrenal crisis a few days to weeks following birth. Girls with simple virilizing 21-hydroxylase deficiency CAH are also born with ambiguous genitalia, but this may be mild enough not to have been diagnosed at birth and may come to attention later because of progressive virilization and signs of

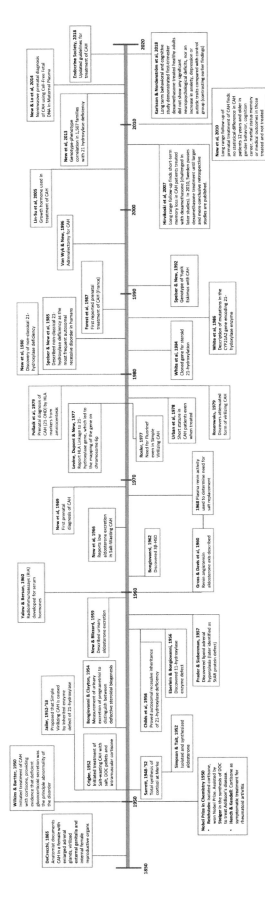

FIG. 47.2 Advances in steroid endocrinology. *(Modified with permission from Fig. 1.2 – Chapter 1 Genetic Steroid Disorders (Copyright Elsevier 2014). New MI, et al. Genetic steroid disorders. Amsterdam; Boston; Heidelberg; London; New York; Oxford; Paris; San Diego; Singapore; Sydney; Tokyo: Elsevier; 2014. xiii, 392 pages.)*

hyperandrogenism. Boys may only present in childhood with rapid somatic growth or sexual precocity. The nonclassical form of 21-hydroxylase deficiency CAH is usually asymptomatic in the newborn period. Other forms of CAH, namely those owing to 11β-hydroxylase and 17-hydroxylase deficiency, do not present with salt wasting; however, patients develop hypertension as they get older. Infants with adrenal hypoplasia congenita may present with mineralocorticoid or glucocorticoid deficiency or hypogonadism. Syndromic forms of adrenal insufficiency, such as Zellweger, IMAGe or Smith-Lemli-Opitz syndrome, have characteristic dysmorphic features. Patients with secondary adrenal insufficiency owing to ACTH deficiency and growth hormone deficiency manifest profound hypoglycemia but do not have hyperpigmentation. If ACTH deficiency is associated with gonadotropin deficiency, the clinical presentation of a microphallus may be the first sign. Aldosterone deficiency disorders usually present with newborn feeding difficulties, failure to thrive, vomiting, dehydration, lethargy, seizures, and electrolyte imbalance (hyponatremia and hyperkalemia). If left untreated, the hypovolemia leads to tachycardia, hypotension, acidosis, and eventual hypovolemic shock and death. Patients with autosomal recessive pseudohypoaldosteronism may have associated pulmonary symptoms[2,5–10] (Table 47.1).

TABLE 47.1 Disorders of the adrenal cortex of fetal and neonatal onset and encoding genes

	Gene (location)	OMIM
Congenital Adrenal Hyperplasia (CAH):		
21-hydroxylase deficiency CAH	CYP21A2 (6p21.33)	613815
11 β-hydroxylase deficiency CAH	CYP11B1 (8q24.3)	610313
3β-hydroxysteroid dehydrogenase 2 deficiency CAH	HSD3B2 (1p12)	613890
StAR protein deficiency (Lipoid CAH)	StAR (8p11.23)	600617
17-hydroxylase17,20-lyase deficiency CAH	CYP17A1(10q24.32)	609300
P450 oxidoreductase deficiency	POR (7q11.23)	613571
X-linked primary adrenal insufficiency:		
DAX-1 deficiency	NR0B1 (Xp21.2)	300473
Adrenoleukodystrophy	ABCD1 (Xq28)	300371
Familial glucocorticoid deficiency:		
Melanocortin 2 receptor	MC2R (18p11.21)	607397
Melanocortin 2 receptor accessory protein	MRAP (22q22.11)	609196
StAR protein deficiency (lipoid CAH)	StAR (8p11.23)	600617
Side chain cleavage enzyme	CYP11A1 (15q24.1)	118485
Minichromosome maintenance complex component 4	MCM4 (8q11.21)	602638
Nicotinamide nucleotide transhydrogenase	NNT (5p12)	607878
Thioredoxin reductase 2	TXNRD2 (22q11.21)	606448
AAA syndrome	AAAS (12q13.13)	605378
Mineralocorticoid pathway defects:		
Glucocorticoid-remediable hyperaldosteronism (GRA)	CYP11B2 (8q24.3)	124080
Autosomal dominant pseudohypoaldosteronism	NR3C2 (4q31.23)	600983
Autosomal recessive pseudohypoaldosteronism	SCNN1A (12p13.31)	600228
	SCNN1B (16p12.2)	600760
	SCNN1G (16p12.2)	600761
Aldosterone synthase deficiency	CYP11B2 (8q24.3)	124080

TABLE 47.1 Disorders of the adrenal cortex of fetal and neonatal onset and encoding genes—cont'd

	Gene (location)	OMIM
Other causes of primary adrenal insufficiency:		
SF-1 deficiency	*NR5A1 (9q33.3)*	*184757*
Zellweger syndrome	*PEX1 (7q21.2)*	*602136*
Wolman syndrome,	*LIPA (10q23.31)*	*613497*
Smith-Lemli-Opitz syndrome	*DHCR7 (11q13.4)*	*602858*
IMAGE syndrome	*CDKN1C (11p15.4)*	*600856*
MIRAGE syndrome	*SAMD9 (7q21.2)*	*610456*
SGPL1 mutations	*SGPL1 (10q22.1)*	*603729*
Secondary adrenal insufficiency:		
T-box transcription factor TBX19	*TPIT (1q23-24)*	*604614*
Proopiomelanocortin	*POMC (2p23.3)*	*176830*
Proprotein convertase subtilisin/kexin type 1	*PCSK1 (5q15)*	*162150*
Homeobox protein prophet of PIT-1	*PROP1 (5q35.3)*	*601538*
Homeobox gene expressed in ES cell	*HESX1 (3p14.3)*	*601802*
Orthodenticle homeobox 2 protein	*OTX2 (14q22.3)*	*600037*
LIM/homeobox protein 4	*LHX4 (1q25.2)*	*602146*

47.4 CONGENITAL ADRENAL HYPERPLASIA

The production of cortisol in the zona fasciculata of the adrenal cortex occurs in five major enzyme-mediated steps (Fig. 47.3). CAH arises from a diminished enzymatic activity at each of the steps of cortisol synthesis with the subsequent increase in ACTH production via the negative feedback system resulting in a distinct hormonal profile. The five different enzymatic defects in CAH are described in the following paragraphs.[2]

47.4.1 21-Hydroxylase Deficiency

CAH occurs as a result of genetic mutations of the ***CYP21A2*** gene (***Cytochrome P450 Family 21 Subfamily A Member 2***), which encodes the 21-hydroxylase enzyme in the adrenal cortex. CAH is transmitted as an autosomal recessive trait. The gene for CAH maps to chromosome 6p21.33 in humans.[11] Several ***CYP21A2*** mutations have been reported to date with variable degrees of associated enzymatic deficiency (Fig. 47.4).

In 21-hydroxylase deficiency, the function of the 21-hydroxylating cytochrome P450 is inadequate, creating a block in the cortisol synthesis. The 21-hydroxylase defect leads to an accumulation of 17-hydroxyprogesterone (17-OHP) and 17-hydroxypregnenolone, the hormone precursors to the 21-hydroxylation step. Excess 17-OHP and 17-hydroxypregnenolone are then shunted into the intact androgen pathway via the 17,20-lyase enzyme.

CAH occurs in a classical and nonclassical form. The classical form includes the salt-wasting form of CAH and the nonsalt wasting form of CAH, the simple virilizing form. The salt-wasting and the simple virilizing form have recognizable different mutations in the steroid 21-hydroxylase gene. The simple virilizing form also has a typical genotype. Both the salt-wasting and simple virilizing forms result in varying degrees of genital ambiguity in the affected female.

The salt-wasting form is considered the most severe phenotype as it also results from mineralocorticoid (aldosterone) deficiency, leading to renal sodium wasting and the risk of fatality unless early treatment is instituted. The newborn may develop an adrenal crisis that requires emergency treatment. The female is usually spared this crisis because of recognition of genital ambiguity at birth. However, male infants do not demonstrate genital ambiguity and therefore may often go

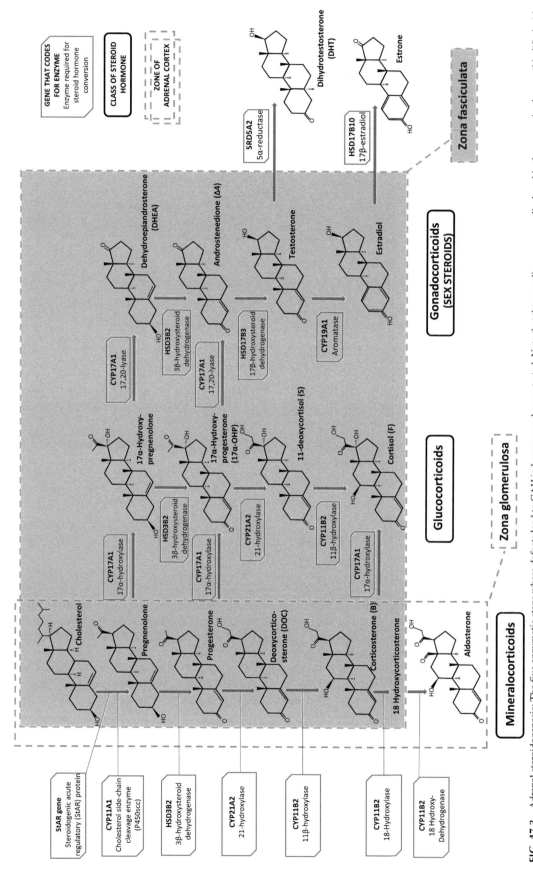

FIG. 47.3 Adrenal steroidogenesis: The five enzymatic steps where defects lead to CAH in human are demonstrated. Note that the encoding genes are displayed in the respective boxes. *(Modified with permission from Fig. 3A.8 – Chapter 3A Genetic Steroid Disorders (Copyright Elsevier 2014). New MI, et al. Genetic steroid disorders. Amsterdam; Boston; Heidelberg; London; New York; Oxford; Paris; San Diego; Singapore; Tokyo: Elsevier; 2014. xiii, 392 pages.)*

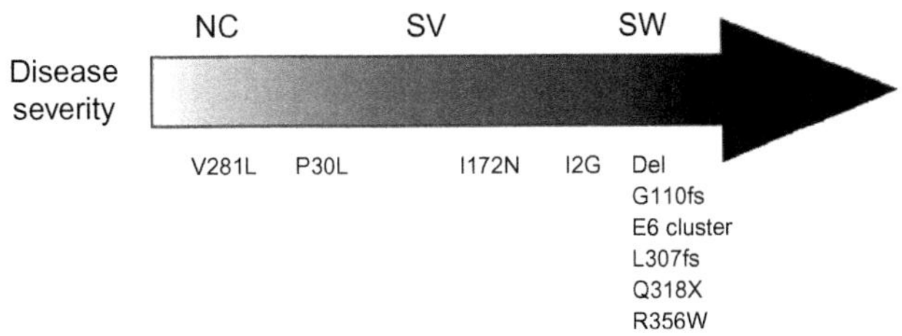

FIG. 47.4 Spectrum of disease severity correlated with CYP21A2 mutations. *(Adapted with permission from Fig. 3A.8 – Chapter 3A* Genetic Steroid Disorders *(Copyright Elsevier 2014).* New MI, et al. Genetic steroid disorders. *Amsterdam; Boston; Heidelberg; London; New York; Oxford; Paris; San Diego; Singapore; Sydney; Tokyo: Elsevier; 2014. xiii, 392 pages.)*

unrecognized and are at risk for adrenal crisis and fatality. The institution of newborn hormonal screening for every baby in the United States has prevented fatality in most cases. In the simple virilizing form, there is no salt wasting but the female is recognized at birth because of genital ambiguity and is diagnosed by newborn screening.[12,13] The 21-hydroxylase enzyme defect in the mild nonclassical form of the disease is only partial and salt wasting does not occur. Salt wasting also does not occur in the simple virilizing form of CAH.[2]

The nonclassical form results from mild genotypic abnormalities and the affected female does not manifest genital ambiguity. Masculinization of the affected female may occur at various times after birth and may require medical treatment. On the other hand, some patients with the nonclassical form of CAH do not manifest masculinizing features until puberty and adulthood. These phenotypic features may include irregular menstruation, impaired fertility, rapid growth with bone age advancement and early fusion of the epiphyses. Boys with the nonclassical form manifest early facial hair, acne, rapid growth, and advanced bone age, which may result in early fusion of epiphyses and short stature.[12,13]

Newborn screening for CAH is carried out in all states in the United States by measuring 17-OHP in blood spots placed on filter paper on the second or third day of life. Unfortunately, newborn screening misses the diagnosis of the nonclassical form of CAH because the 17-OHP is not as elevated in the blood spot as it is in the classical form. Until newborn screening is developed based on genetics rather than hormonal levels, the nonclassical form will be missed based on newborn hormonal screening.[14]

Fortunately, the correlations of the form of CAH and the genotype have been published and the correlation is strong (Fig. 47.5).[15] Thus based on prenatal genetic diagnosis of the fetus, the diagnosis of the specific form of CAH may be determined. The strong correlation of phenotype to genotype may also be used for diagnosis in infancy, childhood, and adulthood, although for milder forms of CAH, this may not always be the case. This may, in part, be explained by the discovery of the "back-door" pathway to androgen synthesis. This pathway is proposed to be an alternative route for the synthesis of dihydrotestosterone (DHT) from 17-α-hydroxyprogesterone (17OHP), which does not involve the intermediate androgens, androstenedione or testosterone, but rather 3α,5α-17-hydropregnanolone and androsterone. Additionally, back-door pathway biomarkers have been suggested in evaluating therapy for CAH.[16–20]

Computational studies have shown the mechanisms by which the mutation alters the phenotype.[11] A nomogram has been constructed to show the response of 17-OHP to ACTH stimulation, which is useful to clinicians for the biochemical diagnosis of CAH. The baseline and 60min after ACTH stimulation concentrations of 17-OHP in ng/dL to the log10 are plotted on the ordinate and the abscissa. A regression line is thereby developed to classify the form of CAH into classical, nonclassical as well as carrier state (Fig. 47.6).[21]

47.4.2   Clinical Features of 21-Hydroxylase Deficiency

External genitalia: Females affected with the classical form of 21-hydroxylase deficiency present at birth with masculinization of external genitalia. Adrenocortical function begins at around the 7th week of gestation; thus a female fetus with classical CAH is exposed to adrenal androgens at the critical time of sexual differentiation, at approximately 9–15 weeks of gestation. Androgens interact with the receptors on the genital skin and induce changes in the developing external female genitalia. This leads to clitoral enlargement, fusion, and scrotalization of the labial folds and rostral migration of the urethral/vaginal perineal orifice, placing the clitoris/phallus in the male position. The degree of genital virilization may range from mild clitoral enlargement alone to, in rare cases, a penile urethra. Degrees of genital virilization have been classically categorized into five Prader stages (Fig. 47.7).[22,23] More recently, more objective scoring systems have been developed that

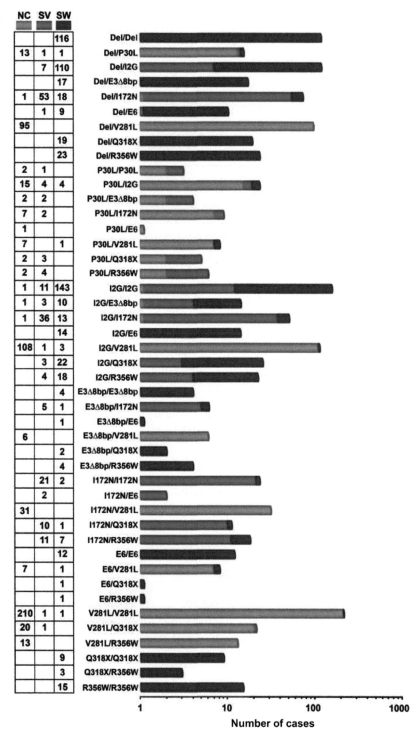

FIG. 47.5 Correlation of the CYP21A2 mutations to the clinical phenotype in 21-OHD CAH. *(Reproduced with permission from New MI, et al. Genotype-phenotype correlation in 1,507 families with congenital adrenal hyperplasia owing to 21-hydroxylase deficiency. Proc Natl Acad Sci USA 2013;110(7):2611–6.)*

describe the genitalia, including the position of the urethral meatus, the extent of posterior fusion and of gonadal descent, and the measurement of the genital tubercle (preferentially used instead of clitoris, phallus, or penis when describing differences/disorders in sex development (DSD)).[24]

Internal genitalia: The internal genitalia of a classical CAH female are normal independent of the degree of external genital masculinization. The patient has capacity for child bearing when treated.[25]

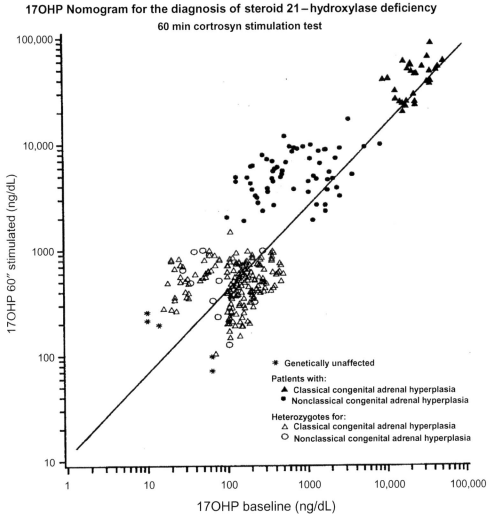

17OHP Nomogram for the diagnosis of steroid 21–hydroxylase deficiency

60 min cortrosyn stimulation test

The data for this nomogram was collected between 1982 and 1991 at the Department of Pediatrics. The New York Hospital–Cornell Medical Center. New York. NY. 10021.

FIG. 47.6 Nomogram relating baseline to ACTH stimulated serum concentrations of 17-OHP. *(Reproduced with permission from Fig. 3A.3 – Chapter 3A Genetic Steroid Disorders (Copyright Elsevier 2014). New MI, et al. Genetic steroid disorders. Amsterdam; Boston; Heidelberg; London; New York; Oxford; Paris; San Diego; Singapore; Sydney; Tokyo: Elsevier; 2014. xiii, 392 pages.)*

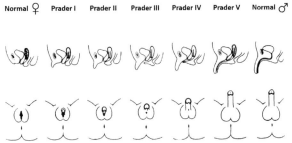

FIG. 47.7 Different degrees of virilization according to the scale developed by Prader: Stage 1: clitoromegaly without labial fusion; Stage 2: clitoromegaly and posterior labial fusion; Stage 3: greater degree of clitoromegaly, single perineal urogenital orifice and almost complete labial fusion; Stage 4: increasingly phallic clitoris, urethra-like urogenital sinus at the base of clitoris and complete labial fusion; Stage 5: penile clitoris, urethral meatus at the tip of phallus and scrotum-like labia (appear like males without palpable gonads). *(Reproduced with permission from Fig. 3A.9 – Chapter 3A Genetic Steroid Disorders (Copyright Elsevier 2014). New MI, et al. Genetic steroid disorders. Amsterdam; Boston; Heidelberg; London; New York; Oxford; Paris; San Diego; Singapore; Sydney; Tokyo: Elsevier; 2014. xiii, 392 pages; New MI, et al. An update on prenatal diagnosis and treatment of congenital adrenal hyperplasia. Semin Reprod Med 2012;30(5):396–9; Ahmed SF, Khwaja O, Hughes IA. The role of a clinical score in the assessment of ambiguous genitalia. BJU Int 2000;85(1):120–124; Prader A, Gurtner HP, The syndrome of male pseudohermaphrodism in congenital adrenocortical hyperplasia without overproduction of androgens (adrenal male pseudohermaphrodism). Helv Paediatr Acta 1955;10(4):397–412.)*

Puberty: Puberty in patients with classical CAH (both girls and boys) occurs at the expected chronological age if properly treated. Those improperly treated and chronically exposed to excess adrenal androgens and aromatized estrogens may have early epiphyseal fusion and an early arrest of growth, leading to short adult height. Other hyperandrogenic signs include male pattern alopecia and acne. Inadequately treated females may develop hirsutism, menstrual irregularities, and impaired fertility. Postpubertal males with inadequate treatment are at a high risk of developing testicular adrenal rest tumors. These represent adrenal rests within the testicular tissue. With proper treatment, adrenal rests may be reduced in size.[25]

Surgery (Genitoplasty): Genitoplasty is the corrective surgery performed by urologists for the correction of genital ambiguity and may involve vaginoplasty and/or clitoroplasty. The timing of genital surgery in the virilized female has been discussed in numerous recent clinical practice guidelines and consensus statements, and it is clear that a more conservative approach is being practiced in many academic centers around the world. Medically necessary surgery to repair the urogenital sinus to prevent hematocolpos and other complications in severely virilized females is not debated; however, it has been argued that the choice of more extensive genitoplasty for minors with CAH be deferred until the patient's age of consent when they can advocate for their gender assignment preference. *The Endocrine Society Clinical Practice Guidelines for Congenital Adrenal Hyperplasia* recommends that "in the treatment of minors with CAH, all surgical decisions remain the prerogative of families (i.e., parents with assent from older children) in joint decision making with experienced surgical consultants" and that "parents be informed about all surgical options, including delaying surgery and/or observation until the child is older." Outcome data cited in the guidelines suggest that early complete surgical repair be performed on virilized females with a low urogenital confluence of the vagina and urethra; whereas, recommended timing is more uncertain for patients with a high confluence of the vagina and urethra close to the bladder neck. A reported advantage to early complete reconstruction is the ability to reconstruct the anterior vaginal wall with excess urogenital sinus tissue. However, at this time, the Endocrine Society states that "there is no objective evidence at this time as to whether early, late or no surgery best preserves overall quality of life or sexual function".[61]

Parents play an important role as caretakers of their infants, and in concert with the healthcare team, they may choose genitoplasty for female infants born with classical CAH, but need to be fully informed about the nonnegligible risk of complications such as enuresis, urinary tract infections, decreased clitoral sensitivity, and vaginal stenosis, as well as the need for long-term follow-up. What is agreed upon by all is that if genital surgery is to be performed, it is critical that the surgical team have demonstrated expertise in genital reconstruction surgery, because the long-term results of treatment depend greatly on the skill and experience of the surgeon.[26–30]

47.4.3 11β-Hydroxylase Deficiency

CAH resulting from mutations in *CYP11B1* (*Cytochrome P450, Family 11, Subfamily B, Member 1*), the gene encoding 11β-hydroxylase, represents a rare autosomal Mendelian disorder resulting in abnormal steroid secretion by the adrenal cortex. Unlike CAH resulting from 21-hydroxylase deficiency, this disease is far more common in the Middle East and North Africa, where consanguinity is common, and results in identical mutations in affected siblings in a family. Clinically affected female newborns are profoundly virilized. Both males and females have significantly advanced bone ages and are frequently hypertensive. The 11-deoxycortisol, which is not frequently assayed, is the most robust biochemical marker of the diagnosis of 11β-hydroxylase deficiency. Computational studies of 25 missense mutations of *CYP11B1* revealed that specific modifications in the heme binding (R374W and 448C) or substrate binding (W116C) site of 11β-hydroxylase or alterations in its stability (L299P and G267S) may predict the severity of disease.[9]

The gene *CYP11B1* is mapped to chromosome 8q 24.3. This gene has nine exons and predominant mutations are found on exon 8 (Fig. 47.8A). In 2017, the largest international cohort of patients with 11β-hydroxylase deficiency CAH demonstrated a worldwide prevalence in Middle Eastern countries, including Turkey, Iran, Pakistan, Saudi Arabia, Yemen, Syria, Lebanon, Egypt, and Tunisia (Fig. 47.8B). The highest rate of consanguinity was demonstrated in Tunisia (Table 47.2). There is a high degree of virilization of genitalia in females affected with 11β-hydroxylase deficiency (Fig. 47.8C), as demonstrated in a genotype-phenotype study where there were 9 females out of 108 with Prader Score 5 (Fig. 47.7). In classical CAH owing to 21-hydroxylase deficiency only 4 patients with Prader score 5 genitalia were observed.[9,31] The international cohort also highlights the bone age advancement, blood pressure elevation, and the significance of 11-deoxycortisol as a biochemical marker for the diagnosis (Fig. 47.8D, E, and F).

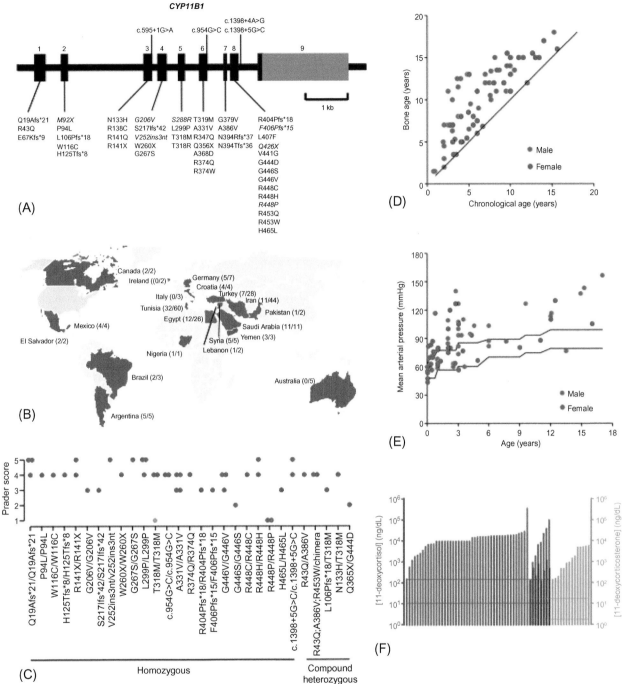

FIG. 47.8 Clinical profile for patients with CAH resulting from 11β-hydroxylase deficiency from 13 nations comprising the International Consortium for Rare Steroid Disorders. (A): Structure of the human CYP11B1 gene that contains nine exons, showing mutations harbored by 108 patients in this international cohort. Previously unreported mutations are shown in italics. (B): Worldwide distribution of our cases of 11β-hydroxylase deficiency. The denominator indicates the number of patients originating from that country with 11β-hydroxylase deficiency. The numerator indicates the number of patients with 11β-hydroxylase deficiencies who have been genotyped. All patients who originated from the Middle East and European countries have been placed in their respective countries. It is evident from this map that the majority of patients with 11β-hydroxylase deficiency originate in the Middle East and North Africa. (C): Prader scores of patients with different genotypes (noted), both as homozygotes and compound heterozygotes. One patient *(green)* has been treated prenatally with dexamethasone. (D): Bone age versus chronological age in male *(blue)* and female *(red)* patients. The *black line* represents a slope of 1 (bone age = chronological age). Of note is that almost all patients show evidence of advanced bone age. (E): Mean arterial pressure (1/3 systolic pressure + 2/3 diastolic pressure) shown for both males and female patients of various ages. The *two lines* indicate the age-appropriate upper and lower limits of the normal range. Blood pressure that is elevated above the normal scores indicates that hypertension is present in both young and old patients. (F): Measurements of 11-deoxycortisol *(red)* and 11-deoxycorticosterone *(green)* in our patient cohort. Shown also are normal reference ranges for both hormones *(horizontal lines)*. *(Reproduced with permission (Copyright Proc Natl Acad Sci USA 2017). Khattab A, et al. Clinical, genetic, and structural basis of congenital adrenal hyperplasia due to 11beta-hydroxylase deficiency. Proc Natl Acad Sci USA 2017;**114**(10):E1933–40.)*

TABLE 47.2 Consanguinity rates in countries with high prevalence of 11β-hydroxylase deficiency CAH[9]

Country	Consanguinity rate
Tunisia	20–39
Iran	39
Egypt	29
Turkey	34
Saudi Arabia	52

47.4.4   3β-Hydroxysteroid Dehydrogenase Deficiency

The enzyme 3β-hydroxysteroid dehydrogenase 2 (3β-HSD2) deficiency is responsible for the translation of $\triangle^5$steroids into $\triangle^4$steroids, which is necessary for the biosynthesis of a class of active steroids, e.g., progesterone, mineralocorticoids, glucocorticoids, androgens, and estrogens. Thus the inactive steroid 17-hydroxypregnenolone is converted to the active steroid 17-OHP (Fig. 47.3). $\triangle^5$steroids are generally not biologically active, while $\triangle^4$steroids are. The classical form of 3β-HSD2 is transmitted as an autosomal recessive trait and is characterized by varying degrees of salt wasting. In genetic males, fetal testicular 3β-HSD2 deficiency causes impaired masculinization of genitalia, while females may exhibit mild virilization of the external genitalia.

The molecular genetics of the severe form of classical 3β-HSD2 deficiency associated with salt wasting has been reported and these mutations are very rare. Review of the specific mutations in the encoding gene, **HSD3B2**, and their phenotype has been reported.[32–35] Although genetic mutations have been documented in the classical form of 3β-HSD2 deficiency, mutations of the mild form of 3β-HSD2 have not been found. It appears that children with premature pubarche and hirsute females do not have decreased adrenal 3β-HSD2 activity resulting from either the severe or mild 3β-HSD2 mutations. As the mild form of 3β-HSD2 deficiency has not been proven to have a genetic basis, the prenatal diagnosis of this defect is uncertain. More studies are required for search for mutations in the mild nonclassical form of 3β-HSD2 deficiency.[36] Of note, **HSD3B1** encodes a distinct enzyme 3β-hydroxysteroid dehydrogenase 1 that is expressed in the placenta and peripheral tissues.[37]

47.4.5   StAR Protein Deficiency

StAR protein deficiency is discussed in further detail under "Familial glucocorticoid deficiency."

47.4.6   17-Hydroxylase/17, 20-Lyase Deficiency

A female with the genetic defect of 17-hydroxylase deficiency was first described by Dr. Edward Biglieri in the early 1960s.[38] Complete deficiency of **CYP17A1 (Cytochrome P450, Family 17, Subfamily A, Member 1)** causes severe disruption of adrenal and gonadal steroidogenesis. The deficiency of 17, 20-lyase results in impaired androgen production and, as a result, estrogen production, as estrogen is formed by the aromatization of androgens. Therefore, neither androgens nor estrogens are produced by the gonads in patients with 17-hydroxylase deficiency (Fig. 47.3). The genes for 17-hydroxylase and 17, 20-lyase have been cloned and mapped (Fig. 47.9).[39–42]

The postnatal deficiency of androgens and estrogens in patients with 17-hydroxylase and 17, 20-lyase leads to sexual infantilism and affected individuals do not develop secondary sexual characteristics. Males have undervirilized external genitalia that are more female appearing and may have a vaginal pouch as a result of failure to produce androgens. Females with 17-hydroxylase deficiency also lack secondary sexual characteristics from estrogen deficiency. The first male described by New et al. was very undervirilized and had breasts.[43–45]

The lack of secreted cortisol results in increased ACTH production via the negative feedback loop, which drives the adrenal to secrete more corticosterone, which compensates for the lack of cortisol. Additionally, the mineralocorticoid, deoxycorticosterone (DOC) levels are elevated and in large amounts raise the blood pressure. Sodium conservation is preserved by the action of DOC, which conserves sodium almost as efficiently as aldosterone. In the untreated patient with 17-hydroxylase deficiency, plasma renin is suppressed owing to volume expansion from increased levels of

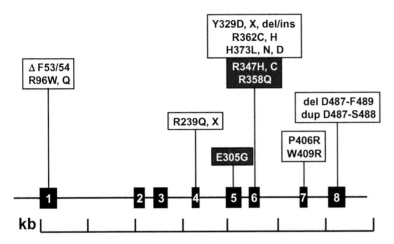

FIG. 47.9 Schematic diagram of CYP17A1 gene, location of common mutations and mutations causing isolated 17,20-lyase deficiency. Exons are shown as black rectangles with white numbers connected by a solid horizontal line, with scale below. Mutations found in isolated 17,20-lyase deficiency are shown in gray boxes with white text. *(Reproduced with permission from Fig. 3G.1– Chapter 3G Genetic Steroid Disorders (Copyright Elsevier 2014). New MI, et al.* Genetic steroid disorders. *Amsterdam; Boston; Heidelberg; London; New York; Oxford; Paris; San Diego; Singapore; Sydney; Tokyo: Elsevier; 2014. xiii, 392 pages.)*

TABLE 47.3 Comparison of different forms of CAH

	Mineralocorticoid	Glucocorticoid	Androgen	Diagnostic adrenal precursor	Clinical features
21 hydroxylase	↓	↓	↑	↑17 OHP ↑ACTH	Virilized 46, XX Salt wasting
StAR protein deficiency	↓	↓	↓	All low ↑ACTH	Undervirilized 46, XY Salt wasting
11 hydroxylase	DOC ↑	↓	↑	↑DOC ↑ACTH	Virilized 46, XX Low renin hypertension
3 β HSD	↓	↓	↑↓	↑17 OH pregneolone	Virilized 46, XX Undervirilized 46, XY Salt wasting
17 hydroxylase	↑	↓	↓	↑ACTH	Undervirilized 46, XY Low renin hypertension

corticosterone and DOC. Because the renin is suppressed, aldosterone is not secreted, resulting in a very low serum aldosterone level.

In conclusion, 17-hydroxylase deficiency causes abnormal elevation of serum hormones in the mineralocorticoid pathway while 17, 20-lyase mostly impairs androgen and estrogen secretion, resulting in abnormal sexual development. Table 47.3 displays a comparison between the different forms of CAH.

47.5 P450 OXIDOREDUCTASE DEFICIENCY

Cytochrome P450 oxidoreductase deficiency (PORD) is the newest form of CAH, first described in 2004.[46] After the classic forms of CAH and their associated genetic defects were identified, there remained patients who demonstrated a metabolic profile of more than one defect—including 21-hydroxylase deficiency and 17-hydroxylase deficiency—but who did not have the genetic defects in *CYP21A2* or *CYP17A1*. Years later, the underlying genetic defect on the *POR* gene was sequenced and described in a Japanese 46, XX girl, who manifested evidence of two defects, 21- and 17-hydroxylase deficiencies. The *POR* gene provides electrons to all microsomal type II P450 steroids and >50 amino acid changes have been reported by various laboratories. *POR* has a major role in the metabolism of drugs, as well as steroids. The gene for *POR* is mapped to chromosome 7q11.23. All microsomal P450 steroidogenic enzymes depend on POR for the supply of electrons from NADPH for their catalytic activities to metabolize drugs and steroid hormones (Fig. 47.10).

FIG. 47.10 Electron donation by cytochrome P450 oxidoreductase to steroidogenic enzymes.

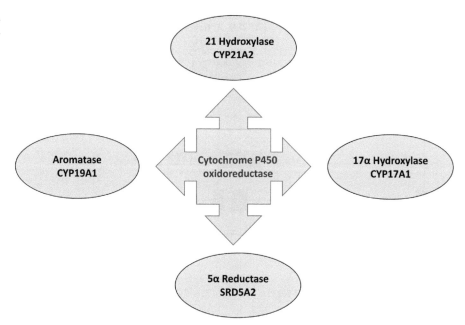

The phenotypic spectrum of PORD is very wide. While PORD definitively disrupts adrenal steroid biosynthesis, the clinical manifestations are quite variable as some patients manifest genital ambiguity at birth in both sexes and some have skeletal malformations, such as craniosynostosis, midface hypoplasia and radio-humeral synostosis, resembling the rare Antley-Bixler syndrome.[46–51]

47.6 PRENATAL DIAGNOSIS AND TREATMENT—NONINVASIVE PRENATAL DIAGNOSIS OF CAH

A major hallmark of classical CAH is genital ambiguity noted at birth in affected females, leading to psychological and psychosexual issues in adult life. Surgical interventions to correct genital ambiguity have been successful only in part, and can result in urinary incontinence and sexual dysfunction.[52–54] Medical management of high-risk expectant mothers with low-dose dexamethasone began in the 1990s.[55] The purpose was to suppress fetal androgen production during urogenital differentiation starting at the 9th gestational week, thereby preventing or attenuating genital virilization. Despite successful outcomes in a cohort of over 500 patients,[55] two sets of concerns have arisen. First, not all high-risk fetuses, namely all males and unaffected (normal or carrier) females, who are being treated from the 9th gestational week benefit from therapy, as they are born with normal genitalia. These unaffected fetuses remain exposed to dexamethasone until therapy is terminated when gender and genetic diagnosis become available 2–3 weeks following chorionic villus sampling (~12 weeks) or amniocentesis (~16 weeks). Thus, 7 out of 8 unaffected fetuses are unnecessarily exposed to dexamethasone for 5–10 weeks. Second, there is an ongoing debate on whether dexamethasone, even when given at fivefold lower doses than that used in the third trimester to enhance lung maturity or prevent premature labor, results in reduced birth weight and mental impairment.[55–61] These issues together have called for a diagnostic test that will establish gender and confirm the diagnosis of CAH definitively before or around the 9th gestational week, and in doing so prevent males and unaffected females from being exposed to dexamethasone unnecessarily.

Treatment must be begun as early as possible, preferentially before 6 weeks, when the external genitalia begin differentiation. Exposure of not-at-risk fetuses can, however, be minimized by the use of cell-free fetal DNA, which can be obtained from maternal blood very early on in gestation (as early as 4 weeks) for the determination of fetal sex through *SRY* testing.

More recently, a method was developed through which inheritance of a CYP21A2 mutation can be established by targeted massively parallel sequencing (MPS) of cell-free fetal DNA in 3.6 mL plasma drawn from an expectant mother as early as ~6 gestational weeks.[62] This technology has been applied with success to the prenatal diagnosis of β-thalassemia, achondroplasia, and cystic fibrosis, and is likely to be used in other monogenic disorders that may benefit from gene or stem cell therapy.[63–67] This technology is not an assay for detecting specific CYP21A2 mutations. Instead, by performing targeted MPS of genomic DNA from the trio (parents and proband), it defines informative SNPs (single nucleotide polymorphisms) around the CYP21A2 locus, so that haplotype blocks can be created to determine paternal and maternal allelic inheritance. Full diagnostic concordance was demonstrated between this noninvasive method and invasive diagnostic procedures, or postnatal genetic testing in 14 families.[62]

47.7   X-LINKED PRIMARY ADRENAL INSUFFICIENCY

47.7.1   Adrenal Hypoplasia Congenita

DAX-1 (dosage-sensitive sex reversal, adrenal hypoplasia critical region, on chromosome X, gene 1) is a nuclear receptor protein that is involved in both gonadal and adrenal development and encoded by the *NR0B1* gene (*nuclear receptor subfamily 0, group B, member 1*).

To date, hundreds of *NR0B1* gene mutations have been reported that give rise to this rare disorder, named adrenal hypoplasia congenita (AHC), usually transmitted in an X-linked fashion, although de novo mutations have been reported.

With a spectrum of variable severity, AHC may present in the newborn period with the picture of adrenal insufficiency and salt-wasting crisis, in addition to characteristics of male hypogonadotropic hypogonadism, namely microphallus and undescended testis, to a less severe phenotype of late onset adrenal insufficiency, delayed puberty, and fertility problems. Of note, AHC with precocious puberty has been previously reported. It is unlikely that a clear genotype–phenotype correlation exists. Management of AHC entails glucocorticoid and mineralocorticoid replacement therapy and appropriate treatment of hypogonadism, if present. Prenatal estriol levels are markers of fetal adrenal well-being and low prenatal estriol levels, although not specific, have been associated with pregnancies carrying fetuses with AHC.[10,68–80]

47.7.2   Adrenoleukodystrophy

Adrenoleukodystrophy is a potentially fatal and progressive peroxisomal disorder with a heterogeneous presentation primarily affecting the central and peripheral nervous system and adrenal gland.[81]

Adrenoleukodystrophy is caused by mutations in the *ATP Binding Cassette Subfamily D Member 1* (*ABCD1*) gene, which is mapped to chromosome Xq28 and encodes very long chain fatty acid (VLCFA) transporter and is inherited in an X-linked fashion. *ABCD1* gene mutations result in accumulation of long chain fatty acids in the central and peripheral nervous systems as well as the adrenal gland, with a resultant damage.[82]

The recent introduction of adrenoleukodystrophy to the newborn screening panel in the United States will allow early diagnosis in the newborn period where early intervention may be lifesaving. The state of New York was the first to screen for adrenoleukodystrophy in 2013.[83]

With onset of symptoms during childhood or later on in adulthood, adrenoleukodystrophy is characterized by its clinical heterogeneity. The most common form, cerebral adrenoleukodystrophy, is associated with significant neurological and adrenal involvement and usually presents during midchildhood with eventual disability in a relatively short period of time.[81]

Adrenomyeloneuropathy (AMN) usually presents in early adulthood and is slowly progressive. A rare form of adrenoleukodystrophy primarily associated with adrenal disease may present any time from early childhood to adulthood. Although female carriers may show some neurological signs and symptoms, adrenal involvement is unlikely.[82,84]

47.8   FAMILIAL GLUCOCORTICOID DEFICIENCY

Familial glucocorticoid deficiency is a group of disorders that results from distinct genetic mutations that are inherited in an autosomal recessive trait—also referred to as ACTH resistance syndromes.

The isolated glucocorticoid insufficiency is secondary to failure of adrenal stimulation by pituitary ACTH while adrenal mineralocorticoid production, primarily under control of the renin angiotensin system, is usually intact. Significant hyperpigmentation occurs due to the action of the markedly elevated levels of ACTH on melanocortin 1 receptors (MC1R), implemented in hair and skin pigmentation.

Markedly elevated ACTH levels combined with a low or undetectable cortisol level in a hyperpigmented newborn is a clinical clue to the diagnosis of ACTH resistance.[85,86]

47.8.1 Pathophysiology of ACTH Resistance

47.8.1.1 Melanocortin 2 Receptor (MC2R) and Melanocortin 2 Receptor Accessory Protein (MRAP) Defects

Mutations in **MC2R**, which encodes the G protein-coupled ACTH transmembrane receptor, are the most common cause of ACTH resistance syndromes, with the pathophysiology being due to the failure of ACTH to bind to its transmembrane adrenal receptor. Additionally, mutations in the **MRAP** gene disrupt the key role of **Melanocortin 2 Receptor Accessory Protein** in facilitating the expression and "trafficking" of the MC2R from the endoplasmic reticulum to the adrenal cell surface. Together, **MC2R** and **MRAP** mutations may be responsible for close to half of the cases of familial glucocorticoid deficiency.[85–87]

47.8.1.2 Lipoid CAH and CYP11A1 Defects

Failure of transmitochondrial cholesterol transport with secondary failure of initiation of steroidogenesis occurs with steroidogenic acute regulatory protein (**StAR**) defects (Fig. 47.3). Lipid accumulation in the cytoplasm with secondary destruction of adrenal cells lead to the disorder lipoid CAH. The expected clinical presentation in the 46, XY newborn with StAR protein defects caused by complete loss of function mutations is that of glucocorticoid deficiency, mineralocorticoid deficiency, and absence of virilization, with female-appearing external genitalia. There have been descriptions of what appears to be a milder or "nonclassical form" of lipoid CAH in which the onset and severity of adrenal insufficiency and gonadal failure may be variable.

Mutations in **CYP11A1** (**Cytochrome P450, Family 11, Subfamily A, Member 1**), which encodes the cytochrome P450 side chain cleavage enzyme, catalyze the conversion of cholesterol to pregnenolone, an early step in adrenal steroidogenesis, and result in a clinical picture of glucocorticoid and mineralocorticoid deficiency and disorder of sexual development similar to that of lipoid CAH; depending on the severity of enzymatic deficiency there is a wide phenotypic spectrum. Adrenal imaging may represent an important clinical pearl in differentiating lipoid CAH from side chain cleavage enzyme deficiency by visualizing enlarged versus small adrenal glands, respectively.[86,88–92]

47.8.1.3 Minichromosome Maintenance Complex Component 4 (MCM4) and Nicotinamide Nucleotide Transhydrogenase (NNT)

MCM4 and **NNT** are two recently described defects in the glucocorticoid resistance family. Defects in minichromosome maintenance-deficient 4 homologue (MCM4) result in alterations in DNA replication and defects in nicotinamide nucleotide transhydrogenase (NNT) with disruption of its presumed role in protection against oxidative stress.[86,93–95] MCM4 defects have been described to be associated with growth defects, immunological dysfunction, and chromosomal fragility. Finally, the first homozygous mutation in **Thioredoxin Reductase 2** (**TXNRD2**), with resultant imbalance between mitochondrial oxidation and reduction and a clinical picture of isolated glucocorticoid deficiency, was reported in a Kashmiri kindred in 2014.[96]

47.8.1.4 Triple-A Syndrome

Triple-A syndrome is caused by mutations in the **AAAS** gene, which encodes a protein **ALADIN** and is implemented in transnuclear molecular transport and is abundant in the adrenal, gastrointestinal, and central nervous system. Patients aff resistance, achalasia of the cardia, and alacrima.[86,97,98]

47.9 MINERALOCORTICOID PATHWAY DEFECTS

47.9.1 Hyperaldosteronism

Hyperaldosteronism occurs in Conn's syndrome owing to a benign adrenal adenoma that secretes aldosterone.[99] Extirpation of the tumor usually results in a cure of the hypertension and muscular weakness, owing to the tumor's secretion of excess aldosterone. In children, however, hyperaldosteronism results from adrenal hyperplasia rather than an adrenal adenoma. In children, an adrenalectomy may not be as successful as the surgery is for Conn's syndrome.

47.9.2   Glucocorticoid-Remediable Hyperaldosteronism

Hyperaldosteronism also occurs in a syndrome known as glucocorticoid-remediable hyperaldosteronism (GRA), a syndrome that was almost simultaneously described by New et al. and Sutherland et al. in 1966.[100,101] The usual physiology of aldosterone is that the mineralocorticoid hormone is secreted by the adrenal cortex in the zona glomerulosa, not in the zona fasciculata. However, in patients with GRA, aldosterone is secreted in the zona fasciculata owing to a chimeric gene. In 1992, Lifton et al.[102] described a large kindred in which the presence of GRA cosegregated with a chimeric gene duplication in the 11β-hydroxylase gene (Fig. 47.11).[103] This results from an unequal crossover of the homologous 11β-hydroxylase (*CYP11B1*) and aldosterone synthase (*CYP11B2-* Cytochrome P450, Family 11, Subfamily B, Member 2) genes, located in close proximity on chromosome 8. As a result, aldosterone is secreted by the zona fasciculata under control of ACTH rather than the zona glomerulosa, which is regulated by angiotensin II. Thus patients with GRA respond to dexamethasone with a fall in aldosterone and improvement of their symptoms of hypertension and hypokalemia. GRA is transmitted as an autosomal dominant trait.[104] Patients with GRA have been observed in many countries, but the syndrome appears to be very rare in Africa. The clinical presentation of GRA can be found in childhood as well as adulthood. Treatment for GRA consists of the administration of glucocorticoid steroids to suppress ACTH and thereby the production of aldosterone. Treatment may also include diuretics and eplerenone.

47.9.3   Pseudohypoaldosteronism

Autosomal dominant pseudohypoaldosteronism (ADPHA) is a rare condition characterized by renal resistance to aldosterone action. Symptomatic newborns present with salt wasting, hyperkalemia, hypotension, metabolic acidosis, and elevated aldosterone levels. While patients respond promptly to dietary salt supplementation, treatment is often not required after childhood. Missense, nonsense, frameshift, and splice mutations in the mineralocorticoid receptor (*MR*) gene encoding the mineralocorticoid receptor, a member of the nuclear receptor superfamily, cause ADPHA. Reports in affected individuals showed initial resistance to aldosterone infusion followed by gradual correction of electrolytes in early childhood with subsequent resolution of symptoms in adulthood. Adults with the autosomal dominant form have been found to be indistinguishable from their relatives except for lifelong elevation of renin, angiotensin II, and aldosterone levels.[105–109]

Autosomal recessive pseudohypoaldosteronism (ARPHA) is the autosomal recessive form of PHA owing to loss of function mutations and deletions in the *alpha ENaC* gene. The neonatal presentation is usually more severe than that of the milder ADPHA. In addition to renal affection, gastrointestinal, pulmonary, salivary, and sweat gland sodium channel involvement is characteristic. Treatment with salt supplementation to correct the hyponatremia, sodium citrate (Bicitra) to correct acidosis, and Kayexalate to correct hyperkalemia is lifesaving and usually continued till adulthood.

Parents of the affected individual are usually heterozygous for the same mutation shown in the proband. An unpublished female patient with genetically confirmed ARPHA had on the first day of life an aldosterone level of 3563 ng/dL (normal aldosterone level 7–175 ng/dL) and very high plasma renin activity levels (>370 ng/mL/h); by the second week of life her aldosterone level was 1674 ng/dL. The patient has grown well and is thriving and has achieved her target height at the age of

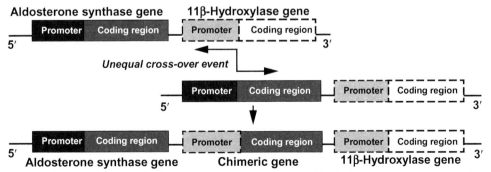

FIG. 47.11   Chimeric gene formation in GRA results form an unequal crossover event, resulting in aldosterone synthesis abnormal regulation by ACTH rather than by the renin-angiotensin system. *(Reproduced with permission from Fig. 6C.3 – Chapter 6C Genetic Steroid Disorders (Copyright Elsevier 2014). New MI, et al. Genetic steroid disorders. Amsterdam; Boston; Heidelberg; London; New York; Oxford; Paris; San Diego; Singapore; Sydney; Tokyo: Elsevier; 2014. xiii, 392 pages; Halperin F, Dluhy RG, Glucocorticoid-remediable aldosteronism. Endocrinol Metab Clin N Am 2011;40 (2):333–341 [viii].)*

16 years. Her electrolyte levels have normalized after treating her with Kayexalate, sodium chloride, and sodium bicarbonate since birth.[107,110]

47.9.4 Hypoaldosteronism

Aldosterone synthase deficiency is an autosomal recessive disorder caused by mutations in the gene *CYP11B2* associated with impaired aldosterone synthesis occurring from defects in aldosterone synthesis from corticosterone. It occurs in two steps: the first step is the 18-hydroxylation of corticosterone to 18-hydroxycorticosterone catalyzed by the 18-hydroxylase enzyme, generally termed *corticosterone methyl oxidase type 1* (*CMO I*). The synthesis of aldosterone from 18 hydroxycorticosterone is catalyzed by the enzyme 18-oxidase, termed *corticosterone methyl oxidase type II* (*CMO II*). CMO type I and II may be collectively termed *aldosterone synthase*. A clinical picture of isolated mineralocorticoid deficiency of variable degree that resolves with age occurs in both CMO type I and type II deficiencies; however, the elevated ratios of corticosterone to 18-hydroxycorticosterone and 18-hydroxycorticosterone to aldosterone respectively may help differentiate both types biochemically.

The impairment of aldosterone synthesis from its precursors was originally documented in the city of Isfahan, Iran,[111] with the most common mutations being *R181W* and *V386A*. These Iranians have aldosterone deficiency owing to CMO type II deficiency.[112,113]

The severity of aldosterone synthase deficiency is dependent on the age, with infants having the most severe form. The deficiency of aldosterone diminishes with age from childhood to adulthood. Although the abnormal biochemical findings do not disappear, the clinical features improve with age. Salt wasting diminishes; the children begin to grow normally and do not require high salt supplementation. There appears to be progressive improvement in renal tubular responsiveness to mineralocorticoids, and serum sodium and potassium progressively normalize. Therapy with salt-retaining steroids can be decreased with age. The infants mostly begin to grow normally and eventually as adults reach a normal height. The cause for the spontaneous remission has not been clearly established.[111,114–116]

47.10 OTHER CAUSES OF PRIMARY ADRENAL INSUFFICIENCY (SEE TABLE 47.4)

47.10.1 Steroidogenic Factor 1 Deficiency

Steroidogenic factor-1 (*SF-1*) is an important transcription factor expressed in the adrenal gland and bipotential gonad in early fetal life; it is encoded by *NR5A1* (*Nuclear receptor subfamily 5 group A member 1*)—mapped to chromosome 9q33.3. Because of its role in steroidogenesis and the development of the hypothalamic pituitary adrenal (and gonadal) axis, SF-1 defects have been associated with primary adrenal insufficiency, 46,XY disorders of sexual development (DSD), and 46,XX ovarian failure, as well as reports of ovotesticular DSD. The role of SF-1 appears to be more crucial in male than in female gonadal development but equally in male and female adrenal development.[117–119]

47.10.2 Zellweger Syndrome

Zellweger syndrome (ZS) is a rare autosomal recessive peroxisomal disorder caused by mutations in the *Peroxins* (*PEX*) genes that encode the peroxisomal assembly proteins. Severe ZS usually presents early in life with a wide spectrum of clinical features including characteristic facial features, ocular abnormalities, musculoskeletal defects, hypotonia, feeding difficulties, cardiac, genitourinary, developmental, neurological, gastrointestinal, and hepatic involvement. Adrenal insufficiency and pancreatic involvement represent the main endocrine features of this progressive and fatal disorder. Biochemical screening is performed by demonstration of elevated plasma levels of VLCFA. ZS is a progressive and fatal disorder with limited treatment options.[6,120,121]

47.10.3 Wolman Syndrome

Deficiency in *lysosomal acid lipase* owing to mutations in the *LIPA* gene results in failure of cleavage of cholesterol esters and its accumulation in the liver, to free cholesterol that is available for adrenal steroidogenesis. This autosomal recessive syndrome may present during the neonatal period but usually during infancy with failure to thrive, vomiting, diarrhea, and, significant enlargement of the liver and spleen. The finding of adrenal calcifications in this context is highly suggestive of the diagnosis. Treatment options include hematopoietic stem cell transplantation and enzyme replacement therapy.[122,123]

TABLE 47.4 Other causes of primary adrenal insufficiency

	Defect	Clinical picture
SF1-deficiency	Transcription factor defect	46,XY disorders of sexual development (DSD), 46,XX ovarian failure Reports of ovotesticular DSD
Zellweger syndrome	Defect in peroxisomal assembly proteins	Characteristic facial features Ocular abnormalities Musculoskeletal defects Hypotonia Feeding difficulties Cardiac defects Genitourinary defects Developmental delays Neurological defects Gastrointestinal & hepatic involvement
Wolman syndrome	Deficiency in lysosomal acid lipase	Failure to thrive Vomiting & diarrhea Significant hepatosplenomegaly
Smith-Lemli-Opitz syndrome	Cholesterol biosynthesis defect	Microcephaly Cognitive & behavioral deficits Cardiac defects Genitourinary defects Skeletal defects Immune defects Genital ambiguity in the 46,XY newborn with a rudimentary uterus Genital malformation of the 46,XX newborn Hypothyroidism and hypoparathyroidism
IMAGe syndrome	Gain of function in proliferating cell nuclear antigen-binding of maternally expressed allele	Intrauterine growth restriction (IUGR) Metaphyseal dysplasia Adrenal hypoplasia congenita Genitourinary abnormalities
MIRAGE syndrome	Sterile alpha motif domain containing 9 mutation	Myelodysplasia, infection, restriction of growth, adrenal hypoplasia, genital phenotypes, and enteropathy
SGPL1 mutations	Intracellular accumulation of sphingosine-1-phosphate	Familial glucocorticoid deficiency Steroid-resistant nephrotic Ichthyosis Primary hypothyroidism Cryptorchidism Immune defects Neurological deficits

47.10.4 Smith-Lemli-Opitz Syndrome

Smith-Lemli-Opitz syndrome (SLOS) is a relatively common autosomal recessive disorder of cholesterol biosynthesis. SLOS is a phenotypically heterogeneous disorder with variable severity caused by >100 different mutations in the *7-dehydroxycholesterolreductase* gene (*DHCR7*) which maps to chromosome 11q13.2–13.5. Clinical features include microcephaly, cognitive and behavioral deficits, and cardiac, genitourinary, skeletal and immune defects. Endocrine features may include adrenal insufficiency, genital ambiguity in the 46,XY newborn with a rudimentary uterus, genital malformation of the 46,XX newborn, hypothyroidism, and hypoparathyroidism.

The clinical picture, elevated plasma 7-dehydrocholesterol (DHC) levels with or without decreased cholesterol levels, and *DHCR7* gene mutational analysis have been used to establish the diagnosis. The mainstay of management is dietary supplementation of cholesterol.[8,124–126]

Prenatal diagnosis of SLOS by demonstrating an *elevated 7-DHC/cholesterol ratio* in the amniotic fluid as well as molecular prenatal analysis of a *DHCR7* gene mutation have been reported.[127–129]

47.10.5 IMAGe Syndrome

The paternal allele of *cyclin dependent kinase inhibitor 1C* (*CDKN1C*), an inhibitor of cellular proliferation, is normally repressed whereas the maternal allele is expressed, a well-established genomic imprinting phenomenon.

Autosomal dominant inheritance of a *CDKN1C* gain of function mutations in the proliferating cell nuclear antigen-binding domain of the maternally expressed allele is associated with the syndromic spectrum of *I*ntrauterine growth restriction (IUGR), *M*etaphyseal dysplasia, *A*drenal hypoplasia congenita, and *Ge*nitourinary abnormalities: IMAGe syndrome. An opposite clinical spectrum of overgrowth and likelihood of malignancies, Beckwith-Wiedemann syndrome, occurs with a loss of function mutations of the same maternally expressed gene.

The main features are IUGR pregnancies with resultant births being small for gestational age infants that may have growth failure with or without GH deficiency, associated with a variable degree of skeletal manifestations and life-threatening primary adrenal failure that may present in the first weeks of life with an adrenal crisis, in addition to microphallus, hypospadias, and bilateral cryptorchidism in the affected male.[7,130–132]

47.10.6 MIRAGE Syndrome

Narumi S et al. recently described the MIRAGE syndrome (acronym for myelodysplasia, infection, restriction of growth, adrenal hypoplasia, genital phenotypes, and enteropathy), which was linked to mutations in *SAMD9* (sterile alpha motif domain containing 9) after sequencing and functional studies in patients with undiagnosed early onset primary adrenal insufficiency.[133,134]

47.10.7 SGPL1 Mutations

This is a recently described syndrome of familial glucocorticoid deficiency and steroid-resistant nephrotic syndrome that may also be associated with ichthyosis, primary hypothyroidism, cryptorchidism, immunodeficiency, and neurological deficits caused by mutations in the gene for *sphingosine-1-phosphate lyase 1* (*SGPL1*).

Pathophysiology is thought to be possibly due to failure to break down S1P due to sphingosine-1-phosphate lyase 1 deficiency and subsequent intracellular accumulation of this important signaling molecule.[131,135]

47.10.8 Secondary Adrenal Insufficiency

Since the glucocorticoid and adrenal androgen pathways are governed by pituitary ACTH, cases of secondary adrenal insufficiency do not manifest with the clinical picture of aldosterone deficiency, as aldosterone is primarily under the control of the renin angiotensin system. ACTH deficiency may be isolated, although rare, or combined with other pituitary hormone deficiencies. The more widespread brain midline defects such as those causing septooptic dysplasia or holoprosencephaly can be associated with phenotypes ranging from subtle craniofacial anomalies to more widespread syndromic features. Mutations in *SHH*, which encodes sonic hedgehog, a critical signaling molecule in embryogenesis, and the *GLI2*, encoding the GLI family zinc finger 2 transcription factor with an activating effect on sonic hedgehog signaling, have been implemented in holoprosencephaly with or without pituitary deficiencies.[136] Affected infants present with signs and symptoms of glucocorticoid deficiency usually without the hyperpigmentation effect of excess ACTH. When ACTH deficiency is combined with other pituitary hormone defects, namely growth hormone deficiency, hypoglycemia and its sequelae in the newborn period may be significant as well as life threatening. Treatment of secondary hypothyroidism may reveal an associated but masked ACTH deficiency; the mechanism of ACTH deficiency masking secondary hypothyroidism is likely due to decreased metabolism of cortisol. On the same note, treatment of secondary adrenal insufficiency may unmask an associated diabetes insipidus.

Mutations in genes encoding transcription factors that orchestrate the hypothalamic pituitary hormone production have been identified in cases of isolated and multiple pituitary hormone deficiencies. The *TPIT* gene (T-box transcription factor TBX19) encodes the T-box transcription factor and is essential for *Proopiomelanocortin (POMC)* transcription. Deletions, missense, nonsense, and splice mutations, inherited in an autosomal recessive fashion, have been identified. Most, but not all, patients with isolated ACTH deficiency who present in the neonatal period have been shown to exhibit TPIT gene mutations.[137–139]

Proopiomelanocortin is normally cleaved by prohormone convertase enzyme to ACTH, α-β-γ MSH, β-γ lipotrophin, and endorphins with a subsequent action upon MC1R (involved in skin pigmentation), MC2R (involved in cortisol production), and MC3R and MC4R (involved in weight control). Mutations in the *POMC* gene are associated with a characteristic picture of lack of pigmentation with red hair, secondary adrenal insufficiency, and obesity and are seen in this rare disorder, which is inherited through an autosomal recessive pattern—another etiology where the only pituitary hormone deficient is ACTH. A clinical picture similar to POMC deficiency, with additional features such as gastrointestinal malabsorption and hypogonadotropic hypogonadism, is seen in patients with prohormone convertase enzyme deficiency secondary to *PCSK1 (Proprotein Convertase Subtilisin/Kexin Type 1)* genetic mutations. Of note, in 2013, Samuels et al. reported a unique case of immunoassayable but bioactive ACTH molecule causing glucocorticoid deficiency.[138,140–142]

ACTH deficiency combined with other pituitary hormone deficiency is by far much more common than isolated ACTH deficiency and work over the years has revealed mutations in genes encoding transcription factors involved in the complex process of pituitary hormone production. The most common etiology behind congenital multiple pituitary hormone deficiencies is mutations in *PROP1 (Homeobox protein prophet of PIT-1)*, which encodes a pituitary-specific paired transcription factor, a disorder inherited in an autosomal recessive fashion and associated with GH, TSH, LH, FSH, prolactin, and ACTH deficiencies. *HESX1 (Homeobox gene expressed in ES cells)* mutations are associated with the syndrome of septooptic dysplasia and its characteristic clinical features (optic nerve hypoplasia, hypoplasia or absence of the septum pellucidum and corpus callosum). *OTX2 (orthodenticle homeobox 2 protein)* mutations are associated with microphthalmia and renal defects. *LHX3 (LIM/homeobox protein 3)* is associated with cervical spine anomalies, deafness, and joint hyperextensibility. In addition to ACTH deficiency, GH, TSH, LH, FSH, and prolactin deficiencies occur in patients with *HESX1*, *OTX2* and *LHX3* mutations. ACTH, GH and TSH deficiencies with cerebellar deficits are described with *LHX4 (LIM/homeobox protein 4)* gene mutations.[138,143,144] Although it was initially thought that pituitary hormone deficiencies were inherited through an autosomal recessive fashion, autosomal dominant and X-linked inheritance patterns are now described. Examples include *LHX4* and *OTX2* mutations, which are transmitted through an autosomal dominant fashion, *HESX1* mutations with both autosomal recessive and dominant inheritance patterns described, and X-linked transmission of *SOX3* mutation, which is associated with anterior pituitary hypoplasia, ectopic posterior pituitary, deficiency in GH, TSH, ACTH, LH, FSH, and variable degrees of developmental delay.[145,146] Table 47.5 summarizes the characteristic clinical and hormonal deficits associated with the multiple pituitary hormone genetic mutations discussed.

TABLE 47.5 Pituitary hormone deficiencies and associated characteristic clinical findings

Gene	Inheritance	Pituitary hormone deficiency	Other clinical manifestations
TPIT	AR	ACTH	
POMC	AR	ACTH	Red hair Obesity
PCSK1	AR	ACTH & LH/FSH	Red hair Obesity Malabsorption
PROP1	AR	ACTH, GH, TSH, LH/FSH & Prolactin	Anterior pituitary hypoplasia or hyperplasia
HESX1	AR, AD	ACTH, GH, TSH, LH/FSH & Prolactin	Optic nerve hypoplasia Hypoplasia or absence of the septum pellucidum and corpus callosum
OTX2	AD	ACTH, GH, TSH, LH/FSH & Prolactin	Microphthalmia Renal defects
LHX4	AD	ACTH, GH, TSH, LH/FSH	Hypoplasia of corpus callosum Cerebellar deficits Ectopic posterior pituitary
LHX3	AR	ACTH, GH, TSH, LH/FSH & Prolactin	Cervical spine anomalies Deafness Joint hyperextensibility
SOX3	XL	ACTH, GH, TSH, & LH/FSH	Anterior pituitary hypoplasia Ectopic posterior pituitary

Abbreviations

17-OHP	17α-hydroxyprogesterone
3βHSD	3β-hydroxysteroid dehydrogenase
AAAS	achalasia-addisonianism-alacrima syndrome
ABCD1	ATP binding cassette subfamily D member 1
ACTH	adrenocorticotropic hormone
ADPHA	autosomal dominant pseudohypoaldosteronism
AHC	adrenal hypoplasia congenita
AMN	adrenomyeloneuropathy
ARPHA	autosomal recessive pseudohypoaldosteronism
bFGF	basic fibroblast growth factor
CAH	congenital adrenal hyperplasia
CDKN1C	cyclin dependent kinase inhibitor 1C
CMO I	corticosterone methyl oxidase type I
CMO II	corticosterone methyl oxidase type II
CYP11A1	cytochrome P450, family 11, subfamily A, member 1
CYP11B1	cytochrome P450, family 11, subfamily B, member 1
CYP11B2	cytochrome P450, family 11, subfamily B, member 2
CYP17A1	cytochrome P450, family 17, subfamily A, member 1
CYP21A2	cytochrome P450 family 21 subfamily A member 2
DAX-1	dosage-sensitive sex reversal, adrenal hypoplasia critical region, on chromosome X, gene 1
DHCR7	7-dehydroxycholesterolreductase
DOC	deoxycorticosterone
DSD	disorder of sexual development
EGF	epidermal growth factor
ENaC	epithelial sodium channel
FSH	follicle stimulating hormone
GH	growth hormone
GRA	glucocorticoid-remediable hyperaldosteronism
HESX1	homeobox gene expressed in ES cells
HSD3B1	hydroxy-delta-5-steroid dehydrogenase, 3 beta- and steroid delta-isomerase 1
HSD3B2	hydroxy-delta-5-steroid dehydrogenase, 3 beta- and steroid delta-isomerase 2
IGF-II	insulin like growth factor II
IUGR	intra uterine growth restriction
LH	luteinizing hormone
LHX4	LIM/homeobox protein 4
LIPA	lysosomal acid lipase
MC1R	melanocortin 1 receptor
MC2R	melanocortin 2 receptor
MC3R	melanocortin 3 receptor
MC4R	melanocortin 4 receptor
MCM4	mini chromosome maintenance-deficient 4 homologue
MPS	massively parallel sequencing
MR	mineralocorticoid receptor
MRAP	melanocortin 2 receptor accessory protein
MSH	melanocyte stimulating hormone
NADPH	nicotinamide adenine dinucleotide phosphate
NNT	nicotinamide nucleotide transhydrogenase
NR0B1	nuclear receptor subfamily 0, group B, member 1
NR5A1	nuclear receptor subfamily 5 group A member 1
OTX2	orthodenticle homeobox 2 protein
PCSK1	proprotein convertase subtilisin/kexin type 1
PEX	peroxins
PHA	pseudohypoaldosteronism
POMC	proopiomelanocortin
PORD	cytochrome P450 oxidoreductase deficiency
PROP1	homeobox protein prophet of PIT-1
SAMD9	sterile alpha motif domain containing 9

SF1	steroidogenic factor 1
SGPL1	sphingosine-1-phosphate lyase 1
SLOS	Smith-Lemli-Opitz syndrome
SNP	single nucleotide polymorphism
StAR	steroidogenic acute regulatory protein
TPIT	T-box transcription factor TBX19
TSH	thyroid stimulating hormone
TXNRD2	thioredoxin reductase 2
VLCFA	very long chain fatty acid
ZS	Zellweger syndrome

REFERENCES

1. Virdis R. Historical milestones in endocrinology. *J Endocrinol Investig* 2005;**28**(10):944–8.

2. New MI, et al. *Genetic steroid disorders.* Amsterdam; Boston; Heidelberg; London; New York; Oxford; Paris; San Diego; Singapore; Sydney; Tokyo: Elsevier; 2014. xiii, 392 pages.

3. Xing Y, Achermann JC, Hammer GD. Chapter 2: Adrenal development. In: *Genetic steroid disorders.* San Diego: Academic Press; 2014. p. 5–27.

4. New MI, Seaman MP. Secretion rates of cortisol and aldosterone precursors in various forms of congenital adrenal hyperplasia. *J Clin Endocrinol Metab* 1970;**30**(3):361–71.

5. White PC. Chapter 3D – Steroid 11β-hydroxylase deficiency and related disorders A2 – New, Maria I. In: Lekarev O, et al., editors. *Genetic steroid disorders.* San Diego: Academic Press; 2014. p. 71–85.

6. Lee PR, Raymond GV. Child neurology: Zellweger syndrome. *Neurology* 2013;**80**(20):e207–10.

7. Eggermann T, et al. CDKN1C mutations: two sides of the same coin. *Trends Mol Med* 2014;**20**(11):614–22.

8. Porter FD. Smith-Lemli-Opitz syndrome: pathogenesis, diagnosis and management. *Eur J Hum Genet* 2008;**16**(5):535–41.

9. Khattab A, et al. Clinical, genetic, and structural basis of congenital adrenal hyperplasia due to 11beta-hydroxylase deficiency. *Proc Natl Acad Sci U S A* 2017;**114**(10):E1933–40.

10. Achermann JC, Meeks JJ, Jameson JL. Phenotypic spectrum of mutations in DAX-1 and SF-1. *Mol Cell Endocrinol* 2001;**185**(1–2):17–25.

11. Haider S, et al. Structure-phenotype correlations of human CYP21A2 mutations in congenital adrenal hyperplasia. *Proc Natl Acad Sci U S A* 2013;**110**(7):2605–10.

12. New MI, et al. Genotype-phenotype correlation in 1,507 families with congenital adrenal hyperplasia owing to 21-hydroxylase deficiency. *Proc Natl Acad Sci U S A* 2013;**110**(7):2611–6.

13. Khattab A, et al. A rare CYP21A2 mutation in a congenital adrenal hyperplasia kindred displaying genotype-phenotype nonconcordance. *Ann N Y Acad Sci* 2016;**1364**:5–10.

14. Therrell Jr BL, et al. Results of screening 1.9 million Texas newborns for 21-hydroxylase-deficient congenital adrenal hyperplasia. *Pediatrics* 1998;**101**(4 Pt 1):583–90.

15. Riedl S, et al. Genotype/phenotype correlations in 538 congenital adrenal hyperplasia patients from Germany and Austria: discordances in milder genotypes and in screened versus prescreening patients. *Endocr Connect* 2019;**8**(2):86–94.

16. Dhayat NA, et al. Androgen biosynthesis during minipuberty favors the backdoor pathway over the classic pathway: Insights into enzyme activities and steroid fluxes in healthy infants during the first year of life from the urinary steroid metabolome. *J Steroid Biochem Mol Biol* 2017;**165**(Pt B):312–22.

17. Fukami M, et al. Backdoor pathway for dihydrotestosterone biosynthesis: implications for normal and abnormal human sex development. *Dev Dyn* 2013;**242**(4):320–9.

18. Kamrath C, et al. Increased activation of the alternative "backdoor" pathway in patients with 21-hydroxylase deficiency: evidence from urinary steroid hormone analysis. *J Clin Endocrinol Metab* 2012;**97**(3):E367–75.

19. O'Shaughnessy PJ, et al. Alternative (backdoor) androgen production and masculinization in the human fetus. *PLoS Biol* 2019;**17**(2):e3000002.

20. Kamrath C, et al. Androgen excess is due to elevated 11-oxygenated androgens in treated children with congenital adrenal hyperplasia. *J Steroid Biochem Mol Biol* 2018;**178**:221–8.

21. Lorenzen F, et al. Hormonal phenotype and HLA-genotype in families of patients with congenital adrenal hyperplasia (21-hydroxylase deficiency). *Pediatr Res* 1979;**13**(12):1356–60.

22. New MI, et al. An update on prenatal diagnosis and treatment of congenital adrenal hyperplasia. *Semin Reprod Med* 2012;**30**(5):396–9.

23. Prader A, Gurtner HP. The syndrome of male pseudohermaphrodism in congenital adrenocortical hyperplasia without overproduction of androgens (adrenal male pseudohermaphrodism). *Helv Paediatr Acta* 1955;**10**(4):397–412.

24. Ahmed SF, Khwaja O, Hughes IA. The role of a clinical score in the assessment of ambiguous genitalia. *BJU Int* 2000;**85**(1):120–4.

25. Nimkarn S, Lin-Su K, New MI. Steroid 21 hydroxylase deficiency congenital adrenal hyperplasia. *Pediatr Clin N Am* 2011;**58**(5):1281–300 [xii].

26. Poppas DP, et al. Nerve sparing ventral clitoroplasty preserves dorsal nerves in congenital adrenal hyperplasia. *J Urol* 2007;**178**(4 Pt 2):1802–6 [discussion 1806].

27. Creighton SM. The adult consequences of feminising genital surgery in infancy. A growing skepticism. *Hormones (Athens)* 2004;**3**(4):228–32.

28. Rink RC. Genitoplasty/Vaginoplasty. *Adv Exp Med Biol* 2011;**707**:51–4.

29. Dangle PP, et al. Surgical complications following early genitourinary reconstructive surgery for congenital adrenal hyperplasia-interim analysis at 6 years. *Urology* 2017;**101**:111–5.

30. Stites J, et al. Urinary continence outcomes following vaginoplasty in patients with congenital adrenal hyperplasia. *J Pediatr Urol* 2017;**13**(1):38 e1–7.

31. Chua SC, et al. Cloning of cDNA encoding steroid 11 beta-hydroxylase (P450c11). *Proc Natl Acad Sci U S A* 1987;**84**(20):7193–7.

32. Simard J, et al. Congenital adrenal hyperplasia caused by a novel homozygous frameshift mutation 273 delta AA in type II 3 beta-hydroxysteroid dehydrogenase gene (HSD3B2) in three male patients of Afghan/Pakistani origin. *Hum Mol Genet* 1994;**3**(2):327–30.

33. Rheaume E, et al. Congenital adrenal hyperplasia due to point mutations in the type II 3 beta-hydroxysteroid dehydrogenase gene. *Nat Genet* 1992;**1**(4):239–45.

34. Rheaume E, et al. Structure and expression of a new complementary DNA encoding the almost exclusive 3 beta-hydroxysteroid dehydrogenase/delta 5-delta 4-isomerase in human adrenals and gonads. *Mol Endocrinol* 1991;**5**(8):1147–57.

35. Simard J, et al. Molecular basis of congenital adrenal hyperplasia due to 3 beta-hydroxysteroid dehydrogenase deficiency. *Mol Endocrinol* 1993;**7**(5):716–28.

36. Zerah M, et al. No evidence of mutations in the genes for type I and type II 3 beta-hydroxysteroid dehydrogenase (3 beta HSD) in nonclassical 3 beta HSD deficiency. *J Clin Endocrinol Metab* 1994;**79**(6):1811–7.

37. Miller W. Mechanisms in endocrinology: rare defects in adrenal steroidogenesis. *Eur J Endocrinol* 2018;.

38. Biglieri EG. 17 alpha-Hydroxylase deficiency: 1963–1966. *J Clin Endocrinol Metab* 1997;**82**(1):48–50.

39. Picado-Leonard J, Miller WL. Cloning and sequence of the human gene for P450c17 (steroid 17 alpha-hydroxylase/17,20 lyase): similarity with the gene for P450c21. *DNA* 1987;**6**(5):439–48.

40. Chung BC, et al. Cytochrome P450c17 (steroid 17 alpha-hydroxylase/17,20 lyase): cloning of human adrenal and testis cDNAs indicates the same gene is expressed in both tissues. *Proc Natl Acad Sci U S A* 1987;**84**(2):407–11.

41. Auchus RJ, Lee TC, Miller WL. Cytochrome b5 augments the 17,20-lyase activity of human P450c17 without direct electron transfer. *J Biol Chem* 1998;**273**(6):3158–65.

42. Katagiri M, Kagawa N, Waterman MR. The role of cytochrome b5 in the biosynthesis of androgens by human P450c17. *Arch Biochem Biophys* 1995;**317**(2):343–7.

43. New MI. Male pseudohermaphroditism due to 17 alpha-hydroxylase deficiency. *J Clin Invest* 1970;**49**(10):1930–41.

44. Biglieri EG, Herron MA, Brust N. 17-hydroxylation deficiency in man. *J Clin Invest* 1966;**45**(12):1946–54.

45. Costenaro F, et al. Combined 17alpha-hydroxylase/17,20-lyase deficiency due to p.R96W mutation in the CYP17 gene in a Brazilian patient. *Arq Bras Endocrinol Metabol* 2010;**54**(8):744–8.

46. Miller WL, et al. P450 oxidoreductase deficiency. *Lancet* 2004;**364**(9446):1663.

47. Fluck CE, et al. Mutant P450 oxidoreductase causes disordered steroidogenesis with and without Antley-Bixler syndrome. *Nat Genet* 2004;**36**(3):228–30.

48. Pandey AV, et al. P450 oxidoreductase deficiency: a new disorder of steroidogenesis affecting all microsomal P450 enzymes. *Endocr Res* 2004;**30**(4):881–8.

49. Huang N, et al. Genetics of P450 oxidoreductase: sequence variation in 842 individuals of four ethnicities and activities of 15 missense mutations. *Proc Natl Acad Sci U S A* 2008;**105**(5):1733–8.

50. McGlaughlin KL, et al. Spectrum of Antley-Bixler syndrome. *J Craniofac Surg* 2010;**21**(5):1560–4.

51. Xie M, et al. Advance in clinical research on Antley-Bixler syndrome. *Zhonghua Yi Xue Yi Chuan Xue Za Zhi* 2018;**35**(2):280–3.

52. Crouch NS, et al. Genital sensation after feminizing genitoplasty for congenital adrenal hyperplasia: a pilot study. *BJU Int* 2004;**93**(1):135–8.

53. Nordenstrom A, et al. Sexual function and surgical outcome in women with congenital adrenal hyperplasia due to CYP21A2 deficiency: clinical perspective and the patients' perception. *J Clin Endocrinol Metab* 2010;**95**(8):3633–40.

54. Crouch NS, et al. Sexual function and genital sensitivity following feminizing genitoplasty for congenital adrenal hyperplasia. *J Urol* 2008;**179**(2):634–8.

55. New MI, et al. Prenatal diagnosis for congenital adrenal hyperplasia in 532 pregnancies. *J Clin Endocrinol Metab* 2001;**86**(12):5651–7.

56. Mercado AB, et al. Prenatal treatment and diagnosis of congenital adrenal hyperplasia owing to steroid 21-hydroxylase deficiency. *J Clin Endocrinol Metab* 1995;**80**(7):2014–20.

57. Hirvikoski T, et al. Long-term follow-up of prenatally treated children at risk for congenital adrenal hyperplasia: does dexamethasone cause behavioural problems? *Eur J Endocrinol* 2008;**159**(3):309–16.

58. Hirvikoski T, et al. Cognitive functions in children at risk for congenital adrenal hyperplasia treated prenatally with dexamethasone. *J Clin Endocrinol Metab* 2007;**92**(2):542–8.

59. Hirvikoski T, et al. Prenatal dexamethasone treatment of children at risk for congenital adrenal hyperplasia: The Swedish experience and standpoint. *J Clin Endocrinol Metab* 2012;**97**(6):1881–3.

60. Bachelot A, et al. Management of endocrine disease: congenital adrenal hyperplasia due to 21-hydroxylase deficiency: update on the management of adult patients and prenatal treatment. *Eur J Endocrinol* 2017;**176**(4):R167–81.

61. Speiser PW, et al. Congenital adrenal hyperplasia due to steroid 21-hydroxylase deficiency: an endocrine society clinical practice guideline. *J Clin Endocrinol Metab* 2018;**103**(11):4043–88.

62. New MI, et al. Noninvasive prenatal diagnosis of congenital adrenal hyperplasia using cell-free fetal DNA in maternal plasma. *J Clin Endocrinol Metab* 2014;**99**(6):E1022–30.

63. Chan J, et al. Human fetal mesenchymal stem cells as vehicles for gene delivery. *Stem Cells* 2005;**23**(1):93–102.

64. Evans MI, et al. Fetal therapy. *Best Pract Res Clin Obstet Gynaecol* 2002;**16**(5):671–83.

65. Mattar CN, et al. Fetal gene therapy: recent advances and current challenges. *Expert Opin Biol Ther* 2011;**11**(10):1257–71.

66. Rahim AA, et al. Perinatal gene delivery to the CNS. *Ther Deliv* 2011;**2**(4):483–91.

67. van Mieghem T, et al. Minimally invasive fetal therapy. *Best Pract Res Clin Obstet Gynaecol* 2012;**26**(5):711–25.

68. Nedumaran B, et al. DAX-1 acts as a novel corepressor of orphan nuclear receptor HNF4alpha and negatively regulates gluconeogenic enzyme gene expression. *J Biol Chem* 2009;**284**(40):27511–23.

69. Tabarin A, et al. A novel mutation in DAX1 causes delayed-onset adrenal insufficiency and incomplete hypogonadotropic hypogonadism. *J Clin Invest* 2000;**105**(3):321–8.

70. Lin L, et al. Analysis of DAX1 (NR0B1) and steroidogenic factor-1 (NR5A1) in children and adults with primary adrenal failure: ten years' experience. *J Clin Endocrinol Metab* 2006;**91**(8):3048–54.

71. Kyriakakis N, et al. Late-onset X-linked adrenal hypoplasia (DAX-1, NR0B1): two new adult-onset cases from a single center. *Pituitary* 2017;**20** (5):585–93.

72. Achermann JC, Vilain EJ. NR0B1-related adrenal hypoplasia congenita. In: Adam MP, et al., editors. *GeneReviews((R))*. Seattle, WA: University of Washington; 1993.

73. Yeste D, et al. ACTH-dependent precocious pseudopuberty in an infant with DAX1 gene mutation. *Eur J Pediatr* 2009;**168**(1):65–9.

74. Domenice S, et al. Adrenocorticotropin-dependent precocious puberty of testicular origin in a boy with X-linked adrenal hypoplasia congenita due to a novel mutation in the DAX1 gene. *J Clin Endocrinol Metab* 2001;**86**(9):4068–71.

75. Loke KY, et al. A case of X-linked adrenal hypoplasia congenita, central precocious puberty and absence of the DAX-1 gene: implications for pubertal regulation. *Horm Res* 2009;**71**(5):298–304.

76. Calliari LE, et al. Mild adrenal insufficiency due to a NROB1 (DAX1) gene mutation in a boy presenting an association of hypogonadotropic hypogonadism, reduced final height and attention deficit disorder. *Arq Bras Endocrinol Metabol* 2013;**57**(7):562–5.

77. Wang CL, Fen ZW, Liang L. A de novo mutation of DAX1 in a boy with congenital adrenal hypoplasia without hypogonadotropic hypogonadism. *J Pediatr Endocrinol Metab* 2014;**27**(3–4):343–7.

78. Phelan JK, McCabe ER. Mutations in NR0B1 (DAX1) and NR5A1 (SF1) responsible for adrenal hypoplasia congenita. *Hum Mutat* 2001;**18** (6):472–87.

79. Durkovic J, et al. Low estriol levels in the maternal marker screen as a predictor of X-linked adrenal hypoplasia congenita: case report. *Srp Arh Celok Lek* 2014;**142**(11 – 12):728–31.

80. Pelissier P, et al. Adrenal hypoplasia congenita: four new cases in children. *Arch Pediatr* 2005;**12**(4):380–4.

81. Gordon HB, Valdez L, Letsou A. Etiology and treatment of adrenoleukodystrophy: new insights from Drosophila. *Dis Model Mech* 2018;.

82. Chen Y, et al. A novel variant in ABCD1 gene presenting as adolescent-onset atypical adrenomyeloneuropathy with spastic ataxia. *Front Neurol* 2018;**9**:271.

83. Rajabi F. Updates in newborn screening. *Pediatr Ann* 2018;**47**(5):e187–90.

84. Raymond GV, Moser AB, Fatemi A. X-linked adrenoleukodystrophy. In: Adam MP, et al., editors. *GeneReviews((R))*. Seattle, WA: University of Washington; 1993.

85. Novoselova TV, Chan LF, Clark AJL. Pathophysiology of melanocortin receptors and their accessory proteins. *Best Pract Res Clin Endocrinol Metab* 2018;**32**(2):93–106.

86. Meimaridou E, et al. Familial glucocorticoid deficiency: new genes and mechanisms. *Mol Cell Endocrinol* 2013;**371**(1–2):195–200.

87. Metherell LA, et al. Mutations in MRAP, encoding a new interacting partner of the ACTH receptor, cause familial glucocorticoid deficiency type 2. *Nat Genet* 2005;**37**(2):166–70.

88. Burget L, et al. A rare cause of primary adrenal insufficiency due to a homozygous Arg188Cys mutation in the STAR gene. *Endocrinol Diabetes Metab Case Rep* 2018;**2018**.

89. Hauffa B, Hiort O. P450 side-chain cleavage deficiency – a rare cause of congenital adrenal hyperplasia. *Endocr Dev* 2011;**20**:54–62.

90. Bizzarri C, et al. Lipoid congenital adrenal hyperplasia by steroidogenic acute regulatory protein (STAR) gene mutation in an Italian infant: an uncommon cause of adrenal insufficiency. *Ital J Pediatr* 2017;**43**(1):57.

91. Lara-Velazquez M, et al. A novel splice site variant in CYP11A1 in trans with the p.E314K variant in a male patient with congenital adrenal insufficiency. *Mol Genet Genomic Med* 2017;**5**(6):781–7.

92. Fluck CE, et al. Characterization of novel StAR (steroidogenic acute regulatory protein) mutations causing non-classic lipoid adrenal hyperplasia. *PLoS One* 2011;**6**(5).

93. Meimaridou E, et al. NNT is a key regulator of adrenal redox homeostasis and steroidogenesis in male mice. *J Endocrinol* 2018;**236** (1):13–28.

94. Meimaridou E, et al. ACTH resistance: genes and mechanisms. *Endocr Dev* 2013;**24**:57–66.

95. Malikova J, Fluck CE. Novel insight into etiology, diagnosis and management of primary adrenal insufficiency. *Horm Res Paediatr* 2014;**82** (3):145–57.

96. Prasad R, et al. Thioredoxin Reductase 2 (TXNRD2) mutation associated with familial glucocorticoid deficiency (FGD). *J Clin Endocrinol Metab* 2014;**99**(8):E1556–63.

97. Shah SWH, et al. AAA Syndrome, case report of a rare disease. *Pak J Med Sci* 2017;**33**(6):1512–6.

98. Cronshaw JM, Matunis MJ. The nuclear pore complex protein ALADIN is mislocalized in triple A syndrome. *Proc Natl Acad Sci U S A* 2003;**100** (10):5823–7.

99. Conn JW, Louis LH. Primary aldosteronism: a new clinical entity. *Trans Assoc Am Phys* 1955;**68**:215–31. discussion, 231–3.

100. New MI, Peterson RE. A new form of congenital adrenal hyperplasia. *J Clin Endocrinol Metab* 1967;**27**(2):300–5.

101. Sutherland DJ, Ruse JL, Laidlaw JC. Hypertension, increased aldosterone secretion and low plasma renin activity relieved by dexamethasone. *Can Med Assoc J* 1966;**95**(22):1109–19.

102. Lifton RP, et al. Hereditary hypertension caused by chimaeric gene duplications and ectopic expression of aldosterone synthase. *Nat Genet* 1992;**2**(1):66–74.

103. Halperin F, Dluhy RG. Glucocorticoid-remediable aldosteronism. *Endocrinol Metab Clin N Am* 2011;**40**(2):333–41 [viii].

104. New MI, et al. Autosomal dominant transmission and absence of HLA linkage in dexamethasone suppressible hyperaldosteronism. *Lancet* 1980;**1**(8167):550–1.

105. Geller DS, et al. Autosomal dominant pseudohypoaldosteronism type 1: mechanisms, evidence for neonatal lethality, and phenotypic expression in adults. *J Am Soc Nephrol* 2006;**17**(5):1429–36.

106. Oberfield SE, et al. Pseudohypoaldosteronism: multiple target organ unresponsiveness to mineralocorticoid hormones. *J Clin Endocrinol Metab* 1979;**48**(2):228–34.

107. Geller DS, et al. Mutations in the mineralocorticoid receptor gene cause autosomal dominant pseudohypoaldosteronism type I. *Nat Genet* 1998;**19**(3):279–81.

108. Sadoughi N, et al. The effect of digitalis on the bladder in man. *J Urol* 1975;**113**(2):178–9.

109. Sartorato P, et al. Different inactivating mutations of the mineralocorticoid receptor in fourteen families affected by type I pseudohypoaldosteronism. *J Clin Endocrinol Metab* 2003;**88**(6):2508–17.

110. Bonnici F. Autosomal recessive transmission of familial pseudohypoaldosteronism. *Arch Fr Pediatr* 1977;**34**(9):915–6.

111. Rosler A. The natural history of salt-wasting disorders of adrenal and renal origin. *J Clin Endocrinol Metab* 1984;**59**(4):689–700.

112. Zhang G, et al. Mutation T318M in the CYP11B2 gene encoding P450c11AS (aldosterone synthase) causes corticosterone methyl oxidase II deficiency. *Am J Hum Genet* 1995;**57**(5):1037–43.

113. Pascoe L, et al. Mutations in the human CYP11B2 (aldosterone synthase) gene causing corticosterone methyloxidase II deficiency. *Proc Natl Acad Sci U S A* 1992;**89**(11):4996–5000.

114. Ulick S. Diagnosis and nomenclature of the disorders of the terminal portion of the aldosterone biosynthetic pathway. *J Clin Endocrinol Metab* 1976;**43**(1):92–6.

115. Lee PD, et al. Biochemical diagnosis and management of corticosterone methyl oxidase type II deficiency. *J Clin Endocrinol Metab* 1986;**62**(1):225–9.

116. Mardesic D, et al. Corticosterone methyloxydase deficiency type II in a Croatian girl. *J Endocrinol Investig* 1992;**15**(3):197–9.

117. Kohler B, Achermann JC. Update – steroidogenic factor 1 (SF-1, NR5A1). *Minerva Endocrinol* 2010;**35**(2):73–86.

118. Ramayya MS, et al. Steroidogenic factor 1 messenger ribonucleic acid expression in steroidogenic and nonsteroidogenic human tissues: Northern blot and in situ hybridization studies. *J Clin Endocrinol Metab* 1997;**82**(6):1799–806.

119. Biason-Lauber A, Schoenle EJ. Apparently normal ovarian differentiation in a prepubertal girl with transcriptionally inactive steroidogenic factor 1 (NR5A1/SF-1) and adrenocortical insufficiency. *Am J Hum Genet* 2000;**67**(6):1563–8.

120. Moser HW. Genotype-phenotype correlations in disorders of peroxisome biogenesis. *Mol Genet Metab* 1999;**68**(2):316–27.

121. Steinberg SJ, et al. Peroxisome biogenesis disorders. *Biochim Biophys Acta* 2006;**1763**(12):1733–48.

122. Tolar J, et al. Long-term metabolic, endocrine, and neuropsychological outcome of hematopoietic cell transplantation for Wolman disease. *Bone Marrow Transplant* 2009;**43**(1):21–7.

123. Hoffman EP, et al. Lysosomal acid lipase deficiency. In: Adam MP, et al., editors. *GeneReviews((R))*. Seattle, WA: University of Washington; 1993.

124. Donoghue SE, et al. Smith-Lemli-Opitz syndrome: clinical and biochemical correlates. *J Pediatr Endocrinol Metab* 2018;**31**(4):451–9.

125. Peng Y, et al. Computational investigation of the missense mutations in DHCR7 gene associated with smith-Lemli-Opitz Syndrome. *Int J Mol Sci* 2018;**19**(1).

126. Nowaczyk MJ, Waye JS. The Smith-Lemli-Opitz syndrome: a novel metabolic way of understanding developmental biology, embryogenesis, and dysmorphology. *Clin Genet* 2001;**59**(6):375–86.

127. Loeffler J, Utermann G, Witsch-Baumgartner M. Molecular prenatal diagnosis of smith-Lemli-Opitz syndrome is reliable and efficient. *Prenat Diagn* 2002;**22**(9):827–30.

128. Kelley RI. Diagnosis of Smith-Lemli-Opitz syndrome by gas chromatography/mass spectrometry of 7-dehydrocholesterol in plasma, amniotic fluid and cultured skin fibroblasts. *Clin Chim Acta* 1995;**236**(1):45–58.

129. Rossiter JP, Hofman KJ, Kelley RI. Smith-Lemli-Opitz syndrome: prenatal diagnosis by quantification of cholesterol precursors in amniotic fluid. *Am J Med Genet* 1995;**56**(3):272–5.

130. Cabrera-Salcedo C, et al. IMAGe and related undergrowth syndromes: the complex spectrum of gain-of-function CDKN1C mutations. *Pediatr Endocrinol Rev* 2017;**14**(3):289–97.

131. Fluck CE. Mechanisms in endocrinology: update on pathogenesis of primary adrenal insufficiency: beyond steroid enzyme deficiency and autoimmune adrenal destruction. *Eur J Endocrinol* 2017;**177**(3):R99–R111.

132. Bennett J, Schrier Vergano SA, Deardorff MA. IMAGe syndrome. In: Adam MP, et al., editors. *GeneReviews((R))*. Seattle, WA: University of Washington; 1993.

133. Narumi S, et al. SAMD9 mutations cause a novel multisystem disorder, MIRAGE syndrome, and are associated with loss of chromosome 7. *Nat Genet* 2016;**48**(7):792–7.

134. Kim YM, et al. A case of an infant suspected as IMAGE syndrome who were finally diagnosed with MIRAGE syndrome by targeted Mendelian exome sequencing. *BMC Med Genet* 2018;**19**(1):35.

135. Reiss U, et al. Sphingosine-phosphate lyase enhances stress-induced ceramide generation and apoptosis. *J Biol Chem* 2004;**279**(2):1281–90.

136. Larson A, Nokoff NJ, Meeks NJ. Genetic causes of pituitary hormone deficiencies. *Discov Med* 2015;**19**(104):175–83.

137. Vallette-Kasic S, et al. The TPIT gene mutation M86R associated with isolated adrenocorticotropin deficiency interferes with protein: protein interactions. *J Clin Endocrinol Metab* 2007;**92**(10):3991–9.

138. Mehta A, Dattani MT. Developmental disorders of the hypothalamus and pituitary gland associated with congenital hypopituitarism. *Best Pract Res Clin Endocrinol Metab* 2008;**22**(1):191–206.

139. Couture C, et al. Phenotypic homogeneity and genotypic variability in a large series of congenital isolated ACTH-deficiency patients with TPIT gene mutations. *J Clin Endocrinol Metab* 2012;**97**(3):E486–95.

140. Cetinkaya S, et al. A patient with Proopiomelanocortin deficiency: an increasingly important diagnosis to make. *J Clin Res Pediatr Endocrinol* 2018;**10**(1):68–73.

141. Martin MG, et al. Congenital proprotein convertase 1/3 deficiency causes malabsorptive diarrhea and other endocrinopathies in a pediatric cohort. *Gastroenterology* 2013;**145**(1):138–48.

142. Samuels ME, et al. Bioinactive ACTH causing glucocorticoid deficiency. *J Clin Endocrinol Metab* 2013;**98**(2):736–42.

143. Gangat M, Radovick S. Pituitary hypoplasia. *Endocrinol Metab Clin N Am* 2017;**46**(2):247–57.

144. Abrao MG, et al. Combined pituitary hormone deficiency (CPHD) due to a complete PROP1 deletion. *Clin Endocrinol* 2006;**65**(3):294–300.

145. Schoenmakers N, et al. Recent advances in central congenital hypothyroidism. *J Endocrinol* 2015;**227**(3):R51–71.

146. Wassner AJ, et al. Isolated central hypothyroidism in young siblings as a manifestation of PROP1 deficiency: clinical impact of whole exome sequencing. *Horm Res Paediatr* 2013;**79**(6):379–86.

Chapter 48

Disorders of Sex Development

Romina P. Grinspon* and Rodolfo A. Rey*,†

*Centro de Investigaciones Endocrinológicas "Dr. César Bergadá" (CEDIE), CONICET-FEI-División de Endocrinología, Hospital de Niños Ricardo Gutiérrez, Buenos Aires, Argentina, †Departamento de Histología, Biología Celular, Embriología y Genética, Facultad de Medicina, Universidad de Buenos Aires, Buenos Aires, Argentina

---

Common Clinical Problems

- Congenital adrenal hyperplasia should be ruled out in all newborns with ambiguous genitalia or completely virilized and non-palpable testes, because it may be life-threatening.
- The aspect of external genitalia rarely suggests an etiology, but rather indicates the severity of the DSD.
- An accurate differential diagnosis between partial androgen insensitivity and 5α-reductase deficiency may be more promptly made using genetic testing than classical endocrine assessment.
- Malformative, nonendocrine DSD may be difficult to rule out, except in newborns with several dysmorphic features.
- Definitions of sex assignment usually take longer than the family and health professionals would like.

48.1 DEFINITIONS

Disorders of sex development (DSDs) are congenital anomalies in which there is a discordance between chromosomal, genetic, gonadal, and/or internal/external genital sex. The acronym DSD and the related nomenclature were coined in a consensus meeting held in 2005 and recently revised and endorsed by all major pediatric endocrine societies;[1] they replaced previously used terms, like hermaphroditism or pseudohermaphroditism, perceived as pejorative. The nomenclature has been generally accepted by medical professionals, though not universally by some patient support groups. The strength of this terminology is that it provides precise biological terms for the communication between professionals, thus facilitating patient access to high-quality healthcare. The negative connotation perceived by some advocacy organizations include the stigma of "disorder" and perceived implications that "sex" involves sexual behavior. Some authors have proposed the use of "differences in sex development". We prefer to keep the term "disorder" in order to maintain a coherence with other medical conditions in which there is a biological divergence from normal development or physiology (e.g., congenital heart disease, congenital malformation of lungs, etc.). In this way, we avoid confusion with psychosocial situations that are not disorders, such as transgender, gender dysphoria and homosexuality.

In this chapter, the complexity of DSD will be approached by describing first a karyotype-based classification deriving from the 2005 consensus and then the developmental pathogenesis of the disorders. Finally, concurring with this book's scope, the diagnosis and management of DSD will be focused on the neonatal patient, with only brief descriptions on presentations and evolution in later periods of life.

48.2 CLASSIFICATION OF DSD BASED ON THE KARYOTYPE

The definition of DSD based on the patient's karyotype, as proposed in 2005, includes atypical sex chromosome conditions for which patients usually do not seek medical help for ambiguous genitalia, like classical Klinefelter syndrome (47,XXY) and Turner syndrome (45,X). These two conditions are far more frequent than all other DSD conditions together. Therefore, the general incidence of DSD is difficult to appraise. A karyotype-based classification of DSD is shown in Table 48.1.

48.2.1 46,XY DSD

The term 46,XY DSD replaced the previously used "male pseudohermaphroditism" and includes all conditions characterized by a complete feminization or an undervirilization of XY individuals, including complete and partial testicular

TABLE 48.1 Karyotype-based classification of DSD

DSD type	Pathogenic classification	Etiology
46,XY DSD	Malformative DSD	Defective morphogenesis of the genital primordia
	Dysgenetic DSD	Complete, partial, or asymmetric gonadal dysgenesis
		Ovotesticular DSD
	Nondysgenetic DSD	Disorders of androgen synthesis
		Disorders of androgen action (AIS)
		Disorders of AMH synthesis or action
46,XX DSD	Malformative DSD	Defective morphogenesis of the genital primordia
	Dysgenetic DSD	Ovotesticular DSD
		Testicular DSD
		Ovarian dysgenesis
	Nondysgenetic DSD	Excessive adrenal androgen synthesis (CAH)
		Decreased placental androgen aromatization (aromatase deficiency)
		Androgen-secreting tumors
		Androgenic drugs
Sex chromosome DSD	Dysgenetic DSD	Ovotesticular DSD (46,XX/46,XY, other mosaicisms with 46,XX and 46,XY lineages)
		Asymmetric gonadal differentiation (45,X/46,XY, other mosaicisms with a 45,X lineage)
		Turner syndrome (45,X and variants)
		Klinefelter syndrome (47,XXY and variants)
		Triple X syndrome (47,XXX and variants)

dysgenesis, defects of testicular hormone synthesis or action, and malformations of the internal or external genitalia not related to gonadal dysgenesis or hormonal defects.

48.2.2   46,XX DSD

The term 46,XX DSD replaced the previously used "female pseudohermaphroditism" and includes all conditions characterized by a virilization of XX individuals, resulting from excessive androgen production, including congenital adrenal hyperplasia (CAH), ovotesticular and testicular disorders, aromatase deficiency, and virilizing tumors. Ovarian dysgenesis is not associated with atypical genitalia but should be considered here from a pathogenic standpoint.

48.2.3   Sex Chromosome DSD

Sex chromosome DSD includes all disorders with an atypical karyotype, like aneuploidies, mosaicisms, and chimeras involving the sex chromosomes, e.g., 45,X/46,XY, 46,XX/46,XY, 47,XXY, 45,X, or any other variant. Their commonality is the existence of gonadal dysgenetic features: from complete to partial forms of gonadal dysgenesis, bisexual (ovotesticular) gonads, and asymmetric gonadal differentiation.

48.3 PATHOGENESIS OF DSD

As described in Chapter 37, normal fetal sexual development involves: (a) the early formation of the urogenital anlage, (b) gonadal differentiation, and (c) sexual differentiation of the internal and external genitalia according to the existence or absence of testicular hormone action. Based on the normal embryo-fetal mechanisms that failed and led to DSD, a pathogenic classification may be established: (1) malformative DSD in eugonadal states, wherein abnormal morphogenesis of the genital primordia occurs in early embryonic life with normal gonadal differentiation; (2) dysgenetic DSD, in patients with abnormal gonadal differentiation leading to fetal-onset primary hypogonadism; and (3) nondysgenetic sex hormone-dependent DSD in patients with a dysfunction limited to Sertoli cells or to Leydig cells but not both, with end-organ insensitivity to testicular hormones or with an excessive exposure to sex hormone agonists or antagonists (Table 48.2).

TABLE 48.2 Pathogenic classification of disorders of sex development

DSD type	Pathogenic mechanism	Examples	Implicated gene	OMIM
Malformative DSD	Defective morphogenesis of the Müllerian ducts or Wolffian ducts	Hand-foot-genital syndrome	HOXA13	140000[a]
		MRKH syndrome	WNT4	277000[a]
		McKusick-Kaufman syndrome	MKKS	236700[a]
	Defective morphogenesis of the urogenital sinus and the primordia of the external genitalia	Isolated aphallia	ROR2	268310[a]
		Isolated hypospadias	GLI3 SPECC1L PITX2	146510[a] 145410[a] 180500[a]
		Cloacal exstrophy Bladder exstrophy	Not known	–
Dysgenetic DSD	Complete or partial gonadal dysgenesis (46,XY)	Swyer syndrome or Partial testicular dysgenesis	SRY	480000[a]
			MAP3K1	613762[a]
			DSS locus including NR0B1 (DAX1)	300018[b]
			ZNRF3	612062[a]
			MAMLD1	300120[a]
		Testicular dysgenesis ± adrenal insufficiency (SF1 deficiency)	NR5A1 (SF1)	612965[a]
		Testicular dysgenesis + mental retardation	DMRT1	602424[a]
		Testicular dysgenesis + minifascicular neuropathy	DHH	607080[a]
		Testicular dysgenesis + clinodactyly, hydrocephaly, and autistic spectrum disorder	FOG2/ZFPM2	603693[a]
		Complete gonadal dysgenesis + craniosynostosis	FGFR2	176943[a]
		ATRX syndrome	ATRX	301040[a]
		Campomelic dysplasia	SOX9	608160[a]
		Denys-Drash syndrome Frasier syndrome	WT1	607102[a]

Continued

TABLE 48.2 Pathogenic classification of disorders of sex development—cont'd

DSD type	Pathogenic mechanism	Examples	Implicated gene	OMIM
	Asymmetric gonadal differentiation (Mixed gonadal dysgenesis)	45,X/46,XY	–	–
		Other mosaicisms with 45,X and Y lineage		
		46,XY (rare)		
	Ovotesticular	46,XX/46,XY	–	–
		Chimerisms/mosaicisms with XX and XY lineages		
		46,XY (extremely rare)		
	Ovotesticular/Testicular	46,XX, SRY+	SRY	400045[b]
		46,XX, SRY-	SOX9	608160[b]
			SOX10	602229[b]
			SOX3	313430[b]
			RSPO1	610644[a]
			WNT4	611812[a]
			NR5A1	184757[a]
Nondysgenetic DSD with testes	Disorders of androgen synthesis	Leydig cell aplasia/hypoplasia	LHCGR	238320[a]
		Smith-Lemli-Opitz syndrome	DHCR7	270400[a]
		Lipoid congenital adrenal hyperplasia	STAR	600617[a]
			CYP11A1	118485[a]
		P450c17 deficiency	CYP17A1	202110[a]
		17,20-lyase deficiency due to the cytochrome b5 mutation	CYB5A	250790[a]
		P450 oxidoreductase deficiency	POR	201750[a]
		3β-HSD type 2 deficiency	HSD3B2	201810[a]
		17β-HSD type 3 deficiency	HSD17B3	264300[a]
		DHT synthesis defects	SRD5A2	264600[a]
			AKR1C2	600450[a]
			AKR1C4	600451[a]
	Disorders of androgen action	Androgen insensitivity syndrome	AR	300068[a]
	Disorders of AMH synthesis or action	Persistent Müllerian duct syndrome	AMH	600957[a]
			AMHR2	600956[a]
Nondysgenetic DSD with ovaries	Excessive adrenal androgen synthesis	Congenital adrenal hyperplasia	CYP21A2	201910[a]
			CYP11B1	202010[a]
			HSD3B2	201810[a]
			POR	201750[a]
		Glucocorticoid resistance	NR3C1	615962[a]
	Impaired placental androgen aromatization	Placental aromatase deficiency	CYP19A1	613456[a]
	Androgen-producing tumors	Luteoma, thecoma, etc.	–	–
	Androgen/progestogen consumption	Norethindrone, ethisterone, norethynodrel, medroxyprogesterone, danazol	–	–

[a]Inactivating mutations.
[b]Gain of function/increased gene dosage mutations.

48.3.1 Malformative DSD

Malformative, nonendocrine-related DSDs are due to defects in the early morphogenesis of the anlagen of the reproductive tract in individuals with normal gonadal differentiation.[2] These disorders are suspected when the genital abnormalities are inconsistent with defective sex hormone secretion or action. The normal embryologic process underlying the formation of the genital primordia in early embryogenesis is impaired due to genetic or environmental causes. In these patients, serum levels of gonadal hormones are usually within the normal range. Malformative DSD includes early defects in the specific morphogenesis of Müllerian ducts, of Wolffian ducts, of the cloaca or the urogenital sinus, or of the anlagen of external genitalia.

48.3.1.1 Defective Morphogenesis of the Müllerian Ducts

Mayer-Rokitansky-Küster-Hauser syndrome (MRKH, OMIM 277000) is a heterogeneous disorder with abnormalities that may range from upper vaginal atresia to total Müllerian agenesis associated with urinary tract abnormalities, and even cervicothoracic somite dysplasia (known as MURCS association, OMIM 601076). Mutations in the WNT4 gene have been identified in a small subset of MRKH patients with hyperandrogenism, but do not seem to be the main etiology of MRKH syndrome.

Vaginal atresia has been described in McKusick-Kaufman syndrome (OMIM 236700), probably caused by mutations in the MKKS gene, hand-foot-genital syndrome due to HOXA13 mutations (OMIM 140000), RCAD (renal cysts and diabetes) syndrome (OMIM 137920), and in patients with velocardiofacial syndrome associated with 22q11.2 deletions (OMIM 192430).

Lack of fusion of the Müllerian ducts results in partial or complete duplication of the uterus. A double vagina occurs when the sinovaginal bulbs fail to fuse, and an atresia of vagina results when they do not develop at all.

Women usually have normal external genitalia at birth and normal development of secondary sexual characteristics, indicating normal endocrine ovarian function, and are referred to the consultation with primary amenorrhea.

48.3.1.2 Defective Morphogenesis of the Wolffian Ducts

Mutations in the *CFTR* gene, usually causative of cystic fibrosis, and in the *ADGRG2* gene can be found in patients with congenital absence of the vas deferens (OMIM 277180), accounting for 1% to 2% of cases of male infertility.

48.3.1.3 Defective Morphogenesis of the Cloaca and the Urogenital Sinus

In cloacal malformations, perineal anatomy may be so affected that the sex of the external genitalia cannot be easily identified. Although urologic and hindgut anomalies are the major problems to be solved in these cases, sex assignment could also be an important issue. Hormone levels are within the normal range for genetic sex, indicating that the gonads are not affected. Depending on severity, cloacal malformations may involve the urinary system, pelvis, abdominal wall, genitalia, spine, and anus.[3]

Persistence of the cloaca. Rarely, failure in the urorectal septum development results in a direct communication between the gastrointestinal, urinary, and genital structures, with a single perineal opening. It is usually associated with urinary tract anomalies, such as hydronephrosis, hydroureter, or dysplastic kidneys.[4]

Cloacal exstrophy. Defects of the closure of the lateral body folds result in an impaired formation of the ventral body wall and lack of completion of the anterior wall of the cloaca. The development of the urorectal septum is also affected, driving to malformations of the anal canal and imperforate anus. Depending on severity, it may also involve malformations of the urinary system, pelvic floor, and spine. Exstrophy of the cloaca may be associated with failure of fusion of the genital tubercle and pubic rami, leading to epispadias (Fig. 48.1). Furthermore, since the body folds do not fuse, the labioscrotal folds are widely spaced. Males also present with cryptorchidism, due to insufficient abdominal pressure for testis descent.[3]

Bladder exstrophy. The pathogenesis is similar to that of cloacal exstrophy, but with a normal development of the urorectal septum. Consequently, the posterior bladder wall is exposed through a midline defect of the abdomen (Fig. 48.1). Genital abnormalities consist of epispadias and a small, split phallus in both sexes. In girls, a bifid uterus and a duplicate or exstrophic vagina are observed. Distinguishing between bifid scrotum and labia majora may prove difficult. In boys, testes usually do not descend to the scrotum.

48.3.1.4 Defective Morphogenesis of the Primordia of the External Genitalia

Aphallia. The isolated absence of the phallus is extremely rare,[5] characterized by a complete absence of the corpora cavernosa and corpus spongiosum, due to a failure in the formation or development of the genital tubercle. The urethra

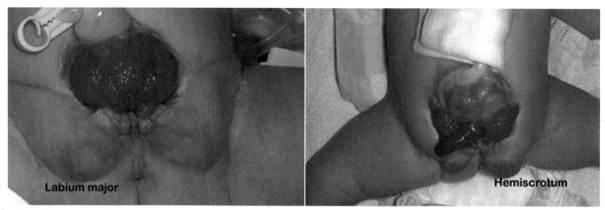

FIG. 48.1 Congenital malformation of the cloacal derivatives hampering the identification of the external genitalia. *Left*: Bladder exstrophy in a female newborn. *Right*: Cloacal exstrophy in a male newborn. Note the difficulty in distinguishing the derivatives of the labioscrotal swellings (labia majora and scrotum), urethral folds, and genital tubercle. *(Reprinted from Ebert AK, Reutter H, Ludwig M, Rosch WH. The exstrophy-epispadias complex.* Orphanet J Rare Dis *2009;4:23. https://doi.org/10.1186/1750-1172-4-23. VC Ebert et al.; licensee BioMed Central Ltd.)*

can open in any position, from prescrotal to high in the rectum, since the penile urethra fails to develop. The scrotum is normal, with descended testes. Clitoris agenesis is a very rare abnormality in XX patients, usually associated with hypoplasia of labia minora.

Micropenis. Defined by a length of <2.5 cm, measured along the dorsal surface from the pubis to the tip with the penis stretched to resistance, micropenis most usually results from insufficient androgen action due to primary or central hypogonadism or to androgen insensitivity. Nonetheless, some cases are due to malformations not explained by androgen defects. This includes the autosomal dominant form of Robinow syndrome (OMIM 180700) due to mutations of *WNT5A*.

Diphallia and Bifid Phallus. True diphallia refers to complete penile duplication, each with two corpora cavernosa and a corpus spongiosum, whereas bifid phallus is characterized by only one corpus cavernosum present in each penis. It is most frequently associated with bladder exstrophy, due to a malformation of the anterior abdominal wall.[6]

Isolated Hypospadias. Hypospadias is the consequence of an incomplete fusion of the urethral folds on the sides of the urethral groove (Fig. 48.2). The urethra abnormally opens along the inferior part of the penis, from the glans (mildest forms) to the perineum (most severe). Hypospadias is found in approximately 1:125 to 1:300 male newborns, representing one of

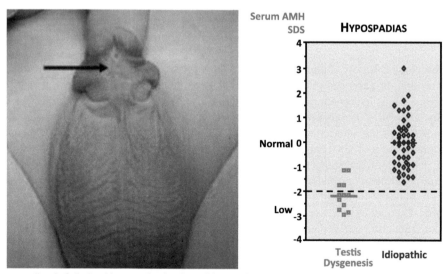

FIG. 48.2 Isolated hypospadias. *Left*: Isolated hypospadias in a boy with normal scrotal configuration. *Right*: In boys with isolated hypospadias, testis hormone secretion (e.g., anti-Müllerian hormone) is normal, as opposed to what is seen in boys with hypospadias because of testicular dysgenesis. *(Left: Reprinted with permission from Yucel S, Dravis C, Garcia N, et al. Hypospadias and anorectal malformations mediated by Eph/ephrin signaling.* J Pediatr Urol *2007;3:354–63. VC Journal of Pediatric Urology. © Elsevier Ltd. doi:10.1016/ j.jpurol.2007.01.199. Right: Reprinted with permission from Grinspon RP, Rey RA. When hormone defects cannot explain it: malformative disorders of sex development.* Birth Defects Res Part C Embryo Today *2014;102(4):359–73. © 2014 Wiley Periodicals, Inc.)*

the most prevalent congenital malformations.[7] The incidence seems to be increasing, probably associated with the effect of environmental endocrine disruptors.[8] Boys with isolated hypospadias, i.e., not associated with other genital malformations, have a low risk of abnormal hormone secretion by the gonads or abnormal end-organ insensitivity.[9] These cases could be explained by a genetic or environmentally induced failure in early morphogenetic events responsible for urethral seam formation and development. Isolated hypospadias is more frequent in boys born preterm, small for gestational age, or conceived with fertility treatments.[10] The underlying pathogenesis is poorly understood. Recent genomewide association analyses have identified 18 genomic regions explaining 9% of cases. In the identified regions, genes with key roles in embryonic development are present, e.g., *DGKK, HOXA4, IRX5, IRX6* and *EYA1*.[11] When hypospadias is associated with other features of impaired virilization (unfused labioscrotal swellings, micropenis, cryptorchidism), a dysgenetic or a hormone-dependent form of DSD is suspected.

Penile-scrotal transposition is a rare malformation, whereby a total or partial exchange of position exists between the scrotum and the penis (Fig. 48.3). The condition is believed to be due to a failure in the caudal migration of labioscrotal folds and/or an abnormal position of the genital tubercle.

48.3.2 Dysgenetic DSD

Gonadal dysgenesis represents a fetal-onset primary hypogonadism affecting all cell lineages—Leydig/theca, Sertoli/granulosa, and germ cells.[12] Dysgenetic DSD may be the underlying etiology in 46,XY DSD, 46,XX DSD, and sex chromosome DSD. While ovarian dysgenesis does not affect fetal genital development, testicular dysgenesis results in atypical differentiation of the genitalia. Complete or "pure" testicular dysgenesis leads to a fully female phenotype of internal and external genitalia because streak gonads secrete neither androgens nor anti-Müllerian hormone (AMH) (Fig. 48.4). Partial forms of testicular dysgenesis are associated with different degrees of Müllerian duct regression, depending on the amount of functional Sertoli cells secreting AMH, and of Wolffian duct development and virilization of the urogenital sinus and the external genitalia, according to the number of functional Leydig cells secreting androgens. One peculiar form of testicular dysgenesis is asymmetric gonadal differentiation (also called mixed gonadal dysgenesis), characterized by the presence of a streak gonad on one side—in association with fallopian tubes and a hemi-uterus—and a dysgenetic testis on the other side—in association with Wolffian duct development and Müllerian duct regression. The karyotype initially described was 45,X/46,XY[13,14] but it can also be 46,XY as described later. Another special type of gonadal dysgenesis consists of the development of both ovarian and testicular tissue in the same individual, called ovotesticular DSD.

Some sex chromosome aneuploidies with gonadal dysgenesis, like Klinefelter syndrome (47,XXY) and Turner syndrome (45,X), do not present with malformations of the external or internal genitalia in the newborn so they will be only briefly described.

48.3.2.1 Dysgenetic DSD in 46,XY Patients

In individuals with a Y chromosome, gonadal dysgenesis is the consequence of defects in the testis determination pathway, normally taking place during the 7th week of embryonic life (Fig. 48.4; Chapter 37).

Clinical features. The typical histological feature of complete or pure gonadal dysgenesis is the existence of a streak of fibrous tissue, with no Sertoli or Leydig cells. Rarely, cord-like structures with abnormal germ cells are observed, which can lead to the formation of gonadoblastoma later in life. The newborn has a normal female aspect, with normal fallopian tubes

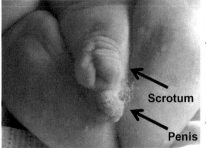

Hormonal laboratory	Patient	Normal values (mean ±SD)
LH (U/l)	3.66	4.81 ± 2.19
FSH (U/l)	0.74	2.30 ± 0.89
Testosterone (ng/dl)	94	76 ± 30
AMH (pmol/l)	550	427 ± 127

FIG. 48.3 Penile-scrotal transposition in a 10-day-old newborn with malformative (nonendocrine) DSD. *Left*: Note that the penis is dorsally positioned with regard to the scrotum. *Right*: Endocrine laboratory results showed hormone serum levels within the reference range for age and sex in this patient. *(Reprinted with permission from Grinspon RP, Rey RA. When hormone defects cannot explain it: Malformative disorders of sex development.* Birth Defects Res Part C Embryo Today *2014;102(4):359–73. © 2014 Wiley Periodicals, Inc.)*

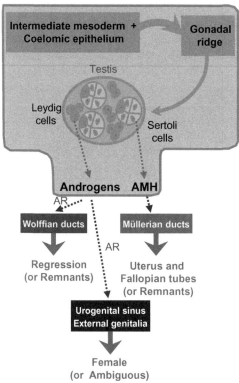

FIG. 48.4 Pathogenesis of dysgenetic disorders of sex development (DSDs) in 46,XY patients. There is a failure of testicular differentiation leading to deficient function of both Sertoli and Leydig cell populations. Lack of AMH results in the existence of uterus and fallopian tubes, whereas lack of androgens results in the regression or Wolffian ducts and feminization of the urogenital sinus and the external genitalia. If gonadal **dysgenesis is not** complete, genitalia are ambiguous. *AR*, androgen receptor. *(Reprinted from Rey RA, Josso N. Diagnosis and treatment of disorders of sexual development. In: Jameson JL, De Groot LJ, de Kretser D, Giudice LC, Grossman A, Melmed S, Potts JT Jr, Weir GC, editors.* Endocrinology: adult and pediatric. *7th ed. Philadelphia, PA: Elsevier Saunders; 2016. pp 2086–2118 e5. ISBN 978-0-323-18907-1, https://doi.org/10.1016/B978-0-323-18907-1.00119-0. © 2016 Saunders, an affiliate of Elsevier Inc.)*

and uterus, owing to the lack of the two testicular hormones involved in fetal sex differentiation. The diagnosis is usually not suspected until the age of puberty, when these girls seek medical advice due to lack of development of secondary sex characteristics. Sex steroids and AMH are undetectable,[12] whereas gonadotropins are extremely high in newborns but may decrease to almost normal levels by the age of 6–9 years,[15] and increase again to extremely high levels in pubertal age. In these cases, the karyotype is 46,XY.

In patients with partial dysgenesis, testes are small, the albuginea is thin, and the seminiferous tubules usually have annular aspect, are dichotomized, and are separated by wide intertubular spaces filled with fibrous connective tissue. Germ cells are absent or scarce and usually abnormal. Gonadal tumor risk is increased.[16,17] The degree of virilization of the external genitalia, Wolffian ducts, and the urogenital sinus, and of regression of Müllerian ducts, is commensurate with the amount of functional testicular tissue. Mild cases may present with a male phenotype and infertility. Androgens and AMH levels are in-between female and male ranges. Gonadotropins are elevated, but not as high as in patients with pure gonadal dysgenesis.

In patients with a mosaicism, the lack of part or all of the Y chromosome is responsible for gonadal dysgenesis. In those with a 46,XY karyotype, different gene defects have been described (reviewed in ref. [18]):

SRY inactivating mutations or deletions (OMIM 480000) are present in approximately 15% of 46,XY females with complete gonadal dysgenesis. Nonreproductive organs are not affected.

MAP3K1 mutations (OMIM 600982) result in increased β-catenin and reduced SOX9/FGF9 expression, resulting in gonadal dysgenesis with no other dysmorphic features in 46,XY patients.

Partial duplications of Xp21.3-p21.2, including *NR0B1*, have been described in XY females with gonadal dysgenesis and no other clinical features. *NR0B1* encodes **DAX1**, suspected to be the underlying cause, although other contiguous genes present in the duplicated region cannot be excluded as causative.[19,20] The locus is known as DSS, standing for dosage-sensitive sex-reversal (OMIM 300018). This phenotype does not occur in 47,XXY patients (e.g., Klinefelter syndrome) because one of the X chromosomes undergoes inactivation.

Four XY females with complete gonadal dysgenesis and one male with hyspospadias and partial gonadal dysgenesis but no other dysmorphic feature were described with variants in *ZNRF3*, an E3 ubiquitin ligase that inhibits canonical WNT signaling.[21]

Two XY females and one patient with ambiguous genitalia due to gonadal dysgenesis were found to carry rearrangements involving the *SOX8* locus at 16p13.[22]

SOX9 mutations or deletions (OMIM 608160) lead to gonadal dysgenesis and campomelic dysplasia (congenital bowing and angulation of long bones), which can also be associated with macrocephaly, micrognathia, low-set ears, flat nasal bridge, congenital dislocation of hips, hypoplastic scapula, small thoracic cage, and cardiac and renal defects.

Heterozygous mutations of *NR5A1*, encoding SF1 (OMIM 612965), have been identified in a wide spectrum of disorders of gonadal and adrenal function.[23] However, in most of the cases adrenal function is normal, and patients present with ambiguous genitalia.

WT1 mutations or deletions (OMIM 607102) are present in patients with Wilms tumor (nephroblastoma), progressive renal diffuse mesangial sclerosis, and/or gonadal dysgenesis.[24] Three distinct forms have been described: (a) Denys-Drash syndrome, defined by the coexistence of gonadal dysgenesis, nephropathy (proteinuria typical of nephrotic syndrome), and Wilms tumor; (b) Frasier syndrome, characterized by gonadal dysgenesis, nephropathy, and gonadoblastoma, and (c) WAGR syndrome, associating Wilms tumor, aniridia, gonadal dysgenesis, and mental retardation.

Chromosome 9p24 deletions (OMIM 154230), encompassing *DMRT1* and *DMRT2*, are associated with gonadal dysgenesis, microcephaly, mental retardation, short stature, and/or bronchial or digestive malformations.

ATRX mutations or deletions (OMIM 301040) have been described in patients with ambiguous genitalia, α-thalassemia, and mental retardation.

DHH mutations or deletions (OMIM 605423) result in gonadal dysgenesis associated with mini-fascicular neuropathy.

In recent years, whole exome sequencing (WES) and whole genome sequencing (WGS) uncovered other genes associated with 46,XY dysgenesis:

FOG2/ZFPM2 mutations result in gonadal dysgenesis and somatic anomalies like clinodactyly and hydrocephaly associated with language, reading and learning difficulties, and autism.[25]

A *FGFR2* mutation was described in one patient with 46,XY complete gonadal dysgenesis and craniosynostosis.[26]

A *TSPYL* defect (OMIM 608800) was identified in a large pedigree with an increased incidence of testicular dysgenesis and sudden death.

48.3.2.2 *Dysgenetic DSD in Patients with Mosaicisms/Chimerism Carrying a Y Chromosome*

Most of the patients with mosaicisms or chimerism involving a Y chromosome develop dysgenetic testes. Partial testicular dysgenesis can be symmetric (dysgenetic testes with similar features bilaterally) or asymmetric (dysgenetic testis on one side, streak gonad contralaterally). In patients with **asymmetric gonadal differentiation** (also called mixed gonadal dysgenesis), the most typical clinical presentation is characterized by asymmetric development of the scrotum, with the testis in scrotal position. As expected, the internal ducts are male on the side of the testis and female (hemi-uterus and fallopian tube) on the side of the streak. The karyotype may be variable: 46,XY with mosaicisms of the sex chromosomes, and frequently 45,X/46,XY in patients with asymmetric gonadal differentiation. However, a 45,X/46,XY karyotype does not always result in asymmetric gonadal differentiation, and it can be an incidental finding in a normally virilized boy.[27] Some patients may also have typical features of Turner syndrome and an increased risk of celiac disease, autoimmune thyroiditis, and cardiovascular defects.[28] Serum levels of androgens and AMH correlate with the amount of functional testicular tissue. The risk of gonadal tumor development is high.[16,17]

When an XX cell line is also present (e.g., 46,XY/46,XX), ovarian tissue may also develop. **Ovotesticular DSD** refers to the existence of testicular tissue—including seminiferous tubules—and ovarian tissue, with the presence of follicular structures containing oocytes. Ovotesticular DSD may present with bilateral ovotestes, one testis, and one ovary, or one ovotestis and one testis or ovary.[29,30] The testicular tissue is usually dysgenetic, whereas the ovarian tissue is most frequently of normal appearance. Ovotesticular DSD can also present in 46,XX individuals (see the following), but is extremely rare in 46,XY patients, and represents 3%–10% of all cases of DSD.[31] Like for all forms of gonadal dysgenesis, the degree of virilization depends on the existing amount of functional testicular tissue.[12] Similarly, serum androgen and

AMH levels are usually between the male and the female ranges. Follicular development and estrogen increase may result in breast development and eventually in vaginal bleeding at the age of puberty. Müllerian derivatives are usually present in less virilized patients, with low AMH. Although the overall risk of gonadal malignancy is low in ovotesticular DSD, it may be higher in the subset of patients carrying a Y chromosome.[16]

48.3.2.3 Dysgenetic DSD in 46,XX Patients

Testicular tissue differentiation can unexpectedly occur in the 46,XX gonadal ridge. When it is the only gonadal tissue present, the condition is called 46,XX testicular DSD, while when it coexists with ovarian tissue it is called 46,XX ovotesticular DSD.[32] The existence of a translocation of the *SRY* gene (SRY-positive cases) to an X chromosome or to an autosome[33] explains the development of testicular tissue in most of the cases. The etiology of 46,XX testicular or ovotesticular DSD in SRY-negative individuals begins to be unveiled and involves overexpression of "pro-testicular" genes or defects of "pro-ovarian" genes.

Overexpression of "pro-testicular" genes includes duplications of *SOX9* (OMIM 608160)[34] or of its regulatory elements,[35] as well as of *SOX10* (OMIM 602229)[36] and *SOX3* (OMIM 300833).[37,38] The particular p.Arg92Gln variant in NR5A1, encoding SF1, has been reported in 46,XX ovotesticular DSD, but the underlying pathogenic mechanism has yet to be identified.[39]

Defects of "pro-ovarian" genes include inactivating mutations in *RSPO1*. Affected individuals also present palmoplantar hyperkeratosis with squamous cell carcinoma of skin (OMIM 610644).[40] A homozygous inactivating mutation in *WNT4* was reported in consanguineous kindred with SERKAL syndrome (OMIM 611812). Some of the patients presented with testicular DSD and others with ovotesticular DSD, in association with renal agenesis, adrenal hypoplasia, and pulmonary and cardiac abnormalities.

Clinical features. Patients with **SRY-positive 46,XX testicular DSD** (or XX males) are completely virilized, with testes and no Müllerian remnants.[41] At birth, they are not noticed, and the diagnosis can be made during childhood, due to mild short stature, in adolescence due to small testis volume, or more frequently in adulthood due to infertility. Sertoli and Leydig cell function is normal in childhood and in the early stages of puberty, as revealed by normal AMH, inhibin B, testosterone, and gonadotropin levels.[42,43] Testis size progresses normally to 4 to 8 mL, mainly due to Sertoli cell proliferation,[44] but then it remains smaller as a consequence of germ cell depletion, as in Klinefelter syndrome,[41] because the existence of two X chromosomes and the absence of a Y chromosome result in meiotic failure.[45] In adulthood, low inhibin B and high FSH reflect seminiferous tubule dysfunction, whereas a mild Leydig cell dysfunction may exist, leading to low-normal testosterone and elevated LH. Increased estrogens may lead to gynecomastia.[41,46]

SRY-negative 46,XX testicular DSD is usually associated with more severe dysgenetic testes, Müllerian remnants, and ambiguous external genitalia.[47] The clinical presentation of patients with **46,XX ovotesticular DSD** is similar to that described in the previous section and depends on the amount of functional testicular and ovarian tissues. In all these cases, tumor risk is low, due to the absence of a Y chromosome.[16]

48.3.2.4 Gonadal Dysgenesis in Sex Chromosome Aneuploidies

Atypical sex chromosome constitution usually does not present with ambiguous genitalia. This includes polysomies of the X chromosome (Klinefelter syndrome) and monosomy of the sex chromosomes (45,X), with their variants.

Klinefelter syndrome, 47,XXY and its variants have a prevalence of approximately 1.5:1000 male newborns, according to population screening studies.[48] However, the clinical reproductive phenotype is completely normal in the vast majority of the cases at birth and during childhood, which explains that it is diagnosed in <10% of the cases before puberty[49]. Gonadal dysgenesis is extremely mild during fetal life, only characterized by a decrease in germ cell numbers, but Leydig and Sertoli cell hormone secretion is normal until midpuberty.[50] Cryptorchidism and learning or behavior disorders are more frequent than in the general population.[48] Pubertal development is usually spontaneous at an appropriate age; however, as in XX males, testicular size rarely progresses beyond 6–8 mL and gynecomastia is more frequent.

Turner syndrome is mainly associated with a 45,X karyotype and has a prevalence of approximately 1:2500 female newborns.[51] However, spontaneous abortion occurs in approximately 98% of pregnancies. Newborns are smaller than average both in length and in weight and may present with congenital lymphedema, cardiovascular defects—especially coarctation or bicuspid aorta—and kidney anomalies. Usually, postnatal growth lies within the normal range for the first 2 to 3 years but then decreases. Later clinical manifestation includes short stature, short, thick and webbed neck, epicanthus and ptosis of the eyelids, hypertelorism, low posterior hairline, broad chest, cubitus valgus, multiple pigmented nevi, recurrent otitis media, and a tendency to keloid formation. Turner syndrome patients have an increased risk of autoimmune disorders, like celiac disease, thyroiditis, diabetes mellitus, rheumatoid arthritis, and inflammatory bowel disease.

Gonads are usually severely dysgenetic, presenting as fibrous streaks,[52] associated in most of the cases with undetectable serum AMH, which predicts the absence of spontaneous pubertal development.[53] Gonadotropin levels are high during infancy but may decrease to normal levels between 6 and 9 years of age.[15]

Variants of Turner syndrome include mosaicisms (e.g., 45,X/46,XX or other variants) or partial loss of the X chromosome (e.g., isochromosomes of the long or the short arms, ring chromosomes). Clinical manifestations are milder. Gonadal dysgenesis is partial, with detectable serum AMH, which indicates the existence of ovarian follicles and predicts a higher probability of spontaneous pubertal development.[53] However, secondary amenorrhea is the rule, due to premature ovarian failure.

48.3.3 Nondysgenetic Sex Hormone-Dependent DSD

48.3.3.1 46,XY Nondysgenetic DSD With Testicular Differentiation

Insufficient virilization of the genitalia may be the result of defects in the production or the action of androgens. In these cases, the pathway of testicular differentiation from the gonadal ridge is not affected. Complete defects in androgen production or action results in a female without uterus, whereas partial deficiencies result in ambiguous genitalia. Defects in the AMH pathway lead to a male with uterus usually associated with cryptorchidism.

48.3.3.1.1 Disorders of Androgen Synthesis

Defects of androgen synthesis represent one form of "dissociated" or "cell-specific" fetal-onset primary hypogonadism, where Leydig cells, but not Sertoli cells, are primarily affected, in contrast with testicular dysgenesis, characterized by an early-onset fetal hypogonadism with whole testicular dysfunction. Serum AMH is within the normal male range or elevated,[43] and Müllerian derivatives are absent (Fig. 48.5). Genetic inheritance of androgen synthesis defects is usually autosomal recessive.

Leydig Cell Aplasia or Hypoplasia (OMIM 238320) is rare and results from inactivating mutations of the luteinizing hormone/chorionic gonadotropin (LHCG) receptor. There is a complete or partial absence of Leydig cell differentiation. Depending on the degree of affectation, clinical manifestations range from mild undervirilization to female external genitalia. Basal and hCG-stimulated testosterone is low or undetectable, plasma LH is elevated, and FSH is normal. Testes are usually cryptorchid with normal seminiferous tubules and absence of Leydig cells.[54]

Smith-Lemli-Opitz syndrome (**SLOS**, OMIM 270400) consists of a dehydrocholesterol reductase (**DHCR**) defect that blocks the last step of cholesterol synthesis, the substrate for steroidogenesis. Since cholesterol participates in signal transduction and processing of sonic hedgehog (SHH), which plays a major role in formation of the nervous system, face, and limbs, this form of DSD is associated with microcephaly, facial malformations, cleft palate, growth retardation, toe syndactyly, pyloric stenosis, and congenital heart defects.[55] Clinical diagnosis of SLOS is suspected by the finding of elevated serum 7–dehydrocholesterol.

Lipoid CAH (OMIM 201710) results from mutations of the gene encoding the steroidogenic acute regulatory protein (StAR), responsible for cholesterol transfer from the cytoplasm into the inner mitochondrial membrane in adrenal and gonadal tissue. Most 46,XY patients are born with a female phenotype with severe glucocorticoid and mineralocorticoid deficiency; however, milder forms with ambiguous or male normal genitalia have been reported. Steroid hormones are extremely low or undetectable in blood and do not respond to hCG and ACTH stimulation. Ultrasound usually reveals massive adrenal enlargement, due to accumulation of cholesterol and cholesterol esters in the adrenal cortex.[56] Lipid accumulation also damages Leydig cells in the fetal testes, but does not affect the fetal ovaries because follicles experience minimal gonadotropin stimulation before the age of puberty; therefore, the ovaries remain undamaged until adolescence in lipoid CAH.

P450scc deficiency (OMIM 118485) is caused by mutation in *CYP11A1*, encoding cytochrome P450 cholesterol side-chain cleavage enzyme cytochrome P450 (P450scc). This enzyme is responsible for pregnenolone synthesis in the mitochondria. Most 46,XY patients are born with female external genitalia, and present subsequently with adrenal mineralocorticoid and glucocorticoid deficiencies. Partial deficiencies presenting with ambiguous genitalia have also been reported. Unlike StAR defects, P450scc deficiency does not present with massive adrenal enlargement.[56,57]

P450c17 deficiency (OMIM 202110) may present as a combined deficiency of 17α-hydroxylase, which hydroxylates pregnenolone or progesterone into 17α-hydroxypregnenolone or 17α-hydroxyprogesterone (17-OHP), and 17,20-lyase, required for the synthesis of dehydroepiandrosterone (DHEA) and △4-androstenedione. Alternatively, isolated 17,20-lyase deficiency has also been described. Lack of production of both gonadal and adrenal sex steroids results in severe undervirilization of 46,XY newborns and absence of puberty and signs of adrenarche in 46,XX patients. Progesterone and 17-OHP accumulate in serum whereas DHEA, △4-androstenedione and testosterone are low. **Combined 17α-hydroxylase/**

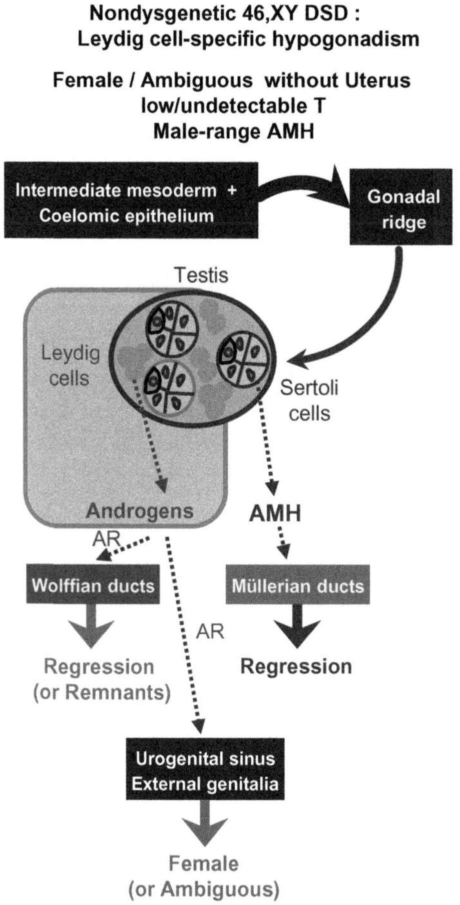

FIG. 48.5 Pathogenesis of nondysgenetic disorders of sex development (DSDs) in 46,XY patients with specific defects of Leydig cell androgen production. Testicular differentiation occurs. Sertoli cells secrete AMH, leading to Müllerian duct regression. Deficient Leydig cell differentiation or function leads to androgen insufficiency, resulting in the regression or Wolffian ducts and feminization of the urogenital sinus and the external genitalia. If the defect is partial, genitalia are ambiguous. *AR*, androgen receptor. *(Reprinted from Rey RA, Josso N. Diagnosis and treatment of disorders of sexual development. In: Jameson JL, De Groot LJ, de Kretser D, Giudice LC, Grossman A, Melmed S, Potts JT Jr, Weir GC, editors. Endocrinology: adult and pediatric, 7th ed. Philadelphia, PA: Elsevier Saunders; 2016. pp 2086–2118 e5. ISBN 978-0-323-18907-1, https://doi.org/10.1016/B978-0-323-18907-1.00119-0. © 2016 Saunders, an affiliate of Elsevier Inc.)*

17,20-lyase deficiency results in a rare form of CAH characterized in both sexes by hypertension and hypokalemia due to the accumulation of deoxycorticosterone and corticosterone. Adrenal crisis is rare, since there are high levels of corticosterone, a weak glucocorticoid; however, glucocorticoid treatment may be necessary for hypertension management. When only **17,20-lyase** activity is affected, androgen, but not glucocorticoid or mineralocorticoid synthesis, is impaired.[57]

Cytochrome b5 deficiency (OMIM 250790): cytochrome *b*5 enhances 17,20-lyase activity of P450c17 without influencing 17-hydroxylase activity. 46,XY DSD was described in patients with impaired 17,20-lyase activity due to mutation in the cytochrome *b*5. The condition is suspected when congenital methemoglobinemia is observed.[57]

P450 oxidoreductase (POR) deficiency (OMIM 613571): POR is an essential redox partner needed for the catalytic activity of three steroidogenic enzymes: P450c17 (preferentially its 17,20-lyase activity), 21-hydroxylase, and aromatase.[57,58] XY newborns are undervirilized but present signs of CAH (e.g., detection of elevated 17-OHP in the neonatal screening), which is suggestive of POR deficiency. Severe forms associated with bone malformations constitute the Antley-Bixler syndrome (ABS, OMIM 201750), characterized by craniosynostosis, fusion of long bones, midface hypoplasia, and choanal stenosis. Laboratory findings are characterized of combined partial deficiencies of 17α-hydroxylase and 21-hydroxylase: elevated serum progesterone and 17-OHP but low DHEA and androstenedione. Basal ACTH is elevated, and cortisol is usually normal with an insufficient response to ACTH stimulation. In puberty, patients develop a hypergonadotropic hypogonadism with elevated 17-OHP, but low or normal androgens and estrogens.

3β-Hydroxysteroid dehydrogenase (HSD) type 2 deficiency (OMIM 201810) is a rare disorder affecting the conversion of △5-steroids to △4-steroids (pregnenolone to progesterone, 17α-hydroxypregnenolone to 17-OHP, DHEA to androstenedione, and androstenediol to testosterone). The *HSD3B2* gene is expressed in the adrenal gland, ovary, and testis and should not be mistaken for *HSD3B1*, expressed in the placenta and peripheral tissues.[57] XY individuals with 3β-HSD type 2 deficiency are born with variable degrees of ambiguous genitalia. XX subjects may also be affected but infants are usually diagnosed later because they may present with absent or minimal virilization. Glucocorticoid and mineralocorticoid production may be compromised and need replacement in severe salt-wasting cases. Increased androgen secretion at puberty may cause premature pubarche in both boys and girls. Laboratory findings are characterized by an elevated Δ5/Δ4 steroids ratio (>10 standard deviations above normal), particularly after ACTH or hCG stimulation. In certain cases, basal levels of Δ4 steroids may be mildly elevated due to the peripheral action of 3β-HSD type 1.[57]

17β-HSD deficiency (OMIM 264300) is caused by mutations in the *HSD17B3* gene, that codes for the 17β-HSD type 3 enzyme that converts △4-androstenedione to testosterone in the testes.[57,59] 46,XY patients present with a female or ambiguous external genital phenotype. Adrenal function is not affected. Virilization at puberty may be explained by peripheral androgen synthesis by other isoforms of the enzyme, like *HSD17B5* (also called *AKR1C3*), which participates in the alternative or "backdoor" steroidogenic pathway.[57] Biochemical findings consist of elevated Δ4-androstenedione, with low/normal testosterone following hCG stimulation. An androstenedione/testosterone ratio above 1.25 is considered diagnostic.[60]

5α-Reductase type 2 deficiency (OMIM 264600), caused by *SRD5A2* mutations, impairs the conversion of testosterone to the more potent androgen dihydrotestosterone (DHT).[61,62] It is a recessive autosomal disorder, observed more frequently in inbred communities in the Dominican Republic, Turkey, and Papua New Guinea. XY patients are poorly virilized at birth, with ambiguous external genitalia. Wolffian ducts, whose development depends on the action of local testosterone, are present. At pubertal age, if the testes have not been removed, virilization occurs due to the action of 5α-reductase type 1 encoded by *SRD5A1*, leading in some cases to the change of the social sex from female to male. In these cases, spontaneous sperm production is achievable when testes are brought to scrotal position. The biochemical profile is characterized by a high testosterone/DHT ratio (usually above 18–20) after hCG stimulation. Elevated 5β/5α urinary metabolite ratio is also useful for diagnosis. In male assigned boys, high doses of testosterone or topic DHT are useful to increase penile size.

3α-HSD type 3 and 3α-HSD type 1 deficiencies are due to mutations in *AKR1C2* (OMIM 600450) and *AKR1C4* (OMIM 600451), respectively, affecting the alternative or "backdoor" pathway of DHT synthesis without the intermediacy of DHEA, androstenedione, or testosterone.[57,63]. XY cases are born with female or ambiguous genitalia. Standard steroid profiles are not informative. Normal urinary excretion of etiocholanolone, androsterone, and other steroids requiring 5α-reduction (e.g., 5α-tetrahydrocortisol) exclude 5α-reductase deficiency. Conversely, increased excretion of pregnenetriol (a urinary metabolite of 17α-hydroxypregnenolone) in response to stimulation with hCG or ACTH, is suggestive of the deficiency of the "backdoor" pathway.

48.3.3.1.2 Disorders of Androgen Action

Alternatively, insufficient virilization may result from defects in the androgen receptor present in target organs (Fig. 48.6). The androgen receptor maps to chromosome Xq12, and >800 gene mutations have been described (http://androgendb.mcgill.ca).

Complete androgen insensitivity syndrome (CAIS) (OMIM 300068) is due to mutations that completely abolish the androgen receptor activity by different mechanisms, affecting the formation of the steroid-receptor-co-regulator complex, its nuclear transport, its binding to DNA, or its transcriptional activation ability. It is the most frequent cause of DSD in completely feminized 46,XY newborns.[64] There is no suspicion at birth, unless a prenatal karyotype has been performed for other reasons. Usually, these patients seek medical attention for primary amenorrhea at pubertal age; breast development occurs normally due to estrogen synthesis from testicular testosterone production. Pubic and axillary hair is absent or very scarce, the vagina is short and blind ending, and the uterus is absent, because AMH production is normal in fetal life. More rarely, the diagnosis is made earlier when a testis is found in the repair of an inguinal hernia in an apparently normal girl. Testicular histology is normal at birth, but germ cell number rapidly declines. Due to androgen insensitivity, meiosis cannot proceed, and spermatozoa are not produced. The risk of germ cell tumor is low, but benign tumors such as Sertoli cell adenomas or hamartomas are frequent.[65] During the first months after birth, basal testosterone and LH do not show the normal postnatal rise.[66] AMH levels are in the normal male range, or slightly elevated, from birth through childhood.[12] At the age of puberty, in nongonadectomized pubertal patients, serum testosterone is in the male range with elevated gonadotropins. AMH levels persist high, because downregulation by androgens does not occur.

Partial androgen insensitivity syndrome (PAIS) (OMIM 312300) results from less severe mutations in the androgen receptor gene. Newborns may present with different degrees of undervirilization of the external genitalia. There are no

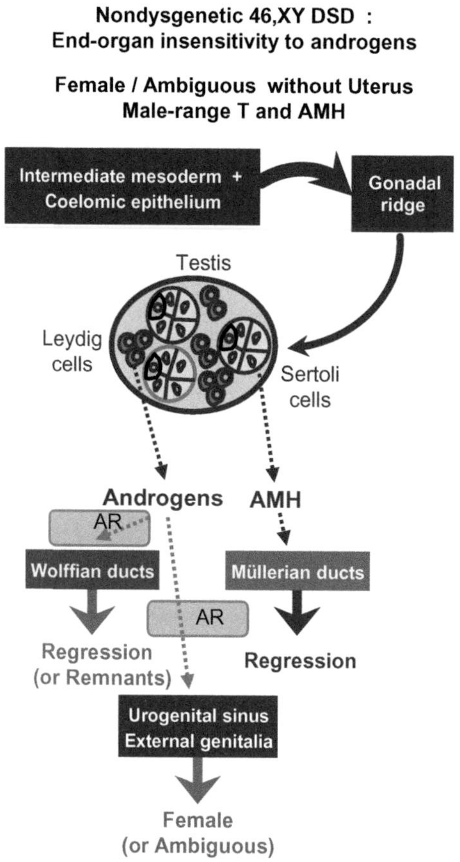

FIG. 48.6 Pathogenesis of nondysgenetic disorders of sex development (DSDs) in 46,XY patients with androgen insensitivity. Testicular differentiation occurs. Sertoli cells secrete AMH, leading to Müllerian duct regression. Leydig cells secrete androgens but androgen receptor (AR) deficiency results in the regression or Wolffian ducts and feminization of the urogenital sinus and the external genitalia. If the defect is partial, genitalia are ambiguous. *AR, androgen receptor. (Reprinted from Rey RA, Josso N. Diagnosis and treatment of disorders of sexual development. In: Jameson JL, De Groot LJ, de Kretser D, Giudice LC, Grossman A, Melmed S, Potts JT Jr, Weir GC, editors.* Endocrinology: adult and pediatric, *7th ed. Philadelphia, PA: Elsevier Saunders, 2016, p. 2086–2118 e5. ISBN 978-0-323-18907-1, https://doi.org/10.1016/B978-0-323-18907-1.00119-0. © 2016 Saunders, an affiliate of Elsevier Inc.)*

fallopian tubes or uterus. Diagnosis is difficult in the absence of family history and cannot easily be distinguished from 5α-reductase type 2 deficiency. Unlike what is observed in CAIS, testosterone and LH are generally elevated during the postnatal activation period.[66] AMH is in the male range.[43] At puberty, pubic and axillary hair development is scant and gynecomastia is frequent. Testosterone increases and AMH may decrease in correlation with the degree of retained androgen action. The correlation genotype/phenotype is poor: the same mutation can result in widely different phenotypes, even within the same pedigree.[67]

48.3.3.1.3 Disorders of AMH Synthesis or Action

The **persistent Müllerian duct syndrome (PMDS)** (OMIM 261550) is characterized by the persistence of the uterus and fallopian tubes, owing to mutations in the genes coding for AMH or its type 2 receptor, in an otherwise normally virilized boy.[68] The existence of ambiguous external genitalia, indicating also a defect in androgen synthesis or action, rules out the diagnosis of PMDS. At birth, cryptorchidism or inguinal hernia are the only clinically evident anomalies. The diagnosis is not anticipated, unless there is a family history, and the presence of Müllerian derivatives is usually discovered when surgery is performed to correct the cryptorchidism or inguinal hernia. Two anatomical forms of PMDS have been described: in one of them patient boys present bilateral cryptorchidism, and both testes are embedded in the broad ligament in an "ovarian" position; in the other form, one testis has descended into the scrotum, dragging the fallopian tube and the contralateral testis, a condition called transverse testicular ectopia. Mutations in the *AMH* or the *AMHR2* genes are found in approximately 85% of PMDS patients. Serum testosterone and gonadotropins are in the male normal range. AMH is undetectable in patients with *AMH* mutations, and within the male range in patients with *AMHR2* mutations.

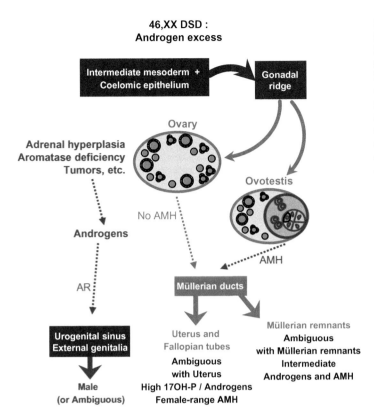

FIG. 48.7 Pathogenesis of disorders of sex development (DSDs) in 46,XX patients with excess androgen. Excess androgen of different sources leads to virilization of the urogenital sinus and external genitalia. Lack of AMH allows the development of fallopian tubes and uterus. *AR*, androgen receptor. *(Reprinted from Rey RA, Josso N. Diagnosis and treatment of disorders of sexual development. In: Jameson JL, De Groot LJ, de Kretser D, Giudice LC, Grossman A, Melmed S, Potts JT Jr, Weir GC, editors. Endocrinology: adult and pediatric, 7th ed. Philadelphia, PA: Elsevier Saunders; 2016. p 2086–2118 e5. ISBN 978-0-323-18907-1, https://doi.org/10.1016/B978-0-323-18907-1.00119-0. © 2016 Saunders, an affiliate of Elsevier Inc.)*

48.3.3.2 46,XX Nondysgenetic DSD With Ovarian Differentiation

Virilization of 46,XX fetuses with normal ovarian differentiation occurs as a consequence of excessive androgen exposure (Fig. 48.7). Since AMH is not produced, the uterus and fallopian tubes develop normally. Excessive androgen sources can be fetal (e.g., CAH), maternal (e.g., steroid secreting tumors) or placental (e.g., aromatase deficiency).

48.3.3.2.1 Disorders of Adrenal Steroidogenesis

CAH represents a group of adrenal steroidogenic disorders where cortisol production is impaired. Insufficient cortisol product leads to increased ACTH secretion, which stimulates the adrenal cortex. Virilization results from the accumulation of adrenal androgens synthesized as a consequence of enzyme blockage. The most common type of CAH is 21-hydroxylase deficiency (21OHD), which represents the most prevalent cause of 46,XX DSD. Deficiencies in 11β-hydroxylase, 3β-HSD, and POR also drive to CAH with virilization in 46,XX patients. Clinical features and laboratory data vary depending on which enzyme is affected, involving excess of androgens and in some cases also deficiency in the production of glucocorticoids and mineralocorticoids. The different forms of CAH are addressed in depth in Chapter 47.

48.3.3.2.2 Generalized Glucocorticoid Resistance

Insensitivity to glucocorticoids (OMIM 615962) is associated with mutations in *NR3C1*, encoding the glucocorticoid receptor. Some mutations act through a dominant negative mechanism to interfere with glucocorticoid signal transduction.[69] Glucocorticoid resistance is characterized by high cortisol concentrations without clinical signs and symptoms of Cushing syndrome but with manifestation of androgen and mineralocorticoid excess. The glucocorticoid resistance of the hypothalamic-pituitary axis leads to increased ACTH secretion, resulting in excessive adrenal cortex hormone production. Most girls are born with normal external genitalia and present with mild signs of virilization during childhood. Hypertension with hypokalemia and metabolic alkalosis could be present due to mineralocorticoid action of compounds as corticosterone, and deoxycorticosterone. Most patients present no clinical manifestations of cortisol deficiency due to the compensation elicited by the elevated levels of glucocorticoids. Biochemical findings include high levels of androgens, corticosterone, deoxycorticosterone, ACTH, and urinary free cortisol.

48.3.3.2.3 Aromatase deficiency

Aromatase is a cytochrome P450 enzyme codified by *CYP19A1*. Aromatase is expressed in the placenta, ovary, testis, and other tissues, and is essential to convert androgens to estrogens. In the human placenta, the conversion of fetal androgens to estrogens protects the mother from the potential virilizing effects of fetal androgens. Placental aromatase deficiency (OMIM 613546) is a rare disorder resulting from deleterious mutations in the coding region or in the promoter of *CYP19A1*.[70] Decreased aromatase activity impairs conversion of androgens to estrogens, resulting in increased androgen concentrations. Affected 46,XX infants present at birth with varying degrees of virilization depending on the residual activity of the enzyme. Maternal history reveals signs of hyperandrogenism during pregnancy, including hirsutism, clitoral hypertrophy, acne, and frontal balding. However, these signs may be absent.[71] In the affected girl, puberty is usually delayed or absent with primary amenorrhea, hypergonadotropic hypogonadism, multicystic ovaries, and decreased bone mineral density.

48.3.3.2.4 Maternal Sources: Androgens and Progestogens

Although the 46,XX fetus is usually protected from excessive androgen exposure by the ability of the fetal-placental unit to aromatize androgens to estrogens, virilization of the external genitalia of a 46,XX fetus can occur due to exposure to high levels of maternal androgens. Elevated androgens may be the result of maternal disorders as CAH, adrenal tumors, ovarian tumors, or hCG-dependent luteoma of pregnancy.[72] Maternal exposure to androgens (testosterone or androgenic steroids) and progestational agents during pregnancy may also induce the virilization of a 46,XX fetus. Norethindrone, ethisterone, norethynodrel, medroxyprogesterone acetate, and danazol have all been implicated in masculinization of the female fetus. Diethylstilbestrol has also been reported to cause not only clear cell adenocarcinoma of the vagina and cervix but also virilization of a 46,XX fetus. Clinical presentation varies between isolated clitoris enlargement to severe genital ambiguity depending on the dose, duration, and period of pregnancy in which the fetus was exposed. The diagnosis of 46,XX DSD arising from transplacental passage of androgenic steroids is largely a diagnosis of exclusion.

48.4 DIAGNOSIS

Owing to their heterogeneity, the diagnostic procedure of DSD may be complex and cannot follow the same systematic rules in all patients. The first issue to consider is the age at presentation: as described earlier, while most conditions may present at birth—or even during intrauterine life—with atypical development of the genitalia, other conditions may remain unapparent until later in childhood or, more probably, pubertal ages. In this chapter, the attention will be focused on the neonatal period of life, with only brief comments on presentations in later periods. The diagnostic approach also varies according to the reason that brought the patient to medical attention: ambiguous genitalia or discordance between fetal karyotype and genital appearance in the newborn, but it could also be pubertal delay or even infertility later in life. The diagnostic workup includes family and prenatal history, physical examination, hormonal laboratory, imaging, histology, and genetic testing. The relative importance and the timeliness of each of them has changed over the last years, especially with the emergence of high throughput technologies like microarrays and next-generation sequencing (NGS).[73] Independently of the approach used, the objectives of reaching an accurate etiologic diagnosis are: (a) to understand the pathogenesis of the disorder, (b) to establish the gonadal sex, functional capacity, and risk of neoplastic degeneration, (c) to assess the anatomical and functional status of the internal and external genitalia and their sensitivity to sex steroids, and (d) to provide genetic counseling.

As may easily be concluded from the knowledge available on normal fetal development of the gonads and genital tract (Chapter 37), anatomical examination gives only a vague hint of the underlying pathophysiology in patients with DSD. Indeed, the existence of ambiguous external genitalia only indicates that androgen activity was insufficient to completely virilize an XY fetus or excessive for an XX fetus. In addition, the probabilistic approach generally used in medicine for differential diagnosis of frequent conditions is not applicable to rare diseases like DSD. Therefore, a pragmatic approach based on the relative incidence of the different etiologies of DSD is not helpful, and a meticulous workup needs to be made to reach a precise diagnosis.

Nonetheless, a clear characterization of the external genitalia gives an idea of the severity of the disorder. Also, the description of other potentially associated malformations may provide useful hints to guide the diagnosis. A careful family history of genital ambiguity or death, consanguinity, infertility, amenorrhea, hirsutism, or other endocrinopathies, as well as information on maternal exposure to exogenous substances or virilization or any other event during pregnancy may be of help.

48.4.1   Assessment During Gestation

Ultrasound assessments during gestation may detect genital ambiguity or a discordance between the external genitalia and the fetal karyotype obtained because of maternal age or due to the existence of a familial history of DSD. The assessment of fetal gonadal hormones in maternal serum or in amniotic fluid gives little information and is not useful for the diagnosis.[74] At this stage, DNA analysis may be useful, as described later (see the section "Genetic Testing").

48.4.2   Newborns with Ambiguous Genitalia

48.4.2.1   Initial Assessment

48.4.2.1.1   Physical Examination

Physical examination of the newborn should include the description of the size and configuration of the phallus. Normal ranges for clitoral and penile size are available, measured fully stretched from the pubic ramus to the tip of the glans over the dorsal side.[75] Description of the trophism of the corpora cavernosa is also useful. Full or incomplete fusion of the urethral folds (hypospadias) should be mentioned together with the position of the meatus, and the existence of only one or two separate urinary and genital orifices. A detailed description should also be provided for the (labio)scrotal folds: whether there is complete fusion of the scrotum, a bifid scrotum, or separate labioscrotal folds (or fused, e.g., in the posterior half or one-third). Presence of structures compatible with testes in the (labio)scrotal folds or in the inguinal canals may be predictive for the differential diagnosis.[76] Anogenital distance reflects exposure to androgens during fetal life; it should be measured from the center of the anus to the posterior junction of the (labio)scrotal folds.[77] In males, the normal distance is 30 ± 7 cm. In females, the anogenital ratio, measured as the distance from anus to base of clitoris/distance from anus to posterior fourchette, should be <0.5; otherwise, excessive androgen exposure is suspected. All these features have been taken into account in different scales, like that of Prader's designed for XX patients with CAH,[78] Quigley's scale for XY patients,[79] or the External Masculinization Score.[80] As already mentioned, when there is a clear dissociation between the degree of masculinization of the various genital structures, a nonendocrine condition due to malformations of particular primordia (e.g., the genital tubercle, the cloacal membrane, etc.) should be considered.

48.4.2.1.2   Laboratory

Genital ambiguity is an endocrine emergency because of the enormous impact on the parents and the need to rapidly eliminate CAH. Indeed, the adrenal insufficiency potentially occurring in newborns with CAH has driven many countries to the establishment of neonatal screening programs designed to detect elevated levels of 17-OHP as a biochemical sign of 21-hydroxylase deficiency.

In the initial assessment, a karyotype is also performed to classify the condition as a 46,XY, 46,XX, or chromosomal DSD.

In the first days of postnatal life, reproductive hormone levels vary significantly (Chapter 37, Table 37.1),[74,81] which needs to be taken into account for the interpretation of the results. Furthermore, there are limitations in the amount of blood that can be drawn in a newborn; therefore, hormonal measurements should be kept to a minimum. The assessment of testosterone and AMH levels may be quite informative in this initial step. When both are below the male range, the amount of functional testicular tissue is scarce, suggesting gonadal dysgenesis (frequently with 46,XY or mosaic karyotypes) or testicular/ovotesticular DSD (frequently with 46,XX or chimeric karyotypes, and no SRY). When testosterone is low but AMH is within the male range, a disorder of testicular Leydig cell development or steroidogenesis is suspected. When both testicular hormones are within the male range, partial androgen insensitivity or defective DHT production are the most probable diagnoses, but malformative, nonendocrine DSD cannot be ruled out. Finally, testosterone in the male range and AMH in the female range is the typical picture of 46,XX DSD due to CAH, aromatase deficiency, or virilizing tumors.[12] Testosterone levels should be assessed after steroid extraction procedures, to avoid falsely elevated results during the first 3 weeks of life.[81] When CAH is suspected, serum electrolytes should be assessed in search for elevated potassium and low sodium, although they may be within the normal range in the first days of life.

Due to the changes in reproductive hormone and electrolyte levels during the first weeks, it is sometimes necessary to repeat their assessment, especially when the first sample was drawn in the first days of life. The presence of ovarian tissue is not easily evidenced because there are not specific markers with diagnostic utility. Although estradiol might be somewhat higher in girls, the sexual dimorphism is not always clear.[74]

48.4.2.1.3 Imaging

The anatomic characteristics of the internal genitalia and the urinary structures need to be established using genitoscopy and/or genitography. The ascertainment of the presence of Müllerian duct remnants and intraabdominal gonads requires an experienced ultrasonographist and equipment with adequate resolution. Otherwise, false positive or false negative results may be frequent. As expected, a combination of male and female internal ducts can be seen. The degree of regression of Müllerian derivatives and of the development of Wolffian ducts depend on the functional capacity of the testes to secrete testosterone and AMH, and of the target organs to respond to them.

48.4.2.2 Following Steps
48.4.2.2.1 46,XY DSD

Once the initial diagnosis of 46,XY DSD is reached, the suspicion of a dysgenetic or a nondysgenetic form warrants further assessment to establish the etiologic diagnosis. As mentioned before, a second blood sample is usually necessary after the second week of life. Measurement of gonadotropins and more gonadal and adrenal steroids in serum[81] or urine[82] may be useful. At this stage, four distinct groups can be recognized: (a) testicular dysgenesis, (b) isolated disorders of androgen synthesis, (c) androgen end-organ disorders, and (d) malformative defects.

(a) Testosterone and AMH are below the male range for age. These features indicate that the development of both testicular somatic cell populations—Leydig and Sertoli cells—are affected, i.e., testes are dysgenetic. The elevation of serum FSH and LH reflects an insufficient negative feedback. Lower testicular hormones and higher gonadotropin levels usually correlate with smaller, more dysgenetic testes, which do not descend to the scrotum, and with higher degree of genital ambiguity. Low adrenal steroids and high ACTH suggest primary adrenal insufficiency, and SF1 defects should be considered. Proteinuria is indicative of renal dysfunction, which is typical of syndromes associated with *WT1* mutations or deletions. Bowing of long bones is typical of campomelic dysplasia due to mutation in *SOX9*. When the genital phenotype is not associated with other anatomic malformations, mutations affecting *SRY* or *MAP3K1* may be the underlying cause of 46,XY dysgenetic DSD. However, other gene defects cannot be excluded at this stage, since the associated phenotypes become evident only later in life, like polyneuropathy due to *DHH* mutations, mental retardation, and α-thalassemia owing to *ATRX* defects, and mental retardation, craniofacial dysmorphism, and delayed motor development found in patients with 9p deletions encompassing *DMRT1*.

(b) Testosterone is below the male range, and AMH is within or above the male range. These features indicate that the testes differentiated and Sertoli cells are normally functional, but there is a disorder in Leydig cell development (LH/CG receptor defects) or function (steroidogenic pathway). LH may be elevated, but FSH is within the normal range for males. To confirm the insufficient capacity of the testes to secrete androgens, a prolonged hCG test should be performed. It consists of six or seven IM injections of 1500 IU every other day, with testicular Δ4 and Δ5 steroids measured 24 to 72 h after the last injection.[83] An ACTH test, consisting of six IM injections 0.5 mg/m^2 of depot ACTH every 12 h, with adrenal Δ4 and Δ5 steroids and cortisol measured before the first injection and 12 h after the last injection may also be necessary.[84] A lack of response to hCG with normal response to ACTH indicates that the defect is in the LH/CG receptor. Defects in specific steroidogenic enzymes or proteins can be deduced from the response patterns to hCG and ACTH (see previous section, "Disorders of Androgen Synthesis"). For specific details concerning CAH, see Chapter 47.

(c) Testosterone and AMH are in the male range, genital abnormalities are consistent with defective androgen action. These 46,XY patients are eugonadal, i.e., both Leydig and Sertoli cell populations developed and function normally. The existence of microphallus, hypospadias, unfused labioscrotal swellings, and/or cryptorchidism are indicative of an insufficient androgen action. Gonadotropins may be elevated. There are two major etiologies, PAIS and 5α-reductase type 2 deficiency, which are not easy to distinguish. An hCG test is sometimes performed with subsequent measurements of testosterone and DHT. An elevated testosterone/DHT ratio is suggestive of 5α-reductase type 2 deficiency, but false negatives may result due to DHT conversion by 5α-reductase type 1 activity at certain ages. Also, false positive results are possible because 5α-reductase activity is regulated by androgens via the androgen receptor; therefore, in PAIS patients DHT production is usually decreased, thus resulting in a falsely elevated testosterone/DHT ratio. Urinary 5β/5α-reduced metabolite ratios have a better diagnostic efficiency: high tetrahydrocorticosterone/allotetrahydrocorticosterone and high etiocholanolone/androsterone ratios confirm 5α-reductase type 2 deficiency, but these assays are not routinely available.

(d) Testosterone and AMH are in the male range, genital abnormalities are inconsistent with androgen defects. These 46,XY patients too are eugonadal, and the genital abnormalities cannot be attributed to a generalized defect of androgen action. Examples are patients with: an isolated hypospadias with normal penile length and testicular volume; or a micropenis associated with a lack of corpora cavernosa in a boy with normally formed scrotum and testes; or epispadias with bladder exstrophy. The condition should be attributed to a defect in a morphogenetic process not due to an endocrine etiology.

48.4.2.2.2 46,XX DSD

Physical examination is helpful to distinguish patients with palpable testes and those without palpable gonads.

Patients with palpable gonads. Ovotesticular and testicular DSD are the most likely diagnoses. As in XY forms of gonadal dysgenesis, testosterone and AMH levels are between the female and the male ranges, reflecting the amount of functional testicular tissue present. The existence of normal FSH levels may be indicative of the existence of ovarian tissue, which usually develops more normally than the testicular counterpart. The diagnosis is confirmed by the histological study. Molecular studies should include the search for *SRY* sequences, for *SOX9, SOX3*, or *SOX10* duplications, or *RSPO1, WNT4*, or *NR5A1* (SF1) mutations in *SRY*-negative cases.[32,39]

Patients with nonpalpable gonads. CAH is the more likely diagnosis. For specific details, see Chapter 47. Ovotesticular DSD is suspected when there is no history of maternal virilization. In these cases, there is less development of testicular tissue than those with palpable gonads. Therefore, testosterone and AMH are closer to the female range. Placental aromatase deficiency is suspected in the existence of a history of maternal virilization during pregnancy. The newborn shows no signs of adrenal dysfunction, estradiol is low, and androgens and gonadotropins are elevated. Molecular studies should point to the *CYP19* gene.[85]

48.4.2.2.3 Chromosomal DSD

The existence of ambiguous genitalia is only exceptionally associated with a 47,XXY or a 45,X karyotype. More frequently, the karyotype shows mosaicisms like 45,X/46,XY, 45,X/46,XY/47,XXY or other variants, or chimerisms 46, XX/46,XY. The presence of a Y chromosome usually results in the development of testicular tissue, which can be more-or-less dysgenetic, leading to the various forms of gonadal dysgenesis, including asymmetric gonadal differentiation (or mixed gonadal dysgenesis), described previously. 45,X lineages are associated with streak gonads, while 46,XX lineages may result in the development of ovarian tissue. Therefore, ovotestes may be present in patients with chromosomal DSD and ambiguous genitalia. The clinical features described earlier for 46,XY and 46,XX dysgenetic DSD apply also for chromosomal DSD.

48.4.3 Newborns with Normal External Genitalia and Discordant Karyotype

DSD patients with completely virilized or feminized external genitalia usually go undiagnosed until the age of puberty, unless there has been a reason for performing a fetal karyotype, e.g., maternal age or familial history of DSD. The newborn's karyotype should be confirmed, and 17-OHP, testosterone, and AMH determined. Physical examination of every newborn must include the palpation of the scrotum and inguinal regions in the search for testes.

48.4.3.1 46,XY DSD

Completely feminized 46,XY newborns may result from complete forms of gonadal dysgenesis (also called pure gonadal dysgenesis or Swyer syndrome), Leydig cell aplasia (due to LH/CG receptor defects), lipoid CAH (due to StAR defects), P450scc defects, or to CAIS (due to androgen receptor mutations). Other steroidogenic defects rarely present with a complete female external phenotype, since the presence of androgens in lower levels or with less potency still provokes some degree of virilization, thus resulting in ambiguous genitalia. The combined assessment of testicular hormones is extremely informative: undetectable testosterone and AMH is typical of pure gonadal dysgenesis, undetectable testosterone and high AMH is characteristic of Leydig cell aplasia and steroidogenic defects, and male-range testosterone and AMH is indicative of androgen insensitivity.[12] However, in some cases, testosterone may be lower than normal in CAIS.[66] Ultrasound examination reveals the existence of a hypoplastic uterus and fallopian tubes in the dysgenetic forms, and their absence in Leydig cell aplasia, testosterone synthesis defects, and CAIS. Nonetheless, microscopic remnants of the Müllerian ducts have been described in some cases.

48.4.3.2 46,XX DSD

Completely virilized 46,XX newborns, with no palpable gonads, may result from the most severe cases of CAH due to 21OH deficiency. They are detected when elevated 17-OHP is found in the neonatal screening program; when the screening is not performed, these patients may present with signs of adrenal crisis, i.e., hypoglycemia and/or salt-wasting, during the second to fourth weeks of life. Uterus and fallopian tubes, together with ovaries, are seen in the ultrasound imaging. Testosterone is in the male range but AMH is in the female range.

Fully virilized 46,XX males with scrotal testes of normal size represent the typical XX males (SRY-positive). They have reproductive hormones in the normal male range, and Müllerian duct derivatives are absent.

48.4.4 Genetic Testing

A step-by-step approach trying to identify the most likely "candidate" gene that could be responsible for the condition under study was the rule until the first decade of the present century. The major breakthrough produced by the Human Genome Project, completed in 2003, and the development of newer, high-throughput technologies in the area of genomics have led not only to an exponential growth in the knowledge of genes involved in sex development but also to a change in the diagnostic approach. Indeed, the classical karyotype and the "candidate" gene approach progressively become less cost-effective—and therefore limited to a restricted number of well-characterized conditions—when compared with comparative genomic hybridization arrays (CGH) and gene panels or whole exome sequencing (WES).

While peripheral blood karyotype analysis remains the main tool to detect balanced chromosomal translocations, such as structural rearrangements of the X chromosome, it is useful to diagnose large chromosome aberrations (>5000 kb). Fluorescent in situ hybridization (FISH) allows the detection of smaller, known sequences of approximately 100 kb. Instead, CGH is a high-resolution method that can detect copy number variants (CNVs), i.e., submicroscopic chromosome insertions or deletions, of 10 kb. Approximately 15% of the cases of DSD can be explained by the presence of CNVs,[86] with rates going up to 25% in syndromic forms of 46,XY gonadal dysgenesis.[87] Chromosomal microarrays are particularly useful in the identification of deletions/duplications of regulatory regions of genes involved in sex development.[32] For instance, deletions upstream of *SOX9* coding regions are responsible for 46,XY dysgenetic DSD,[88] whereas duplications of *SOX9* regulatory regions lead to 46,XX ovotesticular DSD in SRY-negative case.[32]

The main limitation of the "candidate" gene approach is that it requires a precise clinical diagnosis, which is not always possible. For instance, as already mentioned, many forms of 46,XY dysgenetic DSDs are clinically similar; also PAIS and partial deficiencies of various steroidogenic enzymes can be very difficult to distinguish by anatomic, biochemical, or imaging studies. Unsuccessfully choosing candidate genes one after another can be time-consuming and costly. With the advent of massive parallel gene sequencing, or NGS, single gene sequencing has gradually evolved into gene panels, which are now widely used in clinical practice for genetic diagnosis. Different reports have described the utility of gene panels designed for the diagnosis of DSD, including 50 to 80 genes, and showing cost-efficiency and diagnostic rates ranging from 28% to 45% in one step.[18,87] WES is even more powerful, since it is a hypothesis-free approach, which does not require knowing which gene could be defective. On the other hand, it generates enormous amounts of information (roughly, the sequences of exons of all genes on an individual's genome). This leads to the detection of approximately 20,000 sequence variants, when compared to reference databases, which need to be filtered and interpreted using bioinformatic tools and labor-intensive manual curation involving a tight interaction between bioinformaticians and clinicians, in order to detect the most likely pathogenic gene variant. An ethical challenge has arisen from the capacity of NGS techniques to identify variants in genes that are not associated with the condition for which the patient is being studied, i.e., incidental findings. Particular concerns exist about those variants that may be associated with life-threatening conditions. Different strategies have been proposed by different guidelines: while the American College of Medical Genetics maintains a list of 59 genes for which pathogenic variants should be sought and reported to the patient, the Canadian College of Medical Genetics recommends against searching, and the European Society of Human Genetics recommends the analysis to be restricted to relevant genes to decrease the chance of incidental findings.[87] Pretest counseling and informed consent are essential components of the process involved in performing genetic studies.

48.5 MANAGEMENT OF THE NEWBORN WITH DSD

Because of their clinical heterogeneity, management of patients with DSD is complex and involves a multidisciplinary team including initially the neonatologist, the endocrinologist, the geneticist, the nurse, the psychologist, and then also the pediatrician, the radiologist, the gynecologist, and the urologist.[80] DSD conditions should be diagnosed as precisely as possible at the time of presentation. Additionally, communication with the family—and the patient as age allows it—is of paramount importance to reach the best possible biological and psychosocial outcomes. A long-term care plan should be formulated in concert with the family. In this chapter we will focus on the management during the neonatal period.

Newborns with ambiguous genitalia or discordance between prenatal karyotype and genital features at birth require thoughtful deliberation concerning sex assignment and the need for treatment, including early genital surgery. The differential diagnosis is categorized on the basis of the karyotype. Emphasis should be given to the fact that the karyotype is only one of the many biological characteristics of an individual and that by itself it does not define the sex of the newborn. An explanation of the genetic and embryological basis of fetal sex differentiation may be very helpful for the parents to understand their child's condition. The common origin of the testes and ovaries, penis and clitoris, scrotum and labia majora should be discussed to let the parents understand the impact of gonadal differentiation and hormone production on genital development.

Except for CAH, DSD is not life-threatening. However, it is crucial to provide parents with timely and increasingly detailed information. For instance, surgical management of genitalia with an atypical appearance is an increasingly controversial issue. Intersex activists have promoted banning of irreversible genital surgery without the patient's informed consent, whereas medical societies have evolved to now propose that surgery should be done early only for medical, not esthetic, reasons, i.e., to relieve outflow tract obstruction. Alternatives should also be promoted, e.g., supporting families in parenting children with atypical genitalia without recurring to esthetic surgical correction and facilitating psychological adjustment.[89] Full disclosure and education are critical, and psychological family support should be provided by a professional with expertise in DSD. Parent/patient support groups are usually helpful, although in some cases nonrepresentative biases may occur. Three primary ethical principles apply to management of DSD patients:[90] (a) to foster the well-being of the child and future adult, (b) to uphold the rights of children and adolescents to participate in and/or self-determine decisions that affect them, and (c) to respect the family and parent-child relationship. The goal of achieving a balance between the rights, needs and interests are outlined in the following nine recommendations: (1) careful weighing of therapeutic decisions, (2) periodic review of recent medical scientific findings, particularly with respect to long-term treatment outcomes, (3) respect of the ultimate rights of the parents, (4) explain to the parents that determining a binary sex does not automatically ensure the child's well-being, (5) respect of the parents' value system, (6) interventions should be based on exhaustive diagnostic studies and the best possible prognosis, (7) explicit reasoning and justification is necessary for any intervention when conclusive scientific evidence is lacking, (8) providing information to the child commensurate with age, and (9) documentation of treatment information to provide to the individual as an adult.

48.5.1 Sex Assignment

The primary goal of sex assignment in a newborn with DSD is an assignment that aligns best with the future gender identity. However, it should be realized that future gender development cannot be predicted with certainty in any individual, even in the majority of newborns having no discordance between genetic, gonadal, and genital sex. The factors considered for sex assignment are the etiologic diagnosis, the degree of virilization or feminization reflecting androgen exposure, surgical options, malignancy risk, anticipated quality of sexual function, fertility potential, and familial/cultural/psychosocial factors.

Evidence for the impact of prenatal androgens has produced a general shift toward male assignment for 46,XY individuals with evidence of androgen exposure in utero and postnatal androgen responsiveness, from 35% of such patients being assigned male before 1990 to 68% since 1999.[91] This shift was heavily influenced by the male gender development among 46,XY patients with cloacal exstrophy who had been assigned female at birth and were then gonadectomized.[92] Additionally, adult males with small penises usually identify as male.

48.5.1.1 46,XY DSD with Female Genitalia

As already noted, general rules cannot be dictated and each patient should be considered individually. Unfortunately, long-term outcome information for 46,XY DSD patients, especially regarding quality of life, is scarce.[93] Female assignment is certainly appropriate for newborns with completely female genitalia due to pure gonadal dysgenesis, Leydig cell aplasia, or severe steroidogenic insufficiency and CAIS. Particularly patients with dysgenetic DSD have internal genitalia that can be stimulated with adequate hormone replacement therapy, leading to menstrual cycles and gestation capacity after oocyte donation. However, it should be acknowledged that psychological distress issues may exist and need to be addressed,[94] particularly in patients with testes (Leydig cell aplasia, severe steroidogenic insufficiency, and CAIS) and without uterus.

48.5.1.2 46,XY DSD with Ambiguous Genitalia

Male assignment seems adequate in 46,XY DSD patients with partial testicular dysgenesis; these patients have good response to exogenous androgen replacement therapy. When gonadal dysgenesis is too severe, and virilization is minimal with persistence of Müllerian derivatives and feminization of the urogenital sinus, the decision might be toward female assignment.

Male assignment is recommended for patients with partial steroidogenic defects, whereas female assignment can be considered in those with more severe defects despite the absence of Müllerian derivatives. Both those raised males and female have indicated satisfactory sexual function, while those raised male have indicated dissatisfaction with penis length and those raised female have been reported to have clinical distress.[95]

The recommended sex assignment for newborns with 5α-reductase deficiency is male based upon the report that the majority develop a male gender identity when gonads are left intact, and fertility may be possible. However, in very severe forms, female assignment could be considered since those raised females and gonadectomized before puberty have indicated satisfactory sexual function.[1]

PAIS certainly poses one of the most difficult dilemmas. Male assignment should occur where acceptable androgen responsiveness has been demonstrated. In its absence, the decision may tilt toward female assignment.

48.5.1.3 46,XX DSD with Male Genitalia

Completely virilized 46,XX newborns with testes should unequivocally be assigned males. When no testes are present, and Prader 5 stage CAH is diagnosed, the general trend is to assign the newborn as female. If the diagnosis is made too late, for instance in childhood, in simple virilizing forms, male assignment has been maintained with satisfactory results.[96,97]

48.5.1.4 46,XX DSD with Ambiguous Genitalia

The consensus statement on DSD indicated that all 46,XX CAH patients should be assigned female based on available outcome data showing that 95% identify as female.[1] Although there is very little experience on other 46,XX conditions, female assignment seems adequate, including in ovotesticular DSD with predominant ovarian tissue and female internal genitalia. Conversely, when testicular tissue is predominant in 46,XX ovotesticular or testicular DSD, male assignment seems adequate.

48.5.1.5 Chromosomal DSD

Male assignment is undoubted in newborns with Klinefelter syndrome (47,XXY and variants), while female assignment is undisputed in newborns with Turner syndrome (45,X and variants) or with triple X syndrome.

Since chromosomal DSD conditions with ambiguous genitalia result from gonadal dysgenesis, the considerations already made for XX or XY dysgenetic DSD, including ovotesticular DSD, also apply here.

48.5.2 Medical Treatment and Surgical Options

Treatment for CAH is dealt with in detail in Chapter 47. In other forms of DSD, hormone replacement is infrequently needed during the neonatal period. Newborns assigned female are never treated with sex steroids, and those assigned male may require testosterone supplementation in the case of micropenis with hypotrophic corpora cavernosa. The usual protocol includes the application of depot testosterone (testosterone enanthate or cypionate) 25–50 mg IM every 4 weeks for 3 consecutive months.[98]

There has been a decreasing trend in surgical treatment over the last decades. An important influence on the decrease in genital surgery was the growing dissatisfaction expressed by patient support groups with genital surgery judged to have been performed at an unnecessarily early age, without their consent/assent. The concern is based on the perspective that genital surgery during infancy is simply cosmetic. This position is, however, not universally accepted, since it does not take into account the unknown role that external genital anatomy plays in gender identity development. In some settings, allowing a child to grow up with genitalia that do not fit sex assignment may be considered as social experimentation, since there is no evidence on when a person has established a permanent gender or when one is old or mature enough to make a decision of this magnitude. In newborns assigned female, surgery became reserved for those with more severe degrees of clitoris enlargement, and techniques have been refined to preserve innervation. Vaginoplasty is certainly less urgent, and the surgical decision may be delayed, without socially affecting the child or the family. In patients assigned male, the need for the repair of hypospadias and/or penile chordee does not require an urgent decision, as far as urinary infections do not occur. However, delaying it until school age may negatively affect the child owing to the difficulty or impossibility to urinate in a stand-up position like his peers.

In dysgenetic forms of DSD, including complete, partial, asymmetric, and ovotesticular forms, there is a primary hypogonadism. Therefore, hormone replacement therapy will be necessary at pubertal age regardless of the assigned sex. In patients reared as females, estrogen therapy is initially given to induce pubertal changes, and subsequently an estrogen/progestin combined treatment, to mimic menstrual cycles. Low-dose supplementation from early childhood in patients with Turner syndrome remains a controversial issue. Surgical removal of dysgenetic testicular tissue should be considered before pubertal age, especially in patients carrying Y chromosome sequences, to avoid masculinization and malignant transformation.[16] Whenever technically feasible, ovarian tissue should be spared in patients with ovotesticular DSD. In patients assigned male, surgical exploration may be needed to find and descend cryptorchid gonads. Removal may prove necessary when testes are very dysgenetic and cannot be brought down to the scrotum, in order to prevent malignant transformation.[16] Testosterone replacement is performed to induce secondary sex characteristics and pubertal growth. Depot testosterone is typically started 50 mg IM each month for 6 to 12 months, followed by a progressive dose escalation up to a full dose of 250 mg/month in 2 to 3 years.

In XY patients with isolated defects of androgen production due to Leydig cell aplasia or steroidogenic blocks assigned female, estrogen replacement therapy is aimed at the development of secondary sex characteristics and pubertal growth. Because Müllerian ducts regressed in response to AMH in early fetal life, there is no uterus and the vagina is shorter than normal. Menstrual cycles cannot be induced with hormone therapy. When androgen insensitivity is the underlying pathogeny, estrogen therapy is usually not necessary as far as gonads are maintained. In patients with milder forms of defects of androgen production or action reared as males, testosterone replacement may be necessary. The risk of malignant tumor development is low, yet follow-up with ultrasonography is warranted.[65]

In 46,XY boys with PMDS, the main goal of surgical treatment is to place the testes in the scrotum. This may prove difficult, especially when the spermatic cord is too short. If the Müllerian structures limit mobility, proximal salpingectomy and excision of the uterine fundus may be needed, but only after meticulous dissection sparing the vas deferens. The cervix and pedicles of the myometrium usually need to be left in place to preserve vascularization of the male tract.[68] In these boys, Leydig cell function is preserved; therefore, androgen replacement is not necessary.

48.6 LONG-TERM OUTCOMES

Long-term outcome studies available on patients with DSD have limitations owing to difficulties in representative patient sampling and to the quality of the information related to medical, surgical, and psychosocial issues. Furthermore, continual changes in the standards of care hamper the possibility of performing long-term studies to assess the results in adult life of decisions taken in the newborn or the child.

Several factors need to be addressed when assessing outcomes in the quality of life of patients with DSD: genital appearance, endocrine, urinary and sexual function, psychosocial adjustment, and associated disorders like hypertension, cancer, etc. Although the definitions of "good" and "poor" outcomes may be greatly debatable, it seems clear that patients' dissatisfaction is usually associated with the degree of genital ambiguity, whereas the best adjustment is observed in XY patients with complete feminization or XX patients with full virilization.

Genital appearance and urinary and sexual function are usually impaired in patients needing surgical repair of the external and internal genitalia. In patients with DSD raised as males, the impaired ability to respond to exogenous testosterone treatment, e.g., that related to partial androgen insensitivity, predicts a poor outcome: although most report heterosexual orientation, reduced penile length and poor outcomes of surgical procedures result in dissatisfaction with sexual life.[99] Most outcome studies in females were performed in patients with CAH: vaginal stenosis and fistulas, together with dissatisfaction of cosmetic appearance of the external genitalia, are the main complaints.[100] Short stature and associated malformations are responsible for the impairment of quality of life in patients with chromosomal DSD, especially those carrying an X chromosome monosomy (45,X or 45,X/46,XY, as the most frequent).

Overall quality of life has been reported as impaired in most studies including both 46,XX and 46,XY DSD patients. Dissatisfaction is related to nonsexuality, intercourse frequency, avoidance, anorgasmia, and penetration difficulties.[101]

Fertility potential is usually poor in DSD patients but may vary according to the clinical form and sex assignment. In 46, XY DSD with pure gonadal dysgenesis, although the uterus and fallopian tubes are present, spontaneous fertility is not possible due to the lack of oocytes and ovarian steroids. Pregnancy might be achieved after replacement therapy and oocyte donation.[102] In severe defects of androgen synthesis or in CAIS, Müllerian derivatives are absent but uterine transplantation followed by successful pregnancy in a patient with congenital absence of the uterus (Rokitansky syndrome) has opened a promising alternative [103]. In 46,XY patients with ambiguous genitalia raised as males, fertility is disturbed due either to primary spermatogenic defects in patients with partial testicular dysgenesis, or to defective spermatogenesis resulting from partial deficiency in androgen production or action. Furthermore, long-standing cryptorchidism and hypospadias or malformations of the epididymis or vas deferens also affect fertility.[104] Patients with 5α-reductase type 2 deficiency virilize spontaneously at puberty and sperm production occurs due to normal intratesticular testosterone concentration.[105] In patients with mutations in *AMH* or its receptor *AMHR2*, azoospermia is frequent due to the long-standing cryptorchidism or to damage of testicular blood supply during surgical procedures.[68] In patients with **aromatase deficiency** long-term consequences on fertility are unknown,[85] In patients with ovotesticular DSD, the testicular tissue is usually dysgenetic but the ovarian tissue is normal, and pregnancy has been reported, either spontaneously or with assisted reproductive techniques, in a limited number of cases.[106] Like patients with Klinefelter syndrome, those with 46,XX testicular DSD usually have normal testicular function until midpuberty but the existence of two X chromosomes and the absence of a Y chromosome drive to massive germ cell degeneration, small testes, and azoospermia.[41] Patients with sex chromosome aneuploidies and/or mosaicisms usually have dysgenetic gonads and are infertile.

REFERENCES

1. Lee PA, Nordenstrom A, Houk CP, Ahmed SF, Auchus R, Baratz A, et al. Global disorders of sex development update since 2006: perceptions, approach and care. *Horm Res Paediatr* 2016;**85**(3):158–80.

2. Grinspon RP, Rey RA. When hormone defects cannot explain it: malformative disorders of sex development. *Birth Defects Res C Embryo Today* 2014;**102**(4):359–73.

3. Ebert AK, Reutter H, Ludwig M, Rosch WH. The exstrophy-epispadias complex. *Orphanet J Rare Dis* 2009;**4**:23.

4. Warne SA, Hiorns MP, Curry J, Mushtaq I. Understanding cloacal anomalies. *Arch Dis Child* 2011;**96**(11):1072–6.

5. Bothra M, Jain V. Absent phallus: issues in management. *J Pediatr Endocrinol Metab* 2012;**25**(9–10):1013–5.

6. Tirtayasa PM, Prasetyo RB, Rodjani A. Diphallia with associated anomalies: a case report and literature review. *Case Rep Urol* 2013;**2013**. https://doi.org/10.1155/2013/192960.

7. Boisen KA, Chellakooty M, Schmidt IM, Kai CM, Damgaard IN, Suomi AM, et al. Hypospadias in a cohort of 1072 Danish newborn boys: prevalence and relationship to placental weight, anthropometrical measurements at birth, and reproductive hormone levels at three months of age. *J Clin Endocrinol Metabol* 2005;**90**(7):4041–6.

8. Main KM, Skakkebæk NE, Virtanen HE, Toppari J. Genital anomalies in boys and the environment. *Best Pract Res Clin Endocrinol Metab* 2010;**24**(2):279–89.

9. Rey RA, Codner E, Iñíguez G, Bedecarrás P, Trigo R, Okuma C, et al. Low risk of impaired testicular Sertoli and Leydig cell functions in boys with isolated hypospadias. *J Clin Endocrinol Metabol* 2005;**90**(11):6035–40.

10. Woud SG, van Rooij IA, van Gelder MM, Olney RS, Carmichael SL, Roeleveld N, et al. Differences in risk factors for second and third degree hypospadias in the national birth defects prevention study. *Birth Defects Res A Clin Mol Teratol* 2014;**100**(9):703–11.

11. Geller F, Feenstra B, Carstensen L, Pers TH, van Rooij IA, Korberg IB, et al. Genome-wide association analyses identify variants in developmental genes associated with hypospadias. *Nat Genet* 2014;**46**(9):957–63.

12. Rey RA, Grinspon RP. Normal male sexual differentiation and aetiology of disorders of sex development. *Best Pract Res Clin Endocrinol Metab* 2011;**25**:221–38.

13. Bergadá C, Cleveland WW, Jones Jr HW, Wilkins L. Gonadal histology in patients with male pseudohermaphroditism and atypical gonadal dysgenesis: relation to theories of sex differentiation. *Acta Endocrinol* 1962;**40**:493–520.

14. Sohval AR. "Mixed" gonadal dysgenesis: a variety of hermaphroditism. *Am J Hum Genet* 1963;**15**:155–8.

15. Conte FA, Grumbach MM, Kaplan SL. A diphasic pattern of gonadotropin secretion in patients with the syndrome of gonadal dysgenesis. *J Clin Endocrinol Metabol* 1975;**40**(4):670–4.

16. Cools M, Looijenga LH, Wolffenbuttel KP, T'Sjoen G. Managing the risk of germ cell tumourigenesis in disorders of sex development patients. *Endocr Dev* 2014;**27**:185–96.

17. Chemes HE, Venara M, Del Rey G, Arcari AJ, Musse MP, Papazian R, et al. Is a CIS phenotype apparent in children with disorders of sex development? Milder testicular dysgenesis is associated with a higher risk of malignancy. *Andrology* 2015;**3**(1):59–69.

18. Bashamboo A, Eozenou C, Rojo S, McElreavey K. Anomalies in human sex determination provide unique insights into the complex genetic interactions of early gonad development. *Clin Genet* 2017;**91**(2):143–56.

19. Barbaro M, Oscarson M, Schoumans J, Staaf J, Ivarsson SA, Wedell A. Isolated 46,XY gonadal dysgenesis in two sisters caused by a Xp21.2 interstitial duplication containing the DAX1 gene. *J Clin Endocrinol Metabol* 2007;**92**(8):3305–13.

20. Bardoni B, Zanaria E, Guioli S, Floridia G, Worley KC, Tonini G, et al. A dosage sensitive locus at chromosome Xp21 is involved in male to female sex reversal. *Nat Genet* 1994;**7**(4):497–501.

21. Harris A, Siggers P, Corrochano S, Warr N, Sagar D, Grimes DT, et al. ZNRF3 functions in mammalian sex determination by inhibiting canonical WNT signaling. *Proc Natl Acad Sci U S A* 2018;**115**(21):5474–9.

22. Portnoi MF, Dumargne MC, Rojo S, Witchel SF, Duncan AJ, Eozenou C, et al. Mutations involving the SRY-related gene SOX8 are associated with a spectrum of human reproductive anomalies. *Hum Mol Genet* 2018;**27**(7):1228–40.

23. Suntharalingham JP, Buonocore F, Duncan AJ, Achermann JC. DAX-1 (NR0B1) and steroidogenic factor-1 (SF-1, NR5A1) in human disease. *Best Pract Res Clin Endocrinol Metab* 2015;**29**(4):607–19.

24. Niaudet P, Gubler MC. WT1 and glomerular diseases. *Pediatr Nephrol* 2006;**21**(11):1653–60.

25. Bashamboo A, Brauner R, Bignon-Topalovic J, Lortat-Jacob S, Karageorgou V, Lourenco D, et al. Mutations in the FOG2/ZFPM2 gene are associated with anomalies of human testis determination. *Hum Mol Genet* 2014;**23**(14):3657–65.

26. Bagheri-Fam S, Bird AD, Zhao L, Ryan JM, Yong M, Wilhelm D, et al. Testis determination requires a specific FGFR2 isoform to repress FOXL2. *Endocrinology* 2017;**158**(11):3832–43.

27. Lindhardt Johansen M, Hagen CP, Rajpert-De Meyts E, Kjærgaard S, Petersen BL, Skakkebæk NE, et al. 45,X/46,XY mosaicism: phenotypic characteristics, growth, and reproductive function: a retrospective longitudinal study. *J Clin Endocrinol Metabol* 2012;**97**(8):E1540–9.

28. Tosson H, Rose SR, Gartner LA. Description of children with 45,X/46,XY karyotype. *Eur J Pediatr* 2012;**171**(3):521–9.

29. Verkauskas G, Jaubert F, Lortat-Jacob S, Malan V, Thibaud E, Nihoul-Fekete C. The long-term followup of 33 cases of true hermaphroditism: a 40-year experience with conservative gonadal surgery. *J Urol* 2007;**177**(2):726–31 [discussion 31].

30. Wiersma R, Ramdial PK. The gonads of 111 South African patients with ovotesticular disorder of sex differentiation. *J Pediatr Surg* 2009;**44**(3):556–60.

31. Vilain E. The genetics of ovotesticular disorders of sex development. *Adv Exp Med Biol* 2011;**707**:105–6.

32. Grinspon RP, Rey RA. Disorders of sex development with testicular differentiation in SRY-negative 46,XX individuals: clinical and genetic aspects. *Sex Dev* 2016;**10**:1–11.

33. Dauwerse JG, Hansson KB, Brouwers AA, Peters DJ, Breuning MH. An XX male with the sex-determining region Y gene inserted in the long arm of chromosome 16. *Fertil Steril* 2006;**86**(2):463 e1–5.

34. Huang B, Wang SB, Ning Y, Lamb AN, Bartley J. Autosomal XX sex reversal caused by duplication of SOX9. *Am J Med Genet* 1999;**87**(4):349–53.

35. Benko S, Gordon CT, Mallet D, Sreenivasan R, Thauvin-Robinet C, Brendehaug A, et al. Disruption of a long distance regulatory region upstream of SOX9 in isolated disorders of sex development. *J Med Genet* 2011;**48**(12):825–30.

36. Polanco JC, Wilhelm D, Davidson TL, Knight D, Koopman P. Sox10 gain-of-function causes XX sex reversal in mice: implications for human 22q-linked disorders of sex development. *Hum Mol Genet* 2010;**19**(3):506–16.

37. Sutton E, Hughes J, White S, Sekido R, Tan J, Arboleda V, et al. Identification of SOX3 as an XX male sex reversal gene in mice and humans. *J Clin Investig* 2011;**121**(1):328–41.

38. Grinspon RP, Nevado J, Mori Alvarez ML, del Rey G, Castera R, Venara M, et al. 46,XX ovotesticular DSD associated with a SOX3 gene duplication in a *SRY*-negative boy. *Clin Endocrinol (Oxf)* 2016;**85**:669–75.

39. Domenice S, Machado AZ, Ferreira FM, Ferraz-de-Souza B, Lerario AM, Lin L, et al. Wide spectrum of NR5A1-related phenotypes in 46,XY and 46,XX individuals. *Birth Defects Res C Embryo Today* 2016;**108**(4):309–20.

40. Parma P, Radi O, Vidal V, Chaboissier MC, Dellambra E, Valentini S, et al. R-spondin1 is essential in sex determination, skin differentiation and malignancy. *Nat Genet* 2006;**38**(11):1304–9.

41. Vorona E, Zitzmann M, Gromoll J, Schuring AN, Nieschlag E. Clinical, endocrinological, and epigenetic features of the 46,XX male syndrome, compared with 47,XXY Klinefelter patients. *J Clin Endocrinol Metabol* 2007;**92**(9):3458–65.

42. Boucekkine C, Toublanc JE, Abbas N, Chaabouni S, Ouahid S, Semrouni M, et al. Clinical and anatomical spectrum in XX sex reversed patients. Relationship to the presence of Y specific DNA-sequences. *Clin Endocrinol (Oxf)* 1994;**40**(6):733–42.

43. Rey RA, Belville C, Nihoul-Fékété C, Michel-Calemard L, Forest MG, Lahlou N, et al. Evaluation of gonadal function in 107 intersex patients by means of serum antimüllerian hormone measurement. *J Clin Endocrinol Metabol* 1999;**84**(2):627–31.

44. Rey RA. Mini-puberty and true puberty: differences in testicular function. *Ann Endocrinol* 2014;**75**(2):58–63.

45. Huang WJ, Yen PH. Genetics of spermatogenic failure. *Sex Dev* 2008;**2**(4–5):251–9.

46. Aksglæde L, Jorgensen N, Skakkebæk NE, Juul A. Low semen volume in 47 adolescents and adults with 47,XXY Klinefelter or 46,XX male syndrome. *Int J Androl* 2009;**32**(4):376–84.

47. Kousta E, Papathanasiou A, Skordis N. Sex determination and disorders of sex development according to the revised nomenclature and classification in 46,XX individuals. *Hormones (Athens)* 2010;**9**(3):131–218.

48. Groth KA, Skakkebæk NE, Host C, Gravholt CH, Bojesen A. Klinefelter syndrome—a clinical update. *J Clin Endocrinol Metabol* 2013;**98**(1):20–30.

49. Abramsky L, Chapple J. 47,XXY (Klinefelter syndrome) and 47,XYY: estimated rates of and indication for postnatal diagnosis with implications for prenatal counselling. see comments, *Prenat Diagn* 1997;**17**(4):363–8.

50. Rey RA, Gottlieb S, Pasqualini T, Bastida MG, Grinspon RP, Campo SM, et al. Are Klinefelter boys hypogonadal? *Acta Paediatr* 2011;**100**(6):830–8.

51. Nielsen J, Wohlert M. Sex chromosome abnormalities found among 34,910 newborn children: results from a 13-year incidence study in Arhus, Denmark. *Birth Defects Orig Artic Ser* 1990;**26**:209–23.

52. Reynaud K, Cortvrindt R, Verlinde F, De Schepper J, Bourgain C, Smitz J. Number of ovarian follicles in human fetuses with the 45,X karyotype. *Fertil Steril* 2004;**81**(4):1112–9.

53. Hagen CP, Aksglæde L, Sorensen K, Main KM, Boas M, Cleemann L, et al. Serum levels of anti-Mullerian hormone as a marker of ovarian function in 926 healthy females from birth to adulthood and in 172 Turner syndrome patients. *J Clin Endocrinol Metabol* 2010;**95**(11):5003–10.

54. Latronico AC, Arnhold IJ. Inactivating mutations of the human luteinizing hormone receptor in both sexes. *Semin Reprod Med* 2012;**30**(5):382–6.

55. Porter FD. Smith-Lemli-Opitz syndrome: pathogenesis, diagnosis and management. *Eur J Hum Genet* 2008;**16**(5):535–41.

56. Miller WL. Disorders in the initial steps of steroid hormone synthesis. *J Steroid Biochem Mol Biol* 2017;**165**(Pt A):18–37.

57. Auchus RJ, Miller WL. Defects in androgen biosynthesis causing 46,XY disorders of sexual development. *Semin Reprod Med* 2012;**30**(5):417–26.

58. Miller WL. P450 oxidoreductase deficiency: a disorder of steroidogenesis with multiple clinical manifestations. *Sci Signal* 2012;**5**(247):pt11.

59. Mendonça BB, Costa EM, Belgorosky A, Rivarola MA, Domenice S. 46,XY DSD due to impaired androgen production. *Best Pract Res Clin Endocrinol Metab* 2010;**24**(2):243–62.

60. Mendonça BB, Inacio M, Arnhold IJ, Costa EM, Bloise W, Martin RM, et al. Male pseudohermaphroditism due to 17 beta-hydroxysteroid dehydrogenase 3 deficiency. Diagnosis, psychological evaluation, and management. *Medicine (Baltimore)* 2000;**79**(5):299–309.

61. Costa EM, Domenice S, Sircili MH, Inacio M, Mendonça BB. DSD due to 5alpha-reductase 2 deficiency—from diagnosis to long term outcome. *Semin Reprod Med* 2012;**30**(5):427–31.

62. Imperato-McGinley J, Zhu YS. Androgens and male physiology the syndrome of 5alpha-reductase-2 deficiency. *Mol Cell Endocrinol* 2002;**198**(1–2):51–9.

63. Flück CE, Meyer-Boni M, Pandey AV, Kempna P, Miller WL, Schoenle EJ, et al. Why boys will be boys: two pathways of fetal testicular androgen biosynthesis are needed for male sexual differentiation. *Am J Hum Genet* 2011;**89**(2):201–18.

64. Hughes IA, Davies JD, Bunch TI, Pasterski V, Mastroyannopoulou K, MacDougall J. Androgen insensitivity syndrome. *Lancet* 2012;**380**(9851):1419–28.

65. Cools M, Looijenga L. Update on the pathophysiology and risk factors for the development of malignant testicular germ cell tumors in complete androgen insensitivity syndrome. *Sex Dev* 2017;**11**(4):175–81.

66. Bouvattier C, Carel JC, Lecointre C, David A, Sultan C, Bertrand AM, et al. Postnatal changes of T, LH, and FSH in 46,XY infants with mutations in the AR gene. *J Clin Endocrinol Metabol* 2002;**87**(1):29–32.

67. Boehmer ALM, Bruggenwirth H, van Assendelft C, Otten BJ, Verleun-Mooijman MCT, Niermeijer MF, et al. Genotype versus phenotype in families with androgen insensitivity syndrome. *J Clin Endocrinol Metabol* 2001;**86**(9):4151–60.

68. Picard JY, Cate RL, Racine C, Josso N. The persistent Mullerian duct syndrome: an update based upon a personal experience of 157 cases. *Sex Dev* 2017;**11**:109–25.

69. Nicolaides NC, Charmandari E. Chrousos syndrome: from molecular pathogenesis to therapeutic management. *Eur J Clin Invest* 2015;**45**(5):504–14.

70. Marino R, Pérez Garrido N, Costanzo M, Guercio G, Juanes M, Rocco C, et al. Five new cases of 46,XX aromatase deficiency: clinical follow-up from birth to puberty, a novel mutation, and a founder effect. *J Clin Endocrinol Metabol* 2015;**100**(2):E301–7.

71. Bouchoucha N, Samara-Boustani D, Pandey AV, Bony-Trifunovic H, Hofer G, Aigrain Y, et al. Characterization of a novel CYP19A1 (aromatase) R192H mutation causing virilization of a 46,XX newborn, undervirilization of the 46,XY brother, but no virilization of the mother during pregnancies. *Mol Cell Endocrinol* 2014;**390**(1–2):8–17.

72. Hakim C, Padmanabhan V, Vyas AK. Gestational hyperandrogenism in developmental programming. *Endocrinology* 2017;**158**(2):199–212.

73. Alhomaidah D, McGowan R, Ahmed SF. The current state of diagnostic genetics for conditions affecting sex development. *Clin Genet* 2017;**91**(2):157–62.

74. Kuijper EA, Ket JC, Caanen MR, Lambalk CB. Reproductive hormone concentrations in pregnancy and neonates: a systematic review. *Reprod Biomed Online* 2013;**27**(1):33–63.

75. Lee PA, Houk CP, Ahmed SF, Hughes IA. In collaboration with the participants in the international consensus conference on intersex organized by the Lawson Wilkins pediatric Endocrine Society and the European Society for paediatric endocrinology. Consensus statement on management of intersex disorders. *Pediatrics* 2006;**118**(2):e488–500.

76. Arcari AJ, Bergadá I, Rey RA, Gottlieb S. Predictive value of anatomical findings and karyotype analysis in the diagnosis of patients with disorders of sexual development. *Sex Dev* 2007;**1**(4):222–9.

77. Thankamony A, Lek N, Carroll D, Williams M, Dunger DB, Acerini CL, et al. Anogenital distance and penile length in infants with hypospadias or cryptorchidism: comparison with normative data. *Environ Health Perspect* 2014;**122**(2):207–11.

78. Prader A. Genital findings in the female pseudo-hermaphroditism of the congenital adrenogenital syndrome; morphology, frequency, development and heredity of the different genital forms. *Helv Paediatr Acta* 1954;**9**(3):231–48.

79. Quigley CA, De Bellis A, Marschke KB, El-Awady MK, Wilson EM, French FS. Androgen receptor defects: historical, clinical, and molecular perspectives. published erratum appears in Endocr Rev 1995 Aug;16(4):546, *Endocr Rev* 1995;**16**(3):271–321.

80. Ahmed SF, Achermann JC, Arlt W, Balen A, Conway G, Edwards Z, et al. Society for endocrinology UK guidance on the initial evaluation of an infant or an adolescent with a suspected disorder of sex development (revised 2015). *Clin Endocrinol (Oxf)* 2016;**84**(5):771–88.

81. Bergadá I, Milani C, Bedecarrás P, Andreone L, Ropelato MG, Gottlieb S, et al. Time course of the serum gonadotropin surge, inhibins, and anti-Mullerian hormone in normal newborn males during the first month of life. *J Clin Endocrinol Metabol* 2006;**91**(10):4092–8.

82. Dhayat NA, Frey AC, Frey BM, d'Uscio CH, Vogt B, Rousson V, et al. Estimation of reference curves for the urinary steroid metabolome in the first year of life in healthy children: tracing the complexity of human postnatal steroidogenesis. *J Steroid Biochem Mol Biol* 2015;**154**:226–36.

83. Feyaerts A, Forest MG, Morel Y, Mure PY, Morel J, Mallet D, et al. Endocrine screening in 32 consecutive patients with hypospadias. *J Urol* 2002;**168**(2):720–5.

84. Forest MG. Age-related response of plasma testosterone, delta 4-androstenedione, and cortisol to adrenocorticotropin in infants, children, and adults. *J Clin Endocrinol Metabol* 1978;**47**(5):931–7.

85. Belgorosky A, Guercio G, Pepe C, Saraco N, Rivarola MA. Genetic and clinical spectrum of aromatase deficiency in infancy, childhood and adolescence. *Horm Res* 2009;**72**(6):321–30.

86. Croft B, Ohnesorg T, Sinclair AH. The role of copy number variants in disorders of sex development. *Sex Dev* 2018;**12**(1–3):19–29.

87. Barseghyan H, Delot EC, Vilain E. New technologies to uncover the molecular basis of disorders of sex development. *Mol Cell Endocrinol* 2018;**468**:60–9.

88. White S, Ohnesorg T, Notini A, Roeszler K, Hewitt J, Daggag H, et al. Copy number variation in patients with disorders of sex development due to 46, XY gonadal dysgenesis. *PLoS One* 2011;**6**(3).

89. Cools M, Nordenström A, Robeva R, Hall J, Westerveld P, Flück C, et al. Caring for individuals with a difference of sex development (DSD): a consensus statement. *Nat Rev Endocrinol* 2018;**14**(7):415–29.

90. Wiesemann C, Ude-Koeller S, Sinnecker GH, Thyen U. Ethical principles and recommendations for the medical management of differences of sex development (DSD)/intersex in children and adolescents. *Eur J Pediatr* 2010;**169**(6):671–9.

91. Kolesinska Z, Ahmed SF, Niedziela M, Bryce J, Molinska-Glura M, Rodie M, et al. Changes over time in sex assignment for disorders of sex development. *Pediatrics* 2014;**134**(3):e710–5.

92. Diamond DA, Burns JP, Huang L, Rosoklija I, Retik AB. Gender assignment for newborns with 46XY cloacal exstrophy: a 6-year followup survey of pediatric urologists. *J Urol* 2011;**186**(4 Suppl):1642–8.

93. Wisniewski AB, Mazur T. 46,XY DSD with female or ambiguous external genitalia at birth due to androgen insensitivity syndrome, 5alpha-reductase-2 deficiency, or 17beta-hydroxysteroid dehydrogenase deficiency: a review of quality of life outcomes. *Int J Pediatr Endocrinol* 2009;**2009**.

94. Schutzmann K, Brinkmann L, Schacht M, Richter-Appelt H. Psychological distress, self-harming behavior, and suicidal tendencies in adults with disorders of sex development. *Arch Sex Behav* 2009;**38**(1):16–33.

95. Schober J, Nordenstrom A, Hoebeke P, Lee P, Houk C, Looijenga L, et al. Disorders of sex development: summaries of long-term outcome studies. *J Pediatr Urol* 2012;**8**(6):616–23.

96. Lee PA, Houk CP, Husmann DA. Should male gender assignment be considered in the markedly virilized patient with 46,XX and congenital adrenal hyperplasia? *J Urol* 2010;**184**(4 Suppl):1786–92.

97. Apostolos RAC, Cangucu-Campinho AK, Lago R, Costa ACS, Oliveira LMB, Toralles MB, et al. Gender identity and sexual function in 46,XX patients with congenital adrenal hyperplasia raised as males. *Arch Sex Behav* 2018;**47**(8):2491–6.

98. Bin-Abbas B, Conte F, Grumbach M, Kaplan S. Congenital hypogonadotropic hypogonadism and micropenis: effect of testosterone treatment on adult penile size—why sex reversal is not indicated. *J Pediatr* 1999;**134**(5):579–83.

99. Bouvattier C, Mignot B, Lefevre H, Morel Y, Bougnères P. Impaired sexual activity in male adults with partial androgen insensitivity. *J Clin Endocrinol Metabol* 2006;**91**(9):3310–5.

100. Lee P, Schober J, Nordenstrom A, Hoebeke P, Houk C, Looijenga L, et al. Review of recent outcome data of disorders of sex development (DSD): emphasis on surgical and sexual outcomes. *J Pediatr Urol* 2012;**8**(6):611–5.

101. Callens N, van der Zwan YG, Drop SL, Cools M, Beerendonk CM, Wolffenbuttel KP, et al. Do surgical interventions influence psychosexual and cosmetic outcomes in women with disorders of sex development? *ISRN Endocrinol* 2012;**2012**. https://doi.org/10.5402/2012/276742.

102. Creatsas G, Deligeoroglou E, Tsimaris P, Pantos K, Kreatsa M. Successful pregnancy in a Swyer syndrome patient with preexisting hypertension. *Fertil Steril* 2011;**96**(2):e83–5.

103. Brännström M, Johannesson L, Bokström H, Kvarnström N, Molne J, Dahm-Kähler P, et al. Livebirth after uterus transplantation. *Lancet* 2015;**385** (9968):607–16.

104. Guercio G, Costanzo M, Grinspon RP, Rey RA. Fertility issues in disorders of sex development. *Endocrinol Metab Clin North Am* 2015;**44** (4):867–81.

105. Nordenskjold A, Ivarsson SA. Molecular characterization of 5 alpha-reductase type 2 deficiency and fertility in a Swedish family. *J Clin Endocrinol Metab* 1998;**83**(9):3236–8.

106. Schultz BA, Roberts S, Rodgers A, Ataya K. Pregnancy in true hermaphrodites and all male offspring to date. *Obstet Gynecol* 2009;**113**(2): 534–6 Pt 2.

Chapter 49

Pathophysiological Roles and Disorders of Renin-Angiotensin-Aldosterone System and Nitric Oxide During Perinatal Periods

Qinqin Gao, Xiang Li, Xiuwen Zhou, Bailin Liu, Jiaqi Tang, Na Li, Mengshu Zhang, Xiyuan Lu, Zhice Xu and Miao Sun

Institute for Fetology, First Hospital of Soochow University, Suzhou, China

Common Clinical Problems

- Preeclampsia and gestational diabetes can result from altered renin-angiotensin-aldosterone system (RAAS) and nitric oxide (NO).
- Disorders of RAAS and NO can also contribute to preterm birth, intrauterine growth restriction, and early embryo loss.
- Neonatal diseases related to RAAS and NO include kidney disease, pulmonary hypertension, and primary hyper- and hypo-aldosteronism.

49.1 RENIN-ANGIOTENSIN-ALDOSTERONE SYSTEM

In humans, the renin-angiotensin-aldosterone system (RAAS) undergoes major changes in response to pregnancy, and plays a key role in regulating blood pressure, salt balance, and subsequent well-being of the mother and fetus. During normal pregnancy, in addition to the classical circulating RAAS, components of the RAAS are synthesized in the placenta and fetal organs, including the kidney, heart, vascular system, and brain.[1] Local RAAS in those fetal organs can function independently or in concert with the circulating RAAS and participates in the regulation of various aspects of fetal development as pregnancy progresses. In human pregnancy, the maternal and fetal RAAS, and local RAAS in various tissues, interact to ensure a satisfactory pregnancy outcome. In the past 4 decades, there has been accelerated progress in understanding of the physiological functions and pathological changes of RAAS during pregnancy and fetal development.

49.1.1 Dysfunction of RAAS in Fetus and Neonate

In adults, RAAS plays important roles in the physiological control of cardiovascular systems and body fluid homeostasis, as well as the pathogenesis of various cardiovascular, metabolic, and renal diseases. During normal pregnancy, the circulating or/and local RAAS in placenta, fetal brain, cardiovascular, and renal systems, play important roles in the development of fetus and neonate.[1,2] On the other hand, abnormal RAAS in the fetus and neonate can be involved in the developmental programming of various chronic diseases in later life.[1,3] For example, higher levels of plasma angiotensin II (Ang II) in low-birth-weight infants appear to be related to the development of chronic lung diseases.[3] As the theory that adult diseases have origins in fetal life has developed and become accepted, the abnormal RAAS patterns in fetuses and neonates have attracted considerable attention.

49.1.1.1 Abnormal RAAS in the Placenta

During normal pregnancy, RAAS plays a vitally important role in water and salt balance and subsequent well-being of mothers and fetuses. This includes not only the classical RAAS in the mother and fetus, but also the local RAAS in the placenta, which is the major extrarenal RAAS during pregnancy. In the placental unit, expression of local RAAS components varies between species, probably due to marked species differences in placental architecture. As early as 1967, Hodari et al. described a placental RAAS and identified a renin-like substance in human placental tissue.[4] Since then, almost all of RAAS components have been identified in the placenta, and an intrinsic RAAS has been well documented in human placenta based on the presence of its major units.[1,2] During normal pregnancy, the placental RAAS is activated, with an increase in levels of angiotensinogen (AGT), renin, angiotensin converting enzymes (ACE), which can ultimately lead to a local increase of Ang II.[2] Ang II is the main effector of the RAAS. Ang II and its receptors are present throughout the human placental unit, indicating the presence of a functional local RAAS. As Ang II is well known to be a potent vasoconstrictor peptide, the placental RAAS is, therefore, important in controlling the placental vascular functions and blood circulation.[2] Ang II also can modulate the production of other vasoactive substances and hormones from the placental bed,[2] such as prostacyclin and estradiol,[5] demonstrating that placental RAAS plays a crucial role in controlling the maternal-fetal circulation and placental secretory functions. Therefore, disturbances of the placental RAAS may lead to a dysfunctional placenta.

The placental RAAS can be subjected to a number of conditions or environmental insults during pregnancy.[6–8] Chronic caffeine exposure during the gestational period can enhance the expression of the placental Ang II receptor 2 (AT2R).[6] Exposure to relatively low concentrations of the pollutant PM2.5 can alter some characteristics of the placenta, affect the expression of placental RAAS units, and compromise the maternal-fetal interaction, all of which in turn can impair fetal nutrition and growth.[7] Maternal protein restriction reduces the expression of angiotensin converting enzyme 2 (ACE2) in the placenta during late pregnancy.[8] The placental RAAS is also sensitive to maternal hypoxic stress and placental insufficiency.[9] In addition, many pregnancy complications are accompanied with a locally abnormal placental RAAS.[2] Pregnant hypertensive disorder (especially preeclampsia) is an example, with abnormal placental RAAS considered to be a major cause of preeclampsia.[2] In brief, quite a few prenatal insults or stresses can result in changes in placental RAAS; in turn, these changes can ultimately lead to dysfunctional placentas and pregnancy complications.

49.1.1.1.1   Placental Abnormal Secretion

As an organ with endocrine functions, the placenta plays a central role in the regulation of physiological alterations in pregnancy, and is a special bridge for communication between the mother and fetus. This action is also related to its ability to synthesize and release a number of signaling substances, including hormones, growth factors, and cytokines during the progression of pregnancy. The local placental RAAS play a physiological role in the regulation of placental endocrine and paracrine activities.[10–12] For example, Ang II stimulates placental prostaglandin production, and decreases thromboxane release in the isolated perfused human placental cotyledon.[5,10] Ang II also can stimulate placental prostacyclin and prostaglandin E2 production in pregnant ewes.[13] In human placental cells, Ang II can modulate the release of immunoreactive corticotropin-releasing factors from cultured placental cells.[13] Ang II stimulates the release of lactogen in human trophoblastic cells, and an increased Ca^{2+} influx is one of the mechanisms that control Ang II-mediated release of placental lactogen.[11] Ang II also can induce the secretion of pregnancy-specific beta 1-glycoprotein secretion and estradiol from human placenta via the AT1 receptors (AT1R).[12] Thus the contribution of the placental local RAAS to regulating placental endocrine secretions during pregnancy is significant, and alterations in the RAAS can result in dysfunctional placental secretory functions.

On the other hand, abnormal secretion of some placental hormones can in turn affect the local RAAS.[14,15] For example, progesterone can downregulate AT1R expression in isolated trophoblast cells from full-term human placenta.[14] The placental AT2R protein is downregulated during pregnancy, most likely mediated by the sex steroids.[14,15] These facts have led to an interesting hypothesis that the placental RAAS controls major placental secretory activities and endocrine functions, and disturbances in those activities and functions may lead to dysfunctional placenta and related diseases.

Preeclampsia is one such disease. It is the most common medical syndrome of human pregnancy, characterized by hypertension, proteinuria, and placental functional abnormalities associated with placental ischemia. Extensive studies have been done to assess placental RAAS in normal and preeclamptic pregnancies, with the finding that several RAAS components in preeclamptic placenta are changed, including Ang II, AGT, and AT1R, as well as ACE activity, although not all studies have been consistent. In general, Ang II, ACE, and AT1R concentrations in the preeclamptic placenta are found to be significantly increased compared to the normal, whereas angiotensin I (Ang I) and angiotensin 1–7 (Ang 1–7) concentrations are unchanged.[2] In addition, the expression of corticotropin-releasing hormone (CRH) receptor type-1 alpha in the preeclamptic placentas is reduced.[16] Meanwhile, regulation of the placental nitric oxide-cyclic guanosine monophosphate pathway by CRH and CRH-related peptides is impaired in preeclampsia.[17] Such evidence suggests that abnormal placental endocrine function, including within the local RAAS, plays an important role in the development of preeclampsia.

49.1.1.1.2 Placental Vascular Dysfunction

A successful outcome of pregnancy is dependent on adequate blood flow across the placental circulation. The placenta is rich in blood vessels, and placental vascular tone is essential for maintaining adequate blood flow and perfusion. Because placental vessels lack automatic innervation, local vasoconstrictors and vasodilators (including prostanoids, endothelins, serotonin, catecholamines, histamine, RAAS, nitric oxide, and others) are important for controlling placental vasoactivities and blood flow. As an organ with endocrine functions, the placenta can produce numerous vasoactivators that are released into the circulation, dominating the regulation of placental vascular reactivity and blood flow. The balance between vasodilators and vasoconstrictors in the placental unit is crucial for the placental circulation. As mentioned previously, Ang II is not only a potent vasoconstrictor peptide, but it also stimulates the release of various vascular factors, such as prostaglandins and prostaglandin E2. In addition, recent progress has been made in demonstrating that placental vessels behave very differently from nonplacental vessels. Placental vascular trees show higher sensitivity to constriction induced by Ang II, suggesting that the placenta relies heavily on RAAS activity to maintain its vessel tone and local circulation.[2] This evidence suggests that placental RAAS, in particular Ang II, should play a crucial role in controlling vascular tone and blood flow in a normal "maternal-placental" circulation. Therefore, compromised and abnormal Ang II in the placenta must influence vascular resistance and placental perfusion, which could result in placental ischemia, and may ultimately lead to abnormalities, such as the development of preeclampsia.

Many varied studies have yielded variable results regarding physiologic and pharmacologic effects of hormones or drugs on placental blood vessels. The major reason for the inconsistencies is likely a sample size that is too small and large variations in the individual responses of human subjects. These issues were addressed recently by using larger sample sizes ($n > 50$ or even 100) in studies of human placental vessels, as well as by using a relatively pure species of animal placenta.[2] Such new methodological approaches have enabled researchers to confirm that human and sheep placental blood vessels, whether of large or small diameter, respond to Ang II stimulation very differently from most nonplacental vessels.[2] In the aorta, mesentery arteries, femoral arteries, umbilical arteries, and vein, catecholamines play a dominant role in the control of nonplacental vascular tone, such that phenylephrine- or norepinephrine-induced vascular constrictions are much greater than those induced by Ang II. However, no matter large or small placental vessels, phenylephrine- or norepinephrine-induced vasocontractions are weaker than those by Ang II, demonstrating that Ang II is critical in placental vascular systems for controlling vessel tone, and not catecholamines. These new findings also demonstrate that placental endocrine physiology in vascular systems is different from that in nonplacental vessels. Changes in Ang II-dominated placental vascular functions can lead to abnormal placental perfusion, in utero ischemia, and hypoxia, all of which will influence fetal growth. These new findings also help explain why maternal Ang II or RAAS components in the circulation are increased in certain cases of preeclampsia.

49.1.1.2 Abnormal RAAS in Fetus and Neonate

Currently, RAAS has been studied extensively in adults, but to a much lesser degree in fetus and neonate. In human embryos, all components of the RAAS are expressed, as early as 30–35 days of gestation. During normal pregnancy, RAAS not only plays an important role in maintaining fetal blood pressure and fluid-electrolyte homeostasis, but it also involves in normal growth, differentiation, and developmental processes in the fetus and neonate.[1] For example, ACE2 deficiency causes fetal growth restriction, leading to small babies in ACE2 knockout mice,[18] suggesting the importance of normal expression and construction of prenatal RAAS in fetal developmental processes. In pregnancy, in addition to the maternal and placental RAAS, local RAAS also exists in many fetal organs and tissue, including the kidney, cardiovascular system, and brain. Abnormal changes in fetal local RAAS can disrupt organ development during prenatal and postnatal periods.

49.1.1.2.1 Abnormal RAAS in the Kidney

In humans, kidney development or nephrogenesis is completed before birth.[19,20] During the early developmental period, the placenta is primarily responsible for maintaining the fetal fluid-electrolyte homeostasis and the excretory requirements for the fetus. The fetal kidneys are largely involved in regulating fetal blood pressure and maintaining amniotic fluid levels.[21] After the fetus reaches the 34th–36th week of gestational age, nephrogenesis is completed; however, the maturation of the kidney continues through the neonate period.[21] Following birth, renal function in the neonate undergoes significant changes over the course of days to weeks.[21]

Clinical and experimental evidence has shown that the RAAS in the developing kidney undergoes major changes in response to pregnancy.[20] All components of RAAS are highly expressed as early as 4 weeks of gestation in the human embryonic kidney.[20] Renin secretion is considered the rate limiting step in the cascade of events that eventually leads to the formation of biologically active Ang II and aldosterone. Renin is strongly expressed in prenatal and neonatal kidneys, and accordingly, there are elevated plasma levels of renin and Ang II. Moreover, physiological analysis has shown that all the components of the RAAS (renin, AGT, ACE, AT1R, and AT2R) in the kidney can be detected from embryonic day (E) 12 to 17 days of gestation in rats, being higher in fetal and newborn rats than in adult rats.[21] All components of RAAS are synthesized locally in the developing kidney in a pattern, suggesting an important role for the intrarenal RAAS in renal development.

These roles of RAAS in renal development have been investigated in humans and animals (including rodents, pig, and sheep).[22–24] In humans, nephrogenesis is completed before gestational week 36, whereas in rodents, nephrogenesis is not completed roughly until 10 days after birth.[21] Thus rats and mice are born with very immature kidneys, and the first two postnatal weeks correspond approximately to mid- and third-trimester in humans. This difference provides a convenient animal model for studying mechanisms underlying the RAAS-mediated renal development in human fetuses and neonates. ACE and AT1R blockers are widely used in the treatment of hypertension, proteinuric disease, and heart failure. However, administration of any of these compounds during pregnancy places the fetal or neonatal animals at risk for abnormalities in renal morphology and functions, suggesting that the developing embryo and fetus require an intact and healthy RAAS for normal renal development[25–27] (Table 49.1).

For example, pharmacological interruption of AT1R signaling in neonatal rats, which have ongoing nephrogenesis, causes decreased pup body weight, increased death rate, specific renal abnormalities including papillary atrophy and tubular atrophy with expansion of the interstitium, and a marked impairment in urinary concentrating ability.[23] The neonatal rat kidney vasculature is also affected by AT1R inhibitors, resulting in fewer, shorter, and thicker afferent renal arteries.[27] Similar lesions have been observed following maternal use of ACE inhibitors during pregnancy. In addition, these pathological changes in the kidney were only observed with the use of ACE or AT1R inhibitors in rats, while kidneys from AT2R antagonist-treated rats and AT2R-deficient mice were histologically normal.[26] These findings indicate that the renal lesions observed after pharmacological interventions could not be attributed to nonspecific drug effects, and confirm that an intact RAAS is a prerequisite for normal renal development.

Interestingly, pigs treated with ACE inhibition from 2 to 24 days, an age-interval corresponding to a period of active nephrogenesis, display renal changes that are almost identical to those found in rats.[24] In late gestation, blockade of RAAS in fetal sheep causes acute fetal renal failure and oligohydramnios. Accumulated evidence demonstrates that an intact RAAS is required for normal renal development in rats, pigs, and sheep. In humans, clinical studies have revealed renal lesions observed in a fetus exposed to AT1R antagonists throughout pregnancy.[22,25] In pregnant women with essential hypertension treated with Cozaar (AT1R antagonist losartan 50 mg), autopsy examination of their fetuses revealed severe renal lesions, including tubular dysgenesis associated with poorly developed vasa recta.[22] Human fetuses exposed to ACE inhibitors are severely hypotensive at birth, and some of them develop irreversible renal lesions responsible for renal failure and anuria.[25] This damage is similar to that observed in the fetuses and neonates of animal models undergoing experimental blockade of the RAAS, indicating a pivotal role of the RAAS in human fetal kidney development.

Although exposure of the fetus to RAAS inhibitors is potentially harmful throughout pregnancy, the effects are greater in late gestation as compared with early stages.[35] Circulating and local RAAS, especially placental RAAS, as well as the timing of renal development, contribute to the different effects of RAAS inhibitors. Recently, many studies, particularly

TABLE 49.1 Renal lesions by RAAS inhibitors or deletion in fetus and neonate

RAAS blocker or knockout	Renal lesions in fetus and neonate
AT1R or ACE blockers	Abnormal renal morphology (e.g., papillary atrophy, tubular atrophy, and disorganization of the medulla)[22,28] Abnormal renal function (e.g., impaired urinary concentrating ability, renal failure and anuria)[23,29] A fewer, shorter, and thicker renal arteries[27]
AT2R blocker	Histologically normal renal[26,30]
Renin knockout	Hydronephrosis, thickening of renal arterial walls, and fibrosis in the kidney[31]
AT1R knockout	Abnormal renal morphology (e.g., delayed maturity in glomerular growth, hypoplastic papilla, and renal arterial hypertrophy)[32]
AGT knockout	Abnormal renal morphology (e.g., delayed maturity in glomerular growth, hypoplastic papilla)[32,33]
ACE knockout	Tubular obstruction, dilatation, and atrophy; grossly distorted renal arteries[34]

those using various transgenic approaches to manipulate intrarenal levels of RAAS components, have determined the roles of intrarenal RAAS in normal renal development (Table 49.1). Pharmacologic inhibition with RAAS inhibitors results in abnormalities in vasculature and nephrogenesis, leading to reduced nephron number and disorganization of the medulla.[22] Similarly, disruption of any of the RAAS component genes results in renal tubular dysgenesis, with reduced number and shortening of renal tubules as well as architectural disorganization.[31,32,34] For example, although AGT is not essential for renal organogenesis, the renal phenotype of AGT knockout mice is similar to that of human fetuses exposed to RAAS inhibitors in utero.[33] Similar lesions develop in mice with targeted deletion of renin, ACE, or AT1R.[31,32,34] Taken together, an intact RAAS is a prerequisite for normal renal development. During development, deficiencies in the activity of developing renal RAAS play a role in determining fetal growth, renal development, and function. Understanding the complex interactions of the RAAS in the perinatal period is essential in the use of RAAS inhibitors in women during childbearing years and in neonates regarding cardiovascular or renal diseases.

The mid- to late gestational period is critical for functional development of organs, including the kidneys, and is an important window for health and diseases of fetal origin. It is well known that the intrauterine environment is critical for fetal development and furthermore for risk of diseases that onset in adulthood. Nearly 3 decades ago, David Barker and colleagues first noted that adverse intrauterine environments during pregnancy are closely associated with an increased risk of abnormal organ development of fetuses and neonates, as well as diseases in adulthood.[1] The stress of intrauterine environments can lead to a number of physiological and pathological changes in both fetuses and neonates, some of which can be linked to alterations in local RAAS in utero.

The most common consequence of perinatal insults, in relation to the kidneys, is a reduction in nephron endowment. In humans, nephrogenesis, the process of nephron formation, is completed during the third trimester, thus emphasizing the importance of the intrauterine environment. Numerous animal studies have demonstrated the risk effects of intrauterine perturbation (including maternal malnutrition, high-salt diets, and glucocorticoid exposure) on the development of fetal renal RAAS and the kidney, as well as the offspring (Fig. 49.1).

Maternal Malnutrition Maternal malnutrition restricts the nutrient supply to the growing fetus, usually leading to a low birth weight.[36,37] The effects of prenatal malnutrition on the development of intrauterine growth restriction (IUGR)-associated adult diseases were first observed using the Dutch famine model.[36] Gestation is a period of a rapid increase in nephron number, which is critical in determining nephron endowment at birth. Fetal undernutrition may lead to lower nephron endowment, an assertion supported by animal experiments. Fetuses exposed to a low protein diet in utero have proportionally lower body weight and smaller kidneys with reduced nephron numbers at birth.[37–39]

Renal development can be affected by maternal undernutrition, and this is associated with altered regulation of RAAS in the developing kidney. In response to the mother receiving a low-protein diet during pregnancy, newborn pups have low birth weight and a reduced kidney/body weight ratio, while the number of glomeruli per kidney are fewer.[37] RAAS is perturbed in the offspring of maternally malnourished rats and sheep.[37] In newborn pups of mothers on low-protein diets, renal renin and Ang II levels are reduced at birth[37]; after weaning, renin, Ang II, and aldosterone concentrations could be restored to the control levels. Maternal protein restriction can also alter AT1R and AT2R expression in the fetal and neonatal kidney in rats.[38] Renal AT1R expression in low protein fetal rats tended to increase from gestational day 18 to postnatal day 10, while AT2R expression declined until postnatal day 10.[38] During the perinatal period, Ang II, acting via its receptors, plays an important role in renal development.[38] Specifically, Ang II binding to AT1R is critical for adequate proliferation of the

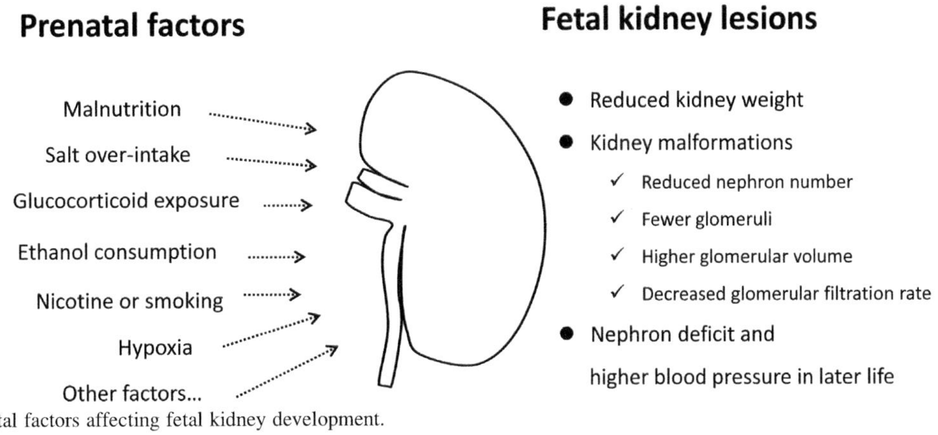

Prenatal factors

Malnutrition

Salt over-intake

Glucocorticoid exposure

Ethanol consumption

Nicotine or smoking

Hypoxia

Other factors...

Fetal kidney lesions

- Reduced kidney weight
- Kidney malformations
  - ✓ Reduced nephron number
  - ✓ Fewer glomeruli
  - ✓ Higher glomerular volume
  - ✓ Decreased glomerular filtration rate
- Nephron deficit and

  higher blood pressure in later life

FIG. 49.1 Prenatal factors affecting fetal kidney development.

renal tubules and branching morphogenesis, while Ang II binding to AT2R controls both the cessation of proliferation and induction of apoptosis in the kidney.[38]

Taken together, the intrarenal RAAS is suppressed at birth in rats born of mothers on a low protein diet, but then RAAS becomes overactive at weaning, associated with a reduced number of glomeruli and glomerular enlargement. The importance of the RAAS in renal development has been demonstrated when the RAAS is interrupted by inadvertent use of ACE inhibitors in humans, or by creating "knockouts" of RAAS genes in mice.

Maternal High-Salt Diets In modern times, salt intake in humans can be excessive. Maternal high salt intake influences organ development such as the fetal kidneys.[40] In rodents, the pups exposed to maternal high-salt diets in utero present lower body weight and disturbances in renal development at birth.[40,41] Prenatally sodium overloaded pups show an increase in 24-h urinary protein and renal oxidative stress, and a reduced glomerular filtration rate. These alterations are associated with reduced plasma levels of Ang II and changes in renal AT1R.[41] Thirty-day-old pups whose mothers received high salt intake during pregnancy show a decrease in glomerular filtration rate compared with the control pups of the same age, and have reduced numbers of Ang II-positive cells in glomeruli and decreased AT1R expression in the renal cortex.[40]

The influence of high-salt diets during pregnancy on renal function and RAAS has also been determined. In ovine fetuses whose mothers were fed high-salt diets for 2 months during mid- to late gestation,[42,43] renal excretion of sodium and urea nitrogen was increased, while urine volume and kidney weight/body weight ratio were decreased. The altered indexes also were observed in the offspring aged 15 and 90 days. Fetal plasma Ang II was decreased, meanwhile, the key elements of fetal renal RAAS were also altered following maternal high salt intake. Expression levels of renal AGT, AT1R, AT2R, ACE, and ACE/ACE2 ratio were significantly increased, while ACE2 expression was decreased in the high-salt diet fetuses.[43] Maternal dietary salt intake during pregnancy affecting fetal renal development is closely associated with altered levels of the key renal elements of RAAS; some of these alterations that develop in the fetus remain after birth as possible risks in developing renal or cardiovascular diseases.

Maternal Glucocorticoid Exposure Glucocorticoids accelerate maturation of organs, especially the lungs, which underpins their widespread use in obstetric and neonatal practice for preterm delivery. However, glucocorticoid administration during pregnancy can exert adverse effects upon organ development,[44] including altered renal development in utero in primate models.[44,45]

Most studies of glucocorticoids have been undertaken using synthetic glucocorticoids dexamethasone and betamethasone, which readily transport across the placental barrier. In rat models, fetuses exposed to glucocorticoid typically show a nephron deficit and higher blood pressure in later life.[45] Pregnant ewes treated with dexamethasone at gestational days 26–28 have been shown to have reduced numbers of nephrons,[44,46] and this is attributable to changes in the renal RAAS.[47] Prenatal exposure to a clinically relevant dose of glucocorticoid during active nephrogenesis has a significant effect on both local and systemic RAAS in the fetus.[46] Administration of betamethasone at gestational days 80–81 resulted in a decrease in plasma renin and renal prorenin concentrations in fetal sheep. Subsequently, 135-day ovine fetuses show an increase in renal renin expression.[47]

These findings suggest that prenatal glucocorticoid has an immediate effect on expression and secretion of renin in the kidney. The downregulation of renin at 80 days of gestation may affect nephron development.[47] When pregnant ewes were treated with dexamethasone in early gestation, the mRNA levels for AGT, AT1R, and AT2R were increased in the fetal kidneys during late gestation.[46] These results provide evidence that using glucocorticoids during pregnancy can alter the renal RAAS in the fetus. The altered expression of RAAS in the developing kidney contributes to a nephron deficit.

Other Factors Many prenatal factors, including ethanol exposure, nicotine exposure, and hypoxia, have also been reported to affect fetal renal development.[48–50] Ethanol consumption remains common during pregnancy; excessive ethanol intake can result in fetal alcohol spectrum disorder. A number of studies involving animals and clinical human reports indicate a close association between prenatal ethanol exposure and fetal renal malformations.[48] If pregnant ewes receive daily intravenous infusions of ethanol from 95 to 133 days of gestational age, fetal glomerular number is reduced.[23] Whether prenatal ethanol exposure affects kidney development in utero via altering RAAS needs further investigation.

Maternal cigarette smoking with fetal nicotine exposure is another common prenatal insult that causes fetal growth restriction in humans and experimental animals.[51] The administration of nicotine in pregnant rats influences the fetal expression of renal Ang II receptors at mRNA and protein levels, as well as kidney weight in 14-day-old pups. Although renal AT1R levels are not significantly changed, the AT1R/AT2R ratio is significantly increased in these 2-week-old newborns, associated with a significant decrease of kidney weight,[51] suggesting that maternal nicotine exposure during pregnancy results in a kidney deficit with altered renal RAAS.

Hypoxia is one of the most important and clinically relevant stresses that can affect fetal development.[49] Hypoxia can be induced by many physiological and pathological factors, including placental insufficiency, umbilical cord around the neck, environmental exposure to toxic chemicals, high altitude, and preeclampsia. In rat models, prenatal hypoxia significantly decreases kidney weight in 21-day fetuses and 7-day neonates. Ovine fetuses exposed to long-term high-altitude hypoxia show a significant decrease in the kidney/body weight ratio, indicating impairment in fetal renal development. Chronic hypoxia also causes a significant increase in AT1R and a decrease in AT2R protein abundance, resulting in a large increase in the AT1R/AT2R ratio in the fetal kidneys.[49]

In addition, environmental chemical exposure also affects kidney development.[50,52] For example, perinatal exposure to di-(2-ethylhexyl) phthalate results in a reduced number of nephrons, higher glomerular volume, and a decrease of renin and Ang II levels in fetal kidney at birth.[52] Prenatal exposure to lipopolysaccharide significantly reduces glomerular numbers and decreases renal cortex renin mRNA expression and the number of Ang II-positive cells in the offspring at 1 day of age.[50]

All these findings suggest that adverse intrauterine environments during pregnancy can affect the kidney development through damaging renal RAAS.

49.1.1.2.2 Altered RAAS in the Cardiovascular System

RAAS in healthy fetuses is critically important for fetal cardiovascular functions, organ development, and maintenance of fetal arterial pressure.[53] Almost all components of RAAS, including renin, ACE, AT1R, and AT2R, have been found in the developing heart and vasculature. Local RAAS is critically important for control of the heart and vasculature during the prenatal period, and for the pathogenesis of cardiovascular diseases.[1,53] However, there has been limited information regarding whether local RAAS is linked to malformations of the cardiovascular system during fetal development. The fact that RAAS regulates several key cellular events, such as proliferation and apoptosis, strongly suggests that RAAS play an important role in cardiovascular development.

During development of the heart, Ang II mediates dextral looping patterns of cardiac embryogenesis via AT1R. Deletion of AT1R leads to a reduction of the heart/body weight ratio and atrophic changes in the myocardium, with reduced coronary flow and lower left ventricular systolic pressure.[53] RAAS is indispensable for development of the vasculature.[54,55] Certain defects or malformations occur if the components of RAAS are lacking.[54,56] Overexpression of AT2R attenuates neointimal formation and negatively regulates DNA synthesis in the developing aorta.[55] During prenatal vasculogenesis, AT1R contributes to vascular smooth cell differentiation by upregulating molecular markers such as smooth muscle α-actin and myosin heavy chain. In general, AT1R and AT2R may synergistically regulate the development of the vasculature during the prenatal periods.[54,55]

Compared with extensive studies on the relationship between RAAS and the cardiovascular system in adults, investigations related to RAAS-mediated cardiovascular regulation in the fetus are limited. However, the development of RAAS in normal and abnormal patterns before birth has attracted considerable attention. Increasing evidence has suggested that changes in expression of RAAS during pregnancy can affect fetal blood pressure[57,58] (Fig. 49.2). Intravenous infusion of

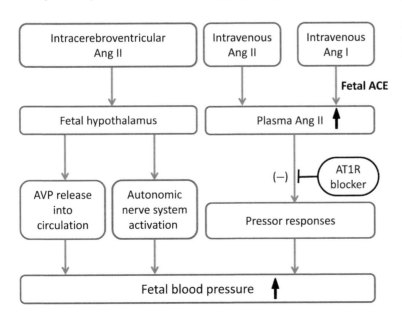

FIG. 49.2 The effects of angiotensin on fetal blood pressure in utero. *Ang I*, angiotensin I; *Ang II*, angiotensin II; *AVP*, arginine vasopressin.

Ang I or Ang II into near-term and preterm ovine fetuses can produce an increase in systolic, diastolic, and mean arterial pressure.[57,58] Intravenous application of Ang I significantly increases fetal blood pressure, accompanied by an increase of fetal plasma arginine vasopressin in sheep.[57] Intracerebroventricular injection of Ang II can significantly increase fetal mean arterial pressure, and decrease heart rate at near term.[59] Application of losartan intracerebroventricularly significantly suppresses the increased fetal blood pressure induced by intravenous infusion of Ang II.[59] These results demonstrate Ang II is critical in controlling fetal cardiovascular responses and plays a central role for RAAS via AT1R pathway in the control of fetal blood pressure.

These lines of evidence provide insight into how local RAAS in the cardiovascular systems may be altered by prenatal insults, including maternal malnutrition, glucocorticoid exposure, and hypoxia.[60–62] A number of epidemiological and experimental studies demonstrate poor nutrition during pregnancy increases cardiovascular risks for the offspring in later life. When ewes were given a 50% reduction in maternal nutrient intake during the last 30 days of pregnancy, fetal arterial blood pressure was higher, and fetal blood pressure responses to application of Ang II were also higher.[63] In isolated femoral arteries, the response curve to noradrenaline was reduced in the fetuses whose mothers were protein-restricted.[64] Maternal nutrient restriction also alters gene expression of RAAS in the fetal heart.[60,65] In fetuses exposed to maternal malnutrition, they showed decreased levels of AT1R and AT2R in the left ventricle.[65] Elevated blood pressure and altered gene expression of key components of the RAAS in the left ventricle have been seen in rats that were subjected to prenatal protein restriction.[60] Thus fetal undernutrition can alter local RAAS-associated bioactive substances, contributing, at least partly, to the development of cardiac and vascular remodeling, and increased blood pressure.

The treatment of pregnant ewes with betamethasone significantly increases fetal mean arterial blood pressure.[66] To determine if antenatal betamethasone alters vascular reactivity, isometric contraction was assessed in endothelium-intact coronary arteries isolated from fetal sheep at 121 to 124 days' gestation.[61] Coronary vessels from betamethasone-treated fetuses exhibited enhanced peak responses to Ang II, accompanied by an increase of AT1R expression in the artery. These findings indicate that antenatal betamethasone exposure enhances coronary vasoconstriction to Ang II by selectively upregulating coronary artery AT1R expression. Moderately elevated maternal cortisol levels late in gestation causes enlargement of the heart of fetal sheep, accompanied by increased AT2R and decreased AT1R,[67] suggesting that glucocorticoid-induced enlargement of the fetal heart may be via RAAS.

The effects of other prenatal insults, such as a high-salt diet and hypoxia on RAAS in the fetal cardiovascular system, have also been tested.[62] Following exposure to high salt, disorganized myofibrillae and loss of mitochondrial cristae are observed in the fetal heart; fetal cardiac Ang II and AT1R are increased, whereas AT2R is not affected. These findings suggest a relationship between high-salt diets in pregnancy and developmental changes of the cardiac RAAS.[62] In addition, prenatal hypoxia can significantly increase Ang II-mediated vessel contractions in fetal thoracic aortas in rodents, associated with altered expression patterns of Ang II receptors.[62] Together, functional changes of cardiovascular or heart RAAS may influence vascular development and blood pressure in the fetuses and neonates, and result in molecular changes in fetal cardiac and vascular tissue that may have long-term impacts.

49.1.1.2.3 Abnormal RAAS in the Central Nervous System

In rodents, renin can be detected in the fetal brain accompanied with AGT, ACE, AT1R, and AT2R from E18 to E19. In ovine fetuses, the brain ACE, AT1R, and AT2R are detected in the developing brain at 70% of gestation. Several neural behaviors during development, such as neuritogenesis processes, cellular migration, and cell survival, can be synergistically regulated by RAAS, and local RAAS in the brain plays an important role in development via binding to AT1R or AT2R.[68]

It is well known that excretion of water and electrolyte from the body occurs mainly via the kidneys, whereas intake of water and salt is controlled by the brain.[69] The brain has its own local RAAS, and this mediates behavioral and endocrine responses that play a critical role in regulation of fluid balance, including water and salt ingestion.[69] Functional studies in the past 2 decades have further confirmed that central application of Ang II or Ang I not only induces an increase in plasma arginine vasopressin concentrations in near-term (~135 gestational days) ovine fetuses, but also increases oxytocin levels in the fetal circulation.[57] Intravenous infusion of Ang I also significantly increased fetal blood pressure, c-fos, and AT1R expression in the supraoptic and paraventricular nuclei in the hypothalamus.[57] Moreover, application of losartan (an inhibitor of AT1R) or captopril (a competitive inhibitor of ACE) significantly suppresses the increased plasma arginine vasopressin in response to intracerebroventricular Ang II in near-term ovine fetuses.[59]

In the developing fetus, the endogenous brain RAAS not only mediates pressor responses and arginine vasopressin release, but also participates in the control of the neuroendocrine responses that are critical in body fluid regulation. RAAS in the fetal brain is important in the control of fetal swallowing activity.[70] Intracerebroventricular Ang II significantly increased swallowing in near-term ovine fetuses, and increased c-fos expression in the dipsogenic regions in the fetal brain.[70] Furthermore, intravenous infusion of Ang II-induced fetal swallowing activity could be blocked by AT1R or ACE inhibitors,[70] indicating that fetal exposure to RAAS inhibitors may have adverse effects on fetal and amniotic fluid homeostasis. The RAAS-mediated central dipsogenic mechanism is intact before birth in sheep, and contributes to fetal and amniotic fluid regulation.

A number of prenatal insults can influence the brain RAAS, including maternal protein restriction, glucocorticoid exposure, cigarette smoking, and water deprivation. When mice dams were given a low protein diet during the second half of the gestation, this caused increased expression of AGT and ACE, and a decreased level of AT2R in the fetal brain.[71] Prenatal dexamethasone administered intravenously to the ewe between 26 and 28 days of gestation increases the expression of AGT and AT1R in the fetal brain in late gestation.[72] The increased expression of brain AT1R after prenatal dexamethasone exposure may be associated with increased cardiovascular activation by exogenous and endogenous Ang II.[73] Prenatal nicotine exposure significantly decreases fetal brain weight, increases AT1R levels at gestation 15 and 21 days, and decreases AT2R levels at gestation day 21 in the fetal brain.[74] Maternal water deprivation in pregnant sheep significantly decreased fetal brain weight, and increased AGT, AT1R, and AT2R protein abundance in the fetal brain.[75] Water deprivation-induced body dehydration is a typical body fluid dysfunction that can influence the expression of the Ang II receptors, as well as other RAAS elements in the fetal brain, and then stimulates release of central arginine vasopressin into the fetal circulation and fetal swallowing activities.

49.1.2 Diseases Related to RAAS Dysfunction

49.1.2.1 Preterm Birth

Preterm birth (PTB) is defined as birth before 37 weeks of gestation, which affects more than 15 million global pregnancies each year and leads to a morbidity of 1 million children every year.[76] Term labor is characterized by the switch of the myometrium from a quiescent to a contractile state, cervical dilatation, and rupture of the membrane, which are accompanied by a shift between anti-inflammatory and proinflammatory pathways. The main difference between preterm and term labor is when labor is initiated. Given that RAAS contributes to vascular remodeling of the spiral arteries[77] and inflammatory signaling pathways, RAAS activity during pregnancy may contribute to PTB.

In fact, there is a growing evidence that abnormal RAAS is involved in preterm birth. Plasma renin activity was markedly increased in preterm infants.[78] Urinary AGT/creatinine ratio was significantly higher in preterm neonates compared with that in full-term neonates in human.[79] Another prospective observational study of 309 pregnant woman indicated that reduced Ang 1–7 in maternal as well as neonatal plasma was independently associated with PTB. Furthermore, the maternal Ang 1–7/Ang II ratio was associated with gestational hypertension and preeclampsia, thereby contributing to PTB.[79]

A substantial body of evidence indicates that maternal genetic influences have a great influence on the risk of PTB. Different genotypes of RAAS in PTB maternal and infant genomes have been discovered. AGT genotypes 174M/M (methionine at amino acid position 174) and 235T/T (threonine at amino acid position 235) contribute to high levels of AGT in plasma. In the blood of women experiencing PTB, the frequency of AGT allele 235M (methionine at amino acid position 235) and two-locus haplotype 174T-235M is increased,[80] indicating a lower AGT level in PTB. As for ACE, a maternal ACE genotype does not appear to contribute to PTB; however, the prevalence of the deletion allele of ACE in PTB infants is increased, associated with higher ACE levels.[81] Variants of AT2R (rs201386833 and rs5950506) in the maternal genome are also associated with PTB.[82] However, there are not enough data to confirm the underlying mechanisms by which RAAS may contribute to PTB.

49.1.2.2 Kidney Disorders

It is well known that the kidneys contain all of the elements of the RAAS, contributing to renal ontogeny, the regulation of blood pressure, and the progression of chronic kidney diseases. Recent evidence has also revealed that inappropriate activation of the intrarenal RAAS plays an important role in the pathogenesis of renal injury and hypertension, and that RAAS blockers such as ACEIs and ARBs have been beneficial in attenuating the progression of chronic kidney diseases in adults.[83] As for neonates and children, RAAS-induced kidney disorders mainly originate from the intrauterine environments and congenital factors.

49.1.2.2.1   Developmental Programming of Kidney Diseases

The fetal origins of adult disease hypothesis (FOAD) states that fetuses exposed to an unfavorable intrauterine environment will adjust the trajectory of organ development to maintain survival. This compensation can increase risks for chronic diseases in adulthood, including cardiovascular, renal, and metabolic diseases.[84] Given that nephron formation is completed prior to birth in human, a reduction in the numbers of nephron will impair renal functions throughout later life.[21] The kidneys participate in the homeostasis of acid-base balance, electrolyte concentrations, and the regulation of blood pressure. Symptoms of kidney dysfunction, such as glomerulosclerosis and decreased urine volume, are usually attributed to aging, poor dietary habits, and medicine application. Prenatal reduction in the total number of nephrons has been shown in experimental induced fetal hypertension.[85] Ontogeny of the intrarenal RAAS is altered throughout the perinatal and postnatal periods. If exposed to prenatal adverse environments, intrarenal Ang II can increase blood pressure independently from systemic RAAS, via inducing vasoconstriction, thereby triggering centrally regulated pressor responses and stimulating aldosterone release.[86]

Prenatal Glucocorticoids Exposure   Endogenous production of glucocorticoids, predominantly cortisol in the human or corticosterone (CORT) in rodents, increases in response to maternal stress. An exogenous glucocorticoid, dexamethasone, is widely used to decrease the risk of prematurity-related chronic lung diseases. Maternal exposure to glucocorticoids in the short term can impair fetal kidney function, reduce nephron endowment, and induce programmed hypertension later in the adult offspring of sheep, rats, and mice.[87,88]

The role of systemic and intrarenal RAAS in glucocorticoids-programmed renal disorders and hypertension has been investigated. Although sex-specific renal dysfunction and hypertension have been observed in the offspring, alteration of RAAS as well as basal intrarenal RAAS is variable among different animal models. In rats receiving intraperitoneal dexamethasone during gestation day 16–22, renal mRNA expression of renin and AGT was lower in the female than in the male, while the female showed higher mRNA expression of AT1R and AT2R in the kidney compared with the male.[89] Another study showed that in rats receiving CORT on gestation day 14 for 48 h, expression of AT1R was also higher in females, while AT2R in females was similar to that in males.[90] The effects of prenatal dexamethasone or CORT on sex-specific blood pressure and expression of RAAS is also variable (shown in Table 49.2). The diversity is related to dose, timing and type of glucocorticoids, sampled parts of the kidney, age of the offspring, and irritation to animals when measuring blood pressure. On the whole, impaired kidney development of offspring is associated with the changes of intrarenal RAAS in multiple models and species. The balance between ACE/Ang II/AT1R axis and Ang 1–7/ACE2/AT2R axis is important in the development of disease.

TABLE 49.2   Changes of RAAS caused by adverse prenatal factors

Prenatal exposure	Species	Age of offspring	Sex	Changes	Reference
Dexamethasone (G16–22)[a]	Rat	4 months	Female	Renal AT2R↑, Mas1↑[b]	89
			Male	BP↑, renal AT2R↑, Mas1↑	89
Corticosterone (E12.5–15)[c]	Mouse	6 months	Female	Renal ACE2↓, AT1Ra↑	91
			Male	Plasma aldosterone↑, renal renin↑, ACE2↑, Mas1↑, Nr3c2↑[d]	91
Corticosterone (E14–15)	Rat	1 month	Female	BP (4 month)↑, renal AT1Rb↑, AT2R↑	90
			Male	BP (4 month)↑, renal AT1Ra↑, AT2R↑	90
High salt (G70–130)	Ewe	15 days and 3 months	Male	Renal ACE2↓, AT1R↑, AGT↑, ACE↑	43
High-salt (G1–21)	Rat	3 months	Male	Plasma Ang I↓, renal AT2R↓	92

[a]G: gestational day.
[b]Mas1: Ang 1–7 receptor.
[c]E: embryonic day.
[d]Nr3c2: aldosterone receptor.

High Salt Intake Maternal high-salt diets during gestation cause glomerulosclerosis, increased proteinuria, and hypertension in the adult offspring.[93] Local renal RAAS plays an important role in cellular proliferation and apoptosis. Thus intrarenal RAAS components mediate nephrogenesis and renal function. For example, growth of the fetal kidney can be regulated via AT1R. The effect of maternal high salt intake on RAAS depends on the age of offspring. Plasma Ang II levels are significantly decreased in the mothers and fetuses of the high-salt diet group, but not in the offspring aged 15 and 90 days. But prenatal high-salt exposure increases the concentration of Ang II[94] and expression of AGT, ACE, ACE2, and AT1R in the kidneys of adult offspring.[43] Furthermore, Ang II increases renal oxidative stress, which may disturb the tubule interstitial microenvironment, leading to structural and functional changes in Na^+ transporters. Therefore, perinatal salt overload leads to renal RAAS overactivity during adulthood, with normal or reduced Ang II levels in plasma.[41] Although the counterregulatory enzymes ACE and ACE2 are both enhanced, ACE/ACE2 is increased in adult offspring exposed to prenatal exposure to high salt, indicating a balance of RAAS is critical to normal renal development. The overactive RAAS appears to be responsible, at least in part, for the aforementioned renal functional alterations produced by perinatal exposure to salt.

Intrauterine Growth Restriction Intrauterine growth retardation (IUGR) is usually defined as impaired growth and development of the fetus and/or its organs during gestation. The effect of maternal malnutrition on the development of IUGR was investigated using the aforementioned Dutch famine model. Children born to these mothers showed an increased albumin/creatinine ratio in adulthood, which is indicative of microalbuminuria. As a result of single nephron hyperfiltration, increased risk for microalbuminuria in children may eventually lead to a reduction in renal function in adults.[36] In animal models, offspring exposed to maternal malnutrition during gestation have reduced body weight, small kidney size, and decreased nephron number at birth.[37] Upregulation of renal AT1R following late gestational protein restriction is observed as early as 4 weeks of age.[38] An increase in plasma renin activity following late gestational protein restriction is also observed as early as 4 weeks of age, or at other periods in postnatal life.[38] Thus temporal alterations of RAAS have been confirmed by gestational protein restriction. More importantly, the critical role of the RAAS in the etiology of hypertension programmed by maternal protein restriction is indicated by RAS blockade.[38] Another IUGR animal model can be created by reducing the flow of both ovarian arteries in pregnant rats. The expression of renal ACE, renin, and AGT are increased in the adult offspring in this experimental model, and the effect of ACE is proved by the ameliorative effect of enalapril on hypertension.[95] The complex alterations of intrarenal RAAS contribute to the etiology of hypertension in IUGR offspring.

Sex differences in Programmed Renal Hypertension Sex differences in blood pressure regulation and in the progression of hypertension have been shown in both clinical and animal models. The renal RAAS functions in a sexually dimorphic manner to regulate renal function and the cardiovascular system. The different RAAS levels in the kidney of normal female and male rodents have been shown in many reports. When evaluating renal function and blood pressure of adult offspring exposed to intrauterine adverse environments, conditions of male offspring seem to be worse than those of females in most cases. The enhanced responsiveness to Ang II is testosterone-dependent in male IUGR offspring.[96] As for females, the sensitivity to Ang II is modulated by ovarian hormones.[97] Sex hormones differentially interact with RAAS pathways, with testosterone increasing expression of renin, AT1R, and upregulating vasopressor responses, while estrogen increases ACE2 and AT2R expression, which are considered beneficial for blood pressure.

49.1.2.2.2 Genetic Renal Disorders

Renal Tubular Dysgenesis (MIM 267430) Autosomal recessive renal tubular dysgenesis is a severe fetal disorder of renal tubular development, characterized by early onset and persistent anuria, ossification defects of the skull, and perinatal death that is likely due to pulmonary hypoplasia from early-onset oligohydramnios (the Potter phenotype).[98] Absence or paucity of differentiated proximal tubules is the histopathologic hallmark of the disorder. Renal tubular dysgenesis is caused by homozygous or compound heterozygous mutations in genes encoding the components of RAAS, including renin on chromosome 1q32, AGT on chromosome 1q42, ACE on chromosome 17q23, or AT1R on chromosome 3q24. Mutations result in either the absence of production or lack of efficacy of Ang II. In addition, secondary renal tubular dysgenesis has been observed in various situations, particularly in fetuses exposed to RAAS blockers,[99] illustrating the importance of a functional RAAS in the maintenance of renal development during fetal life in humans.

Hyperuricemic Nephropathy, Familial Juvenile 2 (MIM 613092) Hyperuricemic nephropathy, familial juvenile 2 (HNFJ2), also named autosomal dominant tubulointerstitial kidney disease, renin-related, is an autosomal dominant hyperuricemic nephropathy. By the age of 1 year, most affected children have mild anemia, slowly progressive renal failure, and hyperuricemia. Most patients have hyperuricemia, gout, and slowly progressive chronic tubulointerstitial kidney disease. Finally, the end-stage renal disease develops during middle-aged life.

The renin gene located on chromosome 1q31–q41 has been identified as the cause of HNFJ2.[100] Both deletion and missense mutations were reported in HNFJ2 families. Due to mutant renin, low plasma renin activity and low plasma concentrations of aldosterone have been found in HNFJ2 patients. It is likely that expression of the mutated proteins has a dominant toxic effect, gradually reducing the viability of renin-expressing cells. This alters intrarenal RAAS and the functionality of the juxtaglomerular apparatus, resulting in nephron dropout and progressive kidney failure.[101]

49.1.2.3 Aldosteronism-Related Diseases

49.1.2.3.1 Primary Aldosteronism

Primary aldosteronism is the most common cause of secondary hypertension. It is due to increased aldosterone production from the adrenal cortex, adrenal hyperplasia, and sometimes adenomas. The amount of aldosterone potentiates renal sodium reabsorption, water retention, and potassium excretion. The increased sodium reabsorption by the kidney results in plasma volume expansion, which is the primary initiating mechanism for hypertension, and subsequent development of fibrosis in vital organs. Various specific genetic alterations identified for rare familial forms of primary aldosteronism include coding genes of cytochrome P450 family 11 subfamily B member, inwardly rectifying potassium channel Kir3.4, Na/K-ATPase, Ca-ATPase, L-type voltage-dependent calcium channel, and mineralocorticoid receptor.[102]

49.1.2.3.2 Primary Hypoaldosteronism

Primary hypoaldosteronism is a rare inborn disorder with life-threatening symptoms in newborns and infants due to an aldosterone synthase defect in adrenal gland, inadequate stimulation of aldosterone secretion, or resistance to the ion transport effects of aldosterone.[103] Primary hypoaldosteronism leads to electrolyte imbalances with hyponatremia and hyperkalemia in newborns and infants, with clinical manifestations that include salt wasting, hypovolemia, and failure to thrive. Mutations of several genes are involved in different types of this disease. For example, genetic alteration of amiloride-sensitive epithelial sodium channel and cytochrome P450 family 11 subfamily B member 2 contribute to pseudohypoaldosteronism type I and aldosterone synthase defects, respectively.[104]

49.2 PATHOPHYSIOLOGICAL ROLES OF NITRIC OXIDE IN MATERNAL, FETAL, AND NEONATAL DISEASES

49.2.1 Pregnant Mother

49.2.1.1 Nitric Oxide (NO) and Preeclampsia

Preeclampsia is a hypertensive disorder of pregnancy, classically defined as new-onset hypertension and proteinuria of at least 300 mg in 24 h. It is among the most common disorders of pregnancy, occurring in up to 8% of all pregnant women worldwide.

Endothelium-derived NO dysfunction has been implicated as a potential cause of preeclampsia. Nitric oxide is a gaseous molecule generated from the conversion of L-arginine to L-citrulline by NO synthase (NOS), and a potent vasodilator and relaxant of vascular smooth muscle. Both increased and reduced NO in the placenta have been reported, as well as changes in the expression or activity of NOS in the preeclamptic placenta, which remain controversial. Some studies reported that there was no difference in the distribution and expression of endothelial nitric oxide synthase (eNOS) in placental tissue between preeclamptic and normal pregnancies.[105] Others showed an increase in eNOS mRNA expression in preeclamptic placenta,[106] and that eNOS immunostaining was intense in the endothelium of terminal villous capillary and stem villous vessels in the preeclampsia group.[107] In addition, other studies demonstrated that human placental NOS activity was markedly reduced in preeclampsia.[108] Endothelial dysfunction is often associated with decreased NO bioavailability, and changes in NO metabolism could be a pathogenic factor in preeclampsia. The NOS activity was diminished, which could be due to the interference of reactive oxygen species (ROS).

In the preeclamptic placenta, increased ROS production seems to suppress the expression and function of eNOS.[109] Moreover, peroxynitrite ($ONOO^-$) is formed as result of NO scavenging by ROS. The $ONOO^-$ not only oxidizes DNA, proteins, and lipids, but also interferes with important vascular signaling pathways. Thus redundant ROS and subsequent increased $ONOO^-$ formation are known to reduce the bioavailability of NO and cause endothelial dysfunction. This leads to lower concentrations of 3′,5′ cyclic Guanosine Monophosphate (cGMP) (the NO intracellular second messenger) in preeclamptic placental circulation compared with normal pregnancy, which could be key elements in the pathogenesis of preeclampsia.

NOS can be also inhibited in vivo by asymmetric dimethylarginine (ADMA). ADMA is an endogenous competitive inhibitor of NOS that could affect NO production. In women with preeclampsia, most investigations reported that plasma ADMA was significantly elevated. Since the release of ADMA by endothelial cells is sufficient to inhibit NO production, it is therefore possible that the concentrations of ADMA could be responsible for the changes of placental NOS activity in preeclampsia, which may be of pathophysiological significance.

Normal pregnancy in rats is accompanied by increased production of NO and its second messenger cGMP with a parallel increase in renal expression of constitutive NOS.[110,111] In pregnant rats, reducing placental blood flow through the administration of NG-nitro-L-arginine methyl ester (L-NAME), an exogenous inhibitor of NOS, can produce the preeclampsia-like syndrome.[112] L-Arginine supplementation[113] or coadministration of sildenafil citrate,[112] which blocks the action of L-NAME, prevented the preeclampsia-like syndrome. However, animal models have failed to provide definitive insights into the pathogenesis of preeclampsia because of their limited applicability to the human form of the disease.

In humans, the role of NO deficiency in the pathogenesis of the hypertension in preeclampsia has been controversial. Although elevated circulating levels of ADMA are consistently found in pregnancies that are complicated by preeclampsia, plasma concentrations are typically, very low with a narrow distribution among healthy adults, making quantification extremely challenging and the clinical significance of the finding uncertain. Furthermore, L-arginine supplementation has not conferred significant benefit in women with pregnancies that are complicated by preeclampsia.

Many vasoactive substances can cause vasodilatation via endothelial-dependent or independent NO-release pathways. The following sections summarize the typical endothelial-dependent and independent NO-donating agents in the preeclamptic placenta.

Bradykinin and acetylcholine (ACh) are classic endothelium-dependent NO donors that mediate vasodilatation. Bradykinin binding to endothelial B2 receptors leads to NO production, prostacyclin formation, elevated intracellular Ca^{2+}, and the formation of hyperpolarizing factor, causing relaxation of the vascular smooth muscle and vasodilatation. Exogenously injected bradykinin can cause hypotension, natriuresis, arterial vasodilatation, increased renal blood flow, and a decrease in total peripheral resistance. Placental arteries already constricted with U46619[114] and vasopressin[115] had a minimal vasodilatory response to bradykinin. There is no significant difference in the bradykinin-induced vasodilatation between normal and preeclamptic placental vessels.

ACh was first reported to be present in the placenta in 1926 and plays an important role in the maturation and development of placental vessels and syncytiotrophoblasts, and the modification of the uterus during labor.[116] Acetylcholine-induced endothelium-dependent vasodilatation has been well confirmed in most blood vessels in the body. However, the effects of ACh on placental vessels were in dispute until 2 years ago, because two studies indicated vasodilatation, two others reported vasoconstriction, and others indicated no effects on vascular tone.[117,118] In an analysis of the reasons for these discrepant experimental results, the researchers found two major causes: large variability as is typical between individual humans, and small sample sizes.

To investigate vascular physiology and pathophysiology in other human vessels such as coronary arteries, a relatively pure species of animal model can help exclude variations from genetic and experimental conditions, which is crucial. However, no functional experiments using animal placental vessels compared with nonplacental vessels were performed until the last few years. Recent studies used a large sample size for human placentas and animal placenta to reveal that unlike most nonplacental blood vessels, ACh has no direct effects on either constriction or dilation in placental vessels in both human and sheep, regardless of normal pregnancy and preeclampsia.[118] This finding suggests that placental vascular dilation based on its own endothelial NO signaling is very limited or weak, which is very different from nonplacental vessels.

In the fetoplacental circulation, the umbilical cord serves as a bridge between the placenta and fetus. Recent progress has demonstrated the effects of ACh on umbilical blood vessels, including veins and arteries. The researchers also used a large size of samples for human umbilical vessels, as well as umbilical cords from sheep, rabbits, and rats, proving that the effect of ACh on umbilical vessels is vasoconstriction, which is different from the dilatory effects of ACh on most of other blood vessels in the body. The evidence of significant differences in the effects of ACh on the placenta and umbilical cord informs us that vascular endocrine physiology has special patterns in placental and umbilical vessels. Since the placental-fetal circulation plays a critical role in fetal development and maternal diseases, further understanding special endocrine physiology and pathophysiology in fetal growth under normal and abnormal conditions should provide new directions for prenatal and developmental studies.

Besides endothelial-dependent agents, vasodilatation may also be triggered by endothelial-independent NO donors. Sodium nitroprusside (SNP), S-nitroso-N-acetylpenicillamine (SNAP), and glyceryl trinitrate (GTN) are endothelial-independent agents that are typically used as NO donators in vasodilatation. Interestingly, even though placental endothelial NO systems seem weak with limited endogenous NO, exogenous NO, from donors such as SNP, can reliably produce vascular dilation in placental blood vessels, in both human and sheep. Notably, placental vascular smooth muscle cells can respond to NO in regulations of vascular relaxation, while its endothelial cells only produced very limited endogenous NO. Thus it seems that placental vascular dilation by NO should be generated from nonendothelial cells in placental vessels or outside blood vessels. Which tissue or cell is a major supply of NO for placental blood vessels is an important and interesting question under investigation.

49.2.1.2   Nitric Oxide and Gestational Diabetes

Gestational diabetes (GDM) is characterized by glucose intolerance with onset or first recognition during pregnancy. GDM exhibits maternal hyperglycemia that usually ends after delivery, and affects the health of the mother and fetus during and after pregnancy. In human endothelial cells, L-arginine is transported via the human cationic amino acid transporters (hCATs), accumulating this amino acid in the intracellular space. L-Arginine is then metabolized by eNOS into L-citrulline and synthesizes NO. Gestational diabetes mellitus is associated with higher expression and activity of hCAT-1, leading to supraphysiological accumulation of L-arginine.[119] This phenomenon results in higher L-arginine metabolism by eNOS due to increased expression and activity of this enzyme, thereby leading to the overproduction of NO.

Early studies indicate that the altered L-arginine/NO pathway in the microvasculature of GDM acts as key factor for GDM-associated fetoplacental vascular dysfunction. The NO level in amniotic fluid and NO synthesis in human placental vein and arteries are increased in GDM pregnancies. Umbilical cord vein endothelial cells isolated from GDM pregnancy show increased NO synthesis and L-arginine transport, associated with higher eNOS mRNA expression, protein abundance, and activity.[120] However, isolated small arteries from women with GDM showed a reduction in the endothelium-mediated vasodilator responses to ACh. This was no longer evident after the administration of the prostaglandin inhibitor indomethacin; relaxation to SNP was similar to both groups.[121] NO synthase inhibitor reduced ACh responsiveness similarly in both groups of women. Since endothelium-dependent dilation of umbilical veins from GDM is blunted, the bioavailability of NO, but not its synthesis by eNOS, is reduced.

Under hyperglycemic conditions, NADPH oxidase (NOX) activity is increased, leading to the generation of superoxide anion (O_2^-), which will cause an oxidative stress environment. The O_2^- generated reacts with NO to produce large amounts of $ONOO^-$ that scavenge NO, thereby reducing its bioavailability. Thus GDM is associated with reduced NO bioavailability and with reduced endothelium-dependent vasodilatation of the fetoplacental vasculature. Therefore, vascular dysfunction resulting from GDM may be a consequence of a functional dissociation between the synthesis of NO and/or its bioavailability to the vascular endothelium and smooth muscle in the human placental circulation.

49.2.2   Fetus and Neonate

49.2.2.1   Nitric Oxide and Intrauterine Growth Restriction (IUGR)

In 1919, all newborns weighing <2500 g (5 lb, 8 oz) were classified as "premature." While the WHO currently defines "low birth weight" as <2500 g (5 lb, 8 oz) or below the 10% of gestational age, "low birth weight" babies can be divided into three categories: (1) healthy but constitutionally small babies, (2) preterm delivery, and (3) IUGR. Intrauterine growth restriction, also called *fetal growth restriction* or *intrauterine growth retardation*, refers to the poor living conditions for the fetus in the mother's womb. IUGR can often lead to fetal and neonatal mortality and morbidity, as well as many pathologic conditions in the offspring, including immediate perinatal adverse events (prematurity, cerebral palsy, intrauterine fetal death, neonatal death), and illnesses with onset delayed as much as decades (obesity, hypertension, type-2 diabetes).[122] IUGR has resulted from many different causes, and is most commonly due to the insufficiency of placenta, which could lead to an inadequate nutrient and oxygen supply to the fetus. Previous studies have reported that the fetus has some recourse to adjust to a limited nutrient supply.[123] However, there are few effective pathways against limited oxygen supply, which is a common occurrence under several obstetric pathological conditions that may lead to IUGR, such as preeclampsia, placenta previa, maternal anemia, smoking, and other causes (Fig. 49.3).

NO, serving as a key signal molecule in both physiological and pathological process, could inhibit platelet aggregation and adhesion to the endothelium and be involved in the control of blood pressure. During pregnancy, NO is generated in placental circulation, regulates vascular tone, and attenuates the actions of vasoconstrictors.[124] The NO synthase of the placental villous vasculature appears to correspond to the type III calcium-calmodulin-dependent endothelial isoform, and is present in umbilical arteries and veins, chorionic arteries and veins, and syncytiotrophoblast. NO synthase appears to be absent from the underlying cytotrophoblast and small blood vessels of the terminal villous capillaries.

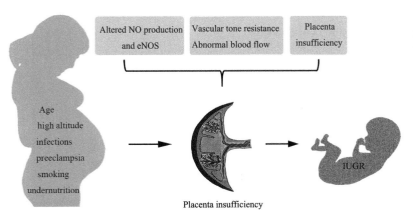

FIG. 49.3 Maternal adverse factors that can lead to placental insufficiency and IUGR through altered NO and eNOS systems.

Placental insufficiency is the most common cause of IUGR, which is characterized by altered expression of vasoactive factors, including NOS. Endothelial NO synthase is an important regulator of vascular tone and blood flow. The inhibition of NO production results in IUGR and preeclampsia-like symptoms in pregnant rodents.[125] In endothelial cells, eNOS mRNA and protein concentrations are increased during development of IUGR, suggesting transcriptional regulation for eNOS in these cells. It is known that during early gestation periods, embryos and the placenta are exposed to a hypoxic environment and the IUGR fetuses are hypoxic at birth. Thus hypoxia may be the stimulus for increased eNOS mRNA and protein in the IUGR placenta.

Doppler flow velocity waveforms showed that vascular resistance was increased in the fetal-placental circulation in pregnancies with preeclampsia and IUGR.[126] This increase has been ascribed to altered vascular activity, which may depend on alterations of NO-mediated vascular functions in the circulation. The fetal circulation in preeclampsia or IUGR is also characterized by abnormal umbilical blood flow velocity waveforms, thought to be indicative of increased placental resistance,[126] which may be linked to abnormal vascular anatomy. Altered eNOS expression in blood vessels in utero is perhaps an adaptive response to increased resistance and poor perfusion during the development of IUGR.

Notably, a number of clinical survey and experimental studies have demonstrated an important relationship between IUGR and the later development of adult diseases. Among those findings, NO-mediated changes have been shown as reduced endothelial function in mesenteric arteries in the offspring with a history of IUGR.[127]

49.2.2.2 Nitric Oxide and Early Embryo Loss

In humans, early embryo loss is defined as losses that occurred before the 3rd week of gestation. Recent studies have shown that NO is associated with this.

The role of macrophage activation in early embryo loss is determined by the release of NO, which is a short-lived mediator that can be induced in a variety of cell types, and produces multiple physiologic and metabolic changes in target tissue and cells.[128] An increase in nitrite oxidation to nitrate by decidual cells could be one way of protecting embryos from the harmful effects of NO/NO^{2-}. Aminoguanidine, a preferential inhibitor of iNOS, may successfully prevent embryo loss, suggesting that NO was the ultimate effector molecule that may cause problems for the growing fetus. Although the primary cause and mechanisms of early embryo loss are still unclear, fetal chromosome anomalies, especially frequently aneuploidy and the intrauterine viral infections, have been considered as the leading causes.[129] Most pregnancy losses have been linked to morphogenetic anomalies of the embryo as maternal specific immune systems rejecting the embryo. Thus abnormal activation of maternal immune effector mechanisms is critical in early embryo loss, and previous studies demonstrated that increased NO production by decidual macrophages was involved. The expression of iNOS and TNF-α mRNA is determined to quantify macrophage activation in murine embryos as a model of spontaneous early embryo loss. Other animal models showed that pregnant mice were induced to abort at a higher rate when iNOS and TNF-α mRNA expression in the embryos was abnormally augmented. These results suggested a correlation between increased iNOS and TNF-α expression with embryo resorption.[130]

In rats with early embryo loss, the loss of macrophages and natural killer-like (NK-like) cells of maternal origin remains relatively constant after gestational day 8, whereas 20%–30% of the embryos show a significant increase in inflammatory cells in the maternal decidua, corresponding to the incidence of early embryo resorption visible at gestational day 12. In resorbing rat embryos, inflammatory macrophages showed evidence of having been primed during early pregnancy, associated with lipopolysaccharide-induced production of TNF-α and NO.[131]

TABLE 49.3 Possible mechanisms of altered NO system and consequences

Possible mechanism for NO abnormality	Consequences	Reference
Decidual macrophages increased NO production	Early embryo loss	129
Macrophage activation	iNOS↑/Early embryo loss	130
Lipopolysaccharide induced the production of TNF-α, NO	More inflammatory cells maternal decidua/Early embryo loss	131
Inhibition of NO synthesis in ovulation	Ovarian blood flow ↓/Ovulatory efficiency ↓/Abnormal oocyte maturation/Early embryo loss	132
Lack of the gene encoding eNOS in placenta	Placental hormone production ↓/Early embryo loss	134

NO is also known to play a functional role in ovulation. Inhibition of NO synthesis has been demonstrated to alter regional ovarian blood flow, inhibit follicle atresia, and reduce ovulatory efficiency and oocyte maturation.[132] Expression of eNOS has also been demonstrated in the placenta and is believed to modulate placental hormone production. Recently, a study has demonstrated that a lack of the gene encoding eNOS negatively impacts early embryonic development and survival in a mouse model.[133] The association between a NOS3 polymorphism and recurrent miscarriage also supports a functional role of NO in early embryonic development.

In cultured macrophages in vitro, estrogen showed no effects on transcription of the iNOS gene and production of NO, whereas in high concentrations, progesterone decreases expression of iNOS. In ovariectomized and hormone-treated mouse uteri, iNOS was induced by estrogens, whereas iNOS in luminal epithelial cells is activated by progesterone[134] (Table 49.3).

Briefly, the provided viewpoints offer the concept of that NO as a physiological mediator in early pregnancy. Identification of a link between idiopathic recurrent miscarriage and a specific variant of a gene involved in the regulation of NO-mediated placental functions and vascular homeostasis allows further insight into the natural history of this syndrome and characterization of susceptible women.

49.2.2.3 NO and Neonatal Pulmonary Hypertension

Pulmonary hypertension is a rare disease in newborns and contributes significantly to morbidity and mortality. Neonatal pulmonary hypertension may be idiopathic or associated with premature closure of the ductus arteriosus, pneumonia, meconium aspiration, prematurity, or lung hypoplasia. Pulmonary vascular remodeling and vasoconstriction are the pathophysiological features of the disease.[135]

During the development of the fetal pulmonary vasculature, many structures and functions change to prepare for the transition to air breathing. At birth, pulmonary hemodynamic differences between the fetus and newborn, including an increase in oxygen tension and blood flow in the pulmonary circulation with a dramatic reduction in pulmonary arterial pressure and resistance, are regulated by various factors. Among them, NO plays a significant role in the normal reduction of pulmonary vascular resistance at birth during the transition from a fetal to a newborn circulatory system.[135] Infants with pulmonary hypertension have low plasma concentrations of arginine and NO metabolites.[136] Upregulation of eNOS is observed in neonatal lung with pulmonary hypertension.[137]

The pulmonary vascular synthesis of an endogenous vasodilator NO can modulate the degree of vascular injury and subsequent fibro-production. Alterations in NO-cGMP signaling pathways may lead to high vascular contractility and persistent pulmonary hypertension in the newborn. In addition to pulmonary vasoconstriction, its pathogenesis includes injury to pulmonary arteries and their structural remodeling.

The US Food and Drug Administration in 1999 and the European Medicine Evaluation Agency and European Commission in 2001 approved the use of inhaled NO for the treatment of newborns with hypoxic respiratory failure associated with clinical or echocardiographic evidence of pulmonary hypertension. Inhaled NO improves systemic oxygenation and lessens the need for extracorporeal membrane oxygenation in neonatal pulmonary hypertension.[138] The supply of NO is effective in reducing pulmonary vascular resistance through an increase in cGMP. It resolves hypoxemia quickly by redistributing pulmonary blood flow away from the shunt, and toward areas with almost normal ventilation/perfusion ratios. Using NO inhalation to treat neonatal PH can significantly reduce mortality.

REFERENCES

1. Mao C, Shi L, Li N, Xu F, Xu Z. Development of local RAS in cardiovascular/body fluid regulatory systems and hypertension in fetal origins. In: De Luca Jr LA, Menani JV, Johnson AK, editors. *Neurobiology of body fluid homeostasis: transduction and integration. Frontiers in neuroscience*, Boca Raton (FL): CRC Press; 2014.

2. Gao Q, Tang J, Li N, Zhou X, Li Y, Liu Y, et al. A novel mechanism of angiotensin II-regulated placental vascular tone in the development of hypertension in preeclampsia. *Oncotarget* 2017;**8**(19):30734–41.

3. Miyawaki M, Okutani T, Higuchi R, Yoshikawa N. The plasma angiotensin II level increases in very low-birth weight infants with neonatal chronic lung disease. *Early Hum Dev* 2008;**84**(6):375–9.

4. Hodari AA, Smeby R, Bumpus FM. A renin-like substance in the human placenta. *Obstet Gynecol* 1967;**29**(3):313–7.

5. Haugen G, Stray-Pedersen S, Bjoro K. The influence of angiotensin II on prostanoid production in preterm human umbilical arteries. *Gynecol Obstet Invest* 1996;**42**(3):159–62.

6. Tanuma A, Saito S, Ide I, Sasahara H, Yazdani M, Gottschalk S, et al. Caffeine enhances the expression of the angiotensin II Type 2 receptor mRNA in BeWo cell culture and in the rat placenta. *Placenta* 2003;**24**(6):638–47.

7. Soto SF, Melo JO, Marchesi GD, Lopes KL, Veras MM, Oliveira IB, et al. Exposure to fine particulate matter in the air alters placental structure and the renin-angiotensin system. *PLoS One* 2017;**12**(8).

8. Gao H, Yallampalli U, Yallampalli C. Maternal protein restriction reduces expression of angiotensin I-converting enzyme 2 in rat placental labyrinth zone in late pregnancy. *Biol Reprod* 2012;**86**(2):31.

9. Goyal R, Lister R, Leitzke A, Goyal D, Gheorghe CP, Longo LD. Antenatal maternal hypoxic stress: adaptations of the placental renin-angiotensin system in the mouse. *Placenta* 2011;**32**(2):134–9.

10. Glance DG, Elder MG, Myatt L. Prostaglandin production and stimulation by angiotensin II in the isolated perfused human placental cotyledon. *Am J Obstet Gynecol* 1985;**151**(3):387–91.

11. Petit A, Gallo-Payet N, Vaillancourt C, Bellabarba D, Lehoux JG, Belisle S. A role for extracellular calcium in the regulation of placental lactogen release by angiotensin-II and dopamine in human term trophoblastic cells. *J Clin Endocrinol Metab* 1993;**77**(3):670–6.

12. Kalenga MK, de Gasparo M, Thomas K, De Hertogh R. Angiotensin II induces human placental lactogen and pregnancy-specific beta 1-glycoprotein secretion via an angiotensin AT1 receptor. *Eur J Pharmacol* 1994;**268**(2):231–6.

13. Petraglia F, Sutton S, Vale W. Neurotransmitters and peptides modulate the release of immunoreactive corticotropin-releasing factor from cultured human placental cells. *Am J Obstet Gynecol* 1989;**160**(1):247–51.

14. Kalenga MK, De Gasparo M, Thomas K, De Hertogh R. Down-regulation of angiotensin AT1 receptor by progesterone in human placenta. *J Clin Endocrinol Metab* 1996;**81**(3):998–1002.

15. Mancina R, Susini T, Renzetti A, Forti G, Razzoli E, Serio M, et al. Sex steroid modulation of AT2 receptors in human myometrium. *J Clin Endocrinol Metab* 1996;**81**(5):1753–7.

16. Karteris E, Goumenou A, Koumantakis E, Hillhouse EW, Grammatopoulos DK. Reduced expression of corticotropin-releasing hormone receptor type-1 alpha in human preeclamptic and growth-restricted placentas. *J Clin Endocrinol Metab* 2003;**88**(1):363–70.

17. Karteris E, Vatish M, Hillhouse EW, Grammatopoulos DK. Preeclampsia is associated with impaired regulation of the placental nitric oxide-cyclic guanosine monophosphate pathway by corticotropin-releasing hormone (CRH) and CRH-related peptides. *J Clin Endocrinol Metab* 2005;**90**(6):3680–7.

18. Bharadwaj MS, Strawn WB, Groban L, Yamaleyeva LM, Chappell MC, Horta C, et al. Angiotensin-converting enzyme 2 deficiency is associated with impaired gestational weight gain and fetal growth restriction. *Hypertension* 2011;**58**(5):852–8.

19. Schutz S, Le Moullec JM, Corvol P, Gasc JM. Early expression of all the components of the renin-angiotensin-system in human development. *Am J Pathol* 1996;**149**(6):2067–79.

20. Mounier F, Hinglais N, Sich M, Gros F, Lacoste M, Deris Y, et al. Ontogenesis of angiotensin-I converting enzyme in human kidney. *Kidney Int* 1987;**32**(5):684–90.

21. Sulemanji M, Vakili K. Neonatal renal physiology. *Semin Pediatr Surg* 2013;**22**(4):195–8.

22. Daikha-Dahmane F, Levy-Beff E, Jugie M, Lenclen R. Foetal kidney maldevelopment in maternal use of angiotensin II type I receptor antagonists. *Pediatr Nephrol* 2006;**21**(5):729–32.

23. Plazanet C, Arrondel C, Chavant F, Gubler MC. Fetal renin-angiotensin-system blockade syndrome: renal lesions. *Pediatr Nephrol* 2014;**29**(7):1221–30.

24. Guron G, Sundelin B, Wickman A, Friberg P. Angiotensin-converting enzyme inhibition in piglets induces persistent renal abnormalities. *Clin Exp Pharmacol Physiol* 1998;**25**(2):88–91.

25. Martinovic J, Benachi A, Laurent N, Daikha-Dahmane F, Gubler MC. Fetal toxic effects and angiotensin-II-receptor antagonists. *Lancet* 2001;**358**(9277):241–2.

26. Friberg P, Sundelin B, Bohman SO, Bobik A, Nilsson H, Wickman A, et al. Renin-angiotensin system in neonatal rats: induction of a renal abnormality in response to ACE inhibition or angiotensin II antagonism. *Kidney Int* 1994;**45**(2):485–92.

27. Tufro-McReddie A, Romano LM, Harris JM, Ferder L, Gomez RA. Angiotensin II regulates nephrogenesis and renal vascular development. *Am J Physiol* 1995;**269**(1 Pt 2):F110–5.

28. Bos-Thompson MA, Hillaire-Buys D, Muller F, Dechaud H, Mazurier E, Boulot P, et al. Fetal toxic effects of angiotensin II receptor antagonists: case report and follow-up after birth. *Ann Pharmacother* 2005;**39**(1):157–61.

29. Lumbers ER, Burrell JH, Menzies RI, Stevens AD. The effects of a converting enzyme inhibitor (captopril) and angiotensin II on fetal renal function. *Br J Pharmacol* 1993;**110**(2):821–7.

30. Hein L, Barsh GS, Pratt RE, Dzau VJ, Kobilka BK. Behavioural and cardiovascular effects of disrupting the angiotensin II type-2 receptor in mice. *Nature* 1995;**377**(6551):744–7.

31. Takahashi N, Lopez ML, Cowhig Jr. JE, Taylor MA, Hatada T, Riggs E, et al. Ren1c homozygous null mice are hypotensive and polyuric, but heterozygotes are indistinguishable from wild-type. *J Am Soc Nephrol* 2005;**16**(1):125–32.

32. Tsuchida S, Matsusaka T, Chen X, Okubo S, Niimura F, Nishimura H, et al. Murine double nullizygotes of the angiotensin type 1A and 1B receptor genes duplicate severe abnormal phenotypes of angiotensinogen nullizygotes. *J Clin Invest* 1998;**101**(4):755–60.

33. Nagata M, Murakami K, Watanabe T. Renal manifestations in angiotensinogen-deficient mice: unexpected phenotypes emerge. *Exp Nephrol* 1997;**5**(6):445–8.

34. Hilgers KF, Reddi V, Krege JH, Smithies O, Gomez RA. Aberrant renal vascular morphology and renin expression in mutant mice lacking angiotensin-converting enzyme. *Hypertension* 1997;**29**(1 Pt 2):216–21.

35. Cooper WO, Hernandez-Diaz S, Arbogast PG, Dudley JA, Dyer S, Gideon PS, et al. Major congenital malformations after first-trimester exposure to ACE inhibitors. *N Engl J Med* 2006;**354**(23):2443–51.

36. Painter RC, Roseboom TJ, van Montfrans GA, Bossuyt PM, Krediet RT, Osmond C, et al. Microalbuminuria in adults after prenatal exposure to the Dutch famine. *J Am Soc Nephrol* 2005;**16**(1):189–94.

37. Woods LL, Ingelfinger JR, Nyengaard JR, Rasch R. Maternal protein restriction suppresses the newborn renin-angiotensin system and programs adult hypertension in rats. *Pediatr Res* 2001;**49**(4):460–7.

38. Sahajpal V, Ashton N. Renal function and angiotensin AT1 receptor expression in young rats following intrauterine exposure to a maternal low-protein diet. *Clin Sci* 2003;**104**(6):607–14.

39. Alwasel SH, Kaleem I, Sahajpal V, Ashton N. Maternal protein restriction reduces angiotensin II AT(1) and AT(2) receptor expression in the fetal rat kidney. *Kidney Blood Press Res* 2010;**33**(4):251–9.

40. Balbi AP, Costa RS, Coimbra TM. Postnatal renal development of rats from mothers that received increased sodium intake. *Pediatr Nephrol* 2004;**19**(11):1212–8.

41. Coimbra TM, Francescato HD, Balbi AP, Marin EC, Costa RS. Renal development and blood pressure in offspring from dams submitted to high-sodium intake during pregnancy and lactation. *Int J Nephrol* 2012;**2012**:919128.

42. Digby SN, Masters DG, Blache D, Hynd PI, Revell DK. Offspring born to ewes fed high salt during pregnancy have altered responses to oral salt loads. *Animal* 2010;**4**(1):81–8.

43. Mao C, Liu R, Bo L, Chen N, Li S, Xia S, et al. High-salt diets during pregnancy affected fetal and offspring renal renin-angiotensin system. *J Endocrinol* 2013;**218**(1):61–73.

44. Moritz KM, De Matteo R, Dodic M, Jefferies AJ, Arena D, Wintour EM, et al. Prenatal glucocorticoid exposure in the sheep alters renal development in utero: implications for adult renal function and blood pressure control. *Am J Physiol Regul Integr Comp Physiol* 2011;**301**(2):R500–9.

45. Ortiz LA, Quan A, Weinberg A, Baum M. Effect of prenatal dexamethasone on rat renal development. *Kidney Int* 2001;**59**(5):1663–9.

46. Moritz KM, Johnson K, Douglas-Denton R, Wintour EM, Dodic M. Maternal glucocorticoid treatment programs alterations in the renin-angiotensin system of the ovine fetal kidney. *Endocrinology* 2002;**143**(11):4455–63.

47. Connors N, Valego NK, Carey LC, Figueroa JP, Rose JC. Fetal and postnatal renin secretion in female sheep exposed to prenatal betamethasone. *Reprod Sci* 2010;**17**(3):239–46.

48. Gray SP, Kenna K, Bertram JF, Hoy WE, Yan EB, Bocking AD, et al. Repeated ethanol exposure during late gestation decreases nephron endowment in fetal sheep. *Am J Physiol Regul Integr Comp Physiol* 2008;**295**(2):R568–74.

49. Mao C, Hou J, Ge J, Hu Y, Ding Y, Zhou Y, et al. Changes of renal AT1/AT2 receptors and structures in ovine fetuses following exposure to long-term hypoxia. *Am J Nephrol* 2010;**31**(2):141–50.

50. Hao XQ, Kong T, Zhang SY, Zhao ZS. Alteration of embryonic AT(2)-R and inflammatory cytokines gene expression induced by prenatal exposure to lipopolysaccharide affects renal development. *Exp Toxicol Pathol* 2013;**65**(4):433–9.

51. Mao C, Wu J, Xiao D, Lv J, Ding Y, Xu Z, et al. The effect of fetal and neonatal nicotine exposure on renal development of AT(1) and AT(2) receptors. *Reprod Toxicol* 2009;**27**(2):149–54.

52. Wei Z, Song L, Wei J, Chen T, Chen J, Lin Y, et al. Maternal exposure to di-(2-ethylhexyl)phthalate alters kidney development through the renin-angiotensin system in offspring. *Toxicol Lett* 2012;**212**(2):212–21.

53. van Esch JH, Gembardt F, Sterner-Kock A, Heringer-Walther S, Le TH, Lassner D, et al. Cardiac phenotype and angiotensin II levels in AT1a, AT1b, and AT2 receptor single, double, and triple knockouts. *Cardiovasc Res* 2010;**86**(3):401–9.

54. Hutchinson HG, Hein L, Fujinaga M, Pratt RE. Modulation of vascular development and injury by angiotensin II. *Cardiovasc Res* 1999;**41**(3):689–700.

55. Nakajima M, Hutchinson HG, Fujinaga M, Hayashida W, Morishita R, Zhang L, et al. The angiotensin II type 2 (AT2) receptor antagonizes the growth effects of the AT1 receptor: gain-of-function study using gene transfer. *Proc Natl Acad Sci USA* 1995;**92**(23):10663–7.

56. Gembardt F, Heringer-Walther S, van Esch JH, Sterner-Kock A, van Veghel R, Le TH, et al. Cardiovascular phenotype of mice lacking all three subtypes of angiotensin II receptors. *FASEB J* 2008;**22**(8):3068–77.

57. Shi L, Mao C, Zeng F, Hou J, Zhang H, Xu Z. Central angiotensin I increases fetal AVP neuron activity and pressor responses. *Am J Physiol Endocrinol Metab* 2010;**298**(6):E1274–82.

58. Xu Z, Shi L, Yao J. Central angiotensin II-induced pressor responses and neural activity in utero and hypothalamic angiotensin receptors in preterm ovine fetus. *Am J Physiol Heart Circ Physiol* 2004;**286**(4):H1507–14.

59. Shi L, Mao C, Wu J, Morrissey P, Lee J, Xu Z. Effects of i.c.v. losartan on the angiotensin II-mediated vasopressin release and hypothalamic fos expression in near-term ovine fetuses. *Peptides* 2006;**27**(9):2230–8.

60. Kawamura M, Itoh H, Yura S, Mogami H, Suga S, Makino H, et al. Undernutrition in utero augments systolic blood pressure and cardiac remodeling in adult mouse offspring: possible involvement of local cardiac angiotensin system in developmental origins of cardiovascular disease. *Endocrinology* 2007;**148**(3):1218–25.

61. Friedrich RH. Ambulatory care: organization and operation. *Bull N Y Acad Med* 1973;**49**(5):379–92.

62. Zhu X, Gao Q, Tu Q, Zhong Y, Zhu D, Mao C, et al. Prenatal hypoxia enhanced angiotensin II-mediated vasoconstriction via increased oxidative signaling in fetal rats. *Reprod Toxicol* 2016;**60**:21–8.

63. Edwards LJ, McMillen IC. Maternal undernutrition increases arterial blood pressure in the sheep fetus during late gestation. *J Physiol* 2001;**533**(Pt 2):561–70.

64. Nishina H, Green LR, McGarrigle HH, Noakes DE, Poston L, Hanson MA. Effect of nutritional restriction in early pregnancy on isolated femoral artery function in mid-gestation fetal sheep. *J Physiol* 2003;**553**(Pt 2):637–47.

65. Gilbert JS, Lang AL, Nijland MJ. Maternal nutrient restriction and the fetal left ventricle: decreased angiotensin receptor expression. *Reprod Biol Endocrinol* 2005;**3**:27.

66. Segar JL, Bedell KA, Smith OJ. Glucocorticoid modulation of cardiovascular and autonomic function in preterm lambs: role of ANG II. *Am J Physiol Regul Integr Comp Physiol* 2001;**280**(3):R646–54.

67. Reini SA, Wood CE, Jensen E, Keller-Wood M. Increased maternal cortisol in late-gestation ewes decreases fetal cardiac expression of 11beta-HSD2 mRNA and the ratio of AT1 to AT2 receptor mRNA. *Am J Physiol Regul Integr Comp Physiol* 2006;**291**(6):R1708–16.

68. Yang H, Wang X, Raizada MK. Characterization of signal transduction pathway in neurotropic action of angiotensin II in brain neurons. *Endocrinology* 2001;**142**(8):3502–11.

69. Fitzsimons JT. Angiotensin, thirst, and sodium appetite. *Physiol Rev* 1998;**78**(3):583–686.

70. El-Haddad MA, Chao CR, Sayed AA, El-Haddad H, Ross MG. Effects of central angiotensin II receptor antagonism on fetal swallowing and cardiovascular activity. *Am J Obstet Gynecol* 2001;**185**(4):828–33.

71. Goyal R, Goyal D, Leitzke A, Gheorghe CP, Longo LD. Brain renin-angiotensin system: fetal epigenetic programming by maternal protein restriction during pregnancy. *Reprod Sci* 2010;**17**(3):227–38.

72. Dodic M, Abouantoun T, O'Connor A, Wintour EM, Moritz KM. Programming effects of short prenatal exposure to dexamethasone in sheep. *Hypertension* 2002;**40**(5):729–34.

73. Dodic M, McAlinden AT, Jefferies AJ, Wintour EM, Cock ML, May CN, et al. Differential effects of prenatal exposure to dexamethasone or cortisol on circulatory control mechanisms mediated by angiotensin II in the central nervous system of adult sheep. *J Physiol* 2006;**571**(Pt 3):651–60.

74. Mao C, Zhang H, Xiao D, Zhu L, Ding Y, Zhang Y, et al. Perinatal nicotine exposure alters AT 1 and AT 2 receptor expression pattern in the brain of fetal and offspring rats. *Brain Res* 2008;**1243**:47–52.

75. Zhang H, Fan Y, Xia F, Geng C, Mao C, Jiang S, et al. Prenatal water deprivation alters brain angiotensin system and dipsogenic changes in the offspring. *Brain Res* 2011;**1382**:128–36.

76. Blencowe H, Cousens S, Chou D, Oestergaard M, Say L, Moller AB, et al. Born too soon: the global epidemiology of 15 million preterm births. *Reprod Health* 2013;**10**(Suppl 1):S2.

77. Kim YM, Bujold E, Chaiworapongsa T, Gomez R, Yoon BH, Thaler HT, et al. Failure of physiologic transformation of the spiral arteries in patients with preterm labor and intact membranes. *Am J Obstet Gynecol* 2003;**189**(4):1063–9.

78. Richer C, Hornych H, Amiel-Tison C, Relier JP, Giudicelli JF. Plasma renin activity and its postnatal development in preterm infants. Preliminary report. *Biol Neonate* 1977;**31**(5–6):301–4.

79. Suzue M, Urushihara M, Nakagawa R, Saijo T, Kagami S. Urinary angiotensinogen level is increased in preterm neonates. *Clin Exp Nephrol* 2015;**19**(2):293–7.

80. Valdez-Velazquez LL, Quintero-Ramos A, Perez SA, Mendoza-Carrera F, Montoya-Fuentes H, Rivas Jr F, et al. Genetic polymorphisms of the renin-angiotensin system in preterm delivery and premature rupture of membranes. *J Renin Angiotensin Aldosterone Syst* 2007;**8**(4):160–8.

81. Uma R, Forsyth JS, Struthers AD, Fraser CG, Godfrey V, Murphy DJ. Correlation of angiotensin converting enzyme activity and the genotypes of the I/D polymorphism in the ACE gene with preterm birth and birth weight. *Eur J Obstet Gynecol Reprod Biol* 2008;**141**(1):27–30.

82. Zhang G, Feenstra B, Bacelis J, Liu X, Muglia LM, Juodakis J, et al. Genetic associations with gestational duration and spontaneous preterm birth. *N Engl J Med* 2017;**377**(12):1156–67.

83. Lee JH, Kwon YE, Park JT, Lee MJ, Oh HJ, Han SH, et al. The effect of renin-angiotensin system blockade on renal protection in chronic kidney disease patients with hyperkalemia. *J Renin Angiotensin Aldosterone Syst* 2014;**15**(4):491–7.

84. Barker DJ. The origins of the developmental origins theory. *J Intern Med* 2007;**261**(5):412–7.

85. Vehaskari VM, Aviles DH, Manning J. Prenatal programming of adult hypertension in the rat. *Kidney Int* 2001;**59**(1):238–45.

86. Navar LG, Harrison-Bernard LM, Nishiyama A, Kobori H. Regulation of intrarenal angiotensin II in hypertension. *Hypertension* 2002;**39**(2 Pt 2):316–22.

87. Ortiz LA, Quan A, Zarzar F, Weinberg A, Baum M. Prenatal dexamethasone programs hypertension and renal injury in the rat. *Hypertension* 2003;**41**(2):328–34.

88. Tain YL, Chen CC, Sheen JM, Yu HR, Tiao MM, Kuo HC, et al. Melatonin attenuates prenatal dexamethasone-induced blood pressure increase in a rat model. *J Am Soc Hypertens* 2014;**8**(4):216–26.

89. Tain YL, Wu MS, Lin YJ. Sex differences in renal transcriptome and programmed hypertension in offspring exposed to prenatal dexamethasone. *Steroids* 2016;**115**:40–6.

90. Singh RR, Cullen-McEwen LA, Kett MM, Boon WM, Dowling J, Bertram JF, et al. Prenatal corticosterone exposure results in altered AT1/AT2, nephron deficit and hypertension in the rat offspring. *J Physiol* 2007;**579**(Pt 2):503–13.

91. Cuffe JS, Burgess DJ, O'Sullivan L, Singh RR, Moritz KM. Maternal corticosterone exposure in the mouse programs sex-specific renal adaptations in the renin-angiotensin-aldosterone system in 6-month offspring. *Physiol Rep* 2016;**4**(8).

92. Cabral EV, Vieira-Filho LD, Silva PA, Nascimento WS, Aires RS, Oliveira FS, et al. Perinatal Na+ overload programs raised renal proximal Na+ transport and enalapril-sensitive alterations of Ang II signaling pathways during adulthood. *PLoS One* 2012;**7**(8).

93. Marin EC, Balbi AP, Francescato HD, Alves da Silva CG, Costa RS, Coimbra TM. Renal structure and function evaluation of rats from dams that received increased sodium intake during pregnancy and lactation submitted or not to 5/6 nephrectomy. *Ren Fail* 2008;**30**(5):547–55.

94. da Silva AA, de Noronha IL, de Oliveira IB, Malheiros DM, Heimann JC. Renin-angiotensin system function and blood pressure in adult rats after perinatal salt overload. *Nutr Metab Cardiovasc Dis* 2003;**13**(3):133–9.

95. Grigore D, Ojeda NB, Robertson EB, Dawson AS, Huffman CA, Bourassa EA, et al. Placental insufficiency results in temporal alterations in the renin angiotensin system in male hypertensive growth restricted offspring. *Am J Physiol Regul Integr Comp Physiol* 2007;**293**(2):R804–11.

96. Ojeda NB, Royals TP, Black JT, Dasinger JH, Johnson JM, Alexander BT. Enhanced sensitivity to acute angiotensin II is testosterone dependent in adult male growth-restricted offspring. *Am J Physiol Regul Integr Comp Physiol* 2010;**298**(5):R1421–7.

97. Ojeda NB, Intapad S, Royals TP, Black JT, Dasinger JH, Tull FL, et al. Hypersensitivity to acute ANG II in female growth-restricted offspring is exacerbated by ovariectomy. *Am J Physiol Regul Integr Comp Physiol* 2011;**301**(4):R1199–205.

98. Gribouval O, Moriniere V, Pawtowski A, Arrondel C, Sallinen SL, Saloranta C, et al. Spectrum of mutations in the renin-angiotensin system genes in autosomal recessive renal tubular dysgenesis. *Hum Mutat* 2012;**33**(2):316–26.

99. Gubler MC. Renal tubular dysgenesis. *Pediatr Nephrol* 2014;**29**(1):51–9.

100. Zivna M, Hulkova H, Matignon M, Hodanova K, Vylet'al P, Kalbacova M, et al. Dominant renin gene mutations associated with early-onset hyperuricemia, anemia, and chronic kidney failure. *Am J Hum Genet* 2009;**85**(2):204–13.

101. Kmoch S, Zivna M, Bleyer AJ. Autosomal dominant tubulointerstitial kidney disease, REN-related. In: Adam MP, Ardinger HH, Pagon RA, Wallace SE, LJH B, Stephens K, et al. editors. *GeneReviews((R))*; 1993. Seattle (WA).

102. Monticone S, Else T, Mulatero P, Williams TA, Rainey WE. Understanding primary aldosteronism: impact of next generation sequencing and expression profiling. *Mol Cell Endocrinol* 2015;**399**:311–20.

103. Torpy DJ, Stratakis CA, Chrousos GP. Hyper- and hypoaldosteronism. *Vitam Horm* 1999;**57**:177–216.

104. Zhang G, Rodriguez H, Fardella CE, Harris DA, Miller WL. Mutation T318M in the CYP11B2 gene encoding P450c11AS (aldosterone synthase) causes corticosterone methyl oxidase II deficiency. *Am J Hum Genet* 1995;**57**(5):1037–43.

105. Mizsak SA, Hoeksema H, Pschigoda LM. The chemistry of rubradirin. II. Rubranitrose. *J Antibiot* 1979;**32**(7):771–2.

106. Smith-Jackson K, Hentschke MR, Poli-de-Figueiredo CE, Pinheiro da Costa BE, Kurlak LO, Broughton Pipkin F, et al. Placental expression of eNOS, iNOS and the major protein components of caveolae in women with pre-eclampsia. *Placenta* 2015;**36**(5):607–10.

107. Myatt L, Eis AL, Brockman DE, Greer IA, Lyall F. Endothelial nitric oxide synthase in placental villous tissue from normal, pre-eclamptic and intrauterine growth restricted pregnancies. *Hum Reprod* 1997;**12**(1):167–72.

108. King RG, Di Iulio JL, Gude NM, Brennecke SP. Effect of asymmetric dimethyl arginine on nitric oxide synthase activity in normal and pre-eclamptic placentae. *Reprod Fertil Dev* 1995;**7**(6):1581–4.

109. Farrow KN, Lakshminrusimha S, Reda WJ, Wedgwood S, Czech L, Gugino SF, et al. Superoxide dismutase restores eNOS expression and function in resistance pulmonary arteries from neonatal lambs with persistent pulmonary hypertension. *Am J Physiol Lung Cell Mol Physiol* 2008;**295**(6): L979–87.

110. Fujiyama S, Matsubara H, Nozawa Y, Maruyama K, Mori Y, Tsutsumi Y, et al. Angiotensin AT(1) and AT(2) receptors differentially regulate angiopoietin-2 and vascular endothelial growth factor expression and angiogenesis by modulating heparin binding-epidermal growth factor (EGF)-mediated EGF receptor transactivation. *Circ Res* 2001;**88**(1):22–9.

111. Conrad KP, Joffe GM, Kruszyna H, Kruszyna R, Rochelle LG, Smith RP, et al. Identification of increased nitric oxide biosynthesis during pregnancy in rats. *FASEB J* 1993;**7**(6):566–71.

112. Ramesar SV, Mackraj I, Gathiram P, Moodley J. Sildenafil citrate improves fetal outcomes in pregnant, L-NAME treated, Sprague-Dawley rats. *Eur J Obstet Gynecol Reprod Biol* 2010;**149**(1):22–6.

113. Helmbrecht GD, Farhat MY, Lochbaum L, Brown HE, Yadgarova KT, Eglinton GS, et al. L-arginine reverses the adverse pregnancy changes induced by nitric oxide synthase inhibition in the rat. *Am J Obstet Gynecol* 1996;**175**(4 Pt 1):800–5.

114. Ong SS, Moore RJ, Warren AY, Crocker IP, Fulford J, Tyler DJ, et al. Myometrial and placental artery reactivity alone cannot explain reduced placental perfusion in pre-eclampsia and intrauterine growth restriction. *BJOG* 2003;**110**(10):909–15.

115. Ong SS, Crocker IP, Warren AY, Baker PN. Functional characteristics of chorionic plate placental arteries from normal pregnant women and women with pre-eclampsia. *Hypertens Pregnancy* 2002;**21**(3):175–83.

116. Sastry BV. Human placental cholinergic system. *Biochem Pharmacol* 1997;**53**(11):1577–86.

117. Gao Q, Tang J, Li N, Liu B, Zhang M, Sun M, Xu Z. What is precise pathophysiology in development of hypertension in pregnancy? Precision medicine requires precise physiology and pathophysiology. *Drug Discov Today* 2018;**23**(2):286–99.

118. Gao Q, Tang J, Li N, Zhou X, Zhu X, Li W, et al. New conception for the development of hypertension in preeclampsia. *Oncotarget* 2016;**7**(48):78387–95.

119. Vasquez G, Sanhueza F, Vasquez R, Gonzalez M, San Martin R, Casanello P, et al. Role of adenosine transport in gestational diabetes-induced L-arginine transport and nitric oxide synthesis in human umbilical vein endothelium. *J Physiol* 2004;**560**(Pt 1):111–22.

120. Westermeier F, Salomon C, Gonzalez M, Puebla C, Guzman-Gutierrez E, Cifuentes F, et al. Insulin restores gestational diabetes mellitus-reduced adenosine transport involving differential expression of insulin receptor isoforms in human umbilical vein endothelium. *Diabetes* 2011;**60**(6):1677–87.

121. Knock GA, McCarthy AL, Lowy C, Poston L. Association of gestational diabetes with abnormal maternal vascular endothelial function. *Br J Obstet Gynaecol* 1997;**104**(2):229–34.

122. Mayer C, Joseph KS. Fetal growth: a review of terms, concepts and issues relevant to obstetrics. *Ultrasound Obstet Gynecol* 2013;**41**(2):136–45.

123. Jobgen WS, Ford SP, Jobgen SC, Feng CP, Hess BW, Nathanielsz PW, et al. Baggs ewes adapt to maternal undernutrition and maintain conceptus growth by maintaining fetal plasma concentrations of amino acids. *J Anim Sci* 2008;**86**(4):820–6.

124. Myatt L, Brockman DE, Langdon G, Pollock JS. Constitutive calcium-dependent isoform of nitric oxide synthase in the human placental villous vascular tree. *Placenta* 1993;**14**(4):373–83.

125. Hefler LA, Reyes CA, O'Brien WE, Gregg AR. Perinatal development of endothelial nitric oxide synthase-deficient mice. *Biol Reprod* 2001;**64**(2):666–73.

126. Thompson RS, Trudinger BJ, Cook CM. Doppler ultrasound waveforms in the fetal umbilical artery: quantitative analysis technique. *Ultrasound Med Biol* 1985;**11**(5):707–18.

127. Hemmings DG, Williams SJ, Davidge ST. Increased myogenic tone in 7-month-old adult male but not female offspring from rat dams exposed to hypoxia during pregnancy. *Am J Physiol Heart Circ Physiol* 2005;**289**(2):H674–82.

128. Ghabour MS, Eis AL, Brockman DE, Pollock JS, Myatt L. Immunohistochemical characterization of placental nitric oxide synthase expression in preeclampsia. *Am J Obstet Gynecol* 1995;**173**(3 Pt 1):687–94.

129. Zhang HK, Luo FW, Geng Q, Li J, Liu QZ, Chen WB, et al. Analysis of fetal chromosomal karyotype and etiology in 252 cases of early spontaneous abortion. *Zhonghua Yi Xue Yi Chuan Xue Za Zhi* 2011;**28**(5):575–8.

130. Weigent DA, Stanton GJ, Johnson HM. Interleukin 2 enhances natural killer cell activity through induction of gamma interferon. *Infect Immun* 1983;**41**(3):992–7.

131. Baines MG, Duclos AJ, Antecka E, Haddad EK. Decidual infiltration and activation of macrophages leads to early embryo loss. *Am J Reprod Immunol* 1997;**37**(6):471–7.

132. Jablonka-Shariff A, Ravi S, Beltsos AN, Murphy LL, Olson LM. Abnormal estrous cyclicity after disruption of endothelial and inducible nitric oxide synthase in mice. *Biol Reprod* 1999;**61**(1):171–7.

133. Tempfer C, Moreno RM, O'Brien WE, Gregg AR. Genetic contributions of the endothelial nitric oxide synthase gene to ovulation and menopause in a mouse model. *Fertil Steril* 2000;**73**(5):1025–31.

134. Huang J, Roby KF, Pace JL, Russell SW, Hunt JS. Cellular localization and hormonal regulation of inducible nitric oxide synthase in cycling mouse uterus. *J Leukoc Biol* 1995;**57**(1):27–35.

135. Madonna R, De Caterina R, Geng YJ. Epigenetic regulation of insulin-like growth factor signaling: a novel insight into the pathophysiology of neonatal pulmonary hypertension. *Vascul Pharmacol* 2015;**73**:4–7.

136. Pearson DL, Dawling S, Walsh WF, Haines JL, Christman BW, Bazyk A, et al. Neonatal pulmonary hypertension–urea-cycle intermediates, nitric oxide production, and carbamoyl-phosphate synthetase function. *N Engl J Med* 2001;**344**(24):1832–8.

137. Sood BG, Wykes S, Landa M, De Jesus L, Rabah R. Expression of eNOS in the lungs of neonates with pulmonary hypertension. *Exp Mol Pathol* 2011;**90**(1):9–12.

138. Clark RH, Kueser TJ, Walker MW, Southgate WM, Huckaby JL, Perez JA, et al. Low-dose nitric oxide therapy for persistent pulmonary hypertension of the newborn. Clinical Inhaled Nitric Oxide Research Group. *N Engl J Med* 2000;**342**(7):469–74.

Chapter 50

Obesity/Perinatal Origins of Obesity

T'ng Chang Kwok*, Shalini Ojha[†,‡] and Michael E. Symonds*

*Division of Child Health, Obstetrics and Gynaecology, University of Nottingham, Nottingham, United Kingdom, [†]Division of Medical Sciences and Graduate Entry Medicine, School of Medicine, University of Nottingham, Derby, United Kingdom, [‡]Neonatal Intensive Care Unit, Derby Teaching Hospitals NHS Foundation Trust, Derby, United Kingdom

Common Clinical Problems

- There is mounting evidence to support the "Developmental Origins of Health and Disease" concept, which depicts the perinatal origins of obesity.
- Dysregulation of the hypothalamus-adipose axis, through changes in the concentrations of circulating factors and potential epigenetic modifications, is considered to cause perinatal programming of obesity in later life in response to perinatal insults such as maternal malnutrition and rapid weight gain postnatally.
- Obesity in early life is not only associated with long-term obesity in adulthood. It is also associated with metabolic, cardiorespiratory, orthopedic, and psychological disorders in childhood.
- A better measure of obesity in early life would be one that discriminates between fat and fat-free mass in order to provide a better understanding of the perinatal programming of obesity and aid in determining the optimum gain in growth parameters.
- Future studies should identify early life modifiable determinants of obesity that could be targeted to prevent long-term obesity and its associated disorders.

50.1 BACKGROUND

Obesity is a global phenomenon and poses a significant public health concern. Worldwide prevalence of obesity has tripled over the last 40 years.[1] In 2016, the World Health Organization (WHO) estimated that 13% of adults (11% of men and 15% of women) or 650 million adults are obese.[1] Obesity is no longer just a problem in high-income countries or the developed world; the rate of obesity is increasing in low- and middle-income countries as well, particularly in the urban setting. Globally, there are more adults who are overweight or obese than underweight. This is a major concern, as more deaths worldwide are linked to obesity than factors associated with being underweight. Obesity is one of the most important risk factors for ischemic heart disease and premature death in adults.[2]

The situation is similar in children. The prevalence of obesity in children less than 5 years of age has increased by more than a quarter in 25 years to 41 million children in 2016.[3] Interestingly, the rate of increase in the prevalence of obesity in these children is 30% faster in developing than in developed countries.[1] In 2016, nearly half of children under 5 years of age living in Asia were overweight or obese.[1] The number of overweight children under 5 years of age has also increased by nearly 50% in Africa over the last 15 years.[1] If the current trend continues, it is estimated that the prevalence of obesity in children less than 5 years of age will reach 70 million by 2025.[3] This is alarming, as epidemiological studies have found that infant and childhood obesity persist to adulthood, alongside the associated health risks.[4]

In view of the significant public health impact of obesity, various international and government agencies have attempted to put in place a wide range of initiatives aimed at reducing and preventing obesity in children and adults with limited success. However, current evidence suggests that these efforts should also be started very early on in life, even before conception. The concept of the "Developmental Origins of Health and Disease," or DOHAD, suggests a perinatal origin of obesity.[5] Changes during the critical period of development very early on in life may permanently alter the physiological function and metabolism, leading to long-term diseases.[4,6]

This chapter aims to explore how perinatal changes lead to the development of obesity, including its pathophysiology and long-term manifestations. A better appreciation of the perinatal origins of obesity will improve efforts aimed to prevent obesity by targeting the critical period of early life development.

Maternal-Fetal and Neonatal Endocrinology. https://doi.org/10.1016/B978-0-12-814823-5.00051-9

50.2 WHAT IS OBESITY?

Obesity occurs when there is an imbalance between the intake and expenditure of energy. This leads to an abnormal accumulation of fat that has important health consequences such as obesity, diabetes, and cardiovascular disorders.

In adults, body mass index (BMI) is a useful epidemiological tool in measuring obesity at a population level. BMI is derived from an individual's weight in kilograms divided by the square value of the height in meters. An adult is defined as obese if the BMI is above 30kg/m^2.[1] As BMI varies with age, the definition of obesity in children is more difficult. The WHO defined obesity in children between 5 and 19 years of age as BMI greater than two standard deviations above the WHO Growth Reference median.[3] In children less than 5 years of age, obesity is defined as weight for height greater than three standard deviations above the WHO Child Growth Standard medians.[3] However, it is important to note that BMI is only a rough guide and not a true measure of the amount of fat in an individual. Obesity is even more difficult and complex to define in the context of the fetus and neonate.

50.2.1 Fetal Macrosomia

Fetal macrosomia is a term often used in obstetrics as a description of excessive fetal growth and refers to an infant who was born large for gestational age. Fetal macrosomia is not only associated with a higher risk of birth complications and metabolic disturbances during the neonatal period; an infant who is macrosomic is also at a greater risk of becoming obese in adulthood, alongside its associated cardiovascular and metabolic diseases.[7]

There is a lack of consensus in defining fetal macrosomia. It is commonly defined either as an absolute birthweight value above 4000, 4500, or 5000 g, or as birthweight above the 90th, 95th, or 97th percentile for the infant's gestational age.[8] However, these definitions do not provide information on fetal obesity, as they do not discriminate between normal and abnormal body compositions. Besides the inconsistency in the definition of *fetal macrosomia*, the measurement of fetal macrosomia antenatally, using either clinical findings or diagnostic imaging, is also fraught with difficulty.

50.2.1.1 Clinical Findings

Prediction of fetal macrosomia based on clinical findings is poor, with detection rates between 40% and 50%.[9] Measurement of symphysis-fundal height was found to predict fetal macrosomia better than just abdominal palpation. Plotting the measured symphysis-fundal height on a customized growth chart improved the detection of fetal macrosomia antenatally. A Cochrane review, however, found insufficient evidence to evaluate the use of symphysis-fundal height measurement in antenatal care,[10] but it may not be prudent to abandon its use unless larger clinical studies find it ineffective.

50.2.1.2 Ultrasonography

Ultrasonography is a commonly used imaging modality during pregnancy to monitor fetal growth. However, the image quality is limited by multiple factors, including the sonographer experience and maternal adiposity. There are various sonographic formulations to estimate fetal weight, such as the Hadlock formula, and recent updates have taken into account measures of fetal adiposity. These include measures of the fetal upper arm or thigh subcutaneous tissue thickness, fetal cheek-to-cheek diameter, and fetal anterior abdominal wall width.[8]

There is a large deviation among the sonographic formulations, as they are derived from a heterogeneous group and are not meant to estimate fetal weight on the upper limit of the scale. Hence there is an ongoing debate as to which is best for predicting fetal macrosomia.[8] A review of 20 studies[11] found the posttest probability for identifying fetal macrosomia sonographically to differ greatly, from 15% to 79%. The variation in accuracy was found to not be affected by the formulation used, the interval between ultrasonography and delivery of the fetus, or the experience of the sonographer. The performance of 36 commonly used sonographic formulations in estimating the fetal weight to identify fetal macrosomia was also recently reviewed.[12] It concluded that there was no sonographic formulation that reached an appropriate detection rate to be recommended in routine clinical practice. Some studies even suggest that these sonographic formulations are no better at predicting fetal macrosomia than clinical predictors.[8]

Apart from identifying fetal macrosomia, sonography could be used to perform Doppler studies on the umbilical cord and ductus venosus blood flow. These may provide an early indicator of the physiological changes leading to obesity. Ductus venosus shunts well-oxygenated placental blood from the liver to the brain and heart. A study of a cohort of 381 women with low-risk pregnancy in Southampton[13] found that women with lower adiposity and healthier diet had lower ductus venosus blood shunting and higher hepatic blood flow on Doppler sonography. This is in contrast to cases of placental insufficiency, where there is reduced hepatic and increased ductus venosus blood shunting, which is characteristic of the brain-sparing response to fetal hypoxemia.

50.2.1.3 Magnetic Resonance Imaging

Magnetic resonance imaging (MRI) has also been used to identify fetal macrosomia. A recent systematic review found MRI to be superior to 2D or 3D ultrasonography to detect fetal macrosomia.[14] Meta-analysis of the three MRI studies of 117 women found a sensitivity of 0.82 (95% confidence interval [CI] of 0.60–0.95) and specificity of 0.98 (95% CI of 0.92–1.00) in using MRI to predict birthweight above the 90th percentile.[14] However, since the finding is based on a small sample size and measurement, a further diagnostic accuracy study is needed.

50.2.2 Neonatal Obesity

The measurement of obesity in neonates is also fraught with difficulties due to the lack of consensus on its definition and the ideal way of measuring obesity.

50.2.2.1 Body Mass Index

BMI can be measured in the newborn and expressed as a Z score or standard deviation score to take into account gestational age and sex. Although BMI provides information on the nutritional status in adult whereby adults with a high BMI are associated with metabolic syndrome and cardiovascular disorder, this relationship in the newborn infant is unclear. Moreover, BMI may not provide a true reflection of body composition, as it does not distinguish between fat and fat-free mass. For example, an infant with low BMI may have higher relative body fat mass with a lower fraction of fat-free mass than another infant with a higher BMI. This is crucial, as it is the abnormal accumulation of body fat in childhood that leads to long-term obesity and health consequences.[15]

50.2.2.2 Body Composition

Body composition measurement provides a better reflection of obesity and its associated long-term health outcomes. However, the lack of reference data makes it hard to interpret individual measurements, so they are not widely used in clinical practice.[16] Furthermore, there are various techniques incorporating a variety of theoretical assumptions in estimating the fat and fat-free mass with variable agreement.[16]

Skinfold thickness is a quick, commonly used method of measuring body composition with low intra- and interobserver variability. Although there are formulas to predict the percentage of total body fat using skinfold thickness, it is a measure of regional adiposity rather than total body fat. Its accuracy and precision are also noted to be reduced in obese children.[17]

The isotope (deuterium) dilution is another method of measuring body composition. Total body water is the main component in fat-free mass. Hence, if the ratio of total body water to fat-free mass is known, fat mass can be estimated. A small amount of water labeled with a nonradioactive trace of deuterium is administered to the infant. Isotope-ratio mass spectrometry is then used to analyze subsequent urine samples to estimate the total body water.[17] The ratio of the total body water to the fat-free mass is fairly constant in healthy infants. However, in diseased states whereby the hydration status of the infants is affected, there may be high variability in the ratio. Besides, this method cannot be carried out easily in clinical practice and is impractical in newborn infants.

Bioelectric impedance analysis (BIA) measures the impedance of body to small electric current. It relies on the fact that the body contains intracellular and extracellular fluid that conducts electric current. By knowing the impedance value of human muscle tissue, body composition can be obtained by estimating the fat-free mass.[17] Hence BIA is similarly affected by clinical hydration status and environmental temperature. BIA is not successfully used in infants, as anthropometry alone was found to be a better predictor of fat-free mass than BIA.[18]

Dual energy X-ray absorptiometry was initially developed to assess bone mineral mass by measuring the differential absorption of two different energy X-rays. Using specific algorithms, relative fat and fat-free mass can be obtained using a similar method. Although useful in identifying the direction of change of fat and fat-free mass, there is bias in quantifying fat and fat-free mass accurately.[17]

Densitometry relies on the concept that fat and fat-free mass have different specific densities. Hence body composition can be obtained by measuring body density. A commonly used technique is air displacement plethysmography, which is useful in monitoring changes in body composition over time. However, it is not accurate in cases whereby fat-free mass may be abnormal. For example, this may be due to fluid retention, which lowers the density of fat-free mass. It also conceals the regional variability of fat mass, which may have important health consequences.[17]

MRI was recently used to estimate the volume of adipose tissue in neonates by analyzing the absorption and emission of electromagnetic energy.[19] However, it is difficult to compare the MRI findings with another method of body composition measurement. This is because assumptions need to be made on the fat content and its density in adipose tissue to convert adipose tissue volume to fat mass.[17] The cost and availability of MRI may also limit its widespread use.

50.3 DEVELOPMENTAL ORIGINS OF HEALTH AND DISEASE

The idea of perinatal origins of obesity and the "Developmental Origins of Health and Disease" concept stem from the perinatal programming hypothesis, which is often called the *Barker hypothesis.*[20] This was initially hypothesized from findings obtained from numerous large epidemiological studies. These studies found that the intrauterine and early postnatal periods are critical for the development of long-term health diseases in adulthood, including obesity.

Changes in the environment during this critical period, especially with regard to the metabolic nutritional state, result in the fetus or infant making predictive adaptations to the metabolic physiology, known as the *thrifty phenotype.*[21] These adaptations were meant to improve the chances of survival and success in the long term if the initial changes were to continue into adulthood. However, these adaptations may have a permanent negative impact on organ and tissue structure as well as function. The epigenetic profile of the fetus and infant may be altered as well, leading to changes in gene expression. As a result, the physiological function of the body is permanently altered, potentially leading to energy balance dysfunction and long-term diseases such as obesity, diabetes, and cardiovascular disorder in adulthood. This situation is especially worsened if there is a mismatch between the initial perinatal environment and the postnatal reality.[22,23]

50.3.1 From Epidemiological Studies to DOHAD

The trio of papers published by Barker et al.[24–26] in the *Lancet* in the late 1980s and early 1990s were among the most influential papers that sparked the Barker or perinatal programming hypothesis.

The first paper[24] found a significant geographical correlation between ischemic heart disease in 1968–1978 with infant mortality rates in 1921–1925 across the local authorities in England and Wales. It was proposed that the relationship reflected the variation in early life nutrition being expressed pathologically on exposure to later dietary influences.

The second paper[25] corroborated the findings of the earlier paper and investigated the individual correlation of birthweight and ischemic heart disease. Retrospective analysis of 5654 adult males born between 1911 and 1930 in Hertfordshire was carried out with good perinatal and death from ischemic heart disease records. Men with the lowest birthweight had a higher death rate from ischemic heart disease. Hence the paper concluded that the risk of ischemic heart disease is determined by the initial environment that led to poor fetal and infant growth, followed by an adult environment that determines high risk for ischemic heart disease.

The third paper[26] found evidence for changes in placental and fetal hormones, such as growth hormone and insulin-like growth factor being associated with fetal undernutrition at different gestation. These adaptations permanently alter the structure, function, and metabolism of the body, leading to metabolic and cardiovascular abnormality in adulthood.

Similar studies, such as the Dutch famine cohort study during the end of World War II[27] and Helsinki birth cohort study from 1934 to 1944,[28] also demonstrated similar findings. Early life growth and nutrition affect the development of chronic diseases in adulthood such as obesity, cardiovascular disorders, and metabolic syndrome. The effect of nutrition on long-term outcome also differs, depending on which part of fetal development malnutrition occurs. This will be discussed in more detail as follows.

50.3.2 "U"-Shaped Relationship

Epidemiological studies also found that perinatal programming operates in a nonlinear "U"-shaped curve manner, whereby overnutrition or high birthweight also leads to adult metabolic syndrome alongside undernutrition or low birthweight.[22] Infants who are large or those who are small for gestational age at birth are both noted to share some similarities, suggesting a potential common mechanism for perinatal programming in these two opposite environmental insults.

The size discrepancies seen in these infants are usually selective,[29] whereby head circumference is usually maintained with a disproportionate abdominal circumference, which is increased in large for gestational age infants and reduced in small for gestational age infants. This is postulated to safeguarding the brain at the expense of subcutaneous fat, liver, and spleen.

In addition, both large and small for gestational age infants developed hypoglycemia and poor carbohydrate tolerance in the newborn period.[29] Large for gestational age infants are exposed to excess nutrition in utero, leading to fetal hyperglycemia. This stimulates the fetal pancreas to secrete insulin, causing fetal hyperinsulinemia. As insulin is a growth promoting factor, these infants are born large for gestational age. As the hyperinsulinemia persists postnatally with cessation of the supply of excess nutrition received in utero, they develop hypoglycemia and poor carbohydrate tolerance at birth. Conversely, small for gestational age infants are exposed to undernutrition in utero, leading to fetal hypoglycemia and hypoinsulinemia. This persists postnatally leading to infants being born small, as well as developing hypoglycemia and poor carbohydrate tolerance at birth.

50.4   HYPOTHALAMUS-ADIPOSE AXIS

The hypothalamus-adipose axis (Fig. 50.1) plays a vital role in maintaining energy homeostasis and controls food intake as well as energy expenditure and storage.[30] The axis is a key target of developmental programming in obesity caused by prenatal and perinatal changes.[31] Hence it is crucial to have a good appreciation of the hypothalamus-adipose axis and how it is regulated. This will aid in the understanding of the pathophysiology of perinatal programming of obesity.

50.4.1   Hypothalamus

The hypothalamus develops from the ventral region of the lateral wall of diencephalon known as the alar plate. A key marker of hypothalamic tissue development is the induction of the Nk2 homeobox transcription factor Nkx2.1. The hypothalamus then differentiates into a number of nuclear areas under the influence of various transcription factors. This neurogenesis in hypothalamus occurs in a "lateral-medial" fashion whereby lateral nuclei developed first.[32]

As a result, the hypothalamus contains several nuclei that produce neuropeptides involved in key physiological functions, including appetite regulation.[33] The perinatal period represents a critical period of organization and development of the appetite regulatory pathway in the hypothalamus.[32] Various genetic and environmental factors during the perinatal period alter the structure and function of the appetite regulatory pathway, leading to obesity and chronic metabolic disease in adulthood.

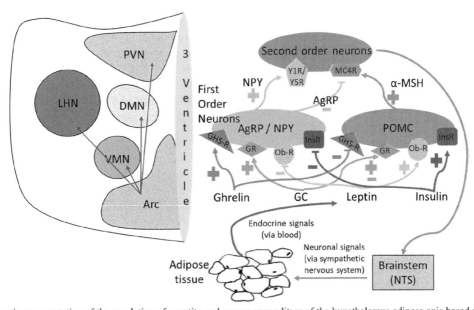

FIG. 50.1   Schematic representation of the regulation of appetite and energy expenditure of the hypothalamus-adipose axis based on data from rodent studies. *α-MSH*, α-melanocyte stimulating hormone; *3 ventricle*, third ventricle; *AgRP*, agouti-related peptide; *Arc*, arcuate nucleus; *DMN*, dorsomedial nucleus; *GC*, glucocorticoids; *GHS-R*, growth hormone secretagogue receptor; *GR*, glucocorticoid receptor; *InsR*, insulin receptor; *LHN*, lateral hypothalamic nucleus; *NPY*, neuropeptide Y; *Ob-R*, leptin receptor; *POMC*, proopiomelanocortin; *PVN*, paraventricular nucleus; *VMN*, ventromedial nucleus. *Modified from Wattez JS, Delahaye F, Lukaszewski MA, Risold PY, Eberle D, Vieau D, et al. Perinatal nutrition programs the hypothalamic melanocortin system in offspring.* Horm Metab Res 2013;**45(13)**:980–90; Ramamoorthy TG, Begum G, Harno E, White A. Developmental programming of hypothalamic neuronal circuits: impact on energy balance control. Front Neurosci 2015;**9**:16.

50.4.1.1 Appetite Regulatory Pathway

The arcuate nucleus in the hypothalamus plays a central role in food intake and energy homeostasis. It is located medio-basally in the hypothalamus next to the third ventricle and medial eminence. The arcuate nucleus integrates peripheral information from hormones such as insulin and ghrelin, adipocytokines such as leptin and adiponectin, as well as nutrients such as glucose and free fatty acid.[30,31] This is possible, as it has a leaky blood brain barrier allowing circulatory factors easy access to the neurons, which also receive peripheral input regarding nutritional status from the vagal nerve.[34]

From the information received, the arcuate nucleus then modulates two neuronal populations, which are characterized by their expression of specific neuropeptides that regulate appetite. These are the anorexigenic neuropeptides, pro-opiomelanocortin (POMC), and cocaine- and amphetamine-regulated transcript (CART), as well as the orexigenic neuropeptides, neuropeptide Y (NPY), agouti-related peptide (AgRP), and γ-aminobutyric acid (GABA).[31,35,36] These two neuronal populations counterregulate each other to modify appetite and energy expenditure, which ultimately regulate body weight. The arcuate nucleus then drives second order neurons in other hypothalamic nuclei such as the ventromedial nucleus (VMN), dorsomedial nucleus (DMN), paraventricular nucleus (PVN), which is also known as the satiety center, and lateral hypothalamic nucleus (LHN), which is also known as the hunger center. Several of the hypothalamic nuclei, especially PVN, regulate appetite and energy expenditure, such as lipolysis and thermogenesis in adipose tissue by the nucleus of solitary tract and sympathetic autonomic nervous system[33] (Fig. 50.1).

50.4.1.2 The Action of Neuropeptides Expressed by Neurons in the Arcuate Nucleus

POMC is broken down into various peptides, including adrenocorticotropic hormone (ACTH), β-endorphin, and α-melanocyte stimulating hormone (α-MSH). α-MSH is the most widely studied derivative of POMC. It has an agonist action at melanocortin-3 (MC3R) and melanocortin-4 receptors (MC4R) expressed on second-order neurons in other hypothalamic nuclei such as the lateral hypothalamic and paraventricular nuclei. This leads to a decrease in the expression of orexigenic peptides such as orexin and melanin concentrating hormone (MCH) in the LHN, but an increase in the expression of anorexigenic peptides such as corticotropin-releasing hormone (CRH) and thyrotropin-releasing hormone (TRH) in the PVN.[31] As a result, energy expenditure is increased while food intake is decreased. CART is a less studied anorexigenic neuropeptide due to the limited understanding of its receptor. It was found to have a similar effect as POMC and is thought to be secreted from the same arcuate neurons as those which secrete POMC,[36] but is more widely expressed throughout the brain and peripheral tissue.[37]

On the other hand, NPY binds selectively to Y1NPY (Y1R) and Y5NPY receptors (Y5R) expressed by second-order neurons located in other hypothalamic nuclei. NPY acts in the opposite way as α-MSH, resulting in decreased energy expenditure with increased food intake.[31] On the other hand, AgRP is an endogenous antagonist for MC4R and regulates signaling events postreceptor.[35] The neuronal projections of both POMC and AgRP areas also overlap indicating cross-interactions between the two neuronal populations. GABA is the least studied of the three orexigenic neuropeptides. It is found to have a similar role as NPY[36]; it regulates the initial phase of appetite and can be a substitute for NPY.

These neurons in the arcuate nucleus are one target of developmental programming of obesity especially induced by changes in maternal nutrition.[35]

50.4.2 Adipose Tissue

Adipose tissue develops from the accretion of fetal fat at 15 to 20 weeks of gestation, with an exponential increase in accumulation from 30 weeks of gestation.[38] In the early phase, adipogenesis is associated with the deposition of subcutaneous fat, especially in the face.[38,39] Visceral fat accumulation occurs later on in the middle of the second and third trimester. It accounts for 50% of maternal weight gain in the third trimester of pregnancy and 46% of the variation in birthweight.[38] Adipocytes in the fetus are plastic and sensitive to various insults. Hence adipogenesis represents a window of vulnerability to insults during gestation and lactation.[30]

50.4.2.1 Role of Adipose Tissue

Adipocytes are specialized cells with energy storage and endocrine roles. Excess energy is stored as triglycerides in lipid droplets in adipocytes during lipogenesis, whereby dietary fatty acids undergo simple esterification. When energy is required, lipolysis occurs, whereby stored triglycerides are hydrolyzed in a pathway driven by the sympathetic autonomic nervous system.[31]

As an endocrine cell, adipocytes produce adipocytokines, hormones, and other appetite-regulating related peptides, which modulates energy homeostasis.[40] Apart from regulating hypothalamic energy balance in an endocrine manner, adipocytes also act in an autocrine or paracrine manner to regulate lipid metabolism.[30]

50.4.2.2 Types of Adipose Tissue

Adipose tissue is composed mostly of mature adipocytes and stromal vascular tissue consisting of preadipocytes, fibroblasts, and endothelial as well as immune cells. There are different types of adipose tissue, such as white adipose tissue (WAT), brown adipose tissue (BAT), and beige adipose tissue.[30]

WAT functions as long-term energy storage. It is derived from preadipocytes recruited from precursor cells with vascular origins from adipogenesis.[41] This is driven by transcription factors like peroxisome proliferator activated receptor alpha (PPARα) and lipid metabolizing enzymes such as fatty acid synthase.[30] Adipocytes in WAT are characterized by a single unilocular lipid droplet that stores excess energy as triglycerides.[30]

BAT plays an important role in energy expenditure through thermogenesis, producing a large amount of heat when maximally stimulated.[42,43] This occurs by the activation of uncoupling protein 1 (UCP1) found within the inner mitochondrial membrane.[44] BAT first appears in the fetus during mid-gestation and gradually declines throughout childhood and adulthood. It has a close developmental relationship with myocytes, where it is derived from the Myf5-positive myoblastic lineage.[45] BAT is characterized by multilocular smaller lipid droplets with a large number of mitochondria and expression of UCP1.[44] BAT is found in small quantities, accounting for up to 4% of the total body weight even at its prominent stage in newborns.[43] Despite so, BAT has great potential in having a significant impact on energy balance.

Beige adipose tissue is found within some WAT depots and shares many morphological and functional features of BAT. However, the amount of UCP1 is only 10% of that of BAT.[46] Beige adipose tissue also has its own unique genetic markers and is thought to share the same origins as WAT, deriving from precursors cells with vascular origins.[30] Hence the presence of beige adipose tissue may suggest a source of adipose tissue found sparsely within WAT, which is potentially converted or recruited into BAT.[47]

50.5 THE MECHANISM LEADING TO PERINATAL ORIGINS OF OBESITY

The programming of obesity is dependent on two closely interacting factors. These are the complex genetic factors that predispose individuals to energy balance dysfunction, as well as the environmental insults during the critical period of development. These may then alter the energy homeostasis pathway with permanent consequences such as obesity.[31,36] The mechanism by which an environmental insult during early development, especially during the perinatal period, affects the programming of obesity remains unclear.

One plausible explanation may be the suboptimal level of circulating factors due to the environmental insults such as malnutrition (Fig. 50.2). This causes permanent changes to the structure and function of organs, especially the hypothalamus-adipose axis, resulting in the perinatal programming of obesity.

Another potential mechanism for developmental programming of obesity is the regulation of gene expression in a spatial and temporal manner due to epigenetic modifications (Fig. 50.2). There is increasing interest in how epigenetic dysregulation of energy homeostasis genes induced by early life environmental insults may account for the persistent changes in metabolic phenotype.[36,48]

50.5.1 Circulating Factors

Metabolomics is a study of the metabolic response to pathological environmental insults and genetic modifications by making quantitative measurements over time. It has generated new hypotheses with regards to mechanisms surrounding the perinatal origins of obesity by describing the biochemical and molecular profile of obesity. The crucial circulating biochemical factors in obesity are hormones such as insulin and ghrelin, as well as adipocytokines such as leptin. The roles of these circulating factors have been previously described in Chapter 39, "Origins of Adipose Tissue and Adipose Regulating Hormones."

Nutrients such as glucose also interact with the arcuate nucleus in the hypothalamus in regulating energy homeostasis. Glucose is taken up by the POMC/CART neurons by glucose transporter GLUT 2. Glucose is then phosphorylated and metabolized to generate ATP, which binds to and block the K_{ATP} channel. As a result, the POMC neuron is depolarized, activating the anorexigenic secondary order neurons.[35]

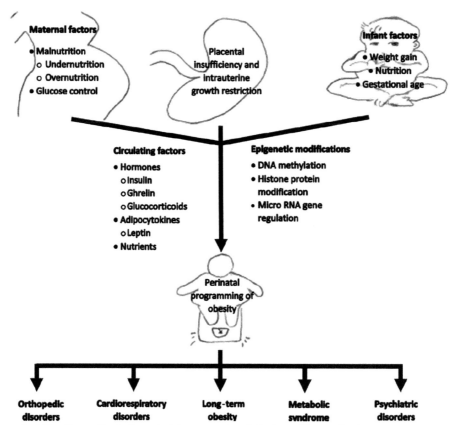

FIG. 50.2   Common perinatal insults resulting in the perinatal programming of obesity and its associated consequences.

50.5.2   Epigenetics

Epigenetics is the study of stable and inheritable changes in gene function without changing the underlying deoxyribonucleic acid (DNA) sequence. Transient environmental insults during prenatal and early postnatal life, especially changes in maternal or perinatal nutrition, may permanently imprint the offspring's genome and alter the transcription of genes crucial in energy homeostasis. This leads to long-term energy homeostasis dysfunction and sensitizes the offspring to obesity and metabolic syndrome in adulthood.[31] The phenotype of some epigenetic modifications may not be present until later in life, especially in genes modulating responses to later environmental changes.[49]

50.5.2.1   Epigenetic Mechanism

There are three postulated mechanisms of epigenetic modification.[36] They are the methylation of DNA, posttranslational histone protein modification, and micro RNA (miRNA) mediated gene regulation.

DNA methylation is the most common and well-understood mechanism for producing highly stable epigenetic modification. It plays an important role in altering gene transcription by methylation of promoter genes, parental imprinting, and X chromosome inactivation.[50] DNA methylation involves a covalent modification by adding a methyl group. The methyl group is commonly added to the C5 position of cytosine residue that is adjacent to the guanine residue. This pair of dinucleotides is called a CpG dinucleotide. DNA methyltransferase catalyzes this process and requires a cofactor and methyl donor in the form of *S*-adenosylmethionine.[36] The methyl group of the *S*-adenosylmethionine is usually obtained from dietary nutrients such as folic acid. Hence dietary modification may alter the process of DNA methylation. DNA methylation subsequently affects gene expression by either preventing transcription factors from binding to recognized sites on the DNA, or stimulates binding of methyl-CpG-binding protein (MBP), which recognizes methylated DNA and recruits transcriptional co-repressor complexes, leading to gene silencing. Hence CpG methylation in the promoter region is generally associated with gene silencing.[51]

Histone packages DNA into nuclear chromatin. Numerous covalent modifications can occur on the N-terminal of the core histone, resulting in alterations of the chromatin organization and gene expression. Hence the epigenetic modification of histone can have a profound effect on gene transcription.[36] Examples of posttranslational histone modifications include acetylation, methylation, phosphorylation, and ubiquitination of histone.[52] Acetylation occurs on the lysine residue of histone, which is generally associated with initiation or elongation of gene transcription. Methylation can occur at either the lysine or arginine residues of histone, which is associated with either transcription activation or silencing, depending on the residue modified.[52] Hence a combination of different epigenetic modifications of histone can regulate the activation and silencing of genes.

MicroRNA (miRNA) is a new class of regulatory molecules that control gene expression at the posttranscriptional level. It exerts an epigenetic effect by being part of a complex network of reciprocal interconnection and regulatory loops, as well as regulating the DNA methylation and histone protein modification. In turn, expression of miRNA is regulated by the DNA methylation and histone protein modification.[53]

These epigenetic modifications to anorexigenic and orexigenic genes in the hypothalamus can alter the appetite regulatory pathway and body weight set point. This leads to the perinatal programming of obesity and metabolic disorder in later life.[36]

50.5.2.2 Examples of Epigenetic Modification

A human twin pair study[54] found DNA methylation and histone modification to diverge strongly in twin pairs with marked differences in life history and environmental insults. Hypothalamic POMC gene is a likely target for epigenetic modification as a result of perinatal programming, as it is regulated by promoter region methylation.[31] Changes in the perinatal nutrition may cause an epigenetic modification in the key regulatory elements of the POMC promoter region. This subsequently affects the appetite regulatory pathway in the hypothalamus, resulting in obesity. Maternal undernutrition during periconception in sheep is associated with hypomethylation of fetal hypothalamic POMC gene.[48] Animal studies in rodents demonstrated that neonatal malnutrition is associated with the hypermethylation of the CpG sites required for leptin and insulin expression of POMC in the hypothalamus.[55] Hence this leads to leptin and insulin resistance, as well as obesity.

Hypomethylation of specific CpG sites and increased acetylation of histones in the promoter region of NPY are observed with feeding newborn rodents a milk high in carbohydrate. This leads to an increased mRNA expression of NPY and subsequently obesity in adulthood.[56] Similarly, undernutrition in maternal sheep is associated with hypomethylation and histone protein modification of the GR promoter region. This leads to an increased GR mRNA expression in the fetal hypothalamus that regulates energy homeostasis,[57] but long-term effects have not been investigated.

Imprinted genes are another target for epigenetic modification and include the insulin like growth factor 2 (IGF2) gene, which controls growth and metabolism in the fetus and early life.[49] Parental imprinting of the IGF2 gene has a labile methylation pattern, which is highly dependent on the nutritional status in early life.[58] The Dutch famine study[59] found hypomethylation of the imprinted IGF2 gene 6 decades later in the offspring of mothers exposed to famine during periconception. This hypomethylation was not noted in unexposed same-sex siblings.

Different epigenetic modifications on identical DNA sequences may permanently alter gene expression levels, leading to long-term hypothalamic dysfunction of energy homeostasis.[35] It remains uncertain as to how epigenetic modification of specific genes associated with obesity is targeted by developmental programming. The timing and intensity of the environmental insult may play a significant role.[36] It is also plausible that dietary factors can influence epigenetic modifications, especially methylation of genes involved in energy homeostasis and obesity. Micronutrients such as dietary folate, vitamin B6, and vitamin B12 are methyl group donors for the methylation of DNA and histone protein.[60] Changes in nutrient and hormone levels may act as the mediator of downstream signals of environmental insults.

Epigenetic modifications such as DNA methylation are potentially reversible. The metabolic changes can be reduced through nutritional intervention. For example, supplementation of folic acid, which is a methyl donor, during the critical period of perinatal development was found to prevent the increase in birthweight in subsequent generations caused by perinatal programming of obesity by epigenetic modification.[61]

50.5.2.3 Transgenerational Epigenetic Modification

Animal studies found epigenetic modifications to extend beyond the first generation, even in the absence of exposure to the adverse environment previously experienced by the first-generation offspring.[62] From an evolutionary point of view, the transgenerational transmission of epigenetic modifications allows future generations to better survive the potential adverse environment experienced by current generations. The mechanism behind this is unclear, but studies found epigenetic inheritance in both maternal and paternal linkages.[49] The Dutch famine study found second-generation offspring to have increased neonatal adiposity and persistent changes in DNA methylation. Although many studies[59] show transgenerational transmission of epigenetic modifications to the second generation, the transmission to the third and subsequent generation remains unclear.[62]

50.5.2.4 *Gender-Specific Effect of Perinatal Programming of Obesity*

There is emerging evidence demonstrating the gender-specific differences seen in the perinatal programming of obesity in offspring, which occurs in response to perinatal environmental insults, especially maternal malnutrition.[30,35,36] This reflects the potential direct interaction between the biological mechanisms of perinatal programming of obesity with sex hormones in the developing fetus and newborn. The difference in sex hormones may modify the perinatal programming of the hypothalamus-adipose axis differently in response to environmental insults.[63]

For example, animal studies using rodents and sheep[36,57] have found that male offspring that were exposed to maternal undernutrition during gestation were more likely to have lower insulin levels and were more sensitive to changes in insulin levels. They also had a higher fat mass than female offspring exposed to the similar environment. This may be because estrogen can regulate the changes in the insulin and leptin as a compensatory mechanism in response to maternal malnutrition. The brain in male offspring is considered to be more sensitive to leptin and insulin resistance associated with maternal malnutrition. The reduced central action of insulin in the male offspring may lower the expression of anorexigenic neuropeptides such as POMC, leading to increased appetite and obesity later on.[36]

The outcomes for male offspring are often noted to be worse than that in females in response to adverse perinatal environmental insults. Hence it is argued that the perinatal programming in male and female offspring differ with timing and outcome.[63] Despite this, few studies currently pay close attention to the gender-specific effects in the perinatal programming mechanism.

50.6 ENVIRONMENTAL INSULTS RESULTING IN THE PERINATAL PROGRAMMING OF OBESITY

Fetal and early postnatal environments have a significant impact on the risk of obesity and metabolic disorder in adulthood, as suggested by DOHAD. This section explores the perinatal environmental factors that lead to programming of obesity using human epidemiological studies (Fig. 50.2). Due to the limitations of human studies, it is difficult to investigate the precise biological mechanism of how these perinatal factors "program" obesity. These factors may exert their impact on the hypothalamus-adipose axis via the mechanisms described previously.

Data from animal models are used to provide further evidence. Different animal models have their own limitations. Many animal studies on the perinatal programming of the hypothalamus-adipose axis use rodents that are an altricial species. The hypothalamus of the rodent is immature at birth and continues to develop by forming axonal projections and synapses to target sites during the first 2 weeks postnatally. Hence the hypothalamus is not fully formed at birth, making the hypothalamus-adipose axis plastic and sensitive to environmental insults postnatally.[64] Different methods have been used to modify the environment during this critical period of hypothalamic development to aid in the understanding and characterizing of perinatal programming of obesity in humans. However, the length of gestation and hypothalamic development in altricial rodents are not comparable to that in humans. The timing of vulnerability of the environmental insults may differ markedly.[64,65] Despite so, many studies show rodents displaying similar developmental programming to precocial species such as sheep and primates.[31] In precocial species, the hypothalamic development and neuronal projection occur prenatally in the fetus stage.

50.6.1 Maternal Nutrition

Prenatal growth trajectory is sensitive to the direct and indirect effects of maternal nutrition.[66] Numerous epidemiological and animal studies have found that maternal malnutrition, which encompasses both undernutrition as well as overnutrition during the perinatal period, creates an adverse environment for the fetus. As a result, persistent physiological changes occur in the fetal hypothalamic appetite regulatory pathway, causing perinatal programming of obesity and metabolic disorder in adulthood.[48] This is especially the case when there is a difference between the prenatal and postnatal environments.[67] Fetal programming induced by maternal malnutrition is thought to involve changes in the hypothalamic appetite regulatory pathway established during early development.

50.6.1.1 *Maternal Undernutrition*

One of the first major epidemiological studies demonstrating a negative impact of maternal undernutrition during pregnancy and disease outcome in offspring is the Dutch famine study from 1944 to 1945.[68] Maternal exposure to undernutrition at different periods of the gestation leads to a slightly different outcome in the offspring. Offspring whose mothers were exposed to famine early on in the gestation had normal birthweight but higher risk of obesity and metabolic disorders.[69]

Offspring had low birthweight if their mothers were exposed to famine later on in gestation.[68] This difference continues into late adulthood. Longitudinal analysis of the Dutch famine cohort found adults at 50 years of age whose mothers were exposed to undernutrition during early gestation had a higher risk of obesity, impaired glucose tolerance, and coronary artery disease, compared with those whose mothers were not exposed to malnutrition.[70]

The finding from human studies corroborated with those from animal studies. Maternal and perinatal undernutrition in rodents were associated with low birthweight and increased appetite postnatally, as well as obesity and insulin resistance in adults.[71]

The use of animal models to mimic maternal undernutrition during gestation has also shed some light on the biological mechanism of action. Maternal undernutrition in rodents was found to affect the structural organization of the hypothalamus in the fetus.[31] Neuronal cell proliferation and axon projection in the hypothalamus were noted to be affected in maternal undernutrition. This alters the density of orexigenic and anorexigenic neurons such as neurons expressing NPY as well as POMC, respectively.[72–74] As a result, regulation of energy homeostasis is impaired, causing obesity and metabolic disorders in adulthood.

Maternal undernutrition also causes long-term programming of the appetite regulatory pathway in the arcuate nucleus of the hypothalamus, favoring the orexigenic pathway.[31] Maternal undernutrition during gestation in rodents consistently demonstrated an increase in orexigenic neuropeptides such as NPY and AgRP, as well as a decrease in anorexigenic neuropeptides such as POMC.[72,73] Similar findings were noted in baboons where offspring who were exposed to maternal undernutrition during gestation have a lower expression of POMC and a higher expression of NPY neuropeptides.[75] In sheep,[57] moderate maternal undernutrition was associated with an increased glucocorticoid receptor expression, which is sustained to adulthood. However, no changes in the POMC and NPY expression were noted at the fetal stage, but a decrease in the POMC expression was found in adulthood.

Adipose tissue in infants of rodents and sheep exposed to maternal undernutrition during gestation was found to have an increased expression of proinflammatory genes and recruitment of macrophages within WAT.[31] This leads to early insulin and/or leptin resistance, causing obesity and metabolic disorders in adulthood.

Offspring of rodents exposed to maternal undernutrition were also found to have increased adipogenesis with an increase in adipocyte number and size. There was also reduced antilipogenic action by leptin noted.[47] The noradrenergic supply to the WAT was also functionally impaired in rodents exposed to maternal undernutrition, potentially causing increased adipogenesis and/or decreased lipolysis.[74]

50.6.1.2 Maternal Overnutrition

Overnutrition is becoming a major public health issue globally with the increasing prevalence of obesity, including obesity rates in pregnant women. Many human epidemiological studies have found that infants who are born to women who have raised BMI, especially in the first trimester, are at an increased risk of obesity and metabolic disorders in adulthood.[66] Interestingly, offspring born to mothers who underwent bariatric surgery have a lower risk of obesity than offspring born before the surgery. However, human studies have their own limitations, as obesity is a lifelong condition that may precede pregnancy. Hence it is difficult to differentiate between gestational obesity and preconception obesity in women. Besides, it is difficult to eliminate all the confounding factors, as offspring may be exposed to the same adverse, obesity-predisposing environment postpartum that their mothers were exposed to during pregnancy.

Animal models of maternal overnutrition, especially in rodents, where a high-fat low carbohydrate maternal diet is given during pregnancy and lactation, is associated with an increased risk of obesity and metabolic disorder in the offspring,[31,36] without any change in birth weight. The neuronal axon projection of the anorexigenic and orexigenic neurons in the arcuate nucleus to the PVN is impaired in the offspring of maternal rodents fed the high-fat diet.[76] An increase in the proliferation of the orexigenic neuropeptide expressing neurons and a reduction in that of the anorexigenic neuropeptides are noted in the offspring of rodents with maternal overnutrition.[31] This subsequently alters the appetite regulatory pathway in the hypothalamus, leading to increased appetite and predisposing the offspring to obesity, which persists into adulthood.

The impact of maternal overnutrition on gene expression of orexigenic and anorexigenic neuropeptides in the hypothalamus is diverse. Various studies have produced conflicting results,[36] making it hard to interpret as compared with that of maternal undernutrition. Some of the changes seen in the neuropeptide levels in the offspring may be a compensatory mechanism for maternal overnutrition, which may change later on in life. Hence further research in this field is needed to provide further clarity on the impact of maternal overnutrition on the expression of these neuropeptides.

Maternal overnutrition in rodents was also found to cause central leptin resistance in the offspring.[31] This leads to an increase in the activity of the orexigenic pathway and a decrease in the activation of the sympathetic nervous system. As a result, the long-term body weight set point is altered, leading to obesity.

Interestingly, obese mothers who lose weight during gestation can increase the risk of intrauterine growth (IUGR) restriction in their offspring, predisposing them to obesity in adulthood.[77] The increased risk of IUGR may be due to a few reasons, including ketosis from the maternal mobilization of WAT; increased maternal cortisol level from weight lost, which inhibits fetal protein synthesis; or reduced fetal nutrient supply as a result of the increased utilization of nutrients by maternal tissue and the reduced uteroplacental blood flow.[66]

50.6.2 Maternal Glucose Control

Maternal diabetes is a common predisposing factor for having infants who are born large for gestational age and subsequently develop an increased risk of obesity and diabetes in adulthood. The direct relationship between birthweight and maternal blood glucose level is noted, even if the maternal glucose level is within the normal range.[8] Interestingly, infants born to mothers after a maternal diagnosis of diabetes have a higher risk of raised BMI and diabetes in adulthood than their siblings born before the diagnosis.[78]

Maternal diabetes during gestation is associated with fetal hyperglycemia, as maternal glucose is transported by the placenta into the fetal circulation. This stimulates the β cell of the fetal pancreas, causing fetal hyperinsulinemia.[79] As insulin is a growth promoting factor, the infant is often born large for gestational age.[29] During the postpartum period, the infant is no longer exposed to the high glucose environment experienced prenatally due to maternal diabetes. Despite this, the hyperinsulinemia persists. As a result, the infant experiences hypoglycemia and subsequent poor carbohydrate tolerance.[80,81]

Animal models of maternal diabetes in rodents using an injection of pancreatic islet toxin streptozotocin early in the pregnancy also confirmed these findings and indicate some potential biological mechanisms.[35] The offspring of diabetic maternal rodents have higher body weight and appetite with hyperglycemia.[36] Structural changes in the hypothalamus are noted, with an altered density of AgRP and POMC expressing neurons in the hypothalamus as well as altered leptin sensitivity.[82] This adverse programming of the appetite regulatory pathway in the hypothalamus predisposes the offspring to obesity and metabolic syndrome in adult life. It can potentially be prevented by normalizing maternal glucose during pregnancy.[36]

50.6.3 Multiple Births

Multiple births present a unique opportunity to investigate the impact of low birthweight on obesity and metabolic disorders. This is because the offspring share many similarities with the programmed offspring from maternal undernutrition, causing low birthweight.[36] It may be because such offspring compete with each other for nutrition and have reduced placental size. Thus the offspring may develop compensatory mechanisms similar to that of the programmed offspring. This is seen in sheep, whereby such offspring can have a higher fat mass in adulthood with altered hypothalamic appetite regulatory pathway, as well as glucose regulation.[83]

50.6.4 Placental Insufficiency

The placenta plays a crucial role in fetal growth and development. It oversees the transfer of nutrients into the fetal circulation and acts as an endocrine structure, secreting hormones needed for fetal growth and development.

The placenta senses changes in the maternal environment, especially maternal nutritional status, through pathways such as the mechanistic target of rapamycin (mTOR). The placenta responds to environmental challenges by altering its structure and function, resulting in changes in uteroplacental blood flow and hence fetal nutrient supply. It also secretes hormones and other signaling molecules in response to the environmental changes.[84] This has a significant impact on fetal growth as well as body composition. Hence, when placental insufficiency occurs, the fetus is at risk of obesity and metabolic disorders in adulthood as a result of fetal programming.

Placental insufficiency is not just purely due to impaired uteroplacental blood flow. It can also be caused by impaired surface area for the placenta to carry out its exchange function effectively, secondary to reduced intervillous space volume or poorly developed peripheral villi.[84] Placental insufficiency predisposes the fetus to impaired transfer of nutrients, disrupting fetal growth and development during gestation, causing IUGR.

The prevalence of IUGR is increasing in high-income countries and accounts for 11% of births in low to middle-income countries.[66] In clinical practice, the term *IUGR* is often used interchangeably with *small for gestational age*, which is defined as having birthweight less than the 10th percentile for gestational age. However, it must be stressed that IUGR refs to the insufficient growth of the fetus. Hence the newer definition of IUGR requires at least two assessments of intra-uterine fetal growth showing inappropriate growth of the fetus before the term IUGR could be used.[85]

IUGR is associated with many chronic diseases in adulthood, including obesity and metabolic syndrome.[66] Animal models using bilateral artery ligation to mimic placental insufficiency and IUGR are often used to explore the biological fetal programming mechanism for nutritional regulation, as well as the development of long-term health outcomes. The induced placental insufficiency leads to a reduced supply of nutrients to the fetus, and hence fetal hypoglycemia and hypoinsulinemia occurs. This accounts for infants being small for gestational age, as insulin is a growth-promoting factor.[36] The fetus then adapts to the adverse environment by altering the metabolic parameters or epigenetic modifications of stem cell population. These mal-adaptations are the basis of perinatal programming of obesity in placental insufficiency and IUGR.[85]

The fetal insulin hypothesis is proposed as a potential explanation for the long-term metabolic risks and obesity observed in infants with IUGR and low birthweight.[85] As a compensatory mechanism for IUGR, there is an increase in expression of insulin-like growth factor 1 (IGF1) and its receptor, IGF1R, to enhance the transfer of nutrients such as glucose and amino acid into the fetus. After birth, a period of increased insulin sensitivity is seen with a reduction in the IGF1 and an increase in insulin-like growth factor binding protein 1 (IGFBP1) level. This increased insulin sensitivity is gradually lost and switches over to insulin resistance over the first 3 years of life at a rate relative to the postnatal weight gain. It has a potential adverse impact on the body composition and metabolic risk in later life.

50.6.5 Birthweight

Birthweight is often used to reflect the intrauterine environment and maternal nutritional status during gestation in human studies. The "thrifty" phenotype[21] describes the fetal adaptation to the adverse intrauterine environment caused by maternal undernutrition and the subsequent low birthweight. The adaptation becomes maladaptive when there is increased nutrient availability postnatally, leading to obesity and metabolic disorders in adulthood. Conversely, emerging studies[86] have found a positive relationship between high birthweight with high adult BMI, reflecting the impact of prenatal and maternal overnutrition on obesity and metabolic disorders in adulthood. Hence a U-shaped relationship between birthweight and adult obesity is seen in human epidemiological studies, with an increased risk in infants with both high and low birthweights.

However, the postnatal environment, especially postnatal weight gain, is noted to have a more significant impact on the development of obesity in adulthood.[85,86] Once postnatal weight gain is taken into account, some human epidemiological studies found that the birthweight is no longer a predictor of obesity in adulthood. It is also crucial to note that BMI is not an accurate surrogate marker of adiposity. The majority of the human epidemiological studies found high birthweight infants to have an increase in fat-free mass in adulthood without impact on the fat mass, as estimated by various means ranging from skinfold thickness to BIA and dual energy X-ray absorptiometry.[4,86]

50.6.6 Gestational Age

Recent advances in neonatal care have seen an increase in the number of premature infants surviving to adulthood. Hence there are a few studies looking at the long-term metabolic impact of prematurity.

Many studies have found that infants who are born prematurely are at an increased risk of obesity, especially central obesity, which carries a poor metabolic risk profile.[87] Reasons behind this finding are unclear at present, and more studies are needed to investigate the biological mechanism. One potential explanation is that many of these preterm infants experience some form of extrauterine growth restriction postnatally, despite potentially having normal fetal growth prior to birth. They are often very unwell, especially in the first few weeks of life, requiring high energy demand for growth and to overcome infection and respiratory distress. However, the amount of nutrient and energy that they received during this period of time often does not match their energy demand, causing extrauterine growth restriction.[88] Hence they may undergo programming in response to this adverse environment. When premature infants recover from this initial period of high energy demand, they are often exposed to a high calorie and high protein milk to improve weight gain. This is because their poor weight gain is associated with poor neurodevelopment. Conversely, the metabolic programming in response to the initial extrauterine growth restriction may become maladaptive when exposed to the excessive weight gain as a result of the high calorie and high protein milk. Hence this may predispose preterm infants to obesity and metabolic disorders in adulthood.[89]

50.6.7 Weight Gain in Early Infancy

Early infancy represents a period of many rapid changes with many of the organs and systems still in the developmentally plastic stage. Studies[4] showed that the weight gain in infants in the first 6 months of life is mainly translated into a gain in the fat mass in relative terms. After that age, the gain in fat-free mass occurs more quickly. Hence excessive weight gain in early infancy, especially in the presence of an adverse prenatal environment or growth restriction, is found to be an important predictor of obesity and metabolic diseases in adulthood. This phenomenon is called *catch-up growth*. Human epidemiological studies found excessive catch-up growth to play a more significant role in predicting long-term obesity than birthweight alone.[85,86]

Rapid catch-up growth is thought to be caused by the increased appetite secondary to a sustained increase in the orexigenic drive, and adaptation or programming to ensure recovery of weight following the prenatal insult. This predisposes infants to obesity and metabolic diseases in later life.

Epidemiological studies and randomized controlled trials conducted in developed countries found excessive weight gain in the early infancy period to play a significant role in predisposing infants to obesity in later life.[4] A review of 10 epidemiological studies found that excessive weight gain in the first year of life is associated with obesity in later life based on BMI with a relative risk between 1.2 and 5.7.[90] Further studies have found that rapid weight gain in early infancy is also associated with a poor body composition of a higher fat mass[4] as well as truncal adiposity.[86] This is crucial, as the BMI may not be a true reflection of adiposity and its metabolic consequences, as previously discussed. The crucial period of weight gain that has a significant impact on long-term obesity risk is unclear at present, with studies suggesting the first 3, 6, or 12 months of life.[4]

The evidence for the role of excessive weight gain in early infancy on obesity risk in developing countries, whereby growth stunting and undernutrition are common, is limited and conflicting. A review of five longitudinal studies from low- and middle-income countries (India, Brazil, Guatemala, Philippines, and South Africa) found that excessive weight gain in the first, second, and third year of life is associated with higher blood pressure in adulthood due to its contribution on the adult BMI rather than the weight gain itself.[91] Hence further studies in developing countries are required, balancing the risk and benefit from excessive weight gain in early infancy.

Preterm infants are another group of infants whereby excessive catch-up growth is noted to have a negative impact on long-term obesity and metabolic risks.[4] However, poor postnatal growth is also a known independent risk factor for adverse neurodevelopmental outcomes.[85] Hence further studies are needed to address the competing risks and benefits of excessive catch-up growth in preterm infants.

50.6.8 Nutrition in Early Infancy

Breastfeeding confers many benefits to both the mother and infant. There is mounting evidence from epidemiological studies that breastfeeding protects the offspring from obesity in later life. Infants who were exclusively breastfed, as well as those breastfed for longer (i.e., weaned later), have a lower BMI and fat mass in adulthood.[92]

The biological mechanism of how breastfeeding lowers the risk of adiposity in adulthood is unclear at present. Breastmilk contains numerous hormones and adipocytokines, such as insulin and leptin, that are crucial for the regulation of the infant's appetite. The macronutrient and biologically active contents of breastmilk may also play a role, with a lower protein and higher docosahexaenoic acid (DHA) content in breastmilk.[92]

In animal models using rodents, breastfeeding was found to alter the expression of genes involved in energy homeostasis in the hypothalamus and WAT. As result, this alters the appetite-regulating pathway in the hypothalamus[31] and increases the proliferation and differentiation of adipocytes.[30] This leads to an increased appetite and perinatal programming of adiposity later on.

50.7 COMPLICATION OF OBESITY

Obesity is associated with complications affecting multiple systems and organs. This section aims to discuss the complications associated with fetal macrosomia and early childhood obesity.

50.7.1 Fetal Macrosomia

50.7.1.1 Maternal Risks

Fetal macrosomia presents an increased maternal risk during labor and delivery. Fetal macrosomia is commonly associated with prolonged first and second stages of labor, with the risk increasing as birth weight increases.[8] Arrest of fetal descent during the second stage of labor may also occur. This impacts the delivery mode of the fetus. Fetal macrosomia is found to increase the risk of Caesarean section as well as instrumental assisted vaginal delivery, especially in cases of primigravida. However, there is a wide variation in the reported overall rates of such delivery methods in fetal macrosomia.[93]

There is also a reported 1.5- to 2.5-fold increase in the risk of perineal tear associated with fetal macrosomia.[93] Post-partum hemorrhage is also noted to be associated with fetal macrosomia. This may be due to a combination of factors, including prolonged labor, assisted vaginal delivery, uterine atony, and perineal tear.

50.7.1.2 Neonatal Risks

Although the literature commonly demonstrates increased morbidity in infants with fetal macrosomia, the overall risk of complications is still low. Some of the commonly associated risks are shoulder dystocia, birth trauma, and metabolic disorders during the early postnatal period.[8]

Macrosomic infants commonly have a higher risk of developing shoulder dystocia at delivery, with variable rates of shoulder dystocia reported. Despite the association with fetal macrosomia, at least half of the infants who developed shoulder dystocia at the delivery are not macrosomic, having birthweights less than 4000 g.[93]

There is also an increased risk of birth trauma associated with fetal macrosomia. Similarly, the risk increases with increasing birthweight. Brachial plexus injury due to traumatic stretching is common in the macrosomic fetus, resulting in paresis of the upper extremity. This may be due to the exogenous traction applied or the endogenous pushing during delivery. A majority of the brachial plexus injuries self-resolve with minimal intervention. Skeletal injuries, especially clavicular fractures, are commonly seen in infants with fetal macrosomia, with an increased risk of up to five times[93] in fetal macrosomia. Similarly, clavicular fractures are managed conservatively with a good long-term outcome.

Neonatal hypoglycemia is common in infants with fetal macrosomia, especially if there is a background of maternal gestational diabetes. The transient fetal hyperinsulinemia associated with maternal gestational diabetes is thought to increase the risk of neonatal hypoglycemia.[8,93]

Fetal macrosomia is also found to be associated with neonatal hyperbilirubinemia during the early postnatal period.[8] This may be partly due to the polycythemia, as well as the increased enterohepatic cycling of bilirubin seen in fetal macrosomia, especially in the presence of maternal gestational diabetes.

Transient electrolyte disturbances are also noted in the early postnatal period in macrosomic infants. The hypomagnesemia and hypocalcemia seen are often asymptomatic and do not require treatment.[8]

50.7.2 Early Childhood Obesity

50.7.2.1 Obesity in Adulthood

Various studies carried out in different population settings have found that infant and early childhood obesity have moderate to strong correlation with obesity in adulthood.[94] This is especially true if the child has higher BMI or has parents who are obese.[94] By 5 years of age, the obesity seen in childhood is noted to be resistant to change, leading to obesity in adulthood.[4,95] This provides further evidence for the perinatal programming of obesity and emphasizes the significance of early life factors in the development of long-term obesity. This is a cause for concern, as obesity in later life is an important risk factor for many chronic disorders, such as cardiovascular diseases, hypertension, stroke, type 2 diabetes mellitus, as well as osteoarthritis.[36] Besides these factors, being obese in early childhood confers a higher risk of multiple cardiometabolic comorbidities in adulthood, even if the obesity does not persist. If the current trend of childhood obesity continues, researchers propose that the current generation of children will have a shorter life-span than their parents due to childhood obesity and its associated complications.[96]

50.7.2.2 Metabolic Syndrome

The basis of metabolic syndrome revolves around the excess energy and mishandling of stored excess energy, resulting in visceral adiposity. This leads to the metabolic derangements seen in metabolic syndrome.[87] In adults, metabolic syndrome is defined as a constellation of symptoms encompassing abdominal obesity, hypertension, hyperglycemia, and dyslipidemia that occur simultaneously and increase the risk of ischemic heart disease, stroke, and fatty liver. Dyslipidemia is characterized by hypertriglyceridemia, as well as a reduced level of high density lipoproteins (HDL). The definition of *metabolic syndrome* in children is fraught with difficulties. Often, the diagnosis is derived from the adult definition, using children percentiles for the features described in the adult definition. However, there is a lack of consensus on its definition in children, with different cutoffs used.[97] This is a major issue, as this definition of metabolic syndrome in children is not outcome-based, unlike the adult definition which is based on the outcome of cardiovascular disease and diabetes.[96]

Despite the difficulty in defining metabolic syndrome in children, it is important to identify these children, as there is emerging evidence that metabolic syndrome tracks into adulthood, leading to nearly twofold increased risk of death by ischemic heart disease in adulthood.[97,98] Components of metabolic syndrome are prevalent in children and seen as early as 5 years of age.[97]

Overall growth in early childhood forms the basis of body composition in adulthood.[99] The amount and location of fat deposition in early childhood affect the cardiometabolic risk profile in adulthood, with higher fat deposition, especially in the visceral region rather than the subcutaneous area conferring the highest risk.[98] With the continuous accumulation of fat, there is increased insulin resistance by skeletal muscle, as well as reduced glucose utilization and insulin degradation by the liver, leading to hyperglycemia as well as hyperinsulinemia and ultimately metabolic syndrome.

A recent review[99] found that obesity in the first 6 years of life is associated with nearly 1.5 times increased risk of metabolic syndrome in an adult. The effect of early childhood obesity on the risk of metabolic syndrome in adulthood increases with increasing age of the child with obesity. Two to six years of life appears to represent the most critical and sensitive time, whereby obesity at this age confers the highest risk of metabolic syndrome in adulthood.[99] Rapid weight gain in infants in the first 2 years of life rather than weight itself was found to increase the risk of metabolic syndrome in adulthood.[100]

50.7.2.3 Insulin Resistance

Insulin resistance is found to be the common denominator of the pathogenesis of the cardiovascular and metabolic complications of obesity. Childhood obesity is associated with reduced insulin sensitivity, which persists into adulthood causing type 2 diabetes mellitus.[95,97] Excess deposition of fat, especially in the intra-abdominal visceral region, leads to increased secretion of proinflammatory cytokines, as well as increased circulatory free fatty acid, which promotes insulin resistance in the liver and skeletal muscle.

Similar to the definition of metabolic syndrome in children, there is a lack of consensus in defining insulin resistance in children, ranging from using fasting insulin levels to using homeostasis model of assessment of insulin resistance (HOMA-IR) with varying cut offs.[97] Unsurprisingly, this leads to wide variations in the reporting of the prevalence of insulin resistance in children, from 5% to 72%, depending on the definition used.[97]

Despite this, it is crucial to identify children with insulin resistance, as this is the initial step in the pathogenesis of type 2 diabetes mellitus. The compensatory hyperinsulinemia from insulin resistance leads to impaired early insulin secretion, causing initially postprandial and then fasting hyperglycemia.[98] Type 2 diabetes mellitus is no longer a disease of adulthood, but is quickly becoming a serious problem in pediatrics with the prevalence of 15%–20% in children and seen as early as 6 years of age.[98]

50.7.2.4 Cardiovascular

Atherosclerosis begins early in childhood.[97] There is a higher risk of endothelial dysfunction, a key step or atherosclerosis, in early childhood obesity, which ultimately leads to hypertension.[98] Atherosclerosis is accelerated by dyslipidemia found in obesity with an increased level of triglyceride and reduced level of high density lipoprotein cholesterol. This may be due to either the direct effect of the dyslipidemia itself or the diet associated with dyslipidemia. Insulin resistance associated with early childhood obesity also contributes to hypertension by increasing renal sodium retention, increasing sympathetic activity, as well as increased vascular smooth muscle growth.[97] These put extra strain on the cardiovascular system, leading to left ventricular hypertrophy and cardiovascular diseases.

50.7.2.5 Nonalcoholic Fatty Liver Disease

Accumulation of macrovesicular fat may also occur in the hepatocytes of up to 70% of obese children, leading to nonalcoholic fatty liver disease (NAFLD).[97] NAFLD shares many similarities with metabolic syndrome and is often described as a hepatic manifestation of metabolic syndrome.[97] Although commonly asymptomatic, initially apart from palpable hepatomegaly in some cases, NAFLD may progress into nonalcoholic steatohepatitis (NASH), which is a progressive form of NAFLD that ultimately leads to liver fibrosis, cirrhosis, hepatocellular carcinoma, as well as liver failure requiring a liver transplant in adulthood.[98] Because of its typical asymptomatic presentation, screening for this condition in obese children is crucial.

50.7.2.6 Respiratory Disorders

Children with obesity often suffer from restrictive lung diseases due to the strain that the excess weight has on the lungs. Nearly a third of overweight and obese children have some form of obstructive sleep apnea,[96] with an increased risk of up to six times in obese children.[98] Obstructive sleep apnea is disordered breathing during sleep with prolonged partial upper airway obstruction and/or intermittent complete airway obstruction, disrupting normal breathing pattern during sleep and the sleeping pattern.[98] As a result, the child will snore and have disturbed sleep. This, in turn, causes daytime tiredness, which may cause neurobehavioral problems and reduce the physical activity of the child, creating a vicious cycle and making it difficult to control obesity. Besides, the strain that obstructive sleep apnea places on the heart leads to pulmonary hypertension and its associated cardiorespiratory long-term complications.

Children with obesity often have increased incidence of asthma and asthmatic attacks. As a result, this reduces the exercise tolerance of the child, limiting the child's physical activity. However, the biological mechanism for this association is unclear at present. It is uncertain if childhood obesity causes asthma or makes the severity of an asthmatic attack worse.

50.7.2.7 Orthopedic Disorder

The effect of weight placed onto the developing skeletal system in obese children leads to various orthopedic growth plate disorders, such as fracture, slipped upper femoral epiphysis (SUFE), and tibia vara, which is known as the Blount disease eponymously.[96]

SUFE is a growth plate disorder that commonly occurs in obese male adolescents. The growth plate of the femur head is displaced from the femur, causing hip and knee pain on walking as well as limited hip internal rotation movement.[98] Tibia vara is a mechanical deficiency of the medial tibial growth plate. As a result, the growth of the medial aspect of the proximal tibial growth plate is disordered, causing pain at the medial aspect of the knee and lower limb deformity such as "bow leg".[98]

50.7.2.8 Psychological Impact

Childhood obesity has a significant psychological impact on the mental health of children. Teasing and bullying are commonly reported by obese children, leading to negative self-image, reduced self-esteem, and social skills. This, in turn, may cause poor educational and financial attainment in later life, as well as mental health disorders such as depression and suicide.[98] Besides this, childhood obesity is also found to lead to loss of control in eating, unhealthy extreme weight control behaviors, and ultimately eating disorders.[98]

50.8 CONCLUSION

The increasing obesity epidemic seen currently may be partly explained by environmental insults, especially malnutrition, in the early life period. The timing and intensity of such events play a significant role in the perinatal programming of obesity. The perinatal period is a sensitive interval for development and programming of the hypothalamus-adipose axis. Various environmental insults with opposing effects, such as overnutrition and undernutrition during the perinatal period, lead to a similar outcome in offspring. This suggests a potential common programming mechanism. However, little is known of the biological mechanism by which the adverse perinatal environment modifies the appetite regulatory pathway and body weight set points, thereby causing obesity in later life. A better understanding of the biological mechanism is needed to help identify early modifiable determinants of obesity in later life. These determinants can then be used to develop intervention strategies during pregnancy and the early postnatal period to prevent obesity and metabolic disorders in adulthood.

The perinatal programming of obesity is a complex pathway. Hence the interventions to tackle obesity should take into account the complexity of the issue. Attempts to simply alter the energy intake or expenditure in infants may be ineffective, especially in infants who are already programmed by circulating factors and epigenetic modifications to gain weight in a certain trajectory. Interventions proposed should also be tailored to different populations, such as preterm infants or infants in developing countries where undernutrition and growth stunting are still common. For example, future studies should explore the impact of proposed interventions on the competing risks of neurodevelopment and cardiometabolic disorders in the preterm infants. This is less of a problem in term infants because weight gain has less of an impact on neurodevelopment compared with preterm infants.

Postnatal weight gain is a significant predisposing factor for obesity in later life. However, there is no consensus on the optimum weight gain that should be achieved by the different infant populations exposed to perinatal insults. Apart from this, a better measure of obesity in infants is needed in the clinical and research settings. Weight alone is no longer an acceptable measure of obesity in infants. At the very least, weight for length should be measured and can be used in clinical practice. Despite this, it does not provide a true reflective measure of adiposity. Hence it does not provide sufficient information in the research setting to explore the biological mechanisms and determinants of perinatal programming of obesity. Longitudinal body composition, and the distinction between the fat as well as the fat-free mass, are crucial in accurately assessing obesity in infants. This will undoubtedly provide more information on the perinatal programming of obesity.

REFERENCES

1. World Health Organisation. *WHO fact sheet: obesity and overweight;* 2017.
2. Smith SC, Collins A, Ferrari R, Holmes DR, Logstrup S, McGhie DV, et al. Our time: a call to save preventable death from cardiovascular disease (heart disease and stroke). *Glob Heart* 2012;**7**(4):297–305.
3. World Health Organisation. *WHO facts and figures on childhood obesity;* 2017.
4. Gillman MW. Early infancy—a critical period for development of obesity. *J Dev Orig Health Dis* 2010;**1**(5):292–9.
5. Gillman MW. Developmental origins of health and disease. *N Engl J Med* 2005;**353**(17):1848–50.
6. Barker DJ. The developmental origins of chronic adult disease. *Acta Paediatr Suppl* 2004;**93**(446):26–33.
7. Boulet SL, Alexander GR, Salihu HM, Pass M. Macrosomic births in the United States: determinants, outcomes, and proposed grades of risk. *Am J Obstet Gynecol* 2003;**188**(5):1372–8.
8. Walsh JM, McAuliffe FM. Prediction and prevention of the macrosomic fetus. *Eur J Obstet Gynecol Reprod Biol* 2012;**162**(2):125–30.
9. Noumi G, Collado-Khoury F, Bombard A, Julliard K, Weiner Z. Clinical and sonographic estimation of fetal weight performed during labor by residents. *Am J Obstet Gynecol* 2005;**192**(5):1407–9.
10. Neilson JP. Symphysis-fundal height measurement in pregnancy. *Cochrane Database Syst Rev* 1998;(1).
11. Chauhan SP, Grobman WA, Gherman RA, Chauhan VB, Chang G, Magann EF, et al. Suspicion and treatment of the macrosomic fetus: a review. *Am J Obstet Gynecol* 2005;**193**(2):332–46.
12. Hoopmann M, Abele H, Wagner N, Wallwiener D, Kagan KO. Performance of 36 different weight estimation formulae in fetuses with macrosomia. *Fetal Diagn Ther* 2010;**27**(4):204–13.
13. Haugen G, Hanson M, Kiserud T, Crozier S, Inskip H, Godfrey KM. Fetal liver-sparing cardiovascular adaptations linked to mother's slimness and diet. *Circ Res* 2005;**96**(1):12–4.
14. Malin G, Bugg G, Takwoingi Y, Thornton J, Jones N. Comparison of MRI and ultrasound to detect fetal macrosomia at term: a systematic review and meta-analysis. *Arch Dis Child Fetal Neonatal Ed* 2014;**99**(S1):A97–A100.
15. Raitakari OT, Juonala M, Viikari JS. Obesity in childhood and vascular changes in adulthood: insights into the Cardiovascular Risk in Young Finns Study. *Int J Obes (Lond)* 2005;**29**(Suppl 2):S101–4.
16. Wells JCK. Toward body composition reference data for infants, children, and adolescents. *Adv Nutr* 2014;**5**(3). 320S–9S.
17. Wells JCK, Fewtrell MS. Measuring body composition. *Arch Dis Child* 2006;**91**(7):612–7.
18. Dung NQ, Fusch G, Armbrust S, Jochum F, Fusch C. Body composition of preterm infants measured during the first months of life: bioelectrical impedance provides insignificant additional information compared to anthropometry alone. *Eur J Pediatr* 2007;**166**(3):215–22.
19. Gale C, Thomas EL, Jeffries S, Durighel G, Logan KM, Parkinson JRC, et al. Adiposity and hepatic lipid in healthy full-term, breastfed, and formula-fed human infants: a prospective short-term longitudinal cohort study. *Am J Clin Nutr* 2014;**99**(5):1034–40.
20. Wadhwa PD, Buss C, Entringer S, Swanson JM. Developmental origins of health and disease: brief history of the approach and current focus on epigenetic mechanisms. *Semin Reprod Med* 2009;**27**(5):358–68.
21. Hales CN, Barker DJP. The thrifty phenotype hypothesis. *Br Med Bull* 2001;**60**:5–20.
22. Gluckman PD, Hanson MA, Cooper C, Thornburg KL. Effect of in utero and early-life conditions on adult health and disease. *N Engl J Med* 2008;**359**(1):61–73.
23. Singhal A, Lucas A. Early origins of cardiovascular disease: is there a unifying hypothesis? *Lancet* 2004;**363**(9421):1642–5.
24. Barker DJ, Osmond C. Infant mortality, childhood nutrition, and ischaemic heart disease in England and Wales. *Lancet* 1986;**1**(8489):1077–81.
25. Barker DJ, Winter PD, Osmond C, Margetts B, Simmonds SJ. Weight in infancy and death from ischaemic heart disease. *Lancet* 1989;**2**(8663):577–80.
26. Barker DJ, Gluckman PD, Godfrey KM, Harding JE, Owens JA, Robinson JS. Fetal nutrition and cardiovascular disease in adult life. *Lancet* 1993;**341**(8850):938–41.
27. Roseboom TJ, van der Meulen JH, Ravelli AC, Osmond C, Barker DJ, Bleker OP. Effects of prenatal exposure to the Dutch famine on adult disease in later life: an overview. *Mol Cell Endocrinol* 2001;**185**(1–2):93–8.
28. Barker DJ, Forsén T, Uutela A, Osmond C, Eriksson JG. Size at birth and resilience to effects of poor living conditions in adult life: longitudinal study. *BMJ* 2001;**323**(7324):1273–6.
29. Dessi A, Puddu M, Ottonello G, Fanos V. Metabolomics and fetal-neonatal nutrition: between "Not Enough" and "Too Much". *Molecules* 2013;**18**(10):11724–32.
30. Lukaszewski MA, Eberle D, Vieau D, Breton C. Nutritional manipulations in the perinatal period program adipose tissue in offspring. *Am J Physiol Endocrinol Metab* 2013;**305**(10):E1195–207.

31. Breton C. The hypothalamus-adipose axis is a key target of developmental programming by maternal nutritional manipulation. *J Endocrinol* 2013;**216**(2):R19–31.

32. MacKay H, Abizaid A. Embryonic development of the hypothalamic feeding circuitry: transcriptional, nutritional, and hormonal influences. *Mol Metab* 2014;**3**(9):813–22.

33. Warchol M, Krauss H, Wojciechowska M, Opala T, Pieta B, Zukiewicz-Sobczak W, et al. The role of ghrelin, leptin and insulin in foetal development. *Ann Agric Environ Med* 2014;**21**(2):349–52.

34. Horvath TL. The hardship of obesity: a soft-wired hypothalamus. *Nat Neurosci* 2005;**8**(5):561–5.

35. Wattez JS, Delahaye F, Lukaszewski MA, Risold PY, Eberle D, Vieau D, et al. Perinatal nutrition programs the hypothalamic melanocortin system in off spring. *Horm Metab Res* 2013;**45**(13):980–90.

36. Ramamoorthy TG, Begum G, Harno E, White A. Developmental programming of hypothalamic neuronal circuits: impact on energy balance control. *Front Neurosci* 2015;**9**:16.

37. Kasacka I, Janiuk I, Lewandowska A, Bekisz A, Lebkowski W. Distribution pattern of CART-containing neurons and cells in the human pancreas. *Acta Histochem* 2012;**114**(7):695–9.

38. Gluckman P, Hanson M. *Developmental origins of health and disease.* 1st ed. Cambridge: Cambridge University Press; 2006. p.519.

39. Poissonnet CM, Burdi AR, Garn SM. The chronology of adipose-tissue appearance and distribution in the human-fetus. *Early Hum Dev* 1984;**10**(1–2):1–11.

40. Wang P, Mariman E, Renes J, Keijer J. The secretory function of adipocytes in the physiology of white adipose tissue. *J Cell Physiol* 2008;**216**(1):3–13.

41. Tang W, Zeve D, Suh JM, Bosnakovski D, Kyba M, Hammer RE, et al. White fat progenitor cells reside in the adipose vasculature. *Science* 2008;**322**(5901):583–6.

42. Aldiss P, Dellschaft N, Sacks H, Budge H, Symonds ME. Beyond obesity—thermogenic adipocytes and cardiometabolic health. *Horm Mol Biol Clin Investig* 2017;**31**(2):1868–91.

43. Symonds ME, Bloor I, Ojha S, Budge H. The placenta, maternal diet and adipose tissue development in the newborn. *Ann Nutr Metab* 2017;**70**(3):232–5.

44. Symonds ME, Pope M, Budge H. The ontogeny of brown adipose tissue. *Ann Rev Nutr* 2015;**35**(1):295–320.

45. Kajimura S, Seale P, Kubota K, Lunsford E, Frangioni JV, Gygi SP, et al. Initiation of myoblast to brown fat switch by a PRDM16-C/EBP-beta transcriptional complex. *Nature* 2009;**460**(7259):1154–U125.

46. Wu J, Cohen P, Spiegelman BM. Adaptive thermogenesis in adipocytes: is beige the new brown? *Genes Dev* 2013;**27**(3):234–50.

47. Lukaszewski MA, Mayeur S, Fajardy I, Delahaye F, Dutriez-Casteloot I, Montel V, et al. Maternal prenatal undernutrition programs adipose tissue gene expression in adult male rat offspring under high-fat diet. *Am J Physiol Endocrinol Metab* 2011;**301**(3). E548–E59.

48. Stevens A, Begum G, White A. Epigenetic changes in the hypothalamic pro-opiomelanocortin gene: a mechanism linking maternal undernutrition to obesity in the offspring? *Eur J Pharmacol* 2011;**660**(1):194–201.

49. Vickers MH. Early life nutrition, epigenetics and programming of later life disease. *Nutrients* 2014;**6**(6):2165–78.

50. Jones PA. Functions of DNA methylation: islands, start sites, gene bodies and beyond. *Nat Rev Genet* 2012;**13**(7):484–92.

51. Bird A. DNA methylation patterns and epigenetic memory. *Genes Dev* 2002;**16**(1):6–21.

52. Kouzarides T. Chromatin modifications and their function. *Cell* 2007;**128**(4):693–705.

53. Iorio MV, Piovan C, Croce CM. Interplay between microRNAs and the epigenetic machinery: an intricate network. *Biochim Biophys Acta* 2010;**1799**(10–12):694–701.

54. Fraga MF, Ballestar E, Paz MF, Ropero S, Setien F, Ballestart ML, et al. Epigenetic differences arise during the lifetime of monozygotic twins. *Proc Natl Acad Sci USA* 2005;**102**(30):10604–9.

55. Coupe B, Amarger V, Grit I, Benani A, Parnet P. Nutritional programming affects hypothalamic organization and early response to leptin. *Endocrinology* 2010;**151**(2):702–13.

56. Mahmood S, Smiraglia DJ, Srinivasan M, Patel MS. Epigenetic changes in hypothalamic appetite regulatory genes may underlie the developmental programming for obesity in rat neonates subjected to a high-carbohydrate dietary modification. *J Dev Orig Health Dis* 2013;**4**(6):479–90.

57. Begum G, Stevens A, Smith EB, Connor K, Challis JRG, Bloomfield F, et al. Epigenetic changes in fetal hypothalamic energy regulating pathways are associated with maternal undernutrition and twinning. *FASEB J* 2012;**26**(4):1694–703.

58. Waterland RA, Lin JR, Smith CA, Jirtle RL. Post-weaning diet affects genomic imprinting at the insulin-like growth factor 2 (Igf2) locus. *Hum Mol Genet* 2006;**15**(5):705–16.

59. Painter RC, Osmond C, Gluckman P, Hanson M, Phillips DIW, Roseboom TJ. Transgenerational effects of prenatal exposure to the Dutch famine on neonatal adiposity and health in later life. *BJOG* 2008;**115**(10):1243–9.

60. Vanhees K, Vonhogen IGC, van Schooten FJ, Godschalk RWL. You are what you eat, and so are your children: the impact of micronutrients on the epigenetic programming of offspring. *Cell Mol Life Sci* 2014;**71**(2):271–85.

61. Waterland RA, Travisano M, Tahiliani KG, Rached MT, Mirza S. Methyl donor supplementation prevents transgenerational amplification of obesity. *Int J Obes (Lond)* 2008;**32**(9):1373–9.

62. Aiken CE, Ozanne SE. Transgenerational developmental programming. *Hum Reprod Update* 2014;**20**(1):63–75.

63. Aiken CE, Ozanne SE. Sex differences in developmental programming models. *Reproduction* 2013;**145**(1):R1–13.

64. Bouret SG. Role of early hormonal and nutritional experiences in shaping feeding behavior and hypothalamic development. *J Nutr* 2010;**140**(3):653–7.

65. Symonds ME, Budge H. Nutritional models of the developmental programming of adult health and disease. *Proc Nutr Soc* 2009;**68**(2):173–8.

66. Wu GY, Imhoff-Kunsch B, Girard AW. Biological mechanisms for nutritional regulation of maternal health and fetal development. *Paediatr Perinat Epidemiol* 2012;**26**:4–26.

67. Hanson MA, Gluckman PD. Early developmental conditioning of later health and disease: physiology or pathophysiology? *Physiol Rev* 2014; **94**(4):1027–76.

68. Ravelli GP, Stein ZA, Susser MW. Obesity in young men after famine exposure in utero and early infancy. *N Engl J Med* 1976;**295**(7):349–53.

69. Roseboom T, de Rooij S, Painter R. The Dutch famine and its long-term consequences for adult health. *Early Hum Dev* 2006;**82**(8):485–91.

70. Ravelli ACJ, van der Meulen JHP, Osmond C, Barker DJP, Bleker OP. Obesity at the age of 50 y in men and women exposed to famine prenatally. *Am J Clin Nutr* 1999;**70**(5):811–6.

71. Yura S, Itoh H, Sagawa N, Yamamoto H, Masuzaki H, Nakao K, et al. Role of premature leptin surge in obesity resulting from intrauterine undernutrition. *Cell Metab* 2005;**1**(6):371–8.

72. Breton C, Lukaszewski MA, Risold PY, Enache M, Guillemot J, Riviere G, et al. Maternal prenatal undernutrition alters the response of POMC neurons to energy status variation in adult male rat offspring. *Am J Physiol Endocrinol Metab* 2009;**296**(3). E462–E72.

73. Delahaye F, Breton C, Risold PY, Enache M, Dutriez-Casteloot I, Laborie C, et al. Maternal perinatal undernutrition drastically reduces postnatal leptin surge and affects the development of arcuate nucleus proopiomelanocortin neurons in neonatal male rat pups. *Endocrinology* 2008; **149**(2):470–5.

74. Garcia AP, Palou M, Priego T, Sanchez J, Palou A, Pico C. Moderate caloric restriction during gestation results in lower arcuate nucleus NPY- and alpha MSH-neurons and impairs hypothalamic response to fed/fasting conditions in weaned rats. *Diabetes Obes Metab* 2010;**12**(5):403–13.

75. Li C, McDonald TJ, Wu GY, Nijland MJ, Nathanielsz PW. Intrauterine growth restriction alters term fetal baboon hypothalamic appetitive peptide balance. *J Endocrinol* 2013;**217**(3):275–82.

76. Bouret SG, Gorski JN, Patterson CM, Chen S, Levin BE, Simerly RB. Hypothalamic neural projections are permanently disrupted in diet-induced obese rats. *Cell Metab* 2008;**7**(2):179–85.

77. McKnight JR, Satterfield MC, Li X, Gao H, Wang J, Li D, et al. Obesity in pregnancy: problems and potential solutions. *Front Biosci (Elite Ed)* 2011;**3**:442–52.

78. Dabelea D, Hanson RL, Lindsay RS, Pettitt DJ, Imperatore G, Gabir MM, et al. Intrauterine exposure to diabetes conveys risks for type 2 diabetes and obesity—a study of discordant sibships. *Diabetes* 2000;**49**(12):2208–11.

79. Lam YY, Hatzinikolas G, Weir JM, Janovska A, McAinch AJ, Game P, et al. Insulin-stimulated glucose uptake and pathways regulating energy metabolism in skeletal muscle cells: the effects of subcutaneous and visceral fat, and long-chain saturated, n-3 and n-6 polyunsaturated fatty acids. *Biochim Biophys Acta* 2011;**1811**(7–8):468–75.

80. Fernandez-Twinn DS, Ozanne SE. Mechanisms by which poor early growth programs type-2 diabetes, obesity and the metabolic syndrome. *Physiol Behav* 2006;**88**(3):234–43.

81. Holemans K, Aerts L, Van Assche FA. Lifetime consequences of abnormal fetal pancreatic development. *J Physiol Lond* 2003;**547**(1):11–20.

82. Steculorum SM, Bouret SG. Maternal diabetes compromises the organization of hypothalamic feeding circuits and impairs leptin sensitivity in offspring. *Endocrinology* 2011;**152**(11):4171–9.

83. Rumball CWH, Oliver MH, Thorstensen EB, Jaquiery AL, Husted SM, Harding JE, et al. Effects of twinning and periconceptional undernutrition on late-gestation hypothalamic-pituitary-adrenal axis function in ovine pregnancy. *Endocrinology* 2008;**149**(3):1163–72.

84. Dimasuay KG, Boeuf P, Powell TL, Jansson T. Placental responses to changes in the maternal environment determine fetal growth. *Front Physiol* 2016;**7**:9.

85. Mericq V, Martinez-Aguayo A, Uauy R, Iniguez G, Van der Steen M, Hokken-Koelega A. Long-term metabolic risk among children born premature or small for gestational age. *Nat Rev Endocrinol* 2017;**13**(1):50–62.

86. Palatianou ME, Simos YV, Andronikou SK, Kiortsis DN. Long-term metabolic effects of high birth weight: a critical review of the literature. *Horm Metab Res* 2014;**46**(13):911–20.

87. Kopec G, Shekhawat PS, Mhanna MJ. Prevalence of diabetes and obesity in association with prematurity and growth restriction. *Diabetes Metab Syndr Obes* 2017;**10**:285–95.

88. Embleton NE, Pang N, Cooke RJ. Postnatal malnutrition and growth retardation: an inevitable consequence of current recommendations in preterm infants? *Pediatrics* 2001;**107**(2):270–3.

89. Embleton ND, Korada M, Wood CL, Pearce MS, Swamy R, Cheetham TD. Catch-up growth and metabolic outcomes in adolescents born preterm. *Arch Dis Child* 2016;**101**:1026–31.

90. Baird J, Fisher D, Lucas P, Kleijnen J, Roberts H, Law C. Being big or growing fast: systematic review of size and growth in infancy and later obesity. *BMJ* 2005;**331**(7522):929–31.

91. Adair LS, Martorell R, Stein AD, Hallal PC, Sachdev HS, Prabhakaran D, et al. Size at birth, weight gain in infancy and childhood, and adult blood pressure in 5 low- and middle-income-country cohorts: when does weight gain matter? *Am J Clin Nutr* 2009;**89**(5):1383–92.

92. Nouri M, Tarighat-Esfanjani A. Mechanisms of breast feeding actions on obesity prevention: a systematic review. *Prog Nutr* 2016;**18**(4):323–33.

93. Cheng Y, Lao T. Foetal and maternal complications in macrosomic pregnancies. *Res Rep Neonatol* 2014;**4**:65–70.

94. Venn AJ, Thomson RJ, Schmidt MD, Cleland VJ, Curry BA, Gennat HC, et al. Overweight and obesity from childhood to adulthood: a follow-up of participants in the 1985 Australian Schools Health and Fitness Survey. *Med J Aust* 2007;**187**(10):599.

95. Steinberger J, Moran A, Hong CP, Jacobs DR, Sinaiko AR. Adiposity in childhood predicts obesity and insulin resistance in young adulthood. *J Pediatr* 2001;**138**(4):469–73.

96. Daniels SR. Complications of obesity in children and adolescents. *Int J Obes (Lond)* 2009;**33**(Suppl 1):S60–5.

97. Vikram NK. Cardiovascular and metabolic complications—diagnosis and management in obese children. *Indian J Pediatr* 2018;**85**(7):535–45.

98. Gungor NK. Overweight and obesity in children and adolescents. *J Clin Res Pediatr Endocrinol* 2014;**6**(3):129–43.

99. Kim J, Lee I, Lim S. Overweight or obesity in children aged 0 to 6 and the risk of adult metabolic syndrome: a systematic review and meta-analysis. *J Clin Nurs* 2017;**26**(23–24):3869–80.

100. Druet C, Stettler N, Sharp S, Simmons RK, Cooper C, Smith GD, et al. Prediction of childhood obesity by infancy weight gain: an individual-level meta-analysis. *Paediatr Perinat Epidemiol* 2012;**26**(1):19–26.

Chapter 51

Abnormal Fetal Growth

Cheri L. Deal

Department of Pediatrics, Université de Montréal, Montreal, QC, Canada; Pediatric Endocrine and Diabetes Service, Centre Hospitalier Universitaire Sainte Justine, Montreal, QC, Canada

Common Clinical Problems

- Fetal growth restriction, sometimes referred to as intrauterine growth restriction (IUGR), includes a wide range of causes of maternal, placental, and/or fetal origin. The majority of fetuses who fail to reach their genetic growth potential in utero will not be diagnosed before birth.
- Fetal overgrowth is most frequently caused by excess maternal weight gain and/or maternal diabetes.
- Associated metabolic and multiorgan morbidities are a concern for physicians caring for small for gestational age (SGA) and large for gestational age (LGA) newborns; the presence of dysmorphisms should prompt a search for congenital defects and a diagnostic workup for a syndromic cause.
- The SGA or LGA infant is at risk for morbidities not only in the postnatal period and in infancy, but also as the child moves into adulthood. This is because the fetal environment, when suboptimal, has the potential to program the fetal epigenome without changing the genome. In this manner, gene activity states can be altered and maintained during the lifespan.
- Many of the syndromes causing abnormal fetal growth involve genes that regulate basic cellular processes, such as growth factor signaling, DNA replication and cell cycle progression, RNA splicing, ubiquitination targeting protein degradation and control of cell death or cell survival.
- Optimal care of infants born with extremes of growth requires prompt diagnostic and therapeutic interventions and should involve a multidisciplinary team.

51.1 INTRODUCTION

Fascination with fetal growth can be documented in many cultures throughout history, dating back to the ancient Egyptians. They speculated that the placenta was the site of the soul, but it was not until Hippocrates that the placenta was viewed as a source of fetal nourishment. Aristotle and Galen also offered their observations on fetal development, but with no formal experimentation, relying on general principles and logic; rather, it was the Islamic culture that encouraged documentation of diseases and their treatment during the Middle Ages. While we generally credit Francis Bacon, lawyer-philosopher (1561–1626) of the Renaissance, with the birth of the scientific method, Leonardo da Vinci (1452–1519) was busy practicing it a century earlier. This artist-scientist-engineer-inventor was using his powers of observation and dissection to understand human fetal development. It was his famous drawings detailing an in situ fetus, as well as his notes with chronological measurements of fetal growth, that truly fueled the science of embryology and our understanding of fetal growth.[1]

Fast forward to our present-day disciplines of embryology, endocrinology, obstetrics, neonatology, and genetics, as well as our access to very powerful genetic and imaging technologies: we are now able to better understand the pathophysiology of fetal growth restriction (FGR) and postnatal growth retardation.

Why are we interested in FGR? First, over recent years, increasing numbers of pregnancies are characterized by FGR, and authors have attributed this to many societal factors (older mothers, professional workload, use of tobacco, maternal malnutrition—even in industrialized countries—and increasing access to assisted reproductive technology). Second, FGR is known to result in an increased risk of perinatal complications, including preterm delivery, with its implications for suboptimal health outcomes in the SGA newborn.[2, 3] Respiratory distress syndrome complicated by bronchopulmonary dysplasia poses a therapeutic dilemma, since supraphysiological doses of glucocorticoids are often used, potentially causing iatrogenic adrenal suppression and impacting on long-term bone health.[4] Perhaps most importantly, the postnatal growth and function of vital organs may be compromised, including that of the lung, the immune system, the brain, the

Maternal-Fetal and Neonatal Endocrinology. https://doi.org/10.1016/B978-0-12-814823-5.00052-0

cardiovascular system, and the organs involved in metabolic regulation. This, in turn, results in the development of potentially multiple morbidities in these babies in the postnatal period.[3] Metabolic complications of FGR can occur in the short term, giving rise to neonatal hypo- or hyperglycemia and hypocalcemia. In the longer term, FGR may lead short stature and/or a host of adult pathologies such as obesity, dyslipidemia, the metabolic syndrome, type 2 diabetes, osteoporosis, coronary artery disease, and hypertension.[5] Although the prevailing theory of the developmental origins of adult health and disease focuses on fetal exposure to environmental/maternal factors, a recent genome-wide association study (GWAS) metaanalysis involving 153,781 subjects from 37 different studies suggests a genetic component must also be considered.[6]

On the other hand, we are also seeing a rise in babies born large for gestational age (LGA), as the obesity epidemic goes global, and this is of great concern to those healthcare professionals caring for these babies and for their mothers. Very large babies bring another set of short-term endocrine complications (such as hyperinsulinemia and hypoglycemia).[7] The U-shaped curve of the relationship of birth weight to childhood obesity has also prompted a look at long-term health risk; studies have now shown that large babies may be at risk for obesity and type 2 diabetes even after adjustment for confounding variables, although this may be population-specific.[8–10]

This chapter will discuss current approaches to the classification and diagnosis of abnormal fetal growth and cover both common and rare etiologies for both SGA and LGA babies. We are, of course, excluding errors in dating conception, but mention it here because of its importance when considering a pre- or postnatal diagnosis of abnormal fetal growth. Emphasis will be put on diagnostic clues to the fetal extremes of growth in the newborn, and their endocrine comorbidities beyond those commonly seen for SGA and LGA babies in the neonatal unit will be discussed.

51.2 DEFINITIONS AND TERMINOLOGY ISSUES FOR THE ABNORMALLY SMALL OR LARGE FETUS AND NEONATE

51.2.1 Small for Gestational Age Fetus and Newborn

The terminology when discussing an abnormally growing fetus has been a source of confusion. The reader is encouraged to consult the review by Mayer and Joseph.[11] This chapter will use the term fetal growth restriction (FGR) to refer to fetuses who have failed to achieve their genetic potential because of an underlying pathology.

While ideally the fetus with growth restriction should be diagnosed before birth, the reality is that up to 80% of growth-restricted fetuses may not have been recognized before birth.[12] This being said, tracking of fetal growth velocity using repeated fetal ultrasounds coupled with use of maternal biomarkers including β-hCG, placental growth factor (PIGF), and pregnancy-associated plasma protein A (PAPP-A) is being investigated in order to improve prenatal diagnosis of abnormal fetal growth.[13] The term IUGR implies that there have been at least two fetal ultrasounds documenting growth below the 10th percentile, performed two or more weeks apart.[14, 15] It is beyond the scope of this chapter to discuss the obstetrical and imaging modalities and the fetal anthropometry currently being used to diagnose FGR, as well as what new technology will bring to diagnosis in the future (see instead Chapter 40 and Refs. 16–18). Nevertheless, it is important that clinicians receiving these newborns can rapidly identify those missed in the prenatal period.

The term *SGA* is used to represent a group of babies just under the normal birth weight, quite possibly for constitutional reasons. This is because we have traditionally used a definition of a birth weight below the 10th percentile based on *fetal growth references*, which include both normal and abnormal pregnancies and/or fetuses with congenital anomalies. While some of these SGA babies may actually have achieved their growth potential (i.e., are constitutionally small), others may be more likely to have a pathological diagnosis, including all those syndromes for which mean birth weight lies well below the normal population reference mean, discussed later, or babies who have actually had inadequate placental blood flow. This may be particularly true for those babies born less than the 3rd percentile. On the other hand, even babies well within the normal growth percentiles may have suffered malnutrition or hypoxia but have gone unrecognized.

When we refer to *fetal growth standards*, we are speaking about children born from normal pregnancies, with no identified growth or medical abnormalities in the (at least) first 2 years of life. Such growth standards have recently been published by the international INTERGROWTH-21st project[19] and they are analogous to the recently published WHO infant growth curves from 0 to 2 years, which are currently the growth curve standard used by many countries. Attempts have also been made to develop customized growth charts, some taking into account many factors that should be considered as covariables in addition to ethnicity (not necessarily synonymous with genetic similarity), such as parental size, parity, gender, and singleton versus twin pregnancies. Although used widely around the world, they are difficult to validate with regards to their clinical usefulness for reasons of sample size.

A recent international consensus group ($N = 57$) has suggested the following criteria for diagnosing FGR, with the numbers in parentheses representing the proportion of the experts in agreement[20]: Birth weight less than the 3rd percentile on population-based or customized growth charts (86%) OR at least 3 out of 5 of the following: (1) birth weight <10th percentile on population-based (78%) or customized growth charts (94%); (2) head circumference <10th percentile (82%); (3) length <10th percentile (82%); (4) prenatal diagnosis of FGR (88%); (5) maternal pregnancy information (e.g., hypertension or preeclampsia) (75%).

The importance of using a uniform definition for SGA is particularly evident when assessing outcomes, as has been shown by Zeve et al.[21] when risk ratios were compared for various morbidities according to the definition used. Using a definition of SGA that includes infants weighing more than 2 SD beneath the mean (<2.3rd percentile) or <3rd percentile, when compared to using a definition of birth weight <10th percentile gives markedly different outcome statistics. This not only includes short-term consequences of SGA but also longer-term complications, such as failure to exhibit catch-up growth or to develop long-term metabolic complications. Pediatric endocrinologists tend to use a definition that includes a newborn weight and/or length less than −2 SD for gestation age, based on reference data from a relevant population as outlined in an international consensus statement on the management of infants born SGA.[22]

Newborns not only can be classified by birth weight centiles (for example, SGA <10th percentile, LGA >90th centile, AGA 10th to 90th centiles) but they can also be classified in low birth weight (LBW) and very low birth weight (VLBW, <1500 g) categories, since the latter bring additional risk for neonatal complications. Generally, birth weights from the 3rd to the 10th percentile for gestational age are considered as moderate FGR, whereas birth weights less than the 3rd percentile for gestational are considered severe FGR. Finally, they can be considered to have either symmetric growth retardation or asymmetric growth retardation, depending on the degree to which the head circumference, and thus brain growth, has been affected relative to the length or weight. Symmetric FGR usually has its origins earlier in gestation and is more likely, but not always, caused by chromosomal/genetic factors. Often, we refer to microcephaly in this context, although it is proportionate to the overall small size of the fetus, for example, in the various syndromes with primary microcephalic dwarfism discussed later. In asymmetric FGR, the head appears proportionately larger (relative macrocephaly) than the length and particularly than the abdomen and extremities. It is the hallmark of inadequate nutrition, with nutrient distribution prioritizing the fetal brain, although it can also be seen in genetic syndromes such as Silver-Russell syndrome (SRS), discussed in following text.[23] The ponderal index, which is a ratio of body weight to length (= weight (g) × 100 ÷ length (cm)), is more useful to detect FGR, particularly in cases of asymmetric FGR.[24]

51.2.2 Large for Gestational Age Fetus and Newborn

Issues similar to percentile considerations are also germane to the discussion of the large newborn, with those greater than the 90th percentile for gestational age qualifying as LGA. Whether using standards of growth or population-based reference curves, weight cut-offs will be different. What is clear is that birth weights greater than the 97th percentile are at the highest risk for neonatal complications.[25] Use of an even more refined grading system for birth weights based on a US population of babies born between 37 and 42 weeks and risk stratified into three categories (grade 1 = those weighing more than 4000 g, grade 2 = those more than 4500 g, and grade 3 = those over 5000 g) shows that babies ≥4000 g have the greatest risk of morbidity and those ≥5000 g are at greatest risk for mortality.[26]

51.3 ACCURATE DETERMINATION OF NEWBORN ANTHROPOMETRY

Whether we are referring to the SGA or the LGA newborn, one of the major challenges is the accurate assessment of newborn anthropometry. The reader is referred to the technical approaches used for the INTERGROWTH 21st project[27] since good clinical decision-making requires accurate data! This requires having a newborn weighing scale with a capacity to measure both the smallest and the largest infant, with increments of 5–10 g depending on weight. Tape measurements should be used for head circumference only, measured to the nearest 0.1 cm, unless in a resource-poor situation where there are no infantometers available. Infantometers typically have a fixed headboard and a movable footboard, with accuracy to the nearest 0.1 cm. Frequent calibration and adequate equipment maintenance and servicing are equally important to insure accurate measurements.

51.4 UNDERSTANDING THE ETIOLOGY OF GROWTH DISORDERS IN THE FETUS

Fetal growth requires a very complex interplay between maternal, placental, and fetal hormonogenesis and metabolism, all of which is influenced by (and may influence) the establishment of adequate placental vascularization and function as well as a normal maternal metabolic and hormonal milieu, as discussed in previous chapters. The intrauterine environment (including uterine pathologies, singleton versus multiple gestation pregnancies, parity) and environmental factors affecting the mother (such as famine, tobacco smoke, antioxidant status, drugs) are also important determinants of fetal growth.[3, 28]

Intrinsic or genetic factors play a role in these interactions, through their orchestration of circulating levels of growth factors (autocrine, paracrine, and endocrine), hormones (maternal, fetal, and placental) and other critical molecules including superoxide dismutase enzymes and detoxification enzyme systems, as well as embryotrophic and embryotoxic cytokines. "Normal" genomes, however, are not enough to ensure normal fetal growth, and it is clear that the epigenome, through modification of the histone proteins (acetylation, methylation, and other modifications) and of DNA (methylation) and lncRNA (long, noncoding) and miRNA (microRNA), are the ultimate determinants of the activity state of genes that affect fetal growth.[29] Indeed, recent genetic analyses using genome-wide methylation arrays in SGA and AGA newborns have shown a variety of methylation abnormalities.[30] Epigenetics also play an important role in the adaptation of the fetus to its environment, referred to as developmental programming. According to this theory, it is the potential mismatch between intrauterine conditions and the environment following birth that sets the newborn infant on the road to health or disease in adulthood, as discussed earlier for the SGA and LGA infant. Evidence over the past 40 years has been accumulating to support this theory, through epidemiological studies in humans, animal models, and elucidation of the molecular mechanisms behind altered gene activity.[31]

51.5 CAUSES AND CONSEQUENCES OF FETAL GROWTH RESTRICTION

Table 51.1 gives the etiologies and risk factors for FGR, according to their cause. The perspectives of the obstetrician and the neonatologist have been outlined recently in reviews by Nardozza et al. and Sharma et al.[32, 33] FGR can also be considered in terms of the timing of growth failure: early onset FGR is recognized before 32 weeks of gestation and is most often due to underlying placental pathology; the causes can be multiple with strong associations with maternal hypertension and preeclampsia (60%). The prevalence has been suggested to be 0.5%–1%, although this obviously depends upon the patient population screened.[34] An onset of FGR after 32 weeks is more frequent, and late FGR is less (15%) associated with preeclampsia. However, given the larger numbers of these births, it potentially represents significant numbers of at-risk neonates even if these babies overall have a much lower mortality and morbidity than do the early FGR babies.[35]

TABLE 51.1 Causes of fetal growth restriction

Fetal	- Constitutionally small fetus Polygenic variants in genes explaining some ethnic and population variation - Chromosomal abnormalities Trisomies 13 (Patau syndrome), 18 (Edward syndrome), and 21 (Down syndrome) Uniparental disomies (e.g., maternal UPD 7, maternal UPD 20, and paternal UPD 6) Sex chromosome deletions or rearrangements (particularly biallelic SHOX deletions causing Langer Mesomelic Dysplasia), classic (45,X) Turner syndrome or Turner syndrome variant karyotypes Autosomal deletions of fetal growth genes and their receptors (IGF-I, IGF-II, IGF1R) (see Table 51.3) - Rare metabolic/endocrine disorders Agenesis of pancreas, congenital absence of islets of langerhans, congenital lipodystrophy, galactosemia, generalized gangliosidosis type I, hypophosphatasia, I-cell disease, leprechaunism, fetal phenylketonuria, transient neonatal diabetes mellitus - Multiple genetic syndromes (see Table 51.2) - Infectious disorders TORCH, syphilis, congenital HIV, congenital rubella, malaria - Congenital anomalies Congenital heart disease, tracheo-esophageal fistula, abdominal wall defects, renal malformations, anorectal malformations, neural tube defects, congenital diaphragmatic hernia
Maternal	- Maternal age—extremes (adolescent, over 35 years) - Parity—first pregnancy or greater than 5 births - Previous history of SGA birth Short interval between subsequent pregnancies—less than 6 months - Maternal hypertension (prior, or pregnancy-associated) - Maternal smoking - Maternal substance abuse - Maternal medications, particularly anticonvulsants, antineoplastic drugs, warfarin - Prolonged exposure to high altitude conditions - Protein calorie malnutrition/poor weight gain/BMI under 20 prior to pregnancy - Maternal congenital heart disease, particularly cyanotic - Maternal asthma, poorly controlled

TABLE 51.1 Causes of fetal growth restriction—cont'd

	- Thrombophilias such as anticardiolipin antibodies - Poorly controlled diabetes, particularly with associated vasculopathy - Preeclampsia - Other chronic maternal conditions (chronic renal disease, sickle cell anemia, systemic lupus erythematosus) - Maternal infections including TORCH, TB, malaria, urinary tract infections, bacterial vaginosis - Uterine malformations, uterine leiomyoma - Assisted reproductive technology

Placental	- Abnormal placental development (abnormal uteroplacental vasculature, avascular placental villi, syncytial knots)
	- Twin (multiple) pregnancies[a]
	   Dichorionic
	   Monochorionic with twin-to-twin transfusion
	- Abnormal umbilical cord insertion
	- Single umbilical artery
	- Multiple gestations
	- Retro-placental hemorrhage/placenta abruption (chronic)
	- Placental hemangioma
	- Placental malaria
	- Chronic villitis of unknown etiology
	- Partial molar pregnancy
	- Confined placental mosaicism

[a]*When discordance exists between the growth of one of the fetuses in a twin pregnancy, infections and fetal factors must be considered, including all the nongenetic and the genetic causes. UPD, uniparental disomy.*

Fetal factors, although less common than placental or maternal, will be the subject of a more detailed discussion in sections below. Their diagnosis can be made prenatally, through current prenatal screening modalities, or only be made in the postnatal period because of newborn phenotype or complications. Of particular interest are those caused by a genetic or epigenetic defect, since they may require long-term follow-up by a pediatric endocrinologist. Some therapies may be optional, such as GH treatment for SGA infants that fail to achieve catch-up growth after birth (see the following text), but some of these conditions have associated endocrinopathies requiring treatment.

51.5.1 Twin or Multiple Gestation Pregnancies

By far the most frequent cause of FGR are twin or multiple gestation pregnancies. Growth (in the absence of all the causes of FGR listed in Table 51.1) tends to slow, particularly in the third trimester. This occurs because of uterine constraints to growth and is proportionate to the mass of the placentae. Preterm birth, morbidity and mortality are higher in these pregnancies, particularly in monochorionic twin pregnancies, where there may be discordant growth of the fetuses because of discordant placental mass and twin-to-twin transfusion.[36] Current efforts aim to identify the pathophysiological causes of selective FGR in twin pregnancies, and fetal therapy, including selective reduction and laser photocoagulation of placental vessels, is now being used and evaluated.[37]

51.5.2 Constitutionally Small Fetus

Infants born at term with population-based birth weights less than the 10th centile are more likely to be constitutionally small compared to those born preterm, based on mortality and morbidity rates in large cohorts of newborns without malformations.[38] As noted previously, maternal size is just one factor that may explain this, particularly if subsequent pregnancies also end in SGA births at term, without perinatal morbidities and without confounding maternal factors such as smoking or drug use. There are no randomized studies available to assess whether taking into account maternal early pregnancy weight, height, parity, or ethnicity will more accurately help in predicting the constitutionally small infant.[39] However, in a GWAS metaanalysis study of birth weights, 15% of the variance in BW could be explained by fetal genetic variation.[6]

While most of our definitions of FGR/SGA are based on weights, because of the inaccuracy of newborn length unless proper techniques are used, it is of interest to have an accurate maternal height. If, with a normal pregnancy history and with no maternal disease or dysmorphisms, maternal height falls at the lower centiles for adult height (under 151 cm, or ≤3rd percentile), constitutional factors may contribute to the SGA term infant. After the second year of life, when the infant is no longer subject to maternal constraints, use of a sex-corrected genetic target range can help predict the appropriate growth corridor for height, again pointing to constitutional factors if in the lower range. Unfortunately, there are no large-scale GWAS studies on birth length. However, given that there are over 400 loci with predominantly minor effects on adult height (less than 1 cm for two variant alleles) according to recent genome data,[40] a polygenic explanation for term SGA fetuses, with minimal to no morbidity and born after a normal pregnancy, is just as likely. Thus the chances of identifying a particular gene with a major effect on prenatal growth are small but not insignificant, particularly for extremes of fetal growth, as discussed in following text and shown in Tables 51.1–51.4.

TABLE 51.2   Rare syndromes with IUGR/SGA birth size[a]

Syndrome name (OMIM #)	Molecular defect(s)[b]	Birth size[c]
With normo- or macrocephaly		
Silver-Russell (180860)[d]	UPD chr 7 mat Chr 11p15 mutations /epimutations of the H19-IGF2 or KCNQ1-CDKN1C domains Mat duplications of 11p15 (AD)	BW and/or BL SDS ≤−2
Temple (616222)[d]	UPD chr 14 mat Pat microdeletions/hypomethylation of DLK1/GTL2 intergenic DMR DLK1 deletion (AD)	Median BW SDS −1.88
3-M (273750)	CUL7, OBSL1 or CCDC8 mutations (AR)	Mean BW SDS −3.1
Mulibrey nanism (253250)	TRIM37 mutations (AR)	Mean BW SDS −2.8
SHORT (269880)	PIK3R1 mutation (AD)	Mean BW SDS −3.3
Floating-Harbor (136140)	SRCAP mutations (AD)	Mean BW SDS −2.5
IMAGe (614732)[d]	Mat CDKN1C mutations	BW SDS range −2.4 to −4.0
MIRAGE (617053)	SAMD9 (AD)	IUGR in 100%
With microcephaly		
Meier-Gorlin, subtypes 1–8 (224690, 613800, 613803, 613804, 613805, 613835, 617063, 617564)	Mutations in ORC1, ORC4, ORC6, CDT1, CDC6, GMNN, CDC25, MCM5 (AR)	Mean BW SDS −3.4
Seckel, subtypes 1–9 (210600, 606744, 613676, 613823, 614728, 614851, 615807, 616777, 617253)	ATR, RBBP8, CENPJ, CEP152, CEP63, NIN, DNA2, TRAIP, NSMCE2 and PCNT mutations (AR)	Mean BW SDS < −4 Mean BW 1500 g (IUGR)
MOPDI/III	RNU4ATAC (AR)	Mean BW SDS < −4
MOPDII (210720)	PCNT mutations (AR)	Mean BW SDS −3.9
Nijmegen Breakage syndrome (251260)	NBN mutations (AR)	Mean BW SDS −1.6
With variable incidence of SGA		
Turner syndrome	Complete/partial loss of one X chromosome	50% with SGA (BW <10th percentile)
SHOX deficiency (127300, 300582, 249700)	SHOX, SHOXY (hemi- or homozygous mutation/del) (Pseudo AD)	Leri-Weill: Mean BL SDS −0.59 ± 1.26 Langer mesomelic dysplasia: reduced BL
Williams-Beuren (194050)	Hemizygous deletion at 7q11.23 (GTF2IRD1/GTF2I) (AD)	IUGR
Smith-Lemli-Opitz (270400)	DHCR7 (AR)	BW <2500 g

TABLE 51.2 Rare syndromes with IUGR/SGA birth size—cont'd

Syndrome name (OMIM #)	Molecular defect(s)	Birth size
Cornelia de Lange (122470, 300882, 610759, 300882)	*NIPBL, SMC1A, SMC3, RAD21 (AD); HDAC8* (XLD)	Mean BW female 2234 g Mean BW male 2454 g
Bloom (210900)	*OBSL1* mutations (AR)	Mean BW female 1841 g Mean BW male 2094 g
Pallister-Hall	*GLI 3* mutations (AD)	IUGR
Microphthalmia 9 (601186)	*STRA6* (AR)	IUGR
Johanson-Blizzard (243800)	*UBR1* (AR)	Low birth weight—SGA
SERKEL(611812)	*MMTV* (AR)	IUGR
Cockayne A (216400)	*ERCC8* (AR)	IUGR
Mitochondrial complex I deficiencies (618238, 618243)	*NUDFAF5, NDUFA10* (AR)	IUGR
Fanconi anemia (0111086)	*FANCA* (AR)	Low birth weight—SGA
IMAGEI (618336)	*POLE* (AR)	IUGR

BW, birth weight; BL, birth length; SDS, standard deviation score; AR, autosomal recessive; AD, adtosomal dominant; XLD, X-linked dominant.
[a]*See text for phenotypic and endocrine features.*
[b]*See OMIM for complete gene name and function: https://www.omim.org/.*
[c]*Where no case series are available for BW data, OMIM clinical synopsis of IUGR/SGA was noted.*
[d]*Syndrome involves genomic imprinting and requires specific parental allele as indicated, to have a phenotype.*

TABLE 51.3 Fetal growth restriction caused by (rare) gene defects involving IGF and insulin

Condition (OMIM #)	Molecular defect(s)	Inheritance	Major clinical features
IGF-I deficiency (608747)	*IGF1* mutation	AD AR	Pre- and postnatal growth retardation, microcephaly, micrognathia, sensorineural deafness, ptosis, delayed bone age, osteopenia, clinodactyly, delayed motor development, intellectual disability
IGF-I resistance/ insensitivity (270450)	*IGF1R* deletion (15q26.3) *IGF1R* mutation	AD (rare AR)	Pre- and postnatal growth retardation, microcephaly, triangular face, thin upper lip, clinodactyly, small hands, short fingers, global developmental delay, intellectual disability. In AR forms, see above with more severe facial dysmorphisms, progeria-like appearance, teeth anomalies, heart defects, vascular anomalies, underdeveloped cerebral gyri, hypoplastic corpus callosum, elevated baseline insulin. With larger 15q contiguous deletion, also see heart defects, cryptorchidism, hypospadias in male, brachydactyly, and developmental delay
15q26-qter deletion (612626)	15q26-qter deletion	AD	
Ring chromosome 15 (no OMIM)[a]	Ring chromosome 15	Sporadic	
IGF-II deficiency (616489)	Paternal *IGF2* mutation	Imprinted gene disorder paternal transmission	Pre- and postnatal growth retardation, relative macrocephaly, triangular face, developmental delay. May have hearing impairment and/or heart defects
Insulin resistance syndrome[b] (246200); Rabson-Mendenhall (262190)	*INSR* mutation	AR	FGR and postnatal failure to thrive with neonatal diabetes, elfin facies, acanthosis nigricans, hypertrichosis, lack of fat tissue, muscle wasting, hyperplasia of gingiva, external genitalia and pancreatic islets, large hands and feet, frequently fatal in early life. Allelic variants give rise to additional symptoms in Rabson-Mendenhall syndrome (see text)

Continued

TABLE 51.3 Fetal growth restriction caused by (rare) gene defects involving IGF and insulin—cont'd

Condition (OMIM #)	Molecular defect(s)	Inheritance	Major clinical features
Transient neonatal diabetes mellitus (601410)	Paternal chromosome 6 UPD	Imprinted gene disorders	FGR and postnatal failure to thrive. Transient neonatal diabetes usually resolving by 3–9 months, with permanent diabetes developing later in life in over 50% of patients. Some patients have macroglossia and/or umbilical hernia
	Paternel duplication 6q24 Hypomethylation, ZAC/PLAGL1 DMR		
	ZFP57 mutations	AR	
Insulin deficiency states			
Pancreatic agenesis Type 1 (260370)	PDX1(IPF1) mutation	AR	FGR/SGA and neonatal diabetes (permanent), +/− exocrine pancreatic deficiency
Pancreatic agenesis Type 2 (615935)	PTF1A mutation	AR	SGA, neonatal diabetes (permanent), +/− exocrine pancreatic deficiency
Mitchell-Riley (615710)	RFX6 mutation	AR	FGR, neonatal diabetes, hypoplastic or annular pancreas, biliary atresia, duodenal/jejunal atresia
Pancreatic and cerebellar agenesis	PTF1A mutation	AR	SGA with microcephaly, neonatal diabetes with pancreatic hypoplasia or agenesis, optic nerve hypoplasia, cerebellar hypoplasia or aplasia, seizures, death in infancy

ZAC/PLAG1, pleomorphic adenoma gene-like 1; ZFP57, zinc finger protein 57; PDX1, pancreas/duodenum homeobox protein 1 gene, also called insulin promoter factor 1 (IPF1); PTF1A, pancreas transcription factor 1 gene; RFX6, regulatory factor X 6; AD, autosomal dominant; AR autosomal recessive.
[a]Several reports describe patients with ring chromosome 15 having IUGR phenotype: see text.
[b]Also called Donohue syndrome or leprechaunism.

51.5.3 Trisomy 13, 18, and 21

Newborn infants with trisomy 18 are more likely to be born SGA than those with trisomy 13 or 21. The Vermont Oxford Network (VON) generated birth weight and head circumference for these three trisomies born between 22 weeks gestation and term, along with anthropometric charts easily used.[41] The authors noted that commonly used population-based growth charts may under- or overestimate SGA/LGA incidence in newborns with trisomies, which may influence medical follow-up of these infants. This same network also studied the incidence of VLBW infants with these trisomies in over 500,000 VLBW babies born in 941 institutions between 1994 and 2009 and found the incidence to be higher than previously reported based on all birth data in the US.[42] While over two-thirds of infants with trisomy 13 or 18 were reported to die by the age of 1 week, current practice suggests that infants with trisomy 21 have a much greater life expectancy even with significant morbidity.

Short-term endocrine considerations in these infants include a higher reported incidence of congenital (primary) hypothyroidism, both compensated and noncompensated, as discussed in Chapter 43. Some authors[43, 44] suggest that earlier follow-up screening should be performed even if the neonatal screen is normal, although current American Academy of Pediatrics recommendations suggest TSH and FT4 measurements at 6 and 12 months and then yearly (Bull Pediatrics 2011). Interpretation of thyroid function in VLBW infants with trisomy 21 is further complicated if other comorbidities are present, particularly congenital heart malformations or gastrointestinal malformations requiring early surgery.

51.5.4 Turner Syndrome and Abnormal Fetal Growth in Sex Chromosome Deletions

Turner syndrome (TS) is the most common cause of spontaneous first-trimester miscarriages. It is diagnosed in 1 in 2000 live-born female births, and the diagnosis is often made in the first trimester by ultrasound. Increased nuchal translucency (also seen in the trisomies discussed earlier) or frank cystic hygroma are highly suggestive, particularly if combined with aortic coarctation or other left-sided heart defects, brachycephaly, renal anomalies such as horseshoe kidney, polyhydramnios, oligohydramnios and FGR.[45] TS arises from partial or complete monosomy for the X chromosome, and in roughly half of cases involves mosaicism with either a normal 46,XX complement, or other cells containing abnormal sex chromosome complements. Complicating prenatal amniocentesis or techniques using cell-free fetal DNA (see Chapter 52) is a lack of specificity owing in part to differing levels of mosaicism for an abnormal sex chromosome complement, since these can be confined to the placenta. In a recent cohort of Turkish individuals with TS, SGA births were found in 33%; the mean birth weight was 0.36 kg lower than that of the non-TS female population and the mean birth length was 1.3 cm shorter.[46] Wisniewski and colleagues investigated the medical records of 468 Polish girls with TS who were delivered at term, and found a mean BW of 2963.[47] Mean BL in an Argentinian cohort of TS females at term was 46.4 ± 3.5 cm,[48] which suggests that roughly half of these babies are below the 10th percentile based on the data from the Intergrowth-21st Project discussed earlier and in Chapter 40.

In addition to FGR, girls with TS also show postnatal growth retardation. This abnormal growth is due to haploinsufficiency for *SHOX*.[49] This gene is located in the pseudoautosomal region of the short arm of both the X and Y chromosomes, and two copies are needed for normal growth. Deletions or mutations in this gene are found in 2% of patients with idiopathic short stature (males and females), and more severe skeletal phenotypes can also be seen such as Léri-Weill dyschondrogenesis and in Langer mesomelic dysplasia. Diagnosis can be made in these latter conditions when ultrasonography demonstrates mesomelia, although birth weight and length may not be SGA. Therapy with GH is now commonly used because of its accepted therapeutic benefits on height, even starting as young as age 2 years.[50]

51.5.5 Unexplained Postnatal Growth and the Importance of a Second Look at BL and BW

Not all diagnoses of TS (or of other syndromes associated with prenatal growth restriction/SGA) are made in the prenatal or early postnatal period, and in a cohort of 55 patients investigated for unexplained short stature with a history of SGA birth, eight genes already associated with postnatal growth disorders were found. Four of the gene mutations found, including in SHOX, are associated with growth plate development (*IHH* in 2 cases, *NPR2* in 2 cases, *SHOX*, and *ACAN*) and two are involved in the RAS/MAPK pathway (*PTPN11*, *NF1*). Of note, seven patients were SGA only for length and one was SGA for both length and weight. Most importantly, none of these patients had findings on clinical examination that led to a diagnostic suspicion in infancy or childhood.[51]

While this chapter will not focus on the more common syndromes potentially causing SGA, the reader should be aware that many exist that may cause FGR, often because of associated congenital malformations or medical conditions, so these will be diagnosed in infancy. Some of those more familiar to the endocrinologist because of concomitant endocrine/metabolic morbidities and postnatal growth retardation include: Williams-Beuren syndrome (OMIM 194050), Smith-Lemli-Opitz syndrome (OMIM 270400), Cornelia de Lange syndrome (OMIM 122470), Bloom syndrome (210900), Pallister-Hall syndrome (146510), microphthalmia syndrome 9 (OMIM 601186), Johnson-Blizzard syndrome (OMIM243800), 46,XX sex reversal with dysgenesis of kidneys, adrenals and lungs, or SERKAL syndrome (OMIM 611812), Cockayne syndrome (OMIM 216400), autosomal recessive microcephaly 10 syndrome (OMIM 615095), mitochondrial complex I deficiencies (multiple types, for examples OMIM 618238, 618243) and some of the defects leading to Fanconi anemia (for example, OMIM 0111086). In fact, an OMIM search for intrauterine growth retardation displayed 399 entries. The syndromes with a genetic or epigenetic etiology deemed important for the pediatric and adult endocrinologist to know about are further discussed in the following paragraphs.

51.5.6 Uniparental Disomy for Chromosomes 6, 7, 11, 14, 15, 16, or 20

Uniparental disomy (UPD) for specific chromosomes has been found in cases of SGA (and LGA; see Section 51.9.1). It can involve an entire chromosome or can be segmental, involving a more restricted chromosomal segment, such as 11p15 because of a mitotic recombination or gene conversion event. Furthermore, somatic mosaicism can be observed for UPD, suggesting a postfertilization error. While there is no justification for routine screening for UPD, fetal findings on ultrasound and/or numeric and/or structural chromosomal aberrations in chorionic villous or amniotic fluid samples may justify further genetic work-up for UPD, with the active presence of a geneticist and/or genetic counselor to explain the findings.[52]

A series of clinical phenotypes of specific UPDs implies the presence of imprinted loci, that is to say, the monoallelic expression in one or more tissues of a limited number of autosomal genes according to their parent of origin. Genomic imprinting involves epigenetic modifications that do not change the DNA sequence but that result in an altered activity state of the gene, such that only the paternally inherited copy is actively transcribed in the case of some genetic loci, and only the maternally inherited copy is actively transcribed at other loci.[53] Imprinted genes giving rise to UPD phenotypes involving growth include the following:

I. Probably the most familiar to endocrinologists is the maternal UPD for chromosome 15, one of the genetic abnormalities associated with Prader-Willi syndrome. Prenatal growth restriction is mild, but these infants are typically born with a birth weight 15% less than their siblings, which may place some of them in the SGA category.[54] However, by far the most common clinical sign is their pre- and postnatal hypotonia and feeding difficulties, and on clinical examination, cryptorchidism and hypoplastic genitalia.

II. The phenotype for paternal UPD 6 is that of FGR with transient neonatal diabetes mellitus (TNDM). This insulin-dependent diabetes has a high probability of becoming permanent later in life and is presumably related to inadequate fetal insulin, one of the major fetal growth factors.[55] Birth weights are consistently below the 2nd percentile. Diabetes is of very early onset.[56] Note that there are other forms of TNDM that involve paternal duplication of the 6q24 region (three copies of the region, but only the two paternal copies are active), reactivation of the maternal allele in this region (through loss of methylation at *PLAGL1* differentially methylated region) or mutations in *ZFP57* (a gene active early after fertilization to maintain normal methylation imprints). This latter gene is located on 6q22, and mutations may give rise to multiple methylation defects (see Table 51.3 and Section 51.7).

III. Maternal UPD 7 is one of the genetic anomalies seen in Russell-Silver syndrome (but at a lower frequency than several specific genetic and epigenetic abnormalities at 11p15.5) and will be discussed in Section 51.6.1. One of the important diagnostic keys is a birth weight and/or birth length for gestational age ≤ -2 SD.[57]

IV. Maternal UPD for chromosome 11 has also been reported in cases of IUGR-SRS,[58, 59] although paternal UPD for this chromosome is more frequent, and results in the overgrowth syndrome of Beckwith-Wiedemann, described in Section 51.9.2.1. Multiple other molecular defects can occur at the 11p15 locus besides UPD (see Section 51.6.1.).

V. Maternal UPD for chromosome 14 is found in Temple syndrome (see Section 51.6.2), and this syndrome has some overlap with Prader-Willi syndrome particularly because of the associated hypotonia, small hands and feet, and development of obesity. Median birth weight SD score (SDS) is -1.88, so many of these patients may be born SGA.[60]

VI. Both maternal UPD 16 and maternal UPD 20 have been reported in patients with pre- and postnatal growth retardation, sometimes described as having SRS.[57]

All of these UPDs are associated with SGA infants with varying degrees of developmental delay and with neurocognitive phenotypes. The associated syndromes and causal genes are discussed in following text and in Table 51.2.

51.6 SPECIFIC SYNDROMES ASSOCIATED WITH BIRTH OF AN SGA INFANT WITH RELATIVE MACROCEPHALY

Although syndromes causing SGA are considered very rare (orphan) diseases, we may see their numbers increase in the future simply because we are now using gene panels or whole exome sequencing to diagnose new cases of the SGA newborn with an accompanying syndromic phenotype, as well as in VLBW patients in the absence of chronic illness and in whom catch-up growth after birth has not occurred. This will help us eventually calculate birth incidence and better frequencies for each of the molecular causes within the same syndrome.

What will become clear in the following section is that many of the gene defects found to be involved include those required for fundamental cellular processes. Some of these genes lie in imprinted domains, which open the door for multiple molecular abnormalities within a syndrome, involving not only the genome but also the epigenome, as briefly discussed earlier in the context of UPD. Some genes clearly have genotype-phenotype correlations to the point that the same gene can give rise to two different syndromes depending on the specific location/type of mutation. Gene mutations can be hypomorphic; in other words, they may conserve partial gene function or they may be dominant negative alleles, which makes it important to explore the functional impact of the mutation. It also calls for good genetic counseling concerning future pregnancies. The multisystemic involvement of many of these conditions also underlines the need for a multidisciplinary team approach, not only for diagnosis, but for subsequent follow-up and treatment.

51.6.1 Silver-Russell Syndrome

According to a recent international consensus,[57] this syndrome should be diagnosed primarily through clinical ascertainment, using a simplified scoring system that includes having at least four of the following: (1) SGA (BW and/or

BL), (2) postnatal growth failure at age 2 years (height ≤ -2 SDS below midparental target height), (3) relative macrocephaly at birth as defined by head circumference ≥ 1.5 SDS above BW and/or BL, (4) protruding forehead, (5) body asymmetry, and (6) feeding difficulties and/or BMI ≤ -2 SDS at age 2 years. Several additional features include facial dysmorphisms, skeletal manifestations, and male genital abnormalities (posterior urethral valves, hypospadias) among others. One of the hallmarks of this syndrome, and many of the others discussed later, is their marked heterogeneity, not only in the molecular causes of the syndrome but also in their phenotype. The incidence of SRS is somewhere between 30,000 and 70,000, but as our diagnostic precision improves with molecular technology, it may be more at the lower end of these figures.

This recent international consensus statement for the diagnosis and management of SRS also proposes an algorithm for determining when and which molecular tests to perform when seeking to confirm a clinical diagnosis. It should be noted, however, that about half of clinically diagnosed children with SRS will not have a known SRS genetic mutation or epimutation (changes in methylation status at particular imprint control regions). By far the most frequent molecular finding in those patients with a clinical score suggesting SRS are disorders involving chromosome 11p15 (approximately 40%–60%), including copy number variations (CNVs) and epimutations. Maternal UPD for chromosome 7 is found in individuals with SRS less than 10% of the time.[57, 61]

Epimutations are very frequent in SRS. They can arise very early in life (even in germ cells) and can be influenced by environmental cues; these cues may affect multiple sites of genome methylation, as has also been found in other syndromes involving imprinted genetic loci, including Beckwith-Wiedemann syndrome[62] and pseudohypoparathyroidism (*GNAS* locus on chromosome 20q).[63] This may partially explain the reportedly increased incidence of SRS in assisted reproductive technology, as shown by a recent metaanalysis.[64] These epimutations can be the result of point mutations or microdeletions at the imprint control regions, or they can be the result of mutations in transactivating factors, such as several recently described proteins with high expression levels in oocytes and cleavage-stage embryos. Mutations in these factors lead to multiple imprint disorders.[65] Mutations in specific enzymes required for establishment and/or maintenance of DNA methylation (DNA methyltransferases) as well as "demethylases" (TET enzymes) have also been described, but are not specifically linked to abnormal fetal growth.[66]

As shown in Fig. 51.1A, there are two areas of interest at chromosome 11p15, a telomeric domain containing the *H19* and *IGF2* genes, and a more centromeric domain including the *KCNQ1* and *CDKN1C* genes, with differentially methylated regions within each domain controlling allelic usage (imprint control region 2 or IRC2 and ICR1, respectively). Thus, the normal situation concerning expression of the growth factor gene *IGF2* is to have only IRC1 methylated on the paternal allele, which permits expression of this gene. The DNA binding protein CTCF can bind at the IRC1 only to the unmethylated maternal allele and block transcription of *IGF2* while permitting expression of H19, a noncoding RNA. Within the other domain, it is the maternal allele which is normally methylated, and both *KCNQ1* (an ion channel gene) and *CDKN1C* (a growth inhibitor gene) are expressed on this allele, while transcription of *KCNQ1OT1 (LIT1)* on the paternal allele participates in the silencing of these same genes. This centromeric domain is more of interest to our understanding of the etiology of Beckwith-Wiedemann syndrome and of IMAGe syndrome, both discussed in following text.

Molecular defects in SRS at 11p15 (Table 51.2) result in decreased expression of *IGF2* and/or increased expression of *H19* and *CDKN1C*—both leading to decreased growth. As there are many conditions that may have a phenotypic overlap with SRS, including 3-M syndrome, Mulibrey nanism, Short syndrome, Floating-Harbor syndrome and IMAGe syndrome among others, a genetic consultation may also help target additional loci for investigation if typical SRS testing does not confirm the diagnosis.

Roughly 25% of patients may undergo recurrent hypoglycemia, so nutritional repletion is a very important part of the care of these infants, as is surveillance for fasting hypoglycemia. Avoidance of excessive weight gain is equally important, so as not to put them at a greater risk for metabolic and cardiovascular complications later in life. In addition, with rare exception, patients with SRS are born SGA and will fail to demonstrate spontaneous catch-up growth, but they are not GH deficient by classic criteria. For this reason, and because of the hypoglycemia risk and poor muscle mass, GH treatment at doses larger than those used for GH deficiency has been recommended and is usually started between 2 and 4 years of age. Interestingly, levels of IGF-I tend to be higher in children with SRS (upper quartile of the normal age-related range) and may rise to very high levels after treatment with GH. This suggests a situation of GH resistance that is not yet understood, and which makes using an IGF-I–based dosing difficult to interpret. While they do not have precocious puberty, children with SRS can have an earlier adrenarche, with a faster progression of peripheral and ultimately central puberty. Bone advancement thus reduces the window for treatment, and therapeutic modalities such as GnRH analogues and aromatase inhibitors are under investigation.[57] Some report success with GH treatment equivalent to responses of other children with a non-SRS diagnosis,[67] but in general, these children do respond nearly as well as children with TS or truly GH deficient patients.

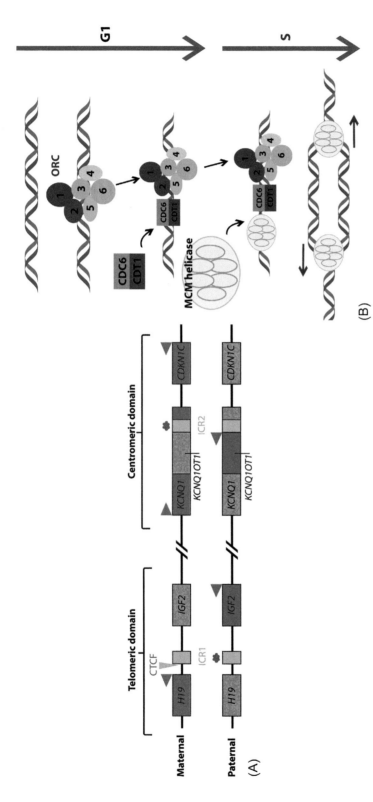

FIG. 51.1   Examples of loci important for regulation of fetal growth. (A) Simplified schematic of an imprinted locus, in this case at chromosome 11p15.5. Only the key elements necessary to understand imprinting at this locus are shown. Two transcriptional domains are important in this region, known for its contribution to syndromes of both fetal undergrowth (Silver-Russell syndrome) and fetal overgrowth (Beckwith-Wiedemann syndrome), one containing the *H19-IGF2* domain, and the other the *KCNQ1-CDKN1* domain. Each of these contains an imprint control region (ICR), whose methylation status (indicated by *) determines which allele of a particular imprinted gene will be actively transcribed. Any perturbation of the methylation status at one or both of these loci can result in expression of a normally silent copy or silencing of a normally active copy. In the diagram, the arrowheads indicate transcription (pink: maternal allele active; blue: paternal gene active). Other proteins play a role in gene expression at imprinted loci—shown here, CTCF, binding to the maternal ICR1. This protein confers a boundary to promoter access to enhancer signals such that in the absence of methylation, CTCF will bind and *H19*, not *IGF2*, will be transcribed. At the other domain, *KCNQ1OT1(LIT1)* codes for a long noncoding RNA that participates in silencing the expression of *KCNQ1* and *CDKN1* on the same, paternal, allele. Methylation of IRC2 is normally found on the maternal chromosome, along with actively transcribed alleles of *KCNQ1* and *CDKN1*. (B) Simplified schematic of one of the cellular processes implicated in primordial microcephalic dwarfism. It shows the steps necessary to permit DNA synthesis in the nucleus, termed licensing of replication origins. A 6-subunit protein complex (ORC1-6, multicolored complex) binds to DNA (red and blue ribbons) and then recruits additional proteins (CDT1 and CDC6, colored squares). This permits another 6-subunit protein complex to bind, the MCM helicase (in yellow), which "unwinds" the DNA double helix in preparation for DNA polymerase to begin synthesizing duplicate strands. The time during the cell cycle (G1, S) at which this occurs is indicated to the right. In Meier-Gorlin syndrome (MGORS), mutations are found in several of the genes involved in this process (see text and Table 51.2). Not shown in the figure but also implicated in MGORS is geminin (coded for by *GMNN*), which interacts with CDT1, and CDC45 (coded for by *CDC45L*), which interacts with specific ORC subunit proteins and helicase MCM subunits. *(Part A: Modified from Wakeling EL, Brioude F, Lokulo-Sodipe O, O'Connell SM, Salem J, Bliek J, et al. Diagnosis and management of Silver-Russell syndrome: first international consensus statement. Nat Rev Endocrinol 2017;13(2):105–24. Part B: Modified from Samuels ME, Deal CL, Skidmore DL. Meier-Gorlin syndrome. Oxford: University Press; 2016.)*

51.6.2 Temple Syndrome

This extremely rare syndrome shows some overlap with SRS, and therefore the involved imprinted genetic locus at 14q32 should be investigated if none of the SRS genetic/epigenetic defects are found when suspecting SRS. The classic features include pre- and postnatal growth retardation with relative macrocephaly, hypotonia, specific facial features that do not always include the frontal bossing seen in SRS, and small hands and feet. In a review of 51 cases, Ioannides et al. described a high incidence of early puberty (86%, age of menarche 10.2 years) and obesity (roughly 50%), so patients and their families should be counseled and followed with this in mind.[60] Retrospective growth data from a limited number of patients treated for 1 year with GH suggested that the response of these patients is similar to that seen in other individuals born SGA. They therefore assert that under the current SGA indications, patients with Temple syndrome could be considered for this treatment option.[68] The genetic and epigenetic defects seen in Temple syndrome are typical of imprinted disorders and are listed in Table 51.1. There may also be an accompanying mosaic trisomy 14.[69]

51.6.3 3-M Syndrome

This syndrome is another cause of FGR with both BW and BL affected, but not head circumference; thus they have relative macrocephaly. They also can share some additional features with SRS, including a triangular-shaped face with a prominent chin and large forehead with bossing. Most patients are also very short at adulthood. Their nose is upturned with a depressed nasal root. Orthopedic features include pectus excavatum, rib hypoplasia and winged scapulae, clinodactyly, pes planis and tall vertebral bodies with lumbar lordosis. They tend to have joint hypermobility. Infertility has been reported in males, so anticipatory guidance should include the need for evaluation of pubertal progression with levels of LH, FHS, and testosterone. Intelligence has been reported as normal. This is an autosomal recessive condition, and three genes have been implicated. *CUL7* was the first and most often implicated in 3-M; it is part of an E3 ligase complex leading to protein ubiquitination and degradation. It interacts with the tumor-suppressor and "guardian of the genome," p53, by decreasing its activity, thus promoting growth. The other two genes, *OBSL1* (cytoskeleton scaffolding) and *CCDC8*, interact with each other and with p53. There may also be links to the growth receptor signaling pathways, since patients with this condition show a very modest response to GH treatment, which suggests resistance.[70]

51.6.4 Mulibrey Nanism

This rare, autosomal recessive condition of pre- and postnatal growth failure is caused by mutations in *TRIM37*. TRIM37 is an E3 ligase, and it is one of a large number of similar molecules that oversee ubiquitin transfer, thus targeting proteins for degradation via the proteasome. Interestingly, excluding Finland, which has reported over 100 cases, about 25 additional cases are reported worldwide. The facial features of these patients include a small triangular face with frontal bossing, mild hypertelorism, a deep, broad nasal bridge, dental crowding, and eye signs that are clinical clues: yellow dotted fundi, decreased retinal pigmentation, choroid hypoplasia, astigmatism, and strabismus. Skeletal findings include a J-shaped sella turcica and slender long bones, some with fibrous dysplasia. Muscular hypotonia and mild speech delays are common, but their intelligence is normal. As patients age, vital organs such as the heart are particularly affected; patients may go on to have constrictive pericarditis, congestive heart failure, and myocardial fibrosis. For the endocrinologist, it is noteworthy that males display small testes and hypergonadotrophic hypogonadism; females rarely menstruate normally. While infants and children can have low fasting glucose, a majority of adults will develop metabolic syndrome and type 2 diabetes, and many have hepatomegaly. Patients also have a risk of developing tumors such as Wilms and gynecological cancers, and much work is now being done to understand how TRIM37 dysregulation contributes to carcinogenesis outside the context of Mulibrey nanism.[71]

51.6.5 Short Syndrome

This acronym stands for short stature, hyperextensibility of joints, ocular depression, Rieger anomaly, and teething delay. FGR, with BW and BL less than the 3rd percentile, is the norm. The facial phenotype resembles those discussed earlier because of the triangular face, micrognathia, and prominent forehead. They may have midface hypoplasia. Sensorineural hearing loss may be present in childhood, along with multiple eye signs and complications, including cataracts, myopia, and glaucoma. Dental signs include a delayed dental age, hypodontia, and malocclusion. Lipoatrophy is described along with thin, wrinkled skin. These patients can develop glucose and type 2 diabetes even during childhood. The disorder is caused by heterozygous mutations in *PIK3R1*, which encodes a subunit of the PI3K holoenzyme. This kinase phosphorylates a number of molecules that are important in growth regulation pathways.[72]

51.6.6 Floating-Harbor Syndrome

This autosomal dominant syndrome is yet another rare syndrome with FGR and adult short stature, for which the literature reveals less than 100 patients. Facial features are very distinct, although as in many of the syndromes causing FGR, the facial gestalt becomes more obvious with age. The face is triangular with deep-set, long-lashed eyes and a prominent nose that broadens at the tip. The lips are thin with frequent eversion of the lower lip, and the ears are posteriorly rotated. Teeth are small with increased spaces. Feet and hands may show broader digits, brachydactyly, and clinodactyly. The voice is high pitched and several have severe receptive and expressive language impairment and an intellectual disability that is mild to moderate. The frequency of the various features was summarized in a cohort of 52 individuals, and while multiple other organ system findings were seen, the frequencies rarely exceeded 10%–20% of the population studied.[73]

Truncated mutations in SRCAP, a chromatin-remodeling ATPase, are responsible for this syndrome. Many protein partners and cellular activities of SRCAP have been described, but perhaps the most interesting is its potential role in DNA methylation, since it was found that individuals with Floating-Harbor syndrome have very specific epigenetic signatures.[74]. GH therapy has been tried in some of these patients, but there is no published analysis of pooled results; response has been described as modest in 2 case reports.

51.6.7 IMAGe Syndrome

This acronym describes the phenotype in these FGR individuals who present with IUGR, metaphyseal dysplasia, adrenal hypoplasia congenita, and genital anomalies. Failure to recognize the adrenal failure and provide glucocorticoids in the neonatal period can result in the death of these infants. They may also have hypo- or hypercalcemia like many of the syndromic SGA infants, as well as craniosynostosis, cleft palate, and scoliosis. Facial features include frontal bossing, low-set ears, a flat nasal bridge, and a short nose. The gene involved in this syndrome, *CDKN1C*, codes for a cyclin-dependent kinase inhibitor (p57^{Kip2}) that suppresses growth by blocking cell cycle progression. It is the same gene that can be found mutated in some patients with an overgrowth phenotype, Beckwith-Wiedemann syndrome, discussed in Section 51.9.2.1. The difference as to whether a mutation will activate this gene, as it does in IMAGe syndrome, depends on its location in the gene and the type of mutation. Point mutations in the C-terminal domain of the protein will enhance its growth suppression potential, whereas truncating mutations or point mutations in the N-terminal domain of the protein reduce its growth inhibiting potential.[75]

51.6.8 MIRAGE Syndrome

Because adrenal gland hypoplasia in an infant born SGA is quite rare and limited to very few genes, it is important to also think of this syndrome when faced with a newborn with the features of the MIRAGE syndrome, namely myelodysplasia, infection, restriction of growth, adrenal hypoplasia, genital phenotypes, and enteropathy. Hyperpigmentation may be a clue to the primary adrenal failure, and the genital anomalies in the absence of bone lesions and with diarrhea, even after cortisol replacement therapy, should alert the clinician to this diagnosis. They may also have thymic hypoplasia. These infants have a proportional growth restriction such that their head circumference is also usually below the 3rd percentile (microcephaly), more like the cases described later. Less than 25 patients have been reported to date, and the gene causing this syndrome is *SAMD9*, which codes for a cytoplasmic protein involved in the regulation of cell proliferation and apoptosis. Gain-of-function mutations lead to growth suppression whereas loss-of-function mutations, or monosomy for chromosome 7 or 7q, causes other diseases with predisposition to ataxia, pancytopenia, and myeloid malignancies, but no FGR.[76, 77]

51.7 Primordial Microcephalic Dwarfism

The major difference between most syndromic causes of FGR discussed earlier and what has been known as primordial microcephalic dwarfism is the relative body proportions. There is a conservation of head size in forms in the former, but in the conditions described that make up this group of FGR causes (Meier-Gorlin syndrome (MGORS), Seckel syndrome, MOPDI/III and MOPDII) pre- and postnatal growth failure is global. As with SRS, the various causes of primordial microcephalic dwarfism are heterogeneous with regards to their etiology and their presentation. Globally, however, they share similarities including autosomal recessive patterns of inheritance and cellular pathways that regulate the number of cells in the individual. The genes involved in these pathways include those that regulate the cell cycle, DNA damage repair, and stability of the genome, centriole/centrosome biogenesis and function, microtubule formation, and spindle organization/orientation. Some of them are found in autosomal recessive cases of microcephaly without pre- and postnatal growth retardation but with a significant impact on brain development and, ultimately, on cognitive disability. Interestingly, many of the genes involved interact with, and lie downstream of, the IGF/mTOR and MAPK signaling pathways, known to be involved in cell growth and differentiation.[78, 79]

It is important to define the precise syndrome and their clinical subtypes of this exceedingly rare condition, in order to better understand the natural history and provide the appropriate counseling to families. Complicating this is the fact that the same gene may be responsible for different subtypes (termed allelism), such as *PCNT* (the gene coding pericentrin and involved in both Seckel syndrome and MOPDII see later). Gene panels are now available to delineate the particular genetic mutations, and this is essential to provide families with reproductive choices. New genes are being detected now that we are using next-generation sequencing paired with our understanding of gene networks.

Several of these syndromes develop an endocrine phenotype including hypergonadotrophic hypogonadism and insulin resistance without the presence of obesity. As with SRS, it is therefore important not to overfeed in early life. Anticipatory guidance for many of the features appearing later, such as the breast hypoplasia/aplasia or orthopedic issues seen in some of the subtypes below, must be given. In the few patients in which GH therapy has been attempted, it was judged to be ineffective and may actually add to the potential for these patients to develop metabolic syndrome.

51.7.1   Meier-Gorlin Syndrome

MGORS is also known as the ear-patella-short stature syndrome, because of its major distinguishing features, which include microtia (small, hypoplastic ears), absent or hypoplastic patellae, and pre- and postnatal growth failure. Intelligence is reported as normal. It is an extremely heterogeneous syndrome, with eight causative genes showing inter- and intragenetic heterogeneity (Table 51.2). It is an autosomal recessive syndrome (with the exception of rare autosomal dominant mutations) that serves to illustrate one of the hallmarks of the general category of microcephalic primordial dwarfism, namely, the involvement of fundamental cell pathways, in this case that of chromosomal (nuclear) replication. Fig. 51.1B shows a simplified schematic of the origin recognition complex including several proteins that are essential to the initiation of DNA synthesis and therefore to cell division. Individuals with mutations in genes involved in the process of DNA replication are thought to have decreased numbers of cells, thus accounting for the smaller body size. The mutations are primarily missense mutations, but truncating mutations are also found, the latter never present in both gene copies because of probable early lethality. Interestingly, one of the mutated proteins (CDC45) is found in the critical region for the highly frequent AD DiGeorge microdeletion syndrome (OMIM 188400); these individuals have a multitude of other congenital abnormalities, so it is difficult to ascertain to what extent this gene contributes to the SGA/short adult stature seen in some.

The phenotype of the various subtypes of MGORS includes many additional features that may or may not be present, including micrognathia, small mouth, structural abnormalities in the respiratory tract (including pulmonary emphysema, laryngo-, trachea- and/or bronchomalacia) and a range of skeletal features (including craniosynostosis, slender ribs and long bones, joint hyperextensibility and scoliosis). Feeding difficulties in infancy are common. Fewer males than females have been reported; they may have cryptorchidism and/or hypospadias. Little information is available about fertility, although girls menstruate normally. Most distressing for female patients is the breast aplasia or hypoplasia. The decreased numbers of cells in individuals with MGORS explains why one would presume that GH therapy, although able to increase growth velocity initially in some patients, does not have significant clinical benefits.[80]

51.7.2   Seckel Syndrome

First of the microcephalic dwarfism syndromes to be described was Seckel syndrome (SS), with a focus on the microcephaly and facial features, which were noted to be "bird-like" with a large, beaked nose, a sloping forehead, and micrognathia. Intellectual disability is described as variable. They may also have malformations of the skeleton, genitourinary tract, heart, and brain although the true frequency of these various clinical manifestations in mutation-proven patients is not available. The phenotype is also complicated by the high incidence of consanguinity in the reported cases, so the contribution of other loci cannot be ignored; deletions of various loci have been found in some SS patients but no clear pattern of digenic inheritance has been reported. OMIM lists nine genes for SS to date, as noted in Table 51.2. Some participate in maintaining telomere integrity and protecting DNA from stress-induced damage or replication errors, while others are important for centriole formation during cell division. Thus they are critical to genome maintenance, and if defective, cells may be targeted to apoptotic pathways.[78, 81]

51.7.3 Microcephalic Osteodysplasitic Primordial Dwarfism, Type I/III (MOPDI/III) or Tabi-Linder Syndrome

The initial classification of microcephalic osteodysplasitic dwarfism was made before the explosion in our knowledge of the genes involved and was therefore based on clinical phenotype. Majewski made great contributions to the classification in the early 1980s and proposed three separate entities. We now define only two MOPDs (see following paragraph for type II), since MOPDI and MOPDIII were found to be caused by the same gene, *RNU4ATAC*, which codes for a small nuclear RNA (snRNA), a component of the minor spliceosome. Spliceosomes are essential large ribonucleoprotein complexes responsible for the removal of introns from pre-RNAs. The phenotype of MOPDI/III is very severe and includes overlap features with the other primary microcephalic dwarfism types, such as small, dysplastic ears, a large fleshy nose, and multiple skeletal abnormalities including short, bowed limbs and brachydactyly, among others. In addition, heart malformations, renal hypoplasia/cysts, cryptorchidism and small genitalia in the male, and severe brain malformations are found. The latter include pachygyria, heterotopias, agenesis of the corpus callosum and hypoplastic frontal lobes. These individuals have an intractable seizure disorder and have profound cognitive deficits as well as neuroendocrine dysfunction. Most individuals that survive until term will die in infancy.[82, 83]

51.7.4 Microcephalic Osteodysplastic Primordial Dwarfism, Type II (MOPDII)

This microcephalic condition with pre- and postnatal growth failure is characterized by relatively short limbs that result in increasingly disproportionate short stature with age. Other distinct skeletal findings and a cognitive function that can be low normal to normal help in separating it from the preceding syndromes, as does the nose, which is large but not as beaked as in Seckel syndrome. They have many dental issues such as hypodontia and enamel hypoplasia. They are particularly susceptible to Moyamoya disease, cerebral aneurisms, and infarctions, and may develop precocious puberty and obesity/type 2 diabetes. MOPDII is caused by homo- or heterozygous mutations in the pericentrin 2 gene (*PCNT2*), which codes for pericentrin. This anchoring protein is critical to the centrosome, from which microtubules radiate and form the spindle apparatus, necessary for the proper alignment and subsequent segregation of chromosomes into daughter cells during cell division.[84]

51.8 SPECIFIC GENETIC DEFECTS IN THE INSULIN-LIKE GROWTH FACTOR AXIS AND INSULIN AXIS ASSOCIATED WITH FGR AND POSTNATAL GROWTH RETARDATION

Fetal production of the IGFs is independent of fetal pituitary growth hormone (GH), although rodent models and human mutations have shown the importance of the autocrine, paracrine, and endocrine effects of the IGFs, both IGF-I and IGF-II, for growth of the fetus. Insulin is also critical for normal fetal growth (see Chapter 40). This said, extreme phenotypes of both congenital GH deficiency and GH insensitivity (Laron syndrome) can be smaller at birth relative to unaffected siblings and/or to population means.[85, 86] However, it is deficient production of IGF-I or IGF-II, or defects in the IGF1R or INSR, that have the largest impact on birth size and clinical phenotype in general. These rare defects will be covered in the following paragraphs and in Table 51.3.

51.8.1 IGF-I Deficiency

To date 10 patients (2 female/8 male) have been described with *IGF1* mutations causing low circulating levels of IGF-I and elevated serum GH. Homozygous deletions or mutations that result in complete loss of IGF-I function have a more severe phenotype: BW/BL SDS ranges from −4.0 to −2.4. The most striking aspect of these patients is their microcephaly/micrognathia, sensorineural deafness, delayed motor development, and intellectual disability. They persist in having severe short stature, which develops rapidly, concomitant with a much-delayed bone age. Some patients have heterozygous mutations and have less severe FGR (BW/BL SDS −3.5 to −1.2). Carriers of an *IGF1* mutation or deletion are on average about 1 SD shorter than noncarriers. They respond poorly to GH treatment, as expected. The recent availability of rhIGF-I with its serum carrier protein, IGFBP-3, in equimolar amounts could prove useful for stimulating growth while preventing IGF-I induced hypoglycemia and other IGF-I side effects sometimes observed in GH insensitivity patients treated with IGF-I alone.[87, 88]

51.8.2 IGF-I Resistance/Insensitivity

Many cases of heterozygous mutations or gene deletions have been reported for the type 1 IGF receptor (IGF1R), which is the functional receptor for both IGF-I and IGF-II and responsible for the stimulation of growth and differentiation. As predicted, their phenotype is similar to IGF-I or IGF-II deficiency, with pre- and postnatal growth failure and microcephaly, and with varying degrees of cognitive disabilities. It has been reported that IGF1R defects leading to haploinsufficiency can be found in as many as 3% of SGA children.[89, 90] The rare autosomal recessive forms have a more severe phenotype and may be confused with progeria. Other larger deletions such as seen with a 15q26.1-qter (a contiguous gene deletion syndrome including the gene for the *IGF1R*) or with ring chromosome 15 have FGR and adult short stature, microcephaly, facial dysmorphisms, renal and lung abnormalities, and developmental delay with intellectual disabilities. In some cases they have been described as having features of Silver-Russell syndrome.[91–93]

51.8.3 IGF-II Deficiency

Epigenetic defects at the 11p15 locus causing Silver-Russell syndrome were discussed earlier; the FGR is presumed to be due to low tissue levels of IGF-II as a result of the ICR1 hypomethylation. Of the six published mutations to date, recently summarized by Rockstroh et al., BW and BL SDS were more severely affected (BW SDS -2.6 to -5.3; BL SDS -3.7 to -5.5) than in IGF-I deficiency, which correlates well with the murine knock-out data. Circulating IGF-II levels ranged from normal to deficient, with normal to frankly elevated IGF-I levels in some patients. The normal levels of IGF-II were seen in the patient with a frameshift mutation leading to the production of an abnormal, but measurable, protein.[94] Also, as expected given the imprinting status of this locus, all mutations reported to date were on the paternal allele and the growth restriction phenotype was only transmitted by the father. Similarly to patients with SRS, head circumference was less affected (relative macrocephaly).[95] It should be noted that the pathophysiology of the growth restriction may have its origins in poor placental growth in these situations, since IGF-II is a major modulator of placental growth as well as fetal growth.[96] What is also interesting in these patients is the persistence of growth retardation during childhood and adolescence, giving credence to the importance of *both* IGF-I and IGF-II for postnatal growth in the human.

Mutations or deletions of the genes mentioned, as well as in other genes in the GH-IGF axis that may or may not give rise to birth weights and/or lengths less than the 10th percentile are summarized in the recent review by Dauber.[97] They include *STAT5B*, coding for a downstream effector of the GH receptor, which is critical for *IGF1* transcription; and IGF Acid labile subunit (*IGFALS*), which codes for a circulating protein found in a ternary complex with the IGF binding protein IGFBP-3 and the IGFs. Very little IGF-I or IGF-II is free in the circulation, and patients with mutations in *IGFALS* have lower serum IGFs and IGFBP3. Although defects in these genes definitely cause postnatal growth failure, it is perhaps too early to ascribe an important role for these proteins in prenatal growth; more data including unaffected sibling data are needed.

51.8.4 Insulin Receptor Gene Defects

Mutations in the gene for the insulin receptor are also linked with FGR and result in severe failure to thrive in postnatal life, given the importance of insulin for the growth and development of the feto-placental unit, and for growth and metabolic regulation ex utero. In their most severe form, autosomal recessive insulin receptor mutations cause the Donohue syndrome, also called leprechaunism. An allelic form is seen with Rabson-Mendenhall syndrome. The features of these patients include a facial phenotype termed elfin with a small face, large ears and eyes, wide nostrils, thick lips, and a large mouth. Certain body parts are hyperplastic, such as the gingiva, the genitalia, the hands and feet, and the islets of Langerhans because of the insulin resistance, resulting in hyperinsulinemia. Acanthosis nigricans is also present. Most striking is the lack of subcutaneous fat tissue and poor muscle mass. They can develop precocious puberty. Their hyperglycemia and ketoacidosis, which is resistant to insulin treatment, has been better controlled with IGF-I through binding to the IGF-I receptor directly, or through binding to hybrid INS-IGF-I receptors. If not controlled, these patients die within the first few years of life.[98–100]

51.8.5 ZFP57 Mutations and Related Molecular Changes Causing TNDM

As stated earlier, paternal chromosome 6 UPD can give rise to TNDM, which is characterized by FGR and infants born SGA. They rapidly develop insulin-requiring (nonimmune) diabetes, which resolves by 3–9 months but then becomes permanent in over 50% of patients. The responsible locus for the UPD phenotype is the *ZAC/PLAGL1* locus; ZAC (also called *PLAGL1*) is expressed only from the paternal allele and is thought to have growth-suppressing properties. An adjacent gene,

HYMAI (hydatidiform mole associated imprinted gene), produces a nontranscribed RNA and is also paternally expressed. There is a differentially methylated region within this locus that, when hypomethylated, results in paternal expression. It is easy to see why UPD or paternal duplications of this region at chromosome 6q24 can lead to overexpression of these genes, which appear to suppress fetal growth, including pancreatic islet cells, and could lead to diabetes.

But what about *ZFP57*? This gene is on the short arm of chromosome 6 (6p22.1), and is not imprinted. When mutated, it can disrupt imprinting at several sites through changes in methylation, including at the TNDM locus *ZAC/PLGL1*, as discussed earlier. Despite the fetal and postnatal growth retardation, infants with this mutation may have macroglossia and/or umbilical hernias, similar to the infants with Beckwith-Wiedemann syndrome.[101] Fourteen mutations in this gene have been described to date, with no clear genotype-phenotype relationship, although all were ascertained because of FGR. All have TNDM and methylation defects at the imprint control regions (differentially methylated regions, DMRs) of several genes, including *PLAGL1, GRB10*, and *PEG3* (the most common), but other DMRs can also be implicated at imprinted gene loci including *MEST, KCNQ1OT1* and *GNAS*.[102]

51.8.6 Defective Genes Involving Pancreatic Development

The hallmark of these rare syndromes is pancreatic aplasia, hypoplasia, or more specifically, hypoplasia of the islets of Langerhans. The phenotype is that of FGR/SGA and neonatal diabetes mellitus (nonimmune), which, unlike the transient forms, is permanent. The genes involved are transcription factors important for pancreatic development. Compound heterozygous or homozygous mutations in two genes, *PDX1* (Pancreatic Agenesis type 1) and *PTF1A* (Pancreatic Agenesis type 2), have been described, and the phenotypes can vary even within the same family. Some patients have exocrine pancreatic insufficiency as well and will have marked failure to thrive if not treated with enzyme supplements in addition to insulin.[103–106] It should be noted that heterozygous mutations in *PDX1* can give rise to MODY 4 or gestational diabetes.[107] More recently, another gene *RFX6* has been described that gives rise to FGR and neonatal diabetes, along with gastrointestinal abnormalities including tracheoesophageal fistula, duodenal atresia, jejunal duplication, Meckel's diverticulum, and biliary atresia. Some patients can present with diabetes later in childhood (Mitchell-Riley syndrome).[108]

51.9 CAUSES AND CONSEQUENCES OF BEING BORN LARGE FOR GESTATIONAL AGE

By far the most common cause of fetal overgrowth is excessive maternal weight gain and/or maternal diabetes. Male infants are more prone to BW > 4000 g, and ethnic differences in LGA risk have been well documented. Being born to a mother who has already carried multiple pregnancies to term, or who had a birthweight > 4000 g is also a risk factor. The differential diagnosis of the LGA infant may imply differences in body composition, for example, newborns of a poorly controlled diabetic mother may have increased body fat, not well measured by ultrasound. Data on newborn body composition reveal that while only 14% is due to adipose tissue, it can account for up to 46% of BW variance.[109] Many LGA fetuses will not be identified until the third trimester; however, unlike the difficulty of identifying fetuses with later-onset FGR clinically, the LGA fetus is more often identified during prenatal visits simply by uterine fundal height measurements and maternal identification.[110, 111]

In addition to birth-related complications for the mother during delivery (protracted labor with increased risk for cesarean delivery or extensive episiotomy, perineal damage, uterine rupture, postpartum hemorrhage), being born LGA carries a higher risk of neonatal hypoglycemia and hematologic or respiratory problems.

Suspicion of a syndromic cause is more likely when fetal ultrasounds reveal detectable malformations. Unfortunately, the majority of syndromes causing prenatal overgrowth are also associated with developmental delay and intellectual disability.[112] Several of these may also carry an increased risk of neoplasia.[113] Fetal overgrowth can be generalized or localized to specific organs and can present with asymmetric body proportions. It can be due to cellular hyperplasia (increased cell numbers) or to cellular hypertrophy, or a combination of the two. Many of the genes involved, as in those causing FGR/SGA, involve intracellular signaling pathways and dysregulation of genes because of an abnormal epigenetic signature. This review will focus on generalized fetal overgrowth; for additional discussion of syndromic fetal overgrowth, the reader is referred to several recent reviews.[114–116]

51.9.1 Chromosomal Abnormalities Associated with Generalized Prenatal Overgrowth

Chromosomal trisomies can be responsible for prenatal overgrowth, including those for trisomy 5p, mosaic trisomy 8 (if not mosaic, complete trisomy 8 is lethal) and trisomy 12p, as well as mosaic tetrasomy 12p (also known as Pallister-Killian syndrome) and paternal UPD 11 (see Beckwith-Wiedemann syndrome, in following text).[117–119] Chromosomal microdeletions or duplications (CNVs), selective translocations, and larger chromosomal deletions or duplications can be found in the LGA infant. In many cases, this has helped to lead to the identification of the causal gene(s), such as those causing Beckwith-Wiedemann syndrome or those belonging to the IGF axis such as the 15q26 overgrowth syndrome due to *IGF1R* duplications.[120] Still others may contain multiple candidate genes, and await the identification of patients with single gene mutations, such as the contiguous gene deletion involving 13q13-q21.[121] Additional examples include translocations involving 2q37, which disrupt the *NPPC* gene and result in its overexpression and an overgrowth phenotype in several patients.[122] This gene codes for C-natriuretic peptide, and mutations in this gene also have been shown to cause autosomal dominant short stature.[123]

51.9.2   Syndromes Associated with Excess Fetal Growth/LGA

Table 51.4 lists the major syndromes that must be considered in the differential diagnosis of the LGA newborn, once maternal and constitutional factors have been eliminated.

TABLE 51.4 Chromosomal findings/syndrome with LGA/birth size[a]

Syndrome/condition (OMIM # if available)	Candidate gene or molecular defect(s)
Chromosome trisomies	
Trisomy 5p	Candidate gene(s) not yet identified
Mosaic trisomy 8	Candidate gene(s) not yet identified
Trisomy 12p	Candidate gene(s) not yet identified
Mosaic tetrasomy 12p (Pallister-Killian) (601803)	Candidate gene(s) not yet identified
Chromosome CNVs/translocations	
Dup15q26/15q25-qter trisomy	*IGF1R* increased gene dosage
Del 13q13-q21	Contiguous gene deletion, candidate gene(s) not yet identified
Del 5q35.3	*NSD1* haploinsufficiency (Sotos Syndrome gene)
Translocations involving 2q37	Overexpression of NPPC
Overgrowth syndromes	
Beckwith-Wiedemann syndrome (130650)	Pat UPD 11 ± mosaicism Dup pat 11p15.5 ICR1 gain of mat methylation ICR2 loss of mat methylations *CDKN1C* mat LOF mutations Mat 11p inversions/translocations activating mat *IGF2* and/or silencing mat *CDKN1C* transcription
Sotos (117550)	*NSD1* haploinsufficiency
Perlman (267000)	Homozygous or compound heterozygous inactivating mutations in *DIS3L2*
Simpson-Golabi-Behmel (312870)	Microdeletions/inactivating mutations/in *GPC3* (X-linked recessive condition; females may be less affected due to random X-inactivation)
Weaver (277590)	*EZH2* haploinsufficiency
Costello (218040)	Heterozygous activating mutations in *HRAS*

[a]*See text for phenotype, gene function, and tumor risk.*

51.9.2.1 Beckwith-Wiedemann Syndrome

BWS is one of the best-known overgrowth syndromes, with an extreme heterogeneity in clinical presentation and in molecular causes and a birth incidence of approximately 1 in 14,000. While BW SDS is frequently >2 SD above the mean, this is not always the case, and overgrowth can be lateralized, leading to hemi-hypertrophy, or can involve only specific tissues and organs, causing macroglossia, nephromegaly, and/or hepatomegaly. Pregnancy findings may include polyhydramnios with or without an abnormally large placenta, and monochorionic, discordant twins are more frequently seen than in other syndromic conditions.[124] Other clinical features include ear pits or creases, exomphalos, umbilical hernia with diastasis recti and facial naevus simplex.

Most concerning is the associated hyperinsulinemic hypoglycemia and the tumor risk in these patients. Hypoglycemia may be transient or may last past the first week of life and be difficult to treat.[125] The embryonal tumors that patients with BWS may develop include neuroblastoma, adrenocortical carcinoma, hepatoblastoma, pheochromocytoma, rhabdomyosarcoma, or Wilms tumor. Wilms tumor may be unilateral and multifocal, or bilateral. Pathological findings can show nephroblastomatosis, pancreatic adenomatosis, adrenal cortex cytomegaly, or placental mesenchymal dysplasia. Because of these very diverse manifestations, birth incidence may actually be higher, since some more discretely dysmorphic infants may not have an appropriate diagnostic workup. This motivated a recent international meeting to develop a scoring system based on phenotype, to guide physicians in their use of diagnostic testing, and if negative, to consider alternative diagnoses.[119]

The genetic and epigenetic mechanisms leading to BWS mirror those seen in SRS. As with SRS, BWS is also associated with assisted reproductive technology and with multilocus methylation defects. Unlike the involvement of other chromosomes in SRS, BWS almost always involves one or more imprinted genes on chromosome 11p15.5, with a few cases within the BWS phenotypic spectrum that may have other diagnoses.[119, 126] The defects are included in Table 51.4, and the reader is again referred to Fig. 51.1 to appreciate the potential for disrupted gene function when the differentially methylated sites are altered. The overgrowth phenotype is believed to be due primarily to IGF-II excess and/or p57^{KIP2} (coded for by *CDKN1C*) deficiency. Interestingly, a recent case report by Giabicani et al.[127] describes a patient who was born with a paternal duplication of *IGF2*, effectively doubling the gene dose for this imprinted growth factor as seen in many cases of BWS, and a simultaneous deletion of the Type 1 IGF receptor gene (*IGF1R*). The fact that the baby was born with an appropriate birth weight and length for gestational age, yet experienced growth failure during early childhood, reinforces our understanding from animal data that IGF-II is the important player during in utero life (along with insulin and the insulin receptor; see Chapter 40). We are also reminded that IGF-II can have its effects independently from the IGF-I receptor, either through autocrine effects or through insulin receptors. Finally, this case emphasizes the point that GH and its receptor and IGF-I and its receptor are mainly important after birth.

We are beginning to better understand the tumorigenesis risk, which differs according to type of genetic/epigenetic diagnosis, and this has helped to refine screening protocols since lifetime risk varies between 3.1% and 28.6%.[119, 128] Prenatal testing is available in some cases where there is a potential risk for recurrence, such as those with loss of function mutations in the maternal copy of *CDKN1C* or paternal duplications of the 11p15.5 locus (50% recurrence risk); genetic counseling is essential. The international consensus meeting also provided guidelines for testing in the case of prenatal ultrasound abnormalities such as fetal macroglossia and abdominal wall defects.[119]

51.9.2.2 Sotos Syndrome

Sotos syndrome, also called cerebral gigantism, is common enough (1 in 10,000–14,000 newborns) for most pediatric endocrinologists to be familiar with the clinical characteristics.[116] Increased BW, BL and macrocephaly/dolichocephaly and a facial phenotype that includes a prominent forehead, mandible, and hypertelorism are the distinguishing features. Brain MRI supports a diagnosis when ventriculomegaly, hypo- or agenesis of the corpus callosum, and other cerebral abnormities are found. Excess postnatal growth with an accelerated bone age eventually leads to tall, but not excessive, adult height. Intellect can be normal, although affected children can also exhibit psychomotor delay. This syndrome is usually sporadic and is caused by haploinsufficiency of the *NSD1* gene (nuclear receptor SET domain containing gene 1). There are many different types of genetic mutations/deletions reported in this gene.[114] Lifetime tumor risk has been calculated as 3% (sacroccygeal teratoma, neuroblastoma, acute lymphoblastic leukemia, retinoblastoma).[115, 128]

51.9.2.3 Perlman Syndrome

This syndrome is caused by autosomal recessive defects in *DIS3L2* (Dis3 mitotic control, S. cerevisiae, homolog-like 2 gene), a nuclear ribonuclease involved in RNA metabolism, and control of cell growth and division. Clinical clues on prenatal ultrasound include polyhydramnios and macrosomia with hepatomegaly, nephromegaly/renal hamartosis/hydronephrosis, and a narrow chest with pulmonary hypoplasia. Facial dysmorphisms include micrognathia and a broad and flat nasal bridge; cryptorchidism is common in male infants. Neonatal mortality is often caused by respiratory distress, and these macrosomic infants may also exhibit hyperinsulinemic hypoglycemia. If they survive the neonatal period, they usually have a moderate developmental delay, but they have a 67% lifetime risk of Wilms tumor.[116]

51.9.2.4 Simpson-Golabi-Behmel Syndrome

Simpson-Golabi-Behmel syndrome (SGBS) is a pre- and postnatal overgrowth syndrome that can be confused with BWS because of the overlapping features and the molecular etiology, which may also involve, indirectly, excess IGF-II signaling. The X-linked causal gene is *GPC3*, which codes for a glycoprotein that attaches to the outer cell membrane and that interacts with growth factors, including IGF-II; in vitro models of tumorigenesis suggest that IGF-IR phosphorylation is stimulated.[129] As in BWS, tumor risk includes hepatoblastoma, Wilms tumor, medulloblastoma, and leukemia, with a lifetime risk of 8%.[130] They must be watched and treated for hyperinsulinemic hypoglycemia, which, if undetected, can exacerbate the intellectual disability seen in about half of patients. Most will have a mild developmental delay or normal intelligence. The following have been found on prenatal ultrasound (in decreasing frequency): polyhydramnios and organomegaly, diaphragmatic hernia, and kidney and heart defects. Postnatal facial features include a coarse-looking face with a large mouth and tongue, short nose, and hypertelorism. Polydactyly/syndactyly and multiple nipples are among the more distinctive findings, along with tongue or lower-lip midline furrows and cleft lip and/or palate. Multiple other skeletal, MRI, and cardiac findings have been reported, in conjunction with the more than 80 different genetic findings involving *GPC3* reported to date.[116, 131]

51.9.2.5 Weaver Syndrome

This pre- and postnatal, autosomal dominant overgrowth syndrome is caused by a defective gene, *EZH2*, which functions as a histone methyltransferase thereby capable of suppressing transcription of specific genes. It is found in a protein complex (Polycomb Repressive Complex 2) essential for normal embryonic development. Macrocephaly is not seen in all patients, although other features overlap with Sotos syndrome such as the broad, depressed nasal bridge. Ears are large and eyes are widely spaced. These infants may also have doughy, loose skin, camptodactyly, joint laxity, umbilical hernia, scoliosis, and hypotonia. Developmental and speech delays are often noted, along with intellectual deficiency. Lifetime tumor risk has been reported as 5% for non-Hodgkins lymphoma, acute lymphoblastic leukemia, and neuroblastoma.[116, 128, 132]

51.9.2.6 Costello Syndrome

Costello syndrome belongs to the RASopathies, and is caused by mutations in *HRAS*, a proto-oncogene that functions as a GTPase. It is found in the 11p15.5 locus but is not among the neighboring imprinted genes. Activating mutations are dominantly transmitted. They result in a phenotype which includes macrocephaly and an LGA BW and/or BL in roughly half of cases reported. This distinguishes it from the other, related syndromes such as Noonan syndrome and cardiofaciocutaneous syndrome where prenatal macrosomia is not seen as frequently.[133] However, failure to thrive is seen postnatally and ultimately these children can be seen for short stature as are children with the other RASopathies. They also require cancer surveillance since lifetime cancer risk is 15%–20% (rhabdomyosarcoma and neuroblastoma).[134] The diagnosis may be suspected on a prenatal echography because of polyhydramnios and macrocephaly, with ventriculomegaly and cardiac malformations and arrhythmias. Facial features are coarse, skin is redundant and wrinkly on the hands with deep palmar creases, and also they have the barrel chest and lymphangiectasias reminiscent of TS.[114, 115]

51.10 CONCLUSION AND FUTURE DIRECTIONS

While amazing gains have been made in our understanding of abnormal fetal growth and of the syndromic causes of fetal growth extremes, it is clear that the next-generation sequencing technologies will allow for further refinements in our diagnoses and in our understanding of phenotype-genotype correlations. It is expected that the prenatal clinical diagnosis of the at-risk growth-restricted or macrosomic fetus will also improve as longitudinal cohorts of fetuses are followed after birth. This will also allow for data collection on the performance of prenatal genetic testing. It is, of course, a primary goal of all healthcare providers and public health authorities to decrease the common causes of the SGA and LGA newborn through prevention, focusing on environmental and nutritional factors that overwhelmingly contribute to a majority of these infants.

REFERENCES

1. Wellner K. *A history of embryology (1959), by Joseph Needham.* Available from: http://embryo.asu.edu/handle/10776/2031; 2010. [Accessed June 2019].

2. Sharma D, Farahbakhsh N, Shastri S, Sharma P. Intrauterine growth restriction—part 2. *J Matern Fetal Neonatal Med* 2016;**29**(24):4037–48.

3. Kesavan K, Devaskar SU. Intrauterine growth restriction: postnatal monitoring and outcomes. *Pediatr Clin N Am* 2019;**66**(2):403–23.

4. Wang D, Vandermeulen J, Atkinson SA. Early life factors predict abnormal growth and bone accretion at prepuberty in former premature infants with/without neonatal dexamethasone exposure. *Pediatr Res* 2007;**61**(1):111–6.

5. Gluckman PD, Hanson MA, Cooper C, Thornburg KL. Effect of in utero and early-life conditions on adult health and disease. *N Engl J Med* 2008;**359**(1):61–73.

6. Horikoshi M, Beaumont RN, Day FR, Warrington NM, Kooijman MN, Fernandez-Tajes J, et al. Genome-wide associations for birth weight and correlations with adult disease. *Nature* 2016;**538**(7624):248–52.

7. Weissmann-Brenner A, Simchen MJ, Zilberberg E, Kalter A, Weisz B, Achiron R, et al. Maternal and neonatal outcomes of large for gestational age pregnancies. *Acta Obstet Gynecol Scand* 2012;**91**(7):844–9.

8. Pettitt DJ, Jovanovic L. Birth weight as a predictor of type 2 diabetes mellitus: the U-shaped curve. *Curr Diab Rep* 2001;**1**(1):78–81.

9. Newby PK, Dickman PW, Adami HO, Wolk A. Early anthropometric measures and reproductive factors as predictors of body mass index and obesity among older women. *Int J Obes* 2005;**29**(9):1084–92.

10. Mi D, Fang H, Zhao Y, Zhong L. Birth weight and type 2 diabetes: a meta-analysis. *Exp Therap Med* 2017;**14**(6):5313–20.

11. Mayer C, Joseph KS. Fetal growth: a review of terms, concepts and issues relevant to obstetrics. *Ultrasound Obstet Gynecol* 2013;**41**(2):136–45.

12. Monier I, Blondel B, Ego A, Kaminiski M, Goffinet F, Zeitlin J. Poor effectiveness of antenatal detection of fetal growth restriction and consequences for obstetric management and neonatal outcomes: a French national study. *BJOG: Int J Obstet Gynaecol* 2015;**122**(4):518–27.

13. Hendrix MLE, Bons JAP, Snellings RRG, Bekers O, van Kuijk SMJ, Spaanderman MEA, et al. Can fetal growth velocity and first trimester maternal biomarkers improve the prediction of small-for-gestational age and adverse neonatal outcome? *Fetal Diagn Ther* 2019;1–11.

14. Lausman A, McCarthy FP, Walker M, Kingdom J. Screening, diagnosis, and management of intrauterine growth restriction. *J Obstet Gynaecol Can* 2012;**34**(1):17–28.

15. Sheridan C. Intrauterine growth restriction—diagnosis and management. *Aust Fam Physician* 2005;**34**(9):717–23.

16. Gordijn SJ, Beune IM, Thilaganathan B, Papageorghiou A, Baschat AA, Baker PN, et al. Consensus definition of fetal growth restriction: a Delphi procedure. *Ultrasound Obstet Gynecol* 2016;**48**(3):333–9.

17. Audette MC, Kingdom JC. Screening for fetal growth restriction and placental insufficiency. *Semin Fetal Neonatal Med* 2018;**23**(2):119–25.

18. Kadji C, Cannie MM, Resta S, Guez D, Abi-Khalil F, De Angelis R, et al. Magnetic resonance imaging for prenatal estimation of birthweight in pregnancy: review of available data, techniques, and future perspectives. *Am J Obstet Gynecol* 2019;**220**(5):428–39.

19. Papageorghiou AT, Ohuma EO, Altman DG, Todros T, Ismail LC, Lambert A, et al. International standards for fetal growth based on serial ultrasound measurements: the Fetal Growth Longitudinal Study of the INTERGROWTH-21st Project. *Lancet* 2014;**384**(9946):869–79.

20. Beune IM, Bloomfield FH, Ganzevoort W, Embleton ND, Rozance PJ, van Wassenaer-Leemhuis AG, et al. Consensus based definition of growth restriction in the newborn. *J Pediatr* 2018;**196**:71–6. e1.

21. Zeve D, Regelmann MO, Holzman IR, Rapaport R. Small at birth, but how small? the definition of SGA revisited. *Hormone Res Paediatr* 2016;**86**(5):357–60.

22. Clayton PE, Cianfarani S, Czernichow P, Johannsson G, Rapaport R, Rogol A. Management of the child born small for gestational age through to adulthood: a consensus statement of the International Societies of Pediatric Endocrinology and the Growth Hormone Research Society. *J Clin Endocrinol Metab* 2007;**92**(3):804–10.

23. Cutland CL, Lackritz EM, Mallett-Moore T, Bardaji A, Chandrasekaran R, Lahariya C, et al. Low birth weight: case definition & guidelines for data collection, analysis, and presentation of maternal immunization safety data. *Vaccine* 2017;**35**(48 Pt A):6492–500.

24. Chard T, Costeloe K, Leaf A. Evidence of growth retardation in neonates of apparently normal weight. *Eur J Obstet Gynecol Reprod Biol* 1992;**45**(1):59–62.

25. Xu H, Simonet F, Luo ZC. Optimal birth weight percentile cut-offs in defining small- or large-for-gestational-age. *Acta Paediatr (Oslo, Norway: 1992)* 2010;**99**(4):550–5.

26. Boulet SL, Alexander GR, Salihu HM, Pass M. Macrosomic births in the united states: determinants, outcomes, and proposed grades of risk. *Am J Obstet Gynecol* 2003;**188**(5):1372–8.

27. Maternal Health Task Force (MHTF), Harvard School of Public Health, Oxford Maternal & Perinatal Health Institute (OMPHI), The Global Health Network, Geneva Foundation for Medical Education and Research (GFMER). *INTERGROWTH-21st course on maternal, fetal and newborn growth monitoring. Module 1. Assesssing newborn size by anthropometry [Course module].* Available from: https://www.gfmer.ch/omphi/intergrowth-course/pdf/Intergrowth-21st-Module1-Assessing-newborn-size%20by-anthropometry-2016.pdf [Accessed June 2019].

28. Burton GJ, Jauniaux E. Pathophysiology of placental-derived fetal growth restriction. *Am J Obstet Gynecol* 2018;**218**(2s):S745–s61.

29. Goyal D, Limesand SW, Goyal R. Epigenetic responses and the developmental origins of health and disease. *J Endocrinol* 2019;**242**(1):T105–t19.

30. Stalman SE, Solanky N, Ishida M, Aleman-Charlet C, Abu-Amero S, Alders M, et al. Genetic analyses in small-for-gestational-age newborns. *J Clin Endocrinol Metab* 2018;**103**(3):917–25.

31. Matthews S, McGowan P. Developmental programming of the HPA axis and related behaviours: epigenetic mechanisms. *J Endocrinol* 2019;.

32. Nardozza LM, Caetano AC, Zamarian AC, Mazzola JB, Silva CP, Marcal VM, et al. Fetal growth restriction: current knowledge. *Arch Gynecol Obstet* 2017;**295**(5):1061–77.

33. Sharma D, Sharma P, Shastri S. Genetic, metabolic and endocrine aspect of intrauterine growth restriction: an update. *J Matern Fetal Neonatal Med* 2017;**30**(19):2263–75.

34. Crovetto F, Triunfo S, Crispi F, Rodriguez-Sureda V, Roma E, Dominguez C, et al. First-trimester screening with specific algorithms for early- and late-onset fetal growth restriction. *Ultrasound Obstet Gynecol* 2016;**48**(3):340–8.

35. Figueras F, Caradeux J, Crispi F, Eixarch E, Peguero A, Gratacos E. Diagnosis and surveillance of late-onset fetal growth restriction. *Am J Obstet Gynecol* 2018;**218**(2s). S790–S802.e1.

36. Townsend R, Khalil A. Fetal growth restriction in twins. *Best Pract Res Clin Obstet Gynaecol* 2018;**49**:79–88.

37. Townsend R, D'Antonio F, Sileo FG, Kumbay H, Thilaganathan B, Khalil A. Perinatal outcome of monochorionic twin pregnancy complicated by selective fetal growth restriction according to management: systematic review and meta-analysis. *Ultrasound Obstet Gynecol* 2019;**53**(1):36–46.

38. Ananth CV, Vintzileos AM. Distinguishing pathological from constitutional small for gestational age births in population-based studies. *Early Hum Dev* 2009;**85**(10):653–8.

39. Carberry AE, Gordon A, Bond DM, Hyett J, Raynes-Greenow CH, Jeffery HE. Customised versus population-based growth charts as a screening tool for detecting small for gestational age infants in low-risk pregnant women. *Cochrane Database Syst Rev* 2014;(5).

40. Guo MH, Hirschhorn JN, Dauber A. Insights and implications of genome-wide association studies of height. *J Clin Endocrinol Metab* 2018;**103** (9):3155–68.

41. Boghossian NS, Horbar JD, Murray JC, Carpenter JH, Vermont ON. Anthropometric charts for infants with trisomies 21, 18, or 13 born between 22 weeks gestation and term: the VON charts. *Am J Med Genet A* 2012;**158A**(2):322–32.

42. Boghossian NS, Horbar JD, Carpenter JH, Murray JC, Bell EF, Vermont ON. Major chromosomal anomalies among very low birth weight infants in the Vermont Oxford Network. *J Pediatr* 2012;**160**(5). 774–80.e11.

43. Purdy IB, Singh N, Brown WL, Vangala S, Devaskar UP. Revisiting early hypothyroidism screening in infants with Down syndrome. *J Perinatol* 2014;**34**(12):936–40.

44. Pierce MJ, LaFranchi SH, Pinter JD. Characterization of thyroid abnormalities in a large cohort of children with down syndrome. *Hormone Res Paediatr* 2017;**87**(3):170–8.

45. Gravholt CH, Andersen NH, Conway GS, Dekkers OM, Geffner ME, Klein KO, et al. Clinical practice guidelines for the care of girls and women with Turner syndrome: proceedings from the 2016 Cincinnati International Turner Syndrome Meeting. *Eur J Endocrinol* 2017;**177**(3): G1–G70.

46. Sari E, Bereket A, Yesilkaya E, Bas F, Bundak R, Aydin BK, et al. Anthropometric findings from birth to adulthood and their relation with karyotpye distribution in Turkish girls with Turner syndrome. *Am J Med Genet A* 2017;**170a**(4):942–8.

47. Wisniewski A, Milde K, Stupnicki R, Szufladowicz-Wozniak J. Weight deficit at birth and Turner's syndrome. *J Pediatr Endocrinol Metabol: JPEM* 2007;**20**(5):607–13.

48. Garcia Rudaz C, Martinez AS, Heinrich JJ, Lejarraga H, Keselman A, Laspiur M, et al. Growth of Argentinian girls with Turner syndrome. *Ann Hum Biol* 1995;**22**(6):533–44.

49. Fiot E, Zenaty D, Boizeau P, Haignere J, Dos Santos S, Leger J. X-chromosome gene dosage as a determinant of impaired pre and postnatal growth and adult height in Turner syndrome. *Eur J Endocrinol* 2016;**174**(3):281–8.

50. Marchini A, Ogata T, Rappold GA. A track record on SHOX: from basic research to complex models and therapy. *Endocr Rev* 2016;**37**(4):417–48.

51. Freire BL, Homma TK, Funari MFA, Lerario AM, Vasques GA, Malaquias AC, et al. Multigene sequencing analysis of children born small for gestational age with isolated short stature. *J Clin Endocrinol Metab* 2019;**104**(6):2023–30.

52. Kotzot D. Prenatal testing for uniparental disomy: indications and clinical relevance. *Ultrasound Obstet Gynecol* 2008;**31**(1):100–5.

53. Mackay DJG, Temple IK. Human imprinting disorders: principles, practice, problems and progress. *Eu J Med Genet* 2017;**60**(11):618–26.

54. Butler MG, Manzardo AM, Forster JL. Prader-Willi syndrome: clinical genetics and diagnostic aspects with treatment approaches. *Curr Pediatr Rev* 2016;**12**(2):136–66.

55. Mackay DJ, Temple IK. Transient neonatal diabetes mellitus type 1. *Am J Med Genet C Semin Med Genet* 2010;**154C**(3):335–42.

56. Temple IK, Gardner RJ, Mackay DJ, Barber JC, Robinson DO, Shield JP. Transient neonatal diabetes: widening the understanding of the etiopathogenesis of diabetes. *Diabetes* 2000;**49**(8):1359–66.

57. Wakeling EL, Brioude F, Lokulo-Sodipe O, O'Connell SM, Salem J, Bliek J, et al. Diagnosis and management of Silver-Russell syndrome: first international consensus statement. *Nat Rev Endocrinol* 2017;**13**(2):105–24.

58. Fisher AM, Thomas NS, Cockwell A, Stecko O, Kerr B, Temple IK, et al. Duplications of chromosome 11p15 of maternal origin result in a phenotype that includes growth retardation. *Hum Genet* 2002;**111**(3):290–6.

59. Eggermann T, Meyer E, Obermann C, Heil I, Schuler H, Ranke MB, et al. Is maternal duplication of 11p15 associated with Silver-Russell syndrome? *J Med Genet* 2005;**42**(5).

60. Ioannides Y, Lokulo-Sodipe K, Mackay DJ, Davies JH, Temple IK. Temple syndrome: improving the recognition of an underdiagnosed chromosome 14 imprinting disorder: an analysis of 51 published cases. *J Med Genet* 2014;**51**(8):495–501.

61. Eggermann T, Buiting K, Temple IK. Clinical utility gene card for: Silver-Russell syndrome. *Eur J Hum Genet: EJHG* 2011;**19**(3).

62. Fontana L, Bedeschi MF, Maitz S, Cereda A, Fare C, Motta S, et al. Characterization of multi-locus imprinting disturbances and underlying genetic defects in patients with chromosome 11p15.5 related imprinting disorders. *Epigenetics* 2018;**13**(9):897–909.

63. Rochtus A, Martin-Trujillo A, Izzi B, Elli F, Garin I, Linglart A, et al. Genome-wide DNA methylation analysis of pseudohypoparathyroidism patients with GNAS imprinting defects. *Clin Epigenetics* 2016;**8**:10.

64. Cortessis VK, Azadian M, Buxbaum J, Sanogo F, Song AY, Sriprasert I, et al. Comprehensive meta-analysis reveals association between multiple imprinting disorders and conception by assisted reproductive technology. *J Assist Reprod Genet* 2018;**35**(6):943–52.

65. Begemann M, Rezwan FI, Beygo J, Docherty LE, Kolarova J, Schroeder C, et al. Maternal variants in NLRP and other maternal effect proteins are associated with multilocus imprinting disturbance in offspring. *J Med Genet* 2018;**55**(7):497–504.

66. Hamidi T, Singh AK, Chen T. Genetic alterations of DNA methylation machinery in human diseases. *Epigenomics* 2015;**7**(2):247–65.

67. Smeets CC, Zandwijken GR, Renes JS, Hokken-Koelega AC. Long-term results of GH treatment in Silver-Russell Syndrome (SRS): do they benefit the same as non-SRS short-SGA? *J Clin Endocrinol Metab* 2016;**101**(5):2105–12.

68. Brightman DS, Lokulo-Sodipe O, Searle BA, Mackay DJG, Davies JH, Temple IK, et al. Growth hormone improves short-term growth in patients with Temple syndrome. *Hormone Res Paediatr* 2018;**90**(6):407–13.

69. Yakoreva M, Kahre T, Pajusalu S, Ilisson P, Zilina O, Tillmann V, et al. A new case of a rare combination of Temple syndrome and mosaic trisomy 14 and a literature review. *Mol Syndromol* 2018;**9**(4):182–9.

70. Clayton PE, Hanson D, Magee L, Murray PG, Saunders E, Abu-Amero SN, et al. Exploring the spectrum of 3-M syndrome, a primordial short stature disorder of disrupted ubiquitination. *Clin Endocrinol* 2012;**77**(3):335–42.

71. Brigant B, Metzinger-Le Meuth V, Rochette J, Metzinger L. TRIMming down to TRIM37: relevance to inflammation, cardiovascular disorders, and cancer in MULIBREY nanism. *Int J Mol Sci* 2018;**20**(1).

72. Innes AM, Dyment DA. SHORT syndrome. In: Adam MP, Ardinger HH, Pagon RA, Wallace SE, LJH B, Stephens K, et al., editors. *GeneReviews((R))*. Seattle (WA): University of Washington; 1993. GeneReviews is a registered trademark of the University of Washington, Seattle. All rights reserved.

73. Nikkel SM, Dauber A, de Munnik S, Connolly M, Hood RL, Caluseriu O, et al. The phenotype of Floating-Harbor syndrome: clinical characterization of 52 individuals with mutations in exon 34 of SRCAP. *Orphanet J Rare Dis* 2013;**8**:63.

74. Hood RL, Schenkel LC, Nikkel SM, Ainsworth PJ, Pare G, Boycott KM, et al. The defining DNA methylation signature of Floating-Harbor syndrome. *Sci Rep* 2016;**6**:38803.

75. Arboleda VA, Lee H, Parnaik R, Fleming A, Banerjee A, Ferraz-de-Souza B, et al. Mutations in the PCNA-binding domain of CDKN1C cause IMAGe syndrome. *Nat Genet* 2012;**44**(7):788–92.

76. Kim YM, Seo GH, Kim GH, Ko JM, Choi JH, Yoo HW. A case of an infant suspected as IMAGE syndrome who were finally diagnosed with MIRAGE syndrome by targeted Mendelian exome sequencing. *BMC Med Genet* 2018;**19**(1):35.

77. Davidsson J, Puschmann A, Tedgard U, Bryder D, Nilsson L, Cammenga J. SAMD9 and SAMD9L in inherited predisposition to ataxia, pancytopenia, and myeloid malignancies. *Leukemia* 2018;**32**(5):1106–15.

78. Klingseisen A, Jackson AP. Mechanisms and pathways of growth failure in primordial dwarfism. *Genes Dev* 2011;**25**(19):2011–24.

79. Morris-Rosendahl DJ, Kaindl AM. What next-generation sequencing (NGS) technology has enabled us to learn about primary autosomal recessive microcephaly (MCPH). *Mol Cell Probes* 2015;**29**(5):271–81.

80. Samuels ME, Deal CL, Skidmore DL. Meier-Gorlin syndrome. In: Erickson RP, Wynshaw-Boris AJ, editors. 3rd ed. *Epstein's inborn errors of development: the molecular basis of clinical disorders of morphogenesis*. Oxford University Press; 2016. ISBN-13: 9780199934522. https://doi.org/10.1093/med/9780199934522.001.0001.

81. Khetarpal P, Das S, Panigrahi I, Munshi A. Primordial dwarfism: overview of clinical and genetic aspects. *Mol Genet Genomics: MGG* 2016; **291**(1):1–15.

82. Pierce MJ, Morse RP. The neurologic findings in Taybi-Linder syndrome (MOPDI/III): case report and review of the literature. *Am J Med Genet A* 2012;**158a**(3):606–10.

83. Putoux A, Alqahtani A, Pinson L, Paulussen AD, Michel J, Besson A, et al. Refining the phenotypical and mutational spectrum of Taybi-Linder syndrome. *Clin Genet* 2016;**90**(6):550–5.

84. Bober MB, Jackson AP. Microcephalic osteodysplastic primordial dwarfism. Type II. A clinical review. *Curr Osteoporosis Rep* 2017;**15**(2):61–9.

85. Gluckman PD, Gunn AJ, Wray A, Cutfield WS, Chatelain PG, Guilbaud O, et al. Congenital idiopathic growth hormone deficiency associated with prenatal and early postnatal growth failure. The International Board of the Kabi Pharmacia International Growth Study. *J Pediatr* 1992;**121**(6):920–3.

86. Laron Z. Laron syndrome (primary growth hormone resistance or insensitivity): the personal experience 1958–2003. *J Clin Endocrinol Metab* 2004;**89**(3):1031–44.

87. Kemp SF, Fowlkes JL, Thrailkill KM. Efficacy and safety of mecasermin rinfabate. *Expert Opin Biol Ther* 2006;**6**(5):533–8.

88. Guevara-Aguirre J, Guevara A, Guevara C. Treatment of growth failure in the absence of GH signaling: the Ecuadorian experience. *Growth Hormon IGF Res* 2018;**38**:53–6.

89. Wit JM, Oostdijk W, Losekoot M, van Duyvenvoorde HA, Ruivenkamp CA, Kant SG. MECHANISMS IN ENDOCRINOLOGY: novel genetic causes of short stature. *Eur J Endocrinol* 2016;**174**(4):R145–73.

90. Krstevska-Konstantinova M, Pfäffle H, Schlicke M, Laban N, Tasic V, et al. *IGF1R* gene alterations in children born small for gestational age (SGA). *Open Access Maced J Med Sci* 2018;**6**(11):2040–4.

91. Cannarella R, Mattina T, Condorelli RA, Mongioi LM, Pandini G, La Vignera S, et al. Chromosome 15 structural abnormalities: effect on IGF1R gene expression and function. *Endocrine Connect* 2017;**6**(7):528–39.

92. Butler MG, Fogo AB, Fuchs DA, Collins FS, Dev VG, Phillips 3rd JA. Two patients with ring chromosome 15 syndrome. *Am J Med Genet* 1988;**29**(1):149–54.

93. Fokstuen S, Kotzot D. Chromosomal rearrangements in patients with clinical features of Silver-Russell syndrome. *Am J Med Genet A* 2014;**164a**(6):1595–605.

94. Rockstroh D, Pfaffle H, Le Duc D, Rossler F, Schlensog-Schuster F, Heiker JT, et al. A new p.(Ile66Serfs*93) IGF2 variant is associated with pre- and postnatal growth retardation. *Eur J Endocrinol* 2019;**180**(1):K1–k13.

95. Begemann M, Zirn B, Santen G, Wirthgen E, Soellner L, Buttel HM, et al. Paternally inherited IGF2 mutation and growth restriction. *N Engl J Med* 2015;**373**(4):349–56.

96. Constancia M, Hemberger M, Hughes J, Dean W, Ferguson-Smith A, Fundele R, et al. Placental-specific IGF-II is a major modulator of placental and fetal growth. *Nature* 2002;**417**(6892):945–8.

97. Dauber A, Rosenfeld RG, Hirschhorn JN. Genetic evaluation of short stature. *J Clin Endocrinol Metab* 2014;**99**(9):3080–92.

98. Takahashi Y, Kadowaki H, Ando A, Quin JD, MacCuish AC, Yazaki Y, et al. Two aberrant splicings caused by mutations in the insulin receptor gene in cultured lymphocytes from a patient with Rabson-Mendenhall's syndrome. *J Clin Invest* 1998;**101**(3):588–94.

99. Nobile S, Semple RK, Carnielli VP. A novel mutation of the insulin receptor gene in a preterm infant with Donohue syndrome and heart failure. *J Pediatr Endocrinol Metabol: JPEM* 2012;**25**(3-4):363–6.

100. Plamper M, Gohlke B, Schreiner F, Woelfle J. Mecasermin in insulin receptor-related severe insulin resistance syndromes: case report and review of the literature. *Int J Mol Sci* 2018;**19**(5).

101. Mackay DJ, Callaway JL, Marks SM, White HE, Acerini CL, Boonen SE, et al. Hypomethylation of multiple imprinted loci in individuals with transient neonatal diabetes is associated with mutations in ZFP57. *Nat Genet* 2008;**40**(8):949–51.

102. Touati A, Errea-Dorronsoro J, Nouri S, Halleb Y, Pereda A, Mahdhaoui N, et al. Transient neonatal diabetes mellitus and hypomethylation at additional imprinted loci: novel ZFP57 mutation and review on the literature. *Acta Diabetol* 2019;**56**(3):301–7.

103. Schwitzgebel VM, Mamin A, Brun T, Ritz-Laser B, Zaiko M, Maret A, et al. Agenesis of human pancreas due to decreased half-life of insulin promoter factor 1. *J Clin Endocrinol Metab* 2003;**88**(9):4398–406.

104. Gonc EN, Ozon A, Alikasifoglu A, Haliloglu M, Ellard S, Shaw-Smith C, et al. Variable phenotype of diabetes mellitus in siblings with a homozygous PTF1A enhancer mutation. *Hormone Res Paediatr* 2015;**84**(3):206–11.

105. Weedon MN, Cebola I, Patch AM, Flanagan SE, De Franco E, Caswell R, et al. Recessive mutations in a distal PTF1A enhancer cause isolated pancreatic agenesis. *Nat Genet* 2014;**46**(1):61–4.

106. De Franco E, Shaw-Smith C, Flanagan SE, Edghill EL, Wolf J, Otte V, et al. Biallelic PDX1 (insulin promoter factor 1) mutations causing neonatal diabetes without exocrine pancreatic insufficiency. *Diabet Med* 2013;**30**(5):e197–200.

107. Gragnoli C, Stanojevic V, Gorini A, Von Preussenthal GM, Thomas MK, Habener JF. IPF-1/MODY4 gene missense mutation in an Italian family with type 2 and gestational diabetes. *Metab Clin Exp* 2005;**54**(8):983–8.

108. Huopio H, Miettinen PJ, Ilonen J, Nykanen P, Veijola R, Keskinen P, et al. Clinical, genetic, and biochemical characteristics of early-onset diabetes in the Finnish population. *J Clin Endocrinol Metab* 2016;**101**(8):3018–26.

109. Bernstein IM, Catalano PM. Influence of fetal fat on the ultrasound estimation of fetal weight in diabetic mothers. *Obstet Gynecol* 1992;**79**(4):561–3.

110. Chauhan SP, Sullivan CA, Lutton TC, Magann EF, Morrison JC. Parous patients' estimate of birth weight in postterm pregnancy. *J Perinatol* 1995;**15**(3):192–4.

111. Hendrix NW, Morrison JC, McLaren RA, Magann EF, Chauhan SP. Clinical and sonographic estimates of birth weight among diabetic parturients. *J Maternal-Fetal Invest* 1998;**8**(1):17–20.

112. Cohen Jr MM. Mental deficiency, alterations in performance, and CNS abnormalities in overgrowth syndromes. *Am J Med Genet C Semin Med Genet* 2003;**117c**(1):49–56.

113. Lapunzina P. Risk of tumorigenesis in overgrowth syndromes: a comprehensive review. *Am J Med Genet C Semin Med Genet* 2005;**137c**(1):53–71.

114. Vora N, Bianchi DW. Genetic considerations in the prenatal diagnosis of overgrowth syndromes. *Prenat Diagn* 2009;**29**(10):923–9.

115. Kamien B, Ronan A, Poke G, Sinnerbrink I, Baynam G, Ward M, et al. A clinical review of generalized overgrowth syndromes in the era of massively parallel sequencing. *Mol Syndromol* 2018;**9**(2):70–82.

116. Yachelevich N. Generalized overgrowth syndromes with prenatal onset. *Curr Probl Pediatr Adolesc Health Care* 2015;**45**(4):97–111.

117. Cohen Jr MM, Neri G, Weksberg R. *Chromosomal disorders with overgrowth. Overgrowth syndromes*. Oxford, UK: Oxford University Press; 2005 p. 161–5.

118. Segel R, Peter I, Demmer LA, Cowan JM, Hoffman JD, Bianchi DW. The natural history of trisomy 12p. *Am J Med Genet A* 2006;**140**(7):695–703.

119. Brioude F, Kalish JM, Mussa A, Foster AC, Bliek J, Ferrero GB, et al. Expert consensus document: clinical and molecular diagnosis, screening and management of Beckwith-Wiedemann syndrome: an international consensus statement. *Nat Rev Endocrinol* 2018;**14**(4):229–49.

120. Tatton-Brown K, Pilz DT, Orstavik KH, Patton M, Barber JC, Collinson MN, et al. 15q overgrowth syndrome: a newly recognized phenotype associated with overgrowth, learning difficulties, characteristic facial appearance, renal anomalies and increased dosage of distal chromosome 15q. *Am J Med Genet A* 2009;**149a**(2):147–54.

121. Kamien B, Digilio MC, Novelli A, O'Donnell S, Bain N, Meldrum C, et al. Narrowing the critical region for overgrowth within 13q14.2-q14.3 microdeletions. *Eu J Med Genet* 2015;**58**(11):629–33.

122. Moncla A, Missirian C, Cacciagli P, Balzamo E, Legeai-Mallet L, Jouve JL, et al. A cluster of translocation breakpoints in 2q37 is associated with overexpression of NPPC in patients with a similar overgrowth phenotype. *Hum Mutat* 2007;**28**(12):1183–8.

123. Hisado-Oliva A, Ruzafa-Martin A, Sentchordi L, Funari MFA, Bezanilla-Lopez C, Alonso-Bernaldez M, et al. Mutations in C-natriuretic peptide (NPPC): a novel cause of autosomal dominant short stature. *Genet Med* 2018;**20**(1):91–7.

124. Barisic I, Boban L, Akhmedzhanova D, Bergman JEH, Cavero-Carbonell C, Grinfelde I, et al. Beckwith Wiedemann syndrome: a population-based study on prevalence, prenatal diagnosis, associated anomalies and survival in Europe. *Eu J Med Genet* 2018;**61**(9):499–507.

125. Munns CF, Batch JA. Hyperinsulinism and Beckwith-Wiedemann syndrome. *Arch Dis Child Fetal Neonatal Ed* 2001;**84**(1):F67–9.

126. Abi Habib W, Brioude F, Azzi S, Rossignol S, Linglart A, Sobrier ML, et al. Transcriptional profiling at the DLK1/MEG3 domain explains clinical overlap between imprinting disorders. *Sci Adv* 2019;**5**(2).

127. Giabicani E, Chantot-Bastaraud S, Bonnard A, Rachid M, Whalen S, Netchine I, et al. Roles of Type 1 insulin-like growth factor (IGF) receptor and IGF-II in growth regulation: evidence from a patient carrying both an 11p paternal duplication and 15q deletion. *Front Endocrinol* 2019;**10**:263.

128. Suri M. Approach to the diagnosis of overgrowth syndromes. *Indian J Pediatr* 2016;**83**(10):1175–87.

129. Cheng W, Tseng CJ, Lin TT, Cheng I, Pan HW, Hsu HC, et al. Glypican-3-mediated oncogenesis involves the Insulin-like growth factor-signaling pathway. *Carcinogenesis* 2008;**29**(7):1319–26.

130. Allen C, Reardon W. Assisted reproduction technology and defects of genomic imprinting. *BJOG: Int J Obstet Gynaecol* 2005;**112**(12):1589–94.

131. Vuillaume ML, Moizard MP, Rossignol S, Cottereau E, Vonwill S, Alessandri JL, et al. Mutation update for the GPC3 gene involved in Simpson-Golabi-Behmel syndrome and review of the literature. *Hum Mutat* 2018;**39**(6):790–805.

132. Edmondson AC, Kalish JM. Overgrowth Syndromes. *J Pediatr Genet* 2015;**4**(3):136–43.

133. Myers A, Bernstein JA, Brennan ML, Curry C, Esplin ED, Fisher J, et al. Perinatal features of the RASopathies: Noonan syndrome, cardiofacio-cutaneous syndrome and Costello syndrome. *Am J Med Genet A* 2014;**164a**(11):2814–21.

134. Rauen KA. The RASopathies. *Annu Rev Genomics Hum Genet* 2013;**14**:355–69.

Part F

New Diagnostic Technologies

Chapter 52

New Technologies in Pre- and Postnatal Diagnosis

Anne-Marie Laberge*, Aspasia Karalis*, Pranesh Chakraborty† and Mark E. Samuels‡

*Medical Genetics, Department of Pediatrics, CHU Sainte-Justine and Université de Montréal, Montreal, QC, Canada, †Department of Pediatrics, Department of Biochemistry, Microbiology and Immunology, Newborn Screening Ontario, Children's Hospital of Eastern Ontario, University of Ottawa, Ottawa, ON, Canada, ‡Department of Medicine, Centre de Recherche du CHU Ste-Justine, Université de Montréal, Montreal, QC, Canada

Clinical Considerations with Current New Technologies

- Genomics technologies promise increased speed of analysis at increasingly lower cost, specifically for diseases with genetic heterogeneity. Not all rare diseases are due to genetics. The molecular pathology of common diseases include environmental factors interacting with multiple rare gene variants.
- Next generation sequencing technologies extends our ability to make the link between rare genomic variants and human disease, but lack of universal standards for analysis and reporting make it difficult to assess accuracy. Large numbers of rare variants within each individual make it challenging to assess genotype-phenotype relationships.
- Proteomic and metabolomics technologies are not contingent on whether the underlying etiology of a patient's condition is genetic or due to environmental factors, and thus should see increasing use in the coming decades.
- RNA sequencing and transcriptome analysis suffer much the same difficulties that diseases with somatic DNA mosaicism present to the diagnostician, namely the difficulty in obtaining the relevant tissue and/or cell types expressing the abnormality.
- Non-invasive prenatal diagnosis using cell-free DNA and newborn screening using newer techniques present challenging financial, ethical and social dilemmas beyond the issues of false positive/false negative considerations; how these are viewed by geographic region can vary enormously.

52.1 BENEFITS AND CAVEATS FOR THE CLINICIAN USING GENOMICS TECHNOLOGIES

Genomics technologies promise two related benefits for the clinician: first, speed of return of relevant biomedical data on the patient's physiological state; and second, the capacity to interrogate much more of the patient's physiological state than pregenomic tests have been capable of. For example, traditional single-gene, Sanger-based deoxyribonucleic acid (DNA) sequencing typically has a several-week turnaround at best, and often several months, and is applied only when preliminary traditional diagnostic tests suggest a particular gene candidate. For some genetic conditions that may be due to mutation in any of several genes (termed genetic heterogeneity), the cost of sequencing all the possible candidates may be prohibitive. In such cases, genes often are sequenced in series, starting with the most frequently mutated gene for a particular phenotype, then in the event of a negative result, continuing with the next most frequently mutated, and so on. This restrains costs, but at the expense of extensive delays before a positive molecular genetic diagnosis is achieved. In contrast, sequencing all genes in the patient's genome at once using next-generation technologies may be more expensive than sequencing a single gene (although depending on the size of the gene, even this is not always the case), but it greatly reduces the turnaround time. Indeed, turnarounds of less than a week are feasible if all the relevant technologies, standard operating procedures, and clinical ethical approvals are already in place.[1] Such a quick turnaround can be critical for patients arriving at a clinic in an acute life-threatening condition, if a positive molecular genetic diagnosis is obtained that permits personalized management. (There is movement for the term *personalized medicine* to be replaced with *precision medicine,* on the reasonable grounds that clinicians have always provided personalized medicine as much as possible. With either term, the often-unstated implication is that genomic technologies are being employed.)

Similar examples could be provided for measuring protein levels or small molecule metabolites in a patient biopsy (whether blood or tissue). In each case, the underlying logic of a "genomic" approach is the measurement of all potentially relevant biomarkers, ideally in a single test. The economic benefit, as already noted, is that faster turnaround times, using

Maternal-Fetal and Neonatal Endocrinology. https://doi.org/10.1016/B978-0-12-814823-5.00053-2

941

TABLE 52.1 Comparison of single-gene/gene-product/metabolite to genome-scale diagnostic tests

Technology	Advantages	Disadvantages
Single-gene sequencing, single protein, RNA, or metabolite measurement	• Simplicity • Cost • Potentially quick turnaround time for a single test, contingent on capacity of the lab (often slow for outsourced, single-gene DNA sequencing)	• Limited information produced • Slow turnaround time, especially if multiple tests must be performed in series • Potentially many different providers required, depending on range of tests that each can provide, requiring complex networks of collaborations/contracts to be developed and maintained
Genome-scale DNA sequencing, RNA sequencing, proteomics, metabolomics	• All genes, proteins, and metabolites potentially interrogated in one step • For each individual technology, only one provider required in principle • Potentially quick turnaround time relative to information content	• Cost • Requires access to sophisticated informatics for primary data analysis • Challenge of meaningfully interpreting large sets of results

Genome-scale may include anything from true whole genome/transcriptome/proteome/metabolome to panels of large numbers of tests.

more comprehensive assays, will minimize unnecessary or redundant traditional clinical diagnostic tests or therapeutic treatments, thereby optimizing patient management as quickly as possible. The trade-off of greater costs of the genomic tests themselves may need to be evaluated on a case-by-case basis, which clearly should take into account nonmedical factors, such as the quality of life of the patient and the patient's family.

In this era of excitement over the use of genomics, especially genomic DNA sequencing, it should be kept in mind that not all rare clinical presentations are genetic simply because they are rare. We do not propose that genomic technologies are a cure-all, in either a diagnostic or therapeutic sense. Nonetheless, especially in pediatric medicine, where genetic disorders are responsible for a much greater proportion of total cases than in adult medicine (reportedly 30% or more of pediatric hospital intakes), genomic technologies are extremely beneficial tools in both a purely medical and also medicoeconomic context. Moreover, proteomic and metabolomics technologies are not contingent on whether the underlying etiology of a patient's condition is genetic or due to environmental factors.

Although some aspects of genomics technologies are already several years old and are well established in many core laboratories around the world, others are newer. The enthusiasm for each new iteration should be tempered with caution. The potential for positive "spin" bias with these technologies is high, among both developers and end users. Nevertheless, the sequencing of clinical patients on genomic scales is now widely applied, in basic biomedical research programs and clinically, especially in the disciplines of pediatrics and oncology. There are many success stories that strongly support the clinical value of genomic diagnostic tests, when applied appropriately (Table 52.1).[2–6]

52.2 DNA SEQUENCING

52.2.1 Next-Generation Sequencing Technology Overview

Sequencing of human genomic DNA, both for research and clinical diagnostic purposes, is decades old. Until recently, technological limitations restricted such assays to very small portions of the genome at a time (such as single genes, or even single coding exons). Since the very beginning of sequencing, we have desired the capability to sequence (and meaningfully interpret) a patient's entire genome with a clinically useful turnaround time. It is worth noting the specific challenges to realizing this dream, as the same ones still constrain the utility of the new sequencing technologies. To understand the bases for the technical limitations (and potential) of high-throughput DNA sequencing, some appreciation for the structure of the human genome and the history of its sequencing by the international research community will be helpful.

The first major issue is simply the size of the human genome. Each somatic cell nucleus contains about 6.2 pg, or approximately 6 billion base pairs of genomic DNA. Because humans are diploid, we typically use the haploid genome as a reference, and so sequencing a new patient's genome requires at least 3 billion bases of usable sequence. In fact, much more is required, partly due to statistical sampling effects; sequencing the genome exactly one time on average would lead to about 37% of the whole genome remaining unsequenced per the Poisson distribution, where $P(0) = e^{-1}$. Moreover, although the haploid genome is used by default as a reference, more than one haploid equivalent is required to capture both alleles at most genomic sites, which coverage is required for variant detection for presumptive genetic disorders, especially dominant ones (with heterozygous causal mutations).

To give a sense of the scale of the size problem, sequencing a new human individual genome to $1 \times$ mean coverage (i.e., 3 billion bases of clean sequence) using traditional Sanger chemistry and one capillary electrophoresis instrument would require 13 years, assuming 365 working days and no instrument down time (both of which are very unrealistic). The solution employed by the Human Genome Projects (both public and private) was to purchase and use many electrophoresis instruments. This is infeasible for clinical patient resequencing. Thus, for routine clinical use, next-generation technologies had to reduce the absolute cost, turnaround time, and instrumentation requirement, by many orders of magnitude. *Next-generation sequencing* as a term is usually taken to mean any technology with major improvements in cost, time, and throughput over Sanger-based capillary electrophoresis sequencing.

The second major problem in human genome sequencing is the large amount of repetitive sequence in the genome. This includes various families of transposon-based repetitive elements, ranging in size from several hundred to several thousand base pairs, presented whole or in fragments in millions of copies dispersed throughout the genome. Overall, such repetitive elements constitute approximately half the entire human genome (and the genomes of most other metazoan organisms as well). These elements, while biologically very interesting, are generally ignored in human medical genetics; it is likely that some genetic conditions may depend on mutations in such elements, but these would be challenging to resolve. Medical resequencing does not require true whole-genome assembly, only alignment of sequence reads to the unique parts of the consensus genome to identify variants. More problematic is the duplication of nominally unique, gene-coding genomic segments. Such duplications include dispersed spliced pseudogenes, presumed to arise via reverse transcription of mature or immature nuclear or cytoplasmic ribonucleic acid (RNA), followed by chromosomal reinsertion of the resulting

TABLE 52.2 First-, second-, and third-generation sequencing platforms (selected)

System	Generation	Bacterial/ viral clones	PCR-generated clones	Typical read length (short <300 bp, medium = about 300–1000 bp, long ≫1000 bp	Capacity for resequencing exomes at acceptable cost	Capacity for resequencing human genomes at acceptable cost
Sanger capillary	First	Yes	Possible	Medium	No	No
Roche/454	Second	No	Yes	Medium	Yes	No
Illumina/ Solexa	Second	No	Yes	Short	Yes	Yes
Thermofisher/ Life Technologies/ ABI SOLiD	Second	No	Yes	Short	Yes	No
Thermofisher/ Life Technologies/ ABI Proton/ Ion Torrent	Second	No	Yes	Short	Yes	Unclear
Complete Genomics (Shenzen)	Third	No	No	Short	Yes	Yes
Pacific Biosciences	Third	No	No	Long	Not appropriate	Not yet
Oxford Nanopore	Third	No	No	Long	Not appropriate	Not yet

For more details, see recent reviews, as well as technical reports from the various manufacturers.[7–9]

complementary DNA (cDNA), as well as true segmental chromosomal duplications that may include some of or all protein-coding genes. New cases of such duplication events occur very rarely, but over evolutionary time frames, the human genome has accrued many of them, which are fixed in the entire population, so that some particular genes are difficult to resequence for variant detection due to the presence of duplicated, presumably nonfunctional copies. Read length plays a key role in analyzing such genes; the longer the individual reads are, the more reliably they can be assigned either to the real coding gene or to a nonfunctional diverging duplicate.

Over the past decade, many next-generation technologies have been explored. Most of these have remained within academic laboratories, but some have gone on to commercialization either of instruments, customized reagents, fee-for-service, or some combination of these. The competition for a "$1000 genome" has been fierce. This chapter will focus on the systems that have captured most of the current market. Competition in this field remains high, so the new technologies of today stand a good chance of becoming outdated technologies tomorrow.

Among next-generation systems, the field distinguishes between second- and third-generation sequencing systems, with *first generation* referring to traditional Sanger-based capillary electrophoresis (see Table 52.2). Second-generation technologies are defined as those that eliminate biological cloning of human genomic DNA in viral or bacterial vectors, and also eliminate the need for electrophoresis during sequencing. Generally, second-generation technologies use polymerase chain reaction (PCR) to amplify fragmented genomic DNA, and some version of real-time parallel sequencing by synthesis to sequence millions to billions of PCR-generated microclones held on a solid support. The requirement for PCR limits the length of genomic DNA fragments that can be sequenced, and makes alignment of individual reads arising from duplicated genomic regions (either segmental duplications, or spliced pseudogenes) problematic with second-generation systems. By far the most successful current technology among second-generation systems is Illumina (originally developed by Solexa); others include Roche/454 pyrosequencing and the ThermoFisher/ABI Ion Proton.

Third-generation technologies are distinguished mainly by the elimination of PCR amplification. This permits much longer individual reads from large, primary patient genomic DNA fragments. The resulting weaker raw signal strengths result in greater error rates, which are overcome with higher coverage but at substantial added cost. However, the longer reads potentially result in much more reliable alignment to the consensus genome, especially in duplicated regions. The current dominant third-generation system is Pacific Biosciences, although Complete Genomics is competitive and Oxford Nanopore is rapidly becoming so. The throughput (hence cost) limitation of the long read systems has forestalled their significant use for human whole-genome sequencing as yet. They have found a major place in agricultural genomics, due to the large amount of repetitive DNA found in most plant genomes and the fact that many agriculturally important plants are polyploid. The high commercial value of food crops justifies the greater cost of third-generation systems, whose very long read lengths greatly facilitate the resulting genomic analyses. Third-generation technology is also used in micro-biomics, the study of microbial organisms, both prokaryotic and eukaryotic, inhabiting both the human body and the environment.

52.2.2   What is Used for the "Reference" or "Normal" Genome?

Up to now, we have mentioned several times the consensus human genome sequence. This is the complete assembled sequence available through public web sites and databases supported at three major international sites: the National Center for Biotechnological Information (NCBI), based in the United States (https://www.ncbi.nlm.nih.gov/projects/genome/guide/human/index.shtml); the University of California at Santa Cruz (UCSC) (http://genome.ucsc.edu/), and Ensembl, based in the European Molecular Biology Laboratory (EMBL) (https://useast.ensembl.org/). These three sites are independently operated, but they now present the same assembled human genome sequence, although with differences in the way that the sequence is presented and the types of genomic annotation provided.

The consensus human genome assembly does not represent any one individual; rather, it was generated from cloned libraries from multiple individuals of varying gender and ethnicity. One important consequence of this is that the consensus sequence contains many variant sites, some of which actually represent minor alleles in the general population. It should also be remembered that at the earlier stages, there were two competing genome projects: the international public consortium and a private company (named Celera at the time). Each of these generated a genomic assembly, but with different names and coming from different sources (multiple individuals for the public project, one individual for the private project). The public project assembly is referred to as the *consensus genome,* whereas the private project sequence is (somewhat confusingly) named *HuRef.* The term *reference genome* is therefore potentially ambiguous, although it is often used in lieu of *consensus genome* to mean the public project version.

Although a patient's genome certainly has a well-defined set of variant sites when compared to the consensus genome sequence defined by the Human Genome Project, the variants actually reported for any patient using high-throughput sequencing technologies represent a subset of the true sites, with some missed variants (false negative calls, type II errors) and some incorrectly defined sites (false positive calls, type I errors), each caused by technical errors at various levels in the physical process of sequencing, variant calling, and annotating.[10,11] To this extent, DNA sequencing is similar to any other medical diagnostic test. However, the cautious practitioner should be aware that at least for the moment, laboratory standards to which all sequencing facilities must adhere have not been universally implemented. It is not impossible to generate such standards and validate all testing laboratories; labs could be required to analyze a universal set of DNA samples, and false positive and negative rates could be measured with respect to a very high quality set of calls generated for the same samples by an international core laboratory.

Although such DNA standards have been proposed,[12–15] a recent survey documented widely varying practices in detailed implementation of genomic/exomic sequencing and reporting.[16] Similarly, although a small number of standard bioinformatics analysis pipelines are available,[17–19] individual sequencing labs are under no obligation to use them. Many sequencing centers have developed their own customized in-house informatics pipelines, while even the publically available pipelines include many tunable parameters that affect error rates differently. Many pipelines regularly resequence potential positive calls using standard Sanger sequencing to eliminate false positives, although this is not formally required. More seriously, false negative rates (missed calls) are not usually defined by individual labs for their particular technology platforms. As yet, therefore, medical sequencing using next-generation technologies lacks the rigorous implementation of universal standards, and clinicians receiving DNA variant reports for their patients with presumptive genetic conditions have no easy way to evaluate the quantitative accuracy of these reports. It is to be hoped that this suboptimal situation will not persist indefinitely.

52.2.3 Whole-Genome, Whole-Exome, and Targeted-Gene Panels

There are three typical implementations of next-generation sequencing: whole-genome, whole-exome, and candidate-gene panels (Table 52.3). All of these may be loosely considered as genomic-sequencing tests because candidate gene panels in a next-generation technology context usually involve large numbers of genes. Each of these tests has advantages and disadvantages, and for a particular patient or a particular potential genetic disorder, any one of these three may be the most efficient choice for a diagnostic test.[5,8,20] The three paradigms will be discussed next.

52.2.3.1 Whole-Genome Sequencing

This paradigm is the easiest to define; all accessible regions of a patient's genome are sequenced. Certain parts of the genome, notably centromeric and telomeric regions, remain effectively inaccessible to all current technologies, mostly

TABLE 52.3 Properties of various next-generation sequencing strategies

Sequencing strategy	Potential turnaround time	Typical burden of rare pathogenic variants	Detection of point mutants and indels	Detection of CNVs and large rearrangements	Cost
Whole-genome sequencing	3–5 days	500–1000	Yes	Yes	High
Whole-exome sequencing	2 weeks	500–1000	Yes	No	Intermediate
Candidate-gene panel	2 weeks	Small, scaling with number of genes tested	Yes	No	Low
Family trios (for recessive or de novo dominant mutations)	Depends on sequencing strategy	0–2	Yes	Depends on sequencing strategy	3 × the individual genome cost

Potential turnaround times refers to extremely optimized setups; typically all strategies take many weeks for routine analysis. *Typical burden* refers to number of potentially causal variants detected in a single proband using each of the strategies. Because only variants in or near protein coding exons are usually flagged, whole-genome and whole-exome strategies generate similar numbers of potential candidate mutations in a single proband, most of which are point variants; whole-genome methods add only a modest number of candidate CNVs in most cases. In analyzing family trios, any of the three strategies may be used, with emphasis on detecting two hits (homozygotes or compound heterozygotes) in the proband, with each parent heterozygous for one hit; or one hit (heterozygote) in the proband, with both parents wild-type.

due to the extremely highly repetitive sequence content. In general, such regions are presumed not to include individual functional genes, but to the extent that some genetic disorders may involve large-scale chromosomal rearrangements in these regions, such disorders cannot be diagnosed using next-generation sequencing. Even now, there remains a useful place for classical and hybridization-based cytology, such as fluorescence in situ hybridization (FISH). That said, chromosomal rearrangements in which breakpoints occur in accessible (especially unique) sequence can be detected, especially with third-generation technologies.

Given the high quality of the consensus human genome reference sequence, whole-genome patient sequencing is straightforward. The total DNA is extracted (usually from fresh whole blood or serum), fragmented, and directly analyzed using a next-generation system. Depending on the technology used (mostly regarding read length), repetitive coding sequences may be incompletely analyzed for genomic variation. By now, whole-genome methods successfully interrogate almost all the protein coding gene repertoire (the total gene number is still uncertain, but probably lies between 20,000 and 22,000 genes). Genes encoding interesting functional or possibly functional molecules, such as transfer ribonucleic acid (tRNA), ribosomal ribonucleic acid (rRNA), other small RNAs, microRNAs, and long noncoding (LNC) RNAs, are also mostly accessible through whole-genome sequencing. Interpretation of called variants is another matter, however. Even now, the functional consequences of variation in most unique but nonprotein coding genomic sequences are difficult or impossible to assess. The most easily interpreted variants are those within or immediately adjacent to exons. Variants that change protein-coding potential [missense, nonsense, and small insertion or deletion (termed indel) variants] are interpretable. Protein-truncating variants (nonsense, frameshifting indels) are usually assumed to be strongly pathogenic unless only the very C-terminus of a protein is affected, and even in these cases, some genes include important functional regions at the very C-terminus. Missense variants, sometimes referred to as *variants of uncertain significance (VUSs)*, are usually interpreted using prediction tools such as SIFT, PolyPhen2, or CADD, which take into account evolutionary conservation of the gene region and specific site in question in other species, and/or biochemical effects of the inferred amino acid change (acidic to basic, hydrophobic to hydrophilic, etc.).[21,22]

Assigning phenotypic consequences to missense variants in a clinical context is challenging but poses no theoretical difference in genomewide sequencing than in single-gene analyses for which standards are well established: variants should be seen in multiple patients, or in experimentally tested functional residues of a protein. The difference in genomewide sequencing is simply the large number of such variants detected in each patient. Coding exon variants that do not change protein coding potential, or synonymous variants, are usually inferred to be benign, although regulatory exonic sequences such as splice enhancers are known, so such variants are at least potentially pathogenic. Our ability to predict functional consequences for synonymous variants is poor at this time. Similarly, prediction of functional consequences of variation in the noncoding regions of messenger RNA (mRNA) (the 5′ and 3′ untranslated regions, or UTRs) is poor. Variants in the 5′ UTR that generate novel out-of-frame start codons, or that interfere with utilization of the normal translational start codon, can potentially be interpreted. Similarly, some well-defined regulatory sequences are known to occur in 3′ UTRs; however, interpretation of variation in these sequences in patients should be made cautiously, if at all.

Here are some basic statistics concerning the individual variant burden, to provide context for the problem of clinical interpretation. Individual human genomes generally contain more than 3 million detectable sequence variants, as compared to the consensus genome assembly, or indeed in comparison to any other individual human genome. This number is slightly (but measurably) higher for individuals of recent African origin (ultimately, we are all of African origin, of course). These 3 + million variants occur in both unique and repetitive sequences, within and without genes, and include point mutations, small insertions and deletions, and large insertions and deletions (copy number variants or CNVs, as discussed later in this chapter). About half of these are heterozygous, and the remainder homozygous. Luckily, most of these variants in individual genomes are fairly common, have modest or no obvious effects on gene function, and are unlikely to contribute to high-penetrance pediatric genetic disorders. If one filters the total set of variants for those that are rare in general populations (e.g., with a 1% minor allele frequency limit) and that occur in unique sequences, the total genomic variant count per individual is reduced substantially. If one further restricts variants to coding exons plus a few bases of adjacent intron sequence (to include potential intron splice site mutations in well-defined essential sequence elements), the number of such rare variants is < 1000, and may be under 500 per patient (depending on the absolute allele frequency threshold and particular version of genomic annotation employed). Almost all of these are typically heterozygous, and hence unlikely to cause recessive genetic disorders (unless as compound heterozygotes with another noncomplementing variant in the same gene, or in extremely rare documented examples of digenic inheritance). Variants in some nonprotein-coding RNAs such as tRNAs can be evaluated for functional significance due to our general level of understanding of function of these molecules; however, while scientifically interesting, variants in microRNAs and lncRNAs are usually not functionally interpretable at this time.

This low rare variant burden per individual has made the discovery of causal genes for rare genetic disorders spectacularly successful during the past decade. In analyzing rare protein-altering variants among patients with a shared, very rare clinical presentation, it is fairly routine to identify a probable causal gene with as few as three such patients. It is actually easier if the patients come from different ethnic backgrounds because they are less likely to share population-restricted variants that can confuse the gene discovery process. Given the high mutation burden in the entire human population, once a strong candidate gene has been proposed and published for a rare phenotype, follow-up replication often ensues within a year.

Despite such successes, the rare variant burden is still typically too high for definitive molecular diagnosis of novel rare phenotypes in single patients. Such diagnoses still live at the interface of clinical and research sequencing. Similarly, genomewide sequencing is inappropriate to use for the diagnosis of less rare medical conditions. The many conditions prevalent at a societal level (e.g., diabetes, asthma, migraine, autism, and autoimmune disorders) are in most cases simply too common to be the result of rare mutations in a single gene in all affected individuals. Nonetheless, rare single-gene (i.e., monogenic) versions of common medical disorders, caused by rare high-penetrance mutations, are well documented for many conditions and often provide useful information regarding the molecular pathology of the disorder, or even novel candidate drug targets.[23] They do not generally explain most of the total population burden of these diseases.

In contrast to the total individual rare variant burden, the burden of completely novel mutations, present in the genome of individuals but not in their parents, is extremely small. These de novo mutations arise either in the germ line (i.e., testes or ovaries) of the parents, and thus they are not detected when DNA is extracted from parental blood, or else early in the embryonic development of the patient. In either case, the medical consequence is a genetic phenotype observed in the patient but in neither parent (of course, such a transmission pattern is also expected for recessive disorders transmitted from carrier unaffected parents). Individual human genomes contain 50–100 de novo variants in the entire accessible genome (excluding highly repetitive sequences). Because protein-coding exons account for only about 1.5% of the total genome, individuals have at most one or two de novo variants in such exons.[24,25] Because some such variants are silent (synonymous—that is, not changing protein-coding potential), the number of pathogenic de novo variants per genome is even smaller. Thus, any pathogenic de novo variant in a patient is a good candidate for causing a novel (i.e., nontransmitted) medical phenotype. In order to find such variants however, trio sequencing is required (patient plus both biological parents). This triples the cost for the test, which is not logistically feasible for some or most medical centers. However, de novo mutations account for a significant proportion of new familial genetic cases, especially in pediatrics and for dominant disorders.[26] In endocrinology, such new mutations in sporadic cases have been reported in various genes, including *CHD7*,[27–30] *SAMD9*,[31] *ARID1B*,[32,33] and *PHEX*,[34–38] and the androgen receptor AR.[39–43]

52.2.3.2 Exome Sequencing

It may seem excessive to sequence the entire genome of a patient if only 1.5% or so of the genome can be functionally interpreted in terms of sequence variation. Whole-genome sequencing represents tremendous technological overkill for the average (pediatric) patient. Because the most interpretable genomic variants lie in protein-coding exons, it was reasonable to propose sequencing only these segments of the genome in the first place. The general term for this paradigm is whole-exome (or just exome) sequencing. The exome is defined as the exonic content of the genome, sometimes restricted to the absolute protein-coding regions and excluding the UTRs, sometimes including noncoding lncRNAs and other small, functional RNAs. Exome sequencing is technically feasible and is currently the most widespread application of next-generation sequencing in medical genetics.

The technical challenge in exome sequencing lies in the fact that coding exons are small and widely dispersed throughout the genome, so they are not easy to separate from the rest of nonexonic DNA in next-generation sequencing protocols. The simplest idea, hugely multiplex PCR just of coding exons, is extremely difficult to implement; if too many different oligonucleotide primers are put in the same PCR reaction, they simply interfere with each other. Using microfluidics, many different PCR reactions can be run in parallel on a chip; currently, this approach is implemented for some exome protocols (such as the Proton instrument). Other exome systems use hybridization capture, with oligonucleotide probe libraries targeting annotated coding exons to physically purify fragments containing exons from patient genomic DNA, followed by next-generation sequencing (often with Illumina second-generation systems). As with whole-genome sequencing, the output from exome sequencing is a set of short sequences, which must be analyzed by a bioinformatics pipeline to generate a set of annotated variants. Exomic data sets are highly simplified compared to the whole genome, as the large majority of reads align with the annotated exons used to design the capture probes. The process of identifying and annotating potential sequence variants in a patient exome is essentially the same as for whole-genome sequencing as described previously.

Because only a small fraction of the genome is sequenced, much less total sequencing is required to achieve deep coverage of a patient's coding genomic regions. This reduces the cost of the sequencing. However, there is a cost for the exon-capture protocol, consisting of the oligo capture library, solid support, and associated consumables, reagents and labor. Although in principle, 30–50 times less total sequence is required per patient, the cost advantage of exome versus whole-genome sequencing is much less—in the 5–$10\times$ cheaper range. This is still greatly advantageous to both research and clinical budgets. Also, the informatics burden for archiving raw exome sequence data is substantially less than for whole-genome data. One caveat to exome sequencing is that some particular genomic regions are difficult or impossible to analyze due to DNA sequence constraints or redundant gene copies. Luckily, such refractory regions are few and well documented.

Exome sequencing is dependent on the current state of annotation of the human genome. A gene that has not yet been annotated as a gene will not be captured using any targeting library because the construction of these libraries uses the genome annotation provided by the public Human Genome Project. Because annotation of the human genome is an ongoing process, exome capture libraries are inevitably out of date to some extent, depending on how often the commercial suppliers of these libraries revise their content of captured sequences. Different suppliers also have somewhat different content based on proprietary aspects of their technologies. Now, exome sequencing is fairly mature, so the content of current libraries is fairly stable.

Because high-penetrance genetic disorders are typically extremely rare, establishing genotype/phenotype correlations poses a significant challenge, as individual centers may only ever see a single case or family for a particular disorder. The obvious solution is to share information among centers. Such information sharing involves some tricky issues regarding patient confidentiality and ethics approvals, but these are not unresolvable. In an academic context, the need to establish priority for publication purposes is another problem, which again is being solved gradually as biologists become more used to large, collaborative projects. New initiatives have been established to encompass the realm of genetic disorders, particularly the International Rare Diseases Research Consortium (IrDiRC), which has a strong focus on clinical utility.[44]

52.2.3.3 Candidate-Gene Panels

Next-generation sequencing of candidate-gene panels is basically a subset of whole-exome gene sequencing. Instead of a library of capture probes (or PCR primers) targeting all annotated coding genes, only genes relevant to a particular medical condition are targeted. These might include all genes known to mutate to cause cardiac disorders (ion channels expressed in the heart, heart-specific myocyte proteins, regulatory genes required for development or maintenance of heart function, etc.). Some genetic disorders are not heterogeneous (e.g., cystic fibrosis), in which case the idea of a gene panel is irrelevant. Alternatively, gene panels have been proposed or developed for large numbers of different and individually rare genetic disorders; OMIM includes on the order of 4000 genes with molecularly characterized disorders; even including only these reduces the sequencing requirement by fivefold over whole-exome sequencing, allowing more patients to be multiplexed and sequenced for the equivalent budget. If clinical genomic-sequencing tests are restricted to previously identified genes, such a "rare phenome"-based test could still be cost effective compared to ordering single-gene tests on individual patients, who may show up at a tertiary care center with any of about 4000 characterized disorders.

52.2.4 Reporting of Genomic-Sequence Data

Clinicians are not normally expected to interpret raw sequence data unless they are trained and/or interested in practicing molecular genetics, as well as their particular medical discipline. The implementation of genomic sequencing for diagnosis implies the availability of a bioinformatics resource to annotate and provide interpretation of the resulting variants.[45] The bioinformatics may be in house or provided by the sequencing lab, dependent on the setup at each care center. In principle, genomic sequencing could be accessible to clinicians who do not work at large care centers; however, to our knowledge, such a system is not widely implemented yet; typically, primary caregivers work through large tertiary care centers that have the resources to carry out and interpret genomic sequencing. It is impossible to know how this is set up in detail at all centers, but in our experience, patients are typically referred to medical genetics before genomic-sequencing tests can be ordered.

Even the relatively modest set of potentially pathogenic rare variants observed in individual patient genomes (500–1000 variants) represents an unrealistic number for interpretation by primary caregivers (such as referring physicians, or even tertiary care center specialists in disciplines like endocrinology). Presumably in specific cases, specialists with extensive experience in genomic genetics could request and receive the complete set of variants, or at least rare pathogenic variants, for patients whom they have referred. More reasonably, tertiary care centers may establish a committee to review the initial set of variants and generate a kind of genomic case report.[2,6] Such a report might note, in decreasing order of utility: (1) specific variants seen in the patient that are already documented in the medical literature to cause the patient phenotype; (2) new and probably pathogenic variants in genes that are already documented to mutate to the patient phenotype; (3) new VUSs occurring in genes already documented to mutate to the patient phenotype; (4) new variants predicted to be highly pathogenic (such as protein truncations) in genes not previously associated with the patient phenotype; and (5) other variants that may be relevant on a case-by-case basis.[5,6,11,46–48]

To generate such a prioritized, very small, set of candidate variants, the review committee requires general expertise in medical genetics, experience in genomic sequencing (at least in a research context), and reasonable familiarity with the various medical specialties that are likely to refer patients for such a diagnostic test. Due to the large number of molecularly characterized genetic syndromes, and the fairly wide range of clinical presentations associated with many of these, it is optimal for the review committee to have significant redundancy in terms of these required kinds of expertise, because different geneticists will almost certainly have had different previous experiences with such patients.

In perspective, the $1000 genome milestone has been achieved in terms of absolute cost (https://www.genome.gov/sequencingcosts/). However, as a diagnostic service provided by outsourced suppliers, medical geneticists can still expect to pay more than this—perhaps as much as $5000—for an interpreted whole genome of a patient. In-house costs may be lower, but they need to take into account equipment purchase, maintenance, and depreciation, as well as the labor required for sample preparation and bioinformatics analysis. Costs are continuing to come down, however, so the real $1000 genome should soon be available.

Despite the fairly high quality of next-generation sequencing, many labs still use Sanger-based traditional sequencing, considering it the gold standard to validate candidate causal variants. The cost of this must be considered in developing a general budget for next-generation sequencing at a large care center.

The decision of which paradigm of genomic sequencing to employ—a whole-genome, whole-exome, or targeted-gene panel, involves multiple aspects, including cost, mandate of the clinical site, state of knowledge in the particular discipline, and support resources available in the local setting.[47] Persani et al. discuss in some detail a recommended diagnostic workflow to determine the optimal genomic sequencing test for patients in endocrinology.[49] Currently, in the entire field of human medical diagnostic genetics, exome sequencing is the most generally used approach. Targeted-gene panels are more prevalent in particular medical areas (such as oncology), whereas whole-genome sequencing is rare, and probably only being used when exome sequencing has failed or is considered likely to fail, or where turnaround time is absolutely critical. Skipping the exon capture hybridization step in principle allows much quicker turnaround for whole-genome sequencing. Patient DNA can be extracted and a complete genome sequence acquired within 24–48 h; with some additional time required for the bioinformatics analysis, a several-day turnaround is feasible. At least one clinical sequencing lab offers a targeted-gene panel specific to endocrine genes and disorders (http://www.exeterlaboratory.com/genetics/endocrine-disorder-ngs-panel-tests/). The test currently includes 75 genes, covering a variety of endocrine disorders such as combined pituitary insufficiency, hypothyroidism, hypoparathyroidism and hyperparathyroidism, glucocorticoid deficiency, pseudohypoaldosteronism type 2, hypophosphatemic rickets, as well as several endocrine gland cancers. GeneDx (https://www.genedx.com/) offers clinical exomes and whole genomes, as well as trios (proband plus parents). There is no doubt that either now or in the near future, there will be other diagnostic providers of genomic tests relevant to endocrinology. We anticipate that eventually, whole-genome sequencing will become the standard clinical test, replacing both exome and targeted-gene panels once costs for actual sample processing, as well as data analysis and long-term archiving, come down sufficiently.

52.2.5 Copy Number Variants and Other Large-Scale Chromosomal Rearrangements

Although large-scale chromosomal rearrangements, including large deletions or duplications (CNVs), are only one of many types of mutational genomic events, they pose a special problem for next-generation technologies and are considered separately here. First, an important bit of nomenclature must be discussed. We have previously mentioned insertion and deletion mutations. In practice, these types of mutations are problematic for the software used to align sequencing reads to the consensus human genome assembly because the alignment requires the introduction of gaps. In practice, insertions or deletions (referred to as *indels* more generally) up to about 30 bases can be called using short read technologies (such as Illumina). Large chromosomal rearrangements, insertions, and deletions are usually identified using nonsequencing based, cytological methods. These include microscopy, as well as quantitative hybridization methods such as FISH or array-comparative genomic hybridization (CGH). These methods have a lower limit of resolution, on the order of a few kilobases to a few dozen kilobases depending on the technology. Thus, there is a large hole between the maximum size of indels easily accessible through second-generation sequencing and the minimum size accessible to nonsequencing methods. This hole can be partially filled by whole-genome sequencing, using specialized software tools that optimize the alignment of gapped sequences, or possibly by third-generation long read systems. Thus whole-genome versus exome sequencing is useful when large indels or other chromosomal rearrangements are suspected (or when point mutants have been excluded by exome sequencing). CNVs are also easier to detect with whole-genome sequencing, as this technology is more generally quantitative and exome data has too much statistical noise for reliable copy number measurement. The gold standard for verifying CNVs is still quantitative PCR (qPCR).

Although for cost and implementation reasons, whole-genome sequencing has not replaced nonsequencing methods for detecting clinical CNVs and chromosomal rearrangements (including the many well-documented contiguous deletion syndromes), such a replacement is likely coming in the not-too-distant future. That said, the complexity of the human genome means that cytological and hybridization-based methods will probably always have some place in medical genetics.[50]

52.2.6 Mosaicism

Throughout the life of an individual, the genome is dynamic, though to only a small extent. This is because new mutations arise during mitosis in the course of normal development and after birth. The genomic replication machinery, while extremely accurate, has a measurable (though small) error rate. Thus, after the initial event of sperm/egg nuclear fusion, the diploid zygotic genome is subject to mutations, leading to mosaicism. Depending on when and in which cells a new mutation arises, it will be restricted to the descendants of that cell in the body. Because the mitotic mutation rate is low, very few mutations are expected to occur early in development, simply due to the small total cell number in the zygote. Such early mutations would result in most cells in the body (or in extraembryonic tissues) carrying the mutation. The more cells there are, the more likely a mutation and the smaller proportion of the total body expected to carry that mutation. The germ line becomes a segregated lineage separate from the somatic body fairly early in development. As a result, it is expected that most mutations will be present either in the germ line or the soma, but not both. This is found true in practice, although not completely, as mutations simultaneously mosaic in both the germ line and soma are documented in the medical literature (albeit rarely).[51]

The genetics literature uses the term *mosaic* somewhat loosely. It may be used to describe the status of an individual (usually a patient) to mean that not all cells in the patient's body carry the mutation. It may also refer to the status of a family, meaning that one of the parental germ lines is mosaic, leading to some offspring carrying a mutation and others receiving the equivalent chromosomal homolog but not carrying the mutation. In the latter case, the implicated parent is a germ-line mosaic individual, but the entire family may be described as displaying mosaicism. Moreover, in some cases, the parental germ line may not actually be mosaic, but it may be completely mutant, so all offspring receiving the chromosomal homolog involved do receive the mutation, but where that parent's somatic cells do not (or at least some of whose cells do not) carry the mutation. The particular meaning of the term *mosaicism* is usually clear in the context of the situation, but it can be ambiguous if information is not provided regarding the genomic status of all family members related to the patient.

The detection of mosaicism in an individual depends on two technical requirements—first, the ability to sample a range of biological tissues; and second, the sensitivity of the assay to a mixture of wild-type and variant sequences in the sample. Typically, only peripheral blood is available for patients and family members. With such samples, mosaicism can only be assessed in the hematopoietic lineage, especially the myeloid cells, as circulating blood erythroid cells contain little or no DNA. Additional tissues that can often be biopsied for genetic diagnostic purposes, without other medical requirements, include saliva (also primarily leukocytes), hair follicles, and skin fibroblasts. DNA can sometimes be recovered usefully from urine, but this is not a reliable source. DNA from more invasive biopies can be obtained when such samples are part of otherwise medically necessary surgical interventions, or at autopsy.

Depending on the specifics of where and when a new mutation arises, DNA from a biopsied sample may contain any fraction of variant sequence, ranging from 0% to 100%. In cases of parental germ-line mosaicism, the patient is expected to carry the causal variant in all cells, making the determination of mosaicism simply a matter of seeing the variant in a patient's blood cells, but not in either parent's blood cells. In such cases, the variant is referred to as de novo, a term that makes no specific implications regarding the mosaic status of any family members. Such a de novo variant may actually have arisen early in the patient's fetal development, not in a parent. Although the majority of cases reported in the literature for mosaicism are assumed to be due to a new variant arising in a parental germ line (and probably rightly so), a small proportion are expected to arise from early zygotic mutation. This distinction has important implications for genetic counseling regarding the potential risk (or lack of same) of recurrence in additional children of these parents. All of this is well documented and understood—the impact of new DNA sequencing technologies is simply to expand the amount of the genome assessed for mosaicism from individual genes or exons to whole exomes or whole genomes. Also, deep (i.e., high-coverage) next-generation sequencing can increase the dynamic range for detection of low proportions of mosaicism.

There are several well-documented endocrine disorders that usually involve mosaicism, such as McCune-Albright syndrome, caused by mosaic gain-of-function-activating mutations in the *GNAS* gene.[52,53] Chromosomal mosaicism involving the X and Y chromosomes is a common observation in endocrinology, with a strong clinical ascertainment for patients displaying intermediate states of sexual development. These can usually be diagnosed by classical or molecular cytology and do not generally require next-generation sequencing. Patients with very small mosaic chromosomal regions (effectively CNVs) below the level of resolution of cytology would benefit from next-generation DNA technologies.

Mosaicism as a molecular mechanism plays a prominent role in cancer genetics. It is now appreciated that many if not most tumors involve some amount of novel genetic variation, often referred to as *somatic mutation*. In some inherited dominant cancer syndromes, a second hit in the relevant gene is found in individual tumors. Moreover, tumor genomes are quite dynamic and evolve during disease progression, with new variants arising and taking over the cell population. This process is especially important in the development of drug resistance in patients. Deep genomic sequencing of tumors, often with comparison to nontumorous tissue from the same patient, has both diagnostic and therapeutic value as cancer medicine becomes increasingly personalized. Mosaicism and somatic mutation can also be involved in the pathology of otherwise familial genetic forms of cancer, including cancers of the endocrine system.[54]

52.2.7 Mitochondrial Genomics

Mitochondria maintain their own, independent genomes, separate from their cell's nuclear genome. The mitochondrial genome is small in humans, containing only 16,569 base pairs, encoding 13 protein genes and a variety of functional RNAs. In contrast, the mitochondrion itself is made up of more than 1000 proteins (the mitochondrial proteome)[55]; hence, most of the protein components of the mitochondrion are now actually encoded by nuclear genes. How this state arose during eukaryotic evolution is unclear, and beyond the scope of this chapter. The important point is that mitochondrial disorders may be defined either by phenotype, mode of transmission, or both. Given the identity of the protein genes encoded by the mitochondrial genome, which all play roles in oxidative phosphorylation, maternally transmitted genetic disorders of the mitochondrial genome itself are often extremely severe. They are very pleiotropic, but they can have an endocrine component to the clinical presentation. It should be kept in mind that the mitochondrial genome itself may not be covered by standard exome capture; either dedicated mitochondrial genomic panels or whole-genome sequencing can be used to screen for mutations in the genome of this organelle.

In contrast, mitochondrial disorders caused by mutations in nuclear genes behave as typical monogenic genetic traits, either dominant or recessive depending on the nature of the mutation, and may be transmitted similarly from either parent. Because most mitochondrial proteins are nuclear genome-encoded, most mitochondrial disorders defined phenotypically are actually caused by nuclear gene mutations. These are also quite pleiotropic disorders, and they sometimes include an endocrine component in the clinical presentation.

52.2.8 RNA-Sequencing and Transcriptomics

Transcriptomics refers to the qualitative and quantitative study of gene expression in different types of cells and tissues under different physiological conditions, specifically by measuring levels of RNA generated from each gene in the genome. A variety of technologies can be used for such measurements, with varying degrees of precision and dynamic range. Recently, RNA sequencing (RNA-Seq) has become the most generally used method of analysis.[56] The underlying concept is extremely simple; RNA extracted from the biological tissue is reverse-transcribed to generate cDNA, which is submitted for next-generation sequencing with any of the technologies previously described in this text. The individual sequence reads are aligned to the consensus human genome, and the depth of coverage is determined simply by counting reads over each exon in the genome and combining results for exons in individual genes. The advantage to RNA-Seq is that it can potentially detect the consequences of genomic variants which affect levels of gene expression, regardless of whether the variants can be meaningfully interpreted at the DNA level. Thus, RNA-Seq complements genome and exome sequencing.

RNA-Seq is also capable of detecting alterations in RNA splicing patterns, due either to changes in cell state or genetic variation in sequences that affect exon choice. Alternative splicing is an almost universal aspect of gene expression. Importantly, genomic variations that affect correct splicing are not necessarily near exons, but they may be deep in intronic sequences. Because mRNAs are relatively long compared to the length of second-generation sequencing reads, third-generation technologies are ideal for RNA-Seq.

The major caveat with RNA-Seq is the availability of relevant clinical material. Unlike the genome, whose sequence is more or less identical, regardless of the tissue source or biopsy used to obtain DNA (aside from situations of mosaicism), very different subsets of the genome are expressed in different cell types or tissues. However, only a few tissues are routinely available from patients with potential genetic disorders: whole blood, for which most DNA is present in leukocytes; saliva, for which most DNA is again present in leukocytes; hair follicles, which represent a fairly specialized cell type; and topical skin biopsy, for which most DNA is present in fibroblasts. If the causal gene of interest is not expressed in one of these cell types, then RNA-Seq is not a useful investigative procedure unless a biopsy can be obtained from the critical tissue. RNA-Seq should be considered as a tool of possible utility in the molecular geneticist's armamentarium, but it is not normally to be considered as a first resort.

52.2.9 The Microbiome

The ecosystem of microorganisms, especially bacteria, colonizing the human body is much more elaborate than was previously understood. Next-generation sequencing has bypassed the need for lab culture, allowing the genomes of mixtures of microorganisms to be sequenced and analyzed directly from bodily samples. A huge number of species of bacteria are regularly present in humans. A large, complex microbiome is a feature not only of humans, but also universally in the world. Moreover, there is not one single microbiome; rather, many microbiomes are present in different microecosystems, including in humans, which have a mouth microbiome, skin microbiome, intestinal microbiome (varying along the gastrointestinal tract), genital microbiome, and others. Not surprisingly, in some tissues, their microbiomes have been shown to change according to disease state, with potential diagnostic and therapeutic potential.

Despite the tremendous interest in microbiomes and the growing spate of research literature, actual examples of clinical utility for definitive diagnostics or treatment are few. Fecal transplants to modify intestinal microbiomes have been proposed, but the clinical utility of these is not yet clear. In the context of endocrinology, we are not aware of specific results or proposals for microbiome application, although there are some intriguing results for effects on neonatal microbiomes after normal vaginal birth versus surgical caesarian section.

52.2.10 Helpful Reference Databases

To assist in the interpretation of the complete set of rare, potentially pathogenic variants in a patient's genome, various entities have established large, publicly accessible databases. These may be organized primarily by phenotype or by gene, but typically not by both simultaneously. It is beyond the scope of this chapter to discuss all of these resources in detail, but they include Online Mendelian Inheritance in Man (OMIM; https://www.omim.org/), Clinical Variants (ClinVar; https://www.ncbi.nlm.nih.gov/clinvar/), Human Genome Variant Database (HGVD; http://www.hgvd.genome.med.kyoto-u.ac.jp/), Orphanet (https://www.orpha.net/), and Human Gene Mutation Database (HGMD; http://www.hgmd.cf.ac.uk/ac/index.php). HGMD is different among these, in that it is now commercially owned and includes both a public and a proprietary version of the database. The public version is deliberately out of date, lacking several years of the most recent findings. The proprietary version has a subscription fee and is complete. These databases are variously restrictive regarding rare versus common variants of rare and common clinical conditions. OMIM and Orphanet are highly biased toward rare, high-penetrance genetic disorders. ClinVar is less biased, and HGMD includes many common variants that show statistical associations of variable strength or reliability to medical conditions. Recently, a new curated database has been announced, ClinGen (https://www.clinicalgenome.org/), which seeks to reconcile some of the limitations of the other databases to improve clinical utility.[57]

Given the enormous genetics literature, these databases do not aspire to complete curation of the literature describing causal variants. OMIM is biased toward clinical and functional descriptions and usually only includes a handful of reported variants for each gene. OMIM also includes genes with no known molecular genetics, as well as syndromes with no known molecular cause but at least potential genetic etiology. Thus, OMIM is more of a medicogenetic than a genomic database. HGMD, on the other hand, tries to curate all variants reported in the medical genetic literature, but with very minimal phenotypic information for each variant. In practice, medical geneticists uses several, if not all, of these resource databases, which can be incorporated into the bioinformatics analysis pipeline so that the initial annotated variant reports include entries for some or most of these databases to the initial review committee. This is essential for timely review of patient genomic variants in practice.

Unfortunately, many human genes have multiple names in the literature, depending on when they were identified and whether the discovery was biochemically, genetically, or genomically based. To resolve these problems, the international HUGO Gene Nomenclature Committee (HGNC; https://www.genenames.org/) was established. This group maintains a web site that provides the definitive name for each human gene, together with annotating various aliases or other gene names that may occur in the literature. For consistency, variant reports for genome sequencing should use the HGNC-approved names, even if review committees may use more familiar alternative gene names.

52.2.11 Next-Generation Sequencing in Endocrinology

There are substantial opportunities for next-generation sequencing as applied to the discipline of endocrinology.[58] We restrict our discussion primarily to diagnostics, or applications for traditional patient management. The field of gene therapy is huge and rapidly evolving and thus is beyond the scope of this chapter. As in most other medical disciplines, DNA sequencing for diagnosis and improved patient management is mostly limited to high-penetrance, single-gene (monogenic) disorders, resulting from severely pathogenic mutations. Such mutations may be either gain or loss of function at the molecular level of the implicated gene and may act either dominantly or recessively (or in some more complicated mode of inheritance). X-chromosome-linked genes yielding endocrine mutation phenotypes show the typical familial pattern of inheritance (sons inheriting a mutant allele from the maternal genome), as do the rare, Y-chromosome-linked genetic disorders (sons inheriting a mutant allele from the paternal genome). Mitochondrial disorders associated with the mitochondrial genome itself show the typical pattern of maternal inheritance. Imprinted genes yielding endocrine genetic disorders show the same atypical pattern of familial transmission as they do for other types of disorders. Mutations causing endocrine disorders may be transmitted from a parent, or may arise as de novo mutations in either a parental germ line or the zygotic soma. All of this is to note that endocrine genetics and genomics generally function similarly to the genetics of other disciplines. To the extent that there are some endocrine-system cancers, the genetics and genomics of these disorders follow similar principles to those of other organ systems.

Tenore et al. and Forlenza et al. have enumerated general types of endocrine dysfunctions, including bone and mineral metabolism, adrenal disorders, gonadal disorders, pituitary and hypothalamic disorders, thyroid disorders, and multiple endocrinopathies, with more than 75 genes known to mutate to yield clinical phenotypes.[59,60] De Sousa et al. discussed high-throughput sequencing for endocrinology, with suggestions for the appropriate workflow from initial presentation through standard diagnostic tests to the application of genomic sequencing. They also commented on the caveats for genomic diagnosis, such as lack of universal quality-control metrics to assess false positive and negative error rates, and the need for counseling to help patients and families understand the implications of molecular diagnosis.[61]

52.2.12 An Example

Two patients were in the care of the Endocrinology Services at CHU Ste-Justine hospital, the University of Sherbrooke and CHU Laval. A boy and a girl, not known to be related, each had hypoglycemia, low cortisol, and high measured adrenocorticotropic hormone (ACTH). The girl initially presented in coma at age 4 years, the boy with seizures at 4 months; both have been followed since for several years. Both had red hair and were somewhat obese. No coding region mutations were detected by Sanger sequencing of the *MC2R* and *MRAP* genes, while sequencing of *POMC* was considered redundant due to the high measured ACTH hormone levels. A tentative diagnosis of adrenal insufficiency with ACTH resistance was made. The patients were placed on glucocorticoid and mineralocorticoid replacement therapy. Although no mineralocorticoid deficiency was observed, replacement was provided in the absence of a clear etiology, as a preventive in case the patients' conditions deteriorated to a condition of combined hormone insufficiency with the potential for life-threatening events.

Whole-exome sequencing was performed for the female patient. Two pathogenic mutations were detected in the *POMC* gene[62]—one a missense variant in the gene segment encoding the mature ACTH peptide (p.R145C), and the second in the 5' UTR, a variant generating a novel out-of-frame methionine start codon that had been previously observed in a homozygous unrelated patient and shown to interfere with normal protein translation.[63] Synthetic ACTH and α-MSH peptides were generated carrying either wild-type or the R145C variant, and the variant peptides showed significantly reduced activity in cell-binding and receptor-mediated signaling assays.[62] The variant peptides showed a reduced but still measurable response in the standard laboratory radioimmunoassay test, indicating that the mutant ACTH peptide was immunoreactive.

The affected boy was subsequently shown to be homozygous for the same p.R145C variant and was presumably distantly related to the female patient.

Nonfunctional immunoreactive proteins or peptides have been well documented for other genes, but never before for ACTH, presumably due to the very small target size of the genomic region encoding the mature peptide. The detection of this material led to the incorrect initial diagnosis of ACTH resistance, rather than deficiency. As a follow-up, mineralo-corticoid therapy was stopped for the patient directly seen by the service; she shows no deleterious consequences after several years. The cost of the exome sequencing and mutation verification (though not all the associated clinical costs and functional research tests) was less than the lifetime cost of mineralocorticoid therapy (which, as hormone treatments go, is relatively inexpensive); moreover, the overtreatment with mineralocorticoid while justified carries its own long-term risks. This was, to our knowledge, one of the first clear cases of genomic-based precision medicine in pediatric endocri-nology, although undoubtedly there are many other examples today.

52.3 PROTEOMICS AND METABOLOMICS

The relationships between the genome, the environment, and the clinical implications for a patient are mediated and reflected in a number of additional -omics. Each of these additional fields has blossomed into its own specific discipline, with common themes as well as unique attributes. The set of individual and measureable environmental factors to which a patient is exposed has been termed the *exposome.* This includes toxic, infectious, iatrogenic, exercise, psychosocial, and other exposures and may be measured in a number of ways. We will not describe the exosome in more detail here, but direct the interested reader to a number of good reviews of this topic. Endogenously, the omics lying between the genome and clinical implications mirror the biological mechanisms by which genes are translated to their functional units. These therefore include the epigenome, transcriptome, proteome, and metabolome. As the study of each of these seeks to under-stand them as a biological network, these individual-omics together are termed *systems biology.*

A *proteome* is the complete set of proteins expressed by an organism, and *proteomics* refers to the study of this pro-teome, including quantitation of proteins, their structures, interactions, and posttranslational modifications. These may be studied in the whole organism, specific tissues, or on a cellular level. Further, while examination in a homeostatic or steady state may be of interest, study of the dynamic changes seen in the proteome in different physiological and pathological states is especially relevant in the medical context.

Similarly, the *metabolome* refers to the complete set of metabolites present in an organism. Practically from a medical perspective, *metabolites* refer to small molecules (typically $<2000\,Da$) that are present in human biofluids such as blood, urine, cerebrospinal fluid (CSF), sweat, and feces. Of course, the true metabolome is much broader and highly compart-mentalized at the levels of organs, cells, and even subcellular compartments. Also, there is a large variation in the concen-tration and abundance of different metabolites. Metabolites may be grouped in a number of ways, including by metabolic pathway, physicochemical properties, abundance, and structural families. Finally, the metabolome encompasses both endogenous compounds, as well as those deriving from exogenous sources. Examples of the latter include xenobiotics, drugs, intestinal bacterial compounds, and environmental pollutants, as well as their metabolites.

While a genome is estimated to have about 20,000 protein-coding genes, these result in many more mRNA transcripts ($>10^6$), proteins, and modified proteins ($>10^7$), due to mechanisms such as alternative splicing and posttranslational protein modification. The biochemical expression of this elaboration of the genetic blueprint results in a more limited set of metabolites. For example, the Human Metabolome Database (HMDB) contains 114,100 metabolites. The meta-bolome, especially that of the accessible body fluid compartments for laboratory analysis, is therefore often viewed as a final common pathway, which may be perturbed in various disease or physiologic states.

Examining the proteome and the metabolome presents numerous challenges not seen in the field of genomic sequencing. Both are dynamic and vary with the physiologic state and environmental conditions. The range of compounds and their physicochemical properties are very broad, and this has significant preanalytical and analytical implications. They are also highly compartmentalized within organs, cells, and subcellular organelles. These are, of course, some of the same properties of the proteome and metabolome that make them useful in clinical medicine and medical research. For example, host responses to infection, physiological and pathophysiological effects of varying diets, and disordered responses to fasting states, are all examples of dynamic processes important in health and disease, which can be associated with dis-turbances in the proteome and metabolome. These associations may be important in understanding causation of disease processes, but the associations may be useful in other ways. For example, perturbations of the metabolome may be useful in the recognition of an associated physiological state (e.g., fasting). They may also be useful for identifying pathways relevant to the pathophysiology of the disease, which may be directly implicated (e.g., carbohydrate and fat metabolic pathways directly regulated by insulin), as well as pathways in the overall metabolic network that are secondarily or more distantly affected. This can provide clinically relevant insights; for example, identification of potential treatment targets, or of biomarkers that may be diagnostically or prognostically useful.

It should be noted that examination of a given -omic need not occur in isolation. For example, it is not uncommon to examine the effect of a stimulus on the transcriptome in order to identify protein families or metabolic pathways to target. Similarly, an -omic study of a cell line may involve knockdown of the expression of a given protein identified through a proteomic study, and examine the effect on the transcriptome and metabolome.

52.3.1 Introduction to Analytical Approaches

Broadly, -omics approaches can be classified as untargeted (exploratory) or targeted (confirmatory) in scope.[64] Untargeted -omics seek to characterize as many metabolites or proteins as possible within a given sample. The ultimate goal of untargeted -omics is to obtain complete and unbiased coverage of the proteome or metabolome.[65,66] Targeted -omics, conversely, focuses on the quantitation of a smaller number of chemically or biochemically related analytes, such as members of a particular pathway. Therefore, the main conceptual difference is that untargeted approaches are inductive and hypothesis-generating (sometimes referred to as *hypothesis-free*), while targeted approaches are reductionist and hypothesis testing.[67,68]

Quantitation in -omics can be relative or absolute. Relative quantitation (semiquantitation) involves the statistical comparison of response data (e.g., peak intensities normalized to an internal standard) to determine differences between sample classes (e.g., control versus treatment or healthy versus disease state).[69,70] This approach is most often used for untargeted, global -omics studies, where a priori information about the sample is limited. While reasons of cost and time may necessitate the use of relative quantitation, absolute quantification is typically reserved for targeted studies, as authentic standards are required for each quantifiable analyte.[64] Absolute and relative quantitation encompass both label-free and label-based techniques, the specifics of which will be described in more detail.

With the appropriate preanalytical workup, virtually any sample can be analyzed in a metabolomics or proteomics context. Biofluids can be easily and/or noninvasively obtained and include whole blood as a liquid sample[71] or as dried blood spots on a filter paper,[72,73] processed blood (i.e., plasma[74] or serum[75,76]), urine,[77,78] CSF,[79] oral fluids,[80] sweat,[81,82] feces and/or fecal water,[83,84] and exhaled breath condensate.[85] Tissues, such as those obtained by biopsy, are more challenging to obtain, and care must be taken to ensure that the sample is homogenous and well preserved in order to reflect the in vitro physiological state most accurately.[86] Finally, cell extracts (e.g., established fibroblast cell lines or patient-derived cell lines) can also be analyzed to assay intracellular molecular mechanisms of disease.[87]

52.3.2 Key Techniques

52.3.2.1 Sample Workup

The sample preparation workflow can be broadly described as analyte extraction with quenching to preserve the physiological state of the sample (e.g., snap-freezing, ice cold solvent addition, protease inhibition), sample enrichment and/or cleanup to remove interfering and noninformative signals [e.g., solid-phase extraction, sodium dodecyl-polyacrylamide gel electrophoresis (SDS-PAGE)] and chemical derivatization/labeling, if necessary.[88] While the exact steps performed will vary depending on the type of experiment (i.e., targeted or untargeted, metabolomics or proteomics) and the downstream analytical platform to be used, minimizing the time from sample collection to analysis is crucial to reduce postcollection alterations such as oxidation or degradation.

52.3.2.2 Separation

Prior to detection and quantification, analytes are typically separated to reduce the number of overlapping features and simplify data analysis and identification. Electrophoretic separations are based on the movement or migration of charged species (ions) within an applied electric field. Separations can be performed in a gel matrix, such as in SDS-PAGE or in solution, such as in capillary electrophoresis. Chromatographic separations, such as liquid chromatography (LC) or gas chromatography (GC), are based on the partitioning of analytes between a stationary phase in the column and the mobile carrier phase (i.e., liquid or gas). Electrophoretic separations are ideal for polar, ionizable analytes such as amino acids, proteins, peptides, and oligonucleotides; however, the high degree of reproducibility and sensitivity of chromatographic approaches have led to their widespread use in metabolomics. While gel-based approaches are still used to purify and fractionate proteins for proteomics,[64,89] gel-free techniques (i.e., chromatography) are increasingly being used either in place of gel-based techniques (often for targeted proteomics) or in addition to them to enhance global proteome coverage.[90]

52.3.2.3 Detection

Mass spectrometry (MS) is the most common detection modality for -omics studies, as it is highly sensitive, requires small sample volumes, and is easily coupled to chromatography.[91] The type of MS used depends on the particular application; however, most untargeted proteomics and metabolomics investigations use high-resolution hybrid instruments, such as a quadrupole time of flight or a quadrupole ion trap or orbitrap, to generate both full-scan and fragmentation data with high mass accuracy.[64,92,93] Data can be acquired by data-dependent methods that will acquire full-scan data on all ions entering the MS and as many fragmentation spectra as possible (e.g., typically the top 10–20 ions). Data-independent methods will isolate a large *m/z* window of precursors and obtain full-fragmentation spectra on them before sliding the *m/z* window over to repeat the analysis. Targeted approaches can utilize triple quadrupole MS (MS/MS), which offers enhanced sensitivity and quantitation by targeting both a precursor ion and a specific ion fragment.[94] Furthermore, MS/MS can be used for analyte identification and structural elucidation, as characteristic fragmentation patterns can reveal information about functional groups and molecular arrangement. The MS can also act as its own separation modality, as compounds that are directly injected or infused into it are thereby separated only by their mass-to-charge ratio (*m/z*). This is often used for metabolome fingerprinting, whereby spectra from different conditions are compared qualitatively or quantitatively to determine class- or treatment-related differences.[91]

Samples must be ionized prior to entering the MS, for detection both electrospray ionization (ESI) and matrix-assisted laser desorption ionization (MALDI) are "soft" ionization techniques that result in minimal fragmentation of the analyte within the ion source.[95] These ionization methods also permit the formation of multiply charged ions, which is crucial in analyzing large-molecular-weight proteins, peptides, and other biopolymers that would otherwise exceed the mass range of the MS.

Nuclear magnetic resonance (NMR) is another common detector used primarily in metabolomics. While it requires minimal sample workup (i.e., solid samples can be analyzed), is inherently quantitative, and is nondestructive, its reduced sensitivity and increased cost relative to MS have led to a decline in popularity.[96] However, the complementary nature of MS and NMR when used in parallel can broaden metabolome coverage.[97]

52.3.3 Proteomics

Proteomics is a broad term describing the study of proteins encoded by the genome, their quantitation, posttranslational modifications (PTMs), and protein-protein interactions.[93] Sample preparation for proteomics requires proteins to be extracted and solubilized from the tissue or biofluid to be profiled. Tissues and cells require homogenization and lysis, while biofluids like serum or plasma can often just be diluted.[98] Protease inhibitors can be added at this stage to preserve PTMs.[64] Samples can also be depleted of a small number of abundant endogenous proteins [i.e., albumin, immunoglobulin G (IgG), and immunoglobulin A (IgA)], which can account for upward of 80% of total protein in a sample and interfere with analysis. Further sample preparation depends on the downstream approach: top-down or bottom-up proteomics.

MS-based proteomics has traditionally been performed with a bottom-up approach. Extracted proteins are digested by enzymes (e.g., trypsin) into a series of peptides prior to separation and analysis by a high-resolution hybrid MS. Here, spectra of both full peptides and their fragments are acquired and searched against known fragment libraries and protein databases to infer the identity of the proteins in the original sample.[2] Despite its widespread use and the ease of handling and separating smaller peptides over large proteins, a bottom-up approach has inherent flaws. Multiple proteins may result in the same peptide, and some peptides may not sample efficiently into the MS, resulting in the potential loss of PTM and incomplete protein sequence coverage.[99] Top-down proteomics ionizes intact proteins prior to fragmentation in the MS, which enhances sequence coverage and allows the identification of the specific proteoform.[100] However, technical limitations such as the challenge of separating large, intact proteins and the difficulties in detecting large-molecular-weight compounds in the MS have relegated top-down approaches to niche applications. As technology continues to improve and the importance of specific proteoforms in biological systems is better understood, it is likely that top-down approaches may become more popular.

Quantitation in proteomics can be label-free or label-based. Label-free approaches are not absolutely quantitative; they use spectral counting or ion intensities to compare protein abundances between independent samples.[101] To reduce inter-sample variability, label-based approaches can be used.

Proteins can be labeled in vivo by growing cells or organisms in the presence of isotopically labeled amino acids. An independent sample of unlabeled proteins can be mixed in, and the two samples can be analyzed simultaneously. The labeled peptides will be detected at a different, typically higher *m/z,* and relative abundances from the different samples can be compared. For biological fluids or liquids that cannot be labeled in culture, stable isotope or isobaric labels can be covalently added to proteins or peptides by chemical or enzymatic reactions.[64,101] Samples can be mixed and analyzed, and the intensities of heavy and light spectral signals can be compared for relative quantification of proteins in the samples. Absolute quantification can only be performed by the addition of labeled peptide standards corresponding to proteins of interest, which represents a significant analytical challenge because a priori sample information may not be known and standards may not be easily obtained. As a result, many proteomics studies use some form of label-based or label-free relative quantitation.

52.3.4 Metabolomics

Metabolomics and proteomics have many preanalytical and analytical similarities. However, the nature of the analytes of interest (i.e., small molecules versus proteins) leads to a unique set of challenges. Metabolites sit at the bottom of the "-omics cascade" and are most closely associated with phenotypes.[102] They are both endogenous and exogenous and represent the real-world end points that are representative of changes at the genomic, transcriptomic, and proteomic levels, as well as external, environmental influences.[103,104] Furthermore, metabolites are composed of chemically diverse compounds that show wide variations in molecular weight, polarity, solubility, and volatility and can span seven to nine orders of magnitude in concentration.[105] As a result, there is no one sample preparation or analytical platform that can be used for untargeted metabolomics. Therefore, global and unbiased metabolome coverage can be obtained only by a series of complementary, orthogonal approaches. For example, the Human Serum Metabolome is a multicentered project as part of the HMDB that used metaanalyses with gas chromatography-mass spectrometry (GC-MS), liquid chromatography (LC-MS), LC-MS/MS, ^{1}H NMR, and direct infusion-tandem mass spectrometry (DI-MS/MS) to identify and quantify over 4000 metabolites.[76]

Metabolomics for human health initiatives often seek to understand or uncover differences or perturbations as a result of disease or treatment. While absolute quantitation is necessary for clinical application, a significant portion of human metabolites remain unidentified or unknown.[39] As a result, many untargeted "discovery" studies are semiquantitative and provide limited actionable information, as data from other -omics cannot be assimilated into a systemswide model,[106] and clinical tests and cutoff concentrations for discriminating metabolites cannot be developed. Targeted metabolomics profiling of predefined expected biochemical pathways can simplify the analytical procedures and provide accurate and precise quantitative results that can be integrated with genomics, transcriptomics, and/or proteomics data.[107] Absolute quantitation is done via an external calibration curve or by stable isotope dilution, whereby isotopically labeled standards are spiked into the sample to account for matrix effects.[108]

52.3.5 Bioinformatics

Obtaining -omics data represents only the initial step in uncovering differentially expressed metabolites or proteins. Modern and sensitive MS instrumentation can generate thousands of mass features, many of which are spurious, unreliable, or redundant.[109] Software is available to convert raw data derived from the instruments (e.g. align chromatographic runs, pick peaks, filter out noise, combine information on related molecules, etc.) into an interpretable matrix of discrete metabolite or protein data.[107] Statistical analyses can indicate differentially expressed metabolites, which can then be identified by accurate mass, chromatographic retention time, spectral matching to databases, authentic standard spiking, or de novo identification by inspection of fragmentation data and/or chemical tests. Unfortunately, metabolite identification is not trivial; no standardized retention time database exists, and fragmentation spectra quality and reproducibility vary by specific mass analyzer and vendor, so database matching (i.e., METLIN, HMDB) is not always straightforward. In silico fragmentation of molecular structures can assist in assigning structural information and/or functional groups to unknown peaks; however, a large number of interesting features can remain unidentified. This limits the biological interpretation and prevents the integration of the metabolomics results with other -omics data.

Proteomics data consists of a large number of fragmentation spectra that must be identified and quantified. Search algorithms aim to match the peptide fragment to sequences in databases and return a match or probability score.[110] Databases can be peptide sequences translated from genome data, mRNA, or even MS/MS spectra. These peptide chunks must then be assembled in silico in the original protein. Redundant or missing sequences, shared peptides, alternative splicing, and an overrepresentation of peptides from abundant proteins can make protein assignment difficult. Peptides are mapped to a protein sequence using various computational tools, and a protein-level score is now computed, reflecting the confidence in the identification. Positive identifications (in either -omics approach) can assist in elucidating biochemical pathways that contribute to observed phenotypes and, when combined with other -omics data, can expand our understanding of molecular models of health and disease, leading to improved diagnosis and more effective and personalized treatments.

52.3.5.1 Clinical Example—Newborn Screening

Newborn screening for inborn errors of metabolism (IMDs) provides an example of relatively small scale targeted metabolomics in clinical practice. The biomarkers for the majority of these are alpha-amino acids and acylcarnitines. Most will be familiar with the former primarily as the monomeric constituents of proteins, while the latter are organic acids derived from fatty acids and amino acid catabolism that are esterified to carnitine. Alpha-amino acids all have an amino group and a carboxyl group attached their alpha carbon, and this common motif results in a specific rearrangement within a tandem mass spectrometer that produces a constant loss of an uncharged fragment with a mass of 102 Da (a neutral loss of 102). Where the alpha amino acids vary is in the moieties attached to the alpha carbon (R groups), and scanning a newborn's dried blood spot sample for compounds with a neutral loss of 102 allows rapid and simultaneous measurement of a number of amino acids. Similarly, butylated acylcarnitines produce a charged fragment with a mass of 85 Da; scanning for all compounds producing a charged fragment of this mass (a parent scan of 85) allows measurement of a large number of acylcarnitines. The neutral loss of 102 Da and the parents of 85-Da methods can be run simultaneously using an extract from a single 3-mm dried blood spot punch, and a sample can be injected onto the tandem mass spectrometer every 2–3 min. Of course, amino acids (e.g., leucine, isoleucine, and allo-isoleucine) or acylcarnitines (e.g., succinylcarnitine and methylmalonylcarnitine) with the same mass (isobaric compounds) cannot be differentiated using this approach. In a typical newborn-screening laboratory, about 10 amino acids and 30 acylcarnitines are measured routinely using this method; it is possible to measure more substances, but only those with utility for screening targeted diseases are usually measured.

The best-known example of diseases targeted by newborn screening using this method is phenylketonuria. This disease results from an inherited deficiency of phenylalnine hydroxylase (PAH), an enzyme that catalyzes the hydroxylation of phenylalanine to form tyrosine—both being amino acids measurable using the "neutral loss of 102 Da" method. Phenyl-alanine accumulates to levels that are toxic to the brain and causes severe developmental disabilities. Tyrosine concentrations, on the other hand, are low, and thus the ratio of phenylalanine to tyrosine is elevated. Treatment involves dietary restriction of phenylalanine and/or pharmacologic provision of tetrahydrobiopterin the PAH cofactor, which can act as a chaperone therapy for patients with certain *PAH* gene variants.

Medium-chain AcylCoA dehydrogenase (MCAD) deficiency is an example of a disease where the relevant biomarkers are acylcarnitines. This enzyme is specific, as the name implies, for medium chain-length fatty acylCoAs, and it is responsible for the first step of the fatty acid beta-oxidation spiral. This is the catabolic pathway necessary for the production of ketone bodies from endogenous fat stores. Patients with MCAD deficiency are unable to produce ketone bodies in the fasting state, resulting in overutilization of glucose and hypoketotic hypoglycemia. Instead, medium-chain (i.e., 6–10 carbon lengths) acylCoAs accumulate and produce high concentrations of corresponding carnitine esters. The 8-carbon octanoylcarnitine accumulation predominates, and together with other saturated and unsaturated medium chain acylcarnitines, they provide a highly sensitive and specific biomarker for neonates with MCAD deficiency. Approximately 25% of patients presenting symptomatically die in their initial presentation, and an additional 25% will be left with a neurodevelopmental disability. Treatment consists of avoidance of fasting, as well as provision of intravenous (IV) glucose when oral intake cannot be maintained (e.g., during a viral gastroenteritis).

These are examples of routine but relatively small-scale metabolomics in routine clinical laboratory practice. Newborn screening also provides two further examples of the relevance of metabolomics and proteomics in clinical medicine. First, the two -omic approaches are important to the discovery and translation of novel biomarkers that can be used to improve screening performance. For example, some biomarkers may be very sensitive, robust, and inexpensive to measure, but they may lack specificity. Other biomarkers may be needed to confer the desired specificity and reduce the number of infants with false-positive screening results. A second example is the secondary hypothesis-independent analysis of the newborn screening-ascertained analytes to find associations with other diseases or health outcomes.

The case of newborn screening for cystic fibrosis provides an excellent example of the first scenario. The blood level of the pancreatically derived immunoreactive trypsinogen (IRT) provides a relatively sensitive biomarker for pancreatic insufficient cystic fibrosis. It is, however, quite nonspecific and leads to a high number of false positives if used in isolation. Two primary strategies have been used to use IRT successfully in newborn screening for CF. First, the IRT concentration in infants typically drops over the first few weeks of life. In infants with CF, they do not drop; indeed, they may even rise. Therefore, many newborn-screening programs will recall babies with an elevated IRT on their newborn-screening sample to obtain a second sample and remeasure IRT (known as the *IRT-IRT strategy*). Unfortunately, in order to achieve adequate sensitivity for CF screening using IRT as a primary marker, IRT cutoffs between the 92nd and 98th percentiles are typically used. This means that 2%–8% of infants may be recalled for a second sample, resulting in potential alarm for a large number of parents, as well as resulting on an additional burden on the screening system.

A widespread alternative strategy is to perform a cystic fibrosis transmembrane conductance regulator (CFTR) mutation panel, and referring a baby for a diagnostic sweat test only if one or two mutations are found (known as the *IRT-DNA strategy*). The mutation panels typically target between 40 and 100 genes. While detection of two pathogenic mutations is essentially diagnostic of CF, some CF patients will not have two mutations included on the panel. In fact, about 1 in 100 babies with only one mutation found on such a panel will prove to have CF. Another way of stating this is that the posttest probability of having CF is 1/100, which is markedly higher than the baseline population risk of about 1/3500 in a mixed North American population. These babies are therefore referred for diagnostic evaluation.

The corollary, however, of a 1/100 probability of disease is that the positive predictive value is only 1%. There is, therefore, much interest in the discovery of additional biomarkers that are more sensitive, specific, or both. Both metabolomics and proteomic approaches have been used for this purpose. For example, metabolomics studies have identified a number of biomarkers, including already routinely measured amino acids, which may prove useful for increasing the specificity as reflexively measured or second-tier biomarkers. Proteomic approaches have identified candidate alternatives to IRT as first-tier biomarkers. A third approach that is gaining traction is third-tier sequencing of the *CFTR* gene in all babies where a mutation panel finds only a single mutation. Unfortunately, genotyping will not ascertain all disease-associated genomic variants (i.e., it is not 100% sensitive), and conversely, variants of unknown significance will be observed, which will impair specificity. Therefore, although there is much promise in this extended genotyping approach, there is a persistent need for additional metabolic or protein biomarkers to allow better phenotyping.[111]

The use of second-tier testing of the same newborn screening blood spot for improving specificity of screening has been applied for both congenital hypothyroidism (CH) and congenital adrenal hyperplasia (CAH). In the case of CH, many algorithms incorporate DBS T4 testing in the second tier when first-tier TSH results are moderately elevated. Only those infants with decreased T4 screen positive and are referred for diagnostic evaluation. Similarly, 17-hydroxyprogesterone is physiologically elevated in the early postnatal period, in stressed neonates, and in preterm infants. The use of second-tier steroid profiling can increase specificity by detecting elevations in other steroids that are elevated (e.g., 4-androstenedione and 21-deoxycortisol), or depressed (e.g., cortisol) in neonates with CAH. The LC/MS approaches used to measure these steroid profiles are amenable to including additional related steroid compounds in the same analysis—they are in essence another example of limited metabolomic analysis. Indeed, more recent research has examined using additional steroids in such profiling to further improve the specificity of CAH screening. Such methods can also be used for the diagnosis and management of patients with CAH.

There are several examples of the secondary analysis of the newborn screening metabolome to seek associations with other health or disease states. It is physiologically expected, and has long been observed, that the metabolome of premature babies differ based on gestational age. Most attention was paid to the screening implications of this variation (e.g., upon screening performance for target diseases), but this is now being investigated as a means to refine gestational age assignment when this is uncertain due to uncertain menstrual dates or lack of first-trimester ultrasound. Predictive models using the routinely measured set of newborn-screening analytes performed better than physical examination based tools (e.g., the Ballard scale), and compared well with ultrasound.[112] Further examples are observed associations between the newborn screening acylcarnitine profiles and risk of early demise,[113] necrotizing enterocolitis,[114] and later-onset kidney disease.[115] Such observations have the potential of leading to the development of clinical risk-prediction tools, but also the identification of pathways relevant to health or disease states, and in addition, they could help clarify the pathophysiology of these states.

52.4 CELL-FREE FETAL DNA TESTING

In recent years, the advent of next-generation sequencing and microarray chromosomal analysis has made it possible to use cell-free fetal DNA (cffDNA) in maternal circulation to test for genetic and chromosomal abnormalities with a noninvasive test. CffDNA testing, then called *noninvasive prenatal testing (NIPT)*, was first offered by a private company in 2011 to look for common aneuploidies (trisomies 21, 13, and 18). Although it was initially targeted for high-risk pregnancies, both pregnant women and practitioners were quickly pushing for more widespread use because of its noninvasive nature and high detection rate for aneuploidies compared to traditional screening options.[116] Currently, cffDNA testing has been integrated into practice mostly for women at high risk of aneuploidy, but there is increasing interest in using it as an alternative to traditional screening strategies for aneuploidies and even, if its reliability is improved further, as a potential alternative to invasive prenatal diagnosis.

Some companies have started offering cffDNA testing for chromosomal microdeletions, but the use of cffDNA testing as a screening tool for these conditions has not been reliably validated and is not recommended at this time.[117]

TABLE 52.4 Risk factors for low-fetal fraction (nonreportable) NIPT[119]

- Early gestational age (prior to 10 weeks' gestation)
- Increased maternal body mass index (BMI)
- Fetal chromosomal anomaly

52.4.1 Methodology of CELL-FREE Fetal DNA Testing

The majority of cell-free DNA (cfDNA) in blood in general comes from hematopoietic cells that release fragments of DNA during cell turnover, as well as from adipose tissue and various solid organs.[118] During pregnancy, cell-free *fetal* DNA (cffDNA) is released from the placenta into the maternal plasma: cffDNA represents a fraction of all cell-free DNA in the maternal circulation.

This fetal fraction increases with gestational age and is reliably >10% as early as 10 weeks' gestation. It needs to be at least 4% for reliable analysis (Table 52.4).

Further, cffDNA testing isolates cell-free DNA fragments from maternal blood and compares the proportion of DNA fragments from target chromosomes[13,18,21] to the proportion of DNA fragments from other chromosomes, used as reference chromosomes. A euploid fetus will have the same proportion of DNA fragments for all chromosomes. Compared with traditional screening for aneuploidies that are based on hormone levels and ultrasound findings, this test looks directly at fetoplacental DNA. For this reason, detection rates are high for aneuploidies compared with traditional screening. Detection rates of cffDNA testing for trisomy 21, 18, 13, and sex chromosome abnormalities (monosomy X) were 99.7%, 98.2%, 99.0%, and 95.8%, respectively.[116] In a recent cohort study, the positive predictive values were 93%, 64%, 44%, and 39%, respectively.[120]

The main limitation of cffDNA testing comes from the fact that the so-called fetal DNA fragments are in fact of placental origin. Detection rate is influenced by the fetal fraction of cell-free DNA, which can be influenced by various fetal, placental, and maternal factors. Explanations for false-negative and false-positive results are twin pregnancies with spontaneous twin reduction early in the pregnancy (a second placenta releases DNA fragments in maternal blood but does not reflect the genetic material of the surviving twin), and confined placental mosaicism (i.e., when the fetus and placenta don't share the exact same genetic material). False-positive results can also be due to interference from abnormal maternal cell-free DNA such as maternal aneuploidy (i.e., 47,XXX), maternal mosaicism, maternal copy number variations (CNVs), maternal malignancy, and maternal prior organ transplant. Other factors may affect test reliability, such as maternal obesity, which leads to lower fetal DNA fraction in maternal blood.

There are several cffDNA techniques available for aneuploidy screening. The main technologies currently used are massive parallel sequencing (MPS), chromosome-selective (or targeted) sequencing (CSS), and single nucleotide polymorphism (SNP)-based sequencing. The purpose of this section is not to go into great detail about the methods themselves, but rather to compare and contrast them to highlight the strengths and weaknesses of each.

MPS is based on the random (or "shotgun") sequencing of cell-free DNA in maternal plasma.[121] MPS methods calculate the standard deviation of the expected count from each chromosome and allocate a z-score for each chromosome. The pregnant woman will be considered at high risk for trisomy 21 if the number of DNA fragments from chromosome 21 in the test sample is more than three standard deviations above the expected number (i.e., z-score > 3).[122] MPS-based analysis can also detect Down syndrome caused by Robertsonian translocations, as well as microdeletions and microduplications.[123,124]

Chromosome-selective (or targeted) sequencing is based on the sequencing of preselected fragments of cell-free DNA from target chromosomes, rather than sequencing the entire mixture of cell-free DNA.[125,126] For example, chromosome 21 represents only 1.3% of the entire genome. Targeted sequencing of chromosomal regions of interest helps reduce cost and increase throughput.[125,126] On the other hand, CSS cannot detect chromosomal aneuploidies in untargeted chromosomal regions. The result of CSS is expressed as a final risk, based on the woman's prior risk of aneuploidy (based on maternal and gestational age), target chromosome counts, and fetal fraction.[125,126]

The SNP-based approach that is used in practice uses targeted amplification of SNPs followed by NGS and sophisticated informatics analysis to identify fetal chromosomal copy number.[127] This method differs from the CSS approach in that it targets specific SNPs instead of nonpolymorphic regions and uses a genotype-based analytic method rather than a counting approach to detect fetal aneuploidy (Table 52.5).

TABLE 52.5 Potential confounders (false positive/false negative results) for NIPT

- Twin or vanishing twin pregnancy
- Mosaicism (true fetal mosaicism, confined placental mosaicism)
- Maternal chromosomal anomaly (e.g., Maternal 47,XXX)
- Maternal CNV (benign or pathogenic)
- Maternal malignancy
- Maternal solid organ transplant

The detection rates for sex chromosome aneuploidies are lower than for autosomal aneuploidies. This is partially attributed to variable amplification that results from different guanosine-cytosine (GC) levels in chromosomes 13 and X, as compared to chromosomes 21 and 18, and is particularly problematic for methods that require a reference chromosome.[128] Because the SNP method analyzes the relative amount of alleles at polymorphic loci and does not utilize a reference chromosome, it is not subject to issues with amplification variation. Thus, it is expected to have consistent sensitivities across all regions interrogated. Indeed, clinical data indicate sensitivities of >99% for trisomy 21, trisomy 18, and trisomy 13. It is also the only method that is capable of detecting triploidy.[129] The targeted approaches (CSS- or SNP-based) will not detect off-target abnormalities, limiting the potential for incidental findings. Higher frequency of feto-placental mosaicism (compared to autosomal aneuploidies) is another explanation for the lower detection rates and positive predictive values for sex chromosome aneuploidies.

For all NIPT methods, test failure due to low fetal fraction poses an additional challenge to clinical management. Patients with low-fetal fraction samples (nonreportable NIPT) may be at increased risk of fetal chromosomal abnormality; such results are warranted either by repeat NIPT (with additional reporting delays) or further investigation by invasive prenatal diagnosis.

In contrast with invasive prenatal diagnostic testing, such as chorionic villous sampling and amniocentesis, cffDNA testing involves no risk to the pregnancy (e.g., risk of miscarriage) and can be done as early as 9–10 weeks of gestation. These are seen as great benefits of this new technology, and many are hoping that it can replace invasive procedures as a diagnostic test. For now, although its sensitivity and specificity are much higher than traditional forms of screening for aneuploidies (based on serum and ultrasound markers), its low positive predictive value, especially for trisomy 13 and 18, explains why cffDNA testing is still considered a first- or second-tier screening test for aneuploidies, not a diagnostic test. On the other hand, because it has a high negative predictive value, its use makes it possible to avoid unnecessary invasive procedures. Unequivocally, international guidelines agree that no irrevocable obstetrical decision should be made in pregnancies with positive NIPT without confirmation by invasive prenatal diagnosis.[119,130,131]

As its use in practice to screen for common aneuploidies increases, there is interest in broadening its use to other indications, including the detection of sex chromosome aneuploidies and monogenic disorders, even though test sensitivity and specificity for these other indications are significantly lower. This currently constitutes a lively debate in the prenatal diagnostics community, both due to clinical and ethical considerations. From a clinical perspective, any expansion toward screening for individually rarer conditions will adversely affect the overall positive predictive value of NIPT; a subsequent increase in invasive diagnostic procedures may jeopardize the goal of NIPT (namely, reducing the risk of iatrogenic pregnancy loss from prenatal diagnostic procedures). Furthermore, when real risk for a rare condition exists (e.g., given family history), personalized genetic counseling should never be replaced by wide-spectrum NIPT. From an ethical perspective, any expansion of prenatal screening should adhere to accepted principles for population screening (such as the widely accepted Wilson and Jungner criteria).

52.4.2 Current Recommendations about the use of Cell-Free Fetal DNA in Practice

In their guidelines about prenatal diagnosis, the Society of Obstetrics and Gynecology of Canada (SOGC) recommends that cffDNA screening be offered as a second-tier screening test to women considered at high risk of aneuploidy based on traditional screening and/or ultrasound findings. For these women, cffDNA screening is considered an alternative to invasive prenatal diagnostic testing.[130]

The American College of Obstetrics and Gynecology (ACOG) recommends that screening for aneuploidies be offered to all pregnant women, and such screening can be performed through traditional screening or cell-free DNA screening. The organization suggests that cffDNA testing should be discouraged as a second-tier screening test in pregnancies considered at high risk for aneuploidy because it will not detect all aneuploidy and delays diagnostic testing.[119] The Society for Maternal-Fetal Medicine (SMFM) also recommends cffDNA testing as the preferred option for first-tier screening and that measurement of AFP and second-trimester ultrasound be performed as well.[131,132]

ACOG and SMFM both recommend against the use of cffDNA testing for microdeletions.[119,131,132] Neither of them recommends specifically for or against testing for fetal sex and fetal sex chromosome aneuploidies, such as Klinefelter syndrome, Turner syndrome, or 47,XXX syndrome. The predictive value of cffDNA testing for sex chromosome aneuploidies is much lower than for autosomal aneuploidies. In terms of using cffDNA testing to confirm fetal sex, the use of cffDNA testing for this purpose is mentioned only in the context of a family history of an X-linked disorder. Most women will be interested to use it to find out the baby's sex early in the pregnancy, but some are considering that practice ethically problematic, citing the possibility that patients will terminate pregnancies based on fetal sex.[133,134] The use of this testing for monogenic disorders is still not commonly available, except to check for fetal Rh status in women who are Rh negative and at risk of developing anti-Rh antibodies.[135]

52.4.3 Ethical and Social Issues Raised by the use of Cell-Free Fetal DNA Testing

Apart from the technical limitations of cffDNA testing, it faces other types of challenges. Ethical and social issues have been raised by the anticipation of widespread use of cffDNA testing, particularly its use for an expanded list of indications.[136]

So long as it remains a screening test, the risk associated with invasive testing will give pause to women at high risk for aneuploidy and will encourage a thorough informed consent process prior to invasive testing. If cffDNA testing reaches the threshold to become a diagnostic test, many fear that diagnostic testing will be made routine in the absence of test risk, and that the consent process will be considered less crucial. Pretest counseling to allow patients to make informed decisions must remain the standard of care for cffDNA testing.

Even though cffDNA testing performs better than traditional screening strategies, it has not yet replaced most traditional screening programs. This is due in great part to the much higher cost of cffDNA testing compared with traditional screening. We expect that cffDNA testing will replace current screening programs within public healthcare systems only if the cost of the technology drops significantly.[137] Meanwhile, most public healthcare systems will either rely on traditional strategies or integrate cffDNA screening as a second-tier test, with the caveat that this may miss some cases of aneuploidy and delay

TABLE 52.6 Positive predictive value calculations for chromosomal anomalies screened by NIPT in a pregnant 35 year-old

	Chromosomal anomaly screened for by NIPT	NIPT sensitivity (pooled methods) (%)	NIPT specificity (pooled methods) (%)	Positive predictive value (%)
Autosomal aneuploidies	Trisomy 21	99.2	99.91	79
	Trisomy 18	96.3	99.87	39
	Trisomy 13	91	99.87	21
Sex chromosome aneuploidies	Monosomy X	90.3	99.77	41
	47,XXX	93.1	99.86	28
	47,XXY	93	99.86	30
	47,XYY	93	99.86	25

Data from Gil MM, Accurti V, Santacruz B, Plana MN, Nicolaides KH. Analysis of cell-free DNA in maternal blood in screening for aneuploidies: updated meta-analysis. Ultrasound Obstet Gynecol 2017; 50(3):302–14.
Positive predictive values generated by the National Society of Genetic Counselors, NIPT/Cell Free DNA Screening Predictive Value Calculator, https://www.perinatalquality.org/Vendors/NSGC/NIPT/ as of March 4, 2019.

invasive diagnostic testing. In this context, many women opt for cffDNA testing offered by private laboratories and paid for either out of pocket or by private insurance plans. This leads to disparities in access to cffDNA testing and raises issues of justice, particularly in countries with public healthcare systems.

Screening for autosomal aneuploidies raises many ethical issues about women's reproductive autonomy, healthcare practitioners' ability to provide up-to-date and balanced information about Down syndrome and other aneuploidies, and the message that such screening sends about the value of living with a disability. The use of cffDNA screening for sex chromosome aneuploidies (Klinefelter syndrome, Turner syndrome, 47,XYY syndrome and 47,XXX syndrome) raises additional significant issues. First, the positive predictive value of cffDNA testing for sex chromosome aneuploidies is estimated at 39%.[119] This means that a positive result on cffDNA testing needs to be confirmed either by invasive prenatal diagnosis or karyotyping in the newborn period. A clinically useful calculator tool was created by the National Society of Genetic Counselors, using the weighted and pooled data from one metaanalysis of NIPT performance metrics in sex-chromosome aneuploidies (see Table 52.6).

Beyond considerations about prenatal screening performance for these conditions, sex chromosome aneuploidies have much less severe health outcomes than autosomal aneuploidies. In some cases, the most clinically significant impact on health is on fertility. The benefits of identifying sex chromosome aneuploidies antenatally are less clear: in most cases, unless there are associated fetal anomalies on ultrasound (e.g., heart defect or cystic hygroma with Turner syndrome), there is no expected impact on fetal or neonatal management. Thus, these children will be labeled from birth with a diagnosis that may not have an impact on their health until puberty, or even into adulthood. While no neonatal screening for sex-chromosome aneuploidies would be considered in asymptomatic neonates, prenatal suspicion raised by NIPT screening could lead to parental request for confirmatory testing either via invasive prenatal testing or postnatal karyotyping. Such requests in turn lead to challenging discussions around social and psychological concerns, consent, and the child's future autonomy and reproductive privacy.[138]

Consequent challenges will include how and when to inform the child that she or he has this sex chromosome aneuploidy, and whether this information is likely to lead to stigmatization outside the healthcare system, considering that some children with sex chromosome aneuploidies may have learning difficulties. Posttest counseling for a positive cffDNA result suggestive of a sex chromosome aneuploidy is a complex and delicate process, and it needs to be done by clinicians who have up-to-date knowledge of the health- and nonhealth-related issues associated with these disorders.

As noted previously, in addition to sex chromosome aneuploidies, cffDNA testing can detect fetal sex. In families with a history of an X-linked disorder, cffDNA testing for early fetal sex determination can be useful to establish whether invasive prenatal diagnosis is warranted and allow earlier invasive testing through chorionic villous sampling, instead of waiting to determine fetal sex on ultrasound and then offer amniocentesis at a later gestational age. In contrast, cffDNA testing to detect fetal sex in the absence of medical indication is considered worrisome because early fetal sex identification raises the issue of sex selection. In Canada, a gender gap at birth has been observed in some communities based on disclosure of fetal sex on ultrasound.[134]

There have been suggestions of implementing a policy to prevent fetal sex selection.[139] In the United Kingdom, there is a push from the Labour Party to ban disclosure of fetal sex.[140] In Canada, the SOGC recognized that pregnant women have the right to know the sex of their fetus as identified during morphological evaluation on ultrasound.[141] Even though no professional organization currently recommends the use of cffDNA testing for fetal sex determination, there is also no statement from any professional society recommending specifically against the use of cffDNA testing for detection of fetal sex. Because cffDNA testing can be accessed directly through private labs, couples who want to know the fetus's sex may be able to find out directly from such a lab. Open discussions about the validity of such testing and the implications for the pregnancy should take place between the pregnant woman, her partner, and the prenatal care provider.

52.4.4 Ethical Issues of Genetic and Genomic Tests in General

Genetic and genomic tests have raised ethical issues since they started being used in clinical practice. Genetic tests have some unique characteristics. First, an individual's genetic characteristics are unlikely to change over time, which means that not only can such a test be done only once in a lifetime, but its result may affect this individual's health, management, and insurability for his or her lifetime. A caveat to this point involves rare examples of somatic mutation-specific genetic disorders, and more generally various cancers. Second, an individual's genetic test result may have implications for family members, if it is inherited, for potential future children, or both. For these reasons, there have long been arguments to support the need for appropriate pretest counseling and informed consent prior to testing.

In the context of cffDNA testing, pregnant women should be counseled in terms of available screening options for aneuploidies, which include traditional screening strategies, cffDNA testing where available (even if not covered by their healthcare system), invasive prenatal diagnosis if she is considered at high risk of aneuploidy, and the option of no screening.[130] Some women are not interested in screening for aneuploidies, and their choice should be respected. The risks and benefits of each alternative should be discussed. Depending on the option selected, there may be a risk of inconclusive results or of identifying an incidental finding, such as maternal malignancy with cffDNA testing or traditional screening (i.e., high AFP levels).

Predictive testing in children is not recommended for adult-onset disorders unless treatment or surveillance should begin in childhood.[142,143] For adult-onset conditions that have no impact during childhood or adolescence, there is no health benefit to early testing. Deferring testing until adulthood respects the person's autonomy to decide whether he or she wants to be tested when old enough to decide on his or her own.

As genomic tests enter general practice, the likelihood of incidental or secondary findings increases. The field of genetics and genomics is still struggling with this issue and how to address these findings. The American College of Medical Genetics and Genomics recommends the disclosure of secondary findings in a list of "actionable" genes, with the caveat that they must be clearly pathogenic findings and there is the possibility of opting out, especially for children.[144,145] Other professional organizations have opted for less directive recommendations. European recommendations are more open-ended, advocating for targeted testing and filtered analysis focusing on the clinical indication, but recommending that the detection of an unsolicited genetic variant indicative of serious health problems that allows treatment or prevention should be reported.[146] For children, European recommendations suggest that "guidelines need to be established as to what unsolicited information should be disclosed in order to balance the autonomy and interests of the child and the parental rights and needs (not) to receive information that may be in the interest of their (future) family."[146]

Taking into consideration the Canadian healthcare context, the Canadian College of Medical Genetics (CCMG) took a more restrained approach by recommending giving competent adults the option prior to testing to choose to receive (or not receive) incidental findings unrelated to the primary test indication.[147] For children, the CCMG recommends the disclosure of incidental findings in the case of highly penetrant disorders that are medically actionable during childhood, but it does not provide a preestablished list of such disorders.[147]

REFERENCES

1. Miller NA, Farrow EG, Gibson M, Willig LK, Twist G, Yoo B, et al. A 26-hour system of highly sensitive whole genome sequencing for emergency management of genetic diseases. *Genome Med* 2015;**7**:100.
2. Petersen BS, Fredrich B, Hoeppner MP, Ellinghaus D, Franke A. Opportunities and challenges of whole-genome and -exome sequencing. *BMC Genet* 2017;**18**(1):14.
3. Adams DR, Eng CM. Next-generation sequencing to diagnose suspected genetic disorders. *N Engl J Med* 2018;**379**(14):1353–62.
4. Rabbani B, Tekin M, Mahdieh N. The promise of whole-exome sequencing in medical genetics. *J Hum Genet* 2014;**59**(1):5–15.
5. Hegde M, Santani A, Mao R, Ferreira-Gonzalez A, Weck KE, Voelkerding KV. Development and validation of clinical whole-exome and whole-genome sequencing for detection of germline variants in inherited disease. *Arch Pathol Lab Med* 2017;**141**(6):798–805.
6. Dewey FE, Grove ME, Pan C, Goldstein BA, Bernstein JA, Chaib H, et al. Clinical interpretation and implications of whole-genome sequencing. *JAMA* 2014;**311**(10):1035–45.
7. Ambardar S, Gupta R, Trakroo D, Lal R, Vakhlu J. High throughput sequencing: an overview of sequencing chemistry. *Indian J Microbiol* 2016;**56**(4):394–404.
8. Goldfeder RL, Wall DP, Khoury MJ, Ioannidis JPA, Ashley EA. Human genome sequencing at the population scale: a primer on high-throughput DNA sequencing and analysis. *Am J Epidemiol* 2017;**186**(8):1000–9.
9. van Dijk EL, Jaszczyszyn Y, Naquin D, Thermes C. The third revolution in sequencing technology. *Trends Genet* 2018;**34**(9):666–81.
10. Goldfeder RL, Priest JR, Zook JM, Grove ME, Waggott D, Wheeler MT, et al. Medical implications of technical accuracy in genome sequencing. *Genome Med* 2016;**8**(1):24.
11. White SJ, Laros JFJ, Bakker E, Cambon-Thomsen A, Eden M, Leonard S, et al. Critical points for an accurate human genome analysis. *Hum Mutat* 2017;**38**(8):912–21.
12. Zook JM, Catoe D, McDaniel J, Vang L, Spies N, Sidow A, et al. Extensive sequencing of seven human genomes to characterize benchmark reference materials. *Sci Data* 2016;**3**.
13. Brownstein CA, Beggs AH, Homer N, Merriman B, Yu TW, Flannery KC, et al. An international effort towards developing standards for best practices in analysis, interpretation and reporting of clinical genome sequencing results in the CLARITY challenge. *Genome Biol* 2014;**15**(3):R53.
14. Oza AM, DiStefano MT, Hemphill SE, Cushman BJ, Grant AR, Siegert RK, et al. Expert specification of the ACMG/AMP variant interpretation guidelines for genetic hearing loss. *Hum Mutat* 2018;**39**(11):1593–613.
15. Richards S, Aziz N, Bale S, Bick D, Das S, Gastier-Foster J, et al. Standards and guidelines for the interpretation of sequence variants: a joint consensus recommendation of the American College of Medical Genetics and Genomics and the Association for Molecular Pathology. *Genet Med* 2015;**17**(5):405–24.

16. O'Daniel JM, McLaughlin HM, Amendola LM, Bale SJ, Berg JS, Bick D, et al. A survey of current practices for genomic sequencing test interpretation and reporting processes in US laboratories. *Genet Med* 2017;**19**(5):575–82.

17. Liu X, Han S, Wang Z, Gelernter J, Yang BZ. Variant callers for next-generation sequencing data: a comparison study. *PLoS ONE* 2013;**8**(9).

18. McKenna A, Hanna M, Banks E, Sivachenko A, Cibulskis K, Kernytsky A, et al. The Genome Analysis Toolkit: a MapReduce framework for analyzing next-generation DNA sequencing data. *Genome Res* 2010;**20**(9):1297–303.

19. Pirooznia M, Kramer M, Parla J, Goes FS, Potash JB, McCombie WR, et al. Validation and assessment of variant calling pipelines for next-generation sequencing. *Hum Genomics* 2014;**8**:14.

20. Chiara M, Pavesi G. Evaluation of quality assessment protocols for high throughput genome resequencing data. *Front Genet* 2017;**8**:94.

21. Castellana S, Mazza T. Congruency in the prediction of pathogenic missense mutations: state-of-the-art web-based tools. *Brief Bioinform* 2013;**14** (4):448–59.

22. Dong C, Wei P, Jian X, Gibbs R, Boerwinkle E, Wang K, et al. Comparison and integration of deleteriousness prediction methods for nonsynonymous SNVs in whole exome sequencing studies. *Hum Mol Genet* 2015;**24**(8):2125–37.

23. Brinkman RR, Dube MP, Rouleau GA, Orr AC, Samuels ME. Human monogenic disorders—a source of novel drug targets. *Nat Rev Genet* 2006;**7** (4):249–60.

24. Awadalla P, Gauthier J, Myers RA, Casals F, Hamdan FF, Griffing AR, et al. Direct measure of the de novo mutation rate in autism and schizophrenia cohorts. *Am J Hum Genet* 2010;**87**(3):316–24.

25. Besenbacher S, Liu S, Izarzugaza JM, Grove J, Belling K, Bork-Jensen J, et al. Novel variation and de novo mutation rates in population-wide de novo assembled Danish trios. *Nat Commun* 2015;**6**:5969.

26. Veltman JA, Brunner HG. De novo mutations in human genetic disease. *Nat Rev Genet* 2012;**13**(8):565–75.

27. Kim Y, Lee HS, Yu JS, Ahn K, Ki CS, Kim J. Identification of a novel mutation in the CHD7 gene in a patient with CHARGE syndrome. *Korean J Pediatr* 2014;**57**(1):46–9.

28. Michelucci A, Ghirri P, Iacopetti P, Conidi ME, Fogli A, Baldinotti F, et al. Identification of three novel mutations in the CHD7 gene in patients with clinical signs of typical or atypical CHARGE syndrome. *Int J Pediatr Otorhinolaryngol* 2010;**74**(12):1441–4.

29. Pauli S, von Velsen N, Burfeind P, Steckel M, Manz J, Buchholz A, et al. CHD7 mutations causing CHARGE syndrome are predominantly of paternal origin. *Clin Genet* 2012;**81**(3):234–9.

30. Wessels K, Bohnhorst B, Luhmer I, Morlot S, Bohring A, Jonasson J, et al. Novel CHD7 mutations contributing to the mutation spectrum in patients with CHARGE syndrome. *Eur J Med Genet* 2010;**53**(5):280–5.

31. Jeffries L, Shima H, Ji W, Panisello-Manterola D, McGrath J, Bird LM, et al. A novel SAMD9 mutation causing MIRAGE syndrome: an expansion and review of phenotype, dysmorphology, and natural history. *Am J Med Genet A* 2018;**176**(2):415–20.

32. Sonmez FM, Uctepe E, Gunduz M, Gormez Z, Erpolat S, Oznur M, et al. Coffin-Siris syndrome with cafe-au-lait spots, obesity and hyperinsulinism caused by a mutation in the ARID1B gene. *Intractable Rare Dis Res* 2016;**5**(3):222–6.

33. Yu Y, Yao R, Wang L, Fan Y, Huang X, Hirschhorn J, et al. De novo mutations in ARID1B associated with both syndromic and non-syndromic short stature. *BMC Genomics* 2015;**16**:701.

34. Acar S, BinEssa HA, Demir K, Al-Rijjal RA, Zou M, Catli G, et al. Clinical and genetic characteristics of 15 families with hereditary hypophosphatemia: novel mutations in PHEX and SLC34A3. *PLoS ONE* 2018;**13**(3).

35. Cheon CK, Lee HS, Kim SY, Kwak MJ, Kim GH, Yoo HW. A novel de novo mutation within PHEX gene in a young girl with hypophosphatemic rickets and review of literature. *Ann Pediatr Endocrinol Metab* 2014;**19**(1):36–41.

36. Durmaz E, Zou M, Al-Rijjal RA, Baitei EY, Hammami S, Bircan I, et al. Novel and de novo PHEX mutations in patients with hypophosphatemic rickets. *Bone* 2013;**52**(1):286–91.

37. Fang C, Li H, Li X, Xiao W, Huang Y, Cai W, et al. De novo mutation of PHEX in a type 1 diabetes patient. *J Pediatr Endocrinol Metab* 2016;**29** (5):621–6.

38. Li SS, Gu JM, Yu WJ, He JW, Fu WZ, Zhang ZL. Seven novel and six de novo PHEX gene mutations in patients with hypophosphatemic rickets. *Int J Mol Med* 2016;**38**(6):1703–14.

39. Chavez B, Mendez JP, Ulloa-Aguirre A, Larrea F, Vilchis F. Eight novel mutations of the androgen receptor gene in patients with androgen insensitivity syndrome. *J Hum Genet* 2001;**46**(10):560–5.

40. Gad YZ, Mazen I, Lumbroso S, Temtamy SA, Sultan C. A novel point mutation of the androgen receptor (F804L) in an Egyptian newborn with complete androgen insensitivity associated with congenital glaucoma and hypertrophic pyloric stenosis. *Clin Genet* 2003;**63**(1):59–63.

41. Leslie ND. Haldane was right: de novo mutations in androgen insensitivity syndrome. *J Pediatr* 1998;**132**(6):917–8.

42. Mongan NP, Jaaskelainen J, Green K, Schwabe JW, Shimura N, Dattani M, et al. Two de novo mutations in the AR gene cause the complete androgen insensitivity syndrome in a pair of monozygotic twins. *J Clin Endocrinol Metab* 2002;**87**(3):1057–61.

43. Sun S, Luo F, Zhou Z, Wu W. A novel androgen receptor gene mutation in a Chinese patient with complete androgen insensitivity syndrome. *Eur J Obstet Gynecol Reprod Biol* 2010;**153**(2):173–5.

44. Boycott KM, Rath A, Chong JX, Hartley T, Alkuraya FS, Baynam G, et al. International cooperation to enable the diagnosis of all rare genetic diseases. *Am J Hum Genet* 2017;**100**(5):695–705.

45. Pabinger S, Dander A, Fischer M, Snajder R, Sperk M, Efremova M, et al. A survey of tools for variant analysis of next-generation genome sequencing data. *Brief Bioinform* 2014;**15**(2):256–78.

46. Hoskinson DC, Dubuc AM, Mason-Suares H. The current state of clinical interpretation of sequence variants. *Curr Opin Genet Dev* 2017;**42**:33–9.

47. Wright CF, FitzPatrick DR, Firth HV. Paediatric genomics: diagnosing rare disease in children. *Nat Rev Genet* 2018;**19**(5):325.

48. Caspar SM, Dubacher N, Kopps AM, Meienberg J, Henggeler C, Matyas G. Clinical sequencing: from raw data to diagnosis with lifetime value. *Clin Genet* 2018;**93**(3):508–19.

49. Persani L, de Filippis T, Colombo C, Gentilini D. GENETICS IN ENDOCRINOLOGY: genetic diagnosis of endocrine diseases by NGS: novel scenarios and unpredictable results and risks. *Eur J Endocrinol* 2018;**179**(3):R111–23.

50. Fukami M, Miyado M. Next generation sequencing and array-based comparative genomic hybridization for molecular diagnosis of pediatric endocrine disorders. *Ann Pediatr Endocrinol Metab* 2017;**22**(2):90–4.

51. Samuels ME, Friedman JM. Genetic mosaics and the germ line lineage. *Genes (Basel)* 2015;**6**(2):216–37.

52. Happle R. The McCune-Albright syndrome: a lethal gene surviving by mosaicism. *Clin Genet* 1986;**29**(4):321–4.

53. Lietman SA, Schwindinger WF, Levine MA. Genetic and molecular aspects of McCune-Albright syndrome. *Pediatr Endocrinol Rev* 2007;**4**(Suppl 4):380–5.

54. Suresh PS, Venkatesh T, Tsutsumi R, Shetty A. Next-generation sequencing for endocrine cancers: recent advances and challenges. *Tumour Biol* 2017;**39**(5).

55. Fasano M, Alberio T, Babu M, Lundberg E, Urbani A. Towards a functional definition of the mitochondrial human proteome. *EuPA Open Proteom* 2016;**10**:24–7.

56. Kremer LS, Wortmann SB, Prokisch H. "Transcriptomics": molecular diagnosis of inborn errors of metabolism via RNA-sequencing. *J Inherit Metab Dis* 2018;**41**(3):525–32.

57. Rivera-Munoz EA, Milko LV, Harrison SM, Azzariti DR, Kurtz CL, Lee K, et al. ClinGen Variant Curation Expert Panel experiences and standardized processes for disease and gene-level specification of the ACMG/AMP guidelines for sequence variant interpretation. *Hum Mutat* 2018;**39**(11):1614–22.

58. Samuels ME, Hasselmann C, Deal CL, Deladoey J, Van Vliet G. Whole-exome sequencing: opportunities in pediatric endocrinology. *Per Med* 2014;**11**(1):63–78.

59. Forlenza GP, Calhoun A, Beckman KB, Halvorsen T, Hamdoun E, Zierhut H, et al. Next generation sequencing in endocrine practice. *Mol Genet Metab* 2015;**115**(2–3):61–71.

60. Tenore A, Driul D. Genomics in pediatric endocrinology-genetic disorders and new techniques. *Pediatr Clin N Am* 2011;**58**(5):1061–81 [ix].

61. De Sousa SM, Hardy TS, Scott HS, Torpy DJ. Genetic testing in endocrinology. *Clin Biochem Rev* 2018;**39**(1):17–28.

62. Samuels ME, Gallo-Payet N, Pinard S, Hasselmann C, Magne F, Patry L, et al. Bioinactive ACTH causing glucocorticoid deficiency. *J Clin Endocrinol Metab* 2013;**98**(2):736–42.

63. Krude H, Biebermann H, Luck W, Horn R, Brabant G, Gruters A. Severe early-onset obesity, adrenal insufficiency and red hair pigmentation caused by POMC mutations in humans. *Nat Genet* 1998;**19**(2):155–7.

64. Bertolla RP. *Proteomics in human reproduction: biomarkers for millenials.* Springer; 2016. p. 9–21.

65. Aebersold R, Mann M. Mass-spectrometric exploration of proteome structure and function. *Nature* 2016;**537**(7620):347–55.

66. Dunn WB, Broadhurst D, Begley P, Zelena E, Francis-McIntyre S, Anderson N, et al. Procedures for large-scale metabolic profiling of serum and plasma using gas chromatography and liquid chromatography coupled to mass spectrometry. *Nat Protoc* 2011;**6**(7):1060–83.

67. Dunn WB, Broadhurst DI, Atherton HJ, Goodacre R, Griffin JL. Systems level studies of mammalian metabolome: the roles of mass spectrometry and nuclear magnetic resonance spectroscopy. *Chem Soc Rev* 2011;**40**(1):387–426.

68. Kell DB, Oliver SG. Here is the evidence, now what is the hypothesis? The complementary roles of inductive and hypothesis-driven science in the post-genomic era. *Bioessays* 2004;**26**(1):99–105.

69. Bird SS, Marur VR, Sniatynski MJ, Greenberg HK, Kristal BS. Lipidomics profiling by high-resolution LC-MS and high-energy collisional dissociation fragmentation: focus on characterization of mitochondrial cardiolipins and monolysocardiolipins. *Anal Chem* 2011;**83**(3):940–9.

70. Kapoore RV, Vaidyanathan S. Towards quantitative mass spectrometry-based metabolomics in microbial and mammalian systems. *Philos Trans A Math Phys Eng Sci* 2016;**374**(2079).

71. Stringer KA, Younger JG, McHugh C, Yeomans L, Finkel MA, Puskarich MA, et al. Whole blood reveals more metabolic detail of the human metabolome than serum as measured by 1H-NMR spectroscopy: implications for sepsis metabolomics. *Shock* 2015;**44**(3):200–8.

72. Chace DH, Millington DS, Terada N, Kahler SG, Roe CR, Hofman LF. Rapid diagnosis of phenylketonuria by quantitative analysis for phenylalanine and tyrosine in neonatal blood spots by tandem mass spectrometry. *Clin Chem* 1993;**39**(1):66–71.

73. Drolet J, Tolstikov V, Williams BA, Greenwood BP, Hill C, Vishnudas VK, et al. Integrated metabolomics assessment of human dried blood spots and urine strips. *Metabolites* 2017;**7**(3):1–14.

74. Trabado S, Al-Salameh A, Croixmarie V, Masson P, Corruble E, Feve B, et al. The human plasma-metabolome: reference values in 800 French healthy volunteers; impact of cholesterol, gender and age. *PLoS ONE* 2017;**12**(3).

75. Dunn WB, Lin W, Broadhurst D, Begley P, Brown M, Zelena E, et al. Molecular phenotyping of a UK population: defining the human serum metabolome. *Metabolomics* 2015;**11**:9–26.

76. Psychogios N, Hau DD, Peng J, Guo AC, Mandal R, Bouatra S, et al. The human serum metabolome. *PLoS ONE* 2011;**6**(2).

77. Bouatra S, Aziat F, Mandal R, Guo AC, Wilson MR, Knox C, et al. The human urine metabolome. *PLoS ONE* 2013;**8**(9).

78. Thevenot EA, Roux A, Xu Y, Ezan E, Junot C. Analysis of the human adult urinary metabolome variations with age, body mass index, and gender by implementing a comprehensive workflow for univariate and OPLS statistical analyses. *J Proteome Res* 2015;**14**(8):3322–35.

79. Wikoff WR, Kalisak E, Trauger S, Manchester M, Siuzdak G. Response and recovery in the plasma metabolome tracks the acute LCMV-induced immune response. *J Proteome Res* 2009;**8**(7):3578–87.

80. Dame ZT, Aziat F, Mandal R, Krishnamurthy R, Bouatra S, Bourzouie S, et al. The human saliva metabolome. *Metabolomics* 2015;**11**(6):1864–83.

81. Calderon-Santiago M, Priego-Capote F, Turck N, Robin X, Jurado-Gamez B, Sanchez JC, et al. Human sweat metabolomics for lung cancer screening. *Anal Bioanal Chem* 2015;**407**(18):5381–92.

82. Macedo AN, Mathiaparanam S, Brick L, Keenan K, Gonska T, Pedder L, et al. The sweat metabolome of screen-positive cystic fibrosis infants: revealing mechanisms beyond impaired chloride transport. *ACS Cent Sci* 2017;**3**(8):904–13.

83. Goedert JJ, Sampson JN, Moore SC, Xiao Q, Xiong X, Hayes RB, et al. Fecal metabolomics: assay performance and association with colorectal cancer. *Carcinogenesis* 2014;**35**(9):2089–96.

84. Marchesi JR, Holmes E, Khan F, Kochhar S, Scanlan P, Shanahan F, et al. Rapid and noninvasive metabonomic characterization of inflammatory bowel disease. *J Proteome Res* 2007;**6**(2):546–51.

85. Carraro S, Giordano G, Reniero F, Carpi D, Stocchero M, Sterk PJ, et al. Asthma severity in childhood and metabolomic profiling of breath condensate. *Allergy* 2013;**68**(1):110–7.

86. Want EJ, Masson P, Michopoulos F, Wilson ID, Theodoridis G, Plumb RS, et al. Global metabolic profiling of animal and human tissues via UPLC-MS. *Nat Protoc* 2013;**8**(1):17–32.

87. Zhang Y, Fonslow BR, Shan B, Baek MC, Yates 3rd JR. Protein analysis by shotgun/bottom-up proteomics. *Chem Rev* 2013;**113**(4):2343–94.

88. Raterink RJ, Lindenburg PW, Vreeken RJ, Ramaautar R, Hankemeier T. Recent developments in sample-pretreatment techniques for mass spectrometry-based metabolomics. *TrAC Trends Anal Chem* 2014;**61**:157–67.

89. Cho WC. Proteomics technologies and challenges. *Genomics Proteomics Bioinformatics* 2007;**5**(2):77–85.

90. Scherp P, Ku G, Coleman L, Kheterpal I. Gel-based and gel-free proteomic technologies. In: Gimble JM, Bunnell BA, editors. *Adipose-derived stem cells: methods and protocols.* Humana Press; 2018.

91. Cajka T, Fiehn O. Toward merging untargeted and targeted methods in mass spectrometry-based metabolomics and lipidomics. *Anal Chem* 2016;**88**(1):524–45.

92. Sande CJ, Mutunga M, Muteti J, Berkley JA, Nokes DJ, Njunge J. Untargeted analysis of the airway proteomes of children with respiratory infections using mass spectrometry based proteomics. *Sci Rep* 2018;**8**(1).

93. Wright PC, Noirel J, Ow SY, Fazeli A. A review of current proteomics technologies with a survey on their widespread use in reproductive biology investigations. *Theriogenology* 2012;**77**(4):738–65. e52.

94. Vidova V, Spacil Z. A review on mass spectrometry-based quantitative proteomics: targeted and data independent acquisition. *Anal Chim Acta* 2017;**964**:7–23.

95. Konermann L, Ahadi E, Rodriguez AD, Vahidi S. Unraveling the mechanism of electrospray ionization. *Anal Chem* 2013;**85**(1):2–9.

96. Mussap M, Antonucci R, Noto A, Fanos V. The role of metabolomics in neonatal and pediatric laboratory medicine. *Clin Chim Acta* 2013;**426**:127–38.

97. Marshall DD, Powers R. Beyond the paradigm: combining mass spectrometry and nuclear magnetic resonance for metabolomics. *Prog Nucl Magn Reson Spectrosc* 2017;**100**:1–16.

98. Rogers JC, Bomgarden RD. Sample preparation for mass spectrometry-based proteomics; from proteomes to peptides. In: Mirzae H, Carrasco M, editors. *Modern proteomics—sample preparation, analysis and practical applications.* Springer; 2016. p. 43–62.

99. Catherman AD, Skinner OS, Kelleher NL. Top down proteomics: facts and perspectives. *Biochem Biophys Res Commun* 2014;**445**(4):683–93.

100. Toby TK, Fornelli L, Kelleher NL. Progress in top-down proteomics and the analysis of proteoforms. *Annu Rev Anal Chem (Palo Alto, Calif)* 2016;**9**(1):499–519.

101. Sap KA, Demmers JAA. Labeling methods in mass spectrometry based quantitative proteomics. In: Leung H-C, Man TK, editors. *Integrative proteomics.* IntechOpen; 2014.

102. Dettmer K, Aronov PA, Hammock B. Mass spectrometry-based metabolomics. *Indian J Exp Biol* 2009;**47**:987–92.

103. Patti GJ, Yanes O, Siuzdak G. Innovation: metabolomics: the apogee of the omics trilogy. *Nat Rev Mol Cell Biol* 2012;**13**(4):263–9.

104. Serkova NJ, Standiford TJ, Stringer KA. The emerging field of quantitative blood metabolomics for biomarker discovery in critical illnesses. *Am J Respir Crit Care Med* 2011;**184**(6):647–55.

105. Dunn WB, Ellis DI. Metabolomics: current analytical platforms and methodologies. *TrAC Trends Anal Chem* 2005;**24**:285–94.

106. Koulman A, Lane GA, Harrison SJ, Volmer DA. From differentiating metabolites to biomarkers. *Anal Bioanal Chem* 2009;**394**(3):663–70.

107. Griffiths WJ, Koal T, Wang Y, Kohl M, Enot DP, Deigner HP. Targeted metabolomics for biomarker discovery. *Angew Chem Int Ed Eng* 2010;**49**(32):5426–45.

108. Chokkathukalam A, Kim DH, Barrett MP, Breitling R, Creek DJ. Stable isotope-labeling studies in metabolomics: new insights into structure and dynamics of metabolic networks. *Bioanalysis* 2014;**6**(4):511–24.

109. Mahieu NG, Patti GJ. Systems-level annotation of a metabolomics data set reduces 25000 features to fewer than 1000 unique metabolites. *Anal Chem* 2017;**89**(19):10397–406.

110. Schmidt JL, Castellanos-Brown K, Childress S, Bonhomme N, Oktay JS, Terry SF, et al. The impact of false-positive newborn screening results on families: a qualitative study. *Genet Med* 2012;**14**(1):76–80.

111. DiBattista A, McIntosh N, Lamoureux M, Al-Dirbashi OY, Chakraborty P, Britz-McKibbin P. Metabolic signatures of cystic fibrosis identified in dried blood spots for newborn screening without carrier identification. *J Proteome Res* 2019;**18**(3):841–54.

112. Wilson K, Hawken S, Potter BK, Chakraborty P, Walker M, Ducharme R, et al. Accurate prediction of gestational age using newborn screening analyte data. *Am J Obstet Gynecol* 2016;**214**(4):513.e1–9.

113. Oltman SP, Rogers EE, Baer RJ, Anderson JG, Steurer MA, Pantell MS, et al. Initial metabolic profiles are associated with 7-day survival among infants born at 22–25 weeks of gestation. *J Pediatr* 2018;**198**:194–200 e3.

114. Sylvester KG, Kastenberg ZJ, Moss RL, Enns GM, Cowan TM, Shaw GM, et al. Acylcarnitine profiles reflect metabolic vulnerability for necrotizing enterocolitis in newborns born premature. *J Pediatr* 2017;**181**:80–5 e1.

115. Sood MM, Murphy MSQ, Hawken S, Wong CA, Potter BK, Burns KD, et al. Association between newborn metabolic profiles and pediatric kidney disease. *Kidney Int Rep* 2018;**3**(3):691–700.

116. Gil MM, Accurti V, Santacruz B, Plana MN, Nicolaides KH. Analysis of cell-free DNA in maternal blood in screening for aneuploidies: updated meta-analysis. *Ultrasound Obstet Gynecol* 2017;**50**(3):302–14.

117. Renga B. Non invasive prenatal diagnosis of fetal aneuploidy using cell free fetal DNA. *Eur J Obstet Gynecol Reprod Biol* 2018;**225**:5–8.

118. Haghiac M, Vora NL, Basu S, Johnson KL, Presley L, Bianchi DW, et al. Increased death of adipose cells, a path to release cell-free DNA into systemic circulation of obese women. *Obesity (Silver Spring)* 2012;**20**(11):2213–9.

119. Committee on Practice Bulletins—Obstetrics, Committee on Genetics, and the Society for Maternal-Fetal Medicine. Practice Bulletin No. 163: screening for fetal aneuploidy. *Obstet Gynecol* 2016;**127**(5):e123–37.

120. Wang JC, Sahoo T, Schonberg S, Kopita KA, Ross L, Patek K, et al. Discordant noninvasive prenatal testing and cytogenetic results: a study of 109 consecutive cases. *Genet Med* 2015;**17**(3):234–6.

121. Chen EZ, Chiu RW, Sun H, Akolekar R, Chan KC, Leung TY, et al. Noninvasive prenatal diagnosis of fetal trisomy 18 and trisomy 13 by maternal plasma DNA sequencing. *PLoS ONE* 2011;**6**(7):e21791.

122. Palomaki GE, Kloza EM, Lambert-Messerlian GM, Haddow JE, Neveux LM, Ehrich M, et al. DNA sequencing of maternal plasma to detect down syndrome: an international clinical validation study. *Genet Med* 2011;**13**(11):913–20.

123. Jensen TJ, Dzakula Z, Deciu C, van den Boom D, Ehrich M. Detection of microdeletion 22q11.2 in a fetus by next-generation sequencing of maternal plasma. *Clin Chem* 2012;**58**(7):1148–51.

124. Lun FM, Jin YY, Sun H, Leung TY, Lau TK, Chiu RW, et al. Noninvasive prenatal diagnosis of a case of down syndrome due to robertsonian translocation by massively parallel sequencing of maternal plasma DNA. *Clin Chem* 2011;**57**(6):917–9.

125. Sparks AB, Struble CA, Wang ET, Song K, Oliphant A. Noninvasive prenatal detection and selective analysis of cell-free DNA obtained from maternal blood: evaluation for trisomy 21 and trisomy 18. *Am J Obstet Gynecol* 2012;**206**(4):319.e1–9.

126. Sparks AB, Wang ET, Struble CA, Barrett W, Stokowski R, McBride C, et al. Selective analysis of cell-free DNA in maternal blood for evaluation of fetal trisomy. *Prenat Diagn* 2012;**32**(1):3–9.

127. Zimmermann B, Hill M, Gemelos G, Demko Z, Banjevic M, Baner J, et al. Noninvasive prenatal aneuploidy testing of chromosomes 13, 18, 21, X, and Y, using targeted sequencing of polymorphic loci. *Prenat Diagn* 2012;**32**(13):1233–41.

128. Fan HC, Blumenfeld YJ, Chitkara U, Hudgins L, Quake SR. Noninvasive diagnosis of fetal aneuploidy by shotgun sequencing DNA from maternal blood. *Proc Natl Acad Sci U S A* 2008;**105**(42):16266–71.

129. Nicolaides KH, Syngelaki A, Gil M, Atanasova V, Markova D. Validation of targeted sequencing of single-nucleotide polymorphisms for non-invasive prenatal detection of aneuploidy of chromosomes 13, 18, 21, X, and Y. *Prenat Diagn* 2013;**33**(6):575–9.

130. Audibert F, De Bie I, Johnson JA, Okun N, Wilson RD, Armour C, et al. No. 348-Joint SOGC-CCMG Guideline: update on prenatal screening for fetal aneuploidy, fetal anomalies, and adverse pregnancy outcomes. *J Obstet Gynaecol Can* 2017;**39**(9):805–17.

131. Society for Maternal-Fetal Medicine (SMFM) Publications Committee. Prenatal aneuploidy screening using cell-free DNA. *Am J Obstet Gynecol* 2015;**212**(6):711–6.

132. Society for Maternal-Fetal Medicine (SMFM) Publications Committee. SMFM Statement: clarification of recommendations regarding cell-free DNA aneuploidy screening. *Am J Obstet Gynecol* 2015;**213**(6):753–4.

133. Browne TK. Why parents should not be told the sex of their fetus. *J Med Ethics* 2017;**43**(1):5–10.

134. Kale R. "It's a girl!"—could be a death sentence. *CMAJ* 2012;**184**(4):387–8.

135. Johnson JA, MacDonald K, Clarke G, Skoll A. No. 343-routine non-invasive prenatal prediction of fetal RHD genotype in Canada: the time is here. *J Obstet Gynaecol Can* 2017;**39**(5):366–73.

136. Chitty LS, Friedman JM, Langlois S. Current controversies in prenatal diagnosis 2: should a fetal exome be used in the assessment of a dysmorphic or malformed fetus? *Prenat Diagn* 2016;**36**(1):15–9.

137. Nshimyumukiza L, Beaumont JA, Duplantie J, Langlois S, Little J, Audibert F, et al. Cell-free DNA-based non-invasive prenatal screening for common aneuploidies in a Canadian Province: a cost-effectiveness analysis. *J Obstet Gynaecol Can* 2018;**40**(1):48–60.

138. Arbour L. *Guidelines for genetic testing of healthy children;* 2003.

139. Thiele AT, Leier B. Towards an ethical policy for the prevention of fetal sex selection in Canada. *J Obstet Gynaecol Can* 2010;**32**(1):54–7.

140. Association P. Labour calls for ban on early foetus sex test. *The Guardian* 2018;(September 17, 2018).

141. Van den Hof MC, Demczuk N, Members of the Diagnostic Imaging Committee. Fetal sex determination and disclosure. *J Obstet Gynaecol Can* 2007;**29**(4):368.

142. Botkin JR, Belmont JW, Berg JS, Berkman BE, Bombard Y, Holm IA, et al. Points to consider: ethical, legal, and psychosocial implications of genetic testing in children and adolescents. *Am J Hum Genet* 2015;**97**(1):6–21.

143. Committee on Bioethics, Committee on Genetics, American College of Medical Genetics, Genomics Social, Ethical, Legal Issues Committee. Ethical and policy issues in genetic testing and screening of children. *Pediatrics* 2013;**131**(3):620–2.

144. Green RC, Berg JS, Grody WW, Kalia SS, Korf BR, Martin CL, et al. ACMG recommendations for reporting of incidental findings in clinical exome and genome sequencing. *Genet Med* 2013;**15**(7):565–74.

145. Kalia SS, Adelman K, Bale SJ, Chung WK, Eng C, Evans JP, et al. Recommendations for reporting of secondary findings in clinical exome and genome sequencing, 2016 update (ACMG SF v2.0): a policy statement of the American College of Medical Genetics and Genomics. *Genet Med* 2017;**19**(2):249–55.
146. van El CG, Cornel MC, Borry P, Hastings RJ, Fellmann F, Hodgson SV, et al. Whole-genome sequencing in health care: recommendations of the European Society of Human Genetics. *Eur J Hum Genet* 2013;**21**(6):580–4.
147. Boycott K, Hartley T, Adam S, Bernier F, Chong K, Fernandez BA, et al. The clinical application of genome-wide sequencing for monogenic diseases in Canada: position statement of the Canadian College of Medical Geneticists. *J Med Genet* 2015;**52**(7):431–7.

Index

Note: Page numbers followed by *f* indicate figures, *t* indicate tables, and *b* indicate boxes.